Welcome to...
Fundamentals of Nursing!
2ND EDITION

Take advantage of all of the resources this unique, two-volume package offers to make learning easier.

Just read through this guide or listen to "**Getting the Most Out of This Learning Package**" podcast on DavisPlus…

http://davisplus.fadavis.com
Keyword Wilkinson

Your Learning Package features…

✓ The Two-Volume Textbook

✓ The Electronic Study Guide—FREE on the BONUS CD-ROM in Volume 1

✓ Resources Online at DavisPlus…
http://davisplus.fadavis.com
Keyword: Wilkinson

✓ The Skills Videos on DVDs (purchase separately)

✓ The Procedure Checklist (purchase separately)

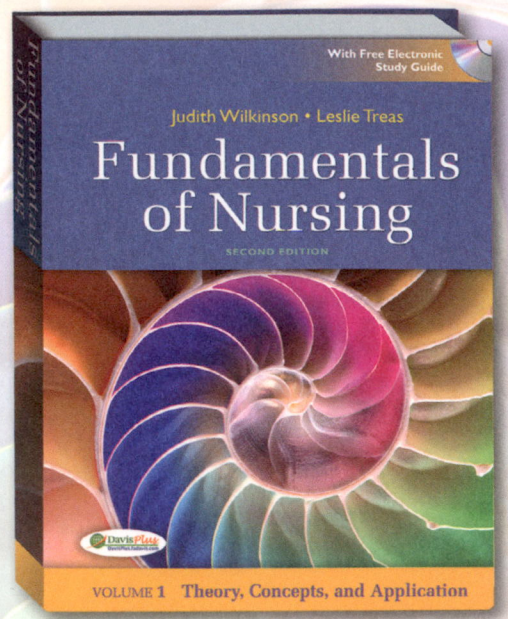

VOLUME 1 Theory, Concepts, and Application

VOLUME 1 is your primary classroom/study textbook.

Learning Outcomes guide your reading and highlight the information you need to know. You can also refer to them later to review each chapter's content.

Learning Outcomes

After completing this chapter, you should be able to:

➤ Describe the normal structure and function of the organs in the urinary system.

➤ Describe the processes of urine formation and elimination.

➤ Discuss factors that affect urinary elimination.

➤ Describe the contents of a nursing assessment and physical ___ focused on urinary elimination.

___ pes of urine

___ ntification of

➤ Discuss common elimination problems: urinary tract infection, urinary retention, and urinary incontinence.

➤ Identify nursing diagnoses associated with altered urinary elimination.

➤ Describe nursing interventions that promote normal urination.

➤ Provide care for clients experiencing urinary problems.

➤ Perform urinary catheterizations following accepted procedures.

➤ Discuss nursing care appropriate for clients who have a urinary diversion.

Meet Your Patient

During your assigned clinical experience at University Hospital, the RN asks you to complete the admission process for Marlena, a 55-year-old woman who is complaining of frequent, painful urination. As you interview her, Marlena becomes embarrassed. "I really don't enjoy talking about this." she admits. Then, she asks to use the bathroom. You ask her to give you a midstream clean-catch urine sample while she is in the restroom. When she returns, she gives you a small specimen of pink-colored, strong-smelling urine. "I feel like I have strong urge to go and then I hardly have any urine. It's a little bloody and burns like crazy during my stream," she reports.

You close the door and interview Marlena in private about her usual urination pattern and current symptoms. Your calm approach and straightforward manner put her at ease. She confides that she is sexually active and that her symptoms began after spending the weekend with her new partner. You take her vital signs: oral temperature 99.4°F (37.4°C), radial pulse 88 beats/min, respiratory rate

20 breaths/min, and blood pressure 108/72 mm Hg.

After you report your assessment data to the RN, the emergency department (ED) physician asks you to perform a dipstick urinalysis on the urine sample and to send the urine sample to the lab for culture and sensitivity. He asks you: "Well, what do you think we need to do next?" How would you answer his question?

As you gain theoretical and practical knowledge in this chapter, we will return to this case study to discuss how you might answer the physician's question and support Marlena's recovery. You will also have the opportunity to ___ your feelings about giving care that patients may ___ personal or even embarrassing.

Meet Your Patient is a real-life patient scenario that opens each chapter in Volume I and continues throughout the chapter, helping you apply theory to practice.

How Does Urinary Elimination Occur?

Where the bladder connects to the urethra is a thickening of smooth muscle, called the **internal urethral sphincter.** When closed, the internal sphincter keeps urine in the bladder from entering the urethra. When the bladder contains 200 to 450 mL of urine (50 to 200 mL in children), the distention activates stretch receptors in the bladder wall. The stretch receptors send sensory impulses to the *voiding reflex center* in the spinal cord, triggering motor impulses that cause the detrusor muscle to contract and the internal sphincter to relax. The internal urethral sphincter is not under voluntary control.

Voiding (also called **urination** or **micturition**) occurs when contraction of the detrusor muscle pushes stored urine through the relaxed internal urethral sphincter into the urethra. This triggers the conscious urge to void. However, voiding may be voluntarily delayed by inhibiting release of a second, **external urethral sphincter.** When the person is ready to urinate, the brain signals the

Headings in the Form of Questions help you to organize your thinking. When you review a chapter for a test, scan the headings and see what you recall about each of them.

Terms in Boldface Type highlight the important concepts when they're defined for the first time. While reviewing the content later, scan the pages for the bold and italicized words. If any seem unfamiliar, read the section again.

Knowledge Check Questions

divide the material into small, manageable sections. Perfect for chapter review now and exam prep later.

KnowledgeCheck 17-5

- For a client whose BP is 150/80, what is the pulse pressure?
- Is that normal? If so, explain. If not, what should the pulse pressure be?

Critical Thinking Questions

prepare you for the "real world" by providing the practice you need in applying the information you have just learned.

Critical Thinking 17-5

- Did you notice that the pulse rates in the preceding two goals are not the same as the full normal range shown in Table 17-1? What do you think might be a reason for this?

Colorful Icons refer you

to Volume 1, Volume 2, the Electronic Study Guide or DavisPlus.

This cross referencing tells you about...

- Additional/enrichment information on the Electronic Study Guide or DavisPlus.
- Review material/forms on the Electronic Study Guide or DavisPlus.
- Clinical information in Volume 2.

HELPFUL HINT: The sentence before the icon tells you what the material is.

You and **your instructor** will determine when or if you will need to use this material.

The Critical Aspects box provides an overview of urinary catheterization. For the complete procedure, Go to Chapter 27, **Procedure 27-2: Inserting a Urinary Catheter**, in Volume 2.

Skills/Procedures are introduced in

Volume 1. **Critical Aspect boxes** describe the principles and rationales for the procedure and explain their relevance.

HELPFUL HINT: An icon shows you where in Volume 2 to find the complete, step-by-step procedure you will use in lab to learn and practice the skill.

Critical Aspects of Procedures 17-1 through 17-6

For steps to follow in all procedures, refer to the inside back cover of Volume 2. Go to the full procedures in Volume 2 to practice and learn a procedure steps. Use these Critical Aspects later to help you review key points.

Procedure 17-1: Assessing Body Temperature

- Clean before and after using if the thermometer is not disposable.
- Select the appropriate site and thermometer type.
- Turn on, or otherwise ready the thermometer.
- Insert the thermometer in its sheath, or use a thermometer designated only for the patient.
- Insert and leave an electronic thermometer in place until it beeps; for other thermometers use the recommended times.
- Cleanse and store in recharging base (store glass thermometers safely to prevent breakage).
- For an oral temperature, obtain a reading 20 to 30 minutes after the patient consumes hot or cold food or fluids or smokes.

Procedure 17-4: Assessing for an Apical-Radial Pulse Deficit

- Palpate and place stethoscope over apex of the heart.
- Palpate the radial pulse.
- Have two nurses carry out the procedure, if possible.
- Count for 60 seconds, simultaneously.
- Compare the pulse rate at both sites; calculate the difference.

Procedure 17-5: Assessing Respirations

- Count unobtrusively (e.g., while palpating the radial pulse).
- Count for 30 seconds if respirations are regular; for 60 seconds if they are irregular.
- Observe the rate, rhythm, and depth of respirations.

Procedure 17-6: Measuring Blood Pressure

- If possible, place the patient in a sitting position, with the feet on the ... the legs ...

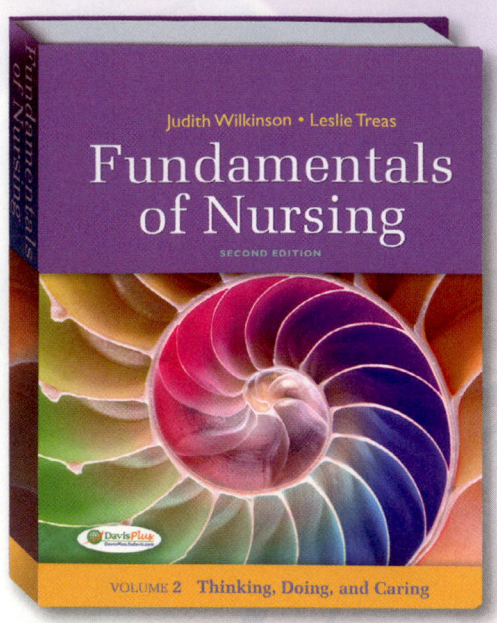

Judith Wilkinson • Leslie Treas

Fundamentals of Nursing

SECOND EDITION

VOLUME 2 Thinking, Doing, and Caring

VOLUME 2 is your primary text for your skills lab and clinical.

THE INFORMATION YOU NEED...

Assessment Guidelines and Tools Boxes
provide a quick review of special assessments your patients may need.

Diagnostic Testing Tables
identify the diagnostic tests required by the condition.

Standardized Language Tables (NANDA, NIC and NOC)
are useful for care planning

THE PROCEDURES YOU NEED...

More than 200 Step-by-Step Procedures

HELPFUL HINT: If you find yourself in lab without Volume 2, use the Critical Aspect Boxes in Volume 1 to review the concepts underlying each procedure.

More than 90 Clinical Insight Boxes
present guidelines for clinical care. These guidelines are based more on principles than step-by-step procedures.

Procedure 17–5 ■ Assessing Respirations

► For steps to follow in all procedures, refer to the inside back cover of this book.

Critical Aspects

- Count unobtrusively (e.g., while palpating the radial pulse).
- Count for 30 seconds if respirations are regular; for 60 seconds if they are irregular. A 60-second count is recommended for increased accuracy, even for regular respirations.
- Observe the rate, rhythm, and depth of respirations.

Equipment
- A watch with a second hand (or a wall clock)

Delegation
You can delegate the counting of respirations to the nursing assistive personnel (NAP) if you conclude that the patient's condition and the NAP's skills allow. Perform the following assessments, and inform the NAP of any special consider-ations (e.g., the need to keep the patient in a certain posi-tion). Ask the NAP to record and report the respirations to you, and to report immediately if they are not within the normal range for this patient (specify the range).

Pre-Procedure Assessments
- Observe for signs of respiratory distress—brea[...] faster or slower than normal, gasping breaths, confusion, circumoral (around the month) cyanosis. Signs of hypoxemia may indicate that the patient is not ad[...] quately oxygenated.
- Determine the baseline respiratory rate and character of respirations.
- Assess for factors that may affect the respiratory rate (e.g., pain, activity, fever, respiratory disorders).

Procedure Steps
When performing the procedure, al-ways identify your patient according to agency policy and be attentive to stan-dard precautions, hand hygie[...] safety and pri[...]

2. Palpate and count the radial pulse; remember that number. Then, kee[...] your hand on the [...]

Clinical Insights

Clinical Insight 27–1 ► Caring for a Patient with an Indwelling Catheter

An indwelling catheter is connected to a drainage tube and collection bag, which constitute a closed system.

Goal 1: Prevent urinary tract infection.
- Do not disconnect the tubing or open the drainage sys-tem (e.g., to obtain specimens or measure the urine). A closed system minimizes the chance for pathogens to enter the system and infect the urinary tract.
- Regularly check connections between the catheter and drainage tubing and the drainage tube and collection bag. Loose connections cause leaks and serve as entry points for pathogens.
- If the system inadvertently becomes disconnected, wipe the ends of both tubes with antiseptic (e.g., alcohol or chlorhexidine-gluconate-alcohol combination product) before reconnecting them.
- If the catheter becomes soiled from drainage or feces, cleanse it w[...] soap and water by cleaning from the the catheter well, and pat it dry. meatu[...] growth of microo[...]

Goal 2: Maintain free flow of urine.
Maintaining free flow of urine prevents backflow of urine into the bladder, which can cause bladder distention and injury. Stasis of urine also provides a medium for growth of micro-organisms. Note that some of the interventions in this sec-tion are the same as those for preventing infection (goal 1).
- Make sure the tubing and bag remain below the level of the bladder to prevent backflow. Urine drains by gravity in this system.
- If the collecting bag must be higher than the bladder at any time, you must clamp the catheter. Clamping prevents backflow of stagnant urine into the bladde[...]
- Frequently inspect the tubing to ensure that urine flow[...] freely in the tubing. Any kinks, coils, or compression of the catheter or tu[...] may impede flow and cause backup into the bladder[...]
- If urine is not flowing, check to be sure the patie[...] lying on the tubing. [...]allow the collection bag to lie on the fl[...]es the effec[...]

THE EXERCISES AND REVIEW YOU NEED…

Caring for the Garcias

The exercises in the following section allow you to practice the kind of thinking you will use as a full-spectrum nurse. Because these are critical-thinking questions, there is usually no single right answer. We do not provide answers for these questions because it is more important for you to think about the questions than to arrive at the "right" answer. These questions are designed to improve your thinking more than to "cover content." Discuss answers with your peers—discussion can stimulate critical thinking. If you have difficulty with any of these questions, consult with your instructor.

Recall that on Joseph Garcia's preliminary visit to the family medicine center, his blood pressure (BP) was 162/94. On subsequent visits, his BP was 168/100 and 174/98. Mr. Garcia was diagnosed with hypertension and prescribed an antihypertension medication, to be taken each morning. This morning Mr. Garcia presents at the clinic for follow-up. The following information is gathered as he checks in for his visit.

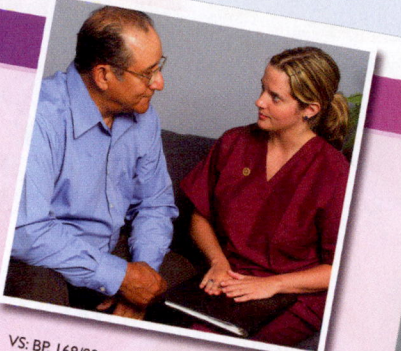

VS: BP, 168/92; pulse, 80; respirations, 20; temperature, 98.4°F (36.9°C)
Weight: 231 lb (105 kg)

Review the preliminary data and the preceding information to answer the following questions:

"Caring for the Garcias"
lets you follow the story of a multi-cultural family and answer questions about their care.

"Applying the Full-Spectrum Nursing Model" Questions
help you develop your clinical reasoning skills by applying the concepts of thinking, doing, and caring.

Critical Thinking and Clinical Reasoning Questions develop the skills you will use in clinical practice.

"What Are the Main Points in This Chapter?"

Knowledge Maps
are visual summaries of the corresponding material in Volume 1.

Applying the Full-Spectrum Nursing Model

PATIENT SITUATION

A patient in the critical care unit had a stable pulse and BP for the first few days. He has become more ill and now his pulse and BP are weak and difficult to palpate. His last BP reading was abnormally low, so it must be monitored frequently. He is receiving intravenous fluids in both arms.

THINKING

1. Critical Thinking (Reflecting and deciding what to do). Which of the patient's vital signs (TPR an BP) might you be able to delegate to nursing assistive personnel?

DOING

2. Practical Knowledge. How would you take the patient's blood pressure? Be specific: (a) Wh site would you use? (b) What equipment would you use?

3. Nursing Process (Assessment).
   a. Will you need to validate any of the vital signs you obtain? If so, why?
   b. How could you validate those vital signs?

CARING

4. Assume that you are very busy. How would you demonstrate caring to this patient w are assessing his vital signs (the ones you did not delegate to a NAP)?

Critical Thinking and Clinical Reasoning

1. Recall the clients you encountered at the community health fair (Meet Your Patient, Volume 1). Two-year-old Jason's oral temperature was 102°F (38.9°C); his skin was warm, dry, and flushed. His mother told you that he had been eating poorly and was very irritable. What cues alert you that something is wrong?

2. You have already established (in Volume 1) what, if any, additional information you need to determine the meaning of Jason's temperature elevation.
   a. What theoretical knowledge may account for Jason's temperature?
   b. Are there any actions you should take while meeting with Jason and his mother? If so, what?
   c. What biases do you have that affect your thinking about this situation? (This requires self-knowledge.)

SECOND EDITION

Fundamentals of Nursing

volume 1

Theory, Concepts, and Applications

Judith M. Wilkinson, PhD, ARNP

Leslie S. Treas, PhD, RN, CPNP-PC, NNP-BC

F.A. Davis Company • Philadelphia

F. A. Davis Company
1915 Arch Street
Philadelphia, PA 19103
www.fadavis.com

Printed in the United States of America

Last digit indicates print number: 10 9 8 7 6 5 4

Publisher, Nursing: Lisa B. Deitch
Special Projects Editor: Shirley A. Kuhn
Director of Content Development: Darlene D. Pedersen
Senior Project Editor: Meghan Ziegler
Design and Ilustrations Manager: Carolyn O'Brien

As new scientific information becomes available through basic and clinical research, recommended treatments and drug therapies undergo changes. The author(s) and publisher have done everything possible to make this book accurate, up to date, and in accord with accepted standards at the time of publication. The author(s), editors, and publisher are not responsible for errors or omissions or for consequences from application of the book, and make no warranty, expressed or implied, in regard to the contents of the book. Any practice described in this book should be applied by the reader in accordance with professional standards of care used in regard to the unique circumstances that may apply in each situation. The reader is advised always to check product information (package inserts) for changes and new information regarding dose and contraindications before administering any drug. Caution is especially urged when using new or infrequently ordered drugs.

Library of Congress Cataloging-in-Publication Data

Wilkinson, Judith M., 1939-
  Fundamentals of nursing / Judith M. Wilkinson, Leslie S. Treas. – 2nd ed.
    p. ; cm.
  Includes bibliographical references and index.
  ISBN-13: 978-0-8036-2264-7
  ISBN-10: 0-8036-2264-3
1. Nursing. I. Treas, Leslie S. II. Title.
  [DNLM: 1. Nursing Process. 2. Nursing Care. 3. Nursing Theory. WY 100]
  RT41.W56 2011
  610.73–dc22   2010037617

Judith M. Wilkinson, PhD, ARNP

Judith Wilkinson taught fundamentals of nursing for 22 years, and more recently, has taught graduate level courses in theory, research, and health policy. She also developed, and taught for many years, an LPN-to-RN transition course. She has given numerous presentations and provided consultation and faculty development workshops for nursing and other schools—primarily in the areas of critical thinking and nursing ethics, but also in standardized nursing languages, teaching strategies, testing, evaluation, and curriculum.

She obtained her PhD in Nursing from the University of Kansas School of Nursing, and master's degrees in Nursing and Education from the University of Missouri-Kansas City School of Nursing. Her basic nursing degree was an ADN from Johnson County Community College, followed by a BSN from Graceland College. She was granted a National Endowment for the Humanities fellowship to study nursing ethics, and a Nurses' Educational Fund (Isabel Hampton Robb) scholarship for her nursing doctoral study. Her master's thesis was a seminal work in moral distress; her doctoral dissertation also studied nursing ethics.

Dr. Wilkinson's clinical background is broad, and includes emergency, critical care, med-surg (float), and obstetric nursing. While engaged in full-time teaching, she maintained certification in inpatient obstetric nursing; her advanced practice license is in nursing care of women.

Her other publications include a nursing process text, a nursing diagnosis handbook (each going into multiple editions), a maternal-newborn care planning book (as a co-author), and journal articles on the topics of curriculum, critical thinking, and nursing ethics. Over the years, she has contributed chapters to several textbooks and authored many ancillary materials, including test banks, learning modules, and review modules.

Judith Wilkinson

Leslie S. Treas, PhD, RN, CPNP-PC, NNP-BC

Dr. Leslie Treas, one of the founders and former vice-president, Research and Development of *Assessment Technologies Institute™, LLC* (ATI) demonstrated leadership and expertise forecasting and directing the design and development of ATI product testing and educational product line since the formation of the company. In this role, Dr. Treas planned and implemented norming, test validation and standard-setting studies to support data-driven product development, creating tests with sound psychometric properties. Under her management, she produced a series of NCLEX-review books and nursing skills DVD set. She has conducted clinical and educational research, publishing in peer reviewed journals of health and education.

Dr. Treas was involved in the start-up of a continuing education company for nurses, physicians, and allied health professionals, serving as Director of Education and Accreditation, *AcaMedic Institute™, LLC*.

Dr. Treas earned a BSN from Pennsylvania State University and MSN degree with emphasis in maternal-child health at the University of Kansas. She obtained a PhD from the University of Kansas in the Educational Psychology and Research Department with dual areas of study of testing and measurement and nursing education. Her primary area of clinical expertise is the care of sick newborns in the NICU and labor and delivery settings in the clinical role of a neonatal nurse practitioner for thirteen years. Dr. Treas obtained dual pediatric and neonatal nurse practitioner certifications at the Cleveland Metropolitan General Hospital, affiliate of Case Western University.

Her journal and textbook publications featured various clinical topics ranging from care of neonatal patients to education-based areas related to nursing licensure preparation and prediction, critical thinking, and others. Leslie has also written articles geared to new graduate readers, addressing contemporary issues involving role change, employment, and communication.

Dr. Treas has presented for annual conferences for Sigma Theta Tau, National Association of Associate Degree Nurses, National Association of Neonatal Nurses, American Association of Colleges of Nursing, National Conference on Professional Nursing Education and Development, Association for the Advancement of Educational Research, to name a few.

She has test writing expertise as a former item writer for the National Certification Examination for Pediatric Nurse Practitioners and Nurses, and also the National Certification Corporation for Neonatal Nurse Practitioner Exam.

Dr. Treas is a member of several professional organizations in the areas of education (e.g., Sigma Theta Tau International Honor Society, National League for Nursing, Pi Lambda Theta International Honor Society and Professional Association in Education), psychometrics and certification (National Organization for Competency Assurance, National Council for Measurement in Education), and clinical nursing (National Association of Neonatal Nurses).

We dedicate this book to:

The creative, dedicated nurse educators, who give so much of themselves to help prepare their students for providing care across the full spectrum of nursing.

My own teachers, who collectively helped to form my perception of, and vision for, nursing and nursing education. To name only four: Dr. Mary Lou Taylor, my teacher and dean at Johnson County Community College, who believed in me and gave me my first teaching job before I was actually qualified to do it; Norma Cole, MSN, my ADN teacher and, later, faculty mentor; she role modeled grace under pressure, to which I aspired but never achieved; Dr. Ann K. Cobb, who taught qualitative research at the University of Kansas, and from whom I first began to understand and appreciate the power of theoretical thinking; and Marie Effingham, MSN, who steered me at an early fork in my career path. She said to me: "A nurse anesthetist has to sit still and be quiet a lot; you'll never be able to do either. Do something else." So I did.

—Judith M. Wilkinson

No work, however seemingly solitary, is ever produced in isolation. I'd like to heartily express my deep gratitude to the many people in my life that made it possible for me to pursue this textbook and arduously see it through to completion. Foremost to my loving husband, Randy, and our children, Megan, Bridget, and Jack, who have supported me with unwavering support in this journey from nurse practitioner to nurse entrepreneur to scholar and writer. Randy tirelessly carried the load and picked up the pieces all along the way. To my mother who always urged me to tackle extraordinary tasks with persistence and diligence. She once said, "How do you eat an elephant? … One bite at a time." This book certainly was just that—one small bite after another, one step at a time, followed by a leap of faith that this important work could be, and would be done. My mother-in-law, Sandy Treas, has been a lifesaver, providing many meals for my family during demanding times over these few years. To Diana Rieser, Nurse Manager of the NICU at Saint Luke's, Kansas City, who walked the walk of what it means to be a thinking, doing, and caring nurse to sick newborns and their families. She mentored "new nurses" with wisdom and care and taught them what it means to be the hands of compassion and competence.

—Leslie S. Treas

Preface

We chose our book title carefully. We have used the words *theory, concepts, application, thinking, doing, and caring* because we believe that excellent nursing requires an equal mix of knowledge, thought, action, and caring. It is knowledge and its application—not just the tasks nurses do—that delineate the various levels of nursing. Even so, skillful performance of tasks is essential to full attainment of the nursing role.

We chose the word *fundamentals* because this text, and its concomitant course, is truly that: the foundation for all that follows. In that sense, and because this basic, fundamental content will be used throughout the nurse's career, we believe it is—or should be—the most important course students take. We want them to say, "Everything I need to know, I learned in fundamentals—all I needed to know about how to think, what to do, and how to be" (at least at a basic level). You will see those themes integrated throughout each chapter.

Among the many additions to the second edition, you will see even more procedures and more illustrations. We have kept the same open, user-friendly, easy-to-read style that students have been telling us they love.

Organization

We have organized the learning package into two volumes to make it easier for on-the-go students to have at hand the material they need in either the classroom or the clinical setting. The content of Volumes 1 and 2 is comprehensive. However, to minimize weight and bulk, and to keep the content manageable for students, we have put some enrichment material to the Electronic Study Guide packaged in Volume 1 for students who need it or who wish to pursue a subject in more depth. This material is also on the DavisPlus Web site. Our chapters are self-contained and rich in cross-references so that teachers and students can use them in any order that fits their needs.

Content within each chapter is generally organized into two major sections: Theoretical Knowledge (Knowing Why) and Practical Knowledge (Knowing How). There is some overlap in these concepts because the two types of knowledge are interdependent. We have made the general distinction because many nursing programs begin with content learned in supporting prerequisite classes and then layer on additional Theoretical Knowledge to explain the rationale for nursing actions and activities (Practical Knowledge). This distinction also affords more flexibility in teaching fundamentals. For example, it is useful to teachers who believe students are more motivated when they present first the concrete (Practical Knowledge), and then the abstract (Theoretical Knowledge); it is equally useful for those who teach from the theoretical to the practical.

We have tried to write a text that can be used as a reference throughout the student's career—one that is comprehensive but not overwhelming. To that end, for example, in Chapter 9 we present a brief overview of growth and development in Volume 1. Many students take a separate growth and development course, and we believe it does not need to be re-taught in fundamentals. But for teachers who wish to teach it, or students who need to review it, we include a comprehensive version of Chapter 9 on the Electronic Study Guide (ESG).

Features

The chapters have numerous pedagogical features to facilitate student learning. These features include:

- *Learning Outcomes and a summary feature entitled "What Are the Main Points in This Chapter?"* – These focus the student's study and provide repetition to facilitate retention of material. In addition, a cross-reference is provided to a "Chapter Overview" podcast on the DavisPlus Web site.
- *Interactive Approach* – The text is written in an engaging style that speaks directly to the student. Recall and critical thinking questions occur frequently in both Volumes 1 and 2 to break chapters up into small, manageable segments and maintain interest.
- *Meet Your Patient* – This chapter-opening feature in Volume 1 introduces one or more patients. The scenario is used throughout the chapter to illustrate theoretical points and make the content "come alive." These patients are often followed in the Critical Thinking activities in Volume 2.
- *Knowledge Checks* – These questions allow students to test their recall of the material presented in the text. Answer sheets and answers are provided on the Electronic Study Guide (ESG).
- *New for Second Edition. Safety Features* – Safety is a big concern in nursing care. To emphasize and help students remember important aspects of safe care, we have specially marked the most important points

about safety to make them visible and memorable. They are shaded in light green and have a cross icon to stand out. We do, of course, have an entire chapter on "Promoting Safety." As well, we have introduced the Quality & Safety Education for Nurses (QSEN) competencies for nurses in the early chapters of Volume 1, and reinforced them where relevant throughout the text.

- *New for Second Edition. What If. . . "* – Volume 2 procedures now include a section to aid students in knowing what to do in special situations that require decisions during a procedure. For example, what if you perform a fingerstick to monitor blood glucose, and the monitor shows a very unusual result or an error message? What should you do? We provide the answer.

- *Critical Thinking Exercises* – Thought-provoking questions in both volumes allow the student to synthesize content and explore personal beliefs. Response sheets are provided on the ESG; suggested responses are found on the Instructors' Resource Disk.

- *Toward Evidenced-based Practice Boxes* – In every chapter, we describe research related to the chapter topic and pose critical thinking exercises for students to examine these findings. The concept of evidence-based practice is introduced in Chapter 6 (Nursing Process: Planning Interventions), further explained in Chapter 8 (Nursing Theory & Research), and mentioned frequently in other chapters as well.

- *Care Plans* – Seventeen care plans integrating NANDA, NIC, and NOC are found in Volume 1 and the ESG. They are based on case studies that allow students to see the nursing process in action. Evidence-based rationales are provided for interventions.

- *New for Second Edition. Care Planning and Care Mapping Exercises* – Several Volume 1 chapters link students to the Student Resource disk and DavisPlus Web site for practice in constructing care plans both in columnar format and as concept maps, using the Concept Map Generator on the Web site. Sample responses are provided.

- *New for Second Edition. Practice Documentation* – Several Volume 2 chapters link students to Practice Documentation exercises on the ESG or DavisPlus.

- *Care Maps* – Care Maps associated with each care plan allow visual learners to grasp the connection between the phases of the nursing process. They also provide an alternative method of care planning.

- *Critical Aspects Boxes* – The critical aspects of all chapter procedures are presented in bullet format in Volume 1 and at the beginning of each procedure in Volume 2. These boxes serve as a reference when studying the Practical Knowledge content in Volume 1; in Volume 2 they provide a quick review just before performing a procedure in the clinical area.

- *Teaching: Self-Care Boxes* – Self-care boxes appear throughout Volume 1. They are similar to the traditional "teaching boxes," but focus on equipping patients to perform self-care.

- *Home Care Boxes* – These provide guidelines for safely modifying care for delivery in the home. Many of the procedures in Volume 2 also have a "Home Care" section for adapting the procedure in the patient's home.

- *Complementary and Alternative Modalities (CAM) Boxes* – Included in several Volume 1 chapters, these describe a complementary therapy related to the chapter topic or present research concerning a complementary therapy (e.g., intercessory prayer in Chapter 14).

- *Caring for the Garcias* – This is an ongoing case study that begins each chapter of Volume 2. It allows students to become familiar with a single family and to experience vicariously the continuity of care they may encounter in outpatient settings. As with all exercises in the 2 volumes, response sheets are provided on the Student Resource disk and DavisPlus Web site.

- *New to Second Edition. Applying the Full-Spectrum Nursing Model* – A part of the critical thinking section of Volume 2, these clinically based exercises guide students to safely practice their thinking skills, and at the same time reinforces the full-spectrum model concepts of thinking, doing, and caring introduced in Volume 1.

- *Critical Thinking and Clinical Reasoning* – These clinically based exercises (in Volume 2) guide students to safely practice their critical thinking skills in preparation for doing so in the clinical area. Frequently, these clinical exercises further analyze material related to the "Meet Your Patient" scenario in Volume 1.

- *New to Second Edition. More Knowledge Maps* – In Volume 2 every chapter now has a knowledge map of Volume 1 theoretical content. This helps students learn the skill of mapping chapter content as a study aid.

- *New to Second Edition. Thinking About the Procedure* – Procedures in Volume 2 include exercises that require students to watch the associated Wilkinson & Treas "Skills Video" to answer the questions. Answers are provided on the Student Resource Disk and DavisPlus.

- *Diagnostic Testing Boxes* – These are found in Volume 2, in applicable chapters. We believe it is more meaningful to place the diagnostic test information near the related content rather than in an isolated chapter. If students need a more comprehensive reference, we recommend a diagnostic testing book.

Themes

The following are themes that are integrated and stressed throughout both volumes of this text, some of them in every chapter:

- *Critical Thinking and the Full Spectrum Model of Nursing.* In addition to the critical thinking questions and exercises in Volumes 1 and 2, concepts in Volume 1 are often presented in an inductive manner, or pose a question to the student (e.g., "What would happen if…..?"). The full spectrum model of nursing is a comprehensive approach to care that uses critical thinking in all aspects of care. It is not rigidly overlaid on each chapter. Because students cannot focus on everything at once, different parts are stressed at different times. Sometimes they are asked, "What theoretical knowledge do you need to . . .?" In other instances they might be asked, "What biases do you have that might interfere with…" The full-spectrum model is reinforced in every chapter of Volume 2 with exercises ("Applying the Full-Spectrum Nursing Model") requiring students to use the model concepts of thinking, doing, and caring.

- **Nursing Process.** Nursing process is related to critical thinking in Chapter 2; Chapters 3 through 7 are a comprehensive presentation of the nursing process, which is presented as reflexive rather than linear. The Practical Knowledge sections of Volume 1 are organized according to the nursing process phases; the procedures in Volume 2 have assessment and evaluation components. In addition, many of the questions and exercises provide opportunity for using the nursing process.

- **NANDA-I, NIC, and NOC Standardized Languages.** Thorough discussion of these taxonomies occurs in the nursing process and other chapters. NOC outcomes and NIC interventions are included in every chapter of Volume 1; many are presented in tables in Volume 2. The Omaha System and the Clinical Care Classification are also used in the community and home health chapters.

- **Caring.** Caring is thoroughly integrated in many chapters and is a part of the Volume 2 book title. Chapter 1 provides historical examples of nursing as a caring profession. Chapter 8 describes the important caring theories. The case study introduces Watson's theory, and that theory is used throughout the chapter to illustrate how theory is applied in nursing. As well, the "Applying the Full-Spectrum Nursing Model" exercises in Volume 2 all have questions involving caring.

- **Wellness.** Many examples used in this text refer to people who are not ill. Chapter 10 emphasizes health; and Chapter 41 talks about the nurse's role in health promotion.

- **Culture.** Cultural diversity is highlighted throughout the text in clinical scenarios, illustrations, and theoretical discussion. Chapter 13 focuses on culturally sensitive nursing care. The *Caring for the Garcias* feature in Volume 2 features a multi-cultural extended family; and ethnic variations are described, as applicable, in procedures.

- *New to Second Edition. Focus on Gerontology.* The Chapter 9 "Expanded Discussion," on the Student Resource Disk, is now divided into Part I, Part II, and Part III, which is entitled "Older Adults." Part III is an in-depth discussion of aging and gerontology, provided by an expert on this topic. Common health problems include dementia, depression, elder abuse, and ageism. Assessments and interventions specifically for

the young-old, middle-old, oldest-old, and frail elderly are provided. We have also included interventions specific to older adults in clinical chapters where they apply. You will also find that many features and exercises use an older adult as the patient.

- **Developmental Stage.** The Theoretical Knowledge in most chapters devotes a section to discussing the effects of lifespan on the chapter topic. In Volume 2, procedures include variations for children and older adults.

- **Spirituality.** Chapter 14 is probably the most extensive presentation of spiritual care available in a fundamentals text. Spirituality is integrated within various chapters in scenarios, examples, and exercises.

- **Documentation.** All chapters include reference to documentation, where relevant. The procedures in Volume 2 all have guidelines for and examples of how to document the procedure. In addition, we have included some "Practice Documentation" exercises on the Student Resource Disk and DavisPlus.

- **Delegation.** Delegation is introduced early, in the nursing process chapters, and is a thread in most Volume 1 chapters. Chapter 38, Leading & Managing, also discusses delegation. In Volume 2, all procedures have guidelines for delegating.

- **ANA Standards.** Nursing and other healthcare standards (e.g., The Joint Commission, Medicare) are frequently referenced. Links to pertinent websites are given so students can keep up with changes to standards.

- **Ethics.** In addition to the comprehensive treatment in Chapter 44, ethical knowledge is an aspect of our full spectrum model. As such, many of the critical thinking exercises ask students to grapple with ethical issues. Good examples are found in Chapter 6, Volume 2, and in the Applying the Full-Spectrum Nursing Model in every chapter.

- **Legal Issues.** Chapter 45 is devoted to legal issues that nurses face every day in their practice. Legal issues are integrated in many other chapters as well (e.g., licensing in Chapter 1; end-of-life legal considerations in Chapter 15).

- **Community and Home Health Care.** Chapters 42 and 43 are devoted exclusively to these topics. Clinical scenarios and examples involve nurses in these settings; Volume 1 has special feature boxes regarding these topics; and procedures in Volume 2 have sections for adapting skills to home care.

- **Complementary Therapies.** Nursing is presented as holistic throughout. Chapter 40 is devoted exclusively to complementary and alternative therapies; and several chapters in Volume 1 (e.g., Chapter 13, Culture & Ethnicity) contain material and/or boxes related to this topic.

- **Contemporary Issues.** We have included information about bioterrorism (Chapter 20, Promoting Asepsis & Preventing Infection; Chapter 42, Community Nursing; and in the Meet Your Nurse Role Model scenario in the informatics chapter). Chapter 20 also includes updated and expanded material on drug-resistant pathogens, emerging infectious diseases, and healthcare-acquired infections. The chapter on safety includes ways to assess for and cope with violence in the healthcare setting.

- *Technology and Computers.* Chapter 39 is an excellent introduction to nursing informatics. Standardized languages and computerized care planning and documentation are interspersed throughout the book (for example, in the nursing process and medications chapters), and especially in standardized language tables in the Volume 2 clinical chapters. We also emphasize electronic documentation in Chapter 16 and in our illustrations for documenting procedures in Volume 2. We further encourage use of technology by providing students with links to material on DavisPlus and many other websites related to the chapter topic.

The Text as a Response to Change

This book was developed to address the needs of today's nursing students and in response to the following changes in nursing education and practice.

Changes in Students

- **Nontraditional Students.** Students range from traditional, younger students to older, second-career students. Many are older and have work or family responsibilities that compete with school. To address this change we have followed two principles of adult learning, that learning must be relevant and efficient. For example, we have divided the content into two volumes devoted to the classroom and clinical setting, respectively. We have made great use of the Electronic Study Guide and DavisPlus to deliver enhancements to the printed text, knowing that highly motivated and computer literate students will welcome the chance to use these technologies to maximize their learning.
- **Variety in Learning Styles.** Students learn in different ways. To address this, we have used over 1400 photos and as many diagrams to assist visual learners. Podcasts, animations and sound files of heart sounds and many other clinical assessment findings are included on the Electronic Study Guide for auditory learners. To teach psychomotor skills, we have, in addition to step-by-step procedures, skills videos, and checklists students can print out for practicing procedures or teachers to use in evaluations.

  Because learning improves when content is meaningful to the learner, each chapter opens with a patient scenario or story of a practicing nurse. This story is woven throughout the chapter to provide context for factual information and to show how concepts are applied and how nurses think. We stress practical application throughout the text because adults want to apply knowledge in real-life circumstances. The Garcia family case, which is introduced in and continues throughout all chapters of Volume 2, is a prime example of this.

- **Reading Comprehension.** Whether because of changes in admission requirements, or because English is a second language, or for other reasons, some schools are finding students' reading abilities to be lower than in the past.

  We addressed this change by writing in an informal style, addressing the student directly ("you will..."). We have not made the content more superficial, but have made reading about it more inviting and user-friendly. We define new terms at their first use in each chapter, and include a glossary on the Student Resource Disk for additional terms the student may not know.

  To aid in retention we have interspersed knowledge checks and critical thinking questions frequently throughout Volume 1 to allow students to check their recall and understanding of the material presented as they progress through the chapters. Recognizing that repetition aids retention, we provide "Learning Outcomes" at the beginning of each chapter in Volume 1. In addition, each chapter in Volume 2 includes a list titled *"What are the Main Points In This Chapter"* and a full-page Knowledge Map of the chapter content. To accompany each chapter, there is also a podcast on the DavisPlus Web site that overviews the chapter content. And finally, the Student Resources contain an Audio Glossary.

- **The Technology Generation.** The newer generation of students is accustomed to using technology and multitasking. To hold their attention, in addition to our easy-to-read style, we have presented information in an interactive manner, and in relatively short segments interspersed with review questions and critical thinking questions. For this same reason, the text frequently directs students to find related information on the Student Resource Disk or DavisPlus and on the Internet, often in the form of podcasts or sound files.

- *New to Second Edition:* New eBooks offer the convenience of accessing the book from wherever the student has Internet access without having to lug around heavy books.

Changes in Curriculum

- **Teachers say they do not have enough time to "cover the content."**

  One way to address this problem is to not re-teach material students have had in other classes. We provide, for example, just enough anatomy and physiology in each chapter to aid students who need to review A&P, or who are taking A&P concurrently with nursing courses. You should not need to "cover" it in class. Most students do take a separate course in growth and development; so we have included most of that material (Chapter 9) on the Student Resource Disk "Expanded Discussion."

  Some curricula have de-emphasized mental health; mental health may be taught in other (e.g.,

medical-surgical) clinical areas, with no separate mental health course.

In response to pleas from educators, we have again expanded the mental health content in Chapter 11 and included tools for psychosocial assessment. In addition to the usual concepts of self-concept and self-esteem, we have included basic assessments and interventions for anxiety and depression, which students will encounter regularly in all areas, not just on mental health units. We have added content specific to older adults (e.g., differentiating between depression and dementia). In Chapter 18, "Communicating & Therapeutic Relationships," we have excellent content on the nurse-patient relationship and communication techniques that mental health teachers find so essential. Chapter 25, Stress & Adaptation, includes information about defense mechanisms.

The curriculum does not include separate pharmacology, nutrition, ethics, or nursing process courses.

Because all nurses need grounding in these topics, we have provided extensive coverage of these topics, both in Volume 1 and the Electronic Study Guide. Chapter 23, Administering Medications, provides in-depth pharmacology information. Chapter 26, Nutrition, provides a good basic foundation for understanding patients' nutritional needs. Chapter 44 is a comprehensive look at nursing ethics. We have, arguably, the most useful and thorough presentation of nursing process available in a fundamentals text. These chapters, as well as most others, will be a valuable reference for students when they take other clinical nursing courses.

Changes in Nursing and Health Care

- *Nursing role is increasingly complex, requiring management, decision-making, delegation, and supervision skills early in the career.*
  To address this change we have included a comprehensive discussion of leadership and management in Chapter 38. The critical thinking exercises, especially in Volume 2, and the Garcias feature help students to develop clinical decision-making skills. Delegation is presented early, in the nursing process chapters, and stressed in the rest of the chapters in Volume 1, as applicable. Each clinical procedure in Volume 2 contains a "Delegation" section.
- *Health care has moved increasingly from the hospital to the home and community.*
  To address this change we have included a provocative discussion about the evolving health care system in the supplementary material for Chapter 1 on the Electronic Study Guide. In addition, Chapters 42 and 43 discuss Home Care and Community Care. Home and community care are integrated throughout Volume 1 (e.g., Healthy People 2020 goals are cited); and the procedures in Volume 2 include home care adaptations, as well as patient teaching points that will enable patients and caregivers to assume more responsibility for care.

- *Nurses need to be critical thinkers and life-long learners.*
  To address this change we have organized the text around a model of Full-Spectrum Nursing, a comprehensive approach to care that uses critical thinking in all aspects of care. The model is reinforced in each chapter of Volume 2 in the feature, "Applying the Full-Spectrum Nursing Model." Critical thinking is integrated throughout both volumes of the text, both in discussion and in critical thinking exercises. Discussion of this model follows.

The Full-Spectrum Model of Nursing

We believe that nursing knowledge is a fusion of theoretical knowledge, practical knowledge, self-knowledge, and ethical knowledge. To function at the highest level, nurses use critical thinking and the nursing process to blend thinking and doing to put caring into action. We refer to this blend as *Full Spectrum Nursing*. We have organized our learning package to reflect this philosophy. This model is presented in Chapter 2 and referred to and used throughout the text.

The Learning Package

This is a well-integrated and cross-referenced package containing a two-volume text, a Student Resource Disk, instructors' materials provided on a CD as well as on DavisPlus, and an associated website. Although any item can be used either in classroom or clinical settings, Volume 1 will usually be used in the classroom setting and in preparing for clinical, whereas Volume 2 will usually be used in the clinical setting or learning lab.

PowerPoint Orientation

Schools who adopt our textbook will have access to a PowerPoint presentation to enable students and new faculty to make the best use of the learning package.

Volume I

Volume 1 contains all the theoretical and conceptual material typically present in a fundamentals text, presented in a clinically focused, user-friendly manner, and incorporating many examples. This presentation allows students to see how the content will be useful to them. In Chapters 8 through 45, the nursing process is used as the model to organize the Practical Knowledge section.

Unit 1—focuses on how nurses think. It begins by showing the evolution of nursing: how our history relates to our present. Chapter 2 focuses on critical thinking, and Chapters 3 through 7 provide an extensive treatment of the nursing process. This unit prepares students to follow the organization of subsequent chapters and provides the thinking tools and processes they need to apply the content of the other chapters. Chapter 8 contains an overview of the processes of theory building, nursing research, and evidence-based practice as they relate to the nurse in practice.

Unit 2—integrates the internal and external factors that affect an individual's health (e.g., family, culture, spirituality, and life stage). Internal factors are personal beliefs or attributes that influence how the client views health, health care, and nursing. A groundbreaking feature is Chapter 10, which describes the health-illness-wellness continuum in an experiential way, encouraging self-knowledge, personal growth, and affective learning of that content.

Unit 3—examines essential nursing interventions. We consider these skills "essential" because nurses use some or all of these skills in <u>all</u> areas of nursing, regardless of setting or patient diagnosis. The unit begins with documentation and includes communication, teaching, taking vital signs, physical assessment, asepsis, safety, hygiene, and medication administration.

Unit 4—concentrates on nursing care that supports physiological function. We examine broad categories of physiological function (e.g., nutrition, elimination, oxygenation) and discuss related nursing care.

Unit 5—explores diverse nursing functions. For example, we look at leadership and management, the use of technology and informatics, and health promotion activities. Chapter 39 is a more thorough introduction to informatics than you will usually find in a fundamentals text. And we are especially proud of Chapter 40, which provides a deeper treatment of holistic healing than you will typically find. We believe that a fundamentals book, overall, provides all concepts needed for a holistic view of the patient—just scan our chapter titles to see what we mean by that. We went one step farther with Chapter 40.

Unit 6—looks at the context for nurses' work. This includes chapters on community and home care, as well as the ethical and legal contexts for nursing work. In addition, we include, on the Electronic Study Guide, an excellent chapter (Chapter 46) on Canadian Healthcare Delivery Systems, written by respected Canadian nurse authors.

Volume 2

Volume 2 is designed primarily, but not exclusively, for use in the skills lab and clinical setting. As does Volume 1, it includes thinking, doing, and caring. The critical thinking exercises require students to use their thinking skills and the nursing process to apply theoretical knowledge to specific patient situations. The clinical procedures, assessment tools, clinical forms, diagnostic testing information, and standardized language tables comprise the practical knowledge sections. Throughout Volume 2, students have access to a simulated experience known as *Caring for the Garcias*, through which they learn about the nursing role, the healthcare system, and the real-world application of the content in Volume 1.

Student Resource Disk

The Student Resource Disk included in Volume 1 and on the DavisPlus Web site at http://davisplus.fadavis.com/Wilkinson2, contains expanded discussions of some of the Volume 1 material, mastery questions, answers to the Volume 1 Knowledge Checks, a panel of NCLEX-style test questions for practice, a glossary, additional care plans and care maps, and procedure checklists. Also included are forms that students can print out to write their answers to Knowledge Checks, Critical Thinking questions, Mastery questions, as well as the Volume 2 critical thinking exercises. It also provides other types of forms that students can print and use in clinical, for example, some assessment tools. The questions themselves have expandable space so that answers can be typed in on the electronic form and then printed out. The large glossary provides definitions of all bolded terms used in the text as well as supplementary terms that may be helpful to students.

Procedure checklists can be used to study for skills lab or clinical, or as a means to assess skill mastery. Checklists are provided in two formats: one is a detailed list of steps for each procedure; another is a generic, principles-based list that instructors can use to evaluate all procedures.

Instructor's Guide

The Instructor's Guide contains everything on the Electronic Study Guide plus additional features to assist faculty. These include an image bank of illustrations from the book, lesson plans, and PowerPoint lecture outlines – now with illustrations. Also included are teaching strategies to accompany each chapter, suggested responses for the critical thinking exercises in Volumes 1 and 2, instructions for using concept mapping, and a test bank of over 1100 NCLEX-style questions, including the newer NCLEX formats.

New for Second Edition: The PowerPoint lecture outlines now include "clicker" questions, a critical thinking question, and illustrations.

Website

The text website, for both students and teachers, is available at www.fadavis.com. The site contains many of the materials you will find on the Student Resource Disk, as well as additional content mastery activities and clinical animations. We have added several new sound files, animations, and mastery activities to the second edition.

- *Podcasts* – For audio learners, podcasts for each chapter summarize the main ideas for convenient prep for class or review for quizzes or exams. There are 12 "stress buster" podcasts: one for each month. You will also find 24 clever and revealing test-taking tips to give you the "one-up" on getting a better test result.

- *NCLEX-style practice questions for students* – We have added more questions to help students right from the beginning of their nursing studies to become comfortable answering NCLEX-style questions.
- *New to Second Edition. E-book.* Tired of lugging around heavy books? Now you can access this two-volume textbook electronically. Log on to the DavisPlus site for on-screen reading—just as though you were turning pages in your own book.

How to Use This Learning Package (for Teachers)

You are fortunate to be working with students at perhaps the most formative point in their nursing education: the fundamentals course. We are certain that each of you will bring your own special style to the teaching of this most-important-of-all nursing courses, and that you will find new and creative ways to use the many teaching and learning features we have provided. We hope your enjoyment of this new and improved learning package is equal to our pride in it.

For suggestions about how to use this integrated learning package.

 Go to "How to Use This Learning Package" on the Instructors Resource Disk.

We have also prepared for you a PowerPoint slide presentation and a podcast explaining how to use the learning package. You can use either or both to orient new teachers and students so they can easily navigate the entire learning package.

 Go to "Getting the Most Out of This Learning Package" podcast on the DavisPlus website.

Getting the Most Out of This Learning Package (for Students)

For ideas about how to use your textbooks and the Electronic Study Guide to get the best results from your studying,

 Go to "Getting the Most Out of This Learning Package" on the Electronic Study Guide.

For when you'd rather listen than read, we now offer podcasts that describe ways for you to use the different components of your learning package—that is, your two-volume book set, nursing skills DVD set, your student Electronic Study Guide, NCLEX-style practice questions, animations, documentation exercises, care mapping exercises, concept map generator, and many more, worthwhile learning tools.

 Go to "Getting the Most Out of This Learning Package" podcast on the DavisPlus website.

We also know that being a student in a nursing program is hard work and can be overwhelming. Log on to the DavisPlus website for 12 useful strategies to reduce your stress while you are on your journey to becoming a nurse.

 Go to "Stress Busters" podcast on the DavisPlus website.

Your goal is to do well in your courses. Knowing testing is an important part of your experience while in school, we now offer clever, test taking tips to help you to take tests with excellence and show what you know!

 Go to "Test-taking Tips" podcast on the DavisPlus website.

Contributors to Second Edition

The following people contributed material that was used in creating this learning package. We are grateful for their assistance.

Julia Aucoin, RN, DNS, BC, CNE
Associate Professor
Kaplan University, Winston-Salem State University,
   and Nova Southeastern University
Durham, North Carolina
Clinical consultant and literature reviews

Linda Blazovich, RN, MSN
Associate Professor, Nursing Program
The College of St. Catherine
St. Paul, Minnesota
Procedure checklists

Diane Bligh, RN, MS, CNS
Associate Professor, Nursing
Front Range Community College
Westminster, Colorado
Knowledge Maps, Instructors Guide, Lecture Outlines,
   Care Planning Exercises

Leanne Cowin, RN, PhD
Professor, School of Nursing & Midwifery
College of Health and Science
University of Western Sydney
Penrith South DC, New South Wales, Australia
Literature searches

Lisa Culliton, MSN, CPN
Pediatric Nurse Practitioner, Silver City Health Center
Faculty, University of Kansas School of Nursing
Kansas City, Kansas
Literature searches

Debbie Ellison, RN, MSN
Professor
Austin Peay State University
Clarksville, Tennessee
Nursing care plans; Chapter 35 procedures

Garrett Fardon
Student, Drake University
Des Moines, Iowa
Clerical assistance

Mary Gant, APN, ACNS-BC, RRT
Performance Improvement Department
Adult Cystic Fibrosis Program
Christiana Care Health System
Newark, Delaware
Chapter 35 procedures

Kathryn Van Dyke Hayes, PhD, RN-BC, CNE
Professor
School of Nursing & Allied Health Professions
Holy Family University
Philadelphia, Pennsylvania
Test bank items

Lisa Lyons, RN, BSN
Nursing Instructor
Bristol-Plymouth Regional Technical School
Taunton, Massachusetts
Chapter 29, 30, 31, and 34 procedures

Lisa LaMothe Melo, RN, BSN
Nursing Instructor
Bristol-Plymouth Regional Technical School
Taunton, Massachusetts
Chapter 29, 30, 31, and 34 procedures

Mary N. Meyer, MSN, ARNP-BC
Director, Learning Lab
University of Kansas School of Nursing
Kansas City, Kansas
Chapter 21 and 28 procedures

Lori Ormsby, MSN, GCNS-BC, APRN, CWOCN
Director, Wound Management Program
Oklahoma State University Medical Center
Oklahoma City, Oklahoma
Chapter 34

Pamela Owen, BSN
Dean of Programs
Canadian Health Care Academy
Vancouver, British Columbia, Canada
Chapter 46

Jessica Pedersen, ARNP, FNP-C
Nurse Practitioner
Kansas City Minute Clinic
Kansas City, Kansas
Chapter 26 procedures

Cynthia Pivec, BS
Instructor, Nursing Laboratory
The College of St. Catherine
St. Paul, Minnesota
Procedure checklists

Linda Puetz, RN, BA, BSN, MEd
Clinical Learning Strategist
Cerner Corporation
Overland Park, Kansas
Chapter 16

Veronica Rempusheski, RN, FAAN, PhD
Jeanne K. Buxbaum Chair of Nursing Science
School of Nursing, College of Health Sciences
University of Delaware
Newark, Delaware
Chapter 9, Part III, Expanded Discussion (ESG)

Elizabeth Richmond, BSN, MEd
Nursing Instructor
Bristol-Plymouth Regional Technical School
Taunton, Massachusetts
Chapter 22 procedures

Sarah Kennedy Roland, RN, MSN
Nursing Instructor
Central Carolina Technical College
Sumter, South Carolina
Documentation exercises, sample nurses notes, test bank items

Susan Simmons, ARNP-BC, PhD
Family Nurse Practitioner
Olathe Medical Services
Overland Park, Kansas
Clinical consultant, literature reviews

Mable H. Smith, RN, JD, PhD
Dean and Professor
University of Southern Nevada
Henderson, Nevada
Chapter 45

Lynne Sullivan, RN, MS
Coordinator of Nursing Programs
Bristol-Plymouth Regional Technical School
Taunton, Massachusetts
Chapter 29, 30, 31, and 34 procedures

Mary Pat Szutenbach, RN, CNS, PhD
Assistant Professor
Loretto Heights School of Nursing
Regis University
Denver, Colorado
Chapter 26

Janet Terra, RN, MSN
Practical Nursing Instructor
Bristol-Plymouth Regional Technical School
Taunton, Massachusetts
Chapter 22 procedures

Cynthia Thompson, RN, BSN
Nursing Instructor
Bristol-Plymouth Regional Technical School
Taunton, Massachusetts
Chapter 22 procedures

Diana Tilton, RN, MSN
Assistant Professor of Nursing
Johnson County Community College
Overland Park, Kansas
Chapter 20 procedures

Lisa Watkins, RN, MS
Associate Dean
Tulsa Community College
Tulsa, Oklahoma
Chapter 27 procedures

Janis Watts, RN, MSN
Manager, Clinical Information Systems & Staff Development
Clarian North Medical Center
Indianapolis, Indiana
Chapter 39

Michelle Williams, RN, MSN
Assistant Professor
School of Nursing
Austin Peay State University
Clarksville, Tennessee
Nursing Care Plans

Contributors from First Edition

Nancy R. Ahern, RN, MSN
Chapters 13 and 14

Rachel E. Albert, RN, PhD
Chapter 18

Mary Ann Andersson, PhD, APRN, BC
Chapter 8

Diane M. Bligh, RN, MS, CNS
Concept Maps, Care Maps, Test Questions, Procedures

Mary Beth Bohli, BSN, MSN
Chapter 4

Christine Dimartile Bolla, RN, DNSC
Chapter 37

Carol Boswell, RN, EdD
Chapter 4

Clara Boyle, RN, EdD
Chapter 25

Mary Anne Bright, EdD, APRN, BC
Chapter 40

Patricia Carroll, RN, CEN, RRT, MS
Care Plans

Traudel B. Cline, AD, BS, MS, PhD
Chapter 22

Pamela Sue Combs, RN, MSN
Chapter 16

Leanne Cowin, BN, MNS, PhD
Chapter 11

Kathleen Crawford, BS, LVN
Chapter 45

Patricia Marie Dillon, RN, DNSc
Procedures

Maggie Thurmond Dorsey, RN, MSN, EdD
Chapter 28

June S. Goyne, RN, MSN, EdD
Chapter 35

Janice Harris, RN, MSN
Chapter 21

Annette Hayes, MSN, RNC, CS
Chapter 9

Collette Bishop Hendler, RN, BS, CCRN
Test Questions, Procedures

Patricia Holden-Huchton, RN, DSN, ACRN
Supplemental Materials for Chapter 1

Anita Huse, RN, MSN, EdD
Chapter 30

Melba Ingram, RN, MSN
Chapter 41

Kathleen Jones MSN, APRN, BC
Procedures

Lori Klingman, RN, MSN
Chapter 9

Susan Jeanne Lamanna, RN, MA, MSN, ANP
Chapter 15

Sandra Dahl McHenry, RN, DNSc
Chapter 32

Gary J. Measom, APRN, PhD, CCRN
Chapter 31

Kristen S. Montgomery, RN, PhD
Chapter 12

Kathleen Ahern Nieubuurt, RN, MS
Test Questions

Barbara Nubile, RN, MSN
Procedures

Mary O'Keefe, RN, PhD, JD
Chapter 45

James C. Pace, DSN, MDiv, APRN-BC, FAANP
Chapter 14

Cindy Parsons DNP, ARNP, BC
Test Questions

Linda Pasto, RN, MS
Chapter 24

Joyce W. Pompey, RN, MSN
Chapter 28

Debbie J. Rahn, RN, MSN, CNE
Chapter 18

Bonnie Raingruber, PhD, MS, BS, CNS
Concept Maps, Mapping Tutorial

Judith P. Ruland, RN, PhD
Chapter 44

Debra Anne Schilleman, RN, BSN, LSAC
Chapter 33

Michelle Seale

Kathy Shepard, RN, CWS
Procedures

Joellen H. Shumway, RN
Chapter 27

Marlene Smadu, RN, BSCN, MADED, EdD
Chapter 46

Pamela Smith, RN, PhD
Chapter 10

Susan Smith, BSN, RNC
Chapter 23

Joanne Thanavaro, DNP, MSN(R), APRN-BC
Chapter 19

Lisa Theriault, RN, MSN, APRN
Chapter 26

Deborah Weaver, RN, PhD
Chapter 3

Diane Whitehead, RN, EdD
Chapter 38

Bruce K. Wilson, RN, PhD, LVN, CNS
Chapter 20

Paige Wimberley, MSN, RN-CS
Chapter 34

Kathleen M. Young, RN, MA
Chapter 39

Steering Committee

Kristen G. Barbee, RN, MSN, CNE
Assistant Professor
Cabarrus College of Health Sciences
Concord, North Carolina

Elaine J. Beaupre, RN, MEd, MSN, CNE
Professor of Nursing
Quincy College
Quincy, Massachusetts

Peg Broadie, RN, MSN
Assistant Professor
Allen College
Waterloo, Iowa

Susan J. Garbutt, RN, DNP, CIC, CNE
Nursing Program Director
Ultimate Medical Academy
Tampa, Florida

Thuy Lam, RN, MSN
Nursing Instructor
J.F. Drake State Technical College
Huntsville, Alabama

Mark W. Longshore, RN, MSN
Nursing Faculty
Front Range Community College
Fort Collins, Colorado

Beatriz C. Nieto, RN, PhD
Associate Professor
The University of Texas – Pan American
Edinburg, Texas

Sarah Roland, RN, MSN
Nursing Instructor
Central Carolina Technical College
Sumter, South Carolina

Caitlin M. Stover, RN, MS, PHCNS-BC
Nursing Instructor
Worcester State College
Worcester, Massachusetts

Reviewers

Jocelyn Amberg, RN, MSN
Nursing Program Director
Albuquerque Public Schools Career Enrichment Center
Albuquerque, New Mexico

Elizabeth M. Andal, PhD, PMHCNS-BC, FAAN
Psychiatric Clinical Nurse Specialist
Truxton Psychiatric Medical Group
Bakersfield, California

Deborah A. Andris, MSN, APNP
Nurse Practitioner, Department of Surgery, Colo-Rectal
    Surgery Program
Medical College of Wisconsin
Milwaukee, Wisconsin

Patrice Balkcom, RN, MSN
Director of Nursing Program, Milledgeville Campus
Central Georgia Technical College
Milledgeville, Georgia

Barbara Bonenberger, RN, MNEd, CNE
Instructor
University of Pittsburgh School of Nursing
Pittsburgh, Pennsylvania

Wanda Bonnel, RN, PhD
Associate Professor
University of Kansas School of Nursing
Kansas City, Kansas

Colette Dieujuste, RNC, MS
Assistant Professor
Simmons College
Boston, Massachusetts

Joyce Arlene Ennis, RN, MSN, ANP-BC
Assistant Professor, Nursing
Carroll University
Waukesha, Wisconsin

Sally Flesch, BSN, MS, EdS, PhD
Coordinator, Professor
Black Hawk College
Moline, Illinois

Deborah L. Galante, RN, MSN, CNOR
Staff Development Specialist
Christiana Care Health System
Newark, Delaware

Lynn Hadaway, RN, MEd, BC, CRNI
Consultant, Infusion Nursing
Lynn Hadaway Associates, Inc.
Milner, Georgia

Deborah B. Hadley, RN, MSN, CNOR
Instructor, Retired
Alcorn State University
PRN Staff Nurse, Postpartum and Medical Units
Natchez Regional Medical Center
Natchez, Mississippi

Linda K. Heitman, RN, PhD, ACNS-BC
Professor
Southeast Missouri State University
Cape Girardeau, Missouri

Gladys L. Husted, RN, PhD, CNE
Professor Emeritus, Distinguished Professor
Duquesne University
Pittsburgh, Pennsylvania

Kathleen C. Jones, RN, MSN, CNS
Associate Professor of Nursing
Walters State Community College
Greeneville, Tennessee

Jeanie Krause-Bachand, RN, EdD, MSN
Associate Professor of Nursing
York College of Pennsylvania
York, Pennsylvania

Janice Garrison Lanham, RN, MS, CCNS, FNP
Nursing Faculty
Clemson University
Seneca, South Carolina

Dawn LaPorte, RN, BSN, CRRN
Faculty
First Choice Training Institute
Nursing Supervisor
Northeast Rehabilitation Hospital
Salem, New Hampshire

Maureen McDonald, RN, MS
Professor, Nurse Education
Massasoit Community College
Brockton, Massachusetts

Laura Smith McKenna, RN, DNSc
College Director
American College of Nursing
Concord, California

Mary N. Meyer, MSN, ARNP-BC
Assistant Professor and Director of Clinical Learning Lab
University of Kansas School of Nursing
Kansas City, Kansas

Pamela S. Miller, RN, MS
Instructor
Mount Carmel College of Nursing
Columbus, Ohio

Christine Ouellette, MS, NP
Adjunct Faculty
Quincy College
Quincy, Massachusetts

Linda Pasto, RN, MS, CNE
Professor of Nursing
Tompkins-Cortland Community College
Dryden, New York

Linda C. Radzvin, RN, PhD, CRNP
Professor and Program Director
Community College of Allegheny County
Monroeville, Pennsylvania

Carla E. Randall, RN, PhD
Assistant Professor
University of Southern Maine College of Nursing and Health
    Professions
Lewiston, Maine

Debra L. Renna, MSN, CCRN
Assistant Professor
Florida International University
North Miami, Florida

Patsy M. Spratling, RN, MSN
Nursing Instructor
Holmes Community College
Ridgeland, Mississippi

Lynn M. Stover, RN, BC, DSN, SANE
Associate Professor of Nursing
Clayton State University School of Nursing
Morrow, Georgia

Mary Pat Szutenbach, RN, PhD, CNS
Assistant Professor
Loretto Heights School of Nursing, Regis University
Denver, Colorado

Marcy Tanner, RN, MSN
Nursing Instructor
Southwestern Oklahoma State University
Weatherford, Oklahoma

Pamela K. Weinberg, RN, MSN
Nursing Instructor
Central Carolina Technical College
Sumter, South Carolina

Acknowledgments

We wish to extend sincere thanks to the exceptional team that helped us create this learning package, and especially to the following people:

- **Lisa Deitch**, Acquisitions Editor and friend, for her vision in helping to create the first edition, and for her continued support throughout its revision.

- **Shirley Kuhn**, Special Projects Editor, for pouring oil on troubled waters (mostly ours) and facilitating communication between the authors and all elements of the production team. We so appreciate her integrity, work ethic, and sense of humor.

- **Meghan Ziegler**, Senior Project Editor, for her amazing ability to organize and retrieve information and files, all the while churning out a mountain of work. She kept chaos at bay, made our lives easier, and never let us down.

- **Darlene Pedersen**, Director of Content Development, for working her magic behind the scenes to support our project. We heartily thank her for throwing us a lifeline, when needed, to make things just a little bit easier.

- **Mary N. Meyer, MSN, ARNP-BC, Shonte′ M. Hutson, MPA,** and the University of Kansas School of Nursing, Kansas City, Kansas, for use of the nursing lab, for models for photos, and for generous assistance with procedures and illustrations.

- **Dean Shepard**, photographer, who blended the science and art of photography to get the job done with excellence and efficiency.

- **Renee Fransen, RN, BSN, David McIntosh,** and **Daniel Tucker**, at NurseSquared, for allowing us to use their documentation software to create electronic documentation illustrations for the procedures. They generously gave of their time teaching us to use the software.

- **Linda Puetz, RN, BA, BSN** and **Cerner Corporation,** for providing screen shots of electronic documentation for the Documenting and Recording chapter.

- **Kathy Carver, MSN, RN**, Professor, and **Kureo Ohta**, Adjunct Faculty, at Johnson County Community College, Overland Park, Kansas; and **Besher Gharaibeh, RN, MSN, CNS,** doctoral candidate and graduate teaching assistant, the University of Kansas School of Nursing, who volunteered their time to serve as photo models.

Contents

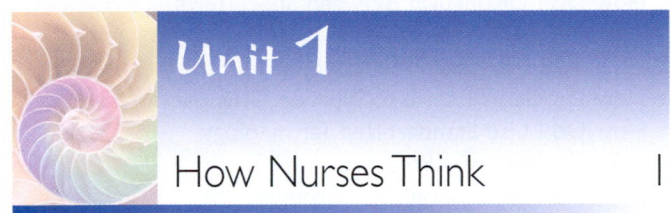

How Nurses Think   1

CHAPTER **4**

Nursing Process: Diagnosis 54

CHAPTER **5**

Nursing Process: Planning Outcomes 80

CHAPTER **6**

Nursing Process: Planning Interventions 101

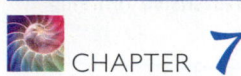

CHAPTER 7

Nursing Process: Implementation & Evaluation   116

CHAPTER 8

Nursing Theory & Research   134

Unit 2

Factors Affecting Health   157

CHAPTER 9

Development Across the Life Span   159

CHAPTER 10

Experiencing Health & Illness   165

CHAPTER **14**

Spirituality   245

CHAPTER **15**

Loss, Grief, & Dying   264

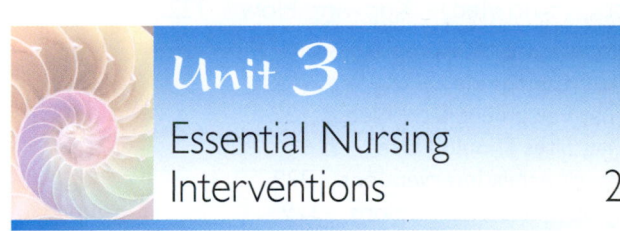

Unit **3**
Essential Nursing Interventions   289

CHAPTER **16**

Documenting & Reporting   291

CHAPTER **17**

Measuring Vital Signs　316

CHAPTER **18**

Communicating & Therapeutic Relationships　351

CHAPTER **19**

Health Assessment: Performing a Physical Examination   370

CHAPTER **20**

Promoting Asepsis & Preventing Infection   408

CHAPTER **21**

Promoting Safety   435

CHAPTER **22**

Facilitating Hygiene   464

CHAPTER **23**

Administering Medications   495

CHAPTER **24**

Teaching Clients   548

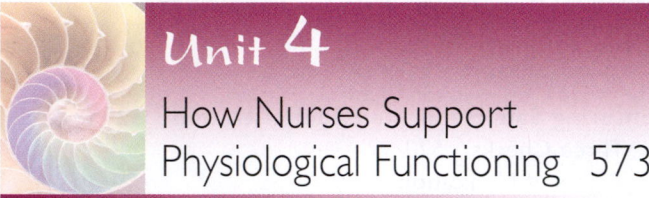

Unit 4
How Nurses Support Physiological Functioning   573

CHAPTER **25**

Stress & Adaptation   575

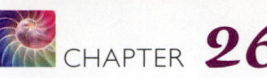

CHAPTER **26**

Nutrition   598

CHAPTER **30**

Pain Management   725

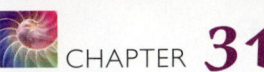

CHAPTER **31**

Activity & Exercise   750

CHAPTER **32**

Sexual Health   781

CHAPTER **33**

Sleep & Rest   812

CHAPTER **34**

Skin Integrity & Wound Healing   830

CHAPTER **35**

Oxygenation 866

 CHAPTER **36**

Fluids, Electrolytes, & Acid-Base Balance 913

 CHAPTER **37**

Perioperative Nursing 950

Unit 5

Nursing Functions   979

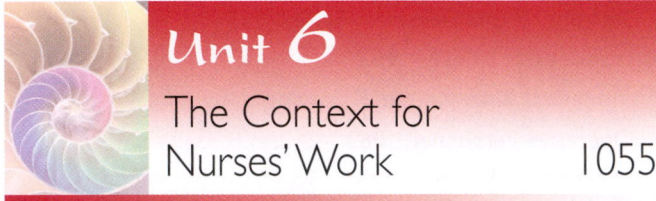

Unit **6**

The Context for
Nurses' Work   1055

CHAPTER **44**

Ethics & Values 1083

 CHAPTER **45**

Legal Issues 1108

 CHAPTER **46**

Healthcare in Canada (Refer to the Student Resource Disk or DavisPlus)

Special Features

How Nurses Think

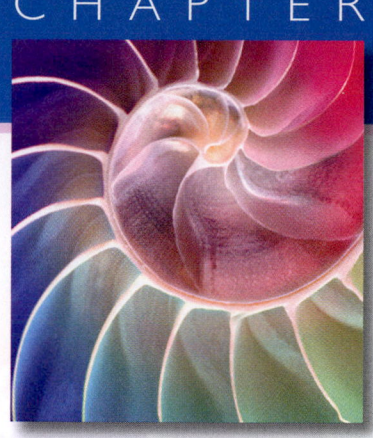

CHAPTER 1

Evolution of Nursing Thought & Action

Learning Outcomes

After completing this chapter, you should be able to:

- ➤ Describe the role of religion in the development of nursing.
- ➤ Identify the factors that led to the change of nursing from a vocation of men and women to a predominantly female profession.
- ➤ Explain the role of the military in the development of the nursing profession.
- ➤ Define *nursing* in your own words.
- ➤ Discuss the transitions nursing education has undergone in the last century.
- ➤ Differentiate among the various forms of nursing education.
- ➤ Explain how nursing practice is regulated.
- ➤ Give four examples of influential nursing organizations.

- ➤ Name and recognize the four purposes of nursing care.
- ➤ Delineate the forces and trends affecting contemporary nursing practice.

If you were assigned the Expanded Discussion on the Electronic Study Guide, you should also be able to demonstrate the following outcomes:

- ➤ Describe the healthcare delivery system in the United States, including sites for care, types of workers, regulation, and financing of healthcare.
- ➤ Name nine expanded roles for nursing.
- ➤ Discuss issues related to healthcare reform.

Nurses Make a Difference ...

Then & Now

Time: 1854, Üsküdar (now part of Istanbul, Turkey) in the Crimea

The hospital tent is set up away from the battlefield. The injured and dying soldiers are lying upon the bare earth, soiled and covered with crusted blood. Outside the air is cool, yet the tent is stifling with the rank odor of disease and death. Scanning the scene, Florence Nightingale gathers her staff of 38 nurses. They review the environmental condition of the hospital tent, the health problems of the soldiers, and the supplies and equipment they have to work with. First, they open the tent to allow in fresh air. Then they clean the tent, bathe the wounded, and provide clean bedding. They assess and dress the wounds, feed the soldiers a nutritious meal, and comfort those dying or in pain. They offer encouragement and emotional care to the healthier soldiers and help them to write letters home.

Within a brief period of time the mortality rate drops from 47% to 2% and morale improves immeasurably.

Time: 2010, Your Local Hospital

While standing at the bedside mixing an antibiotic solution, Susan listens to the ventilator cycle. She notes that her patient has begun to trigger breaths on his own. In the background she hears the cardiac monitor. The sounds have become increasingly irregular over the last hour. She mentally runs through her assessment of the patient. "Why is his heart so irritable?" she thinks. She calls the lab for the morning blood work results. When the lab technician e-mails

(continued on next page)

Nurses Make a Difference ... (continued)

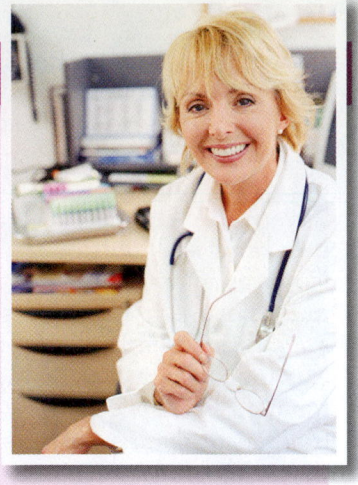

the results to the unit, she notes that the potassium level is low at 2.9 mEq/L. She notifies the attending physician of the lab results and the cardiac irritability. Susan tells the physician, "The patient's potassium is low from the diarrhea he's had since we began the antibiotics." Together they develop a plan to raise the potassium level and check it every 8 hours. Susan administers intravenous (IV) potassium chloride to raise the serum potassium level. Several hours later she documents that the *ectopy* (irregular heartbeat) has decreased to less than 2 beats/min.

Time: 2030, A Local Home

Yesterday, Mr. Samuels underwent cardiac surgery. He was discharged home this morning and is now under your care. As a home health nurse, your role is to assess his condition; provide skilled care; teach Mr. Samuels how to care for himself; instruct his family about his care; and coordinate any required additional services. Mrs. Samuels greets you at the front door. She tells you that her husband is in a lot of pain and that the chest drainage system appears full. She looks frightened as she says, "When my father had cardiac surgery 25 years ago, he spent 4 days in the hospital. The nurses took care of him in the hospital. I don't understand why my husband got sent home so quickly." You explain that changes in technology and the healthcare system allow you to take care of clients in the home who would previously have been in the hospital. As you begin your assessments, you tell Mrs. Samuels, "After I've gathered more information, we'll make a plan for his care that will make all of us more comfortable."

In each of these scenarios, the nurses engaged in *full-spectrum nursing;* that is, they used their minds and their hands to improve the client's comfort and condition. As the scenarios illustrate, nursing roles have changed over time. Yet nursing remains a profession dedicated to care of the client.

Critical Thinking 1-1

The Quality and Safety Education for Nurses (QSEN) project and the Institute of Medicine (IOM) have identified quality and safety competencies for nurses: (1) patient-centered care, (2) teamwork and collaboration, (3) evidence-based practice, (4) quality improvement, (5) safety, and (6) informatics (Cronenwett, Sherwood, Barnsteiner, et al., 2007). Which of these did Florence Nightingale demonstrate? Explain your thinking.

Nursing Images Throughout History

An understanding of the past can lend insight into the present. In the next few pages we will see how nursing has been portrayed in art and popular culture at different periods in history, and relate those images to the practice of contemporary nursing. This will help you appreciate the rich traditions of nursing and the forces that have shaped nursing as it is today. Pay close attention to the rate of change in recent years, and keep in mind that nursing and healthcare are likely to change even more rapidly in the future.

When you think of nursing, what images come to mind? As you think of each of the three scenarios at the opening of this chapter, what do you see when you try to picture the story? Is this the same image you get when you imagine yourself as a nurse?

Artwork, television, popular stories, advertisements, and greeting cards have all portrayed nurses in many ways. Whether the images are flattering or demeaning, accurate or inaccurate, they influence how people view nursing. Some of these images may have, in either a positive or negative way, influenced your decision to become a nurse. In the next section we discuss these images and explore the truth and fiction behind them.

The Angel of Mercy

One common image is the nurse as an angelic creature. The angel-nurse is serene and content and shown with a halo or other religious symbol. This image is so pervasive that uniform shops and medical supply houses sell cups, T-shirts, and pins that feature the angelic nurse. And there is some truth to this stereotype.

History demonstrates a strong link between nursing and religious orders. In ancient Egypt, Greece, and Rome, the temples were health centers as well as places of worship. Priests and priestesses treated the ill with a combination of physical care, prayer, and magic spells.

The Vedas, the most ancient sacred books of the Hindu faith (circa 1200 B.C.E.), provide a detailed description of Indian healthcare practices and are some of the earliest writings to describe a distinct nursing occupation. In these texts, Charaka and Samhita, a physician and surgeon team, detail the roles of the physician, drugs, nurse, and the patient. Their writings indicate that nurses of that period were always men who were part of a priestly order. Nursing responsibilities and attributes included knowledge of the preparation, compounding, and administration of drugs; wisdom; purity; and devotion to the patient.

From the first to the tenth centuries, lay deacons and deaconesses in the Christian church visited the sick in their homes and functioned as nurses. Initially the sick were brought to the local bishop's house for care, but as care of the sick outside the home became popular, this led to overcrowding. Eventually early Christian hospitals developed. The earliest known Christian hospital appeared in the first century. The oldest continuously existing hospital, Hôtel Dieu in Lyons, France, was founded in 542 B.C.E. (Fig. 1-1). In the United States, all training programs for nurses were affiliated with religious orders until well after the Civil War.

The association of nursing with religion has not always been positive. Early Christianity did benefit nursing by creating nursing orders, establishing hospitals, and honoring the service provided by nurses. However, during the 15th to the 19th centuries, the influence of Christianity in general society began to wane. This period marked a transition from medieval to modern civilization. Art, music, literature, and science flourished, but as the Protestant Reformation began to challenge the influence of the Roman Catholic Church, Catholic religious orders were often persecuted and monasteries were closed. Many nurses within religious orders fled to avoid imprisonment or death. In medicine this period was associated with a move from the monasteries to the universities, with major advances in theoretical knowledge of anatomy and physiology, and with a growing understanding of communicable disease.

From the 19th century onward, religious groups gradually reemerged as influential in society and in nursing. Today many nursing programs, universities, colleges, and healthcare institutions are affiliated with religious groups. Examples include the University of Notre Dame, the Seventh Day Adventist hospital system, and the American Baptist nursing home system. Although most of these organizations have mission statements or guidelines that incorporate charitable values, such as compassion and caring, they no longer require religious dedication from their nursing students.

Until about 100 years ago, nurses cared for patients at great risk to their own lives. This is another reason for the association between nursing and spirituality. Today we have an advanced understanding of germ theory, infectious diseases, and sanitation. But this information is relatively new. Before the development of microscopes and techniques for culturing microorganisms in the 19th century, people who entered nursing placed themselves at risk for exposure to diseases that were poorly understood and often could not be cured. Providing care in spite of these risks was considered self-sacrificing, much like the call to serve in religious life. Even as recently as the 1950s, antibiotics were not readily available, and the chief cause of mortality (death) was infectious disease.

Critical Thinking 1-2

Which aspects of the nurse-as-angel appeal to you most when you think about the way you will practice nursing? Why?

The Handmaiden

Another widely recognized stereotype is that of the nurse as handmaiden to the physician. This stereotype portrays the male physician in the dominant role, with the female nurse waiting in anticipation for the physician's orders or supporting the patient at the bedside while the physician provides care (Fig. 1-2).

FIGURE 1-1 Hôtel Dieu in Lyons, France, the oldest continuously existing hospital.

UNE SALLE DE L'HOTEL-DIEU AU XVIᵉ SIÈCLE

FIGURE 1-2 Handmaiden image of nursing.

The validity of this image has changed over time. Initially, the nurse's role was limited to bathing, feeding, and supporting the patient; keeping the patient's environment clean and orderly; and assisting the physician. However, nurses now collaborate with all members of the healthcare team, planning and providing care not only at the direction of physicians but also along with them (Table 1-1). Many activities that nurses now do independently were once performed only by physicians. For example, can you imagine a nurse not being permitted to use a stethoscope or take a blood pressure reading? There was, indeed, a time when only physicians performed those assessments. Today nurses give IV and other injectable medications; but this was not the case as recently as 60 years ago. Injectable penicillin came into use during World War II, allowing many soldiers to survive injuries that would have been fatal in the past; but only physicians and medics in the battlefield hospitals were allowed to administer it. One retired nurse vividly recounts how proud she was to administer her first penicillin injection without direct physician supervision—several years after the war. Today this story seems almost unbelievable because nurses perform so many complex and critical tasks. Nevertheless, the physician remains the final decision-maker for most patient care, even though the practice of nursing has become more complex and autonomous.

Physicians derive much of their power from legal and financial authority. Put simply, the legal definition of medicine has carved out a broad role for physicians, including the supervision of nurses and other health professionals. In contrast, nursing practice acts are not as broad and inclusive. Barbara Safriet, a legal expert on healthcare issues, has extensively studied the boundaries between healthcare providers and the effects of these boundaries when attempting to reform healthcare. She states that physicians, who traditionally came from the wealthy and educated classes, wrote and lobbied early in the history of the medical discipline for legislation that awarded them extensive power and ensured control of healthcare (Quadagno, 2004; Rockwell, 1994). Now it is very difficult to change these laws (Safriet, 1994). To learn more about circumstances that have made it difficult to expand the role of nursing,

 Go to Chapter 1, **Reading More About Evolution of Nursing Thought & Action,** on the Student Resource Disk or DavisPlus at http://davisplus.fadavis.com/Wilkinson2

Table 1-1 ➤ Examples of Nursing Activities	
DEPENDENT ACTIVITIES	**INDEPENDENT ACTIVITIES**
Administering prescribed medication	Evaluating the patient's response to medication and withholding the next dose if the patient has a negative reaction
Assisting with a diagnostic test (e.g., opening trays, handing instruments to the physician)	Teaching the patient what to expect from the diagnostic test; preparing the patient for the test (e.g., shaving a site); supporting the patient during the test
Administering IV fluids	Evaluating the patient's response to treatment; monitoring the flow rate; evaluating the site for redness or leakage
Ensuring that the patient receives the prescribed diet	Teaching a pregnant woman about additional nutrients needed in her diet

Physicians also retain significant power because they generate income for healthcare institutions. People enter a hospital, nursing home, or home service as patients of physicians. The patients—or their insurers—then pay the facility to deliver care that is ordered by the physician. Without physicians, the institution does not generate income. In contrast, nurses are usually employees of healthcare institutions and therefore are usually considered a healthcare expense. Many advanced practice nurses are authorized to order care and bill for services and as a result have some power in healthcare decision making; however, this is not true for most nurses.

Although the handmaiden image was more widespread in the past, even then not all nurses considered themselves to be subservient to physicians. For example, the publications, letters, and diaries of Florence Nightingale, who is revered as the founder of modern nursing, indicate that she considered nurses the colleagues of physicians rather than their servants. In a letter to Elizabeth Blackwell, who later went on to become the first female physician, Nightingale wrote:

No man, not even a doctor, ever gives any other definition of what a nurse should be than this—'devoted and obedient'. This definition would do well for a porter. It might even do for a horse. . . . (Chambers, 1958, p. 130)

At the age of 24, Florence Nightingale was convinced that her mission in life was to be with the sick (Fig. 1-3). She met resistance from her wealthy, upper-class family, who believed that nursing was beneath her social station. Hospitals at that time were dirty and unsanitary,

and provided care only for the poor; the affluent cared for their sick in the home by hiring private care providers. In spite of her family's protests, Nightingale went on to study nursing in Germany.

When Nightingale returned to England to begin her work as a nurse, she immediately set out to lobby politicians and physicians about the importance of nursing and the need for public health reform. She was able to illustrate the importance of nursing and public health through her work during the Crimean War. In Scutari, now Turkey, Nightingale and her staff completely revamped the services offered to the wounded. It was at Crimea that Nightingale became known as the "Lady of the Lamp" because she walked through the camp at night providing care to the sick and wounded. Nightingale's major contributions include:

- The establishment of nursing as a distinct profession
- Introduction of a broad-based liberal education for nurses
- Major reform in the delivery of care in hospitals
- The introduction of standards to control the spread of disease in hospitals
- Major reforms in healthcare for the military

If you would like more information about other historical nursing leaders,

 Go to Chapter 1, **Supplemental Materials: Nursing Leaders,** on the Student Resource Disk or DavisPlus at http://davisplus.fadavis.com/Wilkinson2

The employment status of most nurses is another factor that must be considered when looking at the validity of the handmaiden image. As we discussed earlier, most nurses work for healthcare institutions rather than directly for physicians. If nurses have indeed been handmaidens, perhaps it has been to the institutions that employ them. Nurses are actively working to combat the handmaiden stereotype; for instance, they are forming unions to improve their working conditions and benefits and to advocate for patient safety. It is interesting that, with changes in the healthcare system, more physicians are becoming employees of healthcare institutions as well—and some, like nurses, are forming unions. The increasing costs of healthcare, coupled with decreasing reimbursement for health services, appear to be driving these changes.

 Critical**Thinking** 1-3

What similarities or differences do you see between the angelic and handmaiden images of nursing?

The Battle-Ax

Ironically, the image of the nurse as a battle-ax is in direct opposition to the image of the angel of mercy. These opposing images have coexisted for centuries. In the 1975 film, *One Flew Over the Cuckoo's Nest*, Nurse Ratched

FIGURE 1-3 Florence Nightingale (1820–1910).

personifies the contemporary image of the nurse as the battle-ax or torturer, treating her patients with cruelty and disdain. Charles Dickens created an earlier version of the abusive nurse in his 1844 novel, *Martin Chuzzlewit*, in the character of Sairy Gamp. Mrs. Gamp personified the view of nurses that many people held at that time: she was corrupt, harsh, and frequently intoxicated. How did these negative images come about? And why does this image persist? Again, history may provide insight.

The values of service and devotion to the patient faded along with the influence of Christianity during the 14th to the 16th centuries (a period known as the Renaissance). Before that time, religious-affiliated nursing orders provided most of the care for the sick. However, as science and philosophy grew more sophisticated and popular, religious orders for nursing became less common, and much of the knowledge of caring for the sick was lost. Municipal authorities took over hospitals. In lieu of sending them to jail, they began to sentence criminals to care for the sick in the hospitals—to assume the nursing role. Forced to care for large numbers of patients without training, supplies, assistance, or time off, these criminals often managed their workload by treating patients harshly and drinking alcohol while on duty. Most patients who entered such hospitals died there. Such practices persisted until the 1860s in Europe and until after the Civil War in the United States. It is no wonder, then, that the battle-ax image of nurses endured so long.

Caregiving activities also contribute to the persistence of the battle-ax image. Nurses give injections, clean and dress wounds, draw blood, and start intravenous lines—all are activities that are performed to improve the patient's health, but they may cause significant pain. Unfortunately, this association with pain helps to perpetuate the image of nurses as unfeeling. Aware of the power of this image, nurses on pediatric units typically wear colorful uniforms with child-friendly patterns, such as cartoon characters or cuddly animals, to avoid frightening children who may associate "nurse" with "pain." Many pediatric facilities, and even some adult units and outpatient surgical centers, are delivering care in "street clothes" without white lab coats in order to reduce patient anxiety.

The Naughty Nurse

The image of the sexy, risqué nurse arose in the early part of the 20th century with burlesque shows and persists in popular culture today. For example, in the 1980s, a prime-time television show called *The Nightingales* portrayed nurses as sexy, mindless women. The long-running (1972–1983) hit series *M*A*S*H* prominently featured Hot Lips Houlihan and other nurses, who were potential dates for the bright and talented surgeons. The same is true in recent television programs, such as *ER*,

Nurse Jackie, and *Grey's Anatomy*. Get-well cards often portray nurses in short skirts, fishnet stockings, high heels, and cap, as do paperback novels, comic books, CDs, and other media.

To see how pervasive this image is, go online and search under the term *nurse images*. Your search will yield links to legitimate sites with realistic pictures of nurses, but also to a large number of cartoons, greeting cards, and pornographic Web sites featuring women who are supposedly nurses. Their role is implied through props—a nursing cap, a stethoscope, or a uniform—in the background.

Why is this so? What gives this image its power? As trusted health professionals, nurses frequently provide care that involves exposing the patient's body, contact with bare skin, and discussion of intimate aspects of the client's life. In addition, hospitalized patients are in a weakened, vulnerable state, and the nurse may seem quite powerful by contrast. Thus, despite the fact that nurse–patient contact is professional and does not involve sexual intimacy, the "naughty nurse" stereotype may express a forbidden desire for intimate contact with a stranger in a position of power.

In addition, the traditionally female nurse's collaboration with traditionally male physicians may reinforce the stereotype of the nurse in a sexual role. In television shows and romance novels, compliant nurses are "rewarded" with marriage to the handsome surgeon, whereupon they "escape" nursing and retire to life as "the doctor's wife." Of course, it is true that nurses work closely with physicians and other healthcare providers. This close association may lead to socialization, friendships, and sometimes even marriages among healthcare professionals, but this is the exception rather than the rule. The "naughty nurse" stereotype may be popular, but it is not founded on truth.

Critical Thinking 1-4

- How do the images of the nurse as a battle-ax or sex object affect your view of nursing?
- As a nurse, what can you do to counteract these images?

The Military Image

Nursing imagery is often military, both in the general public and within the profession itself. Throughout the last century, nurses were frequently portrayed in uniform providing support at the battlefield, and nurses are still often depicted as warriors fighting disease. What is the history of these two military images?

Nurses on the Battlefield

Nurses' involvement in the military dates from 27 B.C.E., as the Roman Empire began to consolidate its dominion. Before this time, wounded soldiers depended on the charity of private citizens or religious persons. However, because the Roman Empire relied on the success of military excursions to extend its domain, the survival and well-being of its soldiers were critical. Thus, one of the great contributions of the Roman Empire was the development of the military hospital and the practice of providing first aid on the battlefield.

The Hospitalers During the Middle Ages the two largest influences on nursing were the military and religion. These two threads fused in the Crusaders, soldiers who went to battle to conquer Islamic lands and spread Christianity throughout the world. Among the Crusaders were **hospitalers,** specialized soldiers who at the end of battle returned to the outposts to care for the sick and injured (Fig. 1-4). Among the hospitalers, three orders predominated: (1) the Knights of St. John of Jerusalem, which established men's and women's branches throughout Europe—one of which still exists in England as the Order of Malta; (2) the Teutonic Knights, a strictly male order; and (3) the Knights of St. Lazarus, which was established to care for lepers.

The Civil War Nursing presence on the battlefield continues in more recent history. In 1861, at the outbreak of the Civil War, the U.S. government established the Army Nursing Service. Its role was to organize nurses and hospitals and coordinate supplies for the soldiers. Many trained nurses joined the Army Nursing Service from religious orders that provided nursing education through a mentorship approach. Thousands of laypersons also volunteered.

- **Clara Barton.** Among the lay nurses was Clara Barton, who organized her own nursing efforts. Rather than providing care in base hospitals, far removed from the battlefield, Barton and her volunteers provided care in tents set up close to the fighting. Barton did not discriminate when giving care, nursing soldiers from both the North and South, black and white. When the

FIGURE 1-4 A hospitaler at the time of the Crusades.

war was over, Barton continued this universal care through the establishment of the American Red Cross.

- **Other laypersons.** Other notable figures who served as nurses include Harriet Tubman, who helped slaves escape to freedom on the Underground Railroad; the poet Walt Whitman; the author Louisa May Alcott; and Dorothea Dix, the Union's Superintendent of Female Nurses during the Civil War.

Nurses also served in World War I, World War II, the Korean and Vietnam wars (Fig. 1-5), the Gulf War, and the conflict in Iraq. In these wars the nurses were all formally trained. Formal training for nurses became widespread in Europe in the 1860s after the widely publicized success of Nightingale in the Crimea. In the United States the first formal training program was established in 1873.

FIGURE 1-5 Women's Memorial for the Vietnam War.

Nurses Fighting Disease

A second military image portrays nurses as warriors in the fight against disease. This image is common in public awareness campaigns against infectious diseases.

- **Florence Nightingale.** Florence Nightingale's contributions in public health and **epidemiology** (the study of the distribution and origins of disease) were among the first nursing efforts to fight disease. In her *Notes on Hospitals* (1863), Nightingale stated that air, light, nutrition, and adequate ventilation and space assist the patient to recuperate. The hospitals she designed to incorporate these ideas were associated with decreased mortality, decreased length of hospital stay, and decreased rate of **nosocomial infection** (an infection associated with a healthcare facility and now more commonly called healthcare-associated infection).

- **Lillian Wald and Mary Brewster.** Another notable event in the fight against disease occurred in 1893 when Lillian Wald and Mary Brewster founded the Henry Street Settlement in New York to improve the health and social conditions of poor immigrants. This is considered the start of public health nursing in the United States. Since then, nurses have played an important role in improving health and preventing illness by promoting safe drinking water, adequate sewage facilities, and proper sanitation measures in communities.

In spite of the historical association of nursing with the military, currently only a small percentage of licensed U.S. nurses work in the armed services. Similarly, despite the powerful image of the nurse slaying tuberculosis, only approximately 15% of nurses work in community and public health agencies (HRSA, 2004).

White Women

As you looked at the preceding images of nurses, did you notice that all of them are white women? Women of various ethnicity and men of any race are rarely shown as nurses.

About 82% of RNs in the United States are white, and only about 6% of nurses in the U.S. and Canada are men (Canadian Institute for Health Information, 2006; HRSA, 2004). Male nurses make up a higher percentage in other countries (12.5% in Great Britain, for example); nevertheless, they are a minority of the total nursing population worldwide (Fig. 1-6) (Pullen, 2006). This is ironic considering that many ancient nursing orders were exclusively male. In early Christianity, deacons provided nursing care to parish men while deaconesses provided care to women. During the Crusades, male hospitalers provided nursing care to fellow soldiers who were injured in battle, and even today the majority of medics and hospital corpsmen who provide battlefront first aid are men.

Popular media tend to reflect cultural beliefs. In the 2000 film *Meet the Parents*, Ben Stiller played the role of

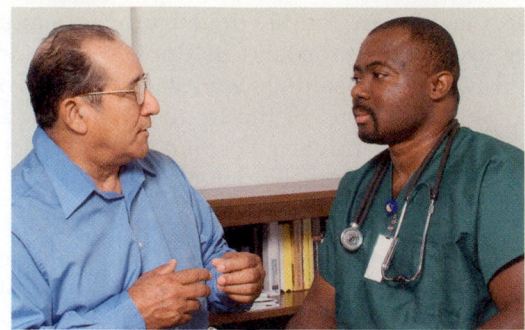

FIGURE 1-6 The roles of men in nursing are now as varied as those for women, and the opportunities for personal and professional fulfillment are as great.

a nurse. His future in-laws, who could not understand why he would choose nursing as a profession, continually challenged him to defend his position and intelligence. This stereotype has not aided in the recruitment of men into the profession. Since the women's movement, women have received support as they moved into traditional male occupations such as physician, engineer, and scientist. However, many men perceive that they have not been welcomed into female-dominated fields (Meadus, 2000).

People of all races and ethnic backgrounds work as nurses around the world. In the United States, Canada, and many European countries, though, most nurses are white. The trend in 2000 and 2004 was toward a slightly more diverse nurse workforce (Table 1-2). Major nursing and healthcare organizations agree on the need to increase diversity in nursing. One proposed solution is to increase the representation of minorities in advanced practice nursing and faculty positions so that they will serve as role models and mentors for incoming nurses. It is encouraging for diversity that more men are being recruited into nursing. For example, in 2006, 8.3% of nursing students in the United States were men (Pullen, 2006). The NLN reported an even higher number: in 2006, men represented 12.1% of nursing graduating students (National League for Nursing, 2008).

Table 1-2 ➤ Race and Ethnicity Among Registered Nurses in the United States		
RACE/ETHNICITY	**2004 (%)**	**2000 (%)**
White	89.3	86.6
Black	4.2	4.9
Asian/Pacific Islander	3.1	3.7
Hispanic/Latino	1.7	2.0
Native American	0.3	0.5
Two or more races	1.4	1.2

Source: March 2004 National Sample Survey of Registered Nurses, Division of Nursing, BHPR, Health Resources and Service Administration (HRSA).

However, it is important that practicing nurses embrace these changes and welcome others into the field.

Critical**Thinking** 1-5

In your opinion, what efforts, if any, should nursing organizations take to recruit a more diverse workforce?

Full-Spectrum Nurse

Nurses are often shown actively caring for the patient—dressing wounds, bathing, giving medications—but the intellectual or thinking side of nursing is rarely portrayed. The angel of mercy and military stereotypes reinforce the idea that nursing is a duty and that nurses are carrying out orders. The naughty nurse, battle-ax, and handmaiden images suggest a woman who is prone to action but may not be carefully considering her actions. To be safe providers, nurses must carefully consider their actions. In reality, a substantial portion of the nursing role involves thinking. Nursing requires careful thought about the patient, the treatment plan, the healthcare environment, the patient's support system, the nurse's support system and resources, and safety. Nurses use clinical judgment, critical thinking, and problem solving as they care for patients.

Clinical judgment involves observing, comparing, contrasting, and evaluating the client's condition to determine whether change has occurred. It also involves careful consideration of the client's health status in light of what is expected based on the client's condition, medications, and treatment. These actions, collectively known as assessment, are discussed in Chapters 3 and 19, and in each of the clinically focused chapters.

Critical thinking is a reflective thinking process that involves collecting information, analyzing the adequacy and accuracy of the information, and carefully considering options for action. Nurses use critical thinking in every aspect of nursing care. Critical thinking is discussed at length in Chapter 2 and applied in every chapter in this text.

Problem solving is a process by which nurses consider an issue and attempt to find a satisfactory solution to achieve the best outcomes. You will often use problem solving in your professional life. The nursing process (see Chapters 2 through 7) is one type of problem-solving process.

Critical**Thinking** 1-6

In the three scenarios of "Nurses Make a Difference: Then & Now," what image of nursing predominates: thinking or doing?

Contemporary Nursing: Education, Regulation, and Organization

As a student about to enter your new professional life, you need to realistically grasp the nature and demands of your chosen career. To help you to better acquaint yourself with nursing today, the remainder of this chapter discusses the current state of nursing, nursing education, and the trends affecting nursing.

How Is Nursing Defined?

As you have seen, there are many images of nursing. These images are only loosely based on fact and sometimes conflict. They make it difficult for the public to know the reality of nursing—and they are confusing to nurses and other members of the healthcare team as well. In addition, the constantly changing nature of nursing, healthcare, and society further complicate the definition of nursing. Therefore, it is important for nurses to articulate clearly, for themselves and for the public, what nursing is and what nurses do. The following are the views of three important nursing organizations on the question, "What is nursing?"

International Council of Nurses Definition

In 1973 the International Council of Nurses (ICN), an organization representing nurses throughout the world, defined nursing according to the beliefs of respected theorist Virginia Henderson:

The unique function of the nurse is to assist the individual, sick or well, in the performance of those activities contributing to health or its recovery (or to peaceful death) that he would perform unaided if he had the necessary strength, will or knowledge. (Henderson, 1966, p. 15)

In the decades since the adoption of this definition, nursing throughout the world has changed. Advances in healthcare have altered the type of care required by clients. Nurses have taken on expanded roles, and once again there is interest in providing care outside the hospital. To reflect these changes, the ICN has revised its definition of nursing, as follows:

Nursing encompasses autonomous and collaborative care of individuals of all ages, families, groups and communities, sick or well and in all settings. Nursing includes the promotion of health, prevention of illness, and the care of ill, disabled and dying people. Advocacy, promotion of a safe environment, research, participation in shaping health policy and in patient and health systems management, and education are also key nursing roles (ICN, 2007).

Critical**Thinking** 1-7

Look at the three scenarios of "Nurses Make a Difference: Then & Now." What nursing actions did the nurses perform that are represented in the ICN definition of nursing?

Nursing Association Definitions

You can see similar changes in the approach of the American Nurses Association (ANA) and the Canadian Nurses Association (CNA). In 1980, the ANA defined nursing as "the diagnosis and treatment of human responses to actual and potential health problems" (p. 2). Attempts to refine this definition have been fraught with difficulty. Nurses are a heterogeneous group of people with varying skills who perform activities designed to provide care ranging from basic to complex in a growing number of settings. It is very difficult to describe the boundaries of the profession. In 2004, the ANA acknowledged six essential features of professional nursing:

- Provision of a caring relationship
- A holistic approach (e.g., human responses to health and illness within the physical and social environments)
- Integration of objective data with knowledge of the patient's subjective experience
- Application of scientific knowledge through the use of judgment and critical thinking
- Advancement of professional nursing knowledge through scholarly inquiry
- Influence of social and public policy to promote social justice (p. 5)

As a result, the ANA redefined professional nursing as:

The protection, promotion, and optimization of health and abilities, prevention of illness and injury, alleviation of suffering through the diagnosis and treatment of human response, and advocacy in the care of individuals, families, communities, and populations (ANA, 2010, in press).

In Canada a task force on the scope of practice stated:

. . . [I]t will never be possible to define, precisely and in great detail, which activities are inside and which are outside the boundaries of nursing. This is partly because the 'state of the art' of health care and nursing are changing so rapidly that such lists become outdated almost before they are completed, and partly because the field has become far too complex to be reduced to lists of tasks and procedures. As the nursing profession matures and the body of nursing knowledge expands, it will become easier to clearly describe the principles, models and functions that are the basis of nursing (CNA, 1993, pp. 17–18).

Although it is not an official CNA definition, a more recent document cites the CNA in providing this description of what nurses do:

RNs are licensed/registered nurses who practice within their province or Territory. An RN uses the nursing process of assessment, diagnosis, planning, implementation and evaluation to serve persons of all ages and at varying levels of illness or wellness. They practice in a variety of settings, including hospitals, long-term care facilities, the community, etc. (Hadley, Graham, & Flannery, 2004).

You may wonder why there has been so much emphasis on creating a definition. Nursing organizations and leaders have pushed for accurate definitions to (1) help the public understand the value of nursing, (2) describe what activities and roles belong to nursing versus other health professions, and (3) help students and practicing nurses understand what is expected of them within their role as nurses.

From our brief review of nursing history, you can see that nursing has undergone tremendous change, from a role limited to providing kindness and support to full-spectrum work that is based in science but still focuses on care and nurturing. Undoubtedly nursing will continue to change as nursing knowledge increases and society changes. Box 1-1 lists several additional definitions of nursing for you to consider.

As a student entering nursing, you can use definitions and descriptions to understand what is expected of you. To aid you in this task, Table 1-3 reviews the essential components of the nursing role. While in the clinical setting, you will observe nurses functioning in each of these capacities. Nursing is a flexible career that requires you to move effortlessly among these areas to meet the needs of the patient.

BOX 1-1 ■ What Is Nursing?

- I use the word nursing, for want of a better word. It has been limited to signify little more than the administration of medicines and the application of poultices. It ought to signify the proper use of fresh air, light, warmth, cleanliness, quiet, and the proper choosing and giving of diet—all at the least expense of vital power to the patient (Nightingale, 1876, p. 5).

- Events that give rise to higher degrees of consideration for those who are helpless or oppressed, kindliness and sympathy for the unfortunate and for those who suffer, tolerance for those of differing religion, race, color, etc.—all tend to promote activities like nursing which are primarily humanitarian (Dock & Stewart, 1938, p. 3).

- Nursing has been called the oldest of the arts and the youngest of the professions. As such, it has gone through many stages and has been an integral part of societal movements. Nursing has been involved in the existing culture—shaped by it and yet helping to develop it (Donahue, 1985, p. 3).

- Nurses provide care for people in the midst of health, pain, loss, fear, disfigurement, death, grieving, challenge, growth, birth, and transition on an intimate front-line basis. Expert nurses call this the privileged place of nursing (Benner & Wrubel, 1989, p. xi).

- Nursing: The care and nurturing of healthy and ill people, individually or in groups and communities. [Taber's also includes as a part of the definition the ANA "essential features" involving holism, use of subjective and objective data, application of scientific knowledge, and provision of a caring relationship.] (Venes, D. Taber's cyclopedic medical dictionary, 2009).

Table 1-3 ➤ Roles and Functions of the Nurse

ROLE	FUNCTION	EXAMPLES
Direct care provider	Addressing the physical, emotional, social, and spiritual needs of the client	Assessing the client Giving medications Patient teaching
Communicator	Using interpersonal and therapeutic communication skills to address the needs of the client, to facilitate communication in the healthcare team, and to advise the community about health promotion and disease prevention	Counseling a client Discussing unit staffing needs at a meeting Providing HIV education at a local school
Client/family educator	Assessing and diagnosing the teaching needs of the client, group, family, or community. Once the diagnosis is made, nurses plan how to meet these needs, implement the teaching plan, and evaluate its effectiveness.	Preoperative teaching Prenatal education for siblings Community classes on nutrition
Client advocate	Supporting clients' right to make healthcare decisions when they are able to voice their opinions and protecting clients from harm when they are unable to make decisions	Helping a client explain to his family that he does not want to have further chemotherapy
Counselor	Using therapeutic communication skills to advise clients about health-related issues	Counseling a client on weight-loss strategies
Change agent	Advocating for change on an individual, family, group, community, or societal level that enhances health. The nurse may use counseling, communication, and educator skills to accomplish this change.	Working to improve the nutritional quality of the lunch program at a preschool
Leader	Inspiring others by setting an example of positive health, assertive communication, and willingness to improve	Florence Nightingale Walt Whitman Harriet Tubman
Manager	Coordinating and managing the activities of all members of the team	Charge nurse on a hospital unit (e.g., assigns patients and work to staff nurses)
Case manager	Coordinating the care delivered to a client	Coordinator of services for clients with tuberculosis
Research consumer	Applying evidence-based practice to provide the most appropriate care, to identify clinical problems that warrant research, and to protect the rights of research subjects	Reading journal articles Attending continuing education; seeking additional education

Knowledge Check 1-1

- What factors make it difficult to define nursing?
- Based on the ICN definition of nursing, what does a nurse do?

 Go to Chapter 1, **Knowledge Check Response Sheet and Answers,** on the Student Resource Disk or DavisPlus at http://davisplus.fadavis.com/Wilkinson2

Is Nursing a Profession, Discipline, or Occupation?

One strategy used to describe a field of work is to categorize it as a profession, discipline, or occupation. Although the term *profession* is freely used, a group must meet the following criteria to be considered a **profession** (Starr, 1982):

- The knowledge of the group must be based on technical and scientific knowledge.
- The knowledge and competence of members of the group must be evaluated by a community of peers.
- The group must have a service orientation and a code of ethics.

Nursing appears to meet all criteria of a profession as defined by Starr. Entry-level nursing education requires coursework in basic and social sciences as well as humanities, arts, and general education. Nursing education and practice are increasingly based on research from nursing and related fields. State or provincial regulatory bodies have defined the criteria that nurses must meet to practice, and they monitor members for adherence to standards. Nursing is clearly focused on providing service to others, and the major professional organizations have developed ethical guidelines to guide the practice of nursing.

To be considered a **discipline,** a profession must have a domain of knowledge that has both theoretical and practical boundaries. The theoretical boundaries of a profession are the questions that arise from clinical practice and are then investigated through research. The practical boundaries are the current state of knowledge and research in the field (Meleis, 1991). This is the known, or the facts that dictate safe practice.

A case can be made that nursing is both a profession and a discipline. It is a scientifically based, self-governed profession that focuses on the ethical care of others. It is also a discipline that is driven by theoretical and practical aspects, demanding thorough knowledge of its scientific basis and clinical skills. Simply stated, nursing requires theoretical knowledge and practical skills.

In spite of meeting criteria for both designations (profession and discipline), nursing is often described as an **occupation** or job. Unlike physicians, most of whom are in control of their practice environment, working conditions, and schedule, most nurses are hourly wage earners. The employer, not the nurse, decides the conditions of practice and the nature of the work. Nurse practice acts do not prevent nurses from functioning more autonomously, however. Rather than continuing to focus on arguments to "prove" that nursing is a profession, the following actions might do more to improve the status of nursing:

- Standardizing the educational requirements for entry into practice
- Enacting uniform continuing education requirements
- Encouraging the participation of more nurses in professional organizations
- Educating the public about the true nature of nursing practice

 Critical**Thinking** 1-8

Evaluate the status of nursing. Is nursing a respected profession? Give examples to support your opinion.

How Do Nurses' Educational Paths Differ?

The transition into the nursing profession involves formal and informal processes. The formal process consists of completing the initial and continuing education required for licensure. The informal process involves a gradual progression in skill and clinical judgment that allows the nurse to advance in the profession.

Formal Education

When the patient calls out "Nurse!" who can respond? To legally use the title *nurse,* a person must be a graduate of an accredited nursing education program and have successfully passed a licensure exam. Students may enter nursing through two paths: as a practical nurse or a registered nurse. Other personnel may respond to the patient's call, but they cannot legally be considered nurses.

Practical and Vocational Nursing Education

Practical nursing education prepares nurses to provide bedside care to clients. Practical nurses are known as licensed practical nurses (LPNs) or licensed vocational nurses (LVNs) in a few states. In the United States a student who wishes to become an LPN/LVN may attend one of approximately 1200 approved programs given at technical schools and community colleges. Educational programs for LPN/LVNs offer both classroom and clinical teaching and usually last 1 year. After completing the practical nursing education program, the student must pass the NCLEX-PN exam. Practical nurses work under the direction of the registered nurse (RN) or the primary care provider.

Registered Nursing Entry Education

Currently, five educational pathways lead to licensure as a registered nurse (RN). Graduates of all these programs must successfully complete the NCLEX-RN exam to practice as RNs.

- *Diploma programs.* Until the 1960s, diploma programs were the mainstay of nursing education. These programs are usually associated with a hospital. The typical program lasts 3 years and focuses on clinical experience in direct patient care. Since the 1960s the number of diploma programs has steadily decreased. In 2004, only about 4% of nursing schools were diploma programs.
- *Associate degree programs.* Most associate degree (AD) programs are offered in community colleges. Although the nursing component typically lasts 2 years, students are required to take numerous other courses in liberal arts and the sciences. Associate degree programs account for about 53% of all RN programs in the United States (Bureau of Labor Statistics, 2006). The student is prepared to provide direct patient care.
- *Baccalaureate degree programs.* Students in baccalaureate programs pursue a course of study like that of other undergraduate students. The course of study lasts at least eight semesters. Students are prepared to provide direct patient care, to work in community care, to use research, and to enter graduate education. About 42% of nursing programs in the United States prepare students at the baccalaureate level (Bureau of Labor Statistics, 2006). Many AD graduates enter RN-to-BSN (or RN "completion") programs to obtain a baccalaureate degree in nursing. The length of time

required to complete the BSN varies according to the program and the number of credits each student can transfer.

- *Master's entry programs.* The typical student in these programs has a baccalaureate degree in another field and has entered nursing as a second career. Programs usually are completed in 3 years of full-time study. At the completion, the student is eligible to take the licensing exam and is awarded a master's degree in nursing.
- *Doctoral entry.* This is the most unusual entry pathway into nursing. The nursing doctorate (ND) path parallels the pathway through which physicians enter the healthcare field. This entry path has very limited enrollment.

For several decades, nursing leaders have debated about the most appropriate educational pathway for entry into the profession. For an overview of this debate,

 Go to Chapter 1, **Supplemental Materials: Entry into Practice Debate,** on the Student Resource Disk or DavisPlus at http://davisplus.fadavis.com/Wilkinson2

Graduate Nursing Education

Graduate nursing education prepares the RN for advanced practice, expanded roles, or research. In master's and doctoral education programs, coursework is concentrated in the nursing major. **Master's degree programs** prepare RNs to function in a more independent role, for example, as advanced practice nurses (APNs) or educators. Programs typically last 2 years or longer and are at the university level. **Doctoral programs** in nursing offer professional degrees. Typically the student has completed a baccalaureate and master's degree before entry into a doctoral program. Degrees awarded are usually the DNS (doctor of nursing science) or PhD (doctor of philosophy). The DNS program prepares the nurse for advanced clinical practice. The PhD is a research degree. For additional discussion on expanded nurse roles,

 Go to Chapter 1, **Supplemental Materials: Expanded Career Roles,** on the Student Resource Disk or DavisPlus at http://davisplus.fadavis.com/Wilkinson2

Other Forms of Formal Education

Advances in healthcare have a strong influence on nursing practice. To stay current after graduating, you must participate in ongoing education. **Continuing education** is a professional strategy to keep up with current clinical knowledge. Continuing education programs are available at work sites, at local colleges and universities, through privately operated educational groups, on the Internet, and in professional journals. In 23 states, renewal of the nursing license requires successful completion of a specified number of continuing education courses. Some states allow nurses to take any approved

coursework, while others have specific requirements in special areas, such as HIV/AIDS and domestic violence. The regulations for continuing education change frequently. When you receive your initial nursing license, you will be notified by your state board of nursing (SBN) about continuing education requirements, if any. Thereafter, the SBN will notify you by mail of any changes in the requirements. For an overview of the continuing education requirements for license renewal in the United States,

 Go to Chapter 1, **Supplemental Materials: Continuing Education Requirements for Nurses,** on the Student Resource Disk or DavisPlus at http://davisplus.fadavis.com/Wilkinson2

Another form of ongoing education is **in-service education.** These programs are offered at the work site, and usually do not count toward meeting the continuing education requirement for license renewal. In-service education is typically institution specific, product specific, or nongeneralizable information. For instance, in-service education might focus on the use of new equipment or the introduction of new policies, or it may resemble traditional continuing education programs.

Informal Education

In addition to formal programs of study, education also requires socialization into the profession. **Socialization** is the informal education that occurs as you move into your new profession. It is the knowledge gained from direct experience, observation in the real world, and informal discussion with peers and colleagues. Professional socialization begins when you enter the educational program and continues as you gain expertise throughout your career. Informal education complements formal education to create clinical competence.

Benner's Model

Patricia Benner (1984) described the process by which a nurse acquires clinical skills and judgment. As this process shows, expertise is not merely a demonstration of skilled application of knowledge, but rather a personal integration of knowledge that requires technical skill, thoughtful application, and insight. This is what we mean in this text when we use the term *full-spectrum nursing*. Expertise requires both thinking and doing skills.

Stage 1: Novice. This phase begins with the onset of education. The novice is typically receptive to education and is "learning the rules" of the profession.

Stage 2: Advanced beginner. After considerable exposure to clinical situations, nurses improve in performance and, through repeated experiences or mentoring, begin to recognize the elements of a situation. The nurse functioning at this level begins to use more facts and is more sophisticated with use of the rules. A new graduate usually functions at this level.

Stage 3: Competence. Nurses achieve competence after a few years of practice. Competent performers have gained additional experience and wrestle with more complex concerns. They are able to handle their patient load and prioritize situations. They are also more involved in their caregiving role and may be emotionally involved in the clinical choices made. Although competent nurses manage clinical care with mastery, they often do not fully grasp the overall scope and most important aspects.

Stage 4: Proficient. Proficient nurses are a resource for less experienced nurses. They are able to see the "big picture" and can coordinate services and forecast needs. They are much more flexible and fluent with their role and able to adapt to nuances of various patient situations. Proficient nurses plan intuitively as much as consciously.

Stage 5: Expert. Expert nurses are able to see what needs to be achieved and how to do it. They trust in and use their intuition while operating with a deep understanding of a situation. They have expert skills and are often consulted when others need advice or assistance.

Benner's model deals with the development of clinical wisdom and competence. Keep in mind that this progression is not automatic. Nurses do not simply move through the stages as they gain experience. Instead, this model assumes that, to improve in skill and judgment, nurses must also be attuned to each clinical situation. This requires an ability to take in information from a variety of sources and to notice subtle variations. Although expertise (Stage 5) is a goal, not everyone can achieve this level of skill.

Nursing Organization Guidelines

The ANA and other organizations are also involved in helping nurses to continue to improve their practice (e.g., by setting standards and articulating nursing values). For example, in the Code for Nurses, the ANA provides guidelines for nurses to conduct themselves in their day-to-day practice. These guidelines describe behaviors and values that help improve practice and participation in the profession. Box 1-2 presents some values and behaviors associated with nursing. See Chapter 44 for further discussion of nursing values and the ANA Code for Nurses.

BOX 1-2 ■ Nursing Values and Behaviors

- The nurse's primary concern is the good of the patient.
- Nurses ought to be competent.
- Nurses demonstrate a strong commitment to service.
- Nurses believe in the dignity and worth of each person.
- Nurses constantly strive to improve their profession.
- Nurses work collaboratively within the profession.

KnowledgeCheck 1-2

- Compare and contrast formal and informal education.
- Name and describe five educational pathways leading to licensure as an RN.

 Go to Chapter 1, **Knowledge Check Response Sheet and Answers,** on the Student Resource Disk or DavisPlus at http://davisplus.fadavis.com/Wilkinson2

How Is Nursing Practice Regulated?

Nurse practice acts are laws that regulate nursing practice. In the United States, each state enacts its own nurse practice act. In Canada, this is done on a provincial level. The state or provincial board of nursing is the agency responsible for regulating nursing practice. Although there are minor variations, each board of nursing is responsible for:

- Defining the practice of nursing
- Establishing criteria that allow a person to be considered a registered nurse (RN) or licensed practical or vocational nurse (LPN/LVN)
- Determining activities that are in the scope of practice of nursing: that nurses may perform (and by implication, those they may not); and those that may be performed only by licensed nurses
- Enforcing the rules that govern nursing

To practice nursing, an individual must be licensed as a nurse. Licenses are issued by the state. All states require graduation from an approved nursing program and successful completion of the National Council Licensure Exam (NCLEX). To receive licensure in another state, the nurse simply applies for reciprocity. For further details about licensing and the regulation of nursing practice, see Chapter 45.

Nursing is also guided by **standards of practice**. Standards "provide a means by which a profession clearly describes the focus of its activities, the recipients of service, and the responsibilities for which its practitioners are accountable" (ANA, 2004, p. vii). Standards are used by individual nurses, employers of nurses, professional organizations, and other professions.

As a student of nursing, you may use the ANA or CNA standards of nursing practice to get a better understanding of nursing. Practicing nurses use the standards to judge their own performance, develop an improvement plan, and understand what employers expect of them. Employers incorporate the standards into annual evaluation tools at hospitals and health facilities. Professional organizations use the standards to educate the public about nursing, to plan for continuing education programs for nurses, and to guide their efforts at lobbying and other activities that advocate for nurses. Finally, other professions read the standards of practice to examine the boundaries between nursing and other health professions. Table 1-4 presents the ANA standards, and Box 1-3 presents examples of provincial standards in Canada.

Table 1-4 ➤ American Nurses Association: Scope and Standards of Clinical Nursing Practice[1]

Standards of Care

Standard 1	Assessment	The registered nurse collects comprehensive data pertinent to the patient's health and/or the situation.
Standard 2	Diagnosis	The registered nurse analyzes the assessment data to determine the diagnoses or issues.
Standard 3	Outcome Identification	The registered nurse identifies expected outcomes for a plan individualized to the patient or situation.
Standard 4	Planning	The registered nurse develops a plan that prescribes strategies and alternatives to attain expected outcomes.
Standard 5	Implementation	The registered nurse implements the identified plan.
Standard 5A	Coordination of Care	The registered nurse coordinates care delivery.
Standard 5B	Health Teaching and Health Promotion	The registered nurse employs strategies to promote health and a safe environment.
Standard 5C	Consultation	The advanced practice registered nurse and the nursing role specialist provide consultation to influence the identified plan, enhance the abilities of others, and effect change.
Standard 5D	Prescriptive Authority and Treatment	The advanced practice registered nurse uses prescriptive authority, procedures, referrals, treatments, and therapies in accordance with state and federal laws and regulations.
Standard 6	Evaluation	The registered nurse evaluates progress toward attainment of outcomes.

Standards of Professional Performance

Standard 7	Ethics	The registered nurse integrates ethical provisions in all areas of practice.
Standard 8	Education	The registered nurse attains knowledge and competency that reflects current nursing practice.
Standard 9	Evidence-Based Practice and Research	The registered nurse integrates evidence and research findings into practice.
Standard 10	Quality of Practice	The registered nurse systematically enhances the quality and effectiveness of nursing practice.
Standard 11	Communication	The registered nurse uses a wide variety of communication skills and formats in all areas of practice.
Standard 12	Leadership	The registered nurse demonstrates leadership in the professional practice setting and the profession.
Standard 13	Collegiality	The registered nurse interacts with and contributes to the professional development of peers and colleagues.
Standard 14	Collaboration	The registered nurse collaborates with patient, family, and others in the conduct of nursing practice.
Standard 15	Professional Practice Evaluation	The registered nurse evaluates one's own nursing practice in relation to professional practice standards and guidelines, relevant statutes, rules, and regulations.
Standard 16	Resource Utilization	The registered nurse utilizes appropriate resources to plan and provide nursing services that are safe, effective and financially responsible.
Standard 17	Environmental Health	The registered nurse integrates the principles of environmental health for nursing in all areas of practice.

Source: American Nurses Association (2010, in press). *Nursing: Scope and Standards of Practice* (2nd ed). Public Comment draft, January 2010. (To be published by August 2010.) Silver Spring, MD: Nursebooks.org.
[1]*Caveat:* This material is from the draft for public comment (ANA, 2010, in press); its wording may be changed somewhat in the final published version. For that version of the ANA Standards of Professional Nursing Practice, go to www.nursingworld.org.

BOX 1-3 ■ Canadian Nurses Association Standards of Nursing Practice

CNA standards are set by the individual provinces and serve as the benchmark to evaluate professional practice. They commonly include these broad standards: accountability; continuing competence; application of knowledge, skills and judgment; professional relationships and advocacy; professional leadership; and self-regulation. Following are some examples:

Professional service to the public. Nursing has a commitment to provide quality care to the public in collaboration with the client, significant others, and other health professionals.

Knowledge-based practice. Each nurse bases his/her practice on nursing science and the related humanities and sciences.

Continuing competence. Each nurse is personally responsible for maintaining current professional knowledge and skills.

Ethical practice. The nurse complies with the CNA Code of Ethics. The registered nurse, in accordance with the *Code of Ethics for Registered Nurses*, establishes professional therapeutic relationships with clients and advocates for and with clients throughout their interactions with the health system.

Professional responsibilities and accountability. The nurse is personally responsible for ensuring his/her practice meets the standards of the profession and legislative requirements.

Self-regulation and professional accountability. The registered nurse assumes responsibility for safe, competent, and ethical practice and is accountable to the client, employer, public, and the profession.

Professional leadership. The registered nurse, in collaboration with clients and other members of the interdisciplinary and/or intersectoral team, demonstrates leadership to improve the profession, health system and/or population health, in the best interests of the client.

Sources: Summarized and adapted from College & Association of Registered Nurses of Alberta. (2005). *Nursing Practice Standards.* Edmonton, Alberta, Canada: Author; Canadian Nurses Association. (1987). *A definition of nursing practice. Standards for nursing practice.* Ottawa, Ontario, Canada: Author; Association for Registered Nurses in Newfoundland and Labrador. (2007). *Standards for nursing practice.* St. John's, Newfoundland, Canada: Author; College of Nurses of Ontario. (1996). *Professional standards for registered nurses and registered practical nurses in Ontario.* Toronto, Ontario, Canada: Author; Registered Nurses Association of the Northwest Territories and Nunavut (2006). *Standards of nursing practice for registered nurses.* Yellowknife, NT, Author; Nurses Association of New Brunswick. (2005). *Standards of practice for registered nurses.* Fredericton, New Brunswick, Canada: Author; Registered Nurses Association of British Columbia. (2003). *Standards for registered nursing practice in British Columbia.* Vancouver: Author; and College of Registered Nurses of Nova Scotia. (2004). *Standards for nursing practice.* Halifax, Nova Scotia, Canada: Author.

Critical Thinking 1-9

What additional information have you learned about nursing from your review of the ANA and CNA standards of practice?

What Are Some Important Nursing Organizations?

Numerous organizations are involved in the profession of nursing. Some of the most influential are discussed here.

American and Canadian Nurses Associations

The American Nurses Association (ANA) and the Canadian Nurses Association (CNA) are the official professional organizations for nurses in their respective countries. Both of these organizations were formed in 1911 from an organization previously known as the Nurses' Associated Alumnae of the United States and Canada.

Originally, these organizations focused on establishing standards of nursing to promote high-quality care and work toward licensure as a means of ensuring adherence to the standards. The ANA and CNA continue to update their standards. Representatives are elected from the local branches of the state organizations to bring their concerns to the national level. As such, they track healthcare legislation, serve as liaisons with national government representatives to inform them of how current and proposed legislation will affect nursing, and develop and sponsor legislation that will have a positive effect on nursing and on patient care. The ANA publishes educational materials on nursing news, issues, and standards.

Similarly, the CNA is composed of a federation of provincial organizations with individual members participating at the provincial level. CNA activities are similar to those of the ANA; however, the CNA is also responsible for administering the nursing licensure exam in Canada (the individual state Boards of Nursing are responsible for this in the United States) and for publishing *Canadian Nurse*.

National League for Nursing

Originally founded as the American Society of Superintendents of Training Schools for Nurses in 1893, the National League for Nursing (NLN) was the first nursing organization with a goal to establish and maintain a universal standard of education. The NLN sets standards for all types of nursing education programs, evaluates nursing education programs, studies the nursing workforce, lobbies and participates with other major healthcare organizations to set policy for the nursing workforce, aids faculty development, funds research on nursing education, and publishes the journal *Nursing Education Perspectives*.

International Council of Nursing

The International Council of Nursing (ICN) represents nursing on a global level. It is composed of a federation of national nursing organizations from more than 120 nations. The ICN aims to ensure quality nursing care for all, supports global health policies that advance nursing and improve worldwide health, and strives to improve working conditions for nurses throughout the world.

National Student Nurses Association

The National Student Nurses Association (NSNA) represents nursing students in the United States. It is the student counterpart of the ANA. Like the ANA, this association comprises elected volunteers who advocate on behalf of student nurses. The NSNA sponsors yearly conventions to address the concerns of nursing students. Local chapters are usually organized at individual schools. The NSNA also publishes *Image,* a journal dedicated to nursing student issues. In Canada, the Canadian University Student Nurses Association serves in the same capacity as the NSNA.

Sigma Theta Tau International

Sigma Theta Tau International (STTI) is the national honor society for nursing. Members are sought from the clinical, educator, and researcher nursing communities as well as from senior level baccalaureate and graduate programs. The goal of this organization is to foster nursing scholarship, leadership, and research.

Specialty Organizations

Numerous specialty organizations have developed around clinical specialties, group identification, or similarly held values. Here are some examples:

- *Clinical specialty.* Association of Operating Room Nurses (AORN); Association of Nurses in AIDS Care (ANAC); Hospice and Palliative Nurses Association (HPNA); Emergency Nurses Association (ENA); American Association of Women's Health, Obstetric and Neonatal Nurses (AWHONN)
- *Group identification.* National Organization for Associate Degree Nursing (NOADN), National Association of Hispanic Nurses (NAHN), American Assembly for Men in Nursing (AMN), National Black Nurses Association (NBNA)
- *Similar values.* Nurses Christian Fellowship (NCF), Nursing Ethics Network (NEN)

Web sites of a variety of nursing organizations are identified on your Electronic Study Guide.

 Go to Chapter I, **Resources for Caregivers and Health Professionals,** on the Student Resource Disk or DavisPlus at http://davisplus.fadavis.com/Wilkinson2

Contemporary Nursing: Caring for Clients

Although a comprehensive definition of nursing is difficult to formulate, all definitions agree that nursing is about caring for clients. Recent studies show that when the proportion of RNs increases in an agency, quality of care rises, death and infection rates drop (Potera, 2007), and length of stay is shorter by at least 30% (Kane, Shamliyan, Mueller, et al., 2007).

Who Are the Recipients of Nursing Care?

The ANA defines the recipients of nursing care as "individuals, groups, families, or communities. . . . The recipient(s) of nursing care can be referred to as patient(s), client(s), or person(s)" (ANA, 1995, p. 2). **Direct care** involves personal interaction between the nurse and clients (e.g., giving medications, dressing a wound, or teaching a client about medicines or care). Nurses deliver **indirect care** when they work on behalf of an individual, group, family, or community to improve their health status (e.g., restocking the code blue cart [an emergency cart], ordering unit supplies, or arranging unit staffing). A nurse may use independent judgment to determine the care needed or may work under the direct order of a primary care provider.

As a nurse, however, you should not view patients as passive recipients of care. On the contrary, nurses should actively encourage patients' involvement in decisions about their care, and facilitate their participation as collaborative members of the healthcare team.

What Are the Purposes of Nursing Care?

Nurses provide care to achieve the goals of health promotion, illness prevention, health restoration, and end-of-life care. Together these aspects of care represent a range of services that cover the spectrum from complete well-being to death.

Health Promotion

In 1948, the World Health Organization (WHO) defined **health** as "a state of complete physical, mental, and social well-being and not merely the absence of disease or infirmity." The definition has not been amended since that time (WHO, 2007). This inclusive definition can be applied to individuals, groups, families, or communities. **Health promotion** activities foster the highest state of well-being of the recipient of the activities. For example, you might counsel a pregnant client about the importance of adequate prenatal nutrition to promote health at the individual level. Group and family-level health promotion activities might include teaching about nutrition during pregnancy in family education programs. On a community level your nursing activities would be focused on reaching a larger number of people. For example, you could advocate for prominent billboards highlighting the importance of prenatal care and nutrition, post signs in grocery stores recommending food sources for pregnant women; and lobby for labeling of substances that should be avoided in pregnancy.

Illness Prevention

Illness prevention focuses on avoidance of disease, infection, and other comorbidities. Activities are targeted to decrease the risk of developing an illness or to minimize the risk of exposure to disease. For example, pneumonia causes many deaths every year. It affects society's most vulnerable: the very young, the very old, and the very ill. Some nursing activities to decrease the risk of pneumonia include:

- Teaching the importance of hand hygiene to decrease the transmission of infection
- Advocating for and administering pneumonia immunizations to those at high risk
- Promoting smoking cessation

Health Restoration

Health restoration activities foster a return to health for those already ill. To restore health, the nurse provides direct care to ill individuals, groups, families, or communities. This aspect of care is what most people think of when they envision the nursing role. Recall that health has physical, mental, and social dimensions. When you engage in health-restoration activities, your care should address each of these dimensions, for example:

- Providing hygiene and nutrition for someone unable to do so independently
- Administering medications or treatments
- Counseling individuals or groups
- Lobbying for policy changes to improve access to care for an underserved group

End-of-Life Care

Not all nursing activities can be directed toward promoting or restoring health, or preventing disease. Death is an inevitable destination on the journey of life. Nurses have been active in promoting the respectful care of those who are terminally ill or dying. Nursing activities for the dying are designed to promote comfort, maintain quality of life, provide culturally relevant spiritual care, and ease the emotional burden of death. Nurses work with dying individuals, their family members and support persons, and organizations that focus on the needs of the terminally ill.

KnowledgeCheck 1-3

Recall the last time that you had a cold. Identify health-promotion, illness-prevention, and health-restoration activities for individuals, families, groups, and communities in relation to the common cold.

 Go to Chapter 1, **Knowledge Check Response Sheet and Answers,** on the Student Resource Disk or DavisPlus at http://davisplus.fadavis.com/Wilkinson2

Where Do Nurses Work?

As a nurse you will have the opportunity to work in a variety of settings. During your education you will have assignments in many settings and clinical units that will allow you to see some of the options available to you upon graduation. Approximately 60% of nurses work in hospitals. The remaining 40% work in extended care facilities, ambulatory care, home health settings, public health, or nursing education (Health Resources and Services Administration, 2004).

Hospitals provide services to patients who require around-the-clock nursing care. This type of care is frequently referred to as *acute care*. Length of stay is limited to the amount of time that the client requires 24-hour observation.

Extended care facilities provide care for clients for an extended period of time—usually longer than 1 month. These facilities include nursing homes, skilled nursing facilities (also known as convalescent hospitals), and rehabilitation facilities. The distinction among them is based primarily on whether they provide skilled or custodial care. **Skilled care** includes services of trained professionals that are needed for a limited period of time after an injury or illness. **Custodial care** consists of help with activities of daily living: bathing, dressing, eating, grooming, ambulation, toileting, and other care that people typically do for themselves (e.g., taking medications, monitoring blood glucose levels).

A **nursing home** provides custodial care for people who cannot live on their own but are not sick enough to require hospitalization. It provides a room, custodial care, and recreation. In the United States approximately 16,000 nursing homes provide care for approximately 1.7 million residents (Centers for Disease Control, 2004). A **skilled nursing facility** primarily provides skilled nursing care for patients who can be expected to improve with treatment. For example, a patient who no longer needs hospitalization may transfer to a skilled nursing facility until she is able to return home.

Ambulatory care is synonymous with outpatient care. Clients live at home or in nonhospital settings and come to the site for care. Ambulatory care sites include private health and medical offices, clinics, and outpatient therapy centers. Recently, low-cost, walk-in, retail clinics have expanded rapidly—in shopping centers, pharmacies, and other retail sites. Typically they treat only common ailments and refer complex or serious illnesses to specialized physicians or emergency rooms (Darcé, 2007).

Home care is provided to clients who are homebound or unable to get to ambulatory care centers for services. Home care services may also be used when the client or family prefers to receive care in the home—particularly when the client is terminally ill. Home care is also appropriate when a client still requires skilled care but is discharged from the hospital because his reimbursable length-of-stay has expired. Services are usually coordinated by a home health or visiting nurse service and include nursing care as well as various therapies and home assistance programs.

Community health deals with care for the community at large. Community health nurses provide services to at-risk populations and devise strategies to improve the health status of the surrounding community. Examples of community health programs include healthcare for the homeless and school-based programs designed to decrease the incidence of teen pregnancies. Community, public health, and home care are discussed separately in Chapters 42 and 43, respectively.

The Healthcare Delivery System

For an expanded discussion of the preceding workplaces and services, as well as the organization and regulation of the healthcare delivery system in the United States,

 Go to Chapter 1, **Supplemental Materials: The Healthcare Delivery System—Expanded Discussion,** on the Student Resource Disk or DavisPlus at http://davisplus.fadavis.com/Wilkinson2

 Go to Chapter 46, **Canadian Healthcare Delivery System,** on the Student Resource Disk or DavisPlus at http://davisplus.fadavis.com/Wilkinson2

QSEN Commission and Quality Improvement

Recall that the Quality and Safety Education for Nurses (QSEN) project and the Institute of Medicine (IOM) have identified the following quality and safety competencies for nurses: patient-centered care, teamwork and collaboration, evidence-based practice, quality improvement, safety, and informatics. Your nursing education should enable you to achieve these competencies.

One important QSEN competency is quality improvement (QI). QSEN defines that competence as the ability to "use data to monitor the outcomes of care processes and use improvement methods to design and test changes to continuously improve the quality and safety of healthcare systems" (Cronenwett et al., 2007). For more detailed information about quality improvement programs and processes,

 Go to Chapter 1, **Supplemental Materials: How Do Providers and Facilities Ensure Quality Care,** on the Student Resource Disk or DavisPlus at http://davisplus.fadavis.com/Wilkinson2

What Factors Influence Contemporary Nursing Practice?

Two types of factors influence contemporary nursing practice: those outside the profession in society at large, and those within nursing and healthcare.

Trends in Society

As you have seen, our historical roots strongly influence current nursing practice and will undoubtedly continue to do so. In addition, nursing is influenced by trends in the economy, the growing number of older adults, increased consumer knowledge, legislation, the women's movement, and collective bargaining.

Toward Evidence-Based Practice

Capezuti, E., Wagner, L., Brush, B., et al. (2007). **Consequences of an intervention to reduce restrictive siderail use in nursing homes.** *Journal of the American Geriatrics Society, 55*(3), 334–341.

This study of more than 700 nursing home residents at 4 sites found that routine use of siderails does not reduce the risk of bed-related falls.

Brush, B. L., & Capezuti, E. (2001). **Historical analysis of siderail use in American hospitals.** *Journal of Nursing Scholarship, 33*(4), 381–385.

This study used social historical research methods to examine the pattern of siderail use, the value attached to siderails, and attitudes about raising siderails over time. Siderails on adult beds were rare until the 1930s; nurses used continual watchfulness to ensure patient safety. Initially siderails were used for temporary protection of confused patients. They were not a part of the bed, but had to be attached to it when they were needed. During the 1930s,

litigation against hospitals and nurses for fall-related injuries, recurrent nurse shortages, and the move away from ward structure toward semiprivate and private rooms all promoted the use of siderails instead of nursing observation. They now have become a permanent fixture of the hospital bed. However, recent research has demonstrated that siderail-induced injuries may occur, and that sustained bedrest has negative physical and emotional consequences. In spite of these recent research-based findings, siderail use remains the norm in promoting patient safety.

1. What trends and factors currently affecting nursing might influence whether siderail use will change in the near future?

2. What additional information would you like to know before advocating for a change in siderail use?

 Go to Chapter 1, **Toward Evidence-Based Practice Suggested Responses,** on the Student Resource Disk or DavisPlus at http://davisplus.fadavis.com/Wilkinson2

The national economy has a tremendous impact on nursing. In many countries outside the United States, healthcare is provided as a benefit of citizenship. In the United States, health insurance coverage is linked to full-time employment with health insurance benefits (although that may change with federal legislation). Thus, when unemployment figures rise, so does the number of people without insurance. Fearing the high cost of healthcare, many uninsured people delay seeking treatment. The effect is that such clients are often sicker when they enter the healthcare system. This taxes the system's resources and raises the level of nursing care required. Another consideration is that the healthcare industry—even in a strong economy—is very expensive to operate. Downturns in the economy affect institutional investments and profits, and the amount of taxes the government can collect; these in turn limit the medications and services that are available. Similarly, the salaries of healthcare providers are influenced by national economic trends.

The growing proportion of older adults in the United States creates a need for more medical and nursing care; at the same time, there are fewer younger people to provide care. The growth rate for adults 65 years and older has greatly outpaced the growth of the population of the country as a whole. It is estimated that by the year 2030, about one in five people will be age 65 and older, and that the oldest old (those 85 years and older) will continue to be the fastest growing part of the population into the next century (Hobbs, 2001; U.S. Census Bureau, 2007, 2008). As people age, they tend to need more assistance with activities of daily living, and they experience more acute and chronic illnesses. In 2007, 13% of the total U.S. population was 65 and older.

The role of the healthcare consumer also affects nursing. Historically, patients relied on the knowledge and decision making of the healthcare team. Now, however, consumers are demanding greater choice in the decisions that affect their health.

- *Patients have access to vast amounts of health and medical information, particularly through the Internet.* Web sites such as WebMD and PubMed and online medical and health journals give consumers accurate, up-to-date health information. Informed consumers tend to be active participants in discussions about their health problems and therapy options.
- *Direct-to-consumer marketing* is another form of health information, in which corporations advertise medications and therapies directed at the potential user. Advertisements appear on the Internet, in magazines, on television, on billboards, and in newspapers. Pharmaceutical and medical device companies rely heavily on this advertising to generate interest in new products. Clients may then request their healthcare providers to prescribe specific trade name therapies they have heard about in the media. So nurses need to be prepared to address the truthfulness of the advertisements and to present balanced information to clients, particularly as they are appropriate for individual clients' conditions.

Consumer interest has also generated legislation that affects nursing care. Legislation directed at the confidentiality of patient records, the patient's right to know (informed consent), and the patient's right to a dignified death (living will/advanced directives) all govern the care that nurses render to patients. These acts are discussed further in Chapters 44 and 45.

The women's movement has been another strong influence. Historically, only unmarried women were allowed to practice nursing. As the women's movement gained momentum, women were no longer forced out of nursing if they chose to have a family. However, the women's movement also opened up more career choices for women, and nursing has become just one of many options as opposed to a preferred career pathway. Also, as you have seen, societal views of nursing as a women's profession influence the decisions of men to enter nursing.

Collective bargaining is a form of negotiating that allows nurses to seek better wages and working conditions as a group rather than individually. A union or organization that represents the nurses usually conducts collective bargaining. Collective bargaining has resulted in significant improvements in wages, benefits, and working conditions for nurses, as well as safer conditions for patients. These improvements have made nursing more attractive as a career choice. Not all states have collective bargaining groups for nurses.

Critical Thinking 1-10

What effect do you think the women's movement has had on the number of women in the nursing work force? Speculate also on the ways in which women entering nursing might have been different before and after the women's movement.

Trends in Nursing and Healthcare

In addition to societal factors, trends in nursing and healthcare also affect contemporary practice. We discuss the most significant trends here.

Increased Use of Complementary and Alternative Medicine

The National Institutes of Health define healthcare treatments or services outside the traditional healthcare system as **complementary and alternative medicine (CAM).** They include medical systems, such as homeopathy, naturopathy, chiropractic, and traditional Chinese medicine, as well as specific treatments, such as herbal medications, dietary changes, massage therapy, yoga, aromatherapy, prayer, and hypnotism (see Chapter 40). The following factors have contributed to this interest in CAM:

- Rising costs of traditional care, including the costs of insurance and medications

- Widespread media reporting of treatment errors. Some people are now uncertain about the safety of traditional healthcare.
- Growing distrust of the role of insurance and managed care organizations in determining treatment options
- Constantly changing health recommendations over the last 20 years. For example, there have been numerous studies to examine the pros and cons of hormone replacement therapy for postmenopausal women.
- Increasing cultural diversity of the population, and the accompanying exchange of information about therapies from different cultural traditions
- Creation of the National Center for Complementary and Alternative Medicine at the National Institutes of Health. This recognition has given CAM a legitimacy it formerly lacked.

Expanded Variety of Settings for Care

More than 30% of registered nurses now work outside the hospital setting, as compared to 20% in 1980 (ANA, 2010, in press; Jonas & Kovner, 2005). This trend is expected to continue. As the site of employment shifts away from the hospital, nurses must be prepared to function in these alternative settings. This change requires entry-level education programs to prepare nurses for this type of work (Wilkinson, 1996). In the hospital, nurses have access to support personnel, consultation with other nurses and healthcare providers, ready access to equipment and diagnostic testing services, and increased access to the patient. As more care is delivered in outpatient, community, or home settings, nurses must be prepared to function more autonomously and creatively. They must adapt care to the equipment available at the site, and they must rely heavily on the skills of patients and family members to detect change and report the need for additional services.

 Critical**Thinking** I-II

What is your nursing program doing to prepare you to work outside the hospital setting?

Interest in Interprofessional Collaboration

The growing role of nursing outside the hospital, the increasing complexity of care, the limited supply of nurses, and the increased use of technology are changing nursing from a largely supportive role to one of increasing responsibility. More and more, leaders in healthcare are finding interprofessional teamwork to be essential to providing safe, high-quality patient outcomes.

Collaboration has been defined as the process of joint decision-making among independent parties, involving joint ownership of decisions and collective responsibility for outcomes (Disch, Bellman, & Ingbar, as cited in Sterchi, 2007). However, in a relationship where there is a power imbalance, true collaboration can occur only if the more powerful parties are willing. Physicians

and nurses tend to have different values and to place different emphases on patient care. This may contribute to strained relationships and disagreements about a patient's plan of care, which may lead to undesired outcomes for patients. True collaboration occurs when institutions state it as a goal and give recognition to those who practice it.

Increased Use of Advanced Practice Nurses

The increased use of advanced practice nurses (APNs) has resulted in greater public exposure for nurses. Professional and public reports (e.g., Tourangeau et al., 2007) demonstrate high patient satisfaction with APNs; comparable, and at times superior, patient outcomes over physician-provided care; better understanding of and compliance with treatment regimen; fewer hospitalizations; and greater cost effectiveness when compared with physician providers. This positive exposure has resulted in increased acceptance and support for all nurses.

Increased Use of Nursing Assistive Personnel

Nursing assistive personnel (NAP) are healthcare providers who help nurses and physicians provide patient care. Common NAP roles include nurse aide, assistant, orderly, and technician. NAPs may perform simple nursing tasks (e.g., bathing, taking temperatures, or making beds) under the direction of the licensed nurse. Some institutions even train NAPs for more complex tasks traditionally reserved for licensed nurses (e.g., inserting urinary catheters, giving certain medications). This redistribution of workload has prompted controversy about safety and quality of care.

Although it may seem appropriate to allow the NAP to assume the simple tasks, this distances the licensed nurse from many aspects of direct patient care. The nurse retains ultimate responsibility for the patient, yet may have to base important patient care decisions on information obtained by the NAP. Unfortunately many nurses now in practice were never taught in their formal nursing programs about delegation and supervision, so they are uncertain about what they can safely and legally delegate and how much responsibility they retain. To remedy this problem, nursing schools are now adding coursework on delegation to their curricula, and textbooks such as this one include information about delegation.

As you progress through your program, you will notice that nurses often gather different information from a client encounter than does someone without nursing experience. For example, after bathing an older adult a nursing assistant will be able to tell the nurse that there are no open areas on the skin. However, a nurse performing the same task would be able to do an extensive client assessment while giving the bath. The nurse would be able to comment on the client's level of cognition (orientation to surroundings and self), the client's tolerance for activity, breath sounds, heart sounds, bowel sounds, and the condition of the skin. The nurse might use the time during the bath to teach the client about his condition or to gather information about the client's home and support system that can be used for discharge planning.

Influence of Nurses on Healthcare Policy

Professional nursing organizations have been actively involved in politics at the local, state, and national levels. Each of the major professional organizations actively lobbies and educates elected and appointed officials about the role of nursing in healthcare. Nursing organizations sponsor legislation that promotes the interest of the profession and supports changes that positively influence health outcomes. Nurse-sponsored legislation has addressed safe staffing in hospitals, needle-exchange programs to decrease the transmission of HIV and other infectious diseases, and funding to increase nursing enrollment during times of nursing shortages.

As individuals, nurses should vote, lobby their elected representatives, and run for political office. Together, nurses represent the largest health professional group; as a voting block, they have strong political power. Many nurses organize local nursing groups to support candidates or legislation, or speak out in the community on health and nursing issues. Nurses are typically trusted and respected political candidates,

running successful campaigns at the local, state, and national level. You should consider all of these political activities as you move into the profession.

Divergence Between High-Tech and High-Touch

Advances in clinical knowledge and technology have contributed to improved care for many patients who are critically ill (e.g., premature newborns and patients with advanced cardiovascular, pulmonary, or renal disease). However, in prolonging life, technology has created numerous legal and ethical dilemmas, particularly about end-of-life care. This trend is in contrast to the concurrent trend toward holism and high-touch therapies, which often avoid technology. One of the challenges in healthcare is integrating these two divergent trends. For an excellent discussion on these colliding values, read *Holistic Health and Healing* by Mary Anne Bright (2002).

 Go to Chapter 1, **Resources for Caregivers and Health Professionals,** on the Student Resource Disk or DavisPlus at http://davisplus.fadavis.com/Wilkinson2

 Suggested Readings: Go to Chapter 1, **Reading More About the Evolution of Nursing Thought & Action,** on the Student Resource Disk or DavisPlus at http://davisplus.fadavis.com/Wilkinson2

 Bibliography: Go to Volume 2, Bibliography.

CHAPTER 2

Critical Thinking & the Nursing Process

Learning Outcomes

After completing this chapter, you should be able to:

➤ Give one definition and one example of critical thinking.

➤ List at least six critical-thinking skills and attitudes.

➤ Review seven attitudes of the critical thinker.

➤ Explain ways in which nurses use critical thinking.

➤ List the six overlapping and interdependent phases of the nursing process.

➤ Describe what the nurse is doing in each phase of the nursing process.

➤ Explain how critical thinking is used in the nursing process.

➤ Explain what is meant in nursing by the concept *caring*.

➤ Discuss, and give examples of, the difference between practical/procedural knowledge and theoretical knowledge.

➤ Name the main concepts of the full-spectrum nursing model.

➤ Explain how nursing knowledge, nursing process, and critical thinking work together in full-spectrum nursing.

Explore Your Nursing Role

It's a pleasant Saturday afternoon, and you're meeting with an old friend whom you haven't seen in 2 years. She asks, "I hear you've decided to become a nurse. What made you choose that? I don't think I could be around people who are sick and in pain. Hospitals are such sad places."

She listens to your answer with interest. To respond to this statement, you will need to consider your motivation for entering nursing and your beliefs about the profession.

Critical Thinking 2-1

How would you reply to her question?

Critical Thinking 2-2

- What factors or persons influenced your decision to be a nurse?
- Have others asked you why you chose to become a nurse? How have the reactions you received before colored your explanation of your career choice?
- What makes this situation similar to or different from your prior experiences?
- What's important in this situation?
- Of the possible answers you are considering, which answer best reflects your true feelings about your career choice? Why are the other answers not appropriate?
- What beliefs and assumptions are coloring your response?

If you are able to answer these questions, then you have used critical thinking to guide your decision making. Critical thinking involves careful consideration of a situation to arrive at a solution, based on analysis of the data. Critical thinking is vital when considering important decisions. It is the kind of thinking you will use as a nurse.

What Is Your View of Nursing?

Chapter 1 introduced you to nursing roles, responsibilities, and activities, and the career of nursing. Throughout this text, you will learn much more. Thus, your view of nursing may change as you progress in your studies. To track your progress, establish a baseline by examining your current view of nursing.

Critical Thinking 2-3

What is your image of nursing? List at least five attributes a nurse should have, and at least five responsibilities that you consider to be a part of nursing.

In the preceding exercise, when you listed some nursing responsibilities, you may have mentioned activities such as "gives medications" or "performs tests and treatments." And you were correct—partially. Much

of nursing is about *doing*, and nursing is activity oriented. But don't forget the importance of *caring*. And now more than ever, the emphasis is on *thinking*. So, another way to describe nursing is to say that *nursing involves thinking, doing,* and *caring*.

The scientific basis for patient care changes constantly. Research continually uncovers new information that alters the practice of all healthcare providers. Therefore, you should know up front that you cannot possibly learn everything about healthcare and nursing in nursing school. In fact, to be a safe and competent nurse you must constantly update your knowledge and skills throughout your career. As a lifelong learner, you will need to develop and refine your critical-thinking skills. Critical thinking helps you to know what is important about each patient's situation, when you need more information, and when you need help to make the best decision.

Theoretical **Knowledge** **knowing** why

What Is Critical Thinking?

If critical thinking is so important, then you might be wondering, what exactly is it? One amusing definition is that critical thinking is "the art of thinking about your thinking while you are thinking in order to make your thinking better: more clear, more accurate, or more defensible" (Paul, 1990). On closer study, this definition makes an important point. It tells us that we should reflect on the thinking process we are using to figure something out: "Why did I ask those particular questions? Do I have enough information to decide, or have I jumped to a conclusion? Have I considered all the possibilities?"

Box 2-1 provides several definitions of critical thinking, or you may want to use the following definition:

Critical thinking is a combination of reasoned thinking, openness to alternatives, an ability to reflect, and a desire to seek truth.

BOX 2-1 ■ Some Definitions of Critical Thinking

- Critical thinking is the disciplined, intellectual process of applying skillful reasoning as a guide to belief or action (Paul, Ennis, & Norris, 1996).
- Critical thinking is careful and deliberate determination of whether to accept, reject, or suspend judgment (Moore & Parker, 2001).
- Critical thinking, as the term is generally used these days, roughly means reasonable and reflective thinking focused on deciding what to believe or do (Ennis, 2006).
- In nursing, critical thinking for clinical decision-making is the ability to think in a systematic and logical manner with openness to questions and to reflect on the reasoning process used to ensure safe nursing practice and quality care (Heaslip, 1992).
- Critical thinking is a purposeful, dynamic, analytic process that contributes to reasoned decisions and sound contextual judgments (Assessment Technologies Institute, 2003).
- Critical thinking is disciplined, self-directed, rational thinking that supports what we know and makes clear what we don't know (Wilkinson, 2007, p. 39).
- The ideal critical thinker is inquisitive, open-minded, flexible, fair-minded, well-informed, persistent in seeking the truth, wise in judgments and decision-making, logical, and honest with facing personal biases. The critical thinker uses sound reasoning and is willing to consider valid alternatives (American Philosophical Association, 1990).

There are many definitions of critical thinking because it is a complex concept and people think about it in different ways—none of them "wrong." In fact, any situation that requires critical thinking is likely to have more than one "right" answer. You do not need critical thinking to add 2 + 2 and come up with the answer. However, you do need critical thinking to problem-solve important decisions.

Critical thinking is linked to evidence-based practice, which you will learn more about later in this book. Evidence-based practice is a research-based method for judging nursing interventions. An important aspect of critical thinking is the process of identifying and checking your assumptions—and this is also an important part of the research process.

Critical thinkers are flexible, nonjudgmental, inquisitive, honest, and interested in seeking the truth. They possess intellectual skills that allow them to use their curiosity to their advantage, and they have critical attitudes that motivate them to use those skills responsibly.

What Are Critical-Thinking Skills?

Skills in critical thinking refer to the cognitive (intellectual) processes used in complex thinking operations such as problem-solving and decision making. In this example, the skills are italicized, and the complex thinking processes are in bold type:

When planning nursing care, nurses *gather information* about the client and then **draw tentative conclusions about the meaning of the information** to *identify the client's problems*. Then they *think of several different actions* they might take to help **solve or relieve the problem**.

The following are a few examples of critical-thinking skills:

- Objectively gathering information on a problem or issue
- Recognizing the need for more information
- Evaluating the credibility and usefulness of sources of information
- Recognizing gaps in one's own knowledge
- Listening carefully; reading thoughtfully
- Separating relevant from irrelevant data and important from unimportant data
- Organizing or grouping information in meaningful ways
- Making inferences (tentative conclusions) about the meaning of the information
- Visualizing potential solutions to a problem
- Exploring the advantages, disadvantages, and consequences of each potential action

What Are Critical-Thinking Attitudes?

Attitudes are not the same as intellectual skills. They are more like feelings and traits of mind. Your attitudes and character determine whether you will use your thinking skills fairly and with an open mind. Without a critical attitude, people tend to use thinking skills to justify narrow-mindedness and prejudice, and to benefit themselves rather than others. The following are some critical-thinking attitudes (Paul, 1990):

- **Independent thinking.** Critical thinkers do not believe everything they are told; they do not just go along with the crowd. They listen to what others think and they learn from new ideas. They do not accept or reject an idea before they understand it. Nurses should challenge actions and policies with little logical support.
- **Intellectual curiosity.** Critical thinkers love to learn new things. They show an attitude of curiosity and inquiry, and frequently think or ask, "What if . . . ," "How could we do this differently?," "How does this work?" or "Why did that happen?"
- **Intellectual humility.** Critical thinkers are aware that they do not know everything, and they are not embarrassed to ask for help when they don't know. They are not too proud to seek the wisdom of mentors with knowledge, skill, and ability. They reevaluate their conclusions or actions in light of new information and are willing to admit when they are wrong.
- **Intellectual empathy.** Critical thinkers try to understand the feelings and perceptions of others. They try to see a situation as the other person sees it.
- **Intellectual courage.** Critical thinkers consider and examine fairly their own values and beliefs, as well as beliefs of others, even when this is uncomfortable. They are willing to rethink, and even reject, previously held beliefs that are not well justified. Without intellectual courage, people become resistant to change.
- **Intellectual perseverance.** Critical thinkers don't jump to conclusions or settle for the quick, obvious answer. Important questions are usually complex, and critical thinkers give them serious thought and research, even when this takes a great deal of effort and time.
- **Fair-mindedness.** Critical thinkers try to make impartial judgments. They treat all viewpoints fairly, realizing that personal biases, customs, and social pressures can influence their thinking. They examine their own biases each time they make a decision.

Critical thinking can be used in all aspects of your life. Any time you are trying to reach an important decision, reasoned action (critical thinking) is called for. Everyday uses of critical thinking might include deciding where you should live, choosing which nursing programs you should apply to, and deciding among several job offers. The rest of this chapter shows you why critical thinking is important to you in your chosen career, nursing.

KnowledgeCheck 2-1

- Define *critical thinking* in your own words.
- List five skills or attitudes that reflect critical thinking.

Go to Chapter 2, **Knowledge Check Response Sheet Answers,** on the Student Resource Disk or DavisPlus at http://davisplus.fadavis.com/Wilkinson2

Why Is Critical Thinking Important for Nurses?

Nurses use complex critical-thinking processes (e.g., problem-solving, decision making, and clinical reasoning) in every aspect of their work (Table 2-1). Because nurses care for a variety of patients with a multitude of concerns, a patient's response to therapy may not always be apparent. Nurses constantly assess their patients and determine how they are responding to nursing interventions and medical treatments. Reasoning and reflection are required for the nurse to decide what interventions to use, determine whether they worked, and, if not, figure out why.

Nurses Deal with Complex Situations

Critical thinking is important for nurses because they deal with complex situations daily. One such situation is that of caring for clients with **comorbidities** (concurrently

Table 2-1 ➤ Complex Thinking Processes	
Problem-solving	Identifying a problem and finding reasonable solutions to it. Requires critical-thinking skills such as organizing data, identifying relevant and important data, making inferences, making decisions, projecting consequences of actions, and applying theoretical knowledge to a specific patient context. The nursing process is a problem-solving process.
Decision making	Choosing the best action to take. In nursing, this is usually the action likely to produce the desired patient outcome. Requires thinking skills such as making judgments (e.g., about what is important) and making choices. Important in problem-solving; however, many decisions are made that are not related to problem-solving.
Clinical Reasoning	Reflective, concurrent, creative thinking about patients and patient care. Clinical reasoning is used in the nursing process. Reasoning is logical thinking that links thoughts together to create meaning.

occurring health problems). For example, if a healthy 9-year-old fell and broke his right arm, he would experience pain and discomfort. However, with proper casting and time to heal, the child would recover. While recovering, he may have to eat using his left hand or limit the use of his injured arm. The child would likely be discharged home from the emergency department or clinic in the care of his parent(s) or guardian(s). The nurse's primary interventions would be to teach the home caregivers the care needed by the child.

The adjustments would be quite different for an older adult who has had a stroke (a comorbidity) that limits the use of his left arm. With decreased function in the left arm, a right-arm fracture would severely affect the older person's ability to care for himself. The nurse would need to evaluate whether the adult requires care in the hospital or in a skilled-care facility and what support services he will need as he convalesces. In the inpatient setting, nursing interventions might initially include assisting the client with eating, bathing, and toileting.

Clients Are Unique

Critical thinking is important because each client is unique. Their *individual differences* (e.g., type of illness, culture, and age) make it impossible to provide strict rules for all client care. Research-based care plans and protocols identify guidelines for providing care; however, nurses must evaluate and modify these guidelines to be sure they are appropriate for each client.

Consider the following example: You have undoubtedly been told to drink plenty of fluid when you have a cough, to keep the secretions moist. Now imagine you are caring for a client in renal failure. Your client no longer urinates and is being considered for dialysis. You notice that this client has a persistent cough. Should you encourage the client to drink as much fluid as possible? Do you see how you could cause harm to a client by unthinkingly doing as you have been told? Nurses must always think, "How will that work in *this* instance?" "How is this like or different from similar situations?"

Culture is another thing that makes a client unique. Ethnic and cultural differences affect a person's view of health and the healthcare system, as well as his responses to health problems. Cultural beliefs influence how people define sickness, at what point they seek healthcare, what type of healthcare provider they see, and the type of treatment they consider acceptable. Critical thinking enables the nurse to assess the client's and family's cultural beliefs and adapt care so that it is culturally sensitive and responsive to their needs.

A client's *roles* also influence when, how, and why a person seeks healthcare. A single mother with young children may ask to be discharged from the hospital early to meet the needs of her family. Clients with extensive support from family or friends may be willing to take more time to convalesce when they are ill. Nurses take these things into consideration, for example, when

determining why a nursing intervention was (or was not) successful.

Other factors may influence how a person responds to illness or to healthcare intervention:

- *Age*. Each of us was raised with a set of beliefs, values, and knowledge that were strongly influenced by the prevailing views of our times.
- *Personal bias*. Clients may have fixed beliefs about health and illness.
- *Personality*. Individuals have unique personalities. This means every person is different; all have individual ways of responding to stress, fear, illness, and pain. Some are hardy and show an attitude of strength, endurance, and high threshold to pain. Others are less tolerant and may outwardly express pain or other conditions associated with illness, hospitalization, and death.
- *Previous experience* with healthcare problems. For example, a boy who has experienced a painful injection in the past may be terrified when he sees the nurse approach with a syringe.

Nurses Apply Knowledge to Provide Holistic Care

In addition to the need to individualize care for each patient, there are some aspects of nursing itself that require the nurse to be a critical thinker.

- *Nursing is an applied discipline.* Nurses deal with complex, ill-defined, and sometimes confusing problems—not well-defined ones such as you find in a math book. This means that nurses must *apply* their knowledge, not just memorize and regurgitate facts.
- *Nursing uses knowledge from other fields.* Nurses use information from chemistry, physiology, psychology, social sciences, and other disciplines to identify and plan interventions for patient problems. Nursing plays an important role within a multidisciplinary approach to patient care.
- *Nursing is fast-paced.* Nurses often deal with demanding situations. A patient's condition may change hour to hour or even minute to minute, so "knowing the routine" may not be adequate. Critical thinking is essential to respond appropriately under stress.

Critical Thinking 2-4

Write a short scenario (story) about a nurse that illustrates one of the reasons why nurses need to be critical thinkers.

A Model for Critical Thinking

A **model** is a set of interrelated concepts that represent a particular way of thinking about something—much in the same way that the shape of a lens affects what you see. For example, you would look through a telescope to view a distant star. Looking at the star through reading glasses or a magnifying glass would give a different view. You will learn more about models in Chapter 8.

The critical thinking model used throughout this book provides one way of making sense of critical thinking. This model organizes critical thinking into five major categories. Table 2-2 defines each category and provides questions to help you focus your thinking in patient care situations. You can use some of the questions when deciding what to think about and do; you can use others when analyzing a situation after it happens (reflecting). Figure 2-1 is a simpler representation of the model, relating it to the nursing process, which is introduced later in this chapter.

This model is not meant to be all-inclusive; there is much more to critical thinking than just the questions listed in Table 2-2. Use it as a guide when you are faced with clinical decisions or unfamiliar situations. The questions can help you to "think about your thinking" as you apply principles and knowledge from various sources to a current problem. This should help you to achieve good outcomes for your patients. You do not need to ask yourself every question in every situation—just those that are relevant. And you do not proceed from top to bottom in the table. The processes do not occur "sequentially," so you may jump back and forth among them.

Let's apply the model to a situation faced by all nursing students. Soon you will begin your clinical rotations, if you have not already done so. Many students find clinical rotations exciting, yet somewhat intimidating. How could you use the five points of the critical-thinking star to approach your first clinical day so that you will be well prepared and able to function safely?

One of the first things you need to consider is your usual response to new experiences. How do you react to change? What other tasks or assignments do you have that will dictate the timing of your preparation? Have you had any previous experiences that will aid or hamper you in your preparation? As you consider these questions, you are addressing the star point of **contextual awareness.**

You need to gather information about the clinical experience. It is important to use **inquiry based on credible sources** as you gather data. For example, you may want to ask your instructor for guidance on how to best prepare. You may also wish to consult a student who has successfully completed the same course. If you have been assigned to provide care for a client, you need to obtain accurate information about the client. You could use the client's chart and your textbooks to prepare. You should use only knowledgeable, reliable sources of information—for example, nursing texts and nursing journals, not lay (nonprofessional) magazines (such as *Parents* magazine) or certain Internet sites. After you have more information, you should go back and analyze your response to the situation. You may find that you are feeling less anxious already! All of this is a part of inquiry.

Now that you know something about the clinical experience, you can plan your day. You need to **consider alternatives** and **analyze your assumptions** about the experience. What is expected of you? What do you expect from the experience? How should you approach your client? How will you introduce yourself? What skills do you have? How will you apply them to caring for your client?

After you feel that you have addressed these concerns, you need to quickly review your preparation **(reflective skepticism).** Have you gathered enough information to feel comfortable in the situation? Have you left anything out? Do you need more information?

This was a demonstration of how you might apply the critical thinking model to a real experience. In this example, you also used theoretical, practical, personal, and ethical knowledge, which are explained in the next section.

KnowledgeCheck 2-2

In the preceding example, identify the actions that demonstrate use of each of the four types of knowledge.

 Go to Chapter 2, **Knowledge Check Response Sheet and Answers,** on the Student Resource Disk or DavisPlus at http://davisplus.fadavis.com/Wilkinson2

What Are the Different Kinds of Nursing Knowledge?

Critical thinking does not occur in a vacuum—you must have something to think about: your knowledge base. Nurses use various kinds of knowledge: theoretical, practical, personal, and ethical. Every chapter of this text is designed to help you gain practical knowledge and theoretical knowledge. Put very simply, that is "knowing what" (to do) and "knowing how" (to do it). In fact, the chapters are organized according to those two types of knowledge.

Each chapter begins by presenting theoretical knowledge. **Theoretical knowledge** consists of information, facts, principles, and evidence-based theories in nursing and related disciplines (e.g., anatomy and psychology). It includes research findings and rationally constructed explanations of phenomena. You will use it to describe your patients, understand their health status, explain your reasoning for choosing interventions, and predict patient responses to interventions and treatments.

Each chapter then provides the practical knowledge that enables you to apply your theoretical knowledge to caring for patients. **Practical knowledge**—knowing what to do and how to do it—consists of processes (e.g., the decision process and the nursing process) and procedures (e.g., how to give an injection), and is an aspect of nursing expertise.

In addition to theoretical and practical knowledge, nurses use **self-knowledge;** that is, self-understanding.

Table 2-2 ➤ Critical-Thinking Model

THINKING PROCESS	DESCRIPTION	QUESTIONS FOR FOCUSING THINKING
Contextual awareness (deciding what to observe and consider)	An awareness of what's happening in the total situation, including values, cultural issues, interpersonal relationships, and environmental influences	▪ What is going on in the situation that may influence the outcome? ▪ What factors may influence my behavior and that of others in this situation (e.g., culture, roles, relationships, economic status)? ▪ What about this situation have I seen before? What is different? ▪ Who should be involved in order to improve the outcome? ▪ What else was happening at the same time that affected me in this situation? ▪ What happened just before this incident that made a difference? ▪ What emotional responses influenced how I reacted in this situation? ▪ What changes in behavior alerted me that something was wrong?
Inquiry (based on credible sources)	Applying standards of good reasoning to your thinking when analyzing a situation and evaluating your actions	▪ How do I go about getting the information I need? ▪ What framework should I use to organize my information? ▪ Do I have enough knowledge to decide? If not, what do I need to know? ▪ Have I used a valid, reliable source of information (e.g., patient, other professionals, references)? ▪ Did I (do I need to) validate the data (e.g., with the client)? ▪ What else do I need to know? What information is missing? ▪ Are the data accurate? Precise? ▪ What's important and what's not important in this situation? ▪ Did I consider professional, ethical, and legal standards? ▪ Have I jumped to conclusions?
Considering alternatives	Exploring and imagining as many alternatives as you can think of for the situation	▪ What is one possible explanation for what is happening or what happened? ▪ What are other explanations for what is happening? What is one thing I could do in this situation? ▪ What are two more possibilities/alternatives? ▪ Are there others who might help me develop more alternatives? ▪ Of the possible actions I am considering, which one is most reasonable? Why are the others not as reasonable? ▪ Of the possible actions I am considering, which one is most likely to achieve the desired outcomes?
Analyzing assumptions	Recognizing and analyzing assumptions you are making about the situation and examining the beliefs that underlie your choices	▪ What have I (or others) taken for granted in this situation? ▪ Which beliefs/values are shaping my assumptions? ▪ What assumptions contributed to the problem in this situation? ▪ What rationale supports my assumptions? ▪ How will I know my assumption is correct? ▪ What biases do I have that may affect my thinking and my decisions in this situation?
Reflecting skeptically and deciding what to do	Questioning, analyzing, and reflecting on the rationale for your decisions	▪ What aspects of this situation require the most careful attention? ▪ What else might work in this situation? ▪ Am I sure of my interpretation of this situation? ▪ Why is (was) it important to intervene? ▪ What rationale do I have for my decisions? ▪ In priority order, what should I do in this situation and why? ▪ Having decided what was wrong/happening, what is the best response? ▪ What might I delegate in this situation? ▪ What got me started taking some action? ▪ What priorities were missed? ▪ What was done? Why was it done? ▪ What would I do differently after reflecting on this situation?

Sources: Model based on Brookfield, S. D. (1991). *Developing critical thinkers.* San Francisco: Jossey-Bass; McDonald, M. E. (2002). *Systematic assessment of learning outcomes: Developing multiple-choice exams.* Boston: Jones and Bartlett Publishers; Paul, R. W. (1993). *Critical thinking: What every person needs to survive in a rapidly changing world* (3rd ed.). Santa Rosa, CA: Foundation for Critical Thinking; Raingruber, B., & Haffer, A. (2001). *Using your head to land on your feet.* Philadelphia: F. A. Davis; and Wilkinson, J. M. (2007). *Nursing process and critical thinking* (4th ed.). Upper Saddle River, NJ: Prentice Hall.

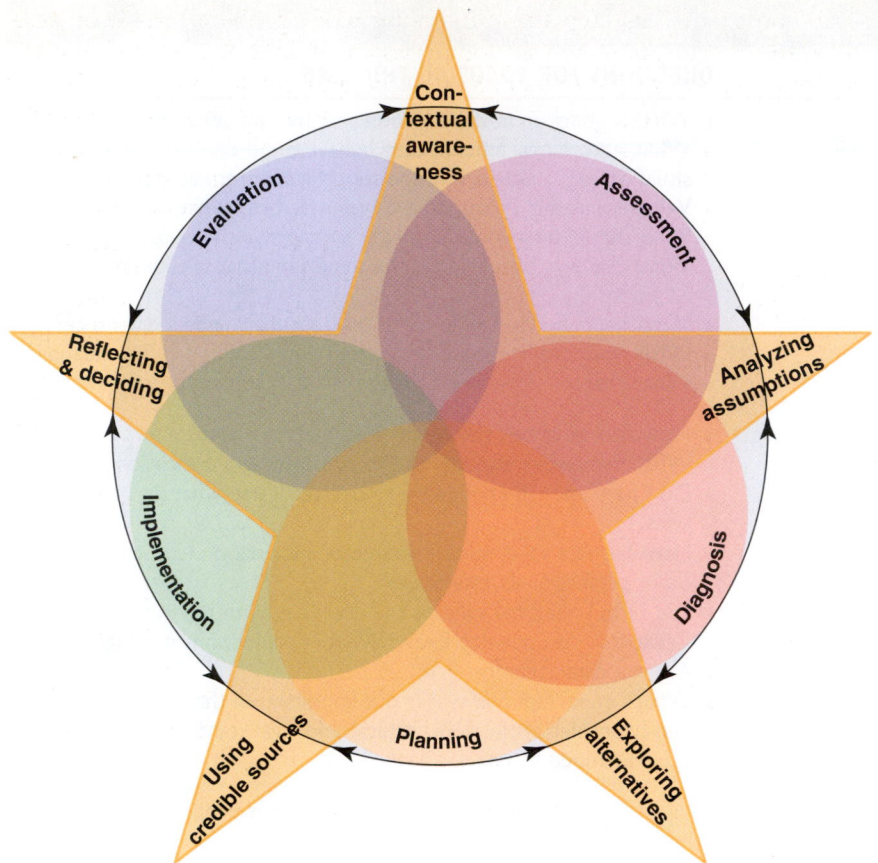

FIGURE 2-1 Model of critical thinking and the nursing process.

To think critically, you must be aware of your beliefs, values, and cultural and religious biases. This kind of knowledge helps you to find errors in your thinking and enables you to "tune in" to your patients. You can gain self-knowledge by developing personal awareness— by reflecting (asking yourself), "Why did I do that?" or "How did I come to think that?"

Finally, nurses use **ethical knowledge;** that is, knowledge of obligation, or right and wrong. Ethical knowledge consists of information about moral principles and processes for making moral decisions. Ethical knowledge helps you to fulfill your ethical obligations to patients and colleagues. Chapter 44 will help expand your ethical knowledge.

Practical **Knowledge** **knowing** how

What Is the Nursing Process?

The **nursing process** is a systematic problem-solving process that guides all nursing actions. It is the type of thinking and doing nurses use in their practice. In fact, the American Nurses Association (ANA) organizes its standards of care around the nursing process (ANA, 2004). The Canadian Nurses Association in 1987 published standards for practice that were also organized around the nursing process. More recently, standards in Canada have been developed by provincial and territorial associations. They, too, usually use the nursing process and critical thinking in their standards for practice (e.g., Alberta Association of Registered Nurses, 2003; Registered Nurses Association of British Columbia, 2003).

Critical**Thinking** 2-5

Practice your critical thinking. What questions should you ask about the last paragraph you have just read? For hints, look at Figure 2-1 and Table 2-2.

When evaluating the last paragraph, you should ask about the credibility of the sources cited, and you should ask yourself whether you have enough information about them to judge their credibility. Do you know what the ANA and the CNA are? What they do? Who belongs to them? What are standards of practice, and who decides what will be included in them? What effect do they have on what you will be doing as a nurse? Those are the kinds of questions you should ask when you see such statements. If you have read Chapter 1, you can probably answer most of these questions. You will see standards of care and practice quoted in chapters throughout this book, beginning in Chapter 3.

All nurses apply the nursing process, to well and ill clients alike, in many settings (e.g., homes, clinics, hospitals). The purpose of the nursing process is to help the nurse provide goal-directed, client-centered care. The nursing process, like nursing itself, involves both thinking and doing. Nurses must have good psychomotor and interpersonal skills, and they must use a sound knowledge base and good judgment to use the nursing process effectively.

What Are the Phases of the Nursing Process?

The nursing process consists of six phases (or steps): assessment, diagnosis, planning outcomes, planning interventions, implementation, and evaluation (Wilkinson, 2007). A model illustrating these phases is shown in Figure 2-2. Note, though, that experts organize the phases in different ways. Many have a five-step process, combining outcomes and interventions into one planning phase. Some even have a four-step process; they combine assessment and diagnosis into one phase that they call "assessment." There is no "right" way to do it because experienced nurses do not use the steps separately anyway. Your text presents them as distinct and separate only to make it easier for you to learn how the process works.

Assessment is the first phase of the nursing process: the data-gathering stage. You will obtain information from many sources: the client via history or physical exam, the client record, lab or test results, other health professionals, the client's family or support system, as well as the professional literature. In this phase, your purpose is to gather data that you will use to draw conclusions about the client's health status.

Diagnosis is the second phase of the nursing process. In this step you will identify the client's health needs (usually stated in the form of a problem) based on careful review of your assessment data. You need to analyze all your data, synthesize and cluster information, and hypothesize about your client's health status. The term *diagnosis* has been thought of as medical, such as a diagnosis of cancer or diabetes. However, nursing diagnoses reflect the client's responses to actual or potential health problems and are different from medical diagnoses, as you will discover in Chapter 4.

Planning is involved in the third and fourth steps of the nursing process. Planning can be divided into two phases: planning (predicting) outcomes and planning interventions. The finished product of the planning phases is a holistic nursing care plan, individualized to reflect the client's problems and strengths. A care plan is a written or electronic document containing detailed instructions for a client's nursing care (see Fig. 5–2).

Planning outcomes is the step in which you work with the client to decide goals for your care—that is, the client outcomes you want to achieve through your nursing activities. These outcomes will drive your choice of interventions. The following is an example of an outcome statement you might find in a care plan:

Nutritional status will improve as evidenced by a weight gain of 3 lb (1.4 kg) by July 1.

See Chapter 5 for more about goals and outcomes.

Planning interventions is the phase in which you develop a list of possible interventions based on your nursing knowledge and then choose those most likely to help the client to achieve the stated goals. The best interventions are evidence based; that is, supported by sound research. See Chapter 6 for more about interventions.

Implementation is the action phase. This is when you carry out or delegate the actions that you previously planned. You may delegate an action to another member of the healthcare team only if it is an action that may safely and legally be carried out by that team member. Delegation is discussed further in Chapters 7 and 38. In the implementation phase, you also document your actions and the client's responses to them.

Evaluation is the final phase of the nursing process. In this phase, you determine whether the desired outcomes have been achieved, and judge whether your actions have successfully treated or prevented the client's health problems. You then modify the care plan as needed. For example, if a problem has been resolved, you delete it from the care plan; if outcomes have not been achieved, you determine why. It may be that a new intervention is needed. If so, you would add it.

Notice that the nursing process is not intended to be linear (one step rigidly following another). Instead it is a *cyclical* process that follows a logical progression. You can see that the evaluation step requires you to begin again using all the other steps. You will find that

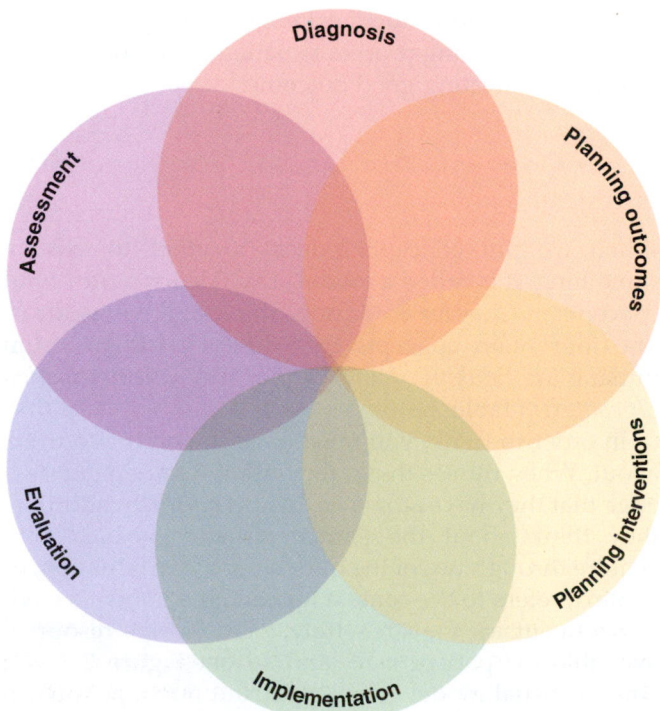

FIGURE 2-2 The phases of the nursing process.

you go back and forth between the steps, especially as you gain nursing experience. In addition to being cyclical, the steps may be *concurrent*. That means that some of the steps may occur at the same time. For example, while inserting a urinary catheter (implementation step), the nurse also observes the urine that returns through the tube (assessment step). You will learn about each nursing process phase in depth in Chapters 3 through 7.

KnowledgeCheck 2-3

- List the six phases of the nursing process.
- In which stage does the nurse collect data?
- Which stage involves problem identification?
- What does the nurse do in the evaluation step?

 Go to Chapter 2, **Knowledge Check Response Sheet and Answers,** on the Student Resource Disk or DavisPlus at http://davisplus.fadavis.com/Wilkinson2

How Is the Nursing Process Related to Critical Thinking?

Critical thinking and the nursing process are interrelated, but not identical:

- Nurses use critical thinking for decisions unrelated to the nursing process (e.g., to decide how many nurses are needed to staff the unit).
- Some nursing activities (e.g., applying a cardiac monitor, inserting a urinary catheter), although they must be done skillfully, do not require reflective critical thinking.

The nursing process is essentially a problem-solving process. As such, it is one of the *complex critical-thinking skills* (see Table 2-1). Complex thinking skills, such as the nursing process, make use of many different critical-thinking skills (see Table 2-2 and Fig. 2-1). The following sections illustrate how nurses use critical thinking, as well as nursing knowledge, in each phase of the nursing process.

What Is Caring?

Caring involves personal concern for people, events, projects, and things. It allows you to connect with others and to give help as well as receive it. One aspect of self-knowledge is to be aware of what and whom you care about. Knowing what the patient cares about reveals what is stressful for the patient, because only things that matter can create stress. Caring also enables the nurse to notice which interventions are effective.

A caring perspective highlights each person as unique and valued, so caring is always specific and relational for each nurse–person encounter. It is not an abstraction. That is, you don't just care for "suffering mankind," but you respond compassionately to *this* patient's needs

right now, in the moment, even if you are busy and tired. Caring involves thinking and acting in ways that preserve human dignity and humanity, and does not treat people as objects. For example, a caring nurse drapes a patient for privacy when inserting a urinary catheter. A caring nurse's actions are never routine or mechanical.

Caring has at least five components:

- *Knowing.* Striving to understand what an event (e.g., an illness) means in the life of the patient
- *Being with.* Being emotionally present for the patient (e.g., making eye contact, actively listening)
- *Doing for.* Doing what the patient would do for himself if he could (e.g., bathing)
- *Enabling.* Supporting the patient through coping with life changes, unfamiliar events, such as hospitalization
- *Maintaining belief.* Having faith in the patient's ability to get through the change or event and to find fulfillment and meaning (Swanson, 1990)

Caring is the central concept in several nursing theories. You will learn more about them in Chapter 8.

KnowledgeCheck 2-4

List all the characteristics of caring that you can remember.

 Go to Chapter 2, **Knowledge Check Response Sheet and Answers,** on the Student Resource Disk or DavisPlus at http://davisplus.fadavis.com/Wilkinson2

What Is Full-Spectrum Nursing?

Full-spectrum nursing is a unique blend of thinking, doing, and caring. It is performed by nurses who fully develop and apply nursing knowledge, critical thinking, and the nursing process to patient situations for the purpose of effecting good outcomes.

What Concepts Are Used in Full-Spectrum Nursing?

When we put concepts (ideas) together to explain something, it is called **a model.** You'll learn more about concepts in Chapter 8; for now, think of them as ideas. The four main concepts that describe full-spectrum nursing are *thinking, doing, caring,* and *patient situation (or context)* (Table 2-3).

In order to think, you must have something to think about. When nurses think, they use the nursing knowledge that they have stored in their memory. In addition, they think about the patient situation, which they acquire through use of the nursing process. Situation, or context, refers to the context for care, the patient's environment outside the care setting, relationships, resources available for patient care, and so on. Figure 2-3 is a simple, visual model of full-spectrum nursing. You can see that the concept's full model involves everything you have learned in this chapter: critical thinking, nursing

Table 2-3 ➤ Full-Spectrum Nursing Concepts			
THINKING	**DOING**	**CARING**	**PATIENT SITUATION**
Critical Thinking Enables you to fully use your knowledge and skills	**Practical Knowledge** Skills, procedures, and processes (including the nursing process)	**Self-Knowledge** Awareness of your values, beliefs, and biases	**Patient Data** Physical, psychosocial, spiritual
Theoretical Knowledge Principles, facts, theories; what you have to think *with*	**Nursing Process** *Assessment and Evaluation:* Everything you know about the patient including context *Planning and Implementation:* What you do for the patient	**Ethical Knowledge** Understanding your obligations; sense of right and wrong	**Patient Preferences Context** Context for care, environment, relationships, culture, resources, supports

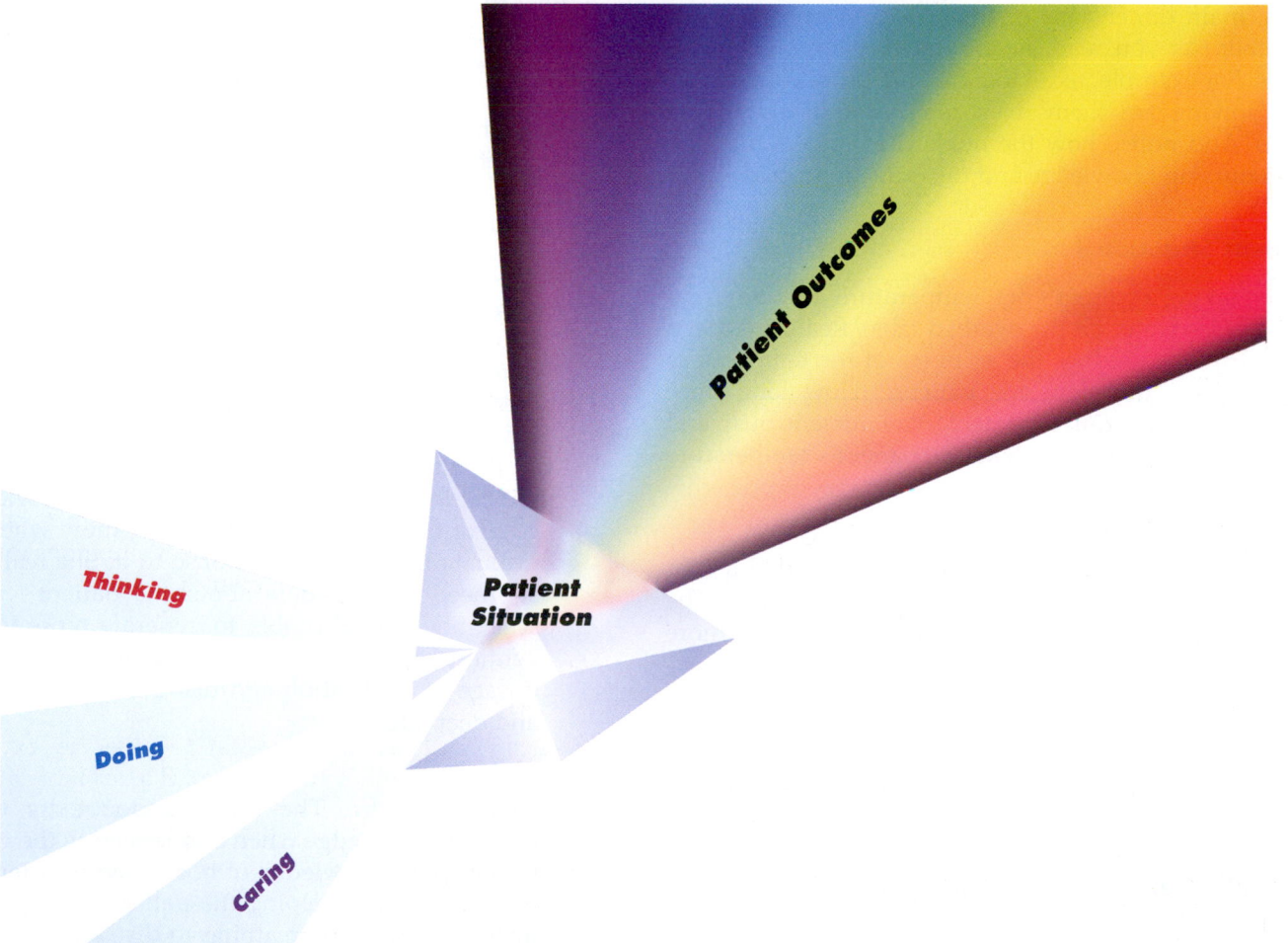

FIGURE 2-3 Model of full-spectrum nursing.

knowledge, and nursing process—but organized under the simple concepts of thinking, doing, caring, and patient situation.

Let's see how the model concepts work together for a full-spectrum nurse. They are all interrelated and overlapping, but we divide them into simple categories to help you understand and remember them. You can see

that a full-spectrum nurse needs excellent thinking skills because there is so much to think *about* and so much to *do*.

KnowledgeCheck 2-5
- What are the four main concepts of the full-spectrum model of nursing?

■ Where do the four types of nursing knowledge fit into the full-spectrum model?

■ What is the ultimate purpose of full-spectrum nursing?

 Go to Chapter 2, **Knowledge Check Response Sheet and Answers,** on the Student Resource Disk or DavisPlus at http://davisplus.fadavis.com/Wilkinson2

How Does the Model Work?

The full-spectrum nursing model is used throughout this text, so it is important that you understand how it works. Nurses use critical *thinking* in all steps of the nursing process. They also apply critical thinking to the four kinds of nursing knowledge, and when they are *doing* for the patient. *Caring* motivates and facilitates the thinking and doing. The goal of all this is to have a positive effect on a patient's health outcomes.

The following patient situations illustrate how the three main dimensions of full-spectrum nursing work together. As you read, notice the overlapping of concepts. For example, recall that nursing process and problem solving are themselves complex critical-thinking skills. And notice how the nurse uses critical thinking with nursing knowledge and the nursing process.

Patient Situation 1

When taking a patient's oral temperature, a nurse sees a glass of ice water on the overbed table. Realizing that a cold drink can reduce the accuracy of the temperature reading, she questions the patient, "How long since you've taken a drink of water?" The nurse is busy and tired, but she returns to take the patient's temperature again at a later time.

Thinking

Theoretical knowledge. The nurse realized that a cold drink can lower the temperature reading. The nurse used interviewing principles to get more information from the patient.

Critical thinking. The nurse recognized relevant information and identified the need for more information. She used the patient's answer to decide what to do. Being aware of context is also critical thinking. The context in this scenario includes ice water within the patient's reach and that the patient was physically capable of reaching it.

Doing

Practical knowledge. The nurse used a psychomotor skill when she measured the patient's temperature to acquire more patient vital sign data and a communication process to question the patient.

Nursing process (Assessment). The nurse observed the glass of ice water on the table. The nurse asked, "How long since you've taken a drink of water?" The nurse also observed the environmental data (e.g., ice water at the bedside). *(Implementation)* The nurse took the patient's temperature.

Caring

The scenario does not say this, but a caring nurse, even a very busy one, would not be annoyed with the patient for the inconvenience of having to come back again to take the temperature. Self-knowledge might include the nurse's awareness that she is tired and feeling irritable. Ethical knowledge would tell her that she has an obligation to get an accurate temperature from the patient rather than thinking, "Oh, I'll just record the reading a degree or two higher, as it doesn't matter that much."

Patient Situation 2

Thirty minutes after giving a pain medication, a nurse checks with the patient to see whether the pain has been relieved. The nurse is using the desired outcome ("States pain relief is adequate . . .") as a criterion for evaluating the effectiveness of the nursing activity. The patient says, "I don't think that medicine is helping a bit." On a scale of 1 to 10, the patient reports her pain as 9. The nurse notifies the primary care provider to request an increase in the dosage of pain medication. She then gives the new medication to the patient and, even though it is the end of her shift, she sits with the patient to help him use guided imagery and deep breathing strategies to reduce his pain until the medication takes effect.

Thinking

Theoretical knowledge. The nurse had theoretical knowledge of the interval needed for the medication to take effect. She also knew facts and principles about pain rating scales and strategies to relieve pain without medication.

Critical thinking. Criterion-based evaluation is a critical-thinking skill. The nurse applied knowledge of the medication's action to know when to evaluate the patient's response to it. She realized she needed more data about the patient's pain scale. She was also able to generate more interventions, such as requesting an adjustment in the dosage of medication and using guided imagery and deep breathing.

Doing

Practical knowledge. The nurse undoubtedly used practical knowledge when administering the medication (e.g., knowledge of how to administer the medication) and helping the patient with guided imagery and deep breathing to distract him from his pain.

Nursing process. The nurse had apparently previously assessed the patient, identified a nursing diagnosis of Acute Pain, set a desired outcome, implemented an intervention, and then evaluated its effect based on new patient data. She also implemented care when she called the primary provider, administered the medications, and used guided imagery and deep breathing. In addition to data about the pain, you might assume that the nurse knew the following about the context: From the way the goal is stated, we can assume that the patient can speak. The patient is most likely hospitalized because he is not administering his own medication, and the nurse plans to check on him in 30 minutes. Certainly the nurse had all that contextual information.

Caring

Ethical knowledge. The nurse served as a patient advocate when she telephoned the care provider for a new prescription. She cared enough about the patient to stay with him and help him reduce the intensity of his pain using nonpharmacological methods until the new medication took effect, even though this meant working late.

Self-knowledge. Perhaps this nurse values a stoic, "tough it out," response to pain. Knowing this about herself, she could put this aside and see the reality of suffering for the patient and how the experience of pain is individual and personal.

As a full-spectrum nurse, you will apply thinking, doing, and caring to patient situations to help benefit patients and bring about good outcomes.

 Go to Chapter 2, **Resources for Caregivers and Health Professionals,** on the Student Resource Disk or DavisPlus at http://davisplus.fadavis.com/Wilkinson2

 Suggested Readings: Go to Chapter 2, **Reading More About Critical Thinking and the Nursing Process,** on the Student Resource Disk or DavisPlus at http://davisplus. fadavis.com/Wilkinson2

 Bibliography: Go to Volume 2, Bibliography.

Toward Evidence-Based Practice

Eisenhauer, L. A., Hurley, A. C., & Dolan, N. (2007). Nurses' reported thinking during medication administration. *Journal of Nursing Scholarship, 39*(1), 82–87.

This study used interviews and real-time tape recordings to document 40 nurses' self-reported thinking processes during medication administration. They identified that nurses used judgment in dosage, timing, and selection of specific medications, and that these situations provided the best data about nurses' use of critical thinking. A key element was the nurses' constant professional vigilance to ensure that patients received the correct medications. Researchers concluded that nurses' thinking processes extended beyond following rules and procedure, and were based on patient data and professional knowledge.

1. What examples of full-spectrum nursing can you see in this brief abstract?

2. Based on this abstract, which of the following questions might this study answer satisfactorily for you? Explain your reasoning.
   a. Do nurses use critical thinking in many aspects of patient care?
   b. Do some nurses use critical thinking when administering medications?
   c. Do all nurses use critical thinking when administering medications?
   d. Which of the 40 nurses demonstrated the highest level of critical thinking?

 Go to Chapter 2, **Toward Evidence-Based Practice Suggested Responses,** on the Student Resource Disk or DavisPlus at http://davisplus.fadavis.com/Wilkinson2

CHAPTER 3

Nursing Process: Assessment

Learning Outcomes

After completing this chapter, you should be able to:

➤ Define nursing assessment, including the four features common to all its definitions.

➤ Explain how assessment is related to each of the other steps of the nursing process.

➤ State the ANA position on delegating assessment.

➤ Name three requirements of The Joint Commission regarding patient assessment

➤ Use assessment skills to gather data during a nursing assessment.

➤ Define initial, ongoing, comprehensive, and focused assessment.

➤ Explain the importance of discharge planning assessment.

➤ List five special needs assessments and state when or why you would use them.

➤ Identify the following types of data: subjective, objective, primary source, secondary source.

➤ Identify at least four components of a nursing health history and state the purpose of each.

➤ Describe the differences between directive and nondirective interviewing.

➤ Compare and contrast open-ended and closed questions, including definitions, uses, advantages, and disadvantages.

➤ Discuss how to prepare for and conduct an interview.

➤ Describe three circumstances in which you should validate data.

➤ Describe two frameworks for organizing data.

➤ State four guidelines for documenting data.

➤ Compose three questions to ask yourself when you are evaluating the quality of your assessments.

Meet Your Patient

As the intake nurse in a community-based clinic in Miami, Florida, your role is to complete a comprehensive nursing assessment and initiate a plan of care for the clients. Your first client is a 24-year-old single woman, Sami, who is requesting clinic services for her general healthcare needs. Sami is Cuban American and lives alone in a one-bedroom apartment. She works as a fitness trainer at the local YMCA while attending college part-time. Her family lives in Tampa, Florida. Sami's earnings place her below the poverty level. In spite of her low income, she realizes that she must have healthcare to prevent illness and to detect and receive treatment of illnesses should they arise. You will be asked to apply full-spectrum thinking to Sami's case throughout the chapter as you learn the concepts of assessment.

Assessment: The First Step of the Nursing Process

Assessment is the systematic gathering of information related to the physical, mental, spiritual, socioeconomic, and cultural status of an individual, group, or community. Although various definitions exist, all definitions of assessment include the following features:

- Collecting data
- Using a systematic and ongoing process
- Categorizing the data
- Recording the data

The purpose of assessment is to obtain enough data to allow you to help the patient. The nursing interview and the physical assessment findings become a part of the **patient database** (all the pertinent patient data obtained by nurses and other health professionals). You will use the facts, impressions, and contextual information obtained in your assessment to develop a plan of care.

How Is Assessment Related to Other Steps of the Nursing Process?

Assessment is the first phase of the nursing process. Data must be accurate and complete, because the remainder of the nursing process rests on this foundation of data. Assessment is related to other nursing process steps as follows (Fig. 3-1):

- *Diagnosis*—Assessment provides the data necessary for identifying the client's actual or potential health problems and strengths.
- *Planning outcomes*—Data about the patient's motivation, family, and available resources help you formulate realistic goals.
- *Planning interventions*—Assessment data also help you to choose the interventions most likely to be acceptable to and effective for the client.
- *Implementation*—You have another opportunity to gather data by observing the client's responses as you perform nursing interventions. For example: While helping a client ambulate, you might observe that she becomes short of breath. If this is new information, you might then identify a new diagnosis of Activity Intolerance.
- *Evaluation*—After performing interventions for existing diagnoses, you assess the patient's responses. This *reassessment* provides the basis for changes in the care plan.

How Does Nursing Assessment Fit into Collaborative Care?

As a nurse, you will focus on your clients' *responses* to illness, which include their physical responses, their understanding of the illness, how it affects their lives and their ability to care for themselves, and their emotional responses and concerns. You will also use assessment with healthy clients, to help identify ways they can maintain their current level of wellness and prevent

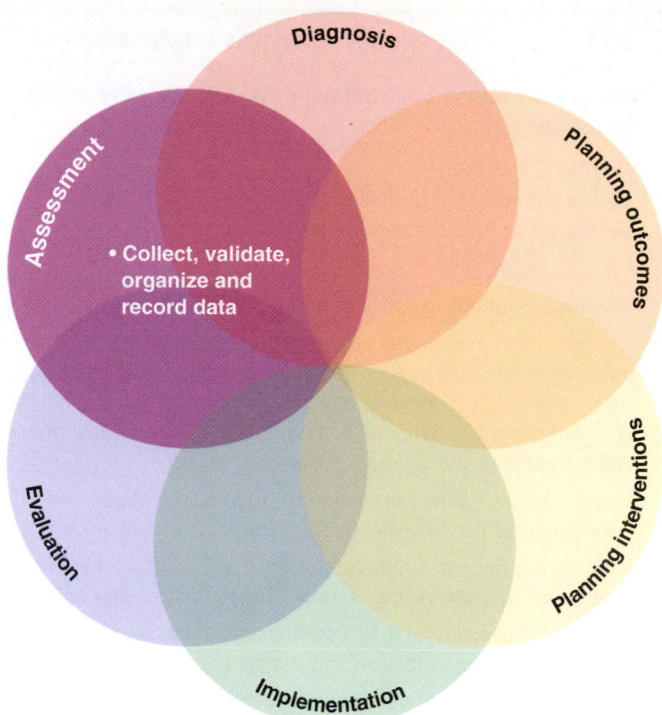

FIGURE 3-1 Nursing process: assessment phase.

disease. This is different from traditional medical assessments, which focus on identifying disease.

Other healthcare professionals can access the database created from the nursing assessment findings. In some settings, the nurse looks at the database and delegates or makes referrals to other professionals with expertise in a particular area of healthcare. This helps ensure that clients receive the proper care by qualified individuals at the time it is needed.

To illustrate, we will use Sami's case: Sami has not had a gynecological (female) examination for 5 years. In the interview, she tells you that her mother has had breast cancer and that her sister is being treated for endometriosis. After asking whether, because of any religious or other beliefs, Sami would be offended by an open discussion, you also ask about her sexual activity, assuring her that you will keep all information confidential. As a result of this interview, you encourage Sami to get a women's health examination as soon as possible. She agrees, and you refer her to a women's clinic, where she will be charged according to her ability to pay.

What Do Professional Standards Say About Assessment?

Complete, skillful, and timely assessment of all clients is an important skill for nurses in all healthcare settings. Standards of governmental agencies, professional organizations, and accrediting bodies, such as the following, all address assessment.

The American Nurses Association (ANA) standards for clinical practice, which apply to all nurses, identify assessment as a professional responsibility (Box 3-1).

BOX 3-1 ■ Professional Standards for Assessment

American Nurses Association Standards of Nursing Practice[1]

Standard 1. Assessment

The registered nurse collects comprehensive data pertinent to the patient's health or the situation.

Competencies

The registered nurse:

Collects comprehensive data including but not limited to physical, functional, psychosocial, emotional, mental, sexual, cultural, age-related, environmental, spiritual/transpersonal, and economic assessments in a systematic and ongoing process while honoring the uniqueness of the person.

Elicits patient values, preferences, expressed needs and their knowledge of the healthcare situation.

Involves the patient, family/support system, other healthcare providers, and environment, as appropriate, in holistic data collection.

Identifies barriers (such as psychosocial, financial, cultural, etc.) to effective communication and makes appropriate adaptations.

Recognizes impact of personal attitudes, values and beliefs when assessing patients with diverse backgrounds or situations.

Assesses family dynamics and impact on patient health and wellness.

Prioritizes data collection activities based on the patient's immediate condition, or anticipated needs of the patient or situation.

Uses appropriate evidence-based assessment techniques and instruments and tools.

Synthesizes available data, information and knowledge relevant to the situation to identify patterns and variances.

Documents relevant data in a retrievable format.

Applies ethical, legal, and privacy guidelines and policies to the collection, maintenance, use, and dissemination of data and information.

Recognizes the person as the authority on his/her own health and honors their preferences in regards to their care.

Source: American Nurses Association (2010, in press). *Nursing: Scope and Standards of Practice* (2nd ed). Public Comment draft, January 2010. (To be published by August 2010.) Silver Spring, MD: Nursebooks.org.
[1]*Caveat:* This material is from the draft for public comment (ANA, 2010, in press); its wording may be changed somewhat in the final published version. For that version of the ANA Standards of Professional Nursing Practice, go to www.nursingworld.org.

Canadian Provincial Standards of Practice (Examples)

In Canada, practice standards are set by each province. The following are examples that apply to assessment.

Province of Alberta

Standard 2. Knowledge-Based Practice: The registered nurse continually strives to acquire knowledge and skills to provide competent, evidence-based nursing practice. The registered nurse:

Indicator 2.1—Demonstrates critical thinking in collecting and interpreting data. . .

Demonstrates critical thinking in collecting and interpreting data, planning, implementing, and evaluating all aspects of nursing care.

Indicator 2.6—Documents timely, accurate reports of data collection. . .

Source: College & Association of Registered Nurses of Alberta. (2003). *Nursing practice: Professional conduct: Nursing practice standards.* https://www.nurses.ab.ca/Carna-Admin/Uploads/Nursing%20Practice%20Standards_1.pdf

Province of Nova Scotia

Standard 3. The registered nurse demonstrates competencies relevant to own scope of nursing practice. Each registered nurse:

Indicator 3.2—Applies appropriate knowledge, skills and judgment to assess, plan, intervene, and evaluate services, and revises plan as needed.

Indicator 3.3—Records and maintains documentation that is clear, timely, accurate, reflective of observations. . .

Source: College of Registered Nurses of Nova Scotia. (2004). *Standards for nursing practice.* http://www.rnans.ns.ca

---

Canadian provincial nursing organizations mention assessment as one dimension of professional practice (see Box 3-1).

Nurse practice acts regulate the practice of nurses in individual states. The National Council of State Boards of Nursing (2006, Article II, Section 2) *Model Nursing Practice Act* also asserts that the scope of nursing includes surveillance and comprehensive assessment of the health status of individuals, families, groups, and communities.

The Joint Commission (2008, Section 1, pp. 171–179) identifies assessment as an essential element of patient care. In agencies where there is an RN on staff, an RN must assess patients' needs for nursing care within 24 hours of inpatient admission. The Joint Commission includes standards that require agencies to provide evidence that:

■ Assessments are written, comprehensive (physical, psychological, and social status), and used to identify and assign priorities for care.
■ Agency policy designates (1) when each patient is to be reassessed and (2) which disciplines can make which assessments.
■ All patients are assessed for pain (p. 186).

KnowledgeCheck 3-1

■ What are the four features common to all definitions of assessment?

- How is a nursing assessment similar to a medical assessment?
- How is it different?

 Go to Chapter 3, **Knowledge Check Response Sheet and Answers,** on the Student Resource Disk or DavisPlus at http://davisplus.fadavis.com/Wilkinson2

Can I Delegate Assessments?

For data to be reliable, someone with education and experience must perform the assessment. Nurse aides or other nursing assistive personnel (NAP) may collect information such as temperature, height, and weight. However, as a nurse, it is your responsibility to assign those tasks, validate the data collected, conduct the interview, and complete the physical assessment. The ANA's *Code of Ethics for Nurses*, Provision 4 (2001) states: "The nurse . . . determines the appropriate delegation of tasks consistent with the nurse's obligation to provide optimum patient care." See Chapters 7 and 38 for a thorough discussion of delegation of tasks to NAPs. The following resources can guide you in deciding which caregivers are qualified to perform parts or all of an assessment.

- *State nurse practice acts.* Each state has a nurse practice act that specifies which portions of the assessment can legally be completed by individuals with different credentials. Look for statements related to delegation. For example, the definitions in the National Council of State Boards of Nursing (NCSBN) *Model Nursing Practice Act* (2006) differentiate between assessments by RNs and LPNs/LVNs (Box 3-2).
- *Agency policies/procedures.* Each facility has policies and procedures that state which caregivers can collect and document specified data.
- *Accrediting agencies.* Agencies, such as The Joint Commission, also provide guidelines on who can perform assessments and document the findings.
- *The American Nurses Association (ANA).* The ANA provides definitions of nursing and *Scope and Standards of Practice* (2004) to guide decisions on who is ultimately responsible and qualified to collect assessment data.

 Critical**Thinking** 3-1

Think about the following situations, then answer the questions. More than one answer may be acceptable. Compare your ideas with those of other students or nurses, or consult your instructor.

- Suppose you are a nurse in a healthcare setting where the policy states that nursing assistive personnel (NAP) can take vital signs (blood pressure, pulse, temperature, and respirations). You have a patient who is critically ill and whose condition is changing rapidly. Would you measure the vital signs or delegate the task to the NAP? Why?
- Imagine that you are a nurse in the same hospital on a different day. All but one NAP have called in sick today because of an influenza outbreak. This NAP is inexperienced and overwhelmed by her tasks. Would you bathe the patients in your caseload (even though that is usually done by an NAP), or would you ask the NAP to do it? Why?

BOX 3-2 ■ NCSBN Model Nursing Practice Act (2007), Selected Definitions Related to Nursing Assessment

Comprehensive Assessment by the RN

An extensive data collection (initial and ongoing) for individuals, families, groups, and communities:

Addressing anticipated changes in client conditions as well as emerging changes in a client's health status

Recognizing alterations to previous client conditions

Synthesizing the biological, psychological, and social aspects of the client's condition

Evaluating the impact of nursing care

Using this broad and complete analysis to make independent decisions and nursing diagnoses

Planning nursing interventions

Evaluating need for different interventions

Communicating the need to communicate and consult with other health team members.

Focused Assessment by the LPN/LVN

An appraisal of an individual's status and situation at hand, contributing to comprehensive assessment by the registered nurse, supporting ongoing data collection, and deciding who needs to be informed of the information and when to inform.

Source: Reproduced from the NCSBN Web site (*www.ncsbn.org*) and used by permission from the National Council of State Boards of Nursing (NCSBN), Chicago, IL © 2006.

It is obvious from those examples that you must use good judgment when applying standards and policies and deciding when to delegate assessments.

Sources of Data

Subjective data (*covert data, symptoms*) is information communicated to the nurse by the client, family, or community. Subjective data reveal the perspective of the person giving the data, and include thoughts, feelings, beliefs, and sensations. Thus, subjective data from two different people can vary. For example, people with insomnia often report getting much less sleep than their sleep partner says they do. Subjective data can be used to clarify objective data (e.g., "How did you get this scar?"). Some people (e.g., infants, adults with mental illness) are unable to provide subjective data. Others can give subjective data, but you might question its accuracy. For example, how credible is a diabetic patient's response about compliance with a diabetic diet and medication regimen when the blood sugar level is markedly elevated? What could you do to double-check the subjective data?

Objective data (*overt data, signs*) are gathered through a physical assessment or from laboratory or diagnostic tests. They can be measured or observed by the nurse or other healthcare providers. Examples are vital signs, x-ray results, skin color, and urine output. One use of objective data is to validate (check) subjective data. In the preceding example, if you thought the report of dietary intake and insulin use was inaccurate, you would measure the blood sugar and ask for a dietary journal. You may also gather objective data when the subjective information seems accurate. For example, when Sami told you her family and sexual history, you learned that she has significant risk factors for breast and cervical cancer and referred her for a gynecological exam. The results of the breast exam and Pap smear (Papanicolaou test, a smear of cervical cells) provide objective data related to these risk factors.

Primary data are the subjective and objective data obtained from the client: what the client says or what you observe. **Secondary data** are obtained "second-hand," for example, from the medical record or from another caregiver. For example, a client's husband may say, "She seems more confused than usual." Or the NAP may report, "Mr. Atlas's heart rate was 100 beats per minute this morning." If you count the heart rate yourself, though, it is primary data. Table 3-1 provides further examples of types and sources of data.

KnowledgeCheck 3-2

During Sami's appointment at the women's clinic, she has a Pap smear, breast exam, and blood work. She also informs the nurse practitioner that her menstrual flow is very heavy and that she experiences severe abdominal cramping. All of these data are

added to the database as references for future visits. Sami's Pap smear results and breast exam are normal, but she is moderately anemic (she has a low hemoglobin level). When the nurse practitioner sees the lab results, she suspects that the heavy flow may be causing Sami's anemia. According to clinic protocol, she prescribes birth control pills for Sami to control her heavy, painful periods and provide contraception. Ongoing assessment will include visits every 6 months to manage her birth control pills and monitor the anemia. State whether the following data are primary or secondary, subjective or objective:

- You see in Sami's health record that her breast exam was normal.
- Sami tells the nurse practitioner that she experiences cramping with her menstrual cycle. *For the nurse practitioner,* is this primary or secondary, subjective or objective data?
- The nurse practitioner tells you that Sami is anemic.
- You check the result of the Pap smear on the computer and see that it is normal.

 Go to Chapter 3, **Knowledge Check Response Sheet and Answers,** on the Student Resource Disk or DavisPlus at http://davisplus.fadavis.com/Wilkinson2

Types of Assessment

Assessment can be broad and general or very specific. The type of assessment you do depends on the client's status. In acute care settings, such as the emergency department, the assessments are rapid and focused on the presenting problem. In inpatient settings, you may perform an initial comprehensive assessment at admission and other, more focused assessments over time, according to the client's needs.

Initial and Ongoing Assessments

An **initial (admission) assessment** is completed when the client first comes to the healthcare agency. First obtain data related to the person's reason for seeking nursing or medical assistance. Then complete a comprehensive assessment if the client's condition permits. Data gathered from the initial assessment provide guidance for care and determine the need for further assessment. Initial assessment data tend to be static; for example, demographic data (marital status, occupation) are not likely to change often.

Ongoing assessment is performed as needed, at any time after the initial database is completed. Ideally, you will make at least some observations at every contact with a client. You use data from ongoing assessments to identify new problems or to follow up on previously identified problems. In comparison to the initial assessment, ongoing assessment reflects the dynamic state of the client. For example, vital signs may change rapidly and serve as important indicators of developing or resolving health problems.

Comprehensive and Focused Assessments

A **comprehensive assessment** (also called a *global assessment, patient database,* or *nursing database*) provides holistic information about the client's overall health

Table 3-1 ➤ Examples of Data Types	
DATA TYPES	
Subjective Data	**Objective Data**
"I have been having a lot of pain in my abdomen."	Suprapubic area firm to light palpation. Lower abdomen semisoft
"My throat hurts when I swallow."	White patches noted at the back of the throat and tonsillar area reddened and swollen
"Our children have no place to go after football games. That is why they get into so much trouble."	In a windshield survey, no public facility was open after football games to allow young people to socialize under supervision.
DATA SOURCES	
Primary Source (Client)	**Secondary Sources (Everything Else)**
Pulse rate 100 beats/min	From chart: WBC count 14,000/mm³.
States feeling short of breath	In transfer report, nurse states that the surgical dressing is dry.
Abdomen tender on palpation	Client's wife states that he has been tired a lot lately.

status. It includes data about the client's body systems and functional abilities, emotional status, spiritual health, and psychosocial situation, including information about the family and community. It enables you to identify client problems and strengths. You need comprehensive data to enhance your sensitivity to a patient's culture, values, beliefs, and economic situation.

A **focused assessment** is performed to obtain data about an actual, potential, or possible problem that has been identified or is suspected. It focuses on a particular topic, body part, or functional ability rather than on overall health status. For example, focused assessments can center on pain, nutrition, spiritual health, social support, lifestyle, and family assessment. These specialized assessments add to the database created by the comprehensive initial assessment.

An *initial focused assessment* is used to follow up on client-reported symptoms or unusual findings during the first exam (e.g., on admission to a hospital). *Ongoing focused assessment* is used to evaluate the status of existing problems and goals. Consider the following examples:

Initial focused assessment. When the nurse asks Mr. Jacobs why he has come to the clinic today, he replies, "I can't get rid of this pain in my foot." The nurse asks questions to get in-depth information about this symptom. For example: When did it begin? On a scale of 1 to 10, how severe is it? What makes it worse? What do you do to make it feel better? She also examines the foot for joint mobility, redness, edema, and tenderness to touch.

Ongoing focused assessment. After surgery, Ms. King has a nursing diagnosis of Acute Pain secondary to abdominal incision. The nurse assesses her pain level at least every 2 hours and before and after administering pain medication.

Critical Thinking 3-2

- Give examples of each type of assessment (initial, ongoing, comprehensive, focused) using patients you have observed or cared for or your own personal experiences as a patient.
- How might age and developmental stage make a difference in your assessment of a patient?
- Suppose you are the triage nurse at the community clinic in the Meet Your Patient scenario. What kind of assessment do you perform at Sami's first visit (initial, ongoing, comprehensive, focused)? What type will the care provider at the women's clinic perform?

Special Needs Assessments

A **special needs assessment** is a type of focused assessment. It provides in-depth information about a particular area of client functioning and often involves using a specially designed form. Some special needs assessments (e.g., of nutrition status and pain) are required by

---

Self-Care

Teaching Self-Assessment

As you learned in Chapters 1 and 2, it is essential for nurses to provide information that will help clients to care for themselves. One important aspect of self-care is performing regular self-assessments to detect symptoms of disease.

Important assessments every person needs to know:

➤ Breast self-exam or testicular self-exam—monthly (Note that this is not presently recommended by all care providers or all best practice guidelines.)

➤ Skin assessment—daily but at least weekly

➤ Feet assessment—daily if diabetic or elderly, otherwise weekly

Before you begin teaching:

➤ Assess the readiness and willingness of your client to learn some type of assessment.

➤ Assess current knowledge or understanding of the topic to be discussed.

See Chapter 19 for details of these assessments.

The Joint Commission for all clients. In some settings, such as hospice, home health, and rehabilitation settings, other special needs assessments (e.g., of functional abilities) are also required. You should perform a special needs assessment any time assessment cues suggest risk factors or problems in an area of client functioning.

Special needs assessments can be quite lengthy; therefore, you need to think carefully about when and how to use them. You need enough data to provide holistic care, but you must balance this need against the need not to intrude on the client's privacy. The data you obtain should enhance the care provided to the client and add to the comprehensive assessment. The following are some special needs assessments:

Nutritional Assessment. Perform a nutritional assessment when data suggest that the client is undernourished, is at risk for Imbalanced Nutrition, or requires nutritional therapy as an intervention (as for a person newly diagnosed with diabetes). In addition to information about food intake, it includes information related to personal, psychosocial, and economic problems that may affect nutrition. See Chapter 26 for more information about nutritional assessment.

Pain Assessment. In addition, good nursing care and accrediting agency standards require you to perform a thorough pain assessment on all patients during the initial assessment and in ongoing assessments (The Joint Commission, Standard PC.8.10, 2008). For more information on pain assessments, see Chapter 30.

Functional Ability Assessment. Health problems and normal aging changes often bring a decline in functional status. Functional ability is especially important in discharge planning and home care. Future rehabilitation needs are derived from initial and ongoing functional ability assessments. The Joint Commission (2008, p. 173) requires a functional ability assessment for all patients "as appropriate." These three functional assessment tools are commonly used:

- **The Katz Index of ADL scale (1963).** This instrument is one of the best for assessing independent performance in very basic areas. It assigns 1 point for independence in each of the following areas: bathing, dressing, toileting, transfer, continence, and feeding (Wallace & Shelkey, 2007). Nurses often use the data to plan staffing and appropriate placement of clients. See Box 3-3 for questions to use when assessing activities of daily living (ADLs). For a link to the Katz scale,

 Go to Chapter 3, **Resources for Caregivers and Health Professionals,** on the Student Resource Disk or DavisPlus at http://davisplus.fadavis.com/Wilkinson2

- **Lawton Instrumental Activities of Daily Living (IADL) scale (1969).** This easy-to-use tool is particularly helpful in assessing a person's ability to independently perform the more sophisticated tasks of everyday life, such as shopping. Identifying early functional decline is important for discharge planning. The Lawton scale is especially useful for older adults, who may begin to experience functional decline within 48 hours of hospital admission (Hirsch, as cited in Graf, 2008). To see the Lawton scale,

 Go to Chapter 3, **Assessment Forms: Lawton IADL,** in Volume 2.

- **The Karnofsky Performance Scale** (Karnofsky & Burchenal, 1949). This tool is used primarily in palliative care settings to assess functional abilities at the end of life. To see this tool,

 Go to Chapter 3, Tables, Boxes, Figures; **Box ESG 3-1, Karnofsky Performance Scale,** on the Student Resource Disk or DavisPlus at http://davisplus.fadavis.com/Wilkinson2

Cultural Assessment. Awareness of cultural influences should guide your assessment and nursing care, but be careful not to stereotype clients based on culture. To be culturally competent, you must be able to assess and honor the diversity among all clients. For content included in a cultural assessment, see Chapter 13.

Spiritual Health Assessment. Spiritual health contributes to overall well-being. For ill persons, spirituality can be a problem or a source of support. To gather useful information, you must do more than ask the client's religious preference. Spiritual health assessment provides insight into how a client interprets life events and health. See Chapter 14 for more detailed information.

BOX 3-3 ■ Questions for Assessing Independence in Activities of Daily Living

Mobility

Does the client require devices (e.g., cane, crutches, walker, wheelchair) for support?

Transfer

Can the client get in and out of bed and in and out of a chair without assistance?

If not, how much help does the client need?

Is the client completely confined to bed?

Bathing

Can the client perform a sponge bath, tub bath, or shower bath with no help?

If not, specifically what assistance does the client need?

Dressing

Can the client get all necessary clothing from drawers and closets and get completely dressed without help?

If not, specifically what assistance does the client need?

Feeding

Can the client feed self without assistance?

If not, specifically what assistance does the client need (e.g., help with cutting meat, tube feeding)?

Toileting

Can the client go to the bathroom, use the toilet, clean self, and rearrange clothing without help?

If a night bedpan or commode is used, can the client empty and clean it independently?

If the client needs help with these activities, specifically what does it include?

Continence

Does the client independently control urination and bowel movements?

If not, how often is the client incontinent of bladder or bowel?

Does the client require an indwelling urinary catheter?

Psychosocial Assessment. A psychosocial assessment includes data about lifestyle, usual coping patterns, understanding of the current illness, personality style, previous psychiatric disorders, recent stressors, major issues related to the illness, and mental status (Gorman, Raines, & Sultan, 2008). Perform a focused psychosocial assessment if initial assessment data indicate that social and emotional needs are not being met (e.g., if the client is very anxious or exhibiting symptoms of stress), or if sociocultural factors (e.g., unemployment) present a risk to health. See Chapter 11.

Wellness Assessment. Health promotion focuses on activities of a well person to achieve a higher level of health. You assume that well people can identify their own health needs, so most assessment tools are self-administered. A wellness assessment includes data about spiritual health, social support, nutrition, physical fitness, health beliefs, and lifestyle, as well as a life-stress review. See Chapter 41 for a more detailed discussion of assessing wellness.

Family Assessment. Health behaviors and beliefs generally have their beginnings in family interactions. Therefore, a family assessment provides a better understanding of the client's health-related values, beliefs, and behaviors. Family assessment is discussed in Chapter 12.

Community Assessment. Community assessment provides information about community demographics, resources, health concerns, points of referral, environmental risks, and community norms and values. See Chapter 42 for more information about community assessment.

 CriticalThinking 3-3

Based on the data you have so far about Sami, consider the need to perform any of the special-purpose assessments. What is your rationale for using or not using a special needs assessment?

What Is Included in a Comprehensive Assessment?

A **comprehensive assessment** consists of a nursing history and physical examination. It contains both subjective and objective data. Figure 3-2 shows what

information is gathered in an initial comprehensive assessment (database) and how it fits into the broad concept of assessment in the nursing process. You will find an example of a form for recording a comprehensive assessment in Volume 2.

VOL 2 Go to Chapter 3, **Assessment Forms: Nursing Admission Data Form,** in Volume 2.

Nurses collect data through the use of all their senses. Whether assessment is initial or ongoing, comprehensive, or focused, you will use the skills of observation, physical examination, and interviewing.

Observation

Observation refers to the deliberate use of all of your senses to gather and interpret patient and environmental data. All that you see, hear, feel, or smell becomes data in the context of assessment. You should try to use the same sequence of observation at each patient contact. By making systematic observations each time you are with a patient, you are less likely to miss an assessment area. The mnemonic (memory aid) in Box 3-4 may help you.

Physical Assessment

Physical assessment (or *physical examination*) produces primarily objective data and makes use of the following techniques, which are described in detail in Chapter 19.

FIGURE 3-2 Overview of assessment content and methods. (*Source:* Wilkinson, J. M. (2007). *Nursing process and critical thinking* (4th ed.), p. 93. Reprinted by permission of Pearson Education, Inc. Upper Saddle River, NJ.)

BOX 3-4 ■ Mnemonic for Systematic Observing

Use the first letter of each word to help you observe systematically as you enter a patient's room.

HELP!!

Help. Observe first signs the patient may need help. Look for signs of distress (e.g., pain, pallor, labored breathing)

Environment and equipment. Next look for safety hazards (spills, equipment cords, sharps). Check to see that all equipment is working: IV line running? Catheter draining? Oxygen working?

Look more closely. Examine the patient thoroughly for appearance, breathing, condition of dressings, correct positioning, skin color and condition, odors, condition of linens, and any other clues that might indicate a need for care.

People. Who are the people in the room? Family? Other caregivers? What are they doing?

FIGURE 3-3 The nurse conducts an informal interview.

- **Inspection.** Observation and visual examination of the client, as well as use of equipment such as an otoscope or ophthalmoscope
- **Palpation.** Light touch, progressing to deeper touch, using the pads of the fingers
- **Percussion.** Striking a body surface with the tip of a finger, which produces different vibrations and sounds depending on what is under the area that is tapped (air, fluid, or solid)
- **Auscultation.** Listening with the unaided ear for sounds made by the client (*direct auscultation*) and listening with the use of a stethoscope (*indirect auscultation*) for normal and abnormal sounds within the body

KnowledgeCheck 3-3

Give at least two more examples of data you might obtain with each of the following senses. One example is provided for each.

- Touch (e.g., bladder distention)
- Vision (e.g., facial expression of pain)
- Smell (e.g., fecal odor)
- Hearing (e.g., bowel sounds)

 Go to Chapter 3, **Knowledge Check Response Sheet and Answers,** on the Student Resource Disk or DavisPlus at http://davisplus.fadavis.com/Wilkinson2

The Nursing Interview

A **nursing interview** is purposeful, structured communication in which you question the patient to gather subjective data for the nursing database (Fig. 3-3). The admission interview is planned, but during ongoing assessment, the interview may be informal, brief, and narrowly focused.

What Are the Components of a Nursing Health History?

Suppose that an elderly man has a fractured hip. The physician is interested in the cause of the fracture, the extent of the injury, and any preexisting medical problems that suggest the client is a poor surgical risk. As the nurse, you would also ask about the cause of the injury but you would want to know what effect the injury has on the man's ability to perform his everyday activities. You would also identify supports and strengths to begin planning for his eventual discharge and self-care. So you see, the nursing health history covers some of the same topics as the medical history, but the rationale for the questions is different.

Health history forms vary among agencies and according to purpose (e.g., inpatient, clinic, surgery, medical, emergency room, or newborn care), but most include the following subjective information:

Biographical Data. This is relatively unchanging information, such as name, address, age, gender, race, religion, marital status, and occupation. The person's responses to these questions reflect his mental status and ability to communicate.

Chief Complaint/Reason for Seeking Healthcare. This is the client's perception of or reason for seeking medical or nursing advice. From this, you will be able to target your assessment to gather the most relevant and important data. Ask, for example, "Tell me why you have come to the hospital today." The client might respond, "I just don't feel right," or "I'm having chest pain." Be sure to document the answer in the client's words, and follow up by asking him specifically what caused him to seek help (e.g., chest pain, a checkup).

History of Present Illness. This an in-depth exploration of the client's chief complaint. Find out when the illness or problem began, whether the onset was sudden or gradual, how often it occurs, what makes it worse, what the person does to relieve it, how the client's health has changed from his usual status, and what effect the illness has had on his daily life.

Client's Perception of Health Status and Expectations for Care. This includes the client's knowledge about his illness and its potential effects on his life. For example, does a client with arterial insufficiency believe his foot will be "normal" again? Also, what does the client expect will be done for him (e.g., does he understand that his foot will be amputated)? And what does he want the nurses to do to help (e.g., leave a light on at night, bring his medication)?

Past Health History. Sometimes called the medical history, this includes childhood diseases and immunizations, previous hospitalizations, and previous surgeries. The past medical history helps guide your assessment and helps you to understand some of the data you obtain. For example, if Sami tells you she had her appendix out when she was 5 years old, you would expect to find a scar on her abdomen.

Family Health History. This includes data on first-degree blood relatives such as mother, father, siblings, and maternal and paternal grandparents. It includes data about diseases they have had, their current state of health and chronic disease, whether or not they are alive, and cause of death if they are not. Risk factors for various illnesses and disorders (e.g., hypertension, allergies) are often tied to multigenerational health problems.

Social History. This includes information about family and other relationships, economic status, occupations, exposure to toxic materials, home and neighborhood conditions, and ethnicity. It also includes data about tobacco, alcohol, and drug use as well as exercise habits.

Medication (Nutritional Supplements, Herbs) History and Device Use. Past and current medication usage may uncover some medical history the client has forgotten to disclose. As you continue with the assessment, you can direct questions toward previous episodes of medical treatment and use of medical devices, such as braces, inhalers, and home oxygen therapy. Also inquire about the use of vitamin and nutritional supplements and alternative-therapy medications such as herbal remedies.

✚ Data about current medications are essential because (1) they may interact with newly prescribed medications and (2) some may affect certain body symptoms, causing abnormalities in your assessment findings (e.g., skin color, laboratory values).

Complementary/Alternative Modalities (CAM). These are therapies used instead of or in addition to the allopathic therapies recommended by physicians—for example, chiropractic care, homeopathy, aromatherapy, music therapy, massage therapy, energy work (therapeutic touch, Reiki), and acupressure or acupuncture. Such therapies can support or interfere with conventional therapies, so this is important information.

Review of Body Systems and Associated Functional Abilities. This is subjective data regarding body systems (e.g., Do you have a productive cough?). It includes functional abilities (e.g., difficulties with dressing, bathing, eating, and elimination). You can obtain these data during the physical assessment as well as in the interview.

Critical Thinking 3-4

The Quality and Safety Education for Nurses (QSEN) competency definitions (2007) identify this skill for competency in patient-centered care: Elicit patient values, preferences, and expressed needs as part of clinical interview. Where do you think this type of patient information fits into the preceding components of a nursing health history? Why?

Types of Interviews

Interviews may be directive or nondirective. Use **directive interviewing** to obtain factual, easily categorized information (e.g., age, sex), or in an emergency situation. In this type of interview, you control the topics and ask mostly closed questions to obtain specific information. **Closed questions** are those that can be answered with a "yes," "no," or other short, factual answer. They usually begin with *who, when, where, what, do (did, does),* and *is (are, were)*. Closed questions are useful for patients who are very anxious or who have communication difficulties.

When you want to promote communication, build rapport, or help the patient to express feelings, use **nondirective interviewing.** This means that you allow the patient to control the subject matter. Your role is to clarify, summarize, and ask mostly open-ended questions that facilitate thought and communication. **Open-ended questions** specify a topic to be explored, but phrase it broadly to encourage the patient to elaborate. Ask open-ended questions when you want to obtain subjective data.

Directive interviewing is efficient but may cause you to miss topics important to the patient. Nondirective interviewing allows you to find out what is important to the patient, but it is time-consuming and can produce much irrelevant data.

A successful interview includes both closed and open-ended questions. Use broad, open-ended questions to guide the patient to talk about certain topics. From the answers to the broad questions, you can decide which topics to clarify or follow up with specific and closed questions. Part of the interview with Sami might have gone like this:

NURSE	When was your last physical examination? *(closed question)*
SAMI	I had a female exam about 5 years ago.
NURSE	What problems have you had in that area? *(open-ended question)*
SAMI	None, really.
NURSE	What about other women in your family? *(open-ended question)*
SAMI	Well, my mother had breast cancer about the same time that I went for my checkup. She's OK now though.
NURSE	Go on . . . *(open-ended question)*
SAMI	And my sister has been taking some pills for endometriosis. She hasn't been able to get pregnant because of that.
NURSE	Are you sexually active? *(closed question)*
SAMI	Yes.
NURSE	Tell me about that. *(open-ended question)*

See Table 3-2 for other examples of closed and open-ended questions.

Preparing for the Interview

While they are learning, some students feel uncomfortable interviewing patients. You may have one of the following concerns:

- You may feel that you are imposing on the patient, who clearly needs rest more than you need information. This may be because you believe a "real nurse" has already obtained the information, or because you

don't have a clear idea of how the information will be used to help the patient.

- You may worry that the patient won't be receptive to answering personal questions from a stranger (you). To help set the tone for the interview, be sure to tell your patients that the information given will be kept confidential and that they can refuse to answer any question. Remember the patient is free to choose what to tell and what to withhold from you. Also, be aware that the patient may have been feeling the need to talk about something, has not known how to bring it up, and is actually relieved you have introduced the topic.

- You may be afraid that some of your questions will upset the patient—that the person will cry or become angry. Remember that patients usually feel better after expressing their emotions. Expressions of strong emotion are hard to accept, but you must learn to do it. You will have large gaps in your data if you avoid difficult topics, and your patients will not get the help they need.

Your interviews will go more smoothly if you take time to prepare yourself and your patient before you begin asking questions. To learn how to do that, and for tips on conducting and closing an interview,

 Go to Chapter 3, **Clinical Insights 3-1, 3-2, and 3-3** in Volume 2.

KnowledgeCheck 3-4

- What are the 10 components of a nursing history and why are they important?
- What are two things you should do to prepare yourself before an interview?
- List several things you could do to be sure the client is comfortable before the interview. To review this information,

 Go to Chapter 3, **Clinical Insight 3-2,** in Volume 2.

- State four guidelines that will help you to obtain complete and accurate data when conducting an interview (these are also in Volume 2).

 Go to Chapter 3, **Knowledge Check Response Sheet and Answers,** on the Student Resource Disk or DavisPlus at http://davisplus.fadavis.com/Wilkinson2

How and When Should I Validate Data?

Suppose a patient has told you that he has never had high blood pressure (BP), but you obtain an abnormal BP reading of 180/98 mm Hg. What would you do? Would you record the 180/98 mm Hg reading, or would you:

- Ask the patient some more questions, such as, "What do you mean when you say you have never had high blood pressure?" or "What have you been doing in the last 15 minutes?"

Table 3-2 ▶ Examples of Closed and Open-Ended Questions	
CLOSED QUESTIONS	**OPEN-ENDED QUESTIONS**
Are you having any pain?	Tell me about your pain.
Do you ever drink excessively?	Tell me about your use of alcohol.
Why did you come to this clinic?	I am glad to see you here today. Could you tell me a little bit about why you decided to come see us?
Do you have any family history of heart disease?	Tell me about your family members and what kind of experiences they may have had with heart disease or problems with circulation.
Are there any parks where you can walk safely?	Tell me about safe places here in your community where you might go to take a walk.

- Ask another nurse to double-check your findings?
- Check when the sphygmomanometer was last calibrated?
- Retake the BP using a different sphygmomanometer?
- Compare the reading to previous entries in the chart?
- Check the BP in the patient's other arm?
- Wait a few minutes and take the reading again in the same arm?

All of those are ways to **validate** your data—to verify it or double-check it. Validating data helps to ensure that it is accurate, complete, and factual and that you have not jumped to conclusions. If the patient tells you that he was running late and has just jogged the two blocks from the parking lot, you would know that 180/98 does not reflect his usual BP and that you need to check it again.

Not all data must be validated. You can usually assume, for example, that laboratory results are correct and that the patient has given you correct information about data such as height, weight, and birth date. You should validate data under the following circumstances (Wilkinson, 2007):

- Subjective and objective data do not agree, or do not make sense together.

  Example: In the preceding situation, the subjective data was "never had high BP," but the objective data, BP 180/98 mm Hg, is a high reading.

- The patient's statements differ at different times in the interview.

  Example: A patient tells you he follows a low-cholesterol diet. However, later when describing his usual daily food pattern, he includes eggs for breakfast, a cheese sandwich for lunch, and a hamburger for dinner.

- The data fall far outside normal range.

  Example: A patient has no symptoms of infection or high fever, but you obtain an elevated oral temperature reading of 106°F (41.1°C). (Hint: Ask him if he has just had something warm to drink.)

- Factors are present that interfere with accurate measurement.

  Example: The patient has very thin arms, and there are no appropriately sized BP cuffs available. Therefore, the BP will probably not be accurate; you should take it again after you can obtain appropriate equipment.

How Can I Organize Data?

Professional standards require systematic data collection (see Box 3-1). This means you collect and record data in predetermined categories, not just at random. Data in most initial (e.g., admission) assessments are automatically categorized by the agency's data-collection form. For ongoing assessments, you may need to provide your own organizing structure, or framework. Because a **framework** represents a particular way of thinking about clients and health, it indicates which information is significant and guides you in deciding which patient data to observe. The major concepts of a model/framework help you to cluster data and find patterns. If you don't understand what a framework is, refer to Chapter 8.

Nonnursing Models

ANA professional standards state that nursing data collection should be holistic. Many agencies use a **body systems (medical) framework** for at least a section of the assessment form. This model is useful for identifying medical problems, but it needs to be combined with other models (e.g., a nursing model or Maslow's Hierarchy of Needs) to provide the holistic data you need to identify both nursing and medical problems.

Maslow's Hierarchy of Needs (Maslow, 1970; Maslow & Lowery, 1998) groups data according to human needs. It states that the basic needs must be met before higher needs can be addressed. Maslow's categories of needs, from most basic to highest, are:

Physiological. Basic survival needs (e.g., oxygen, water, food, and shelter)
Safety and security. The need to be safe and comfortable (e.g., safe from falls and treatment side effects as well as the need for psychological security)
Love and belonging. The need for love and affection (e.g., family, social supports)
Esteem and self-esteem. The need to feel good about oneself (e.g., body image, pride in achievements, admiration from others)
Cognitive. The need for knowledge, understanding, and exploration
Aesthetic. The need for symmetry, order, and beauty
Self-actualization. The need to achieve one's potential; the need for growth and change (e.g., extent to which goals are achieved, role performance)

See Chapter 8 for a more complete discussion of Maslow's model.

Nursing Models

Nurse theorists have developed many different theories and models for thinking about nursing, clients, health, and the environment. Nursing models produce a holistic database that is useful in identifying nursing rather than medical diagnoses. Several nursing theories are described in Chapter 8. Box 3-5 identifies the major concepts of five models frequently used to structure nursing assessments. The concepts are the categories that you would use to gather and cluster data.

BOX 3-5 ■ Assessment Models: Major Concepts

Gordon's Functional Health Patterns

Describe common patterns of behavior that can be functional or dysfunctional. Gordon intended the model for nursing assessment. The functional health patterns are major model concepts:

Health perception/health management

Nutritional/metabolic

Elimination

Activity/exercise

Cognitive/perceptual

Self-perception/self-concept

Sleep/rest

Role/relationship

Sexual/reproductive

Coping/stress tolerance

Value-belief

Source: Adapted from Gordon, M. (1994). Nursing diagnosis: Process and application (3rd ed.). St. Louis, MO: Mosby, p. 70.

The NANDA Nursing Diagnosis Taxonomy II

Consists of functional patterns and is a modified version of the Gordon model. It is intended as a model for categorizing nursing diagnoses, not as a fully developed theory of nursing. The NANDA-I domains (categories) are:

Health Promotion

Nutrition

Elimination and Exchange

Activity/Rest

Perception/Cognition

Self-Perception

Role Relationships

Sexuality

Coping/Stress Tolerance

Life Principles

Safety/Protection

Comfort

Growth/Development

Source: Adapted from NANDA International. (2007). NANDA nursing diagnoses: Definitions & classification 2007–2008. Philadelphia: Author.

The Taxonomy of Nursing Practice (NANDA/NOC/NIC)

Intended as a model for categorizing nursing diagnoses, client outcomes, and nursing interventions. It consists of four domains and 28 classes.

Functional Domain Activity exercise, comfort, growth and development, nutrition, self-care, sexuality, sleep/rest, values/beliefs

Physiological Domain Cardiac function, elimination, fluids and electrolytes, neurocognition, pharmacological function, physical regulation, reproduction, respiratory function, sensation/perception, tissue integrity

Psychosocial Domain Behavior, communication, coping, emotional, knowledge, roles/relationships, self-perception

Environmental Domain Healthcare system, populations, risk management

Source: Dochterman, J. M., & Jones, D. A. (Eds.). (2003). Unifying nursing languages: The harmonization of NANDA, NIC, and NOC. Washington, DC: American Nurses Association, NursesBooks.org.

The Roy Adaptation Model

Conceptualizes patients as adapting constantly to internal and external demands within a biological and psychosocial context. Using this model, you would look at the person's ability to achieve balance in the following "adaptive modes":

Activity and rest

Nutrition

Elimination

Fluid and electrolytes

Oxygenation

Protection

Temperature regulation

Regulation of the senses

Physical self-concept

Personal self-concept

Role function

Interdependence

Source: Adapted from Roy, C., & Andrews, H. (1991). The Roy adaptation model: The definitive statement. Norwalk, CT: Appleton & Lange, pp. 15–17.

Orem's Self-Care Model

Conceptualizes health as the ability to perform self-care. Using this model, you would gather data to identify the following universal self-care deficits that require nursing assistance:

Maintenance of a sufficient intake of air, water, and food

Maintenance of a balance between activity and rest

Maintenance of a balance between time alone and time with others

Provision of care associated with elimination processes and excrements

Prevention of hazards to human life, functioning, and well-being

Promotion of human functioning and development within social groups in accord with human potential, limitations, and desire to be normal (as determined by science, culture, and social values)

Source: Adapted from Orem, D. (1991). Nursing: Concepts of practice (4th ed.). St. Louis, MO: Mosby-Year Book, p. 126.

How Should I Document Data?

The ANA *Scope and Standards of Practice* (2010, in press) and The Joint Commission standards (2008) stress the importance of documenting patient information, including assessment data, in a retrievable format. Accurate, timely, and clear documentation of all assessment findings benefits patients by providing the basis for planning effective nursing care. Furthermore, since the nursing database is a permanent part of the client's record, documentation protects you, the nurse, by establishing that you actually performed the needed assessments. Malpractice suits are not unusual in our society, and court cases may be presented years after you provide care for a patient. Your documentation is the only evidence supporting the care you gave. The assumption in malpractice cases is, "If it isn't documented, it wasn't done."

Guidelines for Recording Assessment Data

Follow these guidelines when recording assessment data:

- *Document as soon as possible* after you perform the assessment.
- *Write neatly, legibly, and in black ink.*
- *Use acronyms sparingly,* using only agency-approved abbreviations.
- *Write the patient's own words, when possible,* in quotation marks. If the comments are too long, summarize what the patient says (e.g., Patient states that he is sleepy).
- *Record only the most important patient words.* If you record everything the patient says, the narrative will probably be too long and contain irrelevant data. For example, write "Patient states, 'I hardly slept at all last night'" even though what the patient actually said was, "I hardly slept at all last night. I tossed and turned and people kept waking me up. Then the thunder and lightning came, and then I had to get up to go to the bathroom, and my wife called early this morning."
- *Use concrete, specific information* rather than vague generalities such as *normal, adequate, good,* and *tolerated well.* For example, what does it mean to say, "Patient slept well"? Did she fall asleep easily and sleep for 6 hours? Did she fall asleep with difficulty, but sleep for 8 hours? Did she sleep only 4 hours, but state that she feels well rested? It is much better to write, "Patient fell asleep before 2100 hr and slept until 0600 hr. She states that she woke up only once during the night and feels rested now. Observed sleeping three times during the night."
- *Record cues, not inferences.* **Cues** are what the client says and what you observe. **Inferences** are judgments and interpretations about what the cues mean. In other words, "just the facts, Jack (or Jill)." When recording cues, you do not need to "waffle" with the words *appears* and *seems.* Don't write "Incision seems red" or "edges appear separated."

For example:

Cues	Inferences
- "My head hurts."	- Patient has a headache.
- Incision red, draining pus, edges separated.	- Incision is infected.
- Tearful. States that father died of a heart attack. Trembling.	- Anxious about scheduled cardiac catheterization.
- States, "I hate my mother. I wish I was dead."	- Patient is angry and suicidal.

Tools for Recording Assessment Data

Each organization has its own forms and formats for documenting initial and ongoing assessments. You will record data on a variety of documents, including nurses' notes and the following:

Graphic flow sheet. Includes vital signs such as blood pressure, pulse, respirations, and temperature so trends over time can be seen clearly (Fig. 3-4).

GRAPHICS

DATE	5/6/2011						
HOSPITAL DAY	2						
POST OP DAY	2						
TIME	0400	0800	1200	1600	2000	2400	0400

C	F							
40.0	104							
39.4	103							
38.8	102							
38.3	101							
37.7	100							
37.2	99			X		X	X	
36.6	98							X
36.1	97							
35.5	96							
35.0	95							

PULSE			88	76	80	74		
RESPIRATIONS			16	14	18	16		
BLOOD PRESSURE			140/84	138/84	130/88	128/82		
HEIGHT 5'2"	WEIGHT	125						
TYPE OF DIET	Clear liquids							

%	B 80%	L 50%	S

INTAKE	11-7	7-3	3-11	24 HR	11-
Oral/Tube	150	450	400	1,000	
Blood/Plasma					
I.V.	650	650	650	1,950	
Other					
Other					
TOTAL	800	1,100	1,050	2,850	

OUTPUT	11-7	7-3	3-11	24 HR	11-7
Liquid Stool					
Urine	100	300	810	1210	
G.I. Suction	10	15	5	30	
Emesis					
Bowel Movement					
Other					
TOTAL				1240	
INITIALS				*(signature)*	

PERMANE

FIGURE 3-4 Graphic flow sheet. (Courtesy of Smith Northview Hospital, Valdosta, GA.)

Intake and output (I&O) sheet. May be on the graphic sheet, as in Figure 3-4, or separate. This form has spaces for all intake: oral, intravenous, and tube feedings. There is also space to record all output: urine, fluid from drainage tubes, wound drainage, and bowel movements.

Nursing admission assessment. Although agency forms differ in organization, all collect similar data as specified by The Joint Commission for standards for initial assessment. For an example of an admission assessment form,

Go to Chapter 3, **Assessment Forms: Nursing Admission Data Form,** in Volume 2.

Nursing discharge summary. This may be a part of the initial assessment form because data obtained at admission are used for discharge planning.

Special-purpose forms. Examples are diabetic flow sheets and medication administration forms.

Computer documentation. In some facilities, initial data and ongoing assessment data are entered into a computer program for organization, shared communication, and easy retrieval (Fig. 3-5).

Toward Evidence-Based Practice

Jones, A. (2007). Admitting hospital patients: A qualitative study of an everyday nursing task. *Nursing Inquiry, 14*(3), 212–223.

This qualitative study explored the everyday work of hospital nurses. It examined the initial assessment of patients being admitted to the hospital to compare what the nursing literature says about assessment with the assessments the researcher observed in practice. The literature clearly states assessments should be patient centered and that they are the important first step to a therapeutic nurse–patient relationship. The researcher concluded that the actual nursing admission assessments were at odds with recommendations in the literature. The nurses used a routinized, bureaucratic approach to assessment as a means of doing the work faster.

Which of the following inferences can you make? State whether the study summary provides *extensive*, *limited*, or no evidence to support each inference.

1. These results occurred because the nurses used a printed form created by the hospital.

2. The nurses did not care about their patients.

3. The nurses were feeling pressured by their workload.

4. The nurses did not know how important the initial assessment is.

5. Nursing practice is not always done according to the literature.

Go to Chapter 3, **Toward Evidence-Based Practice Suggested Responses,** on the Student Resource Disk or DavisPlus at http://davisplus.fadavis.com/Wilkinson2

Shore Memorial Hospital - Clinical Documentation - Production LAN

Thu Jun 24 16:25 Eclipsys continuum User: CMUFFERI	JANE DOE	Unit/Bed: ICU/IC267A

Login	Logout	Census	Patient	Config	Utility

MP %: / Account #:

Admit Physician: M.D., HOWARD M.
Attend Physician: M.D., HOWARD M.
Status:

Age: 46 yrs
Gender: F

Adm Wt: kg
Wt for Calcs: 63.50 kg

Visits

| Section: | Flowsheets | Review | 180 | Notes | ICU Labs | Special | Medications | Care Plans | | | |
| Forms: | Vitals | 180 Detail | Tx/Cares | Assess F/S | Notes | Respiratory | Medications | | | | |

Vital Signs Flowsheet

			06/24 08:00	09:00	10:00	11:00	12:00	13:00	14:00	15:00	16:00	17:00
TEMP	Temperature	F / C	97.8 po / 36.6				98.0 po / 36.7					
HR	Heart Rate		70	69	76	70		77	75	71	80	
RESP	Respiratory Rate	br/min	25	27	21	14	17	19	15	14	23	
BP	Manual BP	S/D (M) Source	/ ( )	/ ( )	/ ( )	/ ( )	/ ( )	/ ( )	/ ( )	/ ( )	/ ( )	/ ( )
	Noninvasive BP	S/D Measured Mean Source	/ ( )	137/59 (86)	/ ( )	122/56 (78)	122/46 (69)	115/58 (76)	96/82 (91)	99/65 (76)	/ ( )	/ ( )
RHYTHM	Rhythm											
	Ectopy	Frequency										
O₂ THERAPY	L/min		3.0	3.0	3.0	3.0	3.0	3.0	3.0	3.0	3.0	
	Device		NC	NC	NC	NC	NC	NC	NC	NC	NC	
MONIT	O₂sat	%										
MISC	Fingerstick Glucose	mg/dl		321								
	Glucose Interventions			Ins bolus 12 units								

Starting Print Screen   ☐ Multi-mark   Newer Data   Sign   Cancel

FIGURE 3-5 Computer screen capture: assessment data. (Courtesy of Shore Memorial Hospital, Somers Point, NJ.)

Reflecting Critically About Assessment

After gathering and recording patient data, use critical thinking to help you evaluate the quality of your assessment. See Chapter 2 for a review of critical thinking, as needed. The following are questions to guide your final judgments about your data.

1. Are my data complete?
   - Have I completed all areas of the assessment form?
   - Is there anything else I need to know to identify or rule out a nursing diagnosis?
   - Have I collected holistic data: physical, emotional, interpersonal, spiritual, and cultural?
2. How do I know the data are accurate?
3. Have I recorded data rather than conclusions (cues, not inferences)?
4. Did I validate any data that do not make sense? Do any of the data conflict with other data?
5. Did I record the data in clear, specific terms, using the patient's own words, when possible, for subjective data? Did I avoid vague terms such as "normal," "good," and "slept well"?
6. Have I followed up with in-depth special needs assessments when appropriate?
7. Have I included only relevant data, taking care to protect the client's privacy?
8. The assessment interview:
   - Did I use therapeutic communication during the assessment?
   - Did I avoid asking too many questions and using too many closed questions?
   - How comfortable was I during the interview?
   - What signals did I get from the client in response to my questions? Did I follow up?
9. Physical assessment, observation, and examination:
   - Did I miss something in the environment?
   - How did the client and significant others respond to me verbally and nonverbally?
   - Did I pay attention to detail?
   - Were my assessment techniques performed skillfully (palpation, percussion, auscultation, inspection)?
10. Memory:
    - Did I have to ask questions in the sequence found on the forms?
    - Did I have to depend on the forms for all aspects of the assessment?
    - Did I have to repeat any area of assessment because I could not remember what I saw, heard, smelled, or felt?

If you have followed the recommended processes and reflected critically on your assessment, you should have the data necessary to create a holistic plan of care individualized to meet the client's needs.

 Go to Chapter 3, **Resources for Caregivers and Health Professionals,** on the Student Resource Disk or DavisPlus at http://davisplus.fadavis.com/Wilkinson2

 Suggested Readings: Go to Chapter 3, **Reading More About Nursing Process: Assessment,** on the Student Resource Disk or DavisPlus at http://davisplus.fadavis.com/Wilkinson2

 Bibliography: Go to Volume 2, Bibliography.

CHAPTER 4

Nursing Process: Diagnosis

Learning Outcomes

After completing this chapter, you should be able to:

➤ Define the following terms: diagnosis, nursing diagnosis, diagnostic reasoning, diagnostic label, defining characteristics, related factors, risk factors, health problem.

➤ Explain how nursing diagnosis is related to the rest of the nursing process.

➤ Relate the history of nursing diagnosis since the 1950s, including the role of the American Nurses Association and NANDA International.

➤ Differentiate between nursing diagnoses, medical diagnoses, and collaborative problems.

➤ Explain the differences between actual, risk, possible, syndrome, and wellness nursing diagnoses.

➤ Describe a process for determining a nursing diagnosis.

➤ Explain why an etiology is always an inference.

➤ Describe at least two frameworks for prioritizing nursing diagnoses.

➤ Describe errors of theoretical and self-knowledge that may occur in diagnostic reasoning.

➤ Use standardized nursing language to write nursing diagnoses.

➤ Write nursing diagnosis statements and collaborative problem statements in correct format.

➤ Explain the relationship between nursing diagnoses and goals/interventions.

➤ State at least five criteria for judging the quality of a diagnostic statement.

➤ Discuss issues associated with the NANDA-I diagnostic labels and with standardized language in general.

Meet Your Patient

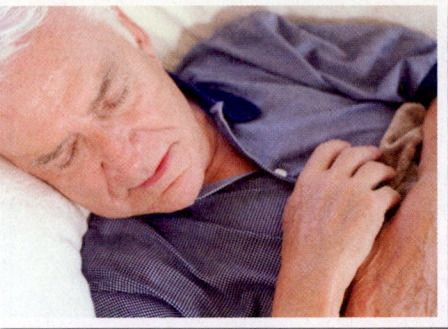

On your unit at an acute care facility, you will be admitting a client, Todd, from the emergency department (ED). Todd's ED nurse telephones you to give a report on his status. The ED nurse tells you that Todd's admitting medical diagnosis is chronic renal failure. He is married, 58 years old, employed, and has a longstanding history of type 2 diabetes mellitus. In the past 3 days, he has developed decreased sensation in his bilateral lower extremities with slight mobility impairment.

You still have many questions concerning Todd's immediate and long-term needs. You will need to ask Todd about his medication regimen, his compliance with his diabetes treatment plan, and the extent to which his family is involved. You will also need to find out what laboratory tests have been completed and how severe his renal dysfunction has become. After you obtain the necessary data, you will organize and analyze it to form some initial impressions about what it means. Some initial impressions might be:

- His admitting diagnosis is chronic renal failure; so you can anticipate a problem with fluid balance.
- He has been admitted to the hospital and is acutely ill, so he may be anxious and fearful.

- He has decreased sensation in his lower extremities, so he may have a mobility or a safety problem.
- He has diabetes, so he is at risk for impaired skin and tissue integrity.
- Because diabetes and renal failure require complex regimens and patient self-care, it is possible that Todd may not be managing his therapy effectively, because he either is not motivated to do so or he lacks the knowledge he needs to comply with treatment.

When Todd and his family arrive on your unit, you begin gathering additional data. Using your comprehensive data, you then make a list of Todd's health problems, in priority order. These actions illustrate the diagnosis phase of the nursing process. The purpose of diagnosing is to identify the client's health status, from which you will create your plan of care.

Theoretical **Knowledge**
knowing why

Professional standards of nursing practice, as well as many state nurse practice acts, identify diagnosing as the unique obligation of the professional nurse (Box 4-1). Although many nursing activities may be delegated, diagnosis cannot. To meet practice expectations and professional obligations as a registered nurse, you will assume the role of diagnostician and make clinical judgments. Most state nurse practice acts limit the role of the licensed practical nurse (LPN/LVN) in diagnosing to a focus on gathering data that will be analyzed by the RN. However, LPN roles vary among states and agencies, and they are subject to change. Furthermore, LPN and RN roles are becoming more closely linked through statewide career ladder programs. So, all clinicians need to stay current with updates in practice acts and standards.

Diagnosis: The Second Step of the Nursing Process

Diagnosis is the second step of the nursing process. It is the phase in which you analyze your assessment data. Using your critical-thinking skills, you identify patterns in the data and draw conclusions about the client's health status, including strengths, problems, and factors contributing to the problems. As in all phases of the nursing process, you should involve the patient and family as much as possible in the diagnostic process.

As you can see in Figure 4-1, diagnosis overlaps with the other nursing process steps. Most nurses actually begin diagnostic reasoning during the assessment phase. For example, you probably formed your initial impressions about Todd while you were still gathering data. On learning the medical diagnosis, chronic renal failure, you would have immediately considered the diagnosis Risk for Imbalanced Fluid Volume, but you would have obtained more data before actually recording that as a nursing diagnosis. So your tentative diagnostic conclusion would actually lead you to collect more data: Is he still producing urine? What is his oral intake? Does he have edema? Do you see how you would move back and forth between assessment and diagnosis? The two stages are not separate at all, but we present them that way to make it easier for you to learn.

Diagnosis is critical because it links the assessment step, which precedes it, to all the steps that follow it (Fig. 4-2). Assessment data must be complete and accurate for you to make an accurate nursing diagnosis. Accuracy is essential because the nursing diagnosis is the basis for planning client-centered goals and interventions.

BOX 4-1 ■ Professional Standards for Diagnosing

American Nurses Association Standards of Nursing Practice[1]

Standard 2. Diagnosis

The registered nurse analyzes the assessment data to determine the diagnoses or issues.

Competencies

The registered nurse:

Derives the diagnoses or issues based on assessment data.

Validates the diagnoses or issues with the patient, family, and other healthcare providers when possible and appropriate.

Documents diagnoses or issues in a manner that facilitates the determination of the expected outcomes and plan.

Identifies actual or potential risks to the patient's health and safety or barriers to health which may include but are not limited to interpersonal, systematic, or environmental circumstances.

Uses standardized classification systems, when available, in naming diagnoses.

Note: There are additional measurement criteria for advanced practice registered nurses.

Source: American Nurses Association (2010, in press). *Nursing: Scope and Standards of Practice* (2nd ed). Public Comment draft, January 2010. (To be published by August 2010.) Silver Spring, MD: Nursebooks.org.
[1]*Caveat:* This material is from the draft for public comment (ANA, 2010, in press); its wording may be changed somewhat in the final published version. For that version of the ANA Standards of Professional Nursing Practice, go to www.nursingworld.org.

Canadian Provincial Standards of Practice (Example)

In Canada, practice standards are set by each province. The following is one example that applies to diagnosis. Note the standards mention interpretation of data but do not specifically use the term *diagnosis*.

Province of Alberta

The registered nurse continually strives to acquire knowledge and skills to provide competent, evidence-based nursing practice. The registered nurse:

Demonstrates critical thinking in collecting and interpreting data, planning, implementing, and evaluating all aspects of nursing care.

Documents timely, accurate reports of data collection, interpretation, planning, implementing, and evaluating care.

Source: College & Association of Registered Nurses of Alberta (2005). *Nursing Practice Standards.* Retrieved from https://www.nurses.ab.ca/Carna-Admin/Uploads/Nursing%20Practice%20Standards.pdf.

Province of New Brunswick

Each nurse:

Indicator 2.4 demonstrates critical thinking in (a) collecting and interpreting data, (b) determining client status and responses to actual or potential health problems.

Source: Nurses Association of New Brunswick. (2005). Standards of practice for registered nurses. Fredericton, Author. http://www.nanb.nb.ca/PDF/practice/StandardsofRegisteredNursesE.pdf

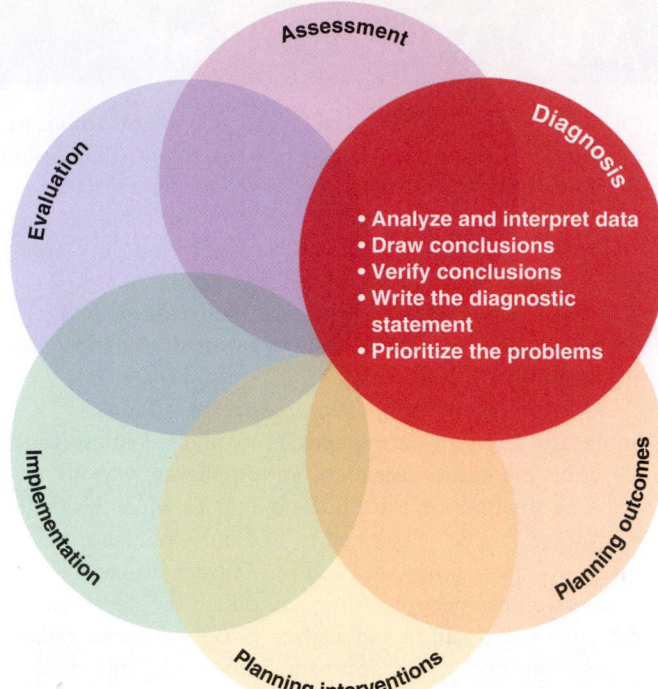

FIGURE 4-1 Nursing diagnosis: Second phase of the nursing process.

You will find the term **diagnosis** used in the nursing literature to refer to:

- The second phase of the nursing process
- The reasoning process used in interpreting assessment data

You will also see the term **nursing diagnosis** used to refer to:

- A formal diagnostic statement of the client's health status, containing both the problem and etiology (factors contributing to the problem)
- The list of standardized terms (labels) used to write diagnostic statements. Those terms are actually problem labels; you must add a second part (etiology) in order to create a complete diagnostic statement.

 VOL 2 Go to Chapter 4, **NANDA-I Taxonomy II: Domains, Classes, and Diagnoses (Labels),** in Volume 2.

Table 4-1 summarizes and provides examples of how nursing diagnosis terminology is used in this text.

What Are the Origins of Nursing Diagnosis?

Before the 1950s, nurses assisted physicians by collecting data to help them diagnose and treat disease. Nursing care was thought of as a set of tasks and organized as a list of "things to do." However, nursing leaders saw the need to describe the knowledge and work that are unique to nursing. The term *nursing diagnosis* was first used in 1953 to differentiate nursing from medicine, when Fry stated that a nursing diagnosis

FIGURE 4-2 Diagnosis links the assessment phase to the rest of the nursing process.

identifies the client's needs for nursing rather than for medical care. During the 1960s, nursing schools began to teach diagnosis as a part of the nursing process but were still careful to explain that nurses were not usurping medical authority by using diagnostic thinking. Until the early 1970s, nursing diagnosis was not widely used in nursing practice, but two major events in 1973 spurred change:

- The First Conference on Nursing Diagnosis was held (Gebbie, 1976). A national task force was formed to begin developing a language to describe the health problems treated by nurses.
- The American Nurses Association (ANA) *Standards of Nursing Practice* included nursing diagnosis as an expectation of professional nurses.

In 1980, the ANA published *Nursing: Social Policy Statement*, which characterized nursing as "the diagnosis and treatment of human response to actual or potential health problems" (ANA, 1980, p. 2). As a result of this definition and the work of the nursing diagnosis task force, most state nurse practice acts began to designate nursing diagnosis as an exclusive

responsibility of registered nurses. Nursing diagnosis (sometimes referred to as *analysis*) is now widely used in nursing education and practice. The formal list of nursing diagnostic labels describes health problems that can be addressed by independent nursing actions and, in that sense, forms the body of knowledge that is unique to nursing.

Since the first conference, the nursing diagnosis group has continued to meet every 2 years. In 1982 it adopted the name North American Nursing Diagnosis Association (NANDA). In 2002 the organization changed its name to NANDA International (NANDA-I), to reflect its large number of members from countries outside the United States and Canada. NANDA-I continues to review and refine the diagnostic labels and to discuss new and revised labels at each biannual conference. The diagnoses on the official list are approved for clinical use and further study; the list is not intended to represent a finished product, because many of the diagnoses are only partially substantiated by research. NANDA-I encourages individual nurses and nursing organizations to submit new and revised diagnoses.

Table 4-1 ➤ Nursing Diagnosis Terminology		
TERM AND EXISTING MEANINGS	**TERMINOLOGY USED IN THIS BOOK**	**EXAMPLE**
Diagnosis		With Todd ("Meet Your Patient"), you used *diagnostic reasoning* to *diagnose* and list his problems. This was the *diagnosis phase* of the nursing process.
1. The second phase of the nursing process	1. Diagnosis	
2. The reasoning process used in identifying patient problems and strengths	2. Diagnostic process, diagnostic reasoning, or diagnosing	
Nursing Diagnosis		For Todd, you might have made a *nursing diagnosis* of Excess Fluid Volume secondary to renal failure. To write that statement, you would have used the *NANDA label* Fluid Excess Volume.
1. The end product of the diagnostic reasoning process: a full diagnostic statement describing client health status. It contains both problem and etiology.	1. Nursing diagnosis, diagnostic statement	
2. A standardized problem label from the NANDA-I taxonomy (e.g., Anxiety)	2. Label, NANDA-I label, problem label, diagnostic label	

KnowledgeCheck 4-1

- Why is the diagnosis step so critical to the other phases of the nursing process?
- Which two nursing organizations have been responsible for making diagnosis a part of the professional nursing role?

 Go to Chapter 4, **Knowledge Check Response Sheet and Answers,** on the Student Resource Disk or DavisPlus at http://davisplus.fadavis.com/Wilkinson2

What Are Health Problems?

A **health problem** is any condition that requires intervention to promote wellness or to prevent or treat disease or illness. After you identify a health problem, you must decide how to treat it: independently or in collaboration with other health professionals. The answer determines whether it is a nursing diagnosis, a medical diagnosis, or a collaborative problem. See Table 4-2 for a comparison of these problem types.

Table 4-2 ▶ Comparison of Nursing Diagnoses, Medical Diagnoses, and Collaborative Problems

	NURSING DIAGNOSIS	MEDICAL DIAGNOSIS	COLLABORATIVE PROBLEM
Definition	A clinical judgment about individual, family, or community responses to a health problem	Disease, illness, injury, or condition validated by signs and symptoms and medical diagnostic studies	Certain potential physiological complications that are always associated with a disease, test, or treatment
Focus	The individual/person	Disease, pathology, and medical treatments/procedures	Pathophysiology (complications caused by the disease process)
Characteristics	Holistic; describes physiological, psychological, social, interpersonal, and spiritual responses	Describes disease or pathology; does not consider the broader range of human responses.	Describes potential physiological complications only; not holistic.
Who Diagnoses?	Professional nurse	Physicians, advanced practice nurses, physician's assistants	Nurses
Who Orders Treatment?	Professional nurse, primarily	Physician, advanced practice nurse, physicians' assistants	Physician prescribes primary interventions; however, the nurse can order some as well.
Problem Status	Can be actual, potential, or possible.	Actual or possible ("rule out")	Always potential; if the problem actually develops, it is then a medical diagnosis.
Purpose of Nursing Interventions	Treat or prevent the problem; relieve the symptoms.	Carry out medical prescriptions for treatment; monitor for improvement or worsening of the condition.	Monitor for development of the complication; institute some, but not all, preventive interventions.
Example of Diagnostic Statement	Ineffective Denial related to difficulty coping with new diagnosis of "heart attack"	Myocardial infarction	Potential Complication of myocardial infarction: congestive heart failure
Example of Data to Support the Diagnosis	Waited more than 6 hours before coming to hospital. Minimizes symptoms, refuses pain medications. States, "I've got to get back to work. I can't stay in the hospital." Laughing, joking, saying, "It's nothing."	Cardiac enzyme levels elevated; has had severe chest pain; elevated white blood cell count; ECG and echocardiogram diagnostic of cardiac muscle ischemia	58-year-old man with diagnosis of myocardial infarction (MI); acknowledges chest pain; ECG and lab work diagnostic of MI

Recognizing Nursing Diagnoses

A **nursing diagnosis** is a statement of client health status that nurses can identify, prevent, or treat independently. It is stated in terms of **human responses** (reactions) to disease, injury, or other stressors, and it can be either a problem or a strength. Human responses can be biological, emotional, interpersonal, social, or spiritual. For example, Todd's medical diagnosis is chronic renal failure. A *physical response* to renal failure might be Excess Fluid Volume. Admission to the ED is also a stressor, to which his *emotional response* might be Anxiety or Fear. What other actual or possible responses were identified for Todd in the situation? Take a moment to write them down.

Recall that Todd has decreased sensation in his lower extremities. This is a stressor, to which he has responded with slight impairment of mobility. Perhaps you identified that because of diminished feeling in his feet, Todd might be at risk for falling (safety), impaired skin or tissue integrity, and ineffective management of his therapy. All of those are responses to disease, illness, or stressors. Also note that besides being a stressor, the decreased sensation in Todd's lower extremities can be considered a physical response to type 2 diabetes mellitus. Was this response on the list you just made?

Critical Thinking 4-1

Imagine you have been in an automobile accident. You have internal injuries and broken bones and will be hospitalized for at least 2 weeks, right before your final exams. What human responses (physical, emotional, interpersonal, social, spiritual) would you have?

In 1990, NANDA-I officially defined *nursing diagnosis* as "a clinical judgment about individual, family, or community responses to actual or potential health problems/life processes. Nursing diagnosis provides the basis for selection of nursing interventions to achieve outcomes for which the nurse is accountable" (NANDA-I, 2007, p. 332). This definition emphasizes the clinical judgment aspect of diagnosing.

Recognizing Medical Diagnoses

A **medical diagnosis** describes a disease, illness, or injury. Its purpose is to identify a pathology so that appropriate treatment can be given. A medical diagnosis is more narrowly focused than a nursing diagnosis. Todd has two medical diagnoses: chronic renal failure and type 2 diabetes mellitus (DM).

Except for advanced practice nurses, nurses cannot legally diagnose or treat medical problems. Your assessment data will help the medical team to identify disease states and evaluate the effects of medical therapies. For example, if your assessment indicates a medication does not adequately relieve a patient's pain, you would inform the primary care provider, who would prescribe a different medication or dosage. You need to know the pathophysiology of the patient's illness to understand and evaluate the effects of medical treatments and to know how to focus your assessments. The following are differences between medical and nursing diagnoses:

You cannot predict a patient's nursing diagnoses just by knowing his medical diagnosis or pathology. Nursing diagnoses are human responses; and human responses are complex and unique to each person. A medical diagnosis, in contrast, remains the same as long as a particular injury or pathology is present. Todd's medical diagnosis of type 2 DM will not change, because the fact that his body cannot use glucose normally will not change. This is not true for his nursing diagnoses. Suppose Todd has a nursing diagnosis of Noncompliance with diabetic diet r/t (related to) lack of knowledge about food groups. If he learned about the foods and began following his diet, he would no longer have this nursing diagnosis. But he would still have the medical diagnosis of type 2 DM.

A medical diagnosis, disease, or pathological condition can have any number of nursing diagnoses associated with it. For example, in response to his type 2 DM, Todd might have nursing diagnoses of Noncompliance and Risk for Impaired Skin Integrity.

Clients with the same medical diagnosis may have different nursing diagnoses. Another client with type 2 DM may not have a diagnosis of Noncompliance, but instead may have a diagnosis of Ineffective Denial because he simply cannot accept that he truly has diabetes. Other patients with type 2 DM might have diagnoses of Anxiety, Deficient Knowledge, Disturbed Body Image, and perhaps others, depending on their unique responses to the stressor, type 2 DM.

Recognizing Collaborative Problems

Collaborative problems are "certain physiologic complications [of diseases, medical treatments, or diagnostic studies] that nurses monitor to detect onset or changes in status" (Carpenito, 2006, p. 19). They have the following characteristics:

All patients who have a certain disease or treatment are at risk for developing the same complications. That is, the collaborative problems (complications) are determined by the medical diagnosis or pathology. Consider these examples:

Todd, because he has type 2 DM, has the collaborative problem Potential Complication of type 2 DM: hyperglycemia and/or hypoglycemia. All other patients with type 2 DM also have those potential complications.

All patients having surgery have the collaborative problem Potential Complication of surgery: infection.

Use your theoretical knowledge of anatomy, physiology, microbiology, pathophysiology, and so on as the basis for identifying the complications associated with a particular disease or treatment.

A collaborative problem is always a potential problem. If it becomes *actual*, then it is no longer a collaborative problem, but a medical diagnosis requiring physician interventions. Consider what would be needed if the preceding potential complications became actual problems:

Actual hyperglycemia (high blood glucose) or actual hypoglycemia (low blood glucose)
Actual infection of a surgical incision

Either condition would require medical intervention to prevent serious harm to the patient.

If you can prevent the complication with independent nursing interventions alone, it is not a collaborative problem. Collaborative problems require both physician-prescribed and independent nursing interventions to prevent them or minimize the complications. The purpose of independent nursing interventions is primarily to monitor for onset of the complication, although nurses can provide some independent preventive measures.

See Figure 4-3 for an algorithm to help you differentiate nursing diagnoses from medical diagnoses and collaborative problems.

KnowledgeCheck 4-2

State whether each of the following represents a nursing diagnosis, medical diagnosis, or collaborative problem:

- After giving birth, all women are at risk for developing postpartum hemorrhage.
- A patient has signs and symptoms of appendicitis, which must be treated with surgery and antibiotics.
- A client is at risk for constipation because he postpones defecation and also does not get enough dietary fiber and fluids. The problem can be prevented by patient teaching, which the nurse is licensed to do.

 Go to Chapter 4, **Knowledge Check Response Sheet and Answers,** on the Student Resource Disk or DavisPlus at http://davisplus.fadavis.com/Wilkinson2

Types of Nursing Diagnoses

You must determine the "status" of each nursing diagnosis—that is, is it an actual, potential, or possible problem; a wellness diagnosis; or a syndrome diagnosis? This is important because each status requires (1) different wording in the diagnostic statement and (2) different nursing interventions (Fig. 4-4).

Actual Nursing Diagnosis: Problem Is Present

An **actual nursing diagnosis** is a problem response that exists at the time of the assessment. You identify it by the signs and symptoms (cues) that are present. Todd ("Meet Your Patient") may have at least one actual nursing diagnosis (Impaired Walking or perhaps Impaired

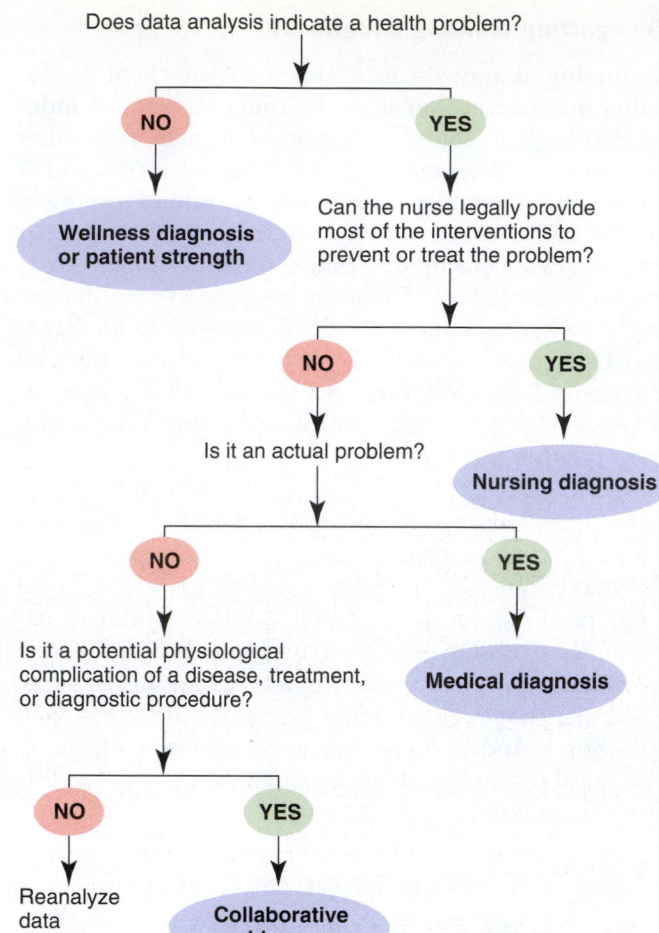

FIGURE 4-3 Algorithm for distinguishing among nursing, medical, and collaborative problems.

Physical Mobility), related to his lack of peripheral sensation; however, no signs and symptoms were given in the scenario to support that diagnosis.

Risk Nursing Diagnosis: Problem May Occur

A **risk nursing diagnosis** describes a problem response that is likely to develop in a vulnerable patient if the nurse and patient do not intervene to prevent it. You will identify a risk diagnosis when the patient does not have signs/symptoms of the problem, but does have risk factors present that increase his vulnerability. For example, Todd's loss of lower limb sensation is a risk factor for a diagnosis of Risk for Falls even though Todd has no symptoms or history of falling.

Use risk nursing diagnoses (also called potential nursing diagnoses) only for patients who have more susceptibility to the problem than others in the same or a comparable setting. For example, all surgical patients have at least some risk for developing infection, so you should not routinely write Risk for Infection on every surgical care plan. You would, instead, write Potential Complication of surgery: infection (incision and systemic). Use the

At the time of assessment, does the patient have enough signs and symptoms (defining characteristics) to identify the specific nursing diagnosis?

YES

Actual nursing diagnosis

Determine etiology

Intervene to treat and/or relieve symptoms

NO

Are there risk factors present that make it likely that a problem will develop if you do not intervene?

YES

Risk (potential) nursing diagnosis

Intervene to remove risk factors

NO

Are there signs and symptoms (defining characteristics) that indicate the possibility of an actual nursing diagnosis, but not enough for you to be certain?

YES

Possible nursing diagnosis

Continue to assess for more defining characteristics

NO

Wellness diagnosis

Institute interventions to promote health

Type of nursing diagnosis
Nursing actions

FIGURE 4-4 Algorithm for determining whether a nursing diagnosis is an actual diagnosis, a risk (potential) diagnosis, a possible diagnosis, or a wellness diagnosis.

nursing diagnosis Risk for Infection for patients who are *unusually* susceptible to infection (e.g., one who is undernourished or one with a compromised immune system).

Possible Nursing Diagnosis: Problem May Be Present

A **possible nursing diagnosis** exists when your intuition and experience direct you to suspect that a diagnosis is present, but you do not have enough data to support the diagnosis. The main reason for including this type of diagnosis on a care plan is to alert other nurses to continue to collect data to confirm or rule out the problem. Todd ("Meet Your Patient") has a symptom of slightly impaired mobility. This could indicate the diagnoses Impaired Physical Mobility, Impaired Walking, or Risk for Falls. You need more data to decide which nursing diagnosis is appropriate, so you might write a nursing diagnosis of Possible Risk for Falls related to decreased sensation in both legs.

Syndrome Nursing Diagnosis: Several Related Problems Are Present

A **syndrome nursing diagnosis** represents a collection of nursing diagnoses that usually occur together. For example, the NANDA label Risk for Disuse Syndrome

is used to represent all the complications that can occur as a result of immobility (e.g., pressure ulcer, constipation, stasis of pulmonary secretions, thrombosis, body image disturbance).

Wellness Nursing Diagnosis: No Problem Is Present

You will use a **wellness diagnosis** when an individual, group, or community is in transition from one level of wellness to a higher level of wellness. A wellness diagnosis describes health status, but it is not a health problem. For you to make a wellness diagnosis, two conditions must be present: (1) The client's present level of wellness is effective and (2) the client wants to move to a higher level of wellness.

KnowledgeCheck 4-3

- What are the five types of nursing diagnoses?
- What kind of nursing diagnosis is each of the following?
  a. Jane Thomas regularly engages in exercise but tells you she would like to increase her endurance.
  b. Mrs. King has several of the signs and symptoms (defining characteristics) of the nursing diagnosis Ineffective Coping.
  c. Alicia Hernandez seems anxious, but you are not sure. You would like to have more data in order to diagnose or rule out a diagnosis of Anxiety.

d. Charles Oberfeldt has no symptoms of constipation. However, he reports that he does not include many fiber-rich foods in his diet and drinks few liquids. In addition, he is now fairly inactive because of a back injury. These are all risk factors for a diagnosis of Constipation.

 Go to Chapter 4, **Knowledge Check Response Sheet and Answers,** on the Student Resource Disk or DavisPlus at http://davisplus.fadavis.com/Wilkinson2

What Is Diagnostic Reasoning?

A comprehensive patient assessment produces a great deal of data. **Diagnostic reasoning** is the thinking process that enables you to make sense of it. This text presents diagnostic reasoning (also referred to as **analysis**) in separate steps so that it is easier to learn, but that is not the way it really occurs (Fig. 4-5). When you first begin to use diagnostic reasoning, use the steps "in order" so that you will not miss anything. But just as you move back and forth between assessing and diagnosing, you will soon find yourself moving back and forth among the steps of diagnostic reasoning, skipping steps, returning to previous steps, and doing some steps simultaneously.

In diagnostic reasoning, you will use your critical thinking to analyze and interpret data, draw conclusions about the patient's health status, verify problems with the patient, prioritize the problems, and record the diagnostic statements.

Analyze and Interpret Data

As you analyze and interpret the data, you will gradually narrow the quantity of data you must deal with. But even as you narrow the field of data to the significant

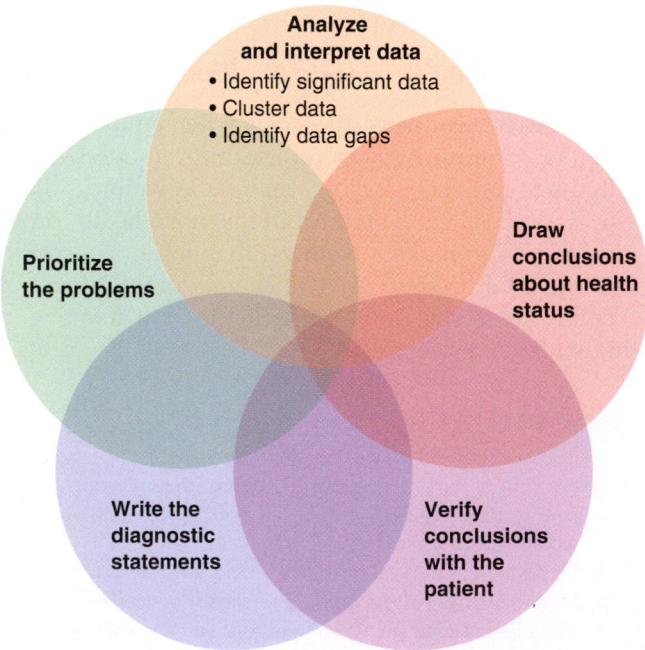

FIGURE 4-5 The diagnostic reasoning process.

points and patterns, you will note the need for new information and further assessments. To analyze and interpret data, follow three steps: (1) identify significant data, (2) cluster cues, and (3) identify data gaps and inconsistencies.

1. Identify Significant Data

Significant data (also called **cues**) are data that influence your conclusions about the client's health status. A cue should alert you to look for other cues that might be related to it (form a pattern). You may be thinking, "How will I recognize a cue?"

A cue is usually an unhealthy response. One way to recognize cues is to draw on your theoretical knowledge (e.g., of anatomy, physiology, psychology, and so on) and compare each piece of data to standards and norms. For example, suppose you have noted that a woman's pulse rate is 110 beats/min (bpm). Is this an unhealthy response—a cue? You would of course use as one standard the average rate (80 beats/min) and normal range (60–100 beats/min) for an adult pulse. But this woman is a long-time cigarette smoker who also drinks coffee and colas containing caffeine. These habits increase pulse rate, so 110 beats/min may be a normal finding for this client. See Box 4-2 for other indications of cues.

KnowledgeCheck 4-4
- What is a cue?
- What are five ways you can recognize a cue?

 Go to Chapter 4, **Knowledge Check Response Sheet and Answers,** on the Student Resource Disk or DavisPlus at http://davisplus.fadavis.com/Wilkinson2

2. Cluster Cues

A **cluster** is a group of cues that are related to each other in some way. The cluster may suggest a health problem. To help ensure accuracy, you should always derive a nursing diagnosis from data clusters rather than from a single cue.

Consider this example. Alma was transferred to the hospital from a long-term care facility. Because of a CVA (cerebrovascular accident, or stroke), Alma can make sounds but cannot speak; and because of joint contractures, she cannot use her hands and arms. Alma is frequently incontinent of urine, so the nurses have diagnosed Overflow Urinary Incontinence and are resigned to the idea that Alma will not be able to control her urine. Because Alma makes loud vocal noises, they have placed her in a room near the nurses' station. When a nursing student is assigned to the care for Alma, the student looks for cues in addition to urinary incontinence. The student assigned to Alma's care notices that urinary incontinence often occurs after Alma's loud vocalizing. She sees a pattern in these cues: urinary incontinence, cannot use hands and arms, and cannot communicate verbally. The

BOX 4-2 ■ Recognizing Cues

The following may indicate cues.

A deviation from population norms
Example: For a well-conditioned athlete who is not a smoker, a heart rate of 120 beats per minute would probably be an unhealthy response (cue). But remember that in addition, you must always consider whether the response is normal for the patient or the situation.

Changes in usual health patterns are not explained by developmental or situational changes
Example: What change has Todd ("Meet Your Patient") experienced in the 3 days before admission to the ED? Is there any developmental or situational explanation for his decreased sensation and mobility? No. It is an unhealthy response: a cue.

Indications of delayed growth and development
Example: A 17-year-old girl has not yet experienced menses, her breasts are just barely developed, and she has very scant pubic and underarm hair.

Changes in usual behaviors in roles or relationships
Example: During her first year at college, a previously successful student begins to skip classes. She stays up late partying and sleeps most of the day. She no longer keeps in contact with her friends, and despite a previous close relationship with her parents, she barely talks to them when they telephone.

Nonproductive or dysfunctional behavior
This may or may not be a change in behavior. It could be a long-standing dysfunctional behavior. *Example:* A man has been abusing alcohol for many years, even though it is causing many problems with his family and job and has begun to damage his liver.

Source: Adapted from Gordon, M. (1994). *Nursing diagnosis: Process and application* (3rd ed.). St. Louis, MO: C.V. Mosby.

student changes the nursing diagnosis to Self-Care Deficit: Toileting related to immobility and inability to communicate the need to void. After the student provides a call device that fits under Alma's arm, Alma is able to press the device and call the nurse when she needs to void. She is no longer incontinent of urine.

Critical Thinking 4-2

For each of the following cue clusters, decide whether the cues represent a pattern; that is, are all the cues related in some way? If so, explain how they are related. If not, state which cue does not fit. If you do not have enough theoretical knowledge to know for sure, draw on your past experiences and discuss the clusters with other students.

a. Dry skin, abnormal return of skin turgor (more than 4 seconds), thirst, and scanty, dark yellow urine
b. Pain and limited range of motion in knees, uses walker, medical diagnosis of osteoarthritis
c. Has hard, painful bowel movement about every 3 days; does not exercise regularly; eats very little dietary fiber; skin is dry.

Clustering data forces you to think about the relationships between the cues. For item (c) in the preceding example, you would think, "What might cause hard, painful bowel movements? I know that dietary fiber promotes peristalsis, so lack of fiber might contribute to constipation. And I remember that lack of exercise is associated with constipation. I don't see how dry skin would be related to constipation."

3. Identify Data Gaps and Inconsistencies

As you cluster and think about relationships among the cues, you will identify the need for data that was not apparent before. In the preceding constipation example (c), you have enough data to support a diagnosis of Constipation. However, you still need to identify factors contributing to the problem. You have two: lack of dietary fiber and lack of exercise. But you should also ask about other causes of Constipation. Does the patient postpone defecation? Does he have a history of relying on laxatives? How much fluid does the client drink? (For example, Todd's skin is dry. Could that be because he is fluid deficient)?

As another example, look again at Todd's data ("Meet Your Patient"). Except for medical diagnoses, there are very few data. The following data gaps exist:

- His admitting diagnosis, chronic renal failure, suggests the possibility of fluid imbalance; however, there are no other data to support that. What is his intake? His output? His skin turgor? The appearance of his urine? Does he have edema? Does he complain of thirst? What are his hemoglobin and hematocrit levels?
- Admission to the ED could cause Anxiety. If you wish to pursue that line of thinking, you will need to observe for physical and verbal symptoms of Anxiety.
- Decreased sensation in his lower extremities might create mobility or safety problems. You would need to know the degree of sensation loss and the exact meaning of "slight loss of mobility" to determine whether to focus on the mobility or the safety issue.
- The effect of diabetes on circulation and skin certainly places Todd at risk for skin problems. However, you need more data to determine whether he has any actual skin problems (e.g., presence or history of sores on his feet).

In addition to missing data, look for inconsistencies in the data. Suppose a client tells you, "I really don't eat much. Three meals a day, and I don't snack between meals." However, she is 5 ft tall and weighs 190 lb. This seems inconsistent because your theoretical knowledge tells you that obesity is usually caused by excessive intake of calories. Even though there are many causes for overweight, you wonder if someone could be so much overweight without "eating much." In this case, you would need more specific data about what the client actually eats; consider having her keep a food diary of everything she eats for a week or two. What else would you want to know? For example, does she have any medical problems that might cause obesity (e.g., hypothyroidism)? Is there any reason she might not want to tell you the truth about her eating pattern? Does she know the number of calories in various foods? Or perhaps, she isn't aware of how much she is eating. More data will help answer your questions.

Draw Conclusions About Health Status

After clustering cues and collecting any missing data, the next step is to begin drawing conclusions about the patient's health status—strengths as well as problems. Decide which one of the following the cluster represents:

- *A patient strength.* If data seem to meet standards and norms, you can conclude the patient has a strength in that area. Using Todd as an example, his strengths might be his marital status, family involvement, and employment status.
- *No problem or a wellness diagnosis.* If data seem to meet standards for normal and no nursing interventions are needed, you can conclude no problem exists in that area. If, in addition, the patient expresses the wish to achieve a higher level of wellness, you would make a wellness diagnosis.
- *A possible problem.* This means there are cues that suggest a problem, but ongoing monitoring will be needed to confirm or rule out the problem.
- *An actual nursing diagnosis.* You will reach this conclusion when a cue cluster contains the signs and symptoms (defining characteristics) of a problem you can treat independently as a nurse.
- *A risk (potential) nursing diagnosis.* You will reach this conclusion when a cue cluster contains risk factors that make nursing interventions necessary to prevent a problem from developing.
- *A collaborative problem.* The client's medical diagnosis or treatment indicates the need to monitor for development of complications and to take some measures to prevent the complication, but you cannot prevent or treat the problem independently.
- *A medical diagnosis.* Nurses are not licensed to make medical diagnoses. If you recognize signs and symptoms suggestive of a medical diagnosis, refer them to a physician for diagnosis and treatment.

1. Make Inferences

Making inferences is a critical thinking skill. Recall that cues are facts (or data), whereas inferences are conclusions (judgments, interpretations) that are based on the data. An inference is not a fact, because you cannot directly check its truth or accuracy. For example:

Fact:	Patient is crying. (You can observe that directly.)
	Patient is trembling. (You can observe that directly.)
Inference:	Patient is anxious. (You cannot observe anxiety, but you know that crying and trembling may be signs of anxiety.)

Even though you cannot ever be completely sure that an inference is accurate, clearly some inferences are supported by more complete and reliable data than others. In the preceding example, suppose you said to the patient, "You seem upset. Can you tell me what's going on?" And the patient replied, "I've never been in the hospital before, and so much has been happening, I guess I'm just anxious about everything." Now you have enough data to support your inference, and you can be reasonably sure that it is accurate (valid). But remember, you can't be absolutely certain. For example, although it is unlikely, the patient might not be telling you the truth. Perhaps she is crying because her husband said cruel things to her, and she is too embarrassed to share that with you. Or perhaps she is a spy and is trying to divert your attention while an accomplice finds the hospital's hidden secrets. Yes, that is far-fetched; but this exaggerated example should convince you that an inference—even one that appears to be more valid than this one—is not a *fact*.

This is an important point in diagnosing. Nursing diagnoses, because they are inferences, are only your reasoned judgment about a patient's health status. So try not to think of a diagnosis as right or wrong, but instead as more accurate or less accurate. Realize that you can never construct a "perfect" diagnosis, but strive to make your diagnostic statements as accurate as possible. Incorrect diagnoses result in ineffective care.

KnowledgeCheck 4-5

- What are the possible conclusions you can draw about a client's health status (e.g., that no problem exists)?
- What is the difference between a cue and an inference?
- How can you be satisfied that you have made a valid inference?

 Go to Chapter 4, **Knowledge Check Response Sheet and Answers,** on the Student Resource Disk or DavisPlus at http://davisplus.fadavis.com/Wilkinson2

2. Identify Problem Etiologies

An **etiology** consists of the factors that are causing or contributing to the problem. Etiologies may be pathophysiological, treatment related, situational, social, spiritual, maturational, or environmental. It is important to correctly identify the etiology because it directs the nursing interventions. Consider this nursing diagnosis:

Constipation related to inadequate intake of dietary fiber

The etiology suggests that you encourage the client to eat more high-fiber foods. You might also teach the client about foods that are high in fiber. But what if that etiology is incomplete? What if you overlooked the fact that the client does not drink enough fluids? Or that he gets very little exercise? And what if you didn't realize that he often postpones defecation when he feels the urge because he is a kindergarten teacher in a crowded, bustling classroom, and he simply cannot leave the children unattended except at scheduled times. In that case, your efforts to increase intake of high-fiber foods would probably not help relieve the person's constipation.

To identify the etiology of a health problem, use your theoretical knowledge (e.g., of psychology, physiology, disease processes) and the patient data to answer questions such as the following:

- What factors are known to cause this problem?
- What patient cues are present that may be contributing to this problem?
- How likely is it that these factors are contributing to the problem?
- What past experiences do I have that support my judgment that these factors are linked to the problem?
- Are these cues *causing* the problem, or are they merely *symptoms* of the problem?

An etiology is always an inference because you can never actually observe the "link" between etiology and problem. You can often be certain that the etiological factors are present. For example, in the preceding Constipation diagnosis, you could measure (observe) the person's fiber intake. You could also observe infrequent, hard stools (Constipation). But you cannot observe that the lack of fiber is the cause of the Constipation. You have to infer that link based on your knowledge of normal elimination and your experiences with other patients.

Critical Thinking 4-3

- How would your nursing interventions be different for the following diagnoses?
  - a. Constipation related to lack of knowledge about laxative use
  - b. Constipation related to weakened abdominal muscles secondary to long-term immobility
- How would your nursing interventions be different for the following diagnoses?
  - a. Ineffective Breastfeeding related to lack of knowledge about breastfeeding techniques
  - b. Ineffective Breastfeeding related to inability of infant to latch on to the breast and to coordinate sucking and swallowing, secondary to prematurity

Verify Problems with the Patient

After identifying problems and etiologies, verify them with the patient. A diagnostic statement is an interpretation of the data, and the patient's interpretations may differ from yours. For example, if you have diagnosed Ineffective Breastfeeding related to lack of knowledge about breastfeeding techniques, you might verify it by saying, "It seems to me you are having difficulty breastfeeding the baby because you are not sure how to position him and get him to latch on to your breast. Does this seem accurate to you?" The woman might confirm your diagnosis, or she might say, "No. I *do* know how to do it; I am just tired and a little nervous with you watching me." Think of nursing diagnoses as tentative, and remain open to changing them based on new data or insights from the patient.

Prioritize Problems

Up to this point, the diagnostic process has focused on identifying and validating health problems. However, clients often have more than one problem, so you must use nursing judgment to decide which ones to address first and which can wait until later. This is **prioritizing.** Prioritizing places the problems in order of importance, but it does not mean you must resolve one problem before attending to another. Problem priority is largely determined by the theoretical framework you use—for example, whether your criteria are human needs, problem urgency, future consequences, or patient preference.

Maslow's Hierarchy of Human Needs

Even though it is not a nursing framework, many nurses use Maslow's hierarchy to prioritize nursing diagnoses (Fig. 4-6). In Maslow's model, basic needs must

Transcendence
of self; helping others self-actualize

Self actualization
Personal growth, reaching potential

Aesthetic
Symmetry, order, beauty

Cognitive
Knowledge, understanding, exploration

Self-esteem
Pride, sense of accomplishment, recognition by others

Love and belonging
Giving and receiving affection, meaningful relationships, belonging to group(s)

Safety and security
Protection, emotional and physical safety and security, order, law, stability, shelter

Physiological
Food, air, water, temperature regulation, elimination, rest, sex, and physical activity

FIGURE 4-6. Maslow's Hierarchy of Human Needs can be used for prioritizing problems. Most nursing diagnoses fall at the cognitive and lower levels. (*Source:* Adapted from Maslow, A. (1971). *The farther reaches of human nature.* New York: The Viking Press; and Maslow, A., & Lowery, R. (Eds.). (1998). *Toward a psychology of being* (3rd ed.). New York: John Wiley & Sons.)

be met before a person can focus on higher needs. Maslow (1970) ranks human needs on eight levels, beginning with the most basic needs. Table 4-3 shows examples of nursing diagnoses at various levels of Maslow's hierarchy. For further information on the Maslow theory, see Chapter 8.

Critical Thinking 4-4

Prioritize the following nursing diagnosis labels (problems) based on the Maslow framework. (1) First assign each diagnosis a high, medium, or low priority. Some may have the same priority. (2) Next rank them in order of importance, with 1 being most important and 5 being least important; use each number only once.

_____ Ineffective Airway Clearance
_____ Ineffective Breathing Pattern
_____ Diarrhea
_____ Risk for Falls
_____ Impaired Memory

Problem Urgency

If you use problem urgency as your ranking criteria, you would rank the problems according to the degree of threat they pose to the patient's life or to the immediacy with which treatment is needed. Assign:

High priority to problems that are life-threatening (e.g., Ineffective Airway Clearance) or that could have a destructive effect on the client (e.g., substance abuse)

Medium priority to problems that do not pose a direct threat to life, but that may cause destructive physical or emotional changes (e.g., Ineffective Denial, Unilateral Neglect)

Low priority to problems that require minimal supportive nursing intervention (e.g., Risk for Delayed Development, Interrupted Breastfeeding, mild Anxiety)

Future Consequences

When assigning priorities, also consider the possible future effects of a problem. Even if a problem is not life-threatening, and even if the patient does not see the problem as a priority, it may result in harmful future consequences for the patient. For example, suppose that Todd ("Meet Your Patient") is hospitalized for 5 days and undergoes inpatient dialysis. His physician prescribes a renal diet and insulin (instead of his previous oral medications) to treat the diabetes mellitus (DM). Todd announces that he would like to go home as soon as possible. "I need to get back to my job and my family," he tells you. He resists learning about his medicines and how to administer his insulin. "Just give me a list of

---

Table 4-3 ➤ Using Maslow's Hierarchy to Prioritize Diagnoses

BASIC NEEDS (MOST BASIC TO HIGHEST LEVEL)	EXAMPLES OF HUMAN NEEDS	EXAMPLES OF NURSING DIAGNOSES
Physiological	Food, air, water, shelter, sleep and rest, elimination, activity, temperature regulation	Imbalanced Nutrition: Less Than Body Requirements Impaired Gas Exchange
Safety and Security	(Includes both physical and psychological safety); law, order, shelter, stability	Risk for Falls Fear Risk for Self-Directed Violence
Love and Belonging	Roles, relationships, the need to give and receive affection, the feeling of belonging	Impaired Social Interaction Ineffective Sexuality Pattern Impaired Parent/Infant/Child Attachment
Self-Esteem	Feelings of confidence, capability, and independence; respect, recognition, and appreciation from others.	Chronic Low Self-Esteem Social Isolation
Cognitive	Knowledge, understanding, exploration	Acute Confusion Impaired Memory Delayed Growth and Development
Aesthetic	Symmetry, order, beauty	It is unusual for nursing diagnoses to fall into this, or the two higher, categories.
Self-Actualization	Personal growth, reaching one's highest potential	
Transcendence	Connecting to something beyond self, helping others reach their potential	Readiness for Enhanced Spirituality Spiritual Distress

Sources: Adapted from Maslow, A. (1971). *The farther reaches of human nature.* New York: The Viking Press; and Maslow, A., & Lowery, R. (Eds.). (1998). *Toward a psychology of being* (3rd ed.). New York: John Wiley & Sons.

my medicines, and I'll take them when I get home," he says. You are aware that his renal failure is secondary to uncontrolled DM and that he was erratic about taking his medication in the past. You suspect that he has not been taking his medicines because he is in denial about his health problems. Clearly his Ineffective Denial may lead to further problems with his treatment plan. You would assign high priority to this problem and address it before attempting to provide teaching for his nursing diagnosis of Deficient Knowledge (insulin).

Patient Preference

Give high priority to problems the patient thinks are most important, provided that this does not conflict with basic/ survival needs or medical treatments. Patients cooperate more fully with interventions they consider important. In addition, they may be more motivated to work on other problems after their own priorities are addressed.

Consider this example. Mr. Amani has had a major surgery within the past 24 hours. His main concern is to obtain pain relief. He refuses to turn, deep-breathe, and cough (TDBC) because it causes pain. However, as his nurse, you realize that these activities are essential for preventing Ineffective Airway Clearance, so you cannot safely support Mr. Amani's priorities. You should of course provide pain medication before helping him TDBC, but it may be impossible for him to be entirely pain-free during these activities. You would explain your actions and continue to emphasize the importance of TDBC. Often when you explain the importance of your priorities, patients come to agree with them.

Documenting Priorities

You will usually prioritize problems as you are recording them. You can indicate the priority by designating each problem as high, medium, or low priority or by ranking all the problems in order from highest to lowest (i.e., 1, 2, 3, and so on). For example:

Labeling Each Problem	Ranking the Problems
Pain (high)	1—Risk for Falls
Risk for Falls (high)	2—Pain
Chronic Low Self-Esteem (low)	3—Imbalanced Nutrition
Imbalanced Nutrition (medium)	4—Chronic Low Self-Esteem

Notice that risk problems can have a higher priority than actual problems. In this example, it is more urgent to prevent falls than to treat low self-esteem.

CriticalThinking 4-5

Suppose that on his transfer from the emergency department, you made the following nursing diagnoses for Todd ("Meet Your Patient"):

- Risk for Imbalanced Fluid Volume secondary to renal failure
- Risk for Falls related to decreased sensation and mobility in legs
- Anxiety r/t unknown prognosis of renal failure and ED environment

- Deficient Knowledge (renal disease process) r/t new diagnosis of renal involvement secondary to type 2 DM
- Using problem urgency as your criterion, assign each of these diagnoses a low, medium, or high priority. You may not have much theoretical knowledge about type 2 DM and chronic renal disease, but use the information provided in the scenario and in the etiologies to prioritize as well as you can. Discuss the case with your classmates and your instructor.

Computer-Assisted Diagnosing

Many institutions use computers for planning and documenting patient care. Some expert (knowledge-based) systems allow you to enter assessment data, and the computer program will generate a list of possible problems. After you choose a problem label, the computer will provide a screen with the definition and defining characteristics of the problem so you can compare them to the actual patient data. After you "accept" the diagnostic label, you complete the problem statement by choosing etiologies from the next computer screen. To see examples of such computer screens,

 Go to Chapter 4, **Tables, Boxes, Figures: ESG Figures 4-1 and 4-2,** on the Student Resource Disk or DavisPlus at http://davisplus.fadavis.com/Wilkinson2

KnowledgeCheck 4-6

List the steps in the diagnostic process.

 Go to Chapter 4, **Knowledge Check Response Sheet and Answers,** on the Student Resource Disk or DavisPlus at http://davisplus.fadavis.com/Wilkinson2

Reflecting Critically on Your Diagnostic Reasoning

An inaccurate diagnosis is useless and can even be harmful. Diagnostic reasoning is complex and vulnerable to error. Yet with the implementation of electronic health records, there is an even greater need for accuracy of nursing diagnoses (Lunney, 2008). Therefore, after you have your prioritized list of problems, you need to evaluate the list for accuracy. When diagnosing, you apply critical thinking to your theoretical and self-knowledge and to the patient data and situation (recall the full-spectrum nursing model in Chapter 2).

Critical thinking + Knowledge + Data = Statement of health status

Think About Your Theoretical Knowledge

The better your knowledge base is, the better is your diagnostic reasoning. Ask yourself the following questions:

- Is my diagnosis based on sound knowledge (e.g., of pathophysiology, psychology, nutrition, and other related disciplines)?

- Do I have sound knowledge about the defining characteristics associated with various nursing diagnoses?
- Do I feel reasonably sure I have interpreted the data correctly?
- Have I identified the problem type correctly—that is, can this problem be treated primarily by nursing interventions?
- Am I qualified to make this diagnosis, or should I ask for consultation (e.g., from a more experienced nurse or other member of the collaborative healthcare team)?

To avoid diagnostic error, build a good knowledge base and learn from your clinical experiences. If you lack knowledge in an area, review the literature. A solid knowledge base will help you (1) to recognize cues and patterns, (2) to associate patterns with the correct problem, (3) give you confidence in your ability to reason, and (4) keep you from relying too much on authority figures (Wilkinson, 2007).

Think About Your Self-Knowledge

Realize that your beliefs, values, and experiences affect your thinking and can be misleading. For example, imagine that a nurse in a labor and delivery unit believes it is important to be strong and uncomplaining, even when experiencing severe pain. When this nurse cares for a woman in early labor who cries out and complains of pain, the nurse sees it as a problem of either Anxiety or Ineffective Coping, not as a problem of Pain. Can you see how that changes the focus of the nurse's care? Ask yourself the following questions (Wilkinson, 2007).

What biases and stereotypes may have influenced my interpretation of the data?   A **bias** is the tendency to slant your judgment based on personal opinion or unfounded beliefs, as the nurse did in the preceding example. **Stereotypes** are judgments and expectations about an individual based on the personal beliefs you have about this group (e.g., men are unemotional; Asians are intelligent; teenagers are irresponsible). Referring to patients by their diagnosis or developmental group is a form of stereotyping (e.g., "the elderly man in room 110"; "the broken hip in 288"). You form stereotypes by making flawed assumptions when you have little or no actual experience with a person or group.

Did I rely too much on past experiences?   This is like stereotyping in that you draw conclusions about an individual based on what you know about people in similar situations. Consider, for example, a nurse who has cared for many first-time mothers (primiparas) during labor. Most of these women experienced moderate anxiety even during early labor. Now each time the nurse cares for a primipara, she expects to see anxiety, and she tends to identify cue clusters as Anxiety, failing to check for other explanations such as Pain or Deficient Knowledge.

Did I rely too much on the client's medical diagnosis, the setting, or what others say about the client (e.g., "He's angry and uncooperative") instead of on the data?   Medical diagnoses and statements from others can help you to think

of possible explanations for your data, but they can also bias your thinking and prevent you from gathering your own data. For example, Ms. Grayson has cancer. She returned to the unit last evening after undergoing a total colectomy and colostomy (removal of the colon and creation of an artificial opening for removal of stool). She had expected to have only an exploratory laparotomy surgery to evaluate abdominal symptoms. This morning in report, the night shift nurse stated, "Ms. Grayson is aware of her cancer and is coping well." While bathing Ms. Grayson, you begin to tell her about her colostomy. She seems shocked. "I didn't know they did that! What's wrong with me?" As you answer her questions, you realize that she has been very groggy from the anesthesia and pain medication and does not recall being told about her surgery and cancer.

Think About Your Analysis and Conclusions

After reflecting on your knowledge, think about how you used the diagnostic process. Be sure your analysis of the data was thorough, that you have accurately identified the patient's problems, and that they are logically linked to the etiologies. Review your interactions with the patient: Do the diagnostic statements reflect his perceptions and priorities, or did he just give you the answers he thought you wanted? Use the questions in Box 4-3 to critique your diagnostic process.

KnowledgeCheck 4-7

To help you fix them in your mind, list at least 10 questions to ask yourself when evaluating your diagnostic reasoning. Refer to Box 4-3 if you need help preparing this list.

 Go to Chapter 4, **Knowledge Check Response Sheet and Answers,** on the Student Resource Disk or DavisPlus at http://davisplus.fadavis.com/Wilkinson2

Practical Knowledge
knowing how

After you have completed the diagnostic reasoning process, the final activity in the diagnosis step is to record the strengths and problem statements. Practical knowledge regarding nursing diagnosis involves selecting the correct standardized problem labels and writing the diagnostic statements.

How Are Diagnostic Statements Written?

This section explains the need for standardized languages, describes the NANDA-I standardized terminology for nursing diagnoses, explains how to choose the correct label, and describes formats for nursing diagnosis and collaborative problem statements.

BOX 4-3 ■ Critiquing Your Diagnostic Reasoning Process

Data Analysis

Did you:

- Identify all the significant data (cues)?
- Omit any important cues from the cluster?
- Include unnecessary cues that may have confused your interpretation?
- Try more than one way of grouping the cues?
- Consider the patient's social, cultural, and spiritual beliefs and needs?
- Identify all the data gaps and inconsistencies?

Drawing Inferences and Interpretations of the Data

- Did you consider all the possible explanations for the cue cluster?
- Is this the best explanation for the cue cluster? Remember that a variety of explanations may be possible.
- Did you have enough data to make that inference? If not, suspend judgment until you gather more data.
- Did you look at patterns, not single cues?
- Did you look at behavior over time, not just isolated incidents?
- Did you jump to conclusions? Or did you take the time to carefully analyze and synthesize the data?

Critiquing the Diagnostic Statement (Problem + Etiology)

- Is the diagnosis relevant, and does it reflect the data?
- Does the diagnostic statement give a clear and accurate picture of the patient's problem or strength?

- When identifying the problem and etiology, did you look beyond medical diagnoses and consider human responses?
- Did you consider strengths and wellness diagnoses?
- Can you explain how the etiology relates to the problem—that is, how it would produce the problem response?
- Does the complete list of problems fully describe the patient's overall health status?

Verifying the Diagnosis

- Did the patient verify this diagnosis?
- When you verified the diagnosis are you certain the patient understood your description of his health status?
- Did you obtain feedback from the patient, or did you just assume that the patient agreed?
- Did you keep an open mind, realizing all diagnoses are tentative and subject to change as you acquire more data?

Prioritizing

- Considering the whole situation, what are the most important problems?
- What aspects of the situation require immediate attention?
- Did you consider patient preferences when setting priorities? If not, was there a good reason?

Standardized Nursing Languages

In order to communicate, people need a shared language. A **standardized language** is one in which the terms are carefully defined and mean the same thing to all who use them. One example is the periodic table for chemical elements. When a chemist in the United States writes Fe or Zn, all other chemists in the world know that she means iron or zinc. Moreover, they know exactly what is meant by iron and zinc, because each is defined by its own atomic number, atomic mass, number of protons, number of neutrons, and so on. There is no confusion. **Standardized nursing languages** are a comparatively recent attempt to bring such clarity to communication about nursing knowledge and nursing thinking.

Nurses need clear, precise, consistent terminology when referring to the same clinical problems and treatments. A uniform language can do the following:

- Support electronic health records
- Define, communicate, and expand nursing knowledge
- Increase visibility of nursing interventions
- Facilitate research to demonstrate the contribution of nurses to healthcare and influence health policy decisions

- Improve patient care by providing better communication among nurses and other healthcare providers and facilitating the testing of nursing interventions

For a full discussion of the benefits of a uniform nursing language

 Go to Chapter 4, **Supplemental Materials: Why Do We Need a Standardized Nursing Language?** on the Student Resource Disk or DavisPlus at http://davisplus.fadavis.com/Wilkinson2

What Is a Taxonomy?

A **taxonomy** is a system for classifying ideas or objects based on characteristics they have in common. Classifications are created and used for various reasons. As mentioned earlier, the periodic table classifies elements according to their atomic mass, number of protons, and so on. Medications are classified in various ways; one way is to classify them according to their use (e.g., analgesics, antibiotics). The following classification systems are widely used in healthcare:

- The American Psychiatric Association (APA) *Diagnostic and Statistical Manual (DSM-IV)* describes mental disorders (e.g., bipolar disorder, schizoaffective disorder; APA, 2000).

- The *International Classification of Disease (ICD-10)* names and classifies medical conditions (World Health Organization [WHO], 1992)
- The *Current Procedural Terminology (CPT)*, used for reimbursement of physician services, names and defines medical services and procedures (American Medical Association [AMA], 2010).

The following are classification systems that the American Nurses Association (ANA) has recognized for describing nursing diagnoses (some describe outcomes and interventions as well):

- *NANDA International.* The first use of standardized nursing language began in the 1970s, with the NANDA classification of nursing diagnoses. This taxonomy includes approximately 200 diagnostic labels with etiologies, risk factors, and defining characteristics. Most chapters of this textbook use NANDA-I terminology.
- *Clinical Care Classification (CCC).* Similar to the NANDA-I system; includes nearly 200 labels. Contains interventions as well as nursing diagnoses. The CCC was developed for home health use, but can be used in any setting.
- *Omaha System.* Contains 42 nursing diagnosis "concepts" (also interventions and outcomes). The Omaha system is primarily for community health use, but can be used in other settings.
- *Perioperative Nursing Data Set (PNDS).* For use in perioperative nursing only. Consists of 64 nursing diagnoses (also includes nursing interventions and patient outcomes). This was the first nursing language developed by a nursing specialty.
- *International Classification for Nursing Practice (ICNP).* Includes diagnoses, outcomes, and nursing actions. The ICNP intends to provide a common language for nurses in various clinical settings worldwide (International Council of Nurses, 2005).

NANDA-I Taxonomy of Diagnostic Terminology

Which of the following could you group together? In what ways are the grouped objects similar?

a five-dollar bill	a penny
weeds (still growing)	new grass
an iron skillet	a needle

You could make these groupings:

- A $5 bill and a penny (because they are both money).
  - A penny, an iron skillet, and a needle (because they are all metal).
    - A $5 bill, grass, and weeds (because they are all green).

Maybe you thought of even other groupings. Any number of principles can be used to classify things and to organize a taxonomy.

The first NANDA taxonomy was simply an alphabetical list. To see that taxonomy,

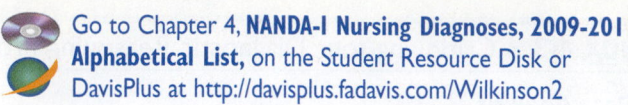
Go to Chapter 4, **NANDA-I Nursing Diagnoses, 2009-2011 Alphabetical List,** on the Student Resource Disk or DavisPlus at http://davisplus.fadavis.com/Wilkinson2

NANDA's *Taxonomy II* (NANDA International, 2007) categorizes nursing diagnoses into 13 domains and 47 classes. A **domain** is an area of activity, study, or interest (e.g., health promotion, nutrition). A **class** is a subdivision of a domain (e.g., health awareness is a class under health promotion; digestion is a class under nutrition).

VOL 2 Go to Chapter 4, **NANDA-I Taxonomy II: Domains, Classes, and Diagnoses (Labels),** in Volume 2.

One strength of the NANDA taxonomy is that it has been developed by nurses from administration, education, practice, and research, and from all specialty areas (e.g., maternity, mental health, medical-surgical, community). Because they represent the thinking of a broad spectrum of nurses, the diagnostic labels can be used in any setting or specialty.

What Are the Components of a NANDA-I Nursing Diagnosis?

Each nursing diagnosis in the NANDA-I taxonomy has four parts: label, definition, defining characteristics, and related or risk factors. You must consider all four parts when formulating a nursing diagnosis.

- The **diagnostic label** (**title** or **name**) is a word or phrase that represents a pattern of related cues and describes a problem or wellness response, such as Disturbed Body Image or Readiness for Enhanced Nutrition. Some labels include descriptors for time, age, and other factors (e.g., acute, deficient, delayed). For the complete list of "Descriptors for NANDA Nursing Diagnoses,"

VOL 2 Go to Chapter 4, **Descriptors for NANDA Nursing Diagnoses,** in Volume 2.

- The **definition** explains the meaning of the label and distinguishes it from similar nursing diagnoses. For example, for a patient with a sleep problem, would you label the problem Sleep Deprivation or Disturbed Sleep Pattern? The following definitions can help you to decide:
Sleep Deprivation: Prolonged periods of time without sleep
Disturbed Sleep Pattern: Time limited disruption of sleep amount and quality
- **Defining characteristics** are the cues (signs and symptoms) that allow you to identify a problem or wellness diagnosis. To use a problem label appropriately, a cluster of defining characteristics must be present in the patient data. For example, you cannot decide to use the label Sleep Deprivation merely by reading the definition. You must be sure the patient actually has some of the defining characteristics for Sleep Deprivation.

- **Related factors** are the cues, conditions, or circumstances that cause, precede, influence, contribute to, or are in some way associated with the problem (label). They can be pathophysiological, psychological, social, treatment-related, situational, maturational, and so on. NANDA-I lists the related factors that are most often associated with each problem label, but keep in mind:

1. *The list is not exhaustive.* Factors other than those listed by NANDA-I could also be associated with the problem. For example, imagine the vast number of factors that might cause someone to have Chronic Low Self-Esteem.
2. *The problem may have more than one related factor.* Human beings are complex, and their problems rarely have one single cause. Nursing diagnoses may have multiple factors as their etiology.
3. *An individual patient will not have all the factors on the list* in the NANDA-I Related Factors for his problem etiology.

- **Risk factors** are events, circumstances, or conditions that increase the vulnerability of a person or group to a health problem. They can be environmental, physiological, psychological, genetic, or chemical. For example, ignoring the urge to defecate and being pregnant increase the risk a person will become constipated. The diagnostic statement would be: Risk for Constipation r/t pregnancy and habitually ignoring the urge to defecate.

For potential (risk) nursing diagnoses, risk factors function as the defining characteristics. They must be present to make the diagnosis, and they almost always form at least a part of the etiology of the diagnostic statement. If **related factors** are present, an actual, rather than potential, problem exists. To help you remember, as a rule:

Related factors are similar to signs and symptoms (of actual problems)
Risk factors are similar to etiologies (of potential problems)

KnowledgeCheck 4-8

- What are the four parts of a NANDA nursing diagnosis?
- What purpose does each part of the nursing diagnosis serve for directing the care of the client?

 Go to Chapter 4, **Knowledge Check Response Sheet and Answers,** on the Student Resource Disk or DavisPlus at http://davisplus.fadavis.com/Wilkinson2

How Do I Know Which Label to Use?

During the diagnostic process, you will already have determined the general topic of the problem and perhaps even have some tentative problem labels in mind.

1. *First, identify the broad topic (or domain) that seems to fit the cue cluster.* You can look at the NANDA-I taxonomy to see which domain the problem seems to fit. For example, suppose that after further assessment, you find that Todd ("Meet Your Patient") has the following defining characteristics:

Intake exceeds output.
Oliguria (low volume of urine)
Generalized edema
Recent rapid weight gain

Which of the following NANDA domains are suggested by those cues?

Health Promotion	Role Relationships
Nutrition	Self–Perception
Elimination	Activity/Rest

The most logical guesses would be Nutrition and Elimination. However, you would need to read the domain definitions in the NANDA-I list (in Volume 2) and look at the classes to be sure.

2. *Narrow your search (to the class or most likely labels).* In the NANDA-I list, read the definitions for the Nutrition and Elimination domains. Then look at the classes in each. Under Elimination, you will find that Class 1 is Urinary Function. Because Todd has renal failure, you may think that his nursing diagnosis will be found in this class. However, remember that renal failure is a pathology or pathological condition; you are looking for Todd's *responses* to renal failure. On examining the diagnosis labels in the Urinary Function class, you will see none of those really represents Todd's defining characteristics.

Now look at the Nutrition domain. You will see the classes Ingestion, Digestion, Absorption, Metabolism, and Hydration. Look at the diagnostic labels listed for the class Hydration. All five of those labels describe fluid balance. You can easily eliminate both "risk" labels because Todd has an actual problem (he has symptoms). You can eliminate Readiness for Enhanced Fluid Balance because it is a wellness diagnosis. So, you must choose between Deficient Fluid Volume and Excess Fluid Volume. From this point, you simply compare Todd's cue cluster to the defining characteristics and definitions of those two labels and choose the best match.

3. *Using a nursing diagnosis handbook, compare definitions and defining characteristics of the diagnostic labels to your cue cluster.* A brief look at the NANDA list should convince you that you cannot know exactly what a diagnostic label means from the label name alone. For example, suppose you have a patient who is not sleeping well at night. As a result, she is too tired to concentrate during the day. Which label would you use to describe this problem: Activity Intolerance, Fatigue, Acute Confusion, or Impaired Thought Processes? You can answer that question only if you know the definition and defining characteristics of those nursing diagnosis labels.

Not all of the defining characteristics need to be present, but recall that the more data you have when you make an inference, the more certain you can be that your inference is correct.

Examples: NANDA-I lists 14 defining characteristics for Ineffective Thermoregulation, including the following:

- Fluctuations in body temperature above and below normal range
- Cyanotic nail beds
- Pallor
- Slow capillary refill
- Tachycardia

You could diagnose Ineffective Thermoregulation on the basis of the first defining characteristic alone, but you might be more certain of your diagnosis if the other cues were also present.

 Critical**Thinking** 4-6

- In the preceding example, what if the first defining characteristic (temperature fluctuations) were not present and you had only 2, 3, and 4 as cues? Could you conclude that Ineffective Thermoregulation is causing those signs? What other explanations might there be for cyanotic nail beds, pallor, and slow capillary refill?
- What if the last defining characteristic were present without the first one? What could cause tachycardia? Do you see the importance of using clusters rather than individual cues?

Formats for Diagnostic Statements

A diagnostic statement consists of a problem and an etiology linked by a connecting phrase.

Problem

The problem describes the client's health status (or a human response to a health problem) and identifies a response that needs to be changed. Use a NANDA-I label when possible. As noted earlier, many NANDA-I labels include a descriptor such as *acute, impaired,* or *deficient*. You will see them arranged in alphabetical lists with the descriptor after the main word (e.g., Physical Mobility, Impaired). However, you should record them as you would say them; for example:

Incorrect: Physical Mobility, Impaired r/t pain in left knee

Correct: Impaired Physical Mobility r/t pain in left knee

Etiology

As discussed earlier, the etiology contains the factors that cause, contribute to, or create a risk for the problem. The etiology may include a NANDA-I label, defining characteristics, related factors, risk factors, or other factors. Remember that an etiology may consist of several factors. The etiology will help you to individualize nursing care because etiologies are unique to the individual. For example, suppose two patients have the following nursing diagnoses:

John: Anxiety r/t lack of knowledge of the treatment procedure

Janet: Anxiety r/t prior negative experiences and lack of trust in health professionals

The problem, Anxiety, is defined the same for both patients. They probably share some of the same defining characteristics, and you would use some of the same interventions for both John and Janet. For example, for all anxious patients, regardless of etiology, a calm, reassuring approach is important. However, to prevent the anxiety from recurring, you would need to treat its cause. To relieve John's anxiety, you would teach him what to expect from the impending procedure. But teaching would do nothing to relieve Janet's anxiety. For her, you would need to spend time building a relationship that demonstrates you can be trusted. You would also encourage her to talk about her fears and feelings.

Because the etiology directs the nursing interventions, include only factors that are influenced by nursing interventions. For example, do not use a medical diagnosis or treatment as an etiology, because you cannot write nursing orders to change it. As another example, there are no independent nursing actions that would change the etiologies in the following diagnosis: Deficient Fluid Volume related to medical order of NPO (nothing by mouth).

Most NANDA-I-related factors are listed in nonspecific terms, so you will usually need to individualize them to reflect each person's unique problem etiology. For example, one of the related factors for Impaired Skin Integrity is "extremes in age." To plan care, you need to know whether this means very old or very young; even better, you should specify the exact age. You would write the diagnostic statement as Impaired Skin Integrity r/t very young age (2 days).

Connecting Phrase (related to)

Most nurses use *related to (r/t)* to connect the problem and etiology, believing that the phrase *due to* implies a direct causal relationship. Because humans are complex, there are usually many factors that combine to "cause" a problem, so it is nearly impossible to prove an exact cause. In fact, even if you eliminate the etiological factors, the problem might remain. For example, even if Janet begins to trust health professionals, she may become anxious for another reason.

A diagnostic statement should describe the client's health status as specifically as possible. The format will vary depending on the type of problem you are describing (Table 4-4).

Table 4-4 ➤ Examples of Diagnostic Statements

FORMAT	PROBLEM TYPE	PROBLEM (CLIENT RESPONSE; NANDA LABEL)	ETIOLOGY (RELATED OR RISK FACTORS)	DEFINING CHARACTERISTICS OR "SECONDARY"
Basic One-Part	Wellness diagnosis	Health-Seeking Behaviors (salt-restricted diet)	None	
	Syndrome diagnosis		None	
	Very specific label	Disuse Syndrome	None	
		Death Anxiety	None	
Basic Two-Part	Actual problem	Impaired Social Interaction	r/t self-consciousness following amputation of bilateral lower extremities	
	Potential problem	Risk for Impaired Parent/Infant/Child Attachment	r/t separation from infant at birth because of mother's illness	
	Possible problem	Possible Impaired Parent/Infant/Child Attachment	r/t separation from infant at birth because of mother's illness	
Basic Three-Part	Actual Problem	Impaired Social Interaction	r/t self-consciousness following amputation of bilateral lower extremities	AEB avoidance of others, social isolation, blaming others for current condition
	Possible Problem	Impaired Social Interaction	r/t self-consciousness following amputation of bilateral lower extremities	AEB blaming others for current condition
Variations	(Specify)	Decisional Conflict (whether to accept chemotherapy)	r/t desire to protect family from financial hardship of a lingering illness	
	Secondary to	Decisional Conflict (whether to accept chemotherapy)	r/t desire to protect family from financial hardship of a lingering illness	Secondary to diagnosis of terminal cancer
	Two-part NANDA-I label	Imbalanced Nutrition: Less Than Body Requirements	r/t loss of appetite from nausea	Secondary to side effects of chemotherapy
	Adding words to the label	Impaired Physical Mobility: Inability to turn self in bed	r/t generalized weakness	Secondary to residual effects of stroke
	Unknown etiology	Parental Role Conflict	r/t unknown etiology or possibly r/t recent divorce	
	Complex etiology	Chronic Low Self-Esteem	r/t complex etiology	
Collaborative Problems	Potential complications of disease, test, or treatment	Potential Complication of preeclampsia: renal failure	None	

AEB = as evidenced by.

Basic Two-Part Statement

The two-part statement is used for actual, risk, and possible diagnoses. The format is:

Problem	r/t	Etiology
Or		
NANDA-I label	r/t	related factors

For actual diagnoses, the etiology consists of related factors; for risk diagnoses, it consists of risk factors. For example, for a client with excessive vomiting you might write Risk for Deficient Fluid Volume r/t excessive losses through vomiting.

Basic Three-Part Statement

The three-part statement is also called the **PES format** (problem, etiology, and symptom). Some nurses use *AEB (as evidenced by)* whereas others use *AMB (as manifested by)*. The format is:

Problem r/t etiology as manifested by (AMB) signs or symptoms

This format adds the patient signs or symptoms that led you to make the diagnosis. For example: Constipation r/t inadequate intake of fluids and fiber-rich foods. AMB painful, hard stool and bowel movement every 3 or 4 days.

This is a good method for students because it helps to ensure that you have enough data to support the problem you have identified.

Although ideally the problem and etiology should thoroughly describe the patient's health status, you can sometimes make the description more clear and useful by including the cues in the statement. However, this method can create a long, unwieldy statement. For example:

Decisional Conflict (whether to accept chemotherapy) r/t desire to protect family from financial hardship of a lingering illness AMB verbalizing uncertainty about what to do and feelings of distress; indecision about having and not having chemotherapy; exhibiting physical signs of anxiety (increased heart rate, restlessness); questioning personal values and beliefs ("I'm not sure what to do. I hate to leave them any sooner than I have to, but I don't want to ruin them financially, either").

For such situations, you can record the cues in the nurses' notes. Another alternative is to list the signs and symptoms below the nursing diagnosis on the care plan instead of including it as part of the statement. For example:

Decisional Conflict (whether to accept chemotherapy) r/t desire to protect family from financial hardship of a lingering illness

Subjective cues: Verbalizes uncertainty about what to do and feelings of distress; vacillates between having and not having chemo; questions personal values and beliefs ("I'm not sure what to do. I hate

to leave them any sooner than I have to, but I don't want to ruin them financially, either").

Objective cues: Exhibits physical signs of anxiety (increased heart rate, restlessness)

Obviously you cannot use the PES format for risk nursing diagnoses, because symptoms are not present with risk diagnoses.

One-Part Statement

You can omit the etiology from certain kinds of diagnostic statements:

Syndrome Diagnoses. Recall that a syndrome diagnosis is a label that represents a collection of several nursing diagnoses. A syndrome diagnosis usually does not need an etiology.

Wellness Diagnoses. As a rule, NANDA-I wellness diagnoses are one-part statements beginning with the phrase Readiness for Enhanced (e.g., Readiness for Enhanced Parenting). However, some of the older labels are stated differently (e.g., Effective Breastfeeding, Health-Seeking Behaviors). Because the wellness label does not represent a problem, no etiology ("cause") is needed.

Very Specific Labels. A few NANDA-I labels are so specific that they imply the etiology, or the only possible etiology is a medical diagnosis (e.g., Death Anxiety, Latex Allergy Response). For Latex Allergy Response, it would be redundant to write Latex Allergy Response r/t sensitivity to latex. The etiology adds nothing to your understanding of the problem, nor does it suggest interventions different from those suggested by the problem label. The same is true for Death Anxiety.

Format Variations

The following are some variations of the basic two- and three-part formats.

"Specify"

You will see the word *specify* in some NANDA labels, for example, Decisional Conflict (specify). This means that the label is useful only if you describe the problem more specifically; for example, Decisional Conflict (whether to accept chemotherapy) r/t desire to protect family from financial hardship of a lingering illness.

"Secondary to"

When the defining characteristics are vague (e.g., Chronic Pain r/t chronic physical disability) you may need to add a second part to the etiology following the words *secondary to* ($2°$). This second part is usually a pathophysiology or disease process (e.g., Chronic Pain r/t chronic physical disability secondary to rheumatoid arthritis). As a rule, you should avoid using pathophysiology or medical diagnoses in the etiology because they cannot be addressed by independent nursing interventions. The words *secondary to* make it clear the nurse is not ultimately responsible for that part of the etiology. Do not use this phrase routinely. Use it only if it adds to the understanding of your diagnostic statement.

Two-Part NANDA-I Label Some NANDA-I labels have two parts. The first part describes a general response; the second part, following a colon, makes it more specific, for example, Imbalanced Nutrition: Less Than Body Requirements.

Adding Words to the NANDA-I Label—The problem phrase must describe the client's health status precisely because general categories are not useful for planning nursing care. For example, what do you think a problem label of Impaired Physical Mobility means? Does it mean that the patient cannot grasp objects with her hands, or that she cannot walk, or that she cannot move at all? For such labels, you will need to add your own words to the label to make it more descriptive, for example, Impaired Physical mobility: inability to turn self in bed r/t generalized weakness secondary to residual effects of stroke.

Other labels that often need to be clarified include: Acute Pain, Chronic Pain, Risk for Infection, and Risk for Injury. Think carefully about whether the clarifying words belong in the problem or the etiology. For example, you may see a pain diagnosis written as: Acute Pain r/t surgical incision. However, surgical incision is a medical treatment and should not be used as the etiology. It would be better to write: Acute Pain (abdominal incision) r/t turning and moving secondary to abdominal surgery. The "rule" for adding words is to first try to make the statement specific or descriptive by writing a good etiology, using the PES format, or adding *secondary to*. If that does not fully describe the health status, add descriptive words to the problem label.

Unknown Etiology Sometimes you will be able to identify the patient's problem but not know the etiology. For example, your patient might have defining characteristics for Parental Role Conflict, but you may need more information to determine the cause. Perhaps there is an impending divorce; perhaps she has just had to take on the care of an elderly parent, and so on. In this case, you could write Parental Role Conflict r/t unknown etiology. Later, when you obtain more data, you will be able to complete the etiology. A similar situation exists when you have some, but not enough, information about the etiology. In this case you would write Parental Role Conflict possibly r/t recent divorce.

Complex Etiology Some problems have too many etiological factors to list, or the etiology is too complex to explain in a brief diagnostic statement. For example, imagine the number of factors that might contribute to problems such as Chronic Low Self-Esteem, Disabled Family Coping, and Adult Failure to Thrive. For such problems you can replace the etiology with the phrase "complex factors" (e.g., Disabled Family Coping r/t complex factors).

Collaborative Problems

A collaborative problem is always a potential problem— a complication of a disease, test, or medical treatment. The disease, test, or treatment is actually the etiology of the problem. Because you cannot treat the etiology with independent nursing interventions, you should not use the "problem + etiology" format. The focus of your interventions is monitoring for and preventing the complication. The format is:

Potential Complication of thrombophlebitis: Pulmonary embolism

As you can see, the word(s) following the colon represent the problem you are monitoring and trying to prevent.

In actual practice, you would not write an etiology for a collaborative problem. However, as a student, you may wish to do so when it clarifies your diagnostic statement or when it helps to suggest nursing interventions (Wilkinson, 2007). For example, a student statement might be:

Potential Complication of magnesium sulfate therapy: Respiratory depression r/t increased blood levels of magnesium because of decreased kidney function secondary to preeclampsia (a pregnancy-related disorder with hypertension as a major pathology).

In addition to alerting you to monitor for respiratory depression, this statement might help remind you to monitor the serum magnesium level, assess for other data related to kidney function, and monitor blood pressure. Again, as a professional nurse, you would *not* write an etiology.

KnowledgeCheck 4-9

Write an example of each of the following diagnostic statement formats, using the listed components—mix and match:
Problem labels: Anxiety, Pain (lower back)
Etiologies: Unknown outcome of surgery; muscle strain and tissue inflammation
Cues: Exhibits physical manifestations of anxiety (e.g., hands shaking); states pain is 9 on a scale of 1 to 10.

- Basic two-part statement
- Basic three-part statement
- Basic two-part statement, using "secondary to" (create your own disease/pathology)
- Statement with unknown etiology
- Possible nursing diagnosis
- Risk nursing diagnosis

 Go to Chapter 4, **Knowledge Check Response Sheet and Answers,** on the Student Resource Disk or DavisPlus at http://davisplus.fadavis.com/Wilkinson2

How Does the Nursing Diagnosis Relate to Outcomes and Interventions?

Keeping in mind there are exceptions, as a general rule: The problem suggests goals, and the etiology suggests interventions.

The Problem Suggests Goals

The problem describes a health status that needs to be changed. From the problem, you can determine the patient outcomes for measuring this change. Consider the following diagnostic statement: Risk for Impaired Skin Integrity r/t complete immobility 2° spinal cord injury. The goal, or outcome, is the opposite of the unhealthy response: Skin will remain intact and healthy.

The goals then suggest assessments, which are actually a type of nursing intervention. The diagnosis Risk for Impaired Skin Integrity tells you to monitor the patient's skin condition. If the problem is not an accurate statement of health status, then your goals and resulting assessments will be wrong. If you incorrectly identified the previous problem as Impaired Physical Mobility 2° spinal cord injury, then the goal would suggest that you monitor the patient's mobility—which would not improve—and you might miss a developing skin problem.

The Etiology Suggests Interventions

The aim of the nursing interventions is to alter the factors contributing to the problem. In the preceding mobility example, you could not cure the spinal cord injury or restore the patient's ability to move about. However, you could provide some mobility by turning and repositioning the patient frequently. This would help prevent Impaired Skin Integrity.

If the etiology is incorrect or incomplete, you might omit important nursing interventions. Suppose there are missing etiological factors in the preceding skin diagnosis and that it should have read: Risk for Impaired Skin Integrity r/t poor nutritional status and complete immobility 2° spinal cord injury. You can see that interventions to support mobility would not be adequate to prevent Impaired Skin Integrity.

Reflecting Critically About Diagnostic Statements

Just as you critiqued your diagnostic reasoning process, you must reflect on the content, format, and meaning of your diagnostic statements.

Guidelines for Judging the Quality of Diagnostic Statements

After you have written your diagnostic statements, use the following criteria to judge their quality (Wilkinson, 2007).

1. *In choosing a NANDA-I label, do not rely on the label definition alone.* Always compare patient data to the defining characteristics of the label as well as to the definition.

   Example: The definition for Parental Role Conflict is "parent experience of role confusion and conflict in response to crisis." You cannot actually observe role confusion and conflict in a patient; however, the defining characteristics for this label include more specific cues, such as "Reluctant to participate in usual caretaking activities."

2. *Include both problem and etiology, with "cause and effect" stated correctly.* A quick check of this is to read your statement backwards: "Etiology causes problem," and see if it makes sense.

   Correct example:
   Diagnostic statement: Ineffective Breastfeeding r/t Deficient Knowledge (positioning infant at breast)
   Read backwards: This statement says deficient knowledge about positioning the infant at breast "causes" Ineffective Breastfeeding. This makes sense.

   Incorrect example:
   Diagnostic statement: Deficient Knowledge r/t Ineffective Breastfeeding (incorrect positioning infant at breast)
   Read backwards: This statement says Ineffective Breastfeeding causes deficient knowledge. This does not make sense.

3. *Be sure that the etiology does not merely restate the problem.*

   Incorrect example: Impaired Physical Mobility r/t inability to walk

   Correct example: Impaired Physical Mobility: Inability to walk r/t weakness and pain in legs

   In the incorrect example, inability to walk is the specific impaired physical mobility. The etiology should state the factors that are causing the inability to walk.

4. *Avoid using medical diagnoses and treatments as etiological factors.* Recall nursing interventions are directed at changing or removing the etiological factors. What could the nurse do to change the following etiology?

   Incorrect example: Risk for Impaired Skin Integrity (ulcers, infection) r/t diabetes mellitus

   The answer, of course, is that the nurse can do nothing to change or get rid of the DM. Try to reword the etiology in terms of something the nurse can change, as follows:

   Correct example: Risk for Impaired Skin Integrity (ulcers, infection) r/t lack of knowledge of self-care measures for inspecting feet and trimming toenails

   If you cannot reword the etiology in terms of something the nurse can change, you may have identified the problem incorrectly; perhaps it is merely the stimulus for another patient problem that you can address independently. In the following example, Risk for Impaired Skin Integrity is one possible "response" to the stimulus, Impaired Physical Mobility.

Incorrect example: Impaired Physical Mobility (total) r/t paralysis secondary to high spinal injury

Correct example: Risk for Impaired Skin Integrity (pressure ulcers) r/t Impaired Physical Mobility (total) secondary to high spinal injury

If none of these seem to work, you can resort to using "secondary to" instead of "related to," as in the following example: Risk for Deficient Fluid Volume secondary to prescribed NPO.

5. **Write the statement clearly.** The statement should give a clear picture of the client's health status, and other health professionals should be able to understand it readily. Avoid abbreviations and jargon as much as possible. For example, do you know what the first statement below means?

Incorrect example: Imp. Phys. Mobility (inability to get OOB w/o assist.) r/t muscle weakness and pain in LL

Correct example: Impaired Physical Mobility (inability to get out of bed without assistance) r/t muscle weakness and pain in left leg

6. **Write the statement concisely.** A wordy statement is likely to be unclear. The following will help limit statement length:
   a. Use "complex etiology" instead of listing numerous etiological factors.
   b. If there are numerous signs and symptoms, either do not use PES format, or describe the signs and symptoms in the nurses' notes.

Incorrect example: Constipation r/t habitually ignoring the urge to defecate, insufficient exercise, weak abdominal muscles, side effects of iron medications, insufficient intake of fluids and fibers, and long-standing reliance on laxatives

Correct example: Constipation r/t complex factors (see nurses' notes)

7. **Be sure the statement is descriptive and specific.** A vaguely stated problem and/or etiology cannot provide guidance for formulating goals and nursing interventions. Follow this guideline even if it means the statement is not as concise as you'd like. You can make the NANDA labels more specific by:
   a. Being sure to include all appropriate etiological factors
   b. Reviewing the label definition. (Do not write the definition, but when you know the meaning of the label, you may find that it is descriptive enough.)
   c. Using PES format to add the patient's signs and symptoms
   d. Adding qualifying words (e.g., "mild," "severe," "occasional," or "constant") to the label

   Example: Severe Neck Pain r/t muscle spasms 2° herniated intervertebral disc

   e. Adding "secondary to" to the etiology.

   Example: Severe Neck Pain r/t muscle spasms 2° herniated intervertebral disc

   f. Adding a colon and descriptors to the label.

   Example: Impaired Physical Mobility: Inability to walk r/t weakness and pain in legs

8. **State the problem as a patient response.**
   a. A problem is not a patient need. As a rule, avoid using the word "need" in a problem statement. A need may cause a problem, but it is not a human response.

   Incorrect example: Needs increased fluids related to . . .

   Correct example: Risk for Deficient Fluid Volume, or Deficient Fluid Volume related to. . .

   b. A problem is not a medical test, treatment, diagnosis, or equipment.

Incorrect examples	Correct examples
Starting on diabetic diet	Deficient Knowledge, Ineffective Denial
Foley catheter in place	Risk for Infection, Urinary Retention
Risk for pneumonia	Risk for Ineffective Airway Clearance
Traction to left leg	Impaired Physical Mobility

   c. A problem is not a nursing goal, a nursing problem, or a nursing action.

Incorrect examples	Correct examples
Prevent urinary tract infection (nursing goal)	Risk for Urinary Tract Infection
Combative, hits caregivers (nursing problem)	Risk for Other-Directed Violence, Ineffective Coping, Confusion
Provide emotional support (nursing action)	Anxiety, Decisional Conflict, Conflict, Anticipatory Grieving

9. **Use nonjudgmental language.** If you examined your biases during the diagnostic process, your statements will probably be neutral. Look for phrases that may imply criticism of a patient, for example:

Incorrect: Risk for Infection r/t poor hygiene and housekeeping

Better: Risk for Infection r/t lack of information about sanitation and hand washing

10. **Avoid legally questionable language.** Be alert for legal implications. Look for phrases that seem to blame caregivers or patients or that refer negatively to patient care. For example, do not write:

Impaired Skin Integrity (excoriated perineum) r/t need for more frequent changes of clothing and linen after incontinence

Risk for Falls r/t lack of staff to adequately supervise ambulation

CriticalThinking 4-7

Rewrite the two preceding diagnostic statements so they contain no legally questionable language. Use imaginary etiological factors if you need to.

Critiquing the NANDA-I System

Despite their potential benefits, critics have pointed out that some NANDA-I labels are too abstract to be useful (e.g., Impaired Adjustment), other labels are merely reworded medical diagnoses (e.g., Decreased Cardiac Output), and few outside nursing knows what the labels mean (e.g., "Why not just say 'tooth decay' or 'missing teeth' instead of 'Impaired Dentition'?") These are legitimate concerns, but as you have learned, when you know the label definition, the term is more meaningful. Also, you can make the labels more specific and useful by adding descriptors, etiological factors, and defining characteristics to the diagnostic statement.

Another criticism is that the NANDA-I diagnoses have not been researched. Historically, this has been true. However, an elected diagnostic review committee evaluates each submitted diagnosis to determine if it complies with the criteria for inclusion in the taxonomy. Moreover, research on the labels has been conducted and is continuing. In 1994, a research team at the University of Iowa (the Nursing Diagnosis Extension Classification [NDEC]) began collaborating with NANDA to extend and refine the NANDA work. They intend to address some of the difficulties with the labels, such as specificity, clinical usefulness, and clinical testing. Also, NANDA-I has formed a research committee. To see that Web site,

 Go to http://www.nanda.org/html/research_committee.html

Compared to the terminology for describing medical diagnoses, the NANDA-I system is relatively new (recall that it was begun just over 30 years ago). Consider that only a little more than 30 years ago AIDS was not a medical diagnosis. All classification systems evolve and change, so many of the difficulties with individual labels will be corrected as the terminology is refined. Meanwhile, try not to reject the idea of standardized language just because of a few problematic labels. You do not need to use the official NANDA-I labels exclusively. If you are uncomfortable with a label, change the wording to make it more useful, or write a completely new label. Remember the point of a standardized language is to more clearly communicate the nature of the patient problem in nursing terms.

The most serious criticisms are leveled by those who say that nurses should not use *any* standardized languages to describe nursing knowledge and nursing work. They contend that using a NANDA-I label to describe health status is "labeling"—that it dehumanizes and stereotypes the person. If this is true, then medical diagnoses would meet the same objection. This objection ignores the fact that we must name objects and ideas in order to communicate them to other people.

Many of the criticisms arise out of disillusionment. It may be that nurses expect too much from nursing diagnosis. Although it is important, it is, after all, merely a process for identifying, naming, and communicating patient health status. We should not expect it to be the "magic bullet" that single-handedly cures all problems of the nursing profession and the patients. For a more comprehensive critique of standardized nursing language, and the NANDA-I system in particular,

 Go to Chapter 4, **Supplemental Materials: Critique of Standardized Nursing Language,** on the Student Resource Disk or DavisPlus at http://davisplus.fadavis.com/Wilkinson2

Toward Evidence-Based Practice

Read about the following study, and then answer the questions at the end of the box.

Müller-Stauber, M., Lavin, M. A., Ian, N., et al. (2006). Nursing diagnoses, interventions and outcomes – application and impact on nursing practice: Systematic review. *Journal of Advanced Nursing, 56(5), 514–531.*

Researchers analyzed the content of 36 published studies to examine the outcomes of using nursing diagnosis. Specifically, they looked at effects on quality of patient assessments, accuracy, and completeness of nursing diagnoses, and on coherence among nursing diagnoses, interventions, and outcomes documented. They found the following:

1. Nursing diagnosis use improved the quality of documented patient assessments.
2. The completeness of nursing diagnoses in practice is problematic; signs and symptoms or etiology were often lacking or incompletely described.
3. There was some evidence for coherent use of documented nursing diagnoses, interventions, and outcomes.
4. There was some evidence that nursing diagnosis improved the quality of interventions documented.
5. There was no evidence that use of nursing diagnosis improved outcomes in patients.

1. What do you think "coherence between nursing diagnoses, interventions, and outcomes" means?

2. From this study, could you reasonably infer that using nursing diagnosis would improve the quality of your nursing assessments? Why or why not?

3. From this study, could you reasonably infer that using nursing diagnosis led to nurses' documenting their interventions better? Why or why not?

 Go to Chapter 4, **Toward Evidence-Based Practice Suggested Responses,** on the Student Resource Disk or DavisPlus at http://davisplus.fadavis.com/Wilkinson2

 Go to Chapter 4, **Resources for Caregivers and Health Professionals,** on the Student Resource Disk or DavisPlus at http://davisplus.fadavis.com/Wilkinson2

 Suggested Readings: Go to Chapter 4, **Reading More About Diagnosis,** on the Student Resource Disk or DavisPlus at http://davisplus.fadavis.com/Wilkinson2

 Bibliography: Go to Volume 2, Bibliography.

CHAPTER 5

Nursing Process: Planning Outcomes

Learning Outcomes

After completing this chapter, you should be able to:

➤ Describe formal, informal, initial, ongoing, and discharge planning.

➤ Identify patients who need a comprehensive, formal discharge plan.

➤ Explain the importance of a written plan of care.

➤ Describe the information contained in a comprehensive nursing care plan.

➤ Compare critical pathways to integrated plans of care (IPOCs) and other standardized care-planning documents.

➤ Discuss the advantages and disadvantages of computerized care planning.

➤ Describe a process for writing an individualized care plan, making use of available standardized care-planning documents.

➤ Define the following terms: goal, outcome, expected outcome, nursing-sensitive outcome.

➤ Differentiate between short-term and long-term goals.

➤ Explain how a goal is derived from a nursing diagnosis.

➤ Differentiate between essential and nonessential goals.

➤ Write appropriate goals for actual, risk, and possible nursing diagnoses.

➤ Use standardized terminology to state patient goals.

➤ Write realistic specific, concrete, and observable goals that do not conflict with the medical plan of care and are stated in terms of patient responses/behaviors.

Meet Your Patient

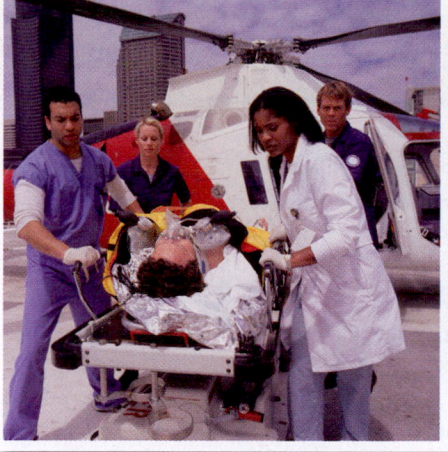

Ben Ivanos has just been admitted to an orthopedic unit after a motorcycle accident. Mr. Ivanos is 24 years old, normally healthy, and taking no medications. He has casts and traction on both legs and a cast on one arm. He is receiving morphine sulfate intravenously via a patient-controlled analgesia (PCA) pump. Imagine that you are an orthopedic nurse and must plan care for Mr. Ivanos. You rank the following nursing diagnoses as highest priority:

1. Acute Pain secondary to musculoskeletal trauma (arms, legs, body) and muscle spasms
2. Risk for Peripheral Neurovascular Dysfunction secondary to casts/traction

You write the following desired outcomes (goals) on the care plan:

Goals for diagnosis 1
Demonstrates correct use of PCA pump.
Rates pain not higher than 4 on a scale of 1 to 10 at all times.
Goals for diagnosis 2
Peripheral pulses palpable

Fingers and toes warm
Fingers and toes without pallor or cyanosis
No edema of fingers and toes
Capillary refill less than 3 seconds

These goals will guide you in choosing nursing interventions for relieving Mr. Ivanos's pain and preventing peripheral neurovascular dysfunction. When the nursing shift changes, the written care plan provides directions for the new caregivers so that they will continue to focus on Mr. Ivanos's most important needs.

Theoretical **Knowledge**
knowing why

What Is Planning?

The professional nurse is responsible for care planning, and cannot delegate it. However, you should be aware that some healthcare facilities list care planning in their job description for licensed practical or vocational nurses. Certainly LPNs can provide valuable input for RNs who are planning the care. Box 5-1 lists American Nurses Association (ANA) and Canadian Nurses Association (CNA) standards that specifically identify planning as the role of the registered nurse.

Planning can be formal or informal. **Formal planning** "is a conscious, deliberate activity involving decision making, critical thinking, and creativity" (Wilkinson, 2007, p. 262). During the planning phases of the nursing process, you will work with the patient and family to derive desired outcomes from identified patient problems (e.g., nursing diagnoses) and then to identify nursing interventions to help achieve those outcomes. The end product of formal planning is a holistic plan of care that addresses the patient's unique problems and strengths.

Not all plans are written. Nurses do **informal planning** while performing other nursing process steps. For example, while performing neurovascular checks for

Ben Ivanos, you might discover that he is not obtaining adequate pain relief. Reflect on this situation. What would you do?

Any response in that scenario would require some mental planning. For example, you might make a mental note (plan) to notify the physician and obtain a prescription for an increase in the analgesic dose.

This text separates the process of planning outcomes from the process of planning interventions because, although related, they are distinctly different activities. This chapter (1) describes planning as a general process, (2) explains how to create a nursing care plan, and (3) discusses how to write patient goals/expected outcomes. Chapter 6 explains how to plan nursing interventions and write nursing orders.

How Is Planning Related to Other Steps of the Nursing Process?

Nursing process steps are overlapping and interdependent. To develop a plan of care with realistic goals and effective nursing orders, you must have accurate, complete *assessment* data and correctly identified and prioritized *nursing diagnoses*. The *goals/desired outcomes* flow logically from the nursing diagnoses. By stating what is to be achieved, the goals then suggest nursing interventions (which are written as nursing orders in the *planning interventions* phase). The plan of care is carried out in the *implementation* phase. In the *evaluation*

BOX 5-1 ■ Professional Standards for Planning Outcomes

American Nurses Association Standards of Nursing Practice[1]

Standard 3. Outcomes Identification

The registered nurse identifies expected outcomes for a plan individualized to the patient or the situation.

Competencies

The registered nurse:

Involves the patient, family, and other healthcare providers in formulating expected outcomes when possible and appropriate.

Derives culturally appropriate expected outcomes from the diagnoses.

Considers associated risks, benefits, costs, current scientific evidence, expected trajectory of the condition, and clinical expertise when formulating expected outcomes.

Defines expected outcomes in terms of the patient, patient values, ethical considerations, environment, or situation with such considerations as associated risks, benefits and costs, and current scientific evidence.

Includes a time estimate for attainment of expected outcomes.

Develops expected outcomes that provide direction for continuity of care.

Modifies expected outcomes based on changes in the status of the patient or evaluation of the situation.

Documents expected outcomes as measurable goals.

Standard 4. Planning

The registered nurse develops a plan that prescribes strategies and alternatives to attain expected outcomes.

Competencies

Uses standardized language or recognized terminology to document the plan.

Note: There are additional standards for advanced practice nurses.

Source: American Nurses Association (2010, in press). *Nursing: Scope and Standards of Practice* (2nd ed). Public Comment draft, January 2010. (To be published by August 2010.) Silver Spring, MD: Nursebooks.org.

[1]*Caveat:* This material is from the draft for public comment (ANA, 2010, in press); its wording may be changed somewhat in the final published version. For that version of the ANA Standards of Professional Nursing Practice, go to www.nursingworld.org.

Canadian Provincial Standards of Practice (Examples)

In Canada, practice standards are set by each province. The following are examples that apply to planning outcomes.

Province of Alberta

Standard 2. Knowledge-Based Practice

Indicator 2.3—The registered nurse demonstrates critical thinking in collecting and interpreting data, planning, implementing, and evaluating all aspects of nursing care.

Standard 4. Provision of Service to the Public

Indicator 4.1—The registered nurse collaborates with the client/significant others and other members of the healthcare team regarding activities of care planning, implementation and evaluation.

Source: College & Association of Registered Nurses of Alberta. (2005). *Nursing practice standards.* 11620 168th Street, Edmonton, AB, Canada, T5M 4A6.

Province of Nova Scotia

Standard 3. Application of Knowledge, Skills, and Judgment

Indicator 3.2—Applies appropriate knowledge and skills to assess, plan, intervene and evaluate services, and revises plan as needed.

Standard 5. Professional Leadership

Indicator 5.1—Coordinates client care and collaborates with other members of the healthcare team.

Source: College of Registered Nurses of Nova Scotia. (2003). *Standards for nursing practice.* 600-1894 Barrington Street, Halifax, NS, Canada B3J 2A8.

---

step, the goals/desired outcomes serve as criteria for evaluating whether the nursing care has been effective. Figure 5-1 illustrates the relationship of planning outcomes to the other stages of the nursing process.

Initial and Ongoing Planning

Initial planning begins with the first patient contact. It refers to the development of the initial comprehensive care plan, which should be written as soon as possible after the initial assessment. The nurse who performs the admission assessment has the benefit of personal contact (rather than relying completely on the written database),

has the best information about the patient, and, ideally, is the one who should initiate the care plan.

You may sometimes need to begin care planning even though the initial database is incomplete. For example, the patient may require emergency care before assessment is complete. Or another patient may need your immediate attention. In such situations, develop a preliminary plan with whatever information you have. You can complete and refine the plan when you are able to perform a more detailed assessment.

Ongoing planning refers to changes made in the plan as you evaluate the patient's responses to care or as you obtain new data and make new nursing diagnoses.

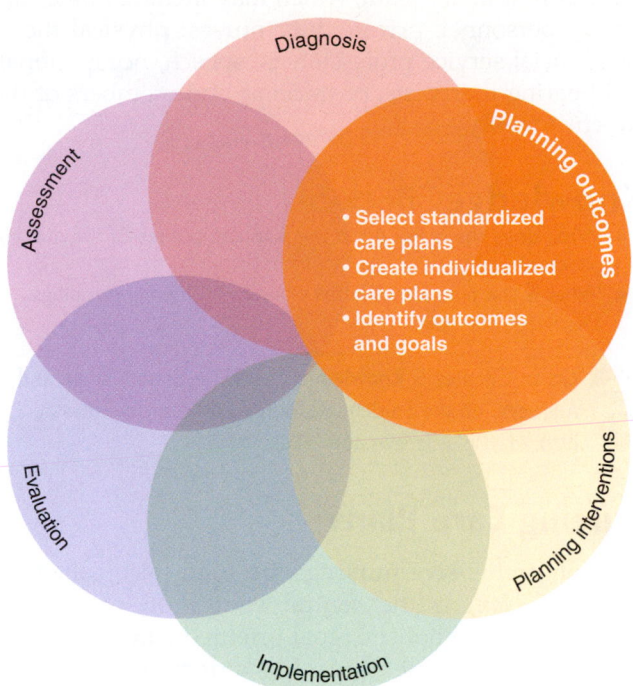

FIGURE 5-1 Nursing process phases: planning outcomes.

For example, after Ben Ivanos's first night on the hospital unit, the nurses discovered that he had not slept well. They identified a new nursing diagnosis for him: Disturbed Sleep Pattern related to unfamiliar environment and pain. They then developed a plan for addressing this problem. Ongoing planning allows you to decide which problems to focus on each day that you care for the patient.

Discharge Planning

In the hospital where Ben Ivanos is being treated, the recommended length of stay for patients with surgical reduction of fractures is 2 days. He will still have casts on his arm and both legs when he leaves the hospital. Obviously, he will not be able to manage his own activities of daily living (shopping, cooking, bathing, and so forth). What questions come to your mind when you think about how he will manage after he leaves the hospital? It is important to stretch your mind, so take a moment now to jot down your ideas.

You may have thought of questions such as the following: Is there anyone who can help Mr. Ivanos with his personal care? Does he live in a house or an apartment? Will he need to go up and down stairs? Who will drive him home from the hospital? Can he be discharged home or will he need to go to a rehabilitation facility? How soon does he need to see his primary care provider again? How will he get to the provider's office? How will he manage his pain at home; what will he use in place of the PCA narcotics?

Discharge planning is the process of planning for self-care and continuity of care after the patient leaves a healthcare setting. Ben Ivanos's case is not unusual. In the United States, outpatient surgeries and short hospital stays are the norm. Many patients are discharged despite ongoing need for nursing care and complex treatments. If appropriate services are not provided or if family members perform care incorrectly, the patient may experience delayed recovery or complications that require further treatment or hospital readmission. This means that nurses must prepare family members to perform tasks such as bathing, changing sterile dressings, and monitoring intravenously administered medications. If family members are not available or if skilled nursing care is needed, arrangements must be made for home healthcare or transfer to a skilled nursing or rehabilitation facility. Sometimes a case manager is assigned, but often staff nurses must plan and coordinate services.

To learn more about the process of discharging patients from an institution, see "Maintaining Trust During Transitions," in Chapter 10 and

Go to Chapter 10, Procedure 10-4, **Discharging a Patient from the Healthcare Facility,** in Volume 2.

Discharge Planning Begins at Assessment

Because patients are in the surgery center or hospital for such a short time, discharge planning must begin at the initial assessment, which should include the following patient data:

- Physical condition and functional and self-care limitations
- Emotional stability and ability to learn
- Financial resources (e.g., personal finances, insurance, community resources such as food stamps, Medicaid)
- Family or other caregivers available
- Caregiving responsibilities the patient may have for others
- Environment, both home and community (e.g., stairs, space for supplies and equipment, availability of transportation to healthcare services)
- Use of community services before admission

Some agencies require that the date of discharge be estimated at the time of admission, except for situations such as admission from the emergency department or a critical care unit. This may require collaborative effort.

Written Discharge Plans

All patients need at least some discharge planning, but you will not always need a separate, written discharge plan. It may be enough to include discharge assessments and teaching as nursing orders on the patient's comprehensive care plan. For example, a middle-aged patient who has been hospitalized for deep vein thrombosis (a blood clot in a major vein, usually the lower leg) will be able to care for herself independently when she goes home. For this patient, you could simply write a nursing order to teach her about the side effects of the warfarin (Coumadin, an anticoagulant) she will be taking at home. In contrast, you will probably need a comprehensive, formal discharge plan if the patient is an older adult (NSW Department of Health, 2007; Walker, Hogstel, & Curry, 2007) or has one or more of the following:

- Difficulty learning or a memory deficit
- A terminal illness
- A complicated major surgery
- No family or significant others to help provide care
- A complex treatment regimen or multiple medications to continue at home
- Self-care deficits (e.g., dressing, feeding, bathing, toileting)
- Incontinence
- An illness with an expected long period of recovery
- Inadequate financial resources
- A newly diagnosed or multiple chronic health problems (e.g., diabetes, chronic pain)
- Emotional or mental illness
- Inadequate services available in the community
- Poor mobility
- Preexisting wound
- Malnutrition

For an example of a discharge planning form, Go to Chapter 5, **Discharge Planning Form**, in Volume 2.

Discharge Planning for Older Adults

The percentage of older adults in hospitals is quite high, and they tend to have complex needs when discharged. Therefore, when an older adult is hospitalized, it is especially important to start discharge planning at the initial admission assessment. This means that assessment of functional abilities, cognition, vision, hearing, social support, and psychological well-being must be a part of the initial assessment so that you can identify needed services at discharge. A comprehensive discharge process for older adults should help to achieve the following objectives:

- Maintain functional ability.
- Lengthen the time between rehospitalizations.
- Involve all concerned parties in decision-making.
- Improve interagency communication (e.g., hospital to nursing home).
- Emphasize client and family involvement and interdisciplinary collaboration (Walker, Hogstel, & Curry, 2007).

Discharge Planning Requires Collaboration

Comprehensive discharge planning involves significant collaboration. The importance of the continuity and quality of discharge patient information has been well researched. Ideally, it is done *with,* not *for,* the patient—patient involvement is important for achieving desired outcomes. In addition, a patient's postdischarge needs, especially for an older adult, often call for services from a multidisciplinary team, which may include home care service personnel; private-duty nurses; physical therapists; social service professionals; speech, occupational, and hearing therapists; physicians; and members of the patient's family.

KnowledgeCheck 5-1

- What does the nurse do in the planning phases of the nursing process?
- What is the purpose of initial planning? Ongoing planning? Discharge planning?

 Go to Chapter 5, **Knowledge Check Response Sheet and Answers,** on the Student Resource Disk or DavisPlus at http://davisplus.fadavis.com/Wilkinson2

Nursing Care Plans

The **comprehensive nursing care plan** (also called *patient care plan*) is the central source of information needed to guide holistic, goal-oriented care to address each patient's unique needs. It is a document—usually several documents—that specify dependent, interdependent, and independent nursing actions necessary for care of a specific patient. It usually combines both standardized and individualized approaches to care.

Why Is a Written Nursing Care Plan Important?

A well-written comprehensive care plan benefits the patient and the healthcare institution by:

Ensuring that Care is Complete. If specific directions are written (e.g., "Turn patient hourly"), they are less likely to be overlooked by busy caregivers.

Providing Continuity of Care. This helps ensure that when an effective intervention is found, all caregivers will use the same approach with the patient. For example, suppose a child who is dehydrated refuses to drink any liquids. The day nurse discovers the child will eat red, and only red, popsicles. If he fails to note that on the care plan, the night nurse may be unable to persuade the child to take liquids orally and may have to administer fluids intravenously to prevent further dehydration.

Promoting Efficient Use of Nursing Efforts. Specific, written instructions help to ensure that nurses do not waste time on ineffective approaches. In the preceding example, the night nurse may waste a great deal of time trying to persuade the child to drink liquids.

Providing a Guide for Assessments and Charting. The nursing orders and goals/expected outcomes on the care plan can help you recall what occurred and ensure nothing is omitted from your documentation.

Meeting the Requirements of Accrediting Agencies. The Joint Commission and professional standards review organizations (PSROs) require a patient-specific plan of care.

What Information Does a Comprehensive Nursing Care Plan Contain?

Regardless of their format, comprehensive care plans include directions for four different kinds of care and include both medical and nursing interventions:

1. *Basic needs and activities of daily living (ADLs).* Whatever the patient's diagnoses, nurses need to know what routine assistance the patient needs with hygiene, nutrition, elimination, and so on.
2. *Medical/multidisciplinary treatment.* Nurses need to know the medical orders for each patient (e.g., prescriptions for intravenous fluids and medications) and the nursing activities necessary for carrying out those orders.
3. *Nursing diagnoses and collaborative problems.* This section may be referred to as the *nursing diagnosis care plan.* It contains goals and nursing orders for the patient's nursing diagnoses and collaborative problems.
4. *Special discharge needs or teaching needs.* Finally, the plan should contain instructions for formal discharge planning and special teaching if they are needed. For example, the client may need to be taught how to self-administer injections or follow a prescribed diet.

What Documents Make Up a Comprehensive Nursing Care Plan?

You will use a variety of documents to create a care plan. Care plans vary widely in format, appearance, and use. In most healthcare organizations, caregivers use preprinted, standardized plans that can be adapted to meet individual needs. Figure 5-2 shows the documents that are most commonly included in a comprehensive nursing care plan.

Form for Client Profile and Basic Needs

Some essential client data either do not change or are used or updated often. This includes the client's profile (e.g., age, providers, drug allergies, and so on), basic needs (e.g., for hygiene, nutrition, and elimination), and diagnostic tests and treatments (e.g., laboratory tests, radiology procedures, and respiratory therapy). To provide quick and easy access, such information is usually recorded on a durable, standardized form and not organized according to medical or nursing diagnoses (see Fig. 5-2A). These are often in electronic format, but may be printed on cardstock and kept in a central location easily accessible to all care providers. For an example of a printed Kardex,

 Go to Chapter 5, **Tables, Boxes, Figures: ESG Figure 5-1,** on the Student Resource Disk or DavisPlus at http://davisplus.fadavis.com/Wilkinson2

FIGURE 5-2 Components of a nursing care plan. *A,* Form for client profile, basic needs, ADLs, and multidisciplinary plans. *B,* Preprinted, standardized plans, both nursing and multidisciplinary. *C,* Individualized care plans to address nursing diagnoses. *D,* Special discharge plan and/or instructions. *E,* Special teaching plan.

For clients who need more than routine attention to their basic needs, you may wish to write a nursing diagnosis care plan. Examples include a client with no appetite and the nursing diagnosis Imbalanced Nutrition: Less Than Body Requirements, or an immobile client with the diagnosis Risk for Impaired Skin Integrity.

Preprinted, Standardized Plans

As shown in Figure 5-2B, a comprehensive care plan usually includes one or more preprinted, standardized documents. It would be too time-consuming to hand-write a complete care plan for every patient. Standardized plans save nursing time, promote consistency of care, and help ensure that nurses do not overlook important interventions. You will find standardized instructions for patient care in a variety of documents within an organization. A document may (1) contain nursing or multidisciplinary interventions and (2) prescribe care for one or more nursing diagnoses (e.g., Anxiety) or a disease or medical condition (e.g., pneumonia). The following are examples of standardized, preprinted instructions for care.

Policies and Procedures
Policies and **procedures** are similar to rules and regulations. When a situation occurs frequently or requires a consistent response regardless of who handles it, management develops a policy to govern how it is to be handled. For example, hospitals have policies about visiting hours. You should consider individual needs and use critical thinking to interpret policies in a caring manner. For example, in some critical care units a patient is allowed one visitor for 10 minutes each hour. Imagine, though, that a patient is expected to die soon, and that his daughter has come from a distant state and brought her three children for one last visit. Would you tell the daughter to take the children in to see their grandfather? Would you insist that she follow the rule and send them in without her, one at a time over a period of 3 hours?

Protocols
Protocols cover specific actions usually required for a clinical problem unique to a subgroup of patients. For example, not every patient on a medical-surgical unit is at risk for falls, but many are. So for a patient in that subgroup (i.e., at risk for falls), the nurse would add a falls protocol, such as in Figure 5-3, to that patient's care plan. Protocols may be written for a particular medical diagnosis (e.g., seizure), treatments (e.g., administration of oxytocin to induce labor), or diagnostic tests (e.g., barium enema). They contain both medical and nursing orders. Some include definitions and rationales for interventions.

Unit Standards of Care
Unit standards of care describe the care that nurses are expected to provide for all patients in defined situations (e.g., all women admitted to a labor unit or all patients admitted to the critical care unit). In this way, they are similar to protocols. Unlike protocols, however, they

(1) apply to every patient in the defined situation, rather than a subgroup; (2) do not become part of the patient's care plan but are kept on file on the unit; and (3) do not usually include specific medical orders. Instead of describing ideal care, standards of care describe the minimum level of care the nurses are expected to achieve given the institution's resources and the client population. Unit standards of care usually are not organized according to nursing diagnoses and usually resemble a list of "things to do" (e.g., complete comprehensive assessment within 2 hours of admission) rather than detailed instructions for care.

Critical Thinking 5-1

- Think of some other "defined situations" for which unit standards of care might be useful.
- Suggest some more subgroups for which a protocol might be appropriate.

Standardized Nursing Care Plans
Standardized (model) nursing care plans detail the nursing care that is usually needed for a particular nursing diagnosis or for all nursing diagnoses that commonly occur with a medical condition. Figure 5-4 is a standardized care plan for a single nursing diagnosis. Although similar to unit standards of care, model care plans are different in that they usually:

- Provide more detailed interventions. They may add to or delete from unit standards of care.
- Are organized by nursing diagnosis and include specific patient goals and nursing orders.
- Are a part of the patient's comprehensive care plan and become a part of the permanent record.
- Describe ideal rather than minimum nursing care.
- Allow you to incorporate addendum care plans.
- Include checklists, blank lines, or empty spaces so that you can individualize goals and interventions.

Students sometimes purchase model care plan books. You can use them as guides, but be aware that they do not address a client's individual needs. For this reason, they may lead you to focus on the common, predictable problems and overlook an unusual—and perhaps more important—problem the person is experiencing. Beginning with the standardized plan may stifle your creativity. It is best to first use the process for writing a nursing care plan (see "What Is the Process for Writing an Individualized Nursing Care Plan?") and then consult the model plan to see whether you have missed anything.

Critical Pathways
Critical pathways are often used in managed care systems. They are outcomes-based, interdisciplinary plans that sequence patient care according to case type. They specify predicted patient outcomes and broad interventions for each day, or in some situations, for each hour (Fig. 5-5). They describe the minimal standard of care required to meet the recommended length of stay for patients with a particular condition or *diagnosis-related group* (*DRG*; e.g., postpartum, myocardial infarction, or

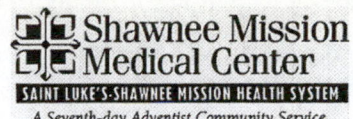

Patient Care Protocol

Title: Fall or Injury/Disruption of Care, Care of the Patient at Risk for   **Effective Date:** 1/9/11

Expected Outcome: The patient at risk for falls will be identified and preventive measures initiated.
                            The patient will not pull out indwelling devices.

Relevant Information: Initiate this protocol for adult patients who have a <u>Conley Fall Scale</u> score of ≥3.

Assessment: 1.   The Conley Fall Scale will be administered on admission to adult inpatients. Further assessment
                           will be based on patient population and identified patient need.

Interventions: Make alterations in environment, such as:
- Avoiding clutter in room.
- Moving patient closer to Nursing Station if indicated.
- Making sure call light, telephone and other personal items are within reach

Educate patient and family about:
- The possibility that family and friends may be called upon to stay with patient with high risk for fall or injury or who attempts to pull out indwelling devices.
- The possibility that, if the above measures are not successful in reducing the patient's fall risk or preventing attempts to pull out indwelling devices, alternative measures such as the use of restraints may have to be considered.

Evaluation: 1.   Evaluate frequently to determine if expected outcome is being met. Change strategies as needed to reduce fall risks or to prevent disruption of indwelling devices.
                      2.   **Criteria for initiation of Restraint Protocol:**
- If interventions have been implemented and patient continues to be at risk of falling or disrupting medical treatment, the protocol <u>Care of the Patient in Restraint for Medical/Surgical Management</u> is initiated.
- The CRN/Supervisor is notified at the time the restraint is initiated for med/surg management and reviews the need for restraint.

FIGURE 5-3 Portion of Patient Care Protocol for patient at risk for falls. (*Source:* Courtesy of Shawnee Mission Health System, Shawnee Mission, KS 66204.)

total hip replacement). An agency usually develops critical pathways for its most frequent case types or for situations in which standardized care can produce predictable outcomes. Although critical pathways are developed by a multidisciplinary team, they tend to emphasize medical problems and interventions.

Integrated Plans of Care

Integrated plans of care (IPOCs) are standardized plans that function as care plans as well as documentation forms. Therefore, there is a different form—or sometimes a different column—for each day of care. Many critical pathways are designed as IPOCs; however, IPOCs do not necessarily (1) organize care according to diagnosis, (2) describe minimal standards of care, or (3) specify a timeline for interventions and outcomes. For an example of an IPOC,

Go to Chapter 5, **Tables, Boxes, Figures: ESG Figure 5-2,** on the Student Resource Disk or DavisPlus at http:// davisplus.fadavis.com/Wilkinson2

Individualized Nursing Care Plans

Nurses use individualized nursing care plans to address nursing diagnoses unique to a particular client (see Fig. 5-2c). These care plans reflect the independent component of nursing practice, and therefore best demonstrate the nurse's critical thinking and clinical expertise. In addition to including goals and nursing orders that you write specifically for a patient, a complete individualized care plan may contain standardized single-problem care plans (see Fig. 5-4).

Standardized plans focus on the common problems and interventions needed by most patients. They do not address unusual problems and may not meet a patient's individual needs. You should always adapt standardized plans by adding the necessary nursing diagnoses, goals/outcomes, and nursing orders not included in the standardized documents. For example, a standardized plan for a client with a myocardial infarction (heart attack) would undoubtedly prescribe care for the nursing diagnosis Pain and the potential complication of heart

PATIENT PLAN OF CARE - GENESIS MEDICAL CENTER - Davenport, Iowa

PAIN, ACUTE: Experience of an unpleasant sensory and emotional sensation for a duration of less than 6 months.
SIGNS & SYMPTOMS: Observed or reported (select at least 2)

☐ Change in BP   ☐ Restlessness   ☐ Grimacing   ☐ Crying
☐ Patients self report of pain   ☐ Diaphoresis   ☐ Increased muscle tension   ☐ Change in pulse rate
☐ Change in respiratory pattern ☐ Whimpering   ☐ Whining

OUTCOME SCORING

RELATED FACTORS	OUTCOMES	ADM				DC	INTERVENTIONS
☐ Physical injuring agent ☐ Psychological injuring agent	[4] Pain control behavior – Recognizes causal factors – Uses non-analgesic relief measures – Uses analgesics appropriately – Reports pain controlled [3] Pain level – Oral/facial expressions of pain – Change in respiratory rate, heart rate BP – Restlessness – Reported pain [3] Comfort level – Reported satisfaction with symptom control – Expressed satisfaction with pain control – Reported physical well-being						☐ Pain management ☐ Analgesic administration ☐ Patient-controlled analgesic (PCA) assistance ☐ Analgesic administration: Intraspinal ☐ Environmental management: comfort ☐ Anxiety reduction ☐ Transcutaneous electrical nerve stimulation (TENS) ☐ Heat/cold application ☐ Distraction ☐ Simple relaxation therapy ☐ Simple massage ☐ Developmental care ☐ Preparatory sensory information ☐ Positioning

Definition of scoring scales	1	2	3	4	5
Pain control — Personal actions to control pain	Never demonstrated	Rarely demonstrated	Sometimes demonstrated	Often demonstrated	Consistently demonstrated
Pain level — Severity of reported pain	Severe	Substantial	Moderate	Slight	None
Comfort level — Extent of physical and psychological ease	None	Limited	Moderate	Substantial	Extensive

Diagnosis _____

Date Initiated _____ RN Initials _____

Date Resolved _____

FIGURE 5-4 Computer printout of standardized care plan for a single nursing diagnosis using standardized language. (*Source:* Adapted from Genesis Medical Center, Davenport, IA 52804. Used with permission.)

HOSPITAL OF THE UNIVERSITY OF PENNSYLVANIA

TOTAL LOWER JOINT (HIP/KNEE)
CLINICAL PATHWAY

ELIGIBILITY CRITERIA: All primary unilateral total hip or total knee
replacements

EXPECTED LOS: 3 Days   ADDRESSOGRAPH

CLINICAL KEYS:

1. Pain managed midpoint on painscale
2. Transfer to chair/commode with assistance POD 1; Ambulate in room, bathroom POD2
3. DVT precautions
4. Discharge plan completed by POD2
5. Patient verbalizes knowledge of hip or knee precautions
6. Knee motion 10 to 70 or better (TKA patients only)

	PACU	IMMED. POST-OP	POD 1	POD 2	POD 3-4
ASSESSMENTS	• NV checks with VS q1h × 4 • Pain • Effects of narcotics/ tolerance • I & 0 × 24hr • Pulse Ox q8 if on O2	• NV check / VS q 4hr → → • S/S DVT →	→ → → → • Pulse Ox × 1 on RA • Dsg/wound status q4	• NV check / VS q 8hr → → → • D/C pulse ox if O2 D/C • Dsg/wound status q8	→ → → → →
CONSULTS		• PT • PMR	→ (If not done already) → (If not done already)		
TESTS	• A/P hip X-ray (THA) • A/P knee X-ray (TKA)		• CBC	→ • INR (if on warfarin)	• A/P hip X-ray →
TREATMENTS	• O2	• D/C O2 if sat 94% • Incentive spirometry • Order walker (hip chair, elevated commode if needed) • Pneumatic compression device (ankle for knees, calf for hips)	→ → • D/C foley • Dressing change (1st dsg change by MD) →	→ → • Dressing change q day and pm	→ → → →
MEDICATIONS	• PCA or epidural	→ • Anticoagulation	• IV heplock • Consider conversion to oral pain meds	• D/C heplock → • D/C PCA/PCEA • PO pain meds	→
ACTIVITY	• Bedrest • Hip precautions if THA • CPM for total knee	→ → →	• OOB to chair BID → → • Weight bear per order • Ambulate with assistive device	• OOB TID → → → → • PT ×2	→ → → → → →
NUTRITION	• NPO	• NPO → ice → advance to full as tolerated	• Regular	→	→
EDUCATION / D/C PLANNING	• Deep breathing exercises	• Pain management • Initiate d/c plan	→ • Home vs rehab decision • Anticoagulation if indicated	→ • S/S wound infection • Medications • Activity level • D/C plan in place	→ → → • Car transfer

Transfer to rehab when:
1. Able to participate in care
2. Tolerating 2 physical therapy sessions
3. Not requiring IV pain medicine
4. Blood values are stable
5. Motivation is commensurate with projected functional status

Discharge to home when:
1. Mobility and ADL's appropriate for degree of assistance at home and home environment
2. Appropriate assistive device and necessary adaptive equipment is used
3. Independent with hip/knee precautions
4. Independent with home exercise program or ongoing PT in the home or outpatient
**IF D/C TO HOME, ENSURE APPROPRIATE CONSULTS TO ARRANGE HOME CARE FOLLOW-UP AND EQUIPMENT

FIGURE 5-5 Portion of a critical pathway. (*Source*: Hospital of the University of Pennsylvania, Philadelphia, PA. Used with permission.)

failure. However, it might not address the needs of a person who is not complying with treatments because he is in denial about his illness (nursing diagnosis: Ineffective Denial). An individualized plan for resolving the patient's denial would improve the likelihood that the rest of the plan will be successful.

You may sometimes include medical orders in a nursing diagnosis or collaborative problem care plan, especially in a student care plan. For example, for a client with a nursing diagnosis of Deficient Fluid Volume, you might list the medical prescription for intravenously administered fluids in the "Nursing Orders" column.

Nursing Diagnosis	Nursing orders
Deficient Fluid Volume related to vomiting and diarrhea	1. Check skin turgor q4hr 2. Medical order: IV normal saline, 150 mL/hr

Special Discharge or Teaching Plans

A nursing plan of care may also contain one or more discharge or teaching plans (see Fig. 5-2d). These are sometimes referred to as *special-purpose* or *addendum* care plans. You can address routine discharge planning and teaching needs by using standardized plans or by including teaching as part of the nursing orders on an individualized care plan. For example, a care plan for the diagnosis Acute Pain might have a nursing order, "Teach patient to splint incision when turning in bed." Chapter 24 shows an example of a teaching plan for the diagnosis Deficient Knowledge.

Computerized Plans of Care

Many healthcare organizations use electronic health records, including *computerized care plans*. The computer stores standardized plans (e.g., for nursing diagnoses, medical diagnoses, or diagnosis-related groups [DRGs]). When you enter a diagnosis or a desired outcome, the computer generates a list of suggested interventions. You then choose appropriate interventions from the list, individualize by choosing from checklists, or type in your own interventions and strategies.

Computer prompts help ensure that you consider a variety of actions and keep you from overlooking common and important interventions. After the initial learning curve, they also reduce the time spent on paperwork. However, computerized planning requires constant use of a step-by-step thinking process, which may cause a decrease in intuition, insight, ability to care, and nursing expertise (Harris, 1990). You must resist the temptation to accept "one size fits all" solutions. Always look for creative approaches that might be more effective for a particular individual. Think, "What would work for *this* person?"

ESG Figure 5-3 in the Student Resource Disk or at DavisPlus shows a computer screen displaying a care plan for the nursing diagnosis Pain. It lists a patient goal

and broadly stated interventions, including assessments and patient education. Most computer programs allow you to print the plan.

 Go to Chapter 5, **Tables, Boxes, Figures: ESG Figure 5-3,** on the Student Resource Disk or DavisPlus at http://davisplus.fadavis.com/Wilkinson2

KnowledgeCheck 5-2

- In addition to care related to the patient's basic needs, what other types of information does a comprehensive care plan contain?
- How are critical pathways different from other standardized care plans?
- What is the main disadvantage of computerized and standardized care plans?

 Go to Chapter 5, **Knowledge Check Response Sheet and Answers,** on the Student Resource Disk or DavisPlus at http://davisplus.fadavis.com/Wilkinson2

 CriticalThinking 5-2

Suppose a nurse sees one of your student care plans and says to you, "You're wasting your time writing those things. We never use the nursing process in the real world." Take a few minutes to write down how you might respond.

Student Care Plans

You may have noticed that the care plans you see in clinical settings look different from the ones you create as a part of your clinical preparation. This is because student care plans are a learning activity as well as a plan of care. They are designed to help you learn and apply concepts from the nursing process, physiology, and psychopathology. For this reason, they may contain more detailed nursing orders as well as other information the instructor may require (e.g., information about lab tests, medications, and assessment data to support the nursing diagnoses). Some instructors may ask you to write rationales and cite references to support them. **Rationales** state the scientific principles or research that supports nursing interventions. Writing rationales helps ensure that you understand the reasons for the interventions—understanding *why* you do *what* you do is one aspect of functioning as a professional. For an example of a student care plan,

 Go to Chapter 5, **Student Care Plan Example,** on the Student Resource Disk or DavisPlus at http://davisplus.fadavis.com/Wilkinson2

Mind-Mapping Student Care Plans

Mind-mapping is a technique for showing relationships among ideas and concepts in a graphical, or pictorial, way. Mind-mapping is thought to stimulate "whole-brain" and critical thinking, and to foster the development of holistic plans of care (Mueller, Johnston, & Bligh, 2002). A mind-mapped care plan uses shapes and pictures to represent the parts of the nursing process (i.e., assessment data, nursing diagnoses, patient goals, interventions, and evaluation), as well as the patient's pathophysiology, medications, and other pertinent information. For complete information about mind-mapping,

Go to Chapter 5, **Supplemental Materials: Mind-Mapping Student Care Plans,** on the Student Resource Disk or DavisPlus at http://davisplus.fadavis.com/Wilkinson2

Practical **Knowledge** **knowing** how

What Is the Process for Writing an Individualized Nursing Care Plan?

Writing an individualized nursing care plan follows in natural sequence from the assessment and diagnosis phases of the nursing process:

Make a Working Problem List. Earlier in the nursing process, you will already have developed and prioritized a list of the patient's nursing diagnoses, collaborative problems, and strengths. Suppose that, after assessment, you prioritized Ben Ivanos's problems as follows:

1. Acute Pain secondary to musculoskeletal trauma (arms, legs, body) and muscle spasms
2. Risk for Peripheral Neurovascular Dysfunction secondary to casts/traction
3. Self-Care Deficit (Total) r/t immobility secondary to casts, especially cast on dominant right arm
4. Potential Complication of fracture: delayed, union, malunion, or nonunion of bone

Decide which problems can be managed with standardized care plans or critical pathways. What institutional documents are available? Suppose that the hospital unit has a critical pathway for "Patients with Casts and/or Traction." This critical pathway would contain goals and interventions to guide the care for problems 2 and 4 above. It would specify regular neurovascular assessments and management of the traction apparatus, for example.

Individualize the standardized plan as needed. Mark off any instructions that do not apply to your patient, and add or adapt nursing orders as appropriate. Many standardized plans provide space for individualizing the goals and interventions. For example, the plan might say "Perform neurovascular checks q_____." You would fill in the frequency of the assessment according to Mr. Ivanos' needs.

Transcribe medical orders to appropriate documents. For example, you might write orders for pain medications on a special medication administration record. Details about Mr. Ivanos' traction would probably go on a Kardex or special section of the critical pathway.

Write ADLs and basic care needs in special sections of the Kardex, care plan, or computer. For Ben Ivanos, you might note on the Kardex that he requires a complete bed bath and help with eating.

Develop individualized care plans for problems not addressed by standardized documents. For Ben Ivanos, you would need to write a plan for problems 1 and 3 above. The critical pathway probably contains some expected outcomes and basic interventions for problem 1, Pain, but you might need to individualize them to make them more effective. If your unit had a Pain protocol, similar to the Falls protocol in Figure 5-3, you would add it to Mr. Ivanos's care plan. If not, you would hand-write goals and interventions for the Pain diagnosis.

Problem 3, Self-Care Deficit, would be partially addressed in the basic care section of Mr. Ivanos' Kardex, but he has special needs. For example, he will need teaching and therapy to increase his ability to care for himself. So you would need to hand-write a plan for this nursing diagnosis.

KnowledgeCheck 5-3

Briefly describe a process for creating a comprehensive, individualized care plan that incorporates collaborative care and standardized planning documents.

Go to Chapter 5, **Knowledge Check Response Sheet and Answers,** on the Student Resource Disk or DavisPlus at http://davisplus.fadavis.com/Wilkinson2

Planning Patient Goals/Outcomes

After assessment and diagnosis, the next step in individualized care planning is to formulate goals for improving or maintaining the patient's health status. **Goals** (also called **expected outcomes, desired outcomes,** or **predicted outcomes**) describe the changes in patient health status that you hope to achieve. **Nursing-sensitive outcomes** are those that can be influenced by nursing interventions. Although critical pathways describe the expected outcomes of multidisciplinary care, they do not provide a way to judge *nursing* effectiveness. The rest of this chapter discusses individualized care planning and nursing-sensitive outcomes.

Goal/expected outcome formulation is the responsibility of the professional nurse (see Box 5-1). You should involve the client as much as possible in goal setting, because goal achievement is more likely if the client believes the goals are important and realistic. Of course, the client must be alert and independent enough to participate. If physical or mental impairments prevent active participation, the nursing team acts on the client's behalf to develop client-centered goals.

What Do the Terms *Goal* and *Outcome* Mean?

Many nurses use the terms *goal* and *outcome* interchangeably. In this text, we usually use the Nursing Outcomes Classification (NOC) terminology: the word *outcome*, used alone, means *any* patient response (positive or negative) to interventions (e.g., the pain could become better or worse; both are outcomes). When referring to desired (positive) patient responses, we use *goals, expected outcomes, desired outcomes,* or *predicted outcomes.* For example:

Outcome	Decision Making
Goals/expected outcomes	Participates in decisions about own care.
	Chooses between two or more alternatives.

Some nurses use the term *goal* to mean a broad, nonspecific statement about the desired results of nursing activities. They use *outcomes* (and other outcome terms such as *expected outcomes*) to mean the more specific, observable responses you would use to judge whether the goal has been met. When goals are defined in this way, you must include both goals and expected outcomes on the care plan because a broad goal does not provide enough guidance for evaluating patient responses to care. You can combine the broad goal and specific expected outcome into a single statement by writing, "as evidenced by," as in the following example:

Broad statement (goal)	Constipation relieved
Specific expected outcome (evaluation criteria)	Will have soft, formed bowel movement within 24 hours
Combined statement (goal + outcome)	Constipation will be relieved *as evidenced by* soft, formed bowel movement within 24 hours

Use of broad goals on the care plan is optional; however, expected outcomes are not optional. You must include them on the care plan.

What Is the Purpose of Goal/Outcome Statements?

Goals are important for planning, implementation, and evaluation. Precise, descriptive, clearly stated goals/expected outcomes:

- Provide a guide for selecting nursing interventions by describing what you wish to achieve.
- Motivate the client and the nurse by providing a sense of achievement when the goals are met. This is especially important when the client must make difficult lifestyle changes.
- Form the criteria you will use in the evaluation phase of the nursing process.

How Do I Distinguish Between Short-Term and Long-Term Goals?

Short-term goals are those you expect the patient to achieve within a few hours or days. They are important:

- In situations in which the patient may be discharged before you can evaluate progress toward long-term goals (e.g., as in a day surgery).
- For providing positive reinforcement to clients who are working toward long-term goals.

Long-term goals are changes in health status that you wish to achieve over a longer period—perhaps a week, a month, or more. They describe the optimum level of functioning you expect the patient to achieve, given health status and available resources. Ideally, this is a return to normal functioning, but that is not always possible. See Table 5-1 for a comparison of short-term and long-term goals.

Table 5-1 ➤ Comparison of Short-Term and Long-Term Goals

	DEFINITION	SITUATIONS FOR USE	EXAMPLES
Short-Term Goals	■ Can be achieved in a few hours or a few days.	■ Acute care ■ Day surgery ■ Clinics ■ Focus on immediate needs ■ Students ■ Evaluation of progress toward long-term goals	■ Describes pain as < 3 on a 1–10 scale within 30 min after receiving analgesic. ■ Limits food intake to 1500 calories per day.
Long-Term Goals	■ Expected changes that occur over a week, a month, or more ■ Optimum level of functioning given health status and resources	■ Home healthcare ■ Extended-care facilities ■ Rehabilitation centers ■ Chronic illness ■ Conditions that are managed, not cured	■ Infant will double birth weight within 5 months. ■ Within 3 months after physical therapy treatments, will dress self except for buttons.

KnowledgeCheck 5-4

Refer to "Meet Your Patient," at the beginning of the chapter. State whether each of Mr. Ivanos's goals was a short-term or long-term goal.

 Go to Chapter 5, **Knowledge Check Response Sheet and Answers,** on the Student Resource Disk or DavisPlus at http://davisplus.fadavis.com/Wilkinson2

What Are the Components of a Goal Statement?

Every expected outcome/goal statement must have the following parts:

- *Subject.* The subject is understood to be the client, but it can also be a function or part of the client. For example:

  [Mrs. Johnson] Will walk to the doorway with the help of one person by 12/13/10.

  Lung sounds will be clear to auscultation within 2 days after receiving antibiotics.

  Assume that the subject is the client unless otherwise stated. Think, "Client will . . ." to help you phrase the goal statement correctly, but do not write it. For example, in the first goal, you should not write "Mrs. Johnson."

- *Action verb.* Use an action verb to indicate the action the client will perform: what the client will learn, do, or say (e.g., Will *walk* to the doorway). Use concrete verbs (i.e., describing actions that you can see, hear, smell, feel, or measure), such as the following:

apply	explain	report
choose	eat	select
demonstrate	list	transfer
describe	measure	turn
drink	prepare	verbalize

- *Performance criteria.* These are the standards for evaluating the client's performance. They describe the extent to which you expect to see the action or behavior. Write them in concrete, observable terms because they indicate what you need to measure in order to evaluate outcomes. Performance criteria specify:

  How, what, when, or where something is to be done
  Amount, quality, accuracy, speed, distance, and so forth

The following example specifies the distance the client is expected to walk: [Client] Will walk *to the doorway* with the help of one person by 12/13/11.

- *Target time.* The realistic date or time by which the performance/behavior should be achieved. The target time is the "when" part of the performance criterion: [Client] will walk to the doorway with the help of one person *by 12/13/11.*

Other examples of target times are *by discharge, within 24 hours, at the next visit, each hour, at all times.* For risk

(potential) nursing diagnoses, the desired outcome is that the problem will not ever occur. You assume that the desired response should occur "at all times," but you may wish to schedule times for evaluating the outcome. For example:

Nursing diagnosis: Risk for Constipation r/t inadequate fluid intake
Expected outcome: Bowel movements will be of normal frequency and consistency.
Target time: At all times
Evaluate: Daily

- *Special conditions.* Describe the amount of assistance or resources needed or the experiences/treatments the client should have to perform the behavior. Include special conditions when it is important for other nurses to know them. For example:

  [Client] Will walk to the doorway *with the help of one person* by 12/13/11.

  After two teaching sessions, [client] will be able to identify foods to avoid on a low-fat diet by 3/1/11.

KnowledgeCheck 5-5

In the following predicted outcomes, identify the subject, action verb, performance criterion, target time, and special conditions (if any). State which components are assumed, if any.

- Will walk to the doorway with the help of one person by 12/13/11.
- After two teaching sessions, (client) will be able to identify foods to avoid on a low-fat diet by 3/1/11.
- Bowel movements will be soft and formed and of his usual frequency.
- Lungs clear to auscultation at all times.

 Go to Chapter 5, **Knowledge Check Response Sheet and Answers,** on the Student Resource Disk or DavisPlus at http://davisplus.fadavis.com/Wilkinson2

How Do Goals Relate to Nursing Diagnoses?

Expected outcomes are derived directly from the nursing diagnosis. Therefore, they will be appropriate only if you identify the nursing diagnosis correctly. The problem clause (the clause at the left) of a nursing diagnosis describes the response or health status you wish to change. A desired outcome states the *opposite* of the problem and implies this response is what the interventions are intended to achieve (Table 5-2).

 Critical**Thinking** 5-3

Answer the following questions for Ben Ivanos's nursing diagnosis of Acute Pain secondary to musculoskeletal trauma (arms, legs, body) and muscle spasms:

- What would be the opposite, healthy response to his problem?
- What changes should you see in appearance, body functions, symptoms, knowledge, and emotions?

Table 5-2 ➤ Comparison of Nursing Diagnoses and Goals

NURSING DIAGNOSIS (PROBLEM SIDE)	GOAL/EXPECTED OUTCOME
Problem response	Opposite of problem response
Present health status	Desired health status
Response that you hope to change	Response that you hope to achieve
Example:	*Examples:*
Ineffective Airway Clearance ───────────────▶	Lungs clear to auscultation
r/t ineffective cough secondary to incision pain ─────▶	Coughs productively

■ If the problem is prevented or solved, how will Mr. Ivanos look or behave? What will you be able to observe (e.g., see, hear, smell, taste, or touch)?

■ What should Mr. Ivanos be able to do to demonstrate a positive change? How well, or how soon, should he be able to do it?

Take a few minutes to think about and write the answers to those questions.

You might have said that the opposite response to pain would be absence of (or relief from) pain, but you couldn't really observe that. "Absence of pain" might serve as a broad goal statement. But how about more specific, observable expected outcomes? How would you know that Mr. Ivanos's pain was relieved?

Specific, observable behaviors that demonstrate absence of pain include the following:

Relaxed body posture
Relaxed facial expression
Does not complain of pain.
States that his pain is relieved (or manageable, or gone).
Rates pain as less than 3 on a scale of 1 to 10.

Essential versus Nonessential Goals

In general, the problem side of the nursing diagnosis suggests the goals, and the etiology suggests nursing interventions. You can also derive some goals from the etiology; however, the **essential patient goals** flow from the problem side of the nursing diagnosis (see the bold print in Table 5-3) because the problem side describes the unhealthy response you intend to change.

Notice in Table 5-3 that the goals derived from the etiology may help resolve the problem, but they could also be achieved without resolution of the problem. Suppose that for a patient with Ineffective Airway Clearance you had written only the goals in regular type. If the patient coughs forcefully and effectively, rates pain as less than 3, and splints his incision while coughing, you might discontinue the interventions for Ineffective Airway Clearance. However, the problem might still exist. Even a client who demonstrates all three of those responses might not be coughing productively enough to clear the airways and might still not have clear lung sounds. This means you should follow this rule:

Table 5-3 ➤ Deriving Goals and Interventions from Nursing Diagnoses

NURSING DIAGNOSIS	GOALS/EXPECTED OUTCOMES	NURSING ACTIVITIES
Problem: ➡	**Lungs clear to auscultation** ➡	Teach deep breathing and coughing
Ineffective Airway	**Coughs productively**	Auscultate lungs q4hr
Clearance	**Respirations 12–20/min**	Assess respiratory rate, breathing, and skin color q4hr
	No pallor or cyanosis	
r/t	**No dyspnea or shortness of breath (SOB)**	
Etiology: ➡	Coughs forcefully/effectively ➡	Teach to splint incision while coughing
Ineffective cough secondary to incisional pain	Rates pain as < 3 on 1–10 scale	Turn, cough, and deep-breathe (TCDB) hourly
	Splints incision while coughing	Medicate for pain 30 minutes before TCDB

For every nursing diagnosis, you must state one goal that, if achieved, would demonstrate resolution or improvement of the problem.

Goals for Actual, Risk, and Possible Nursing Diagnoses

You will develop expected outcomes to promote, maintain, or restore health, depending on the status of the nursing diagnosis. See Table 5-4 for explanations and examples. Review Chapter 4 as needed.

Goals for Collaborative Problems

Recall that collaborative problems are physiological complications of diseases (e.g., diabetes) or medical treatments (e.g., cardiac catheterization) that nurses monitor to detect onset or changes in status. Always, the desired outcome is that the complication will not develop. However, unlike outcomes for nursing diagnoses, these outcomes are not nurse-sensitive; that is, they do not result primarily from nursing interventions. They occur as a result of interventions by several disciplines. Consider the following example:

> *Collaborative problem:* Potential Complication of abdominal surgery: paralytic ileus (paralysis of the ileum of the small intestine)
> *Goal:* Patient will not develop paralytic ileus

Suppose that 36 hours after the surgery, the patient's bowel sounds are absent, his abdomen is distended and painful, and he begins vomiting. What could the nurse have done to prevent this situation? What can the nurse do to relieve the ileus and bring about return of peristalsis? Very little, actually. The primary interventions are medical and, if there is obstruction, probably surgical. Therefore, it would not be appropriate to include a goal for this problem on a nursing care plan, because that would imply that nurses are primarily accountable for the outcome.

Table 5-4 ➤ Expected Outcomes for Various Problem Types

TYPE OF PROBLEM	EXAMPLE OF DIAGNOSIS	EXPLANATION OF DIAGNOSIS	NURSING INTERVENTIONS	EXAMPLE OF EXPECTED PATIENT OUTCOME
Actual Nursing Diagnosis	Constipation r/t inadequate dietary fiber and fluids	Symptoms of constipation present (e.g., no bowel movement [BM])	Resolution or reduction of problem; prevention of complications	Will have normal, formed BM within 24 hours after receiving stool softener.
Risk (Potential) Nursing Diagnosis	Risk for Constipation r/t inadequate dietary fiber and fluids	Risk factors present (e.g., not drinking enough or eating adequate fiber)	Prevention and early detection problem	Will have bowel function within normal limits for patient (e.g., daily bowel movement with no need for stool softener or laxative).
Possible Nursing Diagnosis	Possible Constipation r/t suspected inadequate intake of dietary fiber and fluids	Not enough data (e.g., no BM for 2 days, but no data on intake or on his usual bowel habits)	Confirm or rule out problem.	No patient goal. The nursing goal is "Confirm or rule out the problem."
Collaborative Problem	Potential Complication of abdominal surgery: ileus	Medical treatment creates risk for complication that is prevented by collaborative care.	Primarily detection; prevention is collaborative.	None. Patient responses depend on collaborative care. The broad nursing goal is early identification of the problem.
Wellness Diagnosis	Readiness for Enhanced Nutrition	Bowel habits and dietary intake within normal limits, but can be improved	Maintain or promote higher level of health.	Reports increased intake of dietary fiber and fluids; reports bowel functioning within normal limits.

All goals on a nursing care plan should be nursing-sensitive goals. For collaborative problems, instead of a patient outcome, you might wish to write a nursing goal such as: "Early detection of complication, should it occur." See Table 5-4. Collaborative goals are appropriate on multidisciplinary care plans and critical pathways, however.

On student care plans, to aid your learning, you can write the symptoms of the complication or the normal physiological response you hope to observe (e.g., Bowel sounds present within 24 hours; no abdominal distention; no vomiting), but these are not appropriate on an institutional care plan.

How Do I Use Standardized Terminology for Outcomes?

In Chapter 4, you learned about the NANDA-I standardized terminology for nursing diagnoses. The ANA has also approved several standardized vocabularies for describing client outcomes. The one used throughout most of this book is the Nursing Outcomes Classification (NOC) (Moorhead, Johnson, Maas, & Swanson, 2008).

What Is the Nursing Outcomes Classification (NOC)?

The NOC is a standardized vocabulary of more than 385 nursing-sensitive outcomes developed by a research team at the University of Iowa. In the NOC vocabulary, an **outcome** is "an individual, family, or community state, behavior, or perception that is measured along a continuum in response to nursing interventions" (Moorhead et al., 2008, p. 35). Thus, the NOC is versatile because it is appropriate for use in all specialty and practice areas.

Components of an NOC Outcome

Each NOC outcome consists of an outcome label, indicators, and a measurement scale. The **outcome label** (usually referred to as "the outcome") is broadly stated (e.g., Decision Making, Mobility Level, Concentration). It is a neutral label (a variable), to allow for positive, negative, or no change in patient health status. Because NOC outcomes are linked to NANDA-I nursing diagnoses, you can look up a nursing diagnosis to see the list of outcomes suggested for it (Box 5-2). You can find suggested outcomes for each NANDA-I diagnosis in the NANDA/NIC/NOC "linkages" book (Johnson et al., 2006). You can find "Additional Associated Outcomes" for each diagnosis in Part IV of the *Nursing Outcomes Classification (NOC)* (Moorhead et al., 2008).

The **indicators** are the observable behaviors and states you can use to evaluate patient status. In Table 5-5 the indicators are in the first (left) column. The first one is "Identifies relevant information." This indicator is one way you could know that Decision Making (the broad outcome) was being achieved. For each outcome, you select the indicators that are appropriate to the patient. You can add to the list of indicators if necessary.

BOX 5-2 ■ Outcomes Linked to NANDA-I Diagnosis

Nursing Diagnosis
Situational Low Self-Esteem

Definition
Development of a negative perception of self-worth in response to a current situation (specify)

Suggested Outcomes
Adaptation to Physical Disability
Grief Resolution
Psychosocial Adjustment: Life Change
Self-Esteem

Sources: Johnson, M., Bulechek, G., Butcher, H., et al. (2006). *Nursing diagnoses, outcomes, & interventions: NANDA, NOC, and NIC linkages* (pp. 377–378). St. Louis, MO: C.V. Mosby, NANDA International (2007). *Nursing diagnoses: Definitions & classification 2007–2008.* Philadelphia: NANDA International, p. 189.

Additional Associated Outcomes
Abuse Recovery Status
Abuse Recovery: Emotional
Abuse Recovery: Physical
Abuse Recovery: Sexual
Anxiety Level
Body Image
Burn Recovery
Coping
Development: Late Adulthood
Development: Middle Adulthood
Development: Young Adulthood
Fear Level
Fear Level: Child
Neglect Recovery
Personal Autonomy
Role Performance
Stress Level

Source: Moorhead, S., Johnson, M., Maas, M., & Swanson, E. (2008). *Nursing outcomes classification* (4th ed.). St. Louis, MO: Mosby/Elsevier.

For each outcome, NOC has a 5-point **measurement scale** (the numbers in Table 5-5) for describing patient status for each indicator. As a rule, 1 is least desirable and 5 is most desirable. If you are using NOC, you do not need to write traditional goal statements. You simply write the label, choose the appropriate indicators, and assign a number from the measurement scale. In your initial assessment, you assign the number that represents the patient's present health status. To form

Table 5-5 ➤ Example of a NOC Outcome

Decision Making (0906)

Domain—Physiologic Health (II)

Class—Neurocognitive (J)

Scale(s)—Severely compromised to Not compromised

Definition: Ability to make judgments and choose between two or more alternatives

DECISION MAKING	SEVERELY COMPROMISED	SUBSTANTIALLY COMPROMISED	MODERATELY COMPROMISED	MILDLY COMPROMISED	NOT COMPROMISED
Overall Rating					
Identifies relevant information.	1	2	3	4	5
Identifies alternatives.	1	2	3	4	5
Identifies potential consequences of each alternative.	1	2	3	4	5
Identifies needed resources to support each alternative.	1	2	3	4	5
Identifies time frame necessary to support each alternative.	1	2	3	4	5
Identifies sequence necessary to support each alternative.	1	2	3	4	5
Recognizes contradiction with others' desires.	1	2	3	4	5
Acknowledges social context of the situation.	1	2	3	4	5
Acknowledges relevant legal implications.	1	2	3	4	5
Weighs alternatives.	1	2	3	4	5
Chooses among alternatives.	1	2	3	4	5

Source: Moorhead, S., Johnson, M., Maas, M., & Swanson, E. (2008). *Nursing outcomes classification* (4th ed.). St. Louis, MO: Mosby/Elsevier.

the "goal," you assign the scale number that the patient can realistically achieve after the interventions. Using Table 5-5, you might assign the following numbers:

(NOC Outcome) **Decision Making**
Goals (Indicators + measurement scale)
Identifies relevant information (4, mildly compromised)
Identifies alternatives (4, mildly compromised)
Identifies potential consequences of each alternative (5, not compromised)

For a list of the NOC measurement scales,

 Go to Chapter 5, **Standardized Language,** in Volume 2.

KnowledgeCheck 5-6

Figure 5-4, a patient plan of care for Acute Pain, uses NOC language.

■ What outcomes did the nurse choose for this patient?
■ List two indicators for each of the outcomes.

■ For which outcome does the nurse expect the highest level of functioning to occur after interventions? (Note that in this care plan the measuring scale has been applied to the outcomes rather than to the indicators.)

 Go to Chapter 5, **Knowledge Check Response Sheet and Answers,** on the Student Resource Disk or DavisPlus at http://davisplus.fadavis.com/Wilkinson2.

 Critical**Thinking** 5-4

In Figure 5-4, what do you think the nurse expects to happen? Why do you think she ranked the outcomes this way?

Using NOC with Computerized Care Plans

Standardized language (e.g., NOC) is especially useful in computerized care systems. To see computer screens for locating and choosing NOC outcomes and for choosing NOC indicators, respectively,

 Go to Chapter 5, **Tables, Boxes, Figures: ESG Figures 5-4 and 5-5,** on the Student Resource Disk or DavisPlus at http://davisplus.fadavis.com/Wilkinson2

In those figures, the nurse chose Circulation Status as a patient outcome, and the program provided the definition and the NOC indicators for that outcome. The nurse would then check the indicators that apply to the patient.

Remember that the computer does not think for you. You are responsible for deciding which outcomes and indicators to use for each patient, and for identifying a target time. Most electronic health records have a screen that allows you to type in your own goals as well.

How Do I Write Goals for Groups?

Home and community health nurses are especially likely to write goals for aggregates (groups), such as families and communities. **Community health goals (public health goals)** are those you would use to specify and evaluate the health of groups, aggregates, or populations. They tend to emphasize health promotion, health maintenance, and disease prevention outcomes. For example, the U.S. Public Health Service (USPHS) has proposed four group goals—the following broad, over-arching goals for improving the health of the nation by a target date of 2020 (*Healthy People 2020*):

- Attain high quality, longer lives free of preventable disease, disability, injury, and premature death.
- Achieve health equity, eliminate disparities, and improve the health of all groups.
- Create social and physical environments that promote good health for all.
- Promote quality of life, healthy development and healthy behaviors across all life stages.

NOC currently includes 10 outcomes targeted to Community Health, which they define as "outcomes that describe the health, well-being, and functioning of a community or population" (Moorhead et al., 2008, pp. 142–143). Two examples are Community Competence and Community Risk Control: Lead Exposure. NOC also has 14 outcomes that describe the health of a family as a unit. Two examples are Family Coping and Family Health Status. NOC outcomes can be used in all settings, including home and community nursing. For further explanation, see Chapters 42 and 43. Also, search for Nursing Outcomes Classification on the Web or

 Go to the NOC Web site at http://www.nursing.uiowa.edu/excellence/nursing_knowledge/clinical_effectiveness/index.htm

The following taxonomies were created specifically for describing family and community outcomes.

The Clinical Care Classification (CCC). The CCC system was developed by Virginia Saba, a nurse researcher from Georgetown University, for use in home health nursing. In the CCC, you form goals by adding modifiers to the nursing diagnoses. This system has four nursing diagnoses that are clearly for family units:

Family Coping Impairment
Compromised Family Coping

Disabled Family Coping
Family Processes Alteration

The CCC includes one diagnosis specifically for communities: Community Coping Impairment. For a complete description of the CCC system,

 Go to the CCC Web site at http://www.sabacare.com

The Omaha System. The Omaha System was developed specifically for community health nursing. In that system, you must label all nursing diagnoses as either *individual, family,* or *group.* You can write aggregate outcomes by specifying a *family* or *group* diagnosis and then creating a goal from it, by using terms in a "Problem Rating Scale for Outcomes," as in the following example.

Omaha Nursing Diagnosis: Personal Hygiene. Family. Deficit (Actual Problem)

Present status	*Expected outcome*
Minimal knowledge of family personal hygiene	Adequate knowledge of family personal hygiene

For a complete description of the Omaha System, and to see the "Problem Rating Scale for Outcomes,"

 Go to the Omaha System Web site at http://www.omahasystem.org

KnowledgeCheck 5-7

- Which standardized classification system was designed specifically for community health nursing?
- Which standardized classification system was designed specifically for home healthcare?
- Which standardized classification system was designed for use in all areas and specialties of nursing?

 Go to Chapter 5, **Knowledge Check Response Sheet and Answers,** on the Student Resource Disk or DavisPlus at http://davisplus.fadavis.com/Wilkinson2

How Do I Write Goals for Wellness Diagnoses?

Whether standardized or individualized, expected outcomes for wellness diagnoses describe behaviors or responses that demonstrate health maintenance or achievement of an even higher level of health. For example: Over the next year, [Mr. Needham] will continue to eat a balanced diet with more emphasis on including whole grains and fiber. By using the highest number (5) on the rating scale, you can use the NOC to write wellness outcomes. For example:

Nursing diagnosis: Readiness for Enhanced Nutrition
Expected outcome: Nutritional Status: (5) Not compromised

In addition, many NOC outcomes can be used to measure health (e.g., Activity Tolerance, Child Development,

Growth, Nutritional Status). See Chapter 41 or go to the NOC Web site for a complete list of wellness outcomes.

Outcomes for Special Teaching Plans

As discussed earlier, some patients need a special teaching plan to address learning needs. Expected outcomes are written in the same way as on any other type of care plan, but they are usually called teaching objectives. **Teaching objectives** describe what the patient is to learn and the observable behaviors that will demonstrate learning, and they should state whether learning is to be cognitive, psychomotor, or affective. An example of a cognitive objective is: "By May 1, will list four foods to avoid on a low-fat diet." An example of an affective objective is: "By May 1, will verbalize feeling less anger about diet limitations." An example of a psychomotor goal is: "By May 1, will demonstrate how to use grasp extender to obtain food from the top shelf." For further information about teaching objectives, see Chapter 24.

Reflecting Critically About Expected Outcomes/Goals

After writing the expected outcomes for a client, use the full-spectrum nursing model to help you evaluate their quality. Use the following questions as a guide.
For each nursing diagnosis:

1. *Is there at least one goal that, when met, would demonstrate problem resolution;* that is, does at least one goal flow from the problem clause? (See "Essential versus Nonessential Goals" in this chapter.)
2. *Do the predicted outcomes completely address the nursing diagnosis?* If you have written outcomes in very specific, measurable terms, you may need several for a single nursing diagnosis. Notice in Table 5-3, that none of the outcomes, alone, would demonstrate that the problem of Ineffective Airway Clearance had been resolved. All of those outcomes are important; the ones in bold print are essential.

For each expected outcome:

3. *Is the outcome appropriate for the nursing diagnosis?* In Table 5-3, for example, "Obtains 8 hrs sleep at night" would not be an appropriate outcome for the nursing diagnosis Ineffective Airway Clearance, because it does not flow from either the problem or etiology clause. It may seem related because Ineffective Airway Clearance would probably cause Disturbed Sleep Pattern. If so, a new nursing diagnosis should be written rather than adding a not-quite-related goal to the existing plan.
4. *Is each outcome derived from only one nursing diagnosis?* That is, does it describe only one patient response? Notice that in the following incorrect example, even though diarrhea may cause excoriation of perianal skin, obtaining a good skin outcome would not tell you anything about the status of the Diarrhea diagnosis.

Incorrect:
For a diagnosis of Diarrhea: Will have no diarrhea in the next 12 hours, and skin will be intact and without redness in the perianal area.

Correct:
For a diagnosis of Diarrhea: Will have no diarrhea in the next 12 hours.

For a diagnosis of Impaired Skin Integrity: Skin will remain intact and without redness in the perianal area.

5. *Does each outcome describe only one patient response or behavior?* Look at the "correct" example in (4), above, for the Impaired Skin Integrity diagnosis. How many patient responses does it contain? Notice that it has two responses: skin will remain intact, and skin will not be red. So our "correct" example meets criteria for (4) but not for (5).

Critical Thinking 5-5

Why is it not a good idea to write the Skin Integrity outcome as shown in (4)?

6. *Is the outcome stated as a patient behavior, not a nurse activity?*

Incorrect (nurse activity): Prevent skin irritation
Correct (patient response): Skin will not show signs of irritation

7. *Is the outcome stated in positive terms?* When possible, state what you intend to occur, rather than what should not occur. For example:

Positive wording:	Incision edges approximated
	Incision dry
Negative wording:	No incision drainage
	No redness of incision

This is not always possible, especially for potential problems. It is better, for example, to write "No redness" (even though it is negative) than to write "Skin color normal," because "normal" is too vague. For potential problems, a negatively worded outcome is actually a list of the patient responses you are trying to prevent.

8. *Is the outcome measurable or observable?*

Correct: *Explains* the actions and side effects of Coumadin, by 8/11
Incorrect: *Understands* the actions and side effects of Coumadin, by 8/11

There is no way to observe someone's understanding, so you could not use the second (incorrect) goal to evaluate client progress. Use action verbs; think, "What do I want to see, hear, feel, or smell?"

9. *Are the performance criteria specific and concrete?* Avoid words such as *normal, sufficient, enough, more, less, adequate, increased.* Vague words can be interpreted differently by different people. Does "*adequate* sleep" mean that the patient will sleep 8 hours per night,

will fall asleep within an hour of going to bed, will feel rested in the morning, or will not become sleepy during the day?

10. *Does each goal include all the necessary parts?* Is there a subject (implied or actual), action verb, performance criterion, target time, and special condition (when needed)?

11. *Is the expected outcome realistic and achievable by this patient, given the available resources?* The outcome "Will rest for an hour twice a day" may not be realistic for a single mother with several small children and no help at home. People usually will not work toward goals unless they believe they are possible to achieve.

Be sure to consider the patient's support system, financial status, available community services, and physical and mental status. Also consider whether institutional resources are adequate. For example, there is no point in writing, "Will express anxieties and questions freely to the nurse" if staffing is inadequate to allow the nurse to spend enough time with the patient to develop a relationship.

12. *Does the outcome conflict with the medical or other collaborative treatment plan?* For example, an outcome of "Will attempt to breastfeed the newborn within the first 2 hours after birth" would not be compatible with the medical treatment plan for a new mother with severe preeclampsia, who is sleepy and lethargic from the side effects of medications.

13. *Does the patient, family, or community value the outcome?* The care plan is more likely to be effective if the goal is important to the client. You may, for example, believe that smoking cessation is an important goal for the patient. However, a patient who has been smoking for 20 years and is having only moderate breathing difficulties might not be motivated to achieve this goal, even when given all the related information. When your goals conflict with the patient's, explore the patient's reasoning. Explain your reasoning and try to find a compromise or an alternative approach.

14. *Does the goal conflict with any religious or cultural values?* You may know that early ambulation (e.g., "Ambulates to bathroom within 4 hours after birth of the baby") promotes circulation and helps to prevent thrombophlebitis. However, in some cultures, childbirth is viewed as an illness, and the mother expects to remain in bed for several days with family members taking care of her needs. When the mother is "noncompliant," the reason may be that she is complying with her cultural beliefs rather than the caregiver's plan of care.

KnowledgeCheck 5-8

List at least eight questions you could use to critically evaluate the quality of your goal/outcome statements.

 Go to Chapter 5, **Knowledge Check Response Sheet and Answers,** on the Student Resource Disk or DavisPlus at http://davisplus.fadavis.com/Wilkinson2

Toward Evidence-Based Practice

Scherb, C.A., Stevens, M. S., & Busman, C. (2007). Outcomes related to dehydration in the pediatric population. *Journal of Pediatric Nursing, 22*(5), 376–382.

The purpose of this pilot study was to: (1) determine whether there was a meaningful difference (in statistical terms) in nursing-sensitive patient outcome ratings from admission to discharge and (2) to describe nursing interventions used for children (younger than age 18 years) admitted with a primary diagnosis of dehydration. During the study period, researchers examined 29 patient care records that were a part of a computerized clinical documentation system in a Midwestern hospital. The documentation system used the standardized nursing languages of NANDA, NOC, and NIC.

Standardized care plans (also using NANDA, NOC, and NIC) were initiated upon a child's admission, and individualized as needed. NOC outcomes were rated upon admission and at discharge. Examples of outcomes on the care plan include: Nutritional Status, Fluid Balance, and Urinary Elimination. Of the eight outcomes on the care plan, seven had statistically significant changes (showing the child's improvement).

1. If you had to decide on the basis of this study alone, would you be for or against using standardized nursing languages for documentation and patient care plans in your organization? Explain your reasoning.

 Go to Chapter 5, **Toward Evidence-Based Practice Suggested Responses,** on the Student Resource Disk or DavisPlus at http://davisplus.fadavis.com/Wilkinson2

 Go to Chapter 5, **Resources for Caregivers and Health Professionals,** on the Student Resource Disk or DavisPlus at http://davisplus.fadavis.com/Wilkinson2

 Suggested Readings: Go to Chapter 5, **Reading More About Nursing Process: Planning Outcomes,** on the Student Resource Disk or DavisPlus at http://davisplus.fadavis.com/Wilkinson2

 VOL 2   Bibliography: Go to Volume 2, Bibliography.

CHAPTER 6

Nursing Process: Planning Interventions

Learning Outcomes

After completing this chapter, you should be able to:

➤ Define the term *nursing intervention*.

➤ Compare and contrast independent, dependent, and interdependent (collaborative) nursing interventions.

➤ Explain how theories and research influence the choice of nursing interventions.

➤ Explain how nursing interventions are determined by problem status (i.e., actual or potential problem).

➤ Describe a process for generating nursing interventions for a client.

➤ Explain how to use a standardized vocabulary for nursing interventions and activities.

➤ Give one example of a standardized wellness (health promotion) intervention and one individualized nursing order for performing that intervention.

➤ Give one example of a standardized spirituality intervention and one individualized nursing order for performing that intervention.

➤ Write complete, detailed nursing orders, in correct format, for patients.

➤ Give examples of some questions for reflecting critically about nursing orders you have written.

Meet Your Patient

Ben Ivanos, whom you met in Chapter 5, is confined to bed after a motorcycle accident. He has casts and traction for both legs and a cast on one arm. Since admission to the hospital 3 days ago, he has been receiving narcotic analgesics for severe pain. He has a new nursing diagnosis today: Constipation related to immobility and decreased gastrointestinal (GI) motility secondary to narcotic analgesics. The nurse enters the diagnosis into a care-planning program. In addition to a list of suggested assessments, the computer database generates the following list of suggested treatment interventions:

1. Institute a program to establish a regular pattern of bowel movements.
2. Administer laxative or stool softener, as ordered.
3. Administer enema.
4. Remove stool manually.
5. Encourage increased fluid intake, including warm liquids.
6. Instruct on and encourage a high-fiber diet.
7. Encourage a regular program of activity and exercise.
8. Perform manual reduction of rectal prolapse.

Which interventions should the nurse choose? Which can he eliminate, based on the information provided? You may not yet have enough nursing knowledge to be sure about your answers to these questions, but before reading on, try to think it through with the information and life experience available to you.

The nurse eliminated interventions 1, 3, 4, 7, and 8. Take a few moments to see if you can explain the nurse's reasons for deleting these interventions.

Theoretical **Knowledge** knowing why_____

Compare your explanations to the following reasons given by the nurse. The nurse eliminated intervention:

- **1** because it is useful for patients who are constipated as a result of irregular bowel habits, whereas Mr. Ivanos's problem is caused by immobility and narcotic side effects.
- **3 and 4** because Mr. Ivanos's symptoms did not seem severe enough to warrant an enema or manual removal of stool.
- **7** because it is not practical: Mr. Ivanos cannot exercise in his present condition.
- **8** because it is not relevant: Mr. Ivanos does not have rectal prolapse.

The nurse chose the following interventions to include in the care plan:

- **2** because it directly addresses the problem, Constipation.
- **5 and 6** because they address the etiology of the problem—fluid and fiber soften the stool and help to stimulate bowel activity.

The nurse also reasoned that because narcotics cause constipation, it would be good to administer them less frequently to Mr. Ivanos—if other satisfactory pain-relief measures could be found. So he added the following nursing orders to the care plan:

> Assist to change position every 1–2 hours.
> Encourage distraction (e.g., watching TV, reading, listening to music).
> Assist with relaxation and visualization techniques.
> Obtain medical order for nonnarcotic analgesics to enhance nonpharmacological pain-relief measures.
> Assess effectiveness of nonpharmacological interventions for pain.
> Give prescribed narcotic analgesics if other measures are ineffective.
> The nurse knows people are often self-conscious or embarrassed about using a bedpan, especially in the presence of others. So he also added to the care plan:
> Encourage Mr. Ivanos to summon the nurse when he feels the urge to defecate (place call light within reach). If he does not, then ask at least every 4 hr whether he needs the bedpan.
> Warm the bedpan and provide privacy: Pull the bed curtain; turn on the TV or radio if he has a roommate; explain that you will leave the room and that he should call when he is ready for you to return; and shut the door.

As you can see, to develop interventions to meet Mr. Ivanos's needs, the nurse needed to do more than just look at a list and follow physician orders. He thought critically about (1) his theoretical knowledge (of narcotics,

bowel elimination, and psychological needs), (2) his past experiences with similar patients, and (3) the patient situation (the data about Mr. Ivanos and the factors contributing to his problem). By thinking of interventions to meet the client's specific needs, this nurse may prevent Mr. Ivanos's constipation from worsening. A nurse with less knowledge and experience might have used only the interventions in the computer database, failing to effectively meet the desired outcomes (goals) for Mr. Ivanos.

What Are Nursing Interventions?

Nursing interventions are actions, based on clinical judgment and nursing knowledge, that nurses perform to achieve client outcomes. Interventions are also referred to as *nursing actions, measures, strategies,* and *activities.* This chapter uses those terms interchangeably except when referring to the Nursing Interventions Classification (NIC) standardized labels (discussed later in the chapter), which are always called *interventions.* Figure 6-1 shows how planning interventions relates to the other phases of the nursing process.

Nursing Interventions Reflect Direct and Indirect Care

No matter what term is used, nursing interventions include a broad range of activities. A **direct-care intervention** is one performed through interaction with the client(s). Direct-care activities include physical care, emotional support, and patient teaching. An **indirect-care intervention** is performed away from the client but on behalf of a client or group of clients. Indirect care activities include advocacy, managing the environment,

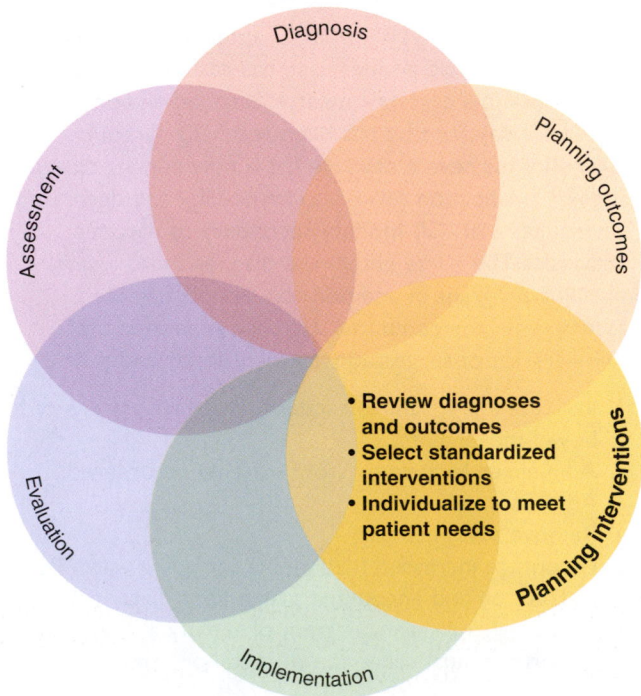

FIGURE 6-1 Nursing process phase: planning interventions.

consulting with other members of the healthcare team, and making referrals.

CriticalThinking 6-1

- Can you think of an example of a direct-care intervention?
- Can you think of an example of an indirect-care intervention?

Nursing Interventions Include Independent, Dependent, and Collaborative Actions

Nurses work collaboratively with other healthcare providers. Some things you do for patients will require a physician's order; many will not. Sometimes the activities of care providers overlap. For example, physicians, nurses, and respiratory therapists may all measure a client's blood pressure; and a nurse and a dietitian may both teach the client about a diet to help manage hypertension. Consider the following scenarios:

- *Nurse A makes a nursing diagnosis of Anxiety related to deficient knowledge about barium enema; she writes a nursing order to teach the patient what to expect from the upcoming diagnostic test.* This is an **independent intervention**—one that registered nurses are licensed to prescribe, perform, or delegate based on their knowledge and skills. It does not require a provider's order. Knowing how, when, and why to perform an activity makes the action **autonomous** (independent). As a rule, nurses prescribe and perform independent interventions in response to a nursing diagnosis. Understand you are **accountable** (answerable) for your decisions and actions with regard to nursing diagnoses and independent interventions. If patient teaching did not relieve the patient's anxiety in this example, it might be the nurse misdiagnosed or chose an ineffective intervention.

- *Nurse B reads a physician's prescription in a patient's chart: Give cephalothin sodium (Keflin) 1 g IV (through the intravenous line) before surgery, and then every 6 hours for 24 hours. She prepares and administers the medication.* This is a **dependent intervention**—one that is prescribed by a physician or advanced practice nurse but carried out by the bedside nurse. Dependent interventions are usually orders for diagnostic tests, medications, treatments, IV therapy, diet, and activity. In addition to carrying out medical orders, you will be responsible for assessing the need for the order, explaining the activities to the patient, and evaluating the effectiveness of the order. For example, after giving the Keflin (an antibiotic), Nurse B observes that the patient has developed a severe rash. Suspecting an allergic reaction, she contacts the physician so the prescription can be changed and antibiotic prophylaxis can be continued after surgery without danger to the patient.

  In addition, you may write nursing orders to individualize a medical order, based on the patient's condition. For example, the provider may prescribe, "Give oral fluids up to 3000 mL every 24 hours." You might individualize the order to give 1500 mL on the day shift, 1000 mL on the evening shift, and 500 mL during the night, so that the patient will not have to be awakened frequently during the night.

- *Nurse C notes that a client newly diagnosed with diabetes has been seen by a dietitian, who taught and provided materials about a diabetic diet. The nurse observes the client's menu choices. She notes that the client is eating candy brought by visitors. She explains to the client how concentrated sugar affects his diabetes; she also communicates her assessments and teaching to the dietitian.* This is an **interdependent (collaborative) intervention**—one that is carried out in collaboration with other health team members (e.g., physical therapists, dietitians, and physicians). Because nurses care for the whole person, their responsibilities often overlap with those of other team members.

CriticalThinking 6-2

- What are some other examples of independent interventions?
- What are some other examples of dependent interventions?
- What are some other examples of interdependent interventions?

How Do I Decide Which Interventions to Use?

Box 6-1 identifies professional standards of care related to planning interventions. Use these standards to guide you in selecting interventions appropriate for the client's nursing diagnoses (or collaborative problems) and the desired outcomes. In addition to these standards, a variety of theories, nursing research, and the client's problem status will all influence your choice of interventions.

As a nurse, you will be responsible for choosing nursing interventions. You cannot delegate this responsibility to nursing assistive personnel. As a rule, licensed practical/vocational nurses (LPN/LVNs) give care according to a plan created by the RN. In many situations, the LPN/LVN contributes to the plan by providing data or by giving feedback about the effectiveness of the interventions. For more information about delegation, see "What Should I Know About Delegation and Supervision?" in Chapter 7.

How Do Theories Influence My Choice of Interventions?

A **theory** is a set of interrelated concepts (ideas) that describes or explains something—nursing, for example. A theory, like a lens, influences your perspective: What you notice, what you consider to be a problem—and how you define a problem—more or less determine what you choose to do about it. For example, suppose a patient is pale and fidgeting and has sweaty palms and a rapid pulse. If you looked at this person through the lens of psychological theory, your first thought might be that the patient is anxious. Your first intervention, then, would probably be to assess for the cause of his anxiety. If you were using a physiological lens, you might suspect pain. Your first intervention, then, might be to ask the patient if he is having pain.

BOX 6-1 ■ Professional Standards for Planning Interventions

American Nurses Association Standards of Nursing Practice[1]

Standard 4. Planning

The registered nurse develops a plan that prescribes strategies and alternatives to attain expected outcomes.

Competencies

The registered nurse:

Develops in partnership with the person, family and others an individualized plan considering the person's characteristics or situation, including but not limited to, values, beliefs, spiritual and health practices, preferences, choices, developmental level, coping style, culture and environment and available technology.

Develops the plan in conjunction with the patient, family, and others, synthesizing patients values and beliefs, developmental level, and coping style.

Includes strategies in the plan of care that address each of the identified diagnoses or issues. These strategies may include, but are not limited to, strategies for promotion and restoration of health and prevention of illness, injury, and disease, the alleviation of suffering and provision of supportive care for those dying.

Provides for continuity within the plan.

Incorporates an implementation pathway or timeline within the plan.

Establishes the plan priorities with the patient, family, and others as appropriate.

Utilizes the plan to provide direction to other members of the healthcare team.

Defines the plan to reflect current statutes, rules and regulations, and standards.

Integrates current scientific evidence, trends and research affecting care in the planning process.

Considers the economic impact of the plan on the patient, family, caregivers, or other affected parties.

Documents the plan of care in a manner that uses standardized language or recognized terminology, and is understood by all participants.

Includes strategies for health, wholeness, and growth from infancy through old age.

Explores practice settings and safe space and time for both the nurse and person/family/significant others to explore suggested, potential and alternative options.

Modifies the plan based on the ongoing assessment of the patient's response and other outcome indicators.

Note: There are additional standards for advanced practice registered nurses.

Source: American Nurses Association (2010, in press). *Nursing: Scope and Standards of Practice* (2nd ed). Public Comment draft, January 2010. (To be published by August 2010.) Silver Spring, MD: Nursebooks.org.
[1]*Caveat:* This material is from the draft for public comment (ANA, 2010, in press); its wording may be changed somewhat in the final published version. For that version of the ANA Standards of Professional Nursing Practice, go to www.nursingworld.org.

Canadian Provincial Standards of Practice

In Canada, practice standards are set by each province. The following are examples that apply to planning interventions.

Province of Alberta

The registered nurse:

Demonstrates critical thinking in collecting and interpreting data, planning, implementing, and evaluating all aspects of nursing care.

Collaborates with the client/significant others and other members of the health-care team regarding activities of care planning, implementation and evaluation.

Sets justifiable priorities when giving care.

Source: College & Association of Registered Nurses of Alberta. (2003). *Nursing practice standards.* CARNA, 11620-168 Street, Edmonton, AB, Canada.

Province of British Nova Scotia

Application of Knowledge, Skills and Judgment

Each registered nurse:

Indicator 3.1—Applies a theoretical and/or evidence-based rationale for nursing decisions.

Indicator 3.2—Applies appropriate knowledge, skills and judgment to assess, plan, intervene and evaluate services, and revises plan as needed.

Source: College of Registered Nurses of Nova Scotia. (2003). *Standards for nursing practice.* Halifax, NS, Canada.

For more information about nursing theories, see Chapter 8.

How Does Nursing Research Influence My Choice of Interventions?

Although much nursing and medical practice is still based on tradition, experience, and professional opinion, these are not an ideal basis for choosing an intervention. Ideally, a nurse would choose an intervention on the basis of firm evidence that it is the best possible

approach for the patient. It stands to reason that such interventions would be those that were developed from a sound body of scientific research. American Nurses Association (ANA) Standards of Nursing Practice (ANA, 2010, in press, p. 45) state that the registered nurse:

- Utilizes current evidence-based nursing knowledge, including research findings, to guide practice decisions.
- Participates in the development of evidence-based practice through research activities. Participation levels occur appropriate to the nurse's education and position.

The ANA standards are expected to change soon after this book is published. This research standard will likely be expanded to emphasize evidence-based practice. To see if you have the most current standards,

 Go to http://www.nursingworld.org/ or http://www. nursingworld.org/MainMenuCategories/ThePracticeof ProfessionalNursing/NursingStandards.aspx

According to the Quality and Safety Education for Nurses (QSEN) group, one competency you should achieve in nursing school is to differentiate clinical opinion from research and evidence summaries. To see an expanded discussion of this competency,

 Go to the Cronenwett, et al. (2007) article, in **Reading More About Nursing Process: Interventions,** in Chapter 6 of the Student Resource Disk or DavisPlus at http:// davisplus.fadavis.com/Wilkinson2

Research-based support for an intervention includes single studies, critical pathways and protocols, clinical practice guidelines, systematic reviews of the literature, and evidence reports. In Chapter 8, you will learn how to ask "PICOT" questions that help you use evidence to decide which interventions to use.

Single Studies

It is not difficult to find individual studies that give you an idea of the effectiveness of an intervention. Research reports are available in research journals, and they are often interpreted and published in such widely circulated journals as the *American Journal of Nursing (AJN), Nursing,* and *RN,* as well as online sites. Unfortunately, there may be only one or two studies of an intervention, and they may have included only a small number of patients. Thus, single studies may not be reliable. To see several examples of single intervention studies,

 Go to Chapter 6, **Reading More About the Nursing Process: Planning Interventions,** on the Student Resource Disk or DavisPlus at http://davisplus.fadavis.com/Wilkinson2

Critical Pathways and Protocols

Critical pathways (also called *clinical pathways* and *collaborative care plans*) are standardized plans of care for frequently occurring conditions (e.g., total hip replacement) for which similar outcomes and interventions are appropriate for all patients who have the condition. They are tools developed by an organization for its own use and are intended to guide best practice at the local level. However, they may not be based on research if the practitioners who develop them are reluctant to change traditional practices they believe to be effective. Furthermore, issues of cost to the organization influence the decision to include an intervention in the plan of care. Nevertheless, critical pathways provide a guide for nursing interventions in that, at the very least, they have been developed on the basis of expert opinion. See Chapter 5 for discussion and examples of critical pathways and protocols.

What Is Evidence-Based Practice?

You can feel more confident about an intervention if several studies have supported it. **Evidence-based practice (EBP)** is an approach that uses firm scientific data rather than anecdote, tradition, intuition, or folklore in making decisions about medical and nursing practice. In nursing it includes blending clinical judgment and expertise with the best available research evidence and patient characteristics and preferences. The goal of evidence-based practice is to identify the most effective and cost-efficient treatments for a particular disease, condition, or problem.

Steps in the EBP process include the following:

- Formulating an answerable question about prevention, diagnosis, prognosis (likely outcome), and interventions
- Conducting a systematic review of published evidence (research) to find studies that shed light on the desired topic
- Evaluating or grading the quality of the evidence obtained. Quality involves validity (closeness to the truth), applicability (usefulness), and impact (extent of the effect). Figure 6-2 lists evidence from strongest to weakest. For more information about "levels of evidence," or how evidence is evaluated,

 Go to **Supplemental Materials, Levels of Evidence,** on the Student Resource Disk or DavisPlus at http:// davisplus.fadavis.com/Wilkinson2

- Compiling and analyzing the data to prepare a structured report of the review
- "Translating" the evidence into guidelines for practice
- Integrating the guidelines and evidence with clinical expertise and the patient's preferences and characteristics

A number of healthcare organizations and groups are devoted to compiling study results that provide evidence to use in formulating guidelines for medical and nursing practice. Online examples include The Joanna Briggs

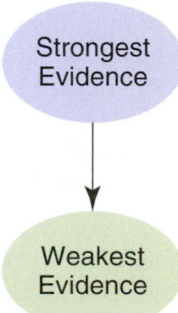

- Meta-analysis of randomized clinical trials
- Individual randomized clinical trials
- Individual cohort study
- Outcomes research
- Individual case-control study
- Case studies
- Expert opinion

Strongest Evidence

Weakest Evidence

FIGURE 6-2 **Hierarchy of research evidence.** (*Source:* Courtesy of Fain, J. A. (2008). *Reading, understanding, and applying nursing research: A text and workbook* (3rd ed., p. 279). Philadelphia: F. A. Davis.)

Institute and the Cochrane Database of Systematic Reviews. You will find such compiled information in clinical practice guidelines, evidence reports, and sometimes in local healthcare agency tools (e.g., clinical pathways and protocols). One example of a compilation of research is found in the March 2003 supplement to the *American Journal of Nursing,* titled "State of the Science on Urinary Incontinence," which is a report from a symposium on incontinence (Newman & Palmer, 2003). For full discussion on the importance of research and evidence-based nursing practice, see Chapter 8.

Evidence Reports

Evidence reports are state-of-the-art, systematic reviews of clinical topics for the purpose of providing evidence for practice guidelines, quality improvement, quality measures, and insurance coverage decisions (Cronenwett, 2002). Evidence reports are usually developed by scientists rather than clinicians, patients, and advocacy groups. Two sources of such reports are (1) the Registered Nurses' Association of Ontario, Canada and (2) the Evidence-Based Practice Center (EPC) Program of the federal Agency for Healthcare Research and Quality (AHRQ). The EPC uses explicit grading systems to review studies and rank the strength of their evidence. For free access to online reviews,

 Go to the AHRQ Web site at http://www.ahrq.gov/

Clinical Practice Guidelines

Evidence reports often form the basis for developing clinical practice guidelines. **Clinical practice guidelines** are systematically developed statements to assist practitioners and patients in making decisions about appropriate healthcare for a particular disease or procedure (Institute of Medicine, 1992). Clinical practice guidelines are usually developed by clinicians, patients, and advocacy groups and are published by specialty organizations, universities, and government agencies. The following are examples:

- The Joanna Briggs Institute (Australia) guidelines on *Topical Skin Care in Aged Care Facilities* (2007)
- University of Iowa research-based guidelines for care of the elderly (Titler, Mentes, Rakel, et al., 1999)
- National Guideline Clearinghouse, initiative of the Agency for Healthcare Research and Quality (AHRQ), U.S. Department of Health and Human Services, is a comprehensive database of guidelines for health professionals (http://www.guideline.gov/)

Clinical practice guidelines form the basis for nursing interventions. One example of clinical practice guidelines is found in Box 6-2. For years, relying on conventional wisdom and word of mouth, nurses tried to prevent pressure ulcers by writing on care plans: "Massage skin over bony prominences." They reasoned that because poor circulation can contribute to the formation of

BOX 6-2 ■ Portion of a Clinical Practice Guideline on Pressure Ulcer Formation

Skin Care and Early Treatment*

Note: This portion of the practice guideline addresses only the interventions related to skin care and early treatment. Other portions of the guideline address positioning, mattresses, education, and other factors contributing to pressure ulcer formation.

Goal: Maintain and improve tissue tolerance to pressure in order to prevent injury.

A. All individuals at risk should have a systematic skin inspection at least once a day, paying particular attention to the bony prominences. Results of skin inspection should be documented. (Strength of evidence = C)

B. Skin assessment should occur at the time of soiling and at routine intervals. . . . Avoid hot water. . . . [and] minimize the force and friction applied to the skin. (Strength of evidence = C)

C. Minimize environmental factors leading to skin drying, such as low humidity (less than 40 percent) and exposure to cold. Dry skin should be treated with moisturizers. (Strength of evidence = C)

D. Avoid massage over bony prominences. . . current evidence suggests this may be harmful. (Strength of evidence = B)

Note: "Strength of evidence" is an AHRQ ranking of the amount and quality of research supporting the guideline. The best ranking is A.

_____

Source: Agency for Healthcare Research and Quality, National Institutes for Health. (2002). Clinical practice guideline. Pressure ulcer formation: Skin care and early treatment. http://hstat.nlm.nih.gov/hq/Hquest/screen/TextBrowse/t/1030737344857/s/58838
   Also available from http://www.ncbi.nlm.nih.gov/books/bv.fcgi?rid=hstat

pressure ulcers, improving circulation to the area would prevent them. But as you can see in item D of the box, research-based practice guidelines show that massage may actually be harmful. This report would certainly motivate you, as a full-spectrum nurse, to remove this "standard" intervention from your practice.

Knowledge Check 6-1

- Explain how theory influences your choice of nursing interventions.
- Why does a clinical practice guideline provide better support for an intervention than does a single study?
- Why does a clinical practice guideline provide better support for an intervention than does an agency's critical pathway?

 Go to Chapter 6, **Knowledge Check Response Sheet and Answers,** on the Student Resource Disk or DavisPlus at http://davisplus.fadavis.com/Wilkinson2

How Does Problem Status Influence Nursing Interventions?

Nursing interventions include activities for observation/assessment, prevention, treatment, and health promotion. As you can see in Table 6-1, the status of the problem (i.e., whether it is a collaborative problem or an actual, potential, possible, or wellness nursing diagnosis) determines which types of activities are required (for a review of problem status, see Chapter 4).

A nursing strategy can be a preventive measure in one situation and a treatment in another. For example, you might write the nursing order, "Refer to a lactation consultant for breastfeeding assistance," to treat a woman with an actual diagnosis of Ineffective Breastfeeding or to help prevent the problem for a woman with a diagnosis of Risk for Ineffective Breastfeeding.

KnowledgeCheck 6-2

Review problem status (actual, potential, or possible nursing diagnosis; collaborative problem; or wellness diagnosis) in Chapter 4. For which type(s) of problem(s) would you write:

- Nursing orders for observation/assessments?
- Nursing orders for treatments?
- Nursing orders for health promotion interventions?
- Preventive nursing orders?

 Go to Chapter 6, **Knowledge Check Response Sheet and Answers,** on the Student Resource Disk or DavisPlus at http://davisplus.fadavis.com/Wilkinson2

What Process Can I Use for Generating and Selecting Interventions?

As you can see from the case of Ben Ivanos, there are usually several nursing measures that might be effective for any one problem. The idea, of course, is to select those most likely to achieve the desired goals. In doing that, you must consider the patient's abilities and preferences; the education, experience, and capabilities of the nursing staff; the resources available (e.g., time, equipment); medical orders; and institutional policies and procedures. When generating interventions, you will use critical thinking skills. For example, imagine you are caring for a hospice patient who has cancer and is dying. She has told you that she is experiencing significant pain, but also that she wants to spend her last hours with her husband and two daughters, who are

Table 6-1 ➤ Relationship of Problem Status to Intervention Type				
PROBLEM STATUS	**INTERVENTION TYPE**			
	Observation	**Prevention**	**Treatment**	**Health Promotion**
Actual nursing diagnosis	To detect change in status (improvement, exacerbation of problem)	To help keep the problem from becoming worse	To relieve symptoms and resolve etiologies (contributing factors)	
Potential (risk) nursing diagnosis	To detect (1) progression to an actual problem or (2) an increase or decrease in risk factors	To remove or reduce risk factors in an effort to keep the problem from developing		
Possible nursing diagnosis	To obtain more data to confirm or rule out a suspected nursing diagnosis			
Collaborative problem	To detect onset of a complication for early physician notification	To implement nursing and medical orders to help prevent development of a complication	To implement nursing and medical orders for relieving or eliminating the underlying condition for which complications may develop	
Wellness diagnosis	To assess a client's wellness practices	To prevent specific diseases (e.g., giving immunizations)	Clients usually manage their own wellness treatment.	To support a client's health promotion efforts and achieve a higher level of wellness

staying with her. Critical thinking skills you might use include the following:

- Making interdisciplinary connections (e.g., "What did I learn in psychology class that might help me here?")
- Predicting (e.g., "If I give morphine to the patient, it should relieve her pain, but she will probably become drowsy.")
- Generalizing (e.g., "I have used touch to relieve anxiety many times in similar situations; perhaps it will also help for this patient.")
- Explaining (e.g., "The morphine causes drowsiness by depressing the central nervous system.")
- Therapeutic judgment (e.g., "The patient wants to spend quality time with her family before she dies. Because the morphine will make her drowsy, I should find out if she wants me to give a smaller dose, even though it will not provide good pain relief, along with some nonpharmacological measures.")

You must always rethink an intervention for each patient. You cannot assume a strategy that was useful in the past will be effective in every situation. In the "Meet Your Patient" scenario, Mr. Ivanos's nurse may have used distraction successfully to relieve the pain of other patients in the past. However, if Mr. Ivanos has severe pain, or if he has difficulty concentrating, then distraction may not be effective. A full-spectrum nurse takes such details into account before choosing an intervention. The following process will help you to select the best interventions (Wilkinson, 2007):

1. Review the nursing diagnosis.
2. Review the desired patient outcomes.
3. Identify several interventions or actions.
4. Choose the best interventions for the patient.
5. Individualize standardized interventions to meet the patient's unique needs.

Review the Nursing Diagnosis

The etiology of a nursing diagnosis describes the factors that contribute to the unhealthy response. Choose strategies you expect will reduce or remove the etiological factors of actual problems, or that will reduce or remove risk factors for potential problems.

- When it is not possible to change the etiology, choose strategies to treat the patient's symptoms (the "A.M.B" part of a diagnosis referred to in Chapter 4). For example, if the cause of pain is a surgical incision, you cannot suddenly "cure" the incision. Your nursing actions should focus on measures to relieve the pain.
- You may not always know the etiology of the problem. However, some interventions may relieve a problem regardless of its cause. For example, when you have a client with Anxiety, regardless of its cause, it is helpful to approach the patient calmly; and when you have a client with Constipation, regardless of its cause, it is always appropriate to assess the frequency

of the bowel movements and the characteristics of the stool. Consider the nursing diagnosis and interventions for Mr. Ivanos in Figure 6-3.

Obviously, some people with constipation do not have pain. The pain-relief nursing order, which flows from the etiology of the problem, is specific to Mr. Ivanos's needs. Administering a stool softener and laxative, however, is a common strategy for constipation, whatever its cause. As a rule, standardized interventions (care common to all patients with a particular condition) flow from the problem side of a nursing diagnosis; individualized interventions, from the etiology.

Critical Thinking 6-3

For the following nursing diagnoses, write one intervention to address the problem and one for the etiology of the problem.

- Ineffective Airway Clearance r/t thick secretions and decreased chest expansion secondary to dehydration and pain
- Self-Care Deficit: Bathing/Hygiene and Dressing/Grooming r/t fatigue secondary to disturbed sleep pattern

Review the Desired Patient Outcomes

Desired outcomes (goals) suggest nursing strategies that are specific to the individual patient. For example, Table 6-2 shows some goals and outcomes for Mr. Ivanos's Constipation diagnosis. For each goal on the care plan, ask "What intervention(s) will help to produce this patient response?"

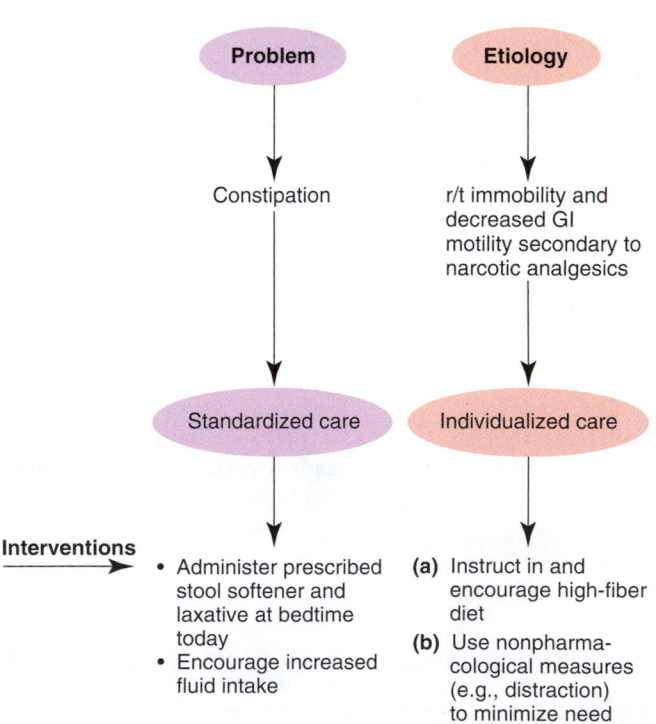

FIGURE 6-3 Nursing interventions flow from the nursing diagnosis.

Table 6-2 ➤ Interventions Flow from Desired Outcomes

GOALS/OUTCOMES	STRATEGIES SUGGESTED BY GOALS
1. Will have bowel movement within 12 hours after receiving stool softener and laxative.	**A. Administer prescribed stool softener and laxative at bedtime today.**
2. Will have daily soft, formed bowel movement during rest of hospital stay.	B. Instruct in and encourage high-fiber diet. C. Encourage increased fluid intake.
3. <u>Within 24 hours, will need narcotics to manage pain < 2×/day.</u>	D. <u>Use nonpharmacological measures (e.g., distraction) to minimize need for narcotics.</u>
4. *Calls nurse when urge to defecate is felt; does not delay defecation.*	E. *Encourage Mr. Ivanos to summon the nurse when he feels the urge to defecate.* F. *Provide privacy (e.g., pull the bed curtain, turn on the TV, leave room).*

Note: Dotted lines indicate indirect contribution to goal.

Strategy A in Table 6-2 would help to achieve goal 1; but because the effects of these medications are short lived, it would do nothing to achieve goals 2 through 4.

Strategies B and C both help to achieve goal 2.

Strategy D (minimize narcotics), in contrast, directly addresses goal 3 and indirectly helps to achieve goal 2.

Strategies E and F both directly address goal 4 and indirectly address goal 2.

As you can see, there may be one or more interventions for each goal, and a single intervention may help to achieve more than one goal. There is no strict one-to-one correspondence between goals and interventions.

Identify Several Interventions or Actions

The next step in choosing interventions is to think of several nursing activities that might achieve the desired outcomes. Don't try to narrow your list at this point; include unusual and creative ideas. You can refer to a standardized list of interventions (e.g., the Nursing Interventions Classification list on your Electronic Study Guide) or choose interventions from standardized care plans and agency protocols. Alternatively, you can generate the interventions yourself, based on your knowledge; experience; and use of nursing texts, journal articles, and professional nurses. To get started, ask yourself: For this nursing diagnosis, (1) What assessments/observations do I need to make? (2) What do I need to do for the patient? Include both dependent and independent activities as appropriate.

Choose the Best Interventions for the Patient

The best interventions are those you expect to be most effective in helping to achieve client goals. When possible, choose interventions based on research and scientific principles. Use the following critical-thinking questions from the full-spectrum nursing model (in Chapter 2) to help you determine the best actions.

Contextual awareness

- Is this intervention acceptable to the client (e.g., congruent with the patient's values and wishes)?
- Is this intervention culturally sensitive?
- What is going on in the patient's life (e.g., family, work situation, financial status) that may enhance or interfere with the effectiveness of the intervention?
- What is going on in the patient's health status (e.g., knowledge, abilities, resources, severity of illness) that may enhance or interfere with the effectiveness of the intervention?

Credible sources

- Have I used valid, reliable sources of information to identify this intervention (e.g., patient, other professionals, references)?
- Did I consider professional, ethical, and legal standards?
- What is the research basis for this intervention, if any?

Considering alternatives

- Is there adequate rationale for this intervention (e.g., principles, theory, facts)?
- Which action(s) is (are) most reasonable? Why are the others not as reasonable?
- Which action(s) is (are) most likely to achieve stated goals?

Analyzing assumptions

- What beliefs, values, or biases do I have that may affect my thinking and my choice of interventions?
- Do I feel any discomfort with this intervention?

Reflecting skeptically

- Are there other interventions I have overlooked?
- What might be the consequences of this intervention? —"What will happen if . . .?"

— Does it have any potential ill effects? If so, how will we manage them?

- Is this intervention feasible (e.g., is it cost-effective, are the time and personnel available for it, can the patient or family manage it at home?)
- How will the intervention interact with medical orders (e.g., you cannot order "elevate head of bed" to facilitate breathing if there is a medical order to keep the patient flat to improve circulation to the neck and head.)
- In priority order, what should I do in this situation and why?
- Do I have the knowledge and skills needed for the intervention, or do I need to consult with someone more qualified in this area?
- What might I delegate in this situation?

Individualize Standardized Interventions

Practice guidelines, systematic reviews of the literature, protocols, critical pathways, and even textbooks describe interventions that are appropriate for most people or the average person. However, they cannot take into account all the individual factors that contribute to a problem or that might affect the effectiveness of an intervention. You must always consider how an intervention can be used with a particular person. For example, after Ben Ivanos's nurse decided which of the computer-generated list of interventions to use, he adapted them to fit Ben's unique needs and preferences. Table 6-3 provides examples of standardized and individualized interventions for Mr. Ivanos.

KnowledgeCheck 6-3

Describe a five-step process for generating and choosing nursing interventions.

Go to Chapter 6, **Knowledge Check Response Sheet and Answers,** on the Student Resource Disk or DavisPlus at http://davisplus.fadavis.com/Wilkinson2

Computer-Generated Interventions

Most computerized care planning programs will generate a list of suggested interventions when you enter either a problem (nursing diagnosis, medical, collaborative) or an outcome (Fig. 6-4). You then choose the interventions appropriate for the patient (as in the case of Ben Ivanos) or type in nursing actions of your own. Computer prompts provide a wide range of interventions for your consideration. However, you must resist the temptation to "settle for" the ready-made solutions. Always look for other, perhaps more effective, strategies based on the patient data. Always think, "Are there other interventions I have overlooked? How should I adapt this for *this* patient?"

To see a computer screen showing how an intervention (Pain Control Techniques Education) is converted to nursing orders,

Table 6-3 ➤ Individualizing Nursing Actions for Ben Ivanos	
STANDARDIZED INTERVENTIONS	**INDIVIDUALIZED NURSING ORDERS**
1. Encourage increased fluid intake.	1. Remind patient to drink a glass of water every hour; also keep ice and tea available at the bedside.
2. Instruct on and encourage a high-fiber diet.	2. Assist with menu choices to obtain more fiber; encourage family to bring salads and fruits from home for snacks.
3. Encourage distraction (e.g., watching TV, reading, listening to music).	3. Provide books from hospital library (he does not enjoy TV); have family bring radio or CD player and headphones from home.
4. Give prescribed narcotic analgesics if other measures are ineffective.	4. Give Tylenol #3 every 4 hr if relaxation, visualization, and distraction are not effective. If orally administered Tylenol #3 is not effective, advise patient to administer IV morphine via patient-controlled analgesia pump.

Go to Chapter 6, **Tables, Boxes, Figures: ESG Figure 6-1,** on the Student Resource Disk or DavisPlus at http://davisplus.fadavis.com/Wilkinson2

How Can I Use Standardized Language to Plan Interventions?

As a review before reading this section, you may wish to do the following:

- See Chapter 4 for a discussion of standardized language to describe nursing diagnoses (NANDA-I).
- See Chapter 5 for a discussion of standardized language to describe patient outcomes (NOC).

Recall that standardized nursing terminologies are important for electronic health records (EHR), for research, and for clear, precise, consistent communication among nurses and with other disciplines. The American Nurses Association (ANA) has recognized 12 standardized vocabularies for recording and tracking the clinical care process (American Nurses Association/Nursing Information & Data Set Evaluation Center [ANA/NIDSEC], 2002). Those most commonly used for describing nursing interventions are the Nursing Interventions Classification (NIC), the Clinical Care Classification (CCC), and the Omaha System. NIC classifies only interventions. The CCC and the Omaha System include nursing diagnoses, outcomes, and interventions.

FIGURE 6-4 Computer care planning: When the nurse selects a nursing diagnosis of Sleep Pattern Disturbance, the computer database generates a list of suggested goals and "procedure options" (interventions); the nurse then chooses those best suited for the patient. *(Source:* Copyright © Ergo Partners, L.C. All rights reserved. Used with permission.)

What Is the Nursing Interventions Classification?

Developed by a research team at the University of Iowa, the Nursing Interventions Classification (NIC) was the first comprehensive standardized classification of nursing interventions (McCloskey & Bulechek, 1992). The fifth edition NIC (Bulechek, Butcher, & Dochterman, 2008) describes 542 direct and indirect-care activities performed by nurses. The NIC is versatile—appropriate for use in all specialty and practice areas, including home health and community nursing.

Each NIC intervention consists of a label, a definition, and a list of the specific **activities** nurses perform in carrying out the intervention (Box 6-3). The **label,** usually consisting of two or three words, is the standardized terminology. The **definition** explains the meaning of the label. You are free to word the activities any way you choose in a care plan or client record. For a complete list of NIC intervention labels and definitions,

 Go to **NIC Interventions** on the Student Resource Disk or DavisPlus at http://davisplus.fadavis.com/Wilkinson2

Locating Appropriate NIC Interventions and Activities

NIC interventions are linked to NANDA-I nursing diagnoses and NOC outcome labels in a "linkages" book, *Nursing Diagnoses, Outcomes, and Interventions: NANDA, NOC, and NIC Linkages,* or, more simply, the NNN linkages book (Johnson, Bulechek, Butcher, et al., 2006). In

---

BOX 6-3 ■ NIC Intervention: Bathing

Definition

Cleaning of the body for the purposes of relaxation, cleanliness, and healing

Activities

Assist with chair shower, tub bath, bedside bath, standing shower, or sitz bath, as appropriate or desired.

Wash hair, as needed and desired.

Bathe in water of a comfortable temperature.

Use fun bathing techniques with children (e.g., wash dolls or toys; pretend a boat is a submarine; punch holes in bottom of plastic cup, fill with water, and let it "rain" on child).

Assist with perineal care, as needed.

Assist with hygiene measures (e.g., use of deodorant or perfume).

Administer foot soaks, as needed.

Shave patient, as indicated.

Apply lubricating ointment and cream to dry skin areas.

Offer hand washing after toileting and before meals.

Apply drying powders to deep skin folds.

Monitor skin condition while bathing.

Monitor functional ability while bathing.

Source: Bulechek, B. M., Butcher, H. K., & Dochterman, J. M. (Eds.). (2008). *Nursing interventions classification (NIC)* (5th ed.). St. Louis, MO: C.V. Mosby, p. 153. Used with permission from Elsevier Science.

this book, you can look up a nursing diagnosis to see the list of outcomes suggested for it and the interventions for achieving each outcome. Refer to Table 6-4 for an example of interventions linked to the nursing diagnosis Risk for Aspiration. Notice there are 5 "major" interventions and 17 "suggested" interventions from which to choose.

Once you have chosen the interventions (based on your knowledge and judgment), you then choose the appropriate activities to carry out the intervention. As you might guess from looking at Box 6-3, you will probably never need to perform all the activities for a client. Choose the best ones for the situation and individualize them to fit the client and the resources (e.g., supplies, equipment) available.

Using NIC in Computerized Care Plans

Standardized language is especially useful in computerized care systems. For a computer screen with suggested NIC interventions for a NANDA-I nursing diagnosis,

 Go to Chapter 6, **Tables, Boxes, Figures: ESG Figure 6-2,** on the Student Resource Disk or DavisPlus at http:// davisplus.fadavis.com/Wilkinson2

For any NIC intervention, the program will also list the more specific nursing activities, which you can individualize as nursing orders.

Table 6-4 ➤ **NIC Interventions Linked to NANDA-I Diagnosis, Risk for Aspiration**

Aspiration, Risk for
The state in which an individual is at risk for entry of gastrointestinal secretions, oropharyngeal secretions, or solids or fluids into tracheobronchial passages.

Major Interventions

Aspiration Precautions	Swallowing Therapy
Airway Management	Vomiting Management
Respiratory Monitoring	

Suggested Interventions

Airway Suctioning	Postanesthesia Care
Amnioinfusion	Respiratory Monitoring
Artificial Airway Management	Resuscitation: Neonate
Enteral Tube Feeding	Sedation Management
Feeding	Self-Care Assistance: Feeding
Gastrointestinal Intubation	Surveillance
Mechanical Ventilation	Teaching: Infant Safety
Oral Health Maintenance	Teaching: Toddler Safety
Positioning	

Source: Johnson, M., Bulechek, G., Butcher, H., et al. (2006). *NANDA, NOC, and NIC Linkages* (2nd ed.). St. Louis, MO: C.V. Mosby, pp. 514–515. Used with permission from Elsevier Science.

 Go to Chapter 6, **Tables, Boxes, Figures: ESG Figure 6-3,** on the Student Resource Disk or DavisPlus at http:// davisplus.fadavis.com/Wilkinson2

Remember that you are responsible for choosing which interventions to use for each patient, when to use them, and which activities to write as specific nursing orders. You can reject *all* of the suggested interventions if they do not fit the patient's unique needs. Most computer programs have a field that allows you to type in your own interventions and activities.

Standardized Languages for Home Health and Community Care

The NIC includes interventions applicable in all settings, including home health and community nursing. However, the following taxonomies were created specifically for those uses:

- **The Clinical Care Classification (CCC).** Previously called the *Home Healthcare Classification,* the CCC was developed for use in home healthcare (Saba, 1995, 2006). In addition to terminology for nursing diagnoses and outcomes, the CCC has 198 interventions. For a complete description of the CCC system, see the nursing process section of Chapter 43 and

 Go to the CCC Web site at http://www.sabacare.com

- **The Omaha system.** The Omaha system was developed for community health nurses to use in caring for individuals, families, and **aggregates** (community groups or entire communities) (Martin, 2005). It includes terminology for diagnoses, outcomes, and interventions. For a complete description of the Omaha system, and for NIC community interventions, see the nursing process section of Chapter 42 and

 Go to the Omaha system Web site at http://www. omahasystem.org

KnowledgeCheck 6-4

- Name and describe three standardized intervention vocabularies recognized by the ANA.
- In the NIC system, what is the difference between interventions and activities?

 Go to Chapter 6, **Knowledge Check Response Sheet and Answers,** on the Student Resource Disk or DavisPlus at http://davisplus.fadavis.com/Wilkinson2

Does Standardized Language Interfere with Holistic Care?

Some nurses have criticized standardized terminologies for focusing on illness and physical interventions. However, NIC, Omaha, and CCC do include interventions to address health promotion, cultural, and spiritual needs. If you have a holistic attitude, you will give holistic care. Using a common language should help rather than hinder your choice of interventions. See Chapter 40 for further discussion of holistic nursing care. The following bulleted items identify interventions focused on wellness, spiritual needs, and culturally sensitive care.

- *Wellness interventions.* When you are caring for a healthy client, the client is the primary decision maker. You will function mainly as a teacher and health counselor. Frequently, the nursing orders outline lifestyle modification or behavior changes the client wants to make, along with self rewards to reinforce the behaviors. For example:

    Specific behavior change: I will consume less than 1400 calories per day for the next week.

    Self reward: I will reward myself with an evening out to hear my favorite band.

    The NIC contains most of the wellness interventions you will need. However, they are not all grouped together in one class. Some examples are Decision-Making Support, Exercise Promotion, and Health Screening. For more information on using standardized languages to describe wellness interventions, see Chapter 41.

- *Spiritual care interventions.* NIC, CCC, and the Omaha system all include terminology to describe spiritual interventions. The following are just a few examples:

NIC:	Spiritual Growth Facilitation, Religious Ritual Enhancement
CCC:	Spiritual Care, Coping Skills
Omaha:	Spiritual Support, Bereavement Support

    Chapter 14 provides full discussion of standardized nursing interventions to address spiritual needs. As you will see, you could also use most of those interventions (e.g., Coping Skills) for other than spiritual problems.

- *Culturally sensitive care.* Except for the NIC Culture Brokerage intervention, there are no standardized interventions that are unique to culturally based needs. All standardized interventions will result in culturally sensitive care if they are delivered by a culturally competent nurse.

Practical **Knowledge** knowing *how*

What Are Nursing Orders, and How Do I Write Them?

Nursing orders are instructions, usually written on a nursing care plan, that describe how and when nursing interventions are to be implemented. Other nurses and nursing assistive personnel are responsible and accountable for implementing nursing orders.

Complementary and Alternative Modalities

Because nursing is a holistic discipline, many nurses are enthusiastic about the techniques and modalities of complementary and alternative care. They believe interventions such as acupressure, aromatherapy, biofeedback, guided imagery, humor, journaling, music therapy, meditation and relaxation, and therapeutic touch help them to address the physical, mental, emotional, and spiritual dimensions of care.

Nursing theories and conceptual models of practice (see Chapter 8) and the current standardized language taxonomies support the use of CAM by nurses.

➤ CAM performed from within a context of a nursing theory takes on meaning as the interventions become part of the purposeful action to achieve goals of care that evolve from the theory.

➤ CAM performed and documented according to one of the standard taxonomies makes clear that the techniques are appropriate as nursing interventions.

Source: Frisch, N. C. (2001, May 31). Nursing as a context for alternative/complementary modalities. *Online Journal of Issues in Nursing,* 6(2), Manuscript 2, p. 2. http://www.nursingworld.org/MainMenuCategories/ANAMarketplace/ANAPeriodicals/OJIN/TableofContents/Volume62001/No2May01/AlternativeComplementaryModalities.aspx

Critical**Thinking** 6-4

Suppose you are caring for a patient 24 hours after a major surgery. You see the following order on the nursing care plan: Ambulate 24 hours postoperatively.

- When you care for the patient, how will you go about implementing this nursing order?
- What else do you need to know to effectively carry out this order?

Components of a Nursing Order

Did you have trouble answering the preceding questions? Even experienced nurses would, because this nursing order is incomplete. As you see from this example, nursing orders must be specific and detailed because many caregivers will use the care plan, and they need to be able to interpret the orders correctly. A well-written nursing order, whether on paper or electronic care plan, contains the following components:

- *Date.* The date the order was written. Change the date each time you review or revise the order. Why do you think it is important to have the date?
- *Subject.* Nursing orders are instructions to nurses, so they are written in terms of *nurse* behaviors. Therefore, the subject of the order is "the nurse." Because anyone reading the care plan should understand this, you do not actually need to write "the nurse" in your orders. For each order, think, but do not write, "The nurse will. . ." or "The nurse should . . ." This will help

you to state the order properly so that it doesn't sound like a goal statement. Goals state patient behaviors; nursing orders state nurse behaviors. For example:

Goal/expected outcome	Nursing order
(Patient) Drinks 100 mL fluids per hour on day shift	(Nurse will) Offer 100 mL water or juice per hour

- **Action verb.** This tells the nurse what action to take—what to do. Examples of action verbs are *assist, assess, auscultate, bathe, change, demonstrate, explain, give, teach,* and *turn.* The following nursing orders show the action verbs in italics:

  Teach the components of a healthy diet, 9/13, day shift

  Offer 100 mL water every hour

  Administer acetaminophen 500 mg orally at least 30 min before dressing change

- **Times and limits.** State when (e.g., which shift, what day), how often, and how long the activity is to be done. Consider the unit routines (e.g., visiting hours, mealtimes), the patient's usual rest times, scheduled tests and procedures (e.g., x-ray studies), and treatments (e.g., physical therapy). The following nursing orders show times and limits

  Teach the components of a healthy diet *on 9/13, day shift.*

  Offer 100 mL water *every hour between 0700 and 1900.*

  Administer acetaminophen 500 mg orally *at least 30 min before dressing change.*

  If you omit specific times, such as "day shift," the order may not be followed. It is easy for a nurse to think, "Perhaps someone else will do it (or has done it)."

- **Signature.** The nurse writing the order should sign it. A signature indicates that you accept legal and ethical accountability for your orders and allows others to know whom to contact if they have questions or comments about the order. If interventions are chosen on an electronic care plan, there may not be an actual signature. However, the name of the nurse who chose the intervention should be indicated in some manner.

Toward Evidence-Based Practice

Orr, P. M., McGinnis, M. A., Hudson, L. R., et al. (2006). A focused telephonic nursing intervention delivers improved adherence to A1c testing. *Disease Management, 9*(5), 277–283.

This 6-month study investigated whether a focused telephone intervention would improve patient adherence to hemoglobin A1c testing (a test of diabetes control). Subjects were patients already enrolled in a diabetes disease management program and were already receiving various types of phone calls and educational materials. During the study, when a routine call was made to a member of the program, the clinician determined whether the A1c had been tested in the past 6 months. If not, a specific goal was created with the member during the conversation (e.g., "I will make an appointment to follow up on my A1c test"); a copy was mailed to the member. Follow-up phone calls were repeated every 2 weeks to check on the member's progress in meeting the goal. Patient records were examined for evidence that an A1c test had been done. At the end of the 6 months, quantitative analysis of data was done. The number of group members who received an A1c test increased significantly, by 12%. Gender did not impact on adherence to A1c testing, but age did. The greatest improvement was observed in the 0–19-year age group (14.9%), those ages 50–59 (12.7%), and those ages 60–69 years (13.4%). All other age categories showed increases ranging from 8.1% to 10.6%. Increases in the number of phone calls made to a member were associated with subsequent increases in A1c testing adherence.

Duhamel, F., Dupuis, F., Reidy, M., et al. (2007). A qualitative evaluation of a family nursing intervention. *Clinical Nurse Specialist, 21*(1), 43–49.

In this qualitative study, a clinical nurse specialist met with each of four couples for four 60-minute therapeutic meetings. Meetings were also audiotaped. The patients were men with congestive heart failure (CHF), with their wives as caregivers. All were retired. Researchers used semistructured interviews before and after the intervention and analyzed them qualitatively. Results showed that both spouses were experiencing a high level of suffering, which was relieved through a family nursing meeting that allowed them to obtain a better understanding of each other's experience.

1. How are these two studies similar? (If you need to do so, read about research in Chapter 8.)

2. Now think about the interventions tested in the two studies. What are their differences?

3. Using these two studies, write two nursing orders for a client who will be discharged tomorrow after being hospitalized for the fourth time for CHF. He will be cared for at home by his wife. (Assume that whatever services you recommend will be available and affordable.)

 Go to Chapter 6, **Toward Evidence-Based Practice Suggested Responses,** on the Student Resource Disk or DavisPlus at http://davisplus.fadavis.com/Wilkinson2

KnowledgeCheck 6-5

List the five components of a nursing order.

 Go to Chapter 6, **Knowledge Check Response Sheet and Answers,** on the Student Resource Disk or DavisPlus at http://davisplus.fadavis.com/Wilkinson2

Reflecting Critically About Nursing Orders

After writing the nursing orders, reflect on the interventions you have chosen. If you followed the process in the section, "What Process Can I Use for Generating and Selecting Interventions?" you will already have thought critically and made some considered decisions as you were choosing the interventions and activities. The following are questions to guide your final judgments about the plan of care.

1. *Is the set of orders complete?* That is, do they address all aspects of the problem?
   — Do they address the etiology of the problem?
   — If the etiology cannot be changed, do the orders focus on the symptoms of the problem?
   — Have I considered physical, emotional, interpersonal, spiritual, and cultural needs?
2. *Is each order technically complete?* That is, does it contain all the required components?
3. *Are the orders clear, specific, and precise?* If you have included all the required components, the orders will usually provide specific enough directions (e.g., when, how often, and so on) to be useful to other nurses. However, you must avoid vague language. For example, an order to "Offer emotional support" is too general to offer direction for care. One nurse might think this means to ask the client about his family, another might sit quietly with the patient, and still another might use a therapeutic statement such as, "This must be difficult for you." Ask yourself, "Would all nurses interpret this order in the same way? Would they all do the same thing after reading it?"

4. *Is the order individualized for this particular patient?* For example, even if you have written an order, "Offer 100 mL fluids every hr," it is even better if you make a note of the kinds of fluids the patient likes or can tolerate.
5. *Are the orders concise?* Long, complex statements may be unclear. Keep the orders as brief as possible without sacrificing clarity and specificity. If the patient requires complex procedures (e.g., insertion of a urinary catheter), don't write the details of the procedure on the care plan. Simply refer to the source of instructions for the procedure: perhaps an agency procedure manual, or a list of instructions to be found at the bedside. Do write in the care plan any modifications to a procedure (e.g., "Do not use alcohol; client's skin is very dry.")
6. *Which orders have priority?* Which nursing orders must be implemented immediately? Which must be done on this shift? Which must be done today? If possible, write them in priority order. In Chapter 4 you learned about frameworks for prioritizing nursing diagnoses (e.g., Maslow's hierarchy, problem urgency, future consequences, and patient preference). You can use these same frameworks to help you prioritize nursing orders.

If you have followed the recommended processes and reflected critically on your interventions, you should have a holistic plan of care individualized to meet the client's needs.

 Go to Chapter 6, **Resources for Caregivers and Health Professionals,** on the Student Resource Disk or DavisPlus at http://davisplus.fadavis.com/Wilkinson2

 Suggested Readings: Go to Chapter 6, **Reading More About the Nursing Process: Planning Interventions,** on the Student Resource Disk or DavisPlus at http://davisplus. fadavis.com/Wilkinson2

 Bibliography: Go to Volume 2, Bibliography.

CHAPTER 7

Nursing Process: Implementation & Evaluation

Learning Outcomes

After completing this chapter, you should be able to:

➤ Define implementation.

➤ State the three broad phases of the implementation process (doing, delegating, recording).

➤ Describe what nurses do in the implementation phase of the nursing process.

➤ Define the terms *delegation* and *supervision*.

➤ Identify and describe the "five rights" of delegation.

➤ Describe the three types of evaluation.

➤ Explain how standards and criteria are used in evaluation.

➤ Explain how structure, process, and outcomes evaluation are related.

➤ Distinguish among ongoing, intermittent, and terminal evaluation.

➤ Describe a process for evaluating client health status (outcomes) after interventions.

➤ Describe a process for evaluating the effectiveness of the nursing care plan.

➤ List variables that may influence the effectiveness of a nursing intervention; state which ones the nurse can and cannot control.

➤ Discuss the importance of nurses' involvement in evaluating the quality of care in an organization.

Meet Your Patients

Patient 1

Jeannette Wu is a very thin 80-year-old woman who is in the hospital after fracturing her hip. Her hip was surgically repaired 4 days ago, but because of her overall fragile health and some postsurgery confusion, her recovery is slower than usual. One of her nursing diagnoses is Self-Care Deficit (Bathing/Hygiene, Dressing/Grooming, and Toileting) related to weakness, pain, confusion, and decreased mobility. Her nursing orders (NIC) include Bathing and Self-Care: Activities of Daily Living (ADLs). As the nurse is helping a newly hired nursing assistive personnel (NAP) with Mrs. Wu's bath, she notices a reddened area on Mrs. Wu's sacrum. Realizing that this may be the beginning of a pressure ulcer, the nurse observes carefully and notes a small skin excoriation (abrasion) in the area. She repositions Mrs. Wu to prevent further pressure on her sacrum. After finishing the bath, the nurse records her findings and enters

on Mrs. Wu's care plan a nursing diagnosis of Impaired Skin Integrity related to impaired bed mobility and minimal subcutaneous tissue. She writes appropriate nursing orders, including an order to observe skin over bony prominences every 4 hours, and then delegates to the NAP the task of turning and repositioning Mrs. Wu every 2 hours. The nurse also sends a consultation request to a wound care nurse specialist.

Meet Your Patients (continued)

Patient 2

Patsy Jimenez is a healthy 25-year-old woman with no medical problems. She eats a balanced diet but does not

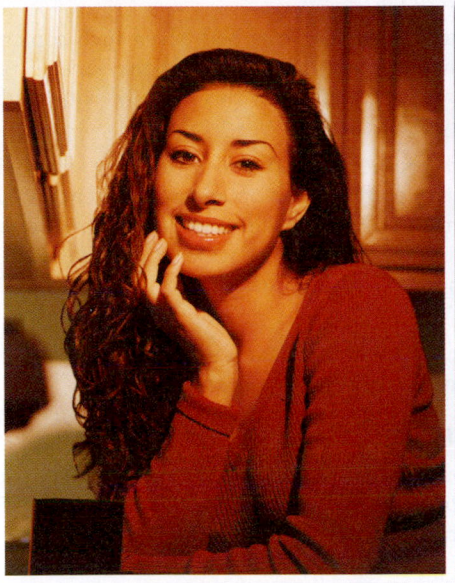

exercise much ("I really hate to exercise!"). She and the nurse have created a plan to help her increase her physical activity. Ms. Jimenez will try to walk for 30 minutes at least 5 days a week. Each week she is successful, she plans to reward herself with a movie or a milkshake, which she usually avoids because of the fat content. The nurse would prefer that Ms. Jimenez not reward herself with food, but respects the patient's decision and realizes that if it is to serve as motivation, the reward must be something that Ms. Jimenez values.

Critical Thinking 7-1

- For Jeannette Wu, which parts of the scenario illustrate *doing* by the nurse?
- For Jeannette Wu, which parts of the scenario illustrate *thinking* by the nurse?
- For Patsy Jimenez, who will be implementing (carrying out) the plan of care?

Implementation: The Action Phase of the Nursing Process

Think of implementation as the action phase of the nursing process. Of course, implementation involves both thinking and doing, but the emphasis is on doing. During **implementation,** you will perform or delegate planned interventions—that is, carry out the care plan. The implementation phase ends when you document the nursing actions in the chart; it evolves into evaluation as you document the resulting client responses (Fig. 7-1). In short, implementation is doing, delegating, and documenting.

As in all phases of the nursing process, think of the client as a collaborative partner. Encourage the client and family to participate as much as possible in the client's care. When Mrs. Wu is less confused and better able to move about, for example, the nurse will encourage her to help bathe herself. Be aware that clients vary in their ability and desire to participate. In the opening scenarios, Mrs. Wu was able to participate very little, but Patsy Jimenez participated fully. Typically, the client implements health-promotion interventions, with little or no involvement by the nurse.

As with other steps of the nursing process, professional nursing organizations have developed standards relating to implementation. These are identified in Box 7-1.

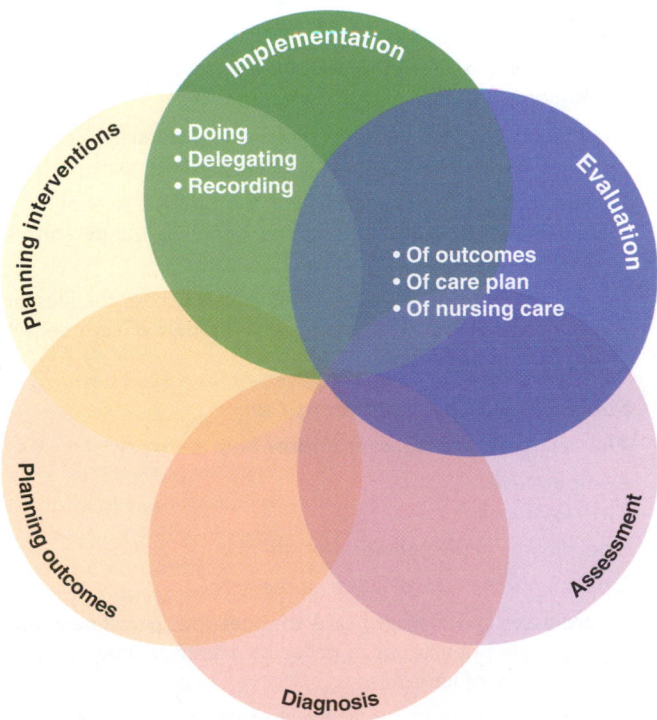

FIGURE 7-1 Nursing process phase: Implementation and evaluation.

BOX 7-1 ■ Professional Standards for Implementation

American Nurses Association Standards of Practice[1]
Standard 5. Implementation
The registered nurse implements the identified plan.

Competencies
The registered nurse:

Partners with the person/family/significant others/caregiver to implement the plan in a safe, realistic, and timely manner.

Demonstrates caring behaviors towards patients, significant others and groups of people receiving care.

Documents implementation and any modifications, including changes or omissions, of the identified plan.

Utilizes technology to measure, record and retrieve patient data, implement the nursing process and enhance nursing practice.

Utilizes evidence-based interventions and treatments specific to the diagnosis or problem.

Provides holistic care that addresses the needs of diverse populations across the lifespan.

Advocates for health care that is sensitive to the needs of patients, with particular emphasis on the needs of diverse populations.

Applies appropriate knowledge of major health problems and cultural diversity in implementing the plan of care.

Applies health care technologies to maximize optimal outcomes for patients.

Utilizes community resources and systems to implement the plan.

Collaborates with health care providers from diverse backgrounds to implement the plan.

Integrates care with other members of the interprofessional healthcare team.

Evaluates and assesses the usefulness in integrating traditional and complementary health care practices.

Implements the plan in a safe and timely manner in accordance with the National Patient Safety goals.

Promotes the person's capacity for the optimal level of participation and problem solving, honoring the person's choices.

Coordinates the health care of individuals across the lifespan using principles of interprofessional models of care delivery and case management.

Standard 5A: Coordination of Care
The registered nurse coordinates care delivery.

Competencies
The registered nurse:

Coordinates implementation of the plan.

Documents the coordination of the care.

Coordinates and manages care to meet the special needs of vulnerable populations in order to maximize independence and quality of life.

Assists the person to recognize alternatives by identifying options for care choices.

Standard 5B: Health Teaching and Health Promotion
The registered nurse employs strategies to promote health and a safe environment.

Competencies
The registered nurse:

Provides health teaching that addresses such topics as healthy lifestyles, risk-reducing behaviors, developmental needs, activities of daily living, and preventive self-care.

Uses health promotion and health teaching methods appropriate to the situation and the patient's values, beliefs, health practices, developmental level, learning needs, readiness and ability to learn, language preference, spirituality, culture, and socioeconomic status.

Seeks opportunities for feedback and evaluation of the effectiveness of the strategies used.

Standard 16. Resource Utilization
The registered nurse utilizes appropriate resources to plan and provide nursing services that are safe, effective and financially responsible.

Competencies
The registered nurse:

Allocates resources based on identified patient care needs, potential for harm, complexity of the task, and desired outcome.

Delegates tasks based on patient need and caregiver competency.

Advocates for the design and implementation of technology that enhances nursing practice and healthcare delivery.

Modifies practice when necessary to promote a positive interface between patients, care providers and technology.

Source: American Nurses Association (2010, in press). *Nursing: Scope and Standards of Practice* (2nd ed.). Public Comment draft, January 2010. (To be published by August, 2010). Silver Spring, MD: Nursebooks.org.
[1]*Caveat:* This material is from the draft for public comment (ANA, 2010, in press); its wording may be changed somewhat in the final published version. For that version of the ANA Standards of Professional Nursing Practice, go to www.nursingworld.org.

Canadian Provincial Standards of Practice

In Canada, each province sets practice standards. The following are examples that apply to implementation.

Province of Alberta
Standard 2. Knowledge-Based Practice

The registered nurse:

Indicator 2.2—Demonstrates critical thinking in collecting and interpreting data, planning, implementing, and evaluating all aspects of nursing care.

BOX 7-1 ■ Professional Standards for Implementation—cont'd

Indicator 2.6—Documents timely, accurate reports of data collection, interpretation, planning, implementing, and evaluating care.

Standard 4. Provision of Service to the Public

The registered nurse:

Indicator 4.1—Collaborates with the client/significant others and other members of the health-care team regarding activities of care planning, implementation, and evaluation.

Indicator 4.3—Is accountable for the supervision of other health-team members, and nursing students when appropriate. . .

Province of New Brunswick

Standard 2. Knowledge-Based Practice

Indicator 2.5—Assigns and delegates care appropriately based on assessment of client needs and competence of care provider.

Source: College and Association of Registered Nurses of Alberta (2003). _Nursing practice standards._ 11620-168 Street, Edmonton, AB T5M 4A6, Canada; Nurses Association of New Brunswick (2005). _Standards of practice for registered nurses._ 65 Regent Street, Fredericton, NB, E3B 7B4, Canada.

How Is Implementation Related to Other Steps of the Nursing Process?

Nursing process phases are interdependent (see Fig. 7-1). Each phase affects and is affected by other phases. Without the assessment, diagnosis, and planning steps, implementation would reflect only dependent functions, such as carrying out policies, protocols, and medical orders. The autonomous nursing activities performed during implementation are built on the nurse's reasoning in the previous three steps. Implementation overlaps in some way with every other phase of the nursing process.

- **Implementation overlaps with assessment.** Nurses use assessment data to individualize interventions for a specific person rather than just giving "routine care." For example, a nursing order may read, "Offer clear liquids hourly; patient likes tea." When taking the tea to the patient, you may discover that she likes sugar in her tea and prefers it without ice. These data allow you to individualize the intervention further. Implementation also provides the opportunity to assess your patients at every contact. In "Meet Your Patients," what data did the nurse obtain while bathing Mrs. Wu? Some nursing orders specifically direct ongoing, focused assessments. When performing an ordered ongoing assessment, you are both implementing and assessing. What ongoing assessment was ordered for Mrs. Wu?
- **Implementation overlaps with diagnosis.** Nurses use data discovered during implementation to identify new diagnoses or to revise existing ones. What new nursing diagnosis did the nurse make for Mrs. Wu after bathing her?
- **Implementation overlaps with planning outcomes and interventions.** When you implement a nursing intervention, it produces patient responses. Patient responses provide the data you need for revising the original goals and nursing orders. As you care for a client, you begin to know her better, and her unique needs become more apparent.
- **Implementation overlaps with evaluation.** When evaluating patient health status and progress toward goals, you will compare the responses you observe during implementation to the existing goals (which were written in the planning outcomes phase).

How Should I Prepare for Implementation?

In addition to "doing, delegating, and documenting," implementation also involves some preparation. Although the care plan will already have been developed in the planning stages of the nursing process, you should do some more planning just before implementing the plan—as explained in the following sections. Notice how important critical thinking and nursing knowledge are to this "doing" phase of the nursing process.

Check Your Knowledge and Abilities

Before beginning a nursing activity, review the care plan and reflect critically on the nursing and medical prescriptions. As a nurse, you will be obligated ethically and legally to clarify or question orders that you believe to be unclear, incorrect, or inappropriate. At the same time, you must decide whether you are qualified to carry out the orders. You should ask for help when:

- You do not have the knowledge or skill needed to implement an order. For example, you may be unfamiliar with a medication, or you may not ever have performed an ordered procedure such as a urinary catheterization.
- You cannot perform the activity safely alone (e.g., helping a heavy, weak patient to ambulate). As another example, when catheterizing Ms. Wu, if she is very weak, the nurse would need someone to help her maintain the desired position during the catheterization.
- Performing the activity alone would cause undue stress for the patient (e.g., giving back care to a patient with multiple fractures).

For a decision tree to help you check whether you are ready to implement care,

 Go to **Resources for Caregivers and Health Professionals,** and follow the link for **"Decision Tree,"** on the Student Resource Disk or DavisPlus at http://davisplus.fadavis.com/ Wilkinson2

Organize Your Work

Because you will be providing care for more than one patient on each shift, you will need to make a time-sequenced work plan ("worksheet") to prioritize your patient care for the day. With the organizational emphasis on cost and efficiency, you may have a great deal of work to accomplish, so you must make the most of every patient contact. Think ahead which interventions you can perform at the same time. Mrs. Wu's nurse performed a skin assessment while she was giving a bed bath. As another example, you might do patient teaching while assisting with breathing exercises. Or while changing a dressing, you might also use that time to show interest and concern for an anxious patient. Many institutions have forms for this type of scheduling, or you may need to write your own list of "things to do" in the order you need to do them. For a worksheet you can use in clinical,

VOL 2 Go to **"Worksheet for Organizing Nursing Care,"** in Chapter 7, Volume 2.

Establish Feedback Points

Establishing feedback points is a part of organizing your work. You cannot assume you will be able to carry out a nursing order in exactly the way it was written. For example, suppose the nursing order states, "Help to ambulate in the hall b.i.d." When you help the patient to stand, he becomes pale, dizzy, diaphoretic, and short of breath. Would you still carry out the order? Of course not. You must always be ready to alter the activity on the spot as the patient's responses demand. This means that you must look for **feedback** (how the patient is responding to the activity) as you perform care. In a sense, this is evaluating. However, because it is done before the intervention is complete, we call it feedback.

When organizing your work, identify points in each intervention where you want to pause for feedback. For example, if you are assisting with range-of-motion exercises, you might plan to assess for pain during movement of each joint and to assess for activity intolerance after exercising both arms and again after exercising the legs. Feedback is not always verbal. For example, it could be a change in vital signs, skin color, or level of consciousness.

Prepare Supplies and Equipment

Preparing supplies and equipment is another aspect of organization. Gather all the supplies and equipment you need before you go to the patient's room. This allows you to work efficiently by eliminating the need to go to the supply room for items you have overlooked. Also, it prevents the stress to your patient that occurs when you interrupt a procedure to go get a needed item.

Suppose you are working alone to insert an intravenous (IV) catheter—a sterile procedure. You have donned your gloves, applied the tourniquet, and done all the steps before inserting the IV catheter. When you insert the catheter, you "blow" the vein and are unable to use it to start the IV fluid. You look in the IV tray, which you had placed just outside the patient's room, and discover that there is not another IV catheter in it; you have used the last one. What are your options at this point? Are there any *good* options?

The answer is that there are no good options. You might call another busy caregiver (provided that one is available) to bring you a sterile IV catheter. Or you could interrupt the procedure and get it yourself, making it necessary to leave the patient, don another pair of gloves, and prep another site. Either way, time and money would be lost, as might your patient's confidence in you. You cannot prevent "blowing" an IV; however, by preparing ahead, you can prevent inefficiency and waste. In this case, that would mean being sure your IV tray is fully stocked before beginning the procedure.

Prepare the Patient

Before performing a nursing activity, identify the patient and reassess him to make sure the activity is still necessary and the patient is physically and psychologically ready for the intervention.

Check your assumptions. This is just good critical thinking. Don't assume that an intervention is still needed simply because it is written on the care plan. For example, on postop day 6 after Jeannette Wu's surgery, the nursing assistant is preparing to give her a bed bath, as instructed on the care plan (Table 7-1, entry for December 18). However, Mrs. Wu has regained some of her strength and is able to sit in a chair. So the nurse and the assistant agree that, with help, Mrs. Wu can bathe at the sink instead of requiring a complete bed bath.

Assess the patient's readiness. To obtain the most benefit from an intervention, a client must be physically and psychologically ready. The hospital's critical pathway for hip fractures recommended a "help bath" on postoperative day 3. However, Mrs. Wu's age and physical condition indicated that she needed a complete bed bath on day 3. The nurse did not assume Mrs. Wu was ready to progress just because the critical pathway dictated it. The following are more examples of ensuring readiness:

- Because her patient was anxious about his test results, a nurse postponed a teaching session until he was feeling calmer.
- While preparing to perform a painful dressing change, a nurse discovered the patient had visitors. The nurse waited until the visitors had gone to do the procedure.

Explain what you will do and what the patient will feel. Clients are collaborative partners, not passive recipients of your care. Many interventions require their participation or cooperation. The following are caring reasons for taking time to explain.

- Explaining the reasons for the action helps to motivate the person to participate.
- Explaining what the person is expected to do gives the person the information she needs to participate.

Table 7-1 ➤ Portions of the Care Plan for Jeannette Wu

Date: 12/16/10 Care Plan Before Implementation on Day 4 Postop

NURSING DIAGNOSIS	DESIRED OUTCOMES	NURSING ORDERS	EVALUATION
12/16 Self-Care Deficit (Bathing/Hygiene, Dressing/Grooming, and Toileting) related to weakness, pain, confusion, and decreased mobility	By day 6 postop (12/18) will assist with bath and oral hygiene.	▪ Complete bedbath daily in A.M. ▪ Give prescribed analgesic 1/2 hr before bath. ▪ Assist with range-of-motion exercises.	

Date: 12/16/06 Care Plan After Implementation on Day 4 Postop

NURSING DIAGNOSIS	DESIRED OUTCOMES	NURSING ORDERS	EVALUATION
12/16 Self-Care Deficit (Bathing/Hygiene, Dressing/Grooming, and Toileting) related to weakness, pain, confusion, and decreased mobility	By day 6 postop (12/18) will assist with bath and oral hygiene.	▪ Complete bedbath daily in A.M. (NAP) ▪ Give Tylenol #3, tabs i by mouth, 1/2 hr before bath ▪ Assist with range-of-motion exercises t.i.d. (RN).	12/16 Too soon to evaluate
12/16 Impaired skin integrity (sacrum) r/t pressure 2° immobility	*By 12/23, skin healed over sacrum; skin intact and normal color over all bony prominences*	▪ *Turn and reposition q2hr; do not place supine (NAP).* ▪ *Observe skin over bony prominences q4hr (RN).*	

Date: 12/18/06 Care Plan After Implementation on Day 6 Postop

NURSING DIAGNOSIS	DESIRED OUTCOMES	NURSING ORDERS	EVALUATION
12/16 Self-Care Deficit (Bathing/Hygiene, Dressing/Grooming, and Toileting) related to weakness, pain, confusion, and decreased mobility	By day 6 postop (12/18) will assist with bath and oral hygiene.	▪ Complete bedbath daily in A.M. *12/18 NAP help with bath at sink daily in A.M. Patient can wash hands and face and perform oral hygiene.* ▪ Give prescribed analgesic 1/2 hr before bath. ▪ Assist with range-of-motion exercises t.i.d. (RN).	*12/18 Goal met. Sat in chair for help with bath. Performed oral hygiene and washed hands and face.*
12/16 Impaired skin integrity (sacrum) r/t pressure 2° immobility	By 12/23, skin healed over sacrum; skin intact and normal color over all bony prominences	▪ Turn and reposition q2hr; do not place supine (NAP). ▪ Observe skin over bony prominences q4hr (RN). ▪ *12/18 Requested foam and fatty mattress pad.* ▪ *12/18 Refer to nutritionist for evaluation.*	*12/18 Skin excoriation over sacrum is larger: now 2 cm × 2 cm, and about 1/2 cm deep*

▪ Explaining what sensations the person can expect helps to relieve anxiety, enables the person to cope with unpleasant or painful sensations, and promotes a trusting relationship.

Provide privacy. This helps to assure psychological readiness.

KnowledgeCheck 7-1

- Why is it important to organize your work before implementing care?
- In addition to organizing your work, what other preparations should you make before implementing care?

  Go to Chapter 7, **Knowledge Check Response Sheet and Answers,** on the Student Resource Disk or DavisPlus at http://davisplus.fadavis.com/Wilkinson2

CriticalThinking 7-2

Suppose your patient, Jeannette Wu, has become incontinent of bowel and bladder. Because she already has Impaired Skin Integrity, the physician writes a new order to insert an indwelling urinary catheter (a drainage tube inserted through her urinary meatus into her bladder). Urinary catheterization is a sterile technique. You have practiced this procedure in the skills lab, but you have never actually performed it on a patient.

- As a student, what should you do?
- If you were a licensed nurse, what are some things you could do to ensure that both you and the patient are prepared for the procedure?

Implementing the Plan: Doing or Delegating

After both you and the patient are prepared, it is time to act. Nursing actions include both those you do yourself and those you delegate to others; and they may be collaborative, independent, or dependent (see Chapter 6 if you do not recall the meaning of these terms). During implementation, you will coordinate and carry out both the nursing orders on the nursing care plan and the medical orders that relate to the patient's medical treatment.

What Knowledge and Skills Do I Need?

There is almost no limit to the number and kinds of nursing interventions you might perform. The *Nursing Interventions Classification* (2008), for example, lists 542 broad interventions (e.g., Hypothermia Treatment), each of which includes approximately 15 to 20 specific activities. For example, one activity for Hypothermia Treatment is "Remove cold, wet clothing and replace with warm, dry clothing" (p. 418). During implementation, then, you can expect to use all the types of knowledge presented in Chapter 2: theoretical, practical, personal, and ethical knowledge, as well as knowledge about the patient situation.

You will also use various combinations of cognitive, interpersonal, and psychomotor skills to perform nursing activities (thinking, doing, caring). For example, when you are inserting an IV catheter, you need cognitive knowledge of sterile procedure, interpersonal skills to reassure the patient, and psychomotor skills to apply the tourniquet and insert the IV catheter.

 Critical**Thinking** 7-3

Use the examples provided in the preceding paragraph to help you write a definition for each of the following terms:
- Cognitive skills
- Interpersonal skills
- Psychomotor skills

How Can I Promote Client Participation and Adherence?

Different interventions require differing levels of participation. However, even a nurse-initiated intervention, such as inserting a urinary catheter, goes more smoothly if the patient participates at least to the extent of holding still while you perform the procedure. Many interventions (e.g., instituting a low-calorie diet) depend almost entirely on the patient's adhering to the therapy. In the case of Ms. Jimenez, implementation of the intervention, walking for 30 minutes five times a week, depends entirely on the client.

People fail to follow therapeutic regimens for various reasons. They may not understand the routine or the reasons for it; there may be cultural objections to the therapy; their lifestyle may make adherence difficult (e.g., no time to exercise); they may be afraid of failing; they may be reluctant to ask questions, either from embarrassment at their lack of knowledge or from hesitance to "bother" a busy nurse or physician. You can promote cooperation with treatments and therapies by following these guidelines:

Assess the client's knowledge. Assess the client's understanding of his illness and the treatments and provide the necessary information. Be as specific as possible with your instructions. Keep instructions simple and clear, and provide a written copy.

Assess the client's supports and resources. You cannot, for example, assume that every patient owns a car or even has other transportation to the clinic. Even if they wish to follow the therapy; some people do not have enough money for food or medicine; some people cannot read printed instructions; some do not have family or friends to help with their care at home, and so on.

Be sensitive to the client's cultural, spiritual, and other needs and viewpoints. For example, regardless of the need for dietary protein, some people do not like the taste of meat, poultry, or fish; others might have religious or cultural objections to eating these foods. You will need to alter your recommendations to reflect client preferences and beliefs.

Realize and accept that some attitudes cannot be changed. For example, regardless of the effects of obesity on blood pressure, a client will not lose weight simply because you tell him it is important. The client must *want* to lose weight. Information alone will not change a person's behavior.

Determine the client's main concerns. For example, you may be concerned that lack of exercise makes it difficult to regulate a client's blood sugar; the client's main concern may be that exercise makes her joints hurt.

Help the client to set realistic goals. Clients usually more readily accept small, rather than drastic, behavioral or lifestyle changes. Perhaps a client with a child who has asthma cannot even imagine that she could stop smoking. But you may be able to convince her it would be better for her child if she would smoke outdoors rather than in the house or in the car (London, 1998).

Talk openly and regularly about adherence. Let the client know you understand how difficult treatment can be and that others struggle with adherence as well.

What Should I Know About Collaborating and Coordinating Care?

For successful implementation, you need the skills of collaboration and coordination. As discussed in Chapter 6, **collaboration** simply means working with patients and other caregivers (e.g., physicians, respiratory therapists) to plan, make decisions, or perform interventions. Unlike delegated activities (discussed in the following section) true collaboration requires shared decision-making.

According to the Quality and Safety Education for Nurses (QSEN) project, one of the competencies you should acquire in nursing school is the ability to function and collaborate on an interdisciplinary team, as well as with other nurses. This means, in part, that you will learn to be assertive in discussions about patient care. At the same time, you should recognize the differences in authority and power that exist on interdisciplinary teams and choose your communication style carefully, taking that into account (Cronenwett, Sherwood, Barnsteiner, et al., 2007).

Coordination of care includes scheduling treatments and activities with other departments (e.g., laboratory, physical therapy, radiology), but it is more than that. In the hospital, nurses are the professionals who have the most frequent and continuous contact with the patient, so they have the most complete picture of the person. Unlike nurses, most other caregivers focus on only a very specific aspect of the patient (e.g., breathing, eating, surgical incision). You will be expected to put together the bits and pieces of information (e.g., the patient's response to physical therapy, dietary intake, emotional status, and vital signs) to provide a holistic view of the person. You will need to read the reports of other professionals; help interpret the results for the patient and family, and make rounds with other professionals to be sure that everyone sees the whole picture.

Outside the hospital, the health professional who has the most contact with the client usually assumes the coordination role. For example, if a client is receiving episodic care for ongoing health problems, the primary care provider (e.g., physician or advanced practice nurse) may coordinate care. For a client discharged home after a hip fracture, the physical therapist may coordinate care.

KnowledgeCheck 7-2

- What are some reasons that a client may not follow a recommended treatment regimen?
- List at least four things you can do to promote client participation in care or adherence to recommendations for treatment.

 Go to Chapter 7, **Knowledge Check Response Sheet and Answers,** on the Student Resource Disk or DavisPlus at http://davisplus.fadavis.com/Wilkinson2

What Should I Know About Delegation and Supervision?

Delegation is the process of directing another person to perform a task or activity; it is a transfer of authority or responsibility. The person delegating retains accountability for the outcome of the activity (ANA & the National Council of State Boards of Nursing [NCSBN], 2006). As a registered nurse, you will frequently delegate patient care activities to licensed vocational (or practical) nurses (LVN/LPNs) and nursing assistive personnel (NAPs), although in some states LVN/LPNs are considered

accountable for their actions because they are licensed. You may also (e.g., as a nurse in charge tasks making unit assignments for the day) *assign* tasks to other RNs; however, this is not delegation because those RNs are accountable for the outcome of their activities. Remember, you can only delegate *down* in the chain of command.

Understand that you cannot delegate nursing care decisions. You can delegate only the responsibility for performing a defined activity in a particular situation. So, even though the nurse has delegated to the NAP the task of turning Mrs. Wu ("Meet Your Patient") every 2 hours, it is *the nurse* who must assess her skin condition and take action if it does not improve.

In some healthcare settings, NAPs are used inappropriately to perform functions that are legally nursing functions (e.g., administering medications) (Dickens, Stubbs, & Haw, 2008). Many nurses are concerned that with a nursing shortage, inappropriate delegation is a threat to patient safety. Nurses may find themselves in a difficult position of caring for sicker patients, using new technologies, administering medications, and juggling these activities with overseeing delegated work. According to the ANA, any nursing intervention that requires critical thinking or professional judgment cannot be delegated. However, the ANA takes the position that RN delegation and direction of specific tasks to NAPs by in accordance with state nurse practice acts, is appropriate, safe, and resource-efficient (ANA, 2007).

 Standard 16 of the Nursing Scope & Standards of Practice (2nd ed) (ANA, 2010, in press) states that the registered nurse "delegates tasks based on patient need and caregiver competency."

When deciding whether to delegate tasks, you should think critically about the task, the circumstance, the person, the direction or communication, and the supervision and evaluation. For a checklist to help you consider these five critical elements, or "five rights" of delegating,

VOL 2 Go to Chapter 7, **Delegation and Evaluation Checklists, The Five Rights of Delegation,** in Volume 2.

Right Task

The first question to ask is, "Can I delegate this task?" As a rule, you should delegate an activity only if it meets *all* of the following criteria (ANA, 1996; ANA/ NCSBN, 2006). The activity:

- Is within your scope of practice to perform and delegate, as defined by your state nurse practice act.
- Is within the LVN/LPN's or NAP's scope of practice.
- Is in accordance with agency policies, if they exist.
- Is performed according to an established sequence of steps and requires little or no modification from one situation to another.
- Does not require ongoing nursing assessments, interpretation, or decision-making.
- Occurs frequently in the daily care of patients on the unit.
- Has reasonably predictable results.

- Is *not* one that requires independent, specialized nursing knowledge, skills, or judgment.
- Is *not* health teaching or counseling.
- Does not endanger a client's life or well-being.

Examples of tasks you might assign to a NAP are bathing a stable patient, ambulating steady patients, obtaining routine vital signs, changing linens, assisting patients with meals, clerical duties, and transporting non-acute patients and specimens. LPNs can usually provide care to medically stable patients according to an established plan of care; they can give you feedback about patient responses for patients who are expected to respond predictably.

Tasks you can usually assign to an LPN include administering some medications (except for IV medications and some controlled substances), starting an IV infusion and administering plain IV solutions, and assisting with identification of blood units for transfusion. You would not assign an LPN to start a blood transfusion, administer chemotherapy, administer or monitor parenteral nutrition, give IV push medications, or create and modify nursing care plans (Ayers & Montgomery, 2008).

Remember that you are assigning staff members to a *task*, not to a patient. You cannot delegate the responsibility for total patient care; and you cannot allow a NAP to delegate care to other NAPs.

Right Circumstance

NAPs are being used in settings where acuity and technology have increased while length of stay has decreased. This means they are caring for sicker patients. We often think of bathing, feeding, and turning patients as tasks appropriate for the NAP; however, such tasks may not be appropriate if the patient is seriously ill. Before deciding to delegate, assess your patient to be certain that her needs match the abilities of the NAP or LPN. It is best if the patient is relatively stable (e.g., with a chronic rather than an acute condition) and does not need extensive help with self-care activities. If the client is very ill or if the results of the task are unpredictable, the task should probably not be delegated. For a tool to help you make appropriate delegation decisions,

 VOL 2 Go to Chapter 7, **Delegation Decision-Making Grid**, in Volume 2.

Right Person

You must also be sure that the LPN or NAP is competent to perform the task and that his workload allows time to do the task properly. Take into consideration the person's experience, training, and cultural competence. The following are evidence of competence:

- The facility has documented proof that the person has demonstrated competence.
- The NAP has performed the task often or has worked with patients with similar diagnoses.

If evidence is lacking, you need to establish the NAP's competence. For example, you might observe and evaluate his performance, or you might ask the NAP, "How many times have you done this procedure?" or "Will you need help with this procedure?" (Also see the next section, "Right Direction/Communication.") Only a professional nurse can evaluate an LPN's or NAP's ability to perform a nursing task.

Right Communication

Right communication means that when you delegate, you should communicate clearly and specifically about each task. You can communicate orally or in writing, but leave no room for misinterpretation.

- **Explain exactly what the task is.** Include what to do and what not to do. For example, "Empty the catheter bag, and measure the amount of urine using the clear, marked plastic container"—not just, "Measure the urine."
- **Include specific times and methods for reporting.** For example, "Come tell me the patient's temperature every hour."
- **Explain the purpose or objective of the task.** For example, "Change Mrs. Wu's position every 2 hours to prevent bedsores; she is not able to turn by herself."
- **Describe the expected results or potential complications to expect.** For example, "She will probably cry out when you turn her, but that is more from fear than from pain," or "I have given her medications, so her temperature should be below 100°F by 0900. If not, let me know immediately."
- **Be specific in your instructions.** For example, "Let me know if Mrs. Wu has any red spots or broken skin areas when you turn her"—not "Tell me what her skin looks like."

Right Supervision

The last item in the checklist involves supervision. **Supervision** is the process of directing, guiding, and influencing the performance of the delegated task. When you delegate tasks to a NAP or LVN/LPN, you or another RN must be available to answer questions and provide help, if necessary. You are responsible for providing supervision and evaluating the outcomes. This includes the following:

- **Monitoring the NAP/LVN/LPN's work.** This is important to be sure it complies with agency policies and procedures and standards of practice. For example, after the NAP bathes a patient, you could check to see whether the patient is clean; or you might choose to observe for a few minutes while the NAP is working. Make frequent patient rounds and get regular reports from those you have assigned to do tasks.
- **Intervening, if necessary.** Many NAPs receive little training, so you may need to demonstrate some caregiving activities.
- **Obtaining and providing feedback from the worker.** Give positive, as well as negative, feedback often. If performance is not acceptable, speak privately with the NAP to explain the specific mistakes that were made. Listen to the NAP's view of the situation.

For example, there may have been too many tasks to complete in the time allowed.

- **Evaluating client outcomes.** Evaluate both the physical response and the relationship with the NAP. Ask the client for input after the care is given.
- **Ensuring proper documentation.** Some agencies permit NAPs to record vital signs and other patient data. You are responsible for seeing that all necessary data are recorded and that they are accurate.

KnowledgeCheck 7-3

- List the "five rights" of delegation.
- List at least four characteristics of a "right task"—that is, a task that would be acceptable to delegate.
- As an RN, how could you establish that a NAP is competent to perform a task?
- List at least three ways to help ensure that the NAP will understand clearly what she needs to do when you delegate a task.
- List at least three things you should do when providing supervision to an unlicensed caregiver.

 Go to Chapter 7, **Knowledge Check Response Sheet and Answers,** on the Student Resource Disk or DavisPlus at http://davisplus.fadavis.com/Wilkinson2

 CriticalThinking 7-4

For your patient, Jeannette Wu:
- Which activity did the nurse delegate to someone else?
- What collaborative activities should the nurse consider?

Documenting: The Final Step of Implementation

After giving care, you will record the nursing activities and the patient's responses. Documentation is a mode of communication among the members of the health team, and it provides the information you need to evaluate the patient's health status and the nursing care plan. For a thorough discussion of documenting, refer to Chapter 16.

Reflecting Critically About Implementation

During the implementation phase, perhaps more than at any other time, nurses combine thinking and doing. You should always be prepared to modify the activity based on the patient's responses. Afterward, when you have some time to reflect, you can think critically about what happened (good or bad) and why. Use the

Toward Evidence-Based Practice

Read about the following studies, and then answer the questions at the end of the box.

Standing, T., Anthony, M., & Hertz, J. (2001). Nurses' narratives of outcomes after delegation to unlicensed assistive personnel. *Outcomes Management for Nursing Practice, 5*(1), 18–23.

The authors of this qualitative study analyzed questionnaires and open-ended responses from 148 licensed nurses. Nurses were asked to write two narratives: one to describe a situation in which delegation of a task to a NAP had a positive outcome, and another that had a negative outcome. In addition, phone interviews were conducted with 27 nurses to expand on those findings. Along with the positive reports, the following negative results were also reported:

- Negative outcomes occurred most often because the NAP (1) did not follow directions or agency procedures, or (2) was overconfident (e.g., carried out activities that had not been delegated).
- With regard to the Five Rights of Delegation, deficiencies were most often related to the right communication or right supervision.

Standing, T., & Anthony, M. K. (2008). Delegation: What it means to acute care nurses. *Applied Nursing Research, 21*(1), 8–14.

The authors of this qualitative study conducted 17 in-depth interviews with acute-care nurses, both novice and

experienced, to examine the nature of delegation. Nurses expressed frustration that they were being held accountable for the NAPs' tasks, while the NAPs themselves were not. Several nurses described NAPs' resentment of RNs. They indicated that the RN-NAP relationship and good communication are at the heart of delegation. The RNs recognized the importance of acknowledging the contribution of the NAP. The RNs pointed out that one negative aspect of delegation is that the NAP sometimes did not perform tasks well, or at all, and sometimes communicated improperly with patients. A positive aspect is that delegation allows the RN time to monitor patient changes, review charts, and focus on "more important things." They concluded nursing education should provide more content on communication and interpersonal relationships.

1. What similarities do you see between the two studies in the authors and the methods?

2. What similarities in results are reported?

3. With your answer to question 2 in mind, what skill do you think you need to learn and practice to prepare for working with and delegating to NAPs?

 Go to Chapter 7, **Toward Evidence-Based Practice Suggested Responses,** on the Student Resource Disk or DavisPlus at http://davisplus.fadavis.com/Wilkinson

following questions, or refer to the critical thinking model. (See Chapter 2, Table 2-2 if you would like other ideas.)

- What was done? Why was it done? What were the patient's responses?
- Did I forget to do anything?
- What was going on in the situation that may have influenced the outcome?
- What factors influenced my behavior (or others' behavior) in this situation?
- Would the activity have been more successful if I had had more knowledge or skill? If so, why did I not realize that ahead of time, and how can I avoid such lack of insight in the future?
- What assumptions or biases (mine or the patient's) contributed to the problem in this situation?
- Did I communicate clearly to the patient?
- Did I convey respect and caring?
- What could I have delegated? What did I delegate that I should *not* have? Why?
- After reflecting on it, what would I do differently in this situation?

Refer to Table 7-2 for examples that demonstrate how the reflection questions might be used in a clinical situation.

Evaluation: The Final Step of the Nursing Process

Evaluation, the final step of the nursing process, is a planned, ongoing, systematic activity in which you will make judgments about:

- The client's progress toward desired health outcomes.
- The effectiveness of the nursing care plan.
- The quality of nursing care in the healthcare setting.

Why Is Evaluation Essential to Full-Spectrum Nursing?

Evaluation is an essential part of full-spectrum nursing for several reasons.

The patient is the nurse's first priority. The aim of all nursing activity is to achieve positive outcomes for patients. Evaluation lets you know whether your interventions are helping the patient as intended. No matter how carefully and conscientiously you perform a procedure, if it does not help the patient achieve desired outcomes, it has "missed the point."

Evaluation helps nurses to conserve scarce resources. Nurses are in short supply. Therefore, nursing time is precious and must be used wisely. Evaluation allows you to discard interventions that are not working well and focus on more effective ones. In addition to saving time, there may be cost savings as well.

Professional standards of practice require evaluation. For example, see the ANA and Canadian practice standards in Box 7-2.

The ANA Code of Ethics requires evaluation. "The nurse's primary commitment is to the recipient of nursing and healthcare services—the patient—whether the recipient is an individual, a family, a group, or a community. . . . The nurse has a responsibility to implement and maintain standards of professional nursing practice. The nurse should participate in planning, establishing, implementing, and evaluating review mechanisms designed to safeguard patients and nurses, such as peer review processes or committees, credentialing processes, quality improvement initiatives, and ethics committees" (ANA, 2001, Section 2.1 and Standard 3.4).

The Joint Commission and professional standards review organizations (PSROs) require evaluation. These organizations use outcomes and performance measures to evaluate the quality of care in healthcare institutions. They conceptualize quality of care as the degree to which health services increase the likelihood of desired health outcomes.

Evaluation helps ensure nursing's survival. Linking nursing interventions to achievement of client outcomes demonstrates the value of nursing. In today's competitive healthcare market, that is essential for ensuring continued funding for nursing services, education, and research.

Table 7-2 ➤ Examples of Reflecting Critically About Implementation		
SITUATION	**QUESTION FOR REFLECTION**	**WHAT MIGHT HAVE HAPPENED?**
The nursing order read, "Assist to ambulate to the end of the hall . . ." However, the patient was able to walk only about half that distance before becoming too weak to stand.	What was going on in the situation that may have influenced the outcome?	Perhaps the patient was weak because he had not slept well the night before; or perhaps he had just had a long, tiring session of physical therapy.
When the patient became too weak to walk, the nurse called for help. Why did she do that instead of helping the patient to sit where he was, or instead of helping him back to the room by herself?	What factors influenced the nurse's behavior in this situation?	Perhaps the patient was very large and the nurse realized she was not strong enough to provide support. Can you think of other reasons the nurse might have chosen that action?

BOX 7-2 ■ Professional Standards of Care: Evaluation

American Nurses Association Standards of Practice[1]
Standard 6. Evaluation

The registered nurse evaluates progress towards attainment of outcomes.

Competencies:

The registered nurse:

Conducts a systematic, ongoing, and criterion-based evaluation of the outcomes in relation to the structures and processes prescribed by the plan of care and the indicated timeline.

Collaborates with the person and others involved in the care or situation in the evaluation process.

Evaluates, in partnership with the person, the effectiveness of the planned strategies in relation to the person's responses and attainment of the expected outcomes.

Documents the results of the evaluation.

Uses ongoing assessment data to revise the diagnoses, outcomes, the plan, and the implementation, as needed.

Disseminates the results to the patient, family, and others involved, in accordance with federal and state regulations.

Actively participates in assessing and assuring the responsible and appropriate use of interventions in order to minimize unwarranted or unwanted treatment and patient suffering.

Source: American Nurses Association (2010, in press). *Nursing: Scope and Standards of Practice* (2nd ed.). Public Comment draft, January 2010. (To be published by August, 2010). Silver Spring, MD: Nursebooks.org.

[1]*Caveat:* This material is from the draft for public comment (ANA, 2010, in press); its wording may be changed somewhat in the final published version. For that version of the ANA Standards of Professional Nursing Practice, go to www.nursingworld.org.

Canadian Provincial Standards of Practice

In Canada, practice standards are set at the provincial level. The following are excerpts from provincial standards that apply to evaluation.

- The registered nurse demonstrates critical thinking in collecting and interpreting data, planning, implementing, *and evaluating all aspects of nursing care.*

- The registered nurse documents timely, accurate reports of data collection, interpretation, planning, implementing, and *evaluating care.*

- The registered nurse initiates and/or participates in quality improvement activities.

Sources: College and Association of Registered Nurses of Alberta. (2003). *Nursing practice standards.* 11620-168 Street, Edmonton, AB T5M 4A6, Canada; College of Registered Nurses of Nova Scotia. (2003). *Standards for nursing practice.* 600-1894 Barrington Street, Halifax, NS B3J 2A8, Canada; Nurses Association of New Brunswick. (2005). *Standards of practice for registered nurses.* 165 Regent Street, Fredericton, NB E3B 7B4, Canada.

Evaluation demonstrates caring and responsibility. Without evaluation, you would not know whether your care was effective. Examining outcomes implies that you care about how your activities affect your clients.

Quality and Safety Education for Nurses (QSEN). This task force includes quality improvement as one of the competencies to be achieved during your education in nursing. Evaluation is essential for this competency.

How Are Standards and Criteria Used in Evaluation?

In a broad sense, evaluation is the systematic process of judging the quality or value of something by comparing it to one or more standards or criteria. In our daily lives, we evaluate many things: for example, a meal, a TV program, an insurance policy we are thinking of buying. However, for formal evaluation, you must decide *in advance* which standards and criteria you will use. As you learned in Chapter 1, **standards** represent expected or accepted levels of performance; they provide a model for what ought to be done. They are established by authority,

custom, or consensus. In nursing, standards are used to describe quality nursing care. The American Nurses Association's standards of practice are a good example of broadly written standards (see Boxes 7-1 and 7-2).

Notice that each of the ANA standards includes a set of measurement criteria, called competencies, to help describe the standard. **Criteria** are measurable or observable characteristics, properties, attributes, or qualities. They describe the specific skills, knowledge, behaviors, and attitudes that are desired or expected. Judges at a diving competition, for example, might evaluate a dive by using criteria for difficulty, technique, and style.

The patient goals and outcomes discussed in Chapter 5 are also examples of criteria. As you learned there, these criteria should be concrete and specific enough to serve as guides for collecting evaluation data. In addition, they should be reliable and valid. A criterion is **reliable** if it yields consistent results—that is, the same results every time, regardless of who uses it. For example, suppose you and another nurse measure a patient's temperature by (1) using an oral thermometer and (2) placing the back of your hand on the patient's forehead. Which method would probably give the same (or nearly same) results every time? As you probably concluded, the oral thermometer is more reliable.

A criterion is **valid** if it is really measuring what it was intended to measure. For example, fever is often used as a criterion for concluding that a person has an infection. However, if used alone, it is not a valid indicator because (1) other conditions, such as dehydration, can cause a fever and (2) elevated temperature is not present in all infections. However, validity of that criterion is increased when you use additional criteria (e.g., elevated white blood cell count, presence of signs of infection such as redness and pus).

CriticalThinking 7-5

- The outcome "Patient will not complain of pain" by itself is not a valid criterion for measuring pain. Why? What would be a more valid criterion for pain?
- A criterion reads, "Measures client vital signs once per shift, or as ordered." For which of the following standards would it be valid (that is, which conclusion could you draw if you knew that a nurse measured the vital signs once per shift, or as ordered)?
  Follows unit policies.
  Performs skills accurately.

Types of Evaluation

Evaluation is categorized according to (1) what is being evaluated (structures, processes, or outcomes) and (2) frequency and time of evaluation.

Evaluation of Structures, Processes, and Outcomes

Structures, processes and outcomes all work together to affect care; however, each requires different criteria and methods of evaluation. **Structure evaluation** focuses on the setting in which care is provided. It explores the effect of organizational characteristics on the quality of care. It requires standards and data about policies, procedures, fiscal resources, physical facilities and equipment, and number and qualifications of personnel. Examples of criteria for structure evaluation include the following:

At least one registered nurse is present on each unit at all times.
A resuscitation cart is available on each floor.

Process evaluation focuses on the manner in which care is given—the activities performed by nurses (and other personnel). It explores whether the care was relevant to patient needs, appropriate, complete, and timely. Your instructor uses process evaluation to evaluate your clinical performance. Your clinical evaluation describes what you did and how well you did it. As a rule, it does not describe the *results* of your activities. Examples of criteria for process evaluation include the following:

Protects patient's privacy when performing procedures.
Washes hands before each patient contact.

Outcomes evaluation focuses on observable or measurable changes in the patient's health status that result from the care given. Although structure and process

are important to quality, the most important aspect is improvement in patient health status. The evaluation step of the nursing process uses outcomes evaluation. Examples of outcomes criteria include:

Patient will walk, assisted, to end of hall by day 5 postop.
Patient reports pain less than 4 on a 1–10 scale within 1 hour after analgesic administration.

Outcomes evaluation is also used when evaluating quality of care in an organization. When used for that purpose, the criteria also state the percentage of clients expected to have the outcome when care is satisfactory. For example:

Post-catheterization urinary tract infection does not occur.
Expected compliance: 100%

This means that the criterion would be met only if no patients developed a urinary tract infection after being catheterized.

Ongoing, Intermittent, and Terminal Evaluation

Evaluation begins as soon as you have completed the first nursing activity and continues during each client contact until all goals are achieved or the client is discharged from nursing care. The client's status determines how often you evaluate. A critically ill patient may need a nurse constantly at the bedside; after a patient undergoes surgery, you may measure vital signs every 15 minutes; as the patient nears discharge, you may evaluate once a day. In long-term care settings, in contrast, residents often have chronic health problems that require evaluation over an extended period of time. Most care is provided by LVN/LPNs and NAPs, and the RN may participate in weekly care conferences to evaluate the resident's response to the current plan of care.

You will perform **ongoing evaluation** while implementing, immediately after an intervention, and at each patient contact. In contrast, **intermittent evaluation** is performed at specified times. Both kinds of evaluation enable you to judge the progress toward goal achievement and to modify the care plan as needed. Goals and expected outcomes should designate times for collecting evaluation data. For example:

Will rate pain as < 3 on 1–10 scale *within 1 hr after medication*.
Will lose 1 lb *per week* until weight of 125 lb is achieved.
By the second home visit, mother will demonstrate proper techniques for breastfeeding.

Terminal evaluation describes the client's health status and progress toward goals at the time of discharge. Most institutions have special discharge forms for terminal evaluation that also include instructions about medications, treatments, and follow-up care.

As in all phases of the nursing process, you should collaborate with the patient and family in evaluation to the extent they are able. As the nurse, you are responsible for drawing evaluative conclusions; however, you should use input from the patient, the family, NAPs and other caregivers (see Box 7-2).

Critical Thinking 7-6

For each of the following goals, when or how often should the nurse collect evaluation data?

- Will rate pain as < 3 on scale of 1 to 10 within *1 hr after medication*.
- Will lose 1 lb *per week* until weight of 125 lb is achieved.
- *By the second home visit*, mother will demonstrate proper techniques for breastfeeding.

How Is Evaluation Related to Other Steps of the Nursing Process?

Evaluation is affected by all other steps of the nursing process. The patient outcomes stated in the *planning outcomes* stage must be concrete, observable, and appropriate for the patient in order to be useful as evaluation criteria. Appropriate outcomes, in turn, depend on complete and accurate *assessment* data and *nursing diagnoses*. You will observe and evaluate client responses during *implementation* in order to make on-the-spot changes in activity. And, of course, *interventions* must be *planned* and *implemented* to produce the patient behaviors that you evaluate.

Evaluation overlaps greatly with the assessment step—both involve data collection. The difference is in *when you collect* and *how you use* the data.

- *Assessment data* are collected before interventions are performed to determine initial or baseline health status and to make nursing diagnoses.
- *Evaluation data* are collected after interventions are performed to determine whether client goals were achieved.

Knowledge Check 7-4

- Explain what is evaluated in each of the following types of evaluation (i.e., the focus of each type of evaluation): structure, process, and outcomes.
- Identify what is evaluated using the following criteria: structure, process, or outcomes.
  In the Emergency Department the time from patient sign-in to assessment by a healthcare worker will be less than 15 minutes.
  A fire extinguisher is located in an accessible spot on each unit.
  No patients with indwelling urinary catheters will develop urinary tract infection.
- Define the following: ongoing evaluation, intermittent evaluation, terminal evaluation.

 Go to Chapter 7, **Knowledge Check Response Sheet and Answers,** on the Student Resource Disk or DavisPlus at http://davisplus.fadavis.com/Wilkinson

How Do I Evaluate Patient Progress?

Evaluation does not "end" the nursing process. It merely provides the information you need to begin another cycle. After giving care, you compare patient responses to the desired outcomes (goals) and use that information to reflect critically on (1) the care plan and (2) each step of the nursing process as it applies to that patient. When evaluating patient progress, you review the desired outcomes, collect reassessment data, judge whether goals have been met, and record the evaluative statement (Wilkinson, 2007). Figure 7-1 illustrates the relationship of the evaluation phase to the rest of the nursing process.

Review Outcomes

First, review the goals/outcomes on the patient's care plan. The goals and indicators you identified in the planning outcomes phase suggest the kind of assessments you need to make and provide criteria by which to judge the data.

Collect Reassessment Data

Next, assess client responses to the interventions. To minimize confusion, assessments made for the purpose of evaluation are called **reassessment.** Reassessments are always focused assessments (see Chapter 3). As already mentioned, the care plan goals determine their focus.

- Suppose, for example, that the nursing care plan lists the following goal: "By 8/24, will walk, unassisted, to the end of the hall without pallor or shortness of breath." What kind of assessments would you make to know whether this goal has been met?
- Suppose the care plan includes the following goal: "By 8/24, will notify nurse as soon as pain begins." How would you obtain the data you need to evaluate this goal?

For the first example, you would observe the patient's skin color as he walked, observe and count his respirations, and ask him if he felt short of breath at any time. The second example is a little less obvious. If the patient doesn't call you, you cannot just assume there is no pain. You would need to ask him whether he has had pain (e.g., "I notice that you have not put your call light on. Have you had any pain at all today?"). If the patient does call you, you still cannot assume it is because of pain, or that he called as soon as the pain began. You must question to clarify, for example: "How can I help you?" "Are you in pain?" "When did it start?"

Critical Thinking 7-7

In the examples in the preceding paragraph, which aspects of critical thinking (in the full-spectrum nursing model in Chapter 2) did you use in order to decide what data you needed?

Goals can be cognitive, psychomotor, or affective, or they may refer to body appearance and function. The nature of the goal determines the kind of data you need to collect. See Table 7-3 for examples of goal types and the kind of reassessment data they require. As in the assessment phase, you will collect data from the client, family, friends, and health team members, as well as from the client's chart (e.g., laboratory results). The RN is responsible for evaluating goal achievement, even though someone else may have supplied the data.

Judge Goal Achievement

Next, compare the reassessment data with the patient's goals. Are the responses (actual outcomes) the same as the expected or desired outcomes? If so, the goal has been met. As always, get the patient's input. Ask her if she thinks the goals have been achieved. Goals or outcomes can be:

- *Achieved.* The actual responses are the same as the desired outcome.
- *Partially achieved.* Some, but not all, of the desired behaviors were observed, or the desired response occurs only some of the time (e.g., the desired heart rate is < 100 beats/min, a goal that is achieved except for one or two episodes a day, when it is 110 beats/min).
- *Not achieved.* The desired response did not occur (actual outcome does not match desired outcome or goal).

Record the Evaluative Statement

Professional standards require that you record your evaluations. You may write an evaluative summary in the nursing notes or on the care plan, depending on the procedure specified by the institution. An evaluative statement should include:

- The conclusion about whether the goal was achieved
- Reassessment data to support the judgment

An evaluative statement for the pain goal "By 8/24, will notify nurse as soon as pain begins" might be:

8/25/06, 0100. Goal not met. Has not used call light at all this A.M. Restless and grimacing with movement during A.M. care. When asked, described pain as 8 on a 1–10 scale. ————————————— J. Hiam, RN

When using standardized outcomes (e.g., NOC) or electronic care plans, your evaluative statements may be different. In the NOC system, each outcome (label) has a scale and indicators (specific patient responses), numbered 1 through 5, which you can use to write goals (see Chapter 5). For example, a patient with a problem of decreased peripheral circulation might have this goal: "Circulation status not compromised." Using standardized language from NOC, you might write a goal (*desired* status) of:

Goal: Circulation Status: 5 (5 means "no deviation from normal range" in the NOC scale).

Each of the indicators could also be made into a goal by adding the desired scale numbers, as follows:

Systolic BP in expected range: 5
Diastolic BP in expected range: 5
Mean BP in expected range: 5

Evaluation statements are written exactly the same as goals, but the scale number describes the patient's *actual* status. So, if on reassessment the patient's blood pressure is quite low and he has orthostatic hypotension, the evaluative statement might be:

Evaluative Statement: Circulation Status: 3 (3 means "moderately compromised" on this NOC scale)

Figure 7-2 is a computer screen showing the NOC outcome of Acceptance: Health Status. The "Initial

Table 7-3 ➤ Reassessments for Different Types of Goals			
TYPE OF GOAL	**INVOLVES**	**EXAMPLE OF GOALS**	**REASSESSMENT TECHNIQUES**
Cognitive	Increases in patient knowledge	■ By 8/24 accurately describes schedule for taking medications. ■ By 8/25 correctly describes the procedure for pouring liquid medications.	Ask the person to repeat information or to apply new knowledge (e.g., to describe to you the schedule for taking her medications).
Affective	Changes in feelings, values, beliefs, and attitudes	■ By 8/24 expresses positive feelings for the newborn. ■ By 8/24 states he is only mildly anxious about changing his own dressing.	Observe client behavior reflecting values and beliefs; talk to the client about feelings and beliefs; observe nonverbal expression of feelings (e.g., laughing, crying).
Psychomotor	Patient's ability to perform skills	■ By 8/24, performs own dressing change, using proper aseptic technique. ■ By 8/24, measures liquid medication accurately.	Ask the person to demonstrate the new skill (e.g., change a dressing, measure a liquid medication).
Body appearance and function	Changes in body systems and functions	■ Heart rate will be 100 beats/min after ambulation to end of hall. ■ By 8/24 can dress self and fasten own zipper.	Observe functioning, examine the body, perform measurements, read laboratory reports (e.g., measure vital signs, observe skin color, assess for pain).

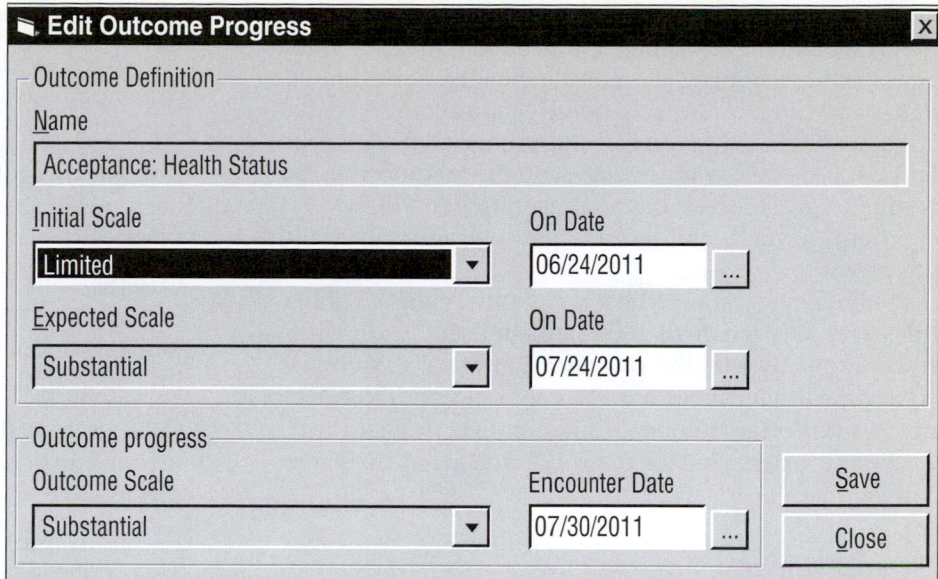

FIGURE 7-2 Computer screen showing outcome progress, using NOC. (*Source:* Courtesy of Ergo Partners, L.C., Boulder, CO. Used with permission.)

Explanation of Figure

Computer field	Nursing process terminology	Represents	Status recorded on computer
Initial scale	Initial assessment	*Actual* status *before* intervention	Limited acceptance of health status
Expected scale	Goal	*Desired* status *after* intervention	Substantial acceptance of health status
Outcome scale	Evaluative statement	*Actual* status *after* intervention	Substantial acceptance of health status

Scale" shows the initial assessment; the "Expected Scale" is the goal; and the "Outcome Scale" is the evaluative statement after intervention and reassessment. Did the interventions achieve the desired effect, or not? If you want to see a computer screen showing a NOC outcome definition and indicators,

Go to Chapter 7, **Tables, Boxes, Figures: ESG Figure 7-1,** on the Student Resource Disk or DavisPlus at http://davisplus.fadavis.com/Wilkinson2

KnowledgeCheck 7-5

Using the following outcomes and reassessment data, determine whether each goal has been met, partially met, or not met.

Goal: By 8/24, will walk, unassisted, to the end of the hall without pallor or shortness of breath.
Reassessment data: 8/24. Walked, unassisted, to end of hall; states no shortness of breath, but skin color was noticeably pale.

Goal: By 8/24, will walk, unassisted, to the end of the hall without pallor or shortness of breath.
Reassessment data: 8/23. Walked, unassisted, to end of hall. Skin color pink; respirations 14/min; no dyspnea observed; states no shortness of breath.

Goal: By 8/24, will walk, unassisted, to the end of the hall without pallor or shortness of breath.

Reassessment data: 8/25. Walked halfway to end of hall before becoming pale and short of breath.

Go to Chapter 7, **Knowledge Check Response Sheet and Answers,** on the Student Resource Disk or DavisPlus at http://davisplus.fadavis.com/Wilkinson2

How Do I Evaluate Collaborative Problems?

For collaborative problems, you will collect reassessment data the same as for nursing diagnoses. However, nurses share the responsibility for preventing complications that occur with collaborative problems with the physician and other members of the health team. The desired outcome for all collaborative problems is that no complication will occur. For example, if a patient's collaborative problem is Potential Complication of myocardial infarction: congestive heart failure (CHF), the logical goal is "CHF will not occur." Clearly, nursing actions alone cannot prevent CHF. Collaborative efforts are required.

Therefore, goals for collaborative problems are not included on the nursing care plan, and the evaluation process is slightly different. Compare the reassessment data to established norms (e.g., normal temperature, normal electrocardiogram pattern, normal blood glucose) and determine whether data are within an acceptable range. If the data indicate the client's condition is worsening (that the complication [e.g., CHF] may be occurring), notify the medical provider. For example, if a patient with the collaborative problem Potential Complication of myocardial infarction: CHF develops fatigue, dyspnea, a productive cough, or abnormal lab results (e.g., elevated blood urea nitrogen [BUN] and creatinine levels), you would suspect CHF and notify the provider.

If the reassessment data are within normal limits, this does not mean that the collaborative problem is resolved—only that the complication has not occurred. As long as the patient has the medical condition (e.g., myocardial infarction), the collaborative problem (e.g., CHF) still exists. See Chapter 4 if you need to review collaborative problems.

Evaluating and Revising the Care Plan

After evaluating patient progress, you will use your conclusions about goal achievement to decide whether to continue, modify, or discontinue the care plan.

Relate Outcomes to Interventions

Even when goals have been met, you cannot assume that the nursing interventions caused the patient outcomes. You need to use critical reflection to identify factors that might have supported or interfered with the effectiveness of an intervention. Recall that organizational structures and processes can also affect patient care. The following are variables that can affect the ability of an intervention to produce the desired outcome:

- The client's ability and motivation to follow directions for treatment
- Availability and support from family and significant others
- Treatments and therapies performed by other healthcare team members
- Client failure to provide complete information during assessment
- Client's lack of experience, knowledge, or ability
- Staffing in the institution (ratio of licensed to unlicensed caregivers; number of patients for whom a nurse is responsible)
- Nurse's physical and mental well-being

Identifying these factors allows you to reinforce or change them. For example, if Jeannette Wu does not achieve a goal of "Intact skin over sacrum" even after being turned every 2 hours by the NAP, you may discover Ms. Wu's skin is more fragile than expected because her hydration and nutrition are not adequate. You could then take measures to support her intake of food and fluids, increasing the effectiveness of the turning intervention. Notice, though, that you cannot control all the variables that might affect the success of an intervention (e.g., the client's lack of experience, staffing in your institution).

Draw Conclusions About Problem Status

Whether you retain or remove a nursing diagnosis from the care plan depends on whether or not goals were met, as follows:

Goals met: If all goals for a nursing diagnosis have been met, you can discontinue the care plan for that diagnosis.

Goals partially met: If some outcomes are met and others not, you may revise the care plan for that problem; or you may continue with the same plan but allow more time for goal achievement.

Goals not met: If goals are not met, you should examine the entire plan and review all steps of the nursing process to decide whether to revise the care plan.

For an example of electronic evaluation of problem status for a client with multiple nursing care needs,

 Go to Chapter 7, **Tables, Boxes, Figures: ESG Figure 7-2,** on the Student Resource Disk or DavisPlus at http://davisplus.fadavis.com/Wilkinson2

Revise the Care Plan

To decide how to revise the care plan, you must review each step of the nursing process. You cannot just discontinue the ineffective interventions and try new ones. The interventions may not need to be changed at all. When goals have not been met, errors in other steps of the nursing process may be the reason. To find a checklist you can use to evaluate the care plan and the process by which it was developed (Wilkinson, 2007),

 Go to Chapter 7, **Delegation and Evaluation Checklists,** in Volume 2.

1. *Review of assessment.* Review all initial and ongoing assessment data. All steps of the nursing process depend on complete and accurate data. So if there are errors or omissions, you may need to revise any or all sections of the care plan (i.e., nursing diagnosis, outcomes, nursing orders). Also, the data may have changed since the care plan was written: the client's condition may have changed, or new data may have been identified.
2. *Review of diagnosis.* Even if there were no errors of assessment, you may need to revise or add new nursing diagnoses. Perhaps the nurse who wrote the diagnostic statement did not communicate the patient's condition clearly, or perhaps it was not validated with the patient. This might have caused an incorrect focus for outcomes and interventions.
3. *Review of planning outcomes.* You will probably need to revise the outcomes if you have added data or revised the nursing diagnosis. If assessment and diagnosis are satisfactory, perhaps the outcomes were unrealistic, written too broadly, or had unrealistic target times.

4. *Review of planning interventions.* If you determine that interventions were not effective in achieving the desired outcomes, or if you have revised nursing diagnoses or outcomes, you will probably need to modify nursing orders.

5. *Review of implementation.* It could be that goals were not met because of a failure to implement the nursing orders or because of the manner in which they were implemented. Get input from the client, significant others, other caregivers, and the client records to find out what went wrong. For example, the person implementing care may have been tired, in a hurry, or abrupt with the client. Or perhaps he did not have the necessary skills. See "Delegating and Supervising Care," earlier in this chapter, if you need a review.

Reflecting Critically About Evaluation

After evaluating the patient's health status and the nursing care plan, you should think critically about your thinking during the evaluation process. That's right: Think about your thinking, not just about your actions. The critical thinking model from Chapter 2 suggests some questions you might use for reflection.

Inquiring
Is my evaluation statement clearly stated (goal met or not met, plus supporting data)?
Were my information sources reliable (e.g., was the patient being honest or merely trying to please me)?
Did I jump to conclusions about goal achievement? Do I need any other data to validate my conclusion?

Noticing context
What was going on either before or during evaluation that might have influenced my ability to gather data or draw conclusions (e.g., Was I in a hurry? Did the patient have visitors?)
What emotional responses influenced my conclusions about goal achievement (e.g., Would I feel as though I had failed if the goal was not met?)

Analyzing assumptions
What biases do I have that may have affected my ability to reassess or evaluate goal achievement?

Reflecting skeptically
Did I make evaluating a priority? Did I schedule time for it, the same as I do for interventions?
Could I have done it better?
What would I do differently next time?

The most common errors of evaluation are failing to:

- Evaluate systematically.
- Record the results.
- Use the reassessment data to examine and modify the care plan.

Because nurses are action oriented, it is easy for most to make a plan and take action. And most nurses regularly observe the patient's responses to the actions. But you will need determined effort to make time to observe *regularly and systematically* and *document the patient's responses* to your actions. Only in that way can you be sure the care has met the client's needs.

Evaluating the Quality of Care in a Healthcare Setting

As a nurse, you may be involved in evaluating and improving the overall quality of nursing care in an organization or a geographical area. At a minimum, your documentation will provide data that regulatory agencies (e.g., The Joint Commission, state boards of nursing) use to determine whether nursing care meets nursing standards.

Quality assurance (QA) programs are specially designed programs to promote excellence in nursing. Variations of quality assurance are quality improvement (QI), continuous quality improvement (CQI), total quality management (TQM), and persistent quality improvement (PQI). Whatever the approach, the goal is to evaluate and improve the care provided in an agency or for a group of patients. One hospital reports reduction in patient falls and medication errors, as well as improvement in nursing documentation after implementation of a quality improvement program chaired by a staff nurse (Johnson, Hallsey, Meredith, et al., 2006).

This chapter has described (1) outcomes evaluation of *client progress* and (2) process evaluation of the *effectiveness of the nursing care plan.* Quality improvement involves evaluation of structures, as well as outcomes and processes. All are important because structures and processes affect patient outcomes. Adequate structures (e.g., staffing, money) and processes (e.g., policies and procedures) do not guarantee desired patient outcomes; however, without them, it is very difficult to obtain good outcomes. For example, a unit could be well staffed (structure) and follow infection-control procedures carefully (process), yet have a higher-than-average rate of urinary tract infections (outcome). The reason may be that most of the patients treated have compromised immune systems, making them especially susceptible to infection. For a full discussion of QA/QI evaluation, see Chapter 1 and

 Go to Chapter 1, **Supplemental Materials,** on the Student Resource Disk or DavisPlus at http://davisplus.fadavis.com/Wilkinson2

 Go to Chapter 7, **Reading More About Implementation & Evaluation,** on the Student Resource Disk or DavisPlus at http://davisplus.fadavis.com/Wilkinson2

 Go to Chapter 7, **Resources for Caregivers and Health Professionals,** on the Student Resource Disk or DavisPlus at http://davisplus.fadavis.com/Wilkinson2

 Bibliography: Go to Volume 2, Bibliography.

CHAPTER 8

Nursing Theory & Research

Learning Outcomes

After completing this chapter, you should be able to:

➤ Define nursing theory.

➤ List four components of a theory.

➤ Describe how a nursing theory is developed.

➤ List the four essential concepts in a nursing theory.

➤ List three ways nurses can use nursing theory.

➤ Discuss the relevance of Florence Nightingale's nursing theory to contemporary nursing practice.

➤ Name three predominant thinkers who proposed theories of caring.

➤ Describe three nonnursing theories and their contributions to nursing.

➤ Define nursing research.

➤ Describe the significance of evidence-based nursing practice.

➤ Describe the history of nursing research in the United States.

➤ Compare and contrast quantitative and qualitative nursing research.

➤ List three components of the research process, and explain their importance.

➤ Name three priorities in the process of protecting research participants, and explain the significance of these to the nursing research process.

➤ Describe the PICO method of formulating a question to guide a literature search.

➤ List at least four steps in the process of analytic reading of research reports, and explain their significance to the appraisal of research.

➤ Describe how to use nursing research in nursing practice.

Meet Your Patient

Imagine you are the charge nurse on the night shift at a long-term care facility. You hear the certified nursing assistant (CNA) and another person speaking loudly down the hall. You immediately go to see what has happened. You are surprised and shocked by what you see. An older patient, Mr. Wilkey, is sitting on the bed of another patient, Mrs. Fredrickson, who is crying and shouting, "Get out! Get out!" Mr. Wilkey is tearful and looks frightened. He keeps repeating, "Where is Momma? Where is Momma?" The CNA is visibly upset and is grabbing at Mr. Wilkey in an effort to get him off the bed.

What are you going to do, and why do you think it will help? Don't be concerned if you don't think you know enough to answer this question. Before you read on, try to answer it based on the knowledge and experience that you *do* have.

There are two general ways to approach this problem. One way is to be upset with Mr. Wilkey and take him from the room immediately, explaining sternly that his behavior is not acceptable and he must stay in his room. Another

possibility is to ask the CNA to calm Mrs. Fredrickson while you talk quietly to Mr. Wilkey and gently guide him out of the room, not rushing him. While you are talking to him, you might ask, "Who is Momma? What does she look like? Do you miss her?" By the time you lead him to his room, you might realize he is exhibiting stage II dementia. You infer that he probably woke up scared and confused and began looking for his long-dead mother. Seeing Mrs. Fredrickson, Mr. Wilkey thought he had found his mother and crawled into her bed.

If you chose the first approach in the scenario, you were demonstrating **mechanistic nursing,** which is based on getting the tasks done. If you chose the second solution, you based your behavior on **holistic nursing,** which requires meeting the needs of the whole person. This scenario demonstrates the powerful impact of nursing theory and research on your daily practice as a nurse. Although there are several theories that guide nursing practice, this chapter draws heavily on theories of caring to illustrate key points. We believe caring is central to nursing and informs all the actions that nurses take. You may recall that it is an important concept in the full-spectrum model introduced in Chapter 2. You will find other theories that pertain to specific aspects of practice in later chapters. For example, developmental theories are discussed in Chapter 9, theories of self-concept in Chapter 11, and family theories in Chapter 12.

The Importance of Nursing Theory and Research

This chapter introduces you to nursing theory and research and how they form the foundations for patient care. Following are three examples that demonstrate how important theory and research are to you in your career as a nurse.

The Framingham Study is a longitudinal, multidisciplinary research project (*longitudinal* means done over a long period of time). It consisted of several studies carried out over 50 years (from 1948 to 1998) to identify the health and healthcare practices of one specific community: Framingham, Massachusetts. The results of the various Framingham studies influenced healthcare practices for diabetes mellitus, breast cancer, heart disease, osteoarthritis in older adults, and other disease entities. For example, one commonly accepted practice that came out of the Framingham study is the use of mammography to screen for breast cancer. There was a time when mammography was considered unreliable and unimportant. The Framingham project changed that attitude and, as a result, improved the healthcare of women.

Dr. Jean Watson (Fig. 8-1) developed a nursing theory called the **Science of Human Caring** (Watson, 1988). This theory describes what *caring* means from a nursing perspective. It may not seem that nurses need to be taught how to care, but Dr. Watson and other nursing theorists found they did. Before the "caring theorists," nurses were somewhat mechanistic in the work they did (much like the first alternative for dealing with Mr. Wilkey). A mechanistic nurse has a list of things to do, completes the list, and does nothing more. The "something more" behaviors often are the caring behaviors, such as singing to a frightened child or taking the time to teach a new mother for the second time how to bathe her baby.

This is not to say that nurses didn't care about their patients before Watson. The point is that a *theory* of caring (such as Watson's) changes the *focus* of nursing. Certainly Nightingale must have cared about the soldiers who

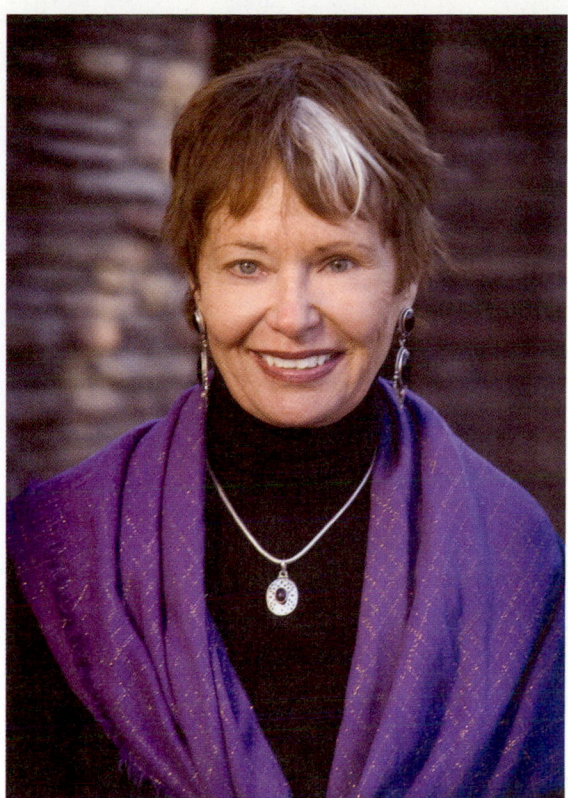

FIGURE 8-1 Dr. Jean Watson, distinguished professor and nursing theorist.

were her patients. But what she wrote about and what she taught the nurses was a set of "things to do." Nurses were valued for the tasks they performed in patient care. Caring theories demonstrate the value of the non–task-oriented aspects of nursing.

Dr. Patricia Benner, in the book *From Novice to Expert* (1984), proposed a theory that should be of special interest to you. This theory, which was explained in Chapter 1, describes the progression of a beginning nurse to increasing levels of expertise. You are a **novice,** or a beginning nurse, simply because you are new to the nursing profession. Benner's theory provides the information necessary to understand how you learn and perform your nursing responsibilities. Benner's theory of caring is discussed later in the chapter. Think of full-spectrum nursing as a jigsaw puzzle (Fig. 8-2). Initially, a nurse has an idea, which usually comes out of experiences in *practice* (the first puzzle piece). Perhaps the idea is something simple like: "Why don't I slow down and spend more time with the patients' families? It would really help them if I took more time."

After seriously considering the new idea, the nurse may decide the idea is worth investigating with *research* (the second puzzle piece). The research question might be: "How does spending more time with family members affect the quality of care the patient receives?" If the research supported the nurse's idea, she could then use the research findings to develop a *theory* (the third puzzle piece). The nurse could even take the research results to nursing administrators to determine whether

FIGURE 8-2 Practice, theory, and research are interrelated: a nurse has an idea, conducts research to test the idea, and finally develops a theory.

the theory could be put into practice in the organization—perhaps as a policy or in a standardized care plan. That would be the beginning of what is called a **clinical practice theory**, a theory that is immediately applicable in the clinical setting.

KnowledgeCheck 8-1

- Compare mechanistic and holistic nursing. Select one of these concepts and describe a scenario in which it is used.
- Briefly describe the Framingham Study, and list three diseases for which this study influenced care.

 Go to Chapter 8, **Knowledge Check Response Sheet and Answers,** on the Student Resource Disk or DavisPlus at http://davisplus.fadavis.com/Wilkinson2

Nursing Theories

Theoretical **Knowledge** knowing why

Florence Nightingale (1859/1992) stated that nursing theories describe and explain what is and what is not nursing. That makes them critical to learn in the beginning of your nursing education. Before focusing on

nursing theory, though, you need to learn a little more about theory in general. Exactly what *is* a theory? And how is a theory created?

A **theory** is an organized set of related ideas and concepts that helps us find meaning in our experiences (such as nursing), organize our thinking around an idea (such as caring), and develop new ideas and insights into the work we do. Put simply, a theory answers the questions: What is this? And how does it work? Although a theory is based on observations of facts, the theory itself is *not* a fact. A theory is merely a way of viewing phenomena (reality); it defines and illustrates concepts and explains how they are related or linked. Theories can be, and are, changed.

What Are the Components of a Theory?

Theories are made up of assumptions, phenomena, concepts, definitions, and statements (or propositions). You can think of these as the building blocks of a theory.

Assumptions

Assumptions are ideas that we take for granted. In a theory, they are the ideas that the theorist or researcher presumes to be true and does not intend to test with research. They are statements about concepts or relationships between concepts. For example, Watson assumed nursing had its own professional concepts and that one of them was caring. Assumptions may or may not be stated. For example, most nursing theorists assume but do not state that human beings are complex. One exception is Martha Rogers (1970), who states outright that human beings are unified wholes that are more than and different from the sum of their parts.

Phenomena

Phenomena are aspects of reality that you can observe and experience. Phenomena are the subject matter of a discipline (when used in this sense, they are often called *phenomena of concern*). Think of phenomena as marking the boundaries (*domain*) of a discipline—making one discipline unique from another. For example, for cartographers (map makers) the phenomena of concern are land formations and land use. For pharmacists, the phenomena of concern are medications: their chemical composition and their effects on the body. For nurses, the phenomena of concern are human beings and, more specifically, their body-mind-spirit responses to illness and injuries. It may seem a subtle difference, but Watson's theory of caring gave us the words and ideas for describing the nursing phenomena of concern in terms of *human beings in their environments*.

Concepts

A **concept** is a mental image of a phenomenon. It is formed by generalizing an abstract idea from your experiences and observations of events, objects, and properties, and it exists as a symbol (e.g., a word or picture) in the mind. For example, what does the word *fever* bring to mind? From your own experience with fever, you know the subjective feeling that fever produces. You have the theoretical knowledge that it is an elevated body temperature; you know the physiology of temperature regulation, so you know what is going on in the body. You may have the visual image of a thermometer or someone who is warm to the touch and possibly perspiring. The word *fever* is a symbol for all of those ideas and images. It is a concept.

Concepts range from simple to complex and from fairly concrete to very abstract. Simple, concrete concepts are those you can observe directly (e.g., height, weight, gender, body type). More abstract and complex concepts are those you observe indirectly (e.g., hematocrit, brain activity, nutritional status). Abstract concepts are those you must infer from many direct and indirect observations (e.g., self esteem, wellness).

A theory usually contains several concepts. For example, Watson includes ten "caring processes" in her original theory (Box 8-1). Each of those is a complex concept. To see how those caring factors have evolved in her theory,

 Go to **Tables, Boxes, Figures: ESG Table 8-2, "Watson's Caritas Processes,"** in Chapter 8 on the Student Resource Disk or DavisPlus at http://davisplus.fadavis.com/Wilkinson2

Definitions

A **definition** is a statement of the meaning of a term or concept that sets forth the concept's characteristics or indicators. A definition may be general or specific. A *theoretical definition* refers to the conceptual meaning of a term, whereas an *operational definition* specifies how you would observe or measure the concept (e.g., when doing research). For example, for pain:

> *Theoretical definition:* Pain is an unpleasant sensory and emotional experience associated with actual or potential tissue damage.
> *Operational definition:* Pain is the patient's verbal statement that he is in pain.

Statements/Propositions

Statements systematically describe the linkages and interactions among the concepts of a theory. The statements, taken as a whole, make up the theory. In Maslow's theory, for example, two concepts are *physiologic needs* and *self-esteem needs.* An example of a statement in that theory would be: "*Physiological needs* must be met to an acceptable degree before a person can attempt to meet his *self-esteem needs*" or perhaps, "*Physiological needs* are more basic (lower level) than *self-esteem needs.*" Maslow's theory is explained fully later in this chapter.

Theory, Framework, Model, or Paradigm?

In any discussion of nursing knowledge, you may hear the terms *theory, framework, model,* or *paradigm.* It may be difficult for you to differentiate among these terms because (1) they are so abstract, (2) they are defined differently by theorists, and (3) you may hear them used interchangeably in general conversation among nurses. As you progress in your career and education, you will need to pay more careful attention to the similarities and differences among these terms. For now, you can use the following definitions (*theory* was defined earlier):

A **paradigm** is the worldview or ideology of a discipline. It is the broadest, most global conceptual framework of a discipline. It includes and guides the values, philosophy, knowledge, theories, and research processes of the discipline. It is a way of thinking that is shared by a community of scholars who are studying and working on the same phenomena. For example, the medical paradigm views a person through a lens that focuses on identifying and treating disease. This lens causes you to look in depth at the person's "parts" (e.g., cells, organs). The nursing paradigm views the person through a lens that focuses more broadly on the entire person and how he responds to isolated changes in his cells and organs. Again, paradigms are not theories; they are just "how we see things."

A **conceptual framework** (also referred to as a *theoretical framework*) is a set of concepts that are related to form a whole or pattern. As a rule, frameworks are not developed using research processes and have not been tested in practice. The relationships among the concepts are described in less detail than in a theory, and assumptions are not stated. Frameworks (and models) tend to be broader and more philosophical than theories. Don't be alarmed if you can't tell the difference

---

BOX 8-1 ■ Watson's Ten Caring Processes

1. Forming a humanistic–altruistic system of values
2. Instilling faith and hope
3. Cultivating sensitivity to self and others
4. Forming helping and trusting relationships
5. Conveying and accepting the expression of positive and negative feelings
6. Systematic use of the scientific problem-solving method that involves caring process
7. Promoting transpersonal teaching–learning
8. Providing for supportive, protective, and corrective mental, physical, sociocultural, and spiritual environment
9. Assisting with gratification of human needs
10. Sensitivity to existential–phenomenological forces

Source: Watson, J. (1988). *Nursing: Human science and human care. A theory of nursing.* Publication No. 15-2236. New York: National League for Nursing Press.

between a theory and a theoretical framework. The experts don't always agree, either. Many theorists, for example, classify the early nursing theories (e.g., Orem's self-care deficit theory and others presented in this chapter) as conceptual frameworks; others classify them as theories.

A **model** is a symbolic representation of a framework or concepts—a diagram, graph, picture, drawing, or physical model. The plastic body parts you have seen in anatomy class are models of the real human body. Models are developed to promote understanding of concepts. Figure 8-2 is a model of the relationships between nursing practice, theory, and research, for example. Some models are more complex. A **conceptual model** (often used interchangeably with *conceptual framework*) is a model that is expressed in language—the symbols are words. In one sense, all models are "conceptual" because they all represent ideas. The full-spectrum model in Chapter 2 is a conceptual model or framework. For now, it is enough to remember that:

1. The terms *theory, model,* and *framework* all refer to a group of related concepts.
2. The terms differ in meaning, depending on the extent to which the set of concepts has been used and tested in practice and on the level of detail and organization of the concepts.
3. A theory has a higher level of research, detail, and organization of concepts than do models and frameworks.

 ## Critical**Thinking** 8-1

 Go to Chapter 4, **NANDA Taxonomy II: Domains, Classes, and Diagnoses (Labels),** in Volume 2.

Do you think this is a theory, a conceptual framework, or a model?

Knowledge**Check** 8-2

- Name the five "building blocks" of a theory.
- How is a paradigm different from a theory?

 Go to Chapter 8, **Knowledge Check Response Sheet and Answers,** on the Student Resource Disk or DavisPlus at http://davisplus.fadavis.com/Wilkinson2

How Are Theories Developed?

To begin developing a theory, a nurse has an idea that seems worth exploring through research. As an example, Dr. Jean Watson had an idea about caring behaviors toward patients. Once the idea was clear in her mind, she performed research to see whether her ideas made sense. She validated her ideas to develop her theory. Once she had a research-based theory, she shared it with others, and it changed nursing practice.

Theories are developed through a specific way of thinking called logical reasoning (Marriner-Tomey & Raile-Alligood, 2006). Generally, you can think of **reasoning** as connecting ideas in a way that makes sense. The purpose of **logical reasoning** is to develop an argument or statement based on evidence that will result in a logical conclusion. Nursing theories cannot be based on guesswork; they must be developed on a solid foundation of logical reasoning. The most commonly used types of logical reasoning are inductive and deductive reasoning.

Inductive reasoning is often used in the nursing process. If you walk into a person's room and note that the patient has a temperature of 101°F (38°C), a pulse of 104 beats/min, and respiration rate of 20 breaths/min, you could reasonably *induce* (conclude) that the person is ill. Induction moves from the specific to the general. You gathered separate pieces of information, recognized a pattern, and formed a generalization. You could not say the person had a *specific* infection (e.g., measles), but you could induce the person is ill. Remember induction by thinking, "I have specific data 'out there,' and I bring it 'in' to make the generalization." Refer to Figure 8-3.

Deductive reasoning is the opposite of inductive reasoning. Deduction starts with a *general premise* and moves to a *specific deduction*. Suppose you receive a call from the emergency department stating they will be admitting a new patient with acute pyelonephritis (kidney infection). Because you know what is involved in the general premise (pyelonephritis), you deduce the patient will probably have an elevated temperature and back pain. You have the "big picture" about what is true in general, and from that you can figure out logically what is likely to be true for a particular individual.

Understanding logical thinking, even on this basic level, will help you understand the thinking that goes into both nursing theory and nursing research. *Caution: Induced and deduced conclusions are not facts. They may or may not accurately reflect reality.*

Critical**Thinking** 8-2

- Your patient is grimacing, groaning, and holding his hands over his abdominal incision. You induce that the patient is having incision pain. How could you be sure your induction is factual (true)?
- Earlier you deduced that your emergency department patient with pyelonephritis will have a temperature and back pain. How confident are you that this is actually so? How could you be more certain your deduction is correct?

The preceding Critical Thinking exercise should demonstrate that inductions and deductions are not "facts" or "truth," but rather that they point you in the direction to go in seeking truth (reality). And they allow you to make connections between ideas when you are developing a theory. The more information you have to support your conclusions, the more confident you can be that they are correct.

FIGURE 8-3 A comparison of inductive and deductive reasoning. Theorists and nurses in practice use both types of reasoning.

What Are the Essential Concepts of a *Nursing* Theory?

There are four basic concepts that are said to represent phenomena of concern for nursing. Any nursing theory should address these four concepts: **person, environment, health,** and **nursing** (Yura & Torres, 1975). Notice this further divides the puzzle piece for nursing theory into four more pieces (Fig. 8-4).

As Watson, Benner, and other theorists considered their questions, research design, and possible outcomes, they undoubtedly kept these four concepts in mind. A meaningful nursing theory defines these four puzzle pieces and explains how they are related to each other. Consider a theory that does not include the concept of person. Such a theory would describe the needs of the nurse and the condition of the environment, as well as the health of the person. However, it would not deal with the person's reaction to her health or lack of health. As a result, the person's learning needs, fears, family concerns, or discharge arrangements would not be considered. That sounds quite mechanistic, doesn't it?

The following illustrates how Watson (1988) viewed the four basic concepts. In her science of human caring, she explored the concept of *caring* as it relates to the person, environment, health, and nursing. Watson focused heavily on the *person* and the *nurse*. She talked about the "transpersonal" caring moments that exist between the two. She presented the *environment* as another way to show caring: by keeping it clean, colorful, or quiet or including whatever promotes health for the person. All of the caring behaviors (see Box 8-1) listed in Watson's theory focus on improving the *health* of the person.

FIGURE 8-4 The four components of a nursing theory are person, nurse, health, and environment.

Critical Thinking 8-3

Think of an experience you have had in clinical. Perhaps it was taking vital signs or bathing a confused patient. Describe how each of the four components of a nursing theory occurred in your clinical situation. Share your thinking with a classmate or co-worker.

- Who was the *person(s)* involved (*person* refers to the patient or resident or the family and support persons)?
- What was the *environment*? A community center? A bathing room in a nursing home? The person's bedside in a hospital?
- What was the *health* condition of the person? For example, was the person seeking information for self-care? Critical? In pain? Ready for discharge?
- How was *nursing* involved? For example, was the nurse compassionate? Angry? Efficient? A novice or an expert?

Observing nursing situations within the framework of the four components of nursing theory will help you understand the importance of each. This is very important because the finished puzzle reflects excellent (full-spectrum) nursing care.

KnowledgeCheck 8-3

- What are the four essential concepts in a nursing theory?
- What is the title of Dr. Watson's theory?
- Caring processes are critical to her theory. What is the purpose of the caring processes?

 Go to Chapter 8, **Knowledge Check Response Sheet and Answers,** on the Student Resource Disk or DavisPlus at http://davisplus.fadavis.com/Wilkinson2

How Do Nurses Use Theories?

Nursing theories try to describe, explain, and predict human behavior. You have already seen in the case of Mr. Wilkey ("Meet Your Patient") how the use of a certain theory could guide the nurse to more compassionate care. Think of a theory as a lens. You can see the stars more clearly if you look at them through a telescope than you can by using binoculars. As another metaphor, the lens of your sunglasses removes glare, allowing you to see more clearly in bright sunlight but decreasing your ability to see in dim light. Theories offer a way of looking at nursing, and in this way they affect your entire perspective. The theory you use influences what you look for, what you notice, what you perceive as a problem, what outcomes you hope to achieve, and what interventions you will choose.

In Practice

Nursing theories serve as a guide for assessment, problem identification, and choosing nursing interventions. They help nurses communicate to other members of the health team what it is that makes nurses unique and important to the interdisciplinary team.

Clinical practice theories very specifically guide what you do each day. They are limited in scope—that is, they

do not attempt to explain all of nursing. A theory on human interaction directs nurse–client communication; another theory provides a guide for teaching people how to be self-reliant. The following are other examples:

1. Nightingale's theory emphasized the importance of the environment in the care of patients. Her work affected the design and building of hospitals for decades.
2. Dr. Imogene Rigdon (Rigdon, Clayton, & Dimond, 1987) developed a theory about bereavement of older women after noticing (and having an idea!) that older women handled grief differently from men and younger women. Hospice organizations all over the country now use this theory to work with older women who have lost a significant other.
3. Nola Pender's theory (Pender, Murdaugh, & Parsons, 2006) on health promotion (see Chapter 41) is the basis for most health promotion teaching done by nurses.
4. Dr. Katharine Kolcaba (1994) developed a theory of holistic comfort in nursing, which provides a more holistic view than earlier theories of pain and anxiety.

In Education

Some schools of nursing use theories to guide curriculum planning, programs, and projects. These are frequently grand theories, such as Watson's theory of caring or Rogers's science of unitary human beings. A **grand theory** covers broad areas of concern within a discipline. A grand theory is usually abstract and does not outline specific nursing interventions. Instead, it tends to deal with the relationships among nurse, person, health, and environment.

A school using Watson's theory, for example, would include aspects of her theory in each class. A course might even be organized around the caring factors listed in Box 8-1. As another example, an inservice education director in a nursing home may choose a narrower and more specific theory (*mid-range* or *practice theory*) of comfort, using it to devise policies and procedures and design educational programs.

In Research

Theories help generate new knowledge by suggesting questions for researchers to study. Researchers also use theories and models as a framework for structuring a study. They provide a systematic way to define the questions for study, identify the variables to measure, and interpret the findings. For example, Kolcaba tested her statement that comfort interventions, as defined in her theory, would improve the health of the whole person.

Who Are Some Important Nurse Theorists?

You will need to thoroughly understand the theories you use in practice and the one (or more) used by your school of nursing. As an educated nurse, you should also have at least a nodding acquaintance with the nurse theorists who have influenced nursing practice. The following three theorists are presented in detail because of their historical significance. The description of their theories is simple and applicable to what you do every day as a nurse.

Florence Nightingale

As you learned in Chapter 1, Florence Nightingale revolutionized nursing. When she went to the Scutari Hospital during the Crimean War, the soldiers slept on mats on the floor, where rats scampered and raw sewage flowed. Nightingale's "idea" was that *more men would survive if they had a clean and healthy environment and nutritious food (so that the body could heal itself).* That may not seem remarkable to you, but consider that the germ theory of infectious disease had not yet been identified.

Nightingale also was an outstanding researcher. She stayed awake late at night to keep records of what was happening at Scutari hospital before and after she introduced her ideas (research). By changing the environment, she dramatically reduced the death rate of the soldiers (Dossey, 1999). She used her research to develop her theory that a clean environment would improve the health of patients. Because of her theory and research, Nightingale changed the way the entire British Army hospital system was managed. For links to more information about Nightingale,

 Go to Chapter 8, **Resources for Caregivers and Health Professionals,** on the Student Resource Disk or DavisPlus at http://davisplus.fadavis.com/Wilkinson2

Virginia Henderson

Virginia Henderson was born in 1897. She began her career as a U.S. Army nurse in 1918. She also was a visiting nurse in New York City and then a teacher of nursing. Her pamphlet, *Basic Principles of Nursing Care,* was published in 1960 by the International Council of Nursing. It was published in 20 languages.

While a nursing student at Walter Reed Army Hospital, Henderson began to question the mechanistic nursing care she was taught to give, as well as the fact she was expected to be the physicians' handmaiden. As a teacher of nursing, she came to recognize there was no clear description of the purpose and function of nursing. She was the first nurse to identify that as a concern. Her "idea" was that *nurses deserve to know what it means to be a nurse.*

Henderson's 1966 book, *The Nature of Nursing,* described her theory of nursing's primary, unique function. She identified 14 basic needs that are addressed by nursing care (Box 8-2). Although the simple things on that list are commonplace today, they had not been identified as components of nursing care until Virginia Henderson did so. Henderson's (1966, p. 3) definition of nursing states: "The unique function of the nurse is to

> ### BOX 8-2 ■ Virginia Henderson's List of Basic Needs
>
> 1. Breathe normally.
> 2. Eat and drink adequately.
> 3. Eliminate body wastes.
> 4. Move and maintain desirable posture.
> 5. Sleep and rest.
> 6. Select suitable clothes—dress and undress.
> 7. Maintain body temperature within normal range by adjusting clothing and modifying the environment.
> 8. Keep the body clean and well groomed, and protect the integument.
> 9. Avoid dangers in the environment and avoid injuring others.
> 10. Communicate with others in expressing emotions, needs, fears, or opinions.
> 11. Worship according to one's faith.
> 12. Work in such a way that there is a sense of accomplishment.
> 13. Play or participate in various forms of recreation.
> 14. Learn, discover, or satisfy the curiosity that leads to normal development and health and use of the available health facilities.
>
> *Source:* Marriner-Tomey, A., & Raile-Alligood, M. (2006). *Nursing theorists and their work* (6th ed.). St. Louis, MO: C.V. Mosby.

assist the individual, sick or well, in the performance of those activities contributing to health or its recovery (or to a peaceful death) that he would perform unaided if he had the necessary strength, will or knowledge. And do this in such a way as to help him gain independence as rapidly as possible." Henderson defined what nursing was in the 20th century. If you would like more information on Henderson,

 Go to Chapter 8, **Resources for Caregivers and Health Professionals,** on the Student Resource Disk or DavisPlus at http://davisplus.fadavis.com/Wilkinson2

Hildegard Peplau

Hildegard E. Peplau was born in 1909 to immigrant parents in Pennsylvania. She was a psychiatric nurse and contributed much to nursing in general. She influenced the advancement of standards in nursing education, promoted self-regulation in nursing through credentialing, and was a strong advocate for advanced nursing practice.

Dr. Peplau's "idea" was that *health could be improved for psychiatric patients if there were a more effective way to communicate with them.* Again, you may feel this is an unnecessary theory because nurses communicate with patients all the time. But remember in the early 1900s, actually talking to and developing a personal relationship with psychiatric patients simply was not done. Psychiatric patients did not have the benefit of psychotropic drugs currently available to manage their symptoms. They were often agitated and extremely difficult to communicate with.

Peplau's research showed that developing a relationship with psychiatric patients does make their treatment more effective. She developed the theory of interpersonal relations, which focuses on the relationship a nurse has with the patient. This is a theory you use every day without even knowing it existed. For more information on Peplau's theory,

 Go to Chapter 8, **Resources for Caregivers and Health Professionals,** on the Student Resource Disk or DavisPlus at http://davisplus.fadavis.com/Wilkinson2

The Caring Theorists

It could be argued that the three leading caring theorists in nursing are Dr. Jean Watson, Dr. Patricia Benner, and Dr. Madeleine Leininger. We have been using Watson's ideas to illustrate principles and concepts of theory. In this section, we discuss Benner and Leininger.

Patricia Benner

Caring is the central concept in Benner and Wrubel's *primacy of caring model.* The nurse's caring helps the client cope. Moreover, it offers opportunity for the nurse to connect with others and to receive as well as give help (Benner & Wrubel, 1989). Caring involves personal concern for persons, events, projects, and things. Therefore, it reveals what is stressful for a person (because if something does not matter to a person, it will not create stress) and provides motivation. Caring also makes the nurse notice which interventions are effective. This theory stresses that each person is unique, so that caring is always specific and relational for each nurse–person encounter.

In Chapter 1, we discussed another of Benner's theories. A critical care nurse, she wanted to find out *what makes an expert nurse.* In this case, the idea took the form of a question. An example of an expert nurse, for her, was an intensive care unit (ICU) nurse who "knew" intuitively when it was time to extubate a critical patient. Benner wanted to know what makes a nurse expert enough to know that and other critical information. She therefore interviewed ICU nurses and, from her research, identified five stages of knowledge development and acquisition of nursing skills. As you may recall, the first level is that of a novice nurse (you). The others are advanced beginner, competent, proficient, and expert nurse (see Chapter 1 if you need to review).

Let's see whether this novice-to-expert theory addresses the four components of a nursing theory. *Person* and *nurse* are very clearly points of focus. Knowing the *nurse's* skill level (novice, advanced beginner, competent, proficient, or expert) provides for an intelligent way to match the nurse's skill with the patient's (*person*) acuity. This is the basis of the theory. The theory also indicates the nurse contributes to the person's *health* according to her skill level.

The *environment* is clearly stated as the ICU. Benner's theory does meet the criteria of the four components of a theory, although some are emphasized more than others. Differences in emphasis are typical of theories, by the way.

Madeleine Leininger

Leininger is the founder of transcultural nursing and was the first nurse in the United States to earn a doctoral degree in cultural and social anthropology. Her theory focuses on caring as **cultural competence** (using knowledge of cultures and of nursing to provide culturally congruent and responsible care). Her "idea" came from working with children from diverse cultures who were under her care in a psychiatric hospital: *Would the psychotherapy for the children be more effective if delivered within the framework of the child's culture* (Marriner-Tomey & Raile-Alligood, 2006)?

Leininger performed the research to confirm her idea that culturally competent care made a difference, and then she developed her theory. She followed the pattern of the puzzle pieces referred to throughout this chapter. The *person* in Leininger's theory is an individual with cultural beliefs that are specific to herself and that may differ from the beliefs of others. Human beings can feel concern for others, but ways of caring vary across cultures. The *nurse* is the professional who values the cultural diversity of the person and is willing to make cultural accommodations for the health benefit of the person. This requires specialized cultural knowledge. The *environment* is wherever the *nurse* and the *person* are together in the healthcare system. *Health* is defined by the *person* and may be culturally specific in its definition. You will learn more about Leininger's theory in Chapter 13.

You may be thinking, "This is all about culture; what does that have to do with caring?"

Leininger's theory brings together the cultures of the *person*, the *nurse*, and the *healthcare system* (indeed, there is a culture of healthcare, as you will discover in Chapter 13) to improve healthcare delivery and its effectiveness. For example, as a nurse, you may need to welcome the Shaman from a Native American tribe who has been asked to perform a sacred dance in the hospital room. This is one way to demonstrate caring and respect for the person who is ill.

This is a true culture-care story: As a young nurse, I was caring for a patient who was a monk from a local religious order. He had just had abdominal surgery, and he would not take any pain medication. He wanted to "offer the pain up to God." That was a serious values clash for me because I believed the patient was jeopardizing his health, yet I did respect his right to live his cultural beliefs. We worked out a compromise. The monk agreed to take pain medication every 8 hours (instead of the prescribed every

3–4 hours), and I was vigilant in attending to ambulation, hygiene, and other needs during the times the medication was in effect. This is an example of applying a theory directly to the needs of the person who is ill.

Other Selected Nurse Theorists

You will find a list of selected nurse theorists and a brief description of their theories in Table 8-1. For a more complete discussion of those theories, you could see the Web sites listed there, and

 Go to Chapter 8, **Supplemental Materials: Other Selected Nurse Theorists,** on the Student Resource Disk or DavisPlus at http://davisplus.fadavis.com/Wilkinson2

Knowledge Check 8-4

Define in a brief conceptual form or title the nursing theory of each theorist listed below:

- Florence Nightingale
- Virginia Henderson
- Hildegard Peplau

Table 8-1 ➤ Selected Nurse Theorists

THEORIST	DATE	THEORY
Peplau, Hildegard E.	1952	Interpersonal relations model: Interpersonal communication can improve mental health.
Henderson, Virginia	1955	14 basic needs addressed by nursing care; definition of nursing; do for the patient what he cannot do for himself
Abdellah, Faye G.	1960	21 nursing problems; deliver care to the whole person.
Orlando, Ida Jean	1961	Interpersonal process; nursing process theory
Wiedenbach, Ernestine	1964	The purpose of nursing is to support and meet patients' needs for help. Nursing is a helping art.
Levine, Myra	1967, 1973	Conservation model; designed to promote adaptation of the person while maintaining wholeness, or health.
Johnson, Dorothy	1968, 1980	The behavioral system model: Incorporates five principles of systems thinking to establish a balance or equilibrium (adaptation) in the person. The patient is a behavioral system consisting of subsystems.
Rogers, Martha	1970	The science of unitary human beings focuses on the betterment of human kind through new and innovative modalities. Maintaining an environment free of negative energy is important.
Orem, Dorothea	1971	The self-care deficit nursing theory explains what nursing care is required when people are not able to care for themselves. Goal is to help client attain total self-care.
King, Imogene	1971	First of two theories was the interacting systems framework, designed to explain the organized wholes within which nurses are expected to function, i.e., society, groups, and individuals. The first theory led to the theory of goal attainment, which focuses on mutual goal setting between a nurse and patient and the process for meeting the goals.
Neuman, Betty	1972	Neuman systems model is based on general system theory (a nonnursing theory) and reflects the nature of living organisms as open systems.
Roy, Sr. Callista	1974	Adaptation model was inspired by the strength and resiliency of children. The model relates to the choices people make as they adapt to illness and wellness.
Leininger, Madeleine M.	1978, 1984	Cultural care diversity and universality theory. Caring theory.
Newman, Margaret	1979	Theory of health as expanding consciousness describes nursing intervention as nonintervention, where the nurse's presence helps patients recognize their own pattern of interacting with the environment.
Watson, Jean	1979	Caring theory. Nursing is an interpersonal process.
Parse, Rosemarie Rizzo	1981	Theory of human becoming focuses on the human–universe–health process and knowledge related to human becoming (or reaching one's potential).
Benner, Patricia and Wrubel, J.	1989	Primacy of caring model. Caring is central to the model and helps the client cope with stressors of illness.

For more information on these theorists,

 Go to Chapter 8, **Supplemental Materials,** on the Student Resource Disk or DavisPlus at http://davisplus.fadavis.com/Wilkinson2

Go to Chapter 8, **Knowledge Check Response Sheet and Answers,** on the Student Resource Disk or DavisPlus at http://davisplus.fadavis.com/Wilkinson2

How Do Nurses Use Theories from Other Disciplines?

Theory development is relatively new in nursing. Except for Nightingale (1859/1992), it was not until the mid-1950s that nursing leaders began to publish their theories about nursing. The profession relied heavily on the theories of other disciplines. Nurses still use knowledge from other disciplines as a part of their scientific knowledge base. The following are a few of the many "borrowed" theories you will use in nursing.

Maslow's Hierarchy of Basic Human Needs

One of the classic theories still used in most nursing education and practice settings is Maslow's hierarchy of needs (1970). Maslow observed that certain human needs are common to all people, but some needs are "more basic" than others. The lower-level (e.g., physiological) needs must be met to some degree before the higher needs (e.g., self-esteem) can be achieved (Fig. 8-5). For example, if you sit down to study but the room is cold, you will likely decide to put on a sweater or turn up the heat before opening your books. Nevertheless, a person may consciously choose to ignore a lower-level need in order to achieve a higher need. For example, the rescuers at the World Trade Center and in Haiti after the earthquake ignored their need for safety and security to help others (transcendence of self). In daily life, most people are partially satisfied and partially unsatisfied at each level.

Everyone has a dominant need, but it varies among individuals. For example, a teenager may have a (self-esteem) need to be accepted by a group. A heroin addict needs to satisfy her cravings for heroin and will not worry much about being accepted by others.

Physiological Needs
Physiological needs, the most basic, are those that must be met to maintain life. They include the needs for food, air, water, temperature regulation, elimination, rest, sex, and physical activity. Most healthy adults meet their physiological needs through self-care. However, many of your nursing interventions will support patients' physiological needs.

Safety and Security Needs
The needs for safety and security are the next priority. Safety and security may refer to either physical or emotional needs. *Physical safety and security* mean protection from physical harm (e.g., falls, infection, and effects of medications) and having adequate shelter (e.g., housing with sanitation, heat, and safety).

Emotional safety and security involve freedom from fear and anxiety—feeling safe in the physical environment

FIGURE 8-5. Maslow's hierarchy of human needs is a theory nurses use every day. (*Sources:* Adapted from Maslow, A. [1970] *The farther reaches of human nature.* New York: Viking Press; and Maslow, A., & Lowery, R. [Eds.]. [1998]. *Toward a psychology of being* (3rd ed.). New York: John Wiley & Sons.)

as well as in relationships. We need the security of a home and family. If there is an abusive husband, for example, the wife will be "stuck" at this level. She will spend an inordinate amount of time attempting to create a safe environment that does not trigger episodes of violence or abuse. This leaves little attention for meeting self-esteem needs, for example.

Love and Belonging Needs
Needs for love and belonging are sometimes called social or affiliation needs. When they dominate, the person strives for meaningful relationships with others. Everyone has a basic need to love and be loved, give and receive affection, and have a feeling of "belonging," for example, in a family, peer group, or community. When these needs are not met, a person may feel isolated and lonely and may withdraw or become demanding and critical.

Self-Esteem Needs
People who have begun to satisfy the need to belong may begin to feel the need for self-esteem. Self-esteem comes through a sense of accomplishment and recognition from others and brings confidence and

independence. As we discuss in Chapter 11, illness can affect self-esteem by causing role changes (e.g., inability to perform one's job), or a change of body image (e.g., loss of a body part). When recognition cannot be obtained through positive behaviors, the person may resort to disruptive or irresponsible actions.

Self-Actualization Needs

The highest level on Maslow's original hierarchy, self-actualization refers to the need to reach your full potential and to act unselfishly. At this level, a person develops wisdom and knows what to do in a variety of situations. Maslow studied self-actualized people to develop a list of their characteristics. To see this list,

 Go to Chapter 8, **Tables, Boxes, Figures: ESG Box 8-1,** on the Student Resource Disk or DavisPlus at http://davisplus. fadavis.com/Wilkinson2

In his later work, Maslow identified two growth needs that must be met before reaching self-actualization (Maslow & Lowery, 1998):

1. *Cognitive needs* to know, understand, and explore
2. *Aesthetic needs* for symmetry, order, and beauty

Transcendence of Self

Later research led Maslow to identify another even higher need (Maslow, 1971): the need for *transcendence of self*. This is the drive to connect to something beyond oneself and to help others realize their potential. Some people include spirituality at this level, which is also the basis for acts of self-sacrifice (for example, donating a kidney so that another person can live).

Applying Maslow's Theory

The following example illustrates how you might use Maslow's theory when teaching patients. Suppose you have been assigned to teach Mrs. Gallegos about her colostomy before her discharge. You put a great deal of effort into obtaining materials in Spanish, Mrs. Gallegos's primary language, and you have arranged for an interpreter in case she has some questions you can't understand or answer. As you walk in the door to begin teaching, you immediately observe that Mrs. Gallegos seems to be in a great deal of pain. What will you do?

Maslow's hierarchy of needs tells you clearly that until the pain (a physiological need) is controlled, Mrs. Gallegos cannot learn. (Maslow considers pursuit of knowledge a self-actualization need.) You arrange for pain medication to be administered and reschedule the teaching session. If you went ahead with the teaching, the experience would be for the sole purpose of "crossing it off your list" (remember mechanistic nursing?) rather than actually teaching Mrs. Gallegos.

Validation Theory

Validation theory (Feil, 2003) arises from social work and provides for a way to communicate with older people with dementia. The theory asks the caregiver to "go where the demented person is in his own mind." For example, if Mr. Wilkey ("Meet Your Patient") is talking about his mother, who has been dead for many years, you would ask questions about her rather than tell him that she is dead. Learning of his mother's death would be a shocking and traumatic experience, which he would relive each time he heard the news. Instead, you would "go where Mr. Wilkey is in his own mind" by asking him, for example, about the color of his mother's eyes, what songs she sings to him, or other personal questions that will likely stimulate meaningful conversation about the mother.

Stress and Adaptation Theory

Hans Selye (1993) developed the stress and adaptation theory. There are many theories about stress, but Selye's was the forerunner of them all. His theory states that a certain amount of stress is good for people; it keeps them motivated and alert. However, too much stress, called *distress*, results in physiological symptoms and eventual illness. Does that happen to you at the end of the semester when you are "distressed" over the number of papers due and the difficulty of the tests for which you are studying? Generally the human body will respond to distress with an illness, such as a cold, that will force the body to slow down or simply go to bed. Selye's theory is discussed more in Chapter 25.

Developmental Theories

Developmental theories look at stages that individuals, groups, families, and communities progress through over time. Several important examples include Erickson's psychosocial developmental theory (discussed in Chapter 9), theories of family development (discussed in Chapters 11 and 12), and Kohlberg's and Gilligan's theories of moral development (discussed in Chapters 9 and 44). These theories are useful in nursing practice because they identify norms and expectations at various stages in development and help you identify activities and interventions that are appropriate for your client.

System Theory

Ludwig von Bertalanffy created system theory in the 1940s (von Bertalanffy, 1976). He intended it to be abstract enough to use for theory and research in any discipline. Today the understanding of systems has evolved to the point that many of the concepts are a part of our everyday language (e.g., healthcare system, body systems, information systems, family systems).

One of the premises of systems theory is that all complex phenomena, regardless of their type, have some principles, laws, and organization in common. A **system** is made up of separate components (or **subsystems**), which constantly interact with each other and with other systems. For example, the cardiovascular and renal systems are subsystems of the body;

the cells are subsystems of those systems. All of those systems and subsystems exchange processes and information with each other and with systems outside the body.

A system maintains some organization even though it is constantly facing internal and external changes. All systems have some common elements. The goal (function) of any system is to process **input** (the energy, information, or materials that enter the system) for use within the system or in the **environment** (everything outside the system) or both. Other common elements include the following:

- **Output** is the product or service that results from the system's throughput (processing of technical, social, financial, and human input). Examples of output are documents, money, nursing diagnoses, and cars.
- **Throughput** consists of the processes the system uses to convert input (raw materials) into output (products to be used by the system or environment). Examples are thinking, planning, sorting, meeting in groups, sterilizing, hammering, and cutting.
- **Feedback** is information about some aspect of the processing that is used to monitor the system and make its performance more effective (e.g., evaluation in the nursing process: how the patient responded to the interventions)
- **Open systems** exchange information and energy freely with the environment. Open systems are capable of growth, development, and adaptation. Examples of open systems include, people, body systems, hospitals, and businesses.
- **Closed systems** have fixed, automatic relationships among their components and little give and take with the environment. One example is a rock. A nursing example is a family that is isolated from the community and resists outside influences.

Several nursing theories have been built on system theory, for example, Johnson's (1968, 1980) behavioral system model, King's (1971) interacting systems framework, and the Neuman systems model (Neuman & Young, 1972), to name a few. For information about these theorists, if you need it,

 Go to Chapter 8, **Supplemental Materials: Other Selected Nurse Theorists,** on the Student Resource Disk or DavisPlus at http://davisplus.fadavis.com/Wilkinson2

KnowledgeCheck 8-5

- Name four theories nurses "borrow" from other disciplines.
- What are the five original levels of Maslow's basic human needs (not including cognitive needs, aesthetic needs, and transcendence)?

 Go to Chapter 8, **Knowledge Check Response Sheet and Answers,** on the Student Resource Disk or DavisPlus at http://davisplus.fadavis.com/Wilkinson2

Practical **Knowledge** **knowing** how

Practical knowledge about theory means using theories to guide you in your use of the nursing process. Recall the lens metaphor: A theory's concepts and principles determine what you look for and what you notice. In the assessment step of the nursing process, your theory tells you what to assess and provides the rationale for the assessments; its major concepts serve as categories for organizing the data. In the diagnosis step, your theory guides you in defining patient problems; in fact, it determines whether you will even recognize a cluster of cues as a problem. The theory helps you to generate appropriate, achievable client outcomes, to choose effective nursing interventions, and to provide rationales for your actions.

There is no reason to discuss theory in this book unless you can apply the information. To show you how, this section applies caring theory to the planning of nursing interventions. Of course you can use *any* theory for this purpose. We use caring theory because of the powerful and positive impact it can have on your nursing care. In reading this chapter, you should have become familiar with two well-known caring theories. Test your recall by writing the theorists' names and basic ideas. If you have difficulty, be sure to review the information about caring theorists before proceeding.

 Critical**Thinking** 8-4

Write a paragraph describing a clinical experience in which you applied or observed one or both of the caring theories. Record your thinking on a piece of paper, and be prepared to share it with your classmates. You may title it "My Experience in Caring."

Planning Theory-Based Interventions/ Implementation

The Nursing Interventions Classification, or NIC (Bulechek, Butcher, & Dochtermak, 2008), introduced in Chapter 6, is theory development in an early stage. Each of the standardized intervention labels (e.g., Exercise Promotion, Infection Control) is a concept, and defining or describing concepts is an important step in theory development.

In this section, we use nine key concepts of Watson's caring theory to describe important nursing activities and approaches.

1. Holistic Nursing Care. The basis of modern nursing, holistic nursing care allows nurses to examine the entire person and the person's world when making healthcare decisions. It goes beyond "just" giving the medication or dressing a wound. These are important tasks, but try to see nursing as giving care to the entire person and all that this entails (e.g., family, friends, fears, cultural beliefs).

2. Honoring Personhood. None of the three caring theorists refers to the person in the healthcare system as a patient unless they need to for clarification. They believe the "patient" is someone who deserves to be honored for individuality in behavior as well as needs. If you accept the need to honor personhood, you will learn the names of the people in your care and will refer to them by name instead of "Room 331," or "the kidney infection down the hall." Honoring personhood requires you to control the fast pace of nursing and hurried care and take time with your patients. You need to look at, talk to, and touch the person to understand what his personhood is.

3. Transpersonal Caring Moments. The concept of transpersonal caring is a moral ideal rather than a task-oriented behavior (remember Mr. Wilkey?). Transpersonal caring moments occur when an actual caring occasion or caring relationship exists between the nurse and the person. This can be a challenge! The current healthcare environment moves people rapidly through the system. How can you find the time to develop authentic caring relationships? The first step is to make a commitment to be a caring nurse: to go to work with the thought, "Today I will be authentic with the people in my care." The word *authentic* simply means to be genuine or real. Or you might think, "I will focus on creating transpersonal caring moments instead of rushed and harried ones." Think back to Mr. Wilkey at the beginning of the chapter. Where did opportunities for transpersonal caring moments with him arise? As a student, you might think, "Today I will practice changing sterile dressings, starting intravenous solutions, or giving intramuscular injections." However, developing the ability to have transpersonal caring moments is just as important.

4. Personal Presence is another phrase for being authentic and "in the moment." If the person in the bed is fearful, you should be fully present, recognize the fear, and support the person experiencing it. Your support may take the form of answering simple questions or providing more in-depth education. It may simply be staying with the person for 2 or 3 minutes while quietly listening and holding the person's hand. The concept of presence suggests that you, the nurse, are emotionally and physically *with* the person for the time you are there. You are not thinking about a medication you need to give or medical orders you need to get. Developing the ability to provide presence is a process. As your psychomotor and nursing process skills become second nature to you, you will find it easier to remain in the moment.

5. Comfort. Most nurses think of comfort as the relief of pain, but it is much more. In Kolcaba's (1994) theory, comfort occurs in four contexts: physical, psychospiritual, social, and environmental. For example, is the person comfortable with you as the caregiver? Some women, especially from Middle Eastern or Asian cultures, are uncomfortable with male nurses. Other questions to consider are whether the patient's modesty is being respected; whether there is too much or too little environmental stimuli; whether the room temperature is right; what cultural values must be respected; whether the patient needs more rest periods in order to heal; and whether the patient needs someone to spend a transpersonal caring moment with him so he can express fears and anxiety. This is the complex picture of comfort.

6. Listening. Listening requires you to quiet your mind and truly listen with your mind and heart. The caring theorists also talk about listening "from within yourself." Some call that *intuition*. Benner believes it is intuition that allows nurses to advance to expert level practice.

7. Spiritual Care is a critical aspect of holistic nursing care (see Boxes 8-1 and 8-2). You need to know what an individual's spiritual needs are and make appropriate plans to meet them. If the person does not want to talk about or deal with her spirituality, you will listen and follow her instructions. However, generally the opposite is true. People who are ill often want to talk about their spiritual needs, but they may be uncomfortable doing so. Helping someone to meet spiritual needs may be as simple as offering to call a clergy member or praying with the person who is sick. Chapter 14 provides more information about spiritual care.

8. Caring for the Family. All nurses who base their practice on caring theories recognize the importance of including the family of the person who is receiving care. Nontraditional family structure (e.g., a same-sex couple, a polygamist family) is not a reason to withdraw support, even if it conflicts with your values. Sometimes in the rush of the day, this can be challenging. What about an older family member with dementia? This person deserves to know what is happening to his loved one even though he most likely will forget the information. If he does forget, patiently repeat what he needs to know. Following the principles of holistic nursing care, respect the need to include all of the family as part of your responsibility. You will find more information about family care in Chapter 12

9. Cultural Competence. This was discussed in the explanation of Leininger's cultural care theory. Also see Chapter 13 if you want more information.

Do you see the value of each of these nine abstract concepts? From them flow very real, concrete nursing actions that make a difference in the lives of patients. Theory is not just "pie in the sky." Understanding nursing theories and applying them throughout your career are essential to full-spectrum nursing care. To perform the essential clinical tasks of nursing within the framework of caring is the highest possible performance of the profession.

KnowledgeCheck 8-6

List and explain three ways to incorporate caring theory into your nursing care.

 Go to Chapter 8, **Knowledge Check Response Sheet and Answers,** on the Student Resource Disk or DavisPlus at http://davisplus.fadavis.com/Wilkinson2

Nursing Research

You now have a good beginning (novice) background in nursing theory. Remember the puzzle pieces (Fig. 8-2)? A nurse has an idea, does research to determine whether the idea is a valid one, and then develops a nursing theory. It is now time to study the research piece of the puzzle.

Theoretical **Knowledge** **knowing** why

Many people, including some nurses, do not know that nurses do research. They see nurses as people who work in hospitals, wear scrubs, and carry a stethoscope in their pocket. Were you aware of the research done in the field of caring before reading this chapter? Most novice nurses would not be. Remember the Framingham Study, which changed medical and nursing practice? Had you heard of that before? To be an effective professional nurse in the 21st century, you need to understand the basic principles of nursing research and their powerful impact on healthcare and the nursing profession. This section of the chapter is designed to show you what research is and how to incorporate it into your practice.

Although there are many definitions of nursing research, this chapter defines **nursing research** as the systematic, objective process of analyzing phenomena of importance to nursing (Nieswiadomy, 2008). Its purpose is to develop knowledge about issues that are important in nursing. Nursing research encompasses all clinical practice arenas, nursing education, and nursing administration.

Nurse researchers currently are making important contributions to the evidence-based practice necessary for professional nursing. Consider this example: When you are in the clinical setting, you will notice that when a nurse discontinues an intravenous (IV) fluid infusion, she sometimes replaces it with a "lock" or "plug" to maintain a route for IV medications, even though the patient no longer needs the fluids. Not many years ago, she would periodically flush the plug with heparin to keep blood from clotting and blocking the IV catheter. But heparin is a drug, and it has side effects. Nurses and other professionals performed several studies to see whether saline (which has no side effects) would work just as well. Goode and others (1991) performed a meta-analysis of those studies showing that saline was indeed just as effective; that is now the standard of care in most institutions. (A **meta-analysis** combines and analyzes the data from several different studies.)

Why Should I Learn About Research?

The best reason, of course, is that the ability to read and use nursing research enhances your ability to give quality patient care. Like theory, research affects you every day you are a nurse. Full-spectrum nurses participate in research by:

- Identifying ideas that should be examined through the research process
- Assisting in, designing, and/or performing research
- Using research as a basis for their practice

In fact, educational and practice standards require that you acquire a degree of research competence.

ANA Standards

The position of the American Nurses Association (ANA) is that all nurses share a commitment to the advancement and ethical conduct of nursing science (ANA, 1994). The following two items from The American Nurses Association (ANA, 2010, in press) Standards of Practice include the ability to use research in planning care:

Standard 4, Planning—Measurement Criterion: The registered nurse integrates current trends and research affecting care in planning.

Standard 5, Implementation—The registered nurse utilizes evidence-based interventions and treatments specific to the diagnosis or problem.

The ANA Standards of Professional Performance include a separate research standard (Standard 9. Evidence-Based Practice and Research). Two criteria for it follow. The registered nurse:

- Utilizes current evidence-based nursing knowledge, including research findings, to guide practice decisions.
- Critically analyzes evidence-based practice and research findings for application to practice.
- Participates in the development of evidence-based practice through research activities. Participation levels occur appropriate to the nurse's education and position.
- Shares research activities and/or findings with peers and others.

Educational Competencies

Recall the Quality and Safety Education for Nurses (QSEN) project has identified quality and safety competencies for nurses. One important competency is the ability to "integrate the best available current evidence with clinical expertise and patient/family preferences and values for delivery of optimal healthcare" (Cronenwett, Sherwood, Barnsteiner, et al., 2007). To see a description of the knowledge, skills, and attitudes you need for achieving this competency,

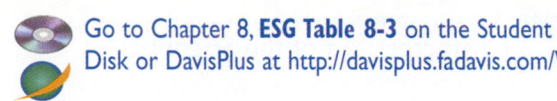 Go to Chapter 8, **ESG Table 8-3** on the Student Resource Disk or DavisPlus at http://davisplus.fadavis.com/Wilkinson2

 Go to Chapter 8, **Knowledge Check Response Sheet and Answers,** on the Student Resource Disk or DavisPlus at http://davisplus.fadavis.com/Wilkinson2

What Is the History of Nursing Research?

The records Florence Nightingale kept while nursing soldiers in the Crimea were the beginning of formalized nursing research. As she developed schools of nursing throughout Britain and the United States, Nightingale urged her students to do clinical research. Yet because she had passed on to them the authoritarian tradition of her time, she found they were not prepared to perform it. Authority-based education does not promote intellectual inquiry or critical thinking, two characteristics essential for research. This is one reason why nursing research was slow to develop.

As baccalaureate, master's, and doctoral programs grew, so did the number and quality of research projects nurses performed. Nursing research is now supported by federal funds and private grants, and results are reported in a growing number of nursing (and other) research journals. Nurses present their research at national and international conferences and publish their results in national and international journals. The preparation of doctoral-level nurses with a strong background in research has enhanced the quality and diversity of nursing research.

How Are Priorities for Nursing Research Developed?

Nursing research provides evidence on which to base nursing care. Ideally, all nursing interventions should be validated through research to show their safety and effectiveness. Professional organizations, such as the ANA and specialty organizations (e.g., the Oncology Nurses Association), have established research priorities that will assist nursing to build a strong knowledge base in areas of importance to society. Brockopp and Hastongs-Tolsma (2003) state that nursing research will continue to be focused on clinical issues. The National Institute of Nursing Research (NINR), a federally funded agency that is a part of the National Institutes of Health (NIH), periodically identifies research themes and priorities for funding (NINR, 2003a, 2003b). For more information about nursing research priorities,

 Go to Chapter 8, **Supplemental Materials: What Are the Priorities for Research in the 21st Century?** on the Student Resource Disk or DavisPlus at http://davisplus. fadavis.com/Wilkinson2

KnowledgeCheck 8-7

- Define nursing research.
- According to the text, why has nursing research been slow to develop?

What Educational Preparation Does a Researcher Need?

At each level of educational preparation, nurses function in different roles in the research process.

Associate Degree and Diploma Nursing. At this educational level, there are three research roles you can fulfill. You can (1) be aware of the importance of research to evidence-based practice, (2) help identify problem areas in nursing, and (3) help collect data with a more experienced nurse researcher.

Baccalaureate Degree in Nursing. If you are a baccalaureate-prepared nurse, you should be able to (1) critique research for application to clinical practice, (2) identify nursing research problems and help implement research studies, and (3) apply research findings to establish sound, evidence-based clinical practice.

Master's Degree in Nursing. Nurses with graduate degrees should be able to (1) analyze problems so that appropriately designed research can be used to solve the problem, (2) through clinical expertise, apply evidence-based practice to nursing care situations, (3) provide support to ongoing research projects, and (4) conduct research for the purpose of assuring quality nursing care.

Doctoral Degree in Nursing or Related Field. Doctorally prepared nurses are specifically educated to be nurse researchers. They are qualified to (1) conduct nursing research, (2) serve as leaders in applying research results to the clinical arena, and (3) develop ways to monitor the quality of nursing care being administered by nurses (adapted from ANA, 1981). In addition, they should disseminate their research findings via publications and conferences.

Practical **Knowledge** **knowing** how

No one expects you to have a sophisticated understanding of research at this point in your career. However, you do need some basic practical knowledge, including information about the scientific method, types of research design, the research process, how to find practice-related research articles, how to identify researchable problems, and how to critique research reports.

What Is the Scientific Method?

Recall that in Chapter 2 you learned the different kinds of nursing knowledge: theoretical, practical, ethical, and self knowledge. There are also various ways to *gain* knowledge.

Trial and Error Plus Common Sense. Suppose a patient has been medicated but is still in pain. You might try repositioning him. If that doesn't help, you might try distraction or visualization techniques. And so on. If visualization provides some relief, you would probably try that technique first when a similar situation occurs with another patient.

Authority and Tradition. This means to rely on an expert or to do "what has always been done." For the patient with unrelieved pain, this would mean you might ask a more experienced nurse what to do. Or you could consult a procedure manual.

Intuition and Inspiration. Intuition is a "feeling" about something—an inner sense. Nurses say, "I just had a feeling something was wrong with the patient, but I can't explain why." For the patient in pain, you might "have a feeling" that a complication was developing, that the pain was due to more than just ineffective pain medication. However, as a novice, you should always check with a more experienced nurse before acting on your intuition.

Logical Reasoning. Using your knowledge and the facts available, you form conclusions (refer to "How Are Theories Developed?"). For the patient in pain, you might think, "This man weighs 300 lb, but I gave him only the standard dose of medication. Probably he needs a higher dose."

Scientific Method. Research is based on the scientific method (or scientific inquiry). **Scientific inquiry** is the process in which the researcher, through use of the senses, systematically collects observable, verifiable data to describe, explain, or predict events. The goals of scientific inquiry are to find solutions to problems and to develop explanations of the world (theories). The scientific method has two unique characteristics that the other ways of gaining knowledge do not:

1. *Objectivity,* or *self-correction.* This means that the researcher uses techniques to keep her personal beliefs, values, and attitudes separate from the research process.
2. *The use of empirical data.* Researchers use their senses to gather empirical data through observation. They attempt to verify the information gathered through a variety of methods so that the research conclusions are based in "reality" rather than on the researcher's beliefs, biases, or hunches.

Box 8-3 summarizes the characteristics of the scientific method.

The scientific method makes use of a variety of procedures and study designs aimed to increase the chances that the data collected will be reliable, relevant, and unbiased. You should recognize the two major categories of research design: quantitative and qualitative. Each category has within it several specific types of research methodologies; however, for now you need to

---

BOX 8-3 ■ Characteristics of the Scientific Method

Begins with an identified problem or need to be studied.

Uses theories, models, and conceptual themes that have been empirically tested.

Uses systematic, orderly methods to acquire empirical evidence to test theories.

Uses methods of control for ruling out other variables that might affect the relationships among the variables they are studying.

Avoids explanations that cannot be empirically tested.

Prefers to generalize the findings (knowledge) so that it can be applied in cases other than those in the study.

Uses built-in mechanisms for self correction.

Source: Adapted from Wilson, H. S. (1993). *Introducing research in nursing* (2nd ed.). Redwood City, CA: Addison-Wesley Nursing.

---

understand only the basic differences (Table 8-2). For an expanded discussion,

 Go to Chapter 8, **Supplemental Materials: Quantitative Research and Qualitative Research,** on the Student Resource Disk or DavisPlus at http://davisplus.fadavis.com/Wilkinson2

Quantitative Research

The main purpose of **quantitative research** is to gather data from enough *subjects* (people being studied) to be able to generalize the results to a similar population. *Generalizing results* means that you think, "What I found to be so for this group of people will probably be the same for all people who are similar" (e.g., "My findings for *this* group of women over age 40 in the United States will probably be useful for *all* women over age 40 in the United States"). In quantitative research, researchers carefully control data collection and are careful to maintain the objectivity of the process. Quantitative data are reported as numbers. The Framingham Study is a classic example of a quantitative study—actually of several quantitative studies. To read more about this landmark research,

 Go to http://www.nhlbi.nih.gov/about/framingham/index.html

Another classic example of quantitative nursing research is the Conduct and Utilization of Research in Nursing (CURN) project, which was intended to increase the use of research by direct-care nurses (Horsley, Crane, & Bingle, 1983). Many of the protocols (procedures) developed from these studies are used today with some modification. The following are some CURN protocol examples:

Clean intermittent catheterization
Intravenous cannula change
Distress reduction through sensory preparation
Preventing decubitus ulcers

Table 8-2 ➤ Comparison of Quantitative and Qualitative Research

	QUANTITATIVE RESEARCH	QUALITATIVE RESEARCH
Data	Numerical data, e.g., questionnaires, number of incidents, or reactions to a medication	Nonnumerical data; data may consist of words from interviews, observations, written documents, and even art or photos.
Persons Studied	Large numbers of *subjects* so it can be generalized to other similar populations	Often uses small numbers of *participants*; is not designed with the intent to generalize.
Hypothesis	Has a hypothesis.	No hypothesis, because it is the research of the "lived experience" of the person or persons being studied; study may be guided by research questions.
Environment	Can be in a laboratory setting; needs to be a controlled environment.	Is often done in the "natural" setting, i.e., the person's home or work setting.
Analysis	Objective data, tested with statistical methods	Subjective data; identifies themes; sometimes converted to numerical data (e.g., by counting categories).

Qualitative Research

Qualitative research focuses on the lived experience of people. The purpose is not to generalize the data, but to share the experience of the person or persons in the study. There is no need for large numbers. A case study of one person can examine the lived experience, for example, of a 19-year-old single mother of triplets or a middle-aged woman with HIV. Qualitative research uses words, quotations from persons interviewed, observations, and other nonnumeric sources of data. The Nun Study, a long-term, multidisciplinary project involving a convent of Catholic nuns in Minnesota, included some qualitative research (e.g., data obtained by interviews and reported in the nuns' own words, and samples of writing from the nuns' diaries, reports, and letters). For more information about the Nun Study,

 Go to http://www.nunstudy.org and http://www.msnbc.msn.com/id/22361498/

KnowledgeCheck 8-8

- Define quantitative research. Name one study presented as an example in this chapter.
- Define qualitative research. Name one study presented as an example in this chapter.

 Go to Chapter 8, **Knowledge Check Response Sheet and Answers,** on the Student Resource Disk or DavisPlus at http://davisplus.fadavis.com/Wilkinson2

What Are the Phases of the Research Process?

At the novice level, you will be using but not performing research. But in order to evaluate the research you read, you should have a general idea of the steps for conducting valid, reliable research. The research process is a problem-solving process, similar to but not the same as the nursing process. Different study designs require different steps, and you will find some variation in how different authors present the research process steps. However, in general, the steps include the following five phases (Fain, 2009):

1. Select and define the problem.
2. Select a research design.
3. Collect data.
4. Analyze data.
5. Use the research findings.

For a more detailed description of those phases,

 Go to Chapter 8, **Supplemental Materials, "What Are the Steps of the Research Process?"** on the Student Resource Disk or DavisPlus at http://davisplus.fadavis.com/Wilkinson2

 Critical**Thinking** 8-5

Take 10 minutes to sit quietly and think about nursing research. Do you have an idea or a problem you would like to see investigated with a research project? If nothing comes to mind quickly, then ponder for a few moments more. Write the information on a sheet of paper. Take the time to do your best thinking. Then share what you have written with your instructor and other students.

- What would you like to have more information about in nursing? Explain why it is a problem or what brought about your idea.
- If you were the research assistant on a nursing research project on your topic, what one-sentence problem statement would you write regarding your research idea?
- What is the purpose of doing this research project? Why should it be done?

You may struggle with this assignment and wonder about its value to you, yet one of the most important things that nurses do is identify problems. Here is your chance to practice.

What Are the Rights of Research Participants?

Every nurse has a moral and legal responsibility to protect research participants from being harmed during the research process. Although research is crucial to the development of the profession, it should never be held in higher regard than the rights of the individuals being studied.

The current ethical standards for research, from all disciplines, are a direct result of the atrocities committed in the name of research in the German prison camps during World War II. After the trials for war crimes committed at that time, the Nuremberg Code was developed in 1949 to protect research participants from unethical behavior. The Nuremberg Code prompted many other codes and standards for performing ethical research (National Institutes of Health, n.d.). The United States government, through the Department of Health and Human Services (DHHS), has a complex set of standards that all researchers must follow.

Informed Consent

As a rule, **informed consent** must be obtained from every participant in a study. Consent is obtained by discussing what is expected of the participant, providing written information on the project to the participant, and obtaining the participant's written consent to be a subject. The following critical concepts are part of the informed consent.

- *Right to not be harmed.* The information given to the participant outlines the safety protocols of the study. If at any time preliminary data indicate potential harm to the participant, the study must be stopped immediately.
- *Right to full disclosure.* Participants have a right to answers to such questions as: What is the purpose of this research? What risks are there? Are there any benefits? Will I be paid? What happens if I get sick or feel worse? Whom do I contact with questions and concerns?
- *Right to self-determination.* This refers to the right to say no. At any time in a study, the participant has the right to stop participating, for any reason. As the nurse, you are responsible to support a participant during the process of withdrawing from a study. Do not allow anyone to coerce the participant into remaining in the study.
- *Rights of privacy and confidentiality.* All research participants have the right to have their identity protected. Generally they are given a code number rather than being identified by name. Once the study is completed and the data are analyzed, the researcher is responsible for protecting the raw data (such as questionnaires and taped interviews).

Institutional Review Boards

The mechanism for overseeing the ethical standards established by the U.S. DHHS is the Institutional Review Board (IRB). Every hospital, university, and other healthcare facility where federal funds are involved has an IRB. It consists of healthcare professionals and people from the community who are willing to review and critique research proposals. The two main responsibilities of the IRB are to (1) protect the research participants from harm and (2) ensure that the research is of value.

KnowledgeCheck 8-9

- List the phases of the research process.
- List four critical concepts that make up informed consent.

 Go to Chapter 8, **Knowledge Check Response Sheet and Answers,** on the Student Resource Disk or DavisPlus at http://davisplus.fadavis.com/Wilkinson2

How Can I Base My Practice on the Best Evidence?

Recall from Chapter 6 that research provides the data for evidence-based practice. When there is a body of research on a topic, experts and professional groups evaluate the quality of the research reports and translate them into guidelines for practice. In your own evidence-based practice, you should use research findings and practice guidelines when they are available. When they are not, you will need to rely on the research reports themselves. The following process should assist you in finding the best evidence for your own interventions. Similar to the phases of research, this process requires you to identify a clinical problem, formulate a searchable question, search the literature, evaluate the quality of the research you find in the literature, and integrate your findings into your practice.

Identify a Clinical Nursing Problem

Even as a novice nurse, you should be prepared to identify clinical problems for research. Identifying a clinical nursing problem comes from being alert and interested in what you are doing each day in your clinical setting. How do you think the tympanic thermometer came into being? Someone became frustrated with the discomfort patients experienced when temperatures were taken rectally. At the same time, there was a great deal of concern over the inaccuracy of axillary temperatures. Someone noticed the problem and wondered: "Is there a better way to do this?"

Common sources of clinical problems are experience, social issues, theories, ideas from others, and the nursing literature (Polit & Beck, 2007). Most of these sources are relevant whether you are identifying a problem for a research study or for doing a literature search.

Experience. As you go about your work, you will notice interventions that may not be working or that require a great deal of effort for the minimal good they do. You will wonder, "How could we do this better?" Or you may notice that for clients with a particular health problem, the outcomes are often not good. You will wonder, "How could we improve the care so the patient's health improves?" Other questions might be, "Why do we do this thing this way? "What do I need to know in order to plan new interventions for patients with this health problem?" You will find plenty of problems if you are curious about why things are done as they are and about what might happen if changes were made. Problems might be related to staffing, equipment, nursing interventions, or coordination among health professionals.

Social Issues. You may be concerned about broader social issues that affect or require nursing care, such as issues of gender equity, sexual harassment, and domestic violence. You may be concerned about patients who do not have access to healthcare or about the health problems of a particular group or subculture.

Theories. Recall that theories must be tested in order to be useful in nursing practice. You might want to suggest research to test a theory you are interested in. If the theory is accurate, what behaviors would you expect to find, or what evidence would you need to support the theory?

Ideas from Others. Your instructor may suggest a topic to research, or perhaps you might brainstorm with nurses or other students. Agencies and organizations that fund research often ask for proposals on certain topics (e.g., the ANA and the National Institute of Nursing Research).

Nursing Literature. Read widely in your field of interest. You may identify clinical problems by reading articles and research reports in nursing journals. This may occur in one of the following ways:

- An article may stimulate your imagination and interest in a topic.
- You may notice a discrepancy in what staff nurses are doing and what the literature recommends.

- You may notice inconsistencies in the findings of two different studies on the same topic.
- You may read a study on a topic of interest to you (e.g., a technique for measuring blood pressure) and wonder whether the results would be the same if the study had been done in a different setting (e.g., a clinic instead of a hospital) or with a different population (e.g., healthy instead of ill people).

Formulate a Searchable Question

When you have found a topic of interest, the next step is to state it in such a way that you can find it in the vast amount of nursing literature that is published. Stated too broadly, the search may yield thousands of irrelevant results. Stated too narrowly, you may get no results. Using the acronym PICO enables you to search efficiently. The acronym stands for *Patient* or *problem*, *Intervention*, *Comparison intervention*, and *Outcomes*. You may not always need a comparison intervention (C). See Box 8-4.

Search the Literature

Once you have stated your guiding question, the next step is to look for research articles related to the question (or problem statement). You may be thinking, "Where do I look for research articles?" As previously stated, evidence reports and practice guidelines may already exist for your clinical problem, so look first for those. If there are none, proceed to search for your topic in research reports in scientific journals.

Indexes and Databases

Obviously you need to go to a library or online and search a database or index for appropriate journal references. A **database** is an electronic bibliographic file that

---

BOX 8-4 ■ PICO Questions

	Sample Questions	Example
P—Patient Population, or Problem	What is the medical diagnosis, nursing diagnosis, patient problem, symptom, situation, or need that requires an intervention?	For patients with Impaired Skin Integrity (perineum) related to urinary incontinence
	How would you describe a group of similar patients?	
I—Intervention, treatment, cause, contributing factor	Which intervention are you considering? Specifically, what might help the problem (improve the situation, etc.)?	Would applying a barrier cream
C—Comparison Intervention	What other interventions are being considered or used?	As compared to washing with soap and water, rinsing well, and air drying after incontinent episodes
O—Outcome	What effect could the intervention realistically have? What do you hope to achieve?	Prevent or achieve less perineal excoriation? Are there any expected undesired effects associated with the intervention?

Sources: University of Southern California, Health Sciences, Los Angeles. Evidence Based Decision Making, "Asking a Good Question (PICO)". Retrieved from www.usc.edu/hsc/ebnet/ebframe/PICO.htm; Center for Evidence Based Medicine, "Asking Focused Clinical Questions." Retrieved from www.cebm.net/index.aspx?o=1036; Sacket, D. L., Richardson, W. S., Rosenberg, W., & Haynes, R. B. (1997). *Evidence-based medicine: How to practice and teach EBM.* New York: Churchill Livingstone.

can be accessed either online or on a CD-ROM. The best database for you, as a novice nurse, is the Cumulative Index to Nursing and Allied Health Literature (CINAHL). This is a comprehensive database that includes more than 1200 nursing and allied health journals. Generally, you will be able to find in CINAHL whatever you are looking for in clinical nursing. Most university libraries have access to CINAHL and other indexes online. If you are an online user, it will be worth your time to get information from the library about conducting online searches. In the library, you will find the printed version of CINAHL in a set of large red books in the reference section.

Once you have access to CINAHL in either format, select words that relate to your topic (e.g., dementia or nursing ethics). The index or database will list journal articles related to the key words. Sometimes, you will get a large number of articles (more than 1000) that carry that word. When that happens, you need to ask the librarian to help you narrow your search. It is beyond the scope of this chapter to provide detailed instructions for literature searches.

For more information about literature databases, see Chapter 39.

KnowledgeCheck 8-10

Where can you go to use CINAHL?

 Go to Chapter 8, **Knowledge Check Response Sheet and Answers,** on the Student Resource Disk or DavisPlus at http://davisplus.fadavis.com/Wilkinson2

Journals

It also is easy to search in a specific journal for articles. The title of a journal provides clues to the content. The critical care journals will have, obviously, articles about critical care. Oncology, orthopedics, and other specialty journals carry information specific to their own specialty. Looking for such journals is another way to do a casual search for articles of interest.

You will find the best research articles in refereed journals. **Refereed journals** are professional journals (not lay magazines, such as *Today's Parent* or *Time*) in which professionals with expertise in the topic review each article and then recommend whether the article should be published. The easiest way to identify a refereed journal is to see whether it has an extensive editorial board listed in the front of the journal. Refereed journals meet a higher standard for publishing, which makes the information you read more credible (and therefore more useful to your work). Two examples of nursing research journals are *Advances in Nursing Science* and *Nursing Research.* For a more extensive list,

 Go to Chapter 8, **Supplemental Materials: Nursing Research Journals,** on the Student Resource Disk or DavisPlus at http://davisplus.fadavis.com/Wilkinson2

How can you tell whether the article you retrieve is a research article? Simply look for the steps in the research process described earlier in this chapter. Does the article have a problem statement and a purpose? Is there a section on the sample and site of the research? And so on.

If your focus is clinical practice, you should not overlook specialty journals, such as *Geriatric Nursing* or the *Journal of Gerontological Nursing,* if you really want information on, say, older adults with dementia. They are not research journals, but they generally have one or two research articles in each issue. If you do not have a specialty interest, review the *American Journal of Nursing* or *RN* for articles of general interest. Again, remember that it is up to you to identify whether the article is research or another form of information sharing.

Evaluate the Quality of the Research

As mentioned previously, you may be fortunate enough to find clinical practice guidelines related to your topic. If so, the related research has already been evaluated by experts, and should have a notation about the level of evidence supporting the guideline. For a description of the different levels of evidence described by guidelines panels,

 Go to Chapter 6, **Supplemental Materials, "Levels of Evidence,"** on the Student Resource Disk or DavisPlus at http://davisplus.fadavis.com/Wilkinson2

If no practice guidelines are available, you will need to critically appraise the individual research articles you find. You can do this by reading analytically and performing a careful appraisal of the research you read.

Analytical Reading

You cannot expect to do a sophisticated critique of a research report at this stage of your education, or probably even on graduation from your basic education. However, you need to know enough to help you decide which articles are worthy of using in your practice. You will make that decision after you have examined the research to determine whether it is well done and meaningful to your work. Begin this process by learning to read analytically. Wilson (1993, p. 25) says that **analytic reading** occurs when you "begin asking questions of what you are reading so that you can truly understand it." For questions to use when reading analytically, see Box 8-5.

Research Appraisal

Not all research is good research. Some published studies contain serious flaws, and you need to be able to recognize them. An effective strategy for conducting a research appraisal is to read the entire article, using the four "analytic reading" questions in Box 8-5 and making notes of questions you have. Then go back and evaluate the article section by section, thinking critically about each (Wilson, 1993).

- *Researcher qualifications* are an easy place to start. Was the researcher qualified as an expert on the study topic? Try to determine whether the author's credentials and background "fit" with the topic.

BOX 8-5 ■ Reading Analytically

When reading analytically, ask yourself the following questions:

1. *What is the book, journal, or article about as a whole?* That is, what is the theme of the article, and how is it developed?

2. *What is being said in detail, and how?* What are the author's main ideas, claims, and arguments? In a research article, you will find this mainly in the abstract and the conclusions.

3. *Is the book, journal, or article "true" in whole or part?* You must decide this for yourself. The strategies in "How Do I Appraise the Research I Read" may help you to determine the truth of a research report.

4. *What of it?* Is it of any significance? Is there any way to use the information to improve patient care, education, or other areas of nursing?

■ *The title* should be concise and clear. Key words in the title should provide clues to the research topic.

■ *The abstract* is a brief (perhaps 500 words) summary of the study. It should be interesting and usually describes at least the purpose, methods, sample, and findings of the study.

■ *The introduction* should catch your interest and set the stage for the rest of the report. The introduction may contain the *review of the literature, theoretical (conceptual) framework, assumptions, and limitations.* At this stage of your expertise, you should primarily check that these are present; however, some explanation follows.

■ *Review of the literature* should be thorough and relevant. The references should logically pertain to the study topic and methods and consist primarily of research and theory articles. The references should support the researcher's variable definitions, methodology, and choices of data-collection tools; it should also present background work on the topic being studied.

■ *Identify the study assumptions.* **Assumptions** are beliefs that you "take for granted" as true but that have not been proven. For example, you assume that when people are in bed, they sleep; and you assume that study participants answer truthfully to the researcher's questions. Assumptions should be clearly stated to avoid confusion regarding the study.

■ *Limitations of the study.* Every study has limitations or weaknesses. Look for the author to admit the things that could not be controlled. For example, a study may test a population of people that would not generalize to other populations, (e.g., testing only white students instead of testing a variety of students who represent the ethnic diversity of the university).

■ *The purpose* should be stated clearly. It should give the reasons for doing the study. Ask these three questions to help you judge it: Will the study (1) solve a problem relevant to nursing, (2) present facts that are useful to nursing, or (3) contribute to nursing knowledge?

■ *The problem statement* should be presented early in the report, and it should be "researchable"; that is, it (1) is stated as a question, (2) involves the relationship between two or more variables, and (3) can be answered by collecting empirical data.

■ *Definition of terms* is essential in a formal research report. However, it often is not included in a published article because of the lack of space.

■ *The research design* indicates the plan for collecting data. As a novice, you probably cannot judge the adequacy of the design, but you should be sure the researcher names and describes it and discusses its strengths and weakness. The researcher should include an explanation of what was done to enhance the validity and reliability of the study. To oversimplify, **validity** means the study actually measures the concept it claims to measure. **Reliability** refers to the accuracy, consistency, and precision of a measure. That is, if someone else repeated the study using the same design, would they obtain similar results? For example, if you weighed the same item on a scale each day and obtained the same *weight* each time, you could say that the scale is reliable. But a scale would not give you a valid measure of *body fat*.

■ *Setting, population, and sample.* The researcher should identify the type of setting where the data was collected, describe the population and sample, and state the criteria that were used for choosing study participants. This section may also contain information about how informed consent was obtained.

■ *Data-collection methods* answer the basic questions of what, how, who, where, and when. Data-collection instruments are the "tools" used to gather the data (e.g., questionnaires or a laboratory instrument). The researcher should provide evidence (pilot tests, literature) that the tools used were reliable and valid.

■ *Data analysis.* A quantitative report would include statistical analyses of the data. A qualitative report would include quotes from the participants. The analyses of both types of data are very specific and beyond the scope of this textbook.

■ *Discussion of findings and conclusion* are the sections of a research report that you may find most interesting. They are the "So what was learned?" sections. All findings should be presented in an objective manner, and compared with information found in the literature. The easiest errors for you to recognize with your present knowledge level are that the researcher:

1. Generalizes beyond the data or the sample. For example, the sample may have been young adult women in a clinic setting, but the researcher might have suggested that the same intervention be used for all women in the clinic, regardless of age.

2. Does not mention any limitations that might have influenced the results.

3. Does not present findings in a clear, logical manner (i.e., you have trouble figuring out what the findings actually are).

■ *Implications and recommendations* are the final pieces of the research critique. The implications are the "shoulds" of the research. In essence, the researcher says, "Now we know this fact; therefore, nurses should . . ." For example, the research "should" be replicated with another population, or the instrument "should" be revised and retested, or that nurses "should" use the study intervention in their practice.

When you read a research article, examine it for each of the preceding items. Although you have limited knowledge and experience, every time you review an article thoroughly, you will learn more about the research process. As you learn, you will be better able to determine the quality of research you will accept as a basis for changing your nursing practice.

KnowledgeCheck 8-11

Explain the difference between analytical reading and research appraisal.
What are the parts of a PICO question?

 Go to Chapter 8 **Knowledge Check Response Sheet and Answers,** on the Student Resource Disk or DavisPlus at http://davisplus.fadavis.com/Wilkinson2

Integrate the Research into Your Practice

True evidence-based practice requires that after discovering and critiquing the best available evidence, nursing expertise be applied to see how the recommended interventions fit into the practice setting and whether they are compatible with patient preferences. If the intervention is to involve more than just an individual nurse, nurse managers must decide to implement the clinical practice guideline in their unit or hospital. They consider costs, barriers to change, facilitators for change, and staff education.

Research is more than just an exercise that nurses engage in to earn master's and doctoral degrees. The ultimate reason for conducting research is to establish an evidence-based practice or to gain greater understanding of a phenomenon. This means that nurses in practice have a responsibility for finding and using the research that others do. Remember the discussion of authority-based practice during Florence Nightingale's era? Even in the 21st century, much nursing practice is still based on authority and tradition. That is not acceptable for full-spectrum professional nurses. You must have reasons for what you do. That is the purpose of research.

According to Nieswiadomy (2008), there are five reasons why nurses *do not* use research as the basis for their practice: (1) lack of knowledge of nursing research, (2) negative attitudes toward research, (3) inadequate forums for disseminating research, (4) lack of support from the employing institution, and (5) study findings that are not ready for the clinical environment. You can utilize nursing research to enhance your practice by acting on the information in this chapter. Learn the content, and read and talk about research with your colleagues and instructors. Once you have a research-based idea clear in your mind, try it out in your clinical setting (with approval from the nurse manager or instructor). Then discuss it with others. You can learn to effectively read and use research, and then you can motivate others to do the same.

 Go to Chapter 8, **Resources for Caregivers and Health Professionals,** on the Student Resource Disk or DavisPlus at http://davisplus.fadavis.com/Wilkinson2

 Suggested Readings: Go to Chapter 8, **Reading More About Nursing Theory and Research,** on the Student Resource Disk or DavisPlus at http://davisplus.fadavis.com/Wilkinson2

 Bibliography: Go to Volume 2, Bibliography.

unit 2

Factors Affecting Health

CHAPTER 9

Development Across the Life Span

Learning Outcomes

After completing Parts I, II, and III of this chapter, you should be able to:

Part I

➤ Discuss the principles of growth and development.

➤ Compare and contrast developmental task theory, psychoanalytic theory, cognitive theory, and the psychosocial theory of growth and development.

➤ Outline the major principles involved in moral and spiritual development.

➤ Identify conditions that influence growth and development at all ages.

Part II

➤ Discuss the cognitive and psychosocial challenges for each age group, infant through middle age.

➤ Identify common health problems seen in each stage of development.

➤ Describe any special assessments unique to each age group.

➤ Discuss age-appropriate interventions for each age group.

➤ Incorporate developmental principles into nursing care.

Part III

➤ Discuss the relationship of life expectancy and livable communities.

➤ Discuss the developmental challenges for each older adult age group.

➤ Identify common health problems seen in each group and for all older adults.

➤ Describe any special assessments unique to each group or older adults.

➤ Discuss age-appropriate interventions for older adults and for each group.

➤ Incorporate developmental principles of aging into nursing care.

Volume 1 provides a brief introduction to development across the life span. For a thorough discussion, including gerontology content,

 Go to Chapter 9, **Development Across the Life Span—Expanded Discussion,** on the Student Resource Disk or DavisPlus at http://davisplus.fadavis.com/Wilkinson2

Meet Your Patients

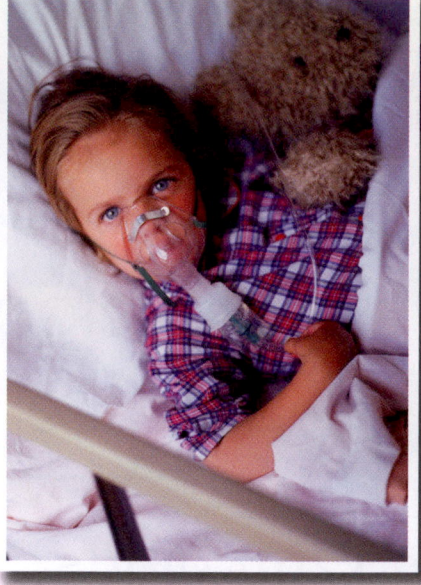

At the end of your first clinical day on the pediatric unit, you reflect on your experiences with the patients for whom you provided care. You were assigned to the care of three children who were diagnosed with pneumonia:

- Tamika, a 3-year-old, lives with her grandparents. Her grandmother is present only during afternoon visiting hours because she must care for her husband, who suffers from numerous health problems.
- Miguel, a 2-month-old, lives with his mother. Since his admission yesterday, Miguel's mother has stayed at his bedside and provided most of her son's care.
- Carrie, a 13-year-old, lives with her parents. Both parents are able to visit only during evening visiting hours, when they leave work.
- Then, you think back to another clinical day when you were assigned to care for Mrs. Higginbotham, an elderly patient with pneumonia who lives alone.

Each of these patients is unique. Although they share the same medical diagnosis, their needs and your nursing care will differ dramatically. These differences stem from a variety of factors, one of the most significant of which is each patient's stage within the life span.

Theoretical Knowledge
knowing why

The Greek philosopher Heraclitus said, "Nothing is permanent but change." We readily see this truth in the dramatic physical, cognitive, and emotional growth that children undergo from one month to another, but it is true also for adults. Throughout the life span, humans are in a constant process of change, not always visible to the eye.

Part I. Concepts of Development: Overview

In this chapter, we present a very brief overview of some principles and theories of growth and development that will serve as the foundation for planning and delivering effective personal care. For a more extensive discussion of normal growth and development across the life span, including common health concerns, nursing assessments, and health promotion interventions,

 Go to Chapter 9, **Development across the Life Span— Expanded Discussion,** on the Student Resource Disk or DavisPlus at http://davisplus.fadavis.com/Wilkinson2

What Is Development?

Growth refers to physical changes that occur over time, such as increases in height, sexual maturation, or gains in weight and muscle tone. **Development** refers to the process of adapting to one's environment over time. Growth is an aspect of development. A few examples of

development are a child who comes to recognize right from wrong, an adolescent who decides on a vocation, or an older adult who recognizes the nearness of death.

What has been the most important force in your becoming the person you are now: characteristics that you inherited from your parents or the environment in which you were raised?

For centuries, scientists have debated the effects of nature versus nurture on growth and development. **Nature** refers to genetic endowment, whereas **nurture** is the influence of the environment on the individual. The birth of a child can be compared to the planting of a tulip. The bulb has all the required factors to produce a beautiful plant, but whether it reaches its full potential is highly dependent on the environment. Is the soil rich in nutrients? Is there enough sunshine? Is there sufficient water? The bulb can grow into a beautiful flower only if it has these necessary ingredients supplied by the environment. A child is similar. The joining of ovum and sperm forms chromosomes that determine appearance, characteristics, and much about how the child will grow and develop. However, environmental factors, such as access to food, love and affection, healthcare and education, also affect how the child develops and thrives throughout the life span.

Principles of Growth and Development

Important principles of growth and development include the following:

Growth and Development Usually Follow an Orderly, Predictable Pattern. However, the timing, rate of change, and response to change are unique for each individual.

For example, all children learn to sit before they walk. One child may learn to sit at 6 months of age and walk at 10 months, whereas another child may first sit at 7 months and not walk until 15 months. Each of these children is developing in the same pattern, and both are progressing within a normal time frame. Similarly, menarche in girls follows a series of bodily changes associated with puberty. In one healthy teen, menstruation might begin at age 9; yet in another, menses might not start until age 15.

Growth Follows a Cephalocaudal Pattern: Beginning at the Head and Progressing Down to the Chest, Trunk, and Lower Extremities. When an infant is born, the head is the largest portion of the body. In the first year, the head, chest, and trunk gain in size, yet the legs remain short. Growth of the legs is readily apparent in the second year.

Development Proceeds in a Proximodistal Pattern: Beginning at the Center of the Body and Moving Outward. For example, the infant first begins to focus his eyes; then lifts the head, later pushing up and rolling over. As the infant grows and gains strength and coordination from head to feet, he will crawl and later walk.

Simple Skills Develop Separately and Independently. Later they are Integrated into More Complex Skills. Many complex skills that we take for granted as adults actually represent a compilation of simple skills. Your ability to feed yourself is an example. This act requires the ability to find your mouth, grasp an object, control movement of that object, coordinate movement of the hand from the plate to the mouth, and swallow solid food. If you have ever tried to learn to play a musical instrument, you are familiar with this principle. You must master simple steps before you are able to play a tune.

Each Body System Grows at its Own Rate. This principle is readily apparent in fetal development; however, it applies throughout life. Perhaps the most noticeable example is the onset of puberty. In the years leading up to puberty, the cardiovascular, respiratory, and nervous systems grow and develop dramatically, yet the reproductive system changes very little. **Puberty** is a series of changes that lead to full development of the reproductive system. The hormone changes that occur with puberty also trigger growth in the musculoskeletal system.

Body System Functions Become Increasingly Differentiated Over Time. Have you ever seen a newborn respond to a loud noise? The newborn's startle response involves the whole body. With maturity, the response becomes more focused, for example, covering the ears. An adult is often able to identify the location of the sound and distinguish the origin of the sound.

Theories of Development

Theories of development attempt to explain and describe patterns of development common to all people. Such theories provide an organizing framework to help you understand and plan for the needs of the patients you will encounter, and they provide a basis for nursing interventions and clinical decision-making. The needs of a 6-year-old differ greatly from those of a 25-year-old or a 65-year-old, even though they may have the same medical diagnosis or even the same nursing diagnosis.

Robert Havighurst, Sigmund Freud, Jean Piaget, Erik Erikson, and others have proposed theories to explain life span development. Each theorist has focused on a domain of human nature to examine how humans develop and has divided the life span into stages. Each stage represents a period of time that shares common characteristics. Most theorists have also identified tasks that are usually accomplished in each stage. As with the caring theories discussed in Chapter 8, an understanding of these key developmental theories is essential to full-spectrum nursing practice. For an expanded discussion on theories of development,

 Go to Chapter 9, **Development Through the Life Span—Expanded Discussion, Theories of Development,** on the Student Resource Disk or DavisPlus at http://davisplus. fadavis.com/Wilkinson2

Developmental Task Theory

Robert Havighurst was an educator who theorized that learning is a lifelong process. He believed a person moves through six life stages, each associated with a number of tasks that must be learned. Havighurst characterizes **developmental task** as "midway between an individual need and societal demand. It assumes an active learner interacting with an active social environment" (1971, p. vi). Failure to master a task leads to imbalance within the individual, unhappiness, and difficulty mastering future tasks and interacting with others.

Psychoanalytic Theory

Sigmund Freud was a pioneer in the science of human development. His psychoanalytic theory focuses on the motivation for human behavior and personality development. Freud believed human development is maintained by instinctual drives, such as libido (sexual instinct), aggression, and survival (Sadock & Sadock, 2007). These drives have varying emphases, depending on the age of the individual. Psychoanalytic theory became the dominant theoretical foundation of early 20th century psychotherapy. However, Freud developed his theory in the Victorian era, when societal norms were very strict. Sexual repression and male dominance over female behavior were the cultural standard. Many of today's social scientists question the relevance of many aspects of his theory to life in the 21st century.

Freud identified several forces that influence the development of our personality. Each has a unique function. The **id** represents instinctual urges, pleasure, and gratification, such as hunger, procreation, pleasure, and aggression. It is dominant in infants and young children. The **ego** begins to develop around 4 to 6 months of age. It strives to balance what is wanted (id) and what is possible to obtain or achieve. The **superego** is sometimes referred to as our conscience. This force develops in early childhood (age 5 to 6). The **unconscious mind** is composed of thoughts and memories that are not readily recalled but unconsciously influence behavior.

In the mid-1950s, Freud's daughter, the psychologist Anna Freud, identified a number of **defense mechanisms,** which she described as thought patterns or behaviors that the ego employs in the face of threat to biological or psychological integrity (Townsend, 2009). In other words, defense mechanisms protect us from excess anxiety. They are discussed more in Chapter 25.

Cognitive Development Theory

Jean Piaget studied his own children to understand how humans develop cognitive abilities. According to Piaget, cognitive development requires three core competencies: adaptation, assimilation, and accommodation. **Adaptation** is the ability to adjust to and interact with one's environment. To be able to adapt, one must assimilate and accommodate. **Assimilation** is the integration of new experiences with one's own system of knowledge. **Accommodation** is the change in one's system of knowledge that results from processing new information. For example, an infant is born with an innate ability to suck. Presented with the mother's nipple, the infant is able to assimilate the nipple to the behavior of sucking. If given a bottle, the infant can learn to accommodate the artificial nipple. However, the baby may adapt by accepting the artificial nipple only from the father, crying and fussing if the mother offers a bottle instead of her breast.

According to Piaget, cognitive development occurs from birth through adolescence in a sequence of four stages: sensorimotor, preoperational thought, concrete operations, and formal operations. A child must complete each stage before moving to the next. The rate at which a child moves through the four stages is determined by inherited intellect and the influence of the environment. Piaget does not address cognitive development after adolescence.

Psychosocial Development Theory

In the 1950s Erik Erikson introduced his theory of psychosocial development. Erikson was strongly influenced by Freud but believed that personality continues to evolve throughout the life span as the individual interacts with the social world. He hypothesized that individuals must negotiate eight stages as they progress through the life span. Most individuals successfully move from stage to stage; however, a person can regress during times of stress to earlier stages or be forced to face tasks of later stages because of unforeseen life events, such as terminal illness. Failure to successfully

master a stage leads to maladjustment. Erikson's theory is widely used in nursing and health care. Below are Erikson's eight stages.

Stage 1: Trust versus mistrust (birth to about 18 months)
Stage 2: Autonomy versus shame and doubt (about 18 months to 3 years)
Stage 3: Initiative versus guilt (3 to 5 years)
Stage 4: Industry versus inferiority (6 to 11 years)
Stage 5: Identity versus role confusion (11 to 21 years)
Stage 6: Intimacy versus isolation (21 to 40 years)
Stage 7: Generativity versus stagnation (40 to 65 years)
Stage 8: Ego integrity versus despair (over 65 years)

Moral Development Theory

Lawrence Kohlberg (1968) developed his theory of moral development by studying the responses to moral dilemmas of 84 boys whose development he followed for a period of 20 years. In this theory, moral reasoning appears to be somewhat age related. According to Kohlberg, moral development is based on one's ability to think at progressively higher levels. Kohlberg believed that, even with maturity, not all people are able to achieve those levels.

As just noted, Kohlberg's research subjects were exclusively male. The validity of his theory for women has been sharply criticized, most prominently by Carol Gilligan (1982, 1993). To address the moral development of women, Gilligan proposed an alternative theory that incorporates the concepts of caring, interpersonal relationships, and responsibility. Gilligan described a three-stage approach to moral development.

Stage 1: Caring for oneself
Stage 2: Caring for others
Stage 3: Caring for oneself and others
See Chapter 44 if you would like a fuller discussion of moral development.

Spiritual Development Theory

James Fowler, a minister, defined faith as a universal human concern and as a process of growing in trust. He noticed that his congregants had very different approaches to faith and that the differences depended on their ages. Basing his studies on the work of Piaget, Erikson, and Kohlberg, he developed a theory of faith development, which includes a pre-stage (Stage 0) and 6 stages of faith (Fowler, 1981). For further explanation,

 Go to Chapter 9, **Development Through the Life Span—Expanded Discussion,** on the Student Resource Disk or DavisPlus at http://davisplus.fadavis.com/Wilkinson2

Part II. Infancy Through Middle Age: Overview

Recall the case of 3-year-old Tamika, who is being raised by her grandmother and has been hospitalized with pneumonia ("Meet Your Patient" scenario). Imagine that Tamika has been abandoned by her mother, who is addicted to heroin. If you observe that Tamika is small for her age and has not met developmental milestones appropriate for a 3-year-old, you could write the following *diagnostic statement*:

Delayed Growth and Development r/t abandonment by mother, recent change in living status, and gestational heroin exposure—as evidenced by underweight status, short stature, limited verbal skills, and onset of walking at 36 months of age

To address Tamika's diagnosis you might use the following *outcomes*:

NOC outcome: Child Development: 3 years
Individualized goal: Tamika will achieve growth between the 35th and 65th percentiles for her age group and be able to walk up steps, verbalize with two- to three-word sentences, and eat a variety of foods within 6 months.

Tamika will need care that helps her catch up developmentally and allows her to establish a strong relationship with her grandmother. Because the grandmother is also caring for an ill husband, you may need to refer this family to community support services for ongoing help. *NIC interventions* appropriate for Tamika are as follows:

Developmental Care
Teaching: Toddler Nutrition
Teaching: Toddler Safety

Specific interventions for Tamika might include therapeutic play with age-appropriate toys, reading stories, and engaging in conversation, as well as teaching the grandmother about these activities. This family may need counseling to assist with this transition.

For a thorough discussion of theoretical and practical knowledge you will need to care for patients from infancy through middle age,

Go to Chapter 9, **Development Through the Life Span— Expanded Discussion, Infancy Through Middle Age,** on the Student Resource Disk or DavisPlus at http://davisplus. fadavis.com/Wilkinson2

Part III. Older Adults: Overview

Ethel Higgenbotham, the 80-year-old woman introduced in the "Meet Your Patient" scenario, has also entered the hospital with pneumonia. Her son tells you that she began to lose weight rapidly, had little appetite, and became withdrawn after the death of her husband. At a recent visit he found his mother confused, with a productive cough, and with small open areas on her lower legs. These problems led to her hospitalization. You observe that she is very thin and frail and refuses to eat. "I just want to die," she tells you. An appropriate *nursing diagnosis* for Mrs. Higgenbotham might be Adult Failure to Thrive.

An appropriate *NOC outcome* would be Will to Live. You might develop the following *individualized goal:*

Mrs. Higgenbotham will gain 1 lb and participate in at least one daily group activity by the first of next month.

Interventions depend on the diagnosis and its etiology. Mrs. Higgenbotham will need care that helps her adjust to widowhood, provides adequate nutrition, and offers activities that provide interaction with others.

Critical Aspects of Procedure 9-1. Assessing for Abuse

VOL 2 For steps to follow in all procedures, refer to the inside back cover of Volume 2. Go to the full procedure in Volume 2 to practice and learn the procedure steps. Use these Critical Aspects later to help you review key points.

Procedure 9-1 Assessing for Abuse

➤ Assess for abuse any time a child or dependent person has an injury.

➤ Use a nonjudgmental approach; do not make assumptions.

➤ Remember, the relationship between suspected abuser and victim is complex. Love, fear, self-doubt, anger, guilt, and many other emotions are common and can influence the report of the abuse and details implicating the abuser.

➤ The key to ruling out abuse is to determine whether the injury was intentional or accidental.

➤ Obtain a focused health history, assessing for physical, sexual, and psychological abuse and neglect.

➤ Determine whether the caregiver of the suspected victim of abuse has a history of mental health disorder, such as anxiety, depression, or dysfunctional coping.

➤ Perform a focused physical assessment; ensure the integrity of evidence that may be needed for criminal prosecution.

➤ For any sexual examination, always have a witness in the room to protect the patient and examiner.

➤ Assess whether injuries are consistent with history.

➤ If appropriate, provide the victim with referrals for help in escaping the abusive situation.

➤ If appropriate, refer the parent, caregiver, or partner involved in abuse to hotlines or agencies focused on stopping the abuse and protecting the victim.

➤ Report abuse according to agency, state, and federal guidelines.

NIC interventions appropriate for Mrs. Higgenbotham are as follows:

Coping Enhancement
Hope Instillation
Self-Care Assistance
Spiritual Support

Individualized Interventions for Mrs. Higgenbotham include grief counseling, nutritional support, and working with her and her family to determine whether it is appropriate for her to continue to live independently.

For a thorough discussion of theoretical and practical knowledge you will need to care for older adults,

 Go to Chapter 9, **Development Through the Life Span— Expanded Discussion, Older Adults,** on the Student Resource Disk or DavisPlus at http://davisplus.fadavis.com/Wilkinson2

Summary

The examples of Tamika and Mrs. Higgenbotham illustrate the importance of theoretical knowledge of growth and development to your nursing care. We have provided a brief review of principles and theories of growth and development. To review information for specific age groups and for suggestions on how to adapt nursing care for various age groups,

 Go to Chapter 9, **Development Through the Life Span— Expanded Discussion,** on the Student Resource Disk or DavisPlus at http://davisplus.fadavis.com/Wilkinson2

As you will learn in the Expanded Discussion on the ESG, abuse is a common problem among children and adults. To learn more about assessing for abuse, see the Critical Aspects box, and

 Go to **Procedure 9-1, Assessing for Abuse,** in Volume 2.

 Suggested Readings: Go to Chapter 9, **Reading More About Growth and Development Through the Life Span,** on the Student Resource Disk or DavisPlus at http://davisplus.fadavis.com/Wilkinson2

 Bibliography: Go to Volume 2, Bibliography.

CHAPTER 10

Experiencing Health & Illness

Learning Outcomes

After completing this chapter, you should be able to:

➤ Explore the concepts of health and illness from a holistic perspective.

➤ Compare and contrast three models of health and illness.

➤ Describe the various ways that people experience health and illness.

➤ Identify factors that disrupt health.

➤ Describe the five stages of illness behavior.

➤ Differentiate between acute and chronic illness.

➤ Identify factors that influence individuals' responses to illness.

➤ Apply the concepts presented in this chapter to a variety of patient care situations.

➤ Explain what the concepts in this chapter mean to you as you work toward becoming a full-spectrum nurse.

Meet Your Patient

Evelyn is 87 years old and has lived in a long-term care facility for the last 5 years. She suffers from congestive heart failure, hypertension, diabetes, macular degeneration resulting in near blindness, a severe hearing deficit, urinary incontinence, and immobility resulting from a hip fracture.

Evelyn was married nearly 60 years to Lloyd, who died 6 years ago. They had 5 children, 17 grandchildren, and 14 great-grandchildren. In these last few years, she has experienced the loss of her husband, home, vision, hearing, mobility, and bladder control. Despite these limitations, she keeps current in the lives of all of her extended family and friends.

She is involved in the lives of the staff of the long-term care facility. She is their confidante and knows about their children, their romances, and the gossip around the institution. She is an avid Minnesota Twins fan and also keeps track of the televised high school basketball tournaments. Whenever there is an election, she makes sure that she votes. She "reads" every talking book she can get her hands on.

Recently Evelyn was admitted to the hospital in severe congestive heart failure. She told her pastor, "I don't want to die yet. I'm having too much fun!"

Evelyn's situation is a far cry from what most people would picture as "good health." However, as you consider the ideas of health presented in this chapter, you might conclude that she is a reasonably healthy person from many standpoints.

Theoretical **Knowledge**
knowing why

Every day there is something in the news about health or illness. Politicians talk about their desire to improve our health and reorganize healthcare. Public schools want students to eat right, exercise, and receive regular immunizations. In an attempt to reduce health insurance claims, employers open on-site fitness centers and employ nurses and counselors to work with employees to improve employee health. Everyone says they want to be healthy.

As a nursing student, you have probably already cared for clients in various stages of health and illness. But have you ever considered what those terms mean? Our understanding of health and illness is influenced by our family, culture, health history, and a host of other factors. As you evolve as a nurse, you'll find that your understanding of these concepts evolves, too. Here we examine some ways that you and your clients might define health and illness and some ways that full-spectrum nurses have come to understand these terms through their thinking, doing, and caring.

You may find this chapter a little different from other chapters in this book and other textbooks. That is because the goal of the chapter is not so much to help you learn facts about health and illness, but to understand how people experience them. Even the language of the chapter is designed for that purpose. Relax and flow with the chapter. Instead of agonizing over each detail, read it in a way that will help you see the "big picture."

How Do We Understand Health and Illness?

What is your image of **health**? Is it the "body beautiful"—an athlete's build, glistening hair, straight white teeth, and a glowing complexion? Being a "picture of health" can depend on whether you were born in the right era—or in the right country, for that matter. Styles of beautiful bodies come and go. For instance, much Indian, African, Greek, and European art portrays ideal women as well-rounded creatures. The perfect body view of health also denies the possibility of health to people who use wheelchairs, prosthetics, or even eyeglasses and hearing aids. Yet many full-spectrum nurses working with disabled clients would indeed describe their clients as healthy.

In describing healthy people, would you disqualify someone with a cold, dandruff, or athlete's foot? What about diabetes, heart disease, or cancer? Doing so would reflect another view of health: that is, *not having illness*. This view may be unfair because it restricts health only to those who do not have some kind of physical impairment.

Another popular concept is that health is *something you can buy*: a weight-loss system, a treadmill, an exercise bicycle, membership in a health club, medicine, liposuction,

coronary bypasses, and so on. In this view, health does not come from within. It's something "out there" that is available if you have enough money or insurance.

Health can also be described as *an ideal state of physical and mental well-being*: something to strive for, but never to attain. Good health is always around the corner but never actually reached, because there is always something more to be achieved. In this view, health is the goal itself, the end instead of one of the means to fulfilling life's purposes.

Theologian Jürgen Moltmann (1983) described health in a different way. He stated that "true health is the strength to live, the strength to suffer, and the strength to die. Health is not a condition of my body; it is *the power of my soul to cope with the varying condition of that body*" (p. 142). Similarly, novelist Robert Louis Stevenson wrote of health, "It is not a matter of holding good cards, *it's playing a poor hand well*." For more traditional definitions of health, refer to Box 10-1.

Now that we've explored some definitions of health, let's consider a definition of illness. When you think of illness, what comes to mind? If you answered with a list of disorders such as heart disease, diabetes, or schizophrenia, you're not alone. Most people have a medical view of illness as disease, which is a pathology affecting an organ or body system. Traditional definitions would

---

BOX 10-1 ■ What Do the Experts Say About Health?

- *The World Health Organization (WHO)* initially defined health as "a state of complete physical, mental and social well-being and not merely the absence of disease or infirmity" (WHO, 1948).

- *In 1986 WHO* redefined health as "a resource for everyday life, not the objective of living. Health is a positive concept emphasizing social and personal resources, as well as physical capacities" (The Ottawa Charter for Health Promotion, 1986).

- *Traditional Chinese medicine* considers health to be a balance between the opposite energy forces of *yin* and *yang*.

- *Ayurveda*, an ancient Indian medical system, describes health as the trinity of body, mind, and spiritual awareness (Sheinfeld-Gorin & Arnold, 2006).

- *Florence Nightingale* believed that health was prevention of disease through the use of fresh air, pure water, efficient drainage, cleanliness, and light (1859).

- *Nursing theorist Jean Watson* (1979) believes that health implies at least three elements: (1) a high level of overall physical, mental, and social functioning; (2) a general adaptive—maintenance level of daily functioning; and (3) the absence of illness (or the presence of efforts that lead to its absence). To Watson, health is a matter of perception. Even an individual with a terminal illness may be considered healthy if he has a high level of functioning, is coping with the diagnosis, and is actively making efforts to improve his status.

also encompass traumatic injury and psychiatric disorders. But is illness merely the sum of these terms?

Nurses Understand Health and Illness as Individual Experiences

If you were the nurse caring for Evelyn in the "Meet Your Patient" scenario, would you understand health as a perfect body or the absence of disease? Probably not. Nurses understand health and illness as individual experiences, emerging from each patient's unique responses. The person with an illness rarely perceives the experience as a medical diagnosis. Instead, people describe their illness in terms of how it makes them *feel*. Think back to the last time you were ill. How did you feel? Did you feel pain, sadness, fatigue, loss? Did you feel overwhelmed? These responses are disruptions to health and, as such, constitute the lived experience of illness. This lived experience is *unique to each patient:* Just as Evelyn might describe herself as "raring to go," another patient who is 10 years younger and on half as many medications may describe herself as "exhausted all the time" and "just waiting to die." In short, nurses honor the client's understanding of his or her state of being.

For many years, nurses have recognized that, like Evelyn, some clients strive to maintain a state of optimal health even when coping with chronic and even terminal disease. Many experience this state as wellness: "a way of life oriented toward optimal health and well-being in which body, mind, and spirit are integrated by the individual to live more fully within the human and natural community" (Myers, Sweeney, & Witmer, 2000, p. 252). This perspective acknowledges the influence of attitude and lifestyle choices on the client's state of being. It also implies that nursing interventions in support of wellness are important for healthy clients, those who are experiencing disease, and even those facing death.

 Critical**Thinking** 10-1

What qualities are essential to your own personal definition of health? How do you define illness?

Knowledge**Check** 10-1

- Provide at least two common definitions of health.
- Explain how full-spectrum nurses define health and illness.
- Define wellness in your own words.

 Go to Chapter 10, **Knowledge Check Response Sheet and Answers,** on the Student Resource Disk or DavisPlus at http://davisplus.fadavis.com/Wilkinson2

Nurses Use Conceptual Models to Understand Health and Illness

You can use a variety of models to understand health and illness. Each emphasizes somewhat different aspects of these complex experiences. Nurses have found the following models particularly useful.

The Health–Illness Continuum

Most of us recognize that our health status changes frequently. For example, although today I feel pretty good and yesterday I was exhausted, I believe I was healthy on both of those days. I know that my exhaustion was related to staying up late enjoying the company of good friends. My medical chart states that I have diabetes and hypertension, but I keep both diseases in control. I take multiple medications, read food labels, exercise aerobically 5 days a week, and lift weights 3 days a week. On the one hand, my mother used to tell me, "You do too much. Relax, take the medicines, and eat treats once in a while. You'll be happier." On the other hand, my father always said, "The more you take care of yourself, the less you rely on medicines, and the better off you are." Am I healthy, ill, or a health nut?

The preceding example illustrates the complex and dynamic nature of human health. In an effort to describe this complex state, many theorists speak of a *health–illness continuum;* that is, they see health and illness as a graduated spectrum that cannot be divided—except arbitrarily—into parts. A person's position on the continuum is constantly changing according to physiological changes, lifestyle choices, and the results of various therapies. As shown in Figure 10-1, the number 1 represents a state of being gravely ill, and 10 represents excellent health, a person in peak form. Notice, however, that a client like Evelyn in the "Meet Your Patient" scenario may view herself at various points on this continuum according to how she feels on any particular day. In other words, the continuum is personal and dynamic: Over the course of time, a client's health will move up and down along this gradient.

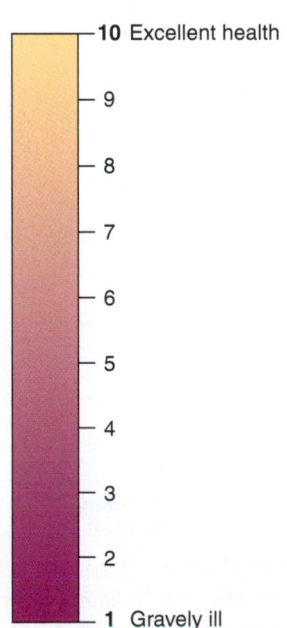

FIGURE 10-1 Over a lifetime, an individual moves up and down on the health-illness continuum.

Dunn's Health Grid

Dunn (1959) created a health grid that plots a person's status on the health–illness continuum against environmental conditions (Fig. 10-2). Many nurses use this grid to help them predict the likelihood that a client will experience a change in health status. For example, Evelyn ("Meet Your Patient") has several problems that are causing a decline in her health status. On a scale of 1 to 10, an independent observer might rate her health as a 3. However, Evelyn has a positive outlook and tells her pastor, "I don't want to die yet. I'm having too much fun!" She also has excellent support from her friends, family, and the facility staff. Clearly, Evelyn is in a favorable environment. This positive setting protects her from harm and provides a good quality of life. On Dunn's grid, Evelyn would probably fall in the area of "protected poor health."

Neuman's Continuum

Nursing theorist Betty Neuman (2002) views health as an expression of living energy available to an individual. The energy is displayed as a continuum with high energy (wellness) at one end and low energy (illness) at the opposite end (Fig. 10-3). The person is said to have varying levels of energy at various stages of life. When more energy is generated than expended, there is wellness. When more energy is expended than is generated, there is illness—possibly death. Although Evelyn ("Meet Your Patient") has several clearly identified health problems, she is engaged in life and active with her family, friends, and long-term care facility staff. We might not

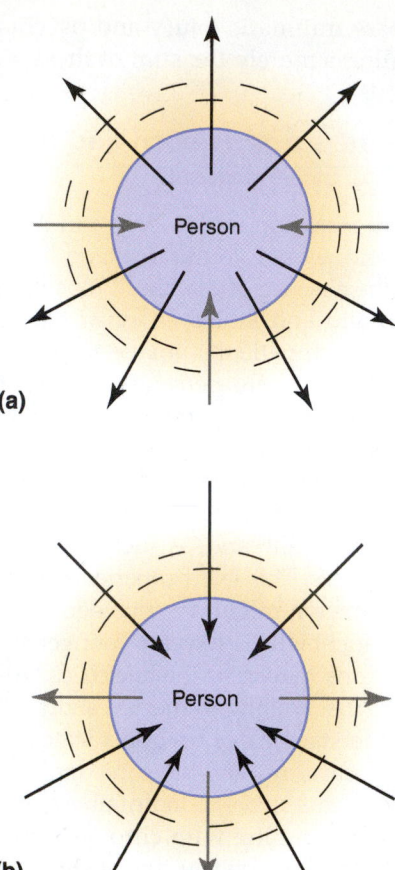

FIGURE 10-3 Neuman's continuum: A balance of input and output. *A,* When energy output exceeds input, illness results. *B,* Wellness occurs when more energy is generated than expended. (*Source:* Neuman, B. (1995). *The Neuman systems model.* In B. Neuman, *The Neuman systems model* (3rd ed., pp. 3–61). East Norwalk, CT: Appleton & Lange.)

all agree on where to place her on Neuman's continuum, but certainly her activity and energy counterbalance her physical frailty.

How Do People Experience Health and Illness?

In envisioning health and illness as a continuum, full-spectrum nurses promote wellness regardless of the circumstances a client faces now or in the future. This approach requires the holistic understanding that health is multidimensional. The following are some of the many dimensions of health that we experience along the health–illness continuum.

Biological Factors

Although biological factors are not entirely within our control, most people consider them when they describe themselves as "well" or "ill." A healthy genetic makeup and freedom from debilitating age-related changes are certainly desired states, and they tip the scale toward the wellness end of the health–illness continuum.

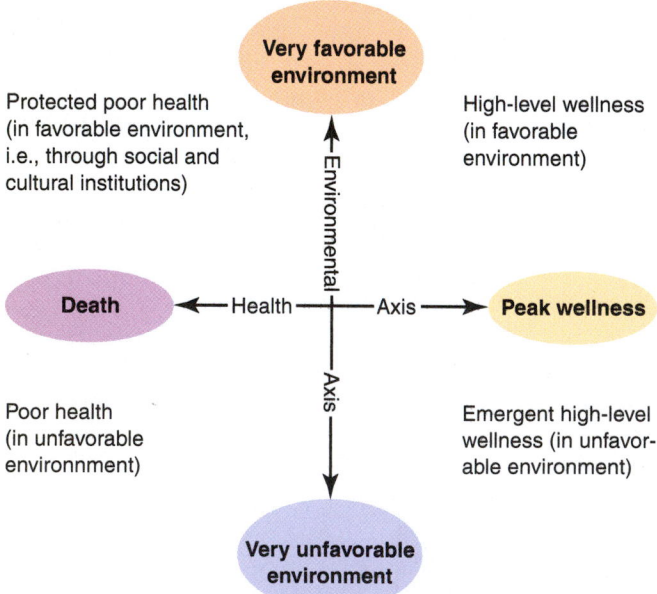

FIGURE 10-2 Dunn's health grid: Health is affected by an individual's status on the health–illness continuum as well as environmental conditions. (*Source:* U.S. Department of Health, Education, and Welfare. Public Health Service. National Office of Vital Statistics.)

Genetic Makeup. For example, the risk of breast cancer increases dramatically in women who have a family history of a mother, sister, or daughter with breast cancer. Recently, a genetic marker for this type of breast cancer has been discovered—that is, some people inherit a tendency to develop breast cancer.

Gender. Many diseases occur more commonly in one gender than another. For example, rheumatoid arthritis, osteoporosis, and breast cancer are more common in women, whereas ulcers, color blindness, and bladder cancer are more common in men.

Age and Developmental Stage. Age and developmental stage influence the likelihood of becoming ill. Certain health problems can be correlated to developmental stage. For example, more than 75% of new breast cancer cases are diagnosed in women older than age 50. As another example, adolescent boys have much higher rates of head injury and spinal cord injury than the general public because of their tendency toward risk-taking behaviors, which peaks during this stage. For further discussion of growth and development, see Chapter 9 in this book and

 Go to **Chapter 9—Expanded Discussion** on the Student Resource Disk.

- **Coping ability.** Developmental stage influences a person's ability to cope with stressors that tend to move him toward the illness end of the continuum. Infants or children who are ill, frightened, or hurt have a limited repertoire of experiences, communication ability, and understanding to help them in their responses. As we progress through the stages of development, we develop understanding and skills to help us deal with illness.
- **Perceptions.** When disease, loss, or other disruptions occur at a younger age than expected, they change our perception of the event and may present a greater challenge to our coping skills than disruptions that are expected. For example, a child's death may seem more tragic than that of an older adult. It is important, though, not to discount the impact of disruptions that occur during the period of a person's life when they might be expected. For example, a client's advanced age does not necessarily make the death of a spouse less traumatic than it would be for a young spouse. Losing someone with whom one has spent most of one's life is an incredible loss, whether or not it is "expected" at that stage of life.

Nutrition

Health requires nourishment, and the most obvious form of nourishment is food. The influence of diet on human health is undeniable: Nutrient-deficiency diseases, such as scurvy and night blindness, are unknown in people who consume a nutritious diet. In addition, many chronic diseases, such as type 2 diabetes mellitus and heart disease, are influenced by our diets, and

nutrition appears to play at least a moderate role in a variety of other diseases, such as osteoporosis and some forms of cancer (Thompson & Manore, 2009). As more studies look at the protective properties of some foods (e.g., antioxidants) and the hazards of others (e.g., refined carbohydrates, *trans*-fatty acids), the phrase "You are what you eat" seems more accurate each day. Chapter 26 discusses nutrition in greater detail.

Physical Activity

Healthy people are usually active people. When they are unable to maintain previous levels of activity, they may perceive themselves as less healthy. Studies support the benefit of moderate physical activity in reducing the risk of chronic disease and promoting longevity (Thompson & Manore, 2009). As little as 30 minutes of gardening or 15 minutes of jogging on most days of the week can lead to these benefits. In addition, certain types of exercise have been shown to reduce the risk of specific diseases, such as osteoporosis and heart disease. For example, weight training has been shown to increase bone density and reduce the risk of osteoporosis in women older than age 40, and aerobic activity, such as walking, decreases the risk of heart disease. Some studies even indicate that regular aerobic exercise helps preserve neurological function as we age.

Sleep and Rest

Sleep nourishes health. Most of the body's growth hormone, which assists in tissue regeneration, synthesis of bone, and formation of red blood cells, is released during sleep. Sleep is also important to mental health because it provides time for the mind to slow down and rejuvenate. Perhaps that is why problems often look much smaller in the morning. In controlled studies, people kept awake for 24 hours experienced difficulty concentrating and performing routine tasks. With increasing levels of sleep deprivation, sensory deficits and mood disturbances occurred. Outside the laboratory, mild but chronic sleep deprivation is common, particularly among students, mothers of infants and young children, and people in pain. Sleep and rest are discussed in more detail in Chapter 33.

Meaningful Work

Many people find that work is a healthy way to cope with stressors. Psychologist Victor Frankl, who survived internment in a Nazi concentration camp, observed in *Man's Search for Meaning* (1959, 1962, 1984, 2004) that engaging in meaningful work promotes health and, even in the midst of horrific stressors, can defend against physical and mental breakdown. The definition of meaningful work varies, but many share the view offered by Morrie Schwartz in *Tuesdays with Morrie:* "You know what really gives you satisfaction?

Offering others what you have to give. . . . [D]evote yourself to your community around you, and devote yourself to creating something that gives you purpose and meaning. You notice, there's nothing in there about a salary" (Albom, 1997).

People also experience meaningful work as a dimension of wellness. For many people, volunteering, pursuing hobbies, and engaging in pleasurable activities can be forms of meaningful work. For example, some find that singing, playing a musical instrument, or listening to music is particularly healing. For others, it may be literature, art, studying the intricacies of the human body, playing basketball, doing counted cross-stitch, gardening, hiking in the wilderness, or even shopping. Remember that being healthy is not all drudgery, such as denying yourself the pleasure of hot fudge sundaes and French fries. Healthful activities can be fun, too. By supporting clients' life work, hobbies, and personal interests, you help them nourish their spirit in their unique way.

Lifestyle Choices

People who consider themselves healthy are usually those who make healthy lifestyle choices. They are aware of the threats to health created by cigarette smoking, alcohol consumption, drug abuse, unprotected sex, and other risky behaviors. Consider the following examples:

- Tobacco use increases recovery time from other illnesses, injuries, and surgery. Smoking also increases the risk of diabetes, infertility, low birth weight and preterm babies, and perinatal death.
- Studies have indicated that drinking a glass of red wine each day can reduce the risk of heart disease and slow bone loss. In contrast, excessive alcohol consumption damages the brain, liver, pancreas, intestines, and neurologic system and can lead to malnutrition. It has also been implicated in several forms of cancer and in fetal alcohol syndrome in newborns. Finally, excessive alcohol consumption is implicated in about half of all motor vehicle accidents and other injuries.
- Substance abuse leads to a deterioration in health, functioning, or social relationships as a result of injection or ingestion of illicit drugs and alcohol. Even prescription drugs can be abused. Drug abuse is a risk factor in many diseases. For example, people who inject illegal drugs are at increased risk of hepatitis and HIV.

You will learn more about effects of lifestyle choices on wellness and safety in Chapters 9, 21, and 41.

Personal Relationships

Living in a healthy family is an important dimension of wellness. Moreover, the family influences a person's view of himself as well or ill. For each of the following contrasting pairs of families, which one in each pair would help you to experience high-level wellness?

- Some families place a high priority on health promotion, whereas others tend to respond to health issues only in times of serious illness.
- Some encourage adventure and risk-taking, whereas others emphasize caution in new situations.
- Some families are very open about expressing feelings and disagreements, whereas others tend to squelch personal feelings to avoid conflict in the family.
- Some families view themselves as capable and successful, others as powerless victims.
- Some families teach good negotiation skills and build a network of family support and community while encouraging the development of independence. In contrast, some parents do not have a large repertoire of coping and communication skills to share with their children.

Especially when clients are coping with life-threatening disease, family relationships can provide critical sustenance and preserve optimal wellness during the experience. Weeks before his death from amyotrophic lateral sclerosis (ALS), a neurological disease, sociologist Morrie Schwartz stated, "It's become quite clear to me as I've been sick. If you don't have the support and love and caring and concern that you get from a family, you don't have much at all. Love is so supremely important" (Albom, 1997). You will learn more about the role of family in human health in Chapter 12.

When illness occurs, some people prefer to be totally independent, priding themselves on never asking for or accepting help. But the reality is that during times of disruption, support from others is crucial. Families, friends, co-workers, healthcare workers, pastors, and counselors may be very effective in helping even rugged individualists deal with difficult life situations. Knowing that support is available, and being willing to accept the support, can greatly affect a person's response to disruptions.

Culture

Culture influences a person's healthcare decisions and health behaviors as well as her view of self as well or ill. Individual and family health may be influenced by ethnicity, the culture of a region or a neighborhood, the culture of a school or work environment, the culture of affluence or poverty, or the culture of a religious group. For example, the cultural group may share health-promoting values, such as a nutritious diet or regular physical activity. This is not to say that individuals can be "profiled" by their cultural background. Just as some clients respond in ways unlike those of their families, some make a conscious decision to break away from culturally conditioned responses.

Our response to illness is also partly determined by our culture. Philosopher Ken Wilber (2000) identifies 11 culturally determined responses to illness. For example, people who belong to fundamentalist religions may interpret illness as a punishment from God and may bear their symptoms stoically (i.e., hide their symptoms) to try to pay for their sins (retribution). People who identify themselves with the New Age movement may believe that illness is a lesson we give ourselves to teach us something we need to learn for our spiritual evolution. They may therefore, try to identify the lesson of their illness—for example, "I need to slow down and be good to myself"—and then attempt to practice it.

The culture of healthcare has traditionally responded to illness with specific therapies aimed at treating a biophysical disorder, whereas nursing, as part of the culture of holism, responds to the physical, emotional, mental, and spiritual dimensions of illness. If you need more information about the influence of culture on health and illness, see Chapter 13.

Religion and Spirituality

Religion and spirituality are closely tied to culture, and clients' religious beliefs and practices can influence their healthcare choices. For example, some people believe that spiritual beliefs influence the mind–body connection to promote wellness and healing. A dramatic example is seemingly spontaneous recovery after a religious rite, as when, for example, a Native American with crippling arthritis is visited by the "false faces" (shamans wearing masks depicting spirits) and then recovers enough to walk across the room.

When healing is not possible because of terminal illness or external circumstances beyond our control, spiritual reserves can help maintain our view of ourselves as "well." Nien Cheng in *Life and Death in Shanghai* (1986) tells her story of surviving 7 years in solitary confinement during China's Cultural Revolution. One of the ways she nourished herself was through reciting scriptures she had memorized. She had nourished her mind during "good" times in her life. When her life became barren, she nourished her mind and spirit through the reserves she had stored. Part of health is having the reserves when you need them, whether physical, mental, or spiritual. You will learn more about the influence of spirituality on health in Chapter 14.

Environmental Factors

The environment can also nourish wellness. For institutionalized clients, a little corner of the room that is uniquely "theirs," with photos and other mementos, can be healing. Other clients may be soothed by the quietness of a chapel, a walk in the country, or even a trip to a shopping mall. Spending time in any place where they feel harmony and peace and draw strength can promote clients' health.

On the other hand, environmental pollutants are a common cause of illness. For example, exposure to secondhand smoke causes an estimated 3000 deaths from lung cancer among American adults each year (Centers for Disease Control and Prevention [CDC], 2006), and carbon monoxide poisoning kills about 480 people (CDC, 2005). Lead poisoning, molds, radon, chemicals (e.g., insecticides), and other pollutants also cause serious disease.

Finances

It is often said that money doesn't buy happiness. Certainly, this is true. However, money does buy access to healthcare and healthcare choices and thus nourishes wellness. In the United States, health insurance is often tied to employment or income level, and health insurance dictates which providers you have access to and what services are available to you. Even in countries with national health programs, such as Canada and some European countries, the standard care available may not include all the services or medications a person desires. The same is true in the United States, for example with Medicare.

Sometimes healthcare providers wonder why people do not take advantage of services that are available to them. Why do they let things go so long before seeking help—or fail to follow up with recommended treatment plans? What may seem very reasonable to us as healthcare professionals may seem totally out of reach or unacceptable to those needing the help. A client's apparent lack of concern or lack of compliance to a treatment regimen may be, in reality, a problem regarding access to healthcare resources. Several factors influence access: distance from the resources; knowledge of available resources; financial ability to access resources; financial ability to make lifestyle adjustments, such as changes in diet or employment; and trust in the resources that are available. Any one or combination of these factors may keep individuals and families from getting the help that they need.

Critical Thinking 10-2

- In what ways could you improve your eating, exercise, and sleep habits?
- How might a hospitalized patient get away from the routine and find peace and harmony?

What Factors Disrupt Health?

We spend much of our lives trying to maintain good health—eating, sleeping, keeping our bodies at a comfortable temperature—in general, tending to our high-maintenance bodily needs. It's a continual process because of the many disruptions to health we face. Not all of these disruptions are incapacitating, but all challenge our ability to function and enjoy our everyday lives, and they tend to move us toward the illness end of the health–illness continuum.

Physical Disease

Disease disrupts our lives in so many ways. It may reduce our ability to perform our life roles effectively or to engage in activities we enjoyed before the illness. The diagnosis of a chronic or life-threatening disease may bring shock, fear, anxiety, anger, or grief: Will I become disabled? How will I support my family? What did I do to deserve this? How can I bear saying good-bye to the people I love? It may also cause clients to question the meaning and purpose of their lives, to become more inwardly focused, or to embrace life even more fully. When she first learned of her diagnosis of breast cancer at age 36, Treya Killam Wilber wrote, "Strange things happen to the mind when catastrophe strikes. It felt like the universe turned into a thin paper tissue, and then someone simply tore the tissue in half right in front of my eyes. I was so stunned that it was as if absolutely nothing had happened. A tremendous strength descended on me, the strength of being both totally jolted and totally stupefied. I was clear, present, and very determined" (Wilber, 2000).

Injury

Injury can cause the same symptoms and emotions as disease, but perhaps its most disruptive aspect is its suddenness. In *Still Me,* actor Christopher Reeve (Superman) described his thoughts in the first days after he recovered consciousness following his cervical spinal cord injury: "The thought that kept going through my mind was: I've ruined my life. I've ruined my life, and you only get one. You can't say, 'I've spoiled this one, so can I have another, please?' There's no counter you can go up to and say, 'I dropped my ice cream cone; could I please have another one?'. . . . Why isn't there a higher authority you can go to and say, 'Wait a minute, you didn't mean for this to happen to *me*'" (Reeve, 1998).

Mental Illness

Clients with mental illness and their families experience a level of pain, suffering, and chronic sorrow that is difficult for healthy people to fully appreciate (Godress, Ozgul, Owen, et al., 2005; Kokanovic, Petersen, & Klimidis, 2006). In addition, if the illness affects work ability, they experience loss of income and altered role relationships, accompanied by the costs of various therapies.

Mental illness carries with it a stigma that has been described as the single most debilitating handicap for people with mental illness (Glod, 1998). This stigmatization can also disrupt the health of family members. For example, an adult sister, whose only sibling has had repeated hospitalizations from exacerbations of schizophrenia, reported overhearing a cousin at a family gathering ask her uncle, "So where is that crazy Dee? Is she in or out of the hospital again? I hope her sister doesn't catch her craziness." The sister stated, "I really feel labeled along with my sister" (Glod, 1998). Family members may also live in constant fear that their loved one may hurt herself or even commit suicide.

Pain

Whether mild or severe, temporary or long-lasting, pain is a disruption. It's not that we can't live with pain—many people do, every day of their lives. However, pain disrupts the smooth operation of our lives; it can change personality, erode coping skills, and interfere with healthy communication. Pain can interfere in life at all levels, particularly when it is chronic or severe. It's hard to concentrate on what we are trying to accomplish when pain is competing for our attention.

Pain that is easily remedied with over-the-counter medications or that is short lived serves only as a minor disruption in our lives. However, pain that is all-encompassing permeates a person's entire existence. Sometimes that pain is physical, sometimes psychological. One young mother of a profoundly mentally disabled 14-year-old girl spoke of "hurting so bad that my bones hurt."

As we discussed in Chapter 1, some of our nursing interventions inflict pain. We ask patients to turn, deep-breathe, and cough after surgery, even though it hurts—a *lot*! We put needles in them, catheterize them, and get them out of bed when they would rather sleep. We pull off tape. We invade their physical personal space. We ask them questions about personal things, such as their bowel movements. It is a challenge to be a comforting, healing presence when we have to do things that cause discomfort.

Loss

Whether the loss of a job; the end of a romantic relationship; the death of a loved one; or the loss of youth, beauty, functioning, or identity, loss cuts to the core of who we are. Most of us cling to a unique identity, which often does *not* include gaining weight or getting wrinkles and gray hair, let alone being a "patient" or losing major bodily functions. When such losses occur, people typically experience a period of significant disintegration that may continue until they either find a way to cope with the loss or succeed in reinterpreting the loss in a meaningful way. Toward the end of her battle with cancer, Treya Killam Wilber lost her near vision. One way she coped with this loss was by replacing her passion for reading with sitting at her window contemplating the mountains beyond (Wilber, 2000).

Many have written about the indignities people suffered in concentration camps, including nakedness, exposure to human excrement, and being treated like children incapable of thoughtful judgment (Bettelheim, 1979; Frankl, 1959, 1962, 1984, 2004; Valladares, 2001). The Nazi guards knew that those three indignities were crucial threats to their prisoners' sense of self. Sadly, patients in hospitals and other institutions may also suffer those three indignities. In situations of illness, think how patients feel who have to don a hospital gown and allow their body to be exposed for various tests or procedures or how it feels to lose control of urination and/or defecation. One woman who was paralyzed as the result of a metastatic lesion on her spine indicated that one of the toughest things she had to deal with was having her daughter give her enemas and clean her up as if she were a baby. As healthcare providers, we may easily forget how humiliating such "routine procedures" may be for the patient. As we have discussed, the disease or injury is a disruption in itself; you can prevent further disruption when you respect patients' dignity by providing for their privacy and allowing them to make choices regarding their care.

If temporary losses are difficult, what about those that are permanent? C. S. Lewis (1961) wrote this about his response to the death of his wife: "I know that the thing I want is exactly the thing I can never get. The old life, the jokes, the drinks, the arguments, the lovemaking, the tiny, heartbreaking commonplace" (p. 22). As nurses, we would like to "fix" everything. Though we can't "fix" the holes that are left when a person suffers a loss, we can be open and sensitive to his heart's cry.

Impending Death

We all know that we have a 100% chance of dying; however, it is easy for most of us to ignore this finality and live as though death were only a remote possibility. Lifton and Olson (1974) state that during middle age, even without the presence of life-threatening illness, people tend to become more aware of the compelling reality of death: "One's life is suddenly felt to be limited. . . . It also becomes apparent that . . . there will not be time for all one's projects" (p. 63).

As a nurse, you will care for clients who are living in the shadow of death. Some may be aware of their condition; others may choose to deny it, ignore it, or "fight it to the end" by trying a series of conventional and alternative therapies. Caring for dying clients makes us painfully aware of our own frailty and is one of the most difficult experiences you will face as a nurse. Chapter 15 provides further discussion of loss, grieving, and dying.

Competing Demands

Even in the normal flow of life, there are many competing demands. Taken independently, they may be easy to handle. Taken together, the cumulative effect wears us down. In times of illness, the other competing demands continue. Children need to be cared for. Aging parents may need care. Bills still need to be paid. Job responsibilities press in. One man with depression reported, "[T]he whole thing bundled together—one caused the other which caused more and it was just a degenerative

loop. . . . [O]ne thing feeds another which feeds another and so forth until you just constantly go down" (Smith, 1992, p. 104).

Sometimes people ignore health issues because the competing demands are too great. Symptoms may even go unnoticed because attention is scattered in so many directions and there is not enough time and energy to research one's symptoms, schedule a doctor's appointment, or follow through with treatments.

When a loved one's illness is acute, such as a broken bone, the stress is usually bearable. It is surprising what people can deal with if they can mark off the days on a calendar, knowing how many days are left of a disruption. Bettleheim (1979) states: "The worst calamity becomes bearable if one believes its end is in sight" (pp. 3–4). But when the illness is chronic, the competing demands can take a heavy toll. One woman who took care of her husband who lived at home on a respirator recounted the overwhelming burden she felt when, after 2 years, he was "no better and no worse. This could go on forever!" Her life was consumed with his care. Although people came in to help, she felt she had to maintain constant alertness in case something went wrong with his respirator. But even in the face of her husband's unrelenting needs, she still had to meet many other demands and challenges each day.

As nurses, we sometimes find it easy to see how people ought to deal with their situations, even to criticize them. But it is so important to realize that the short amount of time that you spend with someone in a hospital or clinic or in a home visit is only one tiny fragment of the cumulative experience that patients and their families experience, sometimes unrelentingly for years on end.

Critical Thinking 10-3

How might you assist your patient to maintain normalcy in spite of illness?

The Unknown

Even normal life changes present challenges. For example, most new parents bringing their first baby home from the hospital are in for plenty of surprises. Every new squeak, twitch, and rash raises concern. Think of the couple who adds to that equation serious health problems in their infant. They go from anticipating a "bundle of joy" to a new world perhaps involving surgery, breathing treatments, seizures, feeding tubes, clinic visits, and keeping track of numerous medications.

With some unknowns, there is time to investigate the potential problem and prepare. For example, if an expectant couple learns via amniocentesis (a prenatal test) that their child has a genetic defect, then during the remaining months of pregnancy they can read about the disorder and meet with other parents who have had children similarly affected. This can help prepare them to anticipate their child's needs. But as we noted earlier, injuries and illnesses can happen abruptly, with no chance to prepare ourselves for new realities. A woman described her experience of finding out she had cancer of the lung with metastasis: "It was on a . . . Friday—I got to feeling kind of bad—kind of like you had the flu or something, you know? . . . so I went to the doctor. . . . And he sent me to the hospital. . . . they started doin' tests on me—all kinds of tests—and found out I had cancer" (Smith, 1992, p. 107).

Imbalance

Our sense of justice tells us that when we are good, good things should happen. When we are bad, bad things should happen. The Buddhist concept of karma suggests that there is a fair balance between what one gives to life and what one receives. Thus, when we perceive that life has violated this rule, we experience the violation as a disruption. Our sense of balance is perhaps most dramatically disturbed by the death of children. Such deaths are sometimes referred to as "out of order" because children (of any age) "should" not die before their parents. Balance is also disrupted when patients, expecting that their painful and harrowing treatments "should" help them get better, do not get better. One young woman under treatment for advanced cancer described it like this: "It's just—you've been working hard, and it's not doin' a . . . bit of good. You know . . . you're doin' what you're supposed to be doin' and focusing and all this and that—and your body is still not responding" (Smith, 1992, p. 111).

Have you seen the bumper sticker "Life is hard. And then you die"? Cynical perhaps, but we do not have to live long before we realize that as much as we would like for everything to be fair, it is not going to happen. Knowing this intellectually, however, does not necessarily reduce the disruptive effect of the imbalance.`

Isolation

How many times have you thought, "No one knows what I'm going through!"? Despite the universality of suffering, a sense of isolation or aloneness seems to accompany it. C. S. Lewis (1961) states, "You can't really share someone else's weakness, or fear or pain" (p. 13). Vanauken (1977), in writing about the death of his young wife, reveals that it was not only suffering his loss, but having to go through the experience *without* her that made it so difficult: "Along with the emptiness . . . I kept wanting to *tell* her about it. We always told each other—that was what sharing was—and now this huge thing was happening to me, and I couldn't tell her" (p. 181).

The sense of aloneness reported by seriously ill clients is related in part to their actual physical separation from loved ones during treatments, hospitalizations, or clinic visits. But it also stems from their feeling that there is no one who is really "in their world." Having

someone physically present does not necessarily remove the sense of aloneness:

> When I lay here it's lonely—very, very lonely. Because [my daughter] can't just sit here and talk to me all the time. She's got wash to do, fold and all that stuff. And then the kids to worry about. . . . The worst thing I've found about this whole disease is the loneliness. . . . Because your family can be with you and if they don't come and sit down and talk to you about different things, you're lonely. It's the loneliness that makes you sad inside. . . . It's like everybody's afraid of you or something. They're afraid that maybe they're gonna catch what you got or something (Smith, 1992).

KnowledgeCheck 10-2

Identify at least four factors that disrupt health.

  Go to Chapter 10, **Knowledge Check Response Sheet and Answers,** on the Student Resource Disk or DavisPlus at http://davisplus.fadavis.com/Wilkinson2

CriticalThinking 10-4

- What impact do disruptions have on your life?
- How could you apply the information about disruptions to the health of a community? To the health of a nation?

Why Do People Experience Illness Differently?

Earlier in this chapter, we mentioned that people vary greatly in terms of their response to life situations. Why is this so? Why do some people react to seemingly insurmountable problems with calmness and grace, while others fall apart over seemingly "small" disruptions? The human experience is so complex and interactive that it is impossible to make neat little categories that we might add up to determine a score predicting how a person will respond to a given situation. There are several factors, however, that may influence an individual's responses to illness.

Stages of Illness Behavior

Illness can be viewed as a social role, in which both the patients and caregivers have duties and expectations that are shaped by the society in which they live. Suchman (1972) identified five stages of illness behaviors that people move through as they cope with disruptions to health: experiencing symptoms, sick role behavior, seeking professional care, dependence on others, and recovery.

Experiencing Symptoms is a signal that illness has begun. If the symptoms are recognizable, such as runny nose, sneezing, and a cough, you may identify the problem as a common cold and turn to previously used remedies. Common problems rarely progress beyond this stage. However, if the symptoms are unusual, severe, or overwhelming, you may progress to the next stage.

Sick Role Behavior is assumed when you have identified yourself as ill. This role relieves you from normal duties, such as work, school, or tasks at home. The severity of the symptoms and anticipated length of illness determine whether you will progress further along the stages of illness. In Western biomedical culture, the prevailing view is that sick persons are not responsible for their illnesses and that a curative process outside the person is needed to restore wellness. We believe that the sick person has the duty to try to get well, to seek healthcare, and to cooperate with the care providers (Cockerham, 2000).

Seeking Professional Care is the next stage. To reach this stage, you must determine that you are ill and that professional care is required to treat the illness. Persons who seek professional care are asking for validation of their illness, explanations for their symptoms, appropriate treatment, and information about the anticipated length of illness. Healthcare professionals often bypass this stage, relying on themselves to identify and treat the problem. This is not always the best course of action because it is difficult to be objective when examining yourself.

Dependence on Others begins when you accept the diagnosis and treatment of the healthcare provider. The severity of the illness and the type of treatment determine the extent of dependence. In some cases, this may be limited to listening to the provider's instructions, filling the prescription, and following directions given in the office. However, illness that requires hospitalization is often associated with dependence on nursing staff and hospital personnel for activities of daily living, medications, and treatments. Some people easily make the transition to dependence; others remain as independent as possible even in the face of severe illness. Personal characteristics and values play a large role in determining how each of us will respond to the challenges of being dependent.

Recovery is the final stage of illness. Dependence is given up, and there is a gradual return to normal roles and functioning. In minor illness, this is usually a return to the status quo. Severe illnesses may require a newly defined level of optimum function. The greater the change, the more difficult this transition will be. Learning to "manage" a chronic illness is the equivalent of a "cure" in an acute illness (Parsons, 1975).

The Nature of the Illness

The nature of the illness affects the way persons react to disruptions. An **acute illness** occurs suddenly and lasts for a limited amount of time. Acute illnesses, such as a cold, flu, or viral infection, may be minor and require no formal healthcare. Some acute illness, such as strep throat, may require a visit to a health provider for treatment or even hospitalization or surgery, as in cholecystitis (gallbladder inflammation secondary to gallstone formation) or pyelonephritis (infection of the kidney).

Although hospitalization and surgery can be quite traumatic, in each case the person is expected to recover. In acute illness, a person may experience the disruptions of pain, competing demands, and the unknown. However, an end is in sight. Relief is expected.

In contrast, **chronic illness** lasts for a long period of time, usually 6 months or more, often for a lifetime. Chronic illness requires the person to make life changes. These changes might be regular visits to the clinic or hospital, daily medications, or lifestyle modifications. Examples of chronic illness include AIDS, diabetes mellitus, rheumatoid arthritis, and hypertension. Because of the lengthy period of illness, people with chronic disease often experience periods of remission or exacerbation. A **remission** occurs when symptoms are minimal to none. An **exacerbation** occurs when symptoms intensify. Clients with chronic illness often complain about the unrelenting nature of their health problems. A person with chronic illness may experience virtually all of the disruptions identified earlier. Box 10-2 identifies some interesting facts about chronic conditions.

Hardiness

Why does one client who drinks, smokes, overeats, and avoids exercise live into his 90s, yet another client who "follows all the rules" dies of a sudden heart attack at age 39? Our bodies do not react to the same stressors in the same way. One factor that may contribute to this difference is the person's hardiness.

Will to Live. **Hardiness** has been described as developing a very strong positive force to live—and enjoying the fight! A man with heart problems said, "I guess everybody that's in the situation, who has to fight to live, and has learned the mental wizardry of it, you know, to make yourself want to live on. But if you want to, you develop this—this very, very strong positive force to make it go" (Smith, 1992, p. 131). Seigel (1986) reported a study by London researchers that revealed a 10-year survival rate of 75% "among cancer patients who reacted to the diagnosis with a 'fighting spirit,'" compared with a 22% survival rate "among those who responded with 'stoic acceptance' or feelings of helplessness or hopelessness" (p. 25)(Fig. 10-4).

A dramatic example is one woman in an advanced stage of cancer and receiving chemotherapy who got up and went to work every day. Even though it was extremely difficult to drag herself out of bed and get ready for work, she felt much better when she could carry on her normal activities instead of dwelling on her constant pain and the threat of impending death. Carrying on normally is not easy to do, however. It takes a concerted, determined effort to persevere.

Adapting to Change. Another aspect of hardiness is the willingness to draw on resources within oneself or from others to break out of old patterns of living when life situations change. Some people find it too difficult to

BOX 10-2 ■ FAQs: Chronic Conditions

- More than 90 million Americans live with chronic conditions.
- Chronic conditions account for about 70% of all deaths in the United States.
- About 80% of older adults have at least one chronic condition; 50% have at least two.
- Approximately 6% of adults older than age 65 have a diagnosable depressive illness.
- The top three risks for functional decline are cognitive impairment, depression, and disease burden.
- The largest declines in functional abilities are associated with these physical conditions: arthritis of the hip or knee; sciatica; and chronic pulmonary diseases.
- Arthritis affects one in five U.S. adults; for more than 40% of those, arthritis limits their activities.
- About 32% of the adult population and 17.1% of children and adolescents were obese in 2003–2004.
- In a large sample of Medicare beneficiaries, the following were the most frequent chronic physical conditions:

Hypertension (50.5%)	Any cancer (other than skin cancer) (12.7%)
Arthritis of the hip or knee (35.5%)	Emphysema, asthma, or COPD (11.2%)
Arthritis of the hand or wrist (35.5%)	Myocardial infarction (8.8%)
Sciatica (21.0%)	Stroke (5.2%)
"Other" heart conditions (19.3%)	Crohn's disease, ulcerative colitis, or inflammatory bowel disease (4.8%)
Angina pectoris or coronary artery disease (14.1%)	Congestive heart failure (4.6%)
Diabetes (13.7%)	

Sources: Centers for Disease Control and Prevention (CDC) (1998, 2001, n.d.); Centers for Medicare & Medicaid Services (2007); Drummond-Dye (2007); Ellis, Shannon, Cox, et al. (2004); National Institute of Mental Health (2003); Stuck, Walthert, Nikolaus, et al., 1999.

FIGURE 10-4 Hardiness has been described as developing a very strong positive force to live—and enjoying the fight!

make life changes, and they just give up. Hardy individuals are willing to seek out information and take initiative in dealing with life situations rather than sitting back and letting someone else control their lives.

Some people don't have many resources to call on. When disruption hits, they lack the cognitive, communicative, creative, and spiritual resources that would support them during difficult times. Ironically, some people blossom during times of adversity. Those who see themselves as hardy tend to approach disruptions with an "I can deal with this" attitude.

The Intensity, Duration, and Multiplicity of the Disruption

Everyone has limits. For healthcare providers, too many demands over too long a period of time can lead to "burnout," a feeling of being overwhelmed and demoralized. For clients and their families, dealing with the cumulative effect of illness and other life disruptions can break down what might otherwise be excellent coping skills. Therefore, their responses may not be typical of what they usually have demonstrated.

KnowledgeCheck 10-3

- Identify the factors that affect how a person responds to the disruptions of illness.
- Define hardiness.

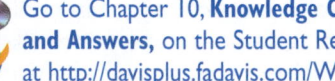 Go to Chapter 10, **Knowledge Check Response Sheet and Answers,** on the Student Resource Disk or DavisPlus at http://davisplus.fadavis.com/Wilkinson2

Toward Evidence-Based Practice

Chan, I. W. S., Lai, J. C. L., & Wong, K. W. N. (2006). Resilience is associated with better recovery in Chinese people diagnosed with coronary heart disease. *Psychology and Health, 21*(3), 335–349.

This study examined the impact of personal resilience (a composite measure of optimism, perceived control, and self-esteem) in 67 Chinese patients in response to an 8-week coronary heart disease rehabilitation program. Results indicated that the patients high in personal resilience achieved better outcomes than those low in personal resilience.

Thompson, C. W., Durrant, L., Barusch, A., & Olson, L. (2006). Fostering coping skills and resilience in home enteral nutrition (HEN) consumers. *Nutrition in Clinical Practice, 21*(6), 557–565.

This qualitative study examined how HEN consumers learned to cope successfully with HEN-related challenges.

Researchers interviewed 12 adult HEN consumers who perceived that they were coping successfully with HEN; they also administered a resilience scale. Results were that these individuals coped successfully by developing an attitude of personal responsibility to accept new life conditions, take charge of their own well-being, seek and accept support, maximize independence and normality, and focus on the positive. In addition, these respondents shared resilient characteristics such as self-efficacy and perseverance.

1. How do the results of these studies apply to the concept of health as presented in this chapter?

2. Can you identify ways in which the methods and findings could be applied to other populations?

 Go to Chapter 10, **Toward Evidence-Based Practice Suggested Responses,** on the Student Resource Disk or DavisPlus at http://davisplus.fadavis.com/Wilkinson2

Practical **Knowledge** knowing *how*

In the preceding section, you have learned how people experience health, wellness, and illness. In this section, we look at how this information can be applied to your nursing practice.

Using the Nursing Process to Promote Health

Throughout this textbook, you will learn to use the nursing process to help clients deal with a variety of health problems. But how does the nursing process relate to the broader aspects of health and illness described in this chapter? Overall, it involves helping clients—regardless of the type of health problem—to look within themselves to develop creative ways to deal with the realities they are facing.

Patients may fail to comply with a proposed healthcare regimen if healthcare providers develop a plan of care that has no cultural or personal relevance for the patient (or family). Perhaps the plan does not consider the knowledge level of the patient or caregiver; or perhaps it is not feasible in terms of available support, time, energy, finances, or location. Patients may leave a hospital setting against medical advice (AMA), thereby endangering their chances of recovery. They may believe that the treatment offered them will not help or that the illness is preferable to the proposed treatment.

Remember that people probably do not refuse to carry out a plan of care simply out of stubbornness, hostility toward healthcare providers, or wanton disregard

for their own welfare. The challenge for nurses is to develop an individualized plan of care in collaboration with patients, based on mutual goals and respect.

◼ ASSESSMENT

In looking at an individual's health status, it is easy to focus on the measurable aspects. Physical needs obviously are crucial, but competing issues may be present and cause the client to view the therapeutic interventions as irrelevant or even disruptive. Obtaining data about the psychosocial, emotional, and spiritual aspects of health requires a level of communication that goes beyond a neat list of skills. Communicating genuine care, concern, and sensitivity comes from who you are as a person, not from assuming a professional persona (putting on your "nurse's hat").

- **Settling in.** Your initial approach to a patient creates a climate that determines the level of communication that takes place. The patient is probably in a new environment, and your tone, words, and facial expressions can bring comfort and ease. Nurses can be in new situations too, and taking a few moments to settle in to the situation can be helpful in facilitating communication.
- **Attuning.** Being maximally attentive is another key factor in facilitating communication. Most people are hungry for someone to listen to them. So often, listeners are so busy thinking about what they want to say that they fail to really listen. Try to focus on what the patient or family has to say instead of thinking ahead to what you want to ask next.
- **Acceptance.** Another vital aspect of communicating is acceptance—acceptance of appearance, lifestyles, ways

of coping, and values. You might ask, "How can I be accepting when there are aspects of this person that go against my entire value system?" Accepting is not the same as "agreeing with." You can accept people as valued, creative, unique individuals, despite their differences from your own ways of being. This view of acceptance does not mean that people will not be held accountable for their actions, for example, in cases of domestic violence and child abuse. It does mean, though, that in your role as a caregiver, you must convey an attitude of accepting the intrinsic value of life—in whatever form that life takes.

■ **Enjoying.** Perhaps even more difficult than accepting is enjoying. You will come into contact with a wide array of individuals, many of whom are different from people you have grown up around and have come to know and enjoy. A challenge for you is to broaden the repertoire of people you enjoy: to see and enjoy commonalities among individuals seemingly so different and to recognize and appreciate the pathos of suffering, in whatever form it takes.

Settling in, attuning, respecting, and enjoying—certainly this is not a step-by-step process, but each is vital to creating a climate for the openness and communication needed for assessment. You might argue that the healthcare environment does not allow time for such a high level of attentiveness. Consider, though, how much time is spent in delivering nursing care. As a full-spectrum nurse, you will assess patients continually during the delivery of all this care. In fact, the physical contact involved in carrying out nursing procedures seems to break down barriers of communication. Nurses hold a unique opportunity in "being with" individuals during difficult life situations; indeed, Benner and Wrubel (1989) state that expert nurses call this the "privileged place of nursing" (p. xi).

One way to approach assessment, whether in outpatient, acute care, long-term care, or home settings, is to ask the patient, "What is the biggest concern you are dealing with today?" You may have a plan of care that addresses areas that you know to be important, but it may fall far short of meeting your patient's needs if you have not addressed the concern that is fundamental to your patient.

In addition to communicating, developing your observation skills will enable you to assess your patients more fully. Watching your patient's responses to you and your care; observing the presence or absence of visitors and the effect on your patients; and observing signs of religious or cultural practices that have significance all provide important information about your patient's strengths and needs.

■ ANALYSIS/NURSING DIAGNOSIS

Several of the nursing diagnosis labels identified by NANDA International relate to health issues discussed in this chapter. Some examples are Anxiety, Caregiver Role Strain, Deficient Knowledge, and Spiritual Distress. An analysis of the assessment data that you gather should also provide the information needed to describe related causal factors, such as Spiritual Distress related to fear of impending death or Situational Low Self-esteem related to loss of job secondary to frequent absences for chemotherapy.

KnowledgeCheck 10-4

Compare and contrast attuning, acceptance, and enjoying.

 Go to Chapter 10, **Knowledge Check Response Sheet and Answers,** on the Student Resource Disk or DavisPlus at http://davisplus.fadavis.com/Wilkinson2

■ PLANNING OUTCOMES/EVALUATION

Goals and outcomes should be both realistic and valued by the patient and family. When you set goals in the broader dimension of health and illness (as in this chapter), it is much harder to be specific in describing expected outcomes and time frames. As a nurse, your role is to help the patient (or family member) envision acceptable outcomes and to set smaller, realistic goals so that the patient recognizes progress. For example, an older woman caring for a spouse with Alzheimer's disease may have a nursing diagnosis of Caregiver Role Strain related to care of spouse with dementia. Together you would establish acceptable goals and break them down into realistic steps. You also would identify outcomes to indicate that the caregiver actually experiences a reduction in strain, such as being able to sleep or having time to pursue meaningful activities.

■ PLANNING INTERVENTIONS/IMPLEMENTATION

The ideal approach is to draw on patient and family strengths to help achieve the desired outcomes. In the preceding example of the older adult caregiver, you would discuss with her the options available to provide support, but she would identify which options were acceptable to her and her spouse. In the heat of the moment, patients and families may not recognize the strengths and creative abilities that they bring to a situation. Part of the art of nursing is to envision strengths and potential in patients and families, just as an artful teacher might recognize a "spark" in a child and encourage that child to learn and grow.

CriticalThinking 10-5

■ How can you use the concepts of health when you are admitting a patient to a hospital setting? To a clinic? To an emergency department? To a rehabilitation or long-term care setting? In initiating home care?

■ What questions can you ask or what observations can you make to help you gain information about individuals' health strategies, disruptions to health, and factors contributing to their responses to disruptions?

- How would you consider health concepts in planning for patients' discharge from healthcare settings?

How Can I Honor Each Client's Unique Health/Illness Experience?

Choosing nursing as a profession means choosing to be an instrument of healing in a hurtful world. However, being an instrument of healing does not come automatically with the title of nurse. Nor does it allow you the luxury of learning just one approach and applying it to every client. It means cultivating a healing presence by listening, being maximally attentive, being aware of your own gifts and limitations of communication, being willing to learn from those in your care, recognizing and respecting others' ways of coping, and enjoying others for who they are.

Nursing care demands a high level of theoretical knowledge: of physiological, psychological, and social principles, as well as savvy knowledge of highly technical equipment. Patients may be impressed, even amazed, by the healthcare technology used to diagnose and treat their illnesses. However, what they most often remember, perhaps through the rest of their lives, is that person who connected with them in a very special way. One man, quadriplegic for 26 years following a car accident in his teens, spoke of a senior nursing student who cared for him during his initial hospitalization. He said that after 26 years, he not only still remembered her, but also still could sense the warmth of her caring presence.

During times of vulnerability, people seem acutely attuned to those who are helpful to them and also to those who slight them in hurtful ways, whether intentionally or not. What a challenge for nurses this makes! In this section, we discuss steps you can take to prepare yourself for responding to your clients in ways that are meaningful and healing to them.

Examine Life's Uncertainties

Wellness is a balancing act between living in the mostly known present and the mostly unknown future. Encourage your clients to make active decisions that positively affect their future. You do not have control over a drunk driver who sails across the median and hits you head on, but you do have control over getting the brakes on your car fixed or wearing your seat belt. Likewise, you do not know whether you will develop cancer or heart disease, but you can take responsibility for learning and practicing prevention and detection of problems.

Making health-promoting lifestyle choices is important, but it cannot protect us from risk. Significant life experiences, such as getting married, having children, investing in friendships, venturing into business, and selecting a profession all involve risk. Making a commitment to *anything* is a risk. Each person has a different "risk-comfort range." Some are willing to risk little, have fewer disappointments, and less sparkling achievements.

Their lives may not glitter, but they may be enjoyable. To others, security is not as important, and they are comfortable taking greater risks.

In *A Severe Mercy*, Sheldon Vanauken (1977) writes about finding and losing a great love. He reasons: "The joy would be worth the pain—if, indeed, they went together. If there were a choice . . . between, on the one hand, the heights and the depths and, on the other hand, some sort of safe, cautious middle way, he, for one, here and now chose the heights and the depths" (p. 9). He did, indeed, find a great love, and when he lost his wife at an early age, he was able to accept their time together as one of his life's greatest blessings. As a nurse, you will face many uncertainties and dilemmas. You will certainly face new experiences and challenges, situations you thought *you* never would have to deal with. You will observe pain, suffering, and death. You may never understand the apparent unfairness of it all. But often life brings new meaning when it takes a different direction from the one planned. For example, a teen whose spinal cord was severed in a motor vehicle accident begins to speak at high schools about the dangers of drinking and driving. Or a couple formerly embittered over their third miscarriage finds joy in adopting two children with disabilities.

As a nurse, you will also be privileged to witness many joys. Some might even qualify as minor triumphs: a patient taking his first steps after major surgery, a pathology report that isn't as bad as feared, or even a peaceful death that brings closure to a grieving family. As you move from novice to expert, you may find that such witnessing causes you to stop questioning life's uncertainties and instead to start treasuring them.

 CriticalThinking 10-6

- What uncertainties have you struggled with?
- What approaches have proven effective for you in dealing with uncertainties?

Envision Wellness for Your Clients and Yourself

Wherever there is a dream, there is someone there to tell you it can't be done, or at least not by you. There is something to be said, however, for "envisioning" wellness for your clients and yourself. Remember Evelyn ("Meet Your Patient")? If her nurses had labeled her as debilitated and close to death, how would that have affected her? In contrast, their acceptance of her vision of herself as well and full of life supports her and aids her healing. In the same way, think of how you view your own health. Is the life you envision for yourself characterized by zest and vigor? What are your family relationships like? What are your values? Does your work give meaning and purpose to your life? The wellness that you envision for yourself can be the blueprint for what you want to become. The skeptic in you might say, "What if I do everything that I know to do to maintain a healthy life and still have a heart attack at 45?" As we have seen, life is full of uncertainties. That does not mean that you have to stop envisioning. Instead, use *flexible envisioning*, adjusting your goals and dreams to each new reality. Health does not mean always getting your first choice. Part of health is being able to dream a new dream, starting over if you need to, but always envisioning that there is something worth striving for.

Establish Trust at Your First Patient Contact

When patients are admitted to a hospital or ambulatory care facility, you will need to support them in their transition from wellness to illness, in dealing with the unknown, and in adjusting to a new environment. The relationship and trust you establish in your first contact with patients can go a long way toward relieving their anxiety and preserving the energy needed for healing. You can make the transition smoother for them if you are prepared. The following activities should be incorporated into your nursing care.

■ *Prepare the room.* A room that is prepared for the client conveys a message of acceptance. Room preparation depends on the type of unit or facility, the client's needs, and the anticipated treatment.

 Go to Chapter 10, **Clinical Insight 10-1: Preparing the Room for an Admission,** in Volume 2.

■ *Greet the client.* Gather basic information ahead of time, such as name, diagnosis, and anticipated length of stay. Imagine how it might feel if you arrived on a gurney for admission and you heard the staff say, "Who's this? I didn't know we were getting an admission. How am I supposed to take care of this one, too?"
■ *Introduce yourself to the client and family.* Explain who you are. Don't be afraid to tell a client that you are a nursing student. Many clients are aware that students have more time to spend with them.
■ *Orient the client to the room and the unit.* Make sure the client knows how to use the bed, the call light, and any equipment that you expect him to use. Show the client the location of the restroom. If you will be measuring the client's intake and output, tell him so during your orientation. If the client is alert, he may be able to assist you with these measures. Remember that one of the disruptions associated with illness is anxiety about the unknown. If you tell your client what to expect, you help to minimize his anxiety.
■ *Gather a health history.* In Chapter 3, you learned about assessment. Chapter 19 provides a step-by-step approach to physical assessment. Be sure to include in your health history the client's expectations and concerns.
■ *Establish a relationship with the client.* Take time to get to know your client. Try to set a tone of caring, respect, and understanding.
For detailed directions on how to admit a client to a hospital unit,

Go to Chapter 10, **Procedure 10-1: Admitting a Patient to a Nursing Unit,** in Volume 2.

The Critical Aspects box provides the highlights of this procedure.

Provide a Healing Presence

Part of what you do as a healing presence will never show up in a written care plan. However, your healing presence may be the most important aspect of care that you have to offer. A statement by a young woman undergoing chemotherapy illustrates the difference the healing presence of a nurse made:

> *The nursing care I got was in response to the physical symptoms I showed. If I was not feeling good, they were sympathetic with me, you know. If I was feeling good, they were cheerful with me, and things like that. But it was nothing further than that. There was no exploration of feelings or anything like that.*
>
> *Some of them were—seemed to be very caring. I remember [one nurse] . . . but she was just a really nice person. And I remember one time that I was throwing up dreadfully for some reason. . . . I rang for her and I said, 'I'm sorry,' and she was almost crying and she said, 'No, I'm sorry you have to do this—you must feel awful.' And she was just very empathetic with it, and I felt like, you know, I wasn't infringing upon her to make her empty my emesis basin or anything like that (Smith, 1992, pp. 233–234).*

Maintain Trust During Transitions

Just as you help patients transition into illness, your support is important in helping them transition to other units within the agency, other agencies, or home. As discussed in Chapter 5, planning for discharge begins with the admission assessment and continues until the patient is well enough to go home or is transferred to another unit or facility.

Handoffs and Transfers. Patients may transfer from one unit to another when their health status changes. For example, a patient on a general nursing unit may be transferred to an intensive care unit when he develops sepsis (a generalized, systemic infection that is often fatal). Patients may transfer from hospital to a long-term care facility or rehabilitation center when they no longer require an acute care hospital. Or a patient in a long-term care facility may be transferred to a hospital when he becomes acutely ill.

When the patient is transferred, he must adjust to a new environment, new routines, and new caregivers. Transfer to a long-term care facility may be necessary because the patient's changed health status means that family members will not be able to care for him at home. This is yet another disruption for the patient and family. You can help by ensuring the transition is smooth and that there is continuity of care. Ensure the patient's comfort and safety, provide for teaching needs, and communicate with the agency or unit sending or receiving

VOL 2 For steps to follow in *all* procedures, refer to the inside back cover of Volume 2. Go to the full procedures in Volume 2 to practice and learn the procedure steps. Use these Critical Aspects later to help you review key points.

Procedure 10-1 Admitting a Patient to a Nursing Unit

➤ Begin the admission: Introduce yourself, assist the patient into a hospital gown, weigh, assist him into the bed.

➤ Validate patient identity.

➤ Obtain a translator if needed.

➤ Complete the nursing assessment, including vital signs and validating the admission list of medications.

➤ Provide information: Room, equipment, routines, Health Insurance Portability and Accountability Act (HIPAA), nurse call system, and advance directives.

➤ Answer any questions; provide printed information.

➤ Complete nursing admission paperwork according to agency policy.

➤ Complete or ensure that admission orders have been completed.

➤ Inventory patient's belongings; send home or lock up valuables.

➤ Finish the admission:

  ➤ Ensure patient comfort (water, positioning, pain).

  ➤ Make one last safety check: Call light, bed position, siderails.

  ➤ Ask: "Is there anything else I can do for you?"

Procedure 10-2 Transferring a Patient to Another Unit in the Agency

➤ Make a final, brief focused assessment.

➤ Plan ahead the amount of help needed.

➤ Schedule time of the transfer.

➤ Make appropriate notifications.

➤ Gather and label patient medications.

➤ Gather the patient's belongings, supplies, and treatment equipment.

➤ Bring the transfer vehicle to the bedside.

➤ Transfer the patient to the new room.

➤ Give oral handoff report and make final nurse's notes entry.

Procedure 10-3 Transferring a Patient to a Long-Term Care Facility

➤ Plan in advance: Notify the patient and family of the impending transfer.

➤ Prepare the patient's records; copy for the new facility if needed.

➤ Pack personal items and treatment supplies.

➤ Coordinate the transfer with the receiving facility and other hospital departments.

➤ Make the final assessment; document and sign.

➤ Move the patient to the transportation vehicle.

➤ Give an oral or telephone report to the receiving nurse; use a standardized form if available.

➤ Notify the long-term care facility if patient is colonized or infected with methicillin-resistant *Staphylococcus aureus* (MRSA) or other contagious microorganisms.

Procedure 10-4 Discharging a Patient from the Healthcare Facility

➤ *Notify the patient and family* well in advance of the discharge.

➤ A day or two before discharge:

  Arrange for or confirm: Transportation and services and equipment needed at home.

  Make referrals.

  Provide teaching about the patient's condition.

  Provide training in use of equipment.

  Ask the caregiver to bring clothing for the patient to wear home.

➤ Day of discharge

  Make and document final assessments.

  Confirm that the patient has house keys, heat is turned on, and food is available.

  Make final notifications (community agencies, transportation).

  Gather and pack the patient's personal items and treatment supplies.

  Label and give take-home medications to the patient.

  Give the patient prescriptions, instruction sheets, appointment cards, and printed discharge instructions.

  Review discharge instructions with the patient.

  Answer questions.

  Document the final nursing note and complete discharge summary.

  Accompany the patient out of the hospital.

  Notify Admissions of the discharge.

  Ensure records are sent to the medical records department.

---

the patient. The process at time of transfer is similar. For information on transfer reports, see Chapter 16. Also refer to the accompanying Critical Aspects box and,

Go to **Procedure 10-2, Transferring a Patient Within the Hospital and Procedure 10-3, Transferring a Patient to a Long-Term Care Facility,** in Volume 2.

Discharge from the Healthcare Facility. As much as patients usually look forward to being discharged, this, too, is a disruption. Patients are discharged when the outcomes of care are met. However, they are often dependent on family members for care and treatments they cannot manage alone. Inability to assume self-care can be stressful and anxiety producing. Successful discharge planning must begin at first patient assessment, on admission to the facility. The same conditions that require a formal discharge plan frequently also indicate the need for referrals for posthospital care in the community. Review "Discharge Planning" in Chapter 5, as needed.

Procedures for discharge vary among agencies. There may be a discharge planner or case manager to coordinate the transition to another agency or to home, but often you will need to manage the discharge. You can help by communicating and coordinating care and services, and by teaching the patient and caregivers about the continuing care the patient needs. For more information, see the accompanying Critical Aspects Box and,

 Go to **Procedure 10-4, Discharging a Patient from the Healthcare Facility,** in Volume 2.

KnowledgeCheck 10-5

Explain how you can promote patient trust during admissions, transfers, and discharges.

 Go to Chapter 10, **Knowledge Check Response Sheet and Answers,** on the Student Resource Disk or DavisPlus at http://davisplus.fadavis.com/Wilkinson2

Is a Healthy Life Attainable?

The themes suggested in this chapter as ways to live a healthy life did not come from people who had easy lives. These themes were teased from literature, autobiographies, and interviews with people who were dealing with life situations that would be viewed as difficult from anyone's standpoint. However, in the midst of their circumstances, they were very much involved in *living*. Ripples or even waves of disruption or despair came into their lives, but through it all they evolved an overriding sense of life worth pursuing. This can be true for you as a nurse and also for those privileged to be under your care.

As a nurse, you offer your personal health and strength to your patients and their families every day. If you barely have enough physical, emotional, and spiritual strength to manage your own stressors, you will not have much available to offer others who are depleted. This is why it is so important for you to nurture yourself in all aspects of your life, to balance learning how to care for others with caring for yourself, to develop yourself as a healing presence in this world.

 Go to Chapter 10, **Resources for Caregivers and Health Professionals,** on the Student Resource Disk or DavisPlus at http://davisplus.fadavis.com/Wilkinson2

 Suggested Readings: Go to Chapter 10, **Reading More About Experiencing Health and Illness,** on the Student Resource Disk or DavisPlus at http://davisplus.fadavis.com/Wilkinson2

 Bibliography: Go to Volume 2, Bibliography.

CHAPTER 11

Psychosocial Health & Illness

Learning Outcomes

After completing this chapter, you should be able to:

➤ Explain the relationship of psychosocial factors to overall health and development.

➤ Identify the factors that influence the development and stability of self-concept.

➤ List the four interrelated components of self-concept.

➤ Identify ten general categories to include in a comprehensive psychosocial assessment.

➤ Perform an assessment using the domains of self-concept, self-esteem, self-identity, and body image.

➤ Develop a nursing care plan for patients exhibiting disturbances in self-concept and self-esteem.

➤ Identify nursing diagnoses, outcomes, and interventions specific to body image disturbance.

➤ Describe interventions for preventing depersonalization.

➤ Describe the anxiety continuum.

➤ List the psychological and physiological effects of anxiety.

➤ Recognize the levels and symptoms of anxiety that are severe enough to merit referral to a mental health professional.

➤ Devise a nursing care plan for the nursing diagnosis of Anxiety.

➤ Identify several ways in which clients manifest depression.

➤ Differentiate between mild depression and that which should be referred to a mental health professional.

➤ Assess older adults for manifestations of depression.

➤ Plan outcomes and nursing interventions for patients who are depressed.

➤ Plan outcomes and nursing interventions for patients with a diagnosis of Risk for Suicide.

Meet Your Patient

You are caring for a 16-year-old patient named Karli who is suffering from fractures to both arms and several ribs, as well as extensive first- and second-degree burns to 30% of her body, following a motor vehicle accident. Karli was driving her parents' car home from her part-time job when she lost control of the car and crashed into a wall. The car exploded in flames. A passerby quickly reported the accident, and fast action by the emergency response team saved Karli's life.

Karli is suffering from a moderate amount of shock and pain. She alternates among outbursts of anger, self-directed sarcasm, and despondence. She tells you that she cannot understand how the accident happened, that one moment she was adjusting the car radio, and the next moment she

awoke in the hospital. Then suddenly she explodes. "It's not fair! I just took my eyes off the road for a second; that's all!" She bursts into tears. Picking at her bandages, she sobs, "No one will ever love me the way I'm going to look. My life is over. I hate myself! You take her hand. "I used to be pretty," she says, "but now I'll look like a freak! What did I do to deserve this? I know plenty of kids who drive drunk or high all the time. I wasn't doing anything wrong! Why did this happen to me?"

Before reading on, jot down a list of the multiple physical, psychological, and social issues that you would need to consider in developing a comprehensive care plan for Karli. You can revisit your list throughout this chapter to compare your answers.

CriticalThinking 11-1

- What theoretical knowledge about Karli's developmental stage will assist you in determining nursing diagnoses, interventions, and outcomes?
- Considering that Karli will need a significant amount of assistance for activities of daily living (ADLs) because of her fractures and burns, how might you use the time to develop your therapeutic relationship?

Theoretical **Knowledge** **knowing** why

This chapter introduces you to the concepts of psychosocial health, self-concept, anxiety, and depression. It is designed to help you provide basic psychosocial care for patients in general practice settings.

Psychosocial Health

Have you ever wondered why some health and life crises are easy to manage whereas others seem like the very last straw? The interactions of the mind and body are continuous and complex. One of the strengths of nursing is that we can go beyond a *biomedical* (disease-oriented) focus to care for the whole person. Nurses recognize that patient responses to illness are influenced not only by the physical pathology but also by the person's psychosocial health and its relationship to her overall wellness.

The term *psychosocial* encompasses both psychological and social factors: A person's psychological state interacts with his social development and position within society to contribute to his overall—or biopsychosocial—well-being (Fig. 11-1). Figure 11-2 illustrates the interlocking psychosocial influences on health and personal development.

Keep in mind that any human dimension may dominate health needs at a given time. For example, a patient suffering from a severe flare-up of psoriasis (a skin disease characterized by red, scaly patches) may require physiological interventions during the acute stage. He may not be ready to deal with body image issues (psychological dimension) until his skin lesions are better. Remember, though, that your patients' psychosocial needs are just as important as, for example, their dietary requirements or their level of pain.

What Is Psychosocial Theory?

You can think of **psychosocial theory** as a method of understanding people as a combination of psychological and social events. Of the many theories of

FIGURE 11-1 In the biopsychosocial view of health, biological, psychological, social, and spiritual factors interact to contribute to health.

FIGURE 11-2 Interlocking psychosocial influences.

psychosocial development, the works of the German psychologist Erik Erikson (1902–1994) are foremost. Using Erikson's theory, you can assess for successful completion of developmental tasks. Refer to Chapter 9 for more information about Erikson's theory. For a summary of developmental tasks,

 Go to Chapter 11, **Tables, Boxes, Figures: ESG Table 11-1,** on the Student Resource Disk or DavisPlus at http:// davisplus.fadavis.com/Wilkinson2

Chapter 8 presents another important psychosocial theory that is relevant for healthcare providers: psychologist Abraham Maslow's theory of self-actualization and self-transcendence. Maslow (1968) developed a widely accepted hierarchy of human needs and motivations, in which essential needs (e.g., air, water, and food)

must be met before higher needs (e.g., learning, creating, understanding, and self-fulfillment). Recall that, in order from most basic to highest need, Maslow's hierarchy includes physiological, safety and security, love and belonging, self-esteem, and self-actualization needs. For more information about psychosocial theories,

 Go to Chapter 11, **Supplemental Materials: Psychosocial Theory,** on the Student Resource Disk or DavisPlus at http://davisplus.fadavis.com/Wilkinson2

KnowledgeCheck 11-1

- Why is psychosocial theory relevant to healthcare?
- What does the term *biopsychosocial* mean?
- Explain the implication of Maslow's hierarchy of human needs for working with a homeless man with gangrene.

 Go to Chapter 11, **Knowledge Check Response Sheet and Answers,** on the Student Resource Disk or DavisPlus at http://davisplus.fadavis.com/Wilkinson2

What Is Self-Concept?

A critical aspect of psychosocial health is self-concept, that is, one's overall view of oneself. **Self-concept** is your complete and unique answer to the question, "Who do you think you are?" (e.g., "I am a student"; "I am successful and competent"). Self-concept forms out of a person's evaluation of his physical appearance, sexual performance, intellectual abilities, success in the workplace, friendship and approval from others, problem-solving and coping abilities, unique talents, and so on. A person with a healthy self-concept has a mostly positive perception of these evaluations of self.

Self-concept both influences and is influenced by social functioning. For example, if it continues, Karli's perception that she is no longer pretty and that she "looks like a freak" (her self-concept) may cause her to withdraw from social interaction and make it difficult to form new relationships (social functioning). Equally, if others—for example, prospective employers—*do* see her as hideously ugly, she may have difficulty finding a place in society.

The "Dynamic Self"

Throughout the ages, mystics, philosophers, anthropologists, and psychologists have observed that the self forms and changes in response to our environment. Thousands of years ago, spiritual texts such as the Hindu *Bhagavad Gita* (or *Song of God*) distinguished between a higher Self, seen as eternal and unchanging, and a lower self that is constantly changing as old ideas are discarded "like worn-out clothes." Centuries later, the Roman Catholic concepts of the soul and body would also reflect this theme.

Anthropologist Margaret Mead (1934) states that we discover who we are through a lifelong process of differentiating from and comparing our self to others.

As we experience life events, we continually reconstruct and develop an understanding of our self. Dickstein (1977) called this idea the **dynamic self,** meaning that who we are (the self) is subject to change through social and environmental influence.

If our concept or our self is changeable, how does it first develop? What factors cause it to change? Can it be harmed, and how? These questions are explored next.

How Is Self-Concept Formed?

Humans are not born with a concept of self; rather, it develops during infancy and childhood as the child interacts with family members, peers, and others. The broad steps of self-concept formation are as follows:

Infant—Learning that the physical self is different from the environment: "me; not me"

Child—Internalizing others' attitudes about the self, primarily parents and peers: "Who do *they* say that I am?"

Child and adult—Internalizing standards of society: "How do I compare to others?"

Adult—Self-actualization and self-adjustment: "This *is* who I am and who I will continue to be."

Change occurs gradually, and the steps overlap. Also, the age at which the stages occur varies widely among individuals. For a summary of the growth of self-concept through the various developmental stages,

 Go to Chapter 11, **Tables, Boxes, Figures: ESG Table 11-2,** on the Student Resource Disk or DavisPlus at http://davisplus.fadavis.com/Wilkinson2

 Critical**Thinking** 11-2

- Explain how each of Maslow's five basic needs is related to psychosocial development; that is, how might each of the needs affect psychosocial health if met or not met?
- To what extent do social relationships help or hinder a person in meeting each need?

What Factors Affect a Person's Self-Concept?

Some factors affecting a person's self-concept cannot be changed, for example, gender and developmental level. Others, such as socioeconomic status and family relationships, can be changed to a degree, but are not fully under the person's control—and certainly not during childhood, when the self-concept is forming. Understanding that such factors are not within a patient's control may help you provide more sensitive, compassionate care to patients experiencing impaired self concept.

Gender

Certain aspects of self-concept differ by gender. Some of the differences appear to be related to the role expectations of boys and girls rather than any actual difference in ability:

Girls typically rate teamwork and cooperation as important to their sense of self, whereas most boys place a higher value on individual achievement.

In elementary and high school, boys have a higher self-concept for mathematical and physical dimensions, and girls have a higher self-concept for verbal and social skills (Bracken, 1996; Hattie, 1992). This does not necessarily mean that their abilities are different, but that their perceptions of their abilities differ.

Physical appearance seems more important to girls, and they may be less satisfied and more self-conscious throughout life because of this.

As role expectations and career choices for both men and women expand, these gender-based differences in self-concept may fade.

Developmental Level

As we mature, our self-concept becomes more inner-guided. That is, others (e.g., friends, the media) have less influence on our ideas about who we are. We become less likely to view our failures and shortcomings as evidence of worthlessness and more likely to see them as challenges common to humans everywhere. A few weeks before his death from a degenerative neurological disease, sociologist Morrie Schwartz reminded his friend Mitch, "We all have the same beginning—birth—and we all have the same end—death. So how different can we be?" (Albom, 1997).

Family and Peer Relationships

The family strongly influences a child's developing self-concept. As an infant's sense of self permanence develops and becomes stable, categories of self begin to emerge (Feiring & Taska, as cited in Bracken, 1996). These include notions of gender, values, and a sense of having a distinct "place" among family members. Self-identity develops as children become familiar with those who consistently interact with them. Social identity is first fostered by interactions between infants and their parents and broadens in toddlerhood through relationships with siblings, grandparents, and extended family members. For older children, peers become more important than family in this respect.

Internal Influences

Whereas the preceding external influences contribute to the *formation* of our self-concept, internal influences help us to *moderate* it. For example, biochemical brain processes influence perceptual acuity, interpretation abilities, and level of insight and judgment.

People who allow their inner "voice" to influence their self-concept have what is called an **internal locus of control**. Such people feel they can exert control over their lives. They take appropriate responsibility for their life experiences and for their responses to them. This enables them to interpret unexpected adverse events

(e.g., injuries and illnesses) in a more positive light. For example, consider a new mother who wanted a natural birth but consented to an emergency cesarean. With an internal locus of control, she might say, "Well, I wanted a natural birth like my sister and my best friend had, but when the nurse midwife told me that my baby wasn't breathing right, the type of birth suddenly didn't seem important. I chose a cesarean, and now I have a beautiful, healthy baby. That's what really matters."

In contrast, when people have an **external locus of control,** they attribute control of their situation to external factors, including other people, institutions, and God. Given the same set of circumstances, a mother with an external locus of control might report: "I wanted a natural birth, but I knew as soon as I walked into the hospital I'd be forced to do things their way. Sure enough, the nurse midwife told me that I had to have a cesarean."

KnowledgeCheck 11-2

- When does self concept become stable?
- What factors have been determined to have an impact on our self concept?

 Go to Chapter 11, **Knowledge Check Response Sheet and Answers,** on the Student Resource Disk or DavisPlus at http://davisplus.fadavis.com/Wilkinson2

What Are the Components of Self-Concept?

Self-concept embraces four interrelated components: body image, role performance, personal identity, and self-esteem.

Body Image

How often do you hear someone say something like the following?

"Look at the muscles on that man. He looks good!"
"Look at her pigging out. She needs that candy like I need a hole in my head."

As a child, you probably grew up overhearing similar statements. Such preoccupations with food, weight, and appearance have led to a prejudice against people who do not have perfect bodies. No wonder that people engage in unhealthy behaviors in order to be thin or that patients like Karli have difficulty coping with disfiguring accidents or with surgeries such as limb amputation and mastectomy.

Body image is your mental image of your physical self, including physical appearance and physical functioning. Both cognitive understanding and sensory input influence body image. For instance, if you understand that darkly tanned skin can indicate harmful exposure to the sun, then you might perceive your own untanned skin as positive, despite media messages to the contrary. Our cognitive understanding is in turn influenced by family, social, ethnic, and cultural norms; education; and exposure to alternative values. The American media portray the ideal male as young, tall, and muscular; nevertheless, many older, short, slender men maintain a positive body image because their cognitive understanding indicates they are in good health, are attractive to their partners, and so on.

Ideal, Perceived, and Actual Body Image. People do not always see their own bodies as objectively as others see them. Some psychological disorders interfere with the ability to interpret sensory data objectively. For example, people with the eating disorders anorexia nervosa and bulimia nervosa see themselves as fat even when their mirror reflects, and other people see, a normal or even an emaciated body. The closer the match between a person's ideal body image and sensory input about his or her body (perceived body image), the more positive the person's body image is likely to be.

For Janalee, thick, luxurious hair is an important component of her ideal body image. Amy hardly thinks about her hair at all; she keeps it very short so that it is easy to care for. Both women have been receiving chemotherapy to treat their cancer, and both are experiencing severe hair loss. Which person do you think will be more likely to experience body image disturbance because of this?

Appearance and Function Influence Body Image. Not surprisingly, a physical disability, such as blindness, deafness, or paraplegia, can interfere with the development of a positive body image. Children born with a physical disability have a high incidence of poor self-concept and depression. This is partially due to social values and the child's inability to form adequate social relationships, but it may also relate to the person's perception that he has low social value. In contrast, an attractive appearance and superior functioning, whether in a career, sports, or academics, contribute to a positive body image. But again, cognitive understanding can increase self-concept even in people who are average in appearance or achievement. For instance, people of average appearance who learn to value integrity, honesty, teamwork, and other social values more than physical attractiveness or success in sports are less likely to suffer from body image disturbance.

Gradual Versus Sudden Body Changes. Gradual changes in physical appearance occur naturally throughout life as the body matures and grows old. Most people adapt to such changes relatively easily, especially because their friends and colleagues are aging, too. In contrast, when changes in appearance or functioning occur abruptly (e.g., following an acute illness or an accident, as happened to your patient, Karli), they are much more difficult to accept. Denial, anger, self-hatred, and despair are a few of many reactions that can follow such an abrupt change in body image. In *Still Me,* actor Christopher Reeve describes the "demons" that haunted him in the first weeks after his cervical spinal cord injury.

"I'd try to go back to sleep, but it wouldn't work, and I'd start to think again, the same tormenting thoughts. It always began with: This can't be me. . . ." (Reeve, 1998).

Body Image Influences Health. Body image influences health and health behaviors. A negative body image has been associated with:

- Depression (McCabe, Ricciardelli, Sitaram, et al., 2006)
- Initiation of smoking among adolescents (Clark, Croghan, Reading, et al., 2005; Stice & Shaw, 2003)
- Increased risk for unintended pregnancy and sexually transmitted infections, including HIV infection (Wingood, DiClemente, Harrington, et al., 2002).

In contrast, a positive body image was found to be a major contributor to overall life happiness in adult women (Stokes & Frederick-Recascino, 2003). There is not yet enough evidence to determine how much of the effect is due to body image alone and how much to body image in combination with other psychosocial issues.

Role Performance

Before you began your nursing program, what were your expectations? What activities did you imagine yourself engaged in, and what behaviors did you think would be expected of you? Together, these expectations make up your conception of the *role* of nursing student. In addition to being a student, you probably play several roles, such as parent, sibling, friend, breadwinner, caregiver, volunteer, and so on.

Role performance can be defined as the actions a person takes and the behaviors he demonstrates in fulfilling a role. Instead of expectations, role performance is the reality. If you expected that you would sail through your nursing program and instead you find yourself so overwhelmed that lately you have begun to skip classes, then you are experiencing **role strain,** a mismatch between role expectations and role performance. In addition, your ideas about how to perform the nursing student role may be very different from those of your instructors. When such a mismatch occurs, you are experiencing an **interpersonal role conflict.** Other types of role conflict are also common. For instance, what if you are a single parent and your child's sudden illness causes you to miss a week of classes and clinicals? When two roles make competing demands on an individual, **interrole conflict** occurs.

Personal Identity

How would you describe yourself to others? Make a list of 10 words or short phrases that describe who you are (e.g., student, motorcycle rider, woman). Then list them in order, with the most important one first. Are you happy with your list? Are you satisfied with who you are? Compare your list with a friend's list. Could you identify her based on her list of identifying labels? Could she identify you?

Your **personal identity** is your view of yourself as a unique human being, different and separate from all others. Identity develops over time, beginning in childhood when you identified with your parents, and then later with teachers, peers, and others. Unlike body image, which is expected to change over time, personal identity is relatively constant and consistent. It is culturally determined and learned through socialization.

People with a strong sense of personal identity are less likely to compare themselves to others or to be unduly influenced by them. They tend to appreciate the unique perspective and contributions of others, yet value their own perspectives and contributions. In contrast, people with a weak sense of personal identity have difficulty distinguishing their boundaries from those of others. They may interpret events in the environment personally, or they may interpret their personal experiences as belonging to everyone. For example, a patient with a weak personal identity may insist that a breakdown in the hospital's air conditioning system is a punishment for his complaint that his room was too cold.

Patients may experience an impaired sense of identity when they are challenged by a serious or chronic illness (e.g., cancer, AIDS, or rheumatoid arthritis). They then place too many limitations on their activities or interpret the responses of others in light of their illness. For instance, a woman with osteoporosis (loss of bone density) might say, "I used to enjoy going bird watching, but I don't go anymore because I might trip and fall."

 Critical**Thinking** 11-3

Think about Karli in the "Meet Your Patient" scenario. If you asked Karli to list 10 labels to identify herself, what do you think they would be? (You may not have enough information to come up with 10, but think of as many as you can.)

Self-Esteem

Self-esteem is, in the simplest terms, how well a person likes himself. It is the difference between the "ideal self" and "actual self," that is, between "what I think I ought (or want) to be" and "what I really am." The area of overlap in Figure 11-3 illustrates the extent of self-esteem. The more overlap, the higher the self-esteem.

The balance between our self-expectations and our true abilities can be precarious. When we succeed beyond our ambitions, we experience a high sense of self-esteem; but when we aim for an ideal self beyond our capabilities, we risk loss of self-esteem. For example, if as a nursing student you find that you are more successful than you expected to be when you enrolled in your nursing program, that is a boost to your self-esteem.

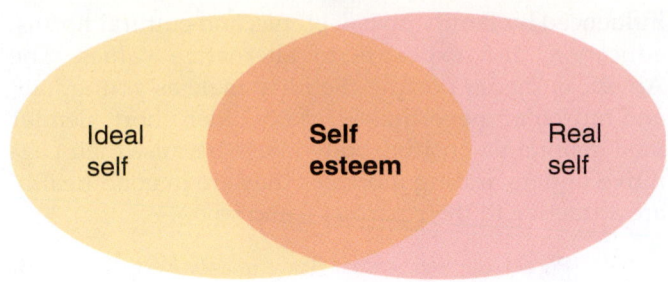

Ideal self: expectations and aspirations; "what I ought to be," "what I wish I were"

Real self: current skills, attributes, and successes; "what I really am"

FIGURE 11-3 Self-esteem is determined by the relationship between an individual's ideal self and real self.

If, however, your expectations of being a skillful nurse outweigh your current abilities, then lower self-esteem is likely.

It is not difficult to imagine how a sudden, disfiguring accident such as Karli's might provoke a crisis in self-esteem, but even mild illnesses and minor setbacks can cause some people to question their self-worth. This is especially true if the problem is interpreted as one incident in a continuing pattern. Consider, for instance, a couple hoping to become parents who experience a third pregnancy loss, or a man who aspires to be a full professor at a leading university who is laid off from his fourth teaching job at a community college.

 Critical**Thinking** 11-4

What if a person does not have any aspirations to success, but is content to meet each day as a learner, vitalized by her daily discoveries? How do you think a high score on an exam would affect her self-esteem? How do you think a poor score on a clinical skills test would affect her self-esteem?

Knowledge Check 11-3

- What four components contribute to an individual's self-concept?
- What is self-esteem?

 Go to Chapter 11, **Knowledge Check Response Sheet and Answers,** on the Student Resource Disk or DavisPlus at http://davisplus.fadavis.com/Wilkinson2

Psychosocial Illness: Anxiety and Depression

Think about the advertisements you've seen recently on TV or in newspapers and magazines. How many times do you recall seeing an ad for a medication for anxiety or depression? These two problems are not confined to mental health settings. They are woven into the fabric of our everyday lives. As a nurse, you should be prepared to recognize and provide care for anxious and depressed patients in all practice settings.

Anxiety

I wake up in the middle of the night with a knot in my stomach and thinking about work. I go over and over my day and worry about my decisions and what I should have done instead. I replay the meetings in my head and think, "I know what that person said, but what did she mean by that?" I wonder whether I can handle the responsibility. My neck and shoulders are so tense that I get headaches. But when I try to relax and watch TV, I can feel my heart racing, and I feel shaky. I can't concentrate well enough to read.

Anxiety is a common emotional response to a stressor. It is a "vague, uneasy feeling of discomfort or dread (the source often nonspecific or unknown to the individual) accompanied by an autonomic response; a feeling of apprehension caused by anticipation of danger. It is an alerting signal that warns of impending danger and enables the individual to take measures to deal with threat" (NANDA International, 2009 p. 242). An anxious person worries; feels nervous, uneasy, and fearful; may be tearful; and often has physical symptoms such as nausea, trembling, and sweating. Anxiety and fear produce similar responses; however, some experts differentiate them as follows:

Fear is a specific, cognitive response to a known threat. It is related to a present event, either physical *or* psychological.

Anxiety is a vague, emotional response to a known or unknown threat. It is related to anticipation of a future event and is the result of psychological conflict rather than physical threat.

Anxiety is one of the most common disturbances in psychosocial health. It is so common, in fact, that mild anxiety is considered normal and even necessary for our survival. No matter what area of nursing you work in, nearly every patient you meet will have at least some degree of anxiety. Chronic anxiety has been associated with physical problems, such as the risk of heart attack (Moser, 2007; Shen, Avivi, Todaro, et al., 2008).

Patients encounter anxiety-producing situations in healthcare settings because of threats to their basic needs (Stuart & Laraia, 2001). Consider the following examples:

- Physiological—anxiety in anticipation of or in response to a diagnosis of cancer
- Safety and security—an upcoming surgery or diagnostic test, such as cardiac catheterization
- Love and belonging—anxiety over potential or actual loss of a loved one
- Esteem—anxiety over potential or actual loss of ability or appearance
- Self-actualization—anxiety over lack of self-fulfillment

Levels of Anxiety

Anxiety ranges from normal to abnormal, depending on its **intensity** and **duration**—how much anxiety is present and how long it has been present. **Normal anxiety** is an essential reaction to a realistic danger or threat to our physical or psychological integrity. In other words, it enables us to survive and, when the threat is no longer present, to move on. For example, anxiety when hiking on a rocky and narrow mountain trail heightens your awareness and quickens your responses, thereby reducing the likelihood of falls. Once you make it to the top, the anxiety leaves, and you can relax and enjoy the view.

Abnormal anxiety is out of proportion to the situation and lasts long after the threat is over, perhaps causing the person to alter her lifestyle. For example, after breaking her ankle in a fall down a short flight of stairs, a young woman moves to a ground-floor apartment. Five years later, she still refuses to use stairs.

You should determine a patient's level of anxiety as accurately as possible because each requires different nursing actions. Peplau (1963) described the following four levels:

Mild Anxiety. This is normal anxiety, experienced in response to the events of day-to-day living. It heightens perception, sharpens the senses, enhances learning, and enables the person to function at his optimal level. Symptoms, if present, may include muscle tension, restlessness, irritability, and a sense of unease. The person rarely experiences it as distressful.

Moderate Anxiety. As anxiety increases, the perceptual field narrows, and the person begins to focus on self and the need to relieve his discomfort. He is less alert to environmental events, may distract easily, and may have a shorter attention span. He may need help with problem solving but can attend to his needs with direction. Physical symptoms may include increased heart and respiratory rate, increased perspiration, gastric discomfort, and increased muscle tension. The person may speak more rapidly, loudly, and at a higher pitch.

Severe Anxiety. At this level, the perceptual field is so narrow that the person can focus on only one particular detail or may shift focus to many extraneous details. Focus is totally on self and the need to relieve the anxiety. Concentration and attention span are severely limited, so the person has difficulty completing simple tasks. The anxiety prevents problem solving and learning. The person may report feelings of dread, confusion, and other unpleasant emotions. Physical symptoms may include headaches, palpitations, tachycardia, insomnia, dizziness, nausea, trembling, hyperventilation, urinary frequency, and diarrhea.

Panic Anxiety. The person becomes unreasonable and irrational and is unable to focus on even one detail in the environment. He may misperceive environmental cues or lose contact with reality (e.g., experience hallucinations or delusions). The person may react wildly (e.g., shouting, screaming, running about, clinging to something) or withdraw completely. At this level of anxiety, the person cannot function or communicate effectively (e.g., may speak incoherently or be unable to speak). He may feel terror and impending doom, believe he has a life-threatening illness, or that he is "going crazy." Physical symptoms include dilated pupils, labored breathing, severe trembling, sleeplessness, palpitations, diaphoresis, pallor, and muscular incoordination (Townsend, 2008).

Coping with Anxiety

People use a variety of coping behaviors to relieve mild anxiety, such as exercising, talking with others, engaging in pleasurable activities, deep-breathing, or using relaxation programs (Bourne, 2005). Less adaptive behaviors include excessive sleeping, eating, smoking, crying, pacing, fidgeting, drinking, laughing, cursing, nail biting, or finger tapping.

When anxiety is more severe, the person attempts to counteract the anxiety in some way. Each person develops unique patterns of coping with anxiety, called **defense mechanisms,** which are used consciously or unconsciously to relieve the anxiety. Examples of defense mechanisms are **denial** (refusing to acknowledge the existence of a real situation or associated feelings) and **displacement** (transferring feelings from one target to another that seems less threatening—for example, kicking the dog when you are angry at your boss). See Chapter 25 for further discussion of defense mechanisms.

When overused, defense mechanisms can be maladaptive and lead to psychological disorders such as phobias, obsessive–compulsive disorders, and dissociative disorders (e.g., amnesia). Excessive or unrelieved anxiety may also contribute to **psychosis,** which is a loss of ability to differentiate self from nonself or by impaired reality testing (that is, knowing what is real and what exists only in one's mind), often accompanied by hallucinations and delusions. Examples of psychotic responses to anxiety include schizophrenia and delusional disorders. These disorders are beyond the scope of this book. If you need more information, refer to a mental health text.

KnowledgeCheck 11-4

- What is anxiety?
- When is anxiety a normal response to life?
- Identify at least three healthcare scenarios that might trigger anxiety in patients.

Go to Chapter 11, **Knowledge Check Response Sheet and Answers,** on the Student Resource Disk or DavisPlus at http://davisplus.fadavis.com/Wilkinson2

Depression

Others imply that they know what it is like to be depressed because they have gone through a divorce, lost a job or broken up with someone. But these experiences carry with them feelings. Depression, instead, is flat, hollow, and unendurable.

—Kay Redfield Jamison, An Unquiet Mind

The term **depression** is commonly used to describe a feeling of sadness or "the blues." But to psychologists, nurses, and other healthcare professionals, it refers to a specific condition with characteristic symptoms and often devastating consequences if left untreated (Steptoe, 2007).

Depression occurs in all age groups, even in very young children. It affects about 11% of the adult population in the United States, and is one of the top three risks for functional decline. The incidence is higher in women than in men (Pleis & Lethbridge-Cejku, 2006). See Table 11-1 for common truths and myths about depression.

Criteria established by the American Psychiatric Association (APA) for **major depressive disorder** include depressed mood most of the day nearly every day for at least 2 weeks, typically accompanied by markedly diminished interest or pleasure in activities the person previously enjoyed. The person may also experience insomnia or hypersomnia, loss of energy, feelings of worthlessness, diminished ability to concentrate, and recurrent thoughts of death (APA, 2000). Unlike the feeling of true sadness, such as might accompany a divorce, death, or other loss, the depressed mood is typically marked by a sense of emptiness. This contributes to the depressed person's tendency to withdraw from social contacts and also explains the characteristically flat affect (Fig. 11-4).

Depression in Older and Middle Adults

The incidence of depression is slightly higher for older adults than for the population as a whole. Of adults 65 to 74 years old, 12% reported that they had feelings associated with depression (sadness, hopelessness, worthlessness, and feeling that everything is an effort)

Table 11-1 ➤ Depression: Truths and Myths	
TRUE	**FALSE**
Depressive disorders are more common among women than men (2:1).	"Getting on with life" will cure depression.
Spiritual distress is associated with depression.	Everyone likes to talk about how they feel.
Depression can be defined as a maladaptive emotional response.	Medication is the answer to depression.
Low socioeconomic circumstances and social isolation correlate with depression.	Once depression has been cured, it does not return.

FIGURE II-4 Depressed affect.

"all or most of the time." For adults 75 and older, this was 15%. The incidence is much higher if you count the people who reported having those feelings only "some of the time" (Pleis & Lethbridge-Cejku, 2006, Table 14).

Depression is a common emotional disorder of older adults. We typically think of older adults as being at higher risk because of their many losses and multiple physical illnesses (e.g., Stanley, Blair, & Beare, 2005). However, at least one recent large, international study found depression to be most common among men and women in their 40s (Blanchflower & Oswald, 2008), and that happiness and sense of well-being reach their lowest in the 40s. This study remains controversial, and more research is needed, but the findings are interesting.

What Causes Depression?

Are our genes responsible for the development of depression? Is depression "anger turned inward"? Depression theories fall into four groupings:

- *Physiological theories* relate depression to biochemical imbalances stemming from hormonal, neurological, or genetic factors.
- *Psychodynamic theories* relate depression to loss, abandonment, and emotional detachment and to diurnal and seasonal mood variations.
- *Cognitive theory* relates depression to negative thinking.
- *Social/environmental theories* relate depression to poor family relationships, difficult interpersonal relationships, and socioeconomic and political factors.

Certainly research has shown that the following factors increase the risk for depression:

Family history of depression
Hormonal or nutritional imbalance

Inability to externalize anger
Low self-esteem
Negative thinking
Learned helplessness and hopelessness
Prior success or failure in coping mechanisms
Traumatic loss
Catastrophic stressors (e.g., unemployment)
Chronic disease
Female sex

What Are the Signs and Symptoms of Depression?

Depression is expressed by changes in thoughts, feelings, and behaviors, as well as physical symptoms and changes in lifestyle. Symptoms may differ in some ways in children and older adults.

Thoughts and Feelings. Depression is characterized by a flat affect; difficulty concentrating; and **anhedonia,** a loss of interest or pleasure in previously enjoyable activities (Steptoe, 2007). Finally, the person may feel worthless, guilt-ridden, or suicidal.

Behaviors. The person may be unable to sleep, or sleep too much, dreading the moment when he has to get out of bed and face family members or responsibilities. Some people lose interest in eating and, therefore, lose weight; others eat frequently but without pleasure in an attempt to keep their "emptiness" at bay. Some people become agitated and restless; others experience slowed thinking and lethargy. Many experience fatigue or feelings of exhaustion throughout the day. Depression may be expressed in children by irritability, tantrums, or not eating.

Physical Symptoms. Like all mental illnesses, depression carries a social stigma; thus, patients who are unwilling to admit—even to themselves—that they might be depressed may present with a physical complaint such as persistent fatigue or a fear of cancer. In such cases, skillful psychosocial assessment is critical. Physical conditions that might accompany depression include headache, migraines, joint aches and pains, stomach ulcers and digestive upsets, lethargy, constipation, sleep deprivation, and weight changes.

Lifestyle Effects. In addition, depression may be masked by attempts to "self-medicate" with alcohol, over-the-counter drugs, or illegal substances; or by disordered eating, participation in dangerous sports, or other forms of reckless behavior. Social isolation is common. In children, depression may manifest in skipping school or difficulty with relationships with others.

What Are the Signs and Symptoms in Older Adults?

Depression is underdiagnosed and undertreated in older adults. It is difficult to diagnose because in older adults:

- Depression is more likely to be masked rather than exhibited by typical symptoms, such as sadness.
- Symptoms are often physical or expressed as personality changes, such as irritability.

- Depression may occur along with, or be mistaken for, dementia and delirium. In older adults, all three conditions may include the symptoms of confusion, distractibility, and memory loss.
- Some of the physical symptoms of depression (e.g., fatigue, anorexia, constipation, and psychomotor retardation) can be confused with physical illness, medication interactions, substance abuse, or "signs of old age" (Gorman & Sultan, 2008).

How Is Depression Treated?

People who are clinically depressed cannot just "snap out of it." If untreated, the symptoms may continue for weeks or even years. Currently, the physiological theory of depression predominates in the medical community, and current evidence shows that biochemical processes determine moods, thought, cognition, and perception. Therefore, treatment of serious depression relies more heavily on antidepressant medication than on psychotherapy. However, the medications have a number of unpleasant, and even serious, side effects, and some patients say that they do not effectively elevate their mood. Psychotherapists acknowledge that individual tolerance of symptoms, coping resources, education, and social support networks all have an important effect on outcomes and treatment.

Of course, you will not be conducting psychotherapy with depressed patients in your general practice. However, you *will* care for patients who are taking antidepressant medications and who have situational or even clinical depressions. Even without being a "psych nurse," there is much you can do to make your care of these patients more effective.

KnowledgeCheck 11-5
- What distinguishes clinical depression from feelings of sadness?
- How might a child manifest depression?
- Why is the nurse–patient (therapeutic) relationship important when caring for depressed individuals?

Go to Chapter 11, **Knowledge Check Response Sheet and Answers,** on the Student Resource Disk or DavisPlus at http://davisplus.fadavis.com/Wilkinson2

Practical **Knowledge** knowing how

Practical knowledge in this chapter consists of planning, implementing, and evaluating care to promote client's mental health and provide support when they experience psychosocial and psychological problems. Remember, the physical body is only one dimension of a person. What patients are thinking and feeling may be equally important to their healing process.

The independent role of the nurse generalist is in assessment and documentation of the patient's behavioral state as it relates to his medical–surgical condition, rather than on the diagnosis and treatment of mental illnesses. Clients who are anxious, for example, may not understand or recall instructions for self-care; and those who are depressed may not have the energy or motivation to follow a medical regimen or keep appointments with their healthcare providers.

Psychosocial Health: Nursing Care

Physical illness may be particularly stressful when it occurs in combination with psychosocial issues. For example, think of Karli ("Meet Your Patient"). Might her condition have been less complicated if (1) she had no disfiguring injuries or (2) if she were an older adult at a developmental stage when appearance is generally less crucial?

ASSESSMENTS: PSYCHOSOCIAL

No matter what the patient's medical diagnosis, you need to perform accurate and ongoing psychosocial assessments to develop holistic nursing diagnoses and interventions. Most admission assessment forms have a few questions to screen psychosocial status. If any of the answers indicate risk for a problem, you may need to conduct a more comprehensive special needs (or system specific) assessment. For an example of a psychosocial assessment tool,

Go to Chapter 11, **Tables, Boxes, Figures: ESG Figure 11-1,** on the Student Resource Disk or DavisPlus at http:// davisplus.fadavis.com/Wilkinson2

A comprehensive psychosocial assessment should include the following categories:

- Biological details
- Recent life changes or stressors (both positive and negative)
- Lifestyle and relationships with the wider social environment
- History of psychiatric disorders
- Functional abilities (behavioral performance)
- Self-efficacy (the belief that you can influence your own behaviors and outcomes)
- Family relationships
- Social resources and network
- Usual coping mechanisms
- Interpersonal communication
- Understanding about current illness
- Major issues raised by current illness
- Health priorities
- Spirituality

When assessing spirituality, consider using the HOPE assessment tool in Chapter 14.

After interviewing the patient, assess her *personality style*. That is, identify any personality traits that may affect her care or compliance, such as a tendency to be dependent, hostile, dramatic, or critical (Gorman & Sultan, 2008).

Psychosocial information is personal and sometimes sensitive. To encourage patients to share this information, you will need to use your developing communication skills. For example:

- Be aware of your own biases and discomforts that could influence your assessment.
- Use active listening through eye contact and verbal response. Be sensitive, though; eye contact is uncomfortable for some people.
- Proceed from general details ("How do you get along with your parents?") to the specific ("Does your mother ever hit you?").
- Use an open and positive voice tone, facial expression, and body language (e.g., avoid frowning, criticizing, or expressing shock).
- Keep the focus on the patient.
- Be respectful and sensitive to cultural and gender-specific details.
- Use open-ended questions (questions that cannot be answered with a yes or no).
- Follow the patient's cues by using reflection and restating.
- Be flexible and use humor as appropriate.
- Provide empathetic feedback and touch as appropriate.

You will learn more about interviewing and communication skills in Chapter 18.

CriticalThinking 11-5

Psychologically, Karli is worried about the unfairness of her situation, and is probably struggling with body image issues. In addition, what do you think her *social* concerns might be?

ANALYSIS/NURSING DIAGNOSIS: PSYCHOSOCIAL

Psychosocial issues involve nearly all areas of patient functioning, so there is overlap between what we are calling "psychosocial" diagnoses and those used in the rest of the chapter to describe the more specific problems of self-concept, anxiety, and depression. That is, you may use some of these psychosocial diagnoses for clients who have problems of self-concept, anxiety, and depression. It would be impossible to list every possible psychosocial diagnosis; the following are but a few.

- *Interrupted Family Processes.* There is a change in family relationships and/or functioning that is significantly affecting the patient's health.
- *Family Coping [Compromised and/or Disabled].* Usual support (comfort and assistance) from a significant other is either compromised (insufficient or withdrawn) or disabled (competing or maladapted), causing a significant health challenge.
- *Parental Role Conflict.* A parent shows significant role confusion and/or conflict in response to crises.
- *Ineffective Coping.* The patient fails to comprehend and effectively judge stressors, when he perceives incorrect

or dangerous life choices as normal, and when there is an inability to use available resources. Inability to identify strengths and resources may be secondary to low self-esteem.

- *Post-Trauma Syndrome.* There is a maladaptive learned response to a traumatic and distressing event.
- *Risk for Loneliness.* The person is separated from persons, culture, objects, or environments to which a person may have ongoing attachments.
- *Social Isolation.* The person experiences significant aloneness that has a negative impact on health, or perceives the isolation as a threat to health.
- *Risk for Other-Directed Violence.* Situations in which a person threatens or uses aggression or violence to harm others. The intention of harm may not be limited to physical harm.
- *Impaired Social Interaction.* The patient shows significant difficulties in social exchange due to an inability to use social skills.

Psychosocial issues can be a problem, a symptom of a problem, or the etiology of a problem. It is important for you to determine what is cause and what is effect, although this can be hard to unravel at times. As you can see in Table 11-2, what you identify significantly affects your choice of goals and nursing activities.

PLANNING PSYCHOSOCIAL OUTCOMES/EVALUATION

As always, the outcomes you identify will serve as guidelines for ongoing assessment and as criteria for evaluation of your patient's responses to care.

NOC standardized outcomes. The Psychosocial Health domain of the NOC taxonomy includes approximately 30 outcomes to describe psychological well-being, psychosocial adaptation, self-control, and social interaction. Other NOC domains also include useful psychosocial outcomes. To see examples of NOC psychosocial outcomes,

VOL 2 Go to Chapter 11, **Standardized Nursing Language, Psychosocial Outcomes: Examples from NOC Taxonomy,** in Volume 2

Individualized goal/outcome statements will depend on the nursing diagnoses used, client input, and realistic expectations of what the client can achieve and agrees to. For example, for Compromised or Disabled Family Coping, examples of goal statements are, "Involves family members in decision making" and "Expresses feelings and emotions freely." If the nursing diagnosis is Impaired Social Interaction, goal statements may call for the client to develop the skills of "engagement, assertiveness, compromise, confrontation, and consideration." For a nursing diagnosis of Parental Role Conflict, goal statements might be, "Reports having a functional support system," "Interacts positively with child," or "Has realistic expectations of parental role."

Table 11-2 ➤ Implications of Identifying a Psychosocial Issue as Problem, Etiology, or Symptom

	AS PROBLEM	AS ETIOLOGY	AS SYMPTOM
Nursing Diagnosis	**Interrupted Family Processes** r/t tumult from parental divorce	Delayed Development r/t lack of stimulation **secondary to Interrupted Family Processes** (parental divorce)	Ineffective Individual Coping (Mother) r/t poor judgment and impaired reality perception, **as manifested by Interrupted Family Processes** and risk-taking behaviors
Sample Goals (based on problem)	*NOC Outcome* Family Functioning	*NOC Outcome* Child Development: 4 years	*NOC Outcomes* Coping, Decision Making, Role Performance, Social Support, Impulse Control
	Goals Members perform expected family roles. Family cares for dependent members.	*Goals* Child demonstrates age-appropriate motor activities. Child uses four- and five-word sentences.	*Goals* Identifies coping strategies that have been effective in the past. Discusses the implications of decision alternatives with family.
Sample Interventions and Activities (based on etiology)	*NIC Interventions* Family Integrity Promotion Family Process Maintenance Normalization Promotion	*NIC Interventions* Developmental Enhancement: Child Parent Education Health Screening	*NIC Interventions* Coping Enhancement Decision-Making Support Impulse Control Training Family Involvement Promotion Support Group Support System Enhancement
	Specific Activities Promote parental involvement in healthcare. Assist the family with skills and education of conflict resolution, coping skills, and problem solving. Link the individual and family to the appropriate support and education services.	*Specific Activities* Establish time for one-on-one care. Provide for creative play (e.g., clay, blocks, painting). Teach parents appropriate stimulation. Teach parents about developmental milestones and expected behaviors. Assess changes in family processes.	*Specific Activities* Identify and discuss alternative behaviors. Encourage delaying decision-making when under stress. Help the mother solve problems constructively. Assist her to evaluate her own behavior. Identify and discuss past successful coping behaviors she has used.

PLANNING PSYCHOSOCIAL INTERVENTIONS/ IMPLEMENTATION

Psychosocial nursing interventions and activities will be determined by the nursing diagnoses you identify, especially by the etiologies.

NIC standardized interventions for psychosocial diagnoses are found primarily in the Behavioral and Family domains of the NIC system. To see examples of these outcomes,

 VOL 2 Go to Chapter 11, **Standardized Nursing Language, Psychosocial Interventions: Examples from NIC Taxonomy,** in Volume 2.

Specific, individualized nursing activities used to help patients maintain a sense of personhood are discussed in the text that follows. For nursing activities in which the nursing goal is to provide conflict mediation, enhance socialization, or strengthen the family,

 Go to Chapter 11, **Supplemental Materials: Psychosocial Nursing Interventions,** on the Student Resource Disk or DavisPlus at http://davisplus.fadavis.com/Wilkinson2

Preventing Depersonalization

Illness, and especially hospitalization, can have a depersonalizing effect that alters the self-concept. The ill person may feel that she has become an object to be examined, poked, prodded, and discussed. You can help patients maintain a sense of personhood by using a caring approach:

- Introduce yourself if the patient does not know you.
- Address the patient by her preferred name each time you enter the room, and always speak respectfully.
- Listen actively when the patient speaks.
- Do not talk *about* the patient to others in the room (e.g., do not say, "He seems to be better today, don't you think?"). Speak *to* the patient.
- Use eye contact and touch, keeping in mind that people vary in their desire to be touched.
- Always offer an explanation before beginning a procedure, and warn the patient before you touch him ("I'm going to touch your leg now").
- Move, turn, and position the patient gently.
- Provide for privacy when performing procedures or discussing something personal or sensitive.

Self-Concept and Self-Esteem: Nursing Care

As is true for psychosocial issues, self-concept and self-esteem issues are a part of the holistic care of well and ill patients in all settings.

ASSESSMENT: SELF-CONCEPT AND SELF-ESTEEM

Psychological tests are typically administered by a clinical psychologist or licensed social worker. However, if you were working in a mental health agency, you might collect in-depth information regarding self-concept by using a psychological measurement tool, to be interpreted by a clinical psychologist or licensed social worker. For an all-purpose assessment you might use screening in any setting,

VOL 2 Go to Chapter 11, **Clinical Insight 11-1: Assessing Self-Concept Problems,** in Volume 2.

Observe for behaviors and comments specifically associated with low self-esteem. People with low self-esteem tend to avoid eye contact and have a stooped posture. They may move slowly and have poor grooming. Their verbal behaviors include speaking hesitantly, being overly critical of others and of self ("I never do anything right."), not accepting positive comments about self ("Oh, anybody could have done it."), apologizing frequently, and verbalizing feelings of powerlessness ("Whatever you say is fine with me."; "It doesn't matter what I do; it won't change anything."). To assess specifically for the self-esteem dimension of a person's self-concept,

VOL 2 Go to Chapter 11, **Clinical Insight 11-2: Performing a Self-Esteem Inventory,** in Volume 2.

When assessing self-concept, keep an open mind. Do not automatically assume, on the basis of a patient's psychosocial history or physical handicaps, that she

suffers from low self-concept. If you suspect serious problems with self-concept, document the patient's responses in your nursing notes and refer the patient for appropriate psychological testing.

Critical Thinking 11-6

In the "Meet Your Patient" scenario, Karli perceives herself as unlovable "looking this way." You should not assume that you know exactly what Karli means by this.
- Which of her words do you need to clarify with her?
- What might you say to her to get her to provide more information about the psychosocial meaning of her statement?

ANALYSIS/NURSING DIAGNOSIS: SELF-CONCEPT AND SELF-ESTEEM

Psychosocial and self-concept issues can be a problem, a symptom of a problem, or the etiology of a problem. It is important for you to determine what is cause and what is effect, although this may not always be clear. As you can see in Table 11-2, your analysis significantly affects your choice of goals and nursing activities.

When analyzing data for self-concept problems, keep the following two guidelines in mind:

- *Avoid seeking simplistic cause-and-effect relationships.* Instead, recognize the complexity of human responses. For example:

  Molly, a 19-year-old student, has just been admitted to your unit and is presenting with clinical depression and low self-esteem. Is Molly depressed because she has low self-esteem? Or is longstanding low self-esteem causing her to feel depressed? Or are the two interrelated?

- *Avoid confusing low self-concept with clinical emotional and/or behavioral psychiatric diagnoses.* There is no recognized diagnosis describing self-concept disorder in the American Psychiatric Association's *Diagnostic and Statistical Manual of Mental Disorders, 4th ed., Text Revision (DSM-IV-TR®*, 2000). Self-concept (particularly self-esteem) plays a secondary role in a number of disorders but is not a primary disorder itself.

As is true of most conditions, a self-concept issue may be described by a NANDA-I problem label, or it may be the etiology (cause) of other problems.

Self-Concept or Body Image as a Problem

You can diagnose a body image or self-concept problem when it is the result of a particular condition and might not exist if not for the condition (e.g., a profoundly deaf adolescent develops self-worth problems). The following nursing diagnoses may be useful for patients with either low overall self-concept or difficulties in specific domains of self-concept (e.g., self-esteem):

Chronic Low Self-Esteem. The person expresses ongoing and longstanding overall self-dissatisfaction and negative self-appraisal (i.e., wide differences between "ideal" and "actual" or "perceived" self). *Etiologies* include but are not limited to depression, mismatch in ideal and perceived self, dysfunctional family, anxiety, or failure to adapt to a change in physical appearance or functioning.

Situational Low Self-Esteem. The person exhibits self-disapproval and negative self-evaluations as a specific reaction to loss or change. *Etiologies:* See Chronic Low Self-Esteem, preceding.

Disturbed Personal Identity. Negative and incorrect assessment of self-identity and inability to determine boundaries between self and others. *Etiologies* include but are not limited to distorted perceptions of self, such as occur in certain mental illnesses; loss of health, limb, physical appearance, or functioning; or dysfunctional family.

Ineffective Role Performance. A person experiences or perceives difficulty in fulfilling a usual role, or there is a mismatch between role expectations and role performance (either perceived or societal expectations). *Etiologies* include but are not limited to job demands exceeding abilities, inadequate resources or support system, family conflicts, domestic violence, unrealistic role expectations, lack of a role model, substance abuse, cognitive deficits, illness or disease, low self-esteem, pain, fatigue, and cognitive deficits.

Disturbed Body Image. An individual has a confused image of his physical self or negatively evaluates his body or an aspect of it. *Etiologies* include but are not limited to loss of functioning or appearance (e.g., acne, scars, breast removal, amputation), eating disorder, gender conflict, or personality disorder.

CriticalThinking 11-7

- Refer to Karli in "Meet Your Patient." Look at the preceding five NANDA-I labels for self-concept problems (Chronic Low Self-Esteem, Situational Low Self-Esteem, Disturbed Personal Identity, Ineffective Role Performance, Disturbed Body Image). Which one most clearly applies to Karli? Explain your thinking.
- Write a nursing diagnosis (problem r/t etiology) for the problem you chose.

Self-Concept or Body Image as Etiology

Self-concept problems are an etiology when they precede a condition such as depression and play a central role in the condition (e.g., low self-esteem causing and maintaining depression or leading to an anxiety disorder). The following are examples of nursing diagnoses with self-concept (e.g., self-esteem) as the etiology:

- *Impaired Adjustment* should be used where a patient experiences difficulties adapting perception and evaluation of self after changes in health status.

- *Complicated Grieving* may develop in anticipation of or following body changes (e.g., hysterectomy) or loss of key roles (e.g., resulting from death of a spouse).
- *Deficient Knowledge* of a healthcare situation may occur because of low self-esteem and lack of confidence in ability to learn or to manage care. Low self-esteem diminishes the motivation to learn.
- *Hopelessness* may occur because of overwhelming role demands, external locus of control, or lack of confidence in abilities.
- *Impaired Social Interaction* may occur when the person's low self-esteem and external locus of control cause him to fear criticism or lack of acceptance from others.
- *Ineffective Health Maintenance* may occur as a result of low self-esteem: not perceiving one's self as capable, or feeling there is no point to making the effort.
- *Sexual Dysfunction* or *Ineffective Sexuality Pattern* may result from negative body image brought about by changes in body structure or function (e.g., pregnancy, medications, surgery, trauma, diseases such as arthritis, or treatments such as radiation).

■ PLANNING SELF-CONCEPT AND SELF-ESTEEM OUTCOMES/EVALUATION

To see *NOC standardized outcomes* and indicators, as well as *individualized goal/outcome statement* examples, for selected self-concept problems,

 Go to Chapter 11, **Standardized Language, Self-Concept Diagnoses: Selected Standardized and Individualized Outcomes,** in Volume 2.

When self-concept is the etiology of other problems (e.g., Sexual Dysfunction related to negative body image), choose outcomes based on the problem label (e.g., Sexual Abuse Recovery, Sexual Functioning, Body Image). The overall goal, in all cases, is that the patient's self-concept (or some aspect of it) will improve.

■ PLANNING SELF-CONCEPT AND SELF-ESTEEM INTERVENTIONS/IMPLEMENTATION

For NIC standardized interventions for self-concept and self-esteem diagnoses, along with examples of nursing activities,

 Go to Chapter 11, **Standardized Nursing Language, Self-Concept Diagnoses: Selected NIC Interventions and Nursing Activities,** in Volume 2.

Although not all-inclusive, those examples should give you an idea of the types of care needed to support self-concept.

Specific, individualized, nursing activities used frequently for patients with psychosocial and self-concept diagnoses are discussed in the text that follows. They include supportive measures to promote self-esteem, self-concept, positive body image, and role satisfaction.

Promoting Self-Esteem and Self-Concept

The dependence that often accompanies illness and aging can bring about loss of self-esteem. Although the foundation for self-esteem is laid in childhood and affected by many sociocultural variables, your nursing approach can help preserve and enhance a patient's self-esteem. Your efforts to preserve self-worth of course promote self-esteem.

It is important to help the client identify past achievements and areas of strength. One way to do that is to point out areas of strength that you observe. Be sure the client considers special aptitudes, such as cooking, arts and crafts, sports, work, and education. Evaluate the client's sense of humor, which can be a strength. Other emotional strengths might include the ability to express emotions, to "feel" for others, to give and receive affection. Relationship strengths include being sensitive to others' needs, being a good listener, and making people feel comfortable. Spiritual strengths may include faith in God and participation in church activities.

Other nursing actions specific to self-esteem include the following:

- Establish a therapeutic nursing relationship emphasizing trust, consistency, honest communication, and unconditional positive regard.
- Encourage the client to be as independent as possible (e.g., by participating in planning his care and performing self-care).
- Monitor for and discourage self-criticism and negative self-talk.
- Teach the client to substitute positive self-talk for negative self-talk. For example, the client says, "I know my blood sugar is high, but I can't seem to stay on my diet. I ate way too much again today." You might say, "But what did you do today that was a good thing?" If necessary, remind the client that she exercised today and has been following her exercise program religiously. Eventually, she should learn to cue herself.
- Use positive and reaffirming language.
- Be supportive and accepting, but do not invade the client's personal space.
- Help the client develop realistic goals that provide achievable challenges (no-fail situations).
- Encourage the client to take part in activities that offer opportunities for success.
- Role-model, and provide opportunities to practice communications skills that will help the person develop interpersonal relationships.
- Refer to self-help and support groups, as needed.
- When possible, ask the client's advice (e.g., "How do you usually do this dressing change?")
- Point out good health practices and healthy aspects of the client's body functions.
- Refer to the Self-Care box for suggestions about teaching parents about promoting self-esteem in their children.

Teaching Parents to Promote Self-Esteem in Children

Demonstrate love and acceptance by:

- Spending some one-on-one time with the child as often as possible: read, play, or just be together
- Being free with touches: A hug, a pat on the back
- Refraining from frequent negative criticism
- Providing nearly total acceptance of the child

Provide security by:

- Having clearly defined limits and consequences for breaking rules
- Being firm and consistent in applying the rules
- Being sure the rules are reasonable
- Allowing some latitude for individual actions within defined limits
- Treating the child with respect
- Establishing routines, such as bedtime activity, homework before play, dressing for school before breakfast in the morning, and so on
- Clearly defining every family member's role

Promote competence by:

- Setting realistic expectations about behaviors
- Assigning a few chores that are within the child's capability (e.g., picking up toys, making the bed)
- Role-modeling values, such as respect for others, honesty, and responsibility
- Providing positive feedback
- Helping the child accomplish goals
- Providing a stimulating and responsive environment
- Providing support in meeting challenges

Promoting Positive Body Image

You can help parents promote a positive body image in their children, and you can help patients develop a different attitude toward their body. Examine your own attitudes about what constitutes a healthy body, and pay attention to the messages you convey to others. Teach clients the following, some of which are the same as for developing self-concept and self-esteem.

Healthy Does Not Mean Perfect. Help clients to accept that healthy bodies come in a wide range of shapes and sizes. Fashion magazines portray an ideal body that is unrealistic and unhealthy for most people. If they make you feel bad by comparison, don't read them! A "perfect" body does not necessarily lead to health, happiness, or success.

Focus on Activity and Healthy Eating. Encourage clients to be active and focus on healthy eating rather than starving and depriving themselves to lose weight.

Don't Make Negative Comments about Your Body. Monitor for negative comments about body functions, weight, or size. Advise the client not to talk negatively about body weight, size, or deformity. Urge clients to be kind to themselves, and point out when they are being unrealistically critical of their body.

Keep a List. Suggest that the client keep a list of things he likes about his body and refer to it when he is feeling down.

Accept Compliments. Provide the client with practice in accepting positive comments about his appearance. Coach his responses as needed (e.g., say, "Thank you" after a compliment).

Challenge Critical Comments. Teach the client to challenge critical comments from others about her appearance.

Surround Yourself with Positive People. Support the client in surrounding herself with positive people who support the changes she is trying to make in her image of her body, not with people who are critical.

Use a Counter. Suggest that the client buy a counter and click it each time he makes a deliberate effort to accept positive feedback about his body or engages in positive body behaviors.

The following are other ideas for helping clients cope with the effects of body changes (e.g., from surgeries or injury):

- Monitor the effects of body changes on self-esteem and overall self-concept.
- Encourage patients to discuss body changes resulting from their illness, surgery, or trauma.
- Provide the opportunity to interact with people who have had similar body changes.

To see a care plan and care map for Body Image Disturbance,

 Go to Student Resources, Chapter 11, **Care Plan and Care Map,** on the Student Resource Disk or at http://davisplus. fadavis.com/Wilkinson2

CriticalThinking 11-8

- Which of the preceding body image interventions would be most appropriate for Karli's nursing diagnosis?
- For the interventions you did not choose, explain why.

Facilitating Role Enhancement

Sometimes the difficulty with self-concept centers on inability to fulfill one's usual or desired role. Specific actions to enhance role satisfaction include the following:

- Help the client distinguish between ideal and actual role performance.
- Help the person to identify her past, present, and future roles. For older adults, encourage reminiscence.

- Discuss boundaries, expectations, and management defined by lifestyle and family networks.
- Facilitate communication between client and significant other regarding the sharing of role responsibilities to accommodate role changes of the ill person.
- Help the client describe realistic roles and expectations tailored to specific health changes.
- Compare realistic roles to previous and less functional roles.
- Help the client examine the difference between previous roles and current role by providing education and a learning environment that focuses on positive and supportive change.
- Help the client identify and role-play behaviors needed in new roles.

KnowledgeCheck 11-6

Without looking back at the preceding material, see whether you can:

- List three interventions for preserving self-worth.
- List three interventions for promoting self-esteem.
- List three interventions for fostering positive body image.
- List three interventions for promoting role enhancement.

 Go to Chapter 11, **Knowledge Check Response Sheet and Answers,** on the Student Resource Disk or DavisPlus at http://davisplus.fadavis.com/Wilkinson2

Nursing Care for Anxiety

In general practice, the focus of nursing care for clients with anxiety is (1) to differentiate between mild anxiety and that which is severe enough to require referral to a mental health professional and (2) to provide interventions to relieve anxiety.

ASSESSMENT: ANXIETY

Your patient assessment should identify the *presence*, *level*, and *cause* of anxiety. It should include data about the following:

- *Observable behaviors*—poor eye contact, restlessness (e.g., pacing, wringing the hands, fidgeting, shuffling the feet), crying, trembling, rapid speech
- *Cognitive changes*—confusion, difficulty concentrating, forgetfulness
- *Objective physical data*—sweating, rapid pulse and respirations, dilated pupils
- *Subjective data*—shortness of breath, nausea, insomnia, worry

As we have said, most ill patients will have at least some level of anxiety. Anxiety becomes a problem when it escalates to a level that interferes with the ability to meet basic needs. You must determine whether the anxiety is normal and adaptive or whether it is severe enough to require nursing interventions, consultation, or referral to a mental health professional. For a checklist to help you make this determination,

Go to Chapter II, **Assessment Guidelines and Tools: Anxiety Assessment Guide,** in Volume 2.

If you suspect severe or disabling anxiety, document the patient's responses in your nursing notes, and refer the person to a physician or mental health clinician. Involve a mental health professional immediately (same day) if you discover any of the following:

- Suicidal thoughts and/or plans that make you uncertain of the patient's safety
- Assaultive or homicidal thoughts and/or plans that make you uncertain about the safety of the patient or others
- Loss of touch with reality (psychosis)
- Significant or prolonged inability to work and care for self or family

Consider a comprehensive physical assessment for anxious patients, to rule out underlying disease or disorders. For example, a patient who suffers from heart palpitations when anxious may be found to have significant cardiac arrhythmias. Other medical conditions that may mimic anxiety symptoms include hormone imbalance, nutritional deficiencies, electrolyte imbalance, and central nervous system disorders. Most anxious patients, even those with diagnosed obsessive–compulsive disorder or panic attacks, are not admitted to the hospital just for their anxiety. You will encounter them more often in community settings or when they are hospitalized for other illnesses.

ANALYSIS/NURSING DIAGNOSIS: ANXIETY

For severe anxiety (neuroses, psychoses), medical treatment includes antianxiety medications and perhaps psychotherapy. The following five NANDA-I labels represent anxiety problems for which nursing interventions may be effective:

- *Anxiety* is a vague, uneasy feeling of discomfort or dread, accompanied by some of the symptoms listed in the preceding "Assessment" section. Anxiety may be unconscious; that is, the patient may not recognize that he is anxious (e.g., "My heart is pounding, and I can't seem to get my breath. What is wrong?").
- *Death Anxiety* is apprehension, worry, or fear related to death or dying.
- *Decisional Conflict* describes a person who is uncertain about what action to take when the choice among the alternatives involves risk, loss, or challenge to personal life values.
- *Fear* is a response to a perceived threat that is consciously recognized as a danger (e.g., "My father died of this same surgery. Truly, I'm scared to death."). Fear is difficulty to differentiate from Anxiety because many of the symptoms are similar.
- *Ineffective Denial* occurs when the person consciously or unconsciously rejects the knowledge or meaning of an event (e.g., a client having a heart attack says or thinks, "They have made a mistake. It's just

sore muscles or pleurisy. I'll go back to work this afternoon.")

Anxiety can be the etiology or a symptom of many other nursing diagnoses, such as Deficient Knowledge, Self-Mutilation, Ineffective Sexuality Pattern, or Insomnia.

KnowledgeCheck 11-7

- List five NANDA-I labels you could use to describe a problem of anxiety.
- List four observations that would alert you that anxiety is severe enough to merit referral to a mental health professional.

 Go to Chapter II, **Knowledge Check Response Sheet and Answers,** on the Student Resource Disk or DavisPlus at http://davisplus.fadavis.com/Wilkinson2

PLANNING OUTCOMES/EVALUATION FOR ANXIETY

You will use outcomes developed in the planning stage as criteria for evaluating patient progress and the success of your nursing interventions. Whether anxiety is a symptom, a problem, or the cause or etiology of a problem, one of the desired outcomes is that the anxiety will be relieved.

For selected NOC standardized outcomes and indicators for anxiety-related diagnoses,

 Go to Chapter II, **Standardized Nursing Language, Anxiety-Related Diagnoses: Selected NOC Outcomes and NIC Interventions,** in Volume 2.

Individualized goal/outcome statements should relate the patient's specific nursing diagnosis, stating behaviors that will indicate that the problem is resolving. The following are some examples.

For Anxiety:
Plans coping strategies for anxious situations.
Uses relaxation techniques as required.
Reports absence of physical and psychological manifestations of anxiety.

For Death Anxiety:
Reports feeling less fearful.
Discusses funeral arrangements with family.

For Decisional Conflict:
Identifies relevant information about the decision and its consequences.
Recognizes how various alternatives conflict with others' desires.

For Fear:
Uses effective coping strategies.
Maintains social relationships and control over life.

For Ineffective Denial:
Verbalizes understanding of the complications that may occur if the disease is not treated.
Follows prescribed regimen for treatments and medications.

Critical**Thinking** 11-9

 Go to Chapter 11, **Standardized Nursing Language, Anxiety-Related Diagnoses: Selected NOC Outcomes and NIC Interventions,** in Volume 2.

Notice that Anxiety Control is listed as a possible outcome for each of the nursing diagnoses. Explain how anxiety relates to each of the diagnoses: Is it a problem, a symptom, or an etiology?

PLANNING INTERVENTIONS/IMPLEMENTATION FOR ANXIETY

Interventions for anxious clients will depend on the cause of the anxiety; however, for *all* anxious clients, regardless of the etiology, the nursing goals in most situations are to help the client to:

- *Recognize that the client is anxious.* Because the symptoms may be varied, subtle, and physical, a person may demonstrate anxious behaviors without even realizing why he is doing so. Or he may attribute his symptoms to a physical illness.
- *Identify the source of the client's anxiety.* This may require a more extended relationship than you might have with a hospitalized client, because it involves the uncovering of emotional conflicts. Nevertheless, a more permanent relief can be obtained once the client recognizes the conflict and can use his conscious, rational mind to deal with it.
- *Deal with the symptoms of the client's anxiety,* for example, with massage, relaxation techniques, and so forth.

NIC standardized interventions and selected activities for anxiety-related diagnoses are listed in Volume 2.

 Go to Chapter 11, **Standardized Nursing Language, Anxiety-Related Diagnoses: Selected NOC Outcomes and NIC Interventions,** in Volume 2.

Specific nursing activities for reducing anxiety include the following:

- Provide a calm and safe environment, including a quiet, reassuring approach to communication and nursing activities. This will help the person remain centered and focused.
- Establish a relationship of trust, caring, and unconditional positive regard (i.e., don't make promises you can't keep; don't make any "judgment" statements such as, "You ought to . . ." or "You shouldn't . . .").
- Be present and stay with the individual to help allay fears, create trust, and promote safety.
- Help the person identify triggers and situations that create anxiety.
- Use clear and factual knowledge tailored to the individual's circumstances.
- Explain and, if necessary, explore details of all healthcare procedures.
- Develop coping strategies and behavior modification techniques.

- Encourage enjoyable, nonstressful activities to give the person an opportunity to think about something other than the anxiety-producing situation.
- Advise regular physical exercise unless contraindicated by a physical condition.
- Control the environment by removing anxiety-provoking equipment and people.
- Administer and monitor antianxiety medication when required.
- Assist the patient in relaxation methods, such as biofeedback, meditation, and therapeutic touch. See Chapter 40 for specific information about these methods.
- In addition, interventions specific for Death Anxiety include the following (also refer to Chapter 15):
  Stay physically close to the patient when he is fearful.
  Obtain spiritual support for the patient and family, as needed.
  Inquire about the patient's and family's specific requests for care.

Nursing Care for Depression

The nurse–patient relationship is vital when you work with a depressed person. Whereas an anxious patient may actively seek your assistance, a depressed person is likely to avoid your approach and may even feel unworthy of your time and effort. Establishing a nurse–patient bond requires a specific, empathetic approach involving warmth, acceptance, and understanding (unconditional positive regard) even in the face of an unresponsive, even angry, reaction.

ASSESSMENT FOR DEPRESSION

You should be alert for signs and symptoms of depression in all healthcare settings. If cues are present, you will need to perform a more thorough screening or comprehensive assessment, such as

 Go to Chapter 11, **Depression Assessment Guide: Patient Health Questionnaire (PHQ),** in Volume 2.

When assessing for depression, observe for symptoms in the following areas:

- *Affective:* Anger, anxiety, guilt, helplessness, powerlessness, hopelessness, sadness; may verbalize lack of feeling; inability to enjoy previously enjoyable activities, low self-esteem, worthlessness
- *Behavioral:* Persistently sad expression, poor eye contact, tearfulness, regression, restlessness, agitation, psychomotor retardation, withdrawal, poor grooming/hygiene, decreased sexual interest, past or current alcohol or substance abuse, past history of suicide attempts
- *Cognitive:* Preoccupation with loss (e.g., of job, of function), self-blame, ambivalence, blaming others, slowed thinking, poor concentration, preoccupation with bodily changes, inability to accept positive comments, guilt, confusion, inability to make decisions

■ *Physiological:* Anorexia or overeating, insomnia or hypersomnia, headache, backache, chest pain, constipation, fatigue, weight loss or weight gain, sleep problems, indigestion, dizziness

For older adults, risk factors for depression include dementia, cancer, alcohol and substance abuse, stroke, myocardial infarction, functional disability, being widowed, being a caregiver, and social isolation (Kurlowicz, 2008). Presence of risk factors should alert you to the need for a system-specific (or special needs) assessment to determine whether depression is present.

Older Adults: Depression, Dementia, or Delirium?

Delirium, also called *acute confusion*, is an acute and potentially reversible disturbance of consciousness and cognition in response to underlying medical or mental illnesses, drug toxicity, and a variety of other causes. **Dementia** is an irreversible decline in mental abilities. It is a permanent progressive decline in cognitive function (APA, 2000). Dementia affects about 22% of adults 65 to 85 years of age, and 40% of those older than age 85 (Howarth, Health, & Snope, 1999). Alzheimer's disease and vascular dementia account for most dementias (53% and 23%, respectively).

Confusion may be present in patients with depression, as well as those who have dementia or delirium. Approximately 10% to 30% of all confusion is reversible (Richardson, 2003). However, because confusion and cognitive difficulties in older adults are so often caused by dementia, care providers often attribute the patient's confusion to Alzheimer's disease and assume that interventions would be useless (Edwards, 2003). This means that for older adults, depression is under-recognized and undertreated. For a comparison of the symptoms of depression and dementia,

 Go to Chapter 11, **Assessment Guidelines and Tools, Differentiating Depression and Dementia,** in Volume 2.

The Geriatric Depression Scale is especially useful in screening for depression in older adults. It requires minimal training to use, and will help you decide whether the patient needs further assessment. To see a short form of the Geriatric Depression Scale,

 Go to Chapter 11, **Tables, Boxes, Figures: ESG Figure 11-2,** on the Student Resource Disk or DavisPlus at http://davisplus. fadavis.com/Wilkinson2

When Should I Refer the Patient to a Mental Health Specialist?

Because depression is so common, many of the patients you see (e.g., medical–surgical, maternity, clinics) will have at least some degree of depression. It will be important for you to differentiate among temporary, situational sadness, low energy, and a psychiatric

diagnosis (clinical depression). Figure 11-5 illustrates the continuum of mild to severe depression incorporating aspects of mood, behavior, thoughts, and physical symptoms.

The presence of any of the following should alert you to make a referral. If you suspect severe depression, document the patient's responses in your nursing notes, and refer the patient to a mental health specialist.

■ Personal history of recurrent depression or bipolar disorder
■ Family history of recurrent depression or bipolar disorder
■ Personal history of recurrence of depression within 1 year after stopping effective treatment
■ Episode of major depression before age 20
■ Severe, sudden, or life-threatening depressive episode (i.e., suicide attempt)

For two alternative methods you can use to identify patients who should be referred to a mental health specialist for evaluation and/or treatment of depression,

 Go to Chapter 11, **Clinical Insight 11-3: Identifying Depressed Patients Who Should Be Referred for Evaluation,** in Volume 2.

✚ If you believe there is a risk for suicide, make the referral immediately (Box 11-1).

■ ANALYSIS/NURSING DIAGNOSIS: DEPRESSION

Depression is a psychiatric diagnosis, so you will not make that diagnosis. Nevertheless, you will need to describe associated problems that are appropriate

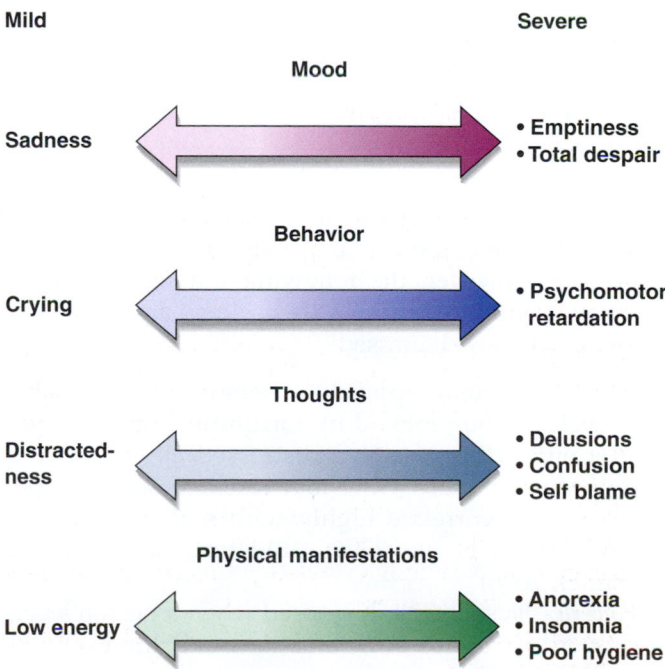

FIGURE 11-5 Depression assessment continuum incorporating mood, behavior, thoughts, and physical state.

BOX 11-1 ■ Cues Indicating a Possible Risk for Suicide

Risk Factors

- Alcohol substance abuse
- Family history of mental disorders or substance abuse
- Family history of suicide
- Firearms in the home
- Family violence, including physical or sexual abuse
- A significant medical illness, such as cancer or chronic pain
- Compulsive gambling
- Recent losses: Physical, financial, personal
- Age, gender, race (elderly or young adult, unmarried, white, male, living alone)
- Recent discharge from an inpatient psychiatry unit

Warning Signs

✚ Patients with risk factors who exhibit any of the following warning signs clearly raise a red flag and merit immediate referral.

- Withdrawal from social contact
- Desire to be left alone
- Preoccupation with death and dying, or violence
- Risky or self-destructive behavior, such as drug use or unsafe driving
- Changes in routine, sleeping patterns
- Changes in eating habits
- Giving away belongings or getting affairs in order
- Personality changes, such as becoming very outgoing after being shy
- Saying goodbye to people as if they won't be seen again
- Talking about suicide (e.g., "I'm going to kill myself," I wish I were dead," or "I wish I hadn't been born.")

Source: Maybury, B. C. (2008). Suicide prevention: Every nurse's responsibility. *Nurse.com,* March 10, 2008. Retrieved from http://news.nurse.com/apps/pbcs.dll/article?AID=200880305017

for nursing intervention. The NANDA-I taxonomy does not have a specific diagnosis that uses the term *depression;* however, the following nursing diagnoses may be useful in describing the feelings and moods of patients who are depressed:

- *Hopelessness* may apply to a person who is unable to seek or comprehend opportunities, options, and alternatives because of a distressed emotional and unmotivated state. Note that research shows hopelessness to correlate highly with suicide (Cheung, Law, Chan, et al., 2006; Goldston, Reboussin, & Daniel, 2006).
- *Powerlessness* may be diagnosed when a person's perception of control over situations and life events is significantly impaired and externally based.

✚ *Risk for Suicide* must always be considered when a patient is depressed, especially when the person has a history of prior attempts or is verbalizing the desire to die or the intent to kill himself.

Remember that depression can cause a variety of physical and behavioral problems, such as the following:

Activity Intolerance
Adult Failure to Thrive
Constipation
Imbalanced Nutrition: Less than Body Requirements
Imbalanced Nutrition: More than Body Requirements
Impaired Social Interaction
Ineffective Health Maintenance
Ineffective Therapeutic Regimen Management
Insomnia
Noncompliance
Self-Care Deficit (Bathing/Hygiene, Dressing/Grooming)
Self-Neglect

The diagnoses of Situational and Chronic Low Self-Esteem are also useful because depressed clients often experience low self-esteem. These diagnoses were presented in the preceding "Self-Concept Diagnoses" section in this chapter.

PLANNING OUTCOMES/EVALUATION FOR DEPRESSION

You will use outcomes developed in the planning stage as criteria for evaluating the patient's progress and the success of your nursing interventions.

For selected NOC standardized outcomes and indicators for depression-related diagnoses,

VOL 2 Go to Chapter 11, **Standardized Nursing Language, Depression-Related Diagnoses: Selected NOC Outcomes and NIC Interventions,** in Volume 2.

Individualized goal/outcome statements should relate to the patient's specific nursing diagnosis, stating behaviors that will indicate that the problem is resolving. The following are some examples:

For Depressed Mood:
Affect is appropriate to the situation.
Refrains from negative self-talk.
Reports feeling less sadness and depression.
Interacts willingly and appropriately with others.
Eats a well-balanced diet to prevent weight loss.
Bathes, washes and combs hair, dresses—maintains grooming and hygiene.

For Hopelessness:
Expresses positive belief in self, others, and meaning of life.
Demonstrates interest in life/activity.
Maintains spiritual belief system or religious affiliation.

For Powerlessness:

Participates in group activities (e.g., church, sports, book group).

Participates in healthcare decisions to the extent possible.

Sets realistic goals for self.

For Risk for Suicide:

Verbalizes any suicidal ideas to staff.

Trusts staff enough to disclose any specific plans for suicide.

PLANNING INTERVENTIONS/IMPLEMENTATION FOR DEPRESSION

For *NIC standardized interventions and selected activities* for depression-related diagnoses,

 VOL 2 Go to Chapter 11, **Standardized Nursing Language, Depression-Related Diagnoses: Selected NOC Outcomes and NIC Interventions,** in Volume 2.

Individualized nursing activities for depression-related diagnoses focus on altering the problem etiologies and relieving symptoms of depression. In general, care of the depressed person involves (1) developing a therapeutic relationship through effective communication and (2) promoting nutrition, exercise, and personal hygiene.

- Use therapeutic communication:
  Be honest and open.
  Be patient.
  Be consistent.
  Do not use false reassurance ("You'll feel better soon").
  Avoid phrases such as "Cheer up" or "Think how lucky you are to have a good family."
  Do make comments such as, "I like the way you look in that dress."
  Do not be overly cheerful.
  Encourage the client to express feelings, including anger.
  Be accepting and nonjudgmental when the client expresses feelings.
  Encourage communication that explores reality, grief, and personal loss.
- Promote activity. Activities in small groups can help build self-esteem.
- Promote and teach good nutrition and hydration.
- Provide support as needed for self-care and decision-making, while promoting as much independence as possible.
- Assess for and provide information about use of complementary and alternative therapies for depression (see Complementary and Alternative Modalities box).

- Monitor for suicide risk. Ask directly: "Have you thought about harming yourself? If so, what do you plan to do?"
- Institute measures to build self-esteem (see "Promoting Self-Esteem and Self-Concept" in this chapter).
- Provide information on support and educational groups.
- Encourage the person to maintain his religious affiliations.

Nursing Interventions for Older Adults

Remember that depression is not a normal part of aging. As mentioned previously, it is important to identify depression in older adults and not mistake it for dementia or "signs of old age."

Team Communication. If you identify signs of depression, be certain to communicate that to other members of the staff and to the primary care provider. You and the other nurses may be the only ones who have repeated contact with the patient, so you may be able to observe cues that are missed by other providers.

Medications. Because metabolism changes with aging, the risk of adverse medication effects is high for older adults. Closely supervise patients being treated with antidepressants because severe side effects are possible. When a patient is admitted to a hospital there is a risk that self-administered medications may be overlooked. If one of those medications is an antidepressant, missed doses combined with a physical illness may cause depression symptoms to worsen.

Reminiscence. Use reminiscence and life review as an intervention. Encourage the patient to talk about significant positive and negative experiences that have occurred during her life.

Suicide Risk. Keep in mind that depression is a significant predictor of suicide in older adults. As an example, the suicide rate among white men age 85 and older is almost double that of the U.S. general population (National Institute of Mental Health, 2008). Older adults often succeed in their suicide attempts. To illustrate: among adults older than age 65 years, there is one suicide for every four attempts; among young adults, there is one suicide for every 100 to 200 attempts (Goldsmith, Pellmar, Kleinman, et al., as cited in Centers for Disease Control and Prevention [CDC], 2007).

Professional Help. Encourage the patient to seek professional help. Older adults are likely to try to "handle it themselves," or even not think of depression as a health problem. Many think that it is normal to be depressed as they grow older.

Many people use herbal therapies to relieve symptoms of anxiety and depression. Patients may self-treat, or herbal therapies may be prescribed by CAM practitioners. You should assess for CAM use to be sure the method is not contraindicated and that the patient has informed the primary care provider about its use.

Depression

CAM	ACTIVE INGREDIENTS	SIDE EFFECTS	CONTRAINDICATIONS	PATIENT TEACHING
Ginkgo Biloba	Ginkgetin, ginkgolic acid, ascorbic acid, flavonols, sterols	Nausea, vomiting, diarrhea (usually mild) Headache	Pregnant or breastfeeding Children Patients using anticoagulants (use with caution) Patients with peptic ulcer disease	Can take 6–8 weeks for patient to feel any better. Mixing with some fruits and nuts could produce poison ivy–like reaction.
Ginseng	Ginsenosides, beta-elemene, sterols, flavonoids, peptides, vitamins B_1, B_2, B_{12}, nicotinic acid, fats, minerals, enzymes	(many) Nausea Vomiting Diarrhea Chest pain Headache Nosebleeds Palpitations Nervousness Insomnia	Cardiovascular disease Hypertension Hypotension Diabetes Pregnancy or breastfeeding Patients with active bleeding Anticoagulants Antiplatelet medications	There are many kinds of ginseng; patient should look up the specific type he is using. ✚ Discourage use by patients who are anticoagulated, or who have hypertension or diabetes.
Kava	Kavapyrones, pypermethystine	Visual disturbances Changes in reflexes and judgment Decreased platelet and lymphocyte counts Hepatotoxicity	Pregnancy Breastfeeding Use of alcohol, alprazolam, or CNS depressants	May experience symptom relief within 1 week. Significant adverse reactions may occur. Kava enhances the effects of alcohol and CNS medications. Because of liver toxicity, the CDC has cautioned consumers against using kava (CDC, 2002). Its use is severely limited and regulated in Australia (Therapeutic Goods Administration, 2005).
St. John's wort	Tannin, naphthodianthrones, flavonoids, bioflavonoids, phloroglucinols	Dry mouth Constipation GI upset Sleep disturbances Restlessness Photosensitivity Interferes with digoxin and indinavir	Pregnancy or lactation Children Use of monoamine oxidase inhibitors (MAOIs), selective serotonin reuptake inhibitors (SSRIs), alcohol, or OTC cold and flu medications	Teach contraindications and side effects. Patients who are depressed should not take this herb without medical supervision

CAM	ACTIVE INGREDIENTS	SIDE EFFECTS	CONTRAINDICATIONS	PATIENT TEACHING
S-Adenosyl Methionine (SAMe)	Amino acid and ATP, which are produced naturally in the body and are now being reproduced artificially as well	Few side effects Gastric upset Hypomania (in patients with bipolar disorder) Anxiety (in patients with depression) Headache		Patients with bipolar disorder should not use this supplement unless under direct supervision of their physician. Use enteric-coated forms to decrease gastric irritation.
Anxiety				
Kava	See "Depression," preceding. Not recommended for use.			

Source: Adapted from Hulisz, D.T. (2008); and Neeb, K. (2001). *Fundamentals of mental health nursing* (2nd ed.). Philadelphia: F. A. Davis, pp. 365–378.

Suicide Prevention Interventions

It is not only patients on psychiatric units who commit suicide. They may be the same patients you care for on a medical–surgical unit or in their homes. Illnesses such as advanced cancer and AIDS are often accompanied by uncontrolled pain and delirium. Because of the suffering and dependency they cause, they are associated with higher suicide rates.

Your most important intervention is assessment. Be alert for risk factors and warning signs that may indicate the possibility of suicide (see Box 11-1). Remember about 80% of those who attempt suicide give some prior verbal or indirect cues.

- Evaluate the patient's medications (e.g., certain antihypertensive agents, steroids, cancer chemotherapeutic agents, amphotericin-B can cause depression).
- If risk factors are present, put them prominently on the care plan and report them to other caregivers.
- Do not avoid the patient because you fear saying the wrong thing. Talking about suicide does not increase the risk.

- Be aware of your personal feelings and anxieties regarding suicide.
- If the patient mentions suicide specifically, be direct. Ask whether he is having thoughts of harming himself.
- If he answers "Yes," do not leave him. Have someone contact his primary care provider so that a psychiatric consult can be ordered, and possibly transfer to a psychiatric unit if the patient is physically stable.
- Ask if the patient has a plan for suicide, and if so, what it is.
- Remove items that might be used for self-harm: for example, razor blades and other sharp objects, shoelaces, belts, intravenous tubing, telephone cords, pills, and glasses. Search the room and the bathroom.
- Make sure the windows cannot be opened.
- Follow agency policy for continuous monitoring, moving to a room close to the nurses' station, and so on. (Gorman & Sultan, 2008; Maybury, 2008).
- Most of all, never attempt to work with a suicidal patient by yourself. Involve other members of the team immediately.

Toward Evidence-Based Practice

(Study A) Smalbrugge, M., Pot, A. M., Jongenelis, L., et al. (2006). **The impact of depression and anxiety on well being, disability and use of healthcare services in nursing home patients.** *International Journal of Geriatric Psychiatry, 21*(4), 325–332.

Researchers studied 350 elderly nursing home patients from 14 nursing homes in the Netherlands to determine the impact of depression and anxiety on well-being, disability, and their use of healthcare services (e.g., the amount of assistance they needed with ADLs). They found the presence of depression and/or anxiety was associated significantly with less well-being, but not with more disability. It was also associated with increased use of

healthcare services: more need for assistance with ADLs, more consultation of medical specialists, a higher mean number of medications, and more use of antidepressants.

(Study B) Wilkinson, S. M., Love, S. B., Westcombe, A. M., et al. (2007). **Effectiveness of aromatherapy massage in the management of anxiety and depression in patients with cancer: A multicenter randomized controlled trial.** *Journal of Clinical Oncology, 25*(5), 532–538

Researchers studied 288 cancer patients who were referred to complementary therapy services with clinical anxiety and/or depression. Patients were randomly assigned

Toward Evidence-Based Practice — cont'd

to a course of aromatherapy massage or usual supportive care alone to determine the effectiveness of supplementing usual supportive care with aromatherapy massage. The researchers concluded that aromatherapy massage does not appear to significantly relieve cancer patients' anxiety and/or depression in the long term, but is associated with clinically important benefit up to 2 weeks after the intervention.

(Study C) Sendelbach, S. E., Halm, M. A., Doran, K. A., et al. (2006). Effects of music therapy on physiological and psychological outcomes for patients undergoing cardiac surgery. *Journal of Cardiovascular Nursing, 21*(3), 194–200.

This study compared the effects of music therapy versus a quiet, uninterrupted rest period on pain intensity, anxiety, physiological parameters, and opioid consumption after cardiac surgery. A total of 86 patients recovering from cardiac surgery were randomly assigned to receive either 20 minutes of rest in bed (control) or 20 minutes of music. Researchers found that patients who listened to music experienced a significant reduction in anxiety, but that there was no effect on blood pressure, heart rate, or

use of opioids. They concluded that patients recovering from cardiac surgery may benefit from music therapy.

1. To help you with your analysis for the following questions, complete this table.

	STUDY A	STUDY B	STUDY C
Intervention			
Type of patient			
Result/conclusion			

2. Which of the studies tested an intervention?

3. Which of the interventions was most successful in relieving anxiety? Explain your thinking.

4. Think about the study that did not test an intervention. What, if anything, is its value to nurses or patients?

 Go to Chapter 11, **Toward Evidence-Based Practice Suggested Responses,** on the Student Resource Disk or DavisPlus at http://davisplus.fadavis.com/Wilkinson2

 Go to Chapter 11, **Resources for Caregivers and Health Professionals,** on the Student Resource Disk or DavisPlus at http://davisplus.fadavis.com/Wilkinson2

 Suggested Readings: Go to Chapter 11, **Reading More About Psychosocial Health and Illness,** on the Student Resource Disk or DavisPlus at http://davisplus.fadavis.com/Wilkinson2

VOL 2 **Bibliography:** Go to Volume 2, Bibliography.

CHAPTER 12

The Family

Learning Outcomes

After completing this chapter, you should be able to:

➤ Distinguish among different family structures.

➤ Describe approaches to working with various types of families to provide optimal care to both well and ill clients.

➤ Explain how family theories provide a framework to understand family functioning.

➤ Identify family risk factors in five different stages of the family life span.

➤ Discuss ways in which economic factors influence nursing practice, family care, and access to services.

➤ Present ways chronic, life-threatening illness can affect families.

➤ Identify populations most at risk for homelessness.

➤ Demonstrate an understanding of family violence.

➤ Conduct a family assessment.

➤ Identify common health beliefs and communication patterns among families.

➤ Identify nursing interventions appropriate when a family member is ill.

➤ Review how risk factors, such as illness and death, substance abuse, violence, mental health disorders, financial hardship, unemployment, and other issues, can change a family's structure, communication, and coping strategies.

➤ Discuss the sandwich generation and assessment and intervention strategies for caregiver burn-out.

Meet Your Patient

J. B. is an 80-year-old man who is hospitalized for end-stage renal disease. His wife died 4 years ago. His remaining family includes two married daughters and four grandchildren. J. B. has several siblings, but they live far away and phone or visit only rarely.

J. B. has lived in the same neighborhood for more than 55 years. When he and his wife, Pamela, first moved into the neighborhood, they lived across the street from Mike and Lena. The two couples socialized, raised their children, and enjoyed many holidays and festivities together. After the children were grown, the two couples sold their homes and each moved into a townhouse near the center of town. They lived next door to each other and continued to spend time together. A year after Pamela died, Mike's wife, Lena, died from liver cancer.

J. B. and Mike now share an apartment to reduce living expenses. They also want the security, support, and

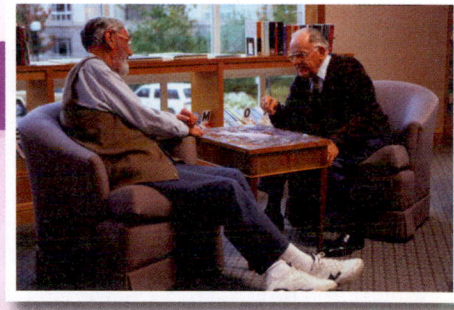

companionship that comes with a roommate situation.

J. B. subscribes to the local paper, and Mike gets a national paper. They read both papers together over breakfast before they start the events of the day. They have season tickets to the baseball games and watch sports together on TV. "Thank goodness we have each other," says Mike. Mike comes to the hospital every morning. He brings both papers and breakfast muffins for J. B., himself, and the nursing unit staff. He spends the day at the hospital and leaves shortly after dinner.

Theoretical **Knowledge**
knowing why_____

What Is a Family?

Traditionally, people have thought of a family as consisting of a husband, wife, and their children. However, as lifestyles have changed, the concept of family has become broader. The U.S. Census Bureau defines the family household as two or more people related by birth, marriage, or adoption (2009). We describe **family** as two or more individuals who provide physical, emotional, economic, or spiritual support while maintaining involvement in each other's lives. They may or may not be related by blood. Most often, people who consider themselves to be family live in the same household; however, adult children living apart from their parents may continue to define themselves as belonging to one family, which may also include siblings, aunts and uncles, and cousins. In short, families come in many forms, living arrangements, and emotional connections.

Changes in Family Structures

Changes in the living arrangements of families in the United States have resulted from a combination of factors, including an aging population, increasing average age at first marriage, high divorce rates, improvements in the health and financial status of the older population, and changing residential preferences. For instance, family households were the norm 30 years ago (81%), whereas in 2007 the percentage dropped to 68%. The percentage of people living alone rose from 17% to 27% in the last three decades, with more being women than men (U.S. Census Bureau, 2009).

Traditional Families American culture has been influenced by a family demographic in which the majority of people lived as married couples with at least one child, the husband in the labor force, and a wife not employed outside the home. The U. S. Census Bureau 2007 Current Population Survey (2009) estimates that 22.5% of American households consist of married couples with children as compared to 40.3% 30 years prior. Of these, the vast majority of "stay-at-home" parents are still women (5.5 million) while only 140,000 fathers "stay-at-home."

The percentage of children living in two-parent homes varies by race:

- Asian—85% of children in live in two-parent home
- White, non-Hispanic—78% live in two-parent home
- Black—38% live in two-parent home

Approximately 23% of children living with a grandparent had no parent present (U.S. Census Bureau, 2009).

Adults who are Married but have no Children This group was once only a small number in American soci-

ety. It now accounts for 28% of households (Population Reference Bureau, 2009).

Dual-Earner Families A dual-earner family is one having both parents in the work force. In contrast to past family structures, trends continue in which nearly two out of three children younger than age 6 live in a dual-earner family (U.S. Census Bureau, 2008).

Single-Parent Families Single-parent families result from divorce, from the death of a partner, or when partners choose not to marry or live together. They make up about 28% of all families with children. This proportion has nearly tripled since 1960. Most single-parent families are headed by women; however, the number of men raising children without a spouse has increased in recent years. The percentage of single-parent households in the United States varies among geographic areas and ethnic groups. Younger children were more likely (10% of children less than 1 year of age) than older children (1% of those between 12 and 17 years) to live with one parent (U.S. Census Bureau, 2009).

Blended and Stepfamilies Single parents commonly remarry to form new family units, such as **stepfamilies** (in which a single parent marries someone who may or may not have children), and **blended families** (in which two single parents marry and raise their children together). Commonly, biological parents who are not living together in the child's home alternate the responsibilities.

Extended Families In many cultural groups, it is common for extended family members (e.g., grandparents, aunts, uncles, cousins) to live within a single dwelling and be considered immediate family. Although J. B.'s siblings are members of his extended family, they do not live with him, and he would not consider them part of his immediate family. The growing number of older adults has created the **sandwiched generation** (Schwartz, 1979), in which middle-aged adults who still have children at home must care for aging parents and often share their household with them. Trends show more grandparent(s) are raising their grandchildren when the parent(s) are unable to do so (e.g., unemployment, divorce, imprisonment, substance abuse, or serious physical or mental illness). The U.S. Census Bureau reports 6.5 million children are raised in grandparent homes.

Other Family Structures In addition to families bound by marriage and blood lines, increasingly other family types exist, such as *heterosexual individuals* who may reside in a common household, or *gay and lesbian couples with or without children*. Although *individuals or couples who adopt children* are not biologically related, nonetheless, they are very much a family as they are emotionally attached and participate in the care and experiences in each other's lives. **Cohabiting adults** choose to live together but not marry or live together as a "trial run" prior to marriage. Cohabiting couples who marry have a higher rate of separation than their counterparts who do not live together before marriage.

Recall that a family is a group of individuals who provide support and assistance to each other. In the scenario, although J. B. and Mike ("Meet Your Patient") are not blood relatives they provide strong support for each other. Many refer to this type of bond as **kith,** persons with a kinship bond. For some people, this bond is stronger than blood-line bonds.

Approaches to Family Nursing

Family nursing refers to nursing care that is holistically directed toward the whole family as well as to individual members (Fig. 12-1). Knowing the family unit is affected by acute or chronic illness, hospitalization, or healthcare interventions, the nurse best cares for the family by involving them in patient care decisions. For J. B., for instance, in the Meet Your Patient scenario the nurses would support Mike's daily visits, and Mike is listed on the Health Insurance Portability and Accountability Act (HIPAA) form for communication of patient information. The staff would involve Mike and J. B.'s adult children in his care, discharge planning, and follow-up care at home. They would also teach Mike about J. B.'s medications and treatments so that he can assist J. B. in his activities of daily living (ADLs).

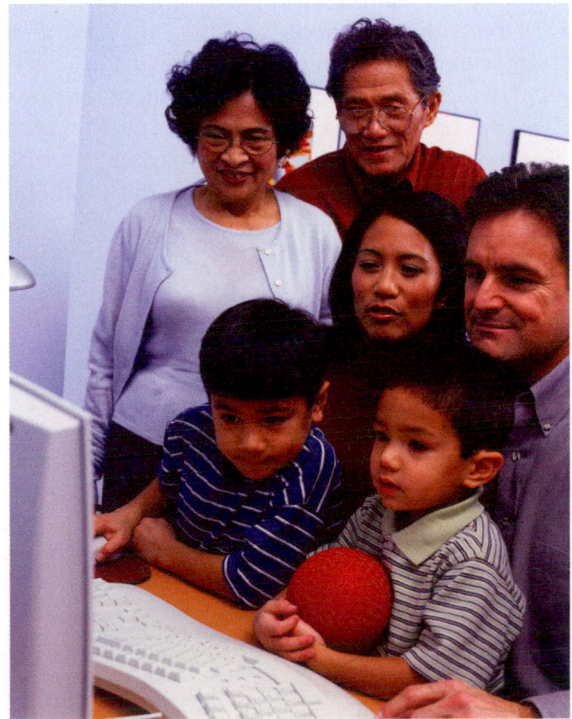

FIGURE 12-1 Family nursing refers to nursing care that is holistically directed toward the whole family as well as to individual members.

Three perspectives on family nursing include the family as (1) context, (2) unit of care, and (3) system. Family nursing is a specialty; to work with the family as a unit of care or as a system, you may need additional preparation. However, as a new graduate, you should be prepared to work, at least, with the **family as the context for care** of an individual person. Your focus in this approach is on one individual (the one who is ill); from this perspective, you view the family as either a resource or a stressor to your patient. Using this approach, you would recognize the importance of J. B.'s friend and roommate, Mike, who is his most important source of support. Before discharge, you would ask J. B., "Will Mike or your daughters be able to help you when you go home?"

A slightly more complex approach views the **family as the unit of care.** Wellness of each member is critical to promoting family health. In this approach, you would view the family as the sum of all individual members and provide assessment and care for all family members; however, you might direct interventions to individual family members rather than the family as a whole. For example, you might provide teaching on nutrition and physical activity to all family members to promote their health. Or, to use our earlier example, you might check Mike's blood pressure when he visits J. B.

The third perspective is the **family as a system.** In this approach, you focus on the family as a whole and as an interactional system. Using this perspective, you direct your assessment and intervention to communications and interactions between family members. The systems approach sees the family as embedded in and interacting with a larger community. Using this approach, you might ask, for example, "How has your family's relationship within the senior's group at your townhouse complex changed since your illness?"

KnowledgeCheck 12-1

- Name at least three types of family structure.
- What are two topics that the nurse can discuss with the family as a unit?

  Go to Chapter 12, **Knowledge Check Response Sheet and Answers,** on the Student Resource Disk or DavisPlus at http://davisplus.fadavis.com/Wilkinson2

CriticalThinking 12-1

- How can you promote family cohesion for a family whose members live great distances from each other?

What Theories Are Useful for Family Care?

Several theories have been proposed to help us understand family functioning. Three such theories are general systems theory, structural–functional theories, family interactional theory, and developmental theory.

General Systems Theory

General systems theory (see Chapter 8) focuses on interactions between systems and the changes that result from these interactions. The family is considered an open system because the members are interdependent on one another, functioning as individuals but also as a family unit as a whole, in maintaining balance from within and by the outside environment. In the case of the family, interaction can occur between members of the family or between multiple families. Healthy families strive to maintain a balance between external stress and internal relationships. Changes in the behaviors or attitudes of an individual member affect the family unit, and changes in family structure and functioning affect individual members. It may help to think of a system as a mobile; if one piece of the mobile is moved, that movement sets the whole mobile in motion.

Other systems surround the family unit (e.g., the community, the city, the state, the healthcare system). Because these systems are broader than the family, they are referred to as **suprasystems.** Smaller components that fit within the family system (e.g., the mother, the marital couple) may be viewed as **subsystems.** Each system has a particular function. For example, one family member might be viewed as the decision maker, another as the peacekeeper, and yet another, the worker, and another as the disciplinarian for the children.

Structural–Functional Theories

Structural–functional family theories are based on the developmental theories of Freud, Erikson, and Havighurst (see Chapter 9 for review) and include the concepts of family roles and interactions. According to Parsons and Bales (1955), the structural–functional approach includes the following assumptions:

- A family is a social system with functional requirements.
- A family is a small group possessing certain features common to small groups.
- The family accomplishes functions that serve both the individual and society.
- Individuals act according to internalized norms that are learned through socialization.

Although they view the family as a social system, structural–functional theories, unlike systems theory, focus on *outcome* rather than process; that is, you would use this theory to assess how well the family functions, both internally among family members and externally with outside systems. Examples of family functions include socialization of children; meeting the physical, financial, and emotional needs of family members; caring for older members; and being productive members of society.

Family Interactional Theory

Family interactional theory views the family as a unit of interacting personalities (Hill and Hansen, 1960). The major emphasis is on family roles. This approach to understanding families de-emphasizes the influence of the external world on what occurs within the family. Nurses working from an interactional perspective focus family healthcare on the interaction and communication between family members; their roles and power; family coping; and relationships with other people outside the direct family unit.

Developmental Theories

Developmental theories focus on the stage of family development. Theorists typically identify eight stages in the family life cycle according to the ages of the children and parents: beginning family, childbearing family, family with preschool children, family with school-age children, family with teenagers and young adults, family launching young adults, postparental family, and aging family. Each stage is associated with developmental tasks the family needs to achieve. Most family development theories do not identify stages and tasks for families who remain childless throughout their lives. To learn about developmental tasks associated with family stages, including those for families without children,

 Go to Chapter 12, **Tables, Family Development,** in Volume 2.

Generally the stages follow one another in a linear progression; however, some families may be in more than one stage at a time or may revert to previous stages. This overlap or reversion is most common in families that have children spaced far apart, in blended families, and in stepfamilies. See Chapter 9 for developmental theories applicable to individual family members.

KnowledgeCheck 12-2

- Which type of theory focuses on interactions among families, family members, and groups in the environment?
- What is the name of the theory that views families as a social system with a focus on outcomes?
- What are some examples of family functions as defined by structural–functional theories?

 Go to Chapter 12, **Knowledge Check Response Sheet and Answers,** on the Student Resource Disk or DavisPlus at http://davisplus.fadavis.com/Wilkinson2

CriticalThinking 12-2

- Using systems theory, you could view J. B., his siblings, his children, and his grandchildren as a system. Refer to the section on family structures—how would you categorize this family structurally?

- Again using systems theory, what or who are the subsystems in the family system described in the preceding question?
- Considering J. B. alone, at what developmental stage is his "family"?

What Are Some Family Health Risk Factors?

Many health risk factors are the same for families as for individuals, and they are similar across age groups and family types. Basically, destructive behaviors remain destructive behaviors, regardless of who is performing them." For a more complete discussion of this topic,

 Go to Chapter 12, **Supplemental Materials: What Are Some Family Health Risk Factors?** on the Student Resource Disk or DavisPlus at http://davisplus.fadavis.com/Wilkinson2

Also see Chapter 9 covering growth and development, Chapter 18 about communicating, Chapter 24 on teaching clients, and Chapter 25 on stress and adaptation, for specific topics as they relate to families.

Childless and Childbearing Couples

Adapting to new roles within the home creates stress for newly married couples, couples who are trying to become pregnant, and new parents who are inexperienced in the challenges and responsibilities of raising a healthy, happy, and safe child (Fig. 12-2). Use of maladaptive coping mechanisms can lead to health problems. For example, someone who uses alcohol to deal with stress is at risk for self-injury and liver disease, and the family may possibly suffer the harmful effects of neglect, family violence, and addiction. In addition, childbearing couples face health risks related to pregnancy, birth, and their children, including the risk for miscarriage, congenital malformations and genetic defects, and concern for the health and safety of the mother and fetus during and after the labor and birth process.

Families with Young Children

Families with young children often experience stress related to finances. For example, dual-earner couples may struggle to pay for child care. Finding safe, nurturing, and affordable child care can be a major source of family stress for parents working outside the home. Common parenting concerns center around child's development, socialization, education, discipline, nutrition, sleeping, toileting, and safety. In addition, the demands of work and childrearing mean less time is available to nurture the couple's relationship, leaving them at increased risk for marital discord.

Injuries and illness create risks to family health. For example, those receiving group child care or who are in school are exposed to other children who might have contagious diseases that can spread to other family members. To reduce the risk for serious infectious

FIGURE 12-2 Newly married couples, couples who are trying to become pregnant, and new parents are vulnerable to stress as they adapt to new roles.

diseases (e.g., mumps or hepatitis B), parents need to be aware of the importance of adhering to the recommended childhood immunization schedule. For families who live with a chronic illness, such as asthma or type 1 diabetes, or a developmental or learning disability, such as autism, the stress related to compromised health, falling behind in school, financial burdens, and even day-to-day living can become overwhelming.

Families with Adolescents

Families with adolescents are often concerned about teen risk-taking behaviors. Adolescents may participate in risky behaviors to belong to a certain clique or to impress others, to feel cool or important, or to experience a feeling of power. Developmentally, adolescents typically do not feel the threat of real danger. Some specific risk-taking behaviors include using tobacco, alcohol, and other illicit drugs; extreme stunts or dares; rebelling against authority; and sexual promiscuity.

At the same time, these families may be dealing with aging parents or grandparents (Fig. 12-3). Families may become "sandwiched" between the needs of the growing adolescents and the needs of grandparents. Women are particularly at risk for stress in these situations

FIGURE 12-3 In families with adolescents or young adults, the parents may become "sandwiched" between the needs of the growing adolescents and the needs of their own parents.

because they are usually the ones who provide the additional care for older relatives.

Families with Young Adults

Young adulthood is a time of transitions that occur in various sequences. Young adults commonly move out of the parental home as their school years end. Many take full-time jobs for the first time, starting professional lives or employment or military careers. This is a time when many marry and begin childbearing and rearing.

Some confront such problems as tight finances, unrealistic expectations for meaningful work and personal relationships, travel, and the responsibility for maintaining property. Financial strain might influence a young adult, alone or with newly formed family, to move back in with his parents until he can "get back on his feet again." This return to the nest, although sensible, can nonetheless be a stress on the family. Role strain and poor communication are common. Although young adults returning to the home of origin can represent a new opportunity for family attachment, the presence of another person in the household is certain to change family dynamics in one way or another

These transitions are common experiences for young adults. Not every young adult will experience or cope with them in the same manner. Also note that not every transition is a permanent accomplishment or marker of social success. Newfound autonomy and independence is exhilarating for some and anxiety-provoking for others. The boundary between adolescence and adulthood is blurred by societal forces (e.g., a contracting economy, changing labor force expectations, and expanding opportunities for women). As this continues, roles within the family will evolve and families will need to find healthy ways to adapt.

Families with Middle-Aged Adults

The middle years are a time of examining life goals and coping with aging and the empty nest. The quality of the spousal relationship might take on a new importance. Satisfaction with work or career accomplishments comes into play for middle-aged adults. Issues related to health and illness for themselves and their aging parents takes a front seat.

The middle years can be a satisfying time of role fulfillment, career success, financial security, and social comfort. It may be a time that the middle adult experiences a new sense of freedom and need for self-exploration and personal growth. Without the time demands of raising children, adults have more time available to pursue other personal interests or professional paths. Increasingly, middle adults are returning to the workforce, changing career pursuits, or enrolling in postsecondary, postgraduate, or professional education.

Nevertheless, some adults experience emotional strain during this period while coping with passing of youth and inevitability of old age. Because the middle years can be a time when career expectations call for peak performance and financial success, it can also be a time of self-doubt triggered by the changes of aging, menopause, empty nest, death of parents, or change in career life or relationships. Some adults in the middle years suffer a **mid-life crisis**, which is a period of intense questioning about the meaning and direction in life, asking what brings personal fulfillment. Adults battling mid-life crisis might display signs of depression, anxiety, or rebellion from the status quo.

The effects of long-standing unhealthy behaviors often become apparent in middle adulthood. For example, people who have used tobacco for many years may now begin to notice an increase in cough and chest congestion; those who have consumed high-fat diets may develop high blood pressure or elevated cholesterol levels. Remember, individual health impacts family health.

Families with Older Adults

Falls and trauma are a common health risk for families with older adults. For more information about this, see Chapters 9 and 21.

Older adults are at risk for social isolation and loneliness because of the loss of relationships that occurs with aging. Family dynamics change as the older person copes with the death of a spouse, sibling, friends, or other loved ones. This can deeply affect an elderly person's quality of life, and even the clarity of thinking. Prolonged grieving can lead to illness and other problems with emotional well-being. At the same time, though retirement can bring the simpler life that many people desire, it does bring a loss of daily contact with colleagues in the workplace and, for some, a reduced sense of responsibility or purpose. Friends can be a significant source of support (Fig. 12-4), but functional losses may cause the person to limit physical activity, volunteer work, church attendance, and other social activities. Isolation, loss, and physical changes increase the risk for depression in this age group.

Maintaining good nutrition and hydration becomes more difficult as a person ages, particularly for the frail elderly. The following are situations that may compromise the nutrition of older adults:

- Forgetting to eat (especially those who live alone)
- Inadequate or unreliable transportation to shop for food
- Lack of money to buy food
- Physical changes that alter taste (e.g., reduced sensitivity in the taste buds and less saliva for taste and swallowing)
- Loss of appetite
- Poorly fitting dentures

For more information about nutrition, see Chapter 26.

Memory and problem-solving are altered with aging. Forgetfulness and confusion can pose risks to safety for older adults, particularly for those living alone or with other aging adults whose mental status is compromised. When older adults, and especially frail elderly, lose their ability to reason, they are vulnerable to physical harm. The demands of keeping the aging adult safe can lead to caregiver role strain and family stress.

FIGURE 12-4 Friends play an important role in the support system of older people.

It is easy to understand from the above scenarios the cascading effect that one deficit, such as lack of transportation, can have on the health of an older adult and her family. Many families are not aware of community resources that can provide help. Be sure to educate them about the availability of community resources, such as Meals on Wheels and home health aides.

Critical Thinking 12-3

- What developmental stage is your family in? How do you know?
- In the Meet Your Patient scenario, what health risks do J. B. and Mike face considering their age and health? What basic attitudes, values, or beliefs influenced you in your childhood family?
- How were decisions made in your childhood family? Were people's feelings and individuals' needs considered?
- Can you remember good times and laughter that bonded you together as a family? In your present family life, how often do you laugh together?

What Are Some Challenges to Family Health?

We have already mentioned the effect of some demographic changes, such as an aging population, on families. This section examines other regional and national trends that affect families.

Poverty and Unemployment

When the economy takes a downturn, families may struggle to provide for basic needs (e.g., food and shelter) and healthcare. In 2005 in the U.S., 46.6 million people did not have health insurance (U.S. Census Bureau, 2006). However, a federal healthcare law passed in 2010 is expected to provide coverage for more people. Approximately one of every seven pregnant women in the United States failed to obtain first-trimester prenatal care. Nearly half of these women gave as their reason lack of money or insurance to pay for the visits. Teenage pregnancy is yet another factor that is strongly associated with poverty and unemployment (Centers for Disease Control and Prevention [CDC], 2007).

Single-parent and low-income families are hardest hit. Most people who are living at or below the federal poverty level are workers with minimum-wage or seasonal jobs. In a sluggish economy nonessential jobs may be eliminated. Furthermore, when the economy spirals downward and fewer workers are paying taxes, state budgets supporting low-income families may be among the first to be cut. Although some people find creative solutions to family poverty (e.g., a woman who is laid off assumes child care for another family whose members remain employed), many families experience extreme hardships when the economy is suffering.

Middle-income families are also affected by corporate downsizing or market fluctuations. Both skilled and unskilled labor can suffer when consumer spending and housing economies are declining. Even families who were living in seeming prosperity may not have sufficient funds to cover a period of unemployment or economic recession. Many people in the United States carry significant credit card debt, a first and possibly second mortgage, car payments, a variety of insurance premiums, and perhaps school loans or other loans.

KnowledgeCheck 12-3

- Which socioeconomic group of families is hardest hit during poor economic periods?
- How are middle-income families affected by poor economic times?

 Go to Chapter 12, **Knowledge Check Response Sheet and Answers,** on the Student Resource Disk or DavisPlus at http://davisplus.fadavis.com/Wilkinson2

Infectious Diseases

Family health may be affected by any number of new or resistant pathogens, such as severe acute respiratory syndrome (SARS), methicillin-resistant staphylococcal aureus (MRSA), West Nile virus, and H1N1 virus. The 2009 H1N1, also called swine flu, is a new pandemic virus, causing illness in humans, especially young children, pregnant women, people 65 years and older, and those with certain chronic diseases.

HIV infection is a devastating event that significantly impacts the family. In addition to the obvious physical and financial stressors, women who infect their infants with HIV bear a tremendous burden of guilt. Some families keep the diagnosis a secret and blame each other, whereas other families support each other and manage the illness as best they can. Advances in treating the infection and preventing its spread have been made through public and patient education, vaccination, antiviral therapy, and other antimicrobial treatments for HIV-related complications.

Even "old" diseases can return to threaten family health. Diseases once managed with immunization are making a comeback, such as polio, mumps, and smallpox. Some infections previously believed to have been eradicated have re-emerged because of failure to comply with immunization in certain populations. As a result, *herd immunity* is reduced. And tuberculosis, which had been cured by antibiotics for more than 50 years, has now resurged in a highly contagious and fatal, multidrug-resistant form.

KnowledgeCheck 12-4

- What age and gender groups are experiencing the fastest rate of growth in new HIV cases?
- Name two previously eradicated diseases that have become a threat again.

 Go to Chapter 12, **Knowledge Check Response Sheet and Answers,** on the Student Resource Disk or DavisPlus at http://davisplus.fadavis.com/Wilkinson2

Chronic Illness and Disability

Chronic illness and disability profoundly change the way families function. Family members' roles evolve over time, especially for the caregiver. Many people with chronic illness and disability require assistance with ADLs, such as getting around the home, feeding, bathing, dressing, toileting, and getting in and out of a chair or bed. Many are not able to work or generate family income, often creating financial strain or poverty. Long-term illness and disability cause mental, emotional, or physical limitations that affect family communication patterns. In addition, relationships within the family may be difficult due to caregiver strain and issues related to dependency. Long-term care of a family member may increase the risk for abuse and neglect, including maltreatment of frail elderly family members.

The Americans with Disabilities Act of 1990 (ADA) defines disability as a substantial limitation in a major life activity. Individuals 15 years and older are determined to have a disability it they meet criteria involving mobility, self-care, physical or sensory limitations, inability to work inside or outside the home, mental or emotional condition that interferes with everyday activities, and receipt of federal benefits based on inability to work. In the United States in 2006:

- 15% of noninstitutionalized people reported one or more disabilities. Slightly more females (15.6%) than males (14.4%) reported a disability.
- The prevalence of disability was lowest for people ages 16 to 20 (6.9%) and highest for those 75 years and older (52.6%).
- The poverty rate of working-age people with disabilities was 25.3%. Among the six types of disabilities, 32.5% were people with mental disability while the lowest group was those with sensory disability (23.3%) (Rehabilitation and Training Research Center on Disability Demographics Statistics, 2007).

Homelessness

Homelessness is a growing problem in many U.S. cities, not only for individuals but for also for families (Fig. 12-5). Many homeless people sleep on the streets, although others live temporarily with relatives or in mission shelters. Homelessness is far more complex than lack of housing. This problem might be explained by a number of factors, such as financial crises, socially dysfunctional relationships, unemployment, lack of job skills, substance abuse, healthcare expenses, or the inability or lack of desire to live within the socially accepted norms of society. In the United States, deep poverty and homelessness often result from mental illness, disability, or misfortune.

Homeless families are often socially isolated. Seeking food and shelter requires a majority of the family's time and effort, threatening family relationships and the long-term physical and emotional health of family members. Many homeless children do not attend school, and those who do tend to perform poorly. Often, homeless families

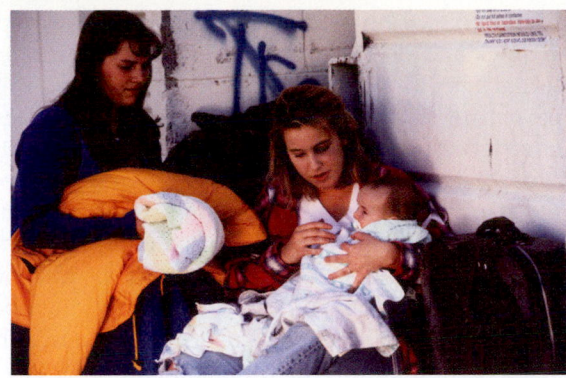

FIGURE 12-5 Many homeless people are single women and children.

do not seek care for significant health problems. Primarily this is because they don't know how to access the healthcare system and qualify for healthcare services.

Single women, members of minority groups, and single-parent families are particularly vulnerable to homelessness and poverty. It is not uncommon for divorced women to end up with less income than their ex-husbands. In addition, many women also might have sole custody of their children, which creates additional expenses for them. In many states, social service departments are so overwhelmed that they are unable to enforce the law for biological fathers struggling to pay child support while keeping up with their own living expenses.

Violence and Neglect Within Families

Domestic violence—including physical, emotional, and sexual abuse—occurs throughout all strata of our society, among all racial, social, and economic groups. As many as one in every four women will be a victim of violence during her lifetime, and more than 3 million children each year are reported to child protective services agencies as alleged abuse victims. The National Child Abuse and Neglect Data Systems estimate that over 500,000 children in the United States are seriously injured each year by various forms of maltreatment. The U.S. Census Bureau (2006) reports cases of substantiated child abuse and neglect have increased 113% between 1990 and 2005. Children ages 3 and younger are the most frequent victims of child fatalities. These children are the most vulnerable for many reasons, including their dependency, small size, and inability to defend themselves.

Any type of violence is likely to have long-lasting effects on the victims and on the family. It may result in the disintegration of the family relationships and structure (e.g., sending the children to foster care, escaping to a battered women's shelter, living with others). Health issues related to domestic violence include physical injury from the assault itself. Chronic health problems commonly emerge either as a complication of traumatic injury or as a physical response to the ongoing stress from violence or neglect. Families experiencing domestic violence have more unintended pregnancies, miscarriages, abortions, and low-birth-weight babies. They

also have more sexually transmitted infections and higher rates of depression, post-traumatic stress syndrome, substance abuse, and suicide. And even though the emotional and physical pain may stop when the victim leaves the family environment, often there are long-term effects involving emotional injury, marred self-esteem, or poor quality relationships. Victims of family violence learn patterns of ineffective coping that can be repeated in successive generations.

KnowledgeCheck 12-5

- Name two causes of homelessness.
- Name two groups of individuals who are vulnerable to homelessness.
- Name two types of violence.
- Describe the effects of family violence that generally endure after the physical injury has healed.

 Go to Chapter 12, **Knowledge Check Response Sheet and Answers,** on the Student Resource Disk or DavisPlus at http://davisplus.fadavis.com/Wilkinson2

Practical **Knowledge**
knowing *how*

A holistic view of family health integrates the biological, social, cultural, and spiritual aspects of life and refers to individual members as well as the whole family. Nurses play a vital role in promoting family wellness across the lifespan. When working with families, you will encourage them to take responsibility for their own family health. Ensuring family privacy is essential for obtaining an accurate and comprehensive family health assessment. Your interactions with families can empower them to practice behaviors that will aid in healing and maintaining good health.

ASSESSMENT

Health assessment for the family is similar to that for individuals. Gather all essential assessment information for each family member. (See Chapter 19 for additional information on physical assessment.) In addition to the individual factors, assess the health of the family unit. For an example of a family assessment form used by a community health agency,

 Go to Chapter 12, **Tables, Boxes, Figures: ESG Figure 12-1,** on the Student Resource Disk or DavisPlus at http://davisplus.fadavis.com/Wilkinson2

In general, a family assessment should include the following:

- Relevant medical data, social and family history for individuals within the family
- Family composition
- Family genogram showing health issues
- Family history and developmental stage

- Description of the home environment and surroundings
- Family structure, including communication patterns and power and role structures
- Family functions
- Health beliefs, values, and behaviors
- Family strengths
- Family stressors and coping
- Abuse and violence within the family. To see an abuse assessment,

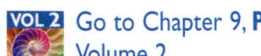 Go to Chapter 9, **Procedure 9–1: Assessing for Abuse,** in Volume 2.

For a more complete description of the context of a family assessment,

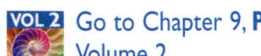 Go to Chapter 12, **Clinical Insights 12-1: Conducting a Family Assessment, and the Family Development table** in Volume 2.

The following sections discuss in more detail the assessment of family health beliefs, communication patterns, coping processes, and caregiver role strain.

Assessing the Family's Health History

The family history can provide clues about a person's health and susceptibility for disease. Genetic differences account for how one person who is predisposed to a health problem may experience the condition or not. Genetic linkages have been discovered for common, complex diseases, such as breast cancer, Alzheimer's' disease, diabetes, macular degeneration, seizures, inflammatory bowel disease, lupus, and heart disease, to name a few.

Genomics is the study of human genes and their function, including the interactions among other genes and the environment. Simply said, it is about the interplay between a person's genetic make-up and other food and environmental toxins, lifestyle, and stress, for example. Genomics can be used to personalize a patient's plan of care by:

- Identifying at-risk individuals for certain conditions so there can be more effective preventative care
- More accurately detecting illness, even before symptoms appear
- Tailoring healthcare to the individual, while reducing a trial-and-error approach
- Evaluating a person's response to the care, considering multiple factors

Genomics helps us to understand how people respond differently to particular drugs and medical treatments. For example, one client with a genetic predisposition for high cholesterol can benefit from a change in diet and exercise to decrease the likelihood that the genetic risk will be expressed. Another person may not respond to lifestyle measures and require cholesterol-reducing drugs.

When assessing the family history, you can use a pictorial tool, called a **genogram,** to display the relationship of family members with pertinent health-related

information (Fig. 12-6). This type of family tree can provide a quick and useful context in which to evaluate an individual's health risks.

To construct a genogram, you will note the causes of death, genetically-linked diseases, and other important health problems. Use a three-generation (or more) genogram to also show environmental (e.g., toxin) and mental health issues (e.g., depression, alcohol abuse, suicide), occupational diseases (e.g., asbestos), infections (e.g., MRSA), and obesity among family members. When developing a genogram, use symbols and abbreviations to denote family members, including a key for interpretation (Box 12-1).

Assessing the Family's Health Beliefs

Health beliefs can vary widely among families and among individuals within families. The differences can be especially great among different generations of a family (e.g., between grandparents and their grandchildren). Some common health beliefs are expressed in such adages as "Doctor knows best," and "Feed a cold, starve a fever." Some families may have an intense skepticism or mistrust of medical care and hospitals and may seek treatment only when absolutely necessary (e.g., when the pain becomes unbearable). Many of these beliefs are passed on from generation to generation.

Even if one family member does not share all of the beliefs of the family, you need to be aware of the family's beliefs because they may influence the individual's decision-making. To illustrate this point, consider a family caring for a member who is frail elderly, confused, and immobile. Say that one family member believes quality of life issues are more important than quantity. Yet another family member who is giving care has a fundamental disagreement with this belief and supports the right of the older adult to receive whatever care is needed for physical safety, emotional fulfillment, and spiritual well-being for any length of time. In a situation like this, the family is at risk for interpersonal conflict, impaired communication, and caregiver strain. If you would like more information on health beliefs, see Chapter 41.

 Critical**Thinking** 12-4

- As a nurse, how can you promote overall wellness in a family with a critically ill member?
- What health beliefs would you want to ask J. B.'s family about?

Assessing the Family's Communication Patterns

To assess family communication patterns, you will need to interview the family and also carefully observe the interactions between family members. Try to uncover the following information:

- Who is the primary decision maker in the family?
- How are family decisions made: by one individual or by family conference?

Family History By Genogram

FIGURE 12-6 Family history by genogram.

BOX 12-1 ■ Family History by Listing Family Members

The following history is for a 37-year-old female patient.

Patient: Age 37, alive and well

Spouse: Age 40, divorced, alcoholism

Daughter: Age 12, alive and well

Son: Age 8, alive and well

Brother: Age 32, alive and well

Sister: Age 30, alive and well

Father: Age 66, hypertension (HTN)

Mother: Age 60, mitral valve prolapse (MVP)

Paternal aunt: Age 65, breast cancer

Maternal uncle: Age 62, HTN

Maternal uncle: Deceased age 28, tuberculosis (TB)

Maternal aunt: Age 64, MVP

Maternal aunt: Age 58, HTN

Maternal aunt: Deceased age 9, ruptured appendix

Paternal grandfather: Deceased age 68, cancer

Paternal grandmother: Age 80, HTN

Maternal grandmother: Age 77, HTN, breast cancer

Maternal grandfather: Deceased age 70, cardiovascular disease (CVD)

■ What is the most frequent means of communication among family members: visits to the home, telephone, e-mail, text messaging and other forms of electronic social networking, in-person social activities (e.g., family get-togethers, going out to dinner), religious activities, church attendance?

Do not rely solely on the information provided by the family members during the interview process. Family members who participate in dysfunctional communication patterns may not come to scheduled family meetings and may not be present during the initial interview. Additionally, when relationships among family members are strained or dysfunctional, they may distort the information they provide about a home situation or another family member. Families usually want to "put on the best face" for healthcare providers, so they may be careful to give socially desirable responses. Carefully observe the words people use and other cues involved in communication, such as body language, direct eye contact, and other nonverbal expressions, particularly among family members.

Assessing the Family's Coping Processes

The physiological manifestations of stress (e.g., anxiety, increased pulse rate) may decrease the effectiveness of interventions and negatively affect a client's health.

Family members who are not coping effectively may cause the client to become stressed or anxious or have problems sleeping. Assessing family coping is a first step to helping the family develop more effective coping patterns. Observe for the following:

- Physical indications of stress, anxiety, or loss of sleep in the client.
- Relationships and communication patterns among family members. As a nurse, you can assess whether family members are irritable and "snap at" (speak harshly or curtly to) one another.
- For inpatients, notice who is visiting. Family members who are not coping well may avoid coming to visit the patient, so this may be an indicator of who is coping and who is not.

KnowledgeCheck 12-6

- Why is it important for you to ask about family health beliefs?
- What factors may impede a family's ability to cope with an individual's illness?

 Go to Chapter 12, **Knowledge Check Response Sheet and Answers,** on the Student Resource Disk or DavisPlus at http://davisplus.fadavis.com/Wilkinson2

Assessing for Caregiver Role Strain

Conflicts between caregiving and other responsibilities can produce tremendous **caregiver role strain** and family stress. The physical, emotional, and time demands involved with taking care of family members who are chronically ill, disabled, or frail can create difficulties among family members. Relationships can be compromised. Financial stress can also be a factor in family functioning. When these stressors add up, family caregivers might suffer from what NANDA-I terms Caregiver Role Strain. This is present when a person has difficulty in performing adequately in the family caregiver role.

To assess for caregiver burnout, observe for dysfunctional communication, such as abusive language and aggression. Look for physical injury to the patient, which may occur when caregivers are overwhelmed and overstressed. On the other hand, you might see the caregiver withdrawing emotionally, which could result in emotional neglect and isolation. Caregivers experiencing role strain might exhibit emotional distress, including depressive symptoms and apathy.

■ ANALYSIS/NURSING DIAGNOSIS

Recall in the diagnostic process you must analyze the data for cues (data that deviate from norms). Therefore, you should be familiar with the characteristics of a healthy family (refer to Box 12-2) so you can use them as your basis for comparison.

For individual family members, of course, any NANDA-I diagnosis may be appropriate for describing

---

BOX 12-2 ■ Characteristics of a Healthy Family

A healthy family requires more than merely the absence of family dysfunction or disease in an individual member. Characteristics of a healthy family are listed, following:

State of family well-being

Sense of belonging and connectedness

Clear boundaries between family members where the responsibilities of adults are clear and separate from responsibilities of growing children

Sense of trust and respect

Honesty and freedom of expression, including different opinions or viewpoints

Spending time together, sharing rituals and traditions

Relaxed body language, physical touch, and frequent eye contact

Flexibility: adaptability and ability to deal with stress, openness to change

Commitment: working together to maintain the family

Spiritual well-being

Respect for privacy of individual members

Balance of giving and receiving

Positive, effective communication

Accountability, including acceptance when mistakes are made

Appreciation and affection for each other

Responding to the needs and interests of all members

Health-promoting lifestyle of individual members

---

a client's health status. **Family diagnoses,** however, are meant to describe the health status of the family as a whole. The following are examples:

Caregiver Role Strain (actual and risk for)
Family Coping: Compromised
Family Coping: Disabled
Dysfunctional Family Processes
Impaired Home Maintenance
Impaired Parenting (actual and risk for)
Ineffective Therapeutic Regimen Management
Ineffective Role Performance
Interrupted Family Processes
Readiness for Enhanced Family Coping
Readiness for Enhanced Parenting
Relocation Stress Syndrome
Risk for Impaired Attachment
Social Isolation

■ PLANNING OUTCOMES AND EVALUATION

NOC outcomes specifically for families as units are found in the NOC domain Family Health, which includes the classes Family Coping, Family Health Status, Family

Integrity, and Parenting Performance. Outcomes from other domains may apply as well, depending on the nursing diagnosis you have made. For a list of NOC outcomes in the Family Health domain, and for Caregiver Role Strain,

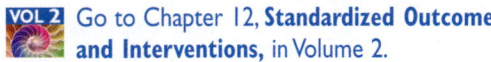 Go to Chapter 12, **Standardized Outcomes and Interventions,** in Volume 2.

Individualized goals/outcome statements you might write for a family include the following examples, which represent some of the traits of healthy families in Box 12-2. The family:

Affirms and supports each member.
Teaches respect for others within and outside the family.
Demonstrates a sense of humor and plays together.
Observes rituals and traditions (e.g., celebrates birthdays).
Respects the privacy of each member.
Communicates effectively and openly.

Remember the outcomes you develop for the care plan serve as the criteria for evaluating your patient's responses to nursing interventions.

PLANNING INTERVENTIONS/IMPLEMENTATION

NIC interventions for families as units are found in the NIC domain Family Integrity Promotion, which includes the classes for the Childbearing Family. Interventions from other domains may apply as well, depending on the nursing diagnosis you have made. For NIC family interventions,

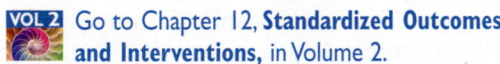 Go to Chapter 12, **Standardized Outcomes and Interventions,** in Volume 2.

Individualized nursing actions you might use with families include the following examples (other interventions are described in succeeding sections):

- Collaborate with family in problem solving and decision making.
- Refer the family to support groups of other families dealing with similar problems.
- Monitor current family relationships.
- Assist with family with conflict resolution.
- Encourage family to maintain positive relationships.
- Establish trusting relationship with family members.
- Counsel family members on additional effective coping skills for their own use.
- Refer for family therapy, as indicated.
- Tell family members it is safe and acceptable to use typical expression of affection when in a hospital setting.

Promoting Family Wellness

Encouraging families to value and incorporate health promotion into their lifestyles will also affect the health of individual members. Health-promotion behaviors are typically learned within the family. You can promote family wellness by addressing both individual and family needs. It is important to identify both strengths and basic weaknesses of the family to adequately meet healthcare needs.

Involving the family in each phase of the nursing process promotes positive health outcomes and helps

Toward Evidence-Based Practice

Huges, M. E., Waite, L. J., LaPierre, T. A., et al. (2007). All in the family: The impact of caring for grandchildren on grandparents' health. *The Journals of Gerontology Series B: Psychological Sciences and Social Sciences, 62,* S108–S119.

Researchers were interested in knowing what effects on the physical and psychological health occur among older adults when caring for grandchildren. Using a sample of 12,872 grandparents ages 50 through 80, they examined the relationship between various types of grandchild care and health of the grandparents. Researchers found no evidence to suggest that caring for grandchildren has dramatic and widespread negative effects on grandparents' health and mental well-being. In fact, the study actually revealed higher level physical health and emotional benefits to grandmothers who babysit. However, there were a small number of grandparents whose health might have been compromised by having children in the home, likely due to infections. This occurred as an exception rather than the rule in a smaller portion of older adults.

The findings were different when the parents are absent or minimally involved with childrearing. When parental involvement was low, grandmothers are more likely to experience poor health behaviors, depression, and lower self-rating of overall health. The findings of this study are important given continuing reliance on grandparents for care of children.

1. Based on this research, if you were the nurse, what kinds of information would you want to gather from families where grandparents provided custodial care to grandchildren?

2. What ways can you think of to support grandparents who assume major roles in raising grandchildren?

 Go to Chapter 12, **Toward Evidence-Based Practice Suggested Responses,** on the Student Resource Disk or DavisPlus at http://davisplus.fadavis.com/Wilkinson2

establish trust between the family and the nurse. Wellness interventions may include contracting, health teaching, anticipatory guidance, and promoting family cohesion during a crisis (e.g., hospitalization of a family member). For specific health promotion activities, see Chapter 41.

Interventions When a Family Member Is Ill

When a family member is ill or hospitalized, the other family members experience a range of emotions—especially when the illness is severe or of sudden onset. Family members may display signs of stress in a variety of ways, for example, by arguing with each other or with healthcare providers, by insisting on immediate care for their loved one, by avoiding the client's room, or by frequently asking that information be repeated. These are normal reactions; do not take them personally.

The patient and family need to understand the medical diagnosis, the plan of care, and what the recovery process will be like. In addition, it is often the nurse who provides extensive discharge instructions to the client and family before they leave the hospital. Specific interventions to help the family cope with the hospitalization of their loved one and manage stress include the following:

- Provide written materials explaining the client's diagnosis or condition.
- Actively involve the family in team meetings.
- Promptly follow up with family concerns or questions.
- Encourage the family to go home and rest.
- Encourage the family to call for updates when they cannot be present.
- Suggest ideas for stress-reducing activities (e.g., walking, meditating).
- Inform the family about on-site availability of a chaplain or chapel.
- Encourage the family to participate in care activities as appropriate.
- Keep the family informed of the client's progress.
- Help the family to identify sources of stress and develop strategies to work through and dissolve the root cause.
- Provide anticipatory guidance regarding outcome and expectations for discharge.

Interventions for Caregiver Role Strain

Interventions specific to caregiver role strain center include the following:

Assessing the caregiver for degree of impaired functioning (e.g., difficult sleeping, weight loss)

Assessing for safety issues that exist for the care receiver

Identifying causes of caregiver strain (e.g., lack of knowledge, frail client with around-the-clock care needs, complex treatments, or conflicts between caregiver and care receiver)

Helping the caregiver to identify and express feelings, including negative ones (e.g., by use of statements such as "This must be hard for you." Or, "I hear you saying you feel angry and confused.")

Supporting the caregiver's ability to manage the situation (e.g., by helping identify community supports, finding someone to share housekeeping activities)

Providing information about and demonstrating caregiving skills and techniques (e.g., dealing with the care receiver's pain)

For a list of NIC interventions for Caregiver Role Strain,

 Go to Chapter 12, **Standardized Outcomes and Interventions,** in Volume 2.

Interventions When There Is a Death in the Family

Death of a close family member is one of the most devastating life experiences. A family needs sensitive and compassionate care during this time, and such care is an appropriate focus for family-centered nursing. Interventions include facilitating the grieving process, encouraging communication, providing spiritual support, and providing compassionate care of the body after death. For more in-depth information about care of the family of a dying patient, see Chapter 15.

 Go to Chapter 12, **Resources for Caregivers and Health Professionals,** on the Student Resource Disk or DavisPlus at http://davisplus.fadavis.com/Wilkinson2

 Suggested Readings: Go to Chapter 12, **Reading More About the Family,** on the Student Resource Disk or DavisPlus at http://davisplus.fadavis.com/Wilkinson2

 Bibliography: Go to Volume 2, Bibliography.

CHAPTER 13

Culture & Ethnicity

Learning Outcomes

After completing this chapter you should be able to:

➤ Explain why cultural competence is important for nurses.

➤ Explain what is meant by "culture."

➤ Discuss concepts pertaining to cultural diversity in nursing.

➤ Identify the characteristics of culture, including their relationship to acculturation.

➤ Discuss patterns of behavior that can reflect cultural and ethnic influences.

➤ Identify vulnerable populations in the United States.

➤ Define and give an example of culture universals and of culture specifics.

➤ Differentiate between cultural archetypes and cultural stereotypes.

➤ Describe the culture of the North American healthcare system, including professional subcultures.

➤ Identify the phenomena of culture, including how they can affect the nursing care needs of clients and families.

➤ Discuss the differing views of culturally diverse clients, including biomedical, holistic, and alternative health systems, such as folk medicine.

➤ Discuss the definitions, theories, and models relating to the provision of culturally competent care.

➤ Explain guidelines for performing a transcultural assessment, including a cultural assessment model.

➤ Recognize the cultural implications inherent in nursing diagnoses.

➤ Describe nursing strategies that promote delivery of culturally competent care to clients and their families.

➤ State some techniques for communicating with clients when there is a language barrier.

Meet Your Patients

Your instructor has given you a clinical assignment. You are to spend the day in a walk-in clinic with a primary care provider and other students from your program. Your initial job is to greet the clients and help them complete a health history form. The first patient you greet is Romano Salvatore. He points to his head and moans. When you ask him what is wrong, he makes a gesture to convey to you that he does not understand what you are saying. He speaks a foreign language that sounds to you like Italian.

The next group to walk in the clinic includes a frantic young mother, Rosanna, with her son, José, 4 years old. José is crying and coughing. Rosanna informs you that José complains of a sore throat and has a fever. She also tells you that she has been to her *curandero,* but José is not getting any better. You also notice that José is wearing a heavy coat and knit hat although it is quite warm outside. When you question Rosanna about the child's clothing, she says that José is cold.

Lee Chan, an elderly Chinese American man, enters the clinic. Mr. Chan is accompanied by eight family members. Because the waiting area is small, all except his daughter Kim are asked to wait outside. Mr. Chan is quiet and does not make eye contact with you. His daughter Kim explains that her father has stomach cancer and is in a lot of pain because of disharmony. When you ask him to rate his pain, he just shakes his head and looks away. Would you wonder what *disharmony* means?

Theoretical **Knowledge knowing** why

Try to answer the following questions about the patients you have just met. You may not have the theoretical knowledge to answer them all—you will acquire that in this chapter—but do your best based on the background you now have.

 ### Critical **Thinking** 13-1

Think about Romano Salvatore.

- If you could speak Italian, what would you ask him?

Think about Rosanna and her child.

- One question that might spring immediately to your mind is, "What is a *curandero?*" How could you find out this information?
- Why do you think that the child is dressed more warmly than you would expect for the weather?

Think about Mr. Chan and his family.

- How would you feel about so many of his family members coming with Mr. Chan to the clinic?
- Why do you think he is not looking at or speaking to you?
- How could you communicate with Mr. Chan? Would you assume that he does not speak your language? Explain your reasoning.

Why Learn About Culture?

The following are some reasons for nurses to learn about culture and cultural competence.

The Population is Diverse. One important reason to learn about culture and ethnicity is that you will almost certainly care for patients who are not from your culture. The United States and Canada are multicultural societies—that is, made up of many cultures. For perhaps 20 years, we have seen increasing immigration from Asian and Spanish-speaking nations, coupled with a higher growth rate among blacks. In 2007, the U.S. Census Bureau classified 66% of the population as non-Hispanic white. In the United States, what were previously referred to as minority groups, when taken together, will soon make up a majority. The number and variety of different cultural and ethnic groups has also increased in the U.S., adding to the diversity. Similarly, population statistics in Canada reveal more than 200 different ethnic groups and a three-fold increase in minority populations since 1981, with Chinese Canadians comprising the largest minority group (Canadian Census, 2007). Figure 13-1 illustrates the change in racial and ethnic makeup expected to occur in the United States by 2050.

Critical **Thinking** 13-2

- With what cultural groups do you identify?
- In the neighborhood where you live, identify the cultural or ethnic groups that are different from your own. How many are there?
- In the school you are now attending, how many different cultural or ethnic groups are represented? What are they?

Health Disparities Exist Among Racial and Ethnic Groups. The Office of Minority Health & Health Disparities (2007) reports evidence that race and ethnicity

**Racial and Ethnic Makeup
2008 and 2050**

		2008	2050
White (not hispanic)		66%	46%
Hispanic		15%	30%
Black		14%	15%
Asian		5%	9%
All other races		1.6%	2%

Racial and ethnic makeup, 2008

Racial and ethnic makeup, 2050

FIGURE 13-1 Racial and ethnic makeup in the United States: 1995 and 2050. (*Source:* Adapted from: Hanson, S. (2001). *Family health care nursing: Theory, practice, and research* (2nd ed.). Philadelphia: F. A. Davis, p. 39; U. S. Census Bureau (2006a). Retrieved from http://www.census.gov/ipc/www/usinterimproj/)

correlate with health disparities in the United States. A *Healthy People 2020* overarching goal is to eliminate disparities and improve the health of all groups. One disparity is that minority groups experience higher rates of illness and death and, in general, poorer health status compared with the white, non-Hispanic population. For example:

The infant death rate among blacks is more than double that of whites. For American Indians and Alaska Natives it is almost double that of whites.

Women of Vietnamese origin suffer nearly five times the rate of cervical cancer as do white women.

Hispanics have higher rates of high blood pressure and obesity than non-Hispanic whites.

In nursing homes, use of physical restraints is higher among Hispanics and Asian/Pacific Islanders than among non-Hispanic whites (*National Healthcare Disparities Report*, 2003).

Nursing is Challenged to Provide Culturally Competent Care. Providing care to a culturally diverse population has become a challenge for nurses. In North America most nurses are white, and the healthcare culture reflects their culture. However, as you saw in the "Meet Your Patients" scenarios, nurses care for patients from many different races and cultures. Nursing care that is appropriate for the dominant cultural group may be ineffective and inappropriate for people with a different cultural heritage. Of course, it is impossible to know about every culture, but it is important to learn about the ones you will encounter most often in your practice. In addition, you will need to delegate and supervise others, ensuring that all clients receive culturally appropriate care. You need a good understanding of culture and ethnicity not only for providing direct care, but also for teaching, supervising, and role-modeling culturally competent care for other care providers.

KnowledgeCheck 13-1

- What do recent demographic trends in North America indicate?
- Why should nurses know more about the culture and ethnicity of clients?

Go to Chapter 13, **Knowledge Check Response Sheet and Answers,** on the Student Resource Disk or DavisPlus at http://davisplus.fadavis.com/Wilkinson2

What Is Meant by Culture?

To provide care in a culturally diverse population, you need to understand what the word *culture* means. Rooted in sociology and more specifically anthropology, we know that culture is both *universal* (everyone has it) and *dynamic* (active). Put simply, **culture** is what people in a group have in common, but it changes over time.

Purnell and Paulanka (2008) define **culture** as "the totality of socially transmitted behavior patterns, arts, beliefs, values, customs, lifeways, and all other products of human work and thought characteristics of a population of people that guides their worldview and decision making" (p. 404). For other definitions of culture,

Go to Chapter 13, **Supplemental Materials: Definitions of Culture,** on the Student Resource Disk or DavisPlus at http://davisplus.fadavis.com/Wilkinson2

Characteristics of Culture

When you are trying to determine what is meant by *culture* or *cultural*, keep in mind the following characteristics:

Culture is Learned. Learning occurs through life experiences shared with other members of the culture.

Culture is Taught. Cultural values, beliefs, and traditions are passed down from generation to generation, either formally (e.g., in schools) or informally (e.g., in families). Some generations totally adopt the values, beliefs, and traditions of their elders; others partially accept the teachings; and some generations move strongly away from them.

Culture is Shared by its Members. Cultural norms are shared through teachings and social interactions.

Culture is Dynamic and Adaptive. Cultural customs, beliefs, and practices are not static. They change over time and at different rates. Cultural change occurs with adaptation in response to the environment.

Culture is Complex. Reread the Purnell and Paulanka (2008) definition to review the many aspects of culture. Cultural assumptions and habits are unconscious and thus may be difficult for members of the culture to explain to others or to identify as different from another culture.

Culture is Diverse. Culture demonstrates the variety that exists among groups and among members of a particular group.

Culture Exists at Many Levels. Culture exists in both the material (art, writings, dress, or artifacts) and the nonmaterial (customs, traditions, language, beliefs, and practices).

Culture has Common Beliefs and Practices. Most members of a culture share the same beliefs, traditions, customs, and practices as long as they continue to be adaptive and satisfy the members' needs. Some members of the group may deviate from cultural norms, but for a norm to be considered cultural, many members must follow it.

Culture is All-encompassing. Culture can influence everything its members think and do.

Culture Provides Identity. Cultural beliefs provide identity and a sense of belonging for its members as long as they do not conflict with the dominant culture and continue to satisfy its members.

Critical Thinking 13-3

Figure 13-2 depicts an example of ways members of particular cultural groups express their cultural uniqueness in dance. Can you think of other ways that people express their culture?

Concepts Related to Culture

The term *bicultural* describes a person who identifies with two cultures and integrates some of the values and lifestyles of each into his life. The person uses more of one cultural base over another when situations call for it. Consider a Jewish man who marries an Italian Catholic woman. Their bicultural children may choose to follow

FIGURE 13-2 Traditional lunar New Year dancer in South Korea.

Jewish tradition while still holding some of the values and beliefs of their Italian heritage. A bicultural person may experience divided loyalties.

In this chapter, multicultural refers to many cultures and is used to describe groups rather than individuals. Many regions of the United States are multicultural, meaning that the region is populated by individuals from many different cultural groups. The same can be said about workplace settings. Remember that culture does not always refer to the ethnicity of a group. Think of a hospital: Caregivers may be members of various ethnic, racial, and religious groups, and the nurses, physicians, physical therapists, and students each comprise a different subculture. A hospital is thus a multicultural setting.

Socialization, Acculturation, and Assimilation

Socialization is the process of learning to become a member of a society or a group. A person becomes socialized by learning social rules and roles, by learning the behaviors, norms, values, and perceptions of others in the same group or role. Families, schools, churches, peer groups, and the media are agents of socialization and foster the development of a culture and its members' identification with it.

Immigrants (new members of a group or country) assume the characteristics of that culture through a learning process called **acculturation.** A person who is acculturated accepts both his own and the new culture, adopting elements of each. Acculturation is the outgrowth of the minority group's need to survive and flourish in the new culture. Many experts theorize that it takes several years, perhaps three generations, for an immigrant group to become acculturated. Some experts view bicultural identity as one level in the acculturation process.

Cultural assimilation occurs when the new members gradually learn and take on the essential values, beliefs, and behaviors of the dominant culture. Assimilation is complete when the newcomer is fully merged into the dominant cultural group. A person becomes assimilated by, for example, learning to speak the dominant language, marrying a member from the new (host) culture, and making close, personal relationships with members of the new group. For example, if you emigrated to Mexico, you would take with you your own language and food preferences. But over time, you would gradually begin to eat more of the local foods and learn to speak Spanish.

Dominant Cultures, Subcultures, and Minority Groups

If you are white, non-Hispanic (e.g., European American) and someone asks you, "What is your culture?" you may reply, "I don't know; I don't think I have one." But that is because you are from what historically has been the mainstream. Because the white culture has been dominant in North America, most white people have been around others similar to themselves. They have not been aware of their culture because they did not see it in contrast to other ways of being. Or, if they did see differences, they assumed their ways were the norm and that everyone else was culturally different.

Ethnocentrism is the tendency to think that your own group (cultural, professional, ethnic, or social) is superior to others and to view behaviors and beliefs that differ greatly from your own as somehow wrong, strange, or unenlightened. The tendency to ethnocentrism exists in all groups, not just in the dominant culture.

What do you think is the dominant culture of the United States and Canada? If you said white or white or European American, you would be only partially correct. The ancestors of most white Americans emigrated from Europe, and many were of Protestant or other Christian religions. We can then say that the dominant culture in the United States and Canada is white Anglo-Saxon Christian of European descent. A **dominant culture** is the group that has the most authority or power to control values and reward or punish behaviors. It is usually, but not always, the largest group.

Subcultures are groups within a larger culture or social system that have some characteristics (e.g., values, behaviors, ancestry, ways of living) that are different from those of the dominant culture. People in subcultures have had different experiences from those in the dominant group because of status, residence, gender, sexual orientation, ethnic background, education, or other factors that unify the group (Purnell & Paulanka, 2008). You may be able to recognize subcultures by their speech patterns, dress, gestures, eating habits, lifestyles, and so on. Some examples of subcultures are street

gangs, physicians, nurses, women, older adults, persons with disabilities, gays and lesbians, people of Appalachian heritage, rural Midwesterners, and people who abuse certain drugs.

Minority groups are also made up of individuals who share race, religion, or ethnic heritage; however, a minority group has fewer members than the majority group. Depending on the type of group, they may or may not share beliefs, practices, or physical characteristics. The term *minority* is sometimes used to refer to a group of people who receive different and unequal treatment from others in society. Some consider it an offensive term because it suggests inferiority and marginalization.

Vulnerable Populations as Subcultures

Vulnerable populations are groups who are more likely to develop health problems and experience poorer outcomes because of limited access to care, high-risk behaviors, and/or multiple and cumulative stressors. Examples include people who are homeless (Fig. 13-3), poor, or mentally ill; people with physical disabilities; the very young; and older adults. Some ethnic and racial minority groups are also vulnerable. For example, among American Indians and Native Alaskans, there is a higher incidence of diabetes, earlier in life, with a higher mortality rate (Urban Indian Health Commission, 2007). Vulnerable populations can be considered subcultures of all of the major cultural groups.

Socioeconomic vulnerability is particularly important. There is probably more variation among people of the same ethnic group but of different social classes than there is among people of different ethnic groups but of the same social class. The subculture of poverty can be found throughout the world.

The public health initiative *Healthy People 2020* addresses the care of vulnerable populations and includes as one of 4 broad goals, the elimination of health inequities. Nursing research is beginning to address these inequities, such as in studying the effectiveness of interventions for treating the mentally ill (Burns, Catty, Becker, et al., 2007; Cloyes, 2007), and in the diagnosis and treatment of heart disease in women of color (Strickland, Giger, Nelson, et al., 2007). When caring for patients from vulnerable populations, it is important that you focus on their strengths and resources, not exclusively on their difficulties and risks. *Healthy People 2020* will be available in 2010. Keep checking for those new initiatives on the U. S. Department of Health & Human Services Web site,

 Go to http://www.healthypeople.gov/HP2020/

Gender as a Subculture

It should come as no surprise that some behaviors are considered acceptable for men but not for women, and vice versa; and that there are values and responses considered more typical of one sex than of the other. For example, in the dominant culture it is more acceptable for women to cry out in pain than for men, who are supposed to "be strong." As another example, the U.S. and Canadian cultures tend to view caring and nurturing as

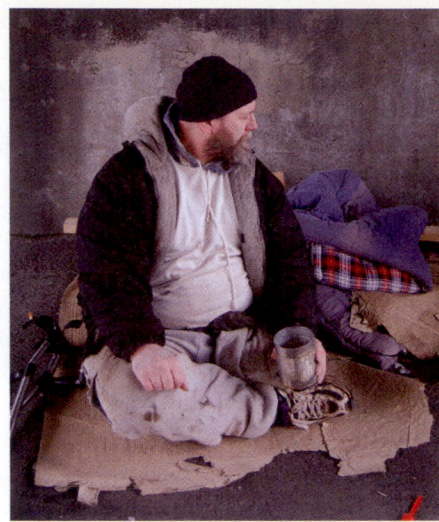

FIGURE 13-3 A homeless man sits on his cardboard begging for spare change.

the province of women, not of men. For example, as cited in Chapter 1, only 6% of registered nurses in the United States and Canada are men, although in 2006 men represented 12.1% of nursing school graduates in the United States.

Ethnicity, Race, and Religion

People sometimes use the terms culture, ethnicity, and race interchangeably, but in fact they have separate, specific meanings.

Ethnicity

Ethnicity is similar to *culture* in that it refers to groups whose members share a common social and cultural heritage that is passed down from generation to generation. However, ethnicity is also similar to *subculture,* in that the members of an **ethnic group** have some characteristics in common (e.g., race, ancestry, physical characteristics, geographic region, lifestyle, religion) that are not shared or understood by outsiders. Examples of ethnic groups include French Canadians, Roman Catholics, Hmongs, and Latinos.

Ethnicity may include race, but it is not the same as race. To demonstrate this statement, the U.S. Census Bureau has numerous categories for race (see the next section). In addition, it identifies two categories for ethnicity: (1) Hispanic, Latino, or Spanish and (2) *Not* Hispanic, Latino, or Spanish. People of Hispanic, Latino, or Spanish origin may be of any race. Subcategories under category (1) are: Mexican, Mexican American, Chicano, Puerto Rican, Cuban, and another Hispanic, Latino, or Spanish origin. The census allows people to choose their race. That is, the people—not the census taker—choose the race with which they identify. Hispanic Americans are people who originally came from any Spanish-speaking country (e.g., Mexico, Spain, and countries in Central and South America). More than 60% of the Hispanic population in the United States are of Mexican origin. **Latino,**

strictly speaking, refers only to people from Latin America (Central or South America). Spanish implies origin in Spain. If you know a client's country of origin, it is more accurate to use it when referring to the client's ethnic origin (e.g., Mexican American, Colombian American) than to use either the term *Hispanic* or *Latino*.

Race

Unlike ethnicity, race is strictly related to biology. **Race** refers to the grouping of people based on biological similarities, such as skin color, blood type, or bone structure (Purnell & Paulanka, 2008). The terms *race* and *ethnicity* overlap somewhat, because race can be a characteristic of a specific ethnic group. The U.S. Census Bureau now divides the population into the following lengthy list of racial categories (U.S. Census Bureau, 2010). Any of the races can be found in the Hispanic/Latino/Spanish category because the Census Bureau does not include Hispanic/Latino/Spanish as a race, but as a sociocultural category. The census form list is as follows:

- White
- Black, black, or Negro
- American Indian or Alaska Native
- [Asian Categories]
  Asian Indian
  Chinese
  Filipino
  Japanese
  Korean
  Vietnamese
  Other Asian
- Native Hawaiian
- [Pacific Islander Categories]
  Guamanian or Chamorro
  Samoan
  Other Pacific Islander (specify, e.g., Tongan)

For definitions of these categories,

 Go to **2010 U.S. Census Questionnaire Guide Book** at http://2010.census.gov/partners/pdf/langfiles/qrb_English.pdf

Remember, those are U.S. Census Bureau terms; if you are culturally sensitive, you will ask people what race they identify with and what name they prefer to use for it. For its purposes, the Census Bureau defines race as reflecting "self-identification by people according to the race or races with which they most closely identify" (U.S. Census Bureau, 2008).

Can you determine a person's race by his appearance? Frequently not. So, then, is race determined by heredity? What race is someone whose father is black and whose mother is white? Historically, most North Americans would say that the person is black. In some other countries (e.g., most of South America), though, that same person would be categorized as white. Although we usually think of race as being based on biological characteristics, anthropologists prefer to think of it as human variation or diversity. Many, including the

U.S. Census Bureau, believe that race is socially rather than biologically determined (U.S. Census Bureau, 2010). For more information on race as a social construct,

 Go to Chapter 13, **Supplemental Materials, "Race as a Social Construct,"** on the Student Resource Disk or DavisPlus at http://davisplus.fadavis.com/Wilkinson2

We all tend to group and categorize data to make it meaningful and useful, but we must be careful to avoid using these categories as the basis for interacting with people or providing care. For example, there are hundreds of subcultures under the broad category of white. When you need to designate a name for a group, be as specific as possible; that is, when you know the client's country of heritage, say, for example, Syrian American instead of white or white .

Religion

Religion may be confused with ethnicity because people within an ethnic group may share the same religion. For example, the Jewish culture overlaps with Jewish faith community. **Religion** refers to an ordered system of beliefs regarding the cause, nature, and purpose of the universe, especially the beliefs related to the worship of a God or gods (Andrews & Boyle, 2007). In many cultures, religion is a high priority (Fig. 13-4).

These distinctions between culture, ethnicity, race, and religion might seem confusing, but think of it this way: You are a member of the subculture of nursing, but you are also a member of an ethnic group (e.g., Portuguese Americans from the Azores), a racial group (e.g., white), and a religion (e.g., Roman Catholicism), each

FIGURE 13-4 Even in this tiny community of rural Appalachia, people have built a place for worship.

with its own sets of beliefs and values. So, your culture is a blend of all of those.

KnowledgeCheck 13-2
- Define culture.
- Give an example of each: ethnic group, race, religion.
- How does culture provide identity for an individual?
- Give an example of acculturation.

 Go to Chapter 13, **Knowledge Check Response Sheet and Answers,** on the Student Resource Disk or DavisPlus at http://davisplus.fadavis.com/Wilkinson2

How Do Cultural Values, Beliefs, and Practices Affect Health?

Values are important because they help shape health-related beliefs and practices. Do you know what values are? Think for a minute about what you "value" in your own life. What are the five ideals, principles, or things that are most important to you?

You may name, for example, learning, family, independence, faith, and cleanliness. Or you may have said something entirely different. Simply put, a personal value is a principle or standard that has meaning or worth to an individual. An example is cleanliness. In contrast, a belief is something that one accepts as true (e.g., "I believe that germs cause disease"), and a practice is a set of behaviors that one follows (e.g., "I always wash my hands before preparing food"). Do you see how values, beliefs, and practices are related?

Cultural values, beliefs, and practices are the principles, standards, ideas, and behaviors that members of a cultural group share. An example of a cultural value is the European American preoccupation with bodily cleanliness. Other values of the dominant U.S. culture include youth, beauty, success, independence, and material belongings. You should not assume a client shares your values, beliefs, and practices—nor those of the dominant culture. Instead, become familiar with the specific values, beliefs, and practices of clients from the different cultural and ethnic (ethnocultural) groups in your community. Remember, though, that individuals within an ethnocultural group vary widely and that *learning commonalities is no substitute for careful assessment of each person*.

What Are Culture Specifics?

Culture universals are the values, beliefs, and practices that people from *all* cultures share. Leininger and McFarland (2006) calls these culture commonalities. In contrast, **culture specifics** (culture diversities in Leininger's theory) are those values, beliefs, and practices that are special or unique to a culture. Let's look at an example. All cultures celebrate the birth of a new baby in some way (a culture universal), but different cultures celebrate "birth rites" in different ways (a culture specific). In Belize, a baby is christened before visitors are allowed, a practice carried out to prevent the *evil eye* (bad spells cast by others); in Greece, *amulets* (objects or charms worn to protect from evil spirits) may be placed on the baby; and in Israel, Jewish male infants are circumcised on the eighth day of life. Similarly, people from all cultures practice marriage rituals in elaborate rituals that are culture specific (Fig. 13-5).

Archetype or Stereotype?

At about this point is where, in your efforts to be culturally sensitive, you might be thinking: "Wait a minute. I went to a Chinese wedding, and it was no different from my own wedding"; or "I know plenty of Greek people who don't put amulets on their babies." Of course you are correct. However, acknowledging that there are commonalities within a group is not the same as saying that *all* people in the group have those characteristics. And that is, more or less, the difference between an archetype and a stereotype.

A **cultural stereotype** is a widely held but oversimplified and unsubstantiated belief that all people of a certain racial or ethnic group are alike in certain respects. Stereotypes are not always negative. Someone may think, for example, that people of a particular heritage are "naturally intelligent" or "naturally athletic." A **cultural archetype** is similar to a model, which you learned about in Chapter 8. An archetype is an *example* of a person or thing—something that is recurrent—and it has its basis in facts. Therefore, it becomes a symbol for remembering some of the culture specifics, and is usually not negative (Campinha-Bacote, 2007). For example, you might think of Mexican Americans as having brown eyes, or of European Americans as having light-colored skin. There is nothing negative about eye color or skin color.

You may encounter cultural archetypes throughout this chapter. Bear in mind there is probably more variation among people *within* an ethnic or cultural group than there is *between* the groups, and that much variation stems from socioeconomic differences or regional origin as much as from race or ethnicity. Each person must be seen as unique—as influenced by his heritage, but not defined by it.

How Do Culture Specifics Affect Health?

Just as they influence our celebrations of births and weddings, culture specifics affect our health beliefs and behaviors. Thus, knowledge of the culture specifics of groups in your community will help explain why clients from different cultures have different expectations of healthcare. And ultimately, it will help you to provide culturally competent care.

Now let's look at six culture specifics that influence health: communication, space, time orientation, social organization, environmental control, and biological variations (Giger & Davidhizar, 2008). We will briefly discuss several other culture specifics: religion and philosophy, politics and the law, the economy, and education.

Communication

Communication includes verbal and nonverbal language (i.e., spoken language, gestures, eye contact, and even silences). Think how difficult it would be if you became ill in a foreign country. How would you tell the caregivers your symptoms? How would you know what they were going to do to treat your illness? Language differences present one of the most difficult obstacles to providing care. Even when you and the client speak the same language, culture influences how feelings and thoughts are expressed and which verbal and nonverbal expressions are appropriate to use. For example, Arabs tend to keep steady eye contact when talking, but not between men and women; Asians and Native Americans usually do not make eye contact (Purnell & Paulanka, 2008). You will learn more about communication strategies when we discuss culturally competent care. Also see Chapter 18 for communication strategies, if you wish.

Space

Space refers to a person's personal space, or how the person relates toward the space around him. Another similar word, **territoriality,** means the behavior and attitude that people exhibit about the area around them they have claimed (Spector, 2004). Both of these ideas are influenced by culture. A person's comfort level is related to space. When an individual's personal space is protected, he feels secure and safe, less anxious, and in control. The following are some examples

FIGURE 13-5 People of all cultures practice marriage rituals.

of culturally influenced attitudes toward personal space:

- Americans, Canadians of Northern European ancestry, and the British keep at least 18 inches of space between themselves and the person with whom they are conversing.
- Arabs and others from the Middle East typically stand quite close when talking.
- Germans usually require a great deal of space, and consider even looking into a room an invasion of privacy.

Within all cultural groups, personal space varies depending on the relationship between the people speaking: intimates versus acquaintances, people of the same versus opposite sex, and people of a different position within the social hierarchy.

Time Orientation

Time orientation varies among people of different cultures. Some persons tend to be present- or future-oriented, whereas others are more rooted in the past. As an example, European Americans tend to be future-oriented. In contrast, Native Americans and Latinos may be more present-oriented. Differences in time orientation can be important as you plan nursing interventions for your clients. For example, for clients who are present-oriented and may tend to show up late (or not at all) for follow-up appointments, you should provide a written or telephone reminder of their appointment.

CriticalThinking 13-4

- Suppose you say to a client, "You will need to exercise and follow a low-calorie diet to lose weight and control your diabetes." What kind of time orientation would a client most likely have in order to follow your directions?
- Suppose a client says, "I know I need to lose weight, but I work so much, and the children take so much time. I just don't have time to shop and cook for the right foods or to exercise." What time orientation does this illustrate?

Social Organization

Social organization includes the family unit (e.g., nuclear, single-parent, or extended family) and the wider organizations (e.g., community, religious, ethnic) with which the individual or family identifies (Spector, 2004). A close social organization can be found in all cultures; however, the specifics vary. For example, in Middle Eastern and Latino cultures, the man is likely to be the dominant family member and the woman the homemaker. But many black families are matriarchal; that is, the decision maker and family leader is a woman.

The social organization of your clients' cultures can provide clues as to how they will act during such life events, as birth, death, illness, grieving, and mourning. For example, imagine a patient who must depend on Medicaid to pay for her healthcare, but who does not

trust large institutions or government agencies. She is likely to use home remedies and to delay seeing a conventional medical physician.

Kinship and social ties also determine who receives healthcare, and in what priority. In the United States, for example, someone of high status (e.g., a celebrity or political figure) is likely to receive better care than a poor person who is unknown in the community. In some cultures, men receive care before women and children.

Environmental Control

Environmental control refers to a person's perception of his ability to plan activities that control nature or direct environmental factors (Spector, 2004). Included in this phenomenon are health and illness beliefs and practices. For example, if a person does not believe he can do anything to "change things," how would this attitude affect his decision to seek medical care? To take medications? To exercise and eat properly? Perception and tolerance of pain is an example of the effect of environmental control. Some people, especially Asian Americans, tend to accept pain stoically, and not demand relief. They do not view circumstances as something to be "controlled." Think again about Mr. Chan ("Meet Your Patients"). Why do you think he just shakes his head and looks away when asked to rate his pain?

Biological Variations

Biological variations include ways in which people are different genetically and physiologically. They create susceptibility to certain diseases and injuries. Biological variations include body build and structure, skin color, vital signs, enzymatic and genetic variations, and drug metabolism (Purnell & Paulanka, 2008; Spector, 2004, p. 23). Most drug studies in the past were based on European American subjects, so "variations" usually refers to differences from those norms (e.g., blacks metabolize antihypertensives differently from European Americans). For more information about assessing biological variations,

 Go to Chapter 13, **Clinical Insights 13-1: Assessing for Biological Variations,** in Volume 2.

To read more about biological susceptibility to diseases,

 Go to Chapter 13, **Supplemental Materials: Disease Risks for Each of the Major Cultural Groups of the United States,** on the Student Resource Disk or DavisPlus at http:// davisplus.fadavis.com/Wilkinson2

Other Culture Specifics

The following may also be culture specifics. The first two, religion/philosophy and education, vary among subcultures in the United States. The other three (technology, politics/law, and the economy) exert broader effects that can be seen among different countries, but less so among subcultures within a country.

Religion and Philosophy. A person's religion may determine what healthcare is acceptable to him. For example, some religions (e.g., Jehovah's Witnesses) do not accept blood transfusions, and many religions forbid abortion.

Education. Education influences the perception of wellness and illness and the knowledge of options that are available for healthcare. These, in turn, affect the person's expectations for care.

Technology. The availability of supplies and equipment determines what is used in the healthcare setting and what comes to be culturally expected. Nurses in most of North America, for example, assume they will have bed linens, water, electricity, necessary medications, and technology such as electrocardiography and x-ray imaging. In many parts of the world, however, these items are not available.

Politics and the Law. Governmental policies affect healthcare. They determine what practitioners will be available and what programs will be funded; for example, the federal government helps fund Medicare, which provides basic medical insurance for people age 65 and older. The legislation passed in 2010 will extend federal funding of healthcare to people of all ages. The legal system defines roles, functions, and standards of health professionals.

Economy. The condition of the economy directly affects the availability of funds for publicly funded services. It also affects the individual's ability to pay for healthcare.

For more information about each of these dimensions of culture,

 Go to Chapter 13, **Tables, Boxes, Figures: ESG Table 13-2,** on the Student Resource Disk or DavisPlus at http:// davisplus.fadavis.com/Wilkinson2

 Critical**Thinking** 13-5

Consider this example: Mrs. Miyagi, a Japanese American, has been admitted to your care on a medical–surgical unit from the postanesthesia care unit (PACU), having undergone a major surgical procedure. She refuses pain medicine, although she appears to you to be in pain. As the hours pass, Mrs. Miyagi continues to refuse the pain medication, so eventually the nurses stop asking.

- Do you assume that she is experiencing no pain?
- Are you or the other nurses stereotyping her for her cultural response to pain?
- What would you do?

KnowledgeCheck 13-3

- Explain the difference between an archetype and a stereotype.
- Identify at least six culture specifics affecting health.
- How could you use this information about culture specifics to provide better care to your clients?

 Go to Chapter 13, **Knowledge Check Response Sheet and Answers,** on the Student Resource Disk or DavisPlus at http://davisplus.fadavis.com/Wilkinson2

What Is the "Culture of Healthcare"?

In any culture, two healthcare systems usually exist side by side: indigenous and professional (Leininger, 1995). Each has its own culture. The **indigenous healthcare system** consists of *folk medicine* and *traditional healing methods,* which may also include over-the-counter (OTC) and self-treatment remedies. Different groups have different folk practices (Table 13-1).

In contrast, the **professional healthcare system** is run by a set of professional healthcare providers who have been formally educated and trained for their appropriate roles and responsibilities. In North America, professional healthcare is dominated by the biomedical healthcare system, which combines Western biomedical beliefs with traditional North American values of self-reliance, individualism, and aggressive action. This system is also known as Western medicine and allopathic medicine. The professional healthcare system also includes practitioners formally trained in alternative healthcare, such as diet therapy, mind–body control methods, therapeutic touch, acupressure, reflexology, naturopathy, kinesiology, and chiropractic. (If you want more information about these, refer to Chapter 40.) All cultural groups probably use the professional healthcare system to at least some degree.

Many professional healthcare providers do not understand the beliefs and practices of the indigenous healthcare systems and traditional healers. For this reason, conflicts arise: The professional provider views the indigenous beliefs and practices as uncivilized and based on the supernatural, and believers in indigenous methods view the professional healthcare culture with distrust. This type of thinking benefits no one. As a nurse, you should become aware of and understand a variety of health beliefs and practices so that you can meet the needs of your clients and families.

What Are Health and Illness Beliefs?

To provide culturally competent care, you need to know how people in various cultural groups understand life processes, how they define health and illness, and what they believe to be the causes of illness (American Nurses Association [ANA], 1997). Generally speaking, people follow one of three major health belief systems: scientific, magico-religious, or holistic (Andrews & Boyle, 2007). You are probably familiar with the **scientific** or **biomedical health system.** Belief in supernatural (mystical) forces dominates the **magico-religious system,** which is considered "alternative" or "indigenous" in the United States and Canada. One example is voodoo, which is practiced in some developing nations in Africa,

Table 13-1 ➤ Folk Healers and Practices

CULTURAL GROUP	FOLK HEALERS	FOLK PRACTICES
White, European American	Nurse	Medicines (OTC and prescribed)
	Physician	Therapeutic or modified diets
	Chiropractor	Exercise
	Acupuncturist	Religious healing rituals (including prayer)
	Massage therapist	Sleep
	Physical therapist	Cleanliness
	Occupational therapist	Amulets
	Respiratory therapist	Herbal therapy
		Naturopathy
		Massage
		Spinal adjustment
		Aromatherapy
Hispanic	*Curandero/curandera*	"Hot" and "cold" therapies
	Espiritualista (spiritualist)	Medals and amulets
	Partera	Prayers
	Yerbero (herbalist)	Herbs and herbal teas
	Sabador	Massage
		Jewelry to ward off the "Evil Eye"
Black	"Old lady" healers	Herbs
	Spiritualist	Oils and poultices
	Hougan, or voodoo priest or priestess	Talismans and amulets (worn or carried to ward off evil)
		Religious rituals ("laying on of hands")
Native American, Eskimo, and Aleut	*Shaman*	Herbs, incantations, and prayers
	Crystal gazer	Rituals and healing ceremonies
	Hand trembler	Blessed medicine bundles or other dried plants or flowers, or burning of dried plants
	Medicine woman or man	
		Stargazing and sandpainting
Asian and Pacific Islander	Herbalist	"Hot" and "cold" foods
	Acupuncturist	Herbs
	Physician	Meditation
	Priest	Acupuncture (inserting needles into meridians or life energy pathways)
		Acupressure
		Energy (Qi) to restore *yin, yang* balance

Sources: Adapted from Andrews, M. M., & Boyle, J. S. (2007). *Transcultural concepts in nursing care* (5th ed.). Philadelphia: Lippincott Williams & Wilkins; Giger, J., & Davidhizar, R. (2008). *Transcultural nursing: Assessment and intervention* (5th ed.). St. Louis, MO: C.V. Mosby; Purnell, L., & Paulanka, B. (2008). *Transcultural healthcare: A culturally competent approach* (3rd ed.). Philadelphia: F. A. Davis; and Spector, R. (2004). *Cultural diversity in health and illness* (6th ed.). Upper Saddle River, NJ: Prentice-Hall.

Latin America, and the Caribbean, and which considers the lion a spiritual symbol (Fig. 13-6). The **holistic belief system** can be similar to magico-religious, but it focuses more on the need for harmony and balance of the body with nature.

What Are Health and Illness Practices?

In addition to knowing the values and beliefs of different cultures, you need to know what people in various cultural groups do to maintain wellness.

FIGURE 13-6 Voodoo is an example of a magico-religious belief system. *Top*, A haitian voodoo shrine (notice the lion). *Bottom*, A haitian man costumed for carnival as the spirit of the lion.

CriticalThinking 13-6

- What do you do to keep yourself healthy?
- What do you do to treat minor illnesses when you do not want to see a physician?

Think about Mr. Chan ("Meet Your Patients"). If he or his daughter asked for a Chinese priest to come to his room and perform a ceremony to restore his harmony, do you think this ceremony would be harmful or helpful to him? Would you support or discourage this? What about Rosanna's dressing her child in a heavy coat and knit hat although it is quite warm outside? Is this harmful or helpful to them? Would you support or discourage this? As you think about those questions,

keep in mind that cultural health practices can be any of the following (Giger & Davidhizar, 2008):

Efficacious (helpful)
Neutral (neither helpful nor causing harm)
Dysfunctional (harmful)
Uncertain (not known)

You should encourage practices that could be helpful and discourage those that may cause harm. There should be no harm in allowing a patient to continue a neutral health practice. For example, people of Arab heritage associate good health with eating properly and fasting to cure disease. Some may treat illness with prayers or simple foods such as dates, honey, salt, and olive oil (Purnell & Paulanka, 2008). You would not want to interfere with these neutral practices. However, you should discourage dysfunctional activities, such as taking herbal remedies along with prescribed drugs without informing the healthcare provider.

KnowledgeCheck 13-4

- List three types of alternative healthcare that are delivered by formally trained practitioners as a part of the professional healthcare system.
- What are magico-religious belief systems?
- As a nurse, in which of the following cultural health practices would you support your client: efficacious, neutral, dysfunctional, uncertain? Why?
- Refer to the "Meet Your Patients" feature. Identify an efficacious practice.

 Go to Chapter 13, **Knowledge Check Response Sheet and Answers,** on the Student Resource Disk or DavisPlus at http://davisplus.fadavis.com/Wilkinson2

CriticalThinking 13-7

What aspects of the indigenous and professional systems have you used for yourself or your family? Give examples.

What Is the Culture of the North American Healthcare System?

Members of the biomedical healthcare system in the United States and Canada belong to a culture with its own set of norms. That culture can be further divided into subcultures, such as those of physicians, nurses, respiratory therapists, and so on. Some of the norms found in these overlapping subcultures include the following (Leppa, 2000):

- Belief in and reliance on the biomedical system
- Valuing of technology
- Desire to conquer disease
- Definition of health as the absence or minimization of disease
- Adherence to a set of ethical standards and codes of conduct

Table 13-2 summarizes the norms of the North American healthcare system.

Table 13-2 ➤ Summary of Cultural Norms of The North American Healthcare System	
NORM	**EXAMPLES**
Beliefs	Standardized definitions of health and illness
	Significance of technology
Practices	Maintaining health and preventing disease through such practices as immunizations and avoidance of stress
	Annual physical examinations and diagnostic tests
Habits	Handwashing
	Use of jargon (e.g., "take your vitals")
	Use of problem-solving methods
	Documentation
Likes	Punctuality
	Neatness and organization
	Compliance (e.g., with medical "orders")
Dislikes	Tardiness
	Disorganization
	Messiness, lack of cleanliness
Customs	Use of procedures (e.g., circumcision, last rites) surrounding birth and death
	Professional respect and observance of hierarchy found in autocratic and bureaucratic systems
Rituals	Annual physical examination
	The surgical procedure

Sources: Adapted from Giger, J., & Davidhizar, R. (2008). *Transcultural nursing: Assessment and intervention* (5th ed.). St. Louis, MO: C.V. Mosby; Munoz, C. & Luckmann, J. (2004). *Transcultural communication In healthcare.* Clifton Park, NY: Thomson Delmar; Purnell, L., & Paulanka, B. (2007). *Transcultural Healthcare: A culturally competent approach* (3rd ed.). Philadelphia: F. A. Davis; and Spector, R. (2004). *Cultural diversity in health and illness* (6th ed.). Upper Saddle River, NJ: Prentice-Hall.

Nursing and Other Professional Subcultures

Nursing is the largest subculture within the healthcare culture. Leininger (1978) defines the **culture of nursing** as the learned and transmitted lifeways, values, symbols, patterns, and normative practices of members of the nursing profession that are not the same as those of the mainstream culture. The nursing subculture's beliefs and values have been formed in part by the society at large, which historically has been dominated by white Anglo-Saxon Protestants. Nursing values include, in addition to those listed in Table 13-2, the following:

- Silent suffering as a response to pain
- Objective reporting and description of pain, but not an emotional response
- Use of the nursing process

- Nursing autonomy
- Caring

In this book, we add *knowledge* and *critical thinking* to the list of nursing values. Although these values may not be consistently rewarded in practice, we believe that a steadily increasing number of nurses realize their importance—that nursing is "knowledge work" and that the nurse's knowledge and thinking are of paramount importance to the well-being of patients.

As you become more socialized into the nursing culture, you should continue to examine professional values to see how strongly you identify with them and how they affect your work with patients. For example, if you value silent suffering in response to pain, how might that cause you to respond to a woman in very early labor who is screaming and crying even though her contractions are very mild on palpation? Would you dismiss her for being a "whiner"? Or scold her ("You can't be hurting that badly this early in labor")? You must be careful not to lose the ability to understand health and illness from the patient's point of view.

Review the case of Rosanna and José ("Meet Your Patients"). After a positive strep test, the primary care provider prescribes an antibiotic for José's fever and sore throat. You observe that Rosanna does not seem to be happy with the medicine, so you stress to her the importance of buying the medicine right away to make him better. On her way out of the clinic, Rosanna throws the prescription in the trash. Why do you think she threw away the prescription?

If you had difficulty thinking of possible answers to the question, see Table 13-3. Also,

 Go to the **Hispanic health cultural specifics** in **ESG Table 13-1** on the Student Resource Disk or DavisPlus at http://davisplus.fadavis.com/Wilkinson2

Some people of Mexican heritage believe that illness is caused by the body's imbalance of "hot" and "cold" (not related to temperature). The scenario doesn't tell you for sure, but it could be that Rosanna did not believe the medication would help her son, so she decided not to spend money on it. Could this problem have been prevented? The answer is yes. You or the primary care provider should have assessed Rosanna's health beliefs and practices and involved her in José's care by discussing treatment options with her. The provider should have asked Rosanna whether the medication was acceptable to her, and if not, asked her to explain her ideas about José's illness. For example, if she considered his ear infection to be "hot," then a "cold" herb or medication would be needed. The provider might have been able to explain that the ordered medication would get rid of the heat and pain that José is experiencing from the infection or find another medication that Rosanna would consider to be "cold."

Table 13-3 ➤ Values and Health and Illness Beliefs and Practices for Selected Ethnocultural Groups in North America

GROUP	DOMINANT VALUES	HEALTH AND ILLNESS BELIEFS	HEALTH AND ILLNESS PRACTICES
Native American	Bonding to family or group Acceptance of nature (Mother Earth) Tradition Sharing Belief in a spiritual power Respect of elders	Health means living in harmony with nature. Surviving under difficult circumstances Body treated with respect Illness is associated with disharmony or evil spirits. Illness is caused by an action that should not have been performed.	Rituals and ceremonies Chanting Purification Meditation Herbs
Asian and Pacific Islander	Extended family Respect for elders Group orientation Subordination to authority Conformity Self-respect and self-control Love of the land	Health is a state of physical and spiritual harmony. Illness is disharmony of basic principles: *yin* and *yang*.	Acupuncture Amulets Moxibustion Meditation Herbs
Black or African American	Family bonding Matrifocal Spiritual orientation Present-oriented	Health is harmony with nature (mind, body, and spirit). Illness is due to disharmony or failure to eat proper foods.	Prayer Laying on of hands Magic rituals Voodoo Herbs
Hispanic or Latino	Extended family Group emphasis Fatalistic Faith and spirituality	Health is good luck or a reward for good behavior, a gift from God. Illness is body imbalance (hot or cold, wet or dry) or punishment.	Prayer Belief in miracles Wearing of religious metals or amulets Religious relics in home Herbs and spices Rituals "Hot" and "cold" therapy
White or European American	Independence Individuality Wealth Comfort Cleanliness Achievement Youth and beauty	Health is a state of physical and emotional well-being. Illness is contagion or contamination that is hereditary, psychosomatic, or supernatural	Biomedical care Home remedies Religious traditions Diet and exercise

Note: Most people in North America use a combination of biomedical and traditional (specific to their culture) healthcare practices.
Sources: Adapted from Giger, J., & Davidhizar, R. (2008). *Transcultural nursing: Assessment and intervention* (5th ed.). St. Louis, MO: C.V. Mosby; Munoz, C. & Luckmann, J. (2004). *Transcultural communication in healthcare.* Clifton Park, NY: Thomson Delmar; Spector, R. (2004). *Cultural diversity in health and illness* (6th ed.). Upper Saddle River, NJ: Prentice-Hall; Andrews, M., & Boyle, J. (1999). *Transcultural concepts in nursing care* (3rd ed.). Philadelphia: Lippincott; and Purnell, L., & Paulanka, B. (2007). *Transcultural healthcare: A culturally competent approach* (3rd ed.). Philadelphia: F.A. Davis.

This is an example of what can happen when healthcare providers are so rigidly grounded in the beliefs of the professional healthcare culture that they fail to recognize and understand the health beliefs and practices of their clients. As you may guess, this way of practicing is a barrier to culturally competent care.

Knowledge Check 13-5

How do the cultural norms of the North American healthcare system differ from those of other cultural groups? Refer to Tables 13-2 and 13-3 in this chapter as needed.

 Go to Chapter 13, **Knowledge Check Response Sheet and Answers,** on the Student Resource Disk or DavisPlus at http://davisplus.fadavis.com/Wilkinson2

Traditional and Alternative Healing

You need to know how healers from various cultures cure and care for members of their group (ANA, 1997). All cultures think of their healthcare system and beliefs as "traditional"; however, we use *traditional* in this chapter to refer to alternative beliefs, those that are not of the Western, North American, biomedical, or professional healthcare systems (previously discussed). You have already learned about different healthcare beliefs and practices clients may have (e.g., biomedical or scientific, holistic, magico-religious). The following section focuses on the types of healing systems that are used in different cultures.

Folk Medicine

When you feel as if you're getting a cold or the flu, what do you do? If you said that you take aspirin or vitamin C or eat chicken soup, then you are practicing folk medicine. You most likely do what your mother or some other relative did for you in similar situations. In North America there is a "pill" for almost everything, and virtually everyone self-medicates with over-the-counter medicines. For many cultures, folk medicine involves natural medicines, such as herbs, plants, minerals, and animal substances. Magico-religious folk medicine involves the use of charms, holy words, rituals, and holy actions for preventing and treating illnesses (Spector, 2004).

Folk medicine is defined as the beliefs and practices that the members of a cultural group follow when they are ill, as opposed to more conventional (i.e., biomedical or professional) standards (Andrews & Boyle, 2007). All cultures throughout the world use folk medicine. These treatments have lasted over time, and knowledge of them is passed down from generation to generation by oral, and sometimes written, tradition. Folk medicine includes both self-treatment and use of folk healers.

Why would someone want to see a folk healer rather than a professional healthcare provider? In the dominant North American culture, the folk healer *is* the professional healthcare provider (i.e., the nurse practitioner, physician, certified nurse midwife, and so on). People of other cultures may seek out folk healers because they speak their native language, share their values and beliefs, charge less money, are readily available, or make house calls. If people perceive that the professional healing system cannot meet their needs, they are likely to seek care from the folk healers within their cultures and avoid the professional system. Table 13-1 identifies folk healers of various cultures and their practices.

Many folk healing traditions are guided not only by cultural practices but also by religious beliefs and rituals. Religious rituals are often associated with births (e.g., circumcision) and deaths (e.g., who is allowed to wash the body and prepare it for burial). It can be almost impossible to separate cultural from religious beliefs. Nevertheless, you cannot assume that because your patient is a member of a certain culture he will also be of a certain religion. It is safer to ask.

Complementary and Alternative Medicine

Complementary medicine is the use of rigorously tested therapies *to complement* those of conventional medicine (Andrews & Boyle, 2007). Examples include chiropractic care, biofeedback, and the use of certain supplements. In contrast, **alternative medicine** is defined as therapies used *instead of* conventional (i.e., biomedical) medicine, and whose reliability has not been validated through clinical testing in the United States. Examples of alternative therapies include iridology, aromatherapy, and magnet therapy.

Some complementary and alternative modalities (CAMs) are derived from the ancient and indigenous healthcare systems of people of other countries, such as traditional Chinese medicine (TCM), and **ayurveda,** the traditional healthcare system of India. As mentioned previously, certain therapies require a healer specially trained in their use (e.g., chiropractic, reflexology, massage therapy). Some alternative and CAM healers (e.g., massage therapists) are licensed by the state. The National Institutes of Health's National Center for Complementary and Alternative Medicine is currently conducting and funding research on a number of CAM therapies.

Knowledge Check 13-6

■ What is folk medicine?
■ What are some common folk medicine practices?
■ Why might members of some cultural groups seek out the local folk healer rather than the conventional healthcare provider?

 Go to Chapter 13, **Knowledge Check Response Sheet and Answers,** on the Student Resource Disk or DavisPlus at http://davisplus.fadavis.com/Wilkinson2

What Is Culturally Competent Care?

The terms *cultural awareness, cultural sensitivity,* and *cultural competence* are often used interchangeably; however, they are different. **Cultural awareness** refers to an appreciation of the external signs of diversity, whereas **cultural sensitivity** has more to do with personal attitudes and being careful not to say or do something that might be offensive to someone from a different culture (Purnell & Paulanka, 2008, p. 6). **Cultural competence** is attained on a continuum ranging from cultural destructiveness (most negative) to cultural proficiency (most positive) (Cross, Bazron, Dennis, et al., 1989). You cannot achieve cultural competence overnight because it is a developmental process. As you become more aware of and sensitive to the needs of individuals from various ethnocultural groups, you will move forward on the journey toward cultural competence: being able to use knowledge and sensitivity in practice. The following are some ideas about cultural competence.

The American Nurses Association (ANA)

The ANA emphasizes in a position paper, "It is important that the nurse consider specific cultural factors impacting on individual clients and recognize that intracultural variation means that each client must be assessed for individual cultural differences" (1997, p. 1). More recently, the ANA *Nursing: Scope and Standards of Practice* (2010, in press) state:

- The nursing needs of human beings are . . . met within the context of a culturally sensitive, caring interpersonal relationship (p. 18).
- Healing is fostered by . . . cultural competence, tolerance, acceptance. . . and conflict resolution (p. 20).
- Nurses have an obligation to promote health to the individual and society regardless of cultural background, value system, religious belief, sexual identity or disability (p. 24).

In addition, standards 1, 3 and 4 require the nurse to provide cultural assessments and formulate culturally appropriate expected outcomes and nursing interventions (pp. 28, 30, 31). *Note:* Revised ANA standards are expected to publish in 2010. To be sure you have the most current version,

 Go to http://www.nursingworld.org/, **Professional Nursing Practice.**

Quality and Safety Education for Nurses (QSEN)

Several of the QSEN competencies also speak to culturally competent care. For example, from the patient-centered care competency, the graduate nurse should be prepared to: (1) provide patient-centered care with sensitivity and respect for the diversity of human experience; (2) seek learning opportunities with patients who represent all aspects of human diversity; and (3) recognize personally held attitudes about working with patients from different ethnic, cultural, and social backgrounds.

Purnell and Paulanka

The Purnell model for cultural competence stresses teamwork in providing culturally sensitive and competent care to improve outcomes for individuals, families, and communities (Purnell, 2000, 2002; Purnell & Paulanka, 2008). The pie-shaped wedges in Figure 13-7 depict the issues all societies and humans share (e.g., pregnancy, nutrition, high-risk behavior, family organization, and death) but that are expressed in ways specific to the culture. These domains provide the organizing framework for the model. The center of the model is empty and represents that which is unknown about a cultural group.

In the context of nursing, Purnell's model (Purnell & Paulanka, 2008, p. 404) defines **cultural competence** as "having the knowledge, abilities, and skills to deliver care congruent with the client's cultural beliefs and practices." Increasing one's consciousness of cultural diversity improves the possibilities for healthcare practitioners to provide culturally competent care.

Leininger

Although Madeline Leininger does not use the specific term *cultural competence,* her theory fits with that concept (Leininger, 2007; Leininger & McFarland, 2006). The goal of her theory is to guide research that will assist nurses to provide culturally congruent care that would contribute to the health or well-being of people using her three modes of nursing care actions and decisions (to be explained later in the chapter). Nurses can achieve this goal by:

- Discovering cultural care and caring beliefs, values, and practices
- Analyzing the similarities and differences of these beliefs among the different cultures

For more information on Leininger's theory of culture care diversity and universality,

 Go to Chapter 13, **Supplemental Materials: Madeline Leininger, and Tables, Boxes, Figures: ESG Figure 13-1,** on the Student Resource Disk or DavisPlus at http://davisplus. fadavis.com/Wilkinson2

Campinha-Bacote

The culturally competent model of care views cultural competence as a process, not an end point. The nurse must see himself as *becoming* culturally competent, rather than *being* culturally competent. The model identifies five components of cultural competence, using the mnemonic ASKED. To be culturally competent, you

| Unconsciously incompetent | Consciously incompetent | Consciously competent | Unconsciously competent |

FIGURE 13-7 Purnell's model for cultural competence. (Source: from Purnell, L., & Paulanka, B. (2007). *Transcultural health care: a culturally competent approach* (3rd ed.). Philadelphia: F. A. Davis, p. 21. Reprinted with permission.)

need cultural: awareness, skills, knowledge, encounters, and desire (Campinha-Bacote, 2003).

- *Awareness* is similar to cultural sensitivity in other models. Take an honest look at your personal biases and prejudices toward cultural groups other than your own.
- *Skills* refers to your ability to conduct with sensitivity a cultural assessment and a culturally based physical assessment.
- *Knowledge* pertains to the information you have about cultural worldviews and theories. You need to know what the patient's view of the world is in order to understand it and work competently with the patient.
- *Encounters* means that it takes practice to become culturally competent. You need as many face-to-face encounters as possible with patients from diverse cultural backgrounds.
- *Desire* suggests that you must *want* to be culturally competent. If there is no genuine desire, you will not be likely to seek out cultural encounters, or work to obtain cultural knowledge and skills.

Critical**Thinking** 13-8

What kind of knowledge do you need to become culturally competent (theoretical, practical, self, ethical)? Explain your answer. See Chapter 2 to review types of knowledge, if necessary.

What Are Some Barriers to Culturally Competent Care?

Your ability to provide culturally competent care may be hampered by various prejudices and language barriers. Self-knowledge and critical thinking are essential in helping you identify and manage them.

Bias, Prejudice, and Discrimination

Ethnocentrism may negatively affect care. People have a tendency to be biased toward their own culture, believing their own beliefs and values are right and that those of other cultures are wrong (or at least bizarre). If you take this attitude, your patient may feel that you disapprove of him or, at the least, you don't understand or respect him. **Bias** is one-sidedness: a tendency to "lean" a certain way, a lack of impartiality. A **cultural stereotype** is the unsubstantiated belief that all people of a certain racial or ethnic group are alike in certain respects. Similar to biases, a stereotype may be positive or negative. **Prejudice** refers to negative attitudes toward other people based on faulty and rigid stereotypes about race, gender, sexual orientation, and so on.

Whereas prejudice refers to people's attitudes, the term **discrimination** refers to the behavioral manifestations of that prejudice. For example, before the 1960s many U.S. hospitals refused treatment to African American. Slightly more subtle discrimination against minority groups still exists in housing, banking, and the job market. It is, in some places, more difficult for a woman, someone who is openly homosexual, or an African American to obtain a loan or to be hired for certain jobs.

Racism

Racism is a form of prejudice and discrimination based on the belief that race is the principal determining factor of human traits and capabilities and that racial differences produce an inherent superiority (or inferiority). The word *race* evokes powerful emotional responses for people who feel that they or their ancestors have been oppressed or exploited, and equally for those who deny such a responsibility. In the United States, the history of discrimination against non-whites has created a focus on differences and racial divisiveness. As a nurse, you must recognize that unconscious racism can play a major role in your ability to communicate with people of other races.

Sexism

Sexism, widespread throughout history, is the assumption that members of one sex are superior to those of the other sex. For example, women have been viewed as more emotional and less rational than men; and assertiveness considered a positive trait in men, may be seen as "pushiness" or aggressiveness in women. Men, too, experience sexism. Male nurses must combat the kind of sexism that asserts that it is "unnatural" for men to engage in caring behaviors. Some female nurses may not accept their male colleagues, and some patients—both male and female—may object to their care, at least initially.

Male chauvinism (assumption of male superiority) is common in many cultures and in healthcare settings. It may be overt or subtle. In the wider society, for example, men may receive higher pay for performing the same work as a woman. In the healthcare setting, you might, even now, hear a male physician calling female nurses or patients "dear," or using a voice tone more appropriate to addressing a child. When you have the opportunity to do so, observe a conversation between a male nurse and a male physician. You may note that the male nurse communicates more directly and uses more eye contact than female nurses do with this same physician. We are not assuming all physicians (or nurses) are

chauvinistic; we are simply stating that you will probably be able to observe this kind of interchange among some professionals. As in other settings, the assumption of equality, by either party, changes the way people communicate.

Language Barriers

By Census Bureau estimates, about 50 million U.S. residents speak a language other than English at home. Another 22 million speak English poorly. A language barrier will obviously affect your ability to communicate with clients. Language barriers can involve foreign languages, dialects, regionalisms (words or pronunciation particular to a specific region), street talk, and jargon (words or expressions used by a subculture, including medicine).

Recall Mr. Salvatore, in "Meet Your Patients." Suppose it is found that he has a brain tumor and needs immediate surgery. You would need to get his consent for surgery even though he and his family do not speak English. You might call the telephone language line to which your hospital subscribes. But suppose that the interpreter has difficulty understanding Mr. Salvatore completely because he uses a different dialect or slang. This is not an unusual situation. In such a case, you would need to explore the resources and policies of your healthcare facility. If there were no other options for translation help, you would have to resort to nonverbal language and pictures to communicate until further resources could be found. It's not the best option, but it may be the only one, at least temporarily. However, if a consent issue is involved, the hospital will almost certainly have a policy to handle the situation.

Street talk, slang, and jargon can be as challenging as a foreign language. For example, the word *bad* can mean bad or good; the meaning changes, and not everyone has the same interpretations. Ebonics (also called black Vernacular English, or AAVE) is a type of English that has, in the past, been spoken primarily by blacks, but many white youth enamored with hip-hop culture now embrace Ebonics as a way to connect with the street culture.

Healthcare jargon can often be distressing to patients. In the healthcare field, we have our own terminology, including abbreviations, which we use so often we may forget that our clients do not understand them. For example, you may frighten some patients if you say to them, "I'm going to take your vitals" before assessing their blood pressure. You may be surprised to learn that many patients will not know what you mean if you ask, "Have you voided today?" Even worse, patients may hesitate to ask for clarification because they don't like admitting that they don't understand a certain word. What other examples of nursing or medical jargon can you think of that might be confusing to clients?

Other Barriers

Lack of knowledge about the cultural and ethnic values, beliefs, and behaviors of people within their community is not unusual among healthcare providers. It can cause them to misinterpret a client's behaviors. *Emotional responses*, such as fear and distrust (both yours and the client's), can arise any time members of different cultural groups meet. If you are aware this may happen, you may be able to avoid this barrier and communicate with your clients effectively. To repeat, self-knowledge is essential in removing barriers.

KnowledgeCheck 13-7

- Define cultural competence.
- How do the barriers of ethnocentricism and language impede nursing care of diverse populations?

 Go to Chapter 13, **Knowledge Check Response Sheet and Answers,** on the Student Resource Disk or DavisPlus at http://davisplus.fadavis.com/Wilkinson2

Practical **Knowledge** knowing how

Each phase of the nursing process presents an opportunity to provide culturally sensitive, congruent, and competent care. Regardless of the patient's cultural group, it is important for you to establish rapport before beginning data collection—especially for sensitive or personal information.

■ ASSESSMENT

Various regulating bodies (e.g., The Joint Commission and the Office of Minority Health) require healthcare organizations to integrate cultural data into a patient's health records. Cultural assessment consists of an interview and a physical assessment. When you perform a cultural assessment, you should gather data directly from your client, but if this is not possible, you may ask for help from a friend or family member of the client.

Toward Evidence-Based Practice

Hagman, L. W. (2004). New Mexico nurses' cultural self-efficacy: A pilot study. *Journal of Cultural Diversity, 11*(4), 146–149.

This study administered a written questionnaire to 15 registered nurses caring for multiethnic patients in New Mexico. They found that the nurses were moderately confident with their cultural knowledge and skills. Because of the small sample, no conclusions could be drawn from the study. Researchers recommended larger, more rigorous studies.

Jackson, A. K. (2007). Cultural competence in health visiting practice: A baseline survey. *Community Practitioner, 80*(2), 1722.

The researcher administered a survey to explore the beliefs, knowledge, and practice in cultural competence of health visitors working in a county in England. Half the respondents were members of a minority ethnic community, with Caribbean origins predominant. Results showed there was a significant difference in respondents' abilities to meet the needs of minority ethnic communities as opposed to those of the white population. They identified language and culture, but not racism, as barriers to culturally competent care. The study concluded that there is a need for cultural competence training.

Broome, B. (2006). Culture 101. *Urologic Nursing, 26*(6), 486–489.

This author states that America is a mix of cultures, ethnic groups, and races; therefore, healthcare

providers need to become more culturally sensitive and competent. She states further that one of the many challenges confronting urologic nurses is learning how culture can influence a patient's response to health and illness.

Instructions: Suppose you are a nurse on a urology unit that serves mainly European Americans, Mexican Americans, and patients of Caribbean origin. You are trying to answer this question: Would knowledge of patients' cultural values and practices enable nurses on our unit to provide care that better meets the needs of our patients, for example, by improving their compliance with treatment regimens. You are looking for the best available research evidence to support your practice. Answer the following questions:

---

1. Thinking of the PICO question format (refer to Chapter 8 if you need to review), who in your question would be represented by "P"?

2. Again using PICO, what is represented by "I"?

3. There is no "C" in the question; what is represented by "O"?

4. Which of the three articles cited provides the best evidence to help answer your question?

 Go to Chapter 13, **Toward Evidence-Based Practice Suggested Responses,** on the Student Resource Disk or DavisPlus at http://davisplus.fadavis.com/Wilkinson2

When you need to use an interpreter, even if it must be a family member, be aware of confidentiality (private information) issues.

The Health History

To encourage clients to talk about themselves, you must convey empathy, show respect, build rapport, establish trust, listen actively, and provide appropriate feedback (Munoz & Luckmann, 2004). Ask open-ended questions when beginning a cultural assessment.

 Always ask clients about their use of alternative medicine and folk remedies so their effects on traditional biomedical medications and treatments can be evaluated. Some remedies may interfere with traditional treatments; others can be dangerous. Many people use folk remedies, but they may be reluctant to tell you so because they fear ridicule or at least disapproval.

You will not need to perform an in-depth cultural assessment on every client, but you will need to recognize situations in which this is needed. Lipson and Meleis (1985) suggest that the following minimum information is important:

Language(s) spoken; proficiency in language of the host
Length of time client has been in the host country
Where client was raised
Ethnic affiliation and identity
Usual religious practices
Nonverbal communication style
Family roles and primary decision-maker about the client's healthcare
Social support in the host country

For a list of questions to help you obtain this information,

 Go to Chapter 13, **Clinical Insights 13-2: Obtaining Minimal Cultural Information,** in Volume 2.

Physical Assessment

Physical assessment may reveal biocultural variations. To assess and evaluate clients accurately, you need to know the normal physiological variations among healthy members of selected populations, for example, body proportions, vital signs, general appearance, skin, musculoskeletal system, illness, and laboratory values. For example, knowledge of biocultural variations in skin is important because of the importance of assessing for pallor, cyanosis, jaundice, erythema, and petechiae, which may be more difficult to evaluate in dark-skinned persons. For more information about assessing the skin, see Chapter 19, and

Go to Chapter 13, **Clinical Insights 13-1: Assessing for Biological Variations,** in Volume 2.

Assessing for Pain

Culture influences the patient's illness behaviors, including responses to pain. Because pain and comfort are subjective responses, you need to quantify your client's pain as objectively as possible by using a pain measurement scale. Regardless of the literature descriptions of cultural responses, it is essential to investigate the meaning of pain to each individual and what they view as acceptable ways to express or cope with pain. For some descriptions of some cultural responses to pain,

 Go to Chapter 13, **Clinical Insights 13-3: Assessing Pain Perception in Selected Cultural Groups,** in Volume 2.

Cultural Assessment Models and Tools

Some agencies have special tools for in-depth cultural assessments. If yours does not, you can structure your assessments using any culture model, such as the following examples.

- Purnell Model for Cultural Competence (2002)
- Andrews and Boyle Transcultural Nursing Assessment Guide (2007)
- Spector's Heritage Assessment Model (2004). Instead of assessing culture specifics, this tool assesses heritage consistency: the degree to which a person's lifestyle reflects his traditional culture (country of origin, race, or ethnic group). This assessment tool also reveals the degree to which the client still identifies with his cultural origins.
- Giger and Davidhizar's Transcultural Assessment Model (2008)

For more information on the preceding cultural assessment models,

 Go to Chapter 13, **Tables, Boxes, Figures: ESG Figures 13-2 and 13-3, and ESG Boxes 13-1 and 13-2,** on the Student Resource Disk or DavisPlus at http://davisplus.fadavis.com/Wilkinson2

For another example of a focused cultural assessment,

 Go to Chapter 13, **Clinical Insights 13-4: Performing a Cultural Assessment...,** in Volume 2.

ANALYSIS/NURSING DIAGNOSIS

There are no NANDA-I diagnoses that specifically address culture. However, cultural factors can be the etiology of various problems. Any of the NANDA-I diagnostic labels can be used for patients of any culture, provided that the defining characteristics are present. Some possible examples include the following:

- *Risk for Imbalanced Nutrition: Less Than Body Requirements* might apply to a patient who is hospitalized and cannot obtain foods prepared in the traditional way of his ethnic group.

- *Impaired Parenting* could occur if the patient's traditional methods of discipline are not acceptable or appropriate in the dominant culture.
- *Spiritual Distress* might occur because a necessary treatment is not congruent with a client's religious beliefs.
- *Powerlessness* might occur when the patient is unable to make healthcare personnel understand the importance of his religious and dietary beliefs.
- *Impaired Verbal Communication* is sometimes used for patients who do not speak or understand the nurse's language. However, this diagnosis is of questionable value in such circumstances. In a classic study, Geissler (1991) found that Impaired Verbal Communication related more to cultural differences between the patient and healthcare provider than to the inability to communicate. So if the patient is verbally "impaired," the nurse is equally "impaired"; that is, communication is as much a "problem" for the nurse as for the patient. It is probably better to use Impaired Verbal Communication as the etiology of other diagnoses, such as Ineffective Therapeutic Regimen Management.
- *Risk for Noncompliance* can be used for clients and/or caregivers who do not follow a health-promoting or therapeutic plan the healthcare provider believes they agreed to. For example, the plan may not "fit" with the client's perception of the cause of his illness. But again, you must use this diagnostic label with care. Geissler (1991) also found that additional defining characteristics are needed before Noncompliance can be appropriately applied to clients not of the dominant U.S. culture. In fact, Geissler suggests the nurse use the term *nonadherence* instead of *Noncompliance*.

The preceding examples illustrate the concern that standardized nursing diagnoses are not always culturally sensitive; that is, they may not apply accurately to patients who are not from the dominant culture. Nursing diagnoses should describe responses that *patients* see as problematic. A nurse and patient who are from different cultures will likely have different perceptions of health and illness. This can lead to misdiagnosis. The nurse may either diagnose a problem that doesn't exist for the patient or diagnose a "real" problem but fail to describe it accurately (Wilkinson, 2007).

Suppose that a 60-year-old woman who works as a hotel maid is repeatedly admitted to your hospital for uncontrolled hypertension. You know uncontrolled hypertension can lead to a stroke. You determine that she does not take her medication, and you diagnose Noncompliance (failure to take prescribed medication). But do you know that an antihypertensive medication can cost more than $100 for a month's supply? Perhaps your patient is raising her grandchildren and paying for

shelter, utilities, food, and clothing uses up her entire income.

Box 13-1 lists some NANDA-I nursing diagnoses that could be interpreted differently by people from different cultures. Undoubtedly there are others. The point is to use all labels carefully and to validate nursing diagnoses with the patient to be sure that the statement describes her health status as *she* sees it.

■ PLANNING OUTCOMES/EVALUATION

The outcomes you choose (whether standardized or individualized) depend on the nursing diagnoses you have identified. If the diagnoses are culturally sensitive, the outcomes should be as well. However, you must involve the patient in order to be certain. For example, suppose your patient is dying. Both you and the patient agree that her diagnosis is Acute Pain, but your goals may be different. You might want the patient to be free from pain. However, the patient's goal may be to stay alert enough to interact with her family, even if it means she must endure some pain. When your cultures differ, it is even more important to validate the goals with the patient. Some individualized goal/outcome statements associated with cultural differences might include the following:

- Agrees to take prescribed analgesic (pain medication) before bedtime and after family leaves for the evening.

BOX 13-1 ■ NANDA-I Nursing Diagnoses With Potential For Cultural Bias

Acute Pain

Anxiety

Chronic Pain

Confusion

Decisional Conflict

Deficient Knowledge

Disabled Family Coping

Effective Breastfeeding

Imbalanced Nutrition: Less Than Body Requirements

Imbalanced Nutrition: More Than Body Requirements

Impaired Social Interaction

Impaired Verbal Communication

Ineffective Breastfeeding

Ineffective Coping

Ineffective Denial

Ineffective Role Performance

Noncompliance

Powerlessness

Social Isolation

- Talks to her spiritual adviser about the possibility of surgery that conflicts with her religious beliefs.
- Freely shares information about folk practices and over-the-counter medications with the primary care provider.
- Asks for clarification from healthcare professional when she does not understand clearly what was said.

PLANNING INTERVENTIONS/IMPLEMENTATION

When planning care for your clients, information about their cultural values, beliefs, and practices will help you identify interventions that will support these practices and incorporate them into their care as much as possible (Wilkinson, 2007). For example, when you are teaching about a specific treatment regimen ordered by the primary care provider, you should find out whether it conflicts with any of the patient's folk beliefs or alternative treatments so you can suggest any necessary modifications. Remember also to identify educational methods that are most appropriate for your client's needs (e.g., translated materials and/or diagrams) and to make community referrals as necessary. Although nursing care depends on the client's specific problems and their etiologies, some nursing interventions and activities can be especially appropriate for providing culturally competent care.

NIC standardized interventions related to culture include the following:

> Active Listening (for Impaired Verbal Communication)
> Family Involvement Promotion (for Readiness for Enhanced Family Coping)
> Self-Responsibility Facilitation (for Powerlessness)
> Culture Brokerage (for Noncompliance)

Culture Brokerage, a Nursing Intervention Classification (NIC) intervention, is defined as "the deliberate use of culturally competent strategies to bridge or mediate between the patient's culture and the biomedical healthcare system" (Bulechek, Butcher, & Dochterman, 2008, p. 245).

Individualized nursing activities and focused assessments are important for all patients. However, patients from different cultural and ethnic groups may have unique needs that can be met by some of the activities included in the following discussion regarding culturally competent care.

KnowledgeCheck 13-8

- Describe, in general, how the nursing process can help you provide culturally competent care.
- How can nursing diagnoses cause bias in the planning of care for patients from different cultures?

Go to Chapter 13, **Knowledge Check Response Sheet and Answers,** on the Student Resource Disk or DavisPlus at http://davisplus.fadavis.com/Wilkinson2

Nursing Strategies for Providing Culturally Competent Care

You should become familiar with the cultural groups you are most likely to encounter. Choose one of the transcultural models to help you to use critical thinking and the nursing process to provide the holistic care your clients deserve.

What Are Leininger's Modes?

Leininger's theory describes the following three "modes" of nursing decisions and actions (Leininger, 1991, Leininger & McFarland, 2006):

1. *Cultural care preservation/maintenance,* which sustains clients' cultural lifestyles in meaningful ways. These are actions that help the client retain or preserve cultural values related to health.
   Example: Encouraging the family to bring ethnic foods that are appropriate for the client's prescribed diet.
2. *Cultural care accommodation/negotiation,* which adapts clients' lifestyles or nurses' actions. The nurse supports and enables the client to adapt to therapies or to negotiate with professionals to achieve satisfying health outcomes. **Negotiation** acknowledges the gap between the nurse's and client's perspectives. You must negotiate when folk or traditional practices might be harmful to the client.
   Example: Negotiating with the client to continue seeing the *curandero,* but to come to the clinic every 6 weeks to have his blood pressure checked. If the client refuses all biomedical or nursing interventions, the only avenue still open is to continue monitoring the client to identify changes in his health status. If a health crisis occurs, it may be possible to renegotiate the care.
3. *Cultural care repatterning/restructuring,* which changes nurses' actions or clients' lifestyles into different patterns. The nurse supports and encourages the client to greatly modify his behaviors and to adopt new, different, and beneficial health behaviors, while still respecting the client's cultural values and beliefs.
   Example 1: When the client absolutely refuses to take the prescribed pain medication, the nurse uses massage, distraction, and other nonpharmacological techniques to help relieve his pain (change in nurse's actions).
   Example 2: A client refuses to see a biomedical doctor for her family's needs. However, when the folk healer is unsuccessful in treating her child's illness and the child becomes critically ill, the nurse convinces the client to bring the child to the emergency department (modification of the client's behaviors).

How Do I Communicate with Clients from Other Cultures?

One of your major considerations as you become more culturally competent is your ability to communicate with clients from different cultures. Become familiar with appropriate verbal and nonverbal communication patterns within the cultural groups, and use them selectively in your communication approaches. Giger and Davidhizar (2008, p. 35) encourage the following guidelines:

- Assess personal beliefs of persons from different cultures.
- Assess communication variables from a cultural perspective.
- Plan care based on the client's communicated needs and cultural background.
- Modify communication approaches to meet cultural needs.
- Understand that respect for the client and communicated needs are central to the therapeutic relationship.
- Communicate in a nonthreatening manner.
- Use validating techniques in communication.
- Be considerate of a client's reluctance to talk when the subject involves sexual matters.
- Adopt special approaches when the client speaks a different language.
- Use interpreters to improve communication.

How Do I Communicate with Clients Who Speak a Different Language?

Communicating with clients who do not speak your language can be especially challenging. The best way to provide culturally competent care to such clients is to use a professional medical interpreter. Largely in response to the changing population composition of the United States, the Office of Minority Health (OMH) developed the National Standards for Culturally and Linguistically Appropriate Services (CLAS) in healthcare. **The CLAS guidelines** require healthcare organizations receiving federal funding to provide language assistance services, including bilingual staff and interpreter services, at no cost to the patient. They must also provide materials and signs in the languages of the commonly encountered groups in their service area (U.S. Department of Health and Human Services, Office of Minority Health 2001). For a complete listing of the CLAS standards,

 Go to Chapter 13, **Supplemental Materials: CLAS Standards,** on the Student Resource Disk or DavisPlus at http://davisplus.fadavis.com/Wilkinson2

An **interpreter** is specially trained to provide the meaning behind the words, whereas a **translator** just restates the words from one language to another. An interpreter can serve as a cultural broker by conveying the client's responses to questions and by providing general information about the client's culture (Munoz & Luckmann, 2004). CLAS standard 6 states that family and friends should not be used as interpreters except on request by the patient. For guidelines when using any type of interpreter,

 Go to Chapter 13, **Clinical Insights 13-5: Communicating with Clients Who Speak a Different Language,** in Volume 2.

Other Strategies

There are several strategies for you to consider and many resources to help you develop strategies specific to various cultural groups (Box 13-2). Consider the

---

BOX 13-2 ■ Being Considerate of Cultural Specifics

Consider verbal and nonverbal communication.

- Know, or find out, whether touch (e.g., a handshake) is expected or prohibited.
- Know, or find out, whether eye contact is expected or avoided. Avoiding eye contact, for some, is a sign of respect.
- Ask the client how he wishes to be addressed.
- Know, or find out, the ways people welcome each other.

Consider the person's need for personal space.

- Know the person's cultural and religious customs regarding touching and contact.
- Know the usual comfortable distance for conversing in the client's culture.

Consider body language.

- Gestures that are acceptable in one culture may be taboo in another. Know what is acceptable to the client.
- Be aware that smiling does not universally indicate friendliness.

Consider time orientation.

- Tell clients when you are coming, and be on time.
- Avoid surprise visits.
- Share your own expectations about time.
- Ask clients what they expect regarding time, appointments, and so on.
- Be sure you know the times for and meanings of the client's religious and ethnic holidays.

Consider social organization.

- Know which person in the family is the leader or decision maker.
- Know what dates are important and whether gifts are expected or not.
- Know how special events, such as births and funerals, are celebrated, whether certain colors have meaning, and what the expected rituals are.

Consider the person's perspective on environmental control.

- Find out what the client's health traditions and practices are.
- Know whether the person believes she has any ability to "change things."
- Know the general influence of the culture on perception and tolerance of pain.
- Know what foods are forbidden, what foods may or may not be eaten together, and what and how utensils are used.

following as you move forward on your journey toward cultural competence:

- Consider each client as a unique individual, influenced but not defined by his culture.
- Understand your own cultural values and practices and appreciate how they may differ from those held by people of other cultures.
- Recognize your own biases about people and groups, and consider how they may affect the care you provide.
- Learn as much as you can about the cultural groups in your community and work area.
- Make an effort to incorporate beliefs and practices from various cultures into your nursing care and teaching materials.
- Encourage helpful or neutral cultural practices, and discourage those that are dysfunctional (harmful).
- Suggest alternatives to harmful practices.
- Accommodate cultural dietary practices when possible. For inpatients, some dietary departments can make special foods, and you can encourage families to bring food from home. In all situations, help patients and families adapt cultural foods to therapeutic diets.
- Respect your clients regardless of cultural background, and never force, pressure, manipulate, or coerce them to participate in care that conflicts with their values and beliefs.
- Advocate for all of your clients, but especially for those not from the dominant culture.
- Consider the cultural role of the family member who makes the primary decisions. To ignore this person is to doom your interventions to failure.
- Work with the folk medicine practitioner in the interest of the client.
- Learn from your mistakes, and don't make them again.

This is by no means an exhaustive list. Most likely, you can think of other strategies. It may help you to "take a trip to BALI":

Be aware of your own cultural heritage
Appreciate that the client is unique: influenced, but not defined by his culture
Learn about the client's cultural group
Incorporate the client's cultural values/behaviors into the care plan.

Knowledge Check 13-9

- List five factors to consider when communicating with clients from different cultures.
- List five factors to consider when communicating with a client using an interpreter.
- List five factors to consider when communicating with a client who does not speak your language, when an interpreter is not available.

 Go to Chapter 13, **Knowledge Check Response Sheet and Answers,** on the Student Resource Disk or DavisPlus at http://davisplus.fadavis.com/Wilkinson2

How Can I Become Culturally Competent?

Of course you can't become culturally competent just by reading. People acquire cultural competence gradually, progressing through the following stages:

Unconscious incompetence—not being aware that you lack knowledge about another culture
Conscious incompetence—being aware that you lack knowledge about another culture
Conscious competence—learning about the client's culture, verifying generalizations about the culture (e.g., archetypes), and providing culture specific interventions
Unconscious competence—automatically providing culturally congruent care to clients of diverse cultures (Purnell & Paulanka, 2008, p. 6)

Theoretical knowledge can increase your awareness and appreciation of cultural differences. But you can achieve cultural competence only if you are motivated to do so, and even then only by interacting with people from cultures different from your own. Carballeira (1997) sums up this process with the LIVE and LEARN model for culturally competent family services:

Like		**L**isten
Inquire		**E**valuate
Visit	and	**A**cknowledge
Experience		**R**ecommend
		Negotiate

If there were only one single intervention you could use in the service of cultural competence, you should routinely ask patients what matters most to them in their illness and treatment. No matter how busy, every nurse can find time to do that. You can then use that information to think through the patient's specific needs for care.

 Go to Chapter 13, **Resources for Caregivers and Health Professionals,** on the Student Resource Disk or DavisPlus at http://davisplus.fadavis.com/Wilkinson2

 Suggested Readings: Go to Chapter 13, **Reading More About Culture and Ethnicity,** on the Student Resource Disk or DavisPlus at http://davisplus.fadavis.com/Wilkinson2

 Bibliography: Go to Volume 2, Bibliography.

CHAPTER 14

Spirituality

Learning Outcomes

After completing this chapter, you should be able to:

➤ Describe the differences and similarities between religion and spirituality.

➤ Discuss what is meant by *spirituality*.

➤ For each of the religions briefly covered in this chapter, describe its major beliefs and their implications for nursing care.

➤ Identify five barriers to spiritual care.

➤ Perform a spiritual assessment.

➤ Distinguish the differences between spiritual care diagnoses and those that may serve as etiologies of other nursing diagnoses.

➤ Plan nursing interventions based on the data obtained in a spiritual assessment.

➤ Examine your own level of comfort in terms of performing spiritual interventions.

➤ Describe collaborative efforts to ensure the spiritual care of the patient or family.

Meet Your Patient

Charles Johnson is a 75-year-old black man with newly diagnosed lung cancer. He began smoking at age 15. His physicians want to start chemotherapy to try to increase his life span. He is unsure whether he wants to have chemotherapy.

Mr. Johnson was brought up in the Baptist Church but has fallen away from practicing his faith over the years. He has been a heavy drinker all of his adult life and, as a young man, became alienated from churchgoing. He explains: "Church folk are all a bunch of hypocrites, if you ask me. I choose not to be a part of any of that." Nevertheless, he says that he tries to be kind to and tolerant of others. "I've messed up my life, so I figure I don't have any business telling other people how to live. I guess I just figure that how a person lives is between them and God."

Mr. Johnson has one surviving relative, a sister, who is concerned about him. His sister is a devout Jehovah's Witness, and she has tried several times to talk to Mr. Johnson about how important Jehovah is in her life. She continually leaves religious pamphlets and materials in his mailbox to encourage him to think about religion again.

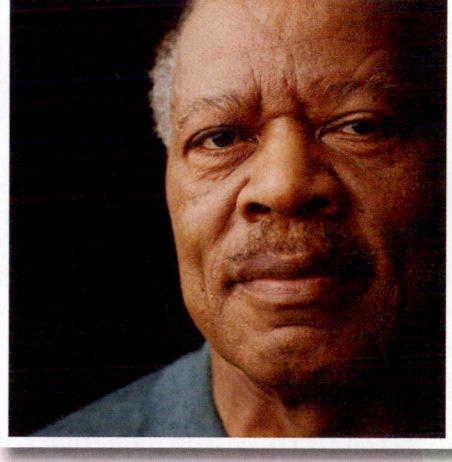

Mr. Johnson's wife divorced him 20 years ago because of his drinking behaviors, and he has alienated his two middle-aged children, a son and a daughter. Mr. Johnson has two grandchildren, whom he rarely sees. He lives alone, is retired, and is having some trouble making ends meet financially. He has one avid hobby: He loves to go out in a boat and fish all day with his buddy, Jim.

- Mr. Johnson clearly has some physical and psychosocial difficulties. Can you identify them?
- Assess Mr. Johnson's support system. Whom can he rely on for help?
- How might you help Mr. Johnson to add some spiritual supports to his available resources?

Theoretical **Knowledge** **knowing** why_____

Spirituality in nursing has multiple layers. Each nurse has her own spirituality that (overtly or covertly) serves as part of the guiding framework for her practice. Furthermore, your patients and families will understand spirituality in a variety of ways. Their spirituality may be deeply ingrained in religious understandings, or it may be separate from formal religion. Many schools of nursing teach spiritual care interventions while emphasizing a philosophy of "not imposing" one's religious beliefs on patients. In addition, nursing practice settings provide multiple levels of care, which impose time constraints on what you can address in day-to-day activities. These layers of competing concerns can lead to confusion and frustration in providing spiritual care or simply avoiding it altogether.

This chapter presents a holistic interpretation of spirituality—one that views spirituality as a component of every person's life. It also encourages you to engage your own spirituality to improve your patients' health and wholeness. It should help you to answer some of the questions posed for Mr. Johnson.

History of Spirituality in Nursing

Through the ages, nurses and other caregivers have demonstrated deep concern for the spiritual as well as the physical and psychological needs of those who are sick and infirm.

In the pre-Christian era, caring for the sick was an expression of the values of hospitality and charity. People prayed to the god(s) for healing and as an adjunct for primitive medical procedures.

In the early Christian era, nursing the sick was honored and respected because it was one of Jesus Christ's primary teachings. Caring for the sick was a vital component of loving one's neighbor. Gradually, religious communities of women and men in the 4th through 12th centuries provided models for combining the healing arts with religious care.

During the post-Reformation period in Europe, nursing orders continued to flourish, among them the Daughters of Charity, the Sisters of Mercy, and the Kaiserswerth Deaconesses (Donahue, 1985). Florence Nightingale trained under Pastor Fliedner at his Deaconess School in Kaiserswerth, as well as under the Daughters of Charity of St. Vincent de Paul in France. For Nightingale, spirituality was at the very heart of human nature and thus was fundamental to healing. Nightingale instilled this idea in her nurses, particularly during their missions in the Crimea where "the lady with the lamp" brought comfort and relief to the sick and the dying (*The Collected Works of Florence Nightingale, 2007;* Macrae, 1995).

By the mid-20th century, nursing in the United States had begun to see spiritual care as less important. As science continued to develop and expand, and as more nurses studied in university settings, nursing joined ranks with the scientific disciplines: Its spiritual underpinnings were replaced by what could be "seen and tested" by the scientific method. Only recently has nursing (and the broader health community) reclaimed the spiritual dimension as a vital part of its identity and recognized its power to influence health.

Today, professional standards of care make clear that patients' spiritual needs are a nursing concern. The Joint Commission (2008) has established standards for spiritual care. In addition, the American Nurses Association (ANA) *Code for Nurses* (2010, in press) states that nurses should consider each patient's lifestyle, value system, and religious beliefs in planning care; and that nursing care measures should enable the patient to live with as much physical, emotional, social, and spiritual well-being as possible.

What Are Religion and Spirituality?

Although there is overlap, spirituality and religion differ in several important ways (Table 14-1). One way to distinguish religion from spirituality is to think of religion as a map and spirituality as a journey. We begin by exploring the map.

What Is Religion?

Many people use a map to get to a certain location. The "map" of religion tells you what to believe and what values are essential. It provides codes of conduct that integrate beliefs and values into a way of living. The map itself may be in the form of a religious tradition (e.g., Christianity) or denomination (e.g., Baptist), which provides an identity and a "lens" for reading the world. The rituals, symbols, sacraments, and holy writings associated with religions serve as bases of authority and provide diverse ways to transcend the physical and access the divine (e.g., God) (Fig. 14-1). Regardless of their differences, many of the world religions have the following in common:

- **Theology**—that is, discussions and theories related to God and God's relation to the world
- Sacred writings that are regarded as authoritative and/or reveal the nature of the divine in some way
- Notion of created order and purpose
- Definition of *human being* that includes important life events
- Notion of sin (primarily in Western religions)
- Explanation of the origin of evil and the nature of suffering
- Conception of either salvation (in Judeo-Christian religions) or enlightenment (in Eastern religions)
- View toward **eschatology,** or doctrines about the human soul and its relation to death, judgment, and eternal life (primarily a Western concept)

Table 14-1 ➤ Comparison of Religion and Spirituality

RELIGION (THE MAP)	SPIRITUALITY (THE JOURNEY)

A "roadmap" that defines:
  Beliefs
  Values
  Code(s) of conduct and ethics
	One's journey through life; a personal quest to define meaning, fulfillment, and satisfaction in life; a will to live; a belief in self

A tradition or system of worship that provides:
  Rituals
  Answers
  Norms
  Connection with God
	A dynamic relationship with that which transcends; a capacity to know and be known (a sense of openness, expectation); connectedness with self, others, nature, and a higher power (Cavendish, Konecny, Mitzeliotis, et al., 2003); belief in a divine being, or infinite source of energy (Beckman, Boxley-Harges, Bruick-Sorge, et al., 2007).

The roadmap and tradition define:
  What is to be believed
  How beliefs affect life
  Self-image and identity
	A lifelong process of growth (which may involve joy and/or struggle); a constant process of taking in "truth" and then adding individual insight to arrive at a way of perceiving and acting in the world

Issues: Faith, belief, trust, the nature of good and evil, the meaning of suffering, judgment, or enlightenment	Issues: Faith, hope, love

- Explanation of the nature of reality, the higher Self or soul, the relationship between humans and the divine, and the purpose of human existence

What Is Spirituality?

If religion serves as the map, spirituality is the day-to-day, moment-by-moment journey in life and living. Like a journey, spirituality takes place over time and involves the accumulation of life experiences combined with the understandings gained (i.e., in terms of finding meaning, value, and purpose in life). Many life events that prompt spiritual growth are fulfilling and joyful, but growth often results from painful life events that cause great internal upheaval, struggle, and challenge.

FIGURE 14-1 Associated with religion are symbols and holy writings, such as this cross and Bible representing Christianity.

You can also think of spirituality as an accumulation of life experiences and insights. They may agree or conflict with traditional religious values and cultural teachings. For example, an American raised in the Episcopal Church, after studying a variety of religions and traveling in Asia for several years, may develop a spirituality that is both universal and highly individual and may feel "at home" in any place of worship in the world.

Like religion, spirituality also allows various ways and means to access the divine in our daily lives, to transcend the physical world, or simply to be still and introspective. For centuries, Eastern traditions have emphasized that spirituality is awareness, paying attention, and being "sensitive to reality" (Krishnamurti, 1989). One Western model of spirituality asserts that we learn to "read" the spiritual in everyday events only when we attain a new "level of literacy." Such literacy enables us to recognize that each day is filled with signs that point to an active Spirit in the world. Life is a process of recognizing this Spirit and understanding its meaning. Being literate in this way allows us to learn about ourselves and others in new and profound ways. This model states that we can engage this Spirit through such sources as nature, animals, leisure, creativity, and service (Brussat & Brussat, 1996).

It is critical for you to recognize and respect the different ways that patients understand religion and spirituality. You need to understand that most people are comfortable with their beliefs (or lack thereof) and that, in providing spiritual care, your primary goal is to support their healing, not convert them to a different view. You must also be able to recognize situations when patients may be experiencing spiritual distress and may need referral to professionals with more specialized training. These aspects of spiritual care are discussed later in this chapter.

KnowledgeCheck 14-1

- Regardless of their differences, what do many world religions have in common?
- Which can be compared to a journey: religion or spirituality?
- True or false? Both religion and spirituality allow a person various ways to access the divine.
- What is Mr. Johnson's religion ("Meet Your Patient")?
- What is his sister's religion?

 Go to Chapter 14, **Knowledge Check Response Sheet and Answers,** on the Student Resource Disk or DavisPlus at http://davisplus.fadavis.com/Wilkinson2

Critical**Thinking** 14-1

- What do you know, or what can you speculate, about Mr. Johnson's ("Meet Your Patient") spirituality?

What are the Core Issues of Spirituality?

As just discussed, spirituality has many dimensions. We limit discussion here to three core issues. In his first letter to the Corinthians in the New Testament of the Bible, Saint Paul identified "three things that last": faith, hope, and love. Following in this tradition, a contemporary manual for nursing care of the dying (Aspen Reference Group, 2002) identifies this same trio as the three core "issues" of spirituality.

Faith

Faith is our ongoing effort to make sense of our lives and purpose for being. Like spirituality itself, faith represents a set of beliefs developed over time, through events that cause us to suffer and those that enable us to rejoice.

Faith struggles are common among people who experience illness and significant loss. People experiencing faith struggles might feel anger, guilt, self-judgment, and worthlessness. C. S. Lewis, a devout Christian, reveals that after the death of his wife, his grief caused him to doubt whether God exists at all, or if so, whether He is perhaps a "Cosmic Sadist" (1961, p. 35) who deliberately tortures us. Finally, Lewis came to understand that such shattering experiences are "one of the marks of His presence" (Lewis, 1961, p. 76).

People who are experiencing the *joys of faith* exhibit a sense of self, as well as insights into their gifts and talents. In his book *Callings,* Gregg Levoy (1997, p. 65) observes that our joy and our enthusiasm move us "toward a kind of divine presence because, through our passions, we are utterly present. . . . We hitch ourselves to something bigger."

Implicit in faith is the idea of *trust:* Trust contributes to a certain confidence in our faith despite the questions that arise along life's way. Trust is so fundamental to faith that a seeming crisis of faith may in truth be a crisis of trust. A patient dying of cancer may claim that she has lost her faith in God, yet still be angry at God for "betraying her" by giving her a terminal illness.

Hope

Hope includes our basic human needs to achieve, create, and to shape something of our life that will endure. If faith is expressed in terms of belief, then hope is rooted in purpose—who am I, what is my purpose, and why have I been created. People who are confronting a debilitating or terminal illness often lose hope. After suffering a near-fatal spinal cord injury, actor Christopher Reeve experienced such a struggle, yet he concluded his second book, *Nothing Is Impossible,* with an essay on hope: "Hope . . . is different from optimism or wishful thinking. When we have hope, we discover powers within ourselves we may have never known—the power to make sacrifices, to endure, to heal, and to love. Once we choose hope, everything is possible" (Reeve, 2002, p. 176).

Love

Many people think of love as a trade: we extend our love because we hope to find that love returned in some way. But relationships can be a source of pain. We want to be loved as we are, yet we may fear what our loved ones think of us, and we compare ourselves with others. Worse, we encounter disappointments, rejection, and feelings of abandonment. Even when our love is shared, we must inevitably face separation at our death or the death of our loved ones. Thus, while active loving in human relationships opens us up to joy and can give life, meaning, and purpose; it also carries with it the certainty of heartbreak (e.g., when a loved one dies).

Illness and sudden injury commonly prompt such "struggles with love." For example, when a man with a debilitating disease loses his ability to work and requires increasing levels of caregiving, he may experience himself as a "burden" and question whether his loved ones would be "better off" if he were to die. When patients question the presence of unconditional love in their lives, family members may be invaluable in reminding them of their inner integrity and worth. Reeve stated that the most powerful words his wife spoke to him in the first days after his injury, "the words that saved my life," were, "You're still you. And I love you" (Reeve, 1998, p. 32).

Cures, Miracles, and Spiritual Healing

The patient, a family member, or a caregiver may ask for a prayer asking God for a cure when your expertise tells you that all curative measures have been exhausted. Certainly you should not say that anything is impossible. But it is equally important to avoid exposing the patient and family to false hope. In such cases, it may be possible for you, as care provider and companion on the spiritual journey, to offer a way to reframe the situation. Perhaps, healing does not necessarily have to imply the elimination of all types of suffering or of the disease.

Rather, it may mean a transformation in a patient's thinking or feeling when that patient has become receptive to the workings of the spirit. In such instances, healing does indeed take place, and the person may experience a miracle.

A **miracle** is anything that allows for the presence of the transcendent (e.g., God, a Higher Being, the experience of one's angel, or any brush with the divine). It is an event that excites wonder and in which we see God at work in our ordinary day-to-day lives (Macquarrie, 1977), but it does not necessarily involve a physical cure. We typically think of miracles as events that break with the natural order of things (e.g., a blind person suddenly can see, with no treatment or explanation); however, miracles more commonly proceed according to natural law. What makes events miracles is the fact that they far exceed our expectations. For instance, an elderly woman, bitter for decades over the death of her daughter during childhood, "feels" her daughter's presence and dies in peace. Miracles are spiritual phenomena. As such, they are mysterious; they are difficult to define and comprehend. In one sense, they can be viewed as perfectly ordinary events; in another, they are extraordinary, for they allow the patient to see and know God is present despite illness or other adversity (Macquarrie, 1977).

 ## Critical**Thinking** 14-2

- Faith is a constant search for comprehension and meaning. What are some of your struggles with faith, and what are some of the "joys" of your faith?

How Might Spiritual Beliefs Affect Health?

Although the preceding sections discussed religion and spirituality as two separate constructs, current research into their influence on health tend to combine the two into one: namely, religion. Most studies have measured both religion and spirituality in terms of *religious involvement*. They tend to use broad measures, such as self-reports of one's own religiousness, denominational affiliation, church attendance or membership, membership in the clergy, and dietary and social habits (e.g., "On a scale of 1 to 5, how religious are you?" "How often do you attend church?"). Despite such limitations, findings have been surprisingly positive in terms of predicting health outcomes. Current research suggests there are many ways religion affects physical and mental health.

- One study found that people who score higher on measures of religious involvement live longer than those with lower religious involvement (McCollough, Hoyt, Larson, et al., 2000).
- Likewise, the literature also suggests that even simplistic measures regarding religion and spirituality (e.g., religious affiliation or church attendance) are significant predictors of health outcomes, including

increased pain tolerance and decreased depression and anxiety (Harrison, Edwards, Koenig et al., 2005; Koenig, McCollough, & Larson, 2001).

- There is a growing body of literature that investigates the possible effects of religion on heart disease, cholesterol, hypertension, cancer, mortality, and health behaviors.

In all of these, the variables studied tend to be broadly stated and nonspecific and thus do not allow for researchers to examine whether there might be potential harmful effects of religion. For a list of other recent studies,

 Go to Chapter 14, **Reading More About Spirituality,** on the Student Resource Disk or DavisPlus at http://davisplus.fadavis.com/Wilkinson2

Although the research suggests that religion has a positive influence on healthcare outcomes, it does not yet answer *how* or *why* religion has this effect. However, there is growing awareness that religion and spirituality are complex variables involving cognitive, emotional, behavioral, interpersonal, and physiological dimensions. For a description of recent research testing more specific variables (e.g., religion as a factor to live a healthy lifestyle),

 Go to Chapter 14, **Supplemental Materials: Religion and Health: Recent Research,** on the Student Resource Disk or DavisPlus at http://davisplus.fadavis.com/Wilkinson2

KnowledgeCheck 14-2
- What are some of the ways that religion might positively influence health?

 Go to Chapter 14, **Knowledge Check Response Sheet and Answers,** on the Student Resource Disk or DavisPlus at http://davisplus.fadavis.com/Wilkinson2

 ## Critical**Thinking** 14-3
- How might religion negatively influence health?
- Has there been a pivotal moment in your life, a moment of crisis or despair that eventually provided an opportunity for spiritual growth?

Major Religions: What Should I Know?

The more you know about the differences and similarities among the world's major religions, the more you will be able to offer comprehensive and compassionate care to patients. Of course, learning about other religions requires you to be open and nonjudgmental. When you care for a patient from a known religious background, you will need to think about how the person's beliefs affect her ideas of health, healing, hospitalization, and the experience of dying. To help you make these connections, the following brief descriptions of several of the world's major religious traditions provide you with several different "worldviews." To learn about the influence of various religions on end-of-life care, see Chapter 15. For more detailed information about each religion,

Go to Chapter 14, **Supplemental Materials: Major Religions: What Should I Know?** and **Reading More About Spirituality,** on the Student Resource Disk or DavisPlus at http://davisplus.fadavis.com/Wilkinson2

Judaism

Judaism is one of the Western world's oldest religions and the foundation on which Christianity and Islam were built. The Jewish Law is set down in the collective writings of the Torah. Judaism is based on the worship of one God (monotheism), obeying the Ten Commandments, and practicing charity and tolerance toward others. The degree to which Jews celebrate rituals and holy days depends on whether the person identifies with the Orthodox, Liberal, Conservative, or Reconstructionist beliefs (Oxtoby & Segal, 2007; Pawlikowski, 1990).

Jews celebrate the Sabbath from sunset on Friday to sunset Saturday evening. For Orthodox Jews, work is prohibited on the Sabbath. This includes writing, traveling, and switching on lights and appliances. During Passover (in March or April), some Jewish patients may require special foods, dinnerware, and utensils. The Day of Atonement, or Yom Kippur (in September or October), is the holiest day of the Jewish calendar. It is a special day of fasting, but fasting is not required if it would be a danger to the patient. A Jewish patient will normally wish to keep that day to pray and rest. For Orthodox patients, you might offer alternatives to oral medication (e.g., injections or suppositories).

Conservative Jews observe strict dietary laws: Only kosher foods are accepted. **Kosher foods** have been prepared under strict guidelines for how animals are slaughtered and do not contain pork, certain types of seafood, or combinations of dairy and meat. If possible, consult a rabbi or dietitian who is knowledgeable about Jewish dietary laws for assistance in planning dietary and activity modifications.

Orthodox Jewish women prefer to have their bodies and limbs covered. They may also prefer to keep their hair covered with a scarf and often wear a wig. Orthodox men keep their head covered with a hat or skullcap (*kappel*). Some Orthodox Jewish sects forbid contraception unless the woman's health is at risk. Nearly all Jewish boys are circumcised, usually 8 days after birth. Orthodox Judaism usually forbids organ transplants, but opinions vary and decisions may rest with the rabbinic authority.

Christianity

Although rituals and practices vary among denominations, Christians are collectively known for their worship of Jesus Christ and their use of the same sacred text, the Bible, which includes the Judaic Old Testament and the New Testament on the life of Christ. However, there are many denominations within Christianity, including Roman Catholicism (with allegiance to the pope in Rome), Orthodoxy (with allegiance to the patriarch of Constantinople), Protestant denominations (e.g., Lutheran, Baptist, United Methodist), and others (e.g., Jehovah's Witnesses, Christian Science). For the most part, Christians hold that Jesus' death atoned for the sins of men and women, providing a way to experience the forgiveness of God and to gain eternal life.

Many denominations practice baptism, so when infants or children are very ill, baptism should be offered. Christians usually have no special dietary requirements, although some choose to abstain from eating meat on Fridays and/or during Lent. Some Christians may wish to abstain from food (fast) before receiving Holy Communion. Some (depending on the denomination) abstain from alcohol.

Family planning varies from religion to religion within Christianity. Some denominations allow artificial birth control methods; others do not. Most denominations do not object to natural family planning methods (e.g., rhythm). Most have no religious objections to blood transfusion or organ transplantation.

Roman Catholicism

In Roman Catholicism, the **sacraments** are a means to obtain grace. A Roman Catholic who is seriously ill might wish to receive the sacrament of *anointing the sick*. This sacrament, once known as the last rites, can be repeated if the person recovers and then becomes ill at a later time. Only a priest can hear the *sacrament of reconciliation* (confession), during which God, through the agency of the priest, grants forgiveness for past sins. The *Eucharist* (communion bread), consecrated at the *mass* (a religious service), may be brought to hospitalized patients by a priest, deacon, or designated lay Eucharistic minister. Other denominations within Christianity (e.g., Episcopalians and Lutherans) observe certain sacraments as well, although the meaning and details of the rituals may vary.

Christian Science

The Christian Science faith is a unique form of Christianity. Established in the United States in 1879, Christian Science teaches a reliance on God for healing rather than on medicine or surgery. Therefore, you might encounter followers as patients only after accidents or because of family or legal pressures.

Christian Scientists do not use alcohol and tobacco; strict Christian Scientists may not drink tea or coffee. Adults will probably not accept a blood transfusion, but parents usually consent to transfusion and other medical care for their child if doctors consider it essential or the law requires them to do so. Adults will not usually consent to donate or receive organs.

Jehovah's Witnesses

Jehovah's Witnesses try to live according to the commands of God as written in both the Old and New Testaments of the Bible. They will accept most medical treatments, but they believe that "taking blood into one's body" is morally wrong. This means that they will not allow transfusions of whole blood or its components. The Jehovah's Witness faith also does not permit donation or receipt of an organ through which blood flows. If blood is not involved (e.g., corneal transplants) they may accept transplantation. As it affects diet, this belief means that meat is not acceptable if an animal has been strangled or shot and not bled properly. Some Jehovah's Witness do not eat meat at all. Jehovah's Witnesses do not celebrate birthdays or holidays, except for the anniversary of the death of Christ. The date of that anniversary varies from year to year. Jehovah's Witnesses abstain from tobacco and other recreational drugs. They may drink alcohol but do not condone drunkenness.

Mormonism

The Mormon Church is also known as the Church of Jesus Christ of Latter-Day Saints. Mormons believe in Jesus and one God; however, they adhere to a more recently revealed sacred writing, the Book of Mormon (which they believe an angel gave to Joseph Smith in the 19th century). Mormons follow a strict health code, known as the Word of Wisdom, which advises healthful living and prohibits the use of tea, coffee, alcohol, and tobacco. Some Mormons (both men and women) wear a sacred undergarment that they remove only for hygiene purposes. Nurses may also remove it before surgery, but it must at all times be considered intensely private and be treated with respect (Keddington, 2007).

Seventh Day Adventism

The Seventh Day Adventist Church is distinguished mostly by observance of Saturday, the original seventh day of the Judeo-Christian week, as the Sabbath, a day of rest and worship. To keep the Sabbath holy, Adventists do no secular work or unnecessary business on Saturday. The church also emphasizes diet, health, and culturally conservative principles (e.g., many Adventists are opposed to body piercing and tattoos. Some even refrain from wearing jewelry). Adventists usually practice communion, which begins with a foot-washing ceremony, four times a year. Regarding dietary practices, the church recommends vegetarianism and adherence to the kosher laws in the Old Testament of the Bible. This includes abstinence from pork, shellfish, and other "unclean" foods. However, most Adventists do eat meat. Most do not use alcohol, tobacco, illegal drugs, and beverages containing caffeine. Although the church is generally anti-abortion, in cases of serious dilemmas (e.g., threat to the woman's life or pregnancy resulting from rape or incest), women are counseled to make their own decisions. The Adventist church is officially against active euthanasia but permits a passive form through withdrawal of medical support to allow the patient to die. Birth control is permitted for married couples.

Islam

The word *Islam* means submission. In particular, a Muslim is one who submits to Allah (God). The principal book of authority in Islam, the Koran (Qu'ran), is the result of a vision received by Muhammad, the founder of Islam, in the early 7th century A.D. Islam teaches that all faiths have essentially one common message: There is a Supreme Being whose sovereignty is acknowledged in worship and whose teaching and commandments must be obeyed.

Muslims are forbidden to eat pork. They may eat other meat, but it has to be *halal* meat, that is, killed in a special manner stated in Islamic law. Fish and eggs are allowed, but not if they are cooked near pork or non-halal meat. During the month of Ramadan, a Muslim fasts between sunrise and sunset; however, those who are sick are not expected to fast. Essential drugs and medicines are allowed at all hours during Ramadan.

Muslims always wash their hands before eating. Patients prefer to wash in free-flowing water, so tub baths are considered unhygienic. If a shower is not available, provide a pitcher to use in the bath.

Women prefer to be treated by female staff. Some women may refuse vaginal examination by a male nurse or physician because they are forbidden to expose their bodies to or be touched by any man other than their husband. Women may wear a locket containing religious writing around the neck in a small leather bag. These are kept for protection and strength, so you should never remove them.

There is no specific religious rule prohibiting blood transfusion or organ transplantation; however, strict Muslims will not usually agree to organ transplants. Orthodox Muslims do not approve of contraception; however, individuals vary widely in their practices. Abortion is frowned on but may be tolerated for medical reasons.

Baha'i

The Baha'i faith was established in 1863 in Persia and has its roots in Babism, a reformist outgrowth of Islam. A Baha'i patient in the hospital will accept usual routines and treatment. Alcohol, including that used in cooking, is not permitted.

Hinduism

Hinduism, which many religious scholars believe is the oldest major religion still practiced today, does not embrace a single body of beliefs and practices. Nor does it maintain the existence of a single deity, believing that no one manifestation of God can possibly capture the limitless nature of God. Thus, Hindus may worship several or even hundreds of gods and goddesses. Even elements in the natural world, such as rivers, fire, and so forth, are considered aspects of God. Sacred Hindu texts include the *Vedas*, the *Bhagavad Gita* (Song of the Blessed One), and the *Ramayana*, the story of the life of the god Rama. Despite commonly held beliefs and texts, Hindu religious practices vary a great deal, depending on areas of origin.

Hindus practice **ayurvedic medicine,** which encompasses all aspects of life, including diet, sleep, elimination, and hygiene. Some believe in the medicinal properties of "hot" and "cold" foods—"hot" and "cold" having nothing to do with either temperature or spicy qualities. Although some Hindus will eat eggs and even chicken, most are lactovegetarians, consuming milk but no eggs. Fasting, which may mean eating only "pure" foods such as fruit or yogurt, is common during major festivals but is not expected of the sick. Tobacco and alcohol may or may not be accepted.

Hindus prefer to wash in free-flowing water (e.g., a shower instead of a tub bath). If a shower is not available, provide a jug of water for the person to use in the bath. Women are modest and usually prefer to be treated by female medical staff. Jewelry often has a religious or cultural significance. Some Hindus wear "sacred thread" around the body or wrist. Do not remove or cut this thread without permission from the patient or next of kin. There is no religious objection to contraception, blood transfusion, or organ donation, as a rule.

Sikhism

Sikhism combines the teachings of Hinduism and Islamic Sufism, which is the mystical branch of Islam. Beliefs of the religion include monotheism and the realization of God through religious exercises and meditation. Many Sikhs are strict vegetarians. Alcohol and tobacco are forbidden. Sikhs may use contraception but do not speak openly about it. They do not generally object to blood transfusions or organ transplantation.

Buddhism

The Buddha, or the "Awakened One," is revered not as a god, but as an example of a way of life (Fig. 14-2). He was born into a royal family in 624 B.C. in a part of northern India that is now in Nepal, gained enlightenment at the age of 35, and then began to teach others how to attain liberation from suffering, not only for themselves, but also for others.

One of the Buddha's core teachings is that suffering can be ended by following the eightfold path: right understanding, right intention, right speech, right action, right livelihood, right effort, right mindfulness, and right contemplation (Bodhi, 2007; Kneirim, 2008). **Nirvana,** similar to the Christian concept of heaven, can

FIGURE 14-2 The Buddha is revered as an example of a way of life.

be attained only through an absence of desire, the achievement of perfection, and the lack of a unique identity.

Many Buddhists follow a vegetarian diet; in some cases, the diet may include both milk and eggs. Fasting customs vary by tradition. Buddhists accept contraception but typically condemn abortion and active euthanasia. They will usually accept blood transfusion and organ transplantation.

Native American Religions

There are more than 400 federally recognized Native American nations or tribes in the United States. Although each has its own traditions and cultural heritage, some general beliefs underlie the more specific tribal ideas. The Earth is considered to be a living organism, the body of a higher individual, and humankind has an intimate relation with this organism through nature. When the Earth is harmed, humankind is harmed, and vice versa. The land belongs to life, life belongs to the land, and the land belongs to itself (Boyd, 1974).

Health is a state of harmony with nature. Whenever disharmony exists, disease or illness can occur. The traditional healer is the medicine man or woman who is wise in the interrelationships of land, humankind, and the universe. Many Native Americans believe that the treatments they receive from medicine men and women and traditional healers are far better than those rendered by the dominant healthcare establishment, which often treats Native Americans with scorn or disrespect (Fig. 14-3). You should know that note-taking by the

FIGURE 14-3 Kokopelli, the humpbacked flute player, has been a sacred figure to Native Americans of the Southwest for thousands of years. He is a legendary symbol of fertility who brought well-being to the people.

professional is forbidden; when you take a history or perform an exam, you must rely on your memory to record findings later. Native Americans tend to converse in a low tone of voice and may maintain long periods of silence. Be sure the setting is quiet enough to allow you to hear the patient because it is impolite to indicate that you did not hear the communications.

Rastafarianism

The Rastafarian movement began in the 1930s in the West Indies. It emphasizes personal dignity and a deep love of God. Rastafarians use the Old and New Testaments of the Bible as their authoritative writings, but they do not consider themselves to be Christian. There are no churches, services, or official clergy.

Rastafarians do not eat pork and shellfish, some are completely vegetarian, and some do not drink milk or coffee. Wearing second-hand clothing is forbidden, so the patient may be unwilling to wear hospital gowns

that have been worn by others. You may need to provide a disposable gown or allow the person to wear her own personal nightclothes. Patients may be anxious about accepting blood transfusion (because of concern about contamination); however, many Rastafarians will accept transfusions after being reassured.

KnowledgeCheck 14-3

- Which major religion believes in the anointing of the sick or dying?
- Which denomination or religion does not believe in blood transfusions?
- In terms of Native American beliefs and healthcare, who is the traditional healer or the person to be consulted in the event of "illness"?
- True or false: Most Hindus are vegetarian.

  Go to Chapter 14, **Knowledge Check Response Sheet and Answers,** on the Student Resource Disk or DavisPlus at http://davisplus.fadavis.com/Wilkinson2

CriticalThinking 14-4

- What are some of the ways that world religions might influence nursing care?

Self-knowledge: What Every Nurse Should Know

As you have seen, your patients' spiritual and religious backgrounds may be diverse and may involve ways of thinking and doing that seem strange to you or that you do not fully understand. Before trying to understand your patients' religious experience, you must give considerable thought to your own spiritual journey. Recall that attaining self-knowledge is an important aspect of becoming a full-spectrum nurse.

What Are Your Personal Biases?

We each carry our own perspectives with us at all times. We tend to view the world through lenses we acquired in childhood, adolescence, and early adulthood. In addition, our religious education is sometimes taught with a certain flavor of "upmanship"; that is, we are taught that our religious beliefs and practices are superior to all others. When you view your own experience as the norm or as the preferred way of organizing the world, you tend to limit the range of care you provide to the patient who believes differently. Spiritual care demands nonjudgmental attitudes and an open manner of thinking that invites rather than excludes.

CriticalThinking 14-5

Consider the following examples. For each person, what moral/spiritual judgments must the nurse be careful *not* to make?

- A nurse is caring for a gay man who is hospitalized with end-stage AIDS.

- A woman has come to the clinic to be treated for gonorrhea (a sexually transmitted disease). She says she has had at least six sexual partners this year.
- A man comes to the emergency department (ED) at least once a month to ask for morphine to treat his back pain. He is known to abuse drugs and to visit other EDs for the same purpose.

If you are aware of your biases, it will be easier to avoid abuses of spiritual care, such as the following:

- **Attempting to convert others to your beliefs.** For example, if a patient is near death, he and his family might be offended if their nurse inquires whether they are "saved" Christians. By remaining focused on the patient's need to talk about meaning, salvation, or other end-of-life issues, you provide full-spectrum spiritual care. As another example, notice that Mr. Johnson's sister (in "Meet Your Patient") seems very close to imposing her religion on him. She may alienate him further if he perceives that he is being "pushed."
- **Trying to be all things to all people,** regardless of their background or the extent of spiritual care needed. Clearly, there are times when you should refer to others with more knowledge and experience in religion and spirituality, with the patient's permission, of course. In addition, whenever a patient requests the services of a rabbi, priest, or other spiritual adviser, you should relay that request to the agency's chaplain so that all disciplines remain informed throughout the care delivery process.

In summary, to work effectively with a diverse population, you must first obtain a greater degree of self-knowledge by (1) being open to the many possibilities for diverse thinking, (2) welcoming challenging experiences that allow for personal growth, and (3) taking time to contemplate how your actions and biases might affect the care of others. The more you know about yourself, the more effectively you care for others.

What Are Some Barriers to Spiritual Care?

Although most nurses would acknowledge that patients have a spiritual dimension, few actually identify spiritual problems or provide spiritual interventions. This may be a result of economic constraints, poor staffing, and high-tech care, which force nurses to focus on physical needs to the exclusion of spiritual needs (Cavendish, Konecny, Mitzeliotis, et al., 2003). You may judge these nurses less harshly after you understand more about the barriers to spiritual interventions by nurses.

Lack of General Awareness of Spirituality

One study of oncology nurses found that more than half incorrectly identified the patient's religion and that only 16% incorporated any kind of spiritual assessment into their care (Sodestrom & Martin, 1987). Highfield's (1992) study confirms the incidence of inaccurate spiritual assessment by nurses of patients in

their care. A greater awareness of spirituality in general will help you tune into the spiritual needs of patients and improve your comfort in communicating about spiritual matters.

Lack of Awareness of Your Own Spiritual Belief System

To feel comfortable making spiritual interventions, you will need more than just theoretical knowledge. You will need introspection and an awareness of your own spiritual journey to integrate the spiritual domain into patient care. Lane (1987) identifies three steps in the spiritual growth of nurses:

1. Developing a "greater awareness of the spirit within self" in order to be a better listener for the patient
2. Opening the self by being totally present with the patient
3. Allowing the patient to share his feelings and emotions without reserve

Activities to heighten your awareness of your own spirituality, gain a broader view of spirituality, and increase sensitivity to others' spiritual needs include the following (Beckman, Boxley-Harges, Bruick-Sorge, et al., 2007):

- Increase your knowledge about spirituality.
- Develop your critical and reflective thinking abilities.
- Explore your own spirituality (e.g., reflection, discussing with others). One technique is to write your own epitaph: one or two lines summing up how you would like to be remembered.
- Reflect on your thoughts and feelings about end-of-life issues. Imagine you have only a few weeks to live; think how you would feel.
- Reflect on your personal experience with grief and loss. For example, what is the first death you can remember? What were your feelings at the time? How do you usually cope with loss? What actions by others comforted you?

You must find ways to take care of and nurture your own spiritual needs; otherwise, providing this aspect of care can be emotionally draining.

Differences in Spirituality Between Nurse and Patient

Patients and nurses can be at different levels in terms of spirituality. When a patient's spiritual beliefs are very different from your own, you must be careful not to impose your beliefs on the patient or discount the importance of the patient's beliefs and rituals. When the patient's views or beliefs are similar to yours, take care not to make false assumptions about his spiritual needs. Just because you agree on some things does not mean you will have the same views or needs in all areas of spirituality or religion.

Critical**Thinking** 14-6

- How does your religion or spirituality differ from Mr. Johnson's?
- How is it similar?
- Can you think of problems these differences and similarities could cause you in caring for him?

Fear that Your Knowledge Base Is Insufficient

Nurses sometimes avoid giving spiritual care because they believe they lack knowledge of spirituality or of the patient's religion. This is a realistic concern. In several studies, nurses were found to be unsure of what constituted spiritual problems and spiritual interventions (Sodestrom & Martin, 1987; Ryan, 1992). In some cases they did not identify the spiritual dimension of care, or they took religious aspects into account but did not place them into a broader spiritual perspective. Highfield and Cason (1983) found that oncology nurses placed greater emphasis on physical and psychosocial nursing care and that they frequently did not identify the patient's spiritual needs. The good news is that spiritual care has never been more welcomed by patients. You can provide truly holistic care for the patient when you address spiritual needs in a plan of care.

Fear of Where Spiritual Discussions May Lead

Many nurses fear that inquiring into the spiritual domain might cause harm to the patient. For example, what if a patient asks you, "Do you think active euthanasia is morally wrong? Would it jeopardize my salvation?" Here are some fears that may arise:

- You may not feel prepared to answer the questions.
- You might have an answer based on your personal religious beliefs but fear the patient may think you are imposing your beliefs on him.
- You might wonder whether communicating your own beliefs (e.g., if you favor active euthanasia) might jeopardize the patient's spiritual life if your ideas turn out to be "wrong."

The following are some ideas that may help counter your fears. First and foremost, keep in mind that the fact that the patient is addressing this concern with you indicates you are open to the spiritual domain of care. Second, the patient in this example is concerned with issues related to euthanasia. This could lead to discussions about the patient's fears of pain, dependence, being a burden on family members, and dying alone. Third, this is an area for which you should seek collaboration with a chaplain, who is more prepared to deal with specific religious issues. You should realize that being open to the spiritual realm and assessing the patient's need for spiritual intervention does not mean that you must be a chaplain or have the extraordinary ability to deal with all spiritual or religious questions or requests. The Practical Knowledge section will provide a more detailed understanding of your role in spiritual care.

KnowledgeCheck 14-4

- What qualities can you demonstrate that may help you improve the quality of spiritual care you provide?
- What common barriers to spiritual interventions do nurses encounter?
- True or false: No matter how nonjudgmental and open we may think ourselves to be, we all carry our own unique biases and prejudices that have the potential to affect patient care.

 Go to Chapter 14, **Knowledge Check Response Sheet and Answers,** on the Student Resource Disk or DavisPlus at http://davisplus.fadavis.com/Wilkinson2

 Critical**Thinking** 14-7

- What are some of the possible abuses of spiritual care provided by nurses?
- What are some ways that you can develop a greater awareness of the "spirit within the self"?
- Discuss ways that nurses (and patients, for that matter) can nurture their own spiritual needs.

Practical **Knowledge**
knowing how

Most hospital admission forms include a place to record the patient's religious preferences, and most nursing assessment forms even include questions such as, "What religious rituals do you practice?" Unfortunately, some nurses believe that by completing such forms, they have addressed the patient's spiritual needs. They may be relieved because they don't feel competent to deal any further with spirituality or because they are afraid to be perceived as imposing their own religion on the patient. However, armed with your basic theoretical knowledge of spirituality and your growing spiritual self-knowledge, you should be able to provide a level of support that extends beyond paperwork to compassion and caring.

Care**Planning** & **Mapping**Practice

To see a care plan and care map for a client with Spiritual Distress,

 Go to Student Resources, **Care Planning and Care Mapping Practice,** at http://davisplus.fadavis.com/Wilkinson2

■ ASSESSMENT

People of the same religion often vary greatly in the degree to which they follow religious practices. It is not enough to "fill in the religion blank" on an assessment form; you must assess each person individually to determine religious needs and practices.

Spiritual Assessment Tools

Some healthcare agencies have focused spiritual assessment tools tailored to their particular setting. Several others have been developed.

HOPE. One easy-to-use screening method is to use HOPE questions. They have not been validated by research, but they do allow for an open-ended exploration of spiritual resources and concerns (Gowri & Hight, 2001). HOPE is a mnemonic, as follows:

H—sources of Hope
O—Organized religion
P—Personal spirituality/Practices
E—Effects on medical care and end-of-life issues

JAREL. The JAREL spiritual well-being scale was developed and is commonly used by nurses (Hungelmann, Kenkel-Rossi, Klassen, et al., 1996). Cutting across religious and atheistic belief systems, it assesses three key dimensions: (1) faith/belief, (2) life/self-responsibility, and (3) life-satisfaction/self-actualization.

SPIRIT. Highfield (2000) has proposed a comprehensive method of spiritual assessment. It involves an interview that is concerned with six key areas designated by the acronym SPIRIT:

SP—**Sp**iritual/religious belief system
I—**I**ntegration within a spiritual community
R—**R**itualized practices and restrictions
I—**I**mplications for medical care
T—**T**erminal events planning.

To see a copy of a spiritual assessment based on this model, and for questions to use for the HOPE approach,

 Go to Chapter 14, **Assessment Guidelines and Tools,** in Volume 2.

You can use the SPIRIT model with the JAREL tool presented in ESG Figure 14-1 and the combined assessment tool and plan of care presented in ESG Figure 14-2. To find these tools,

 Go to Chapter 14, **Tables, Boxes, Figures: ESG Figures 14-1 and 14-2,** on the Student Resource Disk or DavisPlus at http://davisplus.fadavis.com/Wilkinson2

KnowledgeCheck 14-5

- What are the six areas for spiritual assessment summarized in Highfield's (2000) acronym SPIRIT?

 Go to Chapter 14, **Knowledge Check Response Sheet and Answers,** on the Student Resource Disk or DavisPlus at http://davisplus.fadavis.com/Wilkinson2

 CriticalThinking 14-8

- Complete the SPIRIT assessment on yourself. Discuss it with your classmates.

 Go to Chapter 14, **Assessment Guidelines and Tools,** in Volume 2.

Levels of Spiritual Assessment

Given the time constraints of the admission process in inpatient facilities, stresses involved with the patient's introduction to a healthcare setting, and the multiple people involved, it is difficult to obtain meaningful information on initial assessment. For this reason, initial data are often limited to the patient's church preference, name of clergy, whom to call in case of emergency, dietary requirements, and any religious implications for medical care (e.g., refusal of organ transplants or blood transfusion). Over time, as you have more contact with the patient and family, trust will develop, and you will be able to obtain more sensitive, complex, and meaningful information.

 ANALYSIS/NURSING DIAGNOSIS

When analyzing spiritual assessment data, consider the person's developmental stage. People progress through stages of spiritual development in much the same way as they develop physically and cognitively. Spiritual behaviors that seem problematic in one stage may not be so in an earlier stage. To review spiritual development,

Go to **Chapter 9—Expanded Discussion** on the Student Resource Disk or DavisPlus at http://davisplus.fadavis.com/Wilkinson2

Spirituality Diagnoses

The following are NANDA-I diagnostic labels that specifically deal with religion and spirituality.

- *Moral Distress* is experienced when the person makes an ethical or moral decision, but then is unable to carry out the chosen action. Defining characteristics include anguish, powerlessness, guilt, frustration, anxiety, self-doubt, and fear over the inability to act on the moral choice.
- *Impaired Religiosity* is difficulty in exercising or impaired ability to exercise reliance on beliefs or to participate in rituals of a faith tradition (e.g., go to church, take communion).
- *Risk for Impaired Religiosity* occurs when risk factors for Impaired Religiosity are present, but symptoms are not. Risk factors may be categorized as developmental, environmental, physical, psychological, sociocultural, or spiritual. Specific examples include life transitions, lack of transportation, pain, depression, social isolation, and suffering.
- *Readiness for Enhanced Religiosity* is the ability to increase reliance on religious beliefs and/or participate in rituals of a particular faith tradition. The patient is not experiencing a problem, but wishes to make a satisfactory situation even better.
- *Spiritual Distress* is "impaired ability to experience and integrate meaning and purpose in life through a

person's connectedness with self, others, art, music, literature, nature, or a power greater than oneself" (NANDA International, 2009, p. 301). Defining characteristics (signs and symptoms) of this diagnosis include the following.

Connections with self: Expressing a lack of hope, love, courage, acceptance, or peace; a lack of meaning and purpose in life; inability to forgive self; feelings of anger or guilt

Connections with others: Refusing to see clergy; refusing to interact with family or friends; reporting lack of support system; expressions of alienation

Connections with art, music, literature, nature: No interest in nature, decrease in previous interest in music, writing, art, no interest in spiritual reading

Connections with power greater than self: Inability to pray, inability or refusal to participate in religious activities, feelings of abandonment by God or other deity, expressions of anger toward God or other deity, requests to see a religious leader, sudden changes in spiritual practices (increased or decreased)

- *Risk for Spiritual Distress* exists when the patient experiences energy-consuming anxiety, low self-esteem, mental illness, physical illness, blocks to self-love, poor relationships, physical or psychological stress, substance abuse, loss of loved one, natural disasters, situational losses, maturational losses, or inability to forgive. Illness creates countless risk factors for spiritual distress.

- *Readiness for Enhanced Spiritual Well-Being* describes healthy spirituality. NANDA-I (2009) defines it as the "ability to experience and integrate meaning and purpose in life through connectedness with self, others, art, music, literature, nature, and/or a "power" greater than oneself that can be strengthened" (p. 292). It is the opposite of Spiritual Distress, so you will see positive expressions of faith, hope, love, courage, acceptance, and peace; healthy connections with others and with art, music, literature, and nature; and prayer and other expressions of a connection with a power higher than oneself.

The following are examples of full diagnostic statements for spiritual problems:

- *Spiritual Distress* related to overwhelming anxiety associated with the need to have a surgical procedure that is not accepted by her religion
- *Risk for Spiritual Distress* related to unremitting pain and loss of hope for relief, as manifested by patient's question about the usefulness of prayer ("God has forgotten about me.")

Critical Thinking 14-9
- Which of these nursing diagnoses would you use for Mr. Johnson ("Meet Your Patient"): Spiritual Distress, Risk for Spiritual Distress, or Readiness for Enhanced Spiritual Well-Being? Why?

Spirituality as Etiology

In the spiritual realm, it is difficult sometimes to determine what is the problem and what is the etiology. Does the patient experience Spiritual Distress because of pain and hopelessness? Or did the patient first lose faith in God, which led to hopelessness and anxiety? Either way, spiritual support is needed.

Several of the NANDA-I diagnoses relate to spirituality as either problem, etiology, or symptom. Non–NANDA-I problems include anger or resentment; feelings of guilt, shame, inadequacy, abandonment, or distrust; depression or sadness; and the inability to find meaning in life. The following are examples of diagnostic statements with spiritual etiologies:

Anxiety related to inability to reconcile decision to use birth control with religious proscriptions

Chronic Sorrow related to loss of faith in spiritual power outside self

Death Anxiety related to feeling unprepared for death and concern about the afterlife

Decisional Conflict related to confusion about the religious implications of the decision to forego heroic treatment measures

Hopelessness related to lack of belief in a power outside self, combined with overwhelming lack of energy

Interrupted Family Processes related to conflicts among family members about the type of spiritual support needed by the patient

Noncompliance (with treatment regimen) related to the belief that the illness is "God's will" and that healing will occur (without treatment) for the same reason

Powerlessness related to perceiving that prayers have not been answered and that God is either not hearing him or is punishing him

Social Isolation related to inability to participate in church activities secondary to chronic illness

A Non–NANDA-I Diagnosis

Millspaugh (2005) has suggested *Spiritual Pain* as a diagnosis. When a person experiences a combination of awareness of death, loss of relationships, loss of self, loss of purpose, and loss of control, Spiritual Pain may occur. However, this combination of negative experiences can be balanced by having a life-affirming and transcending purpose and an internal sense of control. The presence and quality of Spiritual Pain is determined by the degree to which the person is experiencing each component, and by the relationship of the components to each other. See Figure 14-4.

KnowledgeCheck 14-6
Consider the following statement: A nursing diagnosis that reflects either an actual or a potential problem may reflect religious and/or spiritual dimensions of the human condition.
- Is this statement true?
- Would it be true for a *physical* diagnosis (e.g., Disturbed Sleep Pattern)? Explain your thinking.

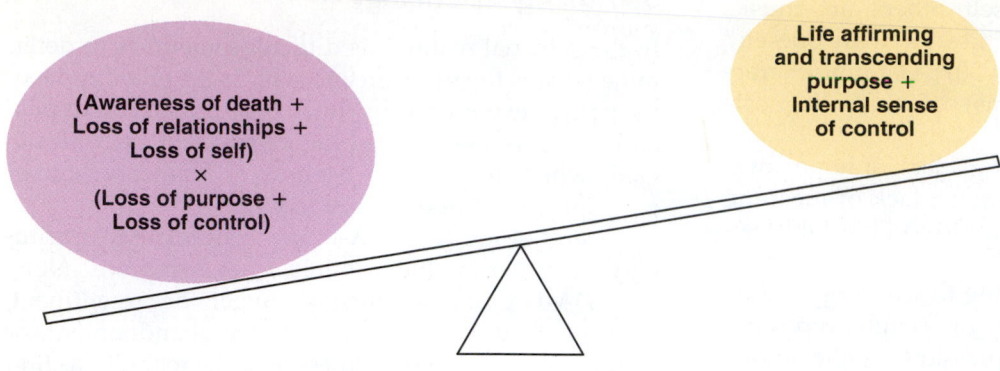

(Awareness of death +
Loss of relationships +
Loss of self)
×
(Loss of purpose +
Loss of control)

Life affirming
and transcending
purpose +
Internal sense
of control

FIGURE 14-4 **Components of spiritual pain.** (*Based on:* C. D. Millspaugh [2005]. Assessment and response to spiritual pain: Part II. *Journal of Palliative Medicine*, 8[6], 1110–1117.)

 Go to Chapter 14, **Knowledge Check Response Sheet and Answers,** on the Student Resource Disk or DavisPlus at http://davisplus.fadavis.com/Wilkinson2

PLANNING OUTCOMES/EVALUATION

The outcomes you establish in the planning stage of the nursing process serve as the criteria for your evaluation of the patient's progress and the success of the nursing interventions.

NOC standardized outcomes associated with spirituality diagnoses include, but are not limited to, the following: Anxiety Level, Comfortable Death, Comfort Status: Psychospiritual, Dignified Life Closure, Hope, Loneliness Severity, Personal Resiliency, Personal Well-Being, Quality of Life, Spiritual Health, and Will to Live (Moorhead, Johnson, Maas, et al., 2008).

Individualized goals/outcome statements you might write for spiritual diagnoses include the following:

For Risk for Spiritual Distress

- Potential spiritual issues are assessed, identified, and explored.
- Exhibits no signs or symptoms of spiritual distress (e.g., finds meaning in life, expresses hope and faith, follows usual religious practices).

For Spiritual Distress

- Returns to previous state of spiritual well-being and comfort (e.g., expresses a sense of peace, asks to see religious adviser).
- Shares spiritual and religious concerns.

For Readiness for Enhanced Spiritual Well-being

- Experiences a higher level of connectedness with self, others, higher power, and/or nature.
- Experiences a nonjudgmental environment in which he feels free to express all questions and concerns.
- Establishes relationship with care provider that promotes the exploration of spiritual issues and their impact on healthcare.

PLANNING INTERVENTIONS/IMPLEMENTATION

Spiritual interventions are interventions to treat and prevent spiritual problems related to the patient's illness.

You will direct some nursing activities to resolving the problem, others at removing the etiology, and still others at relieving symptoms. You will, of course, base your nursing activities on the patient's symptoms and the problem etiologies. However, there are some nursing interventions that address spiritual problems in general.

Standardized (NIC) Spirituality Interventions

Clinical Insight 14-1 includes Nursing Interventions Classification (NIC) interventions and selected activities for the spirituality and religiosity diagnoses discussed in the preceding text.

 Go to **Clinical Insight 14-1** in Volume 2.

NIC standardized interventions to promote spirituality are discussed in this section. The evidence base for these is specific to older adults (National Guidelines Clearinghouse, 2005); however, they would seem to be indicated for other age groups, as well.

When you are performing interventions of a spiritual nature, remember that you absolutely must follow the patient's lead and be caring and respectful without inserting your own beliefs into the conversation. Choose your language carefully—words such as "saved," "repentance," and so on, which may be a part of everyday conversation for people who follow some religions, may cause some patients to feel pressured or uncomfortable. Try to mirror, and not go beyond, the patient's religious terminology. It requires knowledge, skill, and practice to provide religious support without imposing your own beliefs. The safest course of action, of course, is to offer to contact a chaplain for the patient. However, patients cannot always—or may not always want to—wait for a chaplain.

Active Listening (NIC)

The Active Listening intervention allows the nurse to establish a trusting relationship and to hear, understand, and interpret what the client is saying. Listening actively involves four NIC interventions, and one nonstandardized activity.

Presence (NIC)

Presence means to be with patient and family in meaningful ways. This requires not only your actual presence at the bedside, but also being open to issues and concerns of the patient and allowing the patient to lead discussions rather than setting the agenda or controlling the conversation. It involves sincere communication and being fully available to the client, and might include listening to the patient's "stories" about his illness.

Touch

Caring touch, such as hand holding or touching an arm or shoulder, facilitates communication. It conveys concern, comfort, and acceptance, especially during stressful experiences. At least one study has shown touch to improve life satisfaction and faith.

Exploring Meaning (non-NIC)

Meaning refers to a clear understanding of the illness or loss (e.g., loss of independence). It also refers to the concepts of finding meaning and purpose in life, or a sense of personal worthiness. You can facilitate the patient's search for meaning by asking probing questions, providing explanations, and reframing maladaptive interpretations of life events. Finding meaning may promote spiritual growth.

Reminiscence Therapy (NIC)

Reminiscence is the recalling and sharing with another person's past life events. It promotes meaning making through rethinking and clarifying previous experiences. As the patient reminisces, he may make spiritual links by expressing personal beliefs that helped him live through difficult life events. This intervention is more effective within a long-term relationship.

Spiritual Support (NIC)

NIC defines Spiritual Support as "assisting the patient to feel balance and connection with a greater power" (Bulechek, Butcher, & Dochterman, 2008, p. 674). Effective Spiritual Support is based on a focused spiritual assessment, including the person's belief system. It may include assisting with forgiveness, encouraging hope, praying, and reading scriptures or other texts the patient requests.

Forgiveness Facilitation (NIC)

Forgiveness is the act of pardoning or being pardoned for an offense, debt, or obligation. Letting go of the resentment felt for another promotes constructive changes in a person's life, as well as a sense of renewal and reconciliation with God, church, and one's inner being. To provide this intervention, you must first assess the patient's needs for reconciliation with self, others, and God. If, like Mr. Johnson ("Meet Your Patient"), the patient has lost contact with family members because of disagreements, you could collaborate with the social worker and chaplain about ways to facilitate a meeting.

Forgiveness is one aspect of love. People have a spiritual need to forgive others and to be forgiven. When a person cannot forgive others, it separates him from them and interferes with giving and receiving love. When a person cannot forgive himself, he may feel the pain of shame, guilt, and anger. Or the person may be hurting because he wants forgiveness from someone he has wronged or from God. Many people interpret their illness as punishment for sins. Some find it difficult to seek forgiveness and to believe that they have been forgiven, but this is important to achieving spiritual peace.

Group sharing of prayer and forgiveness experiences foster the progress in forgiving others. You can help by listening when the person expresses self-doubt or guilt, providing guidance, praying with the patient if the patient asks you to, asking him if he is ready to forgive someone else, or offering to contact his chosen spiritual leader if intensive spiritual support is needed.

Hope Inspiration (NIC)

Hope is a subjective state of confidence in the possibility of a better future. It includes a positive orientation, faith, and will to live. It has also been described as looking forward with eager expectation. Hopelessness is a state in which the person perceives limited or no alternatives or personal choices. To intervene effectively, it is important to know the source of the person's hope and the factors underlying the feelings of hopelessness. As a nurse, you can encourage spiritual growth, which is thought to facilitate hope, and you can refer your patient to a support group to help in stress reduction, coping, and hope.

Prayer (non-NIC)

Prayer is an integral component of almost every religion. A recent study found that about one-third of U.S. adults use prayer for health concerns; 69% found it "very helpful" (McCaffrey, Eisenberg, Legedza, et al., 2004). The numbers are even higher for older adults, 84% of whom reported using prayer as a form of complementary healing treatment, and 96% using it to cope with stress (Dunn & Horgas, 2000). So, it is quite possible that a patient or a family member may ask you to pray for him or with him.

It is important to distinguish between *praying with* and *praying for*. If the patient asks you to pray *with* him, you must determine whether he simply wants you to be present while he or another person leads the prayer. Ask whether he wants you to begin the prayer or whether he wants to begin the prayer. If a patient asks you to pray *for* him, assess what it is that he wants you to pray for. Often the patient is merely asking you to pray for him on your own time, as frequently as your schedule allows.

Regardless of the situation, if you feel comfortable doing so, then you should enter the experience of prayer with confidence; after all, the patient or family

Complementary & Alternative Modalities (CAM)

Intercessory Prayer

Many people pray when they are ill, and prayer seems to have positive effects. But what about the effects of *intercessory prayer*—the prayers of people for *others* who are ill? How useful is intercessory prayer? The following studies, except for Harris, Gowda, Kilb, et al. (1999), and Matthews, Marlowe, and MacNutt (2000), provide little support for the use of intercessory prayer as a CAM. However, this is not an exhaustive list of studies of intercessory prayer, and research is ongoing.

➤ **Matthews, Conti, & Sireci (2001).** For 95 adult hemodialysis subjects with end-stage renal disease, this study found no appreciable improvement in physiological and psychological well-being.

➤ **Palmer, Katerndahl, & Morgan-Kidd (2004).** Researchers studied 86 community-dwelling persons, ages 18 to 88 years. Intercessory prayer was used for 1 month to intervene with a life concern or problem the participant disclosed at the beginning. No effect on problem resolution was found. However, prayer did effectively reduce the subject's level of concern, but only if the subject initially believed that the problem could be resolved. Also, better physical functioning was

observed among those who had a high belief in prayer.

➤ **Roberts, Ahmed, & Hall (2000).** In a study performed in the United Kingdom, no evidence was found that intercessory prayer affected the numbers of people dying from leukemia or heart disease. Nor did it decrease the odds of a poor outcome for people with heart problems.

➤ **Harris, Gowda, Kilb, et al. (1999).** Remote, intercessory prayer was associated with reduced overall adverse events and shorter length of stay for hospitalized cardiac patients when used as an adjunct to standard medical care.

➤ **Matthews, Marlowe, & MacNutt (2000).** In patients with rheumatoid arthritis, 6 hours of direct-contact intercessory prayer produced overall improvement during a 1-year follow-up. However, there were no additional effects from the supplemental, distant intercessory prayers.

➤ **Benson, Dusek, Sherwood, et al. (2006).** In patients recovering after coronary artery bypass graft (CABG) surgery, this study found that intercessory prayer itself had no effect on complication-free recovery from CABG, but certainty of receiving intercessory prayer was associated with a higher incidence of complications.

member has asked you to be present because he feels at ease with you and trusts in your abilities. However, if you feel at all uncomfortable about offering prayer, then you should state those feelings and offer to find someone who is comfortable with prayer. For example, you might say either of the following to the patient or family, "Thank you for asking me to pray with you; there is another nurse on the floor who is better at this than I am. May I have your permission to seek that person out for you?" Or, you might reply as follows: "I am confident that the chaplain can help you in many ways with your request. May I make a referral to the chaplain for you?"

If you do wish to pray with patients, understanding the different types of prayer may help. **Prayer** consists of those ways that we respond to and interact with the Supreme Being, whether by words, thoughts, or actions. People tend to think of prayer in its narrowest sense as being requests for something. And though this is a very important and useful type of prayer, there are actually at least seven types of prayer (*Book of Common Prayer*, 1979):

- *Adoration* is the directing of our focus and our thoughts to God, asking nothing but to enjoy the presence of God in our lives. This might take the form of meditation.
- *Praise* involves the belief that the love of God draws our praises forth, not to obtain anything, but simply to offer words of praise.

- *Thanksgiving* is offered to God for all the blessings of life and living and whatever draws our attention to God's presence in our lives.
- *Penitence* is the desire to confess one's sins, with an intention to change.
- *Offering* is the offering of all that we have (our life, our work, our hopes and dreams) to God for the purposes that God envisions for us.
- *Intercession* is praying for the needs of others.
- *Petition* is prayer that presents our own needs to God.

As you see, prayer has a variety of purposes, expressions, and meanings to patients and their families, as well as to nurses themselves. For many people, prayer provides for periods of intimacy with God, reveals the presence and love of God, and serves as a powerful source of comfort and hope. For those who embrace the power and influence of prayer, it supports their spiritual journeys and may help them experience forgiveness, love, hope, trust, and meaning. Symbolically, a nurse engaged in prayer manifests the reality of God's presence with that patient.

You can support patients' prayer needs by offering to pray, meditate, or read spiritual text with them, or by providing literature, music, or other items the patient uses in prayer. If you wish to pray with a patient and would like some helpful guidelines,

VOL 2 Go to **Clinical Insight 14-2: Praying with Patients,** in Volume 2.

Other Nursing Activities

Spiritual care involves you in relationships with people who have come face to face with a significant life event that calls forth a new sense of meaning and purpose. To provide excellent spiritual care, you will need to adopt a supportive approach to the patient; a sense of benevolence (a wish to benefit) toward the patient; awareness of the patient, yourself, and the impact of family and significant others; empathy; and nonjudgmental understanding (Dickenson, 1975). Specific nursing activities, to be individualized to each client's needs, are discussed in the text that follows.

Make Referrals When Needed. There are times when you should refer a patient to others with more knowledge and experience in religion and spirituality. For example, a patient may be experiencing Spiritual Distress because he believes he needs forgiveness for a past act, or a patient may refuse medical treatment because she thinks her church would not approve. For hospitalized and hospice patients, you can usually ask the chaplain's office to refer the patient and family to clergy or religious counselors in the community. If you are working in a home or community setting, look in the telephone or other directory for local churches. Priests, ministers, rabbis, and other spiritual advisers are all resources for you and the patient.

Encourage Expression of Feelings. The best way to do this is simply to ask the patient how he is feeling or what he thinks about a particular situation.

Help the Patient Identify Feelings of Guilt. You might ask the following after a patient has voiced a concern: "How do you feel about that?" or "You seem to feel bad about saying/doing that."

Help Significant Others Understand the Patient's Feelings and Needs. Encourage family members to talk with the patient or simply to have a seat at the bedside. Periods of silence often lead into the most therapeutic of discussions.

Maximize the Patient's Comfort and Relief From Pain. This is one of the most important spiritual activities a nurse can perform. A patient cannot think about spiritual issues when plagued with physical pain or discomfort.

Listen to the Patient's "Stories." These tell the life history surrounding the person's illness.

Assess the Patient's Needs for Reconciliation. This may include reconciliation with self, others, and God. If, like Mr. Johnson ("Meet Your Patient"), the patient has lost contact with family members because of disagreements related to past events, you could collaborate with the social worker and chaplain about ways to facilitate a meeting.

Explore with the Client the Possible Meanings of Healing, Miracle, and Cure. Refer to the discussion of miracles earlier in this chapter.

Collaborate with the Dietary Department. Provide foods compatible with the person's religious needs. Encourage family members to bring foods from home, as appropriate.

Respect the Patient's Dress (and other) Requirements as Determined by His Religion. This may include wearing religious icons, jewelry, or special clothes.

Do not Make Assumptions About the Patient's and Family's Beliefs. When a patient dies, for example, a seemingly harmless statement such as "He's gone to a better place" assumes the family believes in an afterlife. If they ask, you can briefly share your beliefs, but reflect their questions back to them (e.g., "Tell me what *you* think happens after death.").

Complementary & Alternative Modalities (CAM)

Spiritual Care

Spiritual interventions, especially prayer, are a frequently used CAM:

- A recent study found that 63% of adult patients with cancer used at least one CAM therapy, which they all believed helped to improve their quality of life by helping them to cope with stress, obtain a sense of control, and decrease the discomforts of treatments and illness (Sparber, Bauer, Curt, et al., 2000).

- In this same study, the CAMs most often used were spiritual, relaxation, imagery, exercise, lifestyle, diet, and nutritional supplementation (Sparber, Bauer, Curt, et al., 2000).

- McCaffrey and colleagues (2004) found that 35% of respondents used prayer for health concerns and reported high levels of perceived helpfulness.

- Keegan (2000) found prayer to be the CAM most frequently practiced by both Mexican and Anglo Americans.

- Dunn and Horgas (2000) found that 96% of community-dwelling elders use prayer to cope with stress and that 84% used prayer as a form of CAM.

- At least one study (le Gallez, Dimmock, & Bird, 2000) found spiritual healing to be ineffective in achieving improved laboratory parameters or clinical symptoms (e.g., pain) in patients with rheumatoid arthritis.

KnowledgeCheck 14-7

- What is prayer?
- Name seven different types of prayer.
- What are the "uses" of prayer by its believers?
- When a patient asks you to pray for him, what might be your most effective first response?

 Go to Chapter 14, **Knowledge Check Response Sheet and Answers,** on the Student Resource Disk or DavisPlus at http://davisplus.fadavis.com/Wilkinson2

CriticalThinking 14-10

- A patient dying of lung cancer asks you to pray with him early one morning. You agree and ask him what he would like you to pray for. He responds: "That I may be cured of my cancer and go back home." He is on oxygen therapy, has pain medications given as prescribed, and is in a room by himself. Construct a prayer that might be meaningful and helpful.

Return to the scenario for Charles Johnson ("Meet Your Patient"). See whether you can answer the three questions more completely now than when you began reading the chapter.

Toward Evidence-Based Practice

Consider the results and/or conclusions from the following studies.

Westlake, C., & Dracup, K. (2001). Role of spirituality in adjustment of patients with advanced heart failure. *Progress in Cardiovascular Nursing, 16*(3), 119–125.

Patients described a process wherein spirituality contributed to their adjustment to advanced heart failure. The process involved regret over past behaviors, the search for meaning in the illness, and the search for hope for the future.

Thomson, J. E. (2000). The place of spiritual well-being in hospice patients' overall quality of life. *Hospital Journal, 15*(2), 13–27.

This study found spiritual well-being to be an important contributor to overall quality of life for hospice patients.

Beery, T., Baas, L., Fowler, C., & Allen G. (2002). Spirituality in persons with heart failure. *Journal of Holistic Nursing, 20*(1), 5–25.

The combined spirituality scores predicted 24% of the variance in total quality of life for people with heart failure being treated medically or via transplant.

Tuck, I., McCain, N., & Elswick, R. (2001). Spirituality and psychosocial factors in persons living with HIV. *Journal of Advanced Nursing, 33*(6), 776–783.

Studying patients with HIV, researchers found spirituality (as measured by a subscale called "existential well-being") was positively related to the patients' quality of life, social support, and effective coping strategies. It was negatively related to perceived stress, uncertainty, psychological distress, and emotional-focused coping.

Bradley, D. (1995). Religious involvement and social resources: Evidence from the data set "Americans' Changing Lives." *Journal for the Scientific Study of Religion, 34*(2), 259–267. (Abstract obtained from International Center for the Integration of Health and Spirituality.)

This research found that frequent attendance at religious services was strongly associated with the extent of a person's social support network.

Touhy, T. A. (2001). Nurturing hope and spirituality in the nursing home. *Holistic Nursing Practice, 15*(4), 45–56.

This study found that spirituality was the only factor, of those studied, that contributed significantly to hope in institutionalized elders.

Oxman, T., Freeman, D., & Mannheimer, E. (1995). Lack of social participation or religious strength or comfort as risk factors for death after cardiac surgery in the elderly. *Psychosomatic Medicine, 57*, 5–15. (Abstract obtained from International Center for the Integration of Health and Spirituality.)

Researchers found that religious faith was the most consistent indicator of survival after heart surgery in older patients. Those without religious faith had almost three times the risk of death; moreover, the more religious the patient, the greater the protective effect the study found.

Koenig, H. G., et al. (1998). The relationship between religious activities and blood pressure in older adults. *International Journal of Psychology in Medicine, 28*(2), 189–213.

This study found that older adults who both attended religious services at least once a week *and* prayed or

Toward Evidence-Based Practice—cont'd

studied the Bible at least daily had consistently lower blood pressure. The study also found that people who tuned in to religious TV or radio shows regularly actually had higher blood pressure than those who were less frequent viewers or listeners.

1. For which of the following do these studies, taken as a whole, provide the stronger support? Explain your reasoning.
   a. Spirituality has a positive effect on physical factors.
   b. Spirituality has a positive effect on psychosocial or emotional factors.

2. Suppose you are a nursing home administrator in an institution where the focus is almost entirely on physical care. You are thinking about a program to teach and encourage your staff to integrate spiritual interventions into their care. Evaluate the findings from each of the studies to see how useful it would be in supporting your idea. Explain your thinking.

 Go to Chapter 14, **Toward Evidence-Based Practice Suggested Responses,** on the Student Resource Disk or DavisPlus at http://davisplus.fadavis.com/Wilkinson2

 Go to Chapter 14, **Resources for Caregivers and Health Professionals,** on the Student Resource Disk or DavisPlus at http://davisplus.fadavis.com/Wilkinson2

 Suggested Readings: Go to Chapter 14, **Reading More About Spirituality,** on the Student Resource Disk or DavisPlus at http://davisplus.fadavis.com/Wilkinson2

 Bibliography: Go to Volume 2, Bibliography.

CHAPTER 15

Loss, Grief, & Dying

Learning Outcomes

After completing this chapter, you should be able to:

➤ Differentiate between loss and grief.

➤ Name and describe at least four types of loss.

➤ Identify the stages of grief as described by Engel, Worden, Rando, and Bowlby.

➤ Compare and contrast four types of grief.

➤ List and discuss at least five factors that affect grieving.

➤ Define *death* according to the Uniform Determination of Death Act.

➤ Give a definition of *higher-brain death*.

➤ Create a timeline of the dying process, indicating the physiological signs and symptoms common to each stage.

➤ List and describe the Kübler-Ross stages of dying and grief.

➤ Define end-of-life care, hospice care, and palliative care.

➤ Identify the legal and ethical issues involved in death and dying.

➤ Assess, diagnose, plan, and implement care of dying patients and their families.

➤ Describe the responsibilities of the nurse regarding postmortem care.

➤ Identify nursing interventions to help clients who are grieving.

Meet Your Patient

Thomas Manning is a 47-year-old man who is in the oncology unit with end-stage cancer of the pancreas. He is married and has three children, ages 18, 15, and 13. His oldest daughter has been away at college for only 6 months. Mr. Manning's father died 3 months ago from complications of alcoholism, and his mother has been withdrawn and grieving. His wife, Mary, tells you that Thomas "just wants to die" and does not want anyone trying to revive him or "jumping on his chest" if he dies. Mary is distressed and wants him to "keep fighting."

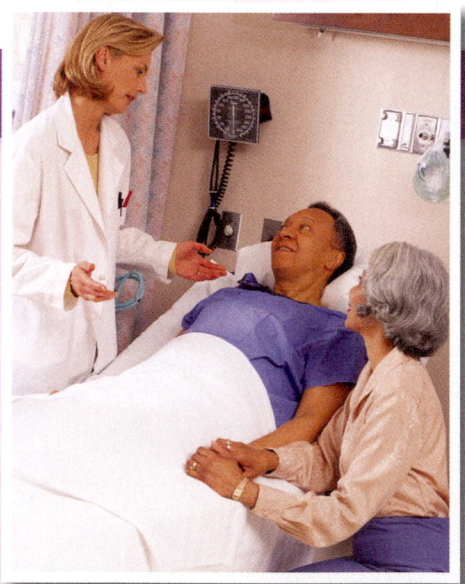

Theoretical **Knowledge**
knowing why_____

Loss and Grief

Throughout your nursing career, you will care for patients coping with loss—of youth, beauty, previous health, functioning, or quality of life. Many of your patients, like Thomas Manning, will be confronting their own approaching death, while family members will be facing loss of their loved one. As their nurse, you can help these people cope with their losses and grieve in a way that is healing, even transformative. But to do so, you need to know how to assess each patient's response to loss, plan appropriate outcomes, and intervene with skill and compassion. As a foundation, you must understand your own feelings and attitudes about loss, grief, and dying. We encourage you to increase your self-knowledge as you work through this chapter.

What Is Loss?

What is the first thing that comes to mind when you think of *loss*? Many people think of losing a loved one through death. Loss, however, is a daily occurrence. Our losses begin at birth when we lose the warmth and security of the womb, and end with the ultimate loss, the death of self. Loss can be defined as the undesired change or removal of a valued object, person, or situation.

Can you think of the first time you experienced a loss and what that felt like? What other losses have you undergone as you matured? For losses that are common at different developmental stages,

  Go to Chapter 15, **Tables, Boxes, Figures: ESG Table 15-1,** on the Student Resource Disk or DavisPlus at http://davisplus.fadavis.com/Wilkinson2

Whenever there is change, there is loss. Because we experience many changes throughout life, we also experience much loss. For example, losses related to changing schools are common in childhood and adolescence, whereas losses related to retirement or changing jobs are common in middle and older adulthood. Loss can be categorized in the following ways:

- *Actual versus perceived loss.* **Actual loss** includes the death of a loved one (or relationship), theft, deterioration, destruction, and natural disaster. Actual loss can be identified by others, not just by the person experiencing it (e.g., hair loss during chemotherapy). In contrast, **perceived loss** is internal; it is identified only by the person experiencing it (e.g., a woman diagnosed with a sexually transmitted infection may perceive herself as having lost her purity).
- *Physical loss versus psychological loss.* **Physical loss** includes (1) injuries (e.g., when a limb is amputated), (2) removal of an organ (e.g., hysterectomy), and (3) loss of function (e.g., loss of mobility).

Psychological losses challenge our belief system. They are commonly seen in the areas of sexuality, control, fairness, meaning, and trust. Some losses may be mixed. For example, after removal of a prostate gland, a man may feel both the physical and psychological loss of sexuality.
- *External versus internal loss.* **External losses** are actual losses of objects that are important to the person because of their cost or sentimental value (e.g., jewelry, pets, a home). These losses can be brought about by theft, destruction, or disasters such as floods and fire. **Internal loss** is another term for perceived or psychological loss.
- *Loss of aspects of self* includes physical losses such as body organs, limbs, body functions, and/or body disfigurement. Psychological and perceived losses in this category include aspects of one's personality, developmental change (as in the aging process), loss of hopes and dreams, and loss of faith.
- *Environmental loss* involves a change in the familiar, even if the change is perceived as positive. Examples include moving to a new home, getting a new job, and going to college. These losses can be perceived or actual.
- *Loss of significant relationships* includes, but is not limited to, actual loss of spouses, siblings, family members, or significant others through death, divorce, or separation (e.g., during war, a move to a foreign country).

  Critical**Thinking** 15-1
Which kinds of loss do you think Thomas Manning is experiencing?

What Is Grief?

Whenever there is loss, there is grieving. Grieving requires energy, so it can interfere with health and delay healing. However, grieving is positive in the sense that it is essential to psychological healing after a loss. Consider the following losses and the different reactions of the women involved.

Both Mrs. Smith and Mrs. Jones have lost a dog. Mrs. Smith's son left his dog with her when he went away to college last year. It has died of old age. Mrs. Jones's dog has been with her for 10 years and has been her only companion since her husband died 5 years ago. Her dog was killed by a car today as they were on their morning walk. Which woman do you think will grieve her loss more? Why? Discuss this situation with a classmate. Do you both have the same opinion about this?

This exercise demonstrates that it is really impossible to decide who would feel "more" grief. The intensity of the grief depends on the *meaning* the person attaches to the loss. Both women probably felt sad. However, the meaning of and attachment to the dog are different for each one. You might have thought Mrs. Smith's loss was minor; however, her dog was owned by her son and may have represented him in her mind. Mrs. Jones's dog was a companion and a protector and may have represented security and friendship. Each woman must grieve what the loss represents to her. This is true for everyone, whether the losses are actual or perceived, physical or psychological.

Grief is the physical, psychological, and spiritual responses to a loss. **Mourning** consists of actions associated with grief (e.g., wailing, wearing black clothing). These processes are normal and natural responses to a loss. The mourning and adjustment time after a loss is the period of **bereavement**. Although each person may express grief differently, some aspects of grief are shared by almost everyone.

KnowledgeCheck 15-1

What types of losses commonly occur in our lives?

 Go to Chapter 15, **Knowledge Check Response Sheet and Answers,** on the Student Resource Disk or DavisPlus at http://davisplus.fadavis.com/Wilkinson2

Stages of Grief

Many authors have focused on the stages or steps people experience in grieving. Remember there is no single, correct way to grieve, nor do people move neatly from one stage or step of grief to the next. Rather, grieving is a fluid, ongoing process. There is constant movement among stages, including recurrences of phases the bereaved person thought were resolved. The following are four major theorists in the field (Table 15-1).

Engel (1961) believed that uncomplicated grief has a clear onset and a predictable course, modified mainly by the abruptness and significance of the loss and how well prepared the bereaved person was. Uncomplicated grief is universal and does not require treatment.

John Bowlby (1982), drawing on attachment theory, suggested that grief occurs when the bereaved learn

that the object of their attachment is lost. Some experts assert that Bowlby's theory does not take into account the individual nature of grief and that it implies loved ones can be replaced. Nevertheless, our understanding of grief is broadened by his idea that grief is a mature way of dealing with loss of attachment. He also provides a slightly different perspective on the stages of grief.

Theresa Rando (1984, 1986, 1993, 2000) identified three processes of grieving (Table 15-1). Rando's (1984) stages are commonly described as the six R's of grieving:

1. *R*ecognizing the loss (awareness)
2. *R*eacting to the separation (feeling the emotions)
3. *R*ecollecting memories of the deceased (remembering, reliving)
4. *R*elinquishing the old attachment (new ways of living without the deceased)
5. *R*eadjusting to the new environment (new coping skills)
6. *R*einvesting self (energy once turned inward on grief begins to be focused outward again).

William Worden (2002) described the tasks a grieving person must achieve. They progress from an initial numbness or denial through experiencing and working through pain and grief and eventually moving on with life.

CriticalThinking 15-2

What are some of the similarities you see in the four theories described?

Grieving as Reconstructing Meaning

Some theorists are moving away from stage models of grieving toward the idea of grieving as a process of reconstructing meaning. For example, Florczak (2008) believes that the sorrow of loss is always present, whether

THEORIST	STAGES	DESCRIPTION
George Engel (1961) Three Stages of Grief	Shock and disbelief	Initial phase; the sufferer denies the loss in an attempt to protect himself against the shock of reality
	Developing awareness of the loss	The sufferer experiences painful feelings of sadness, guilt, shame, helplessness, hopelessness, loss, and emptiness. The person may lose interest in usual activities and experience impaired work performance. She may also experience loss of appetite, sleep disturbances, and even physical symptoms of pain or other discomfort.
	Restitution and recovery	The final phase, which is prolonged and gradual. The person carries on the work of mourning and overcomes the trauma of the loss, and a state of health and well-being is reestablished.

Table 15-1 ▶ Theories of Grief. A Comparison

Table 15-1 ➤ Theories of Grief. A Comparison—cont'd

THEORIST	STAGES	DESCRIPTION
John Bowlby (1982) Phases of Grief	Shock and numbness	Initial stage, in which the person experiences disorientation and feelings of helplessness
	Yearning and searching	The grieving person yearns to be reconnected with the deceased and searches for connections
	Disorganization and despair	The permanence of the loss becomes real. The person feels the pain and emotions of grief to their fullest and feels there is no hope of reconnection.
	Reorganization	Adjusting to life without the deceased (or lost object); developing new coping skills
Theresa Rando (1984, 1986, 1993, 2000) Three Phases of Grieving	Avoidance	Includes shock, disbelief, denial, anger, and bargaining
	Confrontation	The person actually begins to face the loss; a very emotional and upsetting time, when the person feels the grief most acutely.
	Accommodation	The person begins to live with the loss, feel better, and resume some routine activities
William Worden (2002) Four Tasks of Grieving	Accepting the reality of the loss	*Realizing that the loved one (or object) is gone.* In the hours and days after a significant loss, the grieving person typically feels numb and unable to accept the fact of the loss. This numbness is thought to be a helpful form of denial, which allows the person to "take in" only what the psyche is capable of handling at that time. So, the task of realizing the loved one or object is gone may take several days or, in the case of a sudden death, weeks.
	Working through the pain and grief	*Feelings and emotions that surface are intense and can change rapidly.* This makes the person feel "out of control." People in this stage may say they feel as if they are "going crazy." This is usually the longest phase for two reasons. First, because none of us likes to be in pain, we become expert at finding ways not to feel it. We overeat, overmedicate, overwork, and drink to excess to avoid feeling the pain, and we thereby prolong the process of grief. Second, caring people do not like to see their loved ones in pain, so they make attempts to remove the pain (e.g., by distraction) rather than letting the person experience it. Like avoidance, this well-meaning behavior also prolongs the process.
	Adjusting to an environment in which the deceased is missing	*Adjusting to the environment without the deceased.* This may mean performing alone activities and tasks, such as going for walks or shopping, that were once shared. Or it may include taking on roles and responsibilities that the deceased previously held. Such experiences can be extremely sad, frustrating and challenging, or very rewarding. However, once the person has established the new pattern, he or she typically feels satisfaction and increased self-esteem.
	Emotionally relocating the deceased and moving on with life	*Investing emotional energy.* Initially all energy is focused on the deceased: thinking about the person, talking about him/her, reliving memories, and so on. It is nearly impossible to think of anything else. Concentration is difficult, so the grieving person finds it hard to engage in activities such as reading. When the person's energy begins to flow toward others or to different or former interests (e.g., working, socializing), the healing process is in progress.

Sources: Engel, G. L. (1961). Is grief a disease? A challenge for medical research. *Psychosomatic Medicine, XXIII*(1), 18–22; Worden, J. W. (2002). *Grief counseling and grief therapy: A handbook for the mental health practitioner* (3rd ed.). New York: Springer; Rando, T. (1984). *Grief, dying and death: Clinical interventions for caregivers.* Champaign, IL: Research Press; and Bowlby, J. (1982). *Attachment and loss.* 3 vols. New York: Basic Books.

in the foreground or the background of a person's life; however, the meaning of the loss is constantly changing for the bereaved. The sorrow becomes "remembered" sorrow, which sometimes resurfaces and at other times sinks in to the background of other sorrows, joys, and everyday life.

Factors Affecting Grief

To begin thinking about factors affecting grieving, consider the following Critical Thinking exercise.

CriticalThinking 15-3

Mr. Klein is an 86-year-old man whose wife died of heart disease 2 months ago. He has two grown children who both visit him regularly. He also has a very supportive pastor, Mr. Owens, who meets him in the park to share stories. Mr. Owens is 30 years old and has been raising his 5-year-old daughter alone for the last 6 months since his wife died suddenly in an automobile accident. His parents and siblings live out of state. Both of these men are missing their wives very much.

- What factors do you think play a role in each man's grief?
- Who do you think will "get over it" faster?
- What are some issues that may make each man's grief uniquely difficult?

No two people ever grieve in the same manner because there are so many factors that play a role in the grieving process. They include the following.

Significance of the Loss. The meaning the person has attached to the person or object lost will be different for each person. The more attachment to the relationship or object, the more difficult is the grieving.

Amount of Support for the Bereaved. People with more emotional and psychosocial support typically have less complicated grief.

Conflicts Existing at the Time of Death. A conflict left unresolved may cause prolonged grief. For example, if a couple had an argument just before one partner died suddenly, the remaining partner's grief may be complicated by guilt.

Circumstances of the Loss. Was this a sudden, unexpected death, or had the person been suffering from a chronic illness? Specifically, was there an opportunity to prepare for it? Was the death a suicide or homicide? Was the death in any sense avoidable? Was the person in pain? If the circumstances of the loss leave the bereaved feeling guilty or responsible, his healing process may be impeded. This can result from losses other than death as well (e.g., loss of valued property by theft or disaster, loss of a relationship, loss of a job, rejection from college).

Previous Loss. If the person has sustained more than one loss in a short period of time, the grieving process can become more complicated. In the hospital, you will frequently care for patients experiencing multiple losses. For example, consider a patient who has suffered a stroke and loss of mobility and then has to move out of his home of many years to a nursing home. The patient's loss of health and functioning is compounded by the loss of his independence and familiar surroundings.

Spiritual/Cultural Beliefs and Practices. Spirituality and religious beliefs can help or hinder the grieving process. One person might believe the deceased is in a place of contentment and happiness, where all suffering is over. Another may believe that the deceased will soon be reborn, possibly into the same extended family. Another may believe that death is final and there is no longer any life after death. How do you think these beliefs might influence the grieving process? Most cultures engage in rituals (e.g., funerals) that help the bereaved begin the grieving process by openly expressing their emotions and pain (Fig. 15-1). Some cultures may emphasize keeping emotions more subdued and limiting expressions of grief to private settings.

Timeliness of the Death. The death of a child or a young person is almost universally more difficult to accept than the death of an older person. In addition to loss of the person, there is a sense of unfairness because of the loss of *potential*—of what the child might have become or achieved. You may hear someone ask, "Why was her life cut short?" or state, "He had so much going for him, but God didn't give him a chance."

Developmental stages are also an important factor in grieving. They are discussed in the text that follows.

Developmental Stages and Grief

Based on Erik Erikson's stages of psychological growth, we all must achieve certain psychological milestones during a lifetime. If you need to review Erikson's theory,

FIGURE 15-1 Rituals are used to facilitate grieving.

Go to Chapter 9, **Expanded Discussion,** on the Student Resource Disk or DavisPlus at http://davisplus.fadavis.com/Wilkinson2.

Grief can affect the healthy development of life stages, and in turn, the person's stage of development affects the grieving process.

Childhood

Because cognitive development is not yet complete, preschool children do not understand death is final. The belief that death is temporary and reversible is reinforced by cartoon characters who "die" and then "come to life" again. Between ages 5 and 9, children begin to understand that death is permanent, but they believe it will never happen to them or anyone they know. During the weeks after a death, a child may feel immediate grief or may continue to believe the person is still alive. Both are normal reactions. A child may display feelings of sadness on and off over a long period of time and often at unexpected moments.

Young children believe they are the cause of what happens around them. This is known as *magical thinking.* Such thinking may cause them to feel guilt when there is a death of someone close to them. Other responses include regressing to a previous developmental stage: "acting like a baby," demanding food and attention, becoming incontinent, and talking "baby talk."

Adolescence

Adolescence is typically a time for dealing with confusion between one's identity and one's role. The adolescent struggles to learn who he is as a person as he breaks away from parental control. An adolescent who experiences the loss of a parent while "pushing the parent away" may feel a sense of guilt and unfinished business.

At the same time, the bereaved teen also faces psychological, physiological, social, and academic pressures. Although teens may look mature, they often lack emotional maturity. Teens are often expected to be "grown up" and support a surviving parent or younger siblings. When they feel this responsibility, they do not have the opportunity, or the permission, to mourn. Coping may be even more difficult for teens if the death comes suddenly and unexpectedly, for example, when a brother dies in an auto accident.

Adulthood

Adults are cognitively able to understand the nature of death, and they have usually experienced other types of loss by this time. Over time, they perceive loss as a normal part of living. How they respond to loss depends on factors such as the person's self-esteem and the availability of supports. The rest of this section refers primarily to factors that affect the adult grieving process.

Older Adulthood

A special difficulty for older adults is that they experience so many losses. Most deaths occur among older adults, so they are likely to lose friends and siblings in rapid succession. Add to those losses the physical and functional losses and the loss of independence, and the cumulative effects may be devastating.

KnowledgeCheck 15-2

- What are the main tasks of the grieving process?
- What factors affect the grieving process?

Go to Chapter 15, **Knowledge Check Response Sheet and Answers,** on the Student Resource Disk or DavisPlus at http://davisplus.fadavis.com/Wilkinson2

CriticalThinking 15-4

Refer to Thomas Manning and his wife in "Meet Your Patient." Apply each of the preceding factors affecting grief to Thomas and to Mary (they may be different for each spouse). If the scenario does not provide enough information for you to comment, say so and then describe how you would obtain the data you need.

Types of Grief

Grief can be categorized in several ways, most of which have to do with timing and intensity.

Uncomplicated grief (normal grief) is the natural response to a loss. The bereaved person experiences the feelings, behaviors, and cognitions that are expected in light of his culture, social status, and relationship to the lost person or object (Table 15-2). The emotions are intense but gradually diminish over time (several months to several years). Some emotions will always be present, but the intensity will change.

Complicated grief is distinguished from uncomplicated grief by length of time and intensity of emotion. The person's responses are maladaptive, dysfunctional, unusually prolonged, or overwhelming. For example, the bereaved may become severely depressed, violent, or suicidal; become a "workaholic"; become socially isolated, or demonstrate addictive behavior. Or, after several years, the person may still be experiencing as much pain and disruption as in the first months after the loss. Prolonged or complicated grief has been associated with depression, suicidal ideation, and hypertension (Prigerson, Frank, Kasl, et al., as cited in Goldsmith, Morrison, Vanderwerker, et al., 2008). Risk factors for complicated grief include sudden death of a significant other, emotional instability, and lack of social support.

Typically, complicated grief results when the grieving process has been impeded for some reason (e.g., something keeps the person "stuck" in the grief process). Usually the bereaved benefits from the assistance of a grief counselor to help establish and work through the problem areas. Chronic, masked, and delayed grief are all examples of complicated grief:

- **Chronic grief** begins as normal grief but continues long term, with little resolution of feelings and inability to rejoin normal life.

Table 15-2 ➤ Common Grief Reactions

PHYSICAL	EMOTIONAL	BEHAVIORS	COGNITIONS
Loss of appetite	Anger	Forgetfulness	Decreased concentration
Weight loss or gain	Sadness	Being withdrawn	Forgetfulness
Fatigue	Guilt	Insomnia or too much sleep	Impaired judgment
Decreased libido	Relief	Dreaming of deceased	Obsessive thoughts of the deceased or lost object
Decreased immune system response	Shock	Verbalizing the loss	Preoccupation
Decreased energy	Numbness	Crying	Confusion
Possible physical symptoms, such as headache or stomach pain	Loneliness	Loss of productivity at work or school	Questioning spiritual beliefs
	Fear		Searching for understanding
	Anxiety		Searching for purpose and meaning
	Powerlessness		
	Helplessness		

■ **Masked grief** occurs when the person is grieving but expressing the grief through other types of behavior. For example, a man whose wife has died may begin drinking heavily, or a couple whose child has died may find themselves engaging in violent arguments with each other. This change in behavior is part of their grief response, but they don't recognize it as such.

■ **Delayed grief** is grief that is put off until a later time (e.g., "I'll think about it later. Right now, I'm busy trying to keep a roof over our heads and care for my children.").

Disenfranchised grief is experienced in connection with a loss that is not socially supported or acknowledged by the usual rites or ceremonies (Corr, Nabe, & Corr, 2003). Disenfranchised grief may be experienced by a man whose wife has had a miscarriage, a mistress whose lover dies, or a bereaved partner in a homosexual relationship not recognized by the families. In each of these instances, the bereaved person lacks the communal support that is helpful in grieving.

Anticipatory grief is experienced before a loss occurs. A wife caring for her husband through a long illness may grieve as she sees the vibrant man she once knew change before her eyes and as she anticipates his death. Family members caring for a loved one with Alzheimer's disease commonly experience anticipatory grief, realizing that as mental capacity diminishes, the person they once knew will become ever more removed from them. The potential negative outcome of anticipatory grief is that the survivor may detach from a dying person too early in the dying process, leaving the person without emotional support during that period. This does not always happen, of course.

Critical**Thinking** 15-5

Thomas Manning ("Meet Your Patient") had a strained relationship with his father for most of his life. His father was an alcoholic and constantly fought with his mother while Thomas

was growing up. A few months ago, his father was hospitalized for the third time for complications of alcoholism, and Thomas visited him. He confronted his father regarding his drinking and the problems and pain it had caused him and the family. The confrontation ended in an argument. That night, Thomas' father slipped into a coma, and a few days later, without recovering consciousness, he died.

■ What issues does Thomas have to deal with?
■ Why might this be a complicated grief process?

Death and Dying

Death is the ultimate loss. The dying person faces the loss of physical control and function, independence, relationships, possibilities, and ultimately life itself. In mainstream North American culture, death is not seen as a natural part of life, but rather as something to avoid at all costs. People even avoid talking or thinking about it.

How Is Death Defined?

The legal definition of death has evolved over the years. Historically, *death* was defined as the cessation of the flow of vital bodily fluids. This evolved into the traditional definition of heart–lung death: the irreversible cessation of spontaneous respirations and circulation. This criterion was used to define death until the 1960s, when it was replaced by **whole-brain death**: the irreversible cessation of all functions of the brain, including the brain stem. Spontaneous respirations cannot continue once the brain stem stops functioning; the heart, however, may continue to beat until it becomes oxygen starved from cessation of respirations.

In the 1970s, many practitioners began using the term **higher-brain death,** which defines death as the irreversible cessation of all "higher" brain functions (e.g., cognitive functioning, consciousness, memory, reasoning, and so on). By this definition, the brain stem can still be functioning, so both respiratory and cardiac activity may continue even though the person does not make purposive responses to external stimuli; cephalic reflexes are absent; and the electroencephalogram shows no activity.

Based on the two preceding definitions of brain death, it is technically possible to keep a person "alive" indefinitely by using a mechanical ventilator. In 1981 the President's Commission for the Study of Ethical Problems in Medicine proposed the **Uniform Determination of Death Act** (Box 15-1). This definition, which includes the loss of brain stem function, provides a highly reliable means of declaring death for respirator-maintained bodies (DeSpelder & Strickland, 1996, p. 328). For criteria for assessing brain stem functioning,

Go to Chapter 15, **Supplemental Materials: Some Criteria for Assessing Brain Stem Functioning,** on the Student Resource Disk or DavisPlus at http://davisplus.fadavis.com/ Wilkinson2

A **coma** is a prolonged, deep state of unconsciousness lasting days or even years. The patient cannot be aroused and may or may not have decreased brain stem reflexes. In a **persistent vegetative state (PVS),** which sometimes follows a coma, the person does not respond to stimuli, is unaware of the environment, and has no cognition or affective mental functions. However, the person has lost only the higher cerebral functions (see the preceding definition of higher-brain death) and so continues to have a sleep–wake cycle, may have some spontaneous movements, and may open her eyes in response to external stimuli. However, the person cannot speak or obey commands. PVS sometimes follows a coma but can also occur after any event that affects cerebrovascular flow. Patients in a PVS may look somewhat normal and may occasionally grimace, cry, or laugh. The family may believe that the patient is responding to the environment and thus not want to give up hope for

recovery. Because they cannot work through the grieving process, they continue to grieve each day.

What Are the Stages of Dying?

To help dying patients and their families understand the dying process, your theoretical knowledge base must include information on both physiological and psychological processes.

Physiological Stages of Dying

The dying process is unique to each person. However, people experience many similar symptoms as they approach the end of life. Fewer than 10% of patients die suddenly and unexpectedly, as in an accident or massive heart attack. Ninety percent die after a long illness, progressively deteriorating until an active dying phase at the end (Emanuel, Ferris, von Gunten, et al., 2008). The following timeline describes the physiological responses of that group (Karnes, 1995).

One to Three Months Before Death. The dying person begins to withdraw from the world and people. Sleep increases; it becomes difficult for the body to digest food, especially meats; and appetite and food intake decrease. Liquids are preferred. Anorexia may be protective. The resulting ketosis can diminish pain and increase the person's sense of well-being.

One to Two Weeks Before Death. A host of physical changes indicates the body is beginning to lose its ability to maintain itself. Cardiovascular deterioration brings reduced blood pressure, changes in pulse and skin color (e.g., a yellowish pallor), and extreme pallor of the extremities. Temperature fluctuates and perspiration increases. Respiratory rate may increase or decrease; during sleep, the dying person may experience brief periods of apnea. Congestion may cause a rattling sound and/or a nonproductive cough.

Days to Hours Before Death. Often a surge of energy brings mental clarity and a desire to eat and talk with family members. However, as death approaches, patients tend to become dehydrated and have difficulty swallowing, which results in decreased blood volume. The tissues of the tongue and soft palate sag, and the gag reflex declines, so secretions accumulate in the oropharynx and/ or bronchi. Often the mucous membranes become dry and tacky and lips become cracked. Dehydration during the last hours of dying is thought to not cause distress, and perhaps to stimulate endorphin release (Emanuel, Ferris, von Gunten, et al., 2008).

Breathing may be shallow, rapid, or irregular: periods of apnea may lengthen to 10 to 30 seconds before breathing resumes. Congestion causes a "death rattle" that can be quite loud. **Cheyne–Stokes respirations** may occur. This is a cyclic pattern consisting of a 10- to 60-second period of apnea and then a gradual increase in depth and rate of respirations. Respirations gradually

---

BOX 15-1 ■ Uniform Determination of Death Act

1. [Determination of Death] An individual who has sustained either (1) irreversible cessation of circulatory and respiratory functions, or (2) irreversible cessation of all functions of the entire brain, including the brain stem, is dead. A determination of death must be made in accordance with accepted medical standards.

2. [Uniformity of Construction and Application] This act shall be applied and construed to effectuate its general purpose to make uniform the law with respect to the subject of this Act among states enacting it.

Source: President's Commission for the Study of Ethical Problems in Medicine and Biomedical and Behavioral Research. (1981). *Defining death: A report on the medical, legal, and ethical issues in the determination of death.* Washington, DC: Government Printing Office, p. 73.

become slow and shallow, and then the cycle begins again with apnea.

Peripheral circulation decreases, and the person perspires and feels "clammy." The blood pressure decreases, and the pulse may be hard to detect. The extremities become cool and mottled, and the underside of the body may be much darker. Decreased circulation also results in reduced kidney function and decreased urinary output.

Muscles throughout the body relax, causing the face to "droop." As peristalsis slows, the patient may retain feces. Urine output reduces and urine often becomes more concentrated and foul smelling. Sphincters relax, and bowel and bladder incontinence can occur. Vision blurs; the eyes may be open or partially open, but unseeing. Instead, the patient may see things that are not visible to others.

In the final hours of life, many patients become restless and agitated. This response may be caused by medications, liver failure, cerebral hypoxia, renal failure, stool impaction, distended bladder, increased pain, or unresolved emotional or spiritual issues. Near to the time of death, some people unexpectedly become more coherent and energized for a time. Others become less communicative, quiet, and withdrawn (Pitorak, 2003). Fatigue is common.

Moments Before Death. The dying person does not respond to touch or sound and cannot be awakened. Typically, there is a short series of long-spaced breaths before breathing ceases entirely and the heart stops beating (Karnes, 1995).

Psychological Stages of Dying

Perhaps the best known author on the psychology of dying is Dr. Elisabeth Kübler-Ross (1969). She felt that if people understood what dying patients are experiencing, they would be more competent in caring for them. From her research with dying patients, she observed that people tend to experience one or more of five psychological stages during the period from the terminal diagnosis to the actual death (Box 15-2). Her theory has become a classic for professional and lay readers alike, and has been applied to losses other than death. However, it has been criticized by people who misinterpreted it or attempted to apply it in the wrong way. When you study the Kübler-Ross stages, it is important to understand that dying people:

- May not go through *every* stage.
- May not go through the stages in a linear fashion, but rather in random order.
- Do not necessarily complete one stage and move on to the next.
- May experience two or three stages simultaneously.

Bear in mind that it is not the nurse's responsibility to move people on to the next stage so that everyone dies accepting death. It *is* our responsibility to accept and

---

BOX 15-2 ■ Kübler-Ross: Stages of Dying and Grief

Stage	Defining Characteristics
Denial	■ "Not me." "This cannot be happening." "I don't believe it." Usually the person is in a state of shock. Denial is not necessarily negative; it gives the person a chance to prepare psychologically for accepting the news.
Anger	■ "Why me?" "Why is this happening?" Anger can be obvious or subtle. It is the person's response to the feeling that the situation is unfair. The person may take his anger out on people who are "safe" (e.g., family, spouse) or from whom there will be no reprisals (e.g., nurses, physician).
Bargaining	■ "If only I can live until . . ." "Yes me, but . . ." Usually this takes the form of a bargain with God or a Higher Power, in which the person asks to live to see a birth, graduation, wedding, and so forth.
Depression	■ A withdrawn sadness, not to be confused with clinical depression. This is a response to the current loss as well as to any accumulated and/or future losses.
Acceptance	■ Not necessarily *wanting* death (or the loss), but coming to terms with it and ceasing to fight it. The person may seem almost void of feelings.

Source: Kübler-Ross, E. (1969). *On death and dying.* New York: Macmillan.

---

support people "where they are" and help them to verbalize their feelings. We need to understand patients, not change them.

What Is End-of-Life Care?

When, precisely, is end of life? There is no set, agreed-upon definition or set of criteria. A recent set of guidelines provides a working definition that includes the following three situations:

- The patient has a fatal condition.
- Death is likely with the next exacerbation of disease.
- The patient acknowledges the seriousness of the situation (Qaseem, Snow, Shekelle, 2008).

In an effort to humanize healthcare, organizations such as the Institute of Medicine, the American Association of Colleges of Nursing, and the Robert Wood Johnson Foundation have identified competencies for nurses that stress compassion, sensitivity, and technical skills during end-of-life care (Ferrell, Grant, & Virani,

Complementary & Alternative Modalities (CAM)

End-of-Life Care

▸ In Australia, **Sloman (2002)** found that *progressive muscle relaxation training* and guided imagery significantly improved depression and quality of life for people with advanced cancer. However, there was no improvement in depression.

▸ **Johnstone, Polston, Niemtzow, and Martin (2002)** studied the use of *acupuncture* to provide palliative symptom relief to patients in an oncology (cancer) clinic. The major symptoms treated were pain, xerostomia, hot flashes, and nausea and loss of appetite. The 89 patients received from one to nine treatments. Most patients (60%) showed at least 30% improvement in symptoms (taken as a whole).

▸ **Thompson and Reilly (2002)** explored the impact of the *homeopathic approach* on symptom control, mood disturbance, and quality of life for 100 patients attending a cancer clinic. The most common symptoms were pain, fatigue, and hot flushes. The symptoms of fatigue and hot flushes improved significantly, but there was no appreciable pain relief.

▸ In England, **Gambles, Crooke, and Wilkinson (2002)** studied the effects of four to six sessions of *reflexology* on the symptoms of 34 patients receiving palliative care. Patients' comments were generally positive. They reported relief from tension and anxiety relief, as well as improved comfort and well-being.

1999). Some of these competencies include the following (Bednash & Ferrell, 2000):

- Holistic assessment of patients and families (i.e., physical, psychological, social, and spiritual)
- Acknowledging diversity in patients' beliefs and customs
- Using both traditional and complementary approaches
- Applying legal and ethical principles to end-of-life care
- Demonstrating respect for the patients' views and wishes during end-of-life care
- Assessing patient, family, colleagues, and one's own success in coping with suffering, grief, loss, and bereavement at the end of life

For end-of-life nursing care competencies recommended by the American Association of Colleges of Nursing (AACN),

Go to Chapter 15, **Tables, Boxes, Figures: ESG Box 15-1,** on the Student Resource Disk or DavisPlus at http://davisplus.fadavis.com/Wilkinson2

End-of-life care includes palliative care and hospice care, which are similar in that both may involve caring for dying patients, and neither focuses on cure. Some people use the terms interchangeably; however, there are subtle differences.

Palliative Care

When patients reach a stage in their illness in which cure is no longer possible, or when they refuse further treatment, they may be eligible to receive "comfort care"—meaning that no further efforts will be made to stop the disease process or prevent the patient from dying, although certain symptoms (e.g., nausea) will be treated. The correct interpretation of the term *comfort care* is, "Nothing more *can* be done to cure your loved one." However, family members sometimes interpret it to mean "Nothing more *will* be done." In this situation, the term *palliative care* may be more acceptable. As a specialty, palliative care is provided by a holistic team of professionals. However, many patients receive palliative care from their general practice provider, and even in acute care hospitals, especially if staff are comfortable and skilled with pain management and end-of-life care.

Palliative care is actually aggressively planned, holistic comfort care. General issues for most end-of-life care patients include the following:

- Supporting families and caregivers
- Ensuring continuity of care
- Ensuring respect for persons
- Ensuring informed decision-making
- Attending to emotional and spiritual concerns
- Supporting function and survival duration
- Managing symptoms (e.g., pain, dyspnea, depression)

A patient does not necessarily have to be "actively dying" to receive palliative care. It is also provided over a long period of time for those who have slowly progressive diseases. Palliative care should not be seen as merely limiting life-sustaining treatment or allowing death. It should result in increased patient satisfaction, improved symptom control, and cost savings for hospitals (Qaseem, Snow, Shekelle, et al., 2008).

Hospice Care

The hospice movement was set in motion in England by Dame Cicely Sanders, who founded the first modern-day hospice within a London hospital in 1968. Currently there are more than 4500 hospice programs in the United States alone (National Hospice and Palliative Care Organization, 2007). Hospice care focuses on holistic care of patients who are dying or debilitated and not expected to improve. For a patient to be eligible for hospice insurance benefits, a physician must certify that the patient is likely to die within 6 months. It is in this way that hospice differs most from palliative care.

Hospice care is based on two key premises: (1) the quality of life is as important as the length of life, and (2) those who are terminally ill should be allowed to face death with dignity and surrounded by the comfort of their homes and families. Thus, hospice providers consider helping family members an essential part of their role.

Treatment is holistic, addressing the patient's emotional, spiritual, and physical needs. Physical care is primarily palliative, involving symptom management. For example, pain management is considered crucial because patients must be relatively free from pain to make the most of the time remaining to them.

An interdisciplinary team plans care with the patient and family. Family members are encouraged to be an active part of the team as much as they are able. Nursing support is available 24 hours a day, and families are taught what to expect as the disease progresses. Psychosocial and spiritual care have high priority. As the patient nears death, hospice workers remain as long as necessary. After the patient dies, there is follow-up bereavement care for the families.

Although you may think of hospice as "home" care, hospice is a *way* of caring rather than a setting. Some hospitals are able to devote some inpatient beds to hospice care, and freestanding hospices also exist. The purpose of admitting a patient is to provide a family with some respite for a period of time or to stabilize a patient who requires symptom management, or to care for a patient who is in the end stage of a disease (e.g., AIDS or cancer) and needs a level of expert care that family members cannot provide at home.

Legal and Ethical Considerations at End of Life

The technology of life support makes it possible to prolong bodily functions almost indefinitely, leaving patients and families struggling to decide whether prolonging life is appropriate. More and more of these clients depend on nurses for education regarding patient rights and choices surrounding end-of-life care. Each situation is unique, and you should be able to explore with clients the various options available. See Chapters 44 and 45, for more information about the ethical and legal aspects of each of the following topics.

Advance Directives

An advance directive is a group of instructions (written or oral) stating a person's wishes relative to his healthcare if he were incapacitated or unable to make that decision. An ordinary power of attorney does not give another person the right to make healthcare decisions for the patient; only a durable power of attorney for healthcare decisions can do that.

The **Patient Self-Determination Act (PSDA),** passed by Congress in 1990, requires that all healthcare providers who receive Medicare funds (e.g., hospitals, home care agencies, hospices, nursing homes) must educate staff and patients and provide an opportunity for all patients to complete an advance directive (see Chapter 45 if you want more information). The Joint Commission (2008) also requires institutions to address the wishes of the patient regarding end-of-life decisions. State laws

regarding advance directives vary. It is important for you to understand the regulations of your own state as well as federal laws and the policies of your institution. Advance directives are of different types and serve different purposes.

- A **living will** is a document prepared by a competent person giving instructions regarding medical care if that person becomes unable to make decisions. The document provides specific instructions about the kinds of healthcare the person would wish or would wish *not* to have in particular situations. For example, it might specify that no artificial food or fluids be administered.
- A **durable power of attorney (DPOA),** or **healthcare proxy,** exists when a competent person names another individual to make decisions regarding his healthcare choices under certain conditions (e.g., irreversible coma, terminal illness) when he is unable to do so. These instructions are usually written and should include specific instructions about the patient's wishes regarding hydration, feeding tubes, medication, resuscitation, and mechanical ventilation. The document must be witnessed by two persons and can be changed or canceled at any time by the patient. For an example of an advance directive,

Go to Chapter 15, **Tables, Boxes, Figures: ESG Figure 15-1,** on the Student Resource Disk or DavisPlus at http://davisplus.fadavis.com/Wilkinson2

For details of the Patient Self-Determination Act,

Go to Chapter 15, **Supplemental Materials: Patient Self-Determination Act,** on the Student Resource Disk or DavisPlus at http://davisplus.fadavis.com/Wilkinson2

Some people fear that once an advance directive is signed, no further care will be provided. Explain to families and patients that this is not true; instead, the directive is to make sure that they will get however much or little care *they* wish. Remind people that everyone should have an advance directive and that they should not wait until they become ill to prepare one. Such explanations are independent nursing activities, for which you are responsible.

Orders for DNAR

A DNAR order is an order to *not* attempt resuscitation of the patient in the event of a cardiac or respiratory failure. The American Heart Association (AHA) is now using the term *DNAR (do not attempt resuscitation)* instead of *DNR (do not resuscitate).* You must pay careful attention to these orders and agency policies, as well as to any advance directives, to be prepared should one of your patients suffer a cardiac arrest. For an example of a DNAR (DNR) order,

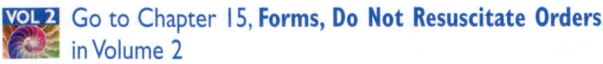

Go to Chapter 15, **Forms, Do Not Resuscitate Orders,** in Volume 2

In many healthcare settings, cardiopulmonary resuscitation (CPR) is performed almost automatically. This practice may be slowly changing, however. It is interesting that the AHA, which has for so long focused on preserving life, has in its more recent publications begun to point out that it is not always appropriate to use CPR. For example, some of their instructor's materials stress that asystole (no cardiac activity) is usually a confirmation of death rather than a rhythm requiring treatment.

Carefully explain to patients and families what CPR involves and what their options are. The patient and/or family has the ultimate say. They have the right to refuse CPR and may request DNAR orders; the physician cannot legally write a DNAR order if the patient or family does not wish it. The American Nurses Association (ANA, 2004) recommendations regarding DNAR are summarized in Box 15-3. For a complete list of the ANA recommendations,

 Go to Chapter 15, **Tables, Boxes, Figures: ESG Box 15-2,** on the Student Resource Disk or DavisPlus at http://davisplus.fadavis.com/Wilkinson2

There is growing evidence that strategies, such as formal and informal family meetings, daily team consensus

---

BOX 15-3 ■ Highlights of ANA Recommendations Concerning DNAR

- The competent patient's choices have highest priority when there is conflict.
- When the patient is not competent, give highest priority to advance directives or the surrogate decision makers.
- DNAR orders should be discussed explicitly with the patient and significant others.
- DNAR orders must be documented, reviewed, and updated.
- DNAR does *not* mean "discontinue care"!
- Nurses should be aware of and have an active role in developing DNAR policies in the institutions where they work; they should participate in interdisciplinary mechanisms for resolving disputes among patients, families, and healthcare practitioners concerning DNAR orders.
- Nurses have a duty to educate patients and families about technologies, termination of treatment decisions, and to encourage them to think about end-of-life preferences and make their wishes known in advance.
- Nurses have a duty to communicate relevant information and to advocate for a patient's end-of-life preferences to be honored.

Source: Adapted from American Nurses Association (ANA). (2004). Position statement: Nursing care and do-not-resuscitate decisions. Retrieved from http://www.nursingworld.org/MainMenuCategories/HealthcareandPolicyIssues/ANAPositionStatements/EthicsandHumanRights/dnr0414405.aspx

---

processes, palliative care team case finding, and ethics consultation improve communication about end-of-life decisions (Boyle, Miller, & Forbes-Thompson, 2005).

Assisted Suicide

Assisted suicide means making available that which is needed for the patient to end his own life (e.g., pharmacological agents or weapons). The patient is physically capable of ending his own life, has expressed the intention to do so, and has turned to the healthcare provider merely to supply the means. The ANA (1994a, 1994b) believes that "the nurse should not participate in active euthanasia (and assisted suicide) because such an act is in direct violation of the Code for Nurses and the ethical traditions of the profession. Nurses have an obligation to provide timely, humane, comprehensive, and compassionate end-of-life care."

Euthanasia

The term **euthanasia** comes from the Greek word *euthanatos,* which means "good death." It refers to the deliberate ending of a life of someone suffering from a terminal or incurable illness. **Active euthanasia** occurs as a result of a direct action (e.g., giving an overdose of medication). Active euthanasia can be *voluntary* (patient consents); *involuntary* (patient refuses); or *nonvoluntary* (patient is unable to consent, or someone else makes the decision and the patient is unaware of it). Active euthanasia goes a step further than assisted suicide. In assisted suicide, the "assistant" makes available the means for the person to take his own life; in euthanasia, the "assistant" also serves as the direct agent of death (e.g., administers the medication).

Passive euthanasia occurs as a result of a *lack* of action (e.g., withholding medications or food necessary to sustain life). Honoring the refusal of treatments that a patient does not desire, that are burdensome, or that will not benefit the patient is not generally considered passive euthanasia and can be ethically and legally permissible. For more information about the ethical and legal issues surrounding euthanasia, see Chapters 44 and 45, respectively.

 Critical**Thinking** 15-6

What are your feelings about assisted suicide and euthanasia? Focus on your feelings, not on principles, explanations, and rationales.

Autopsy

An autopsy is a medical examination of the body to determine the cause of death. Autopsies have also provided relevant data about disease processes and causes. The pathologist performs a detailed internal and external evaluation of the body, removes body organs, and extracts sample tissues for further examination. The organs are then replaced in the body, and the body cavities are closed with sutures. An autopsy requires signed permission from the next of kin, except in cases in which autopsy is required by law (e.g., deaths that are suspicious or unwitnessed).

Organ Donation

People sometimes wish to donate their organs to someone else when they die. Currently all 50 states have adopted some form of the Uniform Anatomical Gift Act (UAGA) for organ donation. However, many states adopted it only in part, or enacted their own unique versions of the UAGA. A revision of the UAGA was proposed in 2006. About half the states have already adopted the 2006 UAGA, and it has been introduced in the legislation of several others. However, there are some ethical concerns that the new UAGA might override an individual's advance directives or result in people becoming donors or kept on life support against their or their family's wishes. (See Box 15-4 for provisions of the document.)

However, even though donor cards are legal in all states, many institutions will not procure organs from the deceased if there is strong family objection (Fig. 15-2). Therefore, if a patient is planning to donate organs or tissues, be sure that he discusses these wishes with family members. The list of persons waiting for organ donations continues to increase. If death is imminent, a healthcare team member (physician or nurse) should ask whether the patient has agreed to be an organ donor. In many institutions, a transplant coordinator contacts the family and makes the request for organ and tissue donation.

KnowledgeCheck 15-3

- What are advance directives?
- What is the ANA position on assisted suicide?

Go to Chapter 15, **Knowledge Check Response Sheet and Answers,** on the Student Resource Disk or DavisPlus at http://davisplus.fadavis.com/Wilkinson2

Practical **Knowledge** knowing how

◼ ASSESSMENT

When a patient is dying or has experienced a loss, you must carefully assess the patient and significant others for the common grief reactions listed in Table 15-2. Other important areas to assess include knowledge base, history of loss, coping patterns and abilities, meaning of the loss or illness, and support systems. For dying patients, you should also make the following assessments:

- When the client and family are ready, encourage them to talk about the client's wishes for burial or cremation or tasks that the client would like taken care of (e.g., giving away valuables, calling family members).

BOX 15-4 ◼ Major Provisions of the Uniform Anatomical Gift Act

- Any person older than age 18, or an emancipated minor, may donate all or part of his or her body for education, research, therapeutic, or transplantation purposes.

- The 2006 UAGA specifies that a parent of a minor, a guardian of an individual, or an agent acting under a healthcare power of attorney can make an anatomical gift on behalf of a living minor, ward, or principal.

- The 2006 UAGA authorizes a minor who is eligible for a driver's license or permit can make a gift without parental consent. However, a parent can revoke the gift if the child dies before age 18.

- The 2006 UAGA says that if the person has not made a donation before death, the next of kin or an agent acting under a healthcare power of attorney can make it when the person dies unless there was a known objection by the deceased. If none of these persons is reasonably available to make the gift, it can be made by the person having authority to dispose of the decedent's body (e.g., a coroner or hospital administrator).

- If the person has made such a gift, the Act says it cannot be revoked by his or her relatives. (However, in actual practice this sometimes happens.) The Revised UAGA (2006) states that if there is a donor card, there is no reason to seek consent from the donor's family, as they have no legal right to give it.

- If there is more than one person of the same degree of kinship (e.g., three sisters), any one of them may make a gift if she is unaware of any objections by the others. If an objection is known, the gift can be made only by a majority of the kin (e.g., sisters) who are reasonably available.

- The gift can be authorized by a card carried by the individual or by written or recorded verbal communication from a relative.

- The gift can be amended or revoked at any time before the death of the donor.

- The time of death must be determined by a physician who is not involved in any transplantation.

- Even if a prospective donor has an advance healthcare directive instructing the withdrawal or withholding of life-support systems, measures to ensure the medical suitability of organs for transplantation or therapy will not be withdrawn or withheld unless the advance directive expressly states this is to be done.

Sources: DeSpelder, L., & Strickland, A. (1996). *The last dance.* Mountain View, CA: Mayfield; Kurtz, S. F., Strong, C.W., & Gerasimow, D. (2007). The 2006 Revised Uniform Anatomical Gift Act—A law to save lives. *Health Law Analysis.* February 2007. Retrieved from http://www.anatomicalgiftact.org/Uploads/kurtzarticle.pdf; National Conference of Commissioners on Uniform State Laws. Revised Uniform Anatomical Gift Act (2006). Retrieved from http://www.anatomicalgiftact.org/DesktopDefault. aspx?tabindex=0&tabid=1; Verheijde, J. L., Rady, M.Y., & McGregor, J. L. (2007). The United States Revised Uniform Anatomical Gift Act (2006): New challenges to balancing patient rights and physician responsibilities. *Philosophy, Ethics, and Humanities in Medicine.* Retrieved from http://www.pubmedcentral. nih.gov/articlerender.fcgi?artid=2001294

Organ/Tissue Donor Card

I wish to donate my organs and tissues. I wish to give:

☐ any needed organs and tissues   ☐ only the following organs and tissues:

_____

Donor
Signature _____ Date _____
Witness _____
Witness _____

FIGURE 15-2 Example of an organ donor card. (*Source:* U.S. Department of Health and Human Services. Retrieved from http://www.organdonor.gov/get_involved/materials.htm)

- Determine whether the dying client has a living will or advance directives.
- Discuss with client and family the possibility of organ donation, if appropriate for the client's circumstances.

Is It Grief or Depression?

When you are performing a focused assessment for grief or loss, you will need to distinguish between grief and depression. Sadness and depression are an integral part of grief. However, depression that lingers beyond what is expected may be a sign that the stress of grieving has triggered a major depressive episode (Ferszt & Leveillee, 2006). Although grief and depression have several symptoms in common (e.g., sadness, insomnia, poor appetite, and weight loss), grief tends to come and go—to be triggered, for example, by a holiday. To differentiate them, and for guidelines to follow when assessing dying and grieving patients,

 Go to Chapter 15, **Assessment Guidelines and Tools,** in Volume 2.

KnowledgeCheck 15-4

What assessments should you make for your terminally ill patient and his or her family?

Go to Chapter 15, **Knowledge Check Response Sheet and Answers,** on the Student Resource Disk or DavisPlus at http://davisplus.fadavis.com/Wilkinson2

■ ANALYSIS/DIAGNOSIS

When you are analyzing patient data, keep in mind that most grief is normal, not complicated or dysfunctional. Do not use a Complicated Grieving diagnosis for every person who is grieving a loss. Complicated Grieving is unusual in some way and is characterized by functional impairment and intense emotion. Pain and grief are

disabling, or the grieving continues over a very long time (perhaps years). The person may deny or have difficulty expressing feelings of loss or may experience physical symptoms as a result of suppressing feelings. Grieving can function as the problem or the etiology of a nursing diagnosis.

Loss and Grieving as Problem

Several nursing diagnoses may be appropriate for a person who is dying or grieving. You must determine whether loss and grieving are the *problem* or the *etiology,* because (as you learned in Chapters 4 and 6) the answer will influence your interventions. Diagnoses related to death and dying and grief and loss overlap, so they are discussed together in the next section. The nursing diagnoses in the table in Volume 2 focus on the emotional responses to loss or impending death—that is, loss and grieving are the *problem.*

 Go to Chapter 15, **Standardized Outcomes and Interventions for Loss and Grieving Diagnoses,** in Volume 2.

 Critical**Thinking** 15-7

Answer the questions in the Standardized Outcomes and Interventions table in Chapter 15 of Volume 2 (see preceding reference).

Loss and Grieving as Etiology

Loss, grief, and dying are an etiology when they create problems in other areas of patient or family function. The following are examples of such nursing diagnoses.

- Acute or Chronic Low Self-Esteem related to inability to change the event for self or significant other; or related to dying while having "unfinished business"
- Anxiety related to possible inability to cope with the loss; or related to unknown outcome of situation
- Death Anxiety (or Fear) related to impending death
- Decisional Conflict related to end-of-life treatment measures (e.g., concern about the expense of "useless" procedures or their effect on the family; knowledge that the treatment may lengthen life but decrease the quality of life)
- Deficient Knowledge related to the new experience of caring for a terminally ill person
- Fatigue related to demands of caring for a dying loved one
- Spiritual Distress related to loss of trust in a loving God

■ PLANNING OUTCOMES/EVALUATION

Encourage the patient and family to play an active role in planning care. Involving family members helps facilitate their acceptance of the diagnosis and may put the patient more at ease. Questions such as the following will help to elicit the patient's goals for end of life (Matzo, Sherman, Sheehan, et al., 2003):

- "What do you still want to accomplish or do?"
- "What are the things you wish you could still do?"
- "If you have pain, what would be an acceptable level for you, on a 0 to 10 scale?"
- "Where do you want to spend the rest of your life? Where are you most comfortable?"
- "If spiritual peace is important to you, what would help you achieve it?"

NOC standardized outcomes are determined by the diagnostic label you use. For examples,

 Go to Chapter 15, **NOC Outcomes and NIC Interventions for Loss and Grieving Diagnoses,** in Volume 2.

Individualized goals/outcome statements you might write for a grieving or dying person include the following examples. The patient and/or family will:

- Communicate openly among themselves and health-care providers (e.g., express fear, concerns, pain).
- Obtain satisfactory pain relief and symptom management.
- Make use of all resources available to assist with coping.
- Exercise control in the management of care to the extent possible.

As always, you will use the goals set in the planning stage as criteria for evaluating the patient's or family's health status.

KnowledgeCheck 15-5

- List three nursing diagnosis labels you might consider when dying or grieving is the primary problem.
- List three nursing diagnoses labels that might occur as a result of dying or grieving.

 Go to Chapter 15, **Knowledge Check Response Sheet and Answers,** on the Student Resource Disk or DavisPlus at http://davisplus.fadavis.com/Wilkinson2

PLANNING INTERVENTIONS/IMPLEMENTATION

NIC standardized interventions associated with death, dying, and bereavement appear in Volume 2.

 Go to Chapter 15, **NOC Outcomes and NIC Interventions for Loss and Grieving Diagnoses,** in Volume 2.

Specific nursing activities are determined by the nursing diagnosis, especially by the etiology. Our ability to help someone who is grieving or dying is largely determined by our attitude. A compassionate approach is essential but challenging. Watching patients struggle with pain, loss, grief, and death may stir our own deepest doubts and fears, and we may reject the challenge to respond from the heart. We may be aware that employers usually reward nurses for what they *do*

rather than who they *are* as people, so it is easy to rationalize that we have other tasks to accomplish that may be equally important. When we do that, we ignore the real gift we may have to offer the suffering patient: our willingness to "walk the walk" with them, if even for a short time. Full-spectrum nurses combine their psychomotor and thinking skills with compassion in ministering to those who are suffering.

Some important nursing interventions, including therapeutic communication, facilitating grief work, helping families, and specific activities involved in care of the dying person are discussed in the following sections. Also see the Nursing Care Plan and Care Map for Grieving.

Therapeutic Communication

It is especially critical to building a trusting relationship with the dying or grieving patient and significant others (Fig. 15-3). Perhaps most important is to listen to the dying patient and to be alert for and respond to nonverbal cues. Encourage patients and family members to express their feelings, and reassure them that their feelings are normal and not "wrong." In discussions about DNAR or withholding or withdrawing treatments, it is important to find out why the patient is seeking that option: Does she wish to avoid suffering, or does she fear being a burden to loved ones?

Physicians and nurses should always work to improve their communication skills because they are essential for achieving better outcomes at end of life (Boyle, Miller, & Forbes-Thompson, 2005). See Box 15-5 for some barriers to end-of-life communication. For tips on communicating with people who are dying or bereaved,

 Go to Chapter 15, **Clinical Insight 15-1: Communicating with People Who Are Grieving,** in Volume 2.

FIGURE 15-3 The nurse encourages and accepts expression of feelings.

Nursing Care Plan

Client Data

Wilma Peterson is caring for her son, Henry, who has AIDS. Henry is 20 years old; his older brother, William, died at home of AIDS-related pneumonia 2 years earlier at age 24. William had left home at 18 to live in Miami and returned to his home in rural Alabama when he became too ill to manage on his own. Henry stayed home to help his mother care for William and learned he was HIV-positive just before his brother died. Henry did not tell his mother of his diagnosis until he was hospitalized for the first time with cytomegalovirus (CMV) infection. Since then, he has not followed nutritional and medical advice and has continued to stay out late and party when he feels well enough. His health has steadily declined.

You are participating in a special Caring for the Caregiver program set up by the public health nurse in your community. In this program, registered nurses visit primary caregivers to assess their needs and offer support services as needed. Thus, your client is Wilma Peterson.

Ms. Peterson is initially cordial when you visit but tells you, "This is a mother's responsibility. I don't stop being his mother because he's grown up. I'm always his mama." As your discussion continues, Ms. Peterson wistfully talks about when William and Henry were boys playing in the backyard. She says, "I didn't really understand this awful disease until William got so sick. Now, I look at Henry and I know what's waiting for him. I know we are going to lose him. Sad . . . just so sad . . ." Her voice trails off as tears well in her eyes.

Nursing Diagnosis

Grieving related to the client's anticipating the loss of a second son, as evidenced by her previous experience caring for her other son who died at home of AIDS and by the client's stating, "I know what's waiting for him."

NOC Outcomes	Individualized Goals / Expected Outcomes
Family Coping (NOC 2600) Psychosocial Adjustment: Life Change (NOC 1305)	*(Short-term goals) At the end of the initial home visit, Ms. Peterson will:* **1.** Identify community resources available to help her care for Henry at home during acute illnesses. **2.** Begin to feel comfortable discussing her concerns with the nurse. *(Long-term goals) Within 6 weeks, Ms. Peterson will:* **1.** Explore activities she would like to participate in once she is no longer caring for Henry. **2.** Talk with Henry to learn what type of funeral he would like.

(continued on next page)

Nursing Care Plan (continued)

Nursing Interventions and Activities*	Rationales

NIC Interventions

Anticipatory Guidance (NIC 5210)

Coping Enhancement (NIC 5230)

Grief Work Facilitation (NIC 5290)

Nursing Activities

1. Encourage Ms. Peterson to talk about her experiences caring for William before he died.

Grieving often occurs in the context of repeated caregiving (Boyle, Bunting, Hodnicki, et al., 2001) or in situations in which the caregiver has other types of previous experience with the same or a similar terminal illness.

2. Ask her to relate similarities and differences between care for William and care for Henry.

Asking the client to discuss previous experiences allows the nurse to validate the nursing diagnosis (O'Connor & Lunney, 1998).

3. Ask Ms. Peterson to describe the elements of Henry's care and to identify which she considers to be the most important.

Clients are holistic and consider more than just medical treatment in the care of a family member. Their actions are often based on cultural and religious beliefs and their own previous experiences instead of a medically based care plan. Clients may operate on a different, parallel track from that of the healthcare providers (Boyle, Bunting, Hodnicki, et al., 2001). By asking what Ms. Peterson does and how she prioritizes Henry's care, the nurse can learn from the client rather than making assumptions based on the healthcare perspective. By showing respect for her experience as a caregiver, the nurse can build a stronger relationship with Ms. Peterson, which will facilitate future nursing interventions and anticipatory guidance.

4. Talk with Ms. Peterson to find out what community resources she used when she cared for William and whether she has accessed them now that she is caring for Henry.

Isolation and loneliness are risk factors for sole caregivers at home. By assessing community resources, the nurse can determine whether Ms. Peterson is "connected" or isolating herself. Isolation puts her at risk for Complicated Grieving (O'Connor & Lunney, 1998). Many community resources provide a sense of belonging and enhance and support coping strategies as well.

5. Promote shared decision-making if this is acceptable to Henry Peterson.

Informing both Ms. Peterson and Henry about the disease, prognosis, treatment, and comfort options allow them to retain some control over their lives together (Teno, Casey, Welch, et al., 2001). Henry's permission must be obtained to preserve his autonomy.

6. Provide nonjudgmental emotional support to Ms. Peterson, and support healthy coping activities she is using.

Establishing a comfortable and emotionally safe environment will allow Ms. Peterson to share her concerns without fear of being judged because of her son's diagnosis (Boyle et al., 2001).

*Interventions are only a sample of those linked to this diagnosis by *NIC*. Activities should be individualized for each client.

Nursing Care Plan (continued)

Evaluation

Review the initial short-term outcomes and goals. Reassess your client to determine whether the goals are achieved in the stated time frame. In this case, long-term goals will fluctuate based on the progression of Henry's illness. In this case, the following occurred as the care plan was implemented:

- Ms. Peterson cried as she described the deterioration in William's health before he died. She worries that Henry will suffer and does not want him to lose his dignity the way she believes William did.

- Ms. Peterson's greatest concern is that Henry is not eating enough. Much of her self-value as a mother arises from her ability to prepare homemade meals to feed her family, and Henry doesn't have much appetite. This is very distressing to her.

- She has not contacted community agencies. She is holding off, hoping Henry will not be "so sick for so long. With these new drugs, he can get better."

- She remains involved in her church, which is the same one she attended as a little girl. However, she will not tell her church group that Henry has AIDS. "They talk too much," she says. Instead, she says he has leukemia.

Only one short-term goal is met at this visit—establishing a comfort level between the client and the nurse. Ms. Peterson has not identified community resources related to caring for Henry at this time.

Plan for Further Evaluation

Additional supportive visits will be needed to help Ms. Peterson understand that contacting community agencies does not mean Henry will die sooner; at this time, denying the need for community help is an important coping mechanism for Ms. Peterson and is not affecting her ability to care for her son. If his condition worsens, this issue will need to be addressed promptly.

References

Boyle, J. S., Bunting, S. M., Hodnicki, D. R., et al. (2001). Critical thinking in black mothers who care for adult children with HIV: A cultural analysis. *Journal of Transcultural Nursing, 12*(3), 193–202.
Bulechek, G., Butcher, H., & Dochterman, J. M. (2008). *Nursing interventions classification (NIC)* (5th ed.). St. Louis, MO: C. V. Mosby.
Johnson, M., Bulechek, G., Butcher, H., et al. (2006). *Nursing diagnoses, outcomes, and interventions: NANDA, NOC, and NIC linkages* (2nd ed.). St. Louis, MO: C. V. Mosby.
Moorhead, S. Johnson, M., Maas, M., et al. (2008). *Nursing outcomes classification (NOC)* (4th ed.). St. Louis, MO: C. V. Mosby
O'Connor, L., & Lunney, M. (1998). Care of the caregiver—Family member with a chronic illness. *Nursing Diagnosis, 9*(4), 152.
Teno, J. M., Casey, V. A., Welch, L. C., et al. (2001). Patient-focused, family-centered end-of-life medical care: Views of the guidelines and bereaved family members. *Journal of Pain and Symptom Management, 22*, 738–751.

Care Map

Son, Henry, with AIDS

Ms. Peterson

First son died from AIDS

Noncompliant with medical advice

"I know what's waiting for him"

"I know we are going to lose him"

Identifies strongly with mom/caregiver role

- Cried when talking about first son's death
- Worried about loss of dignity for Henry

Grieving r/t anticipating loss of second son

NIC intervention: Coping Enhancement

NIC interventions: Anticipatory Guidance, Grief Work Facilitation

- Ask Ms. Peterson what elements of care she thinks are most important
- Ask what community resources she used in the past and whether she has accessed them now
- Promote shared decision making with Henry
- Provide nonjudgmental support; support healthy coping activities

- Encourage Ms. Peterson to talk about her experiences in caring for William before he died
- Ask her to relate similarities and differences between care for William and Henry

NOC outcome: Family Coping
- Identifies community resources for son's home care
- Talks with Henry about funeral

NOC outcomes: Psychosocial Adjustment and Life Change
- States she feels comfortable discussing concerns with nurse
- Explores activities she would like to participate in after son's death

evaluation

Key:

- Data
- Nursing diagnosis
- NIC interventions
- Nursing actions
- NOC outcomes
- Evaluation

BOX 15-5 ■ Barriers to End-of-Life Communication

- Fear of one's own mortality
- Unresolved personal grief issues (e.g., the loss of one's own parent)
- Lack of experience with death and dying
- Fear of expressing emotion (i.e., crying)
- Fear of not knowing the answer to a question
- Not knowing whether to give an honest (and possibly unwelcome) answer to a question
- Not understanding the family's culture
- Keeping physical distance (e.g., standing away from the person or avoiding eye contact)
- Insensitivity: interrupting communication, patronizing, giving false reassurance

Source: Matzo, M., Shermann, D., Sheehan, D., et al. (2003). Teaching strategies from the ELNEC curriculum. *Nursing Education Perspectives, (21)*1,176–183.

If you need more information on communication and therapeutic relationships, refer to Chapter 18.

Facilitating Grief Work

Whether grief results from a loss of health, from an impending death, or from some other loss, you can help patients and families work through their grief by helping them express their feelings, recall memories, and find meaning in their lives. Later in this chapter, we discuss interventions for helping families after the death of a loved one. This section focuses more generally on grieving *any* loss.

Expressing Feelings

Your theoretical knowledge already includes the fact that it is the family, not just an individual patient, who is grieving, whether because of death or some other loss. And you also know that for people to deal with grief in a healthy way, they need to communicate their feelings. Sometimes people are uncomfortable with expressing their feelings and hold them in. This reserve will interfere with their grief resolution, so you may have to facilitate the process. Therapeutic communication will be needed (see Chapter 18). The following are some ways to facilitate expression of feelings:

- Encourage questions, and respond to them within a reasonable time.
- Sit beside the head of the bed; do not appear rushed.
- When you observe the patient or family member expressing feelings, either verbally or nonverbally, encourage them to continue.
- Expect and accept a wide range of feelings, including anger, fear, and loneliness.
- Ask, "How can I help?" "What do you need?" "What would you like for me to do?"

- Be sure that everyone on the healthcare team understands and follows the care plan.
- Ask yourself what you would do if this were your family member.
- Do not compare another person's loss to your own experience. For example, avoid comments such as, "I know how you feel." Instead, say, "Tell me how you feel."

Recalling Memories

Grieving patients and family members may need to recall memories, both good and difficult. One way to encourage recall is to go through photo albums with them and ask questions about the people in the pictures. Also look for objects of sentiment (e.g., a family heirloom) in the environment and ask the dying or bereaved person to share their significance.

Finding Meaning

Another way to facilitate grief work is to help the patient or family find meaning in their lives or in their past. Talking through this meaning is a healthy way to cope. Facilitating life review is one technique to help the patient and/or family recognize the unique contributions this person has made to family, friends, and society. You can begin by asking about the various aspects of the patient's life, commenting on pictures in the room, or picking up on verbal cues that are expressed.

Bibliotherapy

Bibliotherapy is a counseling technique used when grief therapy is indicated. It uses guided reading of self-help or fiction literature to increase client awareness and understanding and promote healing. Poems, novels, and essays can help produce new insights, either as the client retells the story or is guided to discuss his feelings and thoughts about the characters in the story (Briggs & Pehrsson, 2008).

Critical Thinking 15-8

- What would you say to Mrs. Manning ("Meet Your Patient") if you walked into a room and found her sitting in a chair and softly weeping while Mr. Manning sleeps?
- What response would you make when Mr. Manning waves his hand in the air and says, "I'm not taking any more of those damn pills" as you bring him his medications?
- A young woman approaches you in the hall and says, "I want to visit Mom and stay with her, but I just can't stand to see her like that. I feel guilty for wanting to leave." What would be your therapeutic response?

Helping Families of Dying Patients

When a patient is dying, it is especially important to view the family as your unit of care. If the patient is unresponsive, you may find yourself spending most of your care time with the family. This time should be spent providing education, support, and a listening ear. Observing their loved one dying can leave family members feeling confused, angry, helpless, and even devastated; thus, sensitive and compassionate care during this time is essential. You can make good use of the interventions in the preceding sections, as you help family members to understand that what they see may be very different from what the patient is experiencing. For more specific interventions for helping families of dying patients,

 Go to Chapter 15, **Clinical Insight 15-2: Helping Families of Dying Patients,** in Volume 2.

KnowledgeCheck 15-6

- Describe four ways to facilitate the grief work of a grieving or dying person.
- List two specific interventions for helping grieving families.

 Go to Chapter 15, **Knowledge Check Response Sheet and Answers,** on the Student Resource Disk or DavisPlus at http://davisplus.fadavis.com/Wilkinson2

Caring for the Dying Person

To effectively care for terminally ill patients, you must use a holistic model. This means meeting physiological, psychological, social, sexual, and spiritual needs. Most hospitals have an interdisciplinary team to provide holistic care to dying patients and their families. This team may be made up of a physician, nurse, social worker, pastoral care worker, dietitian, physical therapist (and sometimes occupational and speech therapists), and volunteers.

Meeting Physiological Needs

Active dying usually occurs over a period of 10 to 14 days (although it can take as little as 24 hours). The "final hours" refers to the last 4 to 48 hours of life, in which failure of body systems results in death (Pitorak, 2003). In the last hours of life, most patients need skilled care around the clock. Physiological needs during this time include mobility, oxygenation, safety, nutrition, fluids, elimination, personal hygiene, and control of pain and symptoms (nausea, vomiting). See the previous discussion of the physiological stages of dying to review signs of impending death. For specific interventions and guidelines to use when caring for a dying patient,

 Go to Chapter 15, **Clinical Insight 15-3: Caring for the Dying Person: Meeting Physiological Needs,** in Volume 2.

Meeting Psychological Needs

When a patient is terminally ill, the physician is usually responsible for deciding what and how much to tell the person. Ideally, other health team members and the family should be involved in this decision. Everyone involved with the patient should know exactly what he and the family have been told. Most patients want to know their prognosis as soon as possible so that they can put personal affairs in order, share their feelings with family members, and come to terms with their life and death. A systematic review of research suggests that rather than protecting patients, efforts to shield patients from the reality of their situation usually creates greater difficulties for them (Hancock, Clayton, Parker, et al., 2007). A "conspiracy of silence" causes fear, anxiety, and confusion, and it denies

---

Toward Evidence-Based Practice

Hancock, K., Claton, J. M., Parker, S. M., et al. (2007). **Truth-telling in discussing prognosis in advanced life-limiting illnesses: A systematic review.** *Palliative Medicine, 21,* 507–517.

This was a systematic review of 46 studies related to truth-telling in discussing prognosis with patients with progressive, advanced life-limiting illnesses and their caregivers. Results included the following:

- Many health professionals expressed discomfort at having to inform the patient and family of limited life expectancy.
- The majority of health professionals thought that patients and their caregivers should be told the truth about the prognosis.
- Nevertheless, many either avoid discussing the topic or withhold information.
- Reasons for not telling the truth include perceived lack of training, stress, no time to attend to the patient's emotional

needs, fear of a negative effect on the patient, uncertainty about the prognosis, requests from family members to withhold information, and a feeling of inadequacy because further curative treatment was not available.

- Studies suggested that patients can discuss this topic without it having a negative impact on them.

1. Based on this systematic review, do you think health professionals should inform patients when they have an advanced life-limiting (terminal) illness? Explain your thinking.

2. Health professionals feared a negative effect on patients of telling them the truth about their condition. What sorts of negative effects do you think they might be anticipating?

 Go to Chapter 15, **Toward Evidence-Based Practice Suggested Responses,** on the Student Resource Disk or DavisPlus at http://davisplus.fadavis.com/Wilkinson2

people the opportunity to make needed life adaptations. However, be aware that culture may determine which family members are to be informed and how much, if any, information is given to the patient. Also, many patients realize without being told that they are dying. For specific interventions to help meet the psychological needs of dying patients,

 Go to Chapter 15, **Clinical Insight 15-4: Caring for the Dying Person: Meeting Psychological Needs,** in Volume 2.

KnowledgeCheck 15-7

- Describe six nursing interventions to use in meeting the physiological needs of a dying person.
- Describe six nursing interventions to use in meeting the psychological needs of a dying person.
- What should be the focus of your interventions when the patient is very near death?

 Go to Chapter 15, **Knowledge Check Response Sheet and Answers,** on the Student Resource Disk or DavisPlus at http://davisplus.fadavis.com/Wilkinson2

Addressing Spiritual Needs

When a person is terminally ill, his spirituality may become very important as he searches for meaning in the illness and suffering. The person may be looking for forgiveness and/or acceptance or be reaching out to feel connected. Ways to address this need include (but are not limited to) empathetic listening, contacting pastoral care or clergy if the patient asks for this service, special rituals, praying with the patient, music, meditation, or special readings.

Information about specific religious practices may help you provide appropriate interventions at end of life. For example, after the death of an Orthodox Jewish patient, you should handle the body as little as possible if you are not Jewish; most Christian denominations will not object to your washing and preparing the body. Remember, though, that there are wide individual differences and that you must assess each patient and family to determine how closely they adhere to the rituals of their religion. Review Chapters 13 and 14, as needed. For detailed information about a variety of religious practices surrounding death,

 Go to Chapter 15, **Supplemental Materials: Addressing Spiritual Needs,** on the Student Resource Disk or DavisPlus at http://davisplus.fadavis.com/Wilkinson2

Addressing Cultural Needs

A recent study found the following end-of-life concerns were important to people regardless of their ethnicity or gender: comfort, physician communication, having responsibilities taken care of, hope and optimism, and honoring spiritual beliefs. Most groups also were concerned about love and compassion, being cared for, expressing feelings, fixing relationships, saying goodbye, having choices, making plans, not being in pain, and being "ready to go" (Duffy, Jackson, Schim, et al., 2006).

There is also some overlap between religious and cultural practices. For example, most cultural groups engage in some type of religious ceremony that helps the bereaved begin the grieving process. Nevertheless, some death rituals and expressions of grief may be culture based but not necessarily involve religion. Consider these examples:

- Some cultures may emphasize keeping emotions more subdued and limiting expressions of grief to private settings, whereas others gauge the value of the deceased by the amount of wailing and crying.
- Blacks and Hispanics may be reluctant to withdraw life-sustaining treatment or to use a hospice, whereas Arab Muslims may be reluctant to prolong life unnecessarily (Duffy, Jackson, Schim, et al., 2006).

Despite the commonalities among groups, there are some culture-specific differences. To provide culturally sensitive care at end of life, you will need some information about specific cultural practices surrounding death. For this information,

 Go to Chapter 15, **Supplemental Materials: Addressing Cultural Needs,** on the Student Resource Disk at http://davisplus.fadavis.com/Wilkinson2

As with spiritual care, remember that you cannot assume that a person follows the practices of her cultural group; you must assess to be sure.

 CriticalThinking 15-9

Reflect on this reading by Theresa Rando in *The Gift of Presence:*

It is one of the most difficult things in the world to do to sit and listen while another's heart is breaking with grief, to hold the hand of a dying patient who cries silently while staring into space. The gift of presence, the gift of being with those in pain, is the only gift we can give. It is the sole armor patients have against the anguish. The very most we can do for dying patients is to make it better, with our presence and concern, than it would be if we were not there. . . . we cannot "do" anything that can get rid of the psychic pain of impending loss and death (Rando, 1984, p. 272).

Close your eyes and visualize yourself sitting quietly beside a dying patient and holding her hand. Visualize the patient crying silently. Can you still your mind and remain silent, or do you feel you must say something to make the patient feel better?

Providing Postmortem Care

Postmortem care includes care of the patient's body after death and fulfilling any legal obligations, such as arranging transportation to the morgue or funeral home and determining the disposition of the patient's belongings. You will follow agency policies and respect cultural and spiritual preferences, along with the care that is commonly provided. In most states and provinces, the physician must pronounce death; in some areas, however, a coroner or a nurse may also perform this task.

Rigor mortis (the stiffening of the body after death) is caused by contraction of the muscles from a lack of adenosine triphosphate (ATP). It occurs about 2 to 4 hours after death. Rigor mortis begins in the involuntary muscles (e.g., the heart). It appears next in the head, neck, and trunk, and finally in the extremities. It disappears about 96 hours after death. **Algor mortis** occurs when the blood stops circulating. The body temperature drops about 1.88°F (1°C) per hour until it reaches room temperature. The dependent parts of the body appear bluish and mottled because when the blood stops circulating, the red blood cells break down, releasing hemoglobin. This is called **livor mortis.**

If the family wishes to be alone with the body, straighten the bedcovers and make the patient look as natural as possible. Give family members whatever time they need before you prepare the body. Ideally, you will have already established a relationship with the family and will have begun to facilitate their grieving during the patient's dying period. And you will have prepared them as the death becomes imminent. For specific guidelines for care of the body and other immediate postmortem interventions to support family members,

 Go to Chapter 15, **Clinical Insight 15-5: Providing Postmortem Care,** in Volume 2.

KnowledgeCheck 15-8

- Why is it important to position the body with a pillow under the head and shoulders soon after death?
- Why is it important to close the eyes and mouth of the deceased and position the body within at least 2 to 4 hours after death?

 Go to Chapter 15, **Knowledge Check Response Sheet and Answers,** on the Student Resource Disk or DavisPlus at http://davisplus.fadavis.com/Wilkinson2

Providing Grief Education

Sometime after the immediate postmortem period, explain the stages of grief and point out that it takes months or even years to resolve. Explain that grief may become more intense on the anniversary of the death (or other loss) and on significant dates (e.g., birthdays).

Recall that once the bereaved person accepts that the loss is real, his feelings may be so intense that he may wonder if he is losing his sanity. The grieving person may be fatigued from not sleeping, may be disoriented or unable to concentrate, and so on; he may be concerned about what such symptoms mean. Reassure the person that such responses are expected and that there is no single right way to grieve (Egan & Arnold, 2003). Also assure him that although the grief process takes time, the symptoms won't last forever.

Helping Children Deal with Loss

Some families may need information about helping children deal with grief, especially when there is a death in the family. You may need to explain that children perceive death differently from adults. See the accompanying Self-Care box for teaching surviving relatives how to help children deal with grief.

Taking Care of Yourself

When caring for dying patients, you will confront your own feelings of mortality. It is important to understand your own attitudes, fears, and beliefs concerning death, so you should think about these in advance: before you encounter dying patients. This will enable you to deal in a more healthy way with patients and their families. In addition, suppressing feelings associated with death of patients can take a heavy toll on you emotionally.

You will probably experience feelings of grief and loss. When you become involved with dying persons and their families at such an intimate time in their lives, you become connected to them. There is nothing wrong with this emotional involvement; it helps you to be effective in your work. But just as you care for these families, you need also to care for yourself during these times.

- Recognize that feelings of grief and loss are normal.
- Talk with other colleagues about your feelings. Nurses are known for being able to take care of everyone but themselves! Don't be afraid to ask for what you need.

Self-Care

Helping Children Deal with Loss

Teach surviving relatives the following:

➤ If a child is frightened about attending a funeral, the family should not force him to go. It is important, however, to include the child in some service or observance, such as lighting a candle, saying a prayer, or visiting the grave site, at a later time.

➤ The surviving relatives should spend as much time as possible with the child, making it clear that the child has permission to show her feelings openly or freely.

➤ Be prepared for intermittent expressions of sadness and anger from the child, over a long period of time.

➤ Be prepared for the possibility of regression to earlier developmental stages (e.g., talking "baby talk").

➤ Assure the child that he was in no way responsible for the death.

➤ The following are warning signs that may indicate the need for professional help, especially if they are prolonged: an extended period in which the child loses interest in daily activities and events, inability to sleep, loss of appetite, fear of being alone, extended regression, repeated statements about wanting to join the dead person, withdrawal from friends, refusal to attend school, or sharp drop in school performance.

- Do not be afraid to confront grief. Some nurses feel they have to be strong and tend to deny their feelings. They overwork and take care of others. If you use this approach, the feelings will accumulate and begin to wear you down physically and emotionally.
- If you wish, it is appropriate for you to attend calling hours and/or funeral services when one of your patients dies. This helps you diffuse some of your feelings of loss. It also is very meaningful to family members to know that you took the time to remember them and their loved one.
- Learn how to get support for yourself and how to support your colleagues when they experience the death of a patient. One idea is a nurses' support group, or grief team, that meets regularly to talk about the feelings and to remember those who have died. If you need or want a facilitator, pastoral care workers and social workers may be available for these services.

- Do some nice things for yourself on a regular basis (e.g., facial, quiet bubble bath, massage, a sports event). Try to set aside a special spot in your home that is only for relaxation; decorate it with items that help you focus on peaceful thoughts (e.g., candles, pictures, religious objects).

Caring for the dying can be very rewarding but is also emotionally draining. To be effective in your practice, learn to care for yourself as well.

 Go to Chapter 15, **Resources for Caregivers and Health Professionals,** on the Student Resource Disk or DavisPlus at http://davisplus.fadavis.com/Wilkinson2

 Suggested Readings: Go to Chapter 15, **Reading More About Loss, Grief, & Dying,** on the Student Resource Disk or DavisPlus at http://davisplus.fadavis.com/Wilkinson2

 Bibliography: Go to Volume 2, Bibliography

Essential Nursing Interventions

CHAPTER 16

Documenting & Reporting

Learning Outcomes

After completing this chapter you should be able to:

➤ Explain the purposes of documentation.

➤ Compare and contrast the differences between electronic and written documentation.

➤ Identify a variety of charting formats and their purposes.

➤ Use paper and electronic documentation in the clinical setting.

➤ Describe guidelines for documentation.

➤ Identify approved abbreviations to use in charting.

➤ Follow documentation guidelines to accurately record patient health status, nursing interventions, and patient outcomes.

➤ Discuss the key elements of giving an oral patient report.

➤ Explain the process for verifying or questioning a medical order.

➤ Critique samples of charting.

Meet Your Patients

Steven Stellanski is a 16-year-old male who has just been released from the post-anesthesia care unit (PACU) after an emergency appendectomy. You are to admit him to your unit. Steven is groggy but moaning in pain. "Help me, help me," he whispers. He is holding his abdomen and grimacing. The PACU nurse tells you that Steven has Down syndrome and functions at a school-age level.

Steven's vital signs are as follows: tympanic membrane temperature 99.9°F (37.7°C); pulse, 104 beats/min; respirations, 24 breaths/min; and blood pressure 104/68 mm Hg. An intravenous (IV) bag of lactated Ringer's solution is infusing at 125 mL/hr. The dressing on Steven's right lower abdomen is dry and intact. An indwelling catheter is draining pale yellow urine.

The postoperative prescriptions for Steven call for starting a patient-controlled analgesia pump that will deliver morphine sulfate at 1 mg every 15 minutes, up to 4 mg per hour. He is to remain NPO (nothing by mouth) for now. The dressing is to be changed tomorrow morning and the nurses are to institute progressive ambulation as tolerated.

Theoretical **Knowledge**
knowing why

When you imagine yourself working as a nurse, what do you think of? Most people picture themselves at the bedside working with patients. When you look at ads for nursing jobs, they often show a nurse hanging an IV bag, listening to heart sounds, or perhaps teaching a patient. Photos rarely show the nurse charting or reporting care. Yet healthcare professionals rely on these two methods of communication to coordinate patient care. In this chapter, we discuss paper, electronic, and oral communication.

Documentation

Documentation is the act of recording patient status and care in written or electronic form, or in a combination of the two forms. Documentation is not limited to "writing nursing notes," but is the act of making a written record. The terms *documenting, recording,* and *charting* are often used to mean the same thing. Oral communication about a patient's status is called **reporting**—that is discussed later in this chapter.

For many years, the collection of documentation, orders, and other care information for a patient had been called the **medical record** or **chart**. However, with the present emphasis on health promotion, the medical record is now more commonly referred to as the **health record**. A patient's health record permanently documents:

- Care, in chronological order, provided by all healthcare providers
- The patient's responses to interventions and treatments
- Important facts about a client's health history, including past and present illnesses, examinations, tests, treatments, and outcomes

As a nurse, you are responsible for managing and implementing the interdisciplinary plan of care. That responsibility includes documenting the care provided and the progress made toward goals. Research shows that nurses routinely spend 15% to 25% of their workday documenting the care they give, and in some cases considerably more.

How Do Healthcare Providers Use Documentation?

Clear, complete, and accurate documentation in a client health record serves the following purposes:

Planning and Evaluation of a Patient's Care. Documentation enables physicians, nurses, and other healthcare professionals to plan and evaluate treatment and monitor health status over time.

Communication and Continuity of Care. Members of the multidisciplinary team use the health record to communicate about the patient's status and care. For example, if it is not possible to speak directly to the respiratory therapist on your shift, you can at least review the progress notes. Likewise, if you are concerned that the patient is at high risk for developing an infection, you can include a nursing diagnosis of Risk for Infection on the written or electronic interdisciplinary plan of care. You would then initiate nursing orders for regular observation for and document signs of infection.

Legal Documentation. The health record will be scrutinized by legal experts if a dispute about a client's care arises. In court, the health record is legal evidence of the care given to a client, and is used to judge whether the interventions were timely and appropriate. To meet minimum legal standards, the health record must show a clear audit trail that starts with the client's baseline status; and then documents changes in status, interpretation of the changes, interventions used, and client responses to interventions.

Quality Improvement. Healthcare organizations and agencies perform manual chart audits (directed reviews of client medical records) of written documentation. In electronic health record (EHR) systems, reports are run to analyze large amounts of data. Results are used to identify ways to improve care, decrease length of stay, control costs, and pinpoint knowledge and practice gaps that can be addressed through continuing professional education and inservice education. Accrediting agencies, such as The Joint Commission, review written and electronic records to ensure delivery of quality care and public safety.

Professional Standards of Care. The American Nurses Association (ANA) *Scope and Standards of Practice* (2010, in press) includes documentation in many of its standards. By the ANA standards, the registered nurse:

- *Documents relevant data* in a retrievable format. (Standard 1, Assessment)
- *Documents diagnoses* or issues in a manner that facilitates the determination of the expected outcomes and plan. (Standard 2, Diagnosis)
- *Documents expected outcomes* as measurable goals. (Standard 3, Outcomes Identification)
- *Documents the plan of care* in a manner that uses standardized language or recognized terminology, and is understood by all participants. (Standard 4, Planning)
- *Documents implementation* and any modifications, including changes or omission, of the identified plan. (Standard 5, Implementation)
- *Documents the coordination of the care.* (Standard 5a, Coordination of Care)
- *Documents the results of the evaluation.* (Standard 6, Evaluation)
- *Communicates effectively* in a variety of written, spoken and technological formats. (Standard 11, Communication)
- Cooperates in *creating a documented plan* focused on outcomes and decisions related to care and delivery of

services that indicates communication with patients, families, and others. (Standard 14 Collaboration)

- *Documents referrals*, including provisions for continuity of care. (Standard 14, Collaboration)
- *Caveat*: This material is from the draft for public comment (ANA, 2010 in press); its wording may be changed somewhat in the final published version. For that version of the ANA Standards of Professional Nursing Practice, go to www.nursingworld.org.

Reimbursement and Utilization Review. Insurance companies, government and third-party payers, budget managers, and organization billing staff use client health records to determine the cost of care. They also use the health record for **utilization review**, the determination of whether the medical treatments and interventions were necessary and appropriate.

Education. As a student, you are well aware of this use of the health record. The record provides a snapshot of what is going on with the client so you are able to research unfamiliar diagnoses, orders, and treatments before direct care begins. This helps you to deliver safe care.

Research. The health record is also used to gather data for clinical research. The increasing use of EHRs enables rapid analysis of large numbers of health records. Use of large samples of health records and clinical data sets is an essential step toward better understanding the cause and progression of disease, treatment methods, and outcomes across varied populations and diseases.

Why Are Standardized Nursing Languages Important?

Nurses have long understood the need for a standardized vocabulary for describing what nurses do and the outcomes that result. Unlike physician diagnoses and procedures, nursing care has historically not generated charges for reimbursement, except in the case of advanced practice nurses. As healthcare costs escalated, healthcare organizations began to question traditional roles, especially those of nurses. It became, and still is, necessary to measure nursing's contribution to care and demonstrate the value of nursing. Standardized nursing terminology helps do that by making nursing care and its effect on patient outcomes more visible in patient records and retrievable by researchers.

Standardized languages are especially important in EHR systems because computers require standardized information that can be converted to numerical codes. Several standardized nursing language models have been created and are used in nursing documentation, for example, NANDA International (NANDA-I), Nursing Interventions Classification (NIC), and Nursing Outcomes Classification (NOC). To review using standardized nursing language models in your own practice, see Chapter 4: "Standardized Nursing Languages,

What Is a Taxonomy?"; Chapter 5: "How Do I Use Standardized Terminology for Outcomes?"; and Chapter 6: "How Can I Use Standardized Language to Plan Interventions?"

The ANA (2005; 2010, in press) has recommended documentation systems use ANA-recognized terminology (e.g., NANDA-I, NIC, NOC). Standardized terminologies allow researchers to retrieve nursing data for aggregation and analysis. Through the use of standardized languages in nursing documentation, a standard for evidence-based nursing care delivery has now been established. This is a step toward closing the gap between what research shows to be the best nursing practices and the interventions nurses actually use in practice.

How Are Health Records Systems Organized?

A **health records system** is the overall process by which all patient records are created, stored, and retrieved in an organization. In a sense, it consists of all the EHRs in an organization. Each healthcare agency determines the health record system that is used. The nursing leaders in each organization usually determine the documentation forms that nurses will use within the records system.

Source-Oriented Record Systems

Patients in hospitals and long-term care facilities receive care from a variety of disciplines, so these institutions commonly use **source-oriented records**. In a source-oriented system, members of each discipline record their findings in a separately labeled section of the chart. In paper records, nurses chart in the nurses' notes section as well as in the graphic data section. A typical source-oriented record includes the following sections:

- *Admission data*—demographic information, insurance data, contact information
- *Advance directive*—information on client's wishes for the extent of care and medical support that should be given in the event of a life-threatening event
- *History and physical*—a detailed summary of the current health problem; past medical, surgical and social history; medications taken; allergies; review of systems, and physical examination data
- *Physician's orders*—orders for medications, treatments, and activities
- *Progress notes*—chronological charting by healthcare team members including patient exams, problem identification, and patient's response to therapy
- *Diagnostic studies*—reports detailing the findings of tests that have been performed, such as x-ray exam, ultrasound, or pulmonary function tests
- *Laboratory data*—a compilation or results from diagnostic test results
- *Nurses' notes*—documentation of patient care and response to treatment recorded by nurses (usually chronological)

- *Graphic data*—numerical data collected over time and displayed visually to allow analysis of trends. Examples include intake and output records, vital sign flowsheets, rating scales, and checklists regarding patient activity, dietary intake, and activities of daily living (ADL) tasks.
- *Rehabilitation and therapy notes*—chronological charting by therapists about assessments, the treatment plan, and patient response to therapy; usually includes physical therapy, occupational therapy, and respiratory therapy
- *Discharge planning*—includes data from utilization review, case managers, or discharge planners on anticipated client needs after discharge

In source-oriented records, you can easily find the care provided by each discipline. However, a drawback of this system is that data may be fragmented and scattered throughout the patient's record. You need to review all sections of the chart to fully understand the client's condition and care.

It is especially difficult with source-oriented records to track the treatments and client outcomes associated with a particular problem. For example, suppose a client with congestive heart failure is retaining fluids, causing her to be short of breath on exertion. To find the interventions for the problem, you would need to look (1) in the primary care providers' (PCP) orders to see whether cardiac drugs or diuretics were prescribed to help with the fluid retention; (2) in the respiratory therapist's notes for breathing treatments and the client's response; and (3) in the nursing notes to see whether the client is being positioned with the head of the bed elevated to facilitate breathing. To see whether the medications were effective, you would need to read the nurse's notes about the client's responses to activity, the PCP progress notes, and the respiratory therapist's notes.

Problem-Oriented Record Systems

Problem-oriented records (PORs) are organized around the patient's problems. There are no separate sections for each discipline. The POR consists of four parts: database, problem list, plan of care, and progress notes.

- The **database** consists of many parts: demographic data, the history and physical, nursing assessment data, and family and social history. As the patient's condition changes, the database is updated to reflect the patient's current status.
- The **problem list** is a concise listing of problems that have been identified from the database. Once a problem is resolved, it is noted on the problem list. If a problem changes or is redefined, the problem list is updated to reflect the change. See Figure 16-1 for an example of a problem list.
- The **plan of care** includes the primary care provider's orders and the nursing care plan for addressing the identified problems. Other disciplines may also contribute to the plan.

Problem number	Date entered	Date resolved	Client problem
1	4/10/11	4/11/11	Abdominal pain (unknown etiology) Redefined 4/11/11
1A	4/11/11		Appendicitis resulting in emergency appendectomy
1B	4/11/11		Acute pain r/t abdominal incision 2 appendectomy
2	4/10/11		Down syndrome — functions at school-age level
3	4/11/11		Risk for constipation r/t opioid use for pain control and h/o appendicitis

FIGURE 16-1 A problem list for Steven Stellanski ("Meet Your Patient"). Note that problem 1 has been redefined now that the cause of Steven's pain has been determined. Note also that the list contains both medical and nursing diagnoses.

- **Progress notes** are organized according to the problem list. Each discipline charts on shared notes. Charting is labeled according to problem number.

The POR system has several advantages. First, there is a common problem list that includes input from all disciplines. Second, it is easy to monitor the patient's progress because each problem is readily identified in the notes. Third, each discipline has ready access to the findings of the other members of the health team. This may encourage greater collaboration. The POR system requires a cooperative spirit among health providers as well as diligence in maintaining a current database and problem list.

Charting by Exception

Charting by exception (CBE) is more than a format; it is a system of charting in which only significant findings or exceptions to standards and norms of care are charted. To use the CBE system effectively, you must know and adhere to professional, legal, and organizational guidelines for nursing assessments and interventions.

CBE uses preprinted flowsheets to document most aspects of care. CBE assumes that unless a separate entry is made (an *exception*) all standards have been met and the patient has responded normally. Normal responses for various assessments are defined on the form, sometimes on the back of the form. CBE flowsheets vary by specialty, and, in some cases, even by diagnosis. Each flowsheet has entries for expected aspects of care.

CBE reduces the amount of time spent on documentation, reduces repetitive charting of routine care, provides a record that is easily read and understood, and clearly highlights any variations from the expected plan of care. In many organizations, CBE records are kept at the bedside, which promotes timely documentation.

Inadvertent omissions are the main problem associated with CBE. Omissions may result from disagreement over what constitutes a significant variation. Critics of CBE believe it: (1) requires nurses to be overly familiar with the organization's documentation standards and policies; (2) makes it difficult to capture the skilled judgment of nurses; and (3) reduces care to such rote repetitions that you may forget to chart an exception to the established standards. Documentation must be time-sensitive, and under this system, false documentation can be created by assuming that care has been done when it has not.

Here is an example of what part of a CBE flowsheet for your patient, Steven Stellanski, might look like. Notice in the first section, the day-shift nurse merely initials that she has made an assessment or taken one of the listed actions at each of the designated times:

DATE: 04/11/11				
Hour	0800	0900	1000	1100
ACTIVITY				
Bed rest		LP		
Ambulate	LP*			
Sleeping				
BRP				
HOB elevated	LP	LP		

	DAY	EVENING	NIGHT	
Neurological		✓		
Cardiovascular		✓		
Pulmonary		✓		
Gastrointestinal		*		Vomited 3×1, 100 mL clear yellow fluid at 0730. Given Compazine 1 mg IV with relief.

Key: ✓ = normal findings, * = significant finding

Notice also the second table (with the check marks) is a summary for the day shift. This is where the nurse describes and discusses any of the significant findings noted at the individual assessment times.

Electronic Health Record Systems

The EHR consists of records that are entered via computer. EHRs typically combine source-oriented and problem-oriented record styles, although the source-oriented system is most common. For example, a client's EHR often contains orders, clinical documentation, laboratory and other test and procedure results, as well as an interdisciplinary plan of care (IPOC), a problem and diagnosis list, and progress notes entered by physicians, nurses, respiratory therapists, and other professional providers.

Figure 16-2 is a section of an electronic form for recording intake and output in source-oriented format. Figure 16-3 is an electronic IPOC in problem-oriented format. As you can see in Figure 16-2, the input and output (I&O) screen records numerical data. It also allows the nurse to add brief narrative comments in each field. The IPOC can be updated at the times specified by the organization and the I&O data can be entered at any time. Both exist within the same electronic records system.

For a summary of the advantages and disadvantages of both electronic and paper health records, see Boxes 16-1 and 16-2, respectively.

KnowledgeCheck 16-1

- Identify the purposes of the client health record.
- What are the key differences in the organization of source-oriented records, problem-oriented records, electronic documentation systems, and CBE systems?
- What are three advantages of paper health records?
- What are three advantages of EHRs?

 Go to Chapter 16, **Knowledge Check Response Sheet and Answers,** on the Student Resource Disk or DavisPlus at http://davisplus.fadavis.com/Wilkinson2

Documentation and the Nursing Process

The goal of all nursing documentation is a clear, concise representation of the client's healthcare experience that is easily accessible and understood by all members of the healthcare team. Effective documentation allows you to help clients to make sound health decisions. It also enables use of current and consistent data, problem statements, diagnoses, goals, and strategies to support continuity of care. Regardless of the type of documentation that is used, you will use or refer to the nursing process as a guideline when you are charting.

Assessment: Document signs and symptoms that may indicate actual or potential client problems. At an initial assessment, document comprehensive data about all client systems.

Diagnosis/Analysis: After analyzing assessment data, document your clinical nursing judgment about the client's response to actual or potential health conditions or needs.

Outcomes/Planning: Document a measurable and achievable short-term and long-term plan of care with goals directed at preventing, minimizing, or resolving identified client problems or issues.

Implementation: After putting the plan of care into effect, document the specific interventions that were used.

Evaluation: Document client responses to nursing care; document whether the plan of care was effective in preventing, minimizing or resolving the identified problems; and then modify the plan as needed.

FIGURE 16-2 An electronic intake and output (I&O) entry form. (Courtesy of Cerner Corporation, Kansas City, MO.)

FIGURE 16-3 A portion of an electronic Interdisciplinary Plan of Care (IPOC) form. (Courtesy of Cerner Corporation, Kansas City, MO.)

BOX 16-1 ■ Advantages and Disadvantages of an Electronic Health Record

ADVANTAGES

Enhanced communication and collaboration: Communication is improved between healthcare providers.

Improved access to information:

- Multiple healthcare providers can access the same information at the same time.
- Authorized persons can access information remotely (e.g., from a patient's home).
- A few EHRs integrate client information between multiple departments so that one area can immediately see information from another. For example, when the laboratory enters a critical result, such as a clotting time, you do not need to wait for the lab to phone or to send a paper result to the nursing unit.

Time savings:

- Nurses spend up to 25% less time documenting.
- Information is stored and retrieved quickly and easily.
- Reports can be created quickly because of the computer's ability to aggregate data (e.g., a 24-hour graph of the patient's vital signs).
- Repetition and duplication are reduced.

Improved quality of care:

- The system can use protocols to automatically enter orders based on the client's condition. For example, most organizations have policies for making falls prevention assessments. Some EHR systems will automatically enter an order to observe and document risk of falls more often when a patient's "falls score" exceeds a certain level.
- Embedded protocols enhance caregiver knowledge and the ability to follow clinical practice guidelines. For example, suppose there is a medical prescription to administer insulin on the basis of a patient's blood glucose results. In some EHR systems, the nurse can activate an immediate link to the tables of information needed to decide how much insulin to give to the patient.
- Medical errors are minimized by programmed alerts that are automatically displayed when a care provider takes an action that could be harmful (e.g., when a provider prescribes a drug to which a patient is allergic or calls for a dose that exceeds the safe range).
- EHRs help organizations more effectively meet regulatory requirements and accreditation goals.
- Data can be analyzed as they are collected, making immediate nursing decision-making possible.
- EHRs facilitate evidence-based practice by making it possible to analyze thousands of records in ways that cannot be done with paper forms. With this aggregated data, nursing practice can be compared across populations and geographic locations to support nursing decisions and guide professional and organization quality improvement.

Information is private and safe:

- Information is permanently stored and not likely to be lost.
- Confidentiality of client information is enhanced by:
  - Tracking everyone who accesses the chart
  - Proper security clearances
  - Unique passwords
  - Restricted access
  - Using screen protectors that require a person to be directly in front of the screen to read it

DISADVANTAGES

Expense: Electronic documentation systems are expensive.

Downtime: Downtime processes must be in place for times when parts of the EHR are not available (e.g., because of power outages, severe weather, and system upgrades).

Difficulties associated change:

- Learning to use some documentation systems can be challenging and time-consuming.
- Some healthcare providers see no reason to change and resist changing to EHR.
- It is not easy to capture narrative nursing content from paper documentation into an electronic format.
- Some EHRs are not user-friendly (e.g., difficult to quickly find information needed to make care decisions).
- Some systems do not control redundancy well, requiring caregivers to ask the patient for the same information over and over.

Lack of integration: Most EHRs are not integrated across the different departments. This means sometimes a person with a legitimate reason to enter the chart cannot see every part of it he is allowed to see from where he is located. For example, you may not be able to access a patient's lab results from the nurses' desk, but must wait for the lab to send a report.

BOX 16-2 ■ Advantages and Disadvantages of a Paper Health Record

ADVANTAGES

- Care providers are comfortable with it because it is familiar. There is little "learning curve."
- Paper records do not require large databases and secure networks to function.
- There is no downtime for system changes, weather, and so on.
- It is relatively inexpensive to create new forms and update old ones.

DISADVANTAGES

Access may be delayed. Only one care provider can access the record at a time; and the provider must be in the same location as the chart.

Retrieving information may be slow.

- Healthcare providers may need to search through multiple pages to find needed information.
- Specific documentation is difficult to retrieve when needed, especially when files are archived in another part of the building.

Documentation is time-consuming.

- Documentation may take more time because hand-writing is slower than computer entry.
- Documentation is often redundant and repetitive.
- Paper records require manual audit of many charts to create reports and collect client data. This is time- and resource-intensive.

There is a relatively high risk for patient care error.

- Narrative documents are hard to read if the handwriting is illegible or messy. This means nurses have to take time from patient care to contact providers to clarify handwritten prescriptions.
- Papers can be lost from the chart or damaged, leading to duplicate assessments or medication errors.
- There is tremendous inconsistency in how the same client information is documented, even within the same organization. Often, standardized terminology is not used.

Storage of paper records is expensive.

Confidentiality is difficult to protect. There is no way to know who may have access to the paper health record without proper authorization.

What Are Some Common Formats for Nursing Progress Notes?

Nursing documentation can take many forms, including paper documents, computerized electronic documents, audio or video files, e-mails, faxes, scanned paper documents, electronically stored photographs, x-ray findings, and other images. Depending on the documentation model your organization selects, you may use one or more of the following charting formats. Choice of format is also influenced by whether your nursing documentation is written on paper, captured and stored electronically, or in a blend of the two. In all formats, you must learn to use abbreviations appropriately.

Use of Abbreviations

Recall the case of Steven Stellanski ("Meet Your Patient"). Below is a brief admission note using narrative charting format. Underline any words or entries that you do not understand:

4/11/11 Pt received on unit from PACU. VSS. TM temp 99.9°F (37.7°C), P 104, and BP 104.68. LOC unstable. Arouses when name called but quickly drifts off to sleep. PERRLA. Moaning, grimacing, holding abd, whispers "Help me. Help me." LR at 125 mL/hr infusing in R forearm. Urinary catheter in place, draining pale yellow urine. Drsg dry & intact. Morphine sulfate PCA ordered. Will initiate. ———————————— Ray Allenby, RN.

You can see from this entry that nurses use many abbreviations in their paper record charting. Every healthcare institution has a list of approved abbreviations that may and may not be used in documentation. Be sure to consult your organization's list before you chart. For a list of commonly used abbreviations in healthcare and another list of abbreviations that pertain to medication administration,

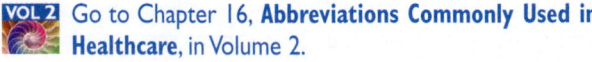

VOL 2 Go to Chapter 16, **Abbreviations Commonly Used in Healthcare**, in Volume 2.

VOL 2 Also go to Chapter 23, **Medication-Related Abbreviations,** in Volume 2.

✚ The Joint Commission (2008c) mandates that healthcare organizations not use the following abbreviations. This is referred to as the "do not use" list.

"U" or "u" for unit
"IU" for International Unit
Q.D., QD, q.d., qd (daily)
Q.O.D., QOD, q.o.d., qod (every other day)
Trailing zero (X.0 mg) and lack of leading zero (.X mg)
MS, MSO4, and MgSO4—could mean morphine sulfate or magnesium sulfate.

The following abbreviations and symbols are under serious consideration for inclusion on The Joint Commission's "do not use" list in the future. Some institutions have already stopped using them:

The symbols ">" and "<" (write "greater than" or "less than")
All abbreviations for drug names (write drug names in full)
Apothecary units (use metric units instead)
The symbol "@" (write "at" or "each")
The abbreviation "cc" (write "mL" or "milliliters")
The abbreviation "μg" (write "mcg" or "micrograms")

✚ The Joint Commission's Patient Safety Goals for 2009 include NPSG.02.–2.01. There is a standardized list of abbreviations, acronyms, symbols, and dose designations that are not to be used throughout the [organization] (Joint Commission, 2008a). This is a very important goal for organizations to meet that ensures patient safety when medications are ordered and administered.

Narrative

Narrative format is used with written source-oriented and problem-oriented charts. The **narrative chart entry** tells the story of the patient's experience in a chronological format. The goal is to track the client's changing health status and progress toward goals. Narrative charting is especially useful when attempting to construct a timeline of events, such as a cardiac arrest or other emergency situations.

In addition to the need to use abbreviations and symbols with caution, some other disadvantages of narrative charting are that it:

- Requires a great deal of time for writing all the details of the client's care—client status, activities, nursing interventions, psychosocial context, and response to treatment may all need to be included.
- Requires you to read the entire note or multiple notes to find client responses and outcomes to interventions.
- Promotes disorganized, repetitive documentation, resulting in a lengthy record with important facts randomly buried in the text. Although subjective and objective data may easily be grouped together, the entry can become difficult to understand if interventions and client responses are also clustered.
- Is inconsistent among healthcare providers. Some believe "if it's not charted, then it's not done." Others document only abnormalities that are relevant to the client's care or change in health status.
- Makes it difficult to track problems from day to day and identify trends.

Problem–Intervention–Evaluation (PIE)

The Problem–Intervention–Evaluation (PIE) system organizes information according to the patient's problems and requires keeping a daily assessment record and progress notes. This eliminates the need for a separate care plan and provides a nursing-focused rather than medical-focused record.

Problem: Use data from your original assessment to identify appropriate nursing diagnoses.
Intervention: Document the nursing actions you take for each nursing diagnosis.
Evaluation: Document the patient's response to interventions and treatments.

Problems are identified from the admission assessment. Subsequent entries begin with identification of the problem number. This type of charting establishes an ongoing care plan. A PIE charting entry for Steven Stellanski might look like this:

4/11/11   1630

P: 1B
I: Pt c̄ 1 mg doses up to 4 mg morphine/hr. Pt groggy yet c/o pain. Has not triggered PCA independently. Rates pain as 8 on scale of 1–10. PCA use reviewed with pt. Demonstrated use c̄ 1st dose at 1615.
E: Pt still moaning & grimacing. Has not initiated another dose via PCA. 2nd dose given as additional demo. Will reevaluate in 1 hr. May need continuous infusion if pt unable to use to control pain. ————————————— Ron Allen, RN

Critics note this style of charting focuses only on the listed problems and not on the client as a whole. However, the primary disadvantage of PIE charting is that it does not document the planning portion of the nursing process. There is no seamless flow of client data, nursing diagnosis, and interventions such as can be seen in a nursing care plan.

SOAP/SOAPIE/SOAPIER

The SOAP format is often used to write nursing and other progress notes. It can be used in source-oriented, problem-oriented, and EHRs. SOAP stands for *Subjective, Objective, Assessment,* and *Plan*. SOAPIE includes these four components plus *Interventions* and *Evaluation*, and SOAPIER adds *Revision* as well. You will refer to those parts when using the SOAP format.

- *Subjective data*—What the patient or family members tell you about the client's signs and symptoms and the reason they are seeking healthcare. Typically this is documented by quoting the actual words said.
- *Objective data*—Factual, measurable clinical findings such as vital signs, test results, and quality of breath sounds. Refer to Chapter 3 to review subjective and objective data.
- *Assessment*—Conclusions drawn from the subjective and objective data, usually patient problems or nursing diagnoses. SOAP terminology is different from the nursing process terminology. In the nursing process chapters we referred to conclusions about data as inferences or problems, and stated that assessment does *not* include conclusions about data. When using SOAP, you *should* document your conclusions about the data under "A."
- *Plan*: Short-term and long-term goals and strategies that will be used to relieve the patient's problems.
- *Interventions*: Actions of the healthcare team that are performed to achieve expected outcomes.
- *Evaluation*: An analysis of the effectiveness of interventions.
- *Revision*: Changes made to the original care plan.

Recall that a POR is organized according to specific patient problems, and has five components: database, problem list, initial plan, progress notes, and a discharge summary. You will refer to and use the following four parts when charting in SOAP format.

Problem List. A numbered list of the patient's current problems in chronological order is compiled so that you can refer to the number when entering your notes.

Initial Plan. This includes expected outcomes and plans for further care interventions and teaching. There is only one initial plan; you update and change the plan in subsequent progress notes.

Progress Notes. This is where you record the SOAP(IER) information. As a rule, you enter a note for each current problem every 24 hours or when the patient's condition changes.

Discharge Summary. At discharge, each problem on the list is covered and a notation made about whether it was resolved. Unresolved problems, with plans for each, are included when communicating with the patient, other facilities, and home health agencies.

Following is an example of SOAP progress notes using the admission data of Steven Stellanski ("Meet Your Patient"). In the previous section, these same data were used to create a narrative note. Notice that the data are similar; however, the narrative note is organized by data source. Steven's SOAPIE® charting entry related to his postoperative nausea and pain could look like this:

4/11/11	0830	#1 – Nausea related to anesthesia
		S – Pt states "I feel sick to my stomach. Help me."
		O – Pt vomited 100 ml clear, light yellow fluid.
		A – Pt is nauseated secondary to anesthesia.
		P – Monitor nausea and give antiemetic as needed.
		I – Pt given Compazine 1 mg IV at 0830.
	0900	E – Pt states he feels less sick to his stomach.—*Ron Allen, RN*
4/11/11	0830	#1B – Acute pain related to abdominal incision 2° appendectomy
		S – States, "help me, help me." Moaning and grimacing.
		O – Moaning and grimacing; holding abd. Drsg dry & intact. BP 104/68, P 104, Resp 24, and TM temp 99.9°F. PERRLA.
		A – Postoperative pain
		P – Give analgesic as needed.
		I – Morphine PCA initiated at 0835. Pt. instructed in use. 1st dose (1 mg) administered as demonstration.
	0900	E – Still moaning & grimacing even after 2nd dose given as additional demo. Still has not initiated additional PCA dose. —*Ron Allen, RN*
	0930	R – Still no pain relief; still has not used PCA independently. Discussed w/ Dr. Jadu. Continuous infusion begun at 2 mg/hr. Will supplement up to 4 mg/hr prn.————— —*Ron Allen, RN*

Disadvantages of SOAP(IE) charting is that it can be inefficient. For example, if the client has overlapping problems, you may find the same interventions and responses repeated in more than one section.

Focus Charting®

The term *focus* is used to encourage you to view the client's status from a positive perspective rather than the negative focus in problem charting. **Focus Charting®** uses assessment data to evaluate client care concerns, problems, or strengths. It also identifies necessary revisions to the care plan as you document each entry.

The focus is often identified as a nursing diagnosis (e.g., Ineffective Breathing Pattern), a sign or symptom (e.g., shortness of breath), a client behavior (e.g., inability to follow inhaler instructions), a special need (e.g., non-English speaking), an acute change in condition (e.g., sudden appearance of chest pain), or a significant event (e.g., surgery). Focus charting® works well in acute care settings and in areas where the same care and procedures are repeated frequently.

The first column contains the time and date. The second column identifies the focus or problem addressed in the note. The third column contains charting in a DAR format. DAR is an acronym for *data, action,* and *response*.

Data. Document subjective and objective information that supports the focus. This aspect reflects the assessment phase of the nursing process and includes other data, such as laboratory results or other diagnostic testing.

Action. Describe interventions performed, such as administering medications or making calls to the physician. This aspect reflects the planning and implementation phases of the nursing process.

Response. Describe the patient's response to your interventions. This aspect reflects the evaluation phase of the nursing process.

Focus Charting® is attractive because it addresses the client's concerns holistically. Critics claim, however, that lack of a common problem list leads to inconsistency in labeling the focus of notes and may cause difficulty in tracking patient progress. The following is an example of a Focus® note.

4/11/11	Focus:	**D:** 16 y.o. rec'd on unit at 1600 from PACU post-appendectomy. Pt w/ Down syndrome. Morphine PCA initiated. Pt unable to use PCA to control pain. Continuous infusion at 2 mg/hr begun at 1745. PERRLA. Alert, drifting in & out of sleep. PACU RNM reports pt functions at school-age level.
1800	Developmental delay	
		A: Will discuss pt status w/ parents and adjust plan of care accordingly.
		———— *Ron Allen, RN*
1830		**R:** Met w/ parents, who report that pt has significant developmental delays & needs supervision w/ all ADLs. Pt comfortable on 2 mg/hr infusion of morphine. Use of PCA for supplementary pain control reviewed with parents. Parents demonstrated understanding and that they will assist pt w/ PCA if add'l meds are needed
		———— *Ron Allen, RN*

FACT

Noted for its individual elements, the FACT documentation model incorporates many CBE principles and includes four key elements:

Flowsheets individualized to specific services
Assessment features standardized with baseline parameters
Concise, integrated progress notes and flowsheets documenting the client's condition and responses
Timely entries documented when care is given

FACT documentation includes only exceptions to the norm or significant information about the patient. It eliminates the need to chart normal findings. The disadvantages of the FACT system are the same as for CBE. The following is a FACT example for Steven.

DATE/TIME	04/12/11 0900	04/12/11 1330
Neurological Alert and oriented to time, place, and person. PERRLA. Symmetry of strength in extremities. No difficulty with coordination. Behavior appropriate to situation. Sensation intact without numbness or paresthesias.	✓	✓
Orient patient		
Refer to neurological flowsheet		
Pain No report of pain. If present, include pain scale intensity choice by patient (0–10) with location, description, duration, radiation, precipitating and alleviating factors.	Abdominal incision pain – score 10	✓
Location	RLQ	
Description	Dull, constant	
Relief measures	Percocet 1 tablet by mouth	
Pain relief: Y = yes / N = no	Y	
Cardiovascular Apical pulse 60 to 100. S_1 and S_2 present. Regular rhythm. Peripheral pulses (radial, pedal) present bilaterally. No edema or calf tenderness. Extremities pink, warm, moveable within patient's ROM.	✓	✓
IV Solution and Rate	D5½ NS at 125 mL/hr	D5½ NS at 125 mL/hr

Electronic Entry

Healthcare is undergoing a technological revolution. Electronic clinical information systems are being used more and more frequently. Streamlining documentation processes makes them more accurate and efficient, and reduces the risk of human error. This frees you to do the expert work that only nurses can do.

The use of electronic documentation requires a shift in how you document your work. The move to EHRs forces change in documentation formats (paper vs. electronic), change in where documentation is done (e.g., at the bedside using a portable wireless device vs. at the nursing station), and change in decision-making processes (immediate vs. gradual).

Electronic documentation forms and flowsheets (such as Fig. 16-2) already include the information that your organization has decided is important to document. Reminders to document specific kinds of information, such as overdue medications and overdue nursing interventions, display automatically to help prevent late or omitted care. Also, the extensive use of clearly named data entry fields, drop-down menus, check boxes, and specially created templates allows you to enter your nursing documentation quickly and efficiently, usually with minimal keyboard typing.

Depending on the EHR system used, progress notes may be documented electronically in prebuilt note formats, in various prebuilt charting forms. In addition, some information traditionally included in written progress notes may be entered as unique comments added to specific data elements as they are entered and electronically signed. In some electronic systems, you may still need to write progress notes on lined paper. Narrative, SOAP, PIE, POC, Focus®, or FACT formats may be used in the progress notes.

Transitioning from paper to electronic documentation can be challenging for some people. It usually takes a few days to know where to document your nursing care and feel confident that you haven't overlooked anything. In addition, the fear of technology still exists for a few nurses who do not use computers in their everyday life. However, EHR software is becoming more logical and user-friendly. Many organizations have printed information, classes, webinars, or electronic learning, such as Web-based tutorials that provide additional information about electronic charting. Take advantage of opportunities to build your knowledge when they arise.

Which Nursing Documentation Format Is Best?

Most charting formats that adequately describe the patient's condition, care given, and response to care are satisfactory and will withstand scrutiny in a court of law. No single paper charting format stands out as better than another. However, recent studies indicate that electronic charting is superior because it typically reduces documentation time; minimizes repetition and redundancy; integrates many parts of the health record

into a single record; and makes the record accessible to multiple care providers at the same time.

Familiarize yourself with the type of documentation you will use in the healthcare area you are assigned. Review notes written or entered electronically by other nurses to become acquainted with different styles, approaches, and approved charting processes. Consult your clinical instructor or other nurses in the area if you have specific questions about charting formats.

KnowledgeCheck 16-2

Summarize the characteristics, advantages, and disadvantages of each of the different kinds of nursing documentation formats (narrative, PIE, SOAP, Focus® CBE, FACT, and electronic entry).

 Go to Chapter 16, **Knowledge Check Response Sheet and Answers** on the Student Resource Disk or DavisPlus at http://davisplus.fadavis.com/Wilkinson2

CriticalThinking 16-1

Compare the documentation examples (narrative, PIE, SOAP, Focus®, CBE and FACT, and electronic documentation). If you have had experience with charting in the clinical setting, apply this experience as well. With which charting format do you feel most comfortable? Why?

What Forms Do Nurses Use to Document Nursing Care?

Documentation forms vary by purpose, institution, and unit. However, regardless of the system or forms used, nursing documentation reflects the nursing process. You record assessments, diagnoses, planning, implementation (what you actually did), and evaluation of client responses. In addition to the nursing progress notes discussed in the preceding text, you will use many other forms. This section discusses the most commonly used paper and electronic documentation forms.

Nursing Admission Data Forms

A separate nursing admission form or a combined interdisciplinary form is completed at the time the patient enters the healthcare system. Creating a baseline assessment is vital for several reasons: (1) It may be used as a benchmark to monitor change; (2) it provides information about the client's support system and helps forecast future needs; (3) it contains critical information: presenting illness or reason for admission, vital signs, allergy information, current medications, activities of daily living (ADL) status, physical assessment data, and discharge planning information. For examples of a paper admission form,

 Go to Chapter 3, **Nursing Admission Data Form,** and

 Go to Chapter 16, **Tables, Boxes, Figures: ESG Figure 16-1 (Adult Inpatient Admission Assessment),** on the Student Resource Disk or DavisPlus at http://davisplus.fadavis.com/Wilkinson2

To see part of an electronic nursing admission data form,

 Go to Chapter 16, **Charting Forms, Adult Admission History Screen,** in Volume 2.

You will use admission forms in all settings, for example, in ambulatory clinics and long-term care facilities. An ambulatory care admission form includes demographic data, allergy information, current medications, family health data, social history, and the client's past medical history. The form completed by Joe Garcia (in Volume 2) at his first clinic visit is an example of an ambulatory care admission form. To see Mr. Garcia's completed form,

 Go to **Meet the Garcias** at the beginning of Volume 2.

Admission forms for long-term care are similar to hospital admission forms. Clients may receive care in long-term care facilities for rehabilitation purposes after a hospital stay or may have extended stays for ongoing care. Whenever possible, this plan is identified on admission.

Discharge data are obtained with the admission assessment, but are often recorded on a separate form. Discharge needs should be evaluated when the patient first enters a healthcare facility, especially in acute-care facilities. Ask yourself what this patient would need if he were to go home in the next few days. For example, would he need help with food preparation? Does he understand how to use his medicines?

Discharge Summary

A **discharge summary** is the last entry made in the paper chart. In the electronic chart, the discharge summary can be begun any time after admission and revised throughout the hospitalization. A summary is completed when the patient is transferred within the same organization, transferred to another facility, or discharged to home. The discharge summary may be a multidisciplinary document or each discipline may write a separate summary. The forms are different in each organization, but they contain similar data. For examples of electronic and paper discharge summaries, respectively, see Figure 16-4 and

 Go to Chapter 10, **Forms, Discharge Assessment/ Instructions,** in Volume 2. Also refer to **Procedure 10-4, Discharging a Patient from the Healthcare Facility,** in Volume 2.

As you can see in Figure 16-4, there is a drop-down menu in which the Nursing Discharge Note is located. It is important to clearly document the patient's condition on discharge. Many patients require follow-up care. The discharge summary serves as baseline data for the healthcare professionals who will follow up on the patient after discharge.

Flowsheets and Graphic Records

You will use flowsheets and graphic records to document assessments and care that are performed frequently, on a recurring schedule, or as a part of unit

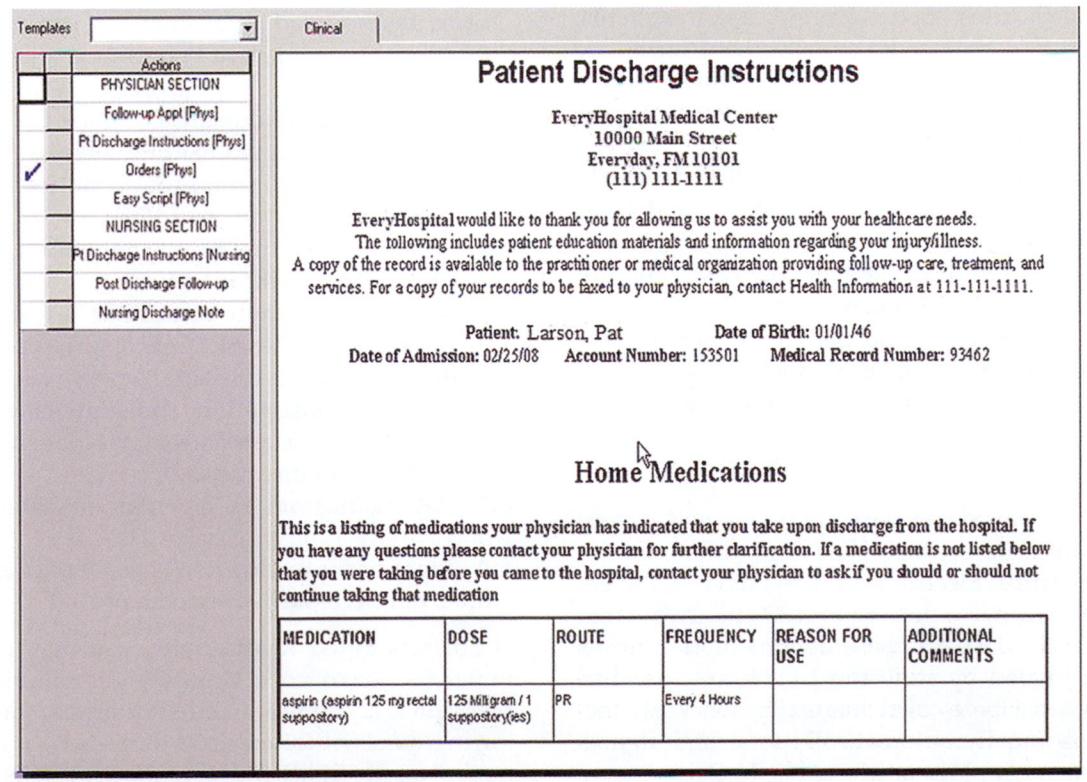

FIGURE 16-4 A portion of an electronic Discharge Planning Form. (Courtesy of Cerner Corporation, Kansas City, MO.)

routines. For example, most hospital units require that vital signs be taken every 8 hours for all patients. How often you perform and document care activities depends on your patient's condition and the unit policy. In the first hour after surgery, for example, you would probably record vital signs every 15 minutes; and after that, every hour for 4 hours.

The simplest paper forms are organized with time on one axis and the activities or patient assessment parameters in columns on the other axis. On electronic forms, the areas (fields) to enter the time and activities are arranged close together. Flowsheets and graphic records allow you to see patterns of change in patient status. For instance, you may view a steady increase in the line representing a patient's blood pressure compared to his pain score on an electronically generated graph. On a paper form, you may scan across a row to see that your patient has not had a bowel movement for several days. Other types of information recorded on flowsheets include intake and output (I&O), weight, hygiene measures, ADLs, and medications administered. For examples of a paper graphic record and an electronic flowsheet, see Figure 3-4 (paper) and Figure 16-2 (electronic).

Checklists

Assessments and care may also be recorded on paper and electronic checklists. Common normal and abnormal findings are commonly organized according to body systems. Figure 16-5 is an example of a paper checklist.

Using a paper form, the nurse checks the box that reflects the current assessment findings. Some checklists include nursing actions, such as wound care, treatments, or IV fluid administration. Essentially these forms are comprehensive charting documents. Exceptions, patient care activities, and patient responses are recorded in the narrative note section of the paper form.

Using an electronic field-based checklist, the nurse enters values or text in the appropriate fields and saves the documentation. Electronic flowsheets typically contain content similar to that on paper checklists, but also include a greater range of potential documentation areas that can be opened as needed. This allows for a more comprehensive record of a patient's assessment, treatments, IV fluid administration, and many other parameters.

Intake and Output Records

You will sometimes use separate intake and output (I&O) paper records to document data about the patient's fluid balance. Electronic systems have flowsheet sections or I&O forms to document I&O and save it into the patient's EHR. Usually these documentation forms contain data totaled by shift and by 24-hour periods. Paper forms must be totaled manually, whereas electronic systems usually automatically total I&O figures for you. For an example of an electronic I&O screen, see Figure 16-2. For a paper I&O record,

VOL 2   Go to Chapter 16, **Charting Forms, Intake and Output Sheet,** in Volume 2.

I&O records are particularly important for clients who have kidney disease, congestive heart failure, or pulmonary edema, or who have undergone major surgery. I&O paper graphics may be kept at the bedside. Patients and families are increasingly active in their own care. If your patient is able to assist with measuring his I&O, teach him how to record data on the paper form. You might also complete electronic I&O documentation at the bedside using a portable wireless computer on wheels or a laptop computer. When appropriate, patients can still track their own intake and output on paper, but you will need to enter the patient's I&O data into the EHR. Chapter 27 provides detailed information about monitoring intake and output.

Medication Administration Records

Medication administration records (MARs) contain information about the medications that have been prescribed for the client. The information and format vary by setting, with significant differences between outpatient and inpatient facilities. Figure 16-6 is a portion of an electronic medication record. Figure 23-7 is a paper MAR.

On the MAR, you will document medications according to the times they are given: scheduled, unscheduled, continuous, prn, stat, and so on.

- **Scheduled medications** are medications that are to be given on a regularly scheduled basis.
- **Unscheduled medications** are medications that are to be given on call at the appropriate time. An example of an unscheduled medication is a preoperative medication to be given right before the patient goes to the operating room.
- **Continuous infusions** are IV fluids that are running consistently unless stopped for a blood transfusion or to give an IV medication that is not compatible with the IV fluid running.
- **prn** is an abbreviation for the Latin term *pro re nata*, or *as needed*. prn medications are given only when the patient meets certain conditions set when the prn medication is ordered. Typical prn medications include those used for pain, fever, mild discomfort, nausea, and constipation. You administer a prn medication when you assess that the patient needs it or when the patient requests it.
- A **stat** medication is given immediately and only once.
- A **single-order** medication is given once at a specified time, not necessarily immediately.

For scheduled medications, you may only have to initial and make a check mark in the column with times preprinted at the top. In circumstances, such as the following, you will often need to record additional information on the MAR and sometimes even in the Progress Notes.

DATE / /

PHYSICAL ASSESSMENT - SHIFT _____

NEURO

LOC	ORIENTATION	SPEECH
❑ ALERT	❑ X3 ❑ FOR AGE	❑ APPROPRIATE
❑ SEDATED	❑ PERSON	❑ APHASIA
❑ LETHARGIC	❑ PLACE	❑ SLURRED
❑ UNRESPONSIVE	❑ TIME	❑ RAMBLING

SENSATION	FONTANELS	
❑ INTACT	❑ FLAT	❑ NA
❑ NUMBNESS	❑ SUNKEN	
❑ TINGLING	❑ BULGING	

CARDIOVASCULAR

RHYTHM	PULSE	EDEMA	CAP. REFILL
❑ REGULAR	❑ STRONG	❑ ABSENT	❑ < 3 SEC.
❑ IRREGULAR	❑ WEAK	❑ _____	❑ > 3 SEC.
❑ MURMUR	❑		

MONITOR RHYTHM

RESPIRATORY

EFFORT   BREATH
                  LU LL SOUNDS RU RL

❑ NORMAL	❑ DYSPNEA	❑❑ CLEAR ❑❑
❑ LABORED	❑ COUGH	❑❑ CRACKLES ❑❑
❑ NASAL FLARING	❑ SPUTUM	❑❑ RHONCHI ❑❑
❑ RETRACTIONS	❑ CRYING	❑❑ WHEEZING ❑❑
❑ IRREGULAR		❑❑ DIMINISHED ❑❑
		❑❑ ABSENT ❑❑

GASTROINTESTINAL

ABDOMEN

❑ FLAT	❑ FIRM	❑ NAUSEA
❑ ROUNDED	❑ TENDER	❑ VOMITING
❑ DISTENDED	❑ NON-TENDER	
❑ SOFT		
❑ GIRTH_____	CM	

BOWEL SOUNDS	STOOL	
❑ ACTIVE	❑ REGULAR	LAST BM
❑ ABSENT	❑ CONSTIPATED	
❑ HYPER	❑ DIARRHEA	_____
❑ HYPO	❑ INCONTINENT	

SUCTION
❑ INTERMITTANT ❑ CONSTANT ❑ CLAMPED
❑ FEEDING TUBE ❑ PATENT
❑ NG ❑ PLACEMENT ✔
DRNG COLOR:

GU

URINE	❑ CATHETER
❑ CLEAR, YELLOW / AMBER ❑ QS	❑ PAIN
❑ OTHER _____ ❑ FREQUENT	
❑ RETENTION	❑ INCONTINENT

MUSCULOSKELETAL

MOBILITY	MUSCLE TONE	ROM
❑ NORMAL	❑ GOOD	❑ FULL
❑ ASSIST X _____	❑ OTHER	❑ LIMITED
❑ AMBULATORY		
❑ BED REST		
❑ OTHER	❑ P.T. CONSULT	

SKIN

CONDITION	TURGOR	MUCOUS MEM
❑ WARM, DRY INTACT	❑ ADEQUATE	❑ MOIST
❑ BREAKDOWN	❑ DECREASED	❑ DRY

COLOR ❑ NORMAL
❑ PALE ❑ CYANOTIC ❑ FLUSHED ❑ _____

WOUND/INCISION/DRESSING

LOCATION/CONDITION/DRAINAGE	HEALING NO S/S INFECTION
_____	❑
_____	❑
_____	❑

TUBES/DRAINS

LOCATION/CONDITION/DRAINAGE	GRAVITY	SUCTION
_____	❑	❑
_____	❑	❑
_____	❑	❑

IV'S

IV SITE / CONDITION	PATENT, NO REDNESS OR SWELLING	PUMP
_____	❑	❑
_____	❑	❑
_____	❑	❑

PAIN

❑ ABSENT PAIN SCALE _____
❑ PRESENT LOCATION _____
❑ CONTROLLED

PSYCHOSOCIAL

EYE CONTACT ❑ YES ❑ NO

❑ APPROPRIATE	❑ RESTLESS	❑ COMBATIVE
❑ FLAT AFFECT	❑ AGITATED	❑ BELLIGERENT
❑ UNCOOPERATIVE	❑ CRYING	❑ ODOR
❑ ANXIOUS	❑ SUBSTANCE USE	

DISCHARGE

DISCHARGE PLAN
❑ NA ❑ ONGOING ❑ COMPLETED
❑ D.P. CONSULT ❑ O.T CONSULT ❑ H.H. CONSULT

EQUIPMENT

❑ BED ALARM	❑ CARDIAC MONITOR
❑ CPM	❑ FEEDING PUMP
❑ IV PUMP X_____	❑ K - PAD
❑ OXIMETER	❑ PCA PUMP
❑ PASSPORT	❑ POLAR ICE
❑ SUCTION	❑ TELEMETRY
❑ _____	❑ _____
❑ _____	❑ _____

SIGN

SIGNATURE X_____ TIME_____
REASSESSED BY X_____ TIME_____

OBSERVATION / INTERVENTION / EVALUATION
(TIME & INITIAL ENTRIES)

PHYSICAL ASSESSMENT - SHIFT _____

NEURO

LOC	ORIENTATION	SPEECH
❑ ALERT	❑ X3 ❑ FOR AGE	❑ APPROPRIATE
❑ SEDATED	❑ PERSON	❑ APHASIA
❑ LETHARGIC	❑ PLACE	❑ SLURRED
❑ UNRESPONSIVE	❑ TIME	❑ RAMBLING

SENSATION	FONTANELS	
❑ INTACT	❑ FLAT	❑ NA
❑ NUMBNESS	❑ SUNKEN	
❑ TINGLING	❑ BULGING	

CARDIOVASCULAR

RHYTHM	PULSE	EDEMA	CAP. REFILL
❑ REGULAR	❑ STRONG	❑ ABSENT	❑ < 3 SEC.
❑ IRREGULAR	❑ WEAK	❑ _____	❑ > 3 SEC.
❑ MURMUR	❑		

MONITOR RHYTHM

RESPIRATORY

EFFORT   BREATH
                  LU LL SOUNDS RU RL

❑ NORMAL	❑ DYSPNEA	❑❑ CLEAR ❑❑
❑ LABORED	❑ COUGH	❑❑ CRACKLES ❑❑
❑ NASAL FLARING	❑ SPUTUM	❑❑ RHONCHI ❑❑
❑ RETRACTIONS	❑ CRYING	❑❑ WHEEZING ❑❑
❑ IRREGULAR		❑❑ DIMINISHED ❑❑
		❑❑ ABSENT ❑❑

GASTROINTESTINAL

ABDOMEN

❑ FLAT	❑ FIRM	❑ NAUSEA
❑ ROUNDED	❑ TENDER	❑ VOMITING
❑ DISTENDED	❑ NON-TENDER	
❑ SOFT		
❑ GIRTH_____	CM	

BOWEL SOUNDS	STOOL	
❑ ACTIVE	❑ REGULAR	LAST BM
❑ ABSENT	❑ CONSTIPATED	
❑ HYPER	❑ DIARRHEA	_____
❑ HYPO	❑ INCONTINENT	

SUCTION
❑ INTERMITTANT ❑ CONSTANT ❑ CLAMPED
❑ FEEDING TUBE ❑ PATENT
❑ NG ❑ PLACEMENT
DRNG COLOR:

GU

URINE	❑ CATHETER
❑ CLEAR, YELLOW / AMBER ❑ QS	❑ PAIN
❑ OTHER _____ ❑ FREQUENT	
❑ RETENTION	❑ INCONTINENT

MUSCULOSKELETAL

MOBILITY	MUSCLE TONE	ROM
❑ NORMAL	❑ GOOD	❑ FULL
❑ ASSIST X _____	❑ OTHER	❑ LIMITED
❑ AMBULATORY		
❑ BED REST		
❑ OTHER	❑ P.T. CONSULT	

SKIN

CONDITION	TURGOR	MUCOUS MEM
❑ WARM, DRY INTACT	❑ ADEQUATE	❑ MOIST
❑ BREAKDOWN	❑ DECREASED	❑ DRY

COLOR ❑ NORMAL
❑ PALE ❑ CYANOTIC ❑ FLUSHED ❑ _____

WOUND/INCISION/DRESSING

LOCATION/CONDITION/DRAINAGE	HEALING NO S/S INFECTION
_____	❑
_____	❑
_____	❑

TUBES/DRAINS

LOCATION/CONDITION/DRAINAGE	GRAVITY	SUCTION
_____	❑	❑
_____	❑	❑
_____	❑	❑

IV'S

IV SITE / CONDITION	PATENT, NO REDNESS OR SWELLING	PUMP
_____	❑	❑
_____	❑	❑
_____	❑	❑

NURSING ASSESSMENT PATIENT NAME

FIGURE 16-5 A portion of a nursing assessment checklist.

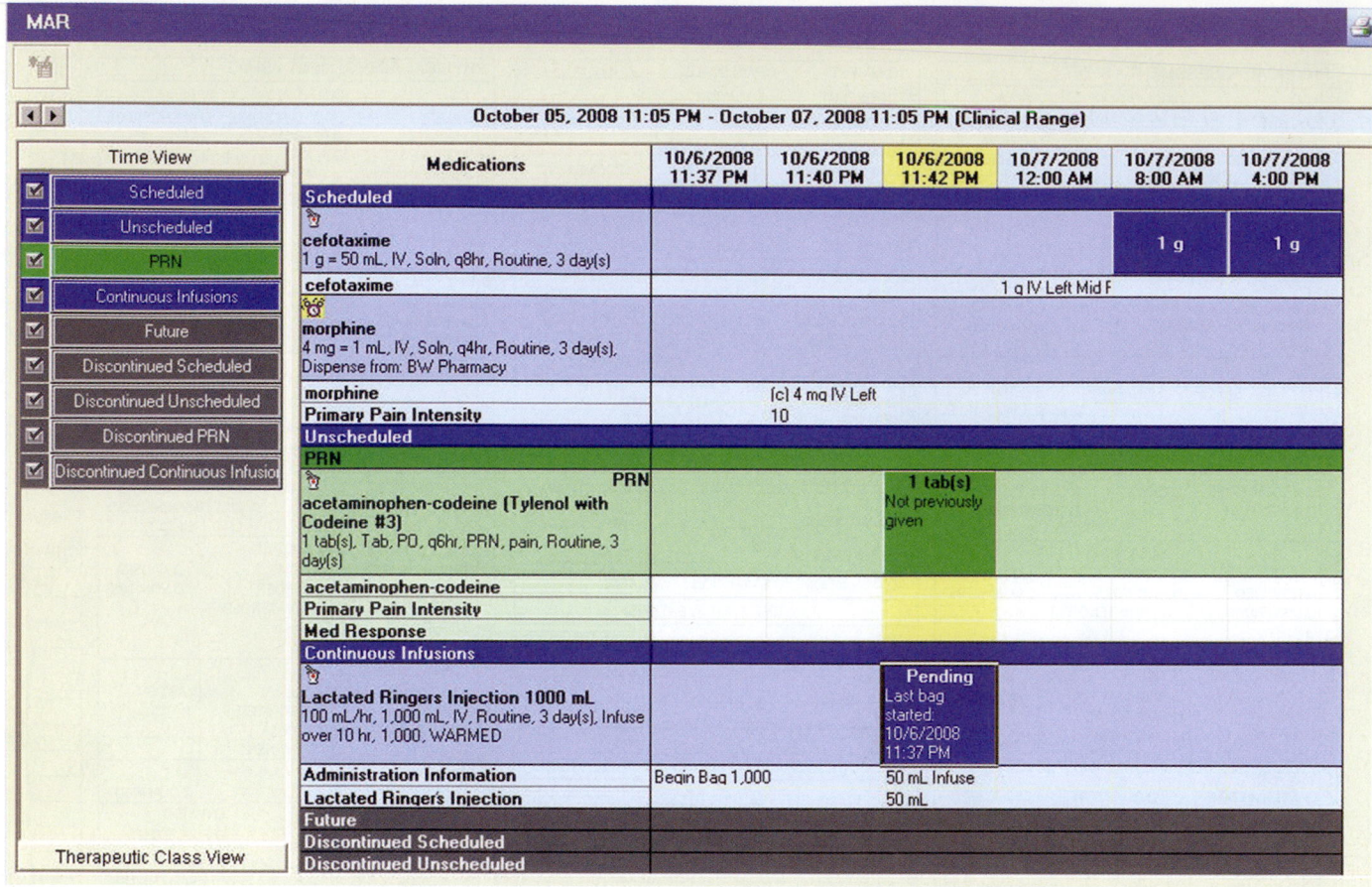

FIGURE 16-6 A portion of an electronic Medication Administration Record. (Courtesy of Cerner Corporation, Kansas City, MO.)

Injections. If you administer an injection, you must chart the site of administration. This documentation protects the patient from repeated injections in the same location.

Assessment Required Before Administration. Some medications require you to make a specific assessment before administering the drug, to ensure that it is safe to give it. For example, according to most protocols, you should not give digoxin (a cardiac medication) if the heart rate is below 60 beats/min. You should hold it and notify the prescriber. Blood pressure and pain medications, insulin, and anticoagulants also require assessments before administration. You will need to document the assessment data directly on the paper MAR or directly into the electronic MAR, along with the time of administration and other required information (see Chapter 23).

Drug Allergies. Drug allergies are always noted on the MAR, whether paper or electronic. This makes them easily visible for caregivers who are ordering and administering medication. If the patient has an allergic reaction to a medicine, be sure to document this response on the medication sheet or electronic form; and make note of this change in the nurses' notes or in the appropriate electronic form. Of course you would notify the prescriber; however, that is reporting, not recording. Reporting is discussed later in this chapter.

prn, Stat, Unscheduled, and Single-Order Medications. Chart on the MAR the time the medication is given. On a paper MAR, make a narrative note that documents your assessment findings and the patient's response to the medication. On an electronic MAR, enter the time of administration and the patient's response to the medication. If necessary, you can also add an electronic comment that briefly describes your assessment findings. Some documented data, such as the pain score before administration of an analgesic, may automatically migrate from other documentation sources to become visible on the MAR.

You may occasionally see a prn order that provides a range of medication to be given based on your assessment of the patient, for example, "Titrate morphine 2 mg IV every 1–2 hours to achieve pain control." In the electronic MAR system, medication range orders (e.g., 1 to 2 mg) are difficult to order, so The Joint Commission and most agency protocols no longer allow dosage range orders.

Patient Refusal. If the patient refuses a medication, note the refusal on the paper or electronic MAR. Your organization's policy will determine how this is recorded. On paper, often you draw a circle around the scheduled time of administration. When documenting electronically, you can click on an option offered in the MAR, such as Not Given, and then select *Patient Refused* from a drop-down field listing multiple reasons why a medication is not given.

Omitted Medication or Delayed Administration. If the patient is not available or is experiencing health changes that require immediate interventions, it may be necessary to withhold a medication or delay its administration. On the paper MAR, some organizations provide a boxed section at the bottom of the MAR with a code to indicate why the medication was withheld or given at a different time. Circle the scheduled time and fill in the symbol. You will also have to document the omission or delay in your nurses' notes. However, in the electronic MAR, often it is possible to reschedule administration times for a single dose or permanently going forward, or to document that a medication could not be given at the scheduled time and will be skipped.

Some electronic medication administration records also allow the care providers to look up detailed information about the medication, including indications, contraindications, expected or adverse effects, and standard dosages for the prescribed drug type (e.g., oral, IV, IM).

MARs for Inpatient Facilities

If you work in an inpatient facility, you will be responsible for administering the patient's medications unless a medication requires special certifications to administer (anesthesia or chemotherapy, for example). An inpatient medication record not only contains a list of medications ordered, but also tracks medication administration and usage for the agency. For a comparison of the content of inpatient and outpatient MARs, see Table 16-1.

MARs for Outpatient Facilities

Outpatient facilities include clinics, primary care offices, and treatment facilities. Because patients do not stay at the facility, usually the medication record primarily contains information about how the patient is to use the medications ordered. Patients retain responsibility for administering their own medications either independently or with the help of family or caregivers.

Kardex or Patient Care Summary

As discussed in Chapter 5, the Kardex® is a special paper form or folding card that briefly summarizes a patient's status and plan of care. Paper Kardex® and electronic patient care summaries typically pull patient data from multiple areas of the health record (medical and nursing diagnoses, orders, treatments, results). Figure 16-7 is an example of an electronic patient care summary screen. To see a paper Kardex®,

 Go to Chapter 5, **Tables, Boxes, Figures: ESG Figure 5-1** on the Student Resource Disk or DavisPlus at http://davisplus. fadavis.com/Wilkinson2

Paper Kardexes are usually kept together in a portable file in a central location in the nurses' station to allow all team members access to patients' summary information. Each patient has a separate electronic summary screen. All authorized members of the care team can access the electronic care summary at the same time, whether they are away from the patient or even outside the organization in a remote location, depending on the institution's permission for access. The paper Kardex and the electronic care summary are not a permanent part of the patient's health record.

Integrated Plan of Care

Integrated plans of care (IPOCs) are a combined charting and care plan form. They are customized to best fit common patient situations in a unit. IPOCs exist in both paper and electronic formats. An IPOC maps out, day by day, the patient goals, outcomes, interventions, and treatments for a specific diagnosis or condition from admission to discharge. Lab work, diagnostic testing, medications, and therapies are all included in the pathway as well as standardized interventions captured in the plan. Administrators applaud IPOCs because they help predict length of stay, monitor costs of care, and can assist with staffing. They also offer other advantages. They eliminate duplicate charting, increase team effort, and enhance the nurse's teaching about what the patient can expect during the hospital stay. Figure 16-3 is an example of an electronic IPOC. For examples of complete printed IPOCs,

Table 16-1 ➤ Comparison of Content of MARs for Inpatient and Outpatient Facilities	
INPATIENT MARS	**OUTPATIENT MARS**
■ Drug name ■ Dosage ■ Route of administration ■ Frequency ■ Duration ■ Scheduled times of administration ■ Charting of medication administration ■ Signatures (written or electronic) of nurses administering medication	■ Drug name ■ Dosage ■ Route of administration ■ Number of pills, patches, and so on, to be dispensed at each prescription refill ■ Number of refills ordered ■ Directions for using the medication, including frequency and duration ■ Historical information about prescriptions, pharmacies used, and refills authorized

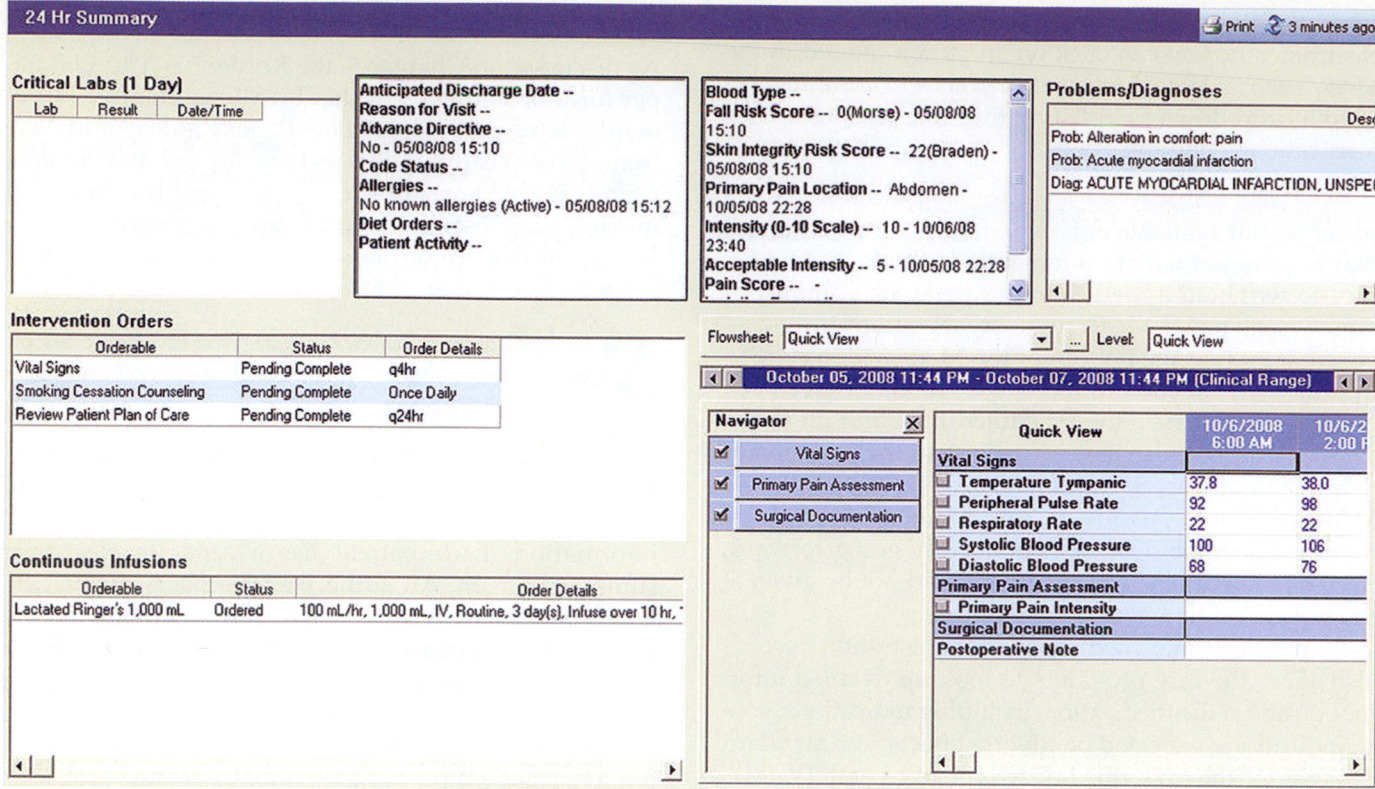

FIGURE 16-7 A portion of an electronic patient care summary screen. (Courtesy of Cerner Corporation, Kansas City, MO.)

 Go to Chapter 5, **Tables, Boxes, Figures: ESG Figure 5-2, Integrated Plan of Care,** or Chapter 16, **Tables, Boxes, Figures: ESG Figure 16-2, Integrated Plan of Care,** on the Student Resource Disk or DavisPlus at http://davisplus.fadavis.com/Wilkinson2

Multiple patient diagnoses can be captured easily in an electronic IPOC. However, in special situations, you may need to adapt the paper IPOC by commenting on special issues in the space provided for narrative comments. Special considerations that may require adaptation of an IPOC include developmental delay (as with our patient, Steven Stellanski), more than one medical diagnosis, mental health concerns, and social issues, such as homelessness. If you find that you are adapting the IPOC frequently for a patient who does not "fit," this may signal a need for the organization to develop a new paper IPOC.

Occurrence Reports

An **occurrence report**, or *incident report*, is a formal record of an unusual occurrence or accident. This is an organizational report and is not part of the client's health record. In Box 16-3 you will see examples of events requiring an occurrence report. Paper occurrence forms and electronic occurrence forms completed online on the organization's secure internal network are both used to track problems and identify areas for quality improvement and to create safer processes and procedures for clients and staff.

BOX 16-3 ■ Events Requiring an Occurrence Report

- Patient fall or other injury
- Medication error
- Incorrect implementation of a prescribed treatment
- Needlestick injury or other injury to staff
- Loss of patient belongings
- Injury of a visitor
- Unsafe staffing situation
- Lack of availability of essential patient care supplies
- Inadequate response to emergency situation

You should report all errors, even if there was no adverse impact on the client. This is important from a safety standpoint and for improving your institution's quality of care. When completing an occurrence form, be sure to clearly identify the client, date, time, and location. Briefly describe the incident in objective terms. Quote the client or persons involved if possible. Avoid drawing conclusions or placing blame. Identify any witnesses to the event and any equipment involved.

Although you would document in the paper nurses' notes or in the client's EHR that a fall, medication error, or similar incident occurred, you usually do not mention the occurrence report itself (e.g., do not chart: "occurrence report completed"). However, you must follow agency policy for documenting reportable incidents. Remember, the nurses' notes or EHR reflect the client's response to the plan of care. Chapter 45 provides additional information on occurrence reports.

The Transition to Electronic Health Records

Although nursing documentation has evolved over time to meet healthcare's changing needs, there was little change in the ways nurses recorded data until the late 20th century, when computers and digital electronic forms began to be widely used in healthcare organizations. Healthcare organizations have been slow to adopt EHR because of the high cost to buy, customize, and maintain systems, and the cost and time involved in training personnel to use a new electronic system.

In 2007, only 11% of community hospitals had fully implemented EHRs, more than half of hospitals reported "partial" implementation, and about one-third indicated no initiation of EHRs (*AMNews*, 2007). In 2006, nearly a third of office-based physicians reported using full or partial EHR systems (Hing, Burt, & Woodwell, 2006). Nevertheless, the shift to EHR is expected to continue as the population continues to become increasingly computer literate. The move to EHRs may occur even faster if the federal government lends its support. At the time this book was written, there was a proposal to make all health records standardized and electronic, and it was anticipated that federal funds would help support this massive task.

How do the numbers in the preceding paragraph compare to the use of EHRs at the time you are reading this book? Has the shift continued as expected? For more discussion of the shift to EHRs,

 Go to Chapter 16, **Supplemental Materials,** on the Student Resource Disk or DavisPlus at http://davisplus.fadavis.com/ Wilkinson2

As a nurse, you will almost certainly need to have computer skills (Fig. 16-8). You will play a crucial role in the development and evaluation of effective EHR systems that make sense to nurses. You may even participate directly in the design–implementation–redesign cycle of the EHR system in your organization.

Whether you document in the client's room, in the hallway or at nurses' station, or on a mobile or handheld device, EHRs promote efficient use of nurses' time, improve interdisciplinary collaboration, streamline processes, make procedures more accurate and efficient, and ensure improved patient safety and care outcomes.

KnowledgeCheck 16-3

- Identify at least five types of paper documentation forms.
- What should you document after administering a prn medication?
- What are some reasons for the slow adoption of electronic documentation and EMRs in the United States?
- What is the purpose of an occurrence report?
- Identify the following abbreviations (see Volume 2):

abd	OOB
BRP	pc
DM	prn
fx	STD
NKDA	tid
q	LUQ

 Go to Chapter 16, **Knowledge Check Response Sheet and Answers,** on the Student Resource Disk or DavisPlus at http://davisplus.fadavis.com/Wilkinson2

What Is Unique About Documentation in Home Healthcare?

Although you will perform many of the same assessments and interventions in home care that you do in other areas of healthcare, the documentation is unique. Healthcare Financing Administration (HCFA) guidelines govern home healthcare documentation. Among the requirements for care are (1) certification of home-bound status, (2) a plan of care, and (3) ongoing assessment of the need for skilled care.

The most commonly used paper home health documentation form is known as OASIS—the Outcome and Assessment Information Set. Due to a federal government mandate that Medicare providers convert to electronic e-prescribing by 2011, home health is now moving toward electronic documentation as well. Many home

FIGURE 16-8 Many healthcare institutions are adopting computerized patient records.

health nurses use laptop computers to retrieve patient data and record progress notes in the home. The computer also allows the nurse to conveniently order supplies needed for home care and to coordinate scheduling of follow-up visits.

In home care, a monthly summary describing the patient's status and ongoing needs is required. The patient's primary care provider signs this form, which is submitted for reimbursement. Chapter 44 provides further information about home care.

Whether your home health documentation is done on paper or electronically, the following will be included:

- Your assessment highlighting changes in the client's condition
- Interventions performed (wound care, dressing changes, teaching, and so on)
- The client's response to interventions
- Any interaction or teaching that you conducted with caregivers
- Any interaction with the patient's primary care provider

If you would like to see an OASIS form,

 Go to Chapter 16, **Tables, Boxes, Figures: ESG Figure 16-3, Outcome and Assessment Information Set (OASIS),** on the Student Resource Disk or DavisPlus at http://davisplus.fadavis.com/Wilkinson2

 Critical**Thinking** 16-2

Why do you think it is essential to document homebound status and the ongoing need for skilled care?

What Is Unique About Documentation in Long-Term Care?

Documentation requirements for long-term care depend on the level of care the client requires. All clients in long-term care facilities must have a comprehensive assessment at admission. Federal law requires that a resident be evaluated using the Minimum Data Set for Resident Assessment and Care Screening (MDS) within 14 days of admission. The MDS must be updated every 3 months and with any significant change in client condition. For an example of an MDS form,

 Go to Chapter 16, **Tables, Boxes, Figures: ESG Figure 16-4, Minimum Data Set** on the Student Resource Disk or DavisPlus at http://davisplus.fadavis.com/Wilkinson2

Legal requirements to protect older adults mandate that you report changes in a client's condition to the primary care provider as well as the client's family. Document your reports in narrative notes on paper or in the appropriate areas of electronic forms. If you are caring for a client receiving Medicare-reimbursed services, such as IV therapy, wound care, or rehabilitation services, documentation is required with each shift. In addition, a summary written by a nurse must be recorded weekly.

The weekly summary for adult clients must include the following:

- A summary of the client's condition
- An evaluation of the client's ability to perform ADLs
- The client's level of consciousness and mood
- Hydration and nutrition status
- Response to medications
- Any treatments provided
- Safety measures (e.g., bed rails, bed alarm, wander guard)

Long-term care facilities also provide intermediate-care services for clients who need assistance with medications, nutrition, and ADLs. These clients require a nursing care summary every 2 weeks. For a nursing assessment flowsheet used in long-term care,

  Go to Chapter 16, **Charting Forms: A flowsheet used in long-term care,** in Volume 2.

KnowledgeCheck 16-4

How do home care and long-term care documentation differ from hospital-based documentation?

 Go to Chapter 16, **Knowledge Check Response Sheet and Answers,** on the Student Resource Disk or DavisPlus at http://davisplus.fadavis.com/Wilkinson2

Critical**Thinking** 16-3

Why do long-term care clients require less frequent charting than clients in acute care settings?

Oral Reporting

The purpose of giving an oral report is to maintain continuity of care. The oral report provides an opportunity for professional communication that assists in organizing your work, and also for learning, building team relationships, and collaborating to improve patient care. Whether the source of the information shared is from a written report form, a paper Kardex®, or a summary view in the EHR, the quality of the report you give and receive influences how you and others plan the day's (or night's) work. Restrict your oral reports to patient-focused discussion and limit extraneous details and social conversation.

How Do I Give a Handoff Report?

The purpose of a **handoff report** (sometimes called a *change-of-shift report* or *handover report*) is to alert the next caregiver about the client's status or recent changes in the client's condition and to discuss planned activities, tests, procedures, or concerns that require follow-up. Handoff report may be given at the bedside or in a conference room using paper notes or a mobile or desktop EHR device.

Handoff reports are usually given orally, although some organizations use written or audio-recorded reports. As a student nurse, you will receive report from either the nurse completing the shift or from the nurse assigned to the client during the shift you will be working. Report any changes to the nurse assigned to the client during your shift, and always give a report before leaving the unit.

Bedside Report, sometimes known as "walking rounds," allows you to observe important aspects of care, such as patient appearance, IV pumps, and wounds. With bedside report, the outgoing nurse can introduce you to the patient and you can begin your assessment. If the patient is alert, give him the opportunity to participate in the report and ask questions. Although this type of report is time-consuming, it encourages continuity of care, team collaboration, and patient/family communication.

Face-to-Face Oral Report may involve only the outgoing and oncoming nurse or may include the entire oncoming shift. When given in a conference room, oral report does not let you directly observe the patient, but it is time-efficient and still allows interaction between nurses.

Audio-Recorded Report is a convenient way to transmit information. The outgoing nurse audio-records a report on the clients under her care. This method can be time-consuming, especially if you must listen to the entire unit report before hearing about your own assigned patients. The main difficulty is that an audio-recorded report does not allow you to ask questions about the client. Occasionally, the audio quality is low and the report is not clear. Unfortunately, a recorded report is often used to allow the outgoing staff to leave promptly, so it may be impossible for you to speak directly with the previously assigned nurse. If you have questions, you must then phone the nurse or review the written notes from the previous shift if you are unable to speak with the nurse directly. Few agencies use audio-recorded handoff reports because The Joint Commission (2008b) recommends using a method that allows for questioning between the giver and receiver of the information.

No matter where or how the handoff report is given, you should use a standardized approach. The PACE format is one example of a standardized approach to handoffs, and was developed specifically for that purpose. The mnemonic stands for Patient/Problem, Assessment/Actions, Continuing/Changes, and Evaluation (Schroeder, 2006).

The **SBAR** (Situation-Background-Assessment-Recommendation) is an easy-to-remember, concrete acronym useful for framing any conversation. Because nurses and physicians communicate in very different ways, SBAR is useful for interdisciplinary communication, especially critical situations requiring a clinician's immediate attention and action. SBAR allows for an easy and focused way to set expectations for what will be communicated and how between members of the team. The SBAR technique can be adapted for handoff reports.

For additional information about communicating with SBAR and PACE,

 Go to Chapter 18, **Clinical Insight 18-3, Communicating with SBAR;** and Chapter 16, **Clinical Insight 16-1, Giving Oral Reports,** in Volume 2.

Regardless of the format used, to prepare to give a handoff report, you need to collect the following information:

- Client progress made during your shift
- Therapies and treatments administered
- Teaching done
- Consultations done or planned with other disciplines
- Status of identified desired outcomes
- Any changes in client status
- Progress made on discharge planning

KnowledgeCheck 16-5

- What data should be included in a handoff report?
- What are the types of handoff reports?

 Go to Chapter 16, **Knowledge Check Response Sheet and Answers,** on the Student Resource Disk or DavisPlus at http://davisplus.fadavis.com/Wilkinson2

What Is a Transfer Report?

Transfer reports are given when a patient is transferred from unit to unit or from facility to facility. For information to include in an oral transfer report,

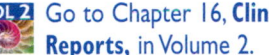 Go to Chapter 16, **Clinical Insight 16-1: Giving Oral Reports,** in Volume 2.

If the patient is being transported to another unit in the same facility, you will need to transport a paper chart with the patient. If both organizations are using an EHR documentation system, then the receiving unit will access the client record electronically. Detailed information about the patient's health history can be communicated between healthcare professionals or transmitted before transfer. Your organization will have a policy on what is to be copied and how materials should be transmitted to the receiving facility. For a review of transfers and discharges, see Chapter 10 in this volume and

 Go to Chapter 10, **Procedures 10-2, 10-3, and 10-4,** in Volume 2.

How Do I Receive and Document Verbal and Telephone Orders?

Although licensed nurses may find it necessary to accept verbal or telephone orders on occasion, verbal and telephone orders increase the risk of hearing or recording the order incorrectly. The Joint Commission addresses how to best avoid the dangers: "For verbal or telephone orders or for telephonic reporting of critical test results, verify the complete order or test result by having the person receiving the information record and 'read-back' the complete order or test result" (The Joint Commission, 2008a).

Telephone Orders

Telephone orders can lead to error because of differences in pronunciation, dialect, or accent; background noise; and unfamiliar terminology. Taking a telephone order may be acceptable when there has been a sudden change for the worse in your patient's condition and the client's primary care provider is not in the hospital, or the physician does not have access to placing orders electronically outside the hospital. Verbal or telephone orders are also acceptable in a life-threatening emergency, but you must apply the "read-back" safeguard. Faxes and e-mail have reduced the need for telephone orders; however, the need for them may never disappear entirely.

For guidelines to use when taking telephone orders,

 Go to Chapter 16, **Clinical Insight 16-2: Receiving Telephone and Verbal Orders,** in Volume 2.

The following is an example of a telephone order transcribed to a paper order sheet:

08/27/11 0805 Morphine 2 mg IV push once for pain now. ———————— T.O. Dr. Kent/S. Hogan R.N.

If the telephone order is entered electronically, the date/time and order remains the same but the order is marked as one entered electronically that will go to the selected physician, Dr. Kent, for his electronic co-signature.

Verbal Orders

Verbal orders are spoken directions for patient care given to you in person, usually during an emergency. Providers should never use verbal orders as a routine method of communicating orders. When recording a verbal order, include the date, time, and the written text of the order or the electronic entry of the order. If you are writing the order on an order sheet, an indicator "V.O." designating verbal orders is then followed by the provider's name and your name. If you are entering the order electronically, then the order will be designated as a verbal order and be routed to the selected physician for co-signature. Follow the Joint Commission safety guidelines, above, and

 Go to Chapter 16, **Clinical Insight 16-2: Receiving Telephone and Verbal Orders,** in Volume 2.

Knowledge Check 16-6

- What important factors should you document when receiving a telephone order?
- What is the purpose of a verbal order? When should it be used?

 Go to Chapter 16, **Knowledge Check Response Sheet and Answers,** on the Student Resource Disk or DavisPlus at http://davisplus.fadavis.com/Wilkinson2

How Do I Question an Order?

If you feel uncertain about an order, you must question it. As a student, you will first want to discuss your concerns with your clinical instructor or the nurse you are working with during your clinical time. Remember, the goal is to provide safe care. If you have concerns, do not remain quiet—act on them.

As a nurse, you will follow your organization's policy for clarifying orders. If an order is written illegibly on a paper order sheet or is entered into the EHR missing details or order components, contact the provider directly to seek clarification. If you believe an order is inappropriate or unsafe, you are legally and ethically required to question the order. Generally, you should contact the provider who wrote the order. If the provider leaves the order as-is and you still don't feel comfortable with it or believe there is an error, you may refuse to carry it out. Inform your chain of command at your organization about your refusal. Usually the person you will speak with is the charge nurse, who may then contact the nurse manager or nursing supervisor. The nature of the order will determine how this situation is handled.

As a new nurse, you may feel uncomfortable about questioning an order. Even experienced nurses sometimes feel uneasy with this challenge. If you are uncertain how to proceed, you can discuss your concerns with your colleagues, the charge nurse, or the supervisor before contacting the provider. Your efforts to clarify the orders help to protect your patient. If you do refuse an order, you must document your refusal and the actions you took to clarify the order.

Practical **Knowledge** **knowing** how

To document care effectively, you need to be familiar with the forms and requirements of your institution. Chart routine nursing actions (e.g., skin care) on the designated paper or electronic flowsheets or forms; and chart your assessments, interventions, and patient responses to care in the format approved by your organization. It is important to chart accurately, completely, and consistently so that the patient's progress can be tracked and appropriate care given.

Whether you are documenting on paper or in an EHR, documentation begins at the start of your shift in a hospital, long-term care facility, or when you first encounter the client during a home visit or at an outpatient facility. Document the condition of your patient when you first observed him. Was he awake? Was he in bed? Did he have any complaints? What did you do? As your shift or visit progressed, you performed your assessment and nursing interventions. What were your findings? Did any abnormalities exist? Finally, what was the patient's response to your intervention? Did any changes from the initial assessment occur?

Remember that the patient's health record is permanent and that information contained in the chart is confidential. As a student, you are granted access to client's charts for educational purposes. You have a duty to keep the information private and confidential. As a student, in most cases, you will be asked to use only the client's initials on school assignments. The Department of Health and Human Services (DHHS) issued updated regulations to protect health information in April 2003. As part of the reform of the Health Insurance Portability and Accountability Act (HIPAA), the regulations affect access, storage, transfer, and discussion of patient information. For more information about privacy, confidentiality, and HIPAA, refer to Chapters 44 and 45.

Guidelines for Documenting Care

Document Accurately, and Use Nonjudgmental Language. Avoid labeling patients. If the patient offers an explanation for refusing a treatment or medication, quote the patient in his own voice. Do not chart personal opinion or judgments, such as "Patient obnoxious and refuses prescribed medication."

Know the Requirements of Reimbursement. Home care, hospitals, and long-term care facilities have specific guidelines for the frequency of charting and the type of data that must be recorded. Clinic and office settings also have requirements that must be met so that services can be reimbursed. Familiarize yourself with these requirements in your work setting.

Provide Details About the Client's Condition. When possible, give specific examples. Including descriptive details allows oncoming staff members and other caregivers to better grasp your patient's individual needs. You should document narrative notes often enough to clearly describe what your client is experiencing, including responses to interventions and treatments.

Document Immediately. Document as soon as possible after making an observation or providing care. The longer you wait, the less you will recall. If you leave your documentation until the end of the shift or until you are back in the home care office, you may forget important details. Whether you are charting on paper at the bedside or electronically, discipline yourself to document promptly.

Never Chart Ahead. It is impossible to see into the future and be sure that what you expect to happen will actually happen. To do this threatens the record's credibility.

If you Chart a Symptom, Also Chart Your Interventions. Do not chart a symptom, such as "c/o pain," without also documenting what you did about it and how the patient responded to your interventions.

Chart Chronologically to Communicate the Changing Status of the Patient. If you forget to make an important entry while charting, you will need to add to or modify your documentation. Record the time and date you are charting, but clearly designate this is a late entry. If you know legal action is pending, do not place a late note in the health record without notifying the nurse manager or risk management officer first. It is a criminal offense to alter a patient record after the organization's approved time limit for doing so has passed.

Date and Time All your Documentation. To avoid confusion between A.M. AND P.M., most organizations use a 24-hour clock or military time (Fig. 16-9). The day begins at 0001 (1 minute past midnight) and ends at 2400 (12 midnight). Most people have little difficulty with early morning hours. However, after 12 noon, the changes are more noticeable.

For example, 1:00 P.M. IS 1300. To convert to military time after 12 NOON, simply add 12 to the clock time. 7:30 P.M. + 12 = 1930 in military time.

For a brief set of documentation tips, see Box 16-4. For detailed guidelines for documentation,

 Go to Chapter 16, **Clinical Insight 16-3**, in Volume 2.

Guidelines for Paper Health Records

Paper health records need to be stored in designated areas to which only healthcare providers have access. In addition, you must not provide written or verbal patient information to anyone not involved in the direct care of the patient, unless the patient has consented to allow that person access.

To ensure your written paper documentation is effective, the forms used must be efficient, comprehensive, and relevant to patient's healthcare needs. The forms

FIGURE 16-9 Many healthcare facilities use the 24-hour clock.

BOX 16-4 ■ Documentation ABCs

Accurate

Bias-free

Complete

Detailed

Easy to read

Factual

Grammatical

Harmless (legally)

must also prompt you to document appropriately so your organization's policies and procedures are met. For detailed guidelines concerning documentation in paper health records,

 Go to Chapter 16, **Clinical Insight 16-4,** in Volume 2.

Guidelines for Electronic Health Records

Well-designed nursing documentation forms and systems help you organize your work, manage your care plans, track client diagnoses and outcomes, and support decision-making by all members of the healthcare team. Initial reluctance to use EHRs usually decreases quickly

as nurses become more comfortable using them (Moody, Slocomb, Berg, et al., 2004). For guidelines specific to the use of electronic documentation,

 Go to Chapter 16, **Clinical Insight 16-5,** in Volume 2.

KnowledgeCheck 16-7
- What aspects of care should be documented?
- When should care be documented?
- How is documentation on paper different than documentation in an EHR or on an electronic digital form?

 Go to Chapter 16, **Knowledge Check Response Sheet and Answers,** on the Student Resource Disk or DavisPlus at http://davisplus.fadavis.com/Wilkinson2

CriticalThinking 16-4

You are caring for two clients on a medical–surgical unit. One of your clients is short of breath and complaining of chest pain. Your other client is recovering from abdominal surgery. He is alert, stable, and free from pain at this time. After stabilizing your first client, you realize you are 45 minutes late administering a medication to the abdominal surgery patient. You are not sure how to proceed.
- What theoretical knowledge do you need?
- You give the medicine as soon as you can (60 minutes late). How and when should you chart the medication administered?
- If you had been aware that you were going to be late with the medication, what might you have done to be sure it was given on time?

Toward Evidence-Based Practice

Smith, K., Smith, V., Krugman, M., et al. (2005). Evaluating the impact of computerized clinical documentation. *CIN: Computers, Informatics, Nursing, 23*(3), 132–138.

A computerized system for planning and documenting patient care was initiated at a western teaching hospital, using the framework of Nursing Interventions Classification (NIC) and Nursing Outcomes Classification (NOC) standardized languages. The software also includes both order entry and a charting application. Staff surveys, observations, and chart audits were conducted before and after the computerized system was implemented. Data demonstrated that after the new system was implemented: (1) staff attitudes toward computers were less positive, (2) the time required for charting was unchanged, and (3) nurses' charting entries were more complete and comprehensive.

Kossman, S., & Scheidenhelm, S. (2008). Nurses' perceptions of the impact of electronic health records on work and patient outcomes. *CIN: Computers, Informatics, Nursing, 26*(2), 69–77.

This study addressed nurses' use of electronic health records (EHR) and their views of the impact of such records on job performance and patient outcomes.

Questionnaires, interviews, and observation data from 46 nurses in medical–surgical and intensive care units at two community hospitals were analyzed. Results indicated that nurses: (1) preferred EHR to paper charts and were comfortable with technology; (2) thought use of EHR impaired critical thinking, decreased interdisciplinary communication, and created a high demand on work time (73% reported spending at least half their shift using the records); (3) believed that EHR improved organization, efficiency, and information access (e.g., helpful alert screens); and (4) thought the use of EHR enabled them to provide safer care but decreased the quality of care.

---

1. Refer to Box 16-1. Compare the Advantages of the EHR in that box to the findings in the above studies. Which EHR advantage is *not* supported by either of these studies? What is the statement in each study that conflicts with the advantage reported in Box 16-1?

2. Which study disagrees with the statement that EHR improves communication between healthcare providers? What does the study say about that?

 Go to Chapter 16, **Toward Evidence-Based Practice Suggested Responses,** on the Student Resource Disk or DavisPlus at http://davisplus.fadavis.com/Wilkinson2

Can I Delegate Charting?

In some facilities, each member of the team is responsible for documenting her part in the care of the client. Nursing assistants or other nursing assistive personnel (NAP) often chart ADLs, activity, and intake and output (I&O) on graphic records. You are responsible for documenting the nursing care you provide. Never chart the actions of others as though you performed them. If an action is crucial to a chain of events, you may document that action on paper or in the EHR, referring to the person who did the action clearly. For example, "Became dizzy; assisted to chair by Nora Roverdale, NAP."

KnowledgeCheck 16-8

- Can charting be delegated?
- You are a student nurse on a medical–surgical unit. You review your client's chart and notice that the physician entered orders that do not appear to be appropriate for your client. The physician is still in the area. How would you handle this situation?

 Go to Chapter 16, **Knowledge Check Response Sheet and Answers,** on the Student Resource Disk or DavisPlus at http://davisplus.fadavis.com/Wilkinson2

Critical**Thinking** 16-5

You note that your client with asthma is having increasing difficulty breathing. You call the physician, who gives you a telephone order for an asthma medication, and then hangs up. When you enter the order electronically as a verbal order, you find out the medication is a nonformulary medication that your pharmacy does not carry.

- Is this an acceptable reason to take a verbal order?
- The physician gets irritated when you call back and says, "I ordered what I wanted." How would you handle this situation?
- You entered the order electronically after the physician hung up. How could this situation have been avoided?

 Suggested Readings: Go to Chapter 16, **Reading More About Documenting and Reporting,** on the Student Resource Disk or DavisPlus at http://davisplus.fadavis.com/Wilkinson2

 Bibliography. Go to Volume 2, Bibliography.

CHAPTER 17

Measuring Vital Signs

Learning Outcomes

After completing this chapter, you should be able to:

➤ State at least one nursing diagnosis that might be used to describe a problem for each of the four vital signs: temperature, pulse, respirations, and blood pressure.

➤ Describe the process of thermoregulation in the body.

➤ Describe the process for taking oral, rectal, axillary, tympanic membrane, and temporal temperatures.

➤ Convert between the Fahrenheit and centigrade temperature scales.

➤ For different patient situations, choose the best way to take the temperature, including site and equipment.

➤ Discuss the concept of a "normal" temperature.

➤ Explain the physiological mechanisms of fever.

➤ Describe at least four nursing interventions for the patient with a fever.

➤ Describe at least six nursing interventions for the patient with temperature alterations other than fever.

➤ Describe methods for obtaining peripheral and apical pulses.

➤ Given a client's age and pulse rate, rhythm, quality, and equality, differentiate between normal findings and those that should be referred to the primary healthcare provider.

➤ Explain how respirations are regulated in the body.

➤ Given a client's age and respiratory rate, depth, and rhythm; chest movement; and associated clinical signs, differentiate between normal findings and those that should be referred to the primary healthcare provider.

➤ Define arterial oxygen saturation, hypoxia, hyperventilation, and hypoventilation.

➤ Discuss at least five nursing interventions for the client with impaired respiratory status.

➤ Describe the physiology of blood pressure, including references to systolic, diastolic, pulse pressure, and mean arterial pressure.

➤ State the normal blood pressure range for the average adult.

➤ Explain why it is important to interpret a client's blood pressure pattern rather than relying on a single reading.

➤ Describe the process of obtaining a brachial blood pressure reading.

➤ Discuss the importance of cuff size when obtaining a blood pressure reading.

➤ Define hypotension, hypertension, essential hypertension, and secondary hypertension.

➤ Identify at least three nursing interventions for the client with hypertension.

Meet Your Patient

Your instructor has scheduled a clinical day at a local community health fair. Students from your program will be available to answer health-related questions, administer flu vaccines, check blood sugar levels, and take vital signs: temperature, pulse, respirations, and blood pressure. You have been asked to check vital signs.

The first person who arrives at the booth is Rosemary, a young mother, with Jason, her 2-year-old son. She tells you he has been eating poorly and is very irritable. You note that the child's skin is warm and dry, and he is flushed. Rosemary explains that she does not have a thermometer, and she would like you to take her son's temperature. Jason's axillary temperature is 101.8°F (38.8°C).

Now it is time to think like a nurse! What may be the meaning of this temperature reading? What, if any, additional data should you collect? How will you explain your findings to Rosemary? What action would you advise Rosemary to take? You may not yet have all the theoretical knowledge you need to answer these questions, but try to do so anyway, based on your present knowledge base and your life experiences.

The next person to arrive at the booth is Ms. Sharma, an active 80-year-old woman who works part time in a local literacy program and walks 3 miles four times per week. Ms. Sharma notes that she has "lost a little pep. I don't feel sick, but I'm tired lately." Her pulse is difficult to feel. The rhythm is irregular, and the strength of the pulse is uneven—some beats are strong, while others are weak. What might this finding mean? What questions do you have for Ms. Sharma? What, if any, additional data should you collect? How will you explain your findings to Ms. Sharma? What action would you advise her to take?

Mr. Jackson stops by to have his vital signs checked. As he sits down next to you, you notice he is short of breath. His respiratory rate is 28 breaths/min, and he appears to be struggling to breathe. What do you think this respiratory rate means? What should be your next action? What would you say to Mr. Jackson?

The next client to arrive is Lucas, a 35-year-old accountant who works for a firm in a nearby office building. Lucas tells you he has been under a lot of stress and is worried about his blood pressure. You measure his blood pressure as 150/98 mm Hg. Is this an acceptable blood pressure? What does this reading mean? What should you discuss with Lucas? What advice should you offer?

You will gain the theoretical knowledge you need to answer the preceding questions as you work through this chapter and learn more about vital signs.

What Are Vital Signs?

The term **vital signs (VS)** suggests assessment of vital or critical physiological functions. Variations in temperature, pulse, respirations, or blood pressure are indicators of a person's state of health and function of the body systems. Therefore, these four measurements are among the most frequent assessments you will make as a nurse. Because of the importance of each of the vital signs, you must be very accurate in your measurements and recordings.

Do not become complacent when a client's vital signs are within normal limits. Although stable vital signs *indicate* physiological well-being, they do not *guarantee* it. Vital signs alone are limited in detecting some important physiological changes; for example, vital signs may sometimes remain stable even when there is moderately large blood loss. Evaluate the vital signs in the context of your overall assessment of the client.

A fifth vital sign, a measure of *pain*, has recently been proposed. See Chapter 30. Some experts recommend that *pulse oximetry* be added to the four traditional measures of physiological status when accurate assessment and monitoring are essential. Pulse oximetry is a technique for assessing oxygenation and is discussed later in this chapter. Also, although it does not fit with the traditional concept, some researchers suggest that *smoking status* be considered a VS during the initial patient encounter ("Vital Signs," 1999). Still others recommend including *emotional distress* as a vital sign. Rather than being overly concerned about whether or not these parameters should be referred to as vital signs, we recommend that nurses include them in all of their ongoing assessments of patients: temperature, pulse, and respirations (TPR); blood pressure; pain; pulse oximetry; emotional status; and (on initial encounter) smoking status.

The rest of this chapter explains the meaning of each of the vital signs and how to assess them.

When Should I Measure a Patient's Vital Signs?

In the community health fair scenario, clients asked you to take their vital signs. However, in many clinical settings you and other care providers will determine how often to measure and record VS. In general, the frequency depends on the patient's condition and the events taking place. The following are common occasions for assessing vital signs:

- On admission to the hospital
- At the beginning of a shift, for inpatients
- At a visit to the healthcare provider's office or clinic
- Before, during, and after surgery or certain procedures
- To monitor the effects of certain medications or activities
- Whenever the patient's condition changes

Although there has been little research to support the optimal frequency for assessing vital signs, agency policies usually require that nurses monitor and record vital signs on a regular basis. The frequency varies by setting and situation. Below are commonly used frequencies:

- In the hospital: once every 4 to 8 hours
- In the home health setting: at each visit
- In the clinic: at each visit
- In skilled nursing facilities, also known as convalescent hospitals: weekly to monthly

When a client's VS vary from their baseline, you should assess and document them more frequently, perhaps every 5 to 15 minutes. As a beginning practitioner, you should validate your clinical assessments with a more experienced nurse.

It is up to the nurse to decide whether vital signs need to be monitored more frequently than the primary care provider has prescribed. Initially, you will measure VS to establish the patient's baseline. A baseline is important because (1) a change in vital signs may be caused by a disease state, the effect of therapies, or merely by changes in activity and environment; and (2) there are normal variations in vital signs among individuals. Table 17-1 shows average or normal findings for adults, but it is important to remember that each person has his or her own baseline for "normal." If a patient's vital signs vary from established norms, compare the finding to that person's baseline to determine the degree and severity of the variation.

How Do I Document Vital Signs?

Most agencies have special flowsheets for documenting vital signs. If the VS are not within normal limits, you will also document them in the nurses' notes, along with any associated symptoms (e.g., cyanosis [blue-gray skin] with abnormal respirations). Document any interventions as well (e.g., elevating the head of the bed when the patient has shortness of breath). For an example of a graphic flowsheet for recording vital signs,

 Go to Chapter 17, **Forms**, in Volume 2.

Table 17-1 ➤ Vital Signs: Average Normal Findings for Adults	
Mean Adult Temperature	
Oral	98°F (36.7°C)*
Rectal	98.6°F (37°C)*
Pulse	
Normal range	60–100 beats/min
Average	80 beats/min
Respirations	
Normal range	12–20 breaths/min
Blood Pressure	
Normal range	100–119 systolic and 60–80 diastolic
Prehypertensive	120–139 systolic and 80–89 diastolic
Average	110/70 (the middle of the "normal" range) (Joint National Committee on Prevention, Detection, Evaluation, and Treatment of High Blood Pressure, 2003)

*This is revised downward from the traditional norms to reflect more recent research (Mackowiak, Wasserman, & Levine, 1992) and a systematic review of the literature (Sund-Levander, Forsberg, & Wahren, 2002). The systematic review reported the following mean normal temperatures: Oral 97.3°F (36.3°C), Rectal 98.3°F (36.9°C). The traditional Wunderlich (1871) average normal temperature is 98.6°F (37.0°C) to 99.5°F (37.5°C), depending on measurement site.

Body Temperature

Body temperature is the degree of heat maintained by the body. It is the difference between heat produced by the body and heat lost to the environment.

Theoretical Knowledge knowing why

To assess and support regulation of body temperature, you will need to know the normal temperature range, how heat is produced by and lost from the body, and factors that influence body temperature.

What Is a Normal Temperature?

No single number can be considered "normal," because body temperature varies among individuals as a result of differences in metabolism. Furthermore, each person's temperature fluctuates with age, exercise, and environmental conditions. However, the body does function optimally within a narrow temperature range.

There is little definitive evidence about what, exactly, is a normal temperature. You may see different values in the many sources you read. We can at least conclude that the traditional belief of 98.6°F (37°C) for an average normal reading is too high, based on available research. A systematic review of the literature found a mean normal oral temperature of 97.3°F (36.3°C) (Sund-Levander, Forsberg, & Wahren, 2002). See Table 17-1. Older adults tend to have lower body temperatures. Pregnant women run higher baseline body temperatures. For age-related variations for all vital signs, including temperature,

Go to Chapter 17, **Tables, Boxes, Figures: ESG Table 17-1,** on the Student Resource Disk or DavisPlus at http:// davisplus.fadavis.com/Wilkinson2

Temporary, slight variations of temperature above or below normal usually are not significant. Greater variations indicate a disturbance of function in some system or region of the body (Fig. 17-1). The degree of temperature elevation does not always indicate the seriousness of the underlying disease or condition. For example, some acute, even fatal, infections may cause only a mild temperature elevation. However, a continuous elevation, even if slight, is cause for concern and indicates a need for further evaluation.

An adult's normal internal temperature, called the **core temperature,** ranges from about 97° to 100.8°F (36.1° to 38.2°C). Most research and clinical practice situations do not report core body temperature because it is not convenient to measure. The core temperature is typically 1° to 2°F (0.6° to 1.2°C) higher than surface (skin) temperature. Rectal and tympanic membrane measurements are used to represent core temperatures; oral and axillary measurements reflect surface temperatures.

How Does the Body Regulate Temperature?

The process of temperature regulation is called **thermoregulation.** To keep the body temperature constant, the body must balance heat production and heat loss. This balance is controlled by the hypothalamus, located between the cerebral hemispheres of the brain. Similar to a thermostat, the hypothalamus recognizes even small changes in body temperature that are sent to it by sensory receptors in the skin.

Decreasing the Body Temperature. When heat sensors in the hypothalamus are stimulated, they send out impulses to reduce the body temperature. This activates compensatory mechanisms, such as peripheral vasodilation, sweating, and inhibition of heat production. Vasodilation diverts core-warmed blood to the body surface, where heat can be transferred to the surrounding environment.

Increasing the Body Temperature. When the sensors in the hypothalamus detect cold, they send out impulses to increase heat production and reduce heat loss. To produce heat, the body responds with shivering and the release of epinephrine, which increases metabolism. To reduce heat loss, the blood vessels constrict. Vasoconstriction conserves heat by shunting blood away from the periphery (where heat is lost) to the core of the body, where the blood is warmed. **Piloerection** (hairs standing on end) also occurs, but it is not an important heat-conserving mechanism in humans.

Behavioral Control of Temperature. In addition, body temperature is under our behavioral control. When people feel cool, they can turn up the thermostat, put on more clothing, or move to a warmer place. When they feel too warm, they can turn on an air conditioner, remove some clothing, or take a cool shower.

How Is Heat Produced in the Body?

The body produces heat through the interaction of three factors: metabolism, the movement of skeletal muscles, and nonshivering thermogenesis.

Metabolism

Metabolism is the sum of all physical and chemical processes and changes that take place in the body. Metabolism uses energy and generates heat. The **basal metabolic rate (BMR)** is the amount of energy required to maintain the body at rest. Body size, lean muscle mass, and numerous hormones influence BMR. For example, hyperthyroidism (an increase in the thyroid hormone thyroxine) increases the BMR. Clients with hyperthyroidism often complain of feeling warm even when they are in a cool environment. By contrast, when

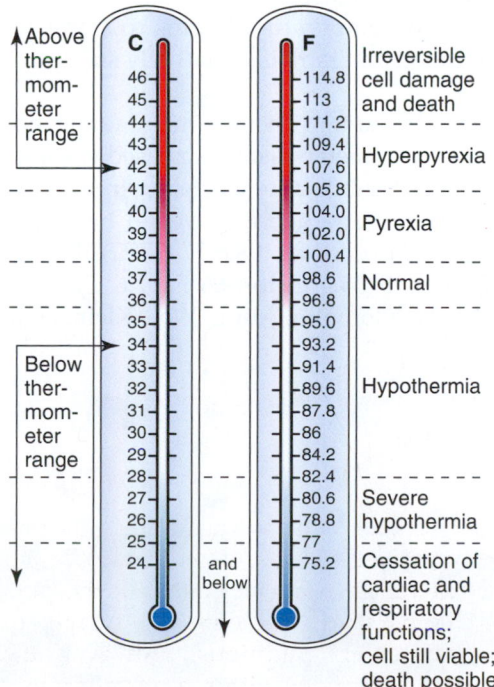

FIGURE 17-1 Ranges of normal and altered body temperatures.

the thyroxine level is low (hypothyroidism), less heat is produced, and clients commonly report feeling cold. Epinephrine and norepinephrine, produced from stimulation of the sympathetic nervous system, also increase BMR and heat production.

Skeletal Muscle Movement

Skeletal muscles are used in all body movements. Muscles need fuel to function. The breakdown (*catabolism*) of fats and carbohydrates in muscle produces energy and heat. It requires very little muscle activity to sit and read this text. However, if you were to go to a local track for a run, you would use more skeletal muscles. After your run, your body temperature would be higher, perhaps as high as 101° to 104°F (38.3° to 40°C). In contrast, if you were to go outside without a coat when the temperature was 35°F (1.6°C), you would begin to feel cold. Your hypothalamus would sense a drop in body temperature and you would begin shivering. This mechanism is so efficient that body heat production can rise to about four times the normal rate in just a few minutes.

Nonshivering Thermogenesis

Nonshivering thermogenesis is the metabolism of brown fat to produce heat. It is used by infants because they cannot produce heat through shivering, as do adults and children. This mechanism disappears in the first few months after birth.

How Is Heat Exchanged Between the Body and the Environment?

Heat moves from an area of higher to an area of lower temperature; that is, cool air and objects "pick up" heat from warmer ones. The mechanisms that effect the exchange of heat between the body and the environment are radiation, convection, evaporation, and conduction (Fig. 17-2).

Radiation is the loss of heat through electromagnetic waves emitting from surfaces that are warmer than the surrounding air. If the uncovered skin is warmer than the air, the body loses heat through the skin. This is why a cool room warms by radiation when it is filled with many people. In contrast, a person can acquire heat by turning on a heat lamp or being in the sunlight. Radiation accounts for almost 50% of body heat loss.

Convection is the transfer of heat through currents of air or water. Nurses use this principle to intentionally effect changes in a patient's body temperature. Immersion in a warm bath may raise body temperature for a hypothermic client. In contrast, the currents of cool air produced by a fan can help reduce a fever. Together, the processes of convection and conduction account for approximately 15% to 20% of all heat loss to the environment.

Evaporation occurs when water is converted to vapor and lost from the skin (as perspiration) or the mucous membranes (through the breath). Evaporation causes cooling. Water loss by evaporation is called **insensible loss.** Evaporation is affected by the relative **humidity** (moisture in the environment). If the air already contains much humidity, then less moisture evaporates from the skin and less cooling occurs.

Conduction is the process whereby heat is transferred from a warm to a cool surface by direct contact. Suppose that a patient's temperature is 98.6°F (37°C) while he is fully dressed in the examination room. If he is dressed in a thin, hospital gown and lying on a cool metal radiology table, his temperature would drop, perhaps as much as a full degree Fahrenheit in the first hour.

What Factors Influence Body Temperature?

The following are some examples of factors involved in the delicate balance of body temperature:

Developmental Level.

Infants and older adults are most susceptible to the effects of environmental temperature extremes. Infants lose approximately 30% of their body heat through the head, which is proportionally larger than the rest of the body compared to adults. This places them at increased risk for decreased body temperature. Body temperature begins to stabilize during early childhood and remains relatively stable until older adulthood.

Older adults have difficulty maintaining body heat because of slower metabolism, decreased vasomotor control, and loss of subcutaneous tissue. In a recent study, older adults (average age 80.7 years) had mean body temperatures lower than 98.6°F (37°C). Temperatures ranged from 94°F (34.4°C) to 99.6°F (37.6°C), but few ever reached 98.6°F (Gomolin, Aung, Wolf-Klein, et al., 2005).

Air conditioning vent

FIGURE 17-2 Mechanisms of heat exchange with the environment: Radiation, convection, evaporation, and conduction.

The average normal temperature for older adults is about 95° to 96.8°F (35° to 36°C). For a comparison of normal VS for various ages,

 Go to Chapter 17, **Tables, Boxes, Figures: ESG Table 17-1,** on the Student Resource Disk or DavisPlus at http://davisplus.fadavis.com/Wilkinson2

Environment. The environment strongly influences body temperature. For example, warm room temperatures, high humidity, or hot baths can increase body temperature. Very high external temperatures can produce high internal temperatures, causing heat stroke. In contrast, cold environments, especially with strong air currents, can lower body temperatures and, in severe cases, lead to hypothermia.

Sex. A woman's body temperature varies (as much as 1°F, or 0.6°C) with her menstrual cycle and pregnancy. Body temperature is lower when progesterone levels are low and increases as progesterone levels increase. Hormonal fluctuations during menopause, when menses stop, often cause temperature fluctuations commonly known as *hot flashes,* which can produce episodes of intense body heat and sweating. At least one study has found differences in the range of normal body temperatures for women and men. However, further studies are needed to confirm these differences (Sund-Levander, Forsberg, & Wahren, 2002).

Exercise. Because it increases metabolism, hard work or strenuous exercise can increase body core temperature to 101° to 104°F (38.3° to 40°C).

Emotions and Stress. Emotional stress, excitement, anxiety, and nervousness stimulate the sympathetic nervous system, causing production of epinephrine and norepinephrine. These biochemical agents trigger an increase in the metabolic rate, which in turn increases body temperature.

Circadian Rhythm. Circadian rhythm is a cyclical repetition of certain physiological processes (e.g., changes in temperature and blood pressure) that occurs every 24 hours. Temperature fluctuates 1° to 2°F (0.6° to 1.2°C) over the course of 24 hours. It is usually lowest in the early morning hours and highest in late afternoon or early evening.

 Critical**Thinking** 17-1

- You notice the following temperature readings in your client's chart:
  0400: 97.4°F
  0800: 97.9°F
  1200: 98.4°F
  1600: 99.6°F
  2000: 100.9°F
  You are working the night shift. When you assess the client's temperature at midnight, it is 101.2°F. What do you notice about the pattern of the temperature readings?
- What is important in this scenario?
- As a nursing student, what should you do?

KnowledgeCheck 17-1

- Which age groups are most susceptible to thermoregulation problems, and why?
- List five factors that affect body temperature.
- What are the compensatory mechanisms for decreasing body temperature?
- What are the compensatory mechanisms for increasing body temperature?

 Go to Chapter 17, **Knowledge Check Response Sheet and Answers,** on the Student Resource Disk or DavisPlus at http://davisplus.fadavis.com/Wilkinson2

What Is Fever (Pyrexia)?

Fever, or **pyrexia,** is a temperature above the person's usual range of normal. Traditionally we have thought of fever as an oral temperature higher than 100°F (37.8°C), or a rectal temperature of 101°F (38.3°C) in an adult. But, remember that many people, especially older adults, have lower normal body temperatures and that a person's normal body temperature changes by as much as 1°F (0.6°C) throughout the day. So it is likely that many people, especially older adults, experience fever at a temperature lower than our traditional definition. A person with a fever is said to be **febrile;** one without fever is **afebrile.** A single high reading may not indicate fever. You need several readings at different times of the day, as well as the person's usual normal reading.

A moderate fever (up to 103°F, or 39.5°C) may be uncomfortable, and it may signal an underlying problem (e.g., influenza or other infection). However, the fever itself does not pose a threat to most clients and is the body's natural defense against infection. Higher fevers can damage body cells and cause delirium and seizures. **Hyperpyrexia** is fever above 105.8°F (41.0°C). Hyperpyrexia is dangerous and requires intervention.

Fever occurs in response to **pyrogens** (fever-producing substances). When bacteria or other foreign substances invade the body, they stimulate **phagocytes** (specialized white blood cells), which ingest the invaders and secrete pyrogens (e.g., interleukin-1). Pyrogens induce secretion of **prostaglandins** (substances that reset the hypothalamic thermostat at a higher temperature). The reset value is called the **set point**. The body's heat-regulating mechanisms then act to bring the core temperature up to this new setting. When the stressor is removed, the set point resets at normal.

Fever occurs in three phases:

- *The initial phase (febrile episode or onset):* The period when body temperature is rising but has not yet reached the new set point. The onset of fever may be sudden or gradual, depending on the condition causing it. The person usually feels chilly and generally uncomfortable and may shiver.
- *The second phase (course):* The period when body temperature reaches its maximum (set point) and remains

fairly constant at the new higher level. The person is flushed and feels warm and dry during this phase, which may last from a few days to a few weeks.

- *The third phase (defervescence or crisis):* The period when the temperature returns to normal. The person feels warm and appears flushed in response to vasodilation. Diaphoresis occurs, which assists with heat loss by evaporation. This phase is commonly referred to as the fever's "breaking."

There are four types of fever:

- **Intermittent fever**: Temperature alternates regularly between periods of fever and periods of normal or below-normal temperature without pharmacological intervention; or the temperature returns to normal at least once every 24 hours.
- **Remittent fever**: Fluctuations in temperature (>3.6°F, or 2°C), all above normal, during a 24-hour period.
- **Constant (sustained) fever**: Temperature may fluctuate slightly (<1°F, or 0.55°C) but is always above normal.
- **Relapsing (or recurrent) fever**: Short periods of fever alternating with periods of normal temperatures, each lasting 1 to 2 days.

At some time in your life, you most likely have taken acetaminophen (Tylenol) or ibuprofen (Advil, Motrin) for a fever. Can you think of a reason why this may or may not be a good idea? Why should you think carefully before administering **antipyretic** (fever-reducing) medications to a client?

The answer is that fever, up to a point, is beneficial. High temperatures (up to 102.2°F, or 39°C) enhance the immune response because they (1) kill or inhibit the growth of many microorganisms, (2) enhance phagocytosis, (3) cause the breakdown of lysosomes and self-destruction of virally infected cells, and (4) cause the release of interferon, a substance that protects cells from viral infection.

This does not mean that you should *never* administer, or take, antipyretic medications. They may be needed to keep the temperature from becoming dangerously high and to promote comfort. Temperatures of 105.8°F (41.0°C) and above can damage cells throughout the body, especially in the brain, causing agitation, confusion, stupor, or coma. Vascular collapse may follow, producing cerebral edema, shock, and death. Death usually results if body temperature becomes higher than 109° to 112°F (43° to 44°C) (McCance & Huether, 2006).

What Is Heat Stroke (Hyperthermia)?

Hyperthermia, like hyperpyrexia (fever), is a body temperature above normal. However, in hyperthermia, the elevated body temperature is higher than the set point. The hypothalamic regulation of body temperature is overwhelmed and does not reset the set point as it does in fever. Hyperthermia occurs because the body cannot promote heat loss fast enough to balance heat production or high environmental temperatures. **Heat exhaustion** and **heat stroke** are common examples. With overexposure to high temperatures and inadequate fluid replacement, the body loses the ability to sweat and is unable to cool down.

Heat exhaustion may occur with a core temperature of 98.6°F (37°C) to 103°F (39.4°C). Warning signs of heat exhaustion vary, but may include weakness, nausea, vomiting, syncope, tachycardia, tachypnea, muscle aches, headache, diaphoresis (heavy sweating), and flushed skin.

Heat stroke occurs if the hyperthermia progresses to a temperature above 103°F (39.4°F). Symptoms include rapid, strong pulse; throbbing headache; delirium; confusion; impaired judgment; red, hot, dry skin; dizziness; seizures; and coma. If emergency treatment is not given, heat stroke can result in death.

What Is Hypothermia?

The Centers for Disease Control and Prevention (CDC) define **hypothermia** as an abnormally low core temperature, less than 95°F (< 35°C). You must know the person's usual normal range of temperature because many, especially older adults, have a normal temperature of less than 95°F. Hypothermia may be associated with extended exposure to cold, such as during surgery, extreme weather conditions, immersion in cold water, or lack of shelter and clothing. As the body temperature drops, metabolic processes slow. Prolonged exposure to the cold is not correctable by shivering and may prove fatal.

Early signs of hypothermia include shivering, cyanosis of lips and fingers, and poor coordination. The person first feels cold, then may feel some pain in the extremities. As body temperature continues to fall, the person experiences mental impairment, confusion, disorientation, slowing of the heart rate and respirations, and inability to take precautions from the cold.

Severe hypothermia occurs when the body temperature drops below 82.4°F (28°C). The person becomes unconscious and stops shivering. The pulse and respirations are irregular and difficult to detect. Although survival has been known to occur at a core temperature of 60.8°F (16°C), death usually results when body temperature falls below 70° to 75°F (21° to 24°C).

Hypothermia is sometimes deliberately induced under close monitoring to decrease the need for oxygen in body tissues (e.g., during cardiac or neurological surgery).

Practical **Knowledge**
knowing *how*

Now that you understand the physiology of temperature regulation, you are ready to gain the practical knowledge of how to assess and support a patient's booy temperature.

ASSESSMENT

In our daily routines, we commonly assess temperature by touch. For example, when you remove a blanket from a warming unit, you can feel that it is warm; however, you probably could not pinpoint the exact temperature of the blanket. The same is true of body temperature. Although some research has shown that people can use simple touch to detect fever, they cannot differentiate *degrees* of fever. Because vital signs are used as indicators of a client's health status, it is essential to have an accurate measure. To see the sequence of steps to take when measuring a patient's temperature, see Critical Aspects for Procedure 17-1 and

 Go to Chapter 17, **Procedure 17-1: Assessing Body Temperature,** in Volume 2.

The Home Care section of Procedure 17-1, in Volume 2, will assist you in teaching clients how to check their temperature at home.

Temperature Measurement Scales: Fahrenheit and Centigrade

Two scales are used for recording temperature: Fahrenheit and centigrade (or Celsius), a metric scale. Most people in the United States are familiar with the Fahrenheit scale; however, some healthcare agencies use centigrade. Electronic and tympanic membrane thermometers can usually measure temperature in either scale; often all you need to do is to flip a switch. Glass thermometers read only one scale (Fig. 17-3), so you may need to convert a reading from one scale to the other. For example, you may have obtained a centigrade reading for a child and plan to explain its significance to the mother, who is familiar only with Fahrenheit. For a chart to use to convert between Fahrenheit and centigrade readings,

 Go to Chapter 17, **Centigrade-Fahrenheit Conversion Chart,** in Volume 2.

 For steps to follow in *all* procedures, refer to the Universal Steps for All Procedures found on the inside back cover of Volume 2. Go to the full procedures in Volume 2 to practice and learn the procedure steps. Use these Critical Aspects later to help you review key points.

Critical Aspects of Procedures 17-1 through 17-6

Procedure 17-1: Assessing Body Temperature

➤ Clean thermometer before and after using if it is not disposable.

➤ Select the appropriate site and thermometer type.

➤ Turn on or otherwise ready the thermometer.

➤ Insert the thermometer in its sheath, or use a thermometer designated only for the patient.

➤ Insert and leave an electronic thermometer in place until it beeps; for other thermometers use the recommended times.

➤ Cleanse and store in recharging base (store glass thermometers safely to prevent breakage).

➤ For an oral temperature, obtain a reading 20 to 30 minutes after the patient consumes hot or cold food or fluids or smokes.

➤ Hold a rectal thermometer securely in place, and never leave it unattended.

Procedure 17-2: Assessing Peripheral Pulses

➤ Make sure the client is resting while you assess the pulse.

➤ Count for 15 or 30 seconds if the pulse is regular; for 60 seconds if it is irregular.

➤ Note pulse rate, rhythm, and quality.

➤ Compare pulses bilaterally.

Procedure 17-3: Assessing Apical Pulse

➤ Position the patient supine or sitting.

➤ Palpate and place the stethoscope at the 5th intercostal space at the midclavicular line.

➤ Count for 60 seconds.

➤ Note pulse rate, rhythm, and quality and the S_1 and S_2 heart sounds.

Procedure 17-4: Assessing for an Apical-Radial Pulse Deficit

➤ Palpate and place stethoscope over apex of the heart.

➤ Palpate the radial pulse.

➤ Have two nurses carry out the procedure, if possible.

➤ Count for 60 seconds, simultaneously.

➤ Compare the pulse rate at both sites; calculate the difference.

Procedure 17-5: Assessing Respirations

➤ Count unobtrusively (e.g., while palpating the radial pulse).

➤ Count for 30 seconds if respirations are regular; for 60 seconds if they are irregular.

➤ Observe the rate, rhythm, and depth of respirations.

Procedure 17-6: Measuring Blood Pressure

➤ If possible, place the patient in a sitting position, with the feet on the floor and the legs uncrossed.

➤ Measure BP after the patient has been inactive for 5 minutes.

➤ Support the patient's arm at the level of the heart.

➤ Use a cuff of the appropriate size.

➤ Wrap the cuff snugly.

➤ Inflate the cuff while palpating the artery. Inflate to 30 mm Hg above the point at which you can no longer feel the artery pulsating.

➤ Place the stethoscope on the artery, and release pressure at 2 to 3 mm Hg per second.

➤ Record systolic/diastolic pressures (first and last sounds heard—e.g., 110/80).

➤ Wait at least 2 minutes before remeasuring.

FIGURE 17-3 Glass thermometers are available with degree markings in Fahrenheit or Centigrade. *Left,* Centigrade scale. *Right,* Fahrenheit scale.

You will probably have access to a conversion chart in clinical settings, but you may sometimes need to convert mathematically. To convert from Fahrenheit to centigrade, subtract 32 from the Fahrenheit temperature and multiply by $\frac{5}{9}$. For example:

A client has a temperature of 102°F. What is his temperature as measured in centigrade?

$$(102 - 32) \times \tfrac{5}{9} = (70 \times 5) \div 9 = 39°C$$

To convert a centigrade reading to Fahrenheit, multiply the centigrade temperature by $\frac{9}{5}$, and add 32. As a cross-check we can verify the preceding example:

Client temperature = 39°C

$$(39 \times \tfrac{9}{5}) + 32 = (351 \div 5) + 32 = 102°F$$

What Equipment Do I Need?

Nurses measure temperature with various kinds of thermometers. Each type has advantages and disadvantages, so you need to think critically about the type of thermometer best suited for each patient situation. See Table 17-2 for photos and a summary of the advantages and disadvantages of various types of thermometers.

Glass Thermometers

Historically, the thermometer was a glass, mercury-filled tube marked in degrees Fahrenheit or centigrade and read visually. Because of the dangers of exposure to mercury (e.g., when thermometers break), the U.S. Environmental Protection Agency and the American Hospital Association now advise against use of equipment containing mercury (USEPA, 2001).

Electronic digital thermometers have replaced glass thermometers in most healthcare agencies. Glass thermometers containing other liquids, such as alcohol or gallium–indium–tin (galinstan), are available and some agencies still use them.

Electronic Thermometers

An electronic thermometer is a rechargeable unit consisting of an electronic probe attached to a portable unit by a thin wire. A beep sounds when the peak temperature is reached. Disposable plastic sheaths are used to cover the probe. To prevent transmission of infection, you discard the sheath after each use. Most units have a separate probe for rectal and oral temperatures, color-coded red and blue, respectively, to be certain the correct probe is used.

Table 17-2 ➤ Advantages and Disadvantages of Various Thermometers		
TYPE OF THERMOMETER	**ADVANTAGES**	**DISADVANTAGES**
Glass Thermometer	■ Flexibility of use: Can be used for measuring oral, rectal, or axillary temperature. ■ Inexpensive initial cost ■ Accuracy, as indicated by several studies ■ Easily disinfected	Do not use glass thermometers containing mercury. If you find one, recommend that it be replaced immediately. ■ Easily broken, so there is ongoing cost of replacement and risk for injury ■ Slow: It takes 3–8 minutes to obtain an accurate reading, depending on the site. ■ Difficult for some people to read accurately

Continued

Table 17-2 ➤ Advantages and Disadvantages of Various Thermometers—cont'd

TYPE OF THERMOMETER	ADVANTAGES	DISADVANTAGES
Electronic Thermometer 	■ Flexibility of use: Can be used for measuring oral, rectal, or axillary temperature. ■ Ease of use ■ Rapid measurement: It takes 2–60 seconds to obtain reading, depending on the unit.	■ Expensive initial cost ■ Requires regular inspection and maintenance to ensure accuracy. ■ Data are conflicting regarding their accuracy compared to other types of thermometer. ■ Need to be kept charged.
Electronic with Infrared Sensor A, Temporal scanner B, Otic thermometer	■ Ease of use ■ Rapid measurement: It takes 2–5 seconds to measure the temperature. ■ May be the most cost-effective method because of time and labor savings from their rapid reading capabilities. ■ Low rate of operator error	■ Expensive initial cost. ■ Less accurate than electronic or glass thermometers when used for tympanic membrane temperatures, as some studies indicate. ■ Requires regular inspection and maintenance to ensure accuracy. ■ Batteries require recharging.
Disposable Chemical Thermometer 	■ Ease of use; requires no special training.	■ Less accurate than glass or electronic thermometers ■ May not reflect true temperature reading; less reliable than other thermometers ■ The skin must be dry ■ Indicates only body surface temperature; does not reflect core.

Electronic Infrared Thermometers

The electronic infrared thermometer is a rechargeable unit that contains a sensor that detects heat in the form of infrared energy given off by the body, for example, at the tympanic membrane or at the temporal artery. The thermometer does not actually touch the tympanic membrane. A beep sounds when the peak temperature is reached.

Disposable Chemical Thermometers

A disposable chemical thermometer is a thin plastic strip, patch, or tape containing a matrix of chemicals that change color at a designated body temperature. Most are used once for an oral or axillary reading, then disposed of. Another form consists of temperature-sensitive tape containing liquid crystals that change color in response to temperature. The tape is applied to the skin of the forehead or abdomen and left for a time specified by the manufacturer (e.g., 15 seconds). Disposable thermometers are useful in the home and for patients in protective isolation. Although there is some conflicting research, they are associated with more errors than glass or electronic thermometers. They are also unreliable, tending to overestimate or underestimate true readings.

Other Types of Thermometers

For special uses, devices have been created to take measurements from the nasopharynx, the pulmonary artery, the bladder, and the skin. A wireless intestinal temperature monitoring system in the form of a pill and an external receiver is sometimes used, for example, during cardiac surgery. Infrared devices have also been used to take thermal measurements of skin surface temperature.

What Sites Should I Use?

Temperatures in the pulmonary artery, esophagus, and bladder accurately measure core temperature. These sites are used in surgery and intensive care, but they are invasive, expensive, and impractical for most clinical settings. Pulmonary artery temperature is considered the "gold standard" to which other sites are compared. A device is placed in the pulmonary artery, and readings are continuously displayed on a monitor.

The usual sites for intermittent measurements are the mouth, rectum, axillae, tympanic membrane, and skin over the temporal artery. These sites allow the thermometer to contact body tissues that are well supplied with blood vessels. This is essential for accurate measurement. Each site has advantages and disadvantages, so you must choose the safest, most accurate, and most reliable site for each client (Table 17-3).

Temperature readings vary depending on the site used. Be aware that research on site differences is conflicting, for example:

1. Temporal artery temperature is usually about the same as rectal temperature.
2. Some researchers report tympanic membrane temperatures to be higher than oral measurements; others have found them to be lower.

Table 17-3 ➤ Disadvantages and Contraindications of Various Sites for Measuring Temperature			
SITE	**ADVANTAGES**	**DISADVANTAGES**	**CONTRAINDICATIONS**
Temporal Artery	▪ Most accurate representation of core temperature ▪ Fast. Most scanners provide a reading in about 3 seconds. ▪ No discomfort is associated with the procedure. ▪ Safe. Can be used even for those who cannot follow instructions (e.g., infants). ▪ Less prone to error than tympanic thermometer	▪ Requires special scanning thermometer. ▪ Any covering, hat, hair, and so forth, prevents heat from dissipating and causes the reading to be falsely high. This is also true for the side of the head lying on a pillow	
Rectal	▪ Most accurately represents core (internal) body temperature. ▪ Use for clients who are unable to follow directions for oral temperature monitoring, or in situations where accuracy is crucial.	▪ Most clients find this method objectionable or embarrassing. ▪ Not recommended as the first choice of site because of the risk for injury to the rectal mucosa, especially infants. ▪ Requires special positioning of the client. ▪ Does not reflect changes in core temperature as rapidly as the oral method. ▪ Presence of stool may cause inaccurate reading.	▪ Clients who may be injured by the method (e.g., clients who have a rectal disease, severe diarrhea, or rectal surgery; newborns, whose rectal mucosa is fragile) ▪ Because it can slow the heart rate by stimulating the vagus nerve, this method is sometimes contraindicated for clients with cardiac surgery and some heart conditions. ▪ Clients with hemorrhoids ▪ Immunosuppressed clients or those with clotting disorders

Continued

Table 17-3 ➤ Disadvantages and Contraindications of Various Sites for Measuring Temperature—cont'd

SITE	ADVANTAGES	DISADVANTAGES	CONTRAINDICATIONS
Oral	▪ Simple, convenient ▪ Comfortable for most patients ▪ Safe for adults and children who are old enough to follow simple directions	▪ Glass thermometers can break if bitten. ▪ Slow; requires up to 8 minutes to ensure an accurate reading (if glass thermometer used). ▪ Patient must keep her mouth closed for several minutes (glass thermometers). ▪ Eating, drinking (e.g., ice water, hot tea), and smoking in the 30 minutes before measurement affect the accuracy of the reading. ▪ Bradypnea may create false temperature elevations.	▪ Clients who cannot cooperate with the instructions or who might be injured (e.g., infants and small children; patients who have had oral surgery, breathe through the mouth, have chills, or are confused or unconscious)
Axillary	▪ Safe ▪ Easy to use ▪ Can be used for children and for uncooperative or unconscious clients. ▪ Recommended over rectal site for routine measurements	▪ Not reflective of core temperature ▪ Considered one of the least accurate sites ▪ Diaphoresis (sweating) can affect the reading. ▪ Thermometer may need to be left in place for a long time (8 minutes if glass is used).	▪ Clients who are perspiring heavily ▪ Does not accurately diagnose fever. If fever is suspected, confirm with measurement from another route.

Tympanic Membrane	▪ Fast (2–5 seconds)
	▪ Can be used for children and for uncooperative or unconscious clients.
		▪ Requires a special thermometer, a relatively expensive initial purchase
		▪ More variable than oral and rectal sites:
		  Must be carefully positioned to ensure accuracy; prone to caregiver measurement errors.
		  Presence of cerumen (earwax) may affect accuracy.
		  Significant differences have been found between readings in left and right ear of same patient.
		▪ Risk of injury to tympanic membrane if not positioned carefully to avoid touching it.
		▪ May be uncomfortable for the client.
		▪ Chemical thermometers (skin temperatures) have been found to be more accurate and reliable than tympanic membrane instruments.
		▪ Hearing aids must be removed.
			▪ Clients who have had recent ear surgery
			▪ Contraindicated in the presence of ear infection

Table 17-3 ➤ Disadvantages and Contraindications of Various Sites for Measuring Temperature—cont'd			
SITE	**ADVANTAGES**	**DISADVANTAGES**	**CONTRAINDICATIONS**
Skin (e.g., forehead)	■ Safe, convenient ■ Easy to use for nonprofessionals ■ Can be used when other sites are contraindicated. ■ Inexpensive (chemical paper or tape is used)	■ Forehead skin temperature is generally 2°–4°F (1°–2°C) less than core temperature; if marked deviations in skin temperatures are detected, the readings must be confirmed via a more reliable route.	■ Should not be used when accurate, reliable readings are required (e.g., in the presence of hypothermia or heatstroke). ■ However, at least one study has shown skin temperatures to be accurate and reliable when obtained with an infrared skin thermometer (DeCurtis, Calzolari, Marciano, et al., 2008).

From lowest to highest readings, the sites are generally thought to be as follows: axillary, oral, tympanic membrane, rectal, and temporal artery. For oral, axillary, and rectal temperatures, there is an approximately 0.8°F or 0.4°C difference between each site and the next higher one. For convenience, nurses tend to round the fraction up to a full 1°F (0.5°C). For example, an axillary temperature of 98.1°F is similar to an oral reading of 99.1°F or a rectal reading of 100.1°F. Use this *only* to help you understand your patient's data. You cannot reliably convert temperatures mathematically between sites. If you take an oral temperature, for instance, record the value you obtain and the site used.

 Critical**Thinking** 17-2

- Convert the following temperatures and analyze the readings. What might they mean?
  - a. 38.5°C _____ °F
  - b. 96.5°F _____ °C
  - c. 37.0°C _____ °F
- Rank the expected early evening temperatures of the following individuals from lowest to highest.
  - a. A 22-year-old college athlete
  - b. A 5-year-old kindergarten student
  - c. An 88-year-old nursing home resident

◼ ANALYSIS/NURSING DIAGNOSIS

Fever and hypothermia may be medical diagnoses, nursing diagnoses, or symptoms of other problems. The following nursing diagnoses may be used when they are considered to be a *client problem* and not just a symptom of an illness or other problem (e.g., fever may be a symptom of problems such as Deficient Fluid Volume, or dehydration). Notice that the nursing diagnosis of Hyperthermia can be used both for temperature elevation from fever (hyperpyrexia) and from heat exhaustion (hyperthermia).

- *Hyperthermia* is diagnosed when a person's body temperature is above normal. Defining characteristics are convulsions, flushed skin, tachycardia, tachypnea, and warmth to touch.

- *Hypothermia* is diagnosed when a person's body temperature is below normal range. Defining characteristics include cool skin, cyanotic nail beds, elevated blood pressure, pallor, piloerection, shivering, slow capillary refill, and tachycardia.
- *Ineffective Thermoregulation* applies when a person's temperature fluctuates above and below the normal range.
- *Risk for Imbalanced Body Temperature* is used when the temperature is normal but the client is at risk for failure to maintain body temperature within the normal range (e.g., newborns and the frail elderly). As you can see, this diagnosis can also apply to risk for either hypothermia or fever.

◼ PLANNING OUTCOMES/EVALUATION

Associated NOC standardized outcomes for Hyperthermia, Hypothermia, Ineffective Thermoregulation, and Risk for Imbalanced Body Temperature include the following: Thermoregulation, Thermoregulation: Newborn, and Vital Signs. Also,

 Go to Chapter 17, **Standardized Language,** in Volume 2.

Individualized goals/outcome statements you might write for a client with Hyperthermia include the following:

- Oral temperature of < 97.6°F (36.4°C) (client's usual normal temperature)
- No clinical signs of fever present (e.g., no chills or flushing)
- Pulse and respiratory rates within normal range for patient

For a client with Hypothermia, the following are examples of goal statements.

- Oral temperature > 97.6°F (36.4°C) (client's usual normal temperature)
- No clinical signs of Hypothermia present (e.g., no disorientation, no decrease in urine output)
- Pulse and respiratory rates within normal range

Use the goals set in the planning outcomes stage to evaluate client responses to interventions.

PLANNING INTERVENTIONS/IMPLEMENTATION

Overall care of the patient depends on the disease causing the fever or hypothermia, and on specific orders from the physician. Nevertheless, there are nursing interventions and activities that address fever and hypothermia, regardless of the cause.

Hyperthermia Interventions

NIC standardized interventions for Hyperthermia and Ineffective Thermoregulation include Fever Treatment, Malignant Hyperthermia Precautions, Newborn Care, Temperature Regulation, Temperature Regulation: Intraoperative, and Vital Signs Monitoring. Also,

 Go to Chapter 17, **Standardized Language,** in Volume 2.

Specific nursing activities for clients with fever and/or nursing diagnoses of Hyperthermia or Ineffective Thermoregulation include the following:

- Provide focused assessments such as the following:
  Help determine the cause of the fever. For example, you may collect specimens from various body sites for culture.
  Monitor the temperature and other VS at least every 2 hours, and more often if the temperature is rising rapidly or if the clinical symptoms are changing. Recall that the increased metabolism accompanying a fever also increases the pulse and respirations. There is conflicting evidence regarding the accuracy and sensitivity of infrared tympanic thermometers and disposable thermometers; therefore, when you suspect fever, it is wise to take a rectal reading with a different type of thermometer for comparison. Obtain an oral reading if the rectal site is contraindicated.
  Observe for the clinical signs that accompany a fever. Symptoms vary, depending on the phase of the fever. The characteristic symptoms include flushed face; dry, hot skin; eyes that appear bright and somewhat apprehensive; rapid, shallow respirations; increased heart rate; unusual thirst; loss of appetite; headache; and complaints of nausea. If the fever is extreme, urine may be concentrated and decreased in volume. Seizures, confusion, or delirium can also be associated with very high fevers.
- Provide collaborative care to treat the underlying cause of the fever. For example, you may administer antibiotics that a physician prescribes to treat a bacterial infection.
- Provide oral or intravenous fluids to replace fluids lost through diaphoresis. They help prevent dehydration or hypovolemia (fluid deficiency) secondary to the fever.
- Use nonpharmacological measures to reduce fever. The following measures are likely to produce shivering, which produces heat; therefore, they can actually raise instead of lower the patient's temperature. When using these measures, be careful not to cause your patient to shiver.
  Cooling blankets that circulate water
  Alcohol or tepid baths
  Cloth-covered ice packs or cool washcloths to the groin, neck, or axillae
  Circulating fan in the room
  Instructing the client to use minimal bed covers
- Provide nutritional support. Food is essential to meet the increased energy needs created by the high metabolic rate accompanying fever. However, lack of appetite often accompanies fever, so food must be made appealing to the patient.
- Provide special mouth care. Apply a water-soluble lip lubricant. Lips may become dry and cracked, the tongue may be swollen, and sores may be present.
- Keep clothing and bed linens dry to promote comfort and help prevent chilling. Recall that diaphoresis occurs during defervescence.
- Provide emergency treatment, if necessary. Heat stroke is a medical emergency because death can occur rapidly. Cooling blankets or cool water baths can be used successfully if the surface temperature is not lowered too quickly. Rapid lowering of the surface temperature causes vasoconstriction, which delays core cooling.
- Teach emergency treatment for hyperthermia and hyperpyrexia at home: Immediately move the person to a shady area if he is outdoors. Cool the victim by placing him in a tub of cool water or a cool shower, or sponging with cool water.
- Advise older adults to stay in air-conditioned buildings when the outside temperature is extremely high; to take cool baths and showers, limit physical activity, and drink plenty of nonalcoholic and noncaffeinated fluids.
- Advise family to check on elderly neighbors and family members at least twice a day, and make sure they have an electric fan.

Hypothermia Interventions

NIC standardized interventions recommended for Hypothermia and Ineffective Thermoregulation include Hypothermia Treatment, Newborn Care, Temperature Regulation, Temperature Regulation: Intraoperative, and Vital Signs Monitoring. Also,

 Go to Chapter 17, **Standardized Language,** in Volume 2.

Specific nursing activities include the following:

- Provide warm, dry clothing, warm drinks, warm blankets, and a warm environment. For mild cases of Hypothermia, this may be enough to restore normal temperature.
- For patients with a temperature below 86°F (30°C), also use warmed intravenous fluids, heating pads or heating blankets, and/or warm baths.
- Give warm, sweet drinks if the person is conscious.

■ Rewarm a patient who is severely hypothermic gradually to prevent complications, such as shock or dysrhythmias (abnormal heartbeats) and to ensure core, as well as surface, warming.

> *Don't* use electric blankets. Vasoconstricted skin burns easily.
>
> *Don't* apply pulse oximetry probes to a vasoconstricted finger.

■ Focused assessments include the following:

> Monitor the temperature and other VS frequently. Hypothermia causes vasoconstriction, coagulation in the microcirculation, and tissue ischemia (lack of oxygen). In the heart, this can lead to dysrhythmias.
>
> Observe for the following symptoms of hypothermia:
>
> Body temperature <95°F (<35°C)
>
> Decreased or irregular pulse, respirations, and blood pressure

A subjective feeling of being cold

Severe shivering (only initially)

Pale, cool, shiny skin

Decreased urine output

Disorientation and/or drowsiness

Critical Thinking 17-3

Recall the clients you encountered at the community health fair. Two-year-old Jason's axillary temperature was 101.8°F (38.8°C); his skin was warm, dry, and flushed. His mother told you that he had been eating poorly and was very irritable.

■ What changes in behavior alert you that something is wrong?

■ Do you have enough theoretical knowledge or patient information to know what is going on?

■ What, if any, additional information about the patient situation do you need?

Toward Evidence-Based Practice

Lawson, L., Bridges, E. J., Ballou, I., et al. (2007). Accuracy and precision of noninvasive temperature measurement in adult intensive care patients. *American Journal of Critical Care*, 16(5), 485–496.

Over a period of 6 months, researchers took repeated measurements at various sites, including the gold standard pulmonary artery catheter, from 60 adults with cardiopulmonary disease in intensive care. They found oral and temporal artery measurements to be the most accurate and precise. Axillary measurements were less accurate, and ear measurements were the least accurate and precise.

Robinson, J. L., Jou, H., & Spady, D. W. (2005). Accuracy of parents in measuring body temperature with a tympanic thermometer. *BMC Family Practice*, 6(1), 3.

Parents and then nurses measured the temperatures of 60 children with a tympanic thermometer designed for home use. Nurses also measured the temperatures with a model of tympanic thermometer commonly used in hospitals. The readings done by parents were significantly different from the readings by nurses using the hospital thermometer a majority of the time, and parents failed to detect fever about 25% of the time.

Heusch, A. I., & McCarthy, P. W. (2005). The patient: A novel source of error in clinical temperature measurement using infrared aural thermometry. *Journal of Alternative & Complementary Medicine*, 11(3), 473–476.

Researchers used an infrared tympanic thermometer to measure the temperatures of 132 subjects, ages 18 to 48 years, who were asymptomatic with no known pathological problems. Temperatures were measured in both ears. There was a significant difference in the temperature in the left compared with the right ear. Also, at temperatures below 36.7°C, the left ear registered a lower temperature than the

right. At temperatures above 36.7°C, the left ear registered a higher temperature than the right ear. Researchers suggested that averaging the temperature in both ears might increase the reliability of infrared tympanic thermometers.

Farnell, S., Maxwell, L., Tan, S., et al. (2005). Temperature measurement: Comparison of non-invasive methods used in adult critical care. *Journal of Clinical Nursing*, 14(5), 632–639.

Researchers took 160 sets of temperature measurements from 25 adult intensive care patients, using a chemical (Tempa·DOT™) and a tympanic thermometer. Patients' temperatures were also being measuring with the gold standard pulmonary artery catheter. They found the chemical thermometer to be more accurate and reliable than the tympanic thermometer. However, compared with the pulmonary artery catheter, both methods were associated with erroneous readings.

1. Make a table containing the following:
   a. The name of the first researcher (e.g., Lawson)
   b. The number and type of subjects in the study
   c. What each study found about *tympanic* temperature measurements

2. Imagine that you are managing a residential long-term care facility that has recently purchased new tympanic thermometers to replace the old mercury-in-glass thermometers. In this facility, VS are routinely taken by nursing assistive personnel. What implications do these four studies have for actions you might need to take? What, in general terms, do you plan to do, and why?

Go to Chapter 17, **Toward Evidence-Based Practice Suggested Responses,** on the Student Resource Disk or DavisPlus at http://davisplus.fadavis.com/Wilkinson2

CarePlanning & MappingPractice

For Care Planning/Care Mapping practice,

Go to Chapter Resources, **Care Planning & Care Mapping Practice**, on DavisPlus at http://davisplus.fadavis.com/Wilkinson2

Pulse

The **pulse** is the rhythmic expansion of an artery produced when a bolus of blood is forced into it by contraction of the heart.

Theoretical Knowledge knowing why

To assess and support regulation of a client's pulse, you will need to know the normal pulse range, how the pulse is produced and regulated, and factors that influence pulse rate. There is little research related to measurement of pulse rate.

What Is a Normal Pulse Rate?

Pulse rate is measured in beats per minute. The normal range for healthy young and middle-aged adults is 60 to 100 beats/min, with an average rate of 70 to 80 beats/min. Table 17-1 identifies average pulse rates for adults. For average pulse rates for other age groups,

Go to Chapter 17, **Tables, Boxes, Figures: ESG Table 17-1,** on the Student Resource Disk or DavisPlus at http://davisplus.fadavis.com/Wilkinson2

An important reason to assess the pulse is to identify when more advanced monitoring is required. When the heart rate is of concern, you will most likely use a cardiac monitor to determine not only the rate, but also the rhythm of the pulse.

How Does the Body Produce and Regulate the Pulse?

The pulse wave begins when the left heart ventricle contracts and ends when it relaxes. Each contraction forces blood into the already filled aorta, increasing pressure within the arterial system. The intermittent pressure and expansion of the arteries causes the blood to move along in a wavelike motion toward the capillaries. You can palpate a light tap at the peak of the wave, when the artery expands. The trough (low point) of a pulse wave occurs when the artery contracts to push the blood along its way. The peak of the wave corresponds to **systole,** or the contraction of the heart; the trough corresponds to **diastole,** or the resting phase of the heart.

Stroke volume is the quantity of blood forced out by each contraction of the left ventricle. You will not usually know your patient's actual stroke volume, though it averages 70 mL in most healthy adults. If stroke volume decreases (as in a large blood loss, or *hemorrhage*), the body tries to maintain the same cardiac output by increasing the pulse rate. The **cardiac output** is the total quantity of blood pumped per minute. It is expressed in liters per minute and calculated as follows:

Cardiac output = stroke volume × pulse (heart) rate

For a person with a pulse of 80 beats/min and an average stroke volume (70 mL), the cardiac output would be about 5600 mL (or 5.6 liters) per minute.

The autonomic nervous system regulates the heart rate. Sympathetic stimulation increases the heart rate (and thus the cardiac output); parasympathetic stimulation decreases it. We discuss this in more detail in Chapter 35.

What Factors Influence the Pulse Rate?

In a healthy adult, the peripheral pulse rate is the same as the heart rate. Therefore, taking the pulse is a quick and simple way to assess the condition of the heart, blood vessels, and circulation. The pulse changes in response to changes in the volume of blood pumped through the heart, variations in heart rate, changes in the elasticity of the arterial walls, or any condition that interferes with heart function. Because the heart and blood vessels are regulated by the nervous system, conditions that interfere with normal functioning of the nervous system also affect the pulse. Other factors that may cause variations in pulse rate, rhythm, or quality include the following:

- *Developmental level.* Newborns have a rapid pulse rate. The rate stabilizes in childhood and gradually slows through old age.
- *Sex.* Adult women have a slightly more rapid pulse rate than do adult men.
- *Exercise.* Muscle activity normally increases the pulse rate. After exercise, a well-conditioned heart returns to normal more quickly than a nonconditioned heart. Also, people who are well conditioned have lower heart rates, both before and during exercise, than those who are not.
- *Food.* Ingestion of food causes a slight increase in pulse rate for several hours.
- *Stress.* Stress triggers the fight-or-flight sympathetic nervous system response, which increases both pulse rate and strength of the heart contractions (stroke volume).
- *Fever.* The pulse rate tends to increase about 10 beats/min for each degree Fahrenheit of temperature elevation. The reasons are that (1) the metabolic rate increases and (2) the body attempts to compensate for the decrease in blood pressure produced by the peripheral vasodilation that occurs with fever.
- *Disease.* Diseases, such as heart disease, hyperthyroidism, respiratory diseases, and infections, are generally associated with increased pulse rates. Hypothyroidism is associated with decreased pulse rates.
- *Blood loss.* Small blood loss is generally well tolerated and produces only a temporary increase in pulse rate. Theoretically, a large blood loss stimulates the

sympathetic nervous system, bringing about an increase in pulse rate to compensate for the decreased blood volume. However, some studies suggest that VS are limited in their ability to detect large blood losses; stable pulse and blood pressure alone do not ensure that there has been no blood loss.

- *Position changes.* Standing and sitting positions generally cause a temporary increase in pulse rate and decrease in blood pressure as a result of blood pooling in the veins of the feet and legs. This decreases blood return to the heart, decreasing blood pressure and subsequently increasing heart rate.
- *Medications.* Stimulant drugs (e.g., epinephrine) increase pulse rate. Cardiotonics (e.g., digitalis) and opioids (e.g., narcotic analgesics) or sedative drugs decrease pulse rate.

Practical **Knowledge**
knowing how

Now that you understand some of the processes and factors that produce and affect the pulse, you are ready to gain the practical knowledge of how to assess and support this aspect of physical functioning.

ASSESSMENT

Assess the pulse by **palpation** (feeling) or **auscultation** (listening with a stethoscope). To palpate the pulse, select the pulse site and lightly compress the client's artery against the underlying bone with the index and middle finger of one of your hands. When a client's pulse is difficult to palpate, you may need to use a Doppler device, which has an ultrasound transducer that transmits the pulse sounds to an audio unit. For a summary of the steps for assessing a client's peripheral pulse, see the Critical Aspects box for Procedure 17-2. For the full procedure,

 Go to Chapter 17, **Procedure 17-2: Assessing Peripheral Pulses,** in Volume 2.

What Equipment Do I Need?

To count the pulse, you need a watch or clock with a second hand or digital display. To auscultate the pulse, you will use a stethoscope. The stethoscope does not magnify sounds, but rather blocks out noise so that you can hear blood pressure and other faint sounds. A **stethoscope** consists of a sound-transmitting device (bell and diaphragm) that is attached to earpieces by rubber tubing and hollow metal tubes (Fig. 17-4). With the earpieces in place, you can use the bell to hear low-frequency sounds (e.g., certain heart sounds). Use the diaphragm to assess high-frequency sounds (e.g., lung sounds).

Stethoscopes can be either single lumen or double lumen. A single-lumen stethoscope has one tube connected to the chestpiece; a double-lumen stethoscope

FIGURE 17-4 *A,* A stethoscope. *B,* The bell, for low-frequency sounds. *C,* The diaphragm, for high-frequency sounds.

has two tubes attached to the chestpiece. Double-lumen stethoscopes are more sensitive than single-lumen instruments.

Most stethoscopes come with soft earpieces that help seal your ear canal to block room noise from interfering with the sound. Stethoscopes have varying lengths of tubing. Short tubing requires you to be close to the patient and to bend more, but the sound may be a bit better than with longer tubing, which is more likely to rub against the body or clothing. Some stethoscopes are made to work effectively through clothing; however, unless you know you are using that type you should place the instrument directly on the skin. Digital stethoscopes are also available, to provide sound clarity in noisy environments and with obese patients.

✚ To prevent cross-contamination, always clean your stethoscope before and after using it to examine a patient. Use a 70% alcohol or benzalkonium chloride wipe. Most stethoscopes are colonized by bacteria, although only a small percentage are pathogenic. Cleaning can reduce the bacterial count by 94% to 100% (CDC, 2005; Kennedy, Dreimanis, Beckingham, et al., 2003; Rutala & Weber, 2004). Antimicrobial stethoscope covers have been developed to prevent surface contamination; however, their effectiveness is still in question. A few agencies have wall-mounted "single swipe" sterilizers for sterilizing stethoscopes. Also, you should not wear a stethoscope around your neck.

What Sites Should I Use?

Nurses assess the pulse at the apex of the heart (**apical pulse**) or at a place where an artery can be pressed by the fingers against a bone (**peripheral pulses**). Peripheral sites are shown in Figure 17-5 and include the radial, brachial, dorsalis pedis, posterior tibial, carotid, femoral, popliteal, and temporal arteries.

The choice of pulse sites depends on the reason for assessing the pulse and/or the accessibility of a site. To measure a peripheral pulse, you would, for example, use the:

- *Radial artery* for routine assessment of vital signs. This is the most commonly used site because it is easily found and readily accessible.
- *Brachial artery* when performing cardiopulmonary resuscitation (CPR) of infants.
- *Carotid artery* when performing CPR of inpatient adults and for assessing circulation to the brain.

✚ Palpate only one side of the neck at a time to avoid interrupting circulation to the head. Palpate lightly so that you don't occlude the artery; and don't massage the area because that can decrease the heart rate and blood pressure. Lay persons should not check the carotid pulse.

- *Dorsalis pedis* (also called *pedal pulse*) and *posterior tibial* arteries for assessing peripheral circulation.
- *Femoral artery* to determine circulation to the legs, in cases of cardiac arrest, and for children.
- *Popliteal artery* for assessing circulation to the lower leg.

Critical Thinking 17-4

- If you obtain a very slow radial pulse, how might you check to be sure your count is accurate?
- What kind of nursing knowledge does this require (i.e., theoretical, practical, self, or ethical knowledge)?

When Should I Take an Apical Pulse?

The apical pulse reading is the most accurate of the pulses. In a healthy person, the apical and peripheral pulses should be about the same. However, in some cardiovascular diseases, they can differ. If the heartbeat is weak, for example, some beats may be too weak to feel in a peripheral site. In this case, you would obtain a lower count for the radial than for the apical pulse. The apical pulse would accurately reflect the heartbeat. Use the apical site when:

- The radial pulse is weak or irregular.
- The rate is <60 beats/min or >100 beats/min.
- The patient is taking cardiac medications (e.g., digitalis).
- Assessing infants and children up to age 3 (because peripheral pulses may be difficult to palpate).

To assess the apical pulse, auscultate and count the number of heartbeats at the apex of the heart. For an adult, this site is on the anterior chest at 3 inches (8 cm) or less to the left of the sternum, at the 4th, 5th, or 6th intercostal space at the midclavicular line. For children, the location is different, depending on age (Fig. 17-6). You will hear two sounds, "lub" and "dub," as the heart valves close. Count each pair of sounds ("lub-dub") as one heartbeat. For step-by-step instructions, see the summary in the Critical Aspects box, and

 VOL 2 Go to Chapter 17, **Procedure 17-3: Assessing the Apical Pulse,** in Volume 2.

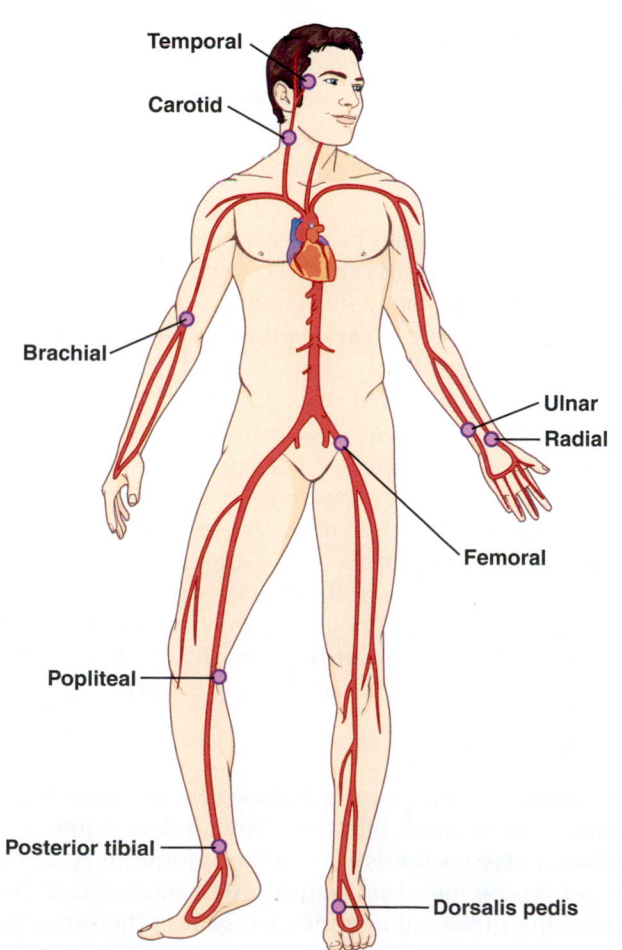

Temporal
Carotid
Brachial
Ulnar
Radial
Femoral
Popliteal
Posterior tibial
Dorsalis pedis

FIGURE 17-5 Sites commonly used for assessing a pulse.

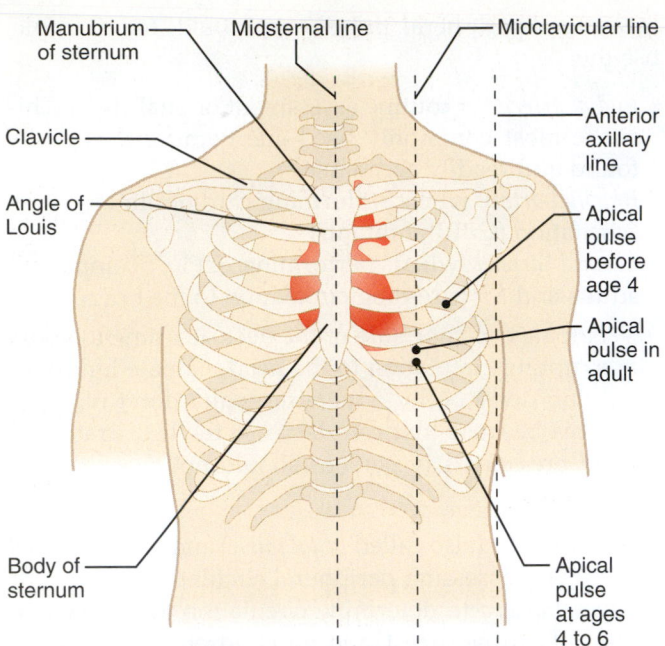

FIGURE 17-6 Location of apical pulse for adults and children.

When Should I Take an Apical–Radial Pulse?

You will sometimes need to obtain a radial and apical pulse reading at the same time to assess for heart function or the presence of heart irregularities. A difference between the two counts **(pulse deficit)** indicates that not all apex beats are being transmitted or felt at the radial artery. As you are listening at the apical site, you will hear a beat without feeling a pulse at the radial artery. You should report pulse deficits promptly to the primary care provider. See the Critical Aspects box for a summary, and

 Go to Chapter 17, **Procedure 17-4: Assessing for an Apical-Radial Pulse Deficit,** in Volume 2.

KnowledgeCheck 17-2

For each of the following, would you expect the pulse rate to be greater or less than the normal adult rate of 80 beats/min?

- A healthy, professional tennis player
- A newborn infant
- An adolescent who has just finished running track
- A client who has just undergone a painful procedure
- A client with a fever
- An accident victim who is hemorrhaging
- A 90-year-old man

 Go to Chapter 17, **Knowledge Check Response Sheet and Answers,** on the Student Resource Disk or DavisPlus at http://davisplus.fadavis.com/Wilkinson2

What Data Should I Collect?

A nurse has documented the following data for five patients:

Patient A: Radial pulse 80 beats/min, strong, regular, and equal bilaterally (the same in both arms)

Patient B: Pedal pulse 96 beats/min, regular, moderate volume, but stronger in the left ankle than the right

Patient C: Brachial pulse 86 beats/min in both arms, slightly irregular; skips about every fifth beat; weak but stronger in left arm

Patient D: Apical pulse 60 beats/min, slightly irregular; heart sounds clearly auscultated

Patient E: Radial pulse 92 beats/min, irregular—beats in triplets—weak, equal bilaterally

What types of information has the nurse gathered about these patients' pulses? (At least three different characteristics of the pulse are represented in the nurse's charting; look for patterns.)

Did you see that for each patient the nurse recorded the rate, rhythm (or pattern), and quality (or volume) of the pulse? If so, well done. Notice also that the nurse compared each patient's left side to the right side.

Rate

To assess the pulse **rate,** count the number of beats per minute while palpating or auscultating. Begin the count with one, rather than zero (Hwu, Coates, & Lin, 2000). For normal, healthy adults, you can determine the rate of a regular heart rhythm by counting the pulse for 15 seconds and multiplying by 4. Research is conflicting, but some studies indicate that a 30-second count is more accurate. If the pulse is irregular or slow, always count for a full minute. Rates below 60 beats/min are known as **bradycardia** (*brady* = slow, *cardia* = heart). Rates in excess of 100 beats/min are known as **tachycardia** (*tachy* = rapid, *cardia* = heart).

Rhythm

The intervals between heartbeats establish a pulse pattern known as the **rhythm.** Normally, the heart beats at regular intervals, much like a metronome. When the intervals between beats vary enough to be noticeable, the rhythm is abnormal **(dysrhythmia).** Abnormal rhythms may be single beats that occur too early or too late, or a group of irregular beats that form a pattern. When assessing an irregular pulse, it is important to determine whether the beat is *regularly irregular* (an irregular rhythm that forms a pattern) or *irregularly irregular* (an unpredictable rhythm). To make this distinction, you must count the rate for a full minute. An irregular heart rhythm can be very serious and may require additional assessment by **electrocardiogram (ECG),** a procedure that traces the electrical pattern of the heart.

Quality

The **quality** of the pulse is assessed by determining the pulse volume and bilateral (both sides) equality of pulses. **Pulse volume** refers to the amount of force produced by the blood pulsing through the arteries. Normally, the pulse volume for each beat is the same. The following terminology refers to pulse volume; numbers are assigned on a scale of 0 to 3.

0—Absent: Pulse cannot be felt.

1—Weak or thready: Pulse is barely felt and can be easily obliterated by pressing with the fingers.

2—Normal quality: Pulse is easily palpated, not weak or bounding.

3—Bounding or full: Pulse is easily felt with little pressure; not easily obliterated.

Bilateral equality is useful in determining whether the blood flow to a body part is adequate. Assess bilateral equality by comparing the pulses on both sides of the body for equal volume. For example, if you are concerned about the circulation to the left hand, assess both the right and left radial arteries to determine whether the volume is the same. If the pulses feel the same, they are said to be *equal in strength bilaterally*. If one pulse is stronger than the other, then the pulses are *unequal bilaterally*. You would record, "Radial pulses unequal in strength bilaterally; weaker in left arm." You may also document the equality by using a pulse volume scale. For example, you might record, "Radial pulses unequal in strength bilaterally; Right 2, Left 1."

If a peripheral pulse is absent or weak, it may be because the circulation is compromised in that extremity. If this is the case, then pallor or cyanosis may be present. **Pallor** refers to the paleness of skin in one area when compared to another part of the body. **Cyanosis** is a bluish or grayish discoloration of the skin due to deficient oxygen in the blood. For example, when circulation to the lower extremities is compromised, the feet often appear pale in comparison to the trunk or arms, the dorsalis pedis and/or posterior tibial pulses may be weak or absent, and the feet may feel cool to the touch.

ANALYSIS/NURSING DIAGNOSIS

An abnormal pulse may present as weak, thready, bounding, irregular, or absent. Pulse changes are symptoms, not problems. Therefore, nursing diagnoses are useful for describing the condition that is *causing* the pulse changes. By itself, a change in pulse (e.g., weak and thready) is not adequate to support the following diagnoses. Other symptoms must also be present.

- Ineffective Tissue Perfusion (Peripheral) can be used when a pulse is absent or weak and cool, pale skin is present.
- Risk for Impaired Skin Integrity and Risk for Impaired Tissue Integrity may be used as secondary diagnoses when Ineffective Tissue Perfusion is present. If tissue is not adequately perfused, tissue ischemia and necrosis (death of tissue) may occur.
- Deficient Fluid Volume may cause the pulse to be weak and thready.
- Excess Fluid Volume may cause the pulse to be bounding and full.
- Decreased Cardiac Output may cause tachycardia, bradycardia, or changes in pulse volume.

PLANNING OUTCOMES/EVALUATION

NOC standardized outcomes include the following:

- Vital Signs Status is the only outcome that directly pertains to assessing the pulse.
- Other outcomes depend upon the nursing diagnosis causing the pulse changes. For example, Ineffective Peripheral Tissue Perfusion can be monitored with the NOC label of Circulation Status.

Some *individualized goal/outcome statements* you might write for pulse status follow:

- Apical pulse will be 60 to 80 beats/min when at rest.
- Pedal pulses will be 80 to 100 beats/min, 2 (on a scale of 0 to 3), and equal bilaterally.

CriticalThinking 17-5

- Did you notice that the pulse rates in the preceding two goals are not the same as the full normal range shown in Table 17-1? What do you think might be a reason for this?

PLANNING INTERVENTIONS/IMPLEMENTATION

NIC standardized interventions include the following:

- Dysrhythmia Management, which applies to monitoring an abnormal pulse
- Vital Signs Monitoring, which may be used for general evaluation of clients who do not have an identified problem with the pulse

VOL 2 Go to Chapter 17, **Standardized Language,** in Volume 2.

Specific nursing activities and focused assessments for a patient with a dysrhythmia depend on the cause of the problem and on specific orders from the physician. For example, a client with a pulse rate of 50 beats/min is usually considered to have bradycardia. However, such a slow resting heart rate would be perfectly normal for a well-trained athlete. Some dysrhythmias are *benign;* that is, they are not dangerous to the client, and they require no interventions. Nursing strategies that address dysrhythmias, regardless of cause, include the following:

- Perform assessments focusing on the dysrhythmia.
  Closely monitor the patient's VS. A reduced heart rate may alter blood pressure and tissue perfusion. The extent of intervention depends on the effect of the dysrhythmia on the client's other vital signs.
  Monitor the patient's activity tolerance. Degree of activity, orientation, and level of fatigue while the dysrhythmia is present are indicators of the patient's ability to tolerate the dysrhythmia.
  Collect and assess laboratory data as prescribed. Cardiac function depends on normal electrolyte balance, particularly potassium, calcium, and magnesium levels. If a client is receiving medications

that affect cardiac rhythm, serum levels of these medications must be checked periodically.

- Help determine the cause of the dysrhythmia. Determine when the client experiences the dysrhythmia. Are there precipitating or alleviating factors?
- Administer antidysrhythmic medications (if prescribed) at regular intervals to control the heart rhythm.
- Provide emotional support. The client experiencing a dysrhythmia may be frightened by the experience. Explain all procedures to the client, and maintain a calm presence. Family members may also be frightened. Be sure to include them in your explanations and teaching.

CriticalThinking 17-6

- Which of the following findings should be referred to the primary healthcare provider so that an electrocardiogram (ECG) can be ordered? Why?
  Patient A, who has a radial pulse of 100 beats/min, regular, and equal bilaterally
  Patient B, who has a regular apical pulse of 100 beats/min
  Patient C, who has a very irregular apical pulse of 78 beats/min
- Recall the clients you encountered at the community health fair. Ms. Sharma is an active 80-year-old woman who works part time and exercises four times per week. She is complaining of feeling tired. You find that her pulse is irregular and uneven.
- What other patient data do you need to know? How would you go about getting this additional information?
- What actions should you consider taking while meeting with Ms. Sharma?
- What theoretical knowledge (rationale) supports your beliefs and actions?

Respiration

Respiration is the exchange of oxygen and carbon dioxide in the body. The process of respiration consists of two separate functions: mechanical and chemical. The mechanical aspects of respirations involve the active movement of air into and out of the respiratory system. This is known as **pulmonary ventilation** or, more commonly, breathing. The chemical aspects of respiration include the exchange of oxygen and carbon dioxide between the alveoli and the pulmonary blood supply **(external respiration),** the transport of these gases throughout the body **(gas transport),** and the exchange of these gases between the capillaries and body tissue cells **(internal respiration).** This chapter focuses on the mechanical aspects of respiration. Chapter 35 explores gas exchange and transport throughout the body. For an animated visual explanation of respiration,

 Go to Student Resources, **Animations: Cardiovascular/ Pulmonary Animations, Carbon Dioxide/Oxygen Transport,** at http://davisplus.fadavis.com/Wilkinson2

Theoretical **Knowledge** knowing why_____

To assess and support clients' respirations, you will need to know the normal range of respiratory rates, how respiration is regulated, the mechanics of breathing, and factors that affect respiration.

What Is a Normal Respiratory Rate?

Like temperature and pulse, respiratory rate normally varies with age, exertion, emotions, and other factors. Normal adult respirations are identified in Table 17-1. For normal respiratory rates at other developmental stages,

 Go to Chapter 17, **Tables, Boxes, Figures: ESG Table 17-1,** on the Student Resource Disk or DavisPlus at http:// davisplus.fadavis.com/Wilkinson2

How Does the Body Regulate Respiration?

Special respiratory centers in the medulla oblongata and pons of the brain, along with nerve fibers of the autonomic nervous system, regulate breathing in response to minute changes in the concentrations of oxygen (O_2) and carbon dioxide (CO_2) in the arterial blood. The primary stimulus for breathing is the level of CO_2 tension in the blood.

- **Central chemoreceptors,** located in the respiratory centers, are sensitive to CO_2 and hydrogen ion (pH) concentrations. Minor increases in either stimulate respirations.
- The partial pressure of oxygen in arterial blood (PaO_2) is normally between 80 and 100. When the PaO_2 falls below normal, **peripheral chemoreceptors** in the carotid and aortic bodies stimulate respirations.

Normally breathing is an involuntary action that requires little effort. However, it is possible to exert conscious control over respiration. For example, a young child who holds his breath during a temper tantrum is exerting conscious control over breathing. Swimming also involves conscious control of breathing.

What are the Mechanics of Breathing?

Pulmonary ventilation depends on changes in the capacity of the chest cavity (Fig. 17-7). In response to impulses sent from the respiratory center along the phrenic nerve, the thoracic muscles and the diaphragm contract. The ribs move upward from midline ½ to 1 inch (1.2 to 2.5 cm), the diaphragm moves downward and out about 0.4 inch (1 cm), and the abdominal organs move downward and forward, expanding the thorax in all directions. As expansion causes airway pressure to decrease below atmospheric pressure, air moves into and expands the lungs. This stage of respiration (drawing air into the lungs) is termed **inspiration.**

During inspiration (diaphragm contracting)

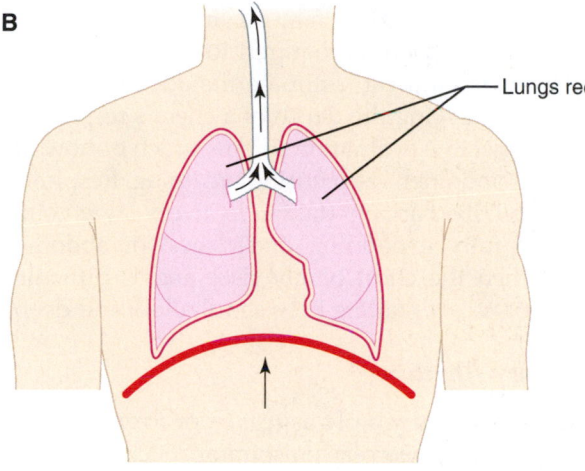

During expiration (diaphragm relaxing)

FIGURE 17-7 Changes in thoracic cavity during inspiration and expiration. *A*, During inspiration. *B*, During expiration.

When the diaphragm and thoracic muscles relax, the chest cavity decreases in size, and the lungs recoil, forcing air from the lungs until the pressure within the lungs again reaches atmospheric pressure. This stage, which involves the expulsion of air from the lungs, is called **expiration.** Expiration is passive and normally takes 2 to 3 seconds, compared to 1 to 1.5 seconds for inspiration. During normal breathing, the chest wall and abdomen gently rise and fall.

KnowledgeCheck 17-3

- Which two gases are exchanged through respiration?
- Which respiratory process involves the movement of air into and out of the lungs?
- What is external respiration?
- What is the primary stimulus for breathing?
- What mechanical forces allow the lungs to expand?

 Go to Chapter 17, **Knowledge Check Response Sheet and Answers,** on the Student Resource Disk or DavisPlus at http://davisplus.fadavis.com/Wilkinson2

What Factors Influence Respiration?

To interpret the meaning of your clients' respiratory data, you need to be aware of factors that influence breathing.

- *Developmental level.* A newborn's respiratory rate ranges from 40 to 90 breaths per minute. As a child ages, the rate gradually decreases until it reaches the normal adult rate of 12 to 20 breaths per minute. The respiratory rate decreases slightly in older adults.
- *Exercise.* Muscular activity causes a temporary increase in respiratory rate and depth so as to increase oxygen availability to the tissues and to rid the body of excess carbon dioxide.
- *Pain.* Acute pain causes an increase in respiratory rate but a decrease in depth.
- *Stress.* Psychological stress, such as anxiety or fear, may markedly influence respiration as a result of sympathetic stimulation. The most common change is an increase in rate.
- *Smoking.* Chronic smoking increases resting respiratory rate as a result of changes in airway compliance (elasticity).
- *Fever.* When heart rate increases because of fever, respiratory rate also increases. For every 1°F (0.6°C) the temperature rises, the respiratory rate may increase up to 4 breaths/min.
- *Hemoglobin.* Respiratory rate and depth increase as a result of anemia (reduced hemoglobin), sickle cell anemia (abnormally shaped red blood cells), and high altitudes. When hemoglobin is decreased or abnormal, the rate and depth of respirations, as well as the heart rate, may increase to maintain adequate tissue oxygenation. High altitudes inhibit the binding of oxygen to hemoglobin and trigger similar compensation efforts.
- *Disease.* The rate of breathing may be increased or decreased by various diseases. For example, brain stem injuries and increased intracranial pressure may interfere with the respiratory center, inhibiting respirations or altering respiratory rhythm.
- *Medications.* Central nervous system depressants, such as morphine or general anesthetics, cause slower, deeper respirations. Caffeine and atropine can cause shallow, fast breathing.
- *Position.* Standing up maximizes respiratory depth; lying flat reduces respiratory depth. Slumping (sitting with shoulders forward, and the back curved in a "C") prevents chest expansion, which impedes breathing.

 CriticalThinking 17-7

Consider the following patient situations. What effect would they have on respirations?

- A client with four fractured ribs
- A woman who is 9 months pregnant
- A young child excited at her birthday party
- An adult who has consumed alcoholic beverages

Practical **Knowledge**
knowing how

Although you will assess the adequacy of external and internal respiration in various ways, it is pulmonary ventilation (breathing) that you assess as a vital sign. Accurate assessment of respirations depends on your ability to recognize normal breathing, abnormal breathing, and factors that affect breathing. This chapter discusses only assessment of respirations. For nursing diagnoses, outcomes, and interventions for respiratory problems, see Chapter 35.

■ ASSESSMENT

Because people can control their breathing rate, it is best to count respirations when the client is unaware of what you are doing. One way to do this is to palpate and count the radial pulse, and then count the respirations before removing your fingers from the client's wrist. For a summary of this procedure, see the Critical Aspects box. For the entire sequence of steps,

 Go to Chapter 17, **Procedure 17-5: Assessing Respirations,** in Volume 2.

What Equipment Do I Need?

The only equipment you need for measuring respiratory rate is a watch with a second hand or digital display. You will need a stethoscope if you auscultate respirations. Many electronic thermometers have counter displays and signals that indicate 15-, 30-, and 60-second time intervals for counting respirations.

What Data Should I Collect?

In addition to measuring the respiratory rate, you will also observe indicators of overall respiratory function, including depth, rhythm, effort, and others. For additional information on respiratory assessment, see Chapter 19 and

 Go to Chapter 19, **Procedure 19–12: Assessing the Chest and Lungs,** in Volume 2.

Rate

The **respiratory rate** is the number of times a person breathes (or completes a cycle of inhalation and exhalation) within a full minute. You can easily count and observe respirations by:

■ Placing your hand on the client's chest (palpation) or observing (inspection) the number of times the client's chest or abdomen rises (inspiration) and falls (expiration)

■ Placing your stethoscope on the client's chest (auscultation) and counting the number of inhalation and exhalation cycles

For a new patient or when you need to ensure accuracy, you must count for 60 seconds ("Vital Signs," 1999). In some situations, for example, for a patient you know well and for whom respiratory rate is not directly relevant

to the assessment, you may count for only 30 seconds and multiply by 2. If respirations vary from normal, you should count for a full minute by auscultation.

Respiratory rate is a measure of the client's general condition, but rate alone is not a good indicator of the adequacy of respiration. You must also assess other characteristics of the respirations. If oxygenation must be carefully monitored, use a pulse oximeter (see Chapter 35).

A person can tolerate **apnea,** cessation of breathing, for only a few minutes. If apnea continues for more than 4 to 6 minutes, brain damage and even death can occur. See Table 17-4 for terminology to describe respiratory rhythms.

Respiratory Depth

Tidal volume is the amount of air taken in on inspiration—about 300 to 500 mL for a healthy adult. Specialized equipment is required to measure tidal volume. However, you can estimate the adequacy of tidal volume by observing the depth of a client's respirations. This is a subjective evaluation of how much or how little the chest or abdomen rises during breathing. Respiratory depth is described as *deep* (taking in a very large volume of air and fully expanding one's chest or abdomen), *shallow* (when the chest barely rises and is difficult to observe), or *normal* (falling between shallow and deep).

Respiratory Rhythm

Rhythm is assessed simply as *regular* or *irregular.* Generally, the period between each respiratory cycle is the same, and there is a regular breathing pattern (see Table 17-4). Infant breathing rhythms are more likely to be irregular than adult rhythms. An abnormal breathing pattern may indicate other health care problems and deserves further assessment. Two abnormal breathing patterns, Cheyne–Stokes and Biot's breathing, are discussed in Chapter 35.

Respiratory Effort

Respiratory effort refers to the degree of work required to breathe. Normal breathing is effortless. When diseases such as asthma or pneumonia are present, the person must work harder to breathe. Increased effort with breathing is called **dyspnea** or labored breathing. It is uncomfortable for the client and frequently produces fatigue and fear. **Orthopnea** is difficulty or inability to breathe when in a horizontal position. As discussed in Chapter 35, you will observe this in some clients with respiratory or cardiac conditions.

Breath Sounds

You will use a stethoscope to listen for breath sounds. Normal respirations are quiet. Abnormal sounds include the following.

■ **Wheezes** are high-pitched, continuous musical sounds, usually heard on expiration. Wheezes are caused by narrowing of the airways. Wheezes can often be heard without a stethoscope.

Table 17-4 ➤ Respiratory Rates and Rhythms

TYPE	DESCRIPTION	ILLUSTRATION
Eupnea	Normal respirations, with equal rate and depth, 12–20 breaths/min	
Bradypnea	Slow respirations, <10 breaths/min	
Tachypnea	Fast respirations, > 24 breaths/min, usually shallow	
Kussmaul's Respirations	Respirations that are regular but abnormally deep and increased in rate	
Biot's Respirations	Irregular respirations of variable depth (usually shallow), alternating with periods of apnea (absence of breathing)	
Cheyne–Stokes Respirations	Gradual increase in depth of respirations, followed by gradual decrease and then a period of apnea	
Apnea	Absence of breathing	

- **Rhonchi** are low-pitched, continuous gurgling sounds caused by secretions in the large airways. They often clear with coughing.
- **Crackles** are caused by fluid in the alveoli. They are discontinuous sounds usually heard on inspiration, but they may be heard throughout the respiratory cycle. They may be high-pitched, popping sounds or low-pitched, bubbling sounds; and have been described as similar to the sound made by rubbing strands of hair together with the fingertips.
- **Stridor** is a piercing, high-pitched sound that is heard without a stethoscope, primarily during inspiration, in infants who are experiencing respiratory distress or in someone with an obstructed airway.
- **Stertor** refers to labored breathing that produces a snoring sound.

See Chapter 19 for further discussion of abnormal breath sounds. To listen to the sounds,

 Go to **Sound File, Breath Sounds,** on the Student Resource Disk or DavisPlus at http://davisplus.fadavis.com/Wilkinson2

Chest and Abdomen Movement

The chest or abdomen normally rises with inspiration and falls with expiration in a gentle and rhythmic pattern. When a person is having difficulty moving air into or out of the lungs, respiratory patterns change. **Intercostal retraction** refers to the visible sinking of tissues around and between the ribs that occurs when the person must use additional effort to breathe. **Substernal retraction** exists when tissues are drawn in beneath the sternum (breastbone), and **suprasternal retraction** exists when tissues are drawn in above the clavicle (shoulder girdle).

Associated Clinical Signs

When you assess respiration, it is important to assess for clinical signs of oxygenation. Signs of **hypoxia** (inadequate cellular oxygenation) include pallor or cyanosis, restlessness, apprehension, confusion, dizziness, fatigue, decreased level of consciousness, tachycardia, tachypnea, and changes in blood pressure. When evaluating cyanosis, the tongue and oral mucosa are the best indicators of hypoxia. Cyanosis of the nails, lips, and skin may be caused by hypoxia, but may also be related to cold or reduced circulation in that area. Chronic hypoxia causes **clubbing** (loss of the nail angle) of the fingers.

A **cough** is a forceful or violent expulsion of air during expiration. Coughs may be *constant* (occurring frequently and consistently) or *intermittent* (occurring occasionally). If secretions are expectorated (coughed up), the cough is *productive*. If no secretions are produced, the cough is *nonproductive* or *dry*. A *hacking cough* is a series of dry coughs that occur together, whereas a *whooping cough* is a sudden, periodic cough that ends with a whooping sound on inspiration. Coughs may be symptoms of allergic reactions, lung disease, respiratory infection, or heart conditions.

KnowledgeCheck 17-4

- How can you estimate a client's tidal volume?
- What is the range of normal for an adult's respiratory rate?
- Besides the rate, what other characteristics of a client's respirations should you observe?
- What are some common clinical signs associated with poor oxygenation?

 Go to Chapter 17, **Knowledge Check Response Sheet and Answers,** on the Student Resource Disk or DavisPlus at http://davisplus.fadavis.com/Wilkinson2

Arterial Oxygen Saturation

The rate, quality, and depth of the respirations are indicators of the general health of the respiratory system. However, they do not measure the amounts of oxygen and carbon dioxide present in the blood—information that is essential for evaluating the effectiveness of respiratory effort. Two methods exist to measure O_2 and CO_2 blood levels. One method is invasive; the other is not.

- **Arterial blood gas (ABG) sampling** directly measures the partial pressures of oxygen and carbon dioxide and blood pH, in other words, the gases in the arterial blood. This method requires the puncture of an artery followed by laboratory testing of the sample. It provides comprehensive data, but it is invasive, painful, time-consuming, and relatively expensive. If you need more information about this diagnostic test, consult a medical–surgical nursing or laboratory tests text.
- **Pulse oximetry** is a noninvasive method of monitoring respiratory status with a device that measures **oxygen saturation** (an indication of the oxygen being carried by hemoglobin in the arterial blood). The oximeter emits light, and a photosensor placed on the client's finger or earlobe measures the light passing through the site and calculates a pulse saturation (SpO_2) that is a good estimate of arterial oxygen saturation. The only risk in pulse oximetry is that clinicians may become overdependent on it or trust erroneous readings. Do not neglect the other aspects of holistic respiratory assessment. In many situations oxygen saturation is monitored routinely along with the other vital signs. For a procedure for applying a pulse oximeter,

VOL 2 Go to Chapter 35, **Procedure 35–2: Monitoring Pulse Oximetry,** in Volume 2.

 Critical**Thinking** 17-8

- Mrs. Dowell has smoked two packs of cigarettes per day for 45 years. She has recently been diagnosed with pneumonia—an infection of the lungs. What VS assessments would be important for Mrs. Dowell, and why?
- Recall the clients you encountered in the community health fair scenario. Mr. Jackson is short of breath and struggling to breathe. His respiratory rate is 28 breaths/min. What else do you need to know about the patient situation? What is important and what is not important in this scenario? What is probably least important?

What Are Some Alterations in Respiration?

As noted earlier, *hypoxia* refers to inadequate cellular oxygenation. It results from decreased oxygen intake, decreased ability of tissues to remove oxygen from blood, impaired ventilation or perfusion, impaired gas exchange between the blood and alveoli, or inadequate levels of hemoglobin.

Hyperventilation occurs when rapid and deep breathing result in excess loss of CO_2 (*hypocapnia*). A client who is hyperventilating may complain of feeling lightheaded and tingly. Causes of hyperventilation include anxiety, infection, shock, hypoxia, drugs (e.g., aspirin, amphetamines), diabetes mellitus, or acid–base imbalance.

Hypoventilation occurs when the rate and depth of respirations are decreased and CO_2 is retained or alveolar ventilation is compromised. Hypoventilation may be related to chronic obstructive pulmonary disease (COPD), general anesthesia, impending respiratory failure, or other conditions that result in decreased respirations.

Blood Pressure

Blood pressure (BP), an important indicator of overall cardiovascular health, is the pressure of the blood as it is forced against arterial walls during cardiac contraction. **Systolic pressure** is the peak pressure exerted against arterial walls as the ventricles contract and eject blood. **Diastolic pressure** is the minimum pressure exerted against arterial walls, between cardiac contractions when the heart is at rest.

Blood pressure is measured in millimeters of mercury (mm Hg) and is recorded as systolic pressure over diastolic pressure (e.g., 110/74 mm Hg). The pulse that can be palpated to determine heart rate is due to the difference between the systolic and diastolic pressures. This difference is known as the **pulse pressure.** The pulse pressure for a BP of 120/80 mm Hg is 40 mm Hg. The pulse pressure is an indication of the volume output of the left ventricle. Generally, the pulse pressure should be no greater than one-third of the systolic pressure, as in the example of a BP of 120/80, with a pulse pressure of 40 ($\frac{1}{3} \times 120 = 40$).

Knowledge**Check 17-5**

- For a client whose BP is 150/80, what is the pulse pressure?
- Is that normal? If so, explain. If not, what should the pulse pressure be?

 Go to Chapter 17, **Knowledge Check Response Sheet and Answers,** on the Student Resource Disk or DavisPlus at http://davisplus.fadavis.com/Wilkinson2

Theoretical **Knowledge** knowing why

To assess and support clients' blood pressure, you will need to know what constitutes a normal reading for a client, how the body regulates blood pressure, and what factors affect the blood pressure.

What Is a Normal Blood Pressure Reading?

For many years, a BP of less than 120 to 129 systolic and less than 80 to 84 diastolic was considered "optimal" for adults; and up to 130 systolic and 85 diastolic was considered "normal" for adults. More recently, an expert panel has classified "normal" as systolic BP below 120 and diastolic BP below 80 (Joint National Committee on Prevention, Detection, Evaluation, and Treatment of High Blood Pressure, 2004). See Table 17-5.

How Does the Body Regulate Blood Pressure?

Blood pressure regulation is a highly complex process. It is influenced by three factors: cardiac function, peripheral vascular resistance, and blood volume. The body constantly regulates and adjusts arterial pressure to supply blood to body tissues via perfusion of the capillary beds. For in-depth discussion, see Chapter 35.

Cardiac Function

Recall that *cardiac output* is the volume of blood pumped by the heart per minute, and that it reflects the functioning of the heart. An increase in cardiac output causes an increase in BP; a decrease in cardiac output causes a decrease in BP (if all other factors remain the same). A change in either stroke volume or heart rate alters cardiac output.

Conditions that *increase* cardiac output by increasing stroke volume include:

- Increased blood volume (as occurs during pregnancy, for example).
- More forceful contraction of the ventricles (as occurs during exercise, for example).

Conditions that *decrease* cardiac output by decreasing stroke volume include:

- Dehydration
- Active bleeding
- Damage to the heart (as seen after myocardial infarction, or heart attack)
- A very rapid heart rate. Up to a point, an increase in heart rate increases cardiac output. However, a very rapid heart rate limits the time allotted for the ventricles to fill, resulting in decreased stroke volume and, ultimately, decreased cardiac output.

Peripheral Resistance

Peripheral resistance refers to arterial and capillary resistance to blood flow as a result of friction between blood and the vessel walls. Increased peripheral resistance creates a temporary increase in BP. The amount of friction or resistance depends on blood **viscosity** (thickness), arterial size, and arterial **compliance** (elasticity). The walls of the veins are thin and very distensible, so they have little influence on peripheral resistance and BP.

Blood viscosity. Blood viscosity influences the ease with which blood flows through the vessels. Viscosity is determined by the **hematocrit** (the percentage of red blood cells in plasma). Any disorder that increases hematocrit (e.g., dehydration) increases blood viscosity and, therefore, BP. Conversely, a low hematocrit, as seen in anemia, lowers viscosity and may reduce BP.

Arterial size. The smaller the radius of a blood vessel, the more resistance it offers to blood flow. Constricted

Table 17-5 ➤ Classification of Adult Blood Pressure*

CATEGORY	SYSTOLIC (MM HG)		DIASTOLIC (MM HG)	FOLLOW-UP
Normal	<120	and	<80	Encourage lifestyle modification if there are risk factors. Recheck in 1–2 years or sooner if there are risk factors.
Prehypertension	120–139	or	80–89	Encourage lifestyle changes; recheck in 1 year or sooner if indicated. Antihypertensives are prescribed only with compelling indications, such as renal disease.
Stage I Hypertension	140–159	or	90–99	Encourage lifestyle modification. Follow up with primary care provider in 1–2 months. (Most patients will be started on thiazide-type diuretics.)
Stage II Hypertension	≥160	or	≥100	Encourage lifestyle modification. Refer for care within 1 week, or immediately if warranted. (Most patients will be given a two-drug combination therapy, e.g., thiazide-type diuretics with angiotensin-converting enzyme [ACE] inhibitors.)

*For adults age 18 and older, based on the average of two or more readings taken at each of two or more visits after an initial screening.
Source: Data from the Joint National Committee on Prevention, Detection, Evaluation, and Treatment of High Blood Pressure. (2004). *JNC 7 Complete Report. The seventh report of the Joint National Committee on Prevention, Detection, Evaluation, and Treatment of High Blood Pressure.* Bethesda, MD: National Institutes of Health. Retrieved May 22, 2008, from http://www.nhlbi.nih.gov/guidelines/hypertension/index.htm

arteries prevent the free flow of blood and, subsequently, increase BP. Dilated arteries allow unrestricted flow of blood, thereby reducing blood pressure. The sympathetic nervous system controls vasoconstriction and vasodilation.

Arterial compliance. Arteries with good elasticity can distend and recoil easily and adequately. When age- or disease-related changes in arterial structure cause a loss of elasticity, peripheral resistance, and possibly BP, increase. **Arteriosclerosis** (hardening of the arteries) is a common contributor to increased BP in middle-aged and older adults.

Blood Volume

The normal volume of blood in the body is about 5 liters (5000 mL). A significant volume decrease, as occurs with hemorrhage or other fluid losses, reduces vascular volume, and BP falls. When vascular volume is increased above the norm, as occurs with renal (kidney) failure and fluid retention, BP increases.

What Factors Influence Blood Pressure?

Blood pressure normally changes from minute to minute with changes in activity or changes in body position. Therefore, you must establish BP *patterns* rather than relying on individual BP readings when determining whether a client's BP is normal or abnormal. This is even more important for older adults because their BP tends to fluctuate even more. The following are some factors that affect the BP:

- *Developmental stage.* An average newborn has a BP of about 40 mm Hg systolic. It increases gradually throughout childhood. A child or adolescent's BP depends on body size; therefore, a smaller child or adolescent has a lower blood pressure than a larger child does. Both systolic and diastolic BP continue to increase with age as a result of decreased arterial compliance. For BP normal ranges,

 Go to Chapter 17, **Tables, Boxes, Figures: ESG Table 17-1,** on the Student Resource Disk or DavisPlus at http://davisplus.fadavis.com/Wilkinson2

- *Sex.* The average BP for men is slightly higher than that for women of comparable age, although the difference is not considered significant. After menopause, a woman's BP tends to increase, possibly due to a decrease in estrogen.
- *Family history.* A family history of hypertension markedly increases the likelihood of an individual's developing hypertension.
- *Lifestyle.* Factors such as increased sodium consumption, smoking, and consumption of three or more alcoholic drinks per day have been shown to elevate BP. Caffeine may raise BP for a short

while after ingestion, but it has no long-term effect on the BP.

- *Exercise.* Physical fitness has been shown to reduce BP in many individuals. However, muscular exertion temporarily increases BP as a result of increased heart rate and cardiac output. You should, therefore, wait about 30 minutes before you assess the BP of someone who has been physically active.
- *Body position.* BP is higher when a person is standing than when sitting or lying down. Readings are higher if taken with the client's arm above heart level or if the arm is unsupported at the client's side. Seated readings are higher if the client's feet are dangling rather than resting on the floor or if the legs are crossed at the knees.
- *Stress.* Fear, worry, excitement, and other stressors cause BP to rise sharply because of sympathetic nervous system stimulation (fight-or-flight response). One example of this is "white-coat hypertension." This occurs when a patient's BP is elevated in the physician's office or clinic—a situation in which he is likely to experience stress—but not at other times. However white-coat hypertension may indicate what happens during other times of stress, so if it is consistently displayed, treatment may be indicated.
- *Pain.* Pain often causes the BP to increase. However, severe or prolonged pain can significantly decrease BP.
- *Race.* Blacks have a higher rate of hypertension than do European Americans, and they have a higher incidence of complications and hypertension-related deaths (McCance & Heuther, 2006).
- *Obesity.* As a rule, obesity increases the BP. This increase is related to the additional vascular supply required to perfuse the large body mass and the resultant increase in peripheral resistance.
- *Diurnal variations.* Generally, BP varies according to the person's daily schedules and routines.
- *Medications.* Many medications alter BP. This effect may be intended, as with antihypertensive medications, or unintended, such as the drop in BP that often results when a client receives pain medication. Many over-the-counter preparations, herbal products, and illicit drugs can affect BP.
- *Diseases.* Diseases that affect the circulatory system or any of the major organs of the body (e.g., the kidneys) may affect BP.

Critical**Thinking** 17-9

- Evaluate the following adult blood pressures. Are they high, low, or normal?
  116/90
  80/50
  184/102
  140/90
  40/0
- What theoretical knowledge did you use in evaluating the blood pressures?

Practical **Knowledge**
knowing how

Now that you understand how blood pressure is maintained and regulated, you are ready to gain the practical knowledge of how to assess and support this aspect of physical functioning.

■ ASSESSMENT

Blood pressure may be assessed directly or indirectly. In the *direct method*, a catheter is threaded into an artery under sterile conditions and attached to tubing that is connected to an electronic monitoring system. The pressure is constantly displayed as a waveform on the monitor screen. Although the direct method of measuring BP is very accurate, its use is confined to critical care areas and surgery because of the risk of sudden arterial blood loss. Usually, you will measure BP via the *indirect*, or *noninvasive, method*. This is an accurate estimate of arterial BP that can be performed in any clinical or community setting. For a summary of a procedure for noninvasive blood pressure monitoring, see the Critical Aspects box. For the complete procedure,

 Go to Chapter 17, **Procedure 17-6: Measuring Blood Pressure,** in Volume 2.

For an animated visual explanation of blood pressure readings,

 Go to Student Resources **Animations: Reading Blood Pressure,** on DavisPlus at http://davisplus.fadavis.com/Wilkinson2

What Equipment Do I Need?

You will need a stethoscope, a blood pressure cuff and sphygmomanometer, or an electronic blood pressure monitor to assess blood pressure. Electronic monitoring is gradually replacing the stethoscope and sphygmomanometer in inpatient settings. However, a common stethoscope and sphygmomanometer are generally sufficient to hear most clients' blood pressures. When blood pressure is weak, ultrasonic stethoscopes are useful for magnifying sound waves occurring during systole.

Evidence-based guidelines suggest that using the bell of the stethoscope enables you to hear blood pressure sounds more accurately, especially at diastolic pressures (Perloff, Grim, Flack, et al., 1993; Vital Signs, 1999). However, most people use the diaphragm because it is easily placed and because some stethoscopes do not have a bell. The key to clarity of sound is to use a high-quality stethoscope with short tubing (National Guideline Clearinghouse, 2005).

A **sphygmomanometer** consists of a vinyl or cloth cuff, a pressure bulb with a regulating valve, and a manometer (Fig. 17-8). Blood pressure cuffs contain an inflatable rubber bladder. The cuff is attached to a gauge or manometer and a valved pressure bulb that inflates

FIGURE 17-8 Types of manometers: top left, aneroid; top right, mercury; bottom, electronic.

the bladder (Fig. 17-9). Cuffs can be placed on either the upper arm or midthigh and are supplied in various sizes.

Sphygmomanometers are either aneroid or mercury. **Aneroid** manometers have dials that register BP by pointers attached to a spring. **Mercury** manometers measure BP using a calibrated upright tube containing mercury (see Fig. 17-8, top). As the bladder of the cuff is inflated, the pressure pushes the column of mercury up the tube. The column of mercury falls as the cuff is

FIGURE 17-9 A blood pressure cuff showing placement of bladder within the cuff.

deflated. Mercury manometers are not as popular as aneroid manometers because they pose a health hazard if the mercury tube is broken. They are, however, easier to maintain and more accurate than aneroid manometers, which require frequent calibration. In 1998, the American Hospital Association and the Environmental Protection Agency recommended that the healthcare industry eliminate mercury-containing waste by the year 2005 (USEPA, 2001). This would include phasing out mercury manometers, and most agencies have done that.

Electronic blood pressure monitors use either microphones to sense sounds or sensors that detect pressure waves as blood flows through arteries (Fig. 17-8, bottom). They can be set to monitor and record BP at timed intervals and do not require the use of a stethoscope. They measure systolic, diastolic, and mean arterial pressures. Electronic monitors are useful when you must monitor BP frequently (e.g., during surgery or when a client is critically ill). However, some evidence suggests that they may be less accurate than auscultated blood pressures, so you should auscultate a baseline BP before initiating automatic monitoring (National Guideline Clearinghouse, 2005).

Many clients use a version of the electronic BP monitor in their homes. These devices can be purchased in grocery stores and pharmacies. They are useful for screening, but clients should seek followup care when readings are not within their normal range. The accompanying Home Care box identifies teaching topics for clients using electronic BP monitors.

Home Care

Teaching Your Client Self-Monitoring of Blood Pressure

Various models of common, acceptable BP devices are available for self-monitoring using the upper arm (finger monitors are inaccurate).

➤ With a portable home device, the client simply pushes a button, and the cuff inflates and deflates automatically. The device provides an electronic digital readout of the BP. Because these devices are sensitive, arm movement or improper cuff placement can cause inaccurate readings. Also, these devices must be recalibrated at least every 6 to 12 months.

➤ Some grocery stores, fitness clubs, and other public places have stationary automatic BP devices for public use. The person places his arm in the cuff, which fits over his clothing. The machine gives a visual display of the BP reading. The accuracy of these machines varies.

Benefits of Self-Monitoring

➤ May detect high BP in those who have not previously had a problem (screening).

➤ Allows for observation of the BP *pattern* in those with high normal BP, rather than a one-time office reading.

➤ Distinguishes "white-coat hypertension" from actual hypertension.

➤ For clients with hypertension, self-monitoring increases participation in treatment and may improve compliance with treatment.

Disadvantages of Self-Monitoring

➤ Possible incorrect use of the BP device

➤ Needless anxiety over a single elevated reading

➤ Clients with hypertension may make adjustments to their medications based on the BP readings without consulting their care provider.

Nursing Implications

➤ Teach proper use of the self-measurement devices.

➤ Periodically evaluate the client's technique.

➤ Teach the meaning of BP readings and the need to look for patterns from multiple readings, not just a single reading.

➤ Explain the need for calibration of the home-monitoring device at least once a year (American Heart Association, n.d.).

➤ Have the client bring the home-monitoring device to clinical visits so that readings can be compared with simultaneously recorded auscultatory readings.

➤ Teach the client to have abnormally high or low readings (occurring on more than one occasion) rechecked by a healthcare provider. Home readings of 135/85 or higher should be considered elevated.

➤ Advise the client to keep a written record of BP readings, including the date and time for each, and bring it to each clinic or office visit.

What Cuff Size Should I Use?

As shown in Figure 17-10, the *width* of the bladder of a properly fitting cuff will cover approximately two-thirds of the *length* of the upper arm (or other extremity) for an adult, and the entire upper arm for a child (National Institutes of Health, 1996). Alternatively, you can check that (1) the *cuff width* is 40% of the arm circumference and (2) the *length* of the bladder encircles 80% of the arm in adults (National Guideline Clearinghouse, 2005; Perloff et al., 1993).

Using a cuff or bladder of the incorrect size can result in a measurement error of as much as 30 mm Hg. If the cuff is too narrow, your reading will be too high; if it is too wide, the reading will be too low. Although cuffs are manufactured in various sizes, in practice, you will

FIGURE 17-10 Determining correct BP cuff size. *A,* The cuff width should be two-thirds of the length of the upper arm, or should encircle 40% of the arm. *B,* The length of the bladder should encircle 80% of the upper arm.

probably have access to only two or three different adult sizes. If you must use a cuff of the improper size, it is better to use one that is too large than one that is too small—be sure to document the cuff size along with the BP reading if you do not have the proper size. Refer to Figure 17-10 and Table 17-6 for information about cuff sizes in centimeters.

Which Site Should I Use?

You usually use the *brachial artery* for assessing BP. However, the condition of the client's arm as well as other factors can interfere with accurate BP measurement. Avoid assessing blood pressure in an arm that has an intravenous access device, renal dialysis fistula, or skin graft; that is paralyzed, diseased, or has extensive trauma; that has a cast or dressings; or that is on the same side of breast or shoulder surgery. In these and similar instances, you can use the forearm, thigh, or calf. Systolic pressure may be 20 to 30 mm Hg higher in the lower extremities than in the arms, but diastolic pressures are similar. Also, forearm and upper arm readings may not be interchangeable. Document the site used. For a summary of the procedure for measuring blood pressure, see the Critical Aspects box. For the entire procedure,

 Go to Chapter 17, **Procedure 17-6: Measuring Blood Pressure,** in Volume 2.

Auscultating Blood Pressure

Blood pressure can be measured indirectly by auscultation or palpation. The preferred, and most commonly used, method is auscultation; however, palpation is useful in certain situations. When auscultating BP, place your stethoscope over an artery, inflate the cuff, and listen for sounds as you deflate the cuff.

As you *inflate* the cuff, the artery is occluded as the pressure of the cuff exceeds the pressure in the artery. At that point, blood flow through the artery is halted, and no sound can be heard. As you *deflate* the cuff, blood begins to flow rapidly through the partially open artery, producing turbulence that you will hear through the stethoscope as a tapping sound.

- *The first sound* you hear when the cuff is slowly deflated is the systolic pressure.
- *The disappearance of sound* identifies the diastolic BP. When the artery is no longer compressed, blood flows freely, and no sound is heard.

The sounds you listen for when you assess BP are called **Korotkoff sounds.** These sounds, described by Russian neurologist Nicolai Korotkoff in 1906, are used to describe the sounds of blood pulsating through arteries (Fig. 17-11).

1st sound—As you deflate the BP cuff, you will initially hear a sound that occurs during systole. It

Table 17-6 ➤ Blood Pressure Cuffs: Acceptable Bladder Sizes*

CUFF TYPE	ARM CIRCUMFERENCE AT MIDPOINT (CM)**	BLADDER WIDTH (CM)	BLADDER LENGTH (CM)
Newborn	<6	3	6
Infant	6–15	5	15
Child	16–21	8	21
Small adult	22–26	12	22
Adult	27–34	16	30
Large adult	35–44	16	36
Adult thigh	45–52	16	42

*The National Heart, Lung, and Blood Institute states that practically speaking, "correct cuff size equals the largest cuff that will fit on the upper arm with room below for the stethoscope head" (2007).
**Arm circumference is half the distance from the acromion to the olecranon process. If correct size not available, use next larger (rather than smaller) size.
Sources: American Heart Association (2005); National Guidelines Clearinghouse (2005); and Perloff, Grim, Flack, et al. (1993).

is a tapping sound that corresponds to the pulse (systolic BP).

2nd sound—Occurs as you further deflate the cuff. It is a soft, swishing sound caused by blood turbulence.

3rd sound—Begins midway through the BP and is a sharp, rhythmic tapping sound.

4th sound—Like the third sound, but softer and fading.

5th sound—Silence; it corresponds with diastole (diastolic BP).

You will not always be able to identify each of the five sounds. In some clients the sounds are distinct, but in others you will note little difference between beginning and ending sounds. To hear these sounds,

 Go to **Sound File, Blood Pressure Sounds,** on the Student Resource Disk or DavisPlus at http://davisplus.fadavis.com/Wilkinson2.

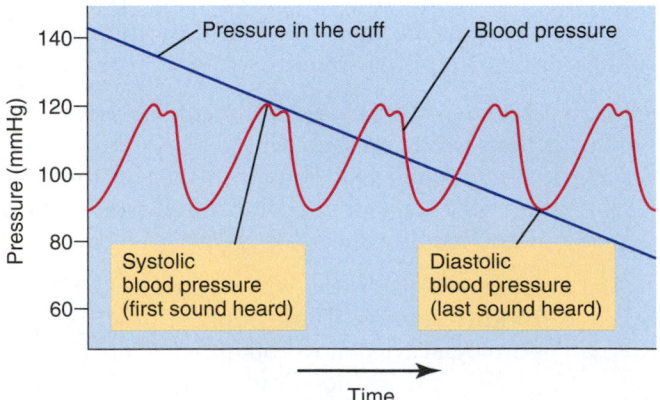

FIGURE 17-11 Relationship of blood pressure to changes in cuff pressure and the first and fifth Korotkoff sounds (BP 120/80).

Palpating Blood Pressure

When the BP is difficult to hear (e.g., when there are cardiac conditions, shock, or other conditions that compromise circulation) you can use palpation alone. You can usually palpate only the systolic BP, because diastolic pressure is difficult to feel. Apply the cuff, and feel for the radial or brachial pulse. Begin to inflate the cuff. When you can no longer feel the pulse, inflate the cuff about 30 mm Hg more. As you release the valve and slowly deflate the cuff, note the reading on the manometer at which you once again feel the pulse. Record the palpated blood pressure according to the way it was assessed (e.g., "Palpated, low Fowler's, left arm 86/——" [or "86 systolic"]).

Using Palpation with Auscultation

You should use palpation with auscultation for calculating the proper cuff inflation pressure before auscultating the BP and for detecting an auscultatory gap, to be discussed shortly.

Calculating Proper Inflation Pressure

The first time you measure a client's BP, you do not know what the systolic BP will be. Should you pump the cuff to 200 mm Hg, just to be sure you don't miss the first sound? The answer is NO. If you overinflate the cuff, the patient will feel discomfort. However, if you underinflate it (e.g., stop inflating at 110 mm Hg), you may miss the first sound and obtain an incorrect reading.

Here is a method that allows you to estimate the systolic BP to ensure that you inflate the cuff to the proper level to obtain an accurate reading. Locate the brachial pulse (alternatively, you can use the radial pulse for this step). Inflate the cuff rapidly to 70 to 80 mm Hg, and then palpate the pulse while you continue inflating the cuff slowly in 10 mm Hg increments until you no longer feel the pulse. Note the pressure at which the pulse disappears. You have two options after that:

1. Continue inflating the cuff to a pressure that is 20 to 30 mm Hg above the level at which the pulse disappeared. Apply the stethoscope to the brachial artery, and deflate the cuff slowly, listening for the BP sounds as you deflate.
2. Or, deflate the cuff rapidly, and note the pressure at which the pulse reappears. Wait 2 minutes, then place the stethoscope over the brachial artery to take the actual measurement. When taking the actual measurement, inflate the cuff to a pressure that is 20 to 30 mm Hg above the palpated level.

Recognizing an Auscultatory Gap

If the client has hypertension, as you auscultate the BP during deflation of the cuff you may note the loss of sounds for as much as 30 mm Hg, followed by the return of sound. This loss and later return of sound is referred to as an **auscultatory gap.** Palpating first and then auscultating (as described in the preceding paragraphs) ensures that you will not miss the isolated first sound. You should record the range of pressures in which the gap occurs (e.g., BP left arm, sitting, 170/90 with an auscultatory gap from 170 to 140). Failure to recognize an auscultatory gap can result in a serious misreading of the systolic BP. For tips that will help ensure the validity of your BP measurements,

 VOL 2 Go to Chapter 17, **Clinical Insight 17-1: Taking an Accurate Blood Pressure,** in Volume 2.

KnowledgeCheck 17-6

- Which of the Korotkoff sounds would you record as the systolic pressure?
- Which of the Korotkoff sounds would you record as the diastolic pressure?
- A nurse is auscultating a BP. He hears the first sound at 170 mm Hg. The sound disappears immediately. At 150 mm Hg, the sound appears again and continues until there is silence at 80 mm Hg. The pressures were taken in the client's right arm while the client was lying down.
  How should the nurse record these pressures?
  How do you explain what happened?

 Go to Chapter 17, **Knowledge Check Response Sheet and Answers,** on the Student Resource Disk or DavisPlus at http://davisplus.fadavis.com/Wilkinson2

■ ANALYSIS/NURSING DIAGNOSIS

Hypotension and hypertension are medical diagnoses or, more commonly, symptoms rather than nursing diagnoses. However, they may be the etiology of nursing diagnoses—for example, Risk for Falls related to orthostatic hypotension.

What Is Hypotension?

Hypotension is diagnosed when systolic blood pressure is less than 100 mm Hg. A low blood pressure is usually not considered a problem. However, further evaluation is always called for if:

- The client is also experiencing dizziness, fatigue, concentration problems, activity intolerance, or shortness of breath, or
- The low blood pressure is of sudden onset.

Hemorrhage and heart failure are two causes of hypotension. Very low BP (hypovolemic shock) is a medical emergency. If you need more information on hypovolemic shock, consult a medical–surgical nursing text.

Orthostatic, or postural, hypotension occurs when a person's BP drops suddenly on moving from a lying position to a sitting or standing position. Orthostatic hypotension is defined as a decrease of 10 mm Hg in standing blood pressure when associated with dizziness and/or fainting is (Joint National Committee, 2004). Postural hypotension results from peripheral vasodilation without a compensatory increase in cardiac output. It is most likely to occur in older adults, pregnant women, clients on prolonged bed rest, and clients with decreased blood volume (e.g., from dehydration or recent blood loss).

The following are examples of nursing diagnoses with hypotension as the etiology.

- Risk for Falls related to dizziness secondary to postural hypotension
- Fear of falling related to fainting secondary to postural hypotension

What Is Hypertension?

A transient elevation in BP is a normal response to physiological or psychological stress (e.g., after eating, after exercise). **Prehypertension** is a BP reading of 120 to 139 mm Hg systolic or 80 to 89 mm Hg diastolic, obtained with two readings taken 6 minutes apart, with the patient sitting. **Hypertension** is a persistently higher than normal BP. It is diagnosed when BP is above 140 mm Hg systolic or above 90 mm Hg diastolic on two or more separate occasions. Physiologically, hypertension is related to thickening of the arterial walls and decreased elasticity of the arteries.

Hypertension is a major cause of illness and death in the United States. Hypertension increases the stress on the heart and blood vessels, and if untreated, it may lead to heart attack, heart failure, peripheral vascular disease, kidney damage, or stroke. The severity of the disorder is directly related to the degree of elevation; however, the latest guidelines (Joint National Committee, 2004) recommend that even prehypertension be treated by lifestyle modifications to prevent coronary artery disease. The diagnosis of hypertension is often delayed because symptoms are mild or absent. Those who experience symptoms may complain of early morning suboccipital headaches, fatigue, and visual changes.

Primary, or **essential, hypertension** is diagnosed when there is no known cause for the BP elevation. Essential hypertension accounts for at least 90% of all cases of hypertension. Although no single cause is identified, family history, age, race, obesity, diet, heavy alcohol consumption, smoking history, high cholesterol levels, and stress all contribute to the development of essential hypertension.

Secondary hypertension occurs when there is a clearly identified cause for the persistent rise in BP. A variety of renal and endocrine disorders may lead to secondary hypertension. Several prescription and non-prescription drugs can also cause BP elevation (e.g., nonsteroidal anti-inflammatory drugs [NSAIDs], oral contraceptives, some decongestants, and adrenal steroid hormones). Nicotine and caffeine cause transient BP increases. Other causes of hypertension include use of cocaine, amphetamines, and other illicit drugs, as well as chronic overuse of alcohol. Treatment is directed at eliminating the underlying cause.

Hypertension is not a nursing diagnosis; it is a medical diagnosis. However, there are nursing diagnoses associated with it, as in the following examples:

- Risk for Decreased Cardiac Output occurs as a response to hypertension (i.e., hypertension is the etiology of this nursing diagnosis). As blood pressure rises, peripheral resistance increases. Over time the heart is unable to compensate, and cardiac output declines.
- Some nursing diagnoses may be the contributing factors for hypertension, for example:
  Imbalanced Nutrition: More than Body Requirements may be used if obesity (> 20% above ideal body weight) is a factor in a patient's hypertension.
  Imbalanced Nutrition: More than Body Requirements (for salt) could be used for a client whose high dietary sodium intake is contributing to hypertension.
- Hypertension may be a defining characteristic (symptom) of some nursing diagnoses, for example: Anxiety and Pain may cause an increase in BP.
- Hypertension may create the need for a diagnosis of Deficient Knowledge related to the need to make lifestyle changes.

PLANNING OUTCOMES/EVALUATION

You may need goals for overall blood pressure monitoring, but more likely you will use them for problems related to hypotension and hypertension.

Outcomes for Hypotension

The *NOC outcomes and goals* you use depend on the nursing diagnosis (the problem caused by the hypotension). For Risk for Falls, you might use NOC's Falls

Occurrence. You might write *an individualized goal* such as, "Patient will have no falls while walking."

Outcomes for Hypertension

The *NOC standardized* outcome for assessing the blood pressure is Vital Signs Status. If it becomes necessary to monitor cardiac output, you could use the labels of Cardiac Pump Effectiveness and Circulation Status.

Individualized goals/outcome statements are developed from the nursing diagnosis. For example, for Decreased Cardiac Output, goals might be, "BP will be at least 110/80," and "Extremities will be warm to the touch with quick capillary refill." If the nursing diagnosis were Imbalanced Nutrition: More Than Body Requirements, the desired outcomes would address the target weight for the client and the ideal number of calories to be consumed.

 Also go to Chapter 17, **Standardized Language**, in Volume 2.

PLANNING INTERVENTIONS/IMPLEMENTATION

NIC standardized interventions for monitoring VS include the following:

Vital Signs Monitoring applies to monitoring an abnormal blood pressure.
Hemodynamic Regulation would be used to evaluate Decreased Cardiac Output.

 Go to Chapter 17, **Standardized Language**, in Volume 2.

Interventions for Hypotension

NIC standardized interventions will be determined by the nursing diagnosis you use. For example, for Risk for Falls related to orthostatic hypotension, you might use the following: Fall Prevention; Self-Care Assistance: Transfer; and Surveillance: Safety.

Specific nursing activities, regardless of the nursing diagnosis used, must address the etiology: for example, the orthostatic hypotension. When you detect orthostatic hypotension:

1. Help the client lie down, and then notify the physician or nurse in charge.
2. Next, obtain *orthostatic vital signs*—that is, take the pulse and BP with the client supine, sitting, and standing. Take each reading 1 to 3 minutes after the client changes position.
3. When documenting orthostatic vital signs, record the client's position in addition to the pulse and BP measurements (e.g., supine P = 80, BP = 150/90; sitting P = 84, BP = 140/84; standing P = 90, BP = 104/60).

Interventions for Hypertension

Specific nursing activities for the patient with hypertension depend on whether hypertension is primary or secondary and on specific orders from the physician. Nursing activities and focused assessments that address hypertension, regardless of its cause, include the following:

- Perform focused assessments:

    Monitor all VS. An elevated BP may affect the client's other VS. Watch for increases in pulse and respiratory rate.

    Monitor the patient's activity tolerance. The patient's degree of involvement in care, orientation, and level of fatigue while experiencing hypertension are all important indicators of decreased cardiac output.

    Accurately measure intake and output. If intake is appreciably greater than output, the increased blood volume will cause the BP to rise further. Pay attention to free fluids as well as fluid in food sources. Also monitor for edema, which is an indicator of fluid retention.

    Weigh the client regularly. Weight loss of as little as 10 lb (4.5 kg) lowers BP in many overweight persons with hypertension. Weight gain may signal poor compliance with the treatment plan and/or indicate fluid retention.

    Collect and assess laboratory data as ordered. Blood urea nitrogen (BUN), creatinine, electrolytes, hemoglobin, hematocrit, and lipid levels must all be assessed regularly.

- *Administer antihypertensive medications* (as prescribed) at regular intervals to control blood pressure.
- *For self-monitoring of BP,* see Home Care: Teaching Your Client Self-Monitoring of Blood Pressure.

One study has found that self-monitoring better predicted clinical outcomes than single office measurements.

- *For client teaching regarding hypertension,* see Self-Care: Teaching Your Client About Hypertension.
- *Teach stress management and relaxation techniques.* Such training has been effective in helping older adults with systolic hypertension to eliminate at least one antihypertensive drug and reduce their BP to target levels.
- *Teach and encourage self-management of behaviors;* provide positive feedback when the patient makes lifestyle changes.

KnowledgeCheck 17-7

- Which of the following patients has hypertension? One with a BP of:

    150/80 on two separate occasions

    180/100 on one occasion

    138/88 on two occasions
- Which of the following client(s) has/have *primary* hypertension?

    Client A, who is obese and has a high sodium intake

    Client B, who is in renal failure

    Client C, who has hypertension induced by pregnancy

    Client D, who has a family history of hypertension

 Go to Chapter 17, **Knowledge Check Response Sheet and Answers,** on the Student Resource Disk or DavisPlus at http://davisplus.fadavis.com/Wilkinson2

Self-Care

Teaching Your Client About Hypertension

Teach the client and family about lifestyle changes for preventing and managing hypertension.

- ➤ Limit salt intake to 1 teaspoon per day (2400 mg of sodium).
- ➤ Consume a diet high in potassium (e.g., fresh fruits and vegetables, such as bananas, potatoes, yogurt, and acorn squash).
- ➤ Consume a diet high in calcium (e.g., milk and milk products, sardines, molasses, tofu).
- ➤ Limit alcohol intake to 1 or 2 drinks per day for men; 1 for women. (One drink is a can of beer, one jigger of liquor, or a glass of wine. Wine is preferred.)
- ➤ Maintain ideal body weight; lose weight if overweight.
- ➤ For overall cardiovascular health, reduce saturated fat and cholesterol intake.
- ➤ Eliminate smoking.
- ➤ Engage in aerobic exercise (30 to 45 minutes, several days a week, or a total of 150 minutes per week).
- ➤ Try to reduce stress and stressful situations.

➤ Teach the client that even one lifestyle change has effects similar to treatment with a single antihypertensive drug. More than one change has an even more positive effect on the BP.

Teach the need for follow-up assessments.

- ➤ If BP is <120/80, recheck at each healthcare encounter or at least every 2 years.
- ➤ If BP is > 120 mm Hg systolic or > 80 mm Hg diastolic, review lifestyle modifications and consult the primary health provider within 1 to 2 months.
- ➤ If BP is > 140 mm Hg systolic or > 90 mm Hg diastolic, review lifestyle modifications and schedule follow-up with a healthcare provider within 1 to 2 months.
- ➤ If BP is 160 mm Hg systolic or higher, or 100 mm Hg diastolic or higher, consult the primary care provider within 1 week, or immediately if the clinical situation warrants.
- ➤ When readings are obtained by self-monitoring, reduce all numbers in the three preceding items by about 5 mm Hg (e.g., a BP > 115 mm Hg systolic or > 75 mm Hg diastolic would merit lifestyle modifications and consultation with the primary health provider).

(National Guideline Clearinghouse, 2007.)

CriticalThinking 17-10

Recall the clients you encountered at the community health fair. Lucas is 35 years old. He has been under a lot of stress. His blood pressure is 150/98.

■ To evaluate his BP, what else do you need to know about Lucas's situation (the context)?

■ What possible actions should you consider while meeting with Lucas?

■ What is the theoretical knowledge (rationale) to support your decisions?

Putting It All Together

In the hospital setting, you will usually take a complete set of VS on patients at regular intervals. In ambulatory care settings, the VS you measure may vary according to the client's chief complaint. Regardless of setting, you will need to use clinical judgment about which VS to measure and how often to measure them.

Evaluating Vital Signs

You should evaluate the client's VS on the basis of known norms as well as the particular client's trends. Suppose your client's BP has consistently been 150 to 160/90 over the last 3 days. This afternoon his BP is 108/60. Although this BP is theoretically normal, it is significantly different from his norm. Therefore, you must evaluate the cause of the change. Has there been a change in the other VS? Has there been a change in the client's medications or condition? How does the client feel? Has his activity level been altered by the change in BP? This change may be positive or negative. You must put all the VS and other clinical signs together to determine your course of action.

A high fever can cause BP to drop precipitously, for instance. Suppose this client's temperature is 103.5°F (39.7°C). In that case, in addition to his drop in BP, you should also anticipate a rise in pulse and respiratory rate. So what should you do? Your action depends on the client's condition and the context. What else is going on in the situation? If medication for the fever has been prescribed for the client, you would administer the medication and evaluate the VS again at frequent intervals. If the VS do not improve, you would then notify the primary care provider.

Now change the context slightly. Add to your preceding data that the client has undergone a surgical procedure and is not taking any antibiotics. Now what should you do? If your answer is to notify the primary care provider, you are correct. Always evaluate the VS as a unit. A sudden change in the client's condition requires you to thoroughly assess the client and report your findings to the primary care provider.

A change in a client's VS may also be a positive sign. For instance, if the client has been in severe pain for 3 days and has finally obtained pain relief, a decrease in BP probably indicates that the current medication regimen has provided better control of the pain. You would still need to monitor the VS at more frequent intervals, however, to ensure that the BP does not continue to fall.

Delegating Vital Signs

In many healthcare settings, several providers interact with the clients. VS may be obtained by nursing assistants or other unlicensed personnel. However, if you are working in a team nursing model as the registered nurse (RN), you are responsible for reviewing and interpreting the findings of all nursing assistive personnel (NAP). This includes evaluating the technique of NAPs and the accuracy of their measurements. The professional nurse *never* relinquishes the responsibility for interpretation of VS trends and decisions based on abnormal VS findings. As a student nurse, you are responsible for functioning within your scope of knowledge. If you are unsure how to interpret the meaning of a patient's VS, you must discuss the findings with your instructor and/or the nurse assigned to care for your client. Even though you are participating in the client's care, the assigned nurse maintains responsibility for client oversight.

 Go to Chapter 17, **Resources for Caregivers and Health Professionals,** on the Student Resource Disk or DavisPlus at http://davisplus.fadavis.com/Wilkinson2

 Suggested Readings: Go to Chapter 17, **Reading More About Vital Signs,** on the Student Resource Disk or DavisPlus at http://davisplus.fadavis.com/Wilkinson2

 Bibliography: Go to Volume 2, Bibliography.

CHAPTER 18

Communicating & Therapeutic Relationships

Learning Outcomes

After completing this chapter, you should be able to:

➤ Define communication.

➤ Identify the three basic levels of communication.

➤ Discuss the elements of the communication process.

➤ List the characteristics of verbal and nonverbal communication.

➤ Analyze factors that influence the communication process.

➤ Describe the elements of collaborative professional communication.

➤ Explain how relationships and roles influence communication.

➤ Describe the role of communication in each of the four phases of the therapeutic relationship.

➤ Compare and contrast techniques that enhance communication to techniques that hinder communication.

➤ Communicate with clients with impaired hearing, speech, or cognition.

➤ Communicate with clients whose culture or language is different from yours.

➤ Write a nursing care plan for a client experiencing impaired communication.

Meet Your Patient

You have been assigned to care for John Barker, a 56-year-old man admitted to the hospital with bleeding in the lower gastrointestinal tract. When you approach Mr. Barker to introduce yourself, you find him in his room with his wife at the bedside. They are holding hands, and clearly both have been crying. You begin by saying, "Good afternoon, Mr. Barker, I am a nursing student from the nearby university. I've been assigned to care for you tomorrow." Mr. Barker swallows hard and says, "I don't think you'll be able to do anything for me!" His wife says, "Don't take it personally. It's not a good time right now. Please just leave us alone."

You leave the room unsure how to respond. When you go to the unit station to review the chart, the charge nurse says, "Oh my! You've been assigned to him? I hope you've got a lot of experience." As you review the chart, you realize that Mr. Barker was just informed that he has metastatic colon cancer and probably has only a few months to live.

Theoretical **Knowledge** **knowing** why

As a nurse, you may encounter situations similar to the one involving Mr. Barker. To respond effectively, you need therapeutic communication skills. The following are examples of professional and regulatory agencies that stress the importance of good communication:

- **Quality and Safety Education for Nurses (QSEN).** To provide for patient safety, nurses need to effectively communicate their concerns about hazards and errors to patients, families, and the healthcare team (Cronenwett, Sherwood, Barnsteiner, et al., 2007).

- **The Joint Commission (2009). The Joint Commission National Patient Safety** Goal 2, aims to improve patient safety by improving communication among caregivers.

- **The Joint Commission (2007).** Performance standards state that patients have the right to receive effective, understandable information.

    As you read this chapter, you will gain theoretical and practical knowledge to help you to communicate effectively with patients, families, and other members of the healthcare team.

What Is Communication?

Communication is a dynamic, reciprocal process of sending and receiving messages. The messages may be verbal, nonverbal, or both, and they may involve two or more people. As such, communication forms the basis for sharing meaning and building effective working relationships among individuals, families, and the healthcare team.

Communication is more than the act of talking and listening (Box 18-1). It is a basic function of human life. From the first cry of a newborn to the whisper of a patient who is dying, the primary purpose of communication is to share information and obtain a response. People use communication to meet their physical, psychosocial, emotional, and spiritual needs.

Communication Occurs on Three Levels

When we think about communication, we usually imagine a dialogue between two individuals. But communication actually occurs on any of three levels. The ability to use all levels of communication improves your effectiveness as a full-spectrum nurse.

Intrapersonal communication is conscious internal dialogue, sometimes known as self-talk. Constructive affirmations, or positive self-talk (e.g., "This will work! I can do it"), promote success in a task. In contrast, negative self-talk (e.g., "I can't do this, it is too difficult") may adversely affect a person's ability to complete a task. Nurses often engage in intrapersonal communication. For example, if you enter a room and notice that your patient is pale, diaphoretic, and moaning, you may ask yourself, "What's happened? This client appears to be in a lot of pain."

Interpersonal communication occurs between two or more people. Face-to-face conversation between two people is the most frequent form of interpersonal communication. Nurses use interpersonal communication to gather information during assessment, to teach about health issues, to explain care, and to provide comfort and support. In addition to communicating directly with clients, professional nurses communicate with other nurses and healthcare team members to provide comprehensive care for clients. Because professional nurses are accountable for appropriate delegation of activities, they must also communicate effectively with nursing assistive personnel (NAP).

Group communication is interaction that occurs among several people. *Small-group communication* occurs when you engage in an exchange of ideas with two or more individuals at the same time. Examples of small-group communication include staff meetings, committee meetings, educational groups, self-help groups, and family teaching sessions. Working with groups requires effective communication skills and a basic understanding of group processes—discussed later in the chapter.

Public speaking is a unique form of group communication. Generally, the speaker addresses a dozen to hundreds of people, with varying degrees of interaction. Speakers may deliver a speech, talk directly with a small group of audience members, or have open discussion with the group. Nurses often engage in public speaking to educate groups of people about health issues, to lobby for legislation related to health promotion, and to address colleagues at professional conferences and conventions.

BOX 18-1 ■ What Is Communication?

Communication is . . . .

- Sharing or transmitting thoughts or feelings

- A way to meet physical, psychosocial, emotional, and spiritual needs

- A process—the act of sending, receiving, interpreting, and reacting to a message

- Content—the actual subject matter, words, gestures, and substance of the message

---

KnowledgeCheck 18-1

- What is the purpose of communication?
- Describe the three levels of communication.
- What level of communication was used in the "Meet Your Patient" scenario?

  Go to Chapter 18, **Knowledge Check Response Sheet and Answers,** on the Student Resource Disk or DavisPlus at http://davisplus.fadavis.com/Wilkinson2

CriticalThinking 18-1

Evaluate your own skills with the three levels of communication.

Communication Involves Both Content and Process

Communication has two major components: content and process. This distinction may seem obvious, but understanding the content and process of your communication helps you communicate more effectively.

The Content of Communication

The **content** of communication describes the actual subject matter, words, gestures, and substance of the message. It is the message that everyone may hear or see. For example, suppose your client said, "I slept through lunch." This statement is open to interpretation. We cannot tell—without also observing him, knowing his history, and so on—whether he thinks this is a good thing because he wanted or needed rest, or a bad thing because he is so exhausted, or a complaint about the staff for not waking him for lunch, or an apology and request for a late lunch. As you can see, the words are just a part of communication. You must also consider the process.

The Process of Communication

Process refers to the act of sending, receiving, interpreting, and reacting to a message. The communication process has five elements: sender, message, receiver, feedback, and channel. Figure 18-1 illustrates the relationship among these elements.

The **sender** begins the conversation to deliver a message (content) to another person. The sender, sometimes called the *source* or the *encoder,* uses verbal and nonverbal methods to transmit the message. **Encoding** refers to the process of selecting the words, gestures, tone of voice, signs, and symbols used to transmit the message. For example, consider the case of Mr. Barker. As a beginning nursing student, you might feel anxious about caring for

Mr. Barker. How could you communicate your concerns to your instructor? You might directly state, "It makes me nervous to be assigned to him," or you might avoid eye contact with your instructor and tell her, "I'm going to need some help today." Both styles communicate your anxiety, but they are encoded differently. Encoding may or may not be done consciously, and it is affected by the nature of the message, the relationship between the sender and receiver, the mood of the sender, and other situational stressors.

The **message** is the verbal and/or nonverbal information the sender communicates. It might be a conversation, a speech, a gesture, a letter, and so forth. Effective messages are complete, clear, concise, organized, timely, and expressed in a manner that the receiver can understand. The message must be appropriate for the situation and for the developmental level of the person receiving the message. For instance, to family members awaiting the results of a life-saving procedure, seeing the patient's nurse walk toward them smiling broadly may give them an immediate nonverbal message about the outcome of the procedure.

The **channel** is the medium used to send the message. Face-to-face communication is a commonly used channel. Nurses frequently use touch as a nonverbal way to communicate caring and concern. Other channels include written pamphlets, audiovisual aids, recordings, telephone and text messages, and the Internet. When choosing the channel that is best suited for communicating a message, consider the type of message, its purpose, and the size of the audience. For example, in the case of Mr. Barker, during this troubled time, touching his hand while remaining silent might send a clearer message of caring than any words you could say.

The **receiver** is the observer, listener, and interpreter of the message. Interpretation, also called **decoding**,

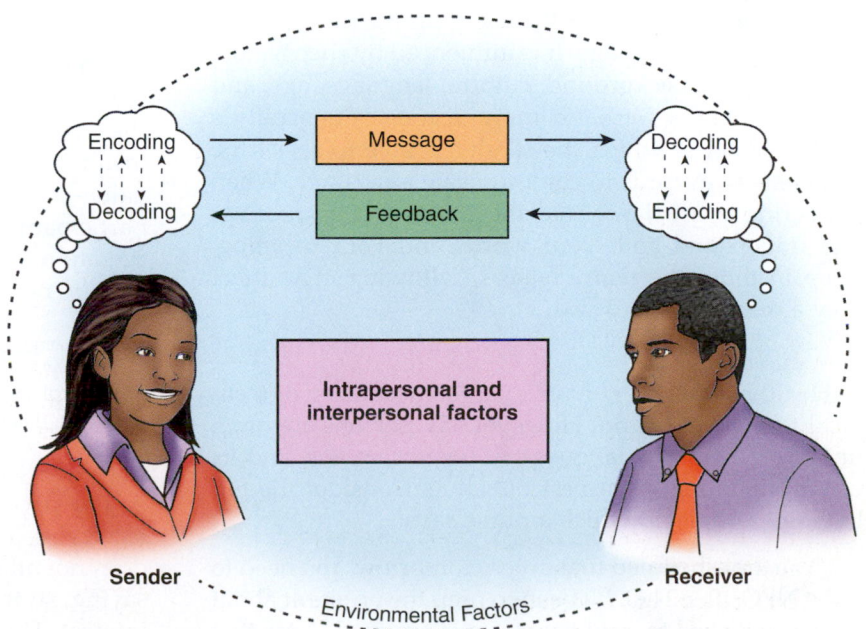

FIGURE 18-1 Communication: A sender encodes and transmits a message to a receiver, who decodes it and transmits feedback.

refers to relating the message to your past experiences to determine the sender's meaning. The receiver uses visual, auditory, and tactile senses to decode the message. If the decoded meaning matches the intended meaning, then the message was effective. However, messages are sometimes misinterpreted, especially when the receiver is not physically or emotionally ready to receive the message. For example, if you approached your instructor to discuss your concerns about Mr. Barker when she was assisting with an emergency on the unit, she might be unable to receive your message.

Once the receiver has received and interpreted the message, he may be stimulated to respond by providing feedback to the sender. **Feedback** validates that the receiver received the message and understood it as the sender intended. Feedback may be verbal, nonverbal, or both. Verifying the message avoids confusion.

KnowledgeCheck 18-2

Using the "Meet Your Patient" scenario, identify at least one sender, one message, one receiver, one channel, and one example of feedback.

 Go to Chapter 18, **Knowledge Check Response Sheet and Answers,** on the Student Resource Disk or DavisPlus at http://davisplus.fadavis.com/Wilkinson2

Communication Can Be Verbal or Nonverbal

People send and receive messages both verbally and nonverbally. The two forms of communication occur spontaneously and simultaneously in interpersonal and group interactions.

Verbal Communication

Verbal communication is the use of spoken and written words to send a message. It is influenced by such factors as educational background, culture, language, age, and past experiences. Verbal communication is generally a conscious act in which the sender is able to select the most effective words to communicate a message. When delivering a verbal message, the goal is that the receiver will understand both your words and your meaning. Keep in mind the many factors, following, that affect how a message is received.

Vocabulary

Healthcare workers have a large vocabulary of technical terms and jargon. However, lay persons are often unfamiliar with the language of healthcare and find its use intimidating, or at best puzzling. Consider the following example, in which a nurse says:

"You are scheduled for surgery tomorrow. You need to be NPO after 2400. I'll be in to prep the op site at about 8. You'll need to void before your pre-med. After that

we'll move you to a gurney and transfer you to the holding area."

Do you think most clients would understand this message? Do you even understand all the words? Clients are often confused by medical terms and technical jargon, but for various reasons (e.g., being embarrassed at not knowing), they often hesitate to ask questions to clarify what was said. How much better it would be if the nurse had said:

"Your surgery will be tomorrow morning. You will not be able to eat or drink anything after midnight. I'll come in about 8 in the morning to clean your hip and get it ready for the operation. Then you'll need to urinate before I give you some medicine to relax you. After that, we'll put you on a cart and roll you up to the operating area."

It is your responsibility to deliver messages that the client can understand; therefore, use medical terms only when you are certain the listener understands them. When encoding a message, consider the receiver's age, knowledge, education, and any cultural differences, including primary language spoken. (These factors are discussed shortly.) Encourage feedback to be sure that the receiver understood the message as you intended.

Denotative and Connotative Meaning

Denotation is the literal (dictionary) meaning of a word. In contrast, **connotation** is the implied or emotional meaning of the word. Consider the following examples:

A mother says to her infant, "Don't cry, baby."
A 40-year-old man says to his nurse, "Would you rub my back, baby?"
A 10-year-old boy says to another boy, "You're a baby!"

The denotative meaning of *baby* is a very young child who is not yet able to walk. However, the connotative meaning is different in each example. In the first example, the connotative meaning is the same as the denotative meaning. In the second example, the nurse might interpret it as a sexist remark; and in the last example, the 10-year-old boy undoubtedly meant *baby* as an insult. As these examples illustrate, words are often value-laden or biased. The situation, qualities of the participants, and the words they choose all affect interpretation. Use terms that provide clear, objective data and are not open for misinterpretation.

CriticalThinking 18-2

Think of two other examples in which the connotative meaning may be different from the denotative meaning.

Pacing

The pace and rhythm of the delivery can alter the receiver's interpretation of the message. A rapid pace does not allow the receiver to track what the speaker is saying, so the receiver may become frustrated and lose interest. The pace must be slow enough for the receiver to interpret one thought before the sender moves on to the next thought. By pausing at intervals, the speaker also gives the listener time to respond. However, the pace must be fast enough to maintain the listener's interest. What happens when a professor talks very slowly during a lecture? Do you find your mind wandering: "I need to take the dog to the vet. . . . What shall we have for dinner? . . ."

Intonation

Intonation, or "tone of voice," reflects the feeling behind the words. We get a sense of a person's intonation by listening to the *pitch* (high or low), *cadence* (rising and falling of the pitch), and *volume* (soft or loud). These variables help a speaker convey confidence, enthusiasm, sadness, fear, anger, anxiety, or boredom. For example, experiment with the variety of ways you might state, "Your test results are in."

Pitch, cadence, and volume can either reinforce or contradict the message. When spoken at a moderate pitch and volume, with a falling cadence, the words, "I understand that I am to report at noon" can be a simple confirmation that the person has received the message. When spoken quietly, hesitantly, and with a rising cadence, it can convey the message that the person actually does not understand at all. Monitor your intonation and that of your clients as you communicate.

People tend to lose interest when someone speaks in a monotone (does not vary the pitch, cadence, and volume). Before presenting lengthy information, whether to an individual or to a group, experiment with these variables to ensure that the listener remains engaged with your topic.

When electronic messaging is used, the receiver does not have the advantage of intonation or body language. This may lead to miscommunication. People sometimes insert *emoticons* (symbols such as "smiley faces") to provide cues to the emotional tone of a message.

Clarity and Brevity

Clarity in communication requires that you select words that convey the intended meaning and that you make sure your spoken words and the nonverbal language send the same message. You can achieve brevity by using the fewest words possible. A conversation that is clear and brief holds the interest of all parties and effectively conveys the intended messages.

Timing and Relevance

Timing is crucial. Before starting a conversation, assess your client. A person who is distracted by pain, hunger, or other physiological needs will not receive the message as you intended it. Similarly, a client attempting to cope with stressors, such as limited finances, an upcoming surgery, or a terminal diagnosis, may be unable to listen effectively.

Also consider the presence of others. For example, asking a client about a personal issue in a public corridor may inhibit his response. You will receive a different response if you ask the same question in a more private setting. In contrast, if you are instructing a client about a recommended diet, be sure that the person who is responsible for shopping and cooking is also present. If your client does neither in his household, he may pay little attention to your instruction—it will not be relevant to him.

Communication is effective when both parties value the interaction and find the discussion relevant. For example, to teach your client about his medicines, choose a time when he is alert, pain-free, and not distracted, and begin by reminding him of the purpose of the discussion: "I'm going to teach you how to take this medication so that it effectively controls your pain." Timing also means that the interaction must allow time for response. A rapid flow of questions or one-sided conversations inhibit interaction.

Credibility

Clients judge the **credibility** (or believability) of the message on the trustworthiness of the sender. Your credibility depends on a pattern of honest and timely response to patient concerns, as well as congruence between your verbal and nonverbal communication.

As a nurse, you will be called on to provide information on a wide range of topics. Give information only if you are certain of the facts. A response such as, "I don't know, but I'll find out and let you know" is far more credible than an incorrect answer or guess. Never lie to the patient. Lying can take many forms, but it always destroys trust. If you tell the patient you will be right back with pain medication but forget to return until she reminds you an hour later, she may doubt your credibility.

If a situation makes you uncomfortable it is better to acknowledge your discomfort than to risk loss of credibility. For example, you may feel uncomfortable talking to Mr. Barker ("Meet Your Patient") about his recent diagnosis. You may be tempted to say, "Maybe the test results are wrong," or "The timeline is just a guess. I think you can beat this." This approach avoids uncomfortable discussion and may make the patient feel better temporarily. However, a more honest approach would be to tell Mr. Barker that you would like him to meet with a counselor or hospital chaplain.

To be credible, your nonverbal communication must match your spoken words. For example, if your client asks you if his wound is "ugly," he will pay attention to your facial expressions as well as your spoken response. If you respond that "The wound looks good," but frown or fail to make eye contact, the client will most likely believe that you are not being completely honest. This may jeopardize future interactions.

Humor

Humor and laughing can have a positive influence on attitude and healing. Laughter can create physiological changes that contribute to well-being and provide an emotional release in a tense situation. However, use humor cautiously. Humor is highly subjective and personal; and it also depends on cultural norms. Never direct humor at the client, disease process, or treatment team. Misused humor can have a negative effect on self-esteem, self-confidence, or the client's confidence in the treatment team. Consider the different effects the following uses of humor might have. Imagine that your patient has had vomiting and diarrhea for the last 8 hours. When you enter the room you jokingly say, "Oh my! You look like you had too much to drink last night." Although the intent was to lighten the mood, this statement may offend your patient. In contrast, imagine that you notice that an older patient thoroughly enjoys visits from his young grandchildren. You might consider sharing with him an amusing story about your own children.

Nonverbal Communication

Nonverbal communication (or body language) is the exchange of messages without the use of words. Verbal communication is a highly conscious activity in which we choose words to communicate. Nonverbal communication occurs on a more unconscious level. Because nonverbal language emerges from how the sender is feeling, it more accurately conveys the true meaning of a message. It may thereby reinforce or contradict the spoken message. For example, in the "Meet Your Patient" scenario, Mr. Barker uses few words. However, he is tearful and distressed. That body language gives you valuable insight into how he is adjusting to the news of his cancer. Let's look at some nonverbal messages.

Facial Expression

Expressions of the face and especially the eyes are some of the most obvious forms of nonverbal communication. Facial expressions communicate joy, anger, sadness, concern, or fear. Raised eyebrows, staring, squinting, or darting eyes all convey meaning.

Smiling is one expression that everyone understands. In contrast, the interpretation of many other facial expressions is culturally dependent. For example, downcast eyes may indicate sadness, poor self-esteem, a desire to avoid the conversation, respect, powerlessness, or submissive behavior. In Western cultures, eye contact usually indicates an interest in the conversation and a willingness to communicate; however, in Eastern cultures, the amount of eye contact considered acceptable varies. Chapter 13 discusses cultural variations.

A mismatch between your verbal message and facial expression may cause the client to doubt your credibility (Fig. 18-2). For example, suppose that a patient states, "I just had my pain pill. Why is my pain still so bad?" You answer, "The medication should take effect within a few more minutes. If it doesn't, call me." Imagine the different effect this reply would have if you were smiling, frowning, raising one eyebrow, or avoiding eye contact.

Posture and Gait

Body position, gait, and posture offer clues to a person's attitudes, emotions, physical well-being, and self-concept. When you see someone with an erect posture,

FIGURE 18-2 The nurse's facial expression is not appropriate because the patient appears to be in distress.

head held high, and a quick gait, what do you think? In Western culture, these are nonverbal indicators of health and a sense of self-assuredness. In contrast, a slow, shuffling gait may signify someone who is ill, is depressed, or has poor self-esteem.

Personal Appearance

Clothing and personal appearance provide clues to a person's feelings, socioeconomic status, culture, and religion. A person who is ill, tired, or depressed may lack energy for hygiene and grooming. Lack of attention to personal appearance is especially significant in a person who typically engages in meticulous grooming. As with all nonverbal data, you need to investigate the meaning of personal appearance to avoid drawing erroneous conclusions.

Dress and accessories are powerful cultural clues. Does the patient dress in a style that differs from local custom? Are pieces of jewelry or religious medallions visible? These are clues to the patient's values, as well as the patient's socioeconomic status. Pay attention to these clues, but do not make assumptions from them. A person who wears an elaborate religious medal may like the ornamentation but not espouse the beliefs that are attached to the symbol.

Have you thought about what your own personal appearance conveys to your patients and colleagues? Most people express their individuality through their dress, hair style, and so on. Nurses, however, must also consider how patients perceive them and whether their appearance helps or hinders their patient relationships. Issues of safety and cleanliness are also essential for nurses, when choosing clothing, hair styles, and body adornment (e.g., jewelry, nail polish, tattoos, body piercings). The traditional white nursing uniform has been almost completely replaced by "scrub clothes" of various colors, which makes it difficult for patients to differentiate nurses from the rest of the healthcare team. To counteract this, some agencies are assigning colors for various workers (e.g., blue for physicians, purple for nurses).

Gestures

Hand and body gestures emphasize and clarify the spoken word. They are good indicators of the feeling tone behind the conversation. Imagine that your client says, "I'm OK." What might it mean if he accompanies his statement with a broad grin and raised arms? What might it mean if, instead, he lowers his head to his hands?

Gestures vary widely among individuals and cultures, so use them with caution. For example, consider the gesture of a "V" made with the second and third fingers of the hand. To some people, this is a peace sign; to others, it is a victory sign; and still others may attach no meaning to it at all. Gestures can help you communicate with individuals with impaired verbal communication. Be careful, however, that you and the patient agree on the meaning of the gestures.

Touch

Touch can convey affection, caring, concern, and encouragement. Avoid using touch when dealing with someone who is angry or mentally disturbed because the touch may be misinterpreted (e.g., as a sign of aggression or sexual attraction). Although touch can be highly effective, use it with conscious awareness of the situation, environment, culture, and receptivity of the patient.

For examples of therapeutic nonverbal behaviors and how patients may interpret them,

 Go to **Clinical Insight 18-1: Enhancing Communication Through Nonverbal Behaviors,** in Volume 2.

KnowledgeCheck 18-3

- Identify the components of verbal and nonverbal communication.
- What action should you take when there is a discrepancy between the client's spoken word and nonverbal body language?

 Go to Chapter 18, **Knowledge Check Response Sheet and Answers,** on the Student Resource Disk or DavisPlus at http://davisplus.fadavis.com/Wilkinson2

CriticalThinking 18-3

- Observe an interaction between family members or your fellow students. Look for congruence between verbal and nonverbal communication. Strategize what you would say to validate the intended meaning when the two modes of communication are not in agreement.
- Recall the brief interaction with the charge nurse in the "Meet Your Patient" scenario. What might you say or do in response?

What Factors Affect Communication?

The following is a discussion of the major factors, in addition to verbal and nonverbal language, that affect communication.

Environment

Communication is most successful in an environment that is quiet, private, free of unpleasant smells, and at a comfortable temperature. As a beginning student, you are aware of the noises and distractions in the clinical setting. However, experienced nurses become accustomed to such distractions. Be sensitive to how the environment is affecting your client. Background noise is distracting, interferes with hearing, and can create confusion. Being around others in pain or distress creates anxiety and fear; lack of privacy may cause embarrassment. All of those feelings may prevent your patient from sharing personal information.

Think creatively to secure the most comfortable environment possible for communicating with patients and families. Hospital chapels, foyers, and activity rooms may be ideal locations for conversation. To discuss private matters, consider talking with the patient in a conference room rather than a shared room. If none of these is possible, at least close privacy curtains and turn off the radio or television.

Developmental Variations

Physical and cognitive development, language skills, level of education, and maturity influence the communication process. Thus, you will need to modify your communication strategies to fit your client's developmental level. By the time you enter nursing practice, your goal should be to communicate effectively, respectfully, and compassionately with patients at all developmental stages. For detailed information on expectations for each developmental stage,

 Go to Chapter 9, **Expanded Discussion,** on the Student Resource Disk or DavisPlus at http://davisplus.fadavis.com/Wilkinson2

Infants and young toddlers with limited language skills communicate nonverbally. Your response may combine verbal and nonverbal communication. For example, if a hospitalized one-year-old cries out for his mother, you might cuddle the child with his favorite toy and explain that "Mama will be back very soon." Older toddlers and preschoolers have more verbal ability. Although they may prefer to have a parent present, they are likely to talk with you and answer questions. School-age children are usually quite comfortable interacting verbally. Pay attention to their vocabulary as they speak, and be sure to match it to the extent possible, using words and phrasing the child will understand. By the time children reach adolescence, most can process abstract concepts. As a result, they are usually able to understand disease processes, treatments, and other health issues. Bear in mind that children with chronic health problems that have required frequent interventions are often more knowledgeable than would be expected for their age.

Older adults may be affected by sensory alterations, such as hearing loss or vision changes, or any of a variety of healthcare problems that affect cognition. Communication strategies for these situations are discussed in the "Planning Interventions/Implementation" section of this chapter.

Gender

Males and females communicate differently and may interpret the same communication differently. Linguist Deborah Tannen, author of *You Just Don't Understand: Women and Men in Conversation* (2001), states that women communicate to form connections and establish relationships. In contrast, male communication styles focus on maintaining independence and favorable positions in a hierarchy. In essence, women want to "be connected," whereas men want to "be one up."

These communication patterns have their roots in early socialization differences. Traditionally, boys are socialized to participate in competitive team sports. Through this play, they learn how to compete, strategize, and win or lose. In contrast, young girls are more likely to engage in one-on-one or fantasy play that requires cooperation and focuses on fairness and negotiation. This early socialization is carried over into communication patterns. Men are more likely to be comfortable in situations that result in a win or loss, whereas women are more likely to attempt to reach consensus. Male communication tends to be purpose driven: more about conveying information and accomplishing a goal, whereas female communication tends to be relationally driven.

Gender differences in communication are important to nurses because male and female patients may communicate their needs very differently. Similarly, the gender of the nurse may affect the response to the patient's requests. For example, a female patient might state, "I feel so lousy today." A female nurse may interpret this as a desire to talk. In contrast, a male nurse may discuss pain control.

Personal Space

People vary in the amount of physical space they are comfortable with when communicating. The distance they maintain between one another is influenced by the relationship of the individuals, the nature of the conversation, the setting, and cultural influences (Fig. 18-3). Also see Chapter 13 for cultural preferences for personal space. Hall (1992) describes four distinct distances influencing communication: intimate distance, personal distance, social distance, and public distance.

Intimate distance is the area immediately surrounding people that they define as their "private space." People prefer to maintain intimate distance between themselves and others during interactions. In Western cultures, intimate distance is within 18 inches of the other person. Within this distance, people can sense each other's smell and body heat and usually can hear

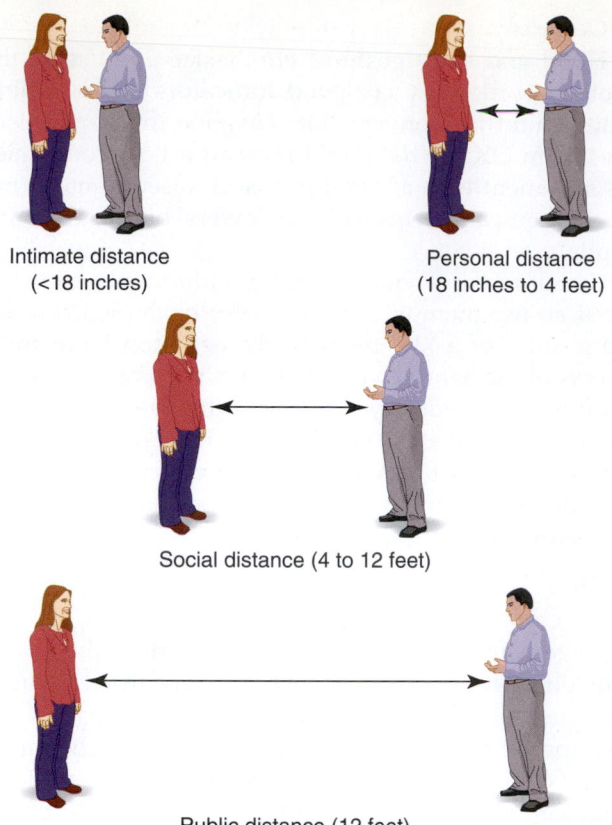

Intimate distance (<18 inches)

Personal distance (18 inches to 4 feet)

Social distance (4 to 12 feet)

Public distance (12 feet)

FIGURE 18-3 The distance that individuals engaged in communication maintain between one another is influenced by their relationship, the nature of the conversation, the setting, and cultural influences.

each other speaking at a low volume. It is also at this distance that body contact occurs. As a nurse, you invade a client's intimate distance to perform assessments and procedures. You even breach a client's intimate distance when touching a hand or shoulder to offer support. It is important to recognize that this may make some clients uncomfortable. Before providing nursing interventions in the client's intimate distance, discuss what you are about to do. It is best to ask the client's permission, even for gentle touch, if you are in the slightest doubt about his receptivity.

Personal distance is from 18 inches to 4 feet. Your interactions with clients and healthcare team members will commonly occur in this range. This distance facilitates sharing of feelings or personal thoughts and is appropriate to maintain when communicating caring or concern.

Social distance is a distance of 4 to 12 feet. It is used in more formal interaction or when communicating with a group of individuals at the same time. At this distance, individuals are not within range to be physically touched. The volume of the spoken words may be loud enough for others to overhear, so people share personal feelings and thoughts less often at this distance. For example, if you stand by a client's door and ask how she is feeling, you will likely receive a more impersonal response than if you were to ask the same question at her bedside.

Public distance is considered to be beyond 12 feet. This distance requires loud and clear enunciation for communication. Public speakers and large educational groups use this form of personal space. This distance is characterized by a lack of individuality and a greater focus on the group or community.

Territoriality

Territoriality refers to the space and things that an individual identifies as belonging to him. Territories may be bounded and visible to others or may be defined by the individual in a way not noticeable to others. In a hospital setting, many clients consider everything within the curtain boundary to be their territory. Clients may be offended if you invade, rearrange, or interfere with this territory by moving furniture, discarding objects, or borrowing items from the room, even if they are institutional property. Be aware of this and request permission to rearrange your client's territory. Also recognize that hospitalized clients are not in their "home" territory and are therefore likely to be less at ease during interactions.

Sociocultural Factors

Culture and socioeconomic status strongly influence communication. Facial expressions, nonverbal communication, and even the selection of whom to interact with are affected. For example, in some cultures it would be unacceptable for a male nurse to address and provide care to a female patient.

Social status also plays a role in communication. Have you ever been present while a physician explained a treatment plan to a patient? Often the client asks no questions or nods approval, yet barrages you with questions when the physician leaves. One reason for this behavior is that many clients perceive less social distance between themselves and the nurse. Consequently, they are more likely to ask you questions or to discuss concerns with you. Social distance can also play a role in how health professionals view clients. For example, you may see impoverished clients being treated with less respect than wealthy members of the community, although this is certainly not an example you will want to follow.

Roles and Relationships

The roles and relationships of the sender and receiver affect communication. They affect the choice of vocabulary, tone of voice, use of gestures, and distance associated with the communication. Think of the way you interact with your instructor. Compare this with the way you interact with your classmates. What are the differences?

Many patients have preconceived notions about nurses. Some may view you as an authority figure. Others may perceive nursing as a lowly occupation and limit conversation with you to matters of comfort and hygiene. Still other patients become confused by the fact that many healthcare workers, such as medical assistants and nursing assistive personnel (NAP), call themselves nurses in spite of the fact that they cannot legally use the title. This makes it unclear whom the patient should speak with about concerns. If you are working with NAP or other team members, be sure to clarify their roles with the patient.

KnowledgeCheck 18-4

- What are the major factors that affect communication?
- In what distance(s) do most nurse–client interactions occur?

 Go to Chapter 18, **Knowledge Check Response Sheet and Answers,** on the Student Resource Disk or DavisPlus at http://davisplus.fadavis.com/Wilkinson2

What Is Collaborative Professional Communication?

Communication is essential to collaborative practice. As a member of the healthcare team, you need to communicate effectively with nurses, physicians, and health professionals from other disciplines. Each of you shares the common goal of providing optimal patient care. This goal should guide the manner in which you communicate—at the bedside, at the nurse's station, in care conferences, or via the patient record. Nurses also need to communicate with peers and colleagues in order to contribute to their professional development. See Box 18-2 for statements from professional organizations about collaborative communication.

Communicating Assertively

Think of communication styles as a continuum from passive, through assertive, to aggressive. A **passive approach** avoids conflict and allows others to take the lead. It tends to be submissive, helpless, indecisive, apologetic, or whining. "Whatever you want. I don't want you to change anything for me," is an example of a passive approach. In contrast, an *aggressive approach* forces others to lose. The goal is to win and be in control. "My way is the correct way. You don't know what you're talking about" typifies an aggressive approach. Other characteristics are that it is bossy, arrogant, opinionated, sarcastic, manipulative, intolerant, or overbearing.

Why might you adopt a **nonassertive style**? As previously discussed, men and women tend to communicate differently. People may also communicate differently with persons of higher or lower status. When speaking to physicians, some nurses still communicate their needs in a style that assures physicians that they are not telling them what to do (e.g., "Do you think Mrs. King's heart rate is a little fast today?" instead of "Mrs. King's heart

BOX 18-2 ■ Collaborative Professional Communication

American Nurses Association (ANA) (2010, in press)

Standards of professional performance (11, 13, and 14), stress the importance of communication to collegiality and collaboration. The following are some of the competencies for these three standards. The registered nurse:

Standard 11. Communication

- Communicates effectively in a variety of written, spoken and technological formats.
- Demonstrates effective communication and information sharing across disciplines and throughout transitions in care.
- Asserts own position/perspective in discussions about patient care.
- Communicates observations or concerns related to hazards and errors to patients, families, and/or health care team.

Standard 13. Collegiality

- Shares knowledge and skills with peers and colleagues as evidenced by such activities as patient care conferences or presentations at formal or informal meetings.
- Provides peers with feedback regarding their practice and/ or role performance.

Standard 14. Collaboration

- Communicates with patient, family, and healthcare providers regarding patient care and the nurse's role in the provision of that care.

Caveat: This material is from the draft for public comment (ANA, 2010, in press); its wording may be changed somewhat in the final published version. For that version of the ANA Standards of Professional Nursing Practice, go to www.nursingworld.org.

American Association of Critical-Care Nurses (AACN)

Skilled communication is necessary to a healthy work environment. Nurses must be proficient in communication skills. Critical elements of communication include the following:

- Focusing on finding solutions and achieving desirable outcomes
- Seeking to protect and advance collaborative relationships among colleagues
- Inviting and hearing all relevant perspectives
- Striving for goodwill and mutual respect
- Building consensus and arriving at common understanding
- Achieving congruence between words and actions, and holding others accountable for doing so
- Developing proficiency with communication technologies (2005)

Quality and Safety Education for Nurses (QSEN)

Communication is essential for teamwork and collaboration. On graduation from nursing school, you should be able to analyze differences in others' communication style preferences and describe the impact of your own communication style on others (Cronenwett, Sherwood, Barnsteiner, et al., 2007).

The Joint Commission (2006)

The 2006 National Patient Safety Goals added Goal 2E, recommending a standardized approach to "hand off" communications, including an opportunity to ask and respond to questions. The broad Goal 2, calls for improving the effectiveness of communication among caregivers.

---

rate was 120 at 8 A.M."). This has been referred to as the doctor–nurse game (Stein, Watts, & Howell, 1990). Such unclear, indirect communication contributes to errors and poor patient outcomes. To advocate for clients, question care decisions, and discuss errors or poor clinical judgment with co-workers, you will need to communicate assertively.

Assertive communication is the expression of a wide range of positive and negative thoughts and feelings in a style that is direct, open, honest, spontaneous, responsible, and nonjudgmental. Assertiveness recognizes your rights while still respecting the rights of others. It allows you to take responsibility for your own thoughts and actions without blaming others, encourages feedback, and enables you to find mutually satisfying solutions to conflict by confronting people constructively. So how do you communicate assertively?

- *Question care decisions openly and honestly.* Refuse to play the doctor–nurse game. Avoid beginning your statements with self-effacing statements that fail to take credit for your contributions (e.g., "You may disagree with this, but. . ."). Be frank, but be flexible and open-minded.

- *Use "I" statements.* An "I" statement should include the elements of behavior (or facts), feeling, and effect (on you). For example, instead of saying, "Why haven't you ordered Mrs. Johnson's pain medications yet?" you might say, "I telephoned you this morning about Mrs. Johnson's lack of pain relief, but I don't see a change in her analgesic order. I am concerned about her discomfort and the effect it may have on her willingness to ambulate."

- *Focus on the issue, not the participants.* For example, "I think this approach might be the best, but I'd like to hear your thoughts."

- *Use effective nonverbal language.* Your body and verbal language should be congruent. Eye contact demonstrates interest and shows sincerity. Use a calm, well modulated voice tone, and add appropriate gestures for emphasis.

- *Don't invite negative responses.* For example, say "I would really appreciate it if you could help me weigh Mr. Max on the bed scale," rather than, "Can you help me weigh him?"

- *Use "fogging" to help you accept criticism without becoming anxious or defensive.* Acknowledge that there may be some truth to it, but remain the judge of your own action Suppose Mrs. Johnson's physician says, "Are you playing pharmacist today?" You might respond, "I agree that I may not be a pharmacist and that I do not know everything there is to know about analgesics. However, Mrs. Johnson needs pain relief and I need your assistance with pain medication."

- *Use negative inquiry.* You might choose, in the preceding situation, to use negative inquiry. You would reply, "So you believe that I do not have adequate knowledge to discuss Mrs. Johnson's pain control?"
- *Strive for a workable compromise*, but not if it affects patient well-being or your feelings of self-respect. Suppose an administrator comes to a patient's room while you are inserting a nasogastric tube and says, "I need to see you right now. Come to the desk immediately." An example of a workable compromise would be to say, "I understand that you need to talk to me right away, and I need to finish what I am doing. So what about meeting you at the desk as soon as I finish, in about 10 minutes?"

It may help to practice ahead of time how you want to look and sound before attempting assertive communication. Assertiveness is a learned skill. Role playing with a colleague can build your confidence. For a summary of assertive communication techniques,

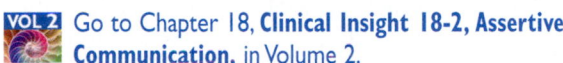 Go to Chapter 18, **Clinical Insight 18-2, Assertive Communication,** in Volume 2.

Using the SBAR Model

Using a standard framework helps you to convey key information clearly and concisely, thus improving interdisciplinary communication and patient outcomes. The SBAR model is designed to overcome differences in nurse-physician communication styles. The acronym represents: Situation, Background, Assessment, Recommendation. For a summary of this model,

 Go to Chapter 18, **Clinical Insight 18-3, Communicating with SBAR,** in Volume 2.

If you need other information about giving a verbal report, also see Chapter 16.

What Is the Role of Communication in Therapeutic Relationships?

A **therapeutic relationship** focuses on improving the health of the client, whether an individual or community. The client gains information and knowledge and works through issues, concerns, and problems related to health status, treatments, and nursing care. **Therapeutic communication** is client-centered communication directed at achieving client goals. It is used to establish the therapeutic relationship, provide and obtain healthcare information, and express interest and concern for the client and family.

Communication Is Essential to All Phases of the Therapeutic Relationship

The therapeutic relationship consists of four phases. As you read about each phase, notice the fundamental role of client-focused communication.

The **pre-interaction phase** occurs before you meet the client. This phase involves gathering information about the client, but the nurse and client do not have direct communication. As a student, you initiate this phase as you prepare for clinical days. The client also experiences a pre-interaction phase, which begins when she identifies the need for healthcare. This can be an anxious time for the client.

The **orientation phase** begins when you meet the client. For Mr. Barker ("Meet Your Patient"), it began when you approached him to introduce yourself. The goal of this phase is to establish rapport and trust through the use of verbal and nonverbal communication. Orientation begins with introductions, followed by an initial exchange of information, such as the client's reason for the visit or chief concerns. Orientation ends when the relationship has been defined. Ideally there is time at the beginning to exchange pleasantries and develop a level of comfort, but in some clinical situations, such as during an emergency, this phase is very brief.

The bulk of therapeutic communication occurs in the **working phase,** the active part of the relationship. During this phase, the nurse communicates caring, the patient expresses thoughts and feelings, mutual respect is maintained, and honest verbal and nonverbal expression occurs. Key communication goals are to assist the client to clarify feelings and concerns. A professional relationship is courteous, trustworthy, and confidential, and accomplished by active listening and other techniques of therapeutic communication presented later in this chapter.

The **termination phase** is the conclusion of the relationship, whether at the end of the nurse's shift or on the client's discharge from the unit, facility, or service. Reviewing and summarizing help to bring the relationship to a comfortable conclusion. If communication has been effective, the termination phase prepares the nurse and client for future interactions. Unsuccessful communication may affect the client's health outcomes or understanding of his disease process, as well as affect the nurse's job satisfaction.

 Critical**Thinking** 18-4

Recall the scenario of Mr. Barker ("Meet Your Patient").
- What phase of the therapeutic relationship is illustrated in the scenario?
- How might the interaction between you and Mr. Barker change if it occurred in a different phase of the therapeutic relationship?
- What could you have done differently?

Therapeutic Communication Has Five Key Characteristics

The therapeutic relationship requires conscious use of your knowledge and skills to effect change in the patient. This is often called the *therapeutic use of self*. Five qualities characterize communication in the therapeutic relationship: empathy, respect, genuineness, concreteness, and confrontation.

Although therapeutic use of self involves empathy and positive regard for patients, it does require some practice for you to recognize the boundaries of a therapeutic relationship and to keep the focus on the patient rather than on your own feelings and experiences. For more information about that, follow the link for Suggested Readings at the end of this chapter.

Empathy

Empathy is the desire to understand and be sensitive to the feelings, beliefs, and situation of another person. Empathy is more than sharing of information. Empathy requires you to be willing to adapt your style, tone, vocabulary, and behavior to create the best approach for each client situation. It is relatively easy to have empathy for people who are like you and who are likeable. It is more difficult to connect with people you see as "difficult" or "different." To empathize with a client, you must look beyond outward appearance or behavior and put yourself, mentally and emotionally, in the client's place. This will help you appreciate the uniqueness of the client.

Respect

In the therapeutic relationship, you communicate respect by valuing the client and being flexible to meet the client's needs. As a nurse, you must be willing to adjust to your client rather than expecting the client to adjust to you, the healthcare environment, or hospital routines. Most healthcare experiences strip the client of power—clothes are removed, roles are discontinued, people are separated from loved ones and familiar surroundings, and schedules are altered. When a relationship is grounded in respect, both parties maintain power and self-esteem. You show your respect for clients in the way you address them, the words and intonation you choose, and in your acknowledgment of their strengths and needs. Making even minor adjustments, such as delaying breakfast for an hour to allow the client to sleep, communicates that you respect the client's wishes.

Genuineness

When interviewing clients, we expect them to respond truthfully. After all, many healthcare decisions are based on the client's responses. Similarly, clients have a right to expect truthful responses from healthcare providers as well. **Genuineness** is the ability to respond honestly. If you are unable to answer a client's question, do not offer guesses. Be honest. Tell the client you need assistance before you can answer the question. Genuineness also involves willingness to self-evaluate. How well did I communicate? Did I handle that situation appropriately? How could I improve my communication?

Concreteness and Confrontation

In a therapeutic relationship, you must offer understandable responses to a client's questions and concerns. To do so requires you to express in concrete, specific terms what you mean. The message must be constructed and delivered in a manner that is suitable for the client. Communication is a reciprocal process. If your client is unable to express his thoughts clearly, you must be willing to confront her to request clarification. Similarly, you must be willing to be confronted if you are unclear.

Therapeutic communication requires practice. A strategy commonly used to improve communication skills is called *process recording*. In **process recording**, two people converse while a third records the conversation. Afterward, the participants analyze the interaction. Audio recording can facilitate process recording. It effectively captures the words and intonation of the conversation, but it must be supplemented by notes on nonverbal communication. Videotaping allows participants to examine both verbal and nonverbal communication. As you examine an interaction, look for the five qualities just discussed. Box 18-3 identifies skills associated with these qualities. Later, the chapter presents specific strategies for enhancing communication, as well as barriers to therapeutic communication. Look for these techniques and barriers in any conversation you analyze.

Communication Is Important in Group Helping Relationships

Most of our previous discussion focused on one-on-one communication. However, nurses frequently communicate with groups. Group communication occurs when you interact with a family, a community, or a committee. Groups can enhance problem solving and creativity, generate understanding and support, enhance morale, and provide affiliation.

BOX 18-3 ■ Skills Needed in a Therapeutic Relationship

The ability to:

- Appreciate experiences and beliefs that differ from your own.
- Recognize and interpret verbal and nonverbal messages.
- Guide the interaction to accomplish goals.
- Determine *whether* communication is taking place.
- Speak when appropriate and remain silent when appropriate.
- Adapt to the pace, tone, and vocabulary of the client.
- Evaluate your own participation in an interaction.

Task Groups

Task groups are developed to address a task or need. Members are chosen based on ability to complete the task. **Short-term groups** dissolve once the task is completed. Short-term groups might include a task force to address holiday scheduling or a panel to critique response to a disaster drill. Because the time together is limited, the focus of communication is on the task at hand. Often time to develop rapport or relationships is limited. Direct verbal communication with congruent nonverbal communication allows the group to function most effectively.

Ongoing Groups

Ongoing groups address issues that are recurrent. Committees are a form of task group. Common ongoing committees in healthcare organizations include quality assurance, infection control, and discharge planning. A committee has a chairperson that may be elected from within or appointed. Members have designated roles within the groups (e.g., recorder, time keeper). In small groups, all members have an opportunity to communicate their opinions. In larger groups, patterns of communication form; some members voice their opinion regularly, whereas others are often silent. When not all members speak, it is essential to examine nonverbal behavior to determine whether the nonspeaking members are in agreement.

Self-help Groups

Self-help groups are voluntary organizations composed of individuals with a common need. Members who have met the goals of the group often run meetings. Alcoholics Anonymous may be the most widely recognized self-help group. Other well-known self-help groups include Weight Watchers, Narcotics Anonymous, and Reach for Recovery (for women with breast cancer). Nurses may be members, facilitators, or consultants for self-help groups. Members are encouraged to share experiences and seek help from other members of the group. The facilitator may serve as a leader of the group or coordinate room arrangements and schedules but acts as a member during sessions. The facilitator is usually chosen by the members. Consultants may be health professionals or experts in the field who offer advice or education to the group. Several channels are available to self-help groups. They may have face-to-face meetings, participate in Internet chat groups, or communicate via newsletters. Communication of shared interests is the link that holds these groups together.

Therapy Groups

Therapy groups are formed to help individual members cope with issues, improve relationships, or address stress. They may be ongoing or have a designated length of operation. Community, public health, and psychiatric nurses sometimes facilitate therapy groups. Group facilitators arrange the time and place of the group and often introduce topics for discussion. Many groups are organized around themes, such as coping with divorce, loss of a spouse, or motherhood. These groups are also called self-awareness or growth groups.

Work-related Social Support Groups

Work-related social support groups help members of a profession cope with the stress associated with their work. The helping professions can be emotionally draining. Social support groups provide an opportunity to share concerns and offer mutual support through formal meetings with a facilitator or informal drop-in events.

Formation of a group does not guarantee its success. To be successful, a group must have characteristics that allow the group to function and achieve its goals (Box 18-4).

KnowledgeCheck 18-5

- Identify and describe the phases of the therapeutic relationship.
- What are the five characteristics of therapeutic communication?
- Describe the difference between a task group and a self-help group.
- Compare and contrast the role of a therapy group with a work-related support group.

  Go to Chapter 18, **Knowledge Check Response Sheet and Answers,** on the Student Resource Disk or DavisPlus at http://davisplus.fadavis.com/Wilkinson2

CriticalThinking 18-5

Review the local newspaper, phone book, hospital bulletin board, and school directory. Identify at least three group helping experiences available. How might you learn more about these organizations? How would you determine whether they are resources that you might make available to your patients?

Practical Knowledge
knowing how

Therapeutic communication is used throughout the nursing process. In the next few sections we will explore communication problems as well as therapeutic interventions.

BOX 18-4 ■ Characteristics of a Successful Group

A successful group has:
- Clearly defined purpose
- Shared set of guidelines under which the group functions
- Sense of shared responsibility
- Shared leadership
- Mutual trust
- Comfort among members
- Climate that is cohesive but does not stifle individuality
- Members who are willing to share feelings, concerns, or beliefs
- Flexibility to change what is not working

ASSESSMENT

Assessment is essential to effective communication. You should assess for factors that alter a client's ability to receive, process, or transmit information, such as the following:

- *Language barrier.* Imagine how difficult it would be if you became ill while traveling in a country where you were unable to speak or read the language. How would you communicate that you were nauseated or in pain; how would you tell them when the symptom started or what makes it worse? Also consider your client's education and literacy. You cannot assume that everyone has an extensive vocabulary, nor that they can read and write.
- *Cognitive skills.* Difficulty understanding or engaging in communication may signal cognitive impairment. Developmental delays and pathology or injury of the central nervous system affect language and cognitive skills.
- *Sensory perceptual alterations.* Assess hearing and vision. Assess for **aphasia** (a difficulty expressing or interpreting messages that may develop after cerebrovascular accident [stroke] or neurological disease).
- *Physiological barriers,* such as respiratory problems, loose-fitting dentures, or cleft palate, which may interfere with speaking.

For guidelines for a focused communication assessment,

 Go to Chapter 18, **Assessment Guidelines and Tools,** in Volume 2.

ANALYSIS/NURSING DIAGNOSIS

Communication can be the problem or the etiology of a nursing diagnosis. The following NANDA-I diagnosis labels describe communication problems. Note that communication problems may involve the inability to receive, interpret, or express spoken, written, and nonverbal messages.

- Readiness for Enhanced Communication is appropriate when the client expresses willingness to enhance communication that is already effective.
- Impaired Verbal Communication is an appropriate diagnosis if the client has (1) expressive aphasia or a physiological problem such as dyspnea, stuttering, or laryngeal cancer that impairs the ability to speak; or (2) receptive aphasia or sensory deficits that impair the ability to receive messages.
- Impaired Communication is the preferred diagnosis if the client is unfamiliar with the dominant language or has some other difficulty receiving and sending messages. Note that this is not a NANDA-I label.

Etiologies of Communication Diagnoses

Your assessment data will help you determine whether communication impairment is the primary problem or whether it is a result of other health problems. Some nursing diagnoses may cause or contribute to communication problems. For example:

- Clients with Acute or Chronic Confusion often have difficulty expressing or receiving verbal and nonverbal messages. Confusion may be related to physical or mental health problems, or may be a side effect of medications or sleep deprivation.
- Mental health problems can also lead to communication problems. For example, Anxiety impairs the ability to deliver and receive messages, and Chronic or Situational Low Self-Esteem often results in limited interaction with others.

Communication as Etiology of Other Nursing Diagnoses

Impaired Verbal Communication may be the etiology of other nursing diagnoses, for example:

- Anxiety r/t inability to communicate needs
- Social Isolation r/t difficulty maintaining relationships secondary to Impaired Verbal Communication
- Impaired Social Interaction r/t inability to carry on conversation
- Chronic Low Self-Esteem r/t fear of conversing with others secondary to stuttering

PLANNING OUTCOMES/EVALUATION

For *NOC standardized outcomes* associated with Impaired Verbal Communication,

 Go to Chapter 18, **Standardized Language,** in Volume 2.

Using NOC indicators with those outcomes, you can develop goals for clients' communication problems.

Individualized client outcomes and goals depend on the nursing diagnosis you identify. For example, for Impaired Verbal Communication, you might write the following desired outcomes. The client:

- Uses alternative methods of communication (e.g., writing, picture board, gestures) effectively (specify time frame).
- Demonstrates minimal frustration with communication difficulties (specify time frame).
- Communicates effectively using a translator or interpreter.
- Interprets messages accurately, as evidenced by appropriate verbal or nonverbal feedback.

PLANNING INTERVENTIONS/IMPLEMENTATION

For *NIC standardized interventions* and selected nursing activities for Impaired Verbal Communication,

 Go to Chapter 18, **Standardized Language,** in Volume 2.

Specific nursing activities for communication problems depend on the etiology of the problem and on the goals selected. The focus of nursing interventions is to

facilitate communication and to resolve or reduce the factors interfering with it.

Enhancing Therapeutic Communication

The following are techniques and activities you can implement immediately to improve your communication with patients and others.

Active Listening

At first glance, the term *active listening* appears to be an oxymoron. People often think of listening as a passive activity. If you have ever been in a one-sided conversation, you are certainly aware that listening can be passive. In contrast, an active listener uses all senses to focus on the sender's message. An active listener gives undivided attention and allows the sender the opportunity to complete comments without interruption. To listen actively, pay attention to verbal and nonverbal communication and look for congruence. If a message is unclear, seek clarification through use of probing questions or reflective comments, such as, "Tell me more," or "When you say . . . what do you mean?"

As a nurse, you can demonstrate active listening by facing your client, making eye contact, and focusing the conversation on issues of importance to the client. If you must take notes during the conversation, record only key words to stimulate your memory at another time. Taking extensive notes distracts you from active listening. Active listening behaviors convey caring, signal a willingness to listen, and provide a comfortable environment for the client to share his concerns.

Failure to listen to your client will result in missed messages or misinterpretation. Consider this example:

Patient: I guess I'm going to surgery tomorrow.
Nurse: (Checking the IV fluids and hanging a medication) Uh-huh.
Patient: The surgeon says I'll be in intensive care for a few days.
Nurse: (Looking at the drainage in the urine collection bag) OK. Your urine looks good.
Patient: I guess this is pretty risky surgery.
Nurse: (Recording on the flowsheet) Yep.

How do you think the patient must feel in this situation? The patient is clearly expressing concern about his upcoming surgery and seems to want to talk about it with the nurse. However, the nurse is busy with a variety of tasks and is not paying attention to the conversation. Undoubtedly, the patient will continue to feel anxious. In fact, his unsuccessful attempts to communicate may even increase his anxiety. If the nurse were listening, this would be an excellent opportunity to discuss the patient's concerns, provide preoperative teaching, and help the patient ease his anxiety.

Establishing Trust

Mutual trust is an essential component not just of professional communication, but also of therapeutic communication because it facilitates disclosure and honesty. As you and the client establish trust, the client can more easily relay information and share feelings. To establish trust, always greet the client by name, listen actively, respond honestly to the client's concerns, and provide care competently and consistently.

Being Assertive

An assertive person is one who is confident and comfortable and remains in charge of where the conversation is going. Assertive communication enables you to deal directly with stressful interpersonal communication, for example, with a client who needs to make some lifestyle changes. An assertive nurse also serves as a role model for the client. The therapeutic relationship is a safe place for clients to practice being assertive and receive feedback about their communication. As needed, review assertiveness and collaborative professional communication, earlier in this chapter.

Restating, Clarifying, and Validating Messages

Restating means using your own words to summarize the message you received from the client. This demonstrates concern, active listening, and understanding of what the patient has said. Below is an example:

Client: I'm so worried about this diabetes. I have young kids. I want to see them grow up. Every diabetic I've known has died young.
Nurse: Diabetes is a serious disease. I understand your worry about its effects on you. However, we want to focus on becoming well controlled so that you can avoid complications.

Clarifying messages helps ensure that you have accurately interpreted the information. For instance, you might state, "I'm not sure what you mean when you say you're so worried about your diabetes." Or, "When you say you're worried, what do you mean?"

To **validate** the message, ask the client whether you are making a correct interpretation: "When you say you're worried about your diabetes, do you mean you are afraid you will die soon?" These techniques help to identify client concerns and focus communication. They are especially helpful if the client is unclear or vague with a message.

Interpreting Body Language and Sharing Observations

Be attentive to what the patient says and how she says it. Note the tone of voice, rate of speech, distance, eye movement, facial expressions, and gestures. Look for congruence between the spoken message and the nonverbal message. If there is inconsistency, share your observations with the patient. You can share your observations by describing the patient's body language or tone of voice. For example, you might state, "I know you said you feel well, but your voice and hands are trembling. How can I help you?" Or more simply, "You're frowning. Has something upset you?"

Exploring Issues

Ask open-ended questions to obtain a clear understanding of an issue and follow your client's thoughts (see Chapter 3). Probing comments such as "Tell me more" encourage your client to share information.

Using Silence

Learn to be comfortable with silence. When you remain attentive, silence demonstrates acceptance and allows clients to compose their thoughts and provide further information. It is especially effective if your client is emotionally upset.

Summarizing the Conversation

At the end of the conversation, summarize what you have heard. For example, you might say, "Today we talked about diet, exercise, and medications for high blood pressure. Your job now is to review the handouts and start taking your medication every morning. I'll see you in 2 weeks when you return for your follow-up visit." Summarizing demonstrates active listening and allows the client to clarify any misunderstandings.

Barriers to Therapeutic Communication

As you learn to communicate therapeutically, you may find yourself thinking, doing, or saying things that seem to close down your conversation. If so, acknowledge your error and return to therapeutic patterns. The following sections describe the most common barriers to therapeutic communication.

Asking Too Many Questions

Asking questions at the appropriate time is important. However, asking too many questions, especially closed questions (requiring only a yes or no answer), can make clients feel they are being interrogated. Excessive questioning may suggest insensitivity or lack of respect to the client's issues, as in the following dialogue:

Patient:	I feel lousy today.
Nurse:	Didn't you sleep well?
Patient:	No, hardly at all.
Nurse:	Did you take anything to help you sleep?
Patient:	No.
Nurse:	Do you think you should have taken something?
Patient:	I guess.
Nurse:	Why didn't you tell the night nurse you needed something?
Patient:	I don't know.

As you can see, this approach controls the range and nature of responses that the client provides. In contrast, open-ended questions stimulate conversation and exploration. Contrast the preceding conversation with the conversation below.

Patient:	I feel lousy today.
Nurse:	Lousy? Tell me more.
Patient:	Well, my back and neck hurt, and I hardly slept at all. I thought it would go away, but I just lay in bed last night worrying.
Nurse:	What kind of things are you worrying about?
Patient:	I'm worried about . . .

In the second conversation, the nurse asked open-ended questions. These prompts encouraged the patient to discuss his concerns.

Asking Why

In many health situations, we want to learn why a patient acted or responded as he did. However, directly asking for reasons suggests criticism to some people. If you ask, "Why did you stop taking your medication?" the patient may become defensive and stop talking. A more subtle approach is usually more comfortable for the patient. You might ask, "What concerns do you have about your medicines?" or "Tell me more about your experience with the medicines." Both of these approaches will help you gather more information about the client's concerns, without suggesting criticism. Review the first dialogue in the previous section, "Asking Too Many Questions," for another example of the effect of "why" questions. How do you think this patient felt?

Changing the Subject Inappropriately

Abruptly changing the topic of discussion makes you seem uninterested. This often occurs when the nurse is intent on one issue and the client is focused on another. For example, imagine that you want to tell the patient about a change in the scheduling for a diagnostic test before you forget. As you enter the room, your patient says, "I am having a lot of pain in my knee today." This situation requires you to address the patient's concern first and postpone discussing the schedule change until the patient can be receptive to the information. In an ongoing dialogue, changing the subject can stop the flow of conversation cold. Both patients and nurses sometime use this tactic to avoid discussing sensitive topics. The following is an example:

Nurse:	This must be a tough time for you. Your wife is very sick. How are you handling this?
Patient's husband:	Yes, it's tough, but I went out to a movie last night. Have you seen that new movie with the avatars? The special effects . . .

Your relationship with the patient's husband and the facts of the patient situation would determine whether you would redirect this conversation back to the original subject or allow him to wander. You may choose to give the husband more time to be comfortable with you before approaching this topic again.

Failing to Probe

Failing to probe can result in incomplete assessment and affect the quality of your care. A thorough assessment requires you to explore issues in detail. Review the following conversations.

Patient: I'm having a lot of discomfort in my back.
Nurse: How much does it hurt?
Patient: Quite a bit. I had trouble sleeping last night.
Nurse: I'll get you something for pain.

Compare that conversation with the next example, in which the nurse gathers additional data.

Patient: I'm having a lot of discomfort in my back.
Nurse: Tell me about the discomfort.
Patient: It hurts a lot. I had trouble sleeping last night.
Nurse: When did you first notice this pain?
Patient: It started in the middle of the night.
Nurse: What does it feel like?
Patient: I feel sore. I'd like to turn over to my side, but I can't because of this heavy cast.
Nurse: Let me help you turn. (Assists patient to turn and uses pillows to hold the patient on her side)
Patient: Oh, that feels better!
Nurse: How is the discomfort now?
Patient: It's pretty much gone.
Nurse: I'm glad you're feeling better. Would you like something for pain as well?
Patient: I think I'm OK now.

In the second example, the nurse followed her original question with additional probing questions. A few additional questions helped clarify what the patient needed and led to immediate comfort.

Expressing Approval or Disapproval

We offer our friends and family members approval when they do something well or disapproval for doing something wrong. But you should exercise caution with this strategy in the nurse–patient relationship. Although it may seem supportive, expressing approval can inhibit further sharing—it puts you in the position of being the judge of what is "right." This often prompts the patient to continue to seek approval. He thinks, "I'd better be careful; she may not approve of the next thing I was going to tell her. She expects me to be *this* way." Consider instead offering recommendations and allowing the patient to choose. Read the following exchange.

Patient: I've decided I'm going to have the surgery.
Nurse: That's great. I think you made the right choice.

Compare that conversation with the following example.

Patient: I've decided I'm going to have the surgery.
Nurse: Tell me about your decision.
Patient: Well, my shoulder has been bothering me for several months now. I know I said I wanted to put off surgery, but I think I'll have a faster recovery if I just get the surgery done now.
Nurse: So your choices are to do a trial of physical therapy and anti-inflammatory medicines, to try a steroid injection, or to have surgery.
Patient: Right. But there's a good chance I'll still need surgery even if I try the therapy or medicines. The only thing that will actually fix the problem is surgery. The others don't guarantee improvement.

Can you see how different the conversation becomes if the nurse does not express approval? By allowing the patient to discuss the choices, the nurse has empowered the patient to make his own healthcare decisions.

Offering Advice

Offering an opinion is rarely helpful. Avoid statements such as, "If I were you . . ." or, "You should . . ." These statements impose your opinion on your clients. In effect, your statements function as approval if they agree with the client's thoughts or disapproval if they do not. As with other forms of approval or disapproval, conversation halts. If the client asks, "What should I do?" help clarify the options, and provide her with information about the choices. Giving the client your solution negates the client's opportunity to participate as a mutual partner in the decision-making process.

Providing False Reassurance

Providing reassurance helps to ease concern, offers comfort, and communicates empathy. So it is an appropriate and therapeutic action—if the reassurance is warranted. For example, consider the client who presents to the emergency department (ED) for treatment of an acute episode of asthma. Because anxiety exacerbates asthma, it is certainly therapeutic to reassure the client that he will be cared for promptly and effectively. In contrast, false reassurance is a barrier to therapeutic communication. When clients or family members ask for information or tell you that they are worried, it is easy to reassure them that everything will be okay. However, such responses are uninformed, inaccurate, and may feel dismissive—even condescending—to the receiver. Examine the following scenario:

> You are a nurse working at the triage station in the local ED. Your role is to evaluate the condition and prioritize the care of all clients presenting for treatment. An ambulance arrives with a man complaining of severe chest pain. He is ashen and short of breath. He tells you his pain is "crushing." Suspecting a heart attack, you immediately move him to the critical care bay of the ED and request urgent evaluation. Several minutes later his wife arrives by private car and approaches the triage station. She anxiously asks, "How is my husband?" How would you respond?

It may be tempting to offer a response such as, "Don't worry, everything will be all right." But do you really know that will be the case? A better approach is to provide accurate information: "I had him immediately taken in for treatment. I'll get you in to see him as soon as I can. Please have a seat, and I'll check on him." This comment is accurate, calming, and avoids misleading the person.

Stereotyping

As discussed in Chapter 13, racial, cultural, religious, age-related, or gender stereotypes distort assessment and prevent you from recognizing the patient's uniqueness. Examples of statements reflecting a stereotype include, "He's old, he won't remember anything you tell him," and "Men are always the biggest crybabies about pain." Such comments may shut down communication and escalate tension. Avoid their use with patients and colleagues.

Stereotypes may be blatant or subtle. Blatant examples, such as those above, are easily recognized and may create an intense reaction. Subtle stereotypes, however, may be equally disruptive to care. Subtle stereotypes common in healthcare include the following:

- Believing a patient will be calm and know what to expect because he has had previous hospitalizations for the same diagnosis, has had previous surgeries or other procedures, or was given information about his condition
- Assuming that patients will understand their healthcare because of their educational level or work experience, for example, expecting that a physician who has suffered a heart attack needs no explanation of her care
- Expecting all patients with the same surgery or diagnosis to experience similar responses

Using Patronizing Language

Patronizing language communicates superiority or disapproval. Statements such as, "You know better than that," are patronizing and offensive to the client. Condescending approaches, such as, "You should have used the call button before you got up. You're lucky you didn't hurt yourself," do not communicate respect for the client.

Patronizing language may seem innocent. Have you heard staff call clients "Sweetie," "Dearie," or "Mama"? The term *elderspeak* describes ways that healthcare workers may unintentionally show disrespect to elderly patients by using such phrases and speaking to them in a high-pitched, slow, repetitive, childlike voice. Staff may also alter pronouns, saying for example, "Are we ready for our bath." Although the intent is communicate caring, many patients are offended because it sounds as though you are speaking to a child. Research indicates mentally competent nursing home residents are irritated by elderspeak, and that people with moderate Alzheimer's disease become more agitated and resistant to care if they are addressed in this manner (Williams, Herman, Gajewski, et al., 2008).

When you first meet your client, use a formal title—Mr., Ms., and so on. This conveys respect, which is essential to a therapeutic relationship. In the orientation phase of the relationship, ask your patient how he would prefer to be addressed. If the patient is unable to respond, ask family members how to address the patient.

KnowledgeCheck 18-6

Identify at least five barriers to communication.

 Go to Chapter 18, **Knowledge Check Response Sheet and Answers,** on the Student Resource Disk or DavisPlus at http://davisplus.fadavis.com/Wilkinson2

Enhancing Communication with Clients from Another Culture

Healthcare facilities should provide interpretation (including translation) services as necessary (The Joint Commission, 2008a, p. 156). Many health facilities have in-house translation services available for communication with non–English-speaking patients. Translators may also be available through telephone contact; and a few are linked via computer to a healthcare interpreter network to enable video teleconferencing.

Use relatives as translators only if there are no other options. It is often culturally unacceptable to have family members ask personal questions. As a result, translations may be altered or questions remain unasked. See Chapter 13 for additional information on the use of translators.

Spanish-speakers currently constitute 1 in 10 U.S. households, so it is not unusual to encounter patients who speak only Spanish. If you do not speak Spanish, most computers have programs for crudely translating English and Spanish terms; however, it is good to learn a few key words to help you communicate until a translator arrives. For a list of a few useful Spanish terms and for guidelines for communicating with clients from other cultures,

 Go to Chapter 18, **Clinical Insight 18-4: Communicating with Clients from Another Culture,** in Volume 2.

Toward Evidence-Based Practice

Ammentorp, J., Sabroe, S., Kofoed, P. E., et al. (2007). The effect of training in communication skills on medical doctors' and nurses' self-efficacy: A randomized controlled trial. *Patient Education and Counseling, 66(3),* 270–277.

This research investigated the effect of communication skills training on doctors' and nurses' self-efficacy. (*Self-efficacy* is the extent to which you believe you are capable of performing actions that influence events and outcomes, for example patient outcomes.) One group of clinicians received a 5-day communication course; the control group did not. Clinicians who participated in the communication course improved their self-efficacy for specific communication tasks by up to 37%. The improvements remained constant for the following 6 months. Researchers concluded that communication skills training can improve clinicians' evaluation of their ability to perform a specific communication task.

Edwards, N., Peterson, W. E., & Davies, B. L. (2006). Evaluation of a multiple component intervention to support the implementation of a "therapeutic relationships" best practice guideline on nurses' communication skills. *Patient Education and Counseling, 63(1-2),* 3–11.

Researchers tested an intervention to assist nurses to implement the Registered Nurses' Association of Ontario best practice guideline for establishing therapeutic relationships. They read client scenarios aloud and asked nurses to respond verbally as though they were interacting with the client. They measured the frequency and quality of nurses' active listening, initiating, and assertiveness skills before and after implementation of the guideline.

After implementation of the guideline, they found a significant decrease in the number of active listening skills used, but a significant improvement in the quality of active listening and initiating skills. They also found increased frequency of initiating skills. They concluded that nurses demonstrated improvements in select communication skills.

1. Which of the following statements is well supported by the evidence in the first report (Ammentorp, Sabroe, Kofoed, et al., 2007)?
   a. Communication courses for healthcare professionals should be at least 5 days long.
   b. If you personally took a 5-day communication course, you would have more faith in your ability to perform specific communication tasks.
   c. People who take a communication course can expect that they will feel more comfortable about performing certain communication tasks.
   d. People who take a communication course can expect some improvement in their ability to perform specific communication tasks.

2. Suppose you are an inservice educator in a hospital. You have decided to institute an inservice program to train nurses in a few specific communication skills. Use the above studies to provide rationale for your decision. Write a brief statement explaining why your decision is reasonable.

 Go to Chapter 18, **Toward Evidence-Based Practice Suggested Responses,** on the Student Resource Disk or DavisPlus at http://davisplus.fadavis.com/Wilkinson2

Enhancing Communication with Clients Who Have Impaired Hearing or Speech

For guidelines to help you communicate with clients who have speech, visual, or hearing deficits, respectively,

 Go to Chapter 18, **Clinical Insight 18-5: Communicating with Clients Who Have Sensory Deficits,** in Volume 2.

 Go to Chapter 29, **Clinical Insight 29-1: Communicating with Visually Impaired Clients,** in Volume 2.

 Go to Chapter 29, **Clinical Insight 29-2: Communicating with Hearing-Impaired Clients,** in Volume 2.

Enhancing Communication with Clients with Impaired Cognition or Reduced Level of Consciousness

Communicating with cognitively impaired clients can be difficult, time-consuming, and frustrating for even the most experienced healthcare provider. Make every effort to communicate regardless of whether or not the client can understand you. For guidelines to help you communicate with clients with impaired cognition or consciousness,

 Go to Chapter 18, **Clinical Insight 18-6: Communicating with Clients Who Have Impaired Cognition or Consciousness,** in Volume 2.

 Go to Chapter 18, **Resources for Caregivers and Health Professionals,** on the Student Resource Disk or DavisPlus at http://davisplus.fadavis.com/Wilkinson2

 Suggested Readings: Go to Chapter 18, **Reading More About Communicating & the Therapeutic Relationship,** on the Student Resource Disk or DavisPlus at http://davisplus.fadavis.com/Wilkinson2

 Bibliography: Go to Volume 2, Bibliography.

CHAPTER 19

Health Assessment: Performing a Physical Examination

Learning Outcomes

After completing this chapter, you should be able to:

➤ Identify the purposes and components of a physical examination.

➤ Discuss the differences among a comprehensive, focused, and ongoing physical examination.

➤ Describe how to prepare for a physical examination.

➤ Demonstrate the skills used in physical examination.

➤ Explain adaptations that may be required when you examine clients of various ages.

➤ Identify the components of the general survey.

➤ Conduct a full physical examination of a client.

➤ Discuss the expected findings of a physical examination.

➤ Document the findings of a physical examination.

➤ Perform a brief bedside physical examination.

Meet Your Patient

Joseph Garcia is scheduled for a comprehensive physical exam at the family health center at 1400 today. As you recall, he has previously been seen and evaluated by Jordan Miller, RN, FNP. Mr. Garcia has medical diagnoses of hypertension, degenerative joint disease, obesity, and heavy tobacco use. During his earlier visit, Jordan instructed Mr. Garcia on a low-salt, low-fat diet and advised him to lose weight and quit smoking. Jordan also ordered lab work to establish a baseline for wellness and detect abnormalities that might indicate illness. Review the results of Mr. Garcia's lab work that follow.

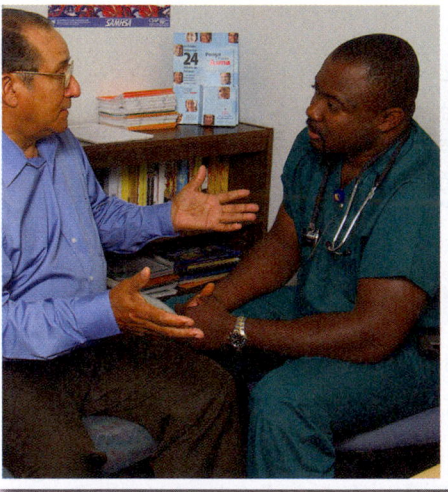

At today's visit, Jordan will perform a comprehensive physical examination of Mr. Garcia and review his lab results. After Joe's appointment, Flordelisa Garcia will also have a comprehensive exam.

Laboratory Data for Joseph Garcia

Name: Joseph Garcia **DOB:** 7/12/50
Acct#: K00205412 Family Medicine Center, J. Miller

Test	Result	Reference Range*
CBC/Differential		
WBC	5.6 x 10³/mm³	5–10 x 10³/mm³
Hemoglobin	14.8 g/dL	M: 14–18 g/dL F: 12–16 g/dL
Hematocrit	45.1%	M: 42–52% F: 37–47%
RBC count	5.1 million/mm³	M: 4.7–5.14 million/mm³ F: 4.2–4.87 million/mm³
MCV	84 mm³	85–95 mm³
MCH	29 pg	28–32 pg
MCHC	34%	33–35%
Neutrophils	57%	59%
Lymphocytes	30%	34%
Monocytes	5%	4%
Eosinophils	2.5%	2.7%
Basophils	0.7%	0.5%
Platelet count	197,000/mm³	150,000–400,000/mm³

Test	Result	Reference Range*
Comprehensive Metabolic Panel		
Sodium	138 mEq/L	135–145 mEq/L
Potassium	4.3 mEq/L	3.5–5.0 mEq/L
Chloride	101 mEq/L	97–107 mEq/L
Carbon dioxide	27 mEq/L	23–29 mEq/L
BUN	16 mg/dL	10–31 mg/dL
Creatinine	0.8 mg/dL	M: 0.6–1.2 mg/dL F: 0.5–1.1 mg/dL
Glucose	156 mg/dL	75–110 mg/dL
Albumin	4.0 g/dL	19–60 years: 3.2–4.8 g/dL
Total protein	7.2 g/dL	6.8–8.0 g/dL
ALT (alanine aminotransferase, also called SGPT)	18 units/L	M: 10–40 units/L F: 7–35 units/L
ALP (alkaline phosphatase)	43 units/L	M: 35–142 units/L F: 25–125 units/L
AST (aspartate aminotranspeptidase, also called SGOT)	26 units/L	M: 19–48 units/L F: 9–36 units/L
Bilirubin, total	0.7 mg/dL	0.3–1.2 mg/dL
Calcium	8.5 mg/dL	8.2–10.2 mg/dL

Test	Result	Reference Range*	
Lipid Panel**			
Total cholesterol	201 mg/dL	<200	-Desirable
		200–239	-Borderline high
		>240	-High
LDL cholesterol (Primary target of therapy)	140 mg/dL	<100 mg/dL	-Optimal
		100–129 mg/dL	-Near optimal/ above optimal
		130–159	-Borderline high
		160–189	-High
		>190	-Very high
HDL cholesterol	34 mg/dL	<40	-Low
Triglycerides	196 mg/dL		

**To interpret lipid panel results, follow the most recent guidelines of the National Cholesterol Education Program (NCEP) Expert Panel on Detection, Evaluation, and Blood Cholesterol in Adults available at www.nhlbi.nih.gov/guidelines/cholesterol/atglance.pdf. The reference range figures in this table will undoubtedly be revised (and lowered) by NCEP in the near future.

Also, the norms for an individual patient's lipid panel depend on the calculation of risk factors. Joe is hypertensive, is obese, and has an elevated blood sugar. His norms reflect high risk for coronary heart disease; they would be about <160 for total cholesterol, <100 for triglycerides, <100 for LDL, and >45 for HDL.

Test	Result	Reference Range*
Urinalysis		
Appearance	Clear	Clear
Color	Amber	Light yellow to amber
Odor	Aromatic	None–aromatic
pH	6.0	5.0–9.0
Specific gravity	1.012	1.001–1.035
Leukocyte esterase	Negative	Negative
Nitrites	Negative	Negative
Ketones	Negative	Negative
Protein	5 mg/dL	<20 mg/dL
Crystals	None	In acid urine: uric acid, calcium oxalate, amorphous urates In alkaline urine: triple phosphate, calcium phosphate, ammonium biurate, calcium carbonate, amorphous phosphates
Casts	None	None, except rare hyaline
Glucose	Negative	Negative
WBC	1/hpf	<5/hpf
RBC	1/hpf	<5/hpf
PSA (prostate-specific antigen)	2.8 ng/mL	<4 ng/mL
Fecal occult blood screen		
Sample #1 — negative Sample #2 — negative Sample #3 — negative		

*For most studies, each laboratory establishes its own reference range.

Theoretical **Knowledge**
knowing why

Health assessment is a comprehensive assessment of the physical, mental, spiritual, socioeconomic, and cultural status of an individual, group, or community. A complete health assessment includes both a nursing history and a physical examination. Nursing assessments focus on the client's functional abilities and physical responses to illness and other stressors. In contrast, medical assessments focus on disease and pathology. As a nurse practitioner, Jordan Miller combines the nursing and medical approaches.

Physical Examination

We usually think of **physical examination,** or **physical assessment,** as the techniques used to gather objective data about the body. However, you will also ask questions to obtain subjective data about each body system or area. This may be done in a separate nursing interview or as you perform the physical examination. Both the interview and the exam require tact and sensitivity.

What Are the Purposes of a Physical Examination?

A physical examination is performed for any of several reasons:

- *To obtain baseline data.* Data about the patient's physical status and functional abilities serve as a baseline for comparison as the patient's health status changes.
- *To identify nursing diagnoses, collaborative problems, and wellness diagnoses.* Problem statements form the basis for the plan of care and help you to address the patient's nursing care needs.
- *To monitor the status of a previously identified problem.* For example, Mr. Garcia has already begun treatment for hypertension. Today's examination will be linked to the lab results to further explore the status of his hypertension.
- *To screen for health problems.* Regular checkups can help to identify health problems at early stages. Because Mr. Garcia has an enlarged prostate, a prostate-specific antigen (PSA) test was done to screen for prostate cancer.

The type of physical examination you perform will depend on the client's health status, the nature of the client encounter, and the setting. For example, at an outpatient appointment for an annual physical, on a client's admission to an inpatient setting, or at the initial home health visit, you would perform a **comprehensive physical assessment,** which includes a health history interview and a complete head-to-toe examination of every body system. Data from a comprehensive physical assessment provide guidance for planning care and determine the need for further assessment.

In an emergency situation, your assessment will be rapid and focused on the presenting problem. A **focused physical assessment** is performed to obtain data about an actual, potential, or possible problem that has been identified. It pertains to a particular topic, body part, or functional ability rather than overall health status, and it adds to the database created by the comprehensive assessment. A **system-specific assessment** is a focused assessment limited to one body system (e.g., the lungs, the peripheral circulation). The following are examples of focused and system-specific physical assessments, respectively:

- Assessing bowel sounds when a client has abdominal pain
- Listening to breath sounds, counting respirations, and obtaining pulse oximetry readings to assess a patient's respiratory status

Ongoing assessment is performed as needed, after the initial database is completed, and, ideally, at every interaction with the patient. For example, on a medical–surgical unit, each nurse who provides care to a client conducts a brief ongoing assessment to determine changes in the client's status. Ongoing assessment data reflect the dynamic state of the client and are used in evaluating client outcomes. For more details on the types of assessment, see Chapter 3. For a form to use in making a brief bedside assessment,

 Go to Chapter 19, **Procedure 19-20, Brief Bedside Assessment,** in Volume 2.

How Do I Prepare to Perform a Physical Examination?

You should develop a systematic approach to physical examination and follow the same order each time you perform an exam. This will help you recall the steps and include all important data. You may use a **head-to-toe approach,** starting at the head and neck, progressing down the body, and examining the feet last. Or you could use a **body systems approach,** examining each system in a predetermined order (e.g., musculoskeletal, cardiovascular, neurological). Before beginning the physical examination, prepare yourself, the environment, and the client.

Prepare Yourself

Preparing for a physical examination requires theoretical knowledge of anatomy and physiology, examination equipment and techniques, therapeutic communication, and documentation. Self-knowledge is also important. How comfortable are you when performing an examination? What skills do you need to review or practice? Will you need assistance to perform some aspects of the exam? Will you need help documenting your findings? Honestly evaluate your strengths as well as areas that need improvement. Be sure to seek help from your instructor, an experienced nurse, fellow students, or other healthcare providers as needed.

Before approaching the patient, familiarize yourself with his situation. What are the patient's main health concerns? What is the purpose of your exam? For instance, if you are doing a focused assessment of a client's wound, you will need to learn about the wound being examined. Is there a dressing over the wound? What supplies will you need to remove and replace the dressing? Has the patient required pain medication before exams in the past? Reviewing previous findings helps you work efficiently and to formulate any questions you might want to ask the patient.

Finally, unless this is an initial assessment, review the nursing plan of care and keep it in mind as you examine the patient. Your assessment data may lead to modification or updating of the care plan.

Prepare the Environment

Physical examination requires you to observe and touch the client's body, so privacy is essential. You will need a room with curtains or a door to shield the client from view. For additional privacy, drape your client and uncover only the area you are examining. For convenience you may use bed linens and/or a gown to drape. Disposable paper drapes are also available.

Because you will need to hear the patient and listen to a variety of sounds during the exam, turn off the television, radio, or other media. You will need good lighting to observe subtle changes in skin and body contours. Adjust the temperature of the room according to patient comfort.

Determine the instruments and equipment you will need. Take everything you need so that you will not have to leave the client to obtain supplies.

Prepare the Client

In most clinical settings, you must examine a client often to evaluate a changing status, and timing will be decided by the client's condition rather than by convenience. However, when possible, it is important to select a time when the client is comfortable and receptive to the examination. Avoid conducting the exam when the client is in pain or is hungry, tired, anxious, or unwilling to cooperate in the assessment.

Take the time to establish rapport with the client, to help him relax and cooperate fully in the assessment. Introduce yourself, ask the client how he wishes to be addressed, and explain what you will be doing. Ask the client to void before the examination; this promotes relaxation and also makes it easier to palpate the abdomen. Always alert the client before touching him. For example, before you start to palpate the neck for lymph nodes, say, "I'm going to feel your neck now." Proper positioning during the exam also promotes comfort (see the following section). Pay attention to the pace of your exam, being careful not to prolong it and tire the client.

Consider developmental and cultural differences. For example, some clients may wish to have a family member present during an exam; some may require a same-sex clinician. If you and the client do not speak the same language, arrange to have an interpreter present.

KnowledgeCheck 19-1

- What are the purposes of a physical examination?
- Describe how you would prepare for a physical exam.

 Go to Chapter 19, **Knowledge Check Response Sheet and Answers,** on the Student Resource Disk or DavisPlus at http://davisplus.fadavis.com/Wilkinson2

CriticalThinking 19-1

- The nurse conducts a physical assessment for Joe and Flordelisa Garcia (see "Meet Your Patients") at an outpatient clinic. Discuss the differences between their planned experience and a focused physical exam of a hospital inpatient.
- Identify a plan to practice and improve your assessment skills.

How Do I Position the Client for a Physical Examination?

The client will need to assume a variety of positions during a comprehensive physical examination. To begin the examination, seat the client on the side of the bed or examination table. Face the client, and establish eye contact. This helps to build rapport and put the client at ease. If your client is unable to sit, assist him to a position on his back with the head of the bed elevated. An upright position allows the client to expand his lungs fully and is useful for assessing vital signs, the head and neck, the heart and lungs, the back, and the upper extremities. As you place your client in positions that allow you to best observe the body system you are examining, be alert to special needs that call for you to modify the position. For example, a patient with a cervical spine problem would need a neck roll when lying supine. Table 19-1 illustrates and describes the major positions you will need to use.

KnowledgeCheck 19-2

Identify the best position for examining the lungs, heart, pulses, and abdomen.

 Go to Chapter 19, **Knowledge Check Response Sheet and Answers,** on the Student Resource Disk or DavisPlus at http://davisplus.fadavis.com/Wilkinson2

What Techniques Do I Need to Perform a Physical Examination?

The skills used in physical examination include inspection, palpation, percussion, auscultation, and sometimes olfaction. You will use these skills in that order except when performing an abdominal assessment, in which case you will perform auscultation before percussion and palpation to avoid disturbing the abdominal sounds.

Inspection

Inspection is the use of sight to gather data. You begin to use inspection the moment you meet the client and continue as you observe the person's gait, personal hygiene, affect, and behavior during the general survey. You will also use inspection as you evaluate each body system. Adequate lighting and proper positioning aid inspection. The otoscope, ophthalmoscope, and penlight also enhance your inspection abilities.

Palpation

Palpation is the use of touch to gather data. Use palpation to assess temperature, skin texture, moisture, anatomical landmarks, and such abnormalities as edema, masses, or areas of tenderness. Following is a list of the most common palpation techniques, using different parts of the hand.

- *Fingertips:* Use for fine tactile discrimination, including assessment of skin texture, swelling, and specific locations of pulsations and masses.

Table 19-1 ➤ Positioning the Client

NAME	DESCRIPTION	COMMENTS
Sitting 	Sitting upright at side of bed or exam table	Use to assess vital signs, head and neck, chest, cardiovascular system, and breasts. If your client is weak, he may need assistance to maintain this position.
Supine (including Fowler's and semi-Fowler's positions) 	Lying flat on the back with arms and legs fully extended	Use to assess the abdomen, breasts, extremities, and pulses. If your client becomes short of breath, raise the head of the bed (HOB). In **Fowler's** position, the head is elevated 60°. In **semi-Fowler's** position, the head is elevated only 30°–45°.
Dorsal Recumbent 	Supine with knees flexed	Use for abdominal assessment if your client has abdominal or pelvic pain. Flexing the knees promotes relaxation of the abdominal muscles.
Lithotomy 	Dorsal recumbent position at end of table with feet in stirrups, legs flexed, and widely open	Use for a female pelvic exam; provides maximum exposure of genitals. Older patients may need support to assume and maintain this position. The patient's legs are exposed here to illustrate position. To see a privacy drape refer to Procedure 22-4 in Volume 2.

Table 19-1 ➤ Positioning the Client—cont'd

NAME	DESCRIPTION	COMMENTS
Sims' 	Flexion of the hip and knees in a side-lying position	Use to examine the rectal area. Use for a female pelvic exam if the patient is unable to assume the lithotomy position. Do *not* use if the client has had total hip replacement.
Prone 	Lying on stomach (A small pillow under the abdomen makes this position more comfortable.)	Use to examine the musculoskeletal system, especially hip extension; may also be used to examine the back and buttocks. May be difficult to assume by clients with respiratory problems.
Lateral Recumbent 	Lying on the side in a straight line	Left lateral recumbent is used to evaluate heart murmur or during a thorough cardiovascular assessment. This position brings the heart closer to the chest wall. If the client cannot assume this position, listen to the heart with the client seated and bending forward.
Knee–Chest 	On hands and knees with head down and buttocks elevated	Provides good visualization for examining the rectal area. However, it is not used often because it is embarrassing and uncomfortable for the client.

Continued

Table 19-1 ➤ **Positioning the Client—cont'd**		
NAME	**DESCRIPTION**	**COMMENTS**
Standing 	Upright posture with both feet flat on the ground	Use to examine the musculoskeletal and neurological systems and to assess gait and cerebellar function. Clients who are weak or who have poor balance may not be able to assume this position.

- *Dorsum of hand:* Use for temperature determination.
- *Palmar surface of hand:* Use for locating general area of pulsations.
- *Grasping with fingers and thumb:* Use to detect the position, shape, and consistency of a mass.

As you begin and move through the assessment of each body system, always advise the client that you are about to touch him, and use a gentle approach. Be certain your hands are warm. Begin with light pressure to detect surface characteristics. Then move to deep palpation to assess the underlying structures. Examine last any areas of discomfort.

Percussion

Percussion is tapping your fingers on the skin using short strokes. Tapping produces vibrations, and the resulting sound allows you to determine location, size, and density of underlying structures. Percussion is especially useful when assessing the abdomen and lungs. For **direct percussion,** tap lightly with the pads of the fingers directly on the skin. **Indirect percussion** is used more frequently and requires two hands. For the best results, keep your fingernails short. Percussion takes practice. To learn more about percussion,

 Go to Chapter 19, **Clinical Insight 19-1: Performing Percussion,** in Volume 2.

A quiet environment allows you to perceive the subtle differences in percussion notes. To learn terminology for the notes you may hear when assessing your clients,

 Go to **Sound Files** on the Student Resource Disk or DavisPlus at http://davisplus.fadavis.com/Wilkinson2

Auscultation

Auscultation is the use of hearing to gather data. **Direct auscultation** is listening without using an instrument. If you have heard wheezing or chest congestion without the use of a stethoscope, you have already performed direct auscultation. **Indirect auscultation** is listening with the help of a stethoscope. The stethoscope has two end pieces, the diaphragm and the bell.

- Use the diaphragm to listen to high-pitched sounds that normally occur in the heart, lungs, and abdomen. Press the diaphragm hard enough to produce an obvious ring on the patient's skin.
- Use the bell to hear low-pitched sounds, such as extra heart sounds (murmurs) or turbulent blood flow, known as bruits. Apply the bell lightly with just enough pressure to produce an air seal with its entire rim.

To improve your skill in indirect auscultation,

 Go to Chapter 19, **Clinical Insight 19-2: Performing Auscultation,** in Volume 2.

Olfaction

Olfaction is the use of the sense of smell to gather data. Some clinicians may not consider this a formal assessment skill; however, you will certainly use this skill in the clinical setting. Olfaction adds information to the data you collect through the other techniques. Consider these examples:

- If a client is slurring his words, you will want to look for data that reveal the cause of the problem. Slurred speech might be caused by a stroke or by sedative medications. However, if the client smells of alcohol you would first investigate recent alcohol use as a probable cause for the slurred words.
- If an older client smells of urine, you would want to assess for problems with leakage of urine or inability to perform self-care.
- If the client's breath has a "fruity" or "acetone" odor, you would suspect ketoacidosis (which may accompany diabetes). You would know to assess the urine for ketones and contact the primary care provider if necessary. You would also ask the client about dietary patterns, because a high-protein, high-fat, low-carbohydrate diet can cause a buildup of ketones in the blood.

KnowledgeCheck 19-3

- Identify five physical assessment skills.
- In what order are these skills performed?

Go to Chapter 19, **Knowledge Check Response Sheet and Answers,** on the Student Resource Disk or DavisPlus at http://davisplus.fadavis.com/Wilkinson2

CriticalThinking 19-2

Think about olfaction as an assessment technique. Give two or three additional examples of data you might collect through the use of smell.

How Do I Modify Assessment for Different Age Groups?

The basic techniques of physical assessment remain the same for all age groups. However, your approach will vary according to the developmental stage of your patient.

Infants

Infants usually feel most secure if a parent holds them during the examination, either against the chest or, for older infants who can sit without support, on the parent's lap. Otherwise, position an infant on a padded examination table.

✚ If there are siderails, raise them to prevent falling. Do not leave the infant's side or turn your back on the infant.

Use the assessment as an opportunity to teach the parent about normal growth and development.

Toddlers

Toddlers can be challenging to examine. They are interested in exploring the environment, but they also like to stay close by a parent, often in the parent's lap. Because they may be fearful of invasive procedures, such as examination of the oral cavity or inner ear, perform these procedures last. Most toddlers enjoy making choices, so use this characteristic to promote the toddler's cooperation. For example, you might provide a choice by saying, "Would you like to sit on the table or in your mother's lap?" or "Should I listen to your chest first, or should we see how much you weigh?" Allow the child to show you his developmental skills. If he needs assistance to remove clothing, have the parent help, and observe how the parent and child interact. Always praise the toddler for his abilities and cooperation. This sets the stage for positive feelings about health care.

Preschoolers

Preschool children are developing initiative and, as a result, usually cooperate with an examination. However, children of this age have fantasies and fears that may arise during the examination. For example, they may object to a noninvasive procedure because they believe it will cause pain or injury, or they may refuse to step on the scale because to them it resembles a monster. In such cases, it may be helpful to demonstrate the procedure on a doll or have the parent step on the scale before you approach the child.

As appropriate, allow the preschool child to sit in a parent's lap if she wishes. By age 5, most children will be comfortable enough to lie on the examination table if a parent is present. Let the child help with the exam. For example, have her hold equipment or remember her height and weight. Give reassurance as you go through the examination: for example, "Your lungs sound very healthy." Always compliment the child on her cooperation.

School-Age Children

The school-age child has a rapidly expanding vocabulary and usually seeks approval of parents, teachers, and healthcare providers. Develop rapport by asking the child about his favorite school or play activities. Allow the child to undress himself and get up and down from the exam table. Demonstrate your equipment before you use it. The school-age child will be interested in how his body works, so use this opportunity for teaching.

Adolescents

The adolescent is self-conscious and introspective and may wish to be examined without parents or siblings present, at least during the more personal aspects of the exam. Offer the adolescent this choice. Adolescents often worry about the "normalcy" of their changing bodies and appreciate respect for their privacy. Be certain to discuss the normal physiological changes that accompany puberty. If you need to review those changes,

 Go to Chapter 9, **Expanded Discussion,** on the Student Resource Disk or DavisPlus at http://davisplus.fadavis.com/Wilkinson2

Adolescent behavior may be strongly influenced by peer values, so emphasize lifestyle habits that promote wellness, including a healthful diet; adequate rest and exercise; and avoidance of tobacco, alcohol, and other drugs. Also discuss sexually transmitted infections and cancer, particularly testicular cancer and human papillomavirus. The first pelvic examination and breast examination usually begin in the teen years. Because suicide is the third leading cause of death among adolescents, you should also use this opportunity to screen for depression and suicide risk (see Chapter 11 for a review of depression and suicide).

Young and Middle Adults

Most young and middle adults are able to cooperate during a physical examination and do not require a modified approach. Modifications may be required if the client has acute or chronic illness or cannot understand or follow instructions.

Older Adults

Older adults are adjusting to changes in physical abilities and health. As part of a comprehensive exam, assess the client's support system and ability to perform activities of daily living. Observe your client's energy level during the physical examination and provide rest periods if needed. If the client tires easily, arrange the exam sequence to limit position changes. Also be aware that stiff muscles and arthritic joints may make it impossible for the client to assume certain positions. Older adults may have impaired vision or hearing, so you may need to adapt your techniques to compensate for this. Obtain feedback to be sure the patient is seeing and hearing you adequately.

The acronym "SPICES" will help you to remember common problems of the elderly that require nursing intervention (Fulmer, 1991, 2007) and to focus your assessment as you perform a comprehensive physical examination:

S—Sleep disorders
P—Problems with eating or feeding
I—Incontinence
C—Confusion
E—Evidence of falls
S—Skin breakdown

KnowledgeCheck 19-4
What exam modifications, based on developmental stage, should you consider for the following clients ("Meet Your Patients"):

- Joe Garcia?
- Joe's 3-year-old granddaughter, Bettina?
- Joe's elderly mother, Katherine?

 Go to Chapter 19, **Knowledge Check Response Sheet and Answers,** on the Student Resource Disk or DavisPlus at http://davisplus.fadavis.com/Wilkinson2

Practical **Knowledge** knowing how

The remainder of the chapter discusses each of the components of a comprehensive physical examination. The Critical Aspects box at the end of the chapter summarizes the entire comprehensive physical assessment, including a summary of the general survey.

For a step-by-step approach to perform each assessment,

 Go to Chapter 19, **Procedures,** in Volume 2.

As you perform your physical assessments, you may wish to refer to laboratory tests associated with each of the systems you are assessing. You can find some normal lab values in the "Laboratory Data for Joseph Garcia (Reference Ranges)" at the beginning of this chapter. For a list of laboratory tests,

 Go to Chapter 19, **Supplemental Materials: Laboratory and Diagnostic Tests by System,** on the Student Resource Disk or DavisPlus at http://davisplus.fadavis.com/Wilkinson2

The General Survey

The general survey is your overall impression of the client. It begins at first contact and continues throughout the exam. When you discover a deviation from normal in the general survey, you will explore it further during focused assessment of that body system. For example, if on meeting the patient you notice a drooping eyelid (ptosis) on one side of her face, you will keep that in mind as you perform the neurological assessment. Ptosis may be caused by a stroke or neurological injury. For a step-by-step approach,

 Go to Chapter 19, **Procedure 19-1: Performing the General Survey,** in Volume 2.

The following are aspects of the general survey.

Appearance and Behavior

Observe the client's general characteristics. Are his speech and behavior appropriate for his developmental stage? Look for indications of his mood and mental status—for instance, does he make eye contact with you? Notice any signs of distress, either physical or emotional.

Observe the condition of your client's face: Are his features symmetrical? Does he look his age? Note the quality of the visible skin; for example, excessive wrinkling of the skin from sun exposure, tobacco use, or illness may make the client appear older than his stated age. Be sure to consider cultural background, because this may influence your findings and interpretation.

Body Type and Posture

Next, observe your client's body size, build, and gait. As you introduce yourself and greet him, assess his muscle strength, mobility, and skin temperature and texture. Posture is also a clue about overall health status. A slumped position may indicate fatigue, depression, osteoporosis, or pain. If your client is immobile, observe his ability to move from side to side and change positions in the bed. Are the client's body movements smooth and coordinated? Does he use a cane or other assistive device? An unsteady gait may be associated with joint, muscle, or neurological disorders. Focused assessments in the remainder of the exam will help to reveal the exact meaning of such cues.

Speech

As you speak with the client and ask health-related questions, look for clues offered by his speech.

- Inappropriate or illogical responses may be associated with psychiatric disorders.
- Difficulty speaking or changes in voice quality may indicate a neurological problem.
- Rapid speech may be a sign of anxiety, hyperactivity, or use of stimulants.
- Hoarseness could indicate inflammation in the throat from infection, overuse, a foreign body, or perhaps a tumor or other obstructive material.
- Slow speech may be due to depression, sedation from medications, or neurological disorders.
- Vocabulary and sentence structure provide information about the client's educational level and comfort with the language.
- A foreign accent with hesitancy and/or sparse verbalization may signal a language barrier and a need for an interpreter.

Dress, Grooming, and Hygiene

A client's ability to dress and perform personal hygiene is affected by physical and emotional well-being. An unkempt appearance may reflect chronic pain, fatigue, depression, or low self-esteem. Poor hygiene may indicate a self-care deficit or physical or mental origin, or lack of easily accessible bathroom facilities.

Mental State

Mental state includes level of consciousness and capacity to interact. Notice whether your client seems awake, alert, and oriented to time, place, person, and self. If the client has an altered mental status, ask a family member about the onset of the change. Keep in mind that many medications, especially in older adults, may contribute to confusion or other changes in mental status.

- Bizarre responses may signal a psychiatric problem.
- Lethargy may be due to medications; depression; or a neurological, thyroid, liver, kidney, or cardiovascular disorder.
- Confusion and irritability may indicate hypoxia or medication side effects.
- Inability to provide a health history or to recall information may indicate a neurological disorder.

Vital Signs

You should assess vital signs as a part of the general survey and with subsequent assessments. Analyze for trends. See Chapter 17 for a complete discussion of vital signs, if needed.

Height and Weight

Height and weight provide valuable information about your client's growth and development, nutritional status, overall general health, and risk for various diseases such as diabetes and heart disease. These data are important for proper dosing of medication. For adults who can stand, measure height and weight using a platform scale with a sliding ruler (Fig. 19-1). When possible, the client should wear minimal clothing (gown) and no shoes. If the client cannot stand safely, use a bed scale. To measure an infant's length, use a stationary measure. Because children have frequent changes in growth, their measurements are documented on growth charts for easy monitoring and comparison to age- and gender-related standards. For growth charts for males and females from birth to 20 years of age,

 Go to Chapter 19, **Supplemental Materials: Growth Charts,** on the Student Resource Disk or DavisPlus at http://davisplus.fadavis.com/Wilkinson2

Body mass index (BMI) evaluates the relationship between height and weight. You can calculate the BMI for adults using a BMI calculator or table. For a BMI table,

 Go to Chapter 19, **Procedure 19-1: Performing the General Survey,** in Volume 2.

Because the proportion of fat to muscle affects BMI calculation, the BMI is not useful for athletes (who have a larger proportion of muscle), for pregnant and lactating women (who have a larger blood and tissue volume), for growing children, or for frail and sedentary older adults.

Once you have completed your general survey of the client, you can begin to focus on each body system. Whether you are doing a complete or focused physical assessment, remember that all body systems

FIGURE 19-1 For adults, measure height with the client's back to the platform scale.

are interrelated. A problem in one system may affect or be affected by other systems.

The Integumentary System

The integumentary system consists of the skin, hair, and nails. In a comprehensive exam, you assess this system briefly in the general survey, and then in greater detail as you move to examine other areas of the body. This allows the client to remain draped as long as possible.

The Skin

To perform a skin assessment, observe skin color, lesions, and other characteristics. Also notice unusual odors. An unpleasant body odor may be a sign of poor hygiene, the presence of a wound, or underlying disease. Excessive sweating may be related to activity (e.g., if the client has just finished exercising), thyroid problems, or overactive sweat glands. An odor of urine or stool may indicate a nursing diagnosis of Self-Care Deficit or Bowel or Urinary Incontinence.

For a summary of skin assessment, refer to the Critical Aspects box at the end of this chapter.

For step-by-step instructions,

 Go to Chapter 19, **Procedure 19-2: Assessing the Skin,** in Volume 2.

Skin Color

Skin color varies according to age and race, although each person's skin color is fairly uniform. Exposed areas, such as the hands, face, and neck, are often darker than unexposed areas, whereas the palms, soles, and nail beds are lighter than the rest of the skin. In people with dark skin, the lips are also usually lighter than surrounding skin. Variations in skin color commonly seen in neonates and infants include the following:

Mongolian Spots are benign, blue-black birthmarks that occur on the lower back and buttocks of black, Hispanic, Native American, and Asian babies. They are due to pigmented cells in the deeper areas of skin. Most fade by age 2 but can persist until early adolescence.

Capillary Hemangiomas, sometimes known as "stork bites," are small, irregular pink-red areas that are often seen around the face and nape of the neck in newborns. They typically disappear in infancy although can persist until age 5.

Café-au-lait Spots are light brown birthmarks that can occur anywhere on the body. The name of these birthmarks is French for "coffee with milk" because of their light-brown color. Most often café-au-lait spots are not associated with medical problems, although they can sometimes signal a genetic disorder.

Table 19-2 discusses the significance of other skin color variations that may be seen in clients of any age.

Skin Characteristics

As does color, the temperature, texture, and turgor of the skin offer clues to the client's health status. Although it is not technically a skin characteristic, you should also check for edema while you are assessing the skin.

Skin Temperature

Use the dorsum of the hand or fingers to assess skin temperature. Compare the temperature of the hands with that of the feet, and compare the right side of the body with the left. The skin should feel warm, but keep in mind that the temperature should be consistent with the room temperature and the patient's activity level. Be sure to check the temperature of the skin over any area of erythema. Erythema accompanied by warmth may indicate infection or inflammatory changes.

If the patient's skin feels excessively warm, validate your data: check her temperature to determine whether she has a fever. Hyperthyroidism stimulates the metabolism and may also elevate skin temperature. Excessive coolness may be due to poor peripheral circulation, shock, exposure to cold, or hypothyroidism.

Skin Moisture

Normally the skin is warm and dry. Excessive moisture may result from hyperthermia, thyroid hyperactivity, anxiety, or hyperhidrosis (excessive sweating). Oily skin is often seen with acne. Dry skin may result from dehydration, chronic renal failure, hypothyroidism, excessive exposure, or overzealous hygiene.

Table 19-2 ➤ Common Skin Color Variations

COLOR VARIATION	DESCRIPTION	SIGNIFICANCE
Pallor	In light-skinned clients: extreme paleness; skin appears white; loss of pink or yellow tones. In dark-skinned clients: a loss of red tones	May be related to poor circulation or a low hemoglobin level (anemia). Best sites to assess for pallor include the oral mucous membranes, conjunctiva, nail beds, palms, and soles of feet.
Cyanosis	A blue-gray coloration of the skin, often described as ashen	If seen in the lips, tongue, mucous membranes, and facial features, it is known as *central cyanosis* and is associated with hypoxia. In newborns, **acrocyanosis**, which is bluish discoloration of palms and soles in the first few hours to days of life, is normal.
		Cold causes the lips to turn blue but the tongue is not affected. Cyanosis may also be seen in the extremities, especially hands and feet, after exposure to extreme cold.
Jaundice	A yellow-orange cast to the skin	Often associated with liver disorders. Best sites to assess for jaundice include the sclera, mucous membranes, hard palate of the mouth, palms, and soles. Jaundice in the newborn is a normal finding in the first few weeks of life unless there is blood incompatibility or a congenital disorder.
Flushing	A widespread, diffuse area of redness	Generalized redness of the face and body may occur as a result of fever, excessive room temperature, sunburn, polycythemia (an abnormal increase in red blood cells), vigorous exercise, or certain skin conditions, such as rosacea.
Erythema	A reddened area	Associated with rashes, skin infections, prolonged pressure on the skin, or application of heat or cold.
Ecchymosis	Bruised (blue-green-yellow) area	May be seen anywhere on the body. The color will vary based on the age of the injury. May indicate physical abuse, internal bleeding, side effect to medication, or bleeding disorder. Refer to Chapter 9 to review assessing for abuse.
Petechiae	Tiny, pinpoint red or reddish-purple spots	Visible in the skin due to extravasation (leakage from vessels) of blood into the skin. May be associated with a variety of disorders and medications.
Mottling	Bluish marbling	Occurs in light-skinned clients, especially when cold. In newborns mottling indicates overstimulation of the autonomic nervous system.

Skin Texture

Normal skin is smooth and soft. The following factors affect skin texture:

- *Exposure.* Exposed areas tend to be drier and coarser in texture, as do the elbows and knees.
- *Age.* The skin of infants and young children is very smooth because of lack of exposure to the environment.
- *Hyperthyroidism and other endocrine disorders* may cause the skin to become coarse, thick, and dry.
- *Impaired circulation.* Peripheral arterial insufficiency is associated with smooth, thin, shiny skin with little to no hair. In contrast, venous insufficiency leads to thick, rough skin that is often hyperpigmented.

Skin Turgor

Turgor refers to the elasticity of the skin, which provides data about hydration status. To assess turgor, lift ("pinch up") a fold of skin (e.g., over the clavicle or on the back of the hand) and allow it to return to its normal position. Normally, skin returns immediately to its original position. Skin that tends to stay pinched for a few seconds **(tenting)** may be a sign of dehydration. Elasticity decreases with age, so tenting may also be seen with normal aging. Edema or scleroderma creates tension, preventing the skin from being pinched up.

Edema

Edema, or an excessive amount of fluid in the tissues, is an abnormal finding. It is common in clients with congestive heart failure, kidney disease, peripheral vascular disease, or low albumin levels. A client with edema may tell you his skin feels "tight" or say, "My shoes don't fit any more." Swollen tissue may feel tender to touch. Edema is not actually a condition of the skin, but it is convenient to assess for it while assessing the skin. Table 19-3 provides a grading system for edema.

Skin Lesions

Any **lesion,** variation in pigment, or break in continuous tissue requires assessment. Lesions considered to be normal variations include **milia**, white raised areas on the nose, chin, and forehead of newborns. These lesions, which resemble "whiteheads," are due to retention of sebum in the maturing sebaceous glands and disappear in infancy. Other normal variations are **nevi** (moles), freckles, birthmarks, **skin tags** (tiny tags or buds of skin usually around skin creases) in middle and older adults, and **striae** (silver-to-pink stretch marks) in pregnant women, women who have had children, and anyone who has experienced significant weight fluctuations. These are not harmful.

Abnormal lesions are classified as primary or secondary. **Primary skin lesions** develop as a result of disease or irritation. The pustules of acne are an example. **Secondary skin lesions** develop from primary lesions as a result of continued illness, exposure, injury, or infection, such as the crusts that form from ruptured pustules. When you observe a lesion, evaluate it for size, shape, pattern, color, distribution, texture, surface relationship, exudate, tenderness, pain, or itching. The table at the end of Procedure 19-2 should help you to categorize lesions. Also see the Abnormal Atlas at the end of Chapter 19 in Volume 2 to view abnormal lesions associated with particular conditions, such as cellulitis and scabies.

VOL 2 Go to Chapter 19, **Procedure 19-2: Assessing the Skin,** and **Abnormal Atlas** in Volume 2.

Table 19-3 ➤ Assessing Edema	
SCALE	**DESCRIPTION**
Trace	A minimal depression is noted with pressure.
+1	Creates a depression of about 2 mm. No visible distortion and rapid return of skin to position.
+2	Creates a depression up to 4 mm in depth that disappears in about 10–15 seconds.
+3	Creates a depression of approximately 6 mm in depth that lasts about 1–2 minutes. The area appears swollen.
+4	Creates a depression up to 8 mm in depth that persists for about 2–3 minutes. The area is grossly edematous.

Evaluate all skin lesions for the possibility of malignancy, especially those located in a site exposed to chronic rubbing or other trauma. Ask the client whether he has any newly developed moles or skin lesions or whether there has been any change in the appearance of existing lesions. You can remember the warning signs of malignant lesions by thinking of the letters ABCDE:

    A—Asymmetry
    B—Border irregularity
    C—Color variation
    D—Diameter greater than 0.5 cm
    E—Elevation above the skin surface

Knowledge Check 19-5

- What aspects of the skin should you assess?
- What assessments should you perform if you find a lesion?
- What warning signs lead you to suspect a malignant lesion?

 Go to Chapter 19, **Knowledge Check Response Sheet and Answers,** on the Student Resource Disk or DavisPlus at http://davisplus.fadavis.com/Wilkinson2

The Hair

When assessing the hair, inspect and palpate for color, texture, and distribution, as well as the condition of the scalp. The hair should be clean and free of debris. A client who does not properly groom her hair may need help with other self-care tasks.

Color. There is a wide range of naturally occurring hair color. Age-related graying of the hair varies among individuals according to their genetic background. White hair accompanied by very pale skin is seen in a condition known as **albinism,** or lack of pigment.

Texture. Normal hair texture varies from fine to coarse. However, hair that is exceptionally dry and coarse hair may be a sign of hypothyroidism; very fine, silky hair may indicate hyperthyroidism.

Distribution. Generally the hair is evenly distributed on the scalp, and fine body hair is present over the body. Men often have more hair on the face, chest, and back. Alterations in hair distribution may be signs of disease.

- **Alopecia** (hair loss) along the temples and in the center of the scalp is considered a normal balding pattern in men and is largely genetically based. Diffuse alopecia can be caused by chemotherapy for the treatment of cancer, by nutritional deficiencies, or by endocrine disorders. Thinning hair can also occur in the perimenopausal period when hormone levels are fluctuating. Patchy hair loss may be due to fungal infections of the scalp, hair pulling, constant wearing of caps, or **alopecia areata**, a benign autoimmune disorder.
- **Hirsutism** (excess facial or trunk hair) may be due to endocrine disorders or steroid use.

Scalp. Normally the scalp is smooth, firm, symmetrical, nontender, and without lesions. Common deviations include an asymmetrical or bumpy scalp due to trauma or lesions, and scaly flakes or patches due to fungal infection (e.g., dandruff), dermatitis, or psoriasis. Tenderness may indicate a localized infection or trauma. In newborns, **cradle cap**—scaly white patches over the scalp due to secretion of sebum—is common. It can be removed with washing and gentle scrubbing

In addition, the hair should be free of debris and **pediculosis** (head lice infestation). Head lice are tiny, very mobile, and difficult to see. You may find it easier to see the eggs, or **nits,** that are deposited on the hair shaft close to the scalp. For a step-by-step description of assessing the hair, see the Critical Aspects box at the end of this chapter, and

 Go to Chapter 19, **Procedure 19-3: Assessing the Hair,** in Volume 2.

The Nails

Healthy nail beds are level, firm, and similar to the color of the skin. The nail is smooth and uniform in texture with a 160° nail plate angle. Examine nails on both hands and feet. However, you may defer examination of the toenails until you are assessing the peripheral circulation. Variations in color, shape, or texture may indicate health problems.

For illustrations of nail variations, go to the Abnormal Atlas at the end of Chapter 19 in Volume 2. For a step-by-step description of nail assessment, see the Critical Aspects box at the end of this chapter, and

 Go to Chapter 19, **Procedure 19-4: Assessing the Nails** and **Abnormal Atlas,** in Volume 2.

Nail Color

Pink nails with rapid capillary refill indicate circulation to the extremities. Pale or cyanotic nail beds are seen in clients with circulatory or respiratory disorders that result in anemia or hypoxia. Other color abnormalities that you may encounter include the following:

- *Half-and-half nails,* in which a distal band of reddish-pink covers 20% to 60% of the nail. These occur in clients with low albumin levels or renal disease.
- *Mees' lines,* which are transverse white lines in the nail bed. They are seen in clients who have experienced severe illnesses or nutritional deficiencies.
- *Splinter hemorrhages,* which are small hemorrhages under the nail bed. They are associated with bacterial endocarditis or trauma.
- *Black nails,* due to blood under the nail, are seen after local trauma. Nails can also drop after blunt trauma.
- *White spots* may indicate zinc deficiency.

Nail Shape

A change in nail shape may indicate underlying disease. Figure 19-2 illustrates the typical nail plate angle of 160°. Clubbing, in which the nail plate angle is 180° or more, is

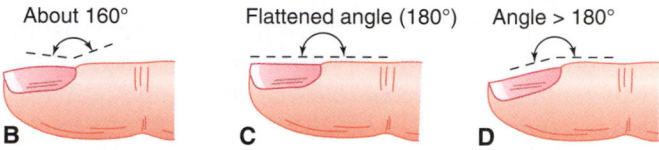

FIGURE 19-2 Nails. *A,* Parts of the nail. *B,* The normal nail plate angle is 160°. *C,* A nail plate angle of 180° or more is known as clubbing. *D,* Late clubbing from long term hypoxia.

associated with long-term hypoxic states, such as occurs with chronic lung disease. Spoon-shaped nails may result from iron deficiency.

Nail Texture

Nails are normally smooth in texture. You may see the following indications of problems:

- Thickened nails may result from poor circulation.
- A thick nail with yellowing is an indication of fungal infection known as *onychomycosis.*
- Brittle nails are seen with hyperthyroidism, malnutrition, calcium and iron deficiency, and repeated use of harsh nail products.
- Soft, boggy nails are seen with poor oxygenation.

The tissue surrounding the nail should be smooth epidermis. Chronic nail-picking results in callus formation around the nail. Occasionally the surrounding skin becomes inflamed. This condition, known as *paronychia,* is painful and may require drainage if infection is present.

 Critical **Thinking** 19-3

You are caring for a woman who has no hair on her head. How might you determine the cause of her hair loss? What other assessments should you perform?

The Head

Assessment of the head is often referred to by the acronym HEENT: head, eyes, ears, nose, and throat. You will use all the assessment techniques—inspection, palpation, percussion, and auscultation—in the HEENT exam.

The Skull and Face

Taking individual variation into account, on inspection the skull should be rounded and the face symmetrical in appearance and movement. Inspect head size; if it seems unusual, measure it.

- A large head in an adolescent or adult may be associated with **acromegaly,** a disorder associated with excess growth hormone. Head size is familial, as well.
- **Microcephaly,** an abnormally small head size, is seen in clients with certain types of mental retardation.
- In infants, abnormal shape or flattening of the skull may result from trauma during a vaginal birth or placing the baby in the same position for several hours every day.
- In infants and children, a head that is growing disproportionally faster than the body may be a sign of **hydrocephalus** (an accumulation of excessive cerebrospinal fluid).
- Asymmetry may be the result of trauma, surgery, neuromuscular disorder, paralysis, or congenital deformity.
- Facial appearance that is inconsistent with gender, age, or racial/ethnic group may indicate an inherited or chronic disorder, such as Graves' disease, hypothyroidism with myxedema, or Cushing's syndrome.

The skull should be smooth to palpation, with no unusual contours or bulges. Jaw motion should be symmetrical with no pain, clicking, or crepitus (cracking). Contour abnormalities, bulging, or tenderness result from trauma, congenital anomalies, or surgery. Irregular jaw movement or cracking of the jaw may indicate **TMJ (temporomandibular joint) syndrome.**

The Critical Aspects box at the end of this chapter summarizes the assessment of the face. For the entire procedure, and an Abnormal Atlas of facial abnormalities,

 Go to Chapter 19, **Procedure 19-5: Assessing the Head and Face,** in Volume 2.

The Eyes

In examining the eyes, you will inspect and palpate the external eye structures, assess vision, and examine the internal eye structures. Have the patient assume a sitting position for the exam. The Critical Aspects box at the end of this chapter summarizes the eye exam. For step-by-step instructions,

 Go to Chapter 19, **Procedure 19-6: Assessing the Eyes,** in Volume 2.

For convenience, you may wish to perform some cranial nerve testing along with the eye exam (e.g., corneal reflex, pupillary reaction, accommodation, and extraocular movements). For instructions on performing a cranial nerve examination,

 Go to Chapter 19, **Procedure 19-16: Assessing the Sensory-Neurological System,** in Volume 2.

External Structures

To review the structure of the external eye, see Figure 19-3. Normal eyelid margins are moist and pink with short

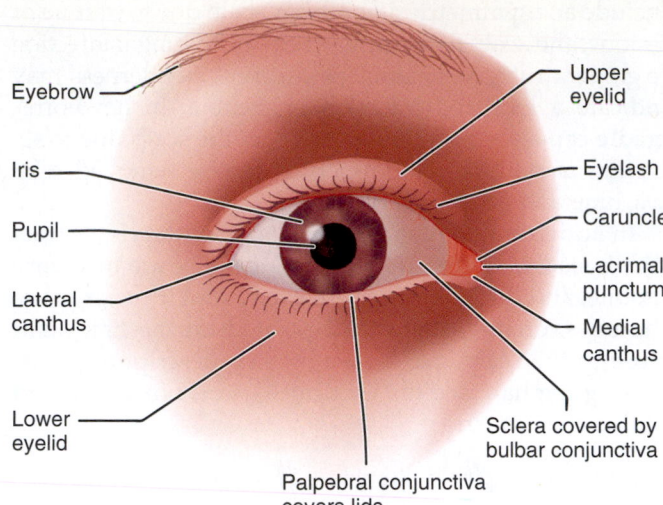

FIGURE 19-3 The external eye and eyelid.

lashes that are evenly spaced and curl outward. The lower eyelid margin appears at the bottom edge of the iris, and the upper eyelid covers half the upper iris. The conjunctiva is smooth, glistening, and peach in color, with minimal blood vessels present. There should be no pallor, dryness, or edema. The following are common abnormal findings on the eyelids:

- Crusting, scales, or swelling of the lid is associated with infection of the eyelids or eyelashes.
- A **pterygium** is a growth or thickening of conjunctiva from the inner canthus toward the iris.
- **Ectropion,** an everted eyelid, is commonly seen in older adults secondary to loss of skin tone. It can lead to excessive dryness of the eyes.
- **Entropion,** an inverted eyelid, can lead to corneal damage.
- **Ptosis,** or drooping of the lid, may be seen in clients who have experienced a stroke (cerebrovascular accident [CVA]) or Bell's palsy (paralysis of the facial nerve). To see ptosis and other abnormalities,

 Go to Chapter 19, **Procedure 19-5: Assessing the Head and Face,** and **Abnormal Atlas,** in Volume 2.

The **sclera** should be smooth, glistening, and blue-white in color with tiny vessels visible. Dark-skinned patients may have a yellowish cast to the peripheral sclera or small brown spots more centrally. Numerous disorders may affect the sclera and conjunctiva, including infection, allergies, injuries, and liver disorders. For example, yellow (**icteric**) sclera may be seen with an elevated bilirubin. Blood visible in the sclera is known as a **subconjunctival hemorrhage** and may be related to trauma or hypertension.

The lens and the **cornea,** or outermost layer of the eyeball, are transparent, smooth, and moist. A white ring encircling the outer rim of the cornea is known as **arcus senilis** and is a normal variant in older adults.

Lens opacities, known as **cataracts,** are frequently seen in older adults and may impair vision. Roughness or irregularity of the cornea is seen with trauma or a corneal abrasion.

The **pupils** should be uniform in color, equal in size, and round. They should **accommodate** equally; that is, the pupils constrict and the eyes converge (cross) as a person attempts to focus on an object moving toward him. This is typically charted as PERRLA: pupils equal, round, reactive to light and accommodation. The following are common pupillary abnormalities:

- Sluggish accommodation may be caused by anticholinergic drugs or advanced age.
- Failure of one or both pupils to accommodate may reflect a cranial nerve III problem or **exophthalmos** (associated with hyperthyroidism). Congenital cataracts, although rare, may be seen in infants and are checked during an eye exam using the "red reflex."
- Cloudy pupils, a finding related to cataracts, are commonly seen in older adults.
- **Mydriasis** (enlarged pupils) may be seen with glaucoma, an increase in intraocular pressure.
- Many medications affect pupil size. Medications called *mydriatics* are used to dilate the pupil to allow better visualization of the internal eye during examination.
- **Miosis** (constricted pupils) often results from medications to treat glaucoma.
- **Anisocoria** (unequal pupils) may be seen with central nervous system disorders such as stroke, head trauma, or cranial nerve injuries. In some individuals, anisocoria may be normal.

Visual Acuity

Visual acuity is a measure of the eye's ability to detect the details of an image. When testing visual acuity, you will assess distant, near, peripheral, and color vision. Nurses usually perform screening tests of visual acuity. Other testing is performed by nurses in advanced or specialty practice or by an optometrist or ophthalmologist as needed.

Distance Vision

Use the Snellen chart from a distance of 20 feet to assess distance vision. Assess each eye separately, and then assess both eyes together. Normal vision is a measure of clear vision at 20 feet (20/20) in the right eye, left eye, and both eyes. If a patient hesitates when reporting the letters or symbols he sees on the Snellen chart, document "with hesitation." If the person misses one or two items in a line, record the number of items missed.

Myopia, or diminished distant vision, is associated with a smaller fraction. For example, 20/100 vision means that to see text a person with normal vision can read at 100 feet, the client has to stand just 20 feet from the Snellen chart. A child's distance vision does not reach 20/20 until around 6 or 7 years of age.

Near Vision

Test near vision by having the client read newsprint from a distance of 35.5 cm (14 in.). A client with normal near vision will be able to read the newsprint without hesitation with either eye and both eyes. With **hyperopia,** or diminished near vision, the client must hold the paper more than 35.5 cm (14 in.) away. As we age, the lens of the eye naturally loses some ability to accommodate to near objects. In clients older than 45 years of age, diminished near vision is known as **presbyopia.**

Color Vision

Color vision is the ability to detect color. **Color blindness** may be genetically inherited (usually seen in males), or it may result from macular degeneration or other diseases that affect the cones of the eye. Use the color bars at the base of the Snellen chart to test color vision. *Ishihara cards* are specialized cards that enable thorough testing for color blindness. They contain embedded figures within a field of color. A person with normal color vision will be able to successfully identify the figures in the cards or the bars on the base of the Snellen chart; one who is color blind will not.

Visual Field

Visual field is the area the eye is able to observe. It is related to peripheral vision and extraocular muscle (EOM) function. **Peripheral vision** describes the boundaries of the visual field while the eye is in a fixed position. The common phrase, "I see you out of the corner of my eye," refers to peripheral vision.

The EOMs control the movement of the eye and eyelids and allow you to track movement. Three cranial nerves (CN) innervate the EOM. They are CN III (oculomotor), CN IV (trochlear), and CN VI (abducens). CN III also works together with CN II (optic) to control the pupillary reaction to light. Figure 19-4 illustrates the eye positions affected by the EOM and the corresponding cranial nerves.

Strabismus (crossed eye) is a condition in which one or both eyes deviate from the object they are looking at. It is normal during the first 1 or 2 months of life. After that, it may be caused by weak intraocular muscles or a lesion on the oculomotor nerve. Constant strabismus of one eye may result in **amblyopia** ("lazy eye"), in which the brain does not fully acknowledge the images seen

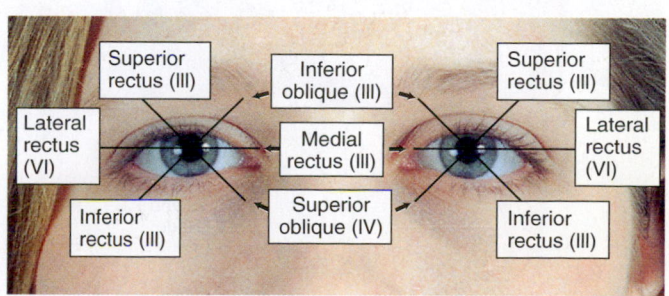

FIGURE 19-4 Cranial nerves and the extraocular muscles.

by the amblyopic eye. This creates reduced vision in that eye, not correctable by glasses or contact lenses.

Visual field abnormalities may be caused by problems with cranial nerves III, IV, and VI or with the retina. Poorly controlled diabetes, cataracts, macular degeneration, and advanced glaucoma are other disorders that limit the visual field.

Internal Structures

To visualize the internal structures of the eye, use an ophthalmoscope in a darkened room. Examine the optic disc, physiological cup, retinal vessels, retinal background, and macula. This is an advanced assessment technique; however, advanced practice nurses and registered nurses on specialty units do perform it with training. Advanced practice nurses use this technique to gain information about certain diseases that affect the eye, such as hypertension and diabetes.

KnowledgeCheck 19-6

- What are the major components of an eye assessment?
- Identify the cranial nerves involved with eye movement and function.

 Go to Chapter 19, **Knowledge Check Response Sheet and Answers,** on the Student Resource Disk or DavisPlus at http://davisplus.fadavis.com/Wilkinson2

The Ears and Hearing

The ears are involved in both hearing and equilibrium. The **external ear** collects and conveys sound waves to the middle ear. It protects the middle ear from environmental factors such as humidity and temperature and prevents entry of foreign matter. The **middle ear** contains the tympanic membrane and cavity, the eustachian tube, and the **ossicles** (the small bones of the middle ear: the malleus, incus, and stapes). The middle ear conducts

sound waves to the inner ear. The **inner ear** is responsible for hearing and equilibrium. Figure 19-5 illustrates the structures of the ear.

You will use an otoscope and tuning fork to examine the ears. For procedure steps and guidelines for using the otoscope and tuning fork, see the Critical Aspects box at the end of this chapter and also

VOL 2 Go to Chapter 19, **Procedure 19-7: Assessing the Ears and Hearing,** in Volume 2.

As with the eyes, nurses are usually responsible only for screening and making referrals. However, in some settings nurses perform advanced assessments.

Examining the External and Middle Ear

On inspection, the ears should be of equal size and similar appearance. Normally the pinna is level with the corner of the eye and within a 10° angle of vertical position (Fig. 19-6). Altered placement of the ear may be a sign of hearing deficit or genetic disorders, including Down syndrome. There should be no lesions or drainage. Bloody drainage may result from trauma. Purulent drainage may be seen with infection.

On palpation, the external structures of the ear are smooth, nontender, pliable, and without nodules. A painful auricle or tragus may be associated with **otitis externa** (an outer ear infection), whereas tenderness behind the ear is seen with **otitis media** (a middle ear infection).

As you begin the otoscopic examination, you may notice that the external auditory canal contains **cerumen** (wax), which protects the middle ear from excessive drying. However, it should not completely obstruct the ear canal. Cerumen may be black, dark red, yellowish, or brown in color and waxy, flaky, soft, or hard, with no odor; all are normal variations. The auditory canal walls are smooth and free of redness or drainage. Be careful as you manipulate the otoscope, because the

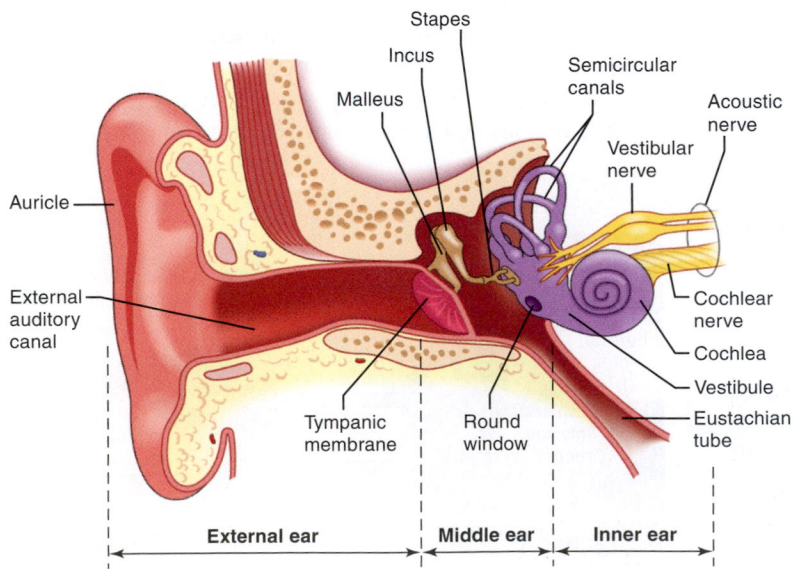

FIGURE 19-5 Cross-section of the ear.

10°   >10°

FIGURE 19-6 Normally the pinna is level with the corner of the eye and within a 108° angle of vertical position.

Normal ear attachment   Deviated alignment   Low-set ear attachment

inner two-thirds of the canal can be tender with the pressure and manipulation of the otoscope head.

Normally the **tympanic membrane (TM)** is pearly gray, shiny, and translucent. The structures of the middle ear should be visible through the membrane. Changes in its appearance arise from abnormalities such as otitis media (which causes a red, bulging TM) and the presence of pressure equalization tubes in young clients with chronic ear infections.

Assessing Hearing

To assess hearing, you will need a quiet room and a tuning fork. Gross hearing ability includes the ability to hear both high- and low-pitched tones. A client who hears low tones will be able to hear and repeat words whispered from 1 to 2 feet behind him. The client can hear high tones if he is able to hear a watch ticking at 5 inches (12 to 13 cm) from each ear.

The Weber and Rinne Tests

Hearing involves transmission of sound vibrations and generation of nerve impulses along CN VIII. The **Weber test** assesses both aspects. When you place a vibrating tuning fork on the center of the client's head, he should be able to sense the vibration equally in both ears. Record a positive Weber test if the vibration is louder in one ear.

If the Weber test is positive, you will need to perform the Rinne test to assess the type of hearing problem. The **Rinne test** also uses a tuning fork to compare air conduction (AC) and bone conduction (BC). Normally AC is twice as long as BC. For step-by-step instructions for performing the Weber and the Rinne tests,

 Go to Chapter 19, **Procedure 19-7: Assessing the Ears and Hearing,** in Volume 2.

The Romberg Test

Along with the cerebellum and midbrain, vestibular cells in the ear are responsible for maintaining equilibrium. To assess equilibrium, perform the Romberg test. Have the client stand with feet together and eyes closed. The client should be able to maintain balance with minimal swaying. Swaying and moving (positive Romberg)

may indicate a vestibular or cerebellar disorder. You may prefer to perform the Romberg test with examination of the neurological system instead of with the ears.

KnowledgeCheck 19-7

Your client has a negative Weber test. What further testing is required?

 Go to Chapter 19, **Knowledge Check Response Sheet and Answers,** on the Student Resource Disk or DavisPlus at http://davisplus.fadavis.com/Wilkinson2

CriticalThinking 19-4

What type of symptoms would you expect a client to be experiencing if he had a positive Romberg test?

The Nose

The nose and sinuses (Fig. 19-7) are part of the respiratory system and are the organs of smell. Vaporized molecules sniffed into the upper nasal cavities trigger receptors that generate impulses along the olfactory nerve (CN I) that travel to olfactory centers in the temporal lobes. The sense of smell diminishes in older adults because of a gradual decrease in and atrophy of the olfactory nerve fibers.

Frontal
Ethmoid
Sphenoid
Maxillary

FIGURE 19-7 Paranasal sinuses: frontal, ethmoid, sphenoid, and maxillary.

The external nose should be smooth, nontender, and symmetrical, with a midline septum. The client should be able to breathe freely through both sides of the nose without obstruction. Normally the mucous membrane inside the nose is pink, moist, and without lesions. To assess the nose and sinuses, you will need a penlight and nasal speculum or an otoscope with broad-tipped speculum. See the Critical Aspects box at the end of this chapter and

 Go to Chapter 19, **Procedure 19-8: Assessing the Nose and Sinuses,** in Volume 2.

The Mouth and Oropharynx

The structures of the mouth include the lips, tongue, teeth, **gingiva** (gums), uvula, hard and soft palate, and salivary glands and ducts (Fig. 19-8). On external inspection, the mouth and lips should be symmetrical and without lesions, swelling, or drooping. For instructions on examining the mouth and oropharynx, see the Critical Aspects box at the end of this chapter and

 Go to Chapter 19, **Procedure 19-9: Assessing the Mouth and Oropharynx,** in Volume 2.

The Lips, Buccal Mucosa, and Gingiva

The lips, **buccal mucosa** (mucous membrane of the cheeks), and gums should be smooth, moist, and pink in color. Increased pigmentation (e.g., bluish or dark patches) occurs in dark-skinned clients. No lesions should be present. The following are abnormal findings:

- Pallor may indicate anemia or inadequate oxygenation.
- **Gingivitis** is a sign of periodontal disease. You will see red, swollen, or spongy, bleeding gingiva and receding gum lines. The gums may be tender.
- **Parotitis** is an inflammation of the parotid salivary gland.

- **Stomatitis** is inflammation of the oral mucosa.
- **Leukoplakia** (thick, elevated white patches) that do not scrape off may be precancerous lesions; white, curdy patches that scrape off and bleed indicate **thrush** (a fungal infection).
- Redness or abrasions of the gingiva may be caused by poorly fitted dentures.
- **Aphthous ulcers** are small, painful vesicles with a reddened periphery and a white or pale yellow base. **Canker sores** are a benign type of aphthous ulcer believed to be caused by viral infection, allergies, stress, or trauma. So-called "major" aphthous ulcers may be caused by herpes simplex virus, human immunodeficiency virus, and bacterial infections.

Be sure to ask your client about use of tobacco, either smoked or chewed. Both forms of tobacco are associated with increased risk for oral cancer.

The Teeth

The upper teeth rest on top of lower teeth, with the upper incisors slightly overriding lower ones. Healthy adults typically have 28 teeth, or 32 if the wisdom teeth are present. The teeth should be fixed to the gum and without obvious debris or darkening that may indicate caries. Tooth decay and periodontal (gum) disease are common. Poor oral hygiene is a major contributing factor for both. As you examine the mouth and teeth, talk to the patient about his oral care. Recommend tooth brushing after each meal, daily flossing, and dental checkups every 6 months. See Chapter 22 for a more complete discussion of oral hygiene and prevention of periodontal disease.

The Tongue

When inspecting the mouth, carefully examine all aspects of the tongue: dorsal, ventral, and lateral. The **tongue** should be moist, symmetrical, slightly rough, smooth, pink, and freely movable. A fissured, or geographic, tongue is a common normal variation (Fig. 19-9). The following are abnormal findings:

- Deviation from the midline, which may be caused by damage to the hypoglossal nerve (CN XII)
- Limited mobility of the tongue

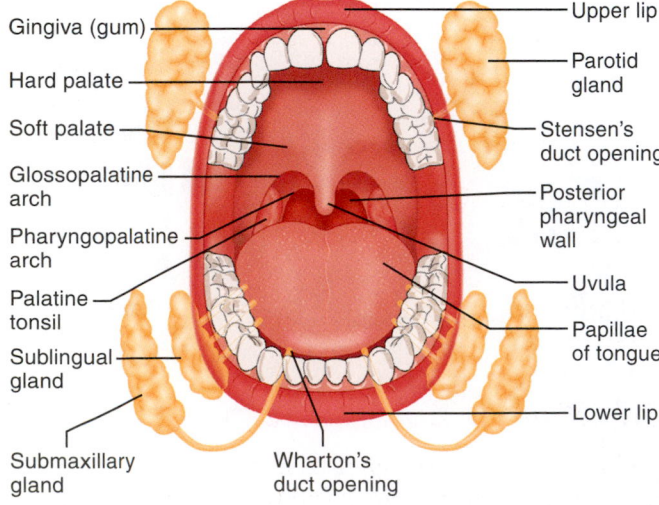

Gingiva (gum)
Hard palate
Soft palate
Glossopalatine arch
Pharyngopalatine arch
Palatine tonsil
Sublingual gland
Submaxillary gland
Wharton's duct opening
Upper lip
Parotid gland
Stensen's duct opening
Posterior pharyngeal wall
Uvula
Papillae of tongue
Lower lip

FIGURE 19-8 Structures of the mouth.

FIGURE 19-9 A geographic tongue is a common normal variant.

- **Glossitis** (inflammation of the tongue)
- A dry, furry tongue, which is associated with dehydration
- A black, "hairy" tongue, which is associated with fungal infections
- Absence of papillae, reddened mucosa, and ulcerations, which may indicate allergy, inflammation, or infection
- Swelling, nodules, or ulcers
- A smooth, red tongue, which may occur in clients who have a deficiency of iron, vitamin B_{12}, or vitamin B_3

The Hard and Soft Palates and Oropharynx

The hard palate, soft palate, and oropharynx should be pink, moist, and intact. No lesions, swelling, erythema, or discharge should be present. If the tonsils are present, they should be symmetrical, small in size, and free of exudate in a healthy person. The uvula is midline and should rise on **phonation** (vocalization).

The Neck

The neck has components of the musculoskeletal, neurological, vascular, respiratory, endocrine, and lymphatic systems. The sternocleidomastoid and trapezius muscles form the landmarks of the neck, known as the **anterior and posterior triangles** (Fig. 19-10). The symmetrical neck muscles center and coordinate movement of the head. Asymmetrical head position may result from damage to the muscles, swelling, or masses. Painful or erratic movement may be due to a benign condition, such as muscle spasm, or to significant problems, including meningitis, neurological injuries, or chronic arthritis.

The trachea, thyroid gland, anterior cervical nodes, and carotid arteries are positioned in the anterior triangle; the posterior cervical nodes are in the posterior triangle. You will palpate the tracheal rings and the cricoid and thyroid cartilage in the midline of the anterior neck (Fig. 19-11).

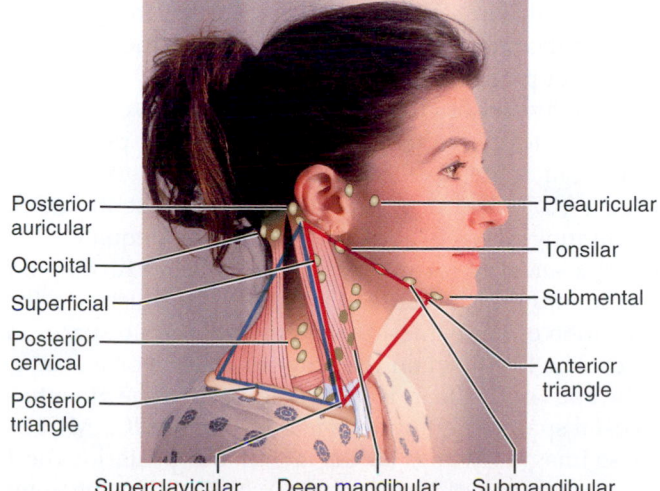

FIGURE 19-10 The anterior and posterior triangles of the neck and the cervical lymph nodes.

Posterior auricular
Occipital
Superficial
Posterior cervical
Posterior triangle
Preauricular
Tonsilar
Submental
Anterior triangle
Superclavicular   Deep mandibular   Submandibular

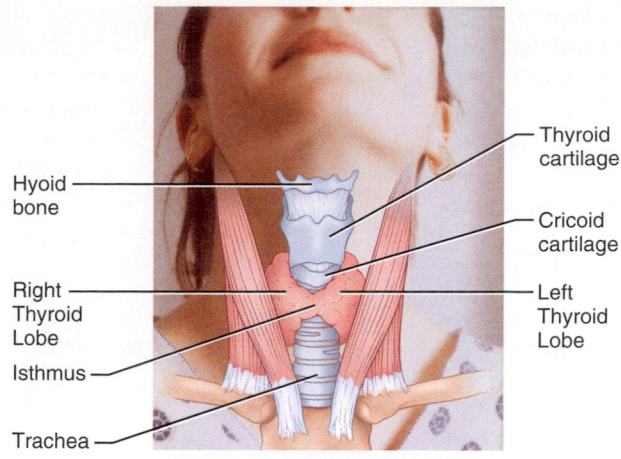

Hyoid bone
Right Thyroid Lobe
Isthmus
Trachea
Thyroid cartilage
Cricoid cartilage
Left Thyroid Lobe

FIGURE 19-11 The tracheal rings and cricoid and thyroid cartilage are palpable in the midline of the anterior neck.

For a summary of instructions for assessing the neck, see the Critical Aspects box at the end of this chapter. Also

 VOL 2 Go to Chapter 19, **Procedure 19-10: Assessing the Neck,** in Volume 2.

The Thyroid Gland

Normally the thyroid is smooth, firm, and nontender. It is often nonpalpable. Thyroid abnormalities are common. An enlarged thyroid may be associated with either hypothyroidism or hyperthyroidism. Thyroid tenderness usually results from inflammation. Thyroid masses may be malignant but are usually benign. If the thyroid is palpable, you will need to auscultate it for bruits.

The Cervical Lymph Nodes

The cervical lymph nodes occur in three chains (Fig. 19-10). The anterior chain is in the anterior triangle, the posterior chain in the posterior triangle. There is a deep cervical chain under the sternocleidomastoid muscle. The lymph nodes are generally not palpable, although occasionally nodes can be felt, especially in young children. Normal nodes are small in size (less than 1 cm), mobile, soft, and nontender. You should describe enlarged nodes (greater than 1 cm in diameter) according to their location, size, shape, consistency, mobility, and tenderness. Enlarged or tender nodes may be caused by infection, malignancy, and other diseases.

 Critical**Thinking** 19-5

A client complains of sore throat, fever, chills, and runny nose. What assessments should you perform?

The Breasts and Axillae

The breasts consist of glandular, adipose, and connective tissue; smooth muscle; and nerves (Fig. 19-12). The functions of the female breast are sexual stimulation

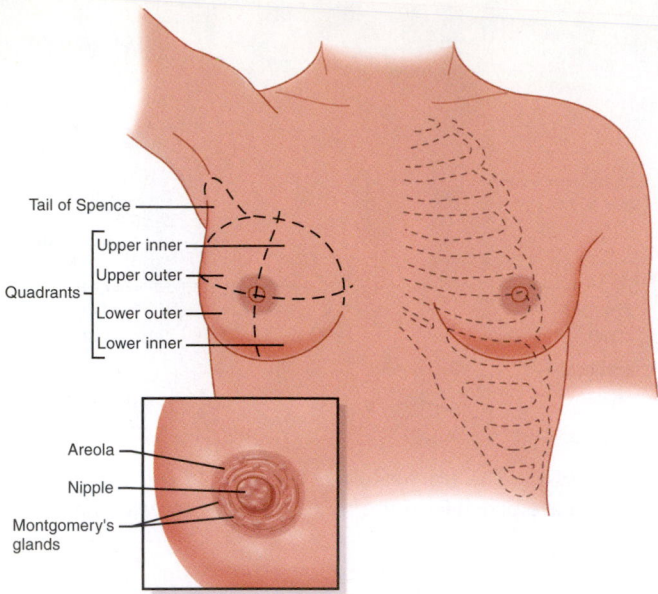

Tail of Spence

Quadrants
- Upper inner
- Upper outer
- Lower outer
- Lower inner

Areola

Nipple

Montgomery's glands

FIGURE 19-12 Breast tissue extends up into the axilla.

and milk production for nourishing offspring. Breast size and shape varies among women, and commonly one breast is slightly larger than the other. At puberty, the ovaries produce estrogen and progesterone, which stimulate the breasts to develop. The menstrual cycle, pregnancy, and breastfeeding also enlarge breast tissue. Although breasts are thought of as female organs, men also have breasts. However, because of limited estrogen and progesterone levels, male breasts develop only minimally.

Breast tissue and lymph drainage for the breast extend up into the axilla. The majority of breast tumors are found in the tail of Spence, in the axilla. A breast exam therefore always includes an exam of the axillae. Many women have breast reconstruction, either after breast removal due to cancer or breast augmentation for cosmetic reasons. These women should not omit breast examination, and it is performed in exactly the same way as for natural breasts.

Currently there is controversy about whether or not we should continue to encourage breast self-examination (BSE) (Tarrant, 2006). Some studies indicate that it does not reduce death rates from breast cancer, but others report increased rates of cancer discovery and earlier detection in groups who perform BSE (Green & Taplin, 2003; Hackshaw & Paul, 2003; Kösters & Gøtzsche, 2003; Thomas et al., 2002; Weiss, 2003). Until there is more evidence, it seems reasonable to continue to use BSE as a screening tool along with the recommended mammograms. Researchers agree patients who perform BSE should be trained to use proper technique in order to avoid false negative findings (ACOG, 2007; Balkaya, Memis, & Demirkiran, 2007; Knutson & Steiner, 2007; Rosolowich, 2006).

You should perform a breast exam for the woman if she cannot do it herself, and demonstrate the procedure

as part of client teaching for self-care. Guidelines vary as to the age at which women should start having clinical breast exams (CBE) and mammograms to screen for breast cancer. However, breast exams are commonly done for adult women. Annual or biennial mammograms or breast thermography most commonly begin after age 40, or at a younger age and more often for those at high risk (ACOG, 2009; American Cancer Society, 2007, 2009). Evidence presently does not support the need for a CBE if a mammogram is done ([USPSTS], 2009b).

Chapter 41 includes a thorough discussion of teaching your client how to perform a breast self-exam. For a summary of breast examination, see the Critical Aspects box at the end of this chapter. For a step-by-step guide to examining the breasts and axillae,

 VOL 2 Go to Chapter 19, **Procedure 19-11: Assessing the Breasts and Axillae,** in Volume 2.

Critical**Thinking** 19-6

What strategies might encourage more women to regularly perform breast self-examination?

The Chest and Lungs

The chest, or thorax, is the bony cage that protects the heart, lungs, and great vessels. The ribs, sternum, and vertebrae form the chest. Be systematic in your assessment: always assess the areas of the chest and lungs in the same order.

Chest Landmarks

Before beginning the thoracic exam, review the following important landmarks that will help you visualize the underlying structures and perform an accurate assessment.

- Identify positions vertically on the anterior chest in relation to the ribs. For example, the space between the 5th and 6th ribs is known as the 5th intercostal space (5th ICS). You can easily palpate the ribs and count the spaces if you remember that the 1st rib is tucked up next to the clavicle (Fig. 19-13A).
- On the posterior chest, identify positions vertically in relation to the vertebra (Fig. 19-14B). The prominent vertebra at the base of the neck is the 7th cervical vertebra (C7). The next one down is T1 (1st thoracic). Counting down to about T9 should be adequate.
- Use a series of imaginary vertical lines to further aid in identifying locations. Figure 19-13B illustrates the location of these lines. Use them with the rib spaces to describe locations on the anterior chest. For instance, the apex of the heart is usually located in the 5th intercostal space at left midclavicular line (5th ICS MCL).
- Use imaginary lines on the lateral and posterior chest as well (see Fig. 19-14A and C). Notice that the anterior axillary line can be used to locate sounds on both the anterior and lateral chest.

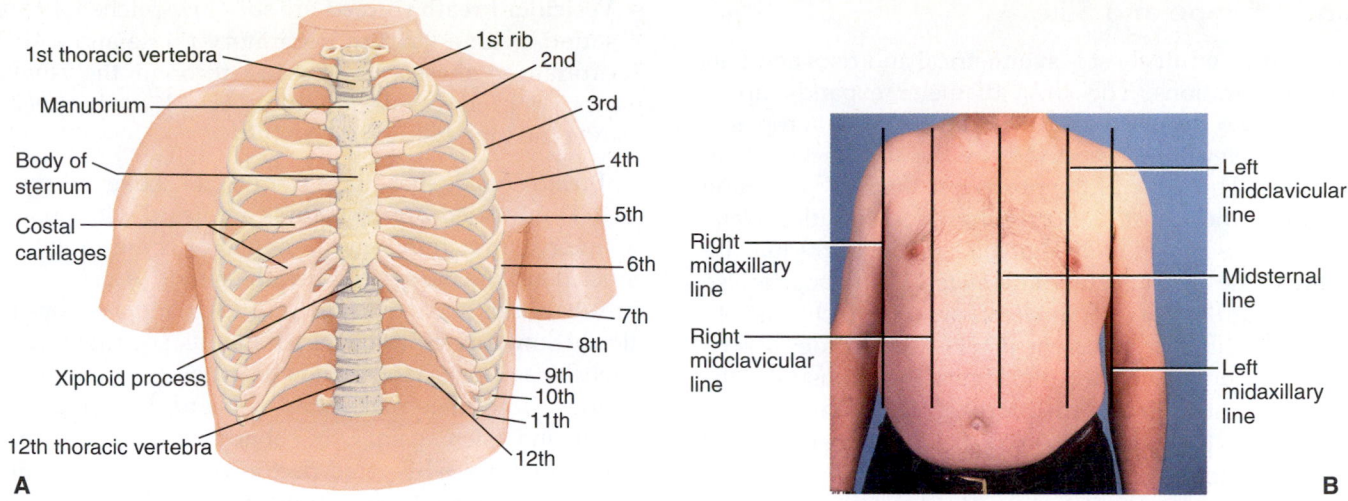

FIGURE 19-13 *A*, The anterior thoracic cage and the bony landmarks. *B*, A series of imaginary vertical lines is used to describe locations on the chest.

FIGURE 19-14 *A*, Lateral chest landmarks. *B*, The vertebrae are the landmarks on the posterior chest. *C*, Landmark lines on the posterior chest.

Chest Shape and Size

The normal adult chest is symmetrical and rises and falls with respirations. The chest diameter expands up to 3 inches (7.6 cm) with deep inspiration. The anteroposterior diameter of the chest is twice the size of the lateral diameter. The slope of the ribs is less than 90°. In young children, the chest is apple-shaped. Musculoskeletal changes associated with aging result in a gradual increase in the anteroposterior diameter. This change is also seen, regardless of age, in clients who have chronic obstructive pulmonary disease (COPD), a disorder associated with long-term smoking. Figure 19-15 illustrates the normal chest ratio and the barrel chest appearance that develops with COPD, in which the anteroposterior and lateral diameters may be equal.

Spinal alterations, such as **kyphosis** (excessive curvature of the thoracic spine) and **scoliosis** (lateral curvature of the spine) alter the shape of the thoracic cage. Osteoporosis, a common disorder associated with aging, is associated with increased porosity of the vertebrae. As a result, vertebrae may compress or collapse, shortening the length of the spine and pushing the ribs forward and downward.

Breath Sounds

Listen to breath sounds in a quiet room by auscultating one full respiratory cycle at each site. Directly apply the stethoscope to the client's skin. Compare breath sounds bilaterally. Three types of breath sounds are heard (Fig. 19-16).

- **Bronchial breath sounds** are loud, high-pitched, tubular sounds; expiration is of longer duration than inspiration. Air moving through the trachea produces these sounds, which you will hear best over the trachea on the anterior chest and below the nape of the neck on the posterior chest.
- **Bronchovesicular breath sounds** are medium-pitched with an equal inspiratory and expiratory phase. Air moving through the large airways of the bronchi produces these sounds, which are best heard over the 1st and 2nd ICS adjacent to the sternum on the anterior chest and between the scapula on the posterior chest.

- **Vesicular breath sounds** are soft, low-pitched, breezy sounds with a lengthy inspiratory phase and a short expiratory phase. Air moving through the smaller airways produces these sounds, which are best heard over the lung fields.

Breath sounds that differ from those above are abnormal. **Diminished breath sounds** are heard with poor inspiratory effort, in the very muscular or obese, or with restricted airflow. **Misplaced breath sounds** (e.g., bronchial breath sounds heard over the lung fields) indicate constriction of flow. **Adventitious breath sounds,** such as wheezes, rhonchi, and rales, are sounds heard over normal breath sounds. If an abnormal sound is heard, have the client cough and listen again. Other abnormal findings include **bronchophony, whispered pectoriloquy, and egophony**. These are abnormal voice sounds that result from consolidation of lung tissue. To find a discussion of these,

 Go to Chapter 19, **Supplemental Materials,** on the Student Resource Disk or DavisPlus at http://davisplus.fadavis.com/ Wilkinson2. Also go to **Sound Files,** to listen to normal and adventitious breath sounds.

For more information about the respiratory system, see Chapter 35. The Critical Aspects box at the end of this chapter summarizes respiratory assessment. For a table describing abnormal lung sounds and the procedure for performing a respiratory assessment,

 VOL 2 Go to Chapter 19, **Procedure 19-12, Assessing the Chest and Lungs,** in Volume 2.

KnowledgeCheck 19-8

- List and describe the location of the horizontal and vertical landmarks of the anterior chest.
- List and describe the location of the horizontal and vertical landmarks of the posterior chest.
- List and describe the location of the vertical landmarks of the lateral chest.

 Go to Chapter 19, **Knowledge Check Response Sheet and Answers,** on the Student Resource Disk or DavisPlus at http://davisplus.fadavis.com/Wilkinson2

Normal adult chest

Posterior

Barrel chest

Posterior

FIGURE 19-15 The normal anteroposterior to lateral ratio is 1:2. The lateral aspect of the chest increases dramatically with COPD, leading to a barrel chest appearance.

FIGURE 19-16 Normal breath sounds.
A, Anterior. *B,* Right lateral. *C,* Left lateral.
D, Posterior.

The Cardiovascular System

The cardiovascular system consists of the heart and the blood vessels. The heart is a muscle that pumps blood throughout the body. In a healthy adult, it is about the size of a clenched fist. The blood vessels, which make up the vascular system, have two main networks: the pulmonary circulation and the systemic circulation. See Chapter 35 if you need to review the anatomy of the cardiovascular system.

Oxygen-depleted blood circulates from the heart into the lungs, where it is oxygenated, then back to the heart. This system is known as the **pulmonary circulation.** From the heart, the blood enters the **systemic circulation.** The left ventricle is the largest chamber of the heart. It pumps blood into the systemic circulation via the arterial system. The arteries subdivide many times, becoming smaller and smaller until they separate, in the tissues and organs, into capillaries. It is at the capillary level that oxygen is delivered to the tissues. The venous system collects the oxygen-depleted blood and returns it to the right atrium of the heart to begin the circuit again. **Coronary circulation,** which circulates blood through the heart itself, is a part of the systemic circulation. For further discussion on pulmonary circulation and oxygenation, see Chapter 35. For animated presentations of the circulatory system and oxygen transport,

 Go to Student Resources, **Animations: Blood Flow** and **Carbon Dioxide/Oxygen Transport,** on DavisPlus at http://davisplus.fadavis.com/Wilkinson2.

The Critical Aspects box at the end of this chapter summarizes assessment of the heart and vascular system. For a complete step-by-step procedure,

 Go to Chapter 19, **Procedure 19-13: Assessing the Heart and Vascular System,** in Volume 2.

The Heart

The heart is positioned at an angle on the left side of the chest in the 3rd, 4th, and 5th intercostal spaces (ICS). To facilitate auscultation of specific heart sounds, perform the cardiac assessment with the client in three positions: sitting, supine, and left lateral recumbent. Clients with chronic heart or lung problems may have little cardiac reserve, so minimize position changes to conserve your client's energy. Be systematic. To keep from missing important parts of the exam, always listen in the same order to all the areas. To help minimize your client's anxiety, explain that it always takes time to examine the heart and circulatory system.

The Cardiac Cycle

During a cardiac cycle, the atria and ventricles alternately contract and relax to fill and empty; while the atria are contracting (emptying), the ventricles are relaxing (filling), and vice versa. **Systole** refers to the contraction, or emptying, of the ventricles. **Diastole** refers to the relaxation, or filling, phase of the ventricles.

Inspecting and Palpating the Heart

Begin your assessment of the heart with the client sitting (Fig. 19-17). Observe the **precordium,** the area of the chest over the heart, for visible pulsations. A small pulsation at the 5th ICS midclavicular line, also known as the **point of maximal impulse (PMI),** is normal. Other visible pulsations on the precordium, known as **heaves** or **lifts,** are associated with an enlarged ventricle.

Also palpate for vibrations. A **thrill** is a vibration or pulsation palpated in any area except the PMI. A thrill is associated with abnormal blood flow and usually has an accompanying **murmur** (additional heart sound).

Auscultating the Heart

Auscultate to establish cardiac rate and rhythm and to identify normal and abnormal heart sounds. A quiet room is essential. You can hear heart sounds from any location on the anterior chest wall. However, the four sites located over the heart valves are the preferred listening areas. Table 19-4 and Figure 19-17 illustrate these locations.

Auscultate in an orderly fashion. Start at the aortic area, and move gradually through each landmark. The

Table 19-4 ➤ Locations for Assessing the Heart		
TITLE	**STRUCTURE ASSESSED**	**LOCATION**
Base Right	Aortic valve	2nd ICS right sternal border
Base Left	Pulmonic valve	2nd ICS left sternal border
Left Lateral	Tricuspid valve	4th ICS left sternal border
Apex	Mitral valve	5th ICS MCL

following is a mnemonic you may use to recall the order of the heart sound landmarks:

Aunt	Aortic
Polly	Pulmonic
Takes	Tricuspid
Meds	Mitral

S_1, S_2, S_3, and S_4 Heart Sounds

Listen carefully at each site to each component of the heart sounds. Listen first with the diaphragm of your stethoscope. Then retrace your steps with the bell.

First Heart Sound. The first heart sound (S_1, or lub) results from the closure of the valves between the atria and ventricles. S_1 ("lub") is a dull, low-pitched sound, loudest over the mitral and tricuspid areas. S_1 marks the beginning of systole.

Second Heart Sound. The second heart sound (S_2, or dub) corresponds to closure of the semilunar valves (between the ventricles and the great arteries exiting the heart). "Dub" is higher in pitch and shorter than the S_1 "lub." The S_2 is loudest at the aortic and pulmonic areas. S_2 marks the beginning of diastole.

Normally, the mitral and tricuspid valves and the aortic and pulmonic valves close within a fraction of a second from each other. This near simultaneous closure results in a singular S_1 and S_2 sound. However, a split sound may occur, at either S_1 or S_2, if there is a delay in closure of one of the valves.

Third Heart Sounds. A third heart sound (S_3), heard immediately after S_2, has a gallop cadence that follows the rhythm of the word KenTUCKy. It is best heard at the apical site with the client lying on his left side. An S_3 is normal in young children and adolescents when they are sitting or lying, but it disappears when they stand or sit up. It is also a normal variant in the third trimester of pregnancy. In adults, an S_3 that does not disappear with position change is abnormal and represents heart failure or volume overload.

Fourth Heart Sounds. A fourth heart sound (S_4), heard immediately before S_1, has a rhythm that follows the

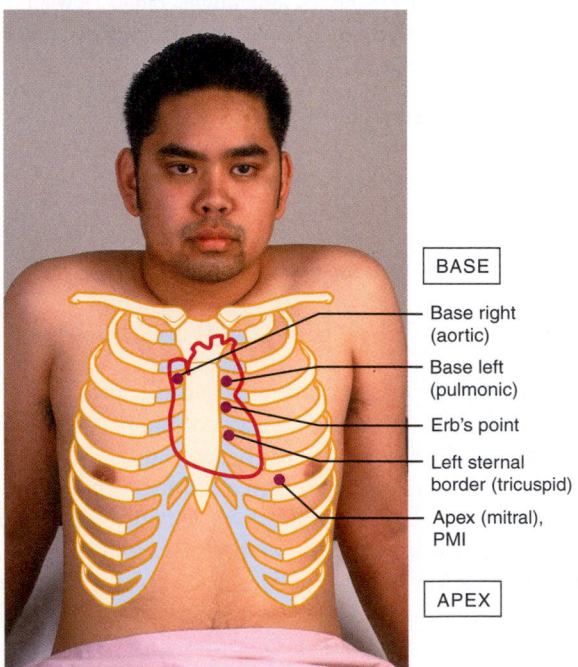

FIGURE 19-17 Cardiac auscultation sites.

BASE

- Base right (aortic)
- Base left (pulmonic)
- Erb's point
- Left sternal border (tricuspid)
- Apex (mitral), PMI

APEX

word FLOrida. S_4 is best heard at the apical site, using the bell of the stethoscope, with the client lying on his left side. An S_4 is normal in athletes and some older clients. It may also be heard in adults with coronary artery disease, hypertension, and pulmonic stenosis. To listen to heart sounds,

 Go to **Sound Files** on the Student Resource Disk or DavisPlus at http://davisplus.fadavis.com/Wilkinson2

Murmurs

Murmurs are additional sounds produced by turbulent flow through the heart. Some murmurs are "innocent," but others represent pathology such as alteration in valve structure. Identifying and classifying a murmur are advanced skills that require practice. To learn more about assessing murmurs, see the Critical Aspects box, and

 Go to Chapter 19, **Procedure 19-13: Assessing the Heart and Vascular System,** in Volume 2.

 Also go to Chapter 19, **Supplemental Materials: Heart Murmurs,** on the Student Resource Disk or DavisPlus at http://davisplus.fadavis.com/Wilkinson2

 Critical**Thinking** 19-7

What findings would you anticipate when assessing Mr. Garcia's ("Meet Your Patient") thorax?

The Vascular System

The vascular system is a network of arteries and veins that transport oxygen, carbon dioxide, and nutrients to the cells of the body. Arteries carry blood away from the heart: The pulmonary arteries carry oxygen-depleted blood from the right ventricle to the lungs, whereas the systemic arteries carry oxygenated blood from the left ventricle to the body periphery. Veins carry blood toward the heart: The pulmonary veins transport oxygenated blood from the lungs to the left atrium, whereas the systemic veins return oxygen-depleted blood from the periphery to the right atrium of the heart.

The Central Vessels

The carotid arteries and internal jugular veins run alongside the sternocleidomastoid muscle on both sides of the neck (Fig. 19-18). These central vessels provide circulation to the brain.

The Carotid Arteries

Because the carotid arteries are large and close to the heart, you can easily feel a pulse over the carotid artery even when it is difficult to palpate a peripheral pulse.

➕ Never palpate both carotid arteries at the same time because bilateral pressure may impair cerebral blood flow. Palpate very lightly and avoid massaging the carotid artery, because pressure on the carotids will cause the pulse rate to drop, and can even lead to cardiac arrest. As a general rule, avoid palpating the carotids except during cardiopulmonary resuscitation or when it is necessary to assess them for a specific reason (such as in a comprehensive physical exam, or when an underlying pathology makes it necessary to establish that circulation to the head is adequate).

Turbulent blood flow through the carotid artery produces a whooshing sound known as a **bruit,** which you can auscultate using a stethoscope. Bruits are common among older adults. The following conditions cause turbulence: **carotid stenosis** (narrowing from plaque), increased cardiac output secondary to fluid overload, use of stimulants, or hyperthyroidism. If you hear a bruit, lightly palpate the neck for thrills (pulsations or vibrations), which further confirm turbulent flow.

FIGURE 19-18 The central vessels.

The Jugular Veins

The jugular veins return blood from the brain to the superior vena cava. The external jugular veins are superficial; the internal jugular veins are deep. Normally the jugular veins are flat when the client is in an upright position and distend when the client lies flat. Jugular venous distention (JVD) is seen when the right side of the heart is congested due to inadequate pump function. The best position for assessment of JVD is semi-Fowler's (30 to 45° angle), as in Figure 19-18. Normally the neck veins are flat at this angle.

The Peripheral Vessels

If you were to lay out all the blood vessels in the peripheral system of an average sized person, you would find more than 60,000 miles of arteries, arterioles, capillaries, and venules. The peripheral vessels supply blood to all the body cells. The **arteries** are a high-pressure system with several palpable pulse sites. The **veins** are a low-pressure system with valves to prevent backflow due to gravity. The veins return blood to the heart via the continuing pressure from the arterial system and pumping action of the adjacent skeletal muscles.

Assess the peripheral vascular system by:

- Measuring the blood pressure (see Chapter 17). Usually you will measure the blood pressure at the start of the exam as part of the general survey.
- Palpating the peripheral pulses (see Chapter 17). In a healthy individual, pulses will be regular, strong, and equal bilaterally. Weak, absent, or asymmetrical pulses may indicate partial or complete occlusion of the artery. Other signs of arterial occlusion include pain, pallor, cool temperature, paresthesia, or paralysis.
- Inspecting and performing tests for adequate perfusion.

The data you obtain when inspecting and palpating the integumentary system provide some information about peripheral tissue perfusion. Recall that when an area is not adequately oxygenated, the skin may be pale, cyanotic, cool, and shiny; hair growth may be sparse, and there may be clubbing of the nails. Inadequate tissue oxygenation may be a result of chronic pulmonary problems; however, it can also result from impaired central or peripheral circulation.

Also assess the venous system. Inspect the veins for signs of distention. Superficial spiderlike veins, especially on the lower extremities, may occur with normal aging. Ropelike distended veins, or **varicosities,** may be painful. If a client has varicosities, assess for valve competence using the **manual compression test** discussed in Volume 2.

KnowledgeCheck 19-9

Identify the precautions to take when evaluating the carotid arteries.

 Go to Chapter 19, **Knowledge Check Response Sheet and Answers,** on the Student Resource Disk or DavisPlus at http://davisplus.fadavis.com/Wilkinson2

The Abdomen

The method most commonly used to identify the location of assessment findings is the four-quadrant method, which divides the abdomen into four sections by "drawing" a line vertically from the xiphoid process to the symphysis pubis and a horizontal line at the level of the umbilicus (Fig. 19-19). For the rarely used nine-region method,

 Go to Chapter 19, **Tables, Boxes, Figures: ESG Table 19-2,** on the Student Resource Disk or DavisPlus at http://davisplus.fadavis.com/Wilkinson2

Examination of the abdomen differs in sequence from all other body systems. Percussion and palpation stimulate the bowel and may alter bowel sounds. Therefore, you should inspect and auscultate before performing percussion and palpation. To promote comfort, ask the client to empty his bladder before the examination. Have the client assume a supine position with flexed knees. This relaxes the abdominal muscles and is usually the most comfortable position. If the client has a painful area, examine that area last to minimize discomfort during the rest of the exam.

Inspecting the Abdomen

The skin over the abdomen is usually paler than that over other parts of the body. The abdomen should be symmetrical with a rounded contour and sunken umbilicus. See Figure 19-20 for normal variations in abdominal shape. You may be able to see peristalsis and aortic pulsations on a very thin client, but in most clients usually you will see no movement. In clients with abdominal distention, the skin will appear taut. Distention may be normal,

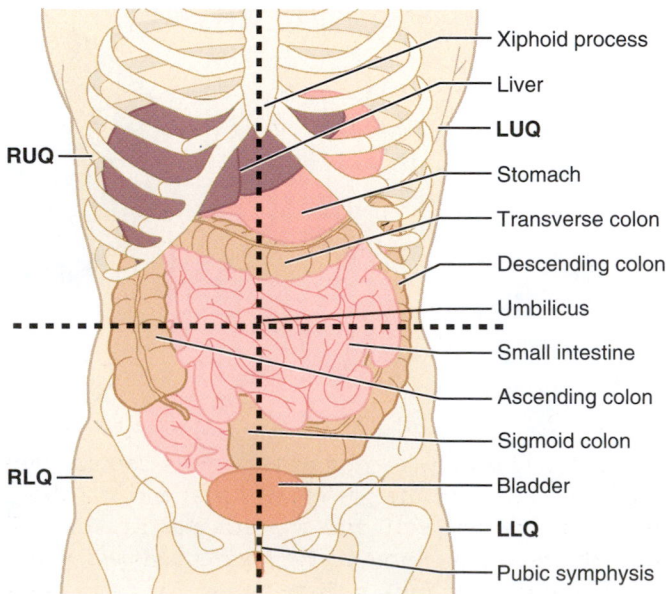

FIGURE 19-19 The four abdominal quadrants.

FIGURE 19-20 Normal variations in abdominal contour.

as with pregnancy, or it may be due to gas or fluid retention or to bowel obstruction.

Auscultating the Abdomen

Proceed in an organized manner, listening in several areas in all four quadrants. Use the same pattern for every examination so that it becomes a habit.

First Auscultate Bowel Sounds. Bowel sounds are high-pitched, irregular gurgles or clicks lasting one to several seconds and occurring every 5 to 15 seconds (or 5 to 30 times per minute) in the average adult. If the client has a nasogastric (NG) tube that is attached to suction, discontinue the suction or clamp off the tube while listening for bowel sounds. Otherwise, you may mistake the sound of suction in the stomach for bowel sounds. Bowel sounds may be:

- **Absent** (none heard after listening for 5 minutes)
- **Hypoactive** (very soft and infrequent, perhaps one per minute) after abdominal surgery or with bowel obstruction, infection, or innervation problems.
- **Hyperactive** (loud rushing sounds occurring every 2 or 3 seconds) with diarrhea, early bowel obstruction, or gastroenteritis (infection of the gastrointestinal tract).

To listen to bowel sounds,

 Go to **Sound Files** on the Student Resource Disk or DavisPlus at http://davisplus.fadavis.com/Wilkinson2

Next Auscultate the Major Arteries. Major arterial vessels lie in the abdomen below the intestines. Listen over the aorta and the renal, iliac, and femoral arteries for the presence of bruits.

Percussing the Abdomen

Use indirect percussion to assess for fluid, air, organs, or masses. Normally there is generalized tympany over the bowels (due to the presence of gas) and the abdomen is nontender, soft, and without masses. You will hear dullness when percussing organs, masses, or fluids. Some practitioners include percussion of the kidney with the abdominal examination.

Palpating the Abdomen

Begin with light palpation to put the patient at ease. Palpate for tenderness and guarding in all four quadrants. Use deep palpation to assess organs and for masses and tenderness. The liver border should be smooth and without masses, and the spleen is not normally palpable. Palpation of the liver and spleen is an advanced technique not usually performed by staff nurses, except perhaps in some specialty areas.

The Critical Aspects box at the end of this chapter summarizes abdominal assessment; for the complete procedure,

 Go to Chapter 19, **Procedure 19-14: Assessing the Abdomen,** in Volume 2.

KnowledgeCheck 19-10

- What strategies can you use to make the client more comfortable during an abdominal assessment?
- Identify the sequence of assessment for the abdominal exam.

 Go to Chapter 19, **Knowledge Check Response Sheet and Answers,** on the Student Resource Disk or DavisPlus at http://davisplus.fadavis.com/Wilkinson2

The Musculoskeletal System

The musculoskeletal system consists of bones, muscles, and joints. Bone is complex living tissue that responds to nutrition, stress, and illness. The bones include *long bones,* such as the humerus and tibia; *flat bones,* such as the sternum and ribs; and *irregular bones,* such as the vertebrae and pelvis. Tendons, ligaments, and cartilage serve as connecting structures. **Bursae,** small disc-shaped, fluid-filled sacs, act as cushions to reduce friction between the joint and the tendons that cross over the joint (Fig. 19-21). The musculoskeletal system provides shape and support to the body, allows movement, protects internal organs, produces red blood cells in the bone marrow, and stores calcium and phosphorus.

Assessment of the musculoskeletal system includes evaluation of the client's posture, gait, bone structure,

Bone

Bursa

Synovial membrane

Joint capsule

Articular cartilage

Joint cavity (synovial fluid)

Tendon

Bone

FIGURE 19-21 Many synovial joints have bursae that act as cushions against friction.

muscle function, and joint mobility. The procedure is summarized in the Critical Aspects box at the end of this chapter. For step-by-step instructions,

 Go to Chapter 19, **Procedure 19-15: Assessing the Musculoskeletal System,** in Volume 2.

Body Shape and Symmetry

To assess bone structure, examine body shape and symmetry. Normally the difference in length between the right and left arm and the right and left leg is less than 1 cm. A greater difference may alter gait and posture or trigger pain.

Major deformities in bone structure affect posture and gait. The client should be able to stand upright with the neck and head midline. There are four normal curvatures of the spine (see Procedure 19-15). The cervical and lumbar are concave, and the thoracic and sacral are convex. Commonly seen abnormalities include **kyphosis** (accentuated thoracic curve), **scoliosis** (lateral "S" deviation of the spine), and **lordosis** (accentuated lumbar curve).

Balance, Coordination, and Movement

Walking is a complex task involving balance, coordination, and movement. Pay attention to the *base of support* and *stride* as the client walks. The average base of support (distance between the feet) in adults is 5 to 10 cm (2 to 4 in.). Stride length (distance between each step) is 30 to 35 cm (12 to 14 in.). A wide base of support or

shortened stride may indicate a balance problem. If the client has an altered gait, try to identify the specific portion of the gait that is abnormal. Abnormal gait may be caused by muscle hypertonicity (e.g., from stroke or brain tumor), lumbar disc problems, muscle atrophy, nerve damage, Parkinson's disease, cerebral palsy, multiple sclerosis, or spinal tumors. If you need additional information on gait, see Chapter 31.

To assess *balance and movement,* have the client perform tandem walking (heel-to-toe), heel-and-toe walking, deep knee bends, and hopping in place. The Romberg test is also used to assess balance; in a comprehensive exam, you may have already performed this test as part of the ear exam.

Two simple measures for assessing *coordination* are finger–thumb opposition and running the heel of one foot down the shin of the other. When performing these activities, the patient's movements should be smooth and controlled.

As you perform each assessment, pay attention to the client's stability and level of comfort. Do not attempt movements that may produce pain or cause the client to fall. For example, recall that Mr. Garcia ("Meet Your Patients") has bilateral knee pain. Before asking him to perform deep knee bends or hop in place, you would want to assess his pain and its triggers.

Joint Mobility and Muscle Function

Healthy joints are smooth, nontender, warm to touch, and of similar color to the surrounding tissue. Any joint deformity requires investigation. Color changes in a joint indicate inflammation or infection. If you see erythema or swelling, investigate further by feeling for warmth. Determine any effect the deformity has on function.

Joints should move freely and without pain or **crepitus** (clicking or grating at a joint). To assess function, test range of motion (ROM) and muscle strength. **Active ROM** requires the client to move the joint through its full ROM. **Passive ROM** is used when the client is unable to exercise each joint independently. Instead, you support the body and move each joint through its ROM. Assess **muscle strength** along with movement by asking the patient to perform ROM while you apply resistance to the part being moved. Muscle strength should be strong (5 on a scale of 0 to 5) and equal bilaterally. For more information about the musculoskeletal system, see Chapter 31.

Critical**Thinking** 19-8

As you recall, Mr. Garcia ("Meet Your Patients") is obese and has been having pain in both of his knees.

- What history questions would you ask him to assess his knee pain?
- What would you do to examine his knees?

The Neurological System

The neurological system controls or affects the function of all body systems and allows interaction with the external world. Its work is carried out through the transmission of chemical and electrical signals between the brain and the rest of the body. The basic functions of the nervous system are cognition, emotion, memory, sensation and perception, and regulation of homeostasis.

A comprehensive neurological assessment takes hours to complete and is usually reserved for clients with symptoms of neurological problems. As a staff nurse in general practice, you usually perform only portions of a neurological exam. In the next few sections, we look at the components of a focused neurological exam. For a summary, see the Critical Aspects box at the end of this chapter. For the complete procedure,

 Go to Chapter 19, **Procedure 19-16: Assessing the Sensory-Neurological System,** in Volume 2.

Developmental Considerations

When interpreting a neurological exam, consider the following developmental changes and modifications:

Infants. Reflexes present at birth include rooting, sucking, palmar grasp, tonic neck reflex (fencing), and Moro. These reflexes disappear during infancy. With neurological injury, as may occur with stroke or trauma, these reflexes may return, indicating severe neurological problems. To review these reflexes,

 Go to Chapter 9, **Expanded Discussion** on the Student Resource Disk or DavisPlus at http://davisplus.fadavis.com/Wilkinson2

Young Children. Because language skills and motor development are age-dependent, the Denver Developmental Screening Test II (DDST) is used as a neurological screen for young children. The DDST examines motor, language, and coordination skills. Chapter 9 Expanded Discussion provides additional information on the DDST. For toddlers and older children, you can usually perform a comprehensive neurological exam with age-appropriate modifications. For example, when testing for smell use materials that a young child knows, such as peanut butter or apples.

Older Adults. With advanced age, changes commonly observed are slower reaction time, a decreased ability for rapid problem-solving, and slower voluntary movement. The number of functioning neurons decreases. However, intelligence, memory, and discrimination do not change with normal aging. Neurological deficits in older adults are usually the result of adverse effects of medications or medication interactions, nutritional deficits, dehydration, cardiovascular changes that alter cerebral blood flow, diabetes, degenerative neurological conditions (e.g., Parkinson's disease or Alzheimer's disease), alcohol or drug use, depression, or abuse.

Cerebral Function

Cerebral function refers to the client's intellectual and behavioral functioning. It includes level of consciousness, orientation, mental status and cognitive function, and communication.

Level of Consciousness

Level of consciousness (LOC) includes arousal and orientation. Arousal may range from alert to deeply comatose. Arousal is classified based on the type of stimuli (auditory, tactile, or painful) required to produce a response from the client. An alert client responds to *auditory stimuli* (e.g., verbal communication or noise). Remember, if your client does not speak your language he may not respond to questions or commands.

If the client does not respond to auditory stimuli, try *tactile stimuli*. Begin with gentle touch to awaken the client and capture attention. Many clients who have hearing deficits lip-read to compensate. If you catch the client's attention by touching her hand, she may be able to respond to the combined auditory and visual stimuli. If the client does not respond to gentle touch, shake her shoulder.

If still no response is obtained, use *painful stimuli*. Painful stimuli include squeezing the trapezius muscle, rubbing on the sternum, putting pressure on the mandible, or putting pressure over the moon of a nail. Clients who respond to painful stimuli withdraw when pressure is applied.

Document LOC by describing the client's response or using the Glasgow Coma Scale (GCS) to grade eye, motor, and verbal responses. The GCS evaluates eye opening, motor responses, and verbal responses. Its limitations are that it relies heavily on vision and verbal interaction, and does not evaluate brain stem reflexes. A systematic review of evidence suggests that best practice should include use of the GCS plus other evaluation of brain stem reflexes, eye examination, vital signs, and respiratory assessment. A new tool, the Full Outline of UnResponsiveness (FOUR), provides additional information beyond that of the GCS. Both scales are included in Volume 2 for you to use in clinical settings.

 Go to Chapter 19, **Procedure 19-16: Assessing the Sensory–Neurological System, Glasgow Coma Scale, and Full Outline of UnResponsiveness Scale,** in Volume 2.

If you are not using the GCS, Box 19-1 identifies commonly used terms to describe LOC. Although these terms are widely used, a thorough description is preferable. Look at the following two chart entries:

Pt. lethargic.
Pt. responds to repeated tactile and verbal stimulation. Quickly drifts off to sleep if stimulation is discontinued.

As you can see, the second charting entry provides significantly more information than the first.

Orientation

Orientation refers to the client's awareness of time, place, and person. **Time orientation** includes awareness of the year, date, and time of day. Older adults who become disoriented to time usually think it is an earlier date. If a client offers a bizarre time or futuristic date, consider psychiatric concerns as the cause of disorientation. Hospitalized patients easily become disoriented to time. They are subjected to lights and noise around the clock; are roused in the middle of the night for medications or time-sensitive treatments; and are given anesthesia and pain medications that alter their sense of awareness.

Orientation to place involves awareness of surroundings. The patient should know that he is, for example, in the hospital and not in church. Patients who have been moved (e.g., from the emergency department to a ward bed) may not recall their room number but are easily re-oriented.

Orientation to person involves recognition of familiar persons and self-identity. The client should be able to state her name or identify people in photographs at the bedside. Because a client may meet many health professionals during a hospitalization, she may not be able to recall your name unless you have had repeated encounters with her.

Mental Status and Cognitive Function

Mental status and cognitive function include behavior, appearance, response to stimuli, speech, memory, communication, and judgment. By this point in the exam, you would have already interviewed the client and talked with him while performing the exam, so you would have a good deal of information about his mental status and cognitive function. You would have already assessed posture, gait, motor movements, dress, and hygiene through the general survey and the musculoskeletal exam; and you would be aware of the client's mood based on his tone of voice, actions, and statements.

Many clinicians choose to screen for mental status and cognitive function by working questions into the interaction with the client as they assess other body systems. The advantage of this type of informal assessment is increased comfort for the client. If you choose this method, observe for clarity of thought, appropriate content, concentration, memory, and ability to perform abstract reasoning. Normal findings include the ability to express and explain realistic thoughts with clear speech; speak with a smooth, natural pattern; follow multistep directions; listen; answer questions; and recall significant past events.

Cranial Nerve Function

Cranial nerve assessment is a key component of the neurological exam. The cranial nerves control a variety of sensory and motor functions (Table 19-5 and Fig. 19-22).

Table 19-5 ➤ Cranial Nerves

CRANIAL NERVE NO.	NAME	TYPE OF NERVE	FUNCTION OF NERVE
I	Olfactory	Sensory	Smell
II	Optic	Sensory	Visual acuity, visual fields, and ocular fundi
III	Oculomotor	Motor	EOM, pupil constriction
IV	Trochlear	Motor	EOM
V	Trigeminal: 3 branches	Sensory and motor	Corneal reflex; scalp, teeth, and facial sensation; and jaw movement
VI	Abducens	Motor	EOM
VII	Facial	Motor and sensory	Facial movement, sense of taste
VIII	Auditory	Sensory	Hearing and equilibrium
IX	Glossopharyngeal	Motor and sensory	Swallowing, gag response, tongue movement, taste, secretion of saliva
X	Vagus	Motor and sensory	Sensation of pharynx and larynx; motor activity of swallowing and vocal cords; sensory in cardiac, respiratory, and blood pressure reflexes; peristalsis; digestive secretions
XI	Spinal accessory	Motor	Head movement and shoulder elevation; motor to larynx (speaking)
XII	Hypoglossal	Motor	Tongue movement

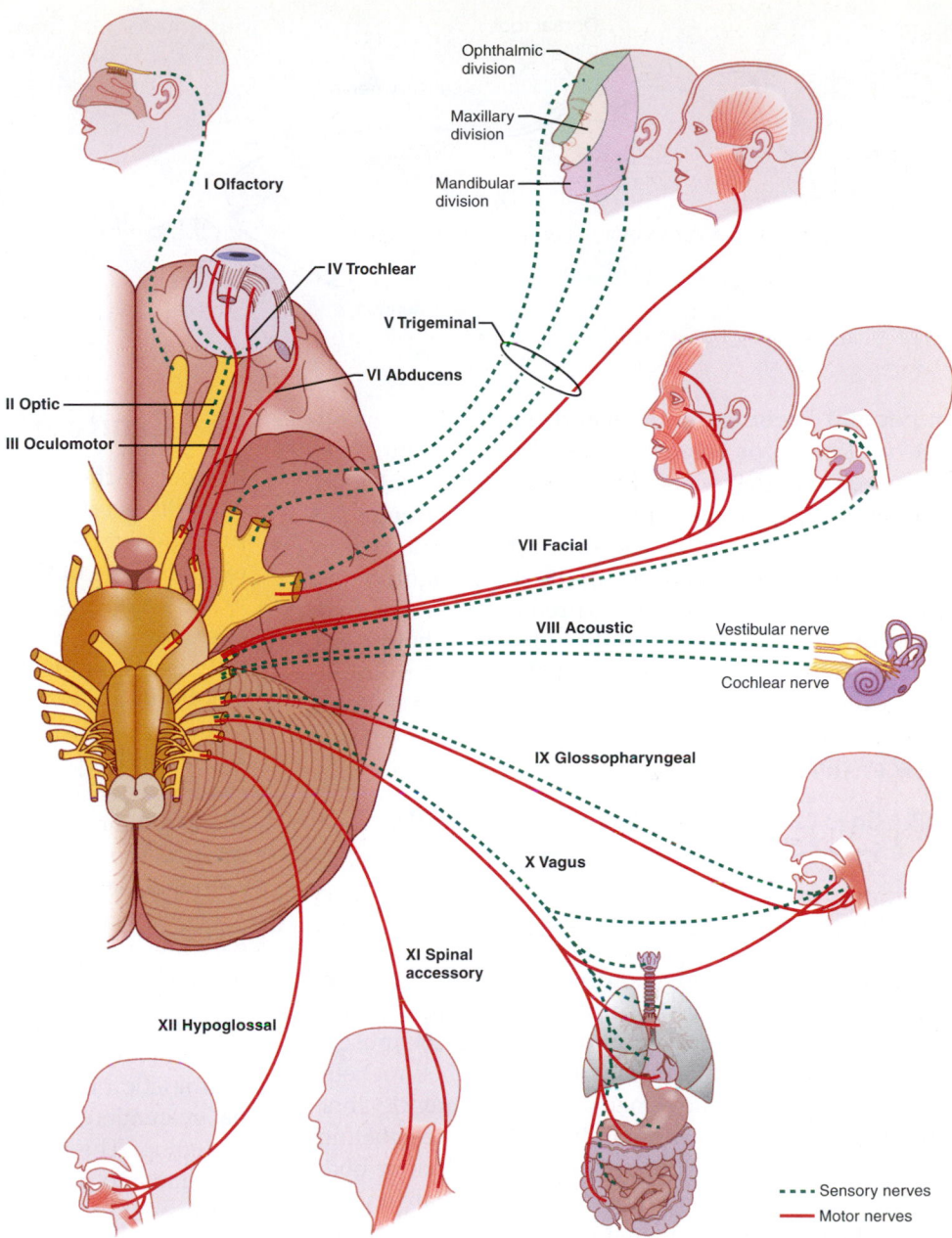

FIGURE 19-22 Origin of cranial nerves.

Reflex Function

Deep tendon reflexes (DTRs) are automatic responses that do not require conscious thought from the brain. A reflex produces a rapid, involuntary response that occurs at the level of the spinal cord (Fig. 19-23). Because the brain is not involved, muscle response is instantaneous. Intact sensory and motor systems are required for a normal reflex response. Each reflex corresponds to a certain level of the cord.

To test DTRs, use a rubber percussion hammer to tap a slightly stretched muscle. A normal response is muscle contraction. Responses are graded on the following scale:

0	No response detected
+1	Diminished response
+2	Response normal
+3	Response somewhat stronger than normal

+4   Response hyperactive with **clonus** (involuntary contractions that continue after the first contraction is elicited by the hammer)

You can elicit **superficial reflexes** by swiftly stroking a body part. Use the base of the reflex hammer or a tongue blade. Avoid pressure. Superficial reflexes are graded as positive or negative.

Sensory Function

To assess sensory function, ask the client to keep his eyes closed as you apply various stimuli. Ask him to indicate when he feels a sensation. Vary your location and approach so that you test sensation, not pattern recognition. If you notice an area of altered sensation, systematically assess the area to define the border of the change. Usually you will limit your testing to the

FIGURE 19-23 Reflex arc.

upper and lower extremities and the trunk. If the client has known or suspected deficits, you should test at numerous other sites. Test light touch, light pain, temperature, vibration, position sense, **stereognosis** (the ability to recognize the form of solid objects by touch), **graphesthesia** (the ability to recognize outlines, numbers, or symbols written on the skin), **two-point discrimination** (the ability to sense whether one or two areas of skin are being touched), **and point localization** (the ability to identify where one is being touched). For techniques for assessing reflexes and sensory function,

 Go to Chapter 19, **Procedure 19-16: Assessing the Sensory–Neurological System,** in Volume 2.

Motor and Cerebellar Function

The neurological system coordinates the function of the skeleton and muscles. Motor pathways transmit information between the brain and muscles and the muscles control movement of the skeleton. The cerebellum helps coordinate muscle movement, regulate muscle tone, and maintain posture and equilibrium. The cerebellum is also largely responsible for **proprioception,** or body positioning. Disorders of motor and cerebellar function result in pain or problems with movement, gait, or posture. Thus, when you assess the musculoskeletal system, you also assess the motor functions of the neurological system.

KnowledgeCheck 19-11

- Identify and describe the components assessed in the neurological exam.
- What approach to assessment should you take if:
  Your client has no neurological problems but you are performing a comprehensive exam?
  Your client is hospitalized for a documented cerebrovascular accident?
  Your client has been admitted with an acute head injury and the extent of neurological injury is unknown?

 Go to Chapter 19, **Knowledge Check Response Sheet and Answers,** on the Student Resource Disk or DavisPlus at http://davisplus.fadavis.com/Wilkinson2

The Genitourinary System

In most practice settings, nurses assess only the patient's external genitalia and inguinal lymph nodes. Nurse practitioners and physicians perform comprehensive examinations of the female and male reproductive and urinary systems, as do nurses working in specialty areas. However, even as a novice nurse you may assist with exams or just be present as a witness or to provide emotional support to the client.

Because a genitourinary (GU) assessment focuses on sexual and reproductive function, it might be embarrassing or uncomfortable for many people. As a result, the assessment requires a competent, professional approach. Your confidence and ease with these topics will help the client to feel more relaxed.

The Male Genitourinary System

The male genitourinary system includes the reproductive system and the urinary system (Fig. 19-24). A complete examination includes assessment of the external genitalia, evaluation for hernias, and a rectal exam for prostate screening. The penis and scrotum are examined by inspection and palpation. You will assess some of the urinary system organs when examining the back (kidneys,

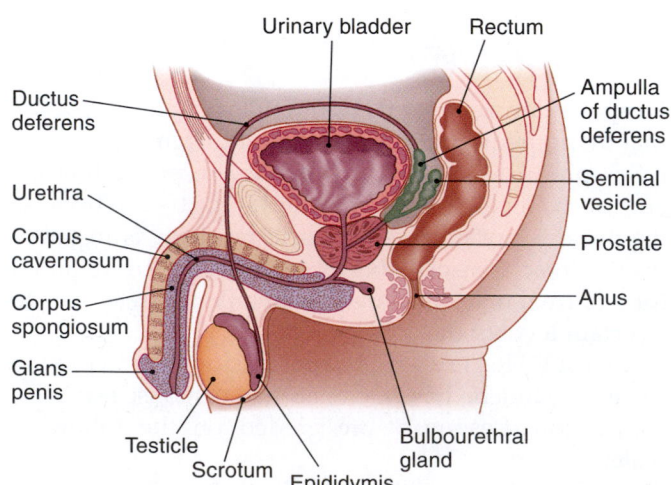

FIGURE 19-24 The male genitourinary system.

ureters) and the abdomen (bladder); the prostate gland is palpated during the exam of the rectum and anus (discussed later in this chapter). For steps to follow in examining the male genitourinary system, see the summary in the Critical Aspects box at the end of this chapter and

 Go to Chapter 19, **Procedure 19-17: Assessing the Male Genitourinary System,** in Volume 2.

Historically in the United States, **circumcision** (excision of the foreskin of the penis) has been a common practice. Circumcision was routinely performed shortly after birth, based on the belief that it had long-term health benefits related to cleanliness of the foreskin. More recently, as a result of the scarcity of clear, scientific evidence, the American Academy of Pediatrics no longer recommends circumcision as a routine practice. However, circumcision is tied to some religious and cultural beliefs (e.g., among Jews and Muslims), so it is still common.

A **hernia** is a protrusion of the intestine (or other organ) through the wall that contains it. In men, this is most likely to be a protrusion of the intestine either through the abdominal wall (**direct hernia**) or into the inguinal canal and possibly into the scrotum (**indirect hernia**). A hernia may be a small protrusion or it may cause pain and distention as a loop of bowel extends into the scrotum. An **umbilical hernia** (fairly common in infants) is an outward bulging due to delayed closure around a small muscle around the umbilicus (belly button). For an illustration of an umbilical hernia,

 Go to **Procedure 19-14: Assessing the Abdomen,** in Volume 2.

During your examination, be sure to reinforce the importance of testicular self-examination (TSE), an important health promotion measure, especially for young men. See Chapter 41 for full discussion of TSE.

KnowledgeCheck 19-12

- What assessment techniques are used when examining the male genitourinary system?
- What is the most common hernia occurring in men?

Go to Chapter 19, **Knowledge Check Response Sheet and Answers,** on the Student Resource Disk or DavisPlus at http://davisplus.fadavis.com/Wilkinson2

The Female Genitourinary System

You may be called upon to assist with a comprehensive examination. For a procedure for inspecting external female genitalia and palpating inguinal lymph nodes, see the Critical Aspects box at the end of this chapter and,

 Go to Chapter 19, **Procedure 19-18: Assessing the Female Genitourinary System,** in Volume 2.

External Examination

For adolescents and young women who are not sexually active, an external GU examination includes the following:

- Inspect the amount and distribution of pubic hair and correlate with stages of sexual maturation.
- Inspect the skin of the pubic area for evidence of swelling, lesions, or pubic lice.
- Inspect the external genitalia: labia, clitoris, urethral orifice, and vaginal orifice. Look for lesions, inflammation, swelling, or discharge.
- Palpate the inguinal lymph nodes.

Internal Examination

Women who are sexually active; who have abnormal findings on external examination; who have abdominal, pelvic, or genitourinary complaints; or who are on hormone therapy require an internal genital examination. The exam includes the following:

- Palpation of Bartholin's glands and Skene's ducts (Fig. 19-25).
- Assessment of vaginal muscle tone and pelvic musculature
- Speculum examination
- Bimanual examination, wherein the examiner palpates the cervix, uterus, and adnexal tissues with the use of one or two fingers within the vagina and the other hand on the outside to help bring the inner structures toward the two hands.

Routine annual Papanicolaou tests (Pap smears) to screen for cervical and uterine cancer are recommended for women by age 21, and for younger women who are sexually active. Women age 30 or older should follow the advice of their provider about spacing out Pap tests

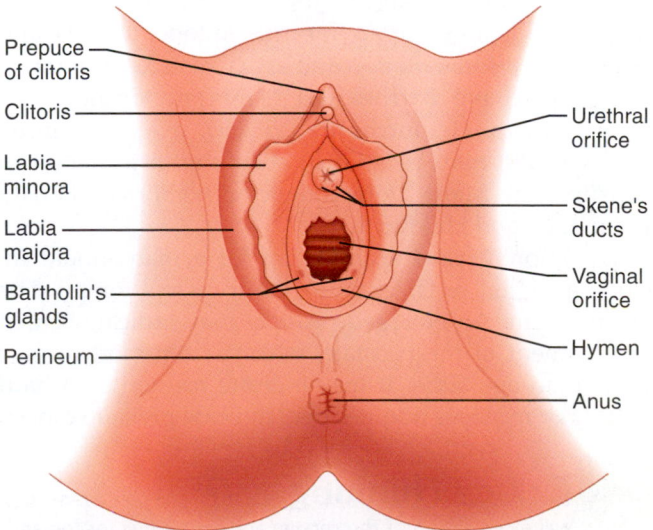

FIGURE 19-25 External female genitalia.

to every 2 or 3 years. Women older than age 65 are not usually routinely screened unless they are at high risk. Of course those with certain vulnerabilities (e.g., weakened immune system, HIV-positive) should have a Pap test every year (American Cancer Society, 2009; U. S. Preventive Services Task Force, 2009a). National screening guidelines vary, and they change frequently.

Additional cultures or screens may be done if there is unusual discharge or risk of sexually transmitted infection. A **speculum examination** is performed to collect specimens and assess the cervix. You will need to gather equipment, explain to the client what will happen, prepare the client, assist the client and examiner during the procedure, assist the client after the procedure, and document your findings.

KnowledgeCheck 19-13

What are the responsibilities of the nurse during an internal exam of the female genitourinary system?

 Go to Chapter 19, **Knowledge Check Response Sheet and Answers,** on the Student Resource Disk or DavisPlus at http://davisplus.fadavis.com/Wilkinson2

The Anus, Rectum, and Prostate

Examining the rectum and anus is the last aspect of a comprehensive examination. For the female client, this exam is usually performed at the end of a bimanual pelvic examination while the client is still in the lithotomy position. Usually a male client assumes the Sims' position, and you perform the exam after completing your examination of the genitals. For a summary of this procedure, see the Critical Aspects box at the end of this chapter. For a step-by-step procedure,

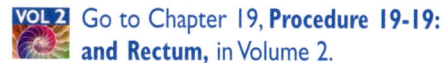 Go to Chapter 19, **Procedure 19-19: Assessing the Anus and Rectum,** in Volume 2.

Inspect the anus and rectum for skin condition and hemorrhoids and palpate for muscle tone, masses, and tenderness. Skin irritation and erythema are common in clients who have diarrhea and infants and toddlers who wear diapers. **Hemorrhoids** (dilated, usually painful, anal vessels) may be seen in clients with a history of constipation. Many women develop hemorrhoids with pregnancy and childbirth.

A comprehensive examination for a man should include a digital rectal examination to assess for prostate enlargement. An enlarged prostate may indicate benign enlargement of the prostate, which is common in men older than age 50; or it may indicate prostatitis. A hard nodule or multiple nodules may indicate prostate cancer.

 CriticalThinking 19-9

How will examination of the rectum and anus differ for Joe and Flordelisa Garcia ("Meet Your Patient")?

Documenting Physical Assessment Findings

Jordan Miller has completed his physical assessment of Joe Garcia ("Meet Your Patient"). Below is his charting entry. Recall that Jordan is an advanced practice nurse and has performed a comprehensive physical assessment. Therefore, this examination and charting entry are more extensive than what would be expected of a staff nurse. Keep in mind that you should use only abbreviations on your clinical agency's approved list.

General Survey. 56-year-old obese man presents to the clinic for a physical exam in no apparent distress. Pt. appears stated age; is well dressed and groomed; and alert and oriented to time, place, and person. Speech is clear, response and affect appropriate. Moves all extremities well, gait steady and balanced. Smells of cigarettes.

Height	5 ft 10 in.
Weight	229 lb (103.9 kg)
BP	166/100
Pulse	88 beats/min
RR	22 breaths/min
Temp	98.5°F (36.9°C), oral
BMI	33

Integumentary. Skin even in color, warm & dry, good turgor, no suspicious lesions. Well healed scar in right inguinal area. Hair clean, coarse, evenly distributed. Some graying. Nails pink, brisk capillary refill, no clubbing.

Head & Neck. Normocephalic, erect, midline. Scalp mobile, no lesions, tenderness, or masses. Facial features symmetrical. Thyroid gland symmetrical and not enlarged; cervical lymph nodes not palpable or tender.

Eyes. Snellen = right eye 20/100, left eye 20/100, both eyes 20/100. Color vision intact. Difficulty noted with near vision. Visual fields normal by confrontation. Extraocular movements intact. PERRLA at 3 mm by direct and consensual. Eyes clear and bright, + blink, no lid lag or abnormalities. Anterior chamber clear. Cornea & iris intact. Sclera white, conjunctiva clear. Lacrimal glands and ducts nontender. + red reflex bilateral, discs flat with sharp margins, vessels intact, retina & macula even in color.

Ears, Nose, & Throat. Skin intact, no masses, lesions, or discharge. Position WNL. External ears nontender to palpation. +whisper test. Weber—no lateralization. External canals clear without redness, swelling, lesions, or discharge. Tympanic membranes intact, light reflex and bony landmarks visible; frontal and maxillary sinuses nontender. Nares patent, able to distinguish familiar odors, mucosa pink, no discharge, septum intact with no deviation.

Mouth. Lips, oral mucosa, gingivae pink with no lesions. All teeth present and in good repair. Pharynx pink, tonsils absent, palate intact. Symmetrical rise of the uvula, + gag and swallow reflex. Tongue smooth, pink, symmetrical, mobile, without lesions, taste intact (correctly identified sweet, salty, and sour).

Respiratory. Respirations 22 breaths/min and unlabored. Trachea midline, AP < transverse chest diameter. Chest expansion symmetrical. No tenderness, scars, masses, or lesions. Diaphragmatic excursion 5 cm. Lungs clear to auscultation.

Cardiovascular. PMI @ MCL at 5th ICS, P 85, regular, no murmurs, gallops, or thrills present; pulses +2, no bruits or thrills, no varicosities; jugular venous pulsation 2 cm at 45°. Carotids without bruits.

Breasts. Symmetrical. No masses, lymphadenopathy, or discharge.

Abdomen. Abdomen soft, rounded, no masses or pulsations. Surgical scar R inguinal area. + bowel sounds, + tympany throughout.

Musculoskeletal. Normal spinal curvature. Joints and muscles symmetrical, no deformity. + Bilateral knee pain (right more than left). Full ROM in upper and lower extremities, + 5 muscle strength, moderate crepitus right knee.

Neurological. Awake, alert, and oriented to time, place and person. CN I–XII intact. Gait steady and coordinated; negative Romberg; unable to do deep knee bends due to pain. Point-point localization, superficial and deep sensation intact, + 2 deep tendon reflexes.

Genitourinary. Circumcised male; penis nontender, no masses, urethral meatus midline, no discharge; testicles descended bilaterally, nontender, inguinal and femoral canals free of masses, prostate small, smooth, mobile, nontender. Rectal wall smooth, no masses, stool hemoccult negative.

 VOL 2 For steps to follow in *all* procedures, refer to the Universal Steps for All Procedures found on the inside back cover of Volume 2. Go to the full procedures in Volume 2 to practice and learn the procedure steps. Use these Critical Aspects later to help you review key points.

Critical Aspects of Procedures 19-1 through 19-20

Comprehensive Physical Examination: Summary

Note: Throughout the assessment, compare findings on both sides of the body.

Procedure 19-1: The General Survey

➤ Observe the patient's apparent age, sex, race, facial expression, body size and type, posture, movements, speech, grooming, dress, hygiene, mental state, and affect.

➤ Identify any signs of distress.

➤ Measure vital signs.

➤ Measure height and weight, and calculate BMI.

➤ Consider the client's cultural/ethnic background, gender, and developmental stage.

➤ Review history data that may influence general survey findings, including usual state of health, current health problem, allergies, and unexplained changes in weight.

➤ Perform functional and SPICES assessments for older adults.

➤ Note verbal and nonverbal responses throughout exam.

Procedure 19-2: Assessing the Skin

➤ Techniques: Inspection, palpation, and olfaction

➤ Assess both exposed and unexposed areas.

➤ Inspect skin color; note any unusual odors.

➤ Inspect and palpate any lesions. Describe their size, shape, color, distribution, texture, surface relationship, and exudate.

➤ Evaluate the lesions for possible malignancy, remembering the mnemonic ABCDE.

➤ Use dorsal aspect of your hand to palpate skin temperature.

➤ Palpate skin turgor by gently pulling up skin, noting its return when you release it.

➤ Palpate skin for texture, moisture, and hydration.

➤ Review history that may influence skin findings.

Procedure 19-3: Assessing the Hair

➤ Techniques: Inspection and palpation

➤ Assess scalp hair and body hair.

➤ Inspect hair for color, quantity, distribution, condition of scalp, and presence of lesions or pediculosis.

➤ Palpate the texture of the hair.

➤ Palpate the scalp for mobility and tenderness.

Procedure 19-4: Assessing the Nails

➤ Techniques: Inspection and palpation

➤ Inspect the nails for color, condition, and shape.

➤ Palpate the texture of the nails.

➤ Assess capillary refill by pressing on the nail and releasing.

➤ Assess factors that may alter nail assessment findings (e.g., a cold environment may slow capillary refill).

➤ Examine nails on both hands and feet.

➤ You may defer examination of the toenails until you assess peripheral circulation.

Procedure 19-5: Assessing the Head and Face

➤ Techniques: Inspection, palpation, auscultation

➤ Inspect the head for size, shape, symmetry, and position.

Continued

➤ Inspect the face for expression and symmetry.

➤ Palpate the head for masses, tenderness, and scalp mobility.

➤ Palpate the face for symmetry, tenderness, muscle tone, and TMJ function.

Procedure 19-6: Assessing the Eyes

➤ Techniques: Inspection and palpation

➤ Assess distance vision using a Snellen chart.

➤ Test near vision by measuring the client's ability to read newsprint at a distance of 14 inches (35.5 cm).

➤ Test color vision by using color plates or the color bars on the Snellen chart.

➤ Assess peripheral vision by determining when an object comes into sight.

➤ Assess EOMs by examining the corneal light reflex, observing the six cardinal gaze positions, and performing the cover/uncover test.

➤ Inspect the external eye structures.

➤ Test the corneal reflex with a cotton wisp, if appropriate.

➤ Check pupil reaction for direct and consensual response.

➤ Assess accommodation by having the patient focus on an approaching object.

➤ Palpate the external eye structures.

Procedure 19-7: Assessing the Ears and Hearing

➤ Techniques: Inspection and palpation

➤ Inspect the external ear for placement, size, shape, symmetry, and the condition of the skin.

➤ Palpate the external structures of the ear for skin condition and tenderness.

➤ Inspect the tympanic membrane and bony landmarks.

➤ Assess gross hearing with the whisper and watch-tick tests.

➤ Perform the Weber test to assess hearing loss.

➤ Perform the Rinne test to identify whether hearing loss is conductive or sensorineural.

Procedure 19-8: Assessing the Nose and the Sinuses

➤ Techniques: Inspection and palpation

➤ Insert the speculum about 1 cm, and then open it as much as possible.

➤ Inspect the external and internal structures of the nose.

➤ Transilluminate and palpate the sinuses.

➤ Palpate the external structures of the nose.

Procedure 19-9: Assessing the Mouth and Oropharynx

➤ Techniques: Inspection and palpation

➤ Inspect the lips, oral mucosa, gums, teeth, and bite.

➤ Inspect the hard/soft palate, tonsils, and uvula.

➤ Inspect the tongue and frenulum; inspect under the tongue.

➤ Palpate the lips and tongue for tenderness and muscle tone.

➤ Test the gag reflex by touching the back of the soft palate with a tongue blade.

Procedure 19-10: Assessing the Neck

➤ Techniques: Inspection and palpation (auscultation as needed)

➤ Inspect the neck. Note symmetry, ROM, and the skin condition.

➤ Palpate the cervical lymph nodes. Note the size, shape, symmetry, consistency, mobility, tenderness, and temperature of any palpable nodes.

➤ Palpate the thyroid. If it is enlarged or if there is a mass, auscultate.

Procedure 19-11: Assessing the Breasts and Axillae

➤ Techniques: Inspection and palpation

➤ Inspect the breasts and axillae for skin condition, size, shape, symmetry, and color.

➤ Inspect the nipples for discharge. Culture any discharge, if present.

➤ If you notice an open lesion or nipple discharge, wear procedure gloves to palpate the breasts.

➤ Palpate the breasts using the vertical strip method, pie wedge method, or concentric circles method.

➤ Palpate the nipples, areolae, and lymph nodes.

Procedure 19-12: Assessing the Chest and Lungs

➤ Techniques: Inspection, palpation, percussion, auscultation

➤ Assess respirations by counting the rate and observing the rhythm, depth, and symmetry of chest movement.

➤ Inspect the chest for anteroposterior: lateral ratio, costal angle, spinal deformity, respiratory effort, and skin condition.

➤ Palpate the trachea.

➤ Palpate the chest for tenderness, masses, or crepitus.

➤ Palpate chest excursion.

➤ Palpate the chest for tactile fremitus.

➤ Percuss the chest.

➤ Percuss diaphragmatic excursion.

➤ Auscultate lung sounds.

Procedure 19-13: Assessing the Heart and Vascular System

➤ Techniques: Inspection, palpation, auscultation

➤ If possible, work from your patient's right side.

➤ Inspect the neck for pulsations.

➤ Measure jugular venous pressure (JVP).

➤ Inspect the precordium for pulsations.

➤ Palpate the carotid arteries.

➤ Palpate the precordium for pulsations, lifts, heaves, or thrills.

➤ Auscultate the carotid arteries with the bell of the stethoscope.

➤ Auscultate the jugular veins with the bell of the stethoscope.

➤ Auscultate the precordium at the apex, left lower sternal border, base left, and base right. Use the bell and then the diaphragm of the stethoscope.

➤ Palpate the peripheral pulses. Any abnormalities require further evaluation.

Procedure 19-14: Assessing the Abdomen

➤ Techniques: Inspection, auscultation, percussion, palpation (in that order)

Critical Aspects of Procedures 19-1 through 19-20

➤ Have the client void before the exam.

➤ Position the client supine with the knees slightly flexed.

➤ Inspect the abdomen.

➤ Auscultate the abdomen for bowel sounds and bruits.

➤ Use indirect percussion to assess at multiple sites in all four quadrants.

➤ Using your fist or blunt percussion, percuss the costovertebral angle bilaterally to assess for kidney tenderness.

➤ Lightly palpate throughout the abdomen by pressing down 1 to 2 cm in a rotating motion. Identify surface characteristics, tenderness, muscle resistance, and turgor.

➤ Use deep palpation to palpate organs and masses.

Procedure 19-15: Assessing the Musculoskeletal System

➤ Techniques: Inspection and palpation

➤ Assess posture, body alignment, and symmetry.

➤ Assess the spinal curvature.

➤ Examine the gait by assessing the base of support, stride, and phases of the gait.

➤ Assess balance through tandem walking, heel-and-toe walking, deep knee bends, hopping, and the Romberg test.

➤ Assess coordination by testing finger–thumb opposition, rhythmic movements of lower and upper extremities, and rapid alternating movements.

➤ Test the accuracy of movements by having the client touch his finger to his nose with his eyes closed.

➤ Measure limb length and circumference. Compare limbs on both sides of the body.

➤ Inspect muscle symmetry.

➤ Perform ROM at all joints.

➤ Assess muscle strength by having the client perform ROM against resistance.

Procedure 19-16: Assessing the Sensory–Neurological System

➤ Assess behavior.

➤ Determine level of arousal.

➤ Determine level of orientation.

➤ Assess memory.

➤ Assess mathematical and calculation skills.

➤ Assess general knowledge.

➤ Evaluate thought processes.

➤ Assess abstract thinking.

➤ Assess judgment.

➤ Assess communication ability.

➤ Test cranial nerves.

➤ Test superficial sensations.

➤ Test deep sensations.

➤ Test discriminatory sensations.

➤ Test deep tendon reflexes.

➤ Test superficial reflexes.

➤ Assess for dementia in institutionalized older adults.

➤ Assess cranial nerves II to XII.

➤ Assess Romberg for balance.

Procedure 19-17: Assessing the Male Genitourinary System

➤ Techniques: Inspection and palpation

➤ Inspect the external genitalia, including color, discharge, and the pattern of hair distribution.

➤ Palpate for lumps, masses, hernias, or enlarged lymph nodes.

Procedure 19-18: Assessing the Female Genitourinary System

➤ Techniques: Inspection and palpation

➤ Inspect the external genitalia.

➤ Palpate lymph nodes and possible hernia sites.

Procedure 19-19: Assessing the Anus and Rectum

➤ Inspect the external anal area, sphincter tone, and stool for occult blood.

➤ Palpate the anus and rectum for muscle tone and masses.

➤ For women, assessment of the anus and rectum is usually performed at the end of the internal pelvic exam; for men, it is done after the genitourinary exam.

Procedure 19-20: Brief Bedside Assessment

➤ Modify the procedure to fit the patient's health status.

➤ Observe the environment and the patient's general appearance.

➤ Measure vital signs, pain status, and pulse oximetry.

➤ Use a systematic (e.g., head-to-toe) approach.

➤ Assess the integument.

➤ Assess the head and neck.

➤ Assess the back with patient sitting.

➤ Assess the anterior chest (heart and lungs).

➤ Assess the abdomen with patient supine.

➤ Assess urinary status.

➤ Assess upper extremities, including edema and capillary refill.

➤ Assess lower extremities, including edema and capillary refill.

➤ Assess for spinal deformities with patient standing.

➤ Assess balance, coordination, ROM, and gait.

➤ Check Babinski reflex and Homans sign.

Go to Chapter 19, **Resources for Caregivers and Health Professionals,** on the Student Resource Disk or DavisPlus at http://davisplus.fadavis.com/Wilkinson2

VOL 2

Bibliography: Go to Volume 2, Bibliography.

CHAPTER 20

Promoting Asepsis & Preventing Infection

Learning Outcomes

After completing this chapter, you should be able to:

➤ Discuss the six links in the chain of infection.

➤ Describe the stages of a typical infectious process.

➤ Summarize the roles of the various barriers involved in the body's primary defenses.

➤ Describe four processes involved in secondary defense.

➤ Compare and contrast humoral and cell-mediated immunity.

➤ Identify activities that promote immune function.

➤ Discuss the factors that place an individual at increased risk for infection.

➤ Explain why it is important to be aware of emerging infectious diseases.

➤ Explain why multiple-drug-resistant pathogens are of special concern in healthcare.

➤ Identify standard precautions to prevent transmission of infection through blood and body fluids.

➤ Describe additional precautions that must be taken when there is concern about contact, droplet, or airborne disease transmission.

➤ Compare and contrast methods of preventing infection by breaking the chain of infection.

➤ Implement measures to prevent healthcare-related infections.

➤ Use medical asepsis when providing care to clients.

➤ Discuss infection prevention and control measures in the home and community.

➤ Implement sterile technique in selected patient care activities.

➤ Discuss the nurse's role in recognizing, preventing, and helping to contain the spread of a biological epidemic.

Meet Your Nursing Role Model

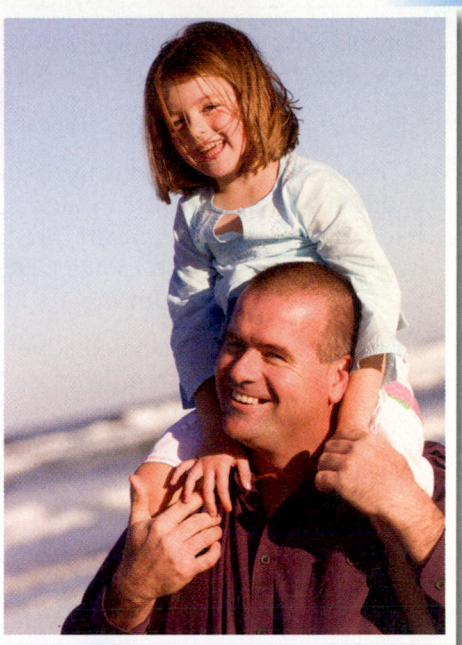

Stephanie Sergi is the 7-year-old daughter of Jason Sergi. Jason works as a nurse on a busy labor and delivery unit in a major medical center. One night at the dinner table, Stephanie asks, "Daddy, what was the most important thing you did at work today?" Jason takes a few minutes to consider his reply. Finally Jason answers, "I washed my hands—a lot."

Jason tells his daughter that he also assisted in the birth of five infants, resuscitated one of the infants who was initially struggling for breath, and identified several problems that prevented complications or even death of mothers in labor. "Daddy, I don't understand why you think washing your hands was so important," Stephanie protested. "Look at all the *really* important things you did today!"

As you read this chapter, think back to Jason's discussion with his daughter. Perhaps you will someday say the same thing to your child or anyone who asks about your day.

Theoretical Knowledge
knowing why

Research continues to lead to the discovery of new infectious microorganisms. Researchers are currently investigating the role of viruses in the development of cancer and other diseases. For example, virally induced cancers include Hodgkin's disease, Kaposi's sarcoma, and cervical cancer. Other research is investigating the role that certain species of bacteria play in producing heart disease (e.g., Spahr, Klein, Khuseyinova, et al., 2006).

Why Must Nurses Know About Infection Processes?

In this chapter, you will learn how infections occur. You will also learn measures to prevent them. We will discuss healthcare-associated infections and related professional standards and guidelines. You will acquire the knowledge of infection processes and protection measures you need to:

- Protect patients from healthcare-related infections.
- Meet professional standards and guidelines.
- Protect yourself from diseases. You must know how to avoid contact with infectious material and exposure to diseases such as AIDS, hepatitis B and C, and drug-resistant tuberculosis, as well as the many common illness-producing microorganisms you will encounter.
- Help lower the cost of healthcare. In hospitals alone, healthcare-associated infections add more than $4.5 billion annually in healthcare costs (McKibben, Horan, & Tokars, 2005).

Healthcare-Associated Infections

Healthcare-associated infections (HAIs), refers to infections associated with healthcare given in any setting (e.g., hospitals, home care, long-term care, and ambulatory settings). **Nosocomial infections** refer more specifically to hospital-acquired infections. Healthcare-associated infections aggravate existing illness and lengthen recovery time. HAIs are the leading complication of hospital care and one of the 10 leading causes of death in the United States (Agency for Healthcare Research and Quality, 2009; Klevens, Morrison, Nadle, et al., 2007; Siegel, Rhinehart, Jackson, et al., 2007). You may be surprised at these facts. After all, healthcare workers are supposed to cure, not harm, people. But when people come to hospitals (and other facilities) for care, they come into contact with many personnel and patients. When they are ill, patients are vulnerable to infection; and they are a source of infection for others. In addition, they undergo needlesticks and other invasive procedures, which can introduce infectious organisms into their bodies.

Professional Standards and Guidelines

Because HAIs seriously increase healthcare costs and patient suffering, many states have enacted laws requiring healthcare organizations to make information about HAIs available to the public. Various government, professional, and accrediting organizations have created quality-control guidelines for healthcare agencies and professionals. The following are important examples:

The Centers for Disease Control and Prevention (CDC), a federal agency, has an extensive Web site devoted to infection control and prevention in healthcare settings. To access this site,

 Go to http://www.cdc.gov/ncidod/dhqp/

The CDC also periodically issues Infection Control Guidelines, which you can access from this site. You will find many of your healthcare facility's policies and procedures to be based on the CDC guidelines. Among the CDC goals for healthcare are to:

- Reduce catheter-associated adverse events [e.g., infections] by 50%. . . in healthcare settings.
- Reduce targeted antimicrobial-resistant bacterial infections by 50%. . . preventing transmission in healthcare settings.

The Agency for Healthcare Research and Quality (AHRQ) has a Web site featuring links to information, tools, and resources on HAIs. The site contains resources for healthcare providers and consumers, and highlights AHRQ-funded research and initiatives to reduce HAIs. To access this site,

 Go to http://www.ahrq.gov/qual/hais.htm

The Joint Commission is a quality oversight agency. Their standards of performance include extensive criteria describing what healthcare organizations must do to minimize the risks of infection. In addition, Goal 7 of their National Patient Safety Goals for 2009 is to "reduce the risk of health care associated infections" (The Joint Commission, 2008b). The Infection Control Initiatives present strategies for healthcare providers to prevent infection in inpatient and community-based settings. To read these initiatives,

 Go to http://www.jointcommission.org/PatientSafety/ InfectionControl/

Quality and Safety Education For Nurses (QSEN) is a group of educators that was formed to address the challenge of preparing nurses with the competencies necessary to improve the quality and safety of their places of work—competencies that you should have on completing your nursing education. Safety is one of the six competencies. Although QSEN does not specifically say so, you should assume safety includes being safe from infection. They make several broad statements regarding knowledge, skills, and attitudes about safety that also apply to infection. For example, you should be able to:

- Demonstrate knowledge of basic scientific methods and processes [e.g., infectious process, inflammatory process].
- Minimize risk of harm to patients and providers [e.g., infectious diseases] through both system effectiveness and individual performance.
- Demonstrate effective use of technology and standardized practice [e.g., CDC guidelines for infection control] that support safety and quality.

To access the QSEN Web site,

 Go to http://www.qsen.org

American Nurses Association (ANA). Using the same broad understanding as for the QSEN competencies, you should assume that the following example criteria from Standard 5 of the *Nursing: Scope & Standards of Practice* apply to infection prevention and control:

- Partners with the person/family/significant others/ caregiver to implement the plan in a safe and timely manner.
- Implements the plan in a safe and timely manner in accordance with the National Patient Safety Goals.

Caveat: This material is from the draft for public comment (ANA, 2010, in press); its wording may be changed somewhat in the final published version. For that version of the ANA Standards of Professional Nursing Practice,

 Go to http://www.nursingworld.org/

How Does Infection Occur?

Imagine that your clinical instructor alerts you to an outbreak of infectious disease in the hospital where you have your assignment. The hospital census is currently more than 200 patients. So far, 14 have become infected, and one has died. Have you ever wondered how infections are spread and why they seem to affect some people more than others?

Infections Develop in Response to a Chain of Factors

The process by which infections spread is commonly referred to as the **chain of infection.** It is made up of six links, all of which must be present for the infection to be transmitted from one individual to another (Fig. 20-1). Here we describe each of the six links. Later in the chapter we discuss how to interrupt the chain to limit the spread of infection. For information about common disease-producing microorganisms and their transmission,

 Go to **ESG Table 20-1, Common Pathogens,** on the Student Resource Disk or DavisPlus at http://davisplus.fadavis.com/ Wilkinson2

Infectious Agent

Some microorganisms live on or in the human body without causing harm. For instance, the *Staphylococcus* bacteria growing on human skin are usually harmless. Other microorganisms are beneficial or even essential for human health and well-being. They are referred to as **normal flora.** Normal flora in the intestine aid in digestion and synthesize vitamin K, and release vitamin B_{12}, thiamine, and riboflavin when they die. In addition, they limit the growth of harmful bacteria by competing with them for available nutrients.

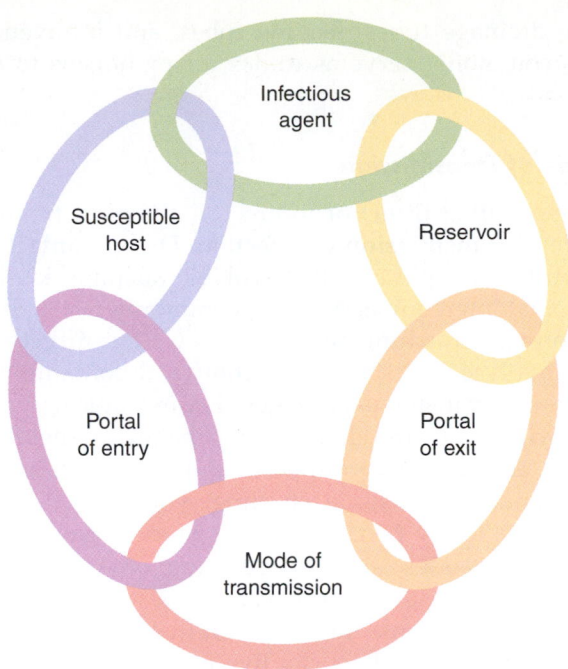

FIGURE 20-1 All six links in the chain of infection must be present for infection to be transmitted from one person to another.

There are two types of normal flora: transient and resident. **Transient flora** are normal microbes that a person picks up by coming in contact with objects or another person (e.g., when you touch a soiled dressing). You can remove these with handwashing. **Resident flora** live deep in skin layers, where they live and multiply harmlessly. They are permanent inhabitants of the skin, and cannot usually be removed with routine handwashing. They are not usually harmful unless they enter the deep tissues (e.g., as through an open wound) or unless the patient is especially vulnerable to disease.

Pathogens are microorganisms capable of causing disease. In fact, the precise definition of the term **infection** is successful invasion of the body by a pathogen (Bauman, Machunis-Masuoka, & Tizard, 2004). The largest groups of pathogenic microorganisms are bacteria, viruses, and fungi (which include yeasts and molds). Less common pathogens are protozoa, helminths (commonly called worms), and *prions*, which are infectious protein particles that cause certain neurological diseases. In addition, normal flora may become pathogenic if disease or injury permit them to enter body regions they do not normally inhabit. For instance, rupture of the bowel through trauma or disease allows intestinal microbes to enter the abdominal cavity or bloodstream, where they cause infection.

Once a pathogen gains entry into a host, four factors determine whether the person develops infection:

- **Virulence** of the organism (its power to cause disease)
- Ability of the organism to survive in the host environment

- Number of organisms (the greater the number, the more likely they are to cause disease)
- Ability of the host's defenses to prevent infection

Reservoir

A **reservoir** is a source of infection: a place where pathogens survive and multiply. The human body is the most common reservoir for pathogens. Animals, insects, and humans are other living reservoirs. Nonliving reservoirs include soil, water, food, and environmental surfaces. Examples include contaminated water, stagnant ponds, garbage, soiled diapers, discarded wound dressings, and raw sewage. In healthcare facilities, many surfaces act as reservoirs. Microorganisms have mass, and they eventually fall to the floor or onto bedside tables, chairs, or equipment. Other surfaces, such as sinks, toilets, bed rails, and bed linens may also become reservoirs because of their proximity to patients, family members, and healthcare providers harboring pathogens.

Some people are capable of defending themselves from active disease but harbor the pathogenic organisms within their bodies. These individuals, called **carriers,** have no symptoms of disease, yet they serve as reservoirs and can pass the disease to others.

Most pathogens prefer a warm, moist, dark environment. To live and thrive in humans, microbes must be able to use the body's precise balance of food, moisture, nutrients, electrolytes, pH, temperature, and light. Food, water, and soil that provide these conditions may serve as nonliving reservoirs, as well.

Nutrients. Bacteria can rapidly multiply in food left at room temperature. For example, the bacteria *Salmonella enteritidis*, which causes salmonellosis ("food poisoning") can multiply in raw and undercooked meat and eggs. To prevent the growth of pathogens, many foods are cooked at high temperatures and stored in a cool environment. Alternatively, many foods are prepared with a concentration of solutes that inhibits the growth of pathogenic microbes. This concept underlies the salting of meats and the production of fruit jellies, jams, and preserves.

Moisture. Pathogens require moisture for survival, for example, the moist environment of wounds, the genitourinary tract, the throat and airways. However, the spores formed by some bacteria allow them to live without water (e.g., the *Bacillus* and *Clostridium* species, both of which cause food-borne disease).

Temperature. For most pathogens, the ideal temperature is 95°F (35°C). Environments that are either too hot or too cold for a particular species will slow its growth or even kill the entire population. In part, the microbes that are pathogenic to humans are so because they thrive at about the same temperature as the human body. Thus, a fever in response to infection can inhibit and even kill invading pathogens.

Oxygen. Many bacteria and most protozoa and fungi are aerobic. That is, they must have oxygen to live and grow. For example, the yeast *Candida albicans* causes infections in the oral mucosa ("thrush") and the vaginal mucosa. Anaerobic organisms do not require oxygen for growth and may even be killed in its presence. One example is *Clostridium tetani*, a spore-forming bacterium, which causes tetanus when a spore enters the body through an open wound.

pH and Electrolytes. To live in humans, pathogens need the body's precise balance of moisture, sugars, pH (acidity), and electrolytes. Most prefer a pH range of 5 to 8. Therefore, they cannot survive in the highly acidic environment of the stomach. When patients take antacids, stomach pH increases and removes this defense. The organisms multiply and can then cause infection in other systems, such as the lungs. Microbes that have a higher or lower pH and electrolyte concentration than the human body are not pathogenic to human beings. That's why, for example, the bacteria that thrive in the Great Salt Lake would not cause infection on your skin.

Light. Microbes grow best in dark environments (e.g., inside the body, deep in wounds, and under dressings). Ultraviolet light is sometimes used to remove pathogens such as *Staphylococcus*, *Salmonella*, and viruses from surgical instruments and other objects. It is also used to disinfect drinking water in developing countries to prevent diseases such as cholera and typhoid fever.

Knowledge Check 20-1

- What is a pathogen?
- What is the role of normal flora?
- Identify at least five reservoirs of infection.

 Go to Chapter 20, **Knowledge Check Response Sheet and Answers,** on the Student Resource Disk or DavisPlus at http://davisplus.fadavis.com/Wilkinson2

Portal of Exit

A contained reservoir is only a potential source of infection. For infection to spread, a pathogen must exit the reservoir. In the case of human or animal reservoirs, the most frequent **portal of exit** is through body fluids, including blood, mucus, saliva, breast milk, urine, feces, vomitus, semen, or other secretions. The body's natural response to foreign materials, including pathogens, is to try to expel them. If you have a pathogen in the respiratory system, you cough and sneeze. If it is in the gastrointestinal system, you vomit or experience intestinal cramping and diarrhea. Microbes responsible for sexually transmitted infections can exit via semen, vaginal secretions, or blood that is present during sex.

Cuts, bites, and abrasions also provide an exit for body fluid. Blood and pus seeping from a wound help transport pathogens away from the broken skin but become a portal by which infection may be transmitted to others. In healthcare-related infections, puncture sites, drainage tubes, feeding tubes, and intravenous lines commonly serve as routes for pathogens to exit the body.

Mode of Transmission

Contact, either direct or indirect, is the most frequent **mode of transmission** of infection. **Direct contact** between two people usually involves touching, kissing, or sexual intercourse. Animals commonly transmit infection via scratching and biting as well. **Indirect contact** involves contact with a **fomite,** a contaminated object that transfers a pathogen. For example, suppose that while you are charting you begin to sneeze or cough. If you cover your nose and mouth with your hand and then resume charting, you may transmit pathogens to the pen, paper, and chart (or keyboard). Shoes, eyeglasses, stethoscopes, and other items we wear also commonly serve as fomites, as do contaminated needles. Some microbes can live only a few seconds on fomites; others can live for years. It depends on the type of microorganism and the environment.

Droplet transmission occurs when the pathogen travels in water droplets expelled as an infected person exhales, coughs, sneezes, or talks. It may also occur during suctioning and oral care. The usual method of transmission is for the droplet to be inhaled or enter the eye of a susceptible person. Although droplets can travel only a few feet from the infectious person, within that distance they may readily contaminate fomites that then transmit the organism by contact.

Airborne transmission occurs with much smaller organisms that can float considerable distances on air currents. Airborne pathogens can travel through heating and air conditioning systems to infect large numbers of people. Sweeping a floor or shaking out contaminated bed linens can stir up airborne microorganisms and launch them on air currents—think of a flying magic carpet (of pathogens). The agents of measles and tuberculosis, as well as many fungal infections, are commonly transmitted in this manner.

A **vector** is an organism that carries a pathogen to a susceptible host, typically by biting or stinging, creating another portal of entry into the body. The mosquito is a common vector for diseases, including malaria, yellow fever, and the West Nile virus. Ticks, fleas, mites, and other insects also carry various diseases.

Portal of Entry

Pathogens can enter the body through various **portals of entry.** Normal body openings, such as the conjunctiva of the eye, the nares (nostrils), mouth, urethra, vagina, and anus are potential portals of entry, as are abnormal openings, such as cuts, scrapes, and surgical incisions. Vectors, such as mosquitos, create portals of entry when they bite through the skin. In healthcare settings, common portals of entry include wounds, surgical sites, and insertion sites for tubes or needles.

Susceptible Host

A **susceptible** (or *compromised*) **host** is a person who is at risk for infection because of inadequate defenses against the invading pathogen. Various factors can increase susceptibility to infection, among them: age (the very young or very old), compromised immune system (as in those receiving immune suppression for organ transplantation or treatment of cancer or chronic illness), and immune deficiency conditions (e.g., HIV, leukemia).

KnowledgeCheck 20-2

- Identify the six links in the chain of infection.
- What kinds of microbes favor the human body as a reservoir of infection?

 Go to Chapter 20, **Knowledge Check Response Sheet and Answers,** on the Student Resource Disk or DavisPlus at http://davisplus.fadavis.com/Wilkinson2

 CriticalThinking 20-1

You are working as a nurse on a medical–surgical unit. What roles might you play in the chain of infection?

Infections Can Be Classified in Various Ways

Infections are classified according to their location in the body, whether it is the patient's first infection, where it was acquired, and how long it lasts.

Local or Systemic. Some infections cause harm in a limited region of the body, such as the upper respiratory tract, the urethra, or a single bone or joint. Such infections are said to be **local.** In contrast, **systemic** infections occur when pathogens invade the blood or lymph and spread throughout the body. **Bacteremia** is the clinical presence of bacteria in the blood, whereas **septicemia** is symptomatic systemic infection spread via the blood.

Primary or Secondary. A **primary infection** is the first infection that occurs in a patient. Especially in immunocompromised patients, one or more **secondary infections** may follow a primary infection. For example, a frail client infected with pneumonia may develop herpes zoster (shingles, a viral infection related to past infection with varicella) related to the stress of illness.

Exogenous or Endogenous. Healthcare providers need to determine the source of pathogens in a patient infected while he is in the facility. In **exogenous healthcare-related infections,** the pathogen is acquired from the healthcare environment. In **endogenous healthcare-related infections,** the pathogen arises from the patient's normal flora, when some form of treatment (e.g., chemotherapy or antibiotics) causes the normally harmless microbe to multiply and cause infection. For example, candidal vaginitis (yeast infection) may develop in a client receiving antibiotics after surgery.

Acute or Chronic. Infections that have a rapid onset but last only a short time, such as the common cold, are said to be **acute.** In contrast, **chronic infections** (e.g., an abscess) develop slowly and last for weeks, months, or even years. Some chronic infections, such as relapsing fever, recur after periods of remission. **Latent infections** cause no symptoms for long periods of time, even decades. Tuberculosis and human immunodeficiency virus (HIV) are examples. HIV typically causes an initial, brief illness that is then followed by about 10 years of latency before the patient begins to experience symptoms of AIDS.

Infections Follow Predictable Stages

Many infections follow a fairly predictable course of events, although the precise duration and intensity of symptoms in each stage vary from one individual to another:

- **Incubation** is the stage between successful invasion of the pathogen into the body and the first appearance of symptoms. In this stage, the person does not suspect that he has been infected but may be capable of infecting others. This stage may last only a day, as with the influenza virus, or as long as several months or even years, as with tuberculosis.
- The **prodromal stage** is characterized by the first appearance of vague symptoms. For example, a person infected with a cold virus may experience a mild throat irritation. Not all infections have a prodromal stage.
- **Illness** is the stage marked by the appearance of the signs and symptoms characteristic of the disease. If the patient's immune defenses and medical treatments (if any) are ineffective, this stage can end in the death of the patient.
- **Decline** is the stage during which the patient's immune defenses, along with any medical therapies, successfully reduce the number of pathogenic microbes. As a result, the signs and symptoms of the infection begin to fade.
- **Convalescence** is characterized by tissue repair and a return to health as the remaining number of microorganisms approaches zero. Convalescence may require only a day or two or, for severe infections, as long as a year or more.

Why Must Nurses Be Aware of Emerging Pathogens and Diseases?

An **epidemic** is an outbreak of a disease that suddenly affects a large group of people in a geographic region (e.g., a city or state) or in a defined population group (e.g., children, healthcare workers). A **pandemic** is an exceptionally widespread epidemic—that is, one that affects a large number of people in an entire country or worldwide. Examples of pandemics are H1N1 influenza ("swine flu") and malaria. You should also know the term, emerging infectious disease. Although there are various definitions, you can think of **emerging infectious diseases** as:

- Newly identified diseases caused by an unrecognized microorganism (e.g., the virus causing AIDS was unknown before 1980) or a known organism (e.g., *Streptococcus* infection causing toxic shock syndrome)
- Diseases occurring in new geographic areas (e.g., West Nile virus in the Western hemisphere) or settings, such as *Clostridium difficele*, which was primarily a hospital-acquired infection and now occurs in the community
- Microorganisms in animals that extend their host range to begin infecting humans (e.g., avian influenza, or "bird flu"; and more recently the H1N1 virus).
- Microbes that evolve to become more virulent (e.g., a strain of *Escherichia coli*, which now causes severe illness)
- Known diseases that dramatically increase in incidence (e.g., mumps and pertussis, also known as whooping cough)
- Organisms that are deliberately altered for bioterrorism (e.g., the contamination of some mail in the United States with *Bacillus anthracis* [anthrax] in 2001).
- Most emerging pathogens are viruses. For a brief discussion of some important emerging infections,

 Go to **Supplemental Materials: Emerging Infectious Diseases,** on the Student Resource Disk or DavisPlus at http://davisplus.fadavis.com/Wilkinson2. Also see **Reading More About Promoting Asepsis & Preventing Infection** on the Student Resource Disk or DavisPlus at http://davisplus.fadavis.com/Wilkinson2.

Continental and intercontinental travel allow for many ways of spreading pathogens. Infected travelers serve as reservoirs for pathogens. The close quarters and recirculated air systems in airplanes provide an ideal environment for the transmission of airborne pathogens and for both direct and indirect contact contamination between passengers. Air travel also enables a person to infect many people headed for widespread locations, often even before the reservoir person shows symptoms of the disease. The 2003 SARS outbreak is a good example of flight travel as a means of transmission: a Chinese physician unknowingly infected at least a dozen guests at a hotel in Hong Kong where he was staying; the guests then flew to Vietnam, Singapore, and Canada, prompting outbreaks in those countries.

Cooperative efforts among many disciplines and organizations worldwide are required to limit the spread of infectious diseases. To this end, the World Health Organization (WHO) has chosen as the first "global patient safety challenge" the reduction of healthcare-associated infection (WHO, 2008). Also, The Joint Commission (2008a) requires hospitals to have an emergency management plan for responding to large numbers of infectious patients who might need to be treated as a result of an epidemic.

What Are Drug-Resistant Pathogens?

Some microorganisms, mostly bacteria, have mutated to develop resistance to one or more classes of antimicrobial drugs. These organisms are said to be **drug-resistant or multidrug-resistant.** Today antibiotic resistance is one of the most significant challenges in treating patients with severe infectious diseases. During the last several decades, the prevalence of multidrug-resistant organisms (MDROs) in U.S. hospitals and medical centers has increased steadily. MDROs are a serious problem because options for treating MDRO infections are limited. Furthermore, they are associated with serious illness, increased mortality, and increased hospital lengths of stay and costs.

A variety of risk factors are associated with MDRO infections (CDC, 2000, last updated 2004). Among them are the following:

- Severe illness
- Previous exposure to antimicrobial agents (e.g., antibiotics)
- Underlying diseases or conditions that make it difficult for the person to fight infection (in particular, chronic renal disease, insulin-dependent diabetes mellitus, peripheral vascular disease, dermatitis, skin lesions)
- Invasive procedures and devices, such as dialysis, urinary catheterization, and intravenous lines
- Repeated contact with the healthcare system, especially acute care facilities, and especially intensive care units (where infection rates tend to be highest)
- Advanced age

MDROs are transmitted by the same routes as other microorganisms. A major factor, though, is transmission in healthcare settings via the hands of healthcare workers, especially for MRSA, *Clostridium difficile*, and vancomycin resistant enterococci (VRE), discussed following. Other significant MDROs include multidrug-resistant tuberculosis (MDR-TB), penicillin-resistant *Streptococcus pneumoniae*, multidrug-resistant *Escherichia coli*, and *Klebsiella pneumoniae*. If you need more information about diseases caused by those organisms, consult a medical–surgical textbook or,

 Go to **Supplemental Materials: What Are Drug-Resistant Pathogens,** on the Student Resource Disk or DavisPlus at http://davisplus.fadavis.com/Wilkinson2

Methicillin-Resistant Staphylococcus aureus

Staphylococcus aureus lives on the skin and in the nose, usually without causing problems. If a person does have a "staph" infection it is normally treated with methicillin, but methicillin-resistant *Staphylococcus aureus* (MRSA) can't be killed by this drug. MRSA is a major cause of complications and death, as well as being a costly problem for the healthcare industry. The incidence of MRSA-related septicemia, pneumonia, and device-associated infections has increased steadily in the past decade; and it increased by 30% from 2004 to 2005. An estimated 1.2 million hospitalized patients acquire a MRSA infection each year in the United States (Association for Professionals in Infection Control and Epidemiology [APIC], 2007; Elixhauser & Steiner, 2007). MRSA is spread by skin-to-skin contact with someone who has it, and by living in crowded conditions.

Although MRSA is associated mainly with hospitalization, new strains are emerging in the community among patients with no apparent MRSA risk factors. These are called community-associated MRSA (CA-MRSA). Usually, CA-MRSA results in minor skin and soft tissue infections, but severe **invasive** disease, including osteomyelitis and a sepsis syndrome with increased mortality also occur. About 14% of all MRSA cases involve CA-MRSA, and it has spread rapidly into hospitals. Some believe you should assume that all suspected *S. aureus* skin and soft-tissue infections are caused by MRSA (Whyte, 2008). For an optional CDC podcast on community associated MRSA risk factors and prevention strategies,

 Go to Chapter 20, **Resources for Caregivers and Health Professionals,** on the Student Resource Disk or DavisPlus at http://davisplus.fadavis.com/Wilkinson2

In 2005, nearly 19,000 people died after being infected with MRSA. Control of MRSA has become a national priority. Because MRSA can survive on hands, clothing, environmental surfaces, and equipment, it is easily spread to vulnerable patients in healthcare settings. Healthcare institutions are targeting MRSA with staff education, aggressive handwashing, increased use of protective gloves and gowns, and targeted screening (Klevens, Morrison, Nadle, et al., 2007).

Vancomycin-Resistant Enterococci

Over the past 20 years, *Enterococcus faecium* strains have developed resistance to the antibiotics vancomycin and ampicillin, and have become an important source of healthcare-related infections throughout the world. Most vancomycin-resistant enterococci (VRE) infections occur in hospitals, and account for about 4% of all hospital infections. Their spread is attributed to failure to follow infection control measures (Rice, 2001). Enterococci, normal residents in the intestines and the female genital tract, also occur in the environment.

VRE are a leading cause of healthcare-acquired bacteremia (bacteria in the blood), surgical wound infection, and urinary tract infection. Patients at increased risk of becoming infected with VRE are those who have previously had long-term antibiotic treatment, are hospitalized, have weakened immune systems, have undergone surgical procedures, have long-term devices such as urinary catheters and central intravenous catheters, or who are colonized with VRE (CDC, 2008a).

Clostridium difficile

In recent years, an unusually virulent strain of *Clostridium difficile* (*C. diff.*), a spore forming organism, has developed. About 3% of healthy adults carry a harmless version of *C. diff.* However, it can become harmful when antibiotics destroy healthy bacteria that normally protect against the disease. The newer *C. diff.* strain is resistant to nearly all antibiotics and virulent enough to cause sepsis, lasting intestinal damage, the need for colon removal, and even death. It thrives in unsanitary hospital environments, so the federal government is pressuring physicians and hospitals to better enforce sanitation standards and overprescription of antibiotics. However, because spores survive for days on surfaces such as doorknobs and toilet seats, at least 10% of *C. diff.* infections are acquired outside the hospital (CDC, 2008b). Prevention of transmission in a healthcare facility focuses on the following:

- Application of contact precautions for patients with diarrhea
- Accurate identification of patients
- Rigorous cleaning of patient rooms and equipment
- Consistent hand hygiene, using soap and water rather than alcohol-based handrubs for mechanical removal of spores.
- Use of a bleach-containing disinfectant for environmental disinfection

 Note that to prevent transmission of *C. diff.* you must wash your hands with soap and water. Alcohol-based hand rubs are not effective because they do not destroy *C. diff.* spores.

Critical Thinking 20-2

Why are emerging infections of special concern in healthcare? Why are multidrug-resistant organisms of special concern in healthcare?

What Are the Body's Defenses Against Infection?

The human body has three "lines of defense" against infectious disease:

- Certain anatomical features limit the entry of pathogens.
- Protective biochemical processes fight pathogens that do enter.
- The presence of pathogens activates immune responses against specific, recognized invaders.

The first two lines of defense are nonspecific; that is, they have no means of adapting their response to each specific invader. Instead, they act in precisely the same way against any and all intruders, from a simple cold virus to deadly fungal spores.

Primary Defenses

The "soldiers" in the first line of defense are the structural barriers of the human body. These **primary defenses** prevent organisms from entering the body. The normal flora of the body provide one such defense. Any treatment that disturbs the balance between the normal flora and other microorganisms can increase the client's risk of developing disease. For example, when broad-spectrum antibiotics are used to treat infection, they may eliminate normal flora in addition to those causing the infection. This allows other kinds of pathogens to multiply, producing a **superinfection.** Other primary defenses are as follows:

- *Skin.* The surface of intact, healthy skin is tough and resilient and prevents entry of many pathogens. The normal flora of the skin inhibit multiplication of other organisms, including pathogens, that land on the skin.
- *The respiratory tree.* The nares, trachea, and bronchi are covered with mucous membranes that trap pathogens, which are then expelled. The nose contains hairs that filter the upper airway; and the nasal passages, sinuses, trachea, and larger bronchi are lined with cilia, tiny hairlike cells that sweep microorganisms upward from the lower airways. Coughing and sneezing forcefully expel organisms from the respiratory tract.
- *Eyes.* The lacrimal glands produce tears that contain lysozyme, an antimicrobial enzyme. Thus, tears help the body wash infective organisms from the eyes.
- *The mouth.* The mouth normally has a large number of pathogenic microorganisms, but saliva, like tears, contains lysozyme and helps continually wash microbes from the teeth and gums. The rich blood supply of the mouth swiftly transports defensive blood cells (discussed later in this section) that keep the microorganisms in check. In addition, normal flora of the mouth compete for nutrition with invading organisms, thereby limiting the number of pathogens.
- *The gastrointestinal tract.* Many pathogens that reach the stomach are destroyed in its acidic environment. Those that successfully enter the small intestine face the antimicrobial action of bile. Simple peristalsis, as well as diarrhea and vomiting, are other first-line defense mechanisms for pathogens that invade the gastrointestinal tract. In addition, normal flora in the intestine secrete antibacterial substances.
- *The genitourinary tract.* Like the respiratory tree, the genitourinary tract is protected with mucous membranes. The epithelial cells lining the urethra and anus secrete mucus, which adheres to pathogens to promote their excretion through urine and stool. Urine itself is highly acidic and contains lysozyme. Mucous membranes lining the vagina also help keep pathogens from establishing colonies there. In addition, the

high acidity and normal flora of the vagina keep pathogens in check.

Secondary Defenses

Pathogens that dodge the primary defenses and gain entry into the body begin to release wastes and secretions and to cause the breakdown of cells and tissues. The presence of such chemicals activates a set of **secondary defenses.**

- **Phagocytosis**—the process by which specialized white blood cells (WBCs), called *phagocytes,* engulf and destroy pathogens directly. Phagocytic white blood cells include neutrophils, monocytes, and eosinophils. *Monocytes* also have the ability to differentiate into **macrophages** that specialize in cleaning up sites of injury or infection by phagocytizing pathogens, used WBCs, and cellular debris. *Eosinophils* are occasionally phagocytic; however, they are responsible mainly for binding to helminths and releasing harmful toxins onto their surface. Table 20-1 summarizes the types of white blood cells and their roles in defending against infection.

Table 20-1 ➤ Types and Functions of White Blood Cells	
TYPE	**FUNCTION**
Granular	
Basophils: 0.5%–1% of total WBCs	Release histamine and heparin granules as part of the inflammatory response. Percentage normal during infections.
Eosinophils: 1%–3% of total WBCs	Destroy helminths; mediate allergic reactions; have limited role in phagocytosis. Percentage increases in parasitic infections.
Neutrophils: 55%–70% of total WBCs	Phagocytize pathogens
Agranular	
Lymphocytes: 20%–35% of total WBCs	T cells—responsible for cell-mediated immunity; recognize, attack, and destroy antigens.
	B cells—responsible for humoral immunity; produce immunoglobulins to attack and destroy antigens. Percentage of total lymphocytes increases in viral infection and chronic bacterial infection; decreases in sepsis.
Monocytes: 3%–8% of total WBCs	Able to phagocytize directly as well as to differentiate into macrophages, which help clean up damaged or injured tissue. Percentage increases in tuberculosis, protozoal, and rickettsial infections.

Note: Laboratory values alone are not adequate for diagnosing infection. Presence of clinical signs (e.g., fever, pus, swelling) must be assessed.

- **The complement cascade**—a process by which a set of blood proteins, called *complement,* triggers the release of chemicals that attack the cell membranes of pathogens, causing them to rupture. Complement also signals white blood cells, called basophils, to release a chemical called histamine, which prompts inflammation.
- **Inflammation**—a process that begins when histamine and other chemicals are released either directly from damaged cells, or from basophils in response to the activation of complement. Histamine and other inflammatory chemicals cause dilation and increased permeability of blood vessels, increasing the flow of phagocytes, antimicrobial chemicals, oxygen, and nutrients to the damaged area. The classic signs and symptoms of inflammation are localized warmth and erythema (redness), which develop as blood flow is increased. In addition, fluid leaking from the more permeable blood vessels accumulates in the surrounding tissue, causing edema, which in turn prompts pain as pressure is exerted on nerve endings (Bauman, Machunis-Masuoka, & Tizard, 2006).
- **Fever**—a rise in core body temperature that increases metabolism, inhibits multiplication of pathogens, and triggers specific immune responses (discussed shortly). Believing that low-grade fevers are a necessary natural defense mechanism, many clinicians do not treat a fever lower than 102°F (38.9°C).

Tertiary Defenses

Why is it that people who recover from an infectious disease like measles or chickenpox never get the disease again, even if they are repeatedly exposed to the virus? The answer lies in **specific immunity:** the process by which the body's immune cells "learn" to recognize and destroy pathogens they have encountered before.

The cells involved in specific immunity are white blood cells called **lymphocytes,** which are produced from stem cells in the red bone marrow. Lymphocytes that grow to maturity in the bone marrow are designated *B lymphocytes,* or *B cells,* whereas those that mature in the thymus are designated *T lymphocytes,* or *T cells.* After they have matured, most B cells and T cells travel to the lymph nodes, spleen, and other sites of lymphatic tissue. Some circulate in blood and lymph. From all of these locations, lymphocytes seek out foreign cells and other matter to target for destruction. Lymphocytes recognize foreign substances by the molecules present on their surfaces. These molecules that trigger a specific immune response are called **antigens.** The two types of specific immunity involving B cells and T cells are discussed next.

Humoral Immunity

The humoral immune response acts directly against antigens. In response to the presence of antigens, macrophages and a class of T cells called *helper T cells* stimulate B cells to become plasma cells and produce **antibodies,**

also called **immunoglobulins (Ig).** Antibodies are proteins with a base region and two arms (somewhat like the letter Y). They bind to target antigens and destroy them by any of the following methods (Fig. 20-2):

- *Phagocytosis.* Antibodies do not phagocytize directly, but instead signal leukocytes (macrophages and neutrophils) to phagocytize the pathogens to which the antibodies are bound.
- *Neutralization.* By binding to a pathogen's attachment sites, antibodies disable the pathogens' machinery for adhering to and invading body cells. Thus, although they are not destroyed, the pathogens are effectively neutralized.
- *Agglutination.* Antibodies have two attachment sites; therefore each antibody can attach to two pathogenic cells in a population. This quality causes the cells to clump together (agglutinate), reducing the cells' activity and increasing the likelihood that the group will be detected by leukocytes and phagocytized.
- *Activation of complement and inflammation.* Antibodies trigger the complement cascade and stimulate the release of inflammatory chemicals to destroy the antigen.

FIGURE 20-2 The humoral immune response produces antibodies to destroy antigens.

Five classes of immunoglobulins (Igs) are secreted by B lymphocytes.

Immunoglobin M (IgM). IgM is produced when an antigen is encountered for the first time. This is a large molecule and cannot pass through the placenta to protect a fetus.

Immunoglobin G (IgG). IgG is the most common immunoglobulin in the body. Once the body recognizes the antigen and produces IgG, special B memory cells are formed that remember the antigen and rapidly produce IgG in response to subsequent infection. However, it takes at least 10 days for IgG to be produced in response to an initial infection. Eventually the IgG response fades. The length of time the body remembers how to produce IgG for a specific pathogen depends on the characteristics of the pathogen, the strength of the initial response, and the health of the person.

IgG is small enough to pass through the placenta. If the mother has developed IgG through previous exposure, IgG will pass through the placenta and protect the fetus from the pathogen. Infants are born with passive immunity from their mother's IgG. They acquire additional IgG through breast milk. Passive immunity can also be given to individuals by administering immune globulins (an injectable medication). Passive immunity is maintained only as long as the IgG molecule exists.

Immunoglobin (IgE). IgE is the immunoglobulin primarily responsible for the allergic response. The body identifies an allergen as a potential pathogen and attempts to destroy or excrete the allergen. Subsequent exposure to the allergen results in a more severe response. Individuals vary in their response to allergens, but a typical allergic response includes some or all of the following symptoms: increased production of mucus, itching (this is actually a defense designed to stimulate the person to rub off the allergen), hives, rashes, eczema, tearing (to flush the eyes of the allergen), sneezing (to clear the upper airway), wheezing (caused by constriction of the airways in an effort to prevent further penetration of the allergen into the lungs), and in the most severe responses, a life-threatening anaphylactic shock.

Immunoglobin A (IgA). The mucous membranes secrete IgA around the body openings. They provide additional protection for these vulnerable portals of entry.

Immunoglobin D (IgD). These antibodies form on the surface of B cells and trap the potential pathogen to prevent it from replicating and causing disease.

Cell-Mediated Immunity

Whereas the humoral immune response acts directly against antigenic cells, the cell-mediated immune response acts to destroy body cells that have become infected, in most cases by viruses. T cells are responsible for the cell-mediated immune response. Four types of T cells play a role (Fig. 20-3):

FIGURE 20-3 The cell-mediated immune response causes white blood cells to attack antigens.

- *Cytotoxic (killer) T cells* directly attack and kill body cells infected with pathogens.
- *Helper T cells* help regulate the action of B cells in humoral immune responses, and of cytotoxic T cells in cell-mediated responses.
- *Memory T cells.* The first time an antigen invades the body, T cells form that respond to that specific antigen. With subsequent infections, the memory T cells are able to increase the speed and amount of the T-cell response.
- *Suppressor T cells* are thought to stop the immune response when the infection has been contained (also see Fig. 20-2).

KnowledgeCheck 20-3

- Identify and describe the purpose of the body's three major lines of defense against infection.
- Mr. Jefferson has an acute infection. If lab work reveals that IgM, but not IgG, is present in his blood, what can you conclude about this infection?

 Go to Chapter 20, **Knowledge Check Response Sheet and Answers,** on the Student Resource Disk or DavisPlus at http://davisplus.fadavis.com/Wilkinson2

What Factors Increase Host Susceptibility?

Anything that weakens the defenses makes a person more susceptible to infection. In addition, any factors that increase the person's exposure to pathogens, such as working at a day care center or being a nurse, increase the risk for infection. Some of the most common factors are discussed below.

Developmental Stage. Young children are vulnerable because their immune systems are immature and have had limited exposure to pathogens. Children frequently begin to have more infections when they start interacting with people outside their family (e.g., when they begin day care or start school). This is a natural process known as acquiring **active immunity.** Older adults are also susceptible hosts because the immune response declines with aging. Skin, a primary defense, becomes less elastic and more prone to breakdown with aging. Elders also tend to be less active, and their nutrition may be inadequate.

Breaks in the First Line of Defense. A break in the skin, whether caused by a surgical procedure, skin breakdown, an insect bite, or insertion of an intravenous device, creates a portal of entry for infectious microorganisms.

Illness or Injury. Recuperation from infection or injury limits the physical resources available to combat a new pathogen.

Tobacco Use. Smoking is a major risk factor for pulmonary infections. Smoking interferes with normal respiratory functioning, including the ability to move the chest, cough, sneeze, or have full air exchange. Chemicals in tobacco paralyze cilia; thus, secretions pool in the lower airways, creating a hospitable environment for bacterial growth. Although tobacco users are most profoundly affected by these changes, people exposed chronically to secondhand smoke (e.g., bartenders, children of smokers) are also affected by these changes and are at increased risk for infection.

Substance Abuse. Alcohol curbs hunger because it contains many calories. As a result, many chronic alcohol users do not consume an adequate diet. Alcohol is also toxic to the liver and to the cells lining the intestinal mucosa. Inhaled substances, such as marijuana and cocaine, affect respiratory cilia in a manner similar to tobacco. Any substances that affect orientation and energy level will diminish food intake, activity, rest, and hygiene—factors that support host defenses. Injecting substances leads to breaks in skin integrity, further increasing the risk of infection.

Multiple Sexual Partners. The number of sexual partners is directly related to the risk of sexually transmitted infections and cervical cancer.

Environmental Factors. Increased exposure to pathogens in one's work situation (e.g., kindergarten teacher, healthcare worker), living situation (e.g., nursing home, parents with young children who are in preschool), and other environmental factors increase one's risk for infection.

Chronic Disease. Many chronic diseases diminish the body's ability to fight infection. Diseases that impair peripheral circulation, such as uncontrolled hypertension (high blood pressure) and diabetes mellitus, make the patient prone to infection in the extremities. Poor circulation prevents antibodies and T cells from reaching the pathogens and damages tissue, making it easier for pathogens to enter. Leukemia, a form of cancer of the blood, increases the production of abnormal white blood cells, but these cells are ineffective in combating infection. Because HIV infects T cells, a patient with AIDS has a reduced ability to fight off secondary infections.

Medications. Some medications are given for the purpose of reducing the immune response, for example, to patients receiving organ or tissue transplants. For most patients, however, decreased immunity is an unwanted side effect of treatment. Even common medications, such as nonsteroidal anti-inflammatory agents (NSAIDs) (e.g., ibuprofen), decrease the immune response. As a side effect, some medications, such as chemotherapeutic agents, decrease the production of white blood cells or cause the cells produced to be abnormal. Even antibiotics can increase the risk for infection. For example, an antibiotic given for a respiratory infection may cause a vaginal yeast infection because it destroys colonies of normal vaginal flora, allowing the harmful microbes to thrive. Such **superinfections** (opportunistic growth of harmful transient pathogens that are normally kept in check), and some can be extremely challenging to treat.

Nursing and Medical Procedures. Several procedures are associated with an increased risk of infection. For example, urinary catheterization may injure the fragile urethral mucosa, provide a direct pathway for pathogens into the bladder, and prevent the normal flushing of the urethra. Also, an IV line inserted to infuse an antibiotic may serve as a portal of entry for pathogens to enter a patient's body.

Knowledge Check 20-4

What factors increase a client's risk for infection?

  Go to Chapter 20, **Knowledge Check Response Sheet and Answers,** on the Student Resource Disk or DavisPlus at http://davisplus.fadavis.com/Wilkinson2

Critical Thinking 20-3

Consider your current lifestyle. How would you evaluate your ability to support your body's defenses?

Critical Thinking 20-4

Recall the scenario of Jason Sergi, the labor and delivery nurse, and his daughter. Why did Jason say that handwashing was the most important thing he did at work that day? Explain your answer by referring to all of the links in the chain of infection.

Practical **Knowledge**
knowing how

As a nurse you will have direct contact with patients who are infected with a variety of pathogens or who are at increased risk for infection. The remainder of this chapter provides practical information for preventing infection in your clients and for caring for clients with infection.

◼ ASSESSMENT

Some elements of the nursing history and physical assessment focus specifically on the risk factors and symptoms of infection.

Nursing History

To elicit information related to infection, ask the client about the following:

- Any exposure to pathogens in the environment, including at work, recent or international travel, contact with people who are ill, and unprotected sexual behavior
- If the patient is febrile, ask "Have you recently traveled outside the country?"
- Any unusual foods or products ingested
- Past and present disease or injury history
- Medications, over-the-counter preparations, herbal products, alcohol intake, and any substances currently in use
- Current level of stress
- Immunization history
- Symptoms of illness

Physical Assessment

Observe the patient's general appearance: Does he seem fatigued? Is he diaphoretic? Is he wrapped in blankets or complaining of feeling chilled? Does the patient appear well nourished? Are the mucous membranes dry? Does the skin have normal elasticity (turgor)? Physical assessment includes a thorough examination of the skin. Look for signs of local infection evidenced by pain, redness, swelling, and warmth. Note the presence or absence of any rashes, along with any breaks or reddened areas of the skin. Patients with poor peripheral circulation often have various skin discolorations, rather than signs of inflammation, when experiencing an infection. Swollen lymph nodes indicate the possible presence of an infection in the area that drains into the nodes. An elevated temperature and pulse rate are classic signs of an infection.

It is important to remember that the presence of one infection does not eliminate the risk for an additional infection. For example, a patient being treated with IV medications for a wound infection is at risk for infection

at the IV site, as well as for a superinfection or an infection related to insufficient immunizations. For a list of tests commonly used to evaluate evidence of or risk for infection,

 Go to Chapter 20, **Diagnostic Testing, Common Tests for Evaluating the Presence of or Risk for Infection,** in Volume 2.

Each specific test should be evaluated based on the patient's condition, age, and coexisting conditions.

◼ ANALYSIS/NURSING DIAGNOSIS

The following two NANDA-I diagnoses directly pertain to infection:

- **Readiness for Enhanced Immunization Status.** This is a wellness diagnosis, used to describe a person who is already following the local, national, and/or international standards of immunization, but who wants to enhance behavior to prevent infectious disease, and learn more about providers of immunizations, possible problems associated with immunizations, knowledge of standards, record-keeping.
- **Risk for Infection.** Virtually any patient in a healthcare setting is at Risk for Infection due to exposure to pathogens in the environment. Use this diagnosis only for patients who are at higher than usual risk (e.g., those with poor nutritional status) and who need nursing interventions to help prevent infection. Do not use it for the generic assessments you do routinely for all patients (e.g., assessing temperature, routine examination of surgical incision). Examples of appropriate use of this diagnosis include the following:
  - Risk for Infection r/t altered immune response secondary to corticosteroid therapy
  - Risk for Infection r/t impaired skin integrity and poor nutritional status

(Patients with actual infection are managed collaboratively with the healthcare team.)

Infection may be a medical diagnosis or the etiology of other nursing diagnoses, such as Fatigue, Risk for Imbalanced Body Temperature, or Pain. Patients with infection may experience other health problems due to their infected status. For example:

Social Isolation r/t communicable disease (e.g., tuberculosis [TB])

Deficient Diversional Activity r/t inability to leave room secondary to protective isolation

Other diagnostic statements may apply, depending upon the patient's condition, treatment ordered, and the patient's response to illness. For a care plan and care map for Risk for Infection,

 Go to Chapter 20, **Care Plan,** on the Student Resource Disk or DavisPlus at http://davisplus.fadavis.com/Wilkinson2

PLANNING OUTCOMES/EVALUATION

For NOC standardized outcomes for Risk for Infection,

 Go to Chapter 20, **Standardized Language,** in Volume 2.

Individualized goals/outcomes statements depend on the specific nursing diagnosis and etiology. For example, for an undernourished woman, if the nursing diagnosis is Risk for Infection r/t intravenous puncture site and probable invasive procedures secondary to active labor, an appropriate goal would be:

Patient will show no signs of localized infection at the infusion site, as evidenced by the absence of swelling, redness, excessive warmth, pain, or drainage.

You will evaluate the nursing care plan by examining the extent to which such goals have been met.

PLANNING INTERVENTIONS/IMPLEMENTATION

When caring for a patient at risk for infection, nursing activities are aimed at breaking the chain of infection at every possible link. Some of the most common reasons patients are diagnosed with Risk for Infection are exposure to pathogens, bypass of their normal defense mechanisms, increased physiological stress, or inadequate immune response. Direct nursing care toward these concerns, and provide the following broad interventions:

- Reduce exposure to pathogens through the use of aseptic technique (discussed shortly).
- Maintain skin integrity and support natural defenses against infection.
- Reduce stress.
- Promote immune function through collaborative care.
- Provide supportive measures to decrease the length of time that invasive devices, such as intravenous lines and urinary catheters, are needed by a patient.

For NIC standardized interventions for Risk for Infection:

 Go to Chapter 20, **Standardized Language,** in Volume 2.

Specific nursing activities will be based on the unique situation of the client, as described in the etiology of the diagnostic statement. For example:

- For clients who have had surgery and general anesthesia or who are at risk for pneumonia, promote coughing and deep breathing on a regular basis.
- For clients who are at risk for disease based on age, debilitated state, community living arrangement, or employment in healthcare facilities, facilitate participation in vaccination programs, which can help them acquire immunity from some communicable diseases.
- Community health nurses can limit disease transmission through surveillance of the community, tracking of disease patterns, and initiation of prompt treatment.

- For clients who have breaks in the skin or incision sites, provide regular assessment for infection status and follow appropriate medical or surgical asepsis guidelines.
- For all clients at risk for infection, provide care that is based on principles of medical asepsis.

Other preventive nursing activities are discussed in the following sections. They include providing client teaching, supporting host defenses, and practicing medical and surgical asepsis.

Providing Client Teaching

Clients and caregivers in their own homes are usually at less risk for infection than they are in the hospital. The client and caregiver share the same potential pathogens and antibodies, and there is limited exposure to others with illness. Nevertheless, to protect their own health and the health of others, clients need to understand basic principles of medical asepsis, personal hygiene, and infection control. You should also teach them to recognize signs and symptoms of infection; and for those who have an infection, help them to understand that particular organism and disease process. For information about teaching infection control in the home and community, see Home Care: Preventing Infection in the Home and Community. To help clients avoid acquiring or spreading CA-MRSA, see Self-Care: Teaching your Patient about Preventing the Spread of CA-MRSA.

Wellness Promotion to Support Host Defenses

Efforts to promote wellness help break the chain of infection by strengthening a person's defenses against invading pathogens. Lifestyle factors essential for promoting host defenses are healthful nutrition, adequate hygiene, rest and exercise, stress reduction, and immunizations.

Nutrition. An acute infection depletes the body's nutritional stores. Therefore, it is important to monitor and support client nutrition, including protein, vitamins, minerals, and water. Nutrients are required to replace lost stores, to maintain production of white blood cells, and to repair damaged tissues. Fever and increased mucus secretions, which are common defenses against infection, increase water loss. Additional water is needed to supplement the lost fluid and to support the increased metabolic rate that occurs with a fever. Chapter 26 further discusses the importance of adequate nutrition.

Hygiene is crucial for maintaining intact skin, a primary host defense. Encourage frequent handwashing, as well as regular showering or bathing, to decreases the bacterial count on the skin. However, be aware that overzealous cleanliness diminishes the skin's natural oils and may lead to cracking of the skin. Chapter 22 focuses on the importance of hygiene for health. Also see the Home Care box.

Home Care

Preventing Infection in the Home and Community

➤ To disinfect the home environment, use and teach caregivers to create a dilute bleach solution. Mix 1 part regular-strength bleach to 50 parts water. The mixture may be stored for a month in an opaque container. ✚ NEVER mix the solution with other household cleaners.

➤ Procedures performed using sterile technique in the hospital (e.g., urinary catheterization) are often performed by clean procedure in the home because of the decreased risk of infection.

➤ Healthcare workers in the home are a potential source of pathogens and should use caution to avoid infecting the client.

➤ If the client or family member is capable and willing to perform the required treatment, provide the necessary teaching; the client will have less exposure to pathogens than he would if a healthcare provider came to the home to provide care.

➤ Assess for subtle signs of infection: temperature increase, fatigue, lymph gland enlargement, delayed healing of wounds, fever, chills, or drainage.

➤ Instruct clients and family members in the signs and symptoms of infection and how and when to contact their primary care provider to report these findings.

➤ Advise those planning international travel to get their vaccinations before departing, especially for travel to Sub-Saharan Africa, South-Central Asia, or Latin America, where they may contract malaria, dengue, rickettsiosis, and influenza.

➤ Teach clients and family members basic hygiene and infection prevention measures in the home, including:

The importance of handwashing before preparing food, before eating, after going to the bathroom, blowing the nose, and before putting the hands near the face.

Keeping the home environment clean to create an optimal environment for care

Safe food preparation and storage (see Chapter 21)

Not sharing personal care items (e.g., towels, washcloths, toothbrushes, combs)

➤ Teach clients and family members actions they can take to help prevent infection when they are outside the home, including:

Washing hands and not touching surfaces in a public bathroom

Carrying and using antibacterial hand gel, as needed while in public places

Using a wet-wipe on the receiver and mouthpiece of public phones before making a call

Washing hands upon returning home (e.g., from shopping)

Asking healthcare providers to wash their hands before touching them, if they have not done so

Using tongs, not fingers, to get food from serving trays in grocery stores and restaurants

Asking for clean silverware or napkins if an item is dropped on the floor in a restaurant

➤ For additional information on home care practices, see Chapter 43.

Rest and Sleep. Rest and sleep renew the body and mind and conserve strength. Sleep needs vary, and there is really no "correct" amount or pattern of sleep. However, sleep of 6 to 9 hours per night is considered fully restorative for most people.

Exercise and Activity. Research demonstrates that exercise is just as important as rest and sleep. Too little activity causes circulation to slow and the lungs to supply less oxygen. Excessive exercise leads to fatigue and joint injury. Chapters 31 and 33 provide in-depth discussion on rest, sleep, activity, and exercise.

Stress Reduction. Whether physical or mental, stress decreases the body's immune defenses. Numerous studies demonstrate a correlation between increased stress and increased disease (Cousins, 1979; Franco, de Barros, Nogueira-Martins, et al., 2003; Schneider, Alexander, Staggers, et al., 2005). Laughing, in contrast, increases oxygenation, promotes body movement, and increases immune responses. See Chapter 25 for further details on the effects of stress, if you wish.

Immunizations. Immunization via vaccination can protect against several infectious diseases (e.g., measles, mumps, and other childhood diseases; pneumonia, influenza, smallpox, and shingles). Unfortunately, some

pathogens, such as the virus that causes the common cold, mutate too rapidly for an immunization to be developed. Encourage clients to follow recommendations for immunizations. For most diseases, at least 85% of the population must be immunized in order to protect the entire population from the disease. If you need specific recommended immunizations throughout the life span and their role in health promotion,

 Go to Chapter 9, **Expanded Discussion,** on the Student Resource Disk or DavisPlus at http://davisplus.fadavis.com/Wilkinson2

KnowledgeCheck 20-5

What actions improve host ability to prevent infection?

 Go to Chapter 20, **Knowledge Check Response Sheet and Answers,** on the Student Resource Disk or DavisPlus at http://davisplus.fadavis.com/Wilkinson2

Practicing Medical Asepsis

Asepsis is a term that means absence of contamination by disease-causing microorganisms. **Medical asepsis** ("clean technique") refers to procedures that decrease the potential for the spread of infections. You probably already practice medical asepsis in other settings without realizing it. For example, at home you wash your hands before and after handling foods. Before chopping food, you make sure the cutting board and utensils you use are clean. After using it, you wash the board with hot, soapy water. In the healthcare setting, medical asepsis includes hand hygiene, environmental cleanliness, standard precautions, and protective isolation. The effectiveness of these measures, and the patient's safety, depend on nurses' rigorously and consistently following the principles of asepsis. When you are hurrying, you may be tempted to take shortcuts, or you may forget to follow a guideline. Remember: You are putting your patient, and possibly yourself, at risk for an infection that could cause serious illness. Assume every patient is potentially infected or colonized with an organism that could be transmitted to others.

Maintaining Clean Hands

Many activities contribute to infection control and prevention, but hand hygiene is the single most important one. The WHO has chosen as the first "global patient safety challenge" the reduction of healthcare-associated infection, with the theme, "clean care is safer care." They have made hand hygiene the cornerstone strategy because it is simple, standardized, low-cost, and based on solid scientific evidence.

Although you may think you already know how to wash your hands, remember that in healthcare settings you are coming in contact with pathogens that are potentially dangerous to you and your patients. Decisions about the type of hand hygiene to use, how long to wash, when to wash, and so on, are based on the amount of contact you have with patients or contaminated objects, as well as the patient's infection status and susceptibility to infection. Handwashing involves five key factors: time, water, soap, friction, and drying (Fig. 20-4). The following briefly summa-

rizes the CDC recommendations for these factors (Boyce & Pittet [CDC], 2002). For more specific details and guidelines to use when making handwashing decisions,

 Go to **Clinical Insight 20-1: Guidelines for Hand Hygiene,** in Volume 2.

- *Time.* In a nonsurgical setting, wash the hands vigorously for at least 15 seconds, longer if hands are visibly soiled. In a surgical setting wash for 2 to 6 minutes, depending on the soap or other product used.
- *Water.* Use warm water and rinse off soap completely. Hot water and soap increase the potential for skin breakdown.
- *Soap.* Use agency-approved soap. The CDC recommends using a 60% alcohol-based solution (rubs, sprays, gels) for routine hand cleansing, and plain or antimicrobial soap and water when hands are visibly dirty. Iodine compounds are also effective, but usually too irritating for regular hand hygiene. If there is a potential for contact with bacterial spores (e.g., when caring for a client with a *C. diff.* infection), you must wash your hands with soap and water; alcohol-based solutions are not effective against spores. If you are interested in a comparison of the effectiveness of various hand-hygiene antiseptic agents,

Go to Chapter 20, **ESG Table 20-2,** on the Student Resource Disk or DavisPlus at http://davisplus.fadavis.com/Wilkinson2

- *Friction.* Rub all surfaces of the hands and wrists vigorously, including the backs of the hands and between the fingers. Remove jewelry and clean areas underneath. Clean underneath the fingernails, using an orangewood stick.
- *Drying.* Use single-use towels or hand dryers to remove all moisture after washing the hands. If using antimicrobial hand gels, apply and rub hands until dry.

Critical Aspects of Procedure 20-1 highlights the essential components of handwashing. For a step-by-step procedure on hand hygiene,

 Go to Chapter 20, **Procedure 20-1: Hand Hygiene,** in Volume 2.

In addition to handwashing, you should keep your fingernails short. According to the CDC, long nails, artificial nails, nail extenders, fingernail polish, watches, and rings with stones can harbor microorganisms. One recent study recommends an even shorter nail length of 2 mm or less (Association of periOperative Registered Nurses [AORN], 2004; Boyce & Pittet, 2002; Pratt, Pellowe, Wilson, et al., 2007; Rupp, Fitzgerald, Puumala, et al., 2008; Ward, 2007).

The most important aspect of medical asepsis is hand cleanliness. Clean hands markedly decrease the transmission of infection. Despite the importance of clean hands, research demonstrates that clinical staff do not consistently observe hand hygiene guidelines (Pratt, Pellowe, Wilson, et al., 2007). In 2008, Medicare

FIGURE 20-4 Clean hands will markedly decrease the transmission of infection.

Critical Aspects of Procedure 20-1

Hand Hygiene

Hand Washing Steps:

1. Wet hands.

2. Soap (at least 15 seconds).

3. Scrub backs of hands, wrists, between fingers, under fingernails.

4. Rinse.

5. Towel-dry.

6. Turn off taps with towel.

If using alcohol-based handrubs:

1. Use alcohol-based handrubs when hands are not soiled.

2. Cover all surfaces of fingers and hands.

3. Rub together until dry.

has stopped paying for patient complications arising from certain hospital-acquired infections, which in many cases result from poor handwashing. You can help improve clinical practice by serving as a role model for good hand hygiene.

Maintaining a Clean Environment

An object is considered **contaminated** if it becomes unclean—that is, if you suspect it may contain pathogens. For example, the floor is contaminated, so anything that comes in contact with the floor becomes contaminated. Soiled dressings, used tissues, sinks, commodes, and bedpans are other examples. Agency policies determine whether a reusable item is cleaned, disinfected, or sterilized, based on how the item is used.

Cleaning

Cleaning is the removal of visible soil (organic and inorganic) from objects and surfaces. It normally is

accomplished manually or mechanically using water with detergents or enzymatic products. A goal of medical asepsis is to keep all public and patient care areas within the facility clean and free from dust, debris, and contamination. Any spilled liquids, dirty surfaces, or potentially contaminated areas should be cleaned immediately. In your home, you use hot water and general cleaning supplies. However, healthcare facilities use special techniques and cleaning solutions formulated to inhibit microbial growth. Items must be cleaned thoroughly before they can be disinfected or sterilized.

Disinfecting

Disinfection removes virtually all pathogens on inanimate objects by physical or chemical means, including steam, gas, chemicals, and ultraviolet light. Disinfection reduces microbial populations, but it does not guarantee that all pathogens are eliminated, because certain viruses, other pathogenic microbes, and spores can remain (Bauman, Machunis-Masuoka, & Tizard, 2006). Chemical germicides can achieve three levels of disinfection. *High-level disinfection* kills all organisms except high levels of bacterial spores. *Intermediate-level disinfection* kills mycobacteria, most viruses, and bacteria. *Low-level disinfection* kills some viruses and bacteria. Disinfection is used for semicritical and noncritical items:

- **Semicritical items** are those that contact mucous membranes or nonintact skin. This category includes reusable devices, such as flexible endoscopes, and respiratory therapy and anesthesia equipment, for example. They must be free of all microorganisms except bacterial spores, so they must at least be disinfected, and sometimes sterilized.
- **Noncritical items** are supplies and equipment that come in contact with intact skin but not mucous membranes. They do not carry a high risk of infection transmission, and they can be decontaminated where they are used. Examples of noncritical patient-care items are bedpans, stethoscopes, and blood pressure cuffs. Examples of noncritical environmental surfaces include floors, food utensils, bed linens, and bed rails (CDC, 2008c). Disinfection is adequate for noncritical items.

Sterilizing

Sterilization is the elimination of all microorganisms (except prions) in or on an object. The major sterilizing methods used in hospitals are (1) autoclaving with moist heat, (2) ethylene oxide gas, and (3) dry heat. Sterilization is used when absolute purity of an object or surface is critical.

- **Critical items** are ones that pose a high risk for infection if they are contaminated with any microorganism. Critical items include those that enter the vascular system or sterile tissue, or through which blood flows. Examples are intravenous catheters, needles for injections, urinary catheters, surgical instruments, some wound dressings, and chest tubes.

If you need more specific information on methods for disinfection and sterilization of patient-care items and environmental surfaces,

 Go to Chapter 20, **ESG Table 20-3, Methods for Disinfection and Sterilization of Patient-Care Items and Surfaces,** on the Student Resource Disk or DavisPlus at http://davisplus.fadavis.com/Wilkinson2

Specially trained personnel carry out disinfection and sterilization in most agencies. As a nurse, you must be familiar with the agency's policies and procedures for cleaning, handling, and transporting items to be disinfected and sterilized, and for working collaboratively with other departments (e.g., the housekeeping department) to keep the patient care area as clean and free of clutter as possible. Clients and caregivers are usually at less risk for infection in their own homes than they are in the hospital. They share the same potential pathogens and antibodies, and there is limited exposure to others with illness and to care providers carrying unusual pathogens, so levels of disinfection and sterilization may differ.

For more specific information about maintaining a clean environment in institutional and home care,

 Go to Chapter 20, **Clinical Insight 20-2, Providing a Clean Patient Environment,** in Volume 2.

CDC Guidelines for Preventing Transmission of Pathogens

In addition to handwashing and maintaining a clean environment, you should follow other precautions to protect yourself and your patients. CDC guidelines provide for two tiers of protection.

- **Standard precautions,** the first tier of protection, apply to care of all patients.
- **Transmission-based precautions**, the second tier of protection, outline precautions to be taken based on the mode of transmission of the infection (Siegel, Rhinehart, Jackson, et al., 2007). Recall from the discussion on the chain of infection that pathogens may be transmitted by contact, droplet, or air. Each mode of transmission requires a different approach to prevent infection.

Table 20-2 provides a summary comparison of standard and transmission-based precautions. For detailed guidelines to aid you in following both types of precautions,

 Go to Chapter 20, **Clinical Insight 20-3, Following CDC Standard Precautions,** and **Clinical Insight 20-4, Following Transmission-Based Precautions,** in Volume 2.

The CDC recommends and the United States Occupational Safety and Health Administration requires employers to provide personal protective equipment (PPE) for healthcare workers (e.g., gloves, gowns, face masks, and eye protection) (U.S. Department of Labor, n.d.). This equipment is to be used in standard precautions as well as transmission-based precautions. Figure 20-5

Table 20-2 ➤ **Comparison of CDC Standard and Transmission-Based Precautions**	
STANDARD PRECAUTIONS	**TRANSMISSION-BASED PRECAUTIONS**
"Tier One" Precautions Use with all clients, in all settings, regardless of suspected or confirmed presence of infection	**"Tier Two" Precautions** Use for patients known or suspected to be infected or colonized with infectious agents.
Principle: All blood, body fluids, secretions, excretions except sweat, nonintact skin, and mucous membranes may contain pathogens.	*Principle:* Routes of transmission for some microorganisms are not completely interrupted using standard precautions alone. Used *in addition to* standard precautions.
Include: hand hygiene; use of gloves, gown, mask, eye protection, or face shield (depending on expected exposure); and safe injection practices.	Three categories of precautions: *Contact Precautions*—For organisms spread by direct contact with the patient or his environment. This is the most common form of transmission.
Does not completely protect against microorganisms spread by contact, droplets, or through the air.	*Droplet Precautions*—For pathogens spread through close respiratory or mucous membrane contact with respiratory secretions (e.g., sneezing, coughing, talking); pathogens that do not remain infectious over long distances.
New Elements of Standard Precautions Added for protection of patients more than of healthcare personnel. They include:	*Airborne Precautions*—For pathogens that are very small and remain infectious over long distances when suspended in the air; and easily transmitted through air currents (e.g., fanning linens, ventilating systems).
Respiratory hygiene and cough etiquette	
Safe injection practices	
Wearing a mask when performing special lumbar puncture procedures	

Source: Siegel, J. D., Rhinehart, E., Jackson, M., Chiarello, L., & the Healthcare Infection Control Practices Advisory Committee (2007). *2007 Guideline for isolation precautions: Preventing transmission of infectious agents in the healthcare setting.* Retrieved from http://www.cdc.gov/ncidod/dhqp/pdf/guidelines/Isolation2007.pdf

provides examples of face masks and eye protection equipment. Critical Aspects for Procedures 20-2 through 20-8 summarizes the procedures for donning and removing PPE. For complete instructions,

 Go to Chapter 20, **Procedure 20-2: Donning Personal Protective Equipment (PPE),** and **Procedure 20-3: Removing Personal Protective Equipment (PPE),** in Volume 2.

FIGURE 20-5 Several types of face masks and eye shields are available.

KnowledgeCheck 20-6

Under what circumstances are standard precautions used?

 Go to Chapter 20, **Knowledge Check Response Sheet and Answers,** on the Student Resource Disk or DavisPlus at http://davisplus.fadavis.com/Wilkinson2

Preventing MDROs

Evidence suggests that MDROs are carried from one person to another via the hands of healthcare personnel. To prevent MDROs, you must adhere strictly to published recommendations for hand hygiene, glove use, and isolation precautions; and for performing invasive procedures such as intravenous and urinary catheterization, and care of central venous ports. Current evidence

---

 VOL 2 For steps to follow in *all* procedures, refer to the Universal Steps for All Procedures found on inside back cover of Volume 2. Go to the full procedures in Volume 2 to practice and learn the procedure steps. Use these Critical Aspects later to help you review key points.

Critical Aspects of Procedures 20-2 through 20-8

Procedure 20-2: Donning Personal Protective Equipment (PPE)

➤ Before exposure, don appropriate personal protective equipment according to standard precautions or transmission guidelines.

➤ Wear an N-95 respirator mask for airborne isolation.

➤ Wear a surgical mask for droplet isolation.

Procedure 20-3: Removing Personal Protective Equipment

➤ Remove PPE at doorway before leaving patient room, or in an anteroom.

➤ Avoid contaminating self, others, or environment when removing equipment.

➤ Considered contaminated: front areas, sleeves, head cover, mask, and gloves of the PPE.

➤ Considered clean: the inside of the gown, gloves, and head cover; the ties on the mask; and ties in the back of the gown.

➤ Always remove gloves first when removing PPE, unless gown ties in front.

Procedure 20-4: Surgical Handwashing: Traditional Method

➤ Don surgical shoe covers, cap, and face mask before the scrub.

➤ Use warm water.

➤ Perform a prewash, using soap and water.

➤ Clean under your fingernails under running water.

➤ Wet the scrub sponge, and apply a generous amount of antimicrobial soap.

➤ Using a circular motion, scrub all surfaces of nails, hands, and forearms at least 10 times, or the length of time specified by agency policy.

➤ Rinse hands and arms by keeping your fingertips higher than your elbow.

➤ Grasp a sterile towel, and back away from the sterile field.

➤ Thoroughly dry your hands before donning sterile gloves.

Procedure 20-5: Surgical Handwashing: Brushless System

➤ Don surgical shoe covers, cap, and face mask before the scrub.

➤ Use warm water.

➤ Perform a prewash, using soap and water.

➤ Clean under your nails under running water.

➤ Apply a generous amount of antimicrobial soap.

➤ Using a circular motion, scrub all surfaces of nails, hands, and forearms at least 10 times, or the length of time specified by agency policy.

➤ Rinse hands and arms by keeping your fingertips higher than your elbow.

➤ Grasp a sterile towel, and back away from the sterile field.

➤ Thoroughly dry your hands before donning sterile gloves.

Procedure 20-6: Sterile Gown and Gloves (Closed Method)

➤ Put on shoe covers, hair covers, and mask before scrub

➤ Perform surgical scrub.

➤ Grasp the gown at the neckline, and slide your arms into the sleeves without extending your hands through the cuffs.

➤ Have a co-worker pull the shoulders of the gown up and tie the neck tie.

➤ Don gloves using the closed method by keeping your hands covered at all times, first with the gown cuffs, and then with the sterile gloves.

➤ Secure the waist tie on your gown by handing it to a co-worker and turning to receive it.

➤ Keep your hands within your field of vision at all times.

➤ Do not turn your back to a sterile field.

Procedure 20-7: Sterile Gloves (Open Method)

➤ Remove all jewelry, including rings and watches.

➤ Place the glove package on a clean, dry surface.

➤ Open the inner package so that the cuffs are closest to you.

➤ Apply the glove of your dominant hand first by touching only the inside of the glove (the folded-over cuff) with your nondominant hand.

➤ Apply the second glove by touching only the outer part of the glove with your already-gloved hand; keep your sterile thumb well away from your bare skin.

➤ Do not touch the gloves to any unsterile items.

Procedure 20-8: Sterile Fields

➤ Prepare the sterile field as close as possible to the time of use.

➤ Do not cover the sterile field once established.

➤ Do not turn away from the sterile field.

➤ Inspect for package integrity, inclusion of sterile indicator, and/or expiration date. Do not use outdated items.

➤ Clear a space and prepare the patient before setting up the sterile field.

➤ Establish the sterile field with a sterile drape or sterile package wrapper.

➤ Add items to the sterile field by gently dropping them onto the sterile field.

➤ Pour sterile solutions into a sterile bowl or receptacle without touching the bowl or splashing onto the sterile field.

➤ Don sterile gloves and perform the procedure.

---

suggests that agencies should place infected patients in private rooms and require care providers to wear gowns and masks, and use antiseptic/disinfectant for handwashing. For a list of actions you can take to help prevent MDROs,

 Go to Chapter 20, **Clinical Insight 20-5, Preventing Multidrug-Resistant Organism Infections,** in Volume 2.

Also refer to the Home Care box and the Self-Care box in this chapter. For extensive information about monitoring these MDROs, consult a medical–surgical or infectious diseases textbook. For the CDC guidelines,

 Go to http://www.cdc.gov

"Protective Environment" in Special Situations

Patients who are immunosuppressed (e.g., receiving chemotherapy) may be placed in a special form of isolation, called protective isolation or reverse isolation. However, the CDC states that standard and transmission-based precautions are adequate protection for most of those patients. They recommend a "protective environment" only for a special class of stem cell transplant patients, who are neutropenic (have a low white blood cell count secondary to chemotherapy). Most of the recommendations are engineering and environmental services rather than nursing measures. To learn more about this,

 Go to Chapter 20, **Clinical Insight 20-6, Maintaining a "Protective Environment" in Special Situations,** in Volume 2.

Patients with compromised immunity are more likely to become infected by pathogens harbored in their own bodies than from pathogens transmitted by other people

(Siegel, Rhinehart, Jackson, et al., 2007). Therefore, except for the special situation described, standard and transmission-based precautions should protect even unusually vulnerable patients from organisms brought in by healthcare workers and visitors.

Nevertheless, you may see what has been called **protective isolation** being used for clients with low WBC counts, clients undergoing chemotherapy, or clients with large open wounds or weak immune systems. Protective isolation usually includes following standard precautions, placing the patient in a private room; restricting visitors; wearing a mask, gown, and gloves for patient care; and special cleaning or disposal of the patient's equipment and supplies. Some units, such as neonatal intensive care units, burn units, and labor and delivery suites, may follow some aspects of protective isolation all the time. Most of these precautions are described by standard and transmission-based precautions.

Control of Potentially Contaminated Equipment and Supplies

Whenever possible, use disposable equipment in an isolation room. Nondisposable equipment and supplies require special handling.

Protective Isolation If a client is in protective isolation, be sure that equipment has been disinfected *before* it is taken into the room. Take linen and dishes directly to the protective isolation room, and hand them to someone wearing the required protective garb.

Transmission-based Isolation If the client is in transmission-based isolation, disinfect the equipment *on removal* from the room. When removing linen or nondisposable

Self-Care

Teaching Your Patient About Preventing the Spread of CA-MRSA

As measures to prevent community-acquired MRSA, everyone should:

➤ Take antibiotics as prescribed. Complete the course of medication as recommended until it is finished.

➤ Contact your healthcare provider if the infection doesn't improve after a few days of taking an antibiotic.

➤ Never use antibiotics prescribed for someone else; and do not give your medication to others.

➤ Follow your healthcare provider's recommendations for influenza and pneumonia vaccinations. Preventing respiratory infections decreases antibiotic use.

➤ Make sure your healthcare providers clean their hands before they touch you. This is one of the most important infection prevention and control measures.

➤ Wash your hands often with soap and water. Wash for 15 to 30 seconds, or as long as it takes to sing the "Happy Birthday" song.

➤ Use alcohol-based hand sanitizer if soap and water are not available or hands are not visibly soiled. Sanitizer should have at least 60% alcohol.

➤ Avoid sharing personal items (e.g., towels, makeup, combs, clothing).

➤ Pay attention to symptoms that may indicate an infection (e.g., drainage from or inflammation of a wound), and contact your healthcare provider immediately.

➤ Cough and sneeze into your elbow and wash your hands after using a tissue.

Clients who have MRSA on their skin or who are infected with MRSA should be taught to:

➤ Keep all sores and cuts clean and covered with bandages.

➤ When changing a bandage:

Don't touch the sore with your bare hands. Wear gloves.

Immediately discard the soiled bandage and gloves in a trashbag where no one else can touch them.

Wash your hands after removing the gloves.

➤ Avoid touching other people's cuts or bandages.

➤ Avoid close-contact activities until your skin infection is healed, unless you can ensure that your sore will not come in contact with another person (e.g., if your sore can be well covered by a bandage and clothing).

➤ Shower daily, using antibacterial soap if your healthcare provider advises it.

➤ Wash your clothing, towels, and bedding separately from other family members' items. Use warm or hot water and bleach, if possible. Use warm or hot setting on the dryer.

➤ Wash exercise clothes after each use.

Sources

Adapted from Centers for Disease Control and Prevention (n.d.), *Tips for adult patients to prevent antimicrobial resistance*. From the Campaign to Prevent Antimicrobial Resistance in Healthcare Settings, CDC, Department of Health and Human Services. Last reviewed April 15, 2004. Retrieved August 4, 2008, from http://www.cdc.gov/drugresistance/healthcare/tools.htm#tips; S. S. Holcomb (2008). MRSA infections. *Nursing 2008, 38*(6): 33; Leung-Chen, P. (2008). Emerging infections. Everybody's crying MRSA. *American Journal of Nursing, 108*(8): 29-31.

---

items from a room with contact, droplet, or airborne isolation, place them in special isolation bags. This process requires two healthcare workers. The worker inside the room wears protective clothing and handles only contaminated items. The second worker stands at the door and holds the isolation bag open. The first worker places items inside the bag without touching the outside of the bag. If the bag contains linens, the isolation bag is closed and placed in a laundry hamper.

Disposing of Used Supplies

Place contaminated disposable equipment and materials containing body fluids in special isolation bags. Securely close the isolation trash bag, and place it in a special isolation trash container. Special disposal methods are used to prevent these objects from going into a landfill, where they could become a reservoir of infection. Because this trash is much more expensive to process, take care to put *only* contaminated materials in the contaminated trash.

Sharps Disposal

Always place disposable needles, syringes, and other sharp items, such as broken glass, in special disposable sharps containers immediately after their use. Never recap a contaminated needle. Refer to Chapters 21 and 23 for further information on preventing needlestick injuries.

Laboratory Specimens

Laboratory specimens contain blood and body fluids and are always considered contaminated. Label the specimen container in a clean area before taking it to the patient. Have the specimen collected by a healthcare worker wearing appropriate protective clothing. Once the specimen is collected, place it in a special transport bag. Do not allow the outside of the bag to touch any contaminated item, including your gloves.

For specific guidelines on care of contaminated equipment and supplies,

 Go to Chapter 20, **Clinical Insight 20-2, Providing a Clean Patient Environment, Clinical Insight 20-3, Following CDC Standard Precautions,** and **Clinical Insight 20-4, Following Transmission-Based Precautions,** in Volume 2.

Supporting the Psychological Needs of Patients in Isolation

Remember, isolation precautions are designed to prevent the spread of disease. It is the disease that is being isolated, *not* the person who has the disease. Patients who are in isolation continue to have a need for human contact. In fact, isolation may produce anxiety and increase the desire for human contact. When caring for a client in isolation, search for ways to reassure and maintain contact with the patient. Possible solutions include the following:

- When wearing the required protective equipment, touch the patient.
- Organize the time you spend in the patient's room to include time for discussion about how the client is coping with isolation.
- If the patient is in droplet isolation, remember that the danger area is 3 feet from the patient. You can go to the door of the room and speak to the patient without a mask.
- Reassure the patient that precautions are temporary.
- Explain that the precautions and the PPE protect you and the patient, as well as family members and other patients.

KnowledgeCheck 20-7

- If you needed to disinfect a sink in a client's home, what would you use?
- List at least three actions clients can take to help avoid infection when they are out in the community.

 Go to Chapter 20, **Knowledge Check Response Sheet and Answers,** on the Student Resource Disk or DavisPlus at http://davisplus.fadavis.com/Wilkinson2

Practicing Surgical Asepsis

Sterile means without life. If an object is sterile, it contains no life and therefore no infectious organisms. The exception is *prions,* the protein particles that cause severe neurological degeneration in animals and humans, such as in bovine spongiform encephalopathy (BSE, also known as "mad cow disease") in cattle and Creutzfeldt–Jakob disease (CJD) in humans. Researchers have not yet determined what types of antimicrobial techniques are successful in destroying prions. Inanimate objects, such as surgical equipment, gauze dressings, or wound irrigation fluid may be sterile. However, humans will always have microorganisms in and on their bodies.

Surgical asepsis, or **sterile technique,** requires creation of a sterile environment and use of sterile equipment. It differs from medical asepsis in that it is more complex and it is not required for use with all patients. Sterilization can be accomplished through the use of special gases or high heat. Surgical equipment and implanted devices are examples of materials that must be sterilized. If you need more information about sterilization processes,

 Go to Chapter 20, **ESG Table 20-3, Methods for Disinfection and Sterilization of Patient-Care Items and Surfaces,** on the Student Resource Disk or DavisPlus at http://davisplus.fadavis.com/Wilkinson2

To create a sterile area, housekeeping personnel perform extensive cleaning using special solutions and

Table 20-3 ▶ A Comparison of Hand Hygiene and Surgical Scrub

	HAND HYGIENE	SURGICAL SCRUB
No visible soil	Use alcohol-based hand rub or soap (plain or antimicrobial) and water.	1. Perform a handwash with soap and water. 2. Then perform the surgical scrub using either an FDA-approved antimicrobial scrub product or an antiseptic hand rub that is FDA-approved for surgical hand asepsis.
Hands visibly soiled	Wash with soap (plain or antimicrobial) and water.	Surgical scrub steps remain the same, even with visible soil.

Sources: AORN (2004); Boyce & Pittet (2002); Pratt, Pellowe, Wilson, et al. (2007).

procedures. All health personnel working in the area must wear appropriate surgical attire and perform a surgical hand scrub.

Performing a Surgical Scrub

A surgical scrub is a modification of the handwashing procedure described earlier (see Table 20-3 for a comparison). It traditionally involves an extended scrub of the hands using a sponge, nail cleaner, and a bactericidal scrubbing agent. A newer method uses a brushless scrub, using a bactericidal scrubbing agent. All methods require a prewash before the surgical scrub. For a summary of the steps involved, see the Critical Aspects box for Procedures 20-4 and 20-5. For the full procedures,

 Go to Chapter 20, **Procedure 20-4: Surgical Handwashing: Traditional Method,** and **Procedure 20-5: Surgical Handwashing: Brushless System,** in Volume 2.

Donning Surgical Attire

Burn units, labor and birth units, and some surgical wards, intensive care units, nurseries, and oncology wards require surgical attire for patient caregiving. In each of these units, nurses care for clients who are at increased risk for infection or are undergoing an invasive procedure that places them at increased risk. The goal on all of these units is to protect the patient from infection transmitted by healthcare workers.

All personnel on these units don *clean* surgical attire, or scrub suits, when they arrive on the unit. These scrub suits should not be worn outside the unit. If you must transport a patient to another area or leave the unit to gather supplies, wear a covering over the scrub suit. Remove the covering on your return to the unit. Additional precautions include a disposable hat to cover the hair, shoe coverings, and face masks.

Personnel engaged in surgery or certain invasive procedures must dress in *sterile* surgical attire. As a beginning student, you will soon find yourself in such a situation. Initially your role will be limited to observation, but you will need to be prepared for these experiences.

First you will change into a scrub suit, apply shoe coverings, and put on a disposable hat. Wash your hands, and apply a face mask. If there is potential for spray of fluids, wear a face mask with eye shield. Be sure to adjust the mask so that it is comfortable to breathe through. Once you have adjusted the mask, perform the surgical scrub. If a surgical gown is required, don it after the hand scrub.

If you are applying full surgical attire, you will need to apply gloves using a closed method, after you have put on your gown. Once you don sterile gloves, you may touch only sterile items. The Critical Aspects box for Procedures 20-2 through 20-8 summarizes how to apply surgical attire. For complete instructions,

VOL 2 Go to Chapter 20, **Procedure 20-6: Donning Sterile Gloves and Gown (Closed Method),** in Volume 2.

You will often wear sterile gloves for procedures that do not require full surgical attire. Open the glove packaging slowly. Avoid fanning the wrapping or touching the gloves. Put the first glove on your dominant hand (Fig. 20-6). This is the open method of gloving.

 A general rule to consider when applying the second glove is to touch glove-to-glove and skin-to-skin. The already-gloved hand may touch any of the sterile surfaces of the second glove. The second hand may touch only the inside of the glove—the portion that will

FIGURE 20-7 When applying the second glove, consider this general rule: glove to glove, skin to skin.

have contact with the skin. Figure 20-7 illustrates the hand positions used to apply the second glove. Although this process sounds awkward, you will develop comfort with practice. The Critical Aspects box for Procedures 20-2 through 20-8 summarizes the open method of gloving. For complete instructions,

VOL 2 Go to Chapter 20, **Procedure 20-7: Sterile Gloves (Open Method),** in Volume 2.

Observing Sterile Technique

Healthcare providers use sterile technique to perform a variety of procedures. Some of the procedures require full surgical attire; others do not. The following procedures, for example, use both sterile technique and principles of medical asepsis: administering an injection, starting an IV line, and performing a sterile dressing change. To clarify, when administering an injection, you prepare the patient, cleanse the injection site, and remove the needle cap using standard precautions. You do not don sterile gloves, but for the rest of the procedure you observe sterile technique by taking care not to touch or otherwise contaminate the exposed needle.

Before performing a sterile procedure, determine what supplies you will need and whether you will need assistance. If the patient is unable to maintain a position required for the procedure, you will need a helper to hold the patient during the procedure.

Wash your hands before gathering materials from the sterile supply area, and then gather the other required supplies and equipment. Check the expiration date on each package. Check the package to make sure it is intact. If it has paper or cloth wrapping, be sure there are no indications that it has ever been wet.

For guidelines related to sterile technique and preparing and maintaining sterile fields,

VOL 2 Go to Chapter 20, **Clinical Insight 20-7: Guidelines for Observing Sterile Technique,** in Volume 2.

FIGURE 20-6 When applying the first glove, touch only the inside cuff of the glove.

Preparing and Maintaining Sterile Fields

There are some variations in how you might set up sterile fields. Sometimes it is as simple as opening a package of supplies wrapped in a sterile disposable cover. The inside of the cover becomes your sterile field; the supplies on it are sterile, as well. At other times, you may work with a larger, reusable or disposable sterile drape (wrapped in an outer wrapping). In that situation, you open the outer wrapping, then pick up the sterile drape grasping only the corners, and allow it to fall open to create a sterile field, perhaps to entirely cover a table surface or to create a sterile field on the patient's bed.

In any sterile field, only the horizontal plane (e.g., the table top) is considered sterile. Consider nonsterile any material that drapes over the horizontal plane. A 1-inch margin around the edges of the sterile field is also considered unsterile because it is in contact with contaminated surfaces.

The Critical Aspects box for Procedures 20-2 through 20-8 summarizes how to prepare and maintain a sterile field, as well as add supplies and sterile liquids to it. For complete procedural steps,

 Go to Chapter 20, **Procedure 20-8A: Preparing and Maintaining a Sterile Field,** in Volume 2.

Adding Supplies to a Sterile Field

Some supplies (e.g., urinary catheter kits) are packaged in a wrapper that can form a sterile field. The outside of these packages is considered clean, and the inside is sterile. You must open these packages in a way that does not contaminate the inside of the wrapping. Be cautious when adding supplies to the sterile field. If they are light and small, gently add them to the sterile field by separating the package flaps and allowing them to fall onto the field. If the object is large, such as an irrigation bowl, slowly unwrap the packaging and, touching only the outside wrapper, place the bowl on the field. If any object falls only partly on the field, it is no longer sterile. For detailed instructions on how to add supplies to a sterile field,

 Go to Chapter 20, **Procedure 20-8B: Adding Supplies to a Sterile Field,** in Volume 2.

Adding Sterile Solutions to a Sterile Field

Add sterile liquids to a sterile field by gently pouring them into a container on the field. Some sterile drapes contain an impermeable membrane between layers. This membrane serves as a barrier to moisture and prevents wicking. With this type of drape, you may pour sterile liquid directly on gauze pads on the field. Pour only an amount of liquid that is sufficient to make the gauze pads damp. Excess fluid may run off the field, causing the field to become contaminated—a wet field is not sterile because it does not provide a barrier to microorganisms on the unsterile surface under the drape. For step-by-step instruction in how to add sterile solutions to a sterile field,

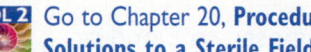 Go to Chapter 20, **Procedure 20-8C: Adding Sterile Solutions to a Sterile Field,** in Volume 2.

KnowledgeCheck 20-8

- When will you need to don sterile gloves using the closed method?
- (True of false) Some procedures require both standard precautions and sterile technique.
- What part(s) of a sterile field are considered to be unsterile?

 Go to Chapter 20, **Knowledge Check Response Sheet and Answers,** on the Student Resource Disk or DavisPlus at http://davisplus.fadavis.com/Wilkinson2

Infection Control and Prevention for Healthcare Workers

It is critical that you learn how to protect yourself from infections. You want not only to avoid personal illness, but also to avoid becoming a reservoir for infection. Nurses and other patient care workers are at great risk of acquiring infections because they come in contact with a large number and variety of pathogens. Skin contact, mucous membrane contact, and puncture wounds often serve as portals of entry.

Nursing assistive personnel (NAP), ancillary personnel, and housekeeping and maintenance workers are often present on nursing units. Visitors, volunteers, and family are also on the unit. It is essential that you protect them from potential hazardous exposure as well as protect yourself and patients from possible microorganisms brought into the unit. As a nurse, you need to monitor other healthcare workers, patients, and visitors for breaks in infection control and prevention.

What Role Does the Infection Preventionist Nurse Play?

The task of the infection prevention nurse is to minimize the number of infections in the healthcare facility. Because it is not possible to provide absolute protection all the time, the nurse must balance the risks for infection with the costs of protective measures and the benefits of various strategies. Infection preventionists must keep current with information about pathogens, antibiotic resistance, and infection control. The nurse also functions as an epidemiologist, tracking down the source of HAIs and strengthening measures to prevent their recurrence. Finally, all members of the infection prevention team enforce compliance with federal, state, and local regulations related to infection control and prevention.

What Should I Do if I Am Exposed to Bloodborne Pathogens?

Exposure to blood, body secretions, or body tissues containing blood or secretions requires immediate action. See Box 20-1 for complete instructions. The first step is

Source: Bloodborne pathogens and needlestick prevention. Post-exposure evaluation. (n.d.) Occupational Safety & Health Administration. U.S. Department of Labor. Retrieved from http:// www.osha.gov/SLTC/bloodbornepathogens/postexposure.html

BOX 20-1 ■ If You Are Exposed to Blood or Other Body Fluids

If you are stuck by a needle or other sharp, or get blood or other potentially infectious materials in your eyes, nose, mouth, or on broken skin:

1. Immediately flood the exposed area with water and clean any wound with soap and water or a skin disinfectant if available.
2. Report the exposure immediately to the appropriate person in the agency. If you are a student, also report immediately to your instructor.
3. Seek immediate medical attention. Consent to testing and follow-up treatment as advised.
4. Complete an incident or injury report.
5. Attend counseling sessions provided by the agency.

to minimize the exposure by washing the area thoroughly. Then notify the appropriate people, complete an injury report, and seek medical attention.

Anyone exposed to bloodborne pathogens should have baseline lab work done to check for hepatitis and HIV. If the patient source is known, the infection preventionist will arrange to have the patient tested. Subsequent testing and possible preventive treatment are based on the type of exposure and what is known about the source and the injured person. To limit risks from the exposure, the infection prevention team will provide counseling and recommendations as soon as possible after the event. Chapters 21 and 23 present information on preventing needlestick injuries.

How Can I Minimize the Effects of Bioterrorism and Epidemics?

In 2001, anthrax spores were sent through the U.S. mail. This incident brought new attention to the possibility of biological agents being used as weapons, especially by terrorists. **Bioterrorism** is the intentional release, or threatened release, of disease-producing organisms or substances for the purpose of causing death, illness, harm, economic damage, or fear. Five diseases with recognized bioterrorism potential are anthrax, botulism, pneumonic plague, smallpox, viral hemorrhagic fevers, and tularemia. The U.S. government has recently funded development of drugs to treat three of these diseases (anthrax, plague, and tularemia).

Recognize an Outbreak

Should a biological event occur, either as a result of bioterrorism or a naturally occurring epidemic, a key factor in minimizing its effects is the ability to quickly recognize unusual disease patterns and detect the presence of infectious diseases. Some electronic patient record systems include special pattern identification programs. The use of these systems supplements, but does not replace, clinical observation skills. Nurses need to assess not only the individual patient's condition, but also clusters of symptoms. Hospital, emergency department, and clinic nurses are in key positions to recognize outbreaks because they see patients from multiple primary care providers. Nurses must keep the following questions in mind:

- Am I seeing an unexpected number of infectious diseases, or diseases possibly caused by infectious organisms?
- Am I seeing similar cases that are not responding to medical treatment?
- Are healthcare workers who come in contact with infectious patients becoming ill?

Notify the Safety Officer

After identifying a suspicious pattern, you should notify the institution's interventionist or safety officer as soon as possible. Appropriate cultures will be needed, and the federal and state health departments should be notified. If the infectious organism is unknown, samples must be preserved for future analysis.

Institute Appropriate Level of Standard Precautions

In the event of an epidemic, the essential principles of hand hygiene and standard precautions will be the core of your infection prevention and control measures. Patients with similar symptoms should be cared for by a minimum number of healthcare personnel, and those personnel must use appropriate isolation precautions. If the etiology and transmission route of the causative organism are unknown, standard, contact, and airborne precautions should be implemented as needed. The Occupational Safety and Health Administration (OSHA) defines types of personal protective equipment and situations in which you are required to wear it (U.S. Department of Labor, n.d.).

Prepare Clients for a Pandemic

Teach clients that preparing for pandemic disease is similar to preparing for other general kinds of emergency preparedness, such as power outages and natural disasters (Self-Care: Teaching Your Patient About Preparing for a Pandemic Disease Outbreak).

Summary

After studying this chapter, you should be armed with the basic knowledge you need to protect yourself and your clients from infection. However, knowledge is not enough. Research continues to show that healthcare professionals too often fail to comply with guidelines for infection prevention, especially the seemingly simple measures such as hand hygiene and standard precautions. Your role as a nurse is to integrate the best current evidence with your clinical expertise and,

Self-Care

Teaching Your Patient About Preparing for a Pandemic Disease Outbreak

➤ Make a preparedness plan with your family and others in the community (e.g., school, business, church groups). Help organize local response planning and be available to help if there is an outbreak. Participate in emergency planning at work and get training if it is available.

➤ Talk with family members about what will be needed to care for them in your home if someone becomes ill.

➤ Expect that usual community services may be disrupted—for example, banks, stores, post offices, and even hospitals and public buildings may be closed

➤ Store a 2-week supply of bottled water and food. Keep extra nonperishable foods. Examples of food and nonperishables include:

　Ready-to-eat canned meats (e.g., ham, tuna)

　Canned fruits, vegetables, beans, soups

　Protein or fruit bars

　Dry cereals

　Peanut butter or nuts

　Dried fruit

　Crackers

　Canned juices

　Canned baby food and formula

　Pet food

➤ Periodically check your regular prescription drugs to keep a continuous supply on hand.

➤ Have nonprescription drugs and health supplies on hand. Examples include:

　Medical supplies, such as blood-pressure and glucose monitors

　Medicines for fever (e.g., acetaminophen, ibuprofen)

　Thermometer

　Soap and water or alcohol-based (60%–95%) handwash

　Antidiarrheal medication

　Vitamins

　Fluids with electrolytes

➤ Keep a 2-week supply of other emergency supplies on hand, such as a flashlight, batteries, portable radio, manual can opener, trash bags, tissues, toilet paper, and disposable diapers.

➤ Keep your family's health information up to date, organized, and accessible.

➤ Make sure you have more than one method to communicate (e.g., telephone and e-mail) and that you can get information from the outside world (including by battery-powered radio).

➤ Be sure everyone in the family washes hands frequently and properly and covers coughs and sneezes with tissues.

➤ Teach family members to stay away from others as much as possible if they are sick. Stay home from work and school if sick.

➤ Get an annual seasonal influenza vaccination.

➤ Explore the possibility of working by telecommuting during a pandemic to avoid unnecessary exposure.

Resources

Davey, V. (2007). Disaster care. Questions and answers on pandemic influenza. *American Journal of Nursing, 107*(7): 50–57; Emergency preparedness and response (2008). New York State Department of Health. Retrieved August 8, 2008, from http://www.health.state.ny.us/ environmental/emergency/Pandemic flu planning checklists for individuals and families. U. S. Department of Health & Human Services. Retrieved August 9, 2008 from http://www.pandemicflu.gov/plan/individual/checklist. html Preparing makes sense. Get ready now (n.d.). U. S. Department of Homeland Security. Retrieved August 8, 2008 from www.ready.gov Veneema, T. G., & Tõke, J. (2006). Early detection and surveillance for biopreparedness and emerging infectious diseases. *Online Journal of Issues in Nursing, 11*(1). Retrieved July 29, 2008 from http://www.nursingworld. org/MainMenuCategories/ANAMarketplace/ANAPeriodicals/OJIN/ TableofContents/Volume112006/No1Jan31/tpc29_2c16059.aspx

through your own individual performance, to minimize harm to patients and others. This includes using technology and standardized practices that support patient safety and quality. Wash your hands! Follow standard precautions!

If you would like to know more about microbiology,

 Go to **Student Resources, A Brief Introduction to Microbiology,** on DavisPlus at http://davisplus.fadavis.com/ Wilkinson2

Toward Evidence-Based Practice

Siegel, J. H., & Korniewicz, D. M. (2007). Keeping patients safe: An interventional hand hygiene study at an oncology center. *Clinical Journal of Oncology Nursing, 11(5), 643–646.*

The purpose of this study was to investigate whether the introduction of a handheld sanitizer spray improved hand hygiene compliance of healthcare workers at an oncology center. Subjects included 25 licensed and 22 unlicensed healthcare professionals. Researchers assessed hand hygiene before and after routine clinical procedures. Participants were observed for 2 weeks before and then for 14 weeks after introduction of the handheld sanitizer spray. Baseline compliance rates were 53% before the sanitizer spray and 49% after it was introduced.

Raskind, C. H., Worley, S., Vinski, J., & Goldfarb, J. (2007). Hand hygiene compliance rates after an educational intervention in a neonatal intensive care unit. *Infection Control & Hospital Epidemiology, 28(9), 1096–1098.*

This observational study assessed the impact of a staff education program to promote hand hygiene. Observations were made before and after the education program. Before the education program, hand hygiene compliance was 89%; 1 month after the education program it increased to 100%. At 3 months, though, the rate decreased to the baseline 89%.

Gammon, J., Morgan-Samuel, H., & Gould, D. (2008). A review of the evidence for suboptimal compliance of healthcare practitioners to standard/universal infection control precautions. *Journal of Clinical Nursing, 17(2), 157–167.*

Internationally standard/universal precautions are regarded as fundamental in infection control and prevention. These researchers examined findings from international research about the extent to which practitioners comply with infection control precautions. They used 37 different studies. They concluded that compliance to infection control precautions is internationally suboptimal, and that compliance does improve after an intervention (e.g., education program). They stated that research fails to indicate whether after a period of time the compliance returns to the prestudy norm.

Ganczak, M., & Szych, Z. (2007). Surgical nurses and compliance with personal protective equipment. *Journal of Hospital Infection, 66(4), 346–351.*

A total of 601 surgical nurses from 18 randomly selected hospitals in Poland were surveyed using a confidential questionnaire. They found that compliance with personal protective equipment (PPE) varied considerably. 83% used gloves, but only 9% used eyewear, and only 5% of respondents routinely used gloves, masks, protective eyewear, and gowns when in contact with potentially infective material. They found higher compliance among those with previous training in infection control or experience of caring for an HIV patient. The most commonly stated reasons for noncompliance (each at about 30%) were nonavailability of PPE, conviction that the patient was not infected, and belief that following the recommended practices actually interfered with providing good patient care. Researchers recommended wider training in and evaluation of infection control.

1. From these abstracts, what do you know about the subjects in the studies?

2. In what way(s) do(es) the Gammon study support the other three studies? Where is the support lacking?

 Go to Chapter 20, **Toward Evidence-Based Practice Suggested Responses,** on the Student Resource Disk or DavisPlus at http://davisplus.fadavis.com/Wilkinson2

 Go to Chapter 20, **Resources for Caregivers and Health Professionals,** on the Student Resource Disk or DavisPlus at http://davisplus.fadavis.com/Wilkinson2

 Suggested Readings: Go to Chapter 20, **Reading More About Promoting Asepsis and Preventing Infection,** on the Student Resource Disk or DavisPlus at http://davisplus.fadavis.com/Wilkinson2.

 Bibliography: Go to Volume 2, Bibliography.

CHAPTER 21

Promoting Safety

Learning Outcomes

After completing this chapter, you should be able to:

➤ List the three leading causes of accidental death in the United States.

➤ Identify factors that create safety risks.

➤ Identify at least five safety hazards in the home environment and interventions to prevent injury from them.

➤ Discuss the steps to follow when you suspect that a client has ingested a poisonous substance.

➤ Describe the choking rescue maneuver, and identify instances when it is appropriate to use it.

➤ Describe the four main physical hazards that are found in the community and interventions to prevent injury from them.

➤ Describe and give examples of hazards that we encounter in the healthcare agency.

➤ Identify four interventions to prevent falls in the healthcare agency.

➤ Discuss when it is appropriate to use siderails in the healthcare agency.

➤ Properly apply restraints and discuss measures to prevent injury in clients who are restrained.

➤ Discuss at least one data collection instrument that is used to assess the client who is at risk for falls.

➤ Formulate a nursing diagnosis in relation to preventing injury in the environment.

➤ Write an individualized goal for clients with a nursing diagnosis of Risk for Falls.

Meet Your Patients

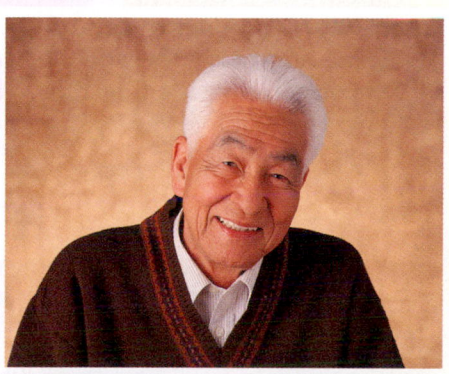

1. Alvin Lin is a 79-year-old man who was just transferred from a long-term care facility to your medical unit. His admitting diagnosis is dehydration and pneumonia. In morning report you were told that he had rested well during the night and was alert and oriented. When you enter his room, he is confused and does not know where he is. He is becoming combative and is trying to get out of bed. How should you respond to the situation?

2. Suppose you are a nurse making a home visit to Teresa, who lives in a rural area. Teresa is 20 years old and has a 2-year-old daughter. She is also responsible for caring for her elderly grandmother, who is recovering from a hip fracture. Teresa states that it is getting more difficult to keep up with her toddler, who is "into everything," and to care for the needs of her grandmother. Her grandmother has a fear of falling and is reluctant to do anything for herself.

Safety is a basic human need, second only to survival needs such as oxygen, nutrition, and fluids. As a nurse, you will be fundamentally concerned with the safety of your clients. You must also be concerned with your own safety and the safety of other care providers. Many accidental injuries can be prevented by being aware of hazards and taking reasonable precautions. This chapter will increase your ability to recognize safety hazards and to plan interventions that promote safety for clients of all ages, such as the two in "Meet Your Patients."

Theoretical **Knowledge** **knowing** why_____

According to the National Safety Council (NSC), accidents, or unintentional injuries, are the fifth leading cause of deaths in the United States. More than 120,000 people die each year as a result of accidents. Expressed another way, one person dies from an accident every 5 minutes. Motor vehicle accidents continue to be the number-one cause of unintentional death, followed by poisonings, falls, choking, fires, and drowning. Of course, the death rate is not the only significant number: approximately 2.8 million people were hospitalized for unintentional injuries in 2005 (NSC, 2008a). See Table 21-1.

Many healthcare organizations are campaigning for safer patient care in an effort to reduce the cost of healthcare and the burden of suffering. The following are examples:

- **The Joint Commission**, the accrediting body for healthcare facilities, each year publishes National Patient Safety Goals. For example, in 2009 the goals include improving the accuracy of patient identification, improving the safety of medication use, and reducing the risk of healthcare associated infections. For a link to the 2009 National Patient Safety Goals,

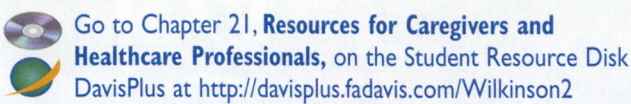 Go to Chapter 21, **Resources for Caregivers and Healthcare Professionals,** on the Student Resource Disk or DavisPlus at http://davisplus.fadavis.com/Wilkinson2

- **Institute of Medicine (IOM).** The IOM report, *To Err Is Human: Building a Safer Health System* brought public attention to patient safety. It stated that it is simply not acceptable for patients to be harmed by the same healthcare system that is supposed to offer healing and comfort. The report identified six major aims that can raise the quality of healthcare. Safety is among these aims (Committee on Quality of Health Care in America, 1999).
- **American Nurses Association (ANA).** *ANA's Health System Reform Agenda* (2008) recommends six major public policy changes that can raise the quality of healthcare. Quality Aim 1 is safe healthcare.
- **Quality and Safety Education for Nurses (QSEN)**, a task force to improve nursing education, identified and described six competencies that all nursing students should have by graduation. Safety is one of those competencies (Cronenwett, Sherwood, Barnsteiner, et al., 2007). For a list of the essential features that demonstrate the safety competence,

 Go to Chapter 21, **ESG Table 21-1, QSEN Safety Competency,** on the Student Resource Disk or DavisPlus at http://davisplus. fadavis.com/Wilkinson2

- **Medicare** has identified "never events": serious and costly errors that cause serious injury or death, and that are mostly preventable. Included in the list of never events are injuries from falls, burns, restraints, or bedrails. Medicare will no longer pay institutions for care required to treat the effects of such errors (Centers for Medicare and Medicaid Services, 2006a, 2008).

What Factors Affect Safety?

To promote client safety, you will need theoretical knowledge about developmental stages and individual risk factors that affect clients' ability to avoid accidental injury. This chapter discusses specific risk factors and describes hazards in three environments: the home, the community, and the healthcare agency. **Environmental hazards** are situations or conditions in which something in the environment can cause human illness or injury. **Environment** includes the physical and psychosocial factors that contribute to each person's life and well-being. You can also define it as any setting in which the nurse and client interact.

Developmental Factors

The type and incidence of accidents vary among age groups. You will find interventions for all age groups integrated into the topics of home, community, and healthcare agency throughout the rest of this chapter. Keep in mind that the descriptions given for each age

Table 21-1 ➤ Leading Causes of Unintentional Deaths in the United States	
MECHANISM OF INJURY	**TOTAL ANNUAL DEATHS, ALL AGE GROUPS**
Motor vehicles	43,432
Poisoning and exposure to noxious substances	30,308
Falls	18,807
Drowning	3,308
Fires, flames, and smoke	3,229

Source: Miniño, A. M., Heron, M. P., Murphy, S. L., et al. (2007). *Deaths: Final data for 2004. National Vital Statistics Reports*, 55(19). Hyattsville, MD: National Center for Health Statistics.

group are characteristics common to most people in that group. However, individuals progress through developmental stages at their own pace, so there will always be some people who do not fit the group description closely. For supplemental discussion of safety needs during different developmental stages,

 Go to Chapter 9, **Expanded Discussion**, on the Student Resource Disk or DavisPlus at http://davisplus.fadavis.com/Wilkinson2

Infant/Toddler. Motor vehicle accidents are the leading cause of death for children ages 1 to 3, followed by drowning. Falls, choking, sudden infant death syndrome (SIDS), and ingesting poisons are other critical safety concerns. Infants and toddlers are completely dependent on others for their care. They have the ability to walk and manipulate objects before they have the judgment to recognize dangers such as falling. In addition, infants and toddlers are curious and tend to explore the environment by putting objects in their mouth. This is why the incidence of choking is highest between 6 months and 3 years of age. As mobility continues to improve, toddlers gain more freedom, and their curiosity leads them to explore cupboards, stairs, open windows, swimming pools, and other hazards (National Center for Injury Prevention and Control, 2007).

Preschooler. Motor vehicle injuries continue to be a major cause of accidental death, along with drowning, fires, and poisoning. However, falls are the primary cause of nonfatal injuries. After age 3, children are a little less prone to falls because their gross and fine motor skills, coordination, and balance have improved. However, the extension of play to the outside environment (playgrounds, pools, front yards, and so on) creates additional safety concerns. Although this age group is more aware of dangers and limitations, adult supervision continues to be essential.

School-age Child. Motor vehicles continue to be the leading cause of accidental death in children in this age group. However, the leading cause of nonfatal injury is falls. School-age children have developed more refined muscle coordination and control, and their decision-making skills have improved. However, because they become more involved in activities outside the home, bone and muscle injuries are common. Injuries are often related to sports, skateboarding, or bicycle riding. Playground injuries are also common. Most school-age children are ready to try any new skill with or without practice or training. They are less fearful than are toddlers. Exposure to the wider school and neighborhood environment also increases the risk for injury inflicted by people outside the home (e.g., abduction).

Adolescent. The leading cause of death in this age group is motor vehicle accidents, followed by homicide. Both of these are frequently associated with alcohol and drug use. Sports and recreational injuries, including diving and drowning incidents are also common, especially when drinking and drug use are involved. Peak physical, sensory, and psychomotor abilities give teenagers a feeling of strength and confidence, yet they lack the wisdom and judgment of adults. This combination, along with feelings of being indestructible, makes them more likely to participate in risk-taking behavior, and, in turn, more prone to injury.

Adult. Motor vehicle accidents continue to be the major cause of death and injury in this age group, along with unintentional poisoning. Workplace injury may also be a significant concern. Other injuries to adults are related to lifestyle (e.g., excessive alcohol use), stress, carelessness, abuse, and decline in strength and stamina. For many, work and family responsibilities often leave little time for regular physical activity, increasing the risk of musculoskeletal injury in the so-called weekend athlete.

Older Adult. Although many older adults have intact senses that enable them to continue to enjoy life as they age, physiological changes do occur. These changes may include reduced muscle strength and joint mobility; slowing of reflexes; decreased ability to respond to multiple stimuli; and sensory losses, particularly hearing and vision. These changes increase the older adult's risk for falls, burns, car accidents, and other injury. Falls are the most common cause of accidental death for adults age 50 and older (Centers for Disease Control and Prevention [CDC], 2004).

Individual Risk Factors

In addition to developmental stage, individual factors also influence a person's risk for unintentional injury. These include lifestyle, cognitive awareness, sensoriperceptual status, ability to communicate, mobility status, physical and emotional health, and awareness of safety measures. Table 21-2 summarizes individual risk factors.

KnowledgeCheck 21-1

- What are some important developmental considerations when providing a safe environment for a preschool child?
- What is the main cause of injuries during the adolescent period?
- What are some ways that the aging process makes the older adult more prone to injury?
- Based on your theoretical knowledge and the scant patient data you have, why do you think Teresa's toddler ("Meet Your Patients") is at risk for accidents? What about Teresa's grandmother?

 Go to Chapter 21, **Knowledge Check Response Sheet and Answers,** on the Student Resource Disk or DavisPlus at http://davisplus.fadavis.com/Wilkinson2

What Safety Hazards Are in the Home?

What safety issues in the home environment would you need to assess with regard to Teresa's toddler and grandmother? If you cannot already answer the question

Table 21-2 ➤ Individual Risk Factors For Injury

RISK FACTORS	BEHAVIOR MANIFESTATION
Lifestyle	Smoking, alcohol abuse, risk-taking behaviors
Cognitive awareness	Confusion due to stress and loss of short-term memory
Sensory and perceptual status	Loss of senses (e.g., vision, hearing, pain), which provide first line of defense
Impaired communication	Language barriers and hearing and speech impairment related to disease processes
Impaired mobility	Impaired strength with accompanying problems in mobility, balance, and endurance
Physical and emotional well-being	Reduced physical stamina and depression, with feelings of loss of control and helplessness
Safety awareness	Reduced cognitive awareness (e.g., of older adult) and immature development of the child

about Teresa's family and home, you should be able to do so after reading this section. The following discussion provides an overview of conditions within the home that increase the risk for injury and death.

Except for motor vehicle accidents, most fatal accidents occur in the home. The leading causes of death in the home are poisonings, falls, fires and burns, and choking. For children, maternal depression, lack of parental social support, and domestic conflict are associated with less safe homes (Rhodes & Iwashyna, 2007).

Poisoning

Poisoning is a leading cause of accidental death; poisoning death rates have more than tripled in the past two decades. Although young children are frequent victims, the increase has been mainly among adults—primarily due to abuse of opioid analgesics. In many cases, the person does not die but becomes ill or suffers other effects. Poisoning exposure accounts for well over 700,000 emergency department visits per year.

Most poisoning of young children occurs because of improper storage of household chemicals, medicines and vitamins, and cosmetics (CDC, n.d., Poisoning...). Box 21-1 lists poisonous agents commonly ingested by children.

Lead poisoning has been a problem in the United States since the 1900s, when white lead was added to paints and tetraethyl lead was added to gasoline. The use of lead in paint has been banned since 1978, but

lead-based paint can still be found in older homes and toys produced in some foreign countries. Some soil (which young children often put in their mouths) contains high lead content. In the United States, poor, urban, and immigrant populations are at higher risk for lead exposure than other groups.

Older children and adolescents may attempt suicide by overdosing with medicines or be poisoned accidentally when experimenting with recreational or prescription drugs intended for adults. In adults, most poisonings occur as a result of illegal drug use or misuse or abuse of prescription drugs, especially narcotic medications, tranquilizers, and antidepressants.

Treatment choice depends on the poison ingested. For most poisonings, the most effective intervention is professional administration of activated charcoal orally or via gastric tube. However, charcoal is not effective for ethanol, alkali, iron, boric acid, lithium, methanol, or cyanide. Depending on the situation, other options for medical treatment include gastric lavage, dialysis, administration of antidotes, and forced diuresis. For a list of medical treatments for commonly ingested poisons,

 Go to Chapter 21, **Tables, Boxes, Figures: ESG Table 21-2,** on the Student Resource Disk or DavisPlus at http://davisplus.fadavis.com/Wilkinson2

✚ Never induce vomiting when the ingested material is acidic or caustic to the esophagus. Although the American Academy of Pediatrics no longer recommends inducing emesis (e.g., with syrup of ipecac), some practitioners may still do so. The National Poison Control Center does not support the routine stocking of ipecac in households with young children. They state that it should be given only on specific recommendation from a poison center or qualified medical personnel (Association of Poison Control Centers, n.d.).

BOX 21-1 ■ Poisonous Agents Commonly Ingested by Children

- Household cleansers, including oven cleaner, drain cleaner, toilet bowl cleaner, and furniture polish
- Medicines, including cough and cold preparations, vitamins, pain medications, antidepressants, anticonvulsants, and iron tablets, which to children may look like M&M candies
- Indoor house plants, including poinsettia, Dieffenbachia, philodendron, and many others
- Cosmetics, hair relaxer, nail products, mouthwash
- Pesticides
- Kerosene, gasoline, lighter fluid, paint thinner, lamp oil, antifreeze, windshield washer fluid, lighter fluid, and other chemicals
- Alcoholic beverages
- Wild plants and mushrooms
- Pesticides, rodent poisons

Carbon Monoxide Exposure

Carbon monoxide (CO) is a colorless, tasteless, odorless, toxic gas. Exposure can cause headaches, weakness, nausea, and vomiting; prolonged exposure leads to seizures, dysrhythmias, unconsciousness, brain damage, and death. Each year in the United States, CO poisoning causes approximately 500 unintentional deaths (Nonfatal, unintentional. . ., 2008). It accounts for a majority of deaths at the scene of fires, and is also a relatively common method of suicide.

The burning of fuel, such as wood, oil, gasoline, natural gas, kerosene, and coal produces CO. Dangerous levels of CO can build up because of a faulty furnace, and it builds up quickly in an unventilated garage when a car is running. Other consumer products involved in CO-related deaths include lawn mowers, charcoal grills, gas water heaters, camp stoves or lanterns, and gas ranges or ovens. Many CO deaths occur during cold weather among older adults and the poor who seek nonconventional heat sources (e.g., gas ranges and ovens) to stay warm.

Scalds and Burns

Scald injuries (e.g., from hot water, steam, or grease) are the most common cause of burns in children younger than the age of 3. Warming food or formula in the microwave may cause the food to become hotter than intended, leading to burns in infants and young children. Sunburn can cause a first- or second-degree burn, and burns may occur from contact with metal surfaces and vinyl seats when cars are parked in the sun. Scalding burns (especially on both feet or both hands) and cigarette burns in children and vulnerable older adults should always prompt you to assess for abuse.

The risk of contact burns in all age groups is greater in the presence of such heating devices as kerosene heaters, wood-burning stoves, and home sauna heating elements. People may use these as alternative heat sources when they cannot afford the cost of traditional furnace fuels. Chemical agents, such as acid, alkali, or other organic compounds, can also cause localized burns.

Fires

Home fires are a major cause of death and injury. Older adults and children younger than the age of 5 years have the greatest risk of fire death. Cooking fires are the number-one cause of home fires and home fire injuries. However, most *fatal* home fires occur while people are asleep, and most fire-related deaths occur from smoke inhalation. Smoking (e.g., cigarettes) is the leading cause of fatal home fires, but during the winter months, heating equipment is equally responsible. Home oxygen administration equipment is also a hazard. In 75% of the home fires involving oxygen, smoking materials are the ignition source; cooking and candles are other common factors. When more oxygen is in the air, items such as hair, plastic, skin oils, clothing, and furniture catch fire at lower temperatures. Any fire that starts will burn hotter and faster. Other causes of fire include unsupervised children playing with matches, improper use of candles, and faulty wiring.

Falls

Falls are the third leading cause of injury-related deaths—the leading cause for older adults. An average of 4 in 100 people experience a nonfatal fall for which they seek medical advice. The rate triples for adults older than age 75 (Adams, Barnes, & Vickerie, 2007). More than half of all falls occur in the home, and about 80% of home falls involve people age 65 years and older. Most injuries caused by falls happen at ground level, not from falls in high places. Falls are more likely to occur when it is dark, when there are spills and clutter, when pets get in the way, and when people are sick, tired, hurrying, or emotionally upset.

Environmental factors that contribute to falls include slippery floors and bathtubs, lack of grab bars, low toilet seats, and high beds. Health issues that increase the risk for falls include poor vision, hypotension (low blood pressure), a history of falls, dizziness, pain, alcohol use, cognitive impairment, polypharmacy, arthritis, gait or balance deficits, and age greater than 80 years (Akyol, 2007; Kenny, Rubenstein, Martin, et al., 2001).

Firearm Injuries

Gun ownership is a controversial issue. Some people keep guns in the home for protection and/or recreation (e.g., hunting, target shooting). However, guns are a source of unintentional injury and death. Gun safety and security are especially important when there are children in the home or someone with a substance abuse problem. Young children may handle a loaded gun with tragic results. Household access to firearms has been implicated as a risk factor for youth suicide and domestic homicide, as well as unintentional injury (Hizel, Ozcebe, Sanli, et al., 2008). Because of the frequency and severity of unintentional firearm injuries involving children, the American Academy of Pediatrics and other groups have mounted efforts to educate parents about firearm safety.

Critical Thinking 21-1

- What are some initial questions you might ask Teresa regarding the home environment?
- What are some basic interventions you might suggest to Teresa to help child-proof her home? To answer this question, you will need to recall information about:
  Safety hazards that we encounter in the home
  Developmental and lifestyle factors that affect safety
  Specific nursing activities that can be used to prevent accidents or injuries related to the environmental hazards (e.g., firearms)

Suffocation/Asphyxiation

Suffocation by smothering is the leading cause of death for infants younger than 1 year. Suffocation may be caused by drowning, choking on a foreign object, or inhaling gas or smoke. Food items, including hot dogs, raw vegetables, popcorn, hard candies, nuts, and grapes, are responsible for most nonfatal choking incidents. Nonfood items, such as latex balloons and plastic bags, cause the majority of suffocation deaths in young children. Suffocation of infants is often related to bed or crib hazards, such as excess bedding or pillows, or toys hung from long ribbons inside the infant's crib. Infants can become entangled in cords from window blinds or in the ribbon or string used to hang a pacifier around an infant's neck.

Drowning is an important cause of accidental death in children 1 to 18 years old. Children up to age 4 are especially at risk for drowning and should never be left unattended in or near a bathtub, hot tub, swimming pool, or other source of water. Even wading pools, toilets, and mop buckets hold enough water to drown a small child.

KnowledgeCheck 21-2

- What are the most common poisonous agents ingested by children?
- Name one source of CO poisoning.

 Go to Chapter 21, **Knowledge Check Response Sheet and Answers,** on the Student Resource Disk or DavisPlus at http://davisplus.fadavis.com/Wilkinson2

Take-Home Toxins

Take-home toxins are hazardous substances transported from the workplace to the home. The National Institute for Occupational Safety and Health (NIOSH, 2003, 2004) reports that pathogenic microorganisms, asbestos, lead, mercury, arsenic, pesticides, caustic farm products, and dozens of other agents cause significant morbidity and mortality in workers' homes (NIOSH, 2003, 2004). These toxins are most likely transported to workers' homes on the workers themselves, on their clothing, or on objects brought from the workplace. In the home, contamination occurs via any of three sources:

- Direct skin-to-skin contact, or direct contact with contaminated clothing
- Arthropod vectors, such as ticks that are responsible for Lyme disease
- Transmission on dust particles that are inhaled (e.g., anthrax spores, arsenic in mine and smelter dust)

Most preventive measures apply to the workplace. However, you can teach clients who are at risk to remove work clothing and to shower, preferably in an open-air shower, before leaving work. If facilities for showering are not available, patient advocacy may be appropriate. (To learn about advocacy, see Chapter 44.)

Before entering their homes, exposed workers who have not showered should remove their clothing. Then they should shower immediately. When handling contaminated clothes or objects, they should wear gloves to reduce the risk of skin transmission. Laundering may not be effective in removing certain toxins in clothes.

What Safety Hazards Are in the Community?

Hazardous agents in the community are a major contributor to illness, disability, and death worldwide. This section discusses four major topics of concern: motor vehicle accidents, pathogens, pollution, and electrical storms.

Motor Vehicle Accidents

Motor vehicle accidents (MVAs) are the leading cause of accidental death in American adults and children older than 1 year of age. They account for about 37% of all accidental deaths. Failure to use seat belts and proper child car seats continues to be the major contributing factor. Severe injuries and death also occur from air bag deployment when young children are improperly placed in the front passenger seat. Many of the fatal MVAs during adolescence involve abuse of alcohol or other substances (CDC, 2006a, 2007; Miniño, Heron, Murphy, et al., 2007; National Safety Council, 2008a). The risk of being injured or killed in a car crash increases for older drivers. Every day, on average, 500 people over age 65 are injured in an automobile accident.

KnowledgeCheck 21-3

List two things a person who works around workplace toxins can do to prevent bringing them into the home.

 Go to Chapter 21, **Knowledge Check Response Sheet and Answers,** on the Student Resource Disk or DavisPlus at http://davisplus.fadavis.com/Wilkinson2

Pathogens

A **pathogen** is any microorganism capable of causing an illness. Pathogens can enter the body through several sources in the environment: food, mosquitoes and other insects, rodents and other animals, and unclean water.

Food-Borne Pathogens

Food poisoning is a nonspecific term that describes illness caused by ingesting bacteria and other microorganisms, or their toxins, in food. Improper food storage and preparation are a major cause of food poisoning. Raw foods are commonly associated with food-borne illness, for example, raw meat, poultry, eggs, shellfish, raw fruits and vegetables, and unpasteurized milk and fruit juice. Poisonous chemicals in the environment, such as mercury, arsenic, zinc, and potassium chlorate, may also contaminate foods. Education is an important intervention for preventing food poisoning. See the section, "Teaching for Safety Self-Care Food-Borne Pathogens," later in the chapter.

Vector-Borne Pathogens

Vectors are organisms that transmit pathogenic bacteria, viruses, and protozoa from one host to another. They include mosquitoes and other insects, rodents, birds, and other animals.

The severity of the reaction to a mosquito bite depends on the degree of allergy to the mosquito's saliva. In addition to the discomfort caused by bites, infected mosquitoes can transmit diseases, such as West Nile virus and malaria. They can also transmit parasites to domestic animals (e.g., dog heartworm, equine encephalitis). Strategies to control mosquito infestation include spraying programs and digging ditches to promote drainage from stagnant areas. All pesticides, whether used by an agency or the consumer, should have the name and amount of active ingredient on the label. No pesticide is 100% safe, so people must use them cautiously.

Other insects, such as roaches, fleas, ticks, sand flies, and lice, can also transmit serious diseases and produce a wide variety of allergens. Allergic sensitivity to cockroaches, for example, is a predictive factor for asthma severity (Lopes, Miranda, & Sarinho, 2006).

Rodents and other animals can also act as vectors and allergens. For example, rabies can be spread through the bite of a rabid animal, some fungal diseases can spread via the inhalation of bird droppings, and mouse proteins have been implicated in occurrence of asthma. Structural defects in a building (e.g., roofs and walls) permit entry of birds, rodents, and other small animals, and dead spaces in walls permit their circulation among apartments in multiunit dwellings (Berg, McConnell, Milam, et al., 2008; Krieger & Higgins, 2002).

Water-Borne Pathogens

Sanitation refers to measures to promote and establish favorable health conditions, especially those related to the community's water supply. People who live in substandard housing may not have safe drinking water, hot water for washing, or adequate methods of waste disposal. People in rural areas often depend on private wells, which may not be adequately maintained and tested for pathogens, such as *Giardia lamblia*, *Cryptosporidium*, and *Escherichia coli*. These are primarily community health problems (see Chapter 42).

Pollution

Pollution is any harmful chemical or waste material discharged into the air, water, or soil. Examples of pollutants are gaseous fumes, asbestos, carbon monoxide, and cigarette smoke. Each year Americans generate millions of tons of waste in their homes and communities (Environmental Protection Agency [EPA], 2008).

- *Air pollution* occurs outdoors and indoors. Motor vehicle emissions are a major cause of *outdoor air pollution* in the United States. Other toxic air pollutants include asbestos; toluene; metals such as mercury, chromium, and lead compounds; and other emissions from factories and power plants. *Indoor pollutants* include radon; carbon monoxide; and allergens from dust mites, cockroaches, mold, rodents, and pets. Allergens are an important health issue because people spend most of their time indoors. Passive exposure to tobacco smoke is associated with respiratory disease and cancer; and environmental air pollution is linked to cardiovascular disease and respiratory viral infection (Ciencewicki & Jaspers, 2007; National Cancer Institute, n.d.; Walker & Mouton, 2008; U.S. Department of Health and Human Services, 2006).
- *Water contamination* in lakes, rivers, and streams ultimately affects both recreation and food production of these waters. Pollution occurs when inadequately treated or inappropriate quantities of human, industrial, or agricultural wastes are released into the water systems. If the pollution is severe enough, the water may become unsafe for human consumption.
- *Noise.* Substantial exposure to noise has been associated with a range of adverse health effects, including hearing loss, stress, elevated blood pressure, and loss of sleep. Noise is pervasive in our society—for example, from road traffic, jet planes, garbage trucks, construction equipment, lawn mowers, and loud music. People who live or work near major roads, bus depots, airports, and trucking routes are at greater risk, as are those in certain work environments (e.g., railroad workers) (U.S. Department of Health and Human Services, 2000).
- *Soil* can become contaminated by improper waste disposal and excessive use of pesticides. Agricultural, industrial, and manufacturing processes create solid and toxic waste. Animal, radioactive, and medical wastes pose special problems. Household products, such as paints, cleaners, oils, batteries, and pesticides, contain corrosive or toxic ingredients that contaminate the environment when disposed of improperly (e.g., in household trash or poured down the drain, on the ground, or into storm sewers).

Electrical Storms

According to the National Weather Service, deaths from lightning strikes lead all other categories of weather-related fatalities. Weather conditions play a major role in outdoor recreation programming. It is important for professionals, participants, and outdoor recreation providers to understand severe weather conditions, specifically thunderstorms and lightning, and the dangers associated with them.

KnowledgeCheck 21-4

- What are the major causes of MVAs?
- List at least three tips for preventing food poisoning.
- What other forms of pollution can invade a healthful environment?

 Go to Chapter 21, **Knowledge Check Response Sheet and Answers,** on the Student Resource Disk or DavisPlus at http://davisplus.fadavis.com/Wilkinson2

 CriticalThinking 21-2

Identify an environmental problem in your neighborhood. What are some possible solutions?

What Safety Hazards Are in the Healthcare Facility?

As many as 98,000 people die from medical injuries each year in U.S. hospitals (Overview of the 100,000. . . n.d.). Several characteristics of healthcare facilities pose safety hazards for residents and workers. We have already discussed the hazard of infection in Chapter 20. Box 21-2 lists the Joint Commission's National Patient Safety Goals for 2009, which should give you an idea of the types of accidents that occur in healthcare agencies. If you would like to see a full explanation of the patient safety goals,

---

BOX 21-2 ■ The Joint Commission 2009 Patient Safety Goals

Goal 1. Improve the accuracy of patient identification.

Goal 2. Improve effectiveness of communication among caregivers.

Goal 3. Improve the safety of using medications.

Goal 7. Reduce the risk of healthcare associated infections.

Goal 8. Accurately and completely reconcile medications across the continuum of care.

Goal 9. Reduce the risk of patient harm resulting from falls.

Goal 13. Encourage patients' active involvement in their own care as a patient safety strategy.

Goal 15. The organization identifies safety risks inherent in its patient population.

Goal 16. Improve recognition and response to changes in a patient's condition.

Universal Protocol: The organization meets the expectations of the Universal Protocol. (This is a preprocedure verification process to make sure that all documents, information, and equipment are available, and that the correct procedure is performed on the correct person and site.)

Source: Adapted from The Joint Commission (2008a). *The Joint Commission Accreditation Program: Hospital. National Patient Safety Goals.* Retrieved from http://www.jointcommission.org/patientsafety/nationalpatientsafetygoals/

 Go to the Joint Commission Web site, in Chapter 21, **Resources for Caregivers and Health Professionals,** on the Student Resource Disk or DavisPlus at http://davisplus.fadavis.com/Wilkinson2

What Are Never Events?

Never events are healthcare-acquired complications for which Medicare will no longer reimburse institutions. Never events can cause serious injury or death to a patient, and should *never* happen in a hospital. You can also gain insight into healthcare facility hazards by examining the following list of never events (Centers for Medicare and Medicaid Services, 2008).

- Foreign object (such as a sponge) left in patients after surgery
- Air embolism
- Administering the wrong type of blood
- Severe pressure ulcers
- Falls and trauma
- Infections associated with urinary catheters
- Infections associated with intravenous catheters
- Symptoms resulting from poorly controlled blood sugar levels
- Surgical site infections following certain elective procedures (e.g., certain orthopedic surgeries, bariatric surgery for obesity)
- Deep vein thrombosis or pulmonary embolism following total knee and total hip replacement procedures.

The Institute for Healthcare Improvement (IHI), an independent, not-for-profit organization, launched the 100,000 Lives Campaign to recommend changes to reduce morbidity and death in American healthcare. At least three of the 100,000 Lives goals support the list of never events: Prevent adverse drug events, prevent central line infections, and prevent surgical site infections. To read the entire list of recommendations,

 Go to Chapter 21, **ESG Box 21-1, The 100,000 Lives Campaign,** in the Student Resource Disk or DavisPlus at http://davisplus.fadavis.com/Wilkinson2

 CriticalThinking 21-3

Many never events can be reduced by good nursing care. By preventing complications and maximizing reimbursement, nurses can prove their value to an organization and make the case for better staffing. Over which of the never events do you think nurses have the most control? Explain your thinking.

Falls

Although anyone can fall, infants and older adults are especially at risk for injury from falls. Most falls occur in the home, but they are a major concern in healthcare facilities, as well. Falls are by far the most common incident reported in hospitals and long-term care facilities (CDC, Falls Among. . . , n.d.). Many patients have risk factors, such as poor vision, cognitive impairment, difficulty with walking or balance, orthostatic hypotension, weakness or dizziness from disease or therapy, and drowsiness from medications. Many cases involve falling from a bed, and falls occur more frequently on nights, weekends, and holidays. Most agencies have established procedures and safety features to prevent falls.

Equipment-Related Accidents

Equipment-related accidents usually occur when equipment malfunctions or is used improperly, for example, when bed alarms fail to work or are set up incorrectly, when suction devices and infusion pumps are not working properly, oxygen cylinders are transported incorrectly, or wheelchairs and beds are not locked during transfer activities. The following interventions help ensure safe use of equipment.

- Seek advice if you are unsure how to operate the equipment.
- Make sure medical equipment has been properly inspected.
- Be alert to signs that the equipment is not functioning properly.
- Make sure that rooms are not cluttered with equipment.
- Follow agency policies regarding equipment brought from the patient's home (e.g., hair dryers, electric shavers, radios); usually these should be inspected for proper grounding and safe cords.

Fires and Electrical Hazards

Because most institutions promote a smoke-free environment, fire in a healthcare agency is more often related to anesthesia or improperly grounded or malfunctioning electrical equipment. Most healthcare agencies have policies for preventing electrical hazards. Nevertheless, patients and visitors do break the rules, so smoking cannot be discounted as a hazard.

When a fire occurs in a public building, an announcement is made over the communication system. Often, words such as "Code Red" or "Code Yellow" are used in an effort to prevent panic among patients and visitors. Depending on the situation, the announcement may ask visitors to leave the building. All personnel must know the fire escape route and follow hospital policy regarding fires.

If you discover a fire, your first instinct may be to contain or put out the fire. Fight that instinct! Your first action is to rescue the patient—move the patient(s) away from the area. Only then should you sound the alarm and attempt to confine the fire. Remember the mnemonic RACE:

Rescue

Activate

Confine

Extinguish

Restraints

A **restraint** is a device or method used for the purpose of restricting a patient's freedom of movement or access to his body, with or without his permission. The most obvious form of restraint is the use of physical force by another person. A restraint may also be (1) a mechanical device, material, or equipment, such as a cloth vest or siderails or (2) a chemical restraint given to control disruptive behavior, for example sedatives and psychotropic agents. Devices such as casts and traction are not considered restraints (Centers for Medicare and Medicaid Services, 2006a; Healthcare Financing Administration [HCFA], 2000; The Joint Commission, 2008b).

Restraints are classified according to the reason for their use: Medical–surgical restraints or restraints used for behavior management. Medicare has specific guidelines for each circumstance. Guidelines are more restrictive when restraints are used for behavior management.

As a safety measure, nurses traditionally restrained highly dependent older adults, patients with poor mobility, those with impaired cognitive status, and those they judged to be at risk for falls. However, they have found that restraints make care more time-consuming and do not reduce falls. Restraints are themselves a safety hazard, and actually increase the likelihood of injury. A restrained person has a natural tendency to struggle and try to remove the restraint and, as a result, can become entangled, suffer nerve damage, circulatory impairment, and even suffocation. Restraint-imposed immobility can cause pressure ulcers, contractures, loss of strength, and other hazards of immobility. Emotionally, the person may suffer anger, fear, humiliation, and diminished self-esteem.

Avoid Restraints When Possible

Research indicates that less restraint use saves time and money, and reduces patient injuries (leBel & Goldstein, 2005; Tilly & Reed, 2008). For those reasons, healthcare facilities are trying to achieve restraint-free environments. When the decision is made to avoid restraints, it is essential to provide alternatives for keeping the patient safe. Multiple approaches are needed, including careful and ongoing assessment and surveillance, finding ways to communicate with the patient, and tailoring exercise programs, medication reviews, and environmental modifications to the needs of individual patients.

To provide the safest possible care environment, the Joint Commission encourages healthcare facilities to:

- Promote among all direct-care staff a commitment to reduce the use of restraints and seclusion.
- Educate caregivers before they take part in any restraint-related activity.
- Document restraint episodes specifically, in detail.
- Maintain one-on-one viewing of patients in restraint and seclusion.

- Include staff members when deciding whether to explore new technology that is considered a safe alternative to traditional restraint devices.
- Budget for an adequate number of qualified staff to attend to patients.

Restraint Is Sometimes Necessary

Restraints may sometimes be necessary. Guidelines are slightly different depending on whether restraints are used to directly support medical healing or for a behavioral health reason (e.g., when a patient is irrational and pulling out his IV lines). Use restraints only as a last resort. As much as possible, use technology (such as bed alarms) and better anticipation of patient needs instead of restraints. If you must use restraints,

 Medicare, The Joint Commission, and other regulators require that restraints be medically prescribed and that you try all less restrictive interventions before using them.

Do Not Depend on Siderails

Siderails are often used in efforts to promote a safe environment or as an aid to independence. It is important to note that, based on the HCFA standards, siderails can be viewed as a restraint. A full-length siderail is a restraint when it is used to prevent the patient from getting out of bed regardless of whether he is able to do so safely. A half- or quarter-length upper siderail can be an aid to independence if it is used by the patient for the purpose of getting into and out of bed. Similarly, split rails are not considered restraints if a client requests them in order to feel more secure (Talerico & Capezuti, 2001; The Joint Commission, 2005).

Remember that older or cognitively impaired adults may regard siderails as a barrier rather than as a reminder that they need assistance. Several studies have shown that siderails may lead to serious falls and injuries. These findings have led healthcare providers to reevaluate the use of restraints and to recommend that siderails not be used routinely (Brusch & Capezuti, 2001; Capezuti, Wagner, Brush, et al., 2007; Evans & Cotter, 2008).

KnowledgeCheck 21-5

- What is a typical cause of fire in healthcare facilities?
- What measures should you take, and in what order, if a fire occurs in the hospital?

 Go to Chapter 21, **Knowledge Check Response Sheet and Answers,** on the Student Resource Disk or DavisPlus at http://davisplus.fadavis.com/Wilkinson2

Mercury Exposure

Mercury is a heavy, odorless, silver-white liquid metal. Mercury is toxic in both acute and chronic exposure. It can be inhaled, ingested, or absorbed through the skin.

It accumulates in muscle tissue and can cause renal and neurological disorders, especially in fetuses and neonates. Because of its shiny color and ability to form beads or balls, mercury is appealing to curious children. See Table 21-3 for potential health effects.

Mercury is most likely to be found in high school and university laboratories, healthcare facilities, and old industrial sites. Products containing mercury include thermometers, thermostats, batteries, fluorescent light bulbs, blood pressure devices, and electrical equipment and switches. For more information about products and devices that may contain mercury,

Go to Chapter 21, **ESG Box 21-2, Products and Devices that May Contain Mercury,** on the Student Resource Disk or DavisPlus at http://davisplus.fadavis.com/Wilkinson2

In 1998, the American Hospital Association (AHA) and the Environmental Protection Agency (EPA) launched a program to eliminate mercury-containing waste in the healthcare industry and prevent it from entering the environment via incinerators, landfills, and wastewater. Mercury thermometers are no longer being made in the United States. However, a very few pharmacies in the United States may still sell them and some people may still have them in their homes. Most, but not all, healthcare facilities have eliminated mercury thermometers and sphygmomanometers. You can help prevent mercury poisoning by taking an active role in

Table 21-3 ➤ Potential Health Effects of Mercury	
PRIMARY ROUTE	**POTENTIAL HEALTH EFFECTS**
	Acute Effects
Toxicity	Symptoms of chills, nausea, malaise, chest tightness and pain, dyspnea, coughing, stomatitis, gingivitis, excess salivation, and diarrhea. High levels can cause severe respiratory irritation, digestive disturbances, and severe renal damage.
Inhalation	Respiratory damage, wakefulness, muscle weakness, anorexia, headache, ringing in the ears, chest pain, inflammation of the mouth, and pneumonitis
Eye	Irritation and corrosion
Skin	Irritation and allergic dermatitis
Ingestion	Intestinal obstruction
	Chronic Effects
Primarily central nervous system	Numbness or tingling of the hands, lips, and feet; behavior and personality changes
Other	Fatigue, weakness, anorexia, weight loss, and gastrointestinal disturbances

eliminating mercury-containing items from your workplace. Some hospitals conduct thermometer exchanges, providing free or low-cost nonmercury thermometers to anyone who brings in a mercury thermometer.

Healthcare facilities must have policies and procedures for hazardous waste spills. These are required by The Joint Commission and federal agencies such as the EPA (2002) and the Occupational Safety and Health Administration (OSHA). You are not likely to encounter mercury exposure in acute care and ambulatory agencies.

Biological Hazards

As a nurse, you will place a high priority on the biological safety of patients. Institutionalized patients are at especially high risk from infectious microorganisms, some of which are highly resistant to antibiotics. To learn about or review healthcare-related infections, asepsis, and infection control, refer to Chapter 20.

Hazards to Healthcare Workers

Nursing is an active profession, and workplace injuries are all too common. Common accidents include back injuries, needlestick injuries, radiation injury, and violence. Nurses sometimes hesitate to report they have been injured because they fear being labeled a complainer or trouble-maker. Some also fear being denied opportunities for promotion and other consequences. However, OSHA requires that employers show employees how to report a workplace injury and prohibits discrimination against employees who make such reports. You should always report an injury. By doing so, you help (1) pinpoint trends and areas of need in safety, and (2) ensure you will receive necessary treatment and follow-up.

Back Injury

Nursing personnel are consistently listed in the top 10 occupations for work-related musculoskeletal disorders (MSDs). Most often the MSD involves the shoulders and back (Bureau of Labor Statistics, 2006). The American Nurses Association (ANA) reports that 52% of nurses report chronic back pain (ANA, 2003), likely because many nursing tasks require bending and twisting of the torso, activities that can cause injury when the nurse does not use correct body mechanics. Among the most stressful activities are transferring patients (e.g., from toilet to chair), weighing patients, lifting a patient in bed, repositioning patients in beds or chairs, and changing bed linens.

In 2003, the American Nurses Association launched the "Handle with Care" campaign, in which they recommended that nurses use assistive equipment and devices for such patient-handling activities in order to prevent injury to themselves and patients. The ANA states that "manual" patient handling should be used only in exceptional situations when it cannot be avoided. For those situations, you can reduce your risk to some degree by

using appropriate body mechanics. Refer to Chapter 31 for information about body mechanics and how to safely lift and move patients. For information about ANA's campaign to prevent musculoskeletal injuries,

 Go to Chapter 21, **Resources for Caregivers and Health Professionals,** on the Student Resource Disk or DavisPlus at http://davisplus.fadavis.com/Wilkinson2

Needlestick Injury

Healthcare workers, mostly nurses and housekeeping staff, suffer up to 1 million injuries per year from needles and other "sharps," putting them at risk for infectious diseases, such as hepatitis B and AIDS. Since 1992 the Occupational Safety and Health Administration (OSHA) has required employers to provide "engineering controls," such as safer medical devices and needleless systems. A federal Needlestick Safety and Prevention Act became law in 2000, and new OSHA standards required employers to maintain a log of sharps injuries and to purchase safer needle devices. Needlestick injury rates declined by more than 36% during the 3-year period following passage of that law. Nevertheless, a recent survey found that 26% of nurses still report having had at least one injury from a sharp, usually a needle, contaminated with a patient's blood (Delahanty & Myers, 2007). Although OSHA has fined hospitals for noncompliance, some employers still have not complied completely with the regulations. For suggestions about how you can prevent needlestick injuries,

 Go to Chapter 21, **Clinical Insight 21-2: Preventing Needlestick Injury,** in Volume 2.

For more discussion on how to handle needles safely,

 Go to Chapter 23, **Procedure 23–10: Recapping Sterile Needles with One-Handed Technique,** in Volume 2.

Radiation Injury

Radiation is the process of emitting radiant energy in the form of waves or particles. Ionizing radiation is used in computerized tomography (CT scans) in diagnostic radiology, linear accelerators in radiotherapy, and positron emission tomography (PET scans) in nuclear medicine. Patients are deliberately exposed to radiation during diagnostic tests and certain medical treatments. Healthcare workers who care for these patients are unavoidably exposed to small doses of radiation.

Take precautions to avoid excessive radiation exposure for the patient and yourself during x-ray procedures. Follow the principles of time, distance, and shielding when caring for a patient who is being treated with an internal radioactive implant:

- Organize nursing care to limit the amount of time with the patient.
- Perform near the patient only the nursing care that is absolutely necessary.

- Wear protective shielding (e.g., a lead apron), if available, and wear a film badge if you deliver care that exposes you to radiation regularly. The film badge will indicate any radiation exposure.

Violence

Hospital security may not be sufficient to protect you from injury if violence breaks out among patients, visitors, and/or staff. This is especially true in the emergency department (ED), which has 24-hour accessibility and may sometimes be crowded and chaotic. Under the stress of an acute illness, patients and family members alike may become anxious and angry and act out in ways that are unpredictable and atypical for them.

Violence typically begins with anxiety and escalates in stages through verbal aggression and then physical aggression. If you can relieve a patient's anxiety, you may be able to halt the progression to physical violence. Certain emotional and physical conditions increase the risk for patient aggression (refer to Practical Knowledge, Assessing the Risk for Violence).

Gang activity, which is widespread in U.S. cities, is another potential source of violence. As gangs spread, so does the likelihood that gang members will be treated in the ED or admitted to the hospital. When a gang member's reputation is threatened or when disrespect is shown, the tendency is to retaliate—sometimes even weeks later—in an effort to restore reputation and respect (Grossman, 2003).

KnowledgeCheck 21-6

- What measures can healthcare workers use to reduce exposure to radiation?
- What safety measures help reduce equipment-related injuries in the healthcare facility?
- As a nurse, what can you do to help prevent injuring your back?

 Go to Chapter 21, **Knowledge Check Response Sheet and Answers,** on the Student Resource Disk or DavisPlus at http://davisplus.fadavis.com/Wilkinson2

Practical **Knowledge** knowing how

This section provides focused assessments for certain safety risks; standardized nursing language for nursing diagnoses, patient outcomes, and general interventions for addressing patient safety; and specific nursing interventions for safety hazards discussed in the "Theoretical Knowledge" section.

■ ASSESSMENT

It is important to assess the client's immediate environment, developmental stage, and individual risk factors. The following will help you to perform focused assessments for falls risk, home safety, and risk for violence.

Assessing for Falls

Assess all inpatients for falls risk when they are admitted to the healthcare setting. For clients at risk for falls, repeat the risk assessment every 8 hours, and increase the frequency of monitoring. Also identify medications that increase the risk for falling (e.g., opioid analgesics, sedatives, and antihypertensives). Most institutions have policies and guidelines for assessing risk for falls. The following are some examples of methods you might use.

Morse Fall Scale

The Morse Fall Scale uses the following questions to assess a person's risk for falls:

1. Does the patient have a history of falling?
2. Does the person have more than one medical diagnosis?
3. Does the person use ambulatory aids, such as crutches or a walker?
4. Does the person have an IV line or a heparin lock?
5. Is the person's gait normal or stooped or otherwise impaired?
6. What is the person's mental status (e.g., disoriented, forgetful)?

You can easily score, tally, and record those six variables on the patient's chart. The risk of falling varies greatly with different patient populations, different times of day, and different stages of the patient's illness. Age alone is not a predictor of falls, but the items scored by the scale are more common in older adults (Morse, 2001). Ideally, the Morse Fall Scale should be calibrated for each particular unit so that fall prevention strategies are targeted to those most at risk. Institutions implementing the Morse Scale should train personnel in the proper use of the scale (Morse, 1997). To see the complete Morse Fall Scale,

 Go to Chapter 21, **Tables, Boxes, Figures: ESG Figure 21-1,** on the Student Resource Disk or DavisPlus at http://davisplus.fadavis.com/Wilkinson2

Assessing Older Adults for Falls

For a flowchart summarizing falls assessment for older adults, refer to Figure 21-1. At least once a year, ask the older adult (or caregivers) about falls. For anyone who reports having had even a single fall, or if you observe any difficulty with ambulation, have the patient perform the Get Up and Go Test. Those who can do this with steadiness need no further assessment. If the person is unsteady or has difficulty performing this test, assess further.

The Get Up and Go Test is simple. Seat the patient in a chair and observe as he follows these instructions:

- Stand up without using your arms for support.
- Walk several paces, turn, and return to the chair.
- Sit back in the chair without using your arms for support.

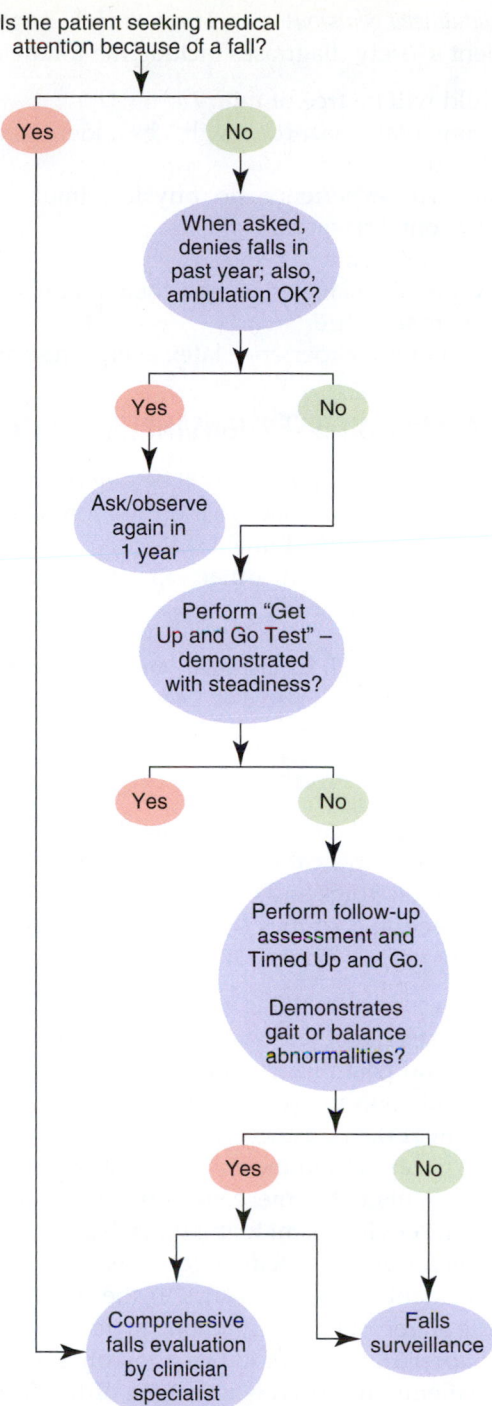

FIGURE 21-1 Falls assessment flowchart.

In any of the following situations, you should refer the patient for a comprehensive fall evaluation. The evaluation should be performed by a practitioner with advanced skills and experience (AHI of Indiana, n.d.; American Academy of Neurology, 2008a, 2008b; Hendrich, 2007; Kenny, Rubenstein, Martin, et al., 2001).

- The patient is seeking care because of a fall.
- The patient or family reports recurrent falls in the past year.
- The patient's gait or balance is abnormal.

To use the Get Up and Go test,

 Go to Chapter 21, **Assessment Guidelines and Tools, Get Up and Go Test,** in Volume 2.

Assessing for Home Safety

As you know, many accidents occur in the home (e.g., fire, poisoning). Everyone should take a few minutes to check for environmental safety hazards.

- A **home safety checklist** is a convenient way for clients to identify potential hazards.

 Go to Chapter 21, **Assessment Guidelines and Tools, Home Safety Checklist,** in Volume 2.

- **The safety assessment scale (SAS)** is an objective way to evaluate the dangers incurred by people with memory and cognitive deficits who live alone at home. The short version of the SAS will enable you to assess the individual's risk status and decide whether she should have an in-depth evaluation. In addition to assessing the person's risk injury, this scale evaluates whether the cognitively impaired person is capable of cooking, taking medications independently, shopping, and performing other activities of daily living by asking questions, such as the following:
  - Does the person live alone?
  - What, if any, are the person's health problems?
  - What is the risk for fire and burns (e.g., does the person smoke; is the stove gas or electric; does the person forget to turn it off)?
  - Is the person capable of cooking, taking medications independently, shopping, and performing other activities of daily living?
  - Can the person recognize food that is fresh and that which is spoiled?
  - Does the person get lost in familiar places? Can he find his way home?

For the complete short form of the SAS,

 Go to Chapter 21, **Tables, Boxes, Figures: ESG Figure 21-2,** on the Student Resource Disk or DavisPlus at http://davisplus.fadavis.com/Wilkinson2

Assessing for Violence

You can be prepared to intervene and perhaps even prevent violence if you recognize risk factors and early warning signs (Flores, 2008).

1. Assess for factors that increase the risk for aggression:

   - Mental disorders, such as dementia, delirium, schizophrenia, and bipolar disorder
   - Being under the influence of alcohol or other drugs
   - Withdrawal from alcohol or other drugs
   - History of violence
   - Clinical conditions such as high fever, epilepsy, head trauma, and hypoglycemia

2. Assess for anxiety:

- Agitation and restlessness
- Pacing
- Talking loudly, speaking rapidly
- Gesturing widely
- Be alert for verbal aggression, such as threats, sarcasm, and swearing.

KnowledgeCheck 21-7

- Which assessment tool would you use for a slightly confused home care client to assess her ability to safely live alone and perform activities of daily living?
- List the six risk factors that are assessed on the Morse Fall Scale.
- How should you screen older adults to see if they need a comprehensive falls evaluation?

 Go to Chapter 21, **Knowledge Check Response Sheet and Answers,** on the Student Resource Disk or DavisPlus at http://davisplus.fadavis.com/Wilkinson2

ANALYSIS/NURSING DIAGNOSIS

Consider the following nursing diagnoses. How would your interventions differ for the two diagnoses?

Risk for Falls related to poor vision secondary to cataracts

Risk for Falls related to muscle weakness, joint instability, and poor sense of balance

The nursing diagnoses listed above illustrate that problem etiologies are important because they affect your choice of interventions. Etiologies may include environmental hazards as well as the developmental and individual risk factors discussed in the preceding sections. Keep in mind that you must state *specific* etiologies for each individual—not just general ones such as "environmental hazards." For example:

Correct: Risk for Falls related to cluttered home environment and joint instability
Incorrect: Risk for Falls related to environmental and physical factors

For NANDA-I labels to use in describing safety problems,

 Go to Chapter 21, **Standardized Language, NANDA-I Diagnoses and NOC Outcomes for Safety Problems,** in Volume 2.

Use the diagnosis Risk for Injury only when the risk cannot be described by one of the more specific nursing diagnoses.

PLANNING OUTCOMES/EVALUATION

The *NOC standardized outcomes* you use will depend on the nursing diagnosis. For some examples,

 Go to Chapter 21, **Standardized Language, NANDA-I Diagnoses and NOC Outcomes for Safety Problems,** in Volume 2.

Individualized goals/outcome statements you might write for a client's safety diagnoses include the following:

- The child will be free of injury.
- Environmental hazards will be identified and eliminated.
- (Client) will experience no physical injury due to environmental hazards.
- Falls will not occur.
- Family members will describe their planned escape routes in case of fire.
- (Client) will not experience latex allergy response.

PLANNING INTERVENTIONS/IMPLEMENTATION

NIC standardized interventions will be determined by the nursing diagnosis you use. To see the more than 50 interventions in the NIC domain (category) of Safety, and some interventions from other NIC domains that are applicable to safety needs,

 Go to Chapter 21, **Standardized Language, Examples of NIC Interventions Related to Safety,** in Volume 2.

General Interventions Related to Safety

Specific nursing activities are designed to monitor and manipulate the physical environment to promote safety in all types of settings and circumstances. The following are some general activities that provide an overview of your role in patient safety:

- Assess and continually monitor the safety needs of patients, based on their level of physical and cognitive function and past history of behavior.
- Assess and continually monitor safety hazards in the environment (i.e., physical, biological, and chemical).
- Remove hazards from the environment, when possible.
- Provide clients with emergency phone numbers.
- Modify the environment to minimize hazards and risk.
- Teach clients about specific safety measures.
- If an accident or injury occurs in the healthcare setting, file an incident report according to agency policy. See Chapter 16 for more information on this topic.
- Urge patients to be active members of the healthcare team (Box 21-3).

The QSEN Safety Competencies should also help you to understand your role in keeping patients safe. To review those competencies,

 Go to Chapter 21, **ESG Table 21-1,** on the Student Resource Disk or DavisPlus at http://davisplus.fadavis.com/Wilkinson2

Home Care Safety Interventions

Specific interventions follow for promoting safety related to particular hazards in home care. After a brief discussion, you will find a series of boxes containing specific home safety interventions.

BOX 21-3 ■ Speak Up®

The Joint Commission encourages patients to become active, involved, and informed participants on the healthcare team, and for parents to do the same to help protect their children from medical errors. The following simple steps are based on research that shows that patients who take part in decisions about their healthcare are more likely to have better outcomes.

Speak up if you have questions or concerns, and if you don't understand, ask again. It's your body and you have a right to know.

Pay attention to the care you are receiving. Make sure you're getting the right treatments and medications by the right healthcare professionals. Don't assume anything.

Educate yourself about your diagnosis, the medical tests you are undergoing, and your treatment plan.

Ask a trusted family member or friend to be your advocate.

Know your medications and why you take them. Medication errors are the most common healthcare errors.

Use a hospital, clinic, surgery center, or other type of healthcare organization that has undergone a rigorous on-site evaluation against established state-of-the-art quality and safety standards, such as that provided by The Joint Commission.

Participate in all decisions about your treatment. You are the center of the healthcare team.

Source: Courtesy of Joint Commission on Accreditation of Healthcare Organizations. The complete Speak Up® document is available at: http://www.jointcommission.org/PatientSafety/SpeakUp/.

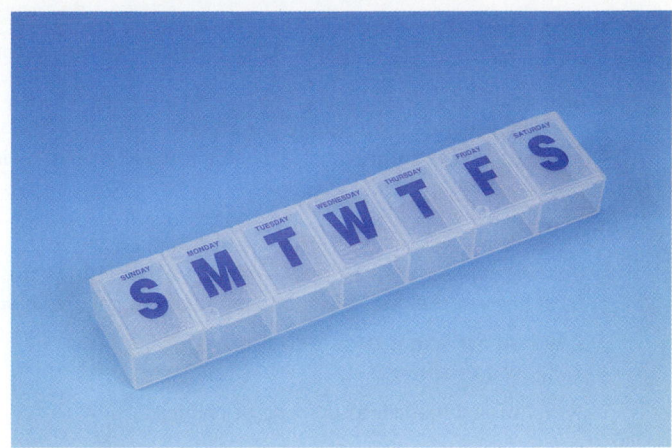

FIGURE 21-2 Medication organizer.

Poisoning. Nursing interventions focus on teaching parents how to childproof the home and what to do if someone ingests a poisonous substance. All homes should be equipped to handle an emergency if poisoning occurs. Teach parents to keep the telephone number for the nearest poison control center easily accessible. If there are no young children in the home, advise families with older adults to prevent accidental overdose or misuse of prescribed medications by using a medication organizer that may be filled once a week by the patient or family member (Fig. 21-2). See the box, Home Care: Preventing Poisoning in the Home and Home Care: If Poisoning Occurs at home at the end of the Choking Rescue section.

Carbon Monoxide Poisoning. If carbon monoxide (CO) intoxication is suspected, the person should be treated with 100% humidified oxygen. A simple blood test may be done to confirm CO levels in the blood. Nursing interventions include teaching prevention measures, such as the following:

- Buy, install, and maintain a home CO detector.
- Never use a gas oven or range to heat a house, even for a short time.
- Ensure that gas or wood-burning appliances are adequately vented to the outside.

- Never operate gasoline-powered engines, such as automobiles, generators, or lawn mowers, in confined spaces, such as garages or basements, or near open doors or windows.
- Never burn charcoal inside a home, cabin, recreational vehicle, or tent—not even in a fireplace.
- Do not use kerosene heaters indoors.
- Repair rust holes or defects in vehicles that could allow exhaust fumes to enter the passenger compartment.

Scalds and Burns. Fire is not the only cause of thermal injuries. Teach clients how to avoid scalds and burns from other causes:

- Turn pot handles toward the back of the stove so that children cannot tip them over.
- Place guardrails in front of radiators and fireplaces.
- Avoid warming infant formula and food in the microwave. You will find that many parents ignore this advice, so also tell them to always check the temperature of formula and food carefully before giving it to the child.
- Do not smoke, use matches, or drink hot liquids while holding an infant. Do not leave burning cigarettes unattended.
- Always check bath water temperature for children and older adults, and set water heater temperature low enough to prevent scalds.
- Remove lids or other coverings from microwaved food carefully.
- Never wear loose-fitting clothing when cooking.
- Wear protective clothing and sunscreen when outside.

Fires. Teach families measures to prevent fires and measures to take should a fire occur. Refer to Home Care: Preventing Injury from Fires in the Home, in the boxes that follow the Choking Rescue section.

Falls. Teach clients, especially older adults, measures for increasing the safety of their home environment. Refer to Home Care: Preventing Falls in the Home, in the boxes that follow the Choking Rescue section.

Home Care

Preventing Poisoning in the Home

Young children will eat and drink almost anything. Most victims of accidental poisoning are children younger than the age of 5. Tips to prevent poisoning include the following:

Careful Words and Actions

➤ Never leave a small child unattended near household cleaning supplies or medicines, even for a moment. If you must answer the phone or doorbell, take the child with you.

➤ Children act fast; it takes only a moment for them to swallow something.

➤ Avoid taking medicines in front of children.

➤ Children tend to imitate adults.

➤ Never call medicines or vitamins "candy." Instead, use the correct name ("cough medicine," and so on).

Careful Storage

➤ Store medicines or household chemicals on high shelves or in locked cabinets and drawers. Never leave them on kitchen or bathroom counters.

➤ Store all household chemicals away from food.

➤ Keep medicines and household chemicals in their original containers. Leave the original labels on. Especially do not store chemicals in containers that normally hold food.

➤ Use child-resistant packaging for medicines and household chemicals. Close the container securely after each use.

➤ Do not assume your child is safe around substances in child-resistant containers; research has shown that many toddlers and preschoolers can open them.

Careful Disposal

➤ Teach clients to take advantage of any community programs that take back unwanted medications for safe disposal (e.g., call the local trash service or a local pharmacy for options in your area).

➤ Teach clients how to safely dispose of outdated prescription medications:

  Crush the medication or add water to dissolve it.

  Mix the drugs with an undesirable substance such as kitty litter or used cooking grease to make it less desirable for pets and children to eat.

  Place the mixture in an empty can or resealable bag and put it in the trash.

➤ Remove all identifying information from prescription labels before throwing containers in the trash or recycling them. It is no longer considered safe to dispose of drugs down the toilet or sink. Wastewater treatment plants are not fully designed to deal with medications, and small amounts have shown up in surface waters. Although there is no evidence of harm to humans or the environment, the long-term effects on people, animals, and the environment are unknown.

Careful Environment Checks

➤ Before purchasing a house plant, verify that it is nontoxic.

➤ Examples of toxic plants are rhododendron, philodendron, English ivy, holly, mistletoe, and lily of the valley.

➤ Find out whether any plants growing in your yard are poisonous, and, if so, remove them.

➤ Teach children that they must never eat berries, wild mushrooms, or other edible-looking plants in yards, fields, and forests.

➤ A wide variety of plants can cause illness and even death in young children.

➤ Warn parents to keep children from chewing on window sills, and so on, and to carefully clean up flakes of paint. Advocate for clients who need to have lead-based paint replaced in their homes.

➤ Lead-based paint can still be found in older homes, and some soil contains a high lead content. Young children often put dirt in their mouths and chew on furniture and window sills, especially when they are teething.

Firearm Injuries. Education is an essential intervention because of the frequency and severity of unintentional firearm injuries involving children. The American Academy of Pediatrics and other groups have mounted efforts to educate parents so that they will be able to make smart choices related to gun safety. Refer to the Home Care: Firearm Safety, in the boxes after the Choking Rescue section.

Suffocation. It is important to teach clients how to prevent suffocation or asphyxiation. They should also recognize the universal sign for choking, shown in the Home Care Box: Preventing Suffocation/Asphyxiation.

Choking Rescue. Teach adults basic first aid for choking, but explain that this is a skill that is best taught using supervised practice with a mannequin. Recommend that clients attend classes presented by organizations such as the Red Cross or the American Heart Association.

The most important thing to remember when someone is choking is to have someone call 9-1-1.

The **choking rescue maneuver** is an emergency procedure for removing a foreign object lodged in the airway. It lifts the diaphragm and forces enough air from the lungs to create an artificial cough. The cough should move and expel the obstruction from the airway. The **Heimlich maneuver** makes use of abdominal thrusts, whereas the American Red Cross (2008) combines back blows with abdominal thrusts, as in the teaching box, "Choking Rescue Maneuver" in the boxes on the following pages. For more detailed instructions about the choking rescue procedure,

 Go to Chapter 21, **ESG Box 21-3, Rescue Maneuver for Choking: Infant or Child Under 12 Months,** and **ESG Box 21-4, Rescue Maneuver for Choking: Adult or Child Over Age 12 Months,** in Volume 2.

Home Care

If Poisoning Occurs at Home

First Aid

➤ Be sure to keep all emergency numbers near the phone. Include your physician's number and the number of the nearest poison control center (PCC). The universal number in the United States is (800) 222-1222. They will connect you to a local PCC. *If you suspect that your child has ingested a poisonous substance, speed is crucial to allow the substance less time to enter the child's system.*

➤ Have this information available:

   Victim's age, weight, and symptoms

   Container of the poison if available

   Time of the poison exposure

   Address where the poisoning occurred

   Telephone number where you can be reached

➤ Have the person sit with his head between his legs or lying on his side. *Prevents aspiration if he vomits.*

➤ Keep the victim as quiet as possible.

Signs of Poisoning

Look for the tell-tale signs of poisoning:

➤ Unusual stains or odors on clothes or skin

➤ Unusual odor on breath

➤ Burns around the mouth

➤ Drowsiness, stomach pain, vomiting, breathing problems, sweating, drooling, irritability, signs of fear, or other sudden changes in behavior

➤ Drugs or chemical containers that are open and/or out of place

Self-Help Actions for Special Situations

If the person:

Has stopped breathing or collapsed: Call 911 or your local emergency number right away. Even if the person seems OK, call the PCC as soon as possible. Assess airway, breathing, and circulation. Initiate emergency resuscitation—CPR (compressions with manual breaths) if trained or cardio-cerebral resuscitation (compressions without respirations) if not trained.

Is having convulsions or loses consciousness: Call 911. Assess breathing and position of the airway. Protect the patient from injury related to falling or involuntary movements related to the seizure. Position the patient on his side to allow secretions to drain out of his mouth; this reduces the risk for aspiration.

Has inhaled poison: (1) Protect yourself from fumes: Take several deep breaths of fresh air, then hold your breath. Hold a wet cloth over your nose and mouth, if possible. (2) Get the person to fresh air right away. (3) Start artificial respirations if you know how. (4) As soon as possible, call 1-800-222-1222, even if the person seems OK.

Has swallowed poisons or medications: (1) Call 1-800-222-1222. If the child is awake and able to swallow, and you suspect that the poison is corrosive, for example, lye or paint solvent, give one-half glassful of water immediately; then call the PCC. (2) Examine the child's mouth, and remove all tablets, powder, or other material. Look for burns, swelling, and so on, and rinse and wipe the mouth with a cloth. (3) Give syrup of ipecac only if advised to do so by the PCC or a qualified medical professional.

Has poisons in the eye: (1) Flood the eye with lukewarm water poured from a cup 2 to 3 inches from the eye. Continue flooding the eye for 15 to 20 minutes. Tell the child to blink as often as possible during flooding. (2) Do not allow the child to rub the eye. (3) Have someone call 1-800-222-1222 as soon as possible.

Has poisons on the skin: (1) Remove contaminated clothing as quickly as possible. (2) Flood the area with lukewarm water for 15 to 20 minutes. Then gently wash the area with soap and water, and rinse. (3) Have someone call 1-800-222-1222 as soon as possible. (4) Later, destroy contaminated clothing.

In all cases of suspected poisoning, if you are unsure of what to do, contact your local poison control center, physician, or emergency personnel (911) immediately.

Sources: First aid tips (n.d.); Injury Center, Centers for Disease Control and Prevention (n.d.).

CriticalThinking 21-4

You are having dinner in a restaurant and notice that the guest at the table beside you seems to be choking.

■ What is the universal sign for choking?

■ What is the first action you should take?

Home Care

Preventing Injury from Fires in the Home

Have a Warning System.

➤ Have working smoke alarms (Fig. 21-3); change batteries every 6 months or more frequently.

➤ Keep a phone near the bed or chair for people who have limited mobility.

FIGURE 21-3 Smoke alarm.

Have an Escape Plan.

➤ Develop and practice a home fire escape plan, and practice it at least twice a year.

➤ Keep a rope or other type of ladder for escape from rooms above ground level.

➤ Have a fire extinguisher in the home, and know where it is located and how to use it; check it regularly and replace it when it becomes outdated.

Have a Preventive Frame of Mind.

➤ When decorating Christmas trees and the exterior of your home, always use fire-safe lights. Do not leave old light sets hung on the outside of your home year after year.

➤ Always unplug Christmas tree lights before leaving home.

➤ Remove the Christmas tree from the home when it becomes dry.

➤ Never leave burning candles unattended. Do not use candles near curtains or other flammable materials.

➤ With charcoal grills, use only charcoal starter fluids designed for barbecue grills.

➤ With gas grills, be sure that the hose connection is tight, and check hoses for leaks.

➤ Store flammable materials (e.g., oil-soaked rags) in appropriate containers.

➤ Do not smoke, especially in bed—and especially in a home where oxygen is in use.

➤ Do not use an open flame when oxygen is in use.

Know What to Do if a Fire Occurs.

➤ Crawl or stay low to the floor to avoid the smoke as much as possible.

➤ Never pour water on a grease fire.

➤ Never discharge a fire extinguisher onto a pan fire.

➤ If it is an oven fire, turn off the heat and keep the door closed.

➤ If it is a microwave fire, keep the door closed, and unplug the microwave.

Promote Electrical Safety in the Home.

➤ Make sure electrical outlets have covers.

➤ Routinely inspect electrical appliances for damaged cords.

➤ Make sure electrical cords do not hang off of tables and countertops.

➤ Do not place electrical cords under carpets.

➤ Replace frayed electrical cords.

Home Care

Firearm Safety

Teach gun owners the following important actions:

➤ Participate in gun safety courses.

➤ Store firearms unloaded and in a secure, locked container when not in use.

➤ Store ammunition in a different location from the firearm.

➤ Know the rules for safe gun handling.

1. Always keep the gun pointed so that even if it were to go off it would not cause injury or damage.

2. Never put your finger on the trigger until you are ready to shoot.

3. Always keep the gun unloaded until ready to use it.

4. Before cleaning a gun, make absolutely sure that it is unloaded. If you do not know how to open the gun and inspect the chamber(s), leave it alone and get help from someone who does.

➤ Even if parents avoid having guns in their own home, it is possible that children will encounter them in other places. Urge parents to teach children safe behavior around firearms, and to be sure children know what to do if they see a gun (e.g., at a friend's house or in school):

1. Stop.

2. Don't touch it.

3. Leave the area.

4. Tell an adult (Kakkuri, 2000).

Preventing Falls in the Home

Exercise Regularly.

➤ Exercise at least 30 minutes every day. Any activity is better than none, but see Chapter 31 for more specific information. The amount of activity depends on age, physical condition, and the intensity of the exercise. Tai chi, yoga, exercise classes, and weight training are helpful ways to improve balance, coordination, flexibility, and strength.

➤ Learn to use assistive devices, such as walkers and canes safely. Be sure rubber tips are not worn. Keep the walking aid by the bed at night.

Take Your Time.

➤ You are more likely to fall when you are tired, sick, rushed, or emotionally upset.

➤ Walk and go up stairs carefully without hurrying; be careful not to be distracted while walking about.

➤ Do one thing at a time; complete it before going on to the next task.

➤ When getting out of bed or a chair, get up slowly and check your balance before standing or walking. Postural hypotension and dizziness on rising are a problem for some people taking medications for high blood pressure and other conditions.

Lighten Loads—Brighten Paths.

➤ Carry things in small loads to be able to see over them, especially on stairs.

➤ Use bags with handles instead of large boxes or laundry baskets to carry items.

➤ Have eyes checked at least once a year.

➤ Clean eyeglasses frequently.

➤ Make sure rooms are adequately lighted, use dim light (e.g., a night light) at night, and turn on the lights before entering a room.

Don't Trip Yourself Up.

➤ Ensure that shoes fit properly, and wear slippers with nonskid soles. Do not go barefoot.

➤ Avoid loose, trailing clothes. Keep hems of clothing at a length to prevent tripping.

➤ Older adults with leg or hip stiffness and pain may shuffle when walking; use of a cane or walker may help.

➤ Check tips of assistive devices, such as canes, walkers, and crutches, for the presence of intact nonskid covers.

➤ Use a ladder or step stool; do not stand on the top step of a stepladder; never climb on a chair.

Clear the Floor.

➤ Tape or otherwise fasten phone and electrical equipment cords to the baseboard.

➤ Arrange furniture to provide wide walking areas.

➤ Keep clutter out of the walkways. Keep floors clear of toys, magazines, and so on.

➤ Remove all scatter or throw rugs (or at least be sure they have nonskid padding under them).

➤ Wipe up all foods and fluids from the floor immediately.

➤ Apply an ice-melt product, salt, or sand to icy sidewalks, steps, and porches.

Use Caution on Stairs.

➤ Keep stairs well lit.

➤ Keep stairs free of clutter. Fasten any stair coverings securely.

➤ Install handrails and slip-resistant floor coverings on staircases.

➤ Provide sturdy handrails on stairs.

➤ Carry several small loads up and down stairs rather than one very large load.

➤ For older adults and those with vision problems, paint the top and bottom steps white or put white stripes on the front edges of steps.

Minimize Bathroom Hazards.

➤ Use shower chairs and raised toilet seats.

➤ Use a bath or shower mat.

➤ Install grab bars and use a nonskid mat in the shower and tub.

➤ Install handheld shower attachments.

Childproof the Home.

➤ Install window guards; never leave a window wide open.

➤ Never leave a child alone on a changing table, even for a moment. Supervise young walkers to protect from falls.

➤ Remove chairs near counters or other areas where young children would be likely to climb. Push chairs all the way under dining table tops.

➤ Use gates at the top and bottom of stairways for small children.

➤ Teach children to pick up their toys.

➤ Be sure that children wear helmets and other appropriate protective gear for bicycling, skateboarding, and other active sports.

For Older Adults or Those with Limited Mobility:

➤ Keep a cordless phone in each room and by the bedside to make it easier to call for help if needed.

➤ Consult a professional.

➤ Ask your doctor or pharmacist to review your medicines—both prescription and over-the-counter—to reduce side effects and interactions. This is especially important for psychotropic medications.

➤ Get treatment for postural hypotension and cardiovascular disorders, including dysrhythmias.

If You Do Fall at Home:

➤ Do not panic.

➤ Stay still for a few minutes to get over the shock.

➤ If you think you are OK, then slide over to a sturdy piece of furniture, get in a kneeling position, and push yourself up; then sit down until you recover.

➤ If you cannot move, try to cover yourself with something to keep warm until help arrives.

Home Care

Preventing Suffocation/Asphyxiation

Instruct parents and caregivers to do the following:

➤ Inspect toys for small, removable parts.

➤ Do not attach pacifiers, rattles, or other infant toys to ribbons or strings.

➤ Do not use sweatshirts or jackets with necktie strings.

➤ Position mobiles well above the crib, out of the infant's reach.

➤ Store plastic bags away from young children in a secure place.

➤ Ensure that the crib is designed to meet federal regulations: Crib slats must be less than 2⅜ inches (6 cm) apart, and the mattress must fit snugly.

➤ When feeding children meat, cheese, or other firm foods, cut the food into very tiny pieces.

➤ Do not give a young child hard candy, chewing gum, nuts, popcorn, grapes, or marshmallows.

➤ Keep venetian blind cords out of the child's reach.

➤ Supervise children's balloon play, and dispose of burst balloons promptly.

➤ Recognize and teach the universal sign for choking (older children): grasping the neck between the thumb and index finger or clutching the neck with both hands (Fig. 21-4).

Measures to Prevent Drowning

➤ Supervise activity when the child is near any source of water, including buckets.

FIGURE 21-4 The universal sign for choking.

➤ Do not allow children to run around a pool or to dive in shallow areas.

➤ If you have a pool, be sure it has a barrier (e.g., tall fence) to prevent children from gaining access.

➤ Insist that children use personal flotation devices (e.g., lifejackets, not float toys). (This is controversial. Some authorities regard flotation devices as toys that provide false security; others say anything that reduces a child's fear of the water is positive, because it is the fear reaction that leads to drowning.)

Sources: National Safety Council (n.d., 2005).

Teaching for Safety Self-Care

Specific interventions follow for promoting safety self-care related to particular hazards in the community and environment. You will find interventions for teaching Safety Self-Care in the five boxes immediately following this page.

Motor Vehicle Accidents. Anticipatory guidance and educational programs are important measures for improving motor vehicle safety for all age groups. Teach families to observe the measures in Self-Care: Teaching Patients About Avoiding Motor Vehicle Injuries.

You may also wish to become politically active on the issue of motor vehicle safety. For instance, you might petition your city council for a stop sign at a particularly dangerous intersection or a reduced speed limit on a highway in your area. Or you might lobby for the enactment of graduated licensing laws in your state to more closely regulate teenage driving or for stronger seat belt laws nationwide.

Food Safety. Teach clients safe food handling and other preventive measures, such as those in the following "4Cs of food safety":

Clean
Cook
Combat cross-contamination
Chill

For further explanation of the 4Cs, refer to the Home Care: Food Safety box.

Vector-Borne Pathogens. To learn about strategies to prevent vector-borne pathogens, see the box, Self-Care: Teaching Clients About Fighting Mosquitoes, Ticks, and Rodents.

Pollution. Teach families that proper disposal and recycling of solid wastes helps to prevent pollution. For teaching tips, refer to the box, Self-Care: Teaching Clients About Reducing Pollution. Also,

 Go to Chapter 21, **The Consumer's Handbook for Reducing Solid Waste,** on the Student Resource Disk or DavisPlus at http://davisplus.fadavis.com/Wilkinson2, or

 Go to http://www.epa.gov/waste/wycd/catbook/index.htm

Electrical Storms. Interventions for preventing injury from electrical storms are found in the Self-Care: Teaching Clients About Safety in Electrical Storms, in the boxes immediately following.

Teaching Clients About Avoiding Motor Vehicle Injuries

➤ Be cautious when walking or bicycling on the roadway, and observe the laws.

➤ Do not drink alcohol or take unprescribed or recreational drugs and drive; have a designated driver.

➤ Do not engage in distracting activities while driving (e.g., use cell phones, read and send text messages, change the music, apply cosmetics).

➤ Observe the speed limits.

➤ Always wear seat belts while driving, and periodically check belts to ensure safe operation.

➤ Make certain children are properly buckled in age-appropriate safety seats in the back seat of the car. If in doubt about the appropriateness or use of safety seats, ask the local police department to check the installation of your child safety seat. See the following table for types of car safety seats.

➤ **Older Adults:** Age-related changes increase the risk for injury or death in a car crash, especially after age 70. But driving helps older adults maintain mobility and independence. Urge them to have regular vision checks, leave a large distance between the car in front of them.

TYPES OF CAR SAFETY SEATS

AGE	TYPE OF SEAT	GUIDELINES
Infants younger than 1 year old	"Infant-only" (These are small, may have carrying handles or be part of a stroller system.)	Use rear-facing seats until the infant is 1 year old and weighs at least 20 lb (Fig. 21-5).

FIGURE 21-5 Infant car seat with infant in rear-facing position in the middle of the back seat.

TYPES OF CAR SAFETY SEATS

AGE	TYPE OF SEAT	GUIDELINES
Toddlers and preschoolers	"Convertible" (can be used rear-facing, then converted to forward-facing) or "forward facing"	Rear-facing seats are safer for toddlers until they are 2 years old. It is best to ride rear-facing as long as possible (until they reach the height and weight maximum specified by the seat manufacturer).
School-age children	Booster seats	After outgrowing their car safety seat, children should stay in a booster seat until the car seat belts fit properly (usually at about 4 ft 9 in. tall and between 8 and 12 years old). Booster seats are safer than a seat belt alone.
Older children	Car lap and shoulder belts.	Children who have outgrown their booster seats should ride in the back seat until 13 years of age. Some experts recommend that anyone weighing <110 lb, regardless of age, ride in the back seat.

Riding in the back seat is associated with a 40% reduction in the risk of fatal injury, and up to 46% in cars with airbags.

Note: These are guidelines, not legal requirements. Some states may also have laws governing types and use of car safety seats. You should be familiar with the laws in your area.

Sources: American Academy of Pediatrics (2009); Centers for Disease Control and Prevention, National Center for Injury Prevention and Control (2006a, 2007); O'Keefe, L. (2009).

For in-depth information about child safety seats,

 Go to the **American Academy of Pediatrics Web site** at http://www.aap.org/healthtopics/carseatsafety.cfm

Home Care

Food Safety

Clean

➤ Wash hands and surfaces often. Always wash your hands with soap and water before handling or preparing food and before eating.

➤ Don't be a source of food-borne illness yourself:

  Avoid preparing food for others if you yourself have a diarrheal illness.

  Avoid changing a baby's diaper while preparing food.

➤ Wash produce. Rinse fresh fruits and vegetables in running tap water to remove visible dirt. Remove and discard the outermost leaves of a head of lettuce or cabbage.

➤ Never use a cutting board, knife, or other object that was used to prepare meat, poultry, or fish for any other purpose until it has been thoroughly washed in hot, soapy water.

➤ Be careful not to contaminate foods while slicing them up on the cutting board. Bacteria grow well on the cut surface of fruits or vegetables.

➤ Wash hands with soap after handling reptiles, birds, or baby chicks, and after contact with pet feces.

Cook

➤ Cook to temperatures sufficient to kill bacteria.

➤ Use a thermometer to measure the internal temperature of meat.

➤ Cook to the following temperatures:

  Ground beef to an internal temperature of 160°F (71°C).

  Leftovers and casseroles, 165°F (74°C)

  Beef, lamb, and veal, 145°F (63°C)

  Pork and ground beef, 160°F (71°C)

  Whole poultry and thighs, 180°F (82°C)

  Poultry breasts, 170°F (77°C)

  Ground chicken or ground beef, 165°F (74°C)

  Stuffed fish, 165°F (74°C)

  Roast meats at an oven temperature of 300°F (149°C) or above

➤ Cook eggs until the yolk is firm. Do not eat raw or partially cooked eggs.

➤ Hold hot food above 140°F (60°C) and for no more than 2 hours.

Combat (Separate)

➤ Avoid cross-contaminating foods by washing hands, utensils, and cutting boards after they have been in contact with raw meat or poultry and before they touch another food.

➤ Put cooked meat on a clean platter, rather than back on one that held the raw meat.

Chill

➤ Refrigerate leftovers within 4 hours. Bacteria multiply quickly at room temperature.

➤ Avoid leaving cut produce (e.g., fruits, vegetables) at room temperature for a prolonged time.

➤ Large volumes of food will cool more quickly if they are divided into several shallow containers for refrigeration.

➤ Do not buy partially thawed items. Be sure they are frozen solid.

➤ Use a cooler to transport foods when the temperature is above 80°F (27°C).

➤ Store deli meat for only 1 or 2 days.

➤ Use thermometers in the refrigerator and freezer.

➤ Keep freezer temperature at 0°F (−18°C) or below.

➤ Keep refrigerator temperature at 40°F (4°C) or below.

➤ Thaw foods in the refrigerator or under cold running water. Use the microwave to thaw foods only if you are going to continue cooking them at that time.

➤ Chill cooked foods rapidly in a shallow (2-inch-deep) container.

➤ Pack lunches in insulated containers. You can refrigerate or freeze sandwiches before packing, to keep them cold.

Store

➤ Cover and date food.

➤ Store vegetables and fruit separately from uncooked meats.

➤ Do not store food in decorative containers unless they are labeled safe for food. Some crystal and pottery, for example, have high lead content.

➤ Store cleaning supplies away from food.

Report

Report suspected food-borne illnesses to your local health department. The local public health department is an important part of the food safety system. Often calls from concerned citizens are how outbreaks are first detected.

Other

➤ Never eat any food that has an odor or that might be spoiled.

➤ Be aware that some imported folk remedies, such as *greta* (which is used by some Hispanic patients for colic), may be contaminated with lead.

➤ Observe sanitation reports for selecting eating establishments in the community.

Sources: Centers for Disease Control and Prevention (2005); U.S. Food and Drug Administration (2007); U.S. Food and Drug Administration. Center for Food Safety and Applied Nutrition (n.d.).

Self-Care

Teaching Clients About Fighting Mosquitoes, Ticks, and Rodents

Mosquitoes

➤ Empty standing water in old tires, buckets, toys, or other outdoor containers.

➤ Change water in bird baths, fountains, wading pools, and potted plant trays at least once a week to destroy mosquito habitats.

➤ Keep rain gutters unclogged.

➤ Keep swimming pools treated with the proper chemicals and circulating.

➤ Use EPA-registered mosquito repellents when necessary, and follow label directions carefully.

➤ Repair holes in window and door screens.

➤ Replace outdoor lights with yellow "bug" lights. They will attract fewer mosquitoes, but are not repellents.

➤ Use head nets, long sleeves, and long pants if you go into areas with high mosquito populations (e.g., salt marshes, deep woods).

➤ Use "bug zappers" or citronella candles for evening outdoor activities.

➤ Contact your local health department if you have questions about mosquitoes or about a spraying program.

➤ If there is a mosquito-borne disease alert, stay indoors during the evening when mosquitoes are active.

Ticks

When walking in tick-infested areas:

➤ Use DEET-containing insect repellant. Reapply it every few hours (or according to the label). DEET formulations as high as 50% are recommended for adults and children over 2 months of age. Use with caution for children. Wash off repellent at night before going to bed.

➤ Treat clothing with permethrin-containing or other insect repellents.

➤ When wearing sunscreen, apply sunscreen first and then repellent.

➤ Wear light-colored clothing. Ticks are attracted to dark colors; also, it is easier to see a tick on light-colored clothing.

➤ Wear long-sleeved shirts, tucked in. Pull socks up over pant legs.

➤ Check your body visually after walking in wooded areas, especially in the hair and skin folds. Use a mirror to view all parts of your body.

➤ Remove ticks right away. This can prevent some infections. For instructions on how to remove attached ticks,

 Go to Chapter 21, **Resources for Caregivers and Health Professionals,** on the Student Resource Disk or DavisPlus at http://davisplus.fadavis.com/Wilkinson2

Rodents

To control rodents, raccoons, and other small animals, remove as many food and water sources as possible. Advise clients to:

➤ Cover food and clean up immediately after meals.

➤ Do not leave unwashed dishes on counters and in sinks.

➤ Keep garbage in closed containers that cannot be overturned.

➤ Repair holes and cracks in the exterior structure of the home, as well as in walls, closets, attic, around sinks and cabinets, and so on.

➤ Use commercial traps or hire professional exterminators.

➤ Participate in neighborhood cleanup projects.

➤ Caution clients that rat and mice poisons and baits can be fatal and should not be used in areas accessible to children and pets.

Sources: Centers for Disease Control and Prevention (2006c); U.S. Environmental Protection Agency (2007).

Self-Care

Teaching Clients About Safety in Electrical Storms

Outside

➤ Seek shelter when you hear thunder.

➤ Stay away from tall objects, particularly individual trees, in the open.

➤ Crouch or sit in the lowest spot possible.

➤ Seek shelter in large buildings.

➤ Stay away from open vehicles, including bicycles and motorcycles.

➤ Move away from water; get out of the water or off small boats.

➤ Drop all metal objects you may have on your body.

Indoors

➤ Do not use corded telephones, computers, or other electrical equipment.

➤ Stay away from plumbing outlets.

➤ Use surge protectors for electrical equipment.

➤ Install ground fault interrupt switches.

Teaching Clients About Reducing Pollution

Hazardous Wastes

➤ Contact the local refuse disposal company for instructions about proper disposal of hazardous wastes (e.g., paints, solvents, pesticides, cleaners, rechargeable batteries).

➤ Encourage the use of products that are nonhazardous or less hazardous, and use only the amount necessary for a project. Share leftover materials with neighbors.

➤ Never dump motor oil into storm drains. For old oil and tires, call your local waste management company, a local quick-lube or tire dealer, or 1-800-MOTOROIL for recommendations regarding disposal.

➤ Talk to an automotive dealer or repair service about recycling or trading in car and other batteries.

Solid Waste

➤ *Reduce* the amount of trash discarded (e.g., don't buy products that have unnecessary packaging).

➤ *Reuse* containers, bags, and products; sell or donate instead of throwing items out.

➤ *Recycle.* Use and buy recyclable and recycled products; compost yard trimmings.

➤ *Respond* by educating others, expressing preferences for less waste (e.g., to manufacturers, merchants).

Air Pollution

➤ Pay attention to air quality warnings, and restrict time spent in high-traffic areas.

➤ Participate in car pools or use public transportation whenever possible.

Noise Pollution

➤ Take actions to help prevent irreversible hearing loss:

  Avoid exposure to continuous high noise levels.

  Wear protective devices (e.g., ear plugs) in environments with a high noise level.

Promoting Safety in the Healthcare Facility

The following interventions will help you to prevent accidents in the healthcare setting.

Preventing Falls. Nursing interventions to prevent falls will, of course, depend on the risk factors that were identified at the initial assessment. Perhaps the single most important thing you can do to prevent falls is to identify those who are at risk for them. You will find other interventions in Box 21-4. For a care plan for Risk for Falls,

 Go to Chapter 21, **Care Plan: Risk for Falls,** on the Student Resource Disk or DavisPlus at http://davisplus.fadavis.com/Wilkinson2

Fires and Electrical Hazards. Electrical hazards are a major cause of fires in healthcare agencies. The following interventions help reduce electrical hazards:

- Before use, have all electrically powered equipment and accessory equipment evaluated by facilities management.
- Participation in education and training programs for electrical safety are mandatory for all employees as established by The Joint Commission standards.
- If an electrical safety hazard is suspected, clearly label the malfunctioning equipment and send it for inspection.
- Use three-pronged electrical plugs whenever possible.
- Observe for breaks or frays in electrical cords.

For other interventions to prevent and respond to fires in the healthcare facility, see Box 21-5.

Avoiding & Using Restraints. The standard of care is to avoid restraints. For a few nursing interventions to help you meet that standard, see Box 21-6. **Ambularms** and bed alarms are used as an alternative for restraints with clients who climb out of bed and are in danger of falling. The Ambularm is worn on the leg and signals when the leg is in a dependent position, such as over the side-rail or on the floor. Another type of alarm is an integral bed alarm, which beeps if the patient's weight is off the mattress for more than a few seconds. The Critical Aspects box for Procedure 21-1 summarizes the key points for using bed monitoring devices. For more specific instructions,

 Go to Chapter 21, **Procedure 21-1: Using a Bed Monitoring Device,** in Volume 2.

Sometimes restraints are necessary. When that occurs, follow organization policies. Also see the Critical Aspects box for Procedure 21-2 and

 Go to Chapter 21, **Procedure 21-2: Using Restraints** and **Clinical Insight 21-1: What You Should Know About Using Restraints,** in Volume 2.

Mercury Spills. If a mercury spill is not properly cleaned, the mercury can remain in cracks and crevices for long periods of time and cause continuous exposure to mercury vapors. Large spills usually must be cleaned by a pollution control agency and can be very costly. It is especially difficult to remove mercury spills from carpets, so they usually have to be disposed of as hazardous waste. If you must clean mercury spills of 25 mL or less (e.g., from a broken, glass thermometer), consult Box 21-7.

Violence. Some agencies have a "public safety room." Patients who have been arrested and brought to the hospital for blood and urine testing for alcohol and drug levels, or any hostile patient who has risk factors for violence, should receive care in the public safety room. For other interventions, see Box 21-8.

BOX 21-4 ■ Preventing Falls In Healthcare Facilities

- Consider instituting hourly rounds on your unit. This has proven effective in reducing the number of falls.
- Provide gait training and advice on the appropriate use of assistive devices.
- Provide review and modification of medications, especially psychotropic medications.
- Place the call light within reach. Have the patient demonstrate the ability to call for the nurse.
- Orient the person to surroundings (e.g., bathroom, chairs; you may need to label items).
- Place disoriented patients in rooms near the nurses' station.
- Provide regular nursing surveillance of hospitalized older adults. Research suggests that this can reduce their falls rate by about 50% (Shever, Titler, Kerr, et al., 2008).
- Keep the bed in a lowered position, except when giving care, with wheels locked (Fig. 21-6A).
- Make sure to lock wheels of wheelchairs, especially during transfer activities (Fig. 21-6B).
- Provide nonskid slippers (Fig. 21-6C).
- Ask patients at risk for falling to wear red or brightly colored socks to alert caregivers.
- Offer to assist with toileting and transfer activities.
- Keep water, urinal, bedpan, and tissues within easy reach of the patient.
- Provide a night light.
- Keep floors dry and free of clutter.
- Educate the patient and family regarding fall prevention strategies.
- For patients at risk for falls, place a warning sticker on the chart or door.
- Communicate falls risk status during handover and transfer reports.
- Document changes in the patient's condition in the patient record.
- Determine the appropriate use of siderails based on the patient's cognitive and functional status. Recent research performed in nursing homes suggests that removing or lowering siderails may help to prevent falls that occur when patients climb over them (Capezuti, Wagner, Brush, et al., 2007).

FIGURE 21-6 Preventing falls. *A*, Locking the bed.

FIGURE 21-6 *B*, Safety locks on wheelchairs.

FIGURE 21-6 *C*, Applying nonskid slippers.

Sources: Adapted from Kenny, Rubenstein, Martin, et al. (2001); Institute for Clinical Systems Improvement (2008); National Guideline Clearinghouse (NGC) (2006); Centers for Disease Control and Prevention, National Center for Injury Prevention and Control (2008); Stevens & Sogolow (2008).

BOX 21-5 ■ Responding to Fire in the Healthcare Facility

You must know your agency's procedures for responding to a fire, including how to evacuate patients from the building. Remember: **R-A-C-E.**

Rescue the patient.

From immediate danger

Move patient(s) into corridor.

Close doors to affected area.

Activate the alarm.

Report fire as to location and kind, and identify yourself.

Activate the nearest alarm.

Confine the fire.

Close all doors and windows.

Turn off all oxygen valves after coordinating with the charge nurse.

Extinguish the fire.

Use the proper extinguisher.

Stay between the fire and the path to safety.

Keep low.

Notes: (1) You should try to extinguish the fire only *after* the R-A-C steps are completed, and only a *small* fire that is contained to one area, such as a trash can. (2) If the fire gets out of control, leave the area immediately.

Extinguisher Classifications

Know where the extinguishers are located and how to use them.

Most agencies use multipurpose (Class ABC) extinguishers.

Class A	Wood, paper, rubber, textiles, plastics
Class B	Flammable liquids, gases, oils, solvents, paints, or greases
Class C	Live electrical wires or equipment
Class D	Combustible metals (e.g., potassium, magnesium, titanium)
Class K	Kitchen fires involving cooking oils and fats

For information about evacuating patients,

 Go to Chapter 21, **Reading More About Promoting Safety,** on the Student Resource Disk or DavisPlus at http://davisplus.fadavis.com/Wilkinson2

Critical Aspects of Procedures 21-1 and 21-2

VOL 2 For steps to follow in *all* procedures, refer to the Universal Steps for All Procedures found on the inside back cover of Volume 2. Go to the full procedures in Volume 2 to practice and learn the procedure steps. Use these Critical Aspects later to help you review key points.

Procedure 21-1: Using a Bed-Monitoring Device

➤ Select the correct type of alarm for your patient.

➤ Explain to the patient and family that the device alerts the staff when the patient tries to get out of the chair or bed.

➤ Apply or place the device; connect the control unit to the sensor pad.

➤ Connect the control unit to the nurse call system, if possible.

➤ Explain that the patient will need to call for assistance when she wants to get up.

➤ Disconnect or turn off the alarm before assisting the patient out of the bed or chair.

➤ Reactivate the alarm after assisting the patient back to the bed or chair.

➤ Understand that bed alarms do not prevent falls by themselves; they are utilized to improve the timeliness of staff response. Patients who are at risk for falls require increased observation and surveillance.

Procedure 21-2: Using Restraints

➤ Follow agency policy, state laws, and professional guidelines.

➤ Try alternative interventions, such as the following, first:

Bed/chair alarms

Patient sitters (nonprofessional staff hired to watch the patient)

➤ Use the least-invasive method among the various types of restraints:

Verbal restraints

Chemical restraints (e.g., antipsychotic or sedative medication)

Seclusion (safe containment to deescalate)

Physical restraints (4-point devices, tie-on, Velcro, leather)

➤ Use restraints only as a last resort to protect a patient and/or caregiver from injury; not for the convenience of the caregiver or as a punishment.

➤ Obtain the required consent form.

➤ Obtain a medical order before restraining, except in an emergency.

➤ Secure restraints in a way that allows for quick release.

➤ Ensure that restraints do not impair circulation, compress nerves, or cause injury to tissue integrity.

➤ Check restraints every 30 minutes.

➤ A prescriber must reassess and reorder the restraints every 24 hours.

➤ Release restraints and assess every 2 hours (more often for behavioral restraints).

BOX 21-6 ■ Avoiding Restraints in Patients with Impaired Cognition

The following nursing interventions provide alternatives to using restraints for patients who are confused or otherwise cognitively impaired.

Provide Consistency

- Keep the environment and the caregivers as consistent as possible.
- Encourage family and friends to remain with the patient around the clock for a few days after admission. This helps relieve anxiety.
- Encourage family and friends to help with care and to bring familiar objects from home.

Medications

Review the patient's medications to determine whether they may affect mental status.

Anxiety

Provide relaxation and relieve anxiety:

- Orient patients and families to their surroundings; reorient as often as necessary. This helps to relieve anxiety and prevent wandering.
- Have family and friends help with activities of daily living (ADLs). This also provides consistency.
- Use therapeutic touch and relaxation techniques, such as massage (see Chapter 40).
- Use the least invasive and most comfortable method to deliver care. For example, use a toileting schedule or provide a bedpan instead of inserting a urinary catheter; or encourage and provide oral fluids to avoid inserting an IV for hydration.
- Discontinue treatments that cause discomfort or agitation as soon as possible. For example, some patients become agitated and pull at or try to escape sensations from indwelling catheters, intravenous catheters, and nasogastric tubes.

Assessment/Surveillance

Provide frequent assessment and surveillance:

- Use one-to-one supervision as needed; encourage family members and friends to stay or to hire sitters for clients who need supervision.
- Place near the nursing station clients with cognitive deficits or who need supervision for other reasons; check on them frequently.
- Assess frequently for cognitive changes.

Communication

Find ways to communicate:

- Assess communication abilities.
- Communicate clearly, calmly, and slowly.
- Smile. Face the patient.
- Can the patient communicate what he needs and wants?
- Be alert for body language, such as gestures, nods, and eye contact. These may be the patient's only way of communicating.
- Ask the patient directly what she needs, for example, "Do you need the bathroom?" Word the question so the patient can answer with a yes or no.

Environment

Modify the environment:

- Use Ambularms and integrated bed alarm systems.
- Reduce noise on the unit.
- Provide adequate light.
- Provide music therapy; this is calming to many patients.
- Use low beds for clients who are likely to fall or wander.
- Remove bed rails.
- Use wedge cushions and body props for patients sitting in chairs to help them maintain good posture in the chair; these help keep them from slumping and falling out of the chair.
- Keep doors to the unit locked if this is feasible and acceptable; in long-term care facilities, also lock outside doors. Have a staff member at main entrances and exits.

Unmet Needs

Identify unmet needs and individualize care to meet them:

- Plan an elimination routine based on the patient's history. Patients often try to get out of bed because they need to go to the toilet.
- Look for the meaning of disruptive behaviors (e.g., wandering). Is it a way of expressing an unmet need? For example, the patient may need to go to the bathroom.
- Provide pain relief and other comfort measures to decrease agitation.
- Provide diversional activities.

BOX 21-7 ■ What to Do if There Is a Mercury Spill

✚ Do not touch mercury droplets. Mercury vaporizes; the toxic vapors can be inhaled or absorbed through the skin.

In the Healthcare Agency

✚ If you are not trained in the procedure, do not attempt to clean up a mercury spill. Notify the environmental services department.

- Keep people and animals away from the area.
- Clean the spill promptly.
- If you are trained, use a commercially made mercury spill kit. All healthcare facilities should have them. Spill kits should contain gloves, protective glasses, mercury-absorbing powder, special mercury sponges, and a disposal bag. Some kits have filtered vacuum equipment.
- Follow agency guidelines and instructions in the kit.
- Clean beads off skin, clothing, and disposable items. Place cleaning materials and disposable items in the disposal bag and seal. Follow agency policy for laundering clothing.
- On hard surfaces, use a flashlight to search for beads.
- Change clothing that has been contaminated.
- Wash well. Shower and wash your hair as soon as possible so you do not unknowingly carry mercury home.
- Ventilate the area well to reduce the concentration of mercury vapors. Promote exhaust ventilation if possible.
- Complete an occurrence report.

In the Home and Community

- If you do not have a spill kit, wear rubber gloves and eye protection; use paper towels for clean-up and a plastic bag for disposal.
- Keep people and pets away from the area.
- Wipe beads off skin, clothing, and disposable items. Place disposable items in the plastic bag and seal with tape.
- On hard surfaces, use cardboard to scrape up the beads and pour them into a can or jar with a lid. Then wash the area.
- Shower or wash well.
- Keep the area well ventilated for several days.
- Do not use a broom or vacuum cleaner. These will just spread the mercury around and be contaminated by it.
- Do not flush mercury or cleaning materials down a toilet or drain.
- Do not wash and reuse contaminated materials.

BOX 21-8 ■ Dealing with Violence

- Intervene to relieve anxiety.
- Treat underlying medical conditions. For example, give medications or check blood glucose levels.
- Administer sedatives such as diazepam or lorazepam. There may be standing orders for these.
- Use a calm, reassuring approach.
- Avoid using threatening, aggressive body language.
- Don't respond to anger with anger.
- Don't defend when the patient is verbally aggressive.
- Don't wear a stethoscope around your neck, dangling jewelry, or anything a patient might use to hurt you.
- Remove from the room objects that could be used as a weapon.
- Don't go into a room alone with an angry patient.
- Remain at least an arm's length away from the angry patient.
- Do not turn your back on an angry patient.
- Do not touch the patient without permission, unless you intend to physically restrain him.
- Keep the room door open; do not let the patient get between you and the door.
- Protect others in the environment. Follow the department's safety guidelines.
- As a last resort, use mechanical restraints if ordered and as necessary.
- Your priority must be your own safety and the safety of others in the area.

 Go to **Procedure 21-2: Using Restraints.**

Sources: Ackley & Ladwig (2007); Bulechek, Butcher, & Dochterman (2008); Doenges, Moorhouse, & Geissler-Murr (2005); Flores (2008); Wilkinson & Ahern (2009).

For guidelines for coping with the presence of gang members in the hospital,

 Go to Chapter 21, **Tables, Boxes, Figures: ESG Box 21-5,** on the Student Resource Disk or DavisPlus at http:// davisplus.fadavis.com/Wilkinson2

Which Safety Interventions Can I Delegate?

As nurse manager on a clinical unit or as a primary care nurse, you may need to delegate safety promotion interventions to nursing assistive personnel (NAP). Which safety interventions would you delegate?

For all delegation decisions, refer to the discussion and guidelines in Chapter 7. One safety activity you might delegate is applying restraints. As in all delegation, you must first be sure that the NAP is competent to perform the skill. You may delegate the application of the restraints; however, you may *not* delegate the assessment of the patient's status nor the evaluation of the patient's response to the restraints. You may assign the NAP to (1) remove and reapply restraints to provide skin care and allow for supervised movement and (2) assess for skin excoriation under or around restraint location and report it to you.

You should be sure assistive personnel are aware of and follow all safety measures and institutional procedures. For example, you can expect the NAPs to remove clutter and spills in patient rooms, to provide patients with nonskid slippers, and to lock beds and wheelchairs.

Toward Evidence-Based Practice

Capezuti, E., Wagner, L., Brush, B., et al. (2007). Consequences of an intervention to reduce restrictive siderail use in nursing homes. *Journal of the American Geriatric Society, 55(3),* 334–341.

Researchers examined the effect of an advanced practice nurse (APN) intervention on restrictive siderail usage in four urban nursing homes and with a sample of 251 residents. A secondary question explored the association between restrictive siderail reduction and bed-related falls. They observed siderail use, and interviewed residents and nurses for functional status, mobility, cognition, behavioral symptoms. They also reviewed the medical record for treatment information and incident reports for fall data. The intervention consisted of the APN consulting with individual residents and providing education and consultation for staff in the facility. Researchers concluded that APN consultation and education intervention can safely reduce siderail use, and that reducing siderail use does not lead to an increase in falls.

Fonad, E., Wahlin, T., Winblad, B., et al. (2008). Falls and fall risk among nursing home residents. *Journal of Clinical Nursing, 17(1),* 126–134.

In this 4-year study, researchers sent questionnaires to staff nurses in five nursing homes in Sweden in order to identify falls risk factors for older adults living in nursing homes. They concluded that neither bed rails nor wheelchairs with safety belts eliminated falls, and that use of antidepressants increased the risk of falls.

1. Which of the following, as fall prevention interventions, have at least some support from either of the two studies, and therefore might be expected to reduce falls?

2. Which study (or studies) support each intervention, and does the study provide direct or indirect support? Explain your thinking.

Interventions:

A. Provide APN consultation with patients.

B. Have an APN teach facility staff about fall prevention.

C. Use siderails on all resident beds.

D. Reduce the use of siderails.

E. Use safety belts for patients in wheelchairs.

F. Avoid using antidepressants when possible.

 Go to Chapter 21, **Toward Evidence-Based Practice Suggested Responses,** on the Student Resource Disk or DavisPlus at http://davisplus.fadavis.com/Wilkinson2

 Go to Chapter 21, **Resources for Caregivers and Health Professionals,** on the Student Resource Disk or DavisPlus at http://davisplus.fadavis.com/Wilkinson2

 Suggested Readings: Go to Chapter 21, **Reading More About Promoting Safety,** on the Student Resource Disk or DavisPlus at http://davisplus.fadavis.com/Wilkinson2

 Bibliography: Go to Volume 2, Bibliography.

CHAPTER 22

Facilitating Hygiene

Learning Outcomes

After completing this chapter, you should be able to:

➤ Explain how personal hygiene relates to health and well-being.

➤ Identify factors influencing personal hygiene practices.

➤ Discuss delegation of hygiene activities to nursing assistive personnel (NAP).

➤ Discuss the nurse's role in determining a client's self-care ability.

➤ Identify nursing diagnoses related to self-care ability and hygiene practices.

➤ Describe normal and abnormal assessment findings of the skin, feet, nails, mouth, hair, eyes, ears, and nose.

➤ State the importance and purpose of bathing.

➤ Describe the following types of baths: complete, assist, partial, towel, bag, shower, tub, and therapeutic.

➤ Apply the nursing process to common hygiene-related problems of the skin, feet, nails, mouth, hair, eyes, ears, and nose.

➤ Demonstrate nursing skills to promote patient hygiene, such as bathing, foot care, and bed making.

➤ Demonstrate care of the eyes, ears, and teeth, including glasses, contacts, hearing aids, and dentures.

➤ Discuss the relationship between a patient's overall well-being and the immediate environment.

Meet Your Patients

Your instructor has assigned you to assist the following patients with their hygiene. You must assess the needs of each person, gather information on their bathing habits and preferences, plan nursing measures necessary to meet individual needs, and together with a NAP (nursing assistive personnel), provide care.

The first person on your assignment is Mrs. Williams, a 76-year-old woman of Indian heritage who was admitted yesterday after suffering a stroke that paralyzed her right side. Since the stroke, she has been unable to speak clearly and becomes frustrated as she attempts to communicate her needs. Her daughter says Mrs. Williams is a proud, independent, and tidy woman who has been living alone since her husband's death last year. She has been driving her car, cleaning the house, doing her grocery shopping, and maintaining the yard and garden. She wears eyeglasses for reading and driving and has a hearing aid, although she rarely uses it.

The second person on your assignment is Mr. Gold, a 68-year-old Orthodox Jewish man admitted last week after he experienced a massive heart attack. Although his eyes are open, he does not respond to external stimuli. Because of Impaired Swallowing, Mr. Gold is unable to take

food or fluid orally. A feeding tube was placed to ensure adequate nutrition and hydration. His oral mucous membranes and lips are dry and crusty. He is incontinent of urine and stool. Mr. Gold's son, Ira, tells you that throughout his life Mr. Gold adhered to Orthodox Jewish law. The son requests that, in honor of his father, certain aspects of these laws be included in the care plan.

What immediate concerns come to your mind about each of these patients? How will you ensure that their hygiene needs are met? Are there any safety issues? Which parts of their hygiene care can you delegate, if any?

Theoretical **Knowledge**
knowing why

This chapter provides the theoretical knowledge you need to answer the preceding questions, as well as others that will arise as you care for patients.

Hygiene and Self-Care

Hygiene describes activities involved in maintaining personal cleanliness and grooming. Personal hygiene contributes to physical and psychological well-being. **Activities of daily living (ADLs),** such as taking a bath or shower, washing hair, or brushing and flossing teeth promote comfort, improve self-image, and decrease infection and disease. When they are healthy, people perform their own personal hygiene; however, some patients need assistance because of illness or injury. As a nurse, you are responsible for providing the necessary assistance and, at the same time, promoting as much self-care as possible. Self-care in ADLs promotes increased activity, independence, and self-esteem.

What Factors Influence Hygiene Practices?

Every patient is unique, so as you would expect, personal hygiene practices vary greatly. The following are a few of the factors that influence a person's hygiene

practices. Respect and accommodate each person's preferences and differences whenever possible. This reflects your caring and promotes maximum participation and independence for your patient.

Personal Preferences. Some people prefer a shower, others a bath. One person may shower in the morning to wake up and feel clean for the day, whereas another bathes in the evening to relax before going to sleep. Choice of soaps, deodorants, shampoos, and moisturizers varies from person to person as well.

Culture and Religion or Spirituality. Cultural and family values and beliefs about hygiene form the foundation for our beliefs as adults. Generally, people in North America consider daily bathing, use of deodorant, and brushing the teeth necessary to eliminate body odors. However, people in some cultures may consider body odors to be completely normal and acceptable, and may find a weekly bath sufficient. Some religious or spiritual beliefs also influence hygiene practices. For example, some religions consider a menstruating woman unclean and require a ritual cleansing bath 7 days after the menstrual bleeding stops. As another example, Orthodox Judaism prohibits receiving personal care from a member of the opposite sex.

Economic Status or Living Environment. Inadequate bathing facilities or lack of money for hygiene supplies can influence how often a person bathes. For example, homeless persons or migrant workers, although they may value cleanliness and grooming, might not have access to running water or soap with which to bathe. People living in poverty must focus on meeting basic needs for food and shelter before they can spend money and energy on hygiene. You may need to be a patient advocate for some people and initiate contact with appropriate community social service agencies.

Developmental Level. Parents and other caregivers perform hygiene care for infants and young children. Older children learn practices that become habits, such as brushing and flossing the teeth. As older children begin to perform their own hygiene independently, they are influenced by the media and societal norms. As a result, they pick and choose hygiene practices that seem important to them. For example, some preteens may avoid water and bathe only under parental duress, but teenagers, who are typically very self-conscious, may begin to take several showers a day. Many teenagers have oily skin and can tolerate frequent bathing, but as we age, the oil-producing sebaceous glands become less active. For adults, frequent bathing and the use of deodorant soap further dries the skin. Older adults may find it necessary to bathe only every 2 or 3 days, use less soap, and increase the use of skin moisturizers.

Knowledge and Cognitive Levels. Not everyone has the knowledge needed to make appropriate decisions. For example, some people who are careful to brush their teeth daily may not know the importance of flossing. Or, some women may not be aware of the importance of cleansing the perineum from front to back after using the toilet. Patient teaching is an important part of your hygiene care because most people will, eventually, take care of their own personal hygiene.

How Does Health Status Affect Self-Care Ability?

Both physiological and emotional factors can interfere with a person's ability or willingness to perform hygiene measures.

Pain. Pain severely limits the person's ability and motivation to perform ADLs. The pain itself, limited mobility caused by the pain, and drowsiness from analgesics used to manage the pain may all contribute to a self-care deficit.

Limited Mobility. Limited mobility (e.g., from joint and muscle problems, injury, weakness, fatigue, surgery, prescribed bedrest, or pain) makes it difficult to perform hygiene activities. For example, a patient may be unable to bend over to wash her lower legs and feet, cut her toenails, or even raise her arms to wash and dry her hair. A patient who is weak or "lightheaded" may be afraid of falling and be reluctant to move about. Such a person needs help, especially getting into the bathtub or shower. Obstacles, such as IV lines, oxygen tubing, nasogastric tubes, indwelling urinary catheters, or casts, may also interfere with the patient's ability to perform self-care.

Sensory Deficits. Sensory deficits diminish a person's ability to perform hygiene measures safely and independently. Safety is a priority for patients with sensory deficits. Consider these examples:

- A patient with macular degeneration (a visual deficit) is admitted to the hospital. Because he is unfamiliar with the new surroundings, he is unable to gather necessary supplies for grooming. You would need to provide direction, assistance, and understanding.
- A patient with a hearing loss is taking an anticoagulant (a medication to delay blood clotting). You may need to provide explicit written instructions about the importance of using an electric razor instead of his preferred double-edged razor.

Cognitive Impairment. Cognitive impairment, such as is found in patients with dementia, delirium, psychoses, stroke, Alzheimer's disease, or traumatic brain injury, may make it impossible for the person to initiate his own grooming. The patient may be unable to determine the need for hygiene, much less know how to accomplish related tasks. For example, a patient with advanced Alzheimer's disease may actually forget how to care for himself and will need step-by-step direction. Because the person may also have difficulty interpreting stimuli in the environment, he may be fearful and resistant to hygiene measures performed by the nurse. Such cognitive deficits may require new or modified hygiene plans.

Emotional or Other Mental Health Disturbances. These may diminish a person's ability to perform hygiene measures. Patients experiencing altered reality states, such as psychoses, delusions, or hallucinations may dress inappropriately for the weather or the situation and have poor hygiene practices. Some are unable to make decisions about "what to do next" when bathing, dressing, and so on. Many people with depression neglect their grooming and hygiene because of a profound lack of energy or motivation.

KnowledgeCheck 22-1

- What are the benefits of personal hygiene?
- Why should you respect and accommodate your patients' hygiene preferences?
- Identify two economic or living environmental factors that may influence how frequently a person bathes.
- Identify one example of a cognitive impairment that may make independent initiation of grooming impossible.
- Why may people experiencing depression neglect their grooming and hygiene?

 Go to Chapter 22, **Knowledge Check Response Sheet and Answers,** on the Student Resource Disk or DavisPlus at http://davisplus.fadavis.com/Wilkinson2

CriticalThinking 22-1

Think about your patients, Mrs. Williams and Mr. Gold ("Meet Your Patients"). After reviewing each of the factors presented determine the following for each patient.

- Which factor(s) will have the most influence on the hygiene practices of this patient?
- Why do you think so?
- How will this factor impact the individual plan of care?

Practical **Knowledge**
knowing how

Although cleanliness can contribute to well-being, comfort, and health, it can also be stressful—for example, to critically ill patients, the frail elderly, and those with dementia. In a study of patients in an intensive care unit, an "adverse event" occurred in 48% of the hygiene interventions performed. Adverse events included decreased oxygenation or ventilation, hypertension, hypotension, intracranial hypertension, and even one cardiorespiratory arrest (Robles, Corcoles, Torres, et al., 2002).

This does not mean you should avoid hygiene care for such patients, but you may need to modify it and evaluate patient responses constantly as you work. You might provide care in small segments, allowing the patient to rest after brushing his teeth, for example.

ASSESSMENT (SELF-CARE)

As a nurse, you must consult with the patient to assess his willingness and ability to perform ADLs. This enables you to determine the type of help needed and to encourage the patient to strive for optimal functioning. Plan hygiene care around the patient's needs, not facility routines or staff convenience. For guidelines for assessing hygiene needs,

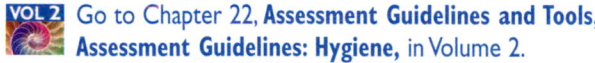

VOL 2 Go to Chapter 22, **Assessment Guidelines and Tools, Assessment Guidelines: Hygiene,** in Volume 2.

Assessing Self-Care Abilities

Begin your assessment of self-care ability by conducting an initial interview with the patient and/or family.

Obtain a Health History. Identify underlying illness, injury, or disease that might contribute to a self-care deficit or affect the person's ability to tolerate hygiene procedures.

Assess the Patient's Cognitive Ability and Physical Functioning. Determining overall grooming and cleanliness, level of consciousness, short- and long-term memory, ability to follow instructions, range of motion and mobility, level of knowledge, and energy level.

Assess for Other Factors. Identify other factors (e.g., cultural, religious) that may influence the patient's hygiene practices and preferences.

Assess for Sensory Disturbances. Assess for auditory, visual, tactile, or olfactory disturbances that interfere

with self-care ability. For example, a person who has decreased tactile sensation (sense of touch) may be at risk for burns because he is not able to determine the temperature of the bath water.

Determine Preferences and Practices. Identify the patient's previous hygiene measures, normal routines, preferences, need for assistive devices, or any other existing problem areas. Assess your patient's functional status regularly to identify the need for care plan modifications. Focus your assessments on the patient's *ability* to perform self-care hygiene measures and the need for assistance, not necessarily on the *quality* of these measures. To assess a patient's self-care abilities, use a standardized functional status rating scale (see Box 22-1), if one is available.

CriticalThinking 22-2

Answer the following questions for Mrs. Williams (from the "Meet Your Patients" scenario).

- What factor(s) may interfere with Mrs. Williams' self-care ability?
- How can you ensure maximum independence with hygiene for her?
- How might you encourage her to strive toward optimal functioning?

ANALYSIS/NURSING DIAGNOSIS (SELF-CARE)

When a person is unable to perform one or more ADLs, a self-care deficit exists. NANDA International self-care diagnoses related to hygiene are Bathing/hygiene, Dressing/grooming, Toileting, and Feeding (2009). Each is described below, except for Feeding Self-Care Deficit, which is included in Chapter 26.

Nursing Diagnoses to Describe Self-Care Abilities

Readiness for Enhanced Self-Care describes a pattern of performing self-care that helps the person to meet health-related goals, and which the person expresses a desire to perform even more independently.

- *Defining Characteristics*: Expresses desire to enhance independence in maintaining life, health, personal development, and well-being; expresses desire to enhance knowledge of and responsibility for self-care; expresses desire to enhance self-care.

Bathing/Hygiene Self-Care Deficit is a state in which a person experiences an impaired ability to perform or complete bathing and hygiene activities independently.

- *Defining Characteristics*. Inability to wash body or body parts, obtain or get to water source, regulate temperature or flow of bath water, get bath supplies, dry body, get in and out of the tub or shower.

Dressing/Grooming Self-Care Deficit is a state in which a person experiences an impaired ability to perform or complete dressing and grooming activities independently.

■ *Defining Characteristics.* Impaired ability to put on or remove necessary items of clothing, fasten clothing, or obtain or replace articles of clothing. Inability to put clothing on upper body or lower body, choose clothing, use assistive devices, use zippers, put on socks and shoes, maintain appearance at satisfactory level, pick up clothes.

Toileting Self-Care Deficit is a state in which the individual experiences an impaired ability to perform or complete toileting activities independently.

■ *Defining Characteristics.* Inability to get to toilet or commode, sit on or rise from toilet or commode, manipulate clothing for toileting, carry out proper toileting hygiene, flush toilet or commode, or get to the bathroom.

Self-Neglect involves culturally framed behaviors in which the patient's performance of one or more self-care activities fails to maintain a culturally accepted standard of health and well-being.

■ *Defining Characteristics.* Inadequate personal or environmental hygiene; nonadherence to health activities.

For common etiologies for self-care diagnoses, see the preceding Theoretical Knowledge section. Also,

 Go to Chapter 22, **Standardized Language, Common Etiologies for Self-Care Diagnoses,** in Volume 2.

When writing self-care diagnoses, classify the patient's functional level if you have access to a standardized scale, such as the one found in Box 22-1. Otherwise, use descriptive terms such as mild, moderate, severe, and total. The following are examples of diagnostic statements you might write:

Using a scale: Bathing/Hygiene Self-Care Deficit **(2)** related to severe knee pain secondary to degenerative joint disease

Using descriptive words: Toileting Self-Care Deficit **(severe)** related to inability to walk to the bathroom secondary to muscle weakness

---

BOX 22-1 ■ Functional Level Classification

Level

1   Requires use of equipment or devices.

2   Requires help from another person(s) for assistance, supervision, teaching.

3   Requires help from another person(s) and equipment or device.

4   Dependent; does not participate in self-care bathing or hygiene.

Source: Gordon, M. (2006). *Manual of nursing diagnosis* (11th ed., p. 175). Sudbury, MA: Jones and Bartlett.

 Critical Thinking 22-3

Which of the preceding NANDA-I self-care diagnoses apply to Mrs. Williams and Mr. Gold ("Meet Your Patients")?

■ Explain the reasoning for your choices.
■ For each patient, what are the related factors for his or her Self-Care Deficit?
■ Write a self-care diagnostic statement for Mrs. Williams and Mr. Gold.

■ PLANNING OUTCOMES/EVALUATION (SELF-CARE)

To see a bathing/hygiene plan of care,

 Go to Chapter 22, **Nursing Care Plan: Bathing/Hygiene Self-Care Deficit,** on the Student Resource Disk or DavisPlus at http://davisplus.fadavis.com/Wilkinson2

The NOC standardized outcome Self-Care: Activities of Daily Living (ADLs) is appropriate for all of the Self-Care Deficit diagnoses. For outcomes for specific diagnoses,

 Go to Chapter 22, **Standardized Language, Selected Standardized Outcomes and Interventions for Self-Care Deficit Diagnoses,** in Volume 2.

Individualized goals/outcome statements you might write for Self-Care Deficits include the following examples:

■ Verbalizes satisfaction with body cleanliness and oral hygiene after A.M. care.
■ Accepts assistance with ADLs or total care, if needed.
■ By October 4, will comb hair unassisted.
■ By October 4, will complete bath independently, except for back and feet, after nurse provides equipment and assists patient to the bathroom.

You will use the outcomes developed in the planning outcomes phase of the nursing process as the criteria for evaluating patient responses to self-care interventions.

■ PLANNING INTERVENTIONS/IMPLEMENTATION (SELF-CARE)

Even when a patient needs assistance with hygiene measures, the overall goal is to promote eventual self-care. Of course, critically ill patients need rest, so you will not push them to perform at their highest level of function. If the patient is able to perform self-care, you might sometimes need to allow him to rest while you perform part of the care, for example, washing his feet and legs.

For *NIC standardized interventions* for Self-Care Deficit diagnoses,

 Go to Chapter 22, **Standardized Language, Selected Standardized Outcomes and Interventions for Self-Care Deficit Diagnoses,** in Volume 2.

Individualized interventions depend on the extent of the client's Self-Care Deficit, as well as the etiology of the problem. The following are some examples:

■ Demonstrate the use of assistive devices (e.g., to help patient grasp and pull on socks).

- Use Velcro® fasteners instead of buttons and zippers.
- Allow sufficient time for all ADLs to prevent fatigue and frustration.
- Offer pain medication before ADLs.

You will find a thorough discussion of specific hygiene-care activities (e.g., care of the skin, oral hygiene) in the remainder of this chapter.

Types of Scheduled Hygiene Care

The following types of scheduled hygiene care are provided in most inpatient facilities (e.g., hospitals and long-term care settings). Although they are scheduled routinely, you should individualize these activities and involve the patient as much as possible.

Hourly rounding (seeing the patient every hour, on schedule) is done to offer help with self-care needs such as pain relief, positioning, and toileting—the most common reasons for medical–surgical patients to use a call light. Hourly rounding, also referred to as *comfort rounds* or *safety rounds*, has been found to improve patient safety and to greatly reduce call light use, freeing up time for staff to complete their tasks without constant interruptions (Meade, Bursell, & Ketelsen, 2007).

Early morning care is provided soon after the patient awakens. It includes preparing the patient for breakfast or other activities, such as diagnostic tests. As needed, assist with toileting, washing the face and hands, giving mouth care, and providing comfort measures.

A.M. (morning) care is hygiene care that occurs after breakfast. Depending on the patient's self-care ability, assist with toileting, bathing, oral hygiene, skin care, hair care (including shaving if needed), dressing, and positioning or helping the patient transfer to a chair. You or the NAP will also change or straighten bed linens, according to agency policy, and tidy the room.

P.M. (afternoon) care consists of preparing patients to receive visitors or afternoon rest. You may assist nonambulatory patients with toileting, hand washing, and oral care; straighten bed linens; reposition the patient; and offer other comfort measures (e.g., pain medications).

H.S. (hour of sleep) care is given before the patient goes to sleep. You should offer the same care as given in the afternoon, adding a back massage to help relax the patient. Also place within easy reach the call light, water glass, urinal, or anything else the patient may need during the night. Turn off lights and TV, and close the door before leaving the room (according to patient needs and preferences). For a back-massage procedure,

 Go to **Procedure 33-1**, in Volume 2.

Delegating Hygiene Care to Nursing Assistive Personnel

In many institutions, nursing assistive personnel (NAP) perform most of the hygiene care. As you have learned, hygiene care can be stressful. Therefore, you will need to carefully assess patients to ensure that it is safe to delegate their care to a NAP. If the patient is unstable or the NAP is inexperienced or unfamiliar with the patient's limitations, you must assist or perform the care yourself. Read "What Should I Know About Delegation and Supervision?" in Chapter 7 for a review of making delegation decisions.

Before assigning a NAP to assist with a bath, shower, or toileting, give instructions about the following:

- Patient's limitations and restrictions, and the amount of assistance necessary
- Use of any assistive devices (e.g., cane, walker, or gait belt)
- Specific safety precautions to follow (e.g., use of gait belt or shower chair)
- Any obstacles present, such as drainage tubes, catheters, IV tubing, or bandages, and how to maintain them during bathing or toileting
- Observations to make during the procedure (e.g., skin condition; the presence of any lesions; areas of special concern over bony prominences and under abdominal folds and breasts; presence, appearance, and amount of urine or stool, or the need to collect a specimen). Explain why the observations are important.

Remember, as the professional nurse, you are responsible for making assessments and determining the meaning of the data reported to you by the NAP. Assisting with or supervising care (especially a bath) is an excellent opportunity for you to assess the patient's level of consciousness, short- and long-term memory, ability to follow instructions, range of motion, skin condition, activity tolerance, and overall self-care ability.

Critical**Thinking** 22-4

Think of Mrs. Williams ("Meet Your Patients"). You have delegated her bathing and oral hygiene to a NAP.

- What information do you need to share with the NAP about this patient's needs, limitations, or preferences?
- What, if any, specific observations will you ask the NAP to make for Mrs. Williams?
- What, if any, specific observations will *you* need to make for Mrs. Williams?
- What action will you take if you determine that the patient's needs and preferences were not met by the NAP?

Care of the Skin

The preceding sections introduced you to the broad topic of hygiene and activities of daily living. The rest of the chapter will deal with specific topics, such as care of the skin.

Theoretical **Knowledge** knowing *why*

To assist patients with skin care, you must have theoretical knowledge about personal hygiene measures and the structure and function of the **integument** (skin).

Anatomy and Physiology of the Skin

The **integumentary system** consists of the skin, the subcutaneous layer directly under the skin, the hair, nails, and the sweat and sebaceous glands. The skin covers the internal structures of the body and protects them from the environment. It has two distinct layers, the epidermis and the dermis (see Fig. 34-1, in Chapter 34).

The **epidermis** (the thicker, outer layer) consists of stratified squamous epithelial tissue composed of keratinized (dead) cells, which are fused to make the skin waterproof. The epidermis continually sheds **(desquamates)** and is completely replaced every 3 to 4 weeks. The epidermis contains **melanin,** a pigment that provides protection against the ultraviolet rays of the sun and that, together with circulating blood, gives skin its color. The **dermis** (the thinner, second layer) contains blood and lymphatic vessels, nerves, bases of hair follicles, and sebaceous and sweat glands.

Functions of the Skin

The skin has five main functions: protection, sensation, regulation, secretion/excretion, and formation of vitamin D.

1. *Protection.* Intact skin is the body's first line of defense against bacteria and other microorganisms that can enter the body and cause infection. It also provides protection from thermal, chemical, and mechanical injury to underlying tissues. **Sebaceous glands** secrete an oily substance called *sebum,* which helps to waterproof and lubricate the skin and decrease bacterial growth.
2. *Sensation.* The skin contains sensory organs or receptors for heat, cold, pressure, touch, and pain.
3. *Regulation.* The skin helps maintain fluid and electrolyte balance by preventing the escape of excess water and electrolytes from the body. It helps to regulate body temperature through the processes of dilating and constricting blood vessels and activating or inactivating sweat glands. **Sweat glands,** concentrated in the axillae and external genitalia, excrete water in the form of perspiration; evaporation produces a cooling effect on the skin.
4. *Secretion/excretion.* The sweat glands secrete fatty acids and proteins and excrete nitrogenous wastes (*urea*), sodium chloride, and water in perspiration.
5. *Vitamin D formation.* The skin contains a form of cholesterol that is changed to vitamin D on exposure to ultraviolet light from the sun. This is why vitamin D is sometimes referred to as the "sunshine vitamin."

See Chapter 34 for more information about the structure and functions of the skin.

Factors Affecting the Skin

In addition to a person's hygiene practices, health status and developmental stage also affect skin condition.

Health Status

Anything that interferes with the hydration, circulation, and nutrition of the skin creates a risk to skin integrity. As you read each of the following factors, think whether it would be present for Mr. Gold ("Meet Your Patients")?

Dampness of the skin is caused by excessive perspiration (e.g., in fever and certain illnesses) and incontinence of urine or bowel. The skin breaks down more easily when it is damp, especially in the skinfolds. This is called **maceration.**

Dehydration is caused by fluid loss (e.g., from vomiting, diarrhea, or fever) and by insufficient fluid intake. This causes the skin to become dry and to crack easily.

Nutritional Status is also a factor. People who are very thin or very obese are more likely to experience skin irritation and injury. *Morbid obesity* makes it physically difficult to reach all areas of the body, and can lead to development of odor and fungal conditions.

Insufficient Circulation may be caused by immobility, vascular disease, and overall inadequate nutritional status. This predisposes the patient to local tissue death and ulceration when skin cells do not receive enough oxygen.

Skin Diseases, such as impetigo (a bacterial infection of the skin), and *systemic diseases,* such as measles and chickenpox, cause lesions that create discomfort and require special hygiene care.

Jaundice, yellow discoloration caused by accumulation of bile pigments in the skin, is a symptom of certain diseases. Jaundice causes the skin to be itchy and dry.

Lifestyle and Personal Choices also affect the skin. For example, people damage their skin by exposure to ultraviolet rays because they want to be tan. Some use sunscreen; some do not. Whether as a matter of style or self-expression, many people have skin tattoos or piercings, creating the risk for systemic and local infection and scarring.

Developmental Stage

Infants have fragile, easily injured skin. As a child matures, the skin becomes more resistant to injury and infection, but children need adults to provide or supervise the cleanliness of their skin. In adolescence, the sebaceous glands enlarge, and secretions increase. The skin becomes oily and susceptible to acne.

With aging, the skin changes in numerous visible ways, increasing the older adult's risk for skin problems, such as pressure ulcers and reduced ability to heal. Refer to Table 22-1 for a description of normal skin changes in older adults.

KnowledgeCheck 22-2

- What are five functions of the skin?
- How does the skin help regulate body temperature?
- What changes take place in the skin as a person ages?

Table 22-1 ➤ Normal Skin Changes in Older Adults

STRUCTURE	CHANGE IN STRUCTURE AND ACTIVITY	CLINICAL EFFECTS
Epidermis	Thinner; decreased rate of cell turnover	Skin appears pale and somewhat translucent; slower healing.
Subcutaneous tissues	Thinner and more fragile, less fat	Decreased protection of bony prominences and thermoregulation
Collagen and elastin fibers in the dermis	Weaken and become less elastic	Skin becomes wrinkled.
Sebaceous and sweat glands	Activity decreases.	Skin becomes dry, scaly, and itchy.
		Temperature regulation in hot weather becomes more difficult.
Hormones (estrogen and progesterone)	Production decreases.	Contributes to drying and thinning of the skin.
Skin	Vascularity decreases.	Skin becomes cool and pale.
Hair follicles	Diminish in number and activity.	Hair becomes thin, grows more slowly.
Melanocytes (pigment cells)	Numbers decrease.	Hair turns gray or white; skin may become unevenly pigmented.
Nails	Thicken, become softer, growth rate diminishes	Nails tear easily.
Skin growths	Become more common (e.g., warts, "liver spots," "age spots")	Most are caused by years of sun exposure; most are harmless (except for skin cancers, which are fairly common but not normal changes).

Go to Chapter 22, **Knowledge Check Response Sheet and Answers,** on the Student Resource Disk or DavisPlus at http://davisplus.fadavis.com/Wilkinson2

Practical **Knowledge** **knowing** how

ASSESSMENT (SKIN)

Assisting with a bath provides an excellent opportunity to assess the patient's skin. Although you can instruct a NAP to report her observations of the patient's skin, you are ultimately responsible for making the assessments. For a thorough discussion of skin assessment, including how to describe and document your observations, see Chapter 19. However, you should routinely make the following assessments as you provide skin care interventions.

Subjective Data

Patients may be sensitive about skin problems or poor hygiene practices, so as you direct your questions to the patient, do so in a nonjudgmental, respectful manner. Ask the patient about:

- Usual bathing and skin care practices and preferences
- Past and current skin problems, including their effects on the patient's life

- Prescription and over-the-counter (OTC) or herbal remedies used to treat any skin problems
- Allergic skin reactions to food, medications, plants, skin care products, or other substances
- History of diseases or other factors that are known to cause skin problems, for example, decreased mobility, decreased circulation, incontinence, inadequate nutrition, or deficient knowledge

Objective Data

Inspect each area of the skin in an orderly, head-to-toe manner, noting overall cleanliness, condition, color, texture, turgor, hydration, and temperature. Also look for rashes, lumps, lesions, and cracking. Look for drainage from wounds or around tubes. Protect the patient's privacy by closing the curtain and exposing only the area being bathed or examined. Be mindful of the room temperature, and try to reduce drafts to avoid chilling the patient. Observe for four significant color changes:

1. **Pallor** in a light-skinned person may appear as pale skin without underlying pink tones. In a dark-skinned person, observe for an ashen gray or yellow color.
2. **Erythema** is redness of the skin. It is related to vasodilation and inflammation. It is difficult to see in dark-skinned people, so you may discover it by palpating the skin for areas of increased warmth.

3. **Jaundice,** a yellow discoloration of the skin, occurs in patients with impaired liver function. It is best seen in the sclerae of the eyes.

4. **Cyanosis,** a bluish coloring of the skin, is caused by decreased peripheral circulation or decreased oxygenation of the blood. It may be related to cardiac, pulmonary, or peripheral vascular problems (e.g., arteriosclerosis). In dark-skinned patients, you can best see cyanosis by examining the conjunctivae, tongue, buccal mucosa, and palms and soles for a dull dark color.

KnowledgeCheck 22-3

- True or False: The professional nurse is responsible for making assessments.
- True or False: Assisting with the bath is an excellent time to assess the patient.
- To inspect for pallor in a dark-skinned person, which areas would you assess for an ashen gray or yellow color?
- What is the term that means "a bluish color of the skin"?
- Name two causes of erythema.
- Where can you best see jaundice?

 Go to Chapter 22, **Knowledge Check Response Sheet and Answers,** on the Student Resource Disk or DavisPlus at http://davisplus.fadavis.com/Wilkinson2

■ ANALYSIS/NURSING DIAGNOSIS (SKIN)

You should be familiar with the following common skin problems:

- **Pruritus** (itching) may lead to scratching and breaks in the skin.
- **Dry skin** tends to crack, burn, or itch.
- **Maceration** is softening of the skin from prolonged moisture (e.g., urinary incontinence). It makes the epidermis more susceptible to injury.
- **Excoriation** is a loss of the superficial layers of the skin caused, for example, by scratching and by the digestive enzymes in feces.
- **Abrasion,** a rubbing away of the epidermal layer of the skin, especially over bony areas or prominences, is often caused by friction or shearing forces that occur when a patient moves or is moved in bed.
- **Pressure ulcers** (decubitus ulcers) are lesions caused by tissue compression and inadequate perfusion. See Chapter 34.
- **Acne** is an inflammation of the sebaceous glands that is common among adolescents and young adults.
- **Burns** are a type of traumatic injury caused by thermal, electrical, chemical, or radioactive agents.

To see illustrations of most of those skin problems,

 Go to Chapter 19, **"Assessing the Skin,"** in Volume 2.

Impaired Skin Integrity as the Problem

When you wish to focus on prevention or treatment of the *skin condition,* use the following NANDA-I (2009) diagnostic labels.

- **Risk for Impaired Skin Integrity.** *Definition:* At risk for skin being adversely altered.
  Risk factors: NANDA-I lists about 20 specific risk factors (e.g., radiation, obesity). It may be easier for you to remember the general conditions that affect the skin: dampness, dehydration, insufficient circulation, nutritional status (thin or obese), skin diseases, systemic diseases, and jaundice.
- **Impaired Skin Integrity.** *Definition:* Altered epidermis or dermis.
  Defining characteristics: Invasion of body structures, destruction of skin layers (dermis), disruption of skin surface (epidermis).

Examples of diagnostic statements for skin problems include the following:

  Risk for Impaired Skin Integrity related to immobility secondary to casts and traction
  Risk for Impaired Skin Integrity related to dehydration and malnutrition
  Impaired Skin Integrity related to decreased peripheral circulation secondary to arteriosclerosis
  Impaired Skin Integrity related to skin fragility secondary to severe peripheral edema

Impaired Skin Integrity as the Etiology

Impaired Skin Integrity may be the etiology of other nursing diagnoses. Certain skin problems place the patient at risk for infection by causing cracks or breaks in the skin. Others may contribute to discomfort and low self-esteem. The following are examples:

  Risk for Infection related to skin lacerations and abrasions
  Situational Low Self-Esteem related to appearance and self-consciousness about skin lesions secondary to severe eczema

CriticalThinking 22-5

- Why are Mrs. Williams and Mr. Gold ("Meet Your Patients") at risk for Impaired Skin Integrity?
- What are the specific kinds of skin integrity problems that pose an increased risk to both patients?

■ PLANNING OUTCOMES/EVALUATION (SKIN)

For *NOC standardized outcomes* for problems of the skin, feet, nails, mouth, teeth, hair, eyes, ears, and nose,

 Go to Chapter 22, **Standardized Language, Selected NOC Outcomes and NIC Interventions for Hygiene Problems,** in Volume 2.

Individualized goals/outcome statements you might write for a patient with skin problems include the following:

- Skin will remain intact and free of secretions.
- Skin will remain free of lesions.
- The patient will follow regimen to improve skin dryness.

PLANNING INTERVENTIONS/IMPLEMENTATION (SKIN)

For *NIC standardized interventions* for skin integrity and skin care,

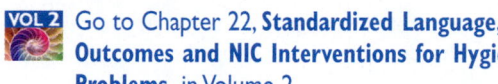 Go to Chapter 22, **Standardized Language, NOC Outcomes and NIC Interventions for Hygiene Problems,** in Volume 2.

Individualized nursing activities for patients with Impaired Skin Integrity include bathing and massage, which are presented in this section. You will usually delegate patient bathing to NAPs. Therefore, your most important interventions may be to be certain that the patient actually gets a bath (see Fig. 22-1).

Rationale for Bathing

Bathing serves three purposes: health, social interaction, and pleasure or relaxation. As the fatty acids, proteins, and nitrogenous waste mix with bacteria on the skin, bacterial growth and odor result. Bathing removes perspiration and bacteria from the skin surface, helping to prevent body odor. The warmth from the bath water and the friction of bathing dilate the blood vessels near the surface of the skin, increasing the circulation. Bathing stimulates depth of respirations and provides sensory input. It can also be a time to strengthen the nurse–patient relationship, promote relaxation and comfort, enhance well-being, and improve self-image. And, as you have already learned, bath time is an excellent time to make a variety of assessments.

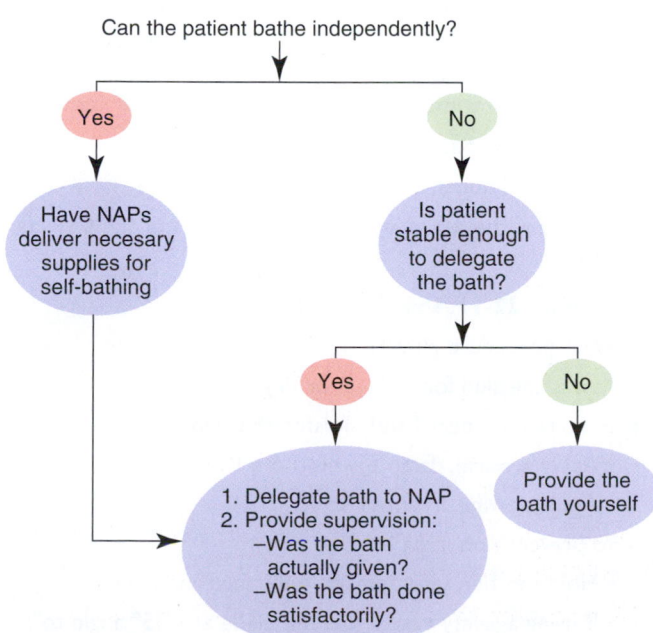

FIGURE 22-1 The RN should assess the patient, delegate bathing as appropriate, and provide supervision.

Choosing the Type of Bath to Meet Patient Needs

The type of bath you give depends on your nursing judgment; the patient's preference, self-care ability, and endurance; and the medical plan of care. As you know, functional ability ranges from completely dependent to completely independent. Different types of baths are appropriate at different levels of ability. **"Assist" bath** is a term commonly used to indicate that the nurse helps the patient with areas that may be difficult to reach, such as the back, feet, and legs. If a complete bath would be stressful to the patient, you may sometimes give a **partial bath;** that is, you will cleanse only the areas that may cause odor or discomfort, such as the axillae and perineum. The following sections discuss other types of baths in detail.

Bed Baths

A **bed bath** is for patients who must remain in bed but who are able to bathe themselves. You will assist by placing supplies on the bedside stand or overbed table. Supplies include a basin of warm water (105°F [41°C]), bath linens, a clean gown, and other bathing supplies such as lotion and cosmetics if desired. Provide privacy, and place the call device within reach. Remove the top linens from the bed, and cover the patient with a bath blanket. If the patient cannot bathe all areas of his body, complete the bath for him.

A **complete bed bath** means you will wash the patient's entire body without assistance from the patient. This is usually performed in a head-to-toe fashion, cleansing from cleanest area to most soiled area. For complete instructions,

 Go to Chapter 22, **Procedure 22-1: Bathing: Providing a Complete Bed Bath,** in Volume 2.

See also the accompanying box, Critical Aspects of Procedures 22-1 through 22-14.

Towel Bath

A **towel bath** is a modification of the bed bath, in which you place a large towel and a bath blanket in a plastic bag, saturate them with a warmed, commercially prepared mixture of moisturizer, disinfectant, nonrinse cleaning agent and use them to bathe the patient. Because the solution dries rapidly, there is no need to towel-dry the patient. Some agencies prefer towel baths because they take less time than a traditional bed bath and because patients find them satisfactory. This is a preferred method for patients who have mild to moderate Impaired Skin Integrity or Activity Intolerance and for patients with dementia (e.g., Alzheimer's disease).

 Go to Chapter 22, **Procedure 22-2: Bathing: Providing a Towel Bath,** in Volume 2.

Bag or Packaged Bath

A **bag bath** is a modification of the towel bath, in which you use 8 to 10 washcloths instead of a towel and

VOL 2 For steps to follow in *all* procedures, refer to the Universal Steps for All Procedures found on the inside back cover of Volume 2. Go to the full procedures in Volume 2 to practice and learn the procedure steps. Use these Critical Aspects later to help you review key points.

Procedures 22-1, 22-2, and 22-3: Bathing: Providing a Complete Bed Bath, Providing a Towel Bath, and Providing a Packaged Bath

➤ Use warm, not hot, water.

➤ Avoid chilling or tiring the patient.

➤ Bathe the patient following the principles of "head to toe" and "clean to dirty."

➤ For extremities, wash and dry from distal to proximal.

➤ Change the water before cleansing the perineum and whenever the water becomes dirty or cool.

➤ Perform hand hygiene when moving from a contaminated body part to bathe a clean body part.

➤ Check the temperature of the packaged bath after microwaving.

Procedure 22-4: Providing Perineal Care

➤ Provide privacy; keep the patient covered as much as possible.

➤ Place waterproof underpad to protect the bed linens.

➤ Use warm water.

➤ Perform perineal care following the principle of "clean to dirty" (front to back).

Procedure 22-5: Providing Foot Care

➤ Inspect the feet thoroughly for skin integrity, circulation, and edema.

➤ Clean the feet with mild soap; clean the toenails; rinse; and dry well.

➤ Trim the nails straight across, unless contraindicated. Check institutional policy; many institutions do not allow nurses to trim nails.

➤ File the nails with an emery board.

➤ Lightly apply lotion, except between the toes.

➤ Ensure that footwear or bedding is not irritating to the feet.

Procedure 22-6: Brushing and Flossing the Teeth

➤ Assess the teeth, mucous membranes, and swallowing ability.

➤ Position the patient to prevent aspiration (sitting or side-lying position).

➤ Hold the brush at a 45° angle, and brush the patient's teeth (or assist).

➤ Floss and rinse.

➤ If the patient is at risk for choking, suction secretions as needed.

Procedure 22-7: Providing Denture Care

➤ Refer to Procedure 22-6, Brushing and Flossing the Teeth.

➤ Remove (and replace) the top denture before the lower denture.

➤ Tilt dentures slightly when removing and replacing.

➤ Handle dentures carefully, and place a towel in the sink to avoid breaking the dentures if you drop them.

➤ Use cool water and a stiff-bristled brush.

Procedure 22-8: Providing Oral Care for an Unconscious Patient

➤ Assess the condition of the teeth (or dentures), gums, and mucous membranes.

➤ Assess for the gag reflex.

➤ Position the patient to prevent aspiration.

➤ Brush and floss the patient's teeth.

➤ Suction secretions as needed.

Procedure 22-9: Shampooing the Hair

➤ Determine the type of procedure needed. Assess the patient's ability to help and the condition of the hair and scalp.

➤ Identify hair care products needed for the procedure.

➤ Protect the bed from getting wet.

➤ Wash the hair with warm water.

➤ Protect the patient's eyes and ears from soap and water.

➤ Towel-dry the hair.

➤ Take care not to burn the patient with the hair dryer, if one is used.

Procedure 22-10: Providing Beard and Mustache Care

➤ Assess the skin for redness, dry areas, or lesions.

➤ Trim the beard and mustache to the desired length with a comb and a scissors or beard trimmer. Follow the manufacturer's instructions if using a trimmer or razor.

➤ Shampoo the beard and mustache.

➤ Apply conditioner, if desired.

➤ Towel-dry the beard and mustache, and comb and style as desired.

Procedure 22-11: Shaving a Patient

➤ Wear procedure gloves.

➤ Assess the skin for redness or dry areas.

➤ To soften the beard and moisten the skin:

  ➤ Apply a warm, damp towel to the face.

  ➤ Apply shaving cream or soap.

➤ To prevent skin irritation:

  ➤ Hold the skin taut, and shave the face and neck.

  ➤ If using a safety razor, hold the blade at a 45° angle to the skin.

  ➤ Apply after-shave product, if desired.

Procedure 22-12: Removing and Caring for Contact Lenses

➤ Instill one or two drops of wetting solution.
➤ Gently remove contact lenses; use your finger pads, not your fingernails.
➤ Clean and store contact lenses in sterile solution.
➤ Mark the containers "L" and "R" to identify the correct eye.

Procedure 22-13: Making an Unoccupied Bed

➤ Remove soiled linens without cross-contaminating other items in the room.
➤ Remake the bed with clean linens.
➤ Do not "shake" or "fan" linens.
➤ Work efficiently and safely.
➤ Ensure that there are no wrinkles in the bottom sheet or drawsheet.

Procedure 22-14: Making an Occupied Bed

➤ Maintain patient safety during the procedure.
➤ Assess the patient's ability to move and need for assistive equipment and patient-handling devices.
➤ Position the patient laterally near the far siderail, and roll soiled linens under him.
➤ Place clean linens on the side nearest you, and then tuck under the soiled linens.
➤ Roll the patient over the "hump," and position him on his other side, near you. Raise the near siderail.
➤ Move to the other side of the bed; pull soiled and clean linens through, and complete the linen change as in Procedure 22-13: Making an Unoccupied Bed.

➤ Place the bed in a low position, raise the siderails, and fasten the call light to the pillow.

Procedure 22-15: Caring for Artificial Eyes

➤ Ask the patient to lie down.
➤ Remove the artificial eye: Raise the upper eyelid; with dominant hand, depress the lower lid and apply slight pressure below the eye (or use a small bulb syringe).
➤ Clean the eye with saline; store in saline or tap water; label the container.
➤ Clean the edge of the eye socket with a moistened cotton ball.
➤ Reinsert the eye: Be sure the prosthesis is wet. Hold it with your dominant hand. Spread the patient's eyelids apart with nondominant hand, and guide prosthesis into the eye socket.

Procedure 22-16: Caring for Hearing Aids

➤ Keep hearing aids away from heat and moisture.
➤ Clean hearing aids with a damp cloth only.
➤ Avoid hairspray and other hair care products.
➤ Turn off hearing aids when not in use.
➤ Replace dead batteries immediately.
➤ Store hearing aids in a case with the battery compartment open.
➤ Keep hearing aids and batteries away from children and pets.
➤ To clean a hearing aid: Turn it off, remove it from the ear, cleanse the outer ear and the hearing aid, check the battery, reinsert it, turn it on, check the volume with the patient.

bath blanket. They are heated in a microwave oven designated for that purpose, and each part of the patient's body is cleansed with a fresh cloth. A **packaged bath** refers to a set of commercially prepared and packaged, premoistened, disposable washcloths that are used in the same way as a bag bath. These too should be warmed. When these are delivered to the bedside, be certain the patient knows what they are for and how to use them.

  Go to Chapter 22, **Procedure 22-3: Bathing: Providing a Packaged or Bag Bath,** in Volume 2.

Critical Thinking 22-6

Suppose you have been providing towel baths to a patient who has mild dementia. One day a visiting family member says, "My father tells me he has not had a bath all week. What's going on here?" What would you do? How could you help to prevent this misunderstanding in the future?

Shower

Most ambulatory patients prefer a shower. It is a time-saver and refreshing as well as cleansing. In a hospital or long-term care facility, some clients can manage a

shower mostly on their own. Even so, you will still need to be sure the shower or tub is clean and safe. Most hospitals and long-term care facilities have safety grab bars and handrails in the bathrooms, but these may need to be installed in the home. You may also need to prepare the client's bathing supplies, assist her to the shower, and help with areas of her body that she cannot reach. For complete information,

 Go to Chapter 22, **Clinical Insight 22-1: Assisting with a Shower or Tub Bath,** in Volume 2.

Tub Bath

If a client is ambulatory but requires much assistance with bathing (e.g., because of pain and stiffness in the hands and arms), you may prefer a tub bath. It will be easier for you to wash and rinse the patient, and you will not get as wet as when you help with a shower. Immersion in the water also helps to soak areas that are crusty, scaly, or soiled and relaxes stiff, sore muscles and joints. Overall, tub baths are thought to be of greater benefit than a sponge or bed bath. Your responsibilities for a tub bath are similar to those for a shower if the patient is ambulatory, and similar to an assist bath if the patient requires a great deal of support.

The tub should have handrails and a nonskid surface to prevent falls. Some patients need assistance getting into and out of a tub. Some kneel or squat first and then sit in the tub. For completely dependent patients, there are specially designed tubs that reduce the effort necessary to lift patients into and out of the tub. You can also use a hydraulic lift and a regular tub (Fig. 22-2). For more information and safety tips for tub baths,

 Go to Chapter 22, **Clinical Insight 22-1: Assisting with a Shower or Tub Bath,** in Volume 2.

Therapeutic Bath

The primary care provider may prescribe **therapeutic baths** for some patients. The prescription will include specific instructions for the type of bath and solution to be used, area of the body to be treated, and water temperature. Oatmeal or coal tar baths are examples of therapeutic baths used to treat specific skin conditions, such as chickenpox lesions or psoriasis. It is your responsibility to add the medically ordered substance, ensure appropriate temperature, assist the patient into the tub, and clean the tub at the end of the bath. A warm sitz bath is another type of therapeutic bath; it helps to cleanse the perineum and soothe inflammation of perineal, vaginal, or rectal tissues.

Perineal Care

The **perineum** (the area between the anus and vulva in a female, or the anus and scrotum in a male) is a dark, warm, moist area that supports bacterial growth. Perineal care promotes comfort and prevents odor, skin excoriation, and infection. You will usually give perineal care (including the external genitalia) along with a complete bed bath, but you may do it at other times as well—for example, when a patient needs only an assist bath. Give perineal care more frequently if the patient is incontinent of urine or feces or has drainage from the area.

Because of personal, cultural, or religious beliefs, some patients may wish to have a same-sex caregiver provide the bath. Whether you and the patient are of the same or opposite sex, perineal care may be embarrassing for you both. Perform care in a professional manner, and provide the patient with privacy (e.g., shut the door, pull bed curtains, drape properly). It may help to have someone of the same sex as the patient present in the room, but a matter-of-fact, sensitive approach puts most patients at ease.

Always wear gloves when providing perineal care because of the possibility of coming in contact with urine, vaginal secretions, or fecal material. As with every patient contact, remember to wash your hands before and after the procedure. For complete information about providing perineal care,

 Go to Chapter 22, **Procedure 22-4: Providing Perineal Care,** in Volume 2.

Also see the Critical Aspects box for Procedures 22-1 through 22-14.

FIGURE 22-2 *A,* A hydraulic lift allows you to transport a patient to a bath or shower. *B,* A tub with a side-opening door enables patients to safely and easily enter the tub. (Courtesy of Carroll Health Care, London, Ontario, Canada.)

KnowledgeCheck 22-4
- What causes body odor?
- What is the best intervention to rid the skin of body odor?
- What is the rationale for providing perineal care?
- How can you protect patient privacy during perineal care?

Go to Chapter 22, **Knowledge Check Response Sheet and Answers,** on the Student Resource Disk or DavisPlus at http://davisplus.fadavis.com/Wilkinson2

Critical Thinking 22-7

- Which of your patients ("Meet Your Patients") will require nurse-assisted perineal care? Explain your reasoning.
- Which patient, if you are a woman, is most likely to be embarrassed by perineal care? Explain your reasoning.
- If you need more theoretical knowledge to answer these questions, what is it? Where could you find the information?

Back Massage

Regardless of the type of bath used, when possible end the bath with a back massage to provide relaxation and stimulate circulation. As with all procedures, be sure there are no contraindications to massage (e.g., fractured ribs, burns, recent heart surgery).

 Go to Chapter 33, **Procedure 33-1: Giving a Back Massage,** in Volume 2.

Bathing Patients with Dementia

Bathing should be a pleasant experience, not a stressful one. However, this is not true for all patients, especially those with dementia. People with dementia tend to become agitated when told it is time to bathe. They commonly yell, scream, pinch, or hit their caregivers (Rasin & Barrick, 2004). The reason for the patients' agitation is usually that they experience pain, cold, fear, and loss of control. When the nurse meets patient comfort needs, the aggressive behavior declines significantly. Simply by adjusting the water temperature or taking special care when washing arthritic joints, you may make the patient more comfortable and less agitated.

Nurses and NAPs sometimes focus, mistakenly, on the need to give a daily tub bath or shower. Caregivers can significantly reduce aggressive behaviors by giving a towel bath or bag bath instead (Rasin & Barrick, 2004). Despite the common myths about bathing, keep in mind that:

- It does not take a large amount of water (e.g., a shower) to get a person clean.
- The bath does not have to be performed at the same time every day, nor in the way "we have always done it here."
- You can educate families that showers and tub baths are not the only ways to get clean.
- The patient will not be at more risk for skin problems or infections if a towel bath is used.
- It is not necessary to bathe a person who is resisting. You can adapt the approach, method, and time.
- Patients who are forced to bathe do not "just forget about it"; many stay upset and agitated for hours.

For more discussion of bathing myths and for instructions about providing a towel bath for a person with dementia,

 Go to Chapter 22, **Clinical Insight 22-2: Bathing a Patient with Dementia,** in Volume 2.

Bathing Morbidly Obese Patients

More than half the adult population is overweight. **Obesity** is traditionally defined as 20% to 40% above one's ideal weight. A person is considered severely, or **morbidly,** obese when he is 100% over ideal weight. In this chapter, we focus only on the special hygiene needs of those who are morbidly obese. Thorough skin assessment is essential, but it is difficult. Be sure to obtain adequate assistance to reposition the patient during the skin exam, so that you do not miss any areas. Pay special attention to skinfolds. Refer to Table 22-2 for etiologies of skin problems in morbidly obese clients, and for interventions to use when providing skin care for severely obese patients. Teach these interventions to NAPs and to patients who bathe independently.

Bathing Older Adults

For older adults, especially the bed-bound and frail elderly, you must provide proper skin care and bathing techniques to prevent skin breakdown. At the same time, you should promote comfort and encourage independence in ADLs. Goals are to prevent drying of and injury to the skin. Bag baths adequately address the problems of skin itching and irritation, improve skin integrity, and are far less distressing to frail older adults (Lentz, 2003). Other interventions include avoiding use of soap, being sure to clean the skin immediately after soiling, and applying skin moisturizer. For further guidelines,

 Go to Chapter 22, **Procedure 22-1: Bathing: Providing a Complete Bed Bath, What if My Patient Is an Older Adult?,** in Volume 2.

Knowledge Check 22-5

- A nurse has given a bath in which he washed a bedridden patient's entire body without assistance from the patient. What is the term for this bath?
- What are the advantages of a towel or bag bath?
- For which type of bath will you most likely have a medical prescription?

 Go to Chapter 22, **Knowledge Check Response Sheet and Answers,** on the Student Resource Disk or DavisPlus at http://davisplus.fadavis.com/Wilkinson2

Critical Thinking 22-8

- Which type of bath would be most appropriate for each of your patients ("Meet Your Patients")?
- Provide rationales for your choices.

Care of the Feet

Foot care is a necessary part of hygiene and essential at any age for tissue health, proper posture, and ambulation.

Table 22-2 ➤ Skin Care for Morbidly Obese Clients

PROBLEM ETIOLOGY	INTERVENTIONS
Hygiene Morbidly obese clients find it physically difficult to reach all areas of the body. In addition, they may have limited mobility. Inability to maintain good hygiene may lead to odor and fungal infections.	Ask how the patient handles skin care at home. Use the same adaptations, if possible. Provide a trapeze to assist the patient to lift and reach difficult areas. Provide a hand-held shower and long-handled brushes. Experts vary on the use of soap. Certainly the skin should be rinsed and dried well.
Moisture Skin in skinfolds stays damp because perspiration cannot evaporate. Moisture contributes to the development of fungal and other skin infections.	Use moisture barrier creams, particularly in skinfolds. Use fans, if permitted. Change linens often. Manage incontinence, including petrolatum barrier creams. If fungal infections occur, you may need a medical prescription for antifungal powders, sprays, cream, or ointment.
Pressure Pressure can be caused by limited mobility, by skin folds where skin rubs on skin, by tight clothing, catheters, and so on.	Reposition the patient frequently to redistribute the pressure of the skinfolds. Reposition catheters and tubes often; use tube holders to prevent rubbing. Separate the skin folds with towels.
Shear and Friction The patient is at risk for friction and shearing injury from pulling skin across the linens when moving in the bed and chair.	The ANA's (2003) position is that you should use specialized lifts and other equipment to move patients safely and avoid injury to yourself. If, in an emergency, you must move the patient, obtain sufficient help to avoid pulling the skin across the sheet or other surfaces. Do not use sheepskins. Use a Gore-Tex® mattress cover. Keep linens wrinkle-free. Provide a trapeze.
Nutrition Morbidly obese patients may have poor nutritional status because of lifestyle factors (e.g., fast food intake and other poor dietary habits) and lack of exercise or mobility.	Recommend evaluation by a nutritionist. Monitor blood sugar. Encourage adequate protein intake.

Source: Adapted from Rose, M., & Drake, D. (2008). Best practices for skin care of the morbidly obese. *Bariatric Nursing and Surgical Patient Care, 3*(2), 129–134.

Theoretical Knowledge
knowing why

When providing foot care, you will need theoretical knowledge about the structure of the feet, life span variations, and common foot problems. The feet provide support for the weight of the entire body and absorb a significant amount of shock during walking. Their musculoskeletal structure is complex, consisting of 26 bones and many muscles, tendons, and ligaments. The feet can be affected by congenital malformations, injuries, improper footwear, and medical conditions. For example, a person with diabetes mellitus or peripheral neuropathy (nerve damage) may experience decreased sensation and delayed healing of open areas on the feet, and people with arthritis experience pain and decreased mobility.

Developmental Variations

The feet are fully grown at about age 20 and, if healthy, change little throughout life. However, problems tend to increase with aging. Because of diseases such as arteriosclerosis and peripheral vascular insufficiency, older adults often have decreased circulation to the lower extremities. This increases their risk for foot ulcers and infection. The incidence of diabetes is high among older adults, further increasing the risk for infection secondary to delayed healing. In addition, the skin becomes dry, predisposing the older adult to cracking of the skin.

Common Foot Problems

More than 43 million people in the United States have foot abnormalities (e.g., pain, deformity, and disability). Many of these problems are the result of improperly fitting shoes (American Academy of Orthopedic Surgeons, 2001).

- **Corns.** A corn is a cone-shaped thickening of the epidermis caused by continuous pressure (e.g., from improperly fitting shoes) over bony prominences, such as the toe joints. Corns are often painful.
- **Calluses.** Calluses are usually found over bony prominences in the weight-bearing part of the foot: the heels, soles, or plantar surfaces of the feet. They are similar to corns but cover a wider area and are not painful.
- **Tinea pedis.** Athlete's foot, a fungal infection of the skin, is aggravated by moisture accumulation in unventilated shoes. Symptoms include itching and burning skin with blisters, scaling, and cracking, especially between the toes. Athlete's foot may be contracted by walking barefoot in public showers.
- **Ingrown toenail.** Improperly trimming the toenails and wearing poorly fitting shoes may cause an ingrown toenail. The toenail grows inward into the soft tissues around it and the tissue at the nail border becomes swollen, inflamed, and painful. The nail may need to be surgically removed.
- **Foot odor.** Microorganisms growing on the feet interact with perspiration to produce foot odor. The warm, moist environment created by shoes encourages both perspiration and bacterial growth.
- **Plantar warts** are painful growths caused by a virus. They may occur on any part of the sole of the foot but often develop under pressure points, such as the heel or ball of the foot.
- **Pressure ulcers** are lesions caused by unrelieved pressure that impairs the circulation; this usually occurs over a bony prominence. In patients confined to bed, the back of the heels, the ankles, and the great toes are common locations; but pressure ulcers do, of course, occur over other bony prominences as well.
- **Bunions** (hallux valgus) are a progressive disorder that begins the enlargement of the first metatarsal

joint at the base of the great toe and then progresses to leaning of the big toe, gradually changing the angle of the bones. A characteristic bump occurs slowly and continues to become increasingly prominent with aging. Tight-fitting shoes (particularly with high heels) are thought to be the cause of bunions in the large majority of patients. Genetics also play a role as do some diseases, such as arthritis. For optional illustrations and more information about bunions,

 Go to the URL of the American College of Foot and Ankle Surgeons, at the link provided in **Resources for Caregivers and Health Professionals,** in Chapter 22 of the Student Resource Disk or DavisPlus at http://davisplus.fadavis.com/Wilkinson2

Practical **Knowledge** **knowing** how

The nursing focus for foot care is on prevention and early identification of problems. For associated *NOC standardized outcomes* and *NIC interventions* for patients with common foot problems,

 Go to Chapter 22, **Standardized Language, Selected NOC Outcomes and NIC Interventions for Hygiene Problems,** in Volume 2.

ASSESSMENT (FEET)

Careful assessment of the feet allows for early detection of common foot problems. For a thorough discussion of foot assessment, see Chapter 19. This chapter describes routine observations that you can make when giving foot care.

You will need information about the patient's normal foot care routine, the type of footwear he usually wears, any foot problems or treatments for them, and any diseases (e.g., diabetes mellitus and peripheral vascular disease) that create risks for foot problems.

As you observe the feet, compare findings for both feet. Assess cleanliness, odor, and skin integrity. Inspect for redness, drainage, and swelling. Palpate for edema, and check for cracks or signs of fungal infection between the toes. The color and temperature of the feet provide data about circulation and oxygenation. For example, cold, dusky, or pale feet may indicate impaired circulation or tissue perfusion secondary to peripheral vascular disease. Check capillary refill. For specific questions to ask,

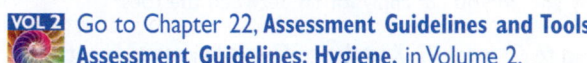 Go to Chapter 22, **Assessment Guidelines and Tools, Assessment Guidelines: Hygiene,** in Volume 2.

ANALYSIS/NURSING DIAGNOSIS (FEET)

The following are examples of nursing diagnoses related to the feet:

- Impaired Skin (or Tissue) Integrity (feet) related to mechanical pressure from wearing shoes that do not fit properly
- Risk for Impaired Skin Integrity (feet) related to (1) decreased sensation secondary to diabetes mellitus and (2) decreased circulation to the feet secondary to arteriosclerosis
- Impaired Walking related to foot pain secondary to arthritis
- Risk for Injury (to feet) related to deficient knowledge of foot hygiene

PLANNING OUTCOMES/EVALUATION (FEET)

Individualized goals/outcome statements you might write for a patient with foot problems include the following:

- Demonstrates proper cleansing, rinsing, and drying of the feet.
- Avoids trimming calluses.
- Wears shoes that fit properly.
- Inspects feet regularly.

PLANNING INTERVENTIONS/IMPLEMENTATION (FEET)

Individualized nursing activities related to care of the feet are those that prevent infection, odor, and trauma to the soft tissues of the feet. While performing foot care, teach the patient about self-care measures for care of the feet (see Self-Care: Teaching Your Client About Foot Care). To learn how to administer foot care see the Critical Aspects box for Procedures 22-1 through 22-14, and

 Go to Chapter 22, **Procedure 22-5: Providing Foot Care,** in Volume 2.

Diabetic Foot Care

Because of impaired circulation and increased risk for infection, people who have diabetes are at high risk for problems with their feet. If they have neuropathy, they may not experience pain with a foot injury, so treatment may be delayed. If untreated, a seemingly minor foot lesion can progress to gangrene and require amputation. The instructions in the box, Self-Care: Teaching Your Client About Foot Care, are especially important for people with diabetes (as well as for those with impaired peripheral circulation).

KnowledgeCheck 22-6

- What are some causes of ingrown toenails?
- What is the cause of foot odor?
- Why should you *not* apply lotion between the toes?

 Go to Chapter 22, **Knowledge Check Response Sheet and Answers,** on the Student Resource Disk or DavisPlus at http://davisplus.fadavis.com/Wilkinson2

Care of the Nails

The nails are part of the integumentary system. They are composed of epithelial tissue. Healthy nail beds are usually clean, pink, smooth, convex, and evenly curved. Present at birth, the nails change very little throughout life; however, as one ages, nails thicken, become ridged, and may yellow or become concave in shape. Other changes are caused by certain pathological conditions. For example, inadequate diet or metabolic changes can cause the nails to become brittle. Also, patients with diabetes mellitus are much more prone to infection and must be vigilant about toenail care. Trauma to the nail can lead to nail bruising or falling out.

For NANDA-I diagnoses, *NOC standardized outcomes,* and *NIC interventions* for patients with common nail problems,

 Go to Chapter 22, **Standardized Language, Selected NOC Outcomes and NIC Interventions for Hygiene Problems,** in Volume 2.

ASSESSMENT (NAILS)

Unclean or rough fingernails may scratch or abrade the skin and create a risk for infection. Other nail changes may reflect an underlying disease process. In addition, the area under the nail can harbor dirt and bacteria, which can be another source for transmitting microbes. When assessing the nails, you should obtain *subjective data* about the patient's usual nail care practices, any history of nail problems, and their treatments. To obtain *objective data,* inspect the nails for shape, contour, and cleanliness. Look for redness or swelling of the skin around the nails, and observe whether they are neatly manicured and trimmed appropriately, straight across.

For more information about physical assessment of the nails, see Chapter 19, and

 Go to Chapter 22, Assessment Guidelines and Tools, **Assessment Guidelines: Hygiene,** in Volume 2.

ANALYSIS/NURSING DIAGNOSIS (NAILS)

There are no NANDA-I labels to describe nail problems. However, the following are some examples of nursing diagnoses related to nail care:

- Risk for Impaired Tissue Integrity related to ingrown nails secondary to trimming too close to the cuticle
- Risk for Infection related to loss of skin integrity secondary to hangnails, cracked cuticles, or trauma from using sharp scissors or nail clippers

PLANNING OUTCOMES/EVALUATION (NAILS)

Individualized goals/outcome statements you might write for a patient with problems related to the care of the nails may include the following:

- Demonstrates proper care of the nails.
- Trims fingernails with supervision.

Self-Care

Teaching Your Client About Foot Care

Use the time during foot care to teach your client the following self-care activities. These measures are good advice for most people, but they are especially important for people who have diabetes or poor peripheral circulation.

Daily Foot Inspection

➤ Inspect the feet daily, using a mirror to view all surfaces. Check between the toes for cracks or redness. Look for calluses, blisters, wounds and lesions, or dry areas. If you cannot check your own feet, have someone else do it.

➤ If you have diabetes, have your feet checked regularly by a professional.

➤ Seek professional help for foot problems, such as poor circulation, corns, and ingrown toenails, and for trimming very thick nails—especially if you have diabetes.

Hygiene for Feet and Nails

➤ Wash, rinse, and dry the feet well.

➤ Avoid soaking the feet (if you are diabetic, or if there is decreased circulation to the feet).

➤ Apply a water-soluble lotion to feet, but do not use lotion between the toes, because it may cause maceration.

➤ Use an antifungal powder, if necessary, for athlete's foot.

➤ Do not cut or file callused areas.

➤ Cut and file toenails straight across. Do not use a razor blade on the nails or feet.

Shoes and Stockings

➤ Wear cotton or wool socks, which absorb perspiration.

➤ Wear well-fitted, sturdy shoes with nonskid soles and arch support. Natural materials, such as canvas and leather, are best because they allow air to circulate and perspiration to evaporate. Shoes should allow ½ to ¾ inch of toe room.

➤ Avoid open-toed shoes, sandals, high heels, and thongs. They do not protect the feet.

➤ Before putting on shoes, check for foreign objects; check that the inside of the shoe is smooth.

Protecting the Feet

➤ Avoid measures that impair circulation to the feet, such as wearing tight garters or knee stockings, or crossing the legs.

➤ Do not go barefoot, even when getting out of bed at night. Wear slippers.

➤ Do not put tape or over-the-counter corn medicines or pads or other medications (e.g., hydrogen peroxide) on the feet.

➤ Do not smoke. This further decreases circulation to the feet.

Seek Medical Attention for the Following:

➤ Pain in the feet or legs. This may be a sign of loss of circulation, serious infection, or nerve damage (neuropathy).

➤ Wounds or ulcers on the feet, especially if they don't seem to be healing

➤ A cut to the feet or lower legs that extends deep into the skin and bleeds significantly

➤ Generalized redness or red streaks surrounding a wound or ulcer on the feet or lower legs. This might be a sign of infection of the tissue (cellulitis).

➤ Fever greater than 101°F (38.5°C).

➤ Confusion. This can be a sign that a wound infection has entered the blood stream (septicemia). A change in mental status might indicate low blood sugar, which occurs with serious infection, or if the patient is diabetic.

■ Seeks care of a **podiatrist** (physician who specializes in foot care) for toenail care.

▮ PLANNING INTERVENTIONS/IMPLEMENTATION (NAILS)

Individualized nursing activities related to proper care of the nails include the following:

■ Teaching for self-care (see the box, Self-Care: Teaching Your Client About Nail Care)
■ Providing nail care for dependent patients (the procedure for care of the fingernails is the same as for care of the toenails). Also,

VOL 2 Go to Chapter 22, **Procedure 22-5: Providing Foot Care,** in Volume 2.

KnowledgeCheck 22-7

■ True or False: Healthy nails are usually clean, smooth, and convexly curved.
■ List at least three nail changes that occur with aging.
■ List at least four things you should teach clients about self-care of their nails.

 Go to Chapter 22, **Knowledge Check Response Sheet and Answers,** on the Student Resource Disk or DavisPlus at http://davisplus.fadavis.com/Wilkinson2

Oral Hygiene

To maintain the integrity of the mucous membranes, teeth, and gums, and to prevent tooth loss and gum disease, it is important to have (1) routine dental check-ups, (2) adequate nutrition, and (3) daily mouth care or oral hygiene. Mouth care removes food particles and

Teaching Your Client About Nail Care

➤ Inspect the nails daily.

➤ Trim nails with a nail clipper. (People with diabetes or circulatory problems should file only, because cutting poses a risk for injury to the tissues.)

➤ File the nails straight across, rounding the corners slightly to prevent scratching. Do not cut deeply into the lateral corners because this may cause ingrown nails.

➤ Remove hangnails by carefully removing them with cuticle clipper.

➤ Clean under the nails with an orangewood stick or other blunt instrument.

➤ Push back the cuticles gently.

➤ Use a moisturizing lotion to soften cuticles.

➤ Avoid biting nails.

➤ Consult a podiatrist for ingrown toenails or other nail problems.

➤ Recommend to patients with diabetes, circulatory insufficiency, or nail problems that they seek nail care from a podiatrist.

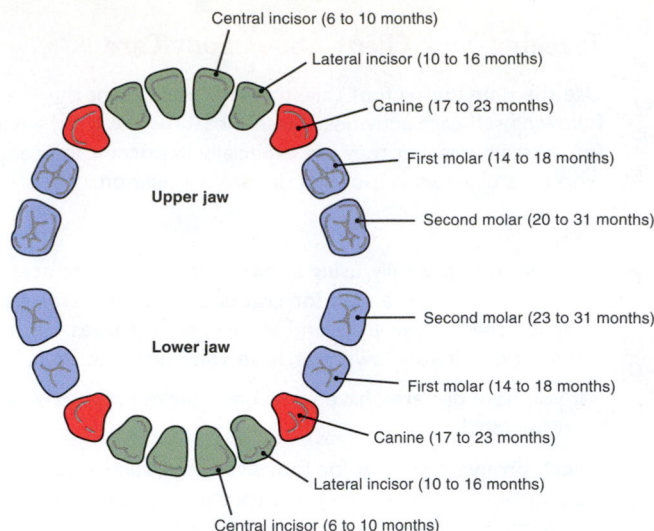

FIGURE 22-3 The 20 deciduous teeth typically erupt by age 2. (Courtesy of P. Dillon [2007]. *Nursing Health Assessment* [2nd ed.]. Philadelphia: F. A. Davis.)

secretions. In addition, a clean mouth helps to promote a better appetite. It also reduces the incidence of health-care-acquired pneumonia in older adults and critically ill patients in acute care settings.

Theoretical **Knowledge** knowing *why*

Digestion of food begins in the mouth (oral cavity). The tongue and teeth begin digestion by breaking up food and mixing it with saliva. Front teeth, also called **incisors**, are for biting and tearing while the teeth in the back of the mouth, known as **molars**, are used for chewing. Saliva, produced by three pairs of salivary glands in the mouth, also acts as a mechanical cleaner of the mouth. The structures of the mouth pertinent to oral hygiene include the tongue, **gingiva** (gums), and teeth.

Developmental Variations

The first set of teeth (the **deciduous teeth**) erupts between 6 months and 2 years of age. By age 2, a child usually has 20 teeth (Fig. 22-3). Between the ages of 6 and 12 years, the deciduous teeth loosen, fall out, and are eventually replaced with 32 permanent teeth (Fig. 22-4). **Wisdom teeth** are the very back molars on either side of each jawbone. Some people have no room for the four wisdom teeth to erupt, so they may need to be extracted to prevent damage to other teeth.

The tooth surface wears away with aging and the gums may begin to recede, resulting in bone and tooth loss and necessitating the use of dentures (false teeth). Poorly fitted or loose dentures can lead to chewing difficulties and even nutritional deficiencies. Other changes that may occur with aging are a brownish pigmentation of the gums and dryness of the oral mucosa, which is caused by decreased saliva production.

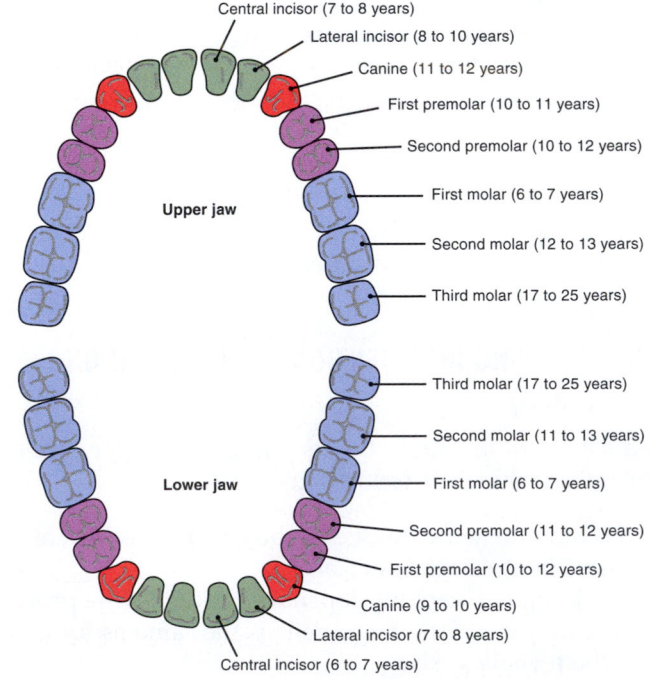

FIGURE 22-4 Most adults have 32 permanent teeth. (Courtesy of P. Dillon [2007]. *Nursing Health Assessment* [2nd ed.]. Philadelphia: F. A. Davis.)

Risk Factors for Oral Problems

Oral health is influenced by heredity, nutrition, and oral hygiene. Therefore, any condition that prevents good oral hygiene can lead to oral problems. Such risk factors include the following:

- *History of periodontal disease*
- *Lack of money or insurance* for dental care
- *Pregnancy.* Increased estrogen during pregnancy increases the vascularity of the gingiva. The gums may bleed easily and become puffy and tender. The condition disappears after the birth, but good hygiene is needed meanwhile to prevent infection.
- *Poor nutrition or eating habits.* Adequate intake of calcium, phosphorus, and vitamin D is essential for healthy teeth and gums. Excessive intake of refined sugars leads to dental decay. One example of this is **baby-bottle tooth decay,** which occurs when parents put an infant or toddler to bed with a bottle or sippy cup of milk, fruit juice, or other sugary beverages. Carbohydrates in the fluid cause demineralization of the tooth enamel, leading to major decay of the upper and lower teeth.
- *Some medications and medical treatments.* The anticonvulsant phenytoin (Dilantin) causes gingival **hyperplasia** (excessive growth of cells). Other medications cause dryness of the mouth. These include diuretics, laxatives (used excessively), medications used to treat cancer, immunosuppressants (cyclosporine), numerous calcium channel blocker agents (especially nifedipine), and tranquilizers such as chlorpromazine (Thorazine) and diazepam (Valium). Medical treatments affecting the oral cavity include the following:

  Jaw surgery, which requires scrupulous oral hygiene to prevent infection

  Radiation treatments of the head and neck. These can permanently damage the salivary glands, resulting in dryness of the mouth. Radiation can also damage teeth and jaw structure.

  Oxygen therapy, which dries the oral mucosa, especially if the client must breathe through the mouth

  Presence of nasogastric tubes, especially if the person breathes through his mouth

- *Any situation that causes dry mouth* predisposes to cracking of the mucosa, including heavy cigarette smoking, excessive alcohol use, inadequate fluid intake or dehydration (e.g., being NPO), and mouth breathing
- *Compromised self-care abilities* may be caused by:

  Decreased level of consciousness (e.g., a person who is comatose or heavily sedated). Such patients are also likely to breathe through the mouth, causing dryness of the mucous membranes.

  Serious illness or injury, weakness, activity intolerance, or paralysis

  Cognitive impairment, as seen in patients with developmental delay, dementia, and certain mental illnesses

Depression

Lack of knowledge or motivation to perform self-care

KnowledgeCheck 22-8

- How do the teeth aid in digesting food?
- How many deciduous teeth does a child usually have?
- List at least three factors that cause dry mouth.
- List at least two medications or medical treatments that can cause oral problems.
- Name four situations that can compromise self-care ability for oral hygiene.

Go to Chapter 22, **Knowledge Check Response Sheet and Answers,** on the Student Resource Disk or DavisPlus at http://davisplus.fadavis.com/Wilkinson2

CriticalThinking 22-9

- For which of your patients, Mrs. Williams or Mr. Gold, does the scenario provide *actual data* to indicate that the patient is at risk for oral problems? What are the data?
- Why is the patient's nursing diagnosis Risk for Impaired Oral Mucous Membrane instead of Impaired Oral Mucous Membrane?

Common Problems of the Mouth

Dental caries (cavities) and periodontal disease are the two most frequent problems affecting the teeth. They are discussed here along with other common mouth problems:

- **Halitosis,** or bad breath, results from poor oral hygiene, eating certain foods (e.g., garlic, onions), tobacco use, dental caries, infections, or even systemic diseases, such as uncontrolled diabetes or liver disease.
- **Dental caries,** or cavities, are caused primarily by a failure to remove **plaque,** an invisible, destructive bacterial film that builds up on the teeth. Plaque buildup eventually leads to destruction of the tooth enamel. Factors that contribute to the formation of cavities include excessive intake of refined sugars, a lack of brushing and flossing, and infrequent visits to the dentist.
- **Gingivitis** is inflammation of the gum tissue surrounding the teeth. If untreated, it may progress to periodontal disease.
- **Periodontal disease (pyorrhea)** is the major cause of tooth loss in adults 35 years and older. It is an inflammation characterized by bleeding and receding gums and destruction of the surrounding bone structure. The patient experiences halitosis and complains of a bad taste in the mouth. When pyorrhea is advanced, the gums become infected, and the teeth loosen and may fall out or need to be removed.

Tooth loss is also the result of untreated plaque, which builds up with dead bacteria and forms hard deposits at the gum lines **(tartar).** The tartar causes deterioration of the supporting structures that hold the teeth in the gums and also attacks the bone tissue, causing the teeth to become loose.

- **Stomatitis,** an inflammation of the oral mucosa, has numerous causes, including bacteria, mechanical trauma, irritants, nutritional deficiencies, and systemic infection. Symptoms may include pain, halitosis, and increased salivation.
- **Glossitis,** an inflammation of the tongue, is caused by deficiencies of vitamin B_{12}, folic acid, and iron.
- **Cheilosis** is a cracking and/or ulceration of the lips, in the form of reddened fissures at the angles of the mouth. It is usually caused by vitamin B-complex deficiencies.
- **Oral malignancies** must be detected as early as possible. Teach patients to see a dentist immediately if any of the following are present in the mouth: lumps, ulcers, white or red patches, bleeding, pain, persistent sores, or numbness.
- **Geographic tongue** is a benign oral condition, not associated with infection or cancer. The tongue has the distinct look of geographic map because some of the **papillae,** which are small bumps on the tongue, are missing from the surface. This causes irregularly shaped smooth, red patches, like a rash. Geographic tongue is usually painless but can sometimes be sensitive to certain substances.

KnowledgeCheck 22-9

- Define and identify several causes of halitosis.
- What are the two most common problems affecting the teeth?
- What is the end result of severe periodontal disease?

 Go to Chapter 22, **Knowledge Check Response Sheet and Answers,** on the Student Resource Disk or DavisPlus at http://davisplus.fadavis.com/Wilkinson2

Practical **Knowledge** knowing how

Oral health status should be a part of every comprehensive assessment. You should also assess the patient's oral cavity when performing or assisting with oral hygiene. Assessment of oral health is particularly important for older adults because of the association between oral health and systemic disease.

For *NANDA-I diagnoses, NOC standardized outcomes,* and *NIC interventions* for patients with problems of the mouth,

 Go to Chapter 22, **Standardized Language, Selected NOC Outcomes and NIC Interventions for Hygiene Problems,** in Volume 2.

◼ ASSESSMENT (ORAL CAVITY)

You might begin your subjective assessment by asking the patient about his usual hygiene practices. You should also interview the patient or examine his records for the risk factors for oral problems discussed in the preceding

section (i.e., history of oral problems, nutritional status, access to dental care, medications such as anticonvulsants or diuretics, radiation therapy, oxygen therapy, NPO status, dehydration, and nasogastric tubes). Ask about tobacco and alcohol use.

As part of your objective assessment during hygiene care, inspect the lips, oral mucosa, gums, and tongue. Mucosa and gums should be pink and moist without lesions or bleeding. Look for loose, missing, or decaying teeth, tartar, stomatitis, and note any unusual odors or halitosis. Check to be sure the tongue is normal in color and without lesions.

The Kayser–Jones Brief Oral Health Status Examination (BOHSE) is used to assess the oral cavity of older adults. It was specifically designed for nursing home residents, with both normal and impaired cognitive functioning, and can be used by a variety of nursing personnel. The tool assigns a numerical rating to findings for: the lymph nodes, lips, tongue, tissue inside the mouth, gums, saliva, condition of natural teeth, condition of artificial teeth, pairs of teeth in chewing position, and oral cleanliness. For a copy of the BOHSE assessment,

 Go to Chapter 22, **ESG Table 22-2,** on the Student Resource Disk or DavisPlus at http://davisplus.fadavis.com/Wilkinson2

To learn more about physical assessment of the oral cavity, refer to Chapter 19. Also,

 Go to Chapter 22, **Assessment Guidelines and Tools,** in Volume 2.

◼ ANALYSIS/NURSING DIAGNOSIS (ORAL CAVITY)

In addition to Self-Care Deficit, discussed in the first part of the chapter, the following are examples of nursing diagnoses that may be useful in describing problems of the mouth:

- Risk for Infection related to mouth lesions
- Impaired Dentition (caries) related to inability to afford dental care
- Impaired Oral Mucous Membrane related to inability to manage mouth care secondary to impaired mobility
- Deficient Knowledge related to lack of interest in learning about oral hygiene

Oral and dental problems can be the etiology of other nursing diagnoses, for example:

- Imbalanced Nutrition related to lack of teeth for mastication
- Pain related to mouth lesions

◼ PLANNING OUTCOMES/EVALUATION (ORAL CAVITY)

Individualized goals/outcome statements you might write for mouth problems include the following:

- Oral mucous membranes will remain pink, moist, and intact.
- Brushes teeth after each meal.

- Flosses daily.
- Demonstrates correct technique for brushing and flossing.
- Makes preventive dental visits every 6 months.

PLANNING INTERVENTIONS/IMPLEMENTATION (ORAL CAVITY)

For some clients, you may need only to provide the necessary supplies for mouth care. For others, you will need to assist or even completely provide care as often as necessary to keep the mouth clean and moist. Rinsing with mouthwash is not a substitute for a thorough cleaning of the teeth and mouth.

Individualized nursing activities related to oral hygiene include (1) teaching for self-care (see the box, Self-Care: Teaching Your Client about Oral Hygiene) and (2) assisting with and providing oral hygiene for dependent patients.

Oral Care for Critically Ill Patients

Patients in long-term care settings and critically ill patients in acute care settings are at high risk for health-care-associated pneumonia. This is especially true for those dependent on a ventilator. Ventilator-associated pneumonia is the most common hospital-acquired infection in critically ill patients. The teeth may be an important reservoir for bacteria that cause pneumonia. A simple and inexpensive way to reduce the risk of pneumonia for these patients is to keep their teeth clean, thus reducing the numbers of bacteria (American Association of Critical-Care Nurses [AACN], 2007). The regimen includes the following:

- Brush the teeth twice a day.
- Use a soft toothbrush.
- Moisturize oral mucosa and lips every 2 to 4 hours.
- Use a chlorhexidine gluconate (0.12%) rinse twice a day during the perioperative period for patients who undergo cardiac surgery (adult patients).
- Use mouthwash inside the mouth twice a day for adult patients who are on a ventilator.

Oral Care for Unconscious Patients

Oral care for unconscious patients is particularly important because they often breathe through the mouth. If the patient is receiving oxygen per cannula or has a nasogastric or feeding tube inserted, the mucous membranes dry out even more. ✚ When providing oral care for an unconscious person, place him on his side, and use a minimal amount of solution to prevent aspiration.

✚ An unconscious patient often responds to oral stimulation by biting down, so use a padded tongue blade instead of your fingers to hold the mouth open. Also use a padded tongue blade when providing oral care for a patient with seizures to avoid the patient biting you.

Follow agency practices for the type and frequency of special mouth care. Some patients may need it every hour or two. You may use commercially packaged applicators or foam swabs to clean the mouth. However, do not use lemon-glycerine swabs because they are drying to the mucosa and may causes changes in tooth enamel. Likewise, do not use hydrogen peroxide because it is irritating to oral mucosa and may alter the balance of normal flora of the mouth. To learn more about how to provide oral care for unconscious patients, see the Critical Aspects box for Procedures 22-1 through 22-14. Also,

VOL 2 Go to Chapter 22, **Procedure 22-6: Brushing and Flossing the Teeth, Procedure 22-7: Providing Denture Care,** and **Procedure 22-8: Providing Oral Hygiene for an Unconscious Patient,** in Volume 2.

Oral Care for Patients with Dementia

Poor oral health and dental pain impact on general well-being—specifically, on the ability to eat, type of diet, weight, speech, hydration, appearance, and social interactions. This is especially true for older adults with dementia, who have many oral diseases and dental problems. Dental disease and pain may be the source of some of the behavior problems in this population. It is a challenge to provide oral hygiene for patients with dementia. Staff sometimes neglect care, giving as reasons a lack of time and the patients' (or residents') behaviors. Residents may be uncooperative: refusing care, refusing to open the mouth, biting the toothbrush, and so on. Research is needed to identify the best interventions (Joanna Briggs Institute, 2004). Meanwhile, for experts' suggestions for ways to provide oral care to patients with dementia,

VOL 2 Go to Chapter 22, **Procedure 22-6: Brushing and Flossing the Teeth,** in Volume 2.

Denture Care

A patient may have a complete set of removable dentures or just an upper or lower plate. Another type of appliance is a **bridge** or partial plate, which consists of one or more artificial teeth. A bridge may be permanently fastened to other teeth, or it may be removable. Artificial teeth are fitted to the individual and should not be used by anyone else. If the person leaves the prosthesis out of his mouth for long periods, the shape of the gums will change, and it will no longer fit properly. The nurse's role is to ensure cleanliness by teaching for self-care (see the box, Self-Care: Teaching Your Client About Oral Hygiene) or to provide denture care for dependent clients. For further information, see the Critical Aspects box for Procedures 22-1 through 22-14, and

VOL 2 Go to Chapter 22, **Procedure 22-7: Providing Denture Care,** in Volume 2.

Self-Care

Teaching Your Client About Oral Hygiene

Measures to promote oral health and prevent periodontal disease and caries include the following:

Preventing Caries and Periodontal Disease

➤ Eliminate high sugar snacks between meals (ice cream, soft drinks, candy, gum, jams and jellies).

➤ Include in the diet cleansing, fibrous foods, such as raw fruits and vegetables.

➤ Include an adequate intake of calcium, phosphorus, and vitamins A, C, and D.

➤ Have regular dental checkups every 6 months.

➤ Brush teeth with a soft brush and toothpaste after each meal and at bedtime (some dentists say twice a day). Bacteria do the most damage to the teeth in the first 24 hours after eating.

➤ Floss between the teeth daily to remove food debris and stimulate the blood flow to the gingiva.

➤ Use a fluoride toothpaste to strengthen tooth enamel.

➤ You can make your own cleanser by combining one part baking soda with two parts salt.

➤ Follow the dentist's recommendations for topical applications of fluoride.

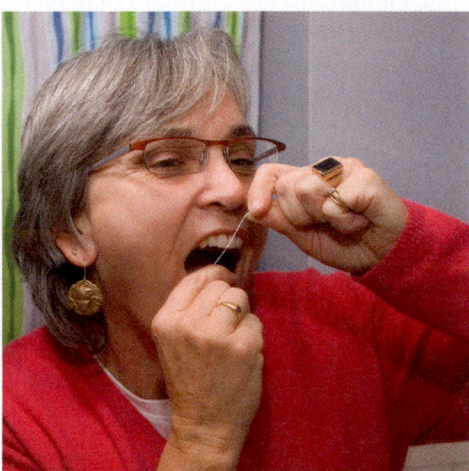

Flossing. Flossing between the teeth is an essential part of oral hygiene.

Brushing and Flossing

➤ Make sure the brush is small enough to reach all teeth. If it is too firm, it can injure enamel and gum tissue.

➤ Electric toothbrushes are effective; however, you should consult your dentist about using waterspray units, because they can force debris into pockets of the gums.

➤ Brush at a 45° angle, from the gum to the tooth crown, using small circular or vibrating motions.

➤ When flossing, (1) wrap one end of the floss around each of your middle fingers. (2) Hold about 1 to 2 inches of floss tightly between the fingers. (3) Insert floss between the teeth by gently moving it back and forth; do not force it. (4) Floss adjacent sides of both teeth to the gum tissue, but not into the gum, because you may injure the tissue. (5) Use a fresh section of floss when it becomes soiled or frayed. (6) Rinse your mouth well when you are finished. A variety of convenient flossing devices are available as an alternative to this method.

Oral Hygiene for Children

➤ Begin oral hygiene when the first tooth erupts. Use a washcloth, cotton ball, or gauze pad moistened with water.

➤ Do not put the child to bed with a bottle or sippy cup. Milk, juice, or any other liquid with sugar can lead to dental caries in the young child when the liquid sits on the teeth at night or for naps.

➤ Begin brushing the child's teeth with a soft toothbrush when she is about 18 months old. Start first using water only. Later, switch to a fluoride-containing toothpaste.

➤ Follow your dentist's instructions for giving a fluoride supplement.

➤ Schedule a visit to the dentist when all 20 deciduous teeth have erupted.

➤ See your dentist if you notice any problems, such as chipping, redness or swelling, caries, or misalignment.

➤ For school-age children, parents may need to supervise mouth care to be sure it is done adequately.

Care of Dentures

➤ If you have dentures or other removable prostheses ("bridges"), wear them. If you do not, the gums are likely to shrink, and you will have further gum loss.

➤ Clean dentures and bridges at least once a day, preferably after each meal.

➤ Remove dentures from the mouth to clean them.

➤ Use regular toothpaste or special denture-cleaning compounds.

➤ Do not use hot water on dentures; it may damage them.

➤ If the dentures have metal parts, do not soak them overnight in cleaning solutions.

➤ Store dentures in a denture cup, in water, to prevent drying. Do not wrap them in tissues because they may accidentally be thrown away.

Self-Care

Patients may have an upper, lower, or partial denture.

Dentures must be cleaned thoroughly as a part of daily oral hygiene.

KnowledgeCheck 22-10

How would you position Mr. Gold ("Meet Your Patients") to perform his oral hygiene?

 Go to Chapter 22, **Knowledge Check Response Sheet and Answers,** on the Student Resource Disk or DavisPlus at http://davisplus.fadavis.com/Wilkinson2

Care of the Hair

Hair is an accessory structure of the skin. The hair helps to maintain body temperature, serves as a receptor for tactile sensation, and influences a person's self-image. **Vellus hair** is the short, fine hair present over much of the body. **Terminal hair,** which is coarser, darker, and longer, is found on the scalp, eyebrows, axillae, perineum, and legs. Sebaceous glands found at the base of the hair follicle secrete sebum, or oil, to lubricate hair and scalp. The condition of the hair is a measure of a person's overall health. See Chapter 19 for more information about changes in hair that occur through the life span and as a result of illness.

For *NOC standardized outcomes* and *NIC standardized interventions* for patients with problems related to care of the hair,

 Go to Chapter 22, **Standardized Language, Selected NOC Outcomes and NIC Interventions for Hygiene Problems,** in Volume 2.

ASSESSMENT (HAIR)

For the purposes of hygiene, you will need information about the patient's history of hair problems or current conditions needing treatment (e.g., pediculosis), diseases or therapy that affect the hair (e.g., chemo-

therapy), and factors influencing the patient's ability to manage her hair and scalp care (e.g., Impaired Mobility). Ask the patient about special products she uses and about her preference for styling her hair. Inspect the condition and cleanliness of the hair, and inspect the scalp for dandruff, lesions, and so forth. For more complete information about assessing the hair, see Chapter 19. Also,

 Go to Chapter 22, **Assessment Guidelines and Tools,** in Volume 2.

ANALYSIS/NURSING DIAGNOSIS (HAIR)

Common problems associated with the hair and scalp include the following (also see Chapter 19):

- **Dandruff** is a condition in which there is excessive shedding of the epidermal layer of the scalp. Primary symptoms include itching and flaking of the scalp, which may be caused by fungal infection.
- **Pediculosis** is an infestation of head lice. Though frequently associated with poor hygiene practices, it knows no socioeconomic boundaries. Head lice spread through sharing of combs, brushes, hair ornaments, hats, and caps.
- **Alopecia,** or hair loss, can be very stressful and affect self-image. Abnormal hair loss, which may be gradual or sudden, can be caused by an autoimmune disorder, hormonal imbalance, thyroid disease, stress, fever, certain medications, or chemotherapy.

There are no NANDA-I labels that apply specifically to the hair. When the difficulty lies with self-care ability, you can of course use Dressing/Grooming Self-Care Deficit and Bathing/Hygiene Self-Care Deficit.

Examples of other nursing diagnoses that may apply include the following:

- Risk for Impaired Skin Integrity related to secretions on the scalp
- Situational Low Self-Esteem related to inability to perform grooming tasks
- Situational Low Self-Esteem related to alopecia secondary to chemotherapy

KnowledgeCheck 22-11

- List at least four assessments you should make of a patient's hair.
- What is pediculosis?
- What is alopecia?

 Go to Chapter 22, **Knowledge Check Response Sheet and Answers,** on the Student Resource Disk or DavisPlus at http://davisplus.fadavis.com/Wilkinson2

PLANNING OUTCOMES/EVALUATION (HAIR)

As always, select outcomes based on the client's nursing diagnoses. *Individualized goals/outcome statements* you might write for a patient with problems related to the hair include the following:

- Scalp and hair are clean.
- States preferences for hair styling.
- By 9/18, brushes own hair.
- Hair and scalp are free from infestation, infection, irritation, or dryness.
- Verbalizes improved comfort and self-esteem.

PLANNING INTERVENTIONS/IMPLEMENTATION (HAIR)

Individualized nursing activities related to the care of the hair include daily brushing and combing of the hair, shampooing, and, for men, shaving and beard care.

Hair Care

Hair should be brushed daily to remove tangles, massage the scalp, stimulate the circulation, and distribute oil down the hair shaft. Use a stiff-bristled brush, but be sure the bristles are not sharp enough to injure the patient's scalp. Likewise, a comb with broken or uneven teeth or one that is too fine can break or snarl the hair or scrape the scalp. Comb tightly curled hair with a wide-toothed comb or pick (Fig. 22-5). Encourage patients to brush and comb their own hair, if they are able to do so. Encouraging family members to assist with hair care will involve them in the patient's care and reduce feelings of helplessness. Do not cut a patient's hair unless he or she consents to the haircut.

Hair Care for Blacks

Hair care is equally important for all patients. However, because white, Hispanic, Asian, and Native American nurses may not know how to do it, they sometimes omit hair care for black

FIGURE 22-5 There are several types of combs for use with various hair types.

patients. The hair of blacks varies in texture—it may be long or short, straight or kinky, thick or thin. Worn naturally, very curly hair can easily become entangled or matted, and it tends to be fragile and easily broken. The scalp also tends to be dry. The hair requires careful handling, especially if it has been chemically straightened, relaxed, or permed. Do not apply chemical relaxers to a patient's hair. Only a licensed beautician should do this.

Shampoo and groom the hair according to the person's preference, of course. In general, though, you should comb and brush the hair daily and apply a light oil to the scalp (e.g., mineral oil or a light moisturizing cream). Ask a family member to bring from home the product the patient prefers to use. If the person's hair is corn-rowed or braided, you can massage, oil, and shampoo it without unbraiding it simply by applying a cloth or net cap to the client's head prior to shampooing.

Shampooing the Hair Shampooing cleans the hair and scalp. It is soothing and relaxing to many patients. Hair can be shampooed while the person is in the shower, standing or sitting over a sink, or in bed. Protect the patient's eyes with a dry washcloth, and make sure the water temperature is appropriate for the patient. For patients who are unable to tolerate a standard shampoo procedure, you can use a dry shampoo as an alternative. However, it is not as effective as shampooing with water. Commercially prepared shampoo caps are available and have, in most institutions, replaced the dry shampoo method. For more information, see the Critical Aspects box for Procedures 22-1 through 22-14 and,

 Go to Chapter 22, **Procedure 22-9: Shampooing Hair for the Patient on Bedrest,** in Volume 2.

Beard and Mustache Care

Beards and mustaches tend to collect food particles. They should be washed daily during a bath or shower and combed and trimmed as necessary. Do not shave a patient's mustache or beard without permission to do so. For details of beard and mustache care, see the Critical Aspects box for Procedures 22-1 through 22-14 and,

 Go to Chapter 22, **Procedure 22-10: Providing Beard and Mustache Care,** in Volume 2.

Shaving

Depending on the culture, shaving is an important part of grooming and helps patients feel better about their appearance. Many men shave their facial hair every day. Women may shave to remove axillary and leg hair. If the patient has a bleeding disorder or is taking anticoagulant medication, you should use an electric razor. For important points about shaving, see the Critical Aspects box for Procedures 22-1 through 22-14 and,

 Go to Chapter 22, **Procedure 22-11: Shaving a Patient,** in Volume 2.

Some dark-haired men (e.g., Blacks and Italians) have tightly curled facial hair, which curls back into the skin when shaved. An inflammatory reaction may occur, resulting in the formation of papules and pustules. In such cases, the man may wish to use a **depilatory** (hair-removing agent) instead of shaving. If you apply a depilatory, be sure to keep the chemical from contacting the patient's eyes, nose, mouth, and ears. Do not use a straight or safety razor to remove the depilatory, because it will irritate the skin. Some men with this condition prefer to grow a beard, especially when they are ill and unable to care for themselves.

Care of the Eyes

Generally you will not need to provide special hygiene care for the eyes. The eyelids and lashes keep dust and debris from entering the eyes, and tears continually cleanse and lubricate them. When necessary, you may gently cleanse the eyes, from the inner to the outer canthus, with a moistened washcloth (but with no soap). If there is drainage or crusting, use a different cloth for each eye to prevent cross-contamination.

ASSESSMENT (EYES)

When performing hygiene care, inspect the eyes for redness, lesions, swelling, crusting, excessive tearing, or discharge. Also check the color of the conjunctivae. You should also ask the patient or check his records to see whether he wears glasses or contact lenses. If the patient wears glasses, ask when he uses them (e.g., for reading, for driving), and ask how well he sees without them. If the patient wears contact lenses, determine:

- The type of lens (hard, soft, long-wearing, disposable)
- How often he wears them (daily, occasionally) and for how long at a time
- Whether they are worn during sleep

- History of or current problems with lens usage (e.g., cleaning, removal)
- Usual practices for cleaning and storage
- History of or current problems with the eyes (e.g., redness, tearing, irritation, dryness, or "scratchy feeling")

These should be adequate data for hygiene care. However, it is not a complete eye assessment. For detailed information about assessing the eyes, see Chapter 19.

ANALYSIS/NURSING DIAGNOSIS (EYES)

Other than Bathing/Hygiene Self-Care Deficit, there is only one NANDA-I label specific to the eyes: Disturbed Sensory Perception: Visual. This label is of limited use for hygiene care. Other diagnoses that might occur include:

- Risk for Infection related to improper hand washing and improper lens cleaning
- Risk for Injury (to eyes) related to wearing lenses longer than recommended

PLANNING OUTCOMES/EVALUATION (EYES)

The only *NOC standardized outcome* specific to the eyes is Sensory Function: Vision. Its use is limited with regard to hygiene care; instead, you would use it if the client has a diagnosis of Disturbed Sensory Perception: Visual.

Individualized goals you might write for eye care include these examples:

- Demonstrates proper cleaning and storage of contact lenses.
- Eyes appear clean and without redness or drainage.

PLANNING INTERVENTIONS/IMPLEMENTATION (EYES)

For *NIC standardized interventions* related to eye care,

 Go to Chapter 22, **Standardized Language, Selected NOC Outcomes and NIC Interventions for Hygiene Problems,** in Volume 2.

Individualized nursing activities related to the care of the eyes include providing eye care to unconscious clients, caring for eyeglasses and contact lenses, and caring for artificial eyes.

Eye Care for the Unconscious Client

Having lost the blink (corneal) reflex, comatose or critically ill patients need more frequent eye care (every 2 to 4 hours). You will need to keep their eyes lubricated with saline or artificial tears to protect them from corneal abrasions and drying. You may also need to use a protective eye shield to keep the patient's eyes closed. Instill eye ointment or drops in the lower lids as ordered.

To review this procedure,

 Go to Chapter 23, **Procedure 23–2: Administering Ophthalmic Medications,** in Volume 2.

Caring for Eyeglasses and Contact Lenses

Eyeglasses need to be cleaned at least once a day. They are expensive, so take care to see that they are not lost or damaged. Using warm water and a soft cloth, clean gently to prevent scratching of the lens. Ask the patient whether the lenses require a special cleaning solution; some patients bring their own. Label each patient's glasses, and store them in a safe place within the patient's reach, preferably in a glasses case in the drawer of the bedside table.

An alternative to glasses, contact lenses are plastic discs worn on the cornea over the pupil. They float on the tears of the eye and stay in place because of surface tension. The cornea is nourished mainly by oxygen from the atmosphere and from tears, so in order to ensure an optimal supply of oxygen, contact lenses must be removed periodically. Wearing time varies from daily wear to up to around 30 days, depending on the type of lens. If you want more information about several different types of contact lenses:

 Go to Chapter 22, **Supplemental Materials, Types of Contact Lenses,** on the Student Resource Disk or DavisPlus at http://davisplus.fadavis.com/Wilkinson2

People usually care for their own contact lenses. Contact lens users must be careful to keep them free of microorganisms that could cause eye infections and to be careful to avoid eye irritation. Teach cleaning and disinfecting measures to clients as needed (see the box, Self-Care: Teaching Clients About Cleaning and Storing Contact Lenses), and follow those measures when you must care for a client's lenses.

If you need to remove a patient's lenses during an emergency, follow universal precautions and handle the lenses as you would any other valuable patient property. ✚ Never use your fingernails to remove a lens, as you may scratch the eye or damage the lens. For hard lenses, if you have a small suction cup available for this purpose, use that instead. For more detailed instructions see the summary in the Critical Aspects box for Procedures 22-1 through 22-14, and

 Go to Chapter 22, **Procedure 22-12: Removing and Caring for Contact Lenses,** in Volume 2.

Caring for Artificial Eyes

An artificial eye is made to look like a natural eye. It can be made of glass or plastic. Some artificial eyes are permanently implanted in the socket, but others must be removed daily for cleaning of the prosthesis and the eye socket. If the patient is not able to perform his own eye care, ask about and follow his usual routines, when possible.

To remove an artificial eye, wear procedure gloves. Using your dominant hand, raise the upper eyelid and depress the lower lid. Apply slight pressure below the eye to release the suction holding it in place

Teaching Clients About Cleaning and Storing Contact Lenses

➤ Cleaning and disinfecting procedures and solutions vary among manufacturers. Depending on the type of lens, use saline solutions or special rinsing and soaking solutions.

➤ Use a special container for the lenses, with a cup labeled for the left and right lens. Some lenses are stored in a solution; others are stored dry. Follow manufacturer's instructions.

➤ Always wash your hands before touching the eyes or the lenses.

➤ Be careful not to allow the lenses to come in contact with soaps, hair sprays, or cosmetics.

➤ Do not wear soft lenses while using eye drops or ointment (wait 1 hour after using drops and at least 4 hours for ointment).

➤ Be aware of the risk for eye irritation when in the presence of smoke or chemical vapors.

To avoid placing a contact lens in the wrong eye, lens cases are marked for the left and right eyes.

(Fig. 22-6). Alternatively, you can use a small bulb syringe, place it directly on the eye, and squeeze to create suction and lift the eye from the socket. For guidelines to remove, clean, and replace an artificial eye,

 Go to Chapter 22, **Procedure 22-15: Caring for Artificial Eyes,** in Volume 2.

KnowledgeCheck 22-12

- True or False: Eyes should be cleansed from the outer to the inner canthus.
- How can a contact lens wearer help prevent eye infections?
- After you have cleaned a prosthetic eye, should you dry it before reinserting it, or leave it wet? To answer this question,

 Go to Chapter 22, **Procedure 22-15: Caring for Artificial Eyes,** in Volume 2.

 Go to Chapter 22, **Knowledge Check Response Sheet and Answers,** on the Student Resource Disk or DavisPlus at http://davisplus.fadavis.com/Wilkinson2

FIGURE 22-6 To remove a prosthetic eye, apply pressure just below the eye.

Care of the Ears

Healthy ears require minimal care. However, you will need to help patients who have limited self-care abilities and teach others about self-care. For example, **cerumen** (wax) impaction is a common cause of hearing loss, especially in older adults. People sometimes believe hearing loss is a normal part of aging and fail to seek treatment. Encourage them to see their primary care provider whenever hearing loss occurs.

✚ Teach patients to avoid using rigid objects, such as bobby pins or toothpicks to clean their ears. Such instruments can traumatize the ear canal and may rupture the **tympanic membrane** (eardrum). Likewise, never use cotton-tipped applicators; they will push the cerumen further into the ear, causing a blockage.

Providing Ear Care

For dependent patients, assess for drainage, excess cerumen, and hearing loss during the bath. Clean the auricle, and remove cerumen from the canal with the tip of the moistened washcloth. If cleansing with a washcloth does not effectively remove excess cerumen buildup, obtain a prescription for **cerumenolytic** drops and water irrigation. You can delegate ear cleaning and hearing aid care to the NAP if you are sure that the NAP knows how to perform these tasks. Describe what you want the NAP to observe and report to you. See Chapter 29 for information about ear irrigations.

Care of Hearing Aids

A hearing aid is a battery-powered device that amplifies sound. Three types of hearing aids are shown in Figure 22-7. In addition to these, some patients wear a hearing aid in the temple pieces of their eyeglasses. People with severe hearing loss may wear a body hearing aid that clips onto the clothing or a harness-type carrier that connects by a cord to the earpiece. Digital hearing aids are rapidly replacing the analog models.

Hearing aids are expensive, so handle and store them properly. They require regular cleaning and replacement of batteries. Even with good care, they usually need to be

FIGURE 22-7 Hearing aids. *A,* The postaural (behind-the-ear) aid is the most widely used. A plastic tube connects it to an earmold. *B,* An in-the-canal aid is the least visible. *C,* The in-the-ear aid is made in one piece; all components are in the earmold.

replaced every 5 to 10 years, and ear molds usually need adjustment more often than that. Never place a hearing aid in water. Even humidity can reduce their effectiveness. For guidelines to remove, clean, and replace a hearing aid,

 Go to Chapter 22, **Procedure 22-16: Caring for Hearing Aids,** in Volume 2.

Care of the Nose

Usually the nose requires no special care. Have the patient remove excess secretions by gently blowing into a tissue with both nostrils open. Holding one nostril shut can force secretions into the eustachian tubes. In debilitated or unconscious patients, dried secretions can interfere with respirations. Remove secretions by gently inserting a moistened cotton-tipped applicator into the nostrils. Occasionally you may need to instill saline into the nares and suction secretions to keep the airway patent. If the patient has a nasogastric (NG) tube, the constant pressure on the skin may cause breakdown. Provide special skin care and a lubricant at the point where the tube touches the nares.

The Client's Environment

A comfortable environment contributes to the client's well-being. It is your responsibility, as a nurse, to see that the bedside unit and surroundings are clean, safe, and comfortable.

ASSESSMENT (SCANNING THE ENVIRONMENT)

Each time you enter a patient's room, you should scan the environment to see whether you need to make adjustments to ensure patient safety and comfort:

- Is the room temperature comfortable?
- Are the siderails up, when indicated?
- Is the bed in low position?
- Are bed wheels locked?
- Are bed linens clean and free of wrinkles?
- Is the patient's call device within reach?
- Is the overbed table clean and uncluttered?
- Is there uncluttered walking space?
- Are there unpleasant odors?

Each time you leave the room, ask, "What else can I do for you?" This ensures that you have not overlooked anything.

PLANNING INTERVENTIONS/IMPLEMENTATION (THE ENVIRONMENT)

Adequate ventilation; proper room temperature; low noise level; and neat, clean surroundings are important to ensure the patient's comfort.

Promoting Ventilation

Body secretions such as urine, feces, vomitus, or draining wounds cause odors in both inpatient facilities and the home. Odors can be offensive, and patients often feel embarrassed by them, so work quickly to free the environment of any sources of odors. Cleanliness is the best way to prevent odors. Other suggestions include the following:

- Provide good ventilation, if this is under your control. For example, open a window or use a fan.
- Empty urinals, bedpans, or emesis basins promptly.
- Dispose of soiled dressings or other malodorous items in appropriate containers, and immediately remove them from the room.

- Unless contraindicated by the patient's illness, you can use a room deodorizer to help eliminate odors.
- Most institutions ban smoking in patient rooms, in part because of the odor.

Controlling Room Temperature

Although preferences may vary, a room temperature between 68° and 74°F (20° and 23°C) is usually comfortable for most patients. Those who are very ill, very young, or very old may need a higher than normal room temperature. If there is no thermostat in the room, you may need to provide blankets, open a window, provide a fan, and so on to adjust the room temperature.

Limiting Noise

People who are ill are often sensitive to various environmental noises, such as an ice machine, suction equipment, paging systems, loud talking, and laughter. In addition, sleeping in a new and strange environment or in the presence of pain may be difficult and interrupted. Make it a priority to control noise in the hospital setting. Keep unnecessary conversations to a minimum, and speak quietly. Some hospitals have instituted a "quiet hour" to promote better rest, for example, in the afternoon or during early morning hours. Others have installed decibel meters to help nurses be mindful of noise escalation during activity in the nurses' station.

Standard Bedside Equipment

In a hospital, standard bedside equipment usually includes a bed, bedside stand (end table), overbed table, and one or two chairs. The wall unit may consist of a call light, oxygen, suction and electrical outlets, and light fixtures and switches. The patient's personal items are usually kept in the bedside stand. Therefore, you should request permission from the patient before opening the stand. A wash basin, soap dish, bedpan, and urinal may also be kept in the lower cabinet of this stand. Keeping these items clean helps to prevent odor and possible infection.

Hospital Beds

Hospitalized patients spend a significant amount of time in bed. Hospital beds can be uncomfortable and may contribute to restlessness and poor sleep. Memory foam and moisture control mattresses are available and provide more comfort. However, they are expensive and not used routinely. Hospital beds are generally standard in size and higher and narrower than a home bed. This allows you to reach the patient more easily and safely.

Hospital beds are usually electronically controlled, so the patient can raise and lower the head and foot separately by the push of a button. You can also raise and

Toward Evidence-Based Practice

American Association of Critical-Care Nurses (AACN). (2007). AACN practice alert. Oral care in the critically ill. Retrieved December 18, 2008 from http://classic.aacn.org/ AACN/practiceAlert.nsf/Files/OC/$file/Oral%20Care%20in% 20the%20Critically%20Ill%20.pdf

This evidence report reviewed 14 references and graded the evidence for the conclusions they drew. They used a I to VI scale, with Level VI being the strongest support and Level I being the weakest (manufacturer's recommendations only). The following are two AACN recommendations for oral care in the critically ill:

■ Use oral chlorhexidine gluconate (0.12%) rinse twice a day for adult patients undergoing cardiac surgery; not routinely for all patients. (Level V)
■ Brush teeth, gums, and tongue at least twice a day. (Level II)

Sona, C., Zack, J., Schallom, M., et al. (2008). The impact of a simple, low-cost oral care protocol on ventilator-associated pneumonia rates in a surgical intensive care unit. *Journal of Intensive Care Medicine*, Nov. 17. Abstract retrieved December 22, 2008, from http://www.ncbi.nlm.nih.gov/ pubmed/19017665

Researchers examined the effects of an oral care protocol on ventilator-pneumonia rates on ventilator patients in a surgical intensive care unit. The protocol included brushing the teeth twice daily with a fluoride toothpaste and brush and applying chlorhexidine gluconate (0.12%) twice daily. They concluded that the oral care protocol led to a significantly decreased risk of acquiring ventilator-associated pneumonia in surgical intensive care patients.

Watando, A., Ebihara, S., Ebihara, T., et al. (2004). Daily oral care and cough reflex sensitivity in elderly nursing home patients. *Chest, 126*(4), 1066–1070.

These researchers explored the effects of intensive oral care on improvement of cough reflex sensitivity in elderly nursing home residents. Caregivers cleaned the subjects' teeth after every meal for 1 month; a control group of patients cleaned their own teeth after every meal. No special paste or solution was used. The intervention significantly improved cough reflex sensitivity in the intervention group. Therefore, researchers concluded that intensive oral care may reduce the incidence of pneumonia by improving cough reflex sensitivity in elderly nursing home residents.

1. Suppose you are a critical-care nurse, using the AACN Practice Alert guidelines. For which of the two AACN recommendations would you most want to have further research evidence?

2. Which of the two studies above provide additional support for that guideline? Explain your thinking.

3. How are the patients in the two studies alike or different from the patients for whom the AACN Practice Alert was designed?

 Go to Chapter 22, **Toward Evidence-Based Practice Suggested Responses,** on the Student Resource Disk or DavisPlus at http://davisplus.fadavis.com/Wilkinson2

Head

Flat   Foot

Semi-Fowler's position
(30° angle)

Trendelenburg's position

Fowler's position
(45° angle)

Reverse Trendelenburg's
position

Sitting position
(special wound-care
beds; also adjust to
sitting position)

FIGURE 22-8 Hospital beds adjust to several positions.

lower the height of the bed electronically (see Fig. 22-8 for bed positions). Patient safety is your priority, so although you should raise the entire bed to a working level that is comfortable for you, be sure to place the bed in the lowest position before leaving the bedside. Long-term care settings usually have low beds to make it easier for ambulatory patients to transfer into and out of bed. As a part of the admission procedure, you will teach patients how to use the bed controls. To review the admission process,

VOL 2 Go to Chapter 10, **Procedure 10–1: Admitting a Patient to a Nursing Unit,** in Volume 2.

Patients may use siderails when moving into and out of bed. Siderails may help to prevent falls by patients with decreased consciousness. However, siderails are considered a passive restraint and may pose risk to a patient with a cognitive impairment. See Chapter 21 for additional information about the safe use of siderails and other equipment.

 Always be sure to lock the wheels on a hospital bed when it is stationary. For example, an unlocked bed could roll out from under an ambulatory patient who is moving from the bed to a chair. Ensure that the wheels are locked when you are helping the patient to a sitting position on the side of the bed or assisting with a transfer to a chair or stretcher.

Mattresses and Linens

Mattresses are usually firm and covered in a water-repellant material that resists staining and soiling and may be easily wiped down with a germicidal cleaner. A variety of special therapeutic mattresses are available to help reduce the effects of pressure over the bony prominences (e.g., sacrum, heels). See Chapter 34 for further discussion of special mattresses.

Using a mattress cover and/or pad promotes patient comfort and prevents soiling of the mattress. Plastic covers, however, do not allow moisture to escape, and

contribute to skin maceration for patients who are incontinent or diaphoretic. If a plastic surface lies directly under the sheet, you should place a cloth or other absorbent pad between the patient and the sheet. Sheets may be fitted or flat. Other linens include draw-sheets, washable incontinence pads, pillowcases, blankets, bedspreads, and gowns.

Bed Making

Clean, wrinkle-free bed linens help to promote comfort and a sense of well-being. In contrast, wrinkled and soiled linen can contribute to skin breakdown and pressure areas. Linens are generally changed daily after the bath and when soiled. If patients are up and about during the day, such as on a rehabilitation unit, beds are made daily, but bed linen may be changed weekly or only when soiled. If the patient is immobile or on bedrest, the bed is made while the patient occupies it. You or the NAP may make an unoccupied bed or an occupied bed. For more information about bed making, see the Critical Aspects box for Procedures 22-1 through 22-14, and

VOL 2 Go to Chapter 22, **Procedure 22-13: Making an Unoccupied Bed,** and **Procedure 22-14: Making an Occupied Bed,** in Volume 2.

 Critical**Thinking** 22-10

For which of your patients ("Meet Your Patients") will you most surely need to make an occupied bed? Why?

 Go to Chapter 22, **Resources for Caregivers and Health Professionals,** on the Student Resource Disk or DavisPlus at http://davisplus.fadavis.com/Wilkinson2

Suggested Readings: Go to Chapter 22, **Reading More About Facilitating Hygiene,** on the Student Resource Disk or DavisPlus at http://davisplus.fadavis.com/Wilkinson2

VOL 2 **Bibliography:** Go to Volume 2, Bibliography.

CHAPTER 23

Administering Medications

Learning Outcomes

After completing this chapter, you should be able to:

➤ Name at least five sources of medication information.

➤ Distinguish among various nomenclature systems for naming and classifying drugs.

➤ Review various systems for storing and distributing medications.

➤ Examine the factors affecting drug absorption.

➤ Present three modes of drug distribution throughout the body.

➤ Determine what factors affect pharmacokinetics.

➤ Discuss the routes by which medications are absorbed in the body, including each one's advantages and disadvantages.

➤ State the primary site of drug metabolism (biotransformation) in the body.

➤ Explain how drug excretion occurs at each of the following sites: kidneys, liver, gastrointestinal tract, lungs, and exocrine glands.

➤ Define onset, peak, and duration of drug action; therapeutic level, peak level, and trough level; and biological half-life.

➤ Compare and contrast primary, secondary, cumulative, and side effects; and adverse, toxic, allergic, anaphylactic, and idiosyncratic reactions.

➤ Define drug-drug interaction, antagonistic drug relationship, synergistic drug relationship, drug incompatibility, and medication contraindications.

➤ Correctly calculate drug dosages, including (1) conversion among the metric, apothecary, and household measurement systems and (2) working with units and milliequivalents (mEq).

➤ List the types of medication prescriptions, including the methods for communicating them.

➤ Discuss the agencies and legislation that help to ensure drug quality and safety.

➤ Describe nursing assessment before, during, and following the administration of a drug.

➤ Plan care for clients with problems of Risk for Injury and Noncompliance related to medications.

➤ Administer medications using the "three checks" and "rights of medication."

➤ Describe appropriate steps you would take if communicating a medication error.

➤ Demonstrate the correct procedure for administering medications by the oral, enteral, inhalant, and parenteral routes.

➤ Perform proper technique for use of a metered-dose inhalant (MDI).

➤ Demonstrate the intramuscular injection procedure at the following sites: ventrogluteal, deltoid, and vastus lateralis.

➤ Explain why the dorsogluteal site is no longer recommended for intramuscular injections.

➤ List five steps you can incorporate in your practice to ensure safe medication administration and prevent a medication error.

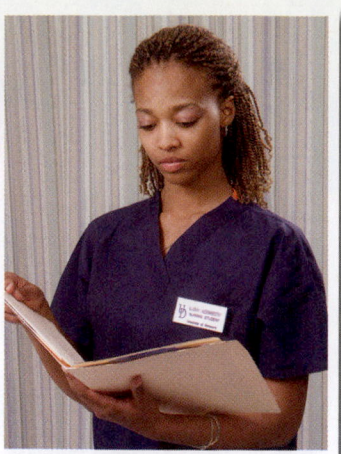

Meet Your Patients

You are scheduled to administer medications to five patients on the medical–surgical unit today. You will be administering medications unsupervised for the first time. Your clinical instructor will be available as a resource. Your patients are:

- Margaret Marks, an 82-year-old woman who has a fractured hip and experiences periods of confusion
- Cary Pearson, a 70-year-old man with feeding and swallowing difficulties who receives his medications through a gastrostomy tube
- Cyndi Early, a 32-year-old woman with diabetes who is scheduled for surgery at 1000 today
- James Bigler, a 44-year-old man who has had a repair of a compound fracture of the right arm and is receiving intravenous fluids and medications
- Rebecca Jones, an 84-year-old woman with compression fractures of two lumbar vertebrae resulting from a fall at a nursing home.

You have reviewed your assignment but are unsure of where to begin. Should you visit your patients first and perform an assessment? Should you review the charts first? What should you do with the MARs (medication administration records)? There are so many questions running through your head, and you are a little nervous

being on your own. Perhaps you could use the model of full-spectrum nursing (Chapter 2) to focus your thinking. In general, any time you give a medication, you will need to incorporate the following:

1. *Theoretical Knowledge*: Find out about the actions and expected effects of the medications you are to give.
2. *Patient Situation*: Assess the health status (e.g., disease process) of each patient as it relates to his medications.
3. *Critical Thinking*: Why is the drug being given? Is there anything about the patient's physiology that may alter his responses to the drug? Do you need to modify the administration procedure in any way?
4. *Practical Knowledge*: Be sure that you know the procedures for administering each medication safely.

By the time you complete this chapter, you will have the information you need to make those kinds of judgments. And remember that while you are a student, your instructor and the staff nurses will be there for support.

Theoretical **Knowledge** **knowing** why _____

Pharmacology is the science of drug effects. It deals with all drugs used in society, legal and illegal, prescription and nonprescription, and "street" drugs. Because of their potential for harm as well as benefit, you should thoroughly understand the medications you administer.

How Are Drugs Named and Classified?

A **drug** is a chemical that interacts with a living organism and alters its activity. In healthcare, drugs are used in diagnosing, treating, or preventing a disease or other medical condition. The term *drug* is used interchangeably with *medication,* although some people think of the term *drug* as meaning an illegal substance.

Drug Names

A drug may have multiple names. The **chemical name,** rarely used in nursing practice, is the exact description of the drug's chemical composition and molecular structure. For example, *2-(p-isobutylphenyl) propionic acid* is the chemical name of the anti-inflammatory drug ibuprofen. When the developing manufacturer is ready

to market a drug, the United States Adopted Name Council (USAN Council) assigns the **generic (nonproprietary) name.** This is usually similar to the chemical name, but it is simpler. The generic name is also the **official name** that is listed in publications such as the *United States Pharmacopeia (USP)* and *National Formulary (NF)*. For example, *ibuprofen* is both a generic and an official name. When the drug is marketed, the manufacturer sells it under a **brand (trade** or **proprietary) name.** The brand name is easily recognized because it begins with a capital letter and sometimes has a registration mark® at the upper right of the name. Different manufacturers of the same medication may give the medication different brand names. For example, Advil, Nuprin, and Motrin are all brand names for ibuprofen.

Prescription drugs require a written order from a healthcare provider (e.g., physician or advanced practice nurse) who is licensed by the state to prescribe or dispense drugs. **Nonprescription,** or **over-the-counter (OTC),** drugs may be purchased without a prescription and are assumed to be safe for the general population if consumers follow the manufacturer's directions. Some drugs are nonprescription at low doses but require a prescription for the consumer to purchase in a higher dose. For example, naproxen sodium 200 mg is sold over the counter as Aleve, whereas naproxen 500 mg is sold as Naprosyn and requires a prescription. Some drugs once available only by prescription may become OTC, such as with loratadine (Claritin).

Drug Classifications

It is not realistic to know everything about every drug, so "looking it up" must become second nature. If you learn the common characteristics for a drug classification, then when you encounter a new drug, you will be able to associate it with its classification and make inferences about its basic characteristics.

- By usage—why the drug is used
- By body system—where the drug works
- By chemical or pharmacological class—what the drug is made of,

To see an explanation and examples of those classifications methods,

Go to **ESG Table 23-1, Drug Classification System,** on the Student Resource Disk or DavisPlus at http://davisplus.fadavis.com/Wilkinson2

A drug can be placed in more than one category in a classification system. Classified by usage, for example, ibuprofen (Motrin) can be an analgesic, anti-inflammatory, and an antipyretic agent. A drug can act on more than one body system, as well; in fact, most do. For example, diazepam (valium) is used for its antianxiety effects, but it also decreases the activity of the intestinal system and other smooth muscles.

KnowledgeCheck 23-1

- Name three ways a drug may be classified.
- List at least four ways a drug could be named.

Go to Chapter 23, **Knowledge Check Response Sheet and Answers,** on the Student Resource Disk or DavisPlus at http://davisplus.fadavis.com/Wilkinson2

What Mechanisms Promote Drug Quality and Safety?

In the United States until the 20th century, there were no mechanisms for publishing drug ingredients, no regulations to govern the contents of drugs, and no limitations regarding their sale. People could buy medicines containing potent and dangerous ingredients, such as opium, morphine, heroin, and alcohol. Besides the money people wasted on ineffective drugs, drug addiction and complications and deaths from drug overdose were common. Now, reliable sources of drug information, state and federal regulations and standards controlling drug administration, and a variety of systems for storing and distributing medications in healthcare agencies all work together to protect consumers.

Drug Listings and Directories

When in doubt, look it up! As a nurse, you are professionally, morally, legally, and personally responsible for every dose of medication you administer. Always use current information when researching a medication. The following references have become the official standards for the healthcare industry:

- *United States Pharmacopoeia (USP).* This directory of drugs approved by the Food and Drug Administration (FDA) lists the physical and chemical composition of each drug. Any drug included in this book has met rigorous standards of quality, strength, and purity and the manufacturer is permitted to use the letters USP after the drug name.
- *National Formulary* (United States). This resource identifies the therapeutic value of drugs as well as their formulas and prescriptions.
- *British Pharmacopoeia.* This is the British version of the USP. Drugs listed in the *British Pharmacopoeia* are considered official and subject to legal control in Great Britain. It is also used in Canada.
- *Canadian Formulary.* This is a listing of all drugs and formulas used in Canada. Not all the drugs listed in this formulary are in the *British Pharmacopoeia.*

In addition to the pharmacopoeia and formularies, the following are reliable resources for medication information:

Nursing Drug Handbooks. Several nursing drug handbooks are available from textbook and other publishers. They serve as a quick resource for information (e.g., dosage, side effects) and nursing interventions associated with a drug.

Physician's Desk Reference (PDR). This book, commercially compiled by the pharmaceutical companies, lists manufacturers' prescribing information and is a standard resource for professionals prescribing and administering medication. The information contained in the PDR is updated annually and is the same information found in drug package inserts. The PDR does not include nursing interventions but does contain information on dosing, routes of administration, and side effects.

Pharmacology Texts. A textbook provides more information about physiology and pathophysiology, and provides broader information, than the drug formulary or a handbook. It may or may not have detailed information about the specific drug you are giving, but it will include a thorough discussion of the drug's classification.

Electronic and Internet-based Formularies. The Internet, computer software, PDAs and other handheld devices offer convenient access to formulary information.

Pharmacist. A clinical pharmacist can assist you with medication-related concerns (e.g., dosage calculations, compatibility, admixture administration, and adverse reactions).

Medication Package Inserts. Most medications are packaged with an insert that provides information identical to that found in the drug formulary. Inserts also contain instructions that are specific for that particular drug.

Institutional Medication Policies and Procedures. Every institution has policies and procedures governing medication administration. You should know the policies and protocols for each institution in which you practice.

CriticalThinking 23-1

Mr. Pearson ("Meet Your Patient") has a medication, metoprolol (Lopressor), due at 0800. You are not familiar with this medication.

- What do you need to know before giving the drug?
- What resources might you use to learn about this medication?
- Which is the generic and which is the brand name of this medication?
- Select a nursing drug handbook and research this medication. What kinds of information are available to you in the book?
- Now look up the drug in a pharmacology text. How is that information similar to and different from the information in the handbook?

Legal Considerations

In the United States and Canada, drug administration is controlled by federal, state or provincial, and local laws. Standards of nursing care, state nurse practice acts, and organizational policies and procedures define your role and responsibilities in administering medications. You must be familiar with them to know what you can and cannot do. In addition, you must recognize the limits of your own experience, skills, and knowledge.

The Food and Drug Administration (FDA) of the U.S. Department of Health and Human Services regulates the manufacture and sale of all medications and monitors their safety and effectiveness. It also regulates, through controlled clinical trials, the testing of any medication that is to be marketed and sold in the United States. This process helps to ensure ineffective or unsafe drugs are not marketed; if later found unsafe, they are subject to a recall. However, many medicinal products are *not* regulated by the FDA. For example, herbal remedies and some naturopathic supplements are considered "food products" and are not regulated. Yet they are advertised as having health benefits.

Nurse Practice Acts

In most states, a nurse (other than an advanced practice nurse, or APN) cannot prescribe or administer medications without an authorized provider's (e.g., physician or APN) order. If you violate the state's nurse practice act by giving medications without an order/prescrip-

tion, your state board of nursing could revoke your license to practice nursing.

CriticalThinking 23-2

Obtain a copy of your nurse practice act for the state in which you work. To find a copy,

Go to the **National Council of State Boards of Nursing** Web site at http://www.ncsbn.org/

What does your state's nurse practice act tell you about administering medications?

For a state-by-state summary of scope of practice regulations for licensed practical nurses (LPNs)/licensed vocational nurses (LVNs) administering intravenous (IV) medications,

Go to **ESG Table 23-2, LPNs State-by State Scope of Practice for IV Administration,** on the Student Resource Disk or DavisPlus at http://davisplus.fadavis.com/Wilkinson2

U.S. Drug Legislation

Various state and federal agencies regulate the manufacture and sale of medications. Each state must conform to federal regulations concerning medications. The states may, in turn, institute additional controls. Finally, local governments may enact regulations for the use of alcohol and tobacco. For a historical list of U.S. laws regulating drug quality and safety,

Go to Chapter 23, **ESG Table 23-3, U.S. Legislation for Drug Quality and Safety,** on the Student Resource Disk or DavisPlus at http://davisplus.fadavis.com/Wilkinson2

Canadian Drug Legislation

Drug regulation is carried out through the Health Protection branch of the Canadian government. Under this branch, the Drugs Directorate oversees the bureaus that deal with specific areas of regulation, such as prescription drugs, nonprescription drugs, biological agents, drug research, and control of drug quality. The Canadian Food and Drugs Act (1953) protects consumers from contaminated, adulterated, and unsafe drugs.

Regulation of Controlled Substances

Controlled substances are drugs considered to have either limited medical use or high potential for abuse or addiction. Under the Controlled Substances Act (CSA) of the Comprehensive Drug Abuse Prevention and Control Act of 1970, it is illegal to possess a controlled substance without a valid prescription. For a summary of categories of controlled substances,

Go to Chapter 23, **Tables, Boxes, Figures: ESG Table 23-4, Schedules for Controlled Substances,** on the Student Resource Disk or DavisPlus at http://davisplus.fadavis.com/Wilkinson2

Controlled substances must be stored, handled, disposed of, and administered according to regulations established by the U.S. Drug Enforcement Agency (DEA). Only prescribers with a *national provider identification number* have the authority to prescribe controlled substances. Facilities using controlled substances must store them in locked drawers within a second locked area. (This process is known as **double locking.**) The facility must also keep a record of every dose administered. A count of all controlled substances is performed at specified times, usually at change of shift. To facilitate counting and tracking inventory, drug manufacturers package many narcotics in sectioned containers, with each tablet separately and consecutively numbered (Fig. 23-1).

The Canadian Narcotic Control Act (1961) regulates the manufacture, distribution, and sale of narcotics in Canada. Possession of narcotics for any reason other than those related to medical use is an offense subject to severe penalties.

Critical Thinking 23-3

Locate the controlled substance area on your nursing unit.

- Is a double-locking system in place?
- Who is responsible for "carrying" the narcotics keys?
- What is done if there is a discrepancy between a narcotic sign-out sheet and the actual number of narcotic doses present?

Systems for Storing and Distributing Medications

Most inpatient healthcare facilities have specific areas designed for preparation of medications. Usually this is a central room ("medication room") or mobile cart. Some nursing units store drugs and supplies in a locked cabinet in or near patient rooms. Whatever the method, all drugs are secured in designated areas accessible only to nurses.

Stock Supply

Medications used most frequently may be kept in **stock supply** (bulk quantity), labeled, and in a central loca-

tion. For example, acetaminophen elixir and cough syrups may be kept in large multidose bottles from which you measure doses for more than one patient. Stock supplies require you to measure the dose each time a patient needs it, so the potential for measurement error is present each time a dose is prepared. However, a bulk supply of medication is often very cost-effective.

Unit-Dose System

A locked, mobile cart is used, with drawers containing separate compartments for each patient's medications (Fig. 23-2). Extra drawers contain supplies, such as medication cups, syringes, and alcohol swabs. The pharmacy staff refills the drawers each shift or every 24 hours. Limited amounts of **prn** ("give according to patient need") medications and stock medications are also kept in the mobile cart.

A **unit dose** is the prescribed amount of drug the patient receives at a single time. For example, if 800 mg of ibuprofen (Motrin) is prescribed to be given every 8 hours, the unit dose is 800 mg. Each unit dose (usually one tablet) is individually packaged and labeled with drug name, dose, and expiration date. The pharmacist checks each unit dose before sending the drug to the nursing unit, and you will recheck the drug and dose when preparing it for administration. The unit-dose system not only saves nursing time, but also is the safest method because of the double-check system.

FIGURE 23-2 Medications may be kept in locked, mobile carts, with a drawer for each patient. Mobile (portable) medication carts are linked to the automated dispensing unit.

FIGURE 23-1 To facilitate counting, many narcotics are packaged in sectioned containers with each tablet numbered consecutively.

Automated Dispensing System

An automated dispensing system is a computerized system similar to a unit–dose system. The locked cart contains all the medications frequently used on a particular nursing unit, and the computer database contains records and counts of the medications, as well as the medication prescriptions for each patient on the unit. Each nurse uses a password to access the machine and enters the data about the needed drug, after which the machine dispenses the medication. The machine tracks dispensed medications for billing and controlled-substances monitoring. The medications are usually packaged in unit doses, but some bulk medications may also be kept on the cart. This method allows for immediate administration of newly prescribed medications, prn medications, controlled substances, and emergency medications because the nurse does not need to wait for the pharmacy to fill a prescription.

Self-Administration

At times while in the hospital, patients may self-administer medications. For example, sublingual nitroglycerin (used for chest pain) is self-administered in the outpatient setting, and some patients can continue self-administration of the drug while in the hospital. The drugs prescribed for self-administration are supplied in individual containers and stored at the bedside. Remind the patient to tell you when he takes the drug. This method promotes independence and allows you to evaluate before discharge the patient's ability to manage medications safely and accurately. Keep in mind that some institutions do not permit patients to administer their own medications. Be sure to check with the policy in your institution.

KnowledgeCheck 23-2

- What legislation defines controlled substances in both the United States and Canada?
- How is medication quality managed?

 Go to Chapter 23, **Knowledge Check Response Sheet and Answers,** on the Student Resource Disk or DavisPlus at http://davisplus.fadavis.com/Wilkinson2

What Is Pharmacokinetics?

Pharmacokinetics refers to the absorption, distribution, metabolism, and excretion of a drug (Fig. 23-3). These four processes determine the intensity and duration of a drug's actions. Each drug has unique pharmacokinetic characteristics.

What Factors Affect Drug Absorption?

Absorption refers to the movement of the drug from the site of administration into the bloodstream. The rate of absorption determines when a drug becomes available to exert its action; thus, absorption also influences metabolism and excretion. Absorption depends on the

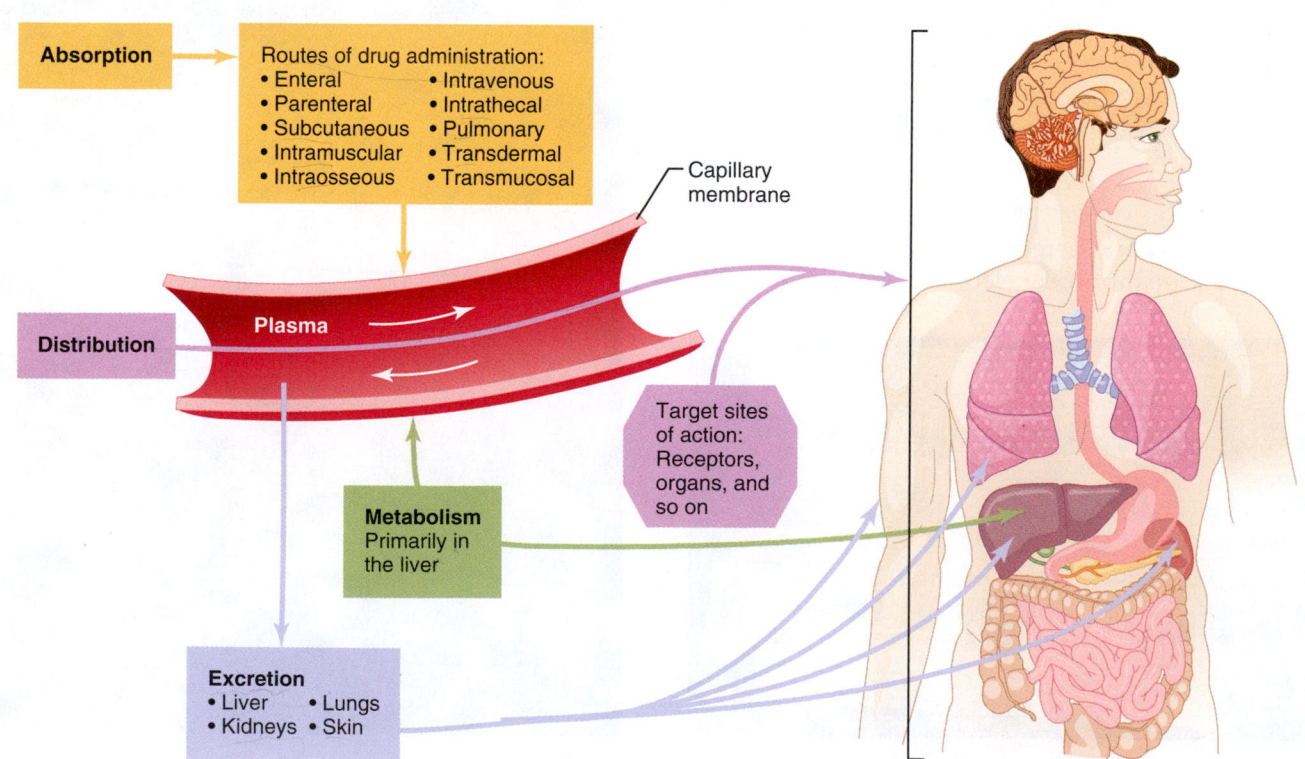

FIGURE 23-3 Pharmacokinetics is the study of drug absorption, distribution, metabolism, and excretion, which determine the intensity and duration of a drug's actions in the body.

route of administration, form of the drug, drug solubility, effects of pH, blood flow to the area, and body surface area.

Route of Administration

Drugs are given for either local or systemic effect. The **local effects** of a drug occur at the site of application (e.g., certain topical applications of drugs to the skin), so no absorption occurs. When a medication is given for a **systemic effect,** the drug must be absorbed into the bloodstream before it can be distributed to a distant location. A drug may enter the circulation either by injection into a vein or by absorption from other areas into which it has been placed (e.g., muscle, stomach lining, mucous membranes, skin).

Drugs are manufactured for a specific route of administration: oral, sublingual, buccal, inhalant, topical, enteral, and parenteral and are absorbed at different rates depending on the route. The form (preparation) of

a drug usually determines its route of administration. Medications are available in a variety of forms.

Table 23-1 summarizes the preparations and the advantages and disadvantages for the various routes of administration. The choice of route is crucial in determining the suitability of the drug for an individual patient. For example, if your patient is vomiting, an oral drug will not be absorbed effectively in the stomach and would likely be expelled during vomiting. If the patient has diarrhea, rapid motility of the gastrointestinal (GI) tract would decrease absorption. If your patient, Cary Pearson ("Meet Your Patient"), has a prescription for an oral medication, would you question the route? Why or why not?

Solubility of the Drug

Solubility refers to the ability of a medication to be transformed into a liquid form that can be absorbed into the bloodstream. **Enteric-coated** drugs cannot be

---

TABLE 23-1 ➤ Preparation Types and Advantages and Routes of Administration

ROUTE: ORAL The drug is swallowed and absorbed from the stomach or small intestines.

PREPARATION TYPES	ADVANTAGES	DISADVANTAGES
Capsule—A gelatinous container that holds the liquid, powder, or oil form of the drug. When swallowed, the gelatin container dissolves in the gastric juices. **Pill**—This term is rarely used now. *Tablet* is the preferred term. **Tablet**—A powdered drug is compressed into a hard, compact form (e.g., round, oval) that is easy to swallow and then breaks up into a fine powder in the stomach. The tablet is the most common oral preparation. *Enteric-coated tablets* have an acid-insoluble coating to keep them from dissolving in the stomach; they disintegrate in the alkaline secretions of the small intestine. **Time-released tablet or capsule**—A tablet or capsule formulated so that it does not dissolve all at once, but gradually releases medication over a few hours **Elixir**—A liquid containing water and about 25% alcohol that is sweetened with volatile oils (e.g., aromatic elixir); not as sticky or as sweet as syrups **Extract**—A very concentrated form of a drug made from animals or vegetables; may be a syrupy liquid or a powder **Fluid extract**—An alcohol-based solution of a drug from a vegetable source (e.g., belladonna); the most concentrated of the fluid preparations **Spirits**—A concentrated alcohol-based solution of a volatile (easily evaporated) substance or oil (e.g., ammonia, peppermint oil, orange oil); contains larger amounts of the substance than can be dissolved in water	■ Convenient ■ Sterility is not needed for oral use. ■ Economical ■ Noninvasive, low-risk procedure ■ Easy to administer, good for self-administration ■ Capsule can mask unpleasant taste of a drug. ■ Capsule can be time-release	■ Unpleasant taste may cause noncompliance. ■ May irritate gastric mucosa. ■ Patient must be conscious. ■ Digestive juices may destroy drug. ■ Cannot use if patient has nausea and vomiting or decreased gastric motility. ■ Cannot use if patient has difficulty swallowing. ■ Potential for aspiration ■ May be harmful to teeth. ■ Onset of action is slow.

Continued

TABLE 23-1 ➤ Preparation Types and Advantages and Routes of Administration—cont'd

PREPARATION TYPES	ADVANTAGES	DISADVANTAGES
Syrup—An aqueous solution of sugar, used to disguise unpleasant taste of drugs		
Tincture—An alcohol or water-and-alcohol (with a high percentage of alcohol) solution made by extracting potent plants; may also be used externally (e.g., tincture of iodine)		
Powder—Finely ground drug(s), usually mixed with a liquid before ingesting; some are used internally, others externally. (Some are mixed with diluents for parenteral injection.)		
Solution—Drug(s) dissolved in a liquid carrier. *Aqueous solutions* are medications dissolved in water. (May be used orally, externally, and parenterally.)		
Suspension—Drug(s) that are suspended (not completely dissolved) in a liquid. *Aqueous suspensions* are suspended in water. *Never used for IV or intra-arterial routes*		

ROUTE: ENTERAL The drug is given directly into the stomach or intestine (e.g., through a nasogastric or gastrostomy tube).

PREPARATION TYPES	ADVANTAGES	DISADVANTAGES
Same as for oral medications.	Can be used for patients with Impaired Swallowing as an alternative to parenteral administration	■ Not all tablets or capsules can be crushed; medications can clog the NG tube. ■ NG tube itself presents some risk of aspiration.

ROUTE: SUBLINGUAL (a variation of transmucosal administration)—The drug is held under the tongue and absorbed across the sublingual mucous membrane.

PREPARATION TYPES	ADVANTAGES	DISADVANTAGES
Lipid-soluble lozenge (troche)—A flat, round preparation that dissolves when held in the mouth. May act locally or be absorbed through mucosa for systemic effect. **Tablet** (See oral route.)	■ Used for local or systemic effects ■ Convenient ■ Sterility not needed ■ Quick delivery to general circulation ■ Bypasses stomach and intestines; absorbed directly into bloodstream	■ May inadvertently be swallowed in the saliva. ■ Not useful for drugs with unpleasant taste ■ May irritate the oral mucosa. ■ Patient must be conscious. ■ Useful only for highly lipid-soluble drugs ■ Patient must hold the drug in place until it is dissolved, which may take a few minutes. ■ Limited period of effectiveness, requiring frequent redosing

ROUTE: BUCCAL/TRANSMUCOSAL ADMINISTRATION Medication is held against the mucous membrane of cheek until it dissolves.

PREPARATION TYPES	ADVANTAGES	DISADVANTAGES
Lipid-soluble lozenge or tablet (See oral and sublingual routes.) **Spray**—Can be dispersed to the nasal or pharyngeal mucosa for rapid absorption.	■ Same as sublingual ■ Rapid, convenient, portable	■ Same as sublingual

ROUTE: TOPICAL (SKIN) The drug acts locally or is absorbed directly through skin (transdermal or percutaneous absorption).

PREPARATION TYPES	ADVANTAGES	DISADVANTAGES
Aerosol spray or foam—A liquid or foam that is sprayed by air pressure onto the skin **Cream**—A non-oily, semisolid substance applied to the skin	■ Continuous dosing ■ Sterility is not needed. ■ For local or systemic effects	■ Effective only for lipid-soluble drugs and must be specially formulated

TABLE 23-1 ➤ Preparation Types and Advantages and Routes of Administration—cont'd

PREPARATION TYPES	ADVANTAGES	DISADVANTAGES
Gel or **jelly**—A clear or translucent semisolid substance that liquefies when applied to the skin **Liniment**—An oily liquid to rub into the skin **Lotion**—An *emollient* (softening or soothing agent) for use on the skin; may be a clear solution, suspension, or emulsion **Ointment**—A semisolid, fatty (usually petroleum jelly- or lanolin-based) substance for skin or mucous membranes; usually not water soluble **Paste**—Similar to an ointment, but thicker and stiffer **Tincture** (see oral route). **Transdermal patch**—Releases constant, controlled amounts of medication, for systemic effect.	■ Long-acting systemic effect ■ Useful if patient is unable to take oral medications ■ Acceptable to most patients	■ May cause local irritation, especially if the patient is allergic to latex or tape. ■ Discarded patches may pose danger of poisoning. ■ Leaves residue on skin. ■ Accurate doses can be difficult to obtain when the drug is in a tube or jar.

ROUTE: TOPICAL: INSTILLATIONS The drug is placed into a body cavity (e.g., urinary bladder, rectum, vagina, ears, nose, eye).

PREPARATION TYPES	ADVANTAGES	DISADVANTAGES
Solutions (for nose, ears, and eyes; enemas per rectum)—Drug(s) dissolved in a liquid carrier **Suppositories** (for bladder, vagina, rectum)—Drug(s) mixed with a glycerin-gelatin or cocoa butter base and shaped for insertion into the body. They dissolve gradually at body temperature. **Jellies, creams** (for vagina and rectum)—See skin route.	■ Continuous dosing ■ Sterility is not needed ■ Useful if patient is unable to take oral medications ■ May be used for local or systemic effects	■ May be embarrassing for the patient. ■ Drugs may be poorly absorbed from the rectum if stool is present or if the patient defecates before the suppository melts.

ROUTE: TOPICAL: INHALATION A device (e.g., nebulizer, face mask) breaks the drug into finely dispersed particles, which are breathed into the respiratory passages. Some drugs are intended for local effects in the respiratory passages; others (e.g., anesthetic gases) are for systemic effects, especially in the brain.

PREPARATION TYPES	ADVANTAGES	DISADVANTAGES
Aerosols—Aerosols are liquids in very fine particles that can be inhaled into the lungs; they are sprayed under air pressure. **Gases**—Gas is a basic form of matter (i.e., solid, liquid, and gas). A gas must be kept in a closed container; otherwise, the fast-moving molecules escape into the air. Examples are oxygen, nitrogen, carbon dioxide, and anesthetic gases.	■ Quick and efficient local and systemic route through the lungs ■ May be given to unconscious patient. ■ Allows continuous dosing, and dosage can be easily modified.	■ Requires special equipment. ■ May irritate lung mucosa. ■ Useful only for drugs that are gases at room temperature. ■ May have unexpected systemic effect when only local effect is desired.

ROUTE: ALL PARENTERAL ROUTES

PREPARATION TYPES	ADVANTAGES	DISADVANTAGES
Depends on route.	■ Patient may be conscious or unconscious.	■ Requires sterile procedures. ■ Poses risk for infection because skin is broken. ■ Requires skill. ■ May cause some pain. ■ Produces anxiety. ■ More expensive than oral administration

ROUTE: PARENTERAL: INTRAVENOUS The drug is injected directly into the vein, either by bolus or slow infusion.

PREPARATION TYPES	ADVANTAGES	DISADVANTAGES
Aqueous solutions—Drug(s) dissolved in water	■ Rapid effect because absorption is bypassed; therefore, good for emergency situations	■ Poses risk of transient drug concentrations if drug is injected too rapidly.

Continued

TABLE 23-1 ➤ Preparation Types and Advantages and Routes of Administration—cont'd

PREPARATION TYPES	ADVANTAGES	DISADVANTAGES
	■ Patient needs only one needlestick, even for multiple doses.	■ Limited to highly soluble medications. ■ Poses risk for sepsis because pathogens may be introduced directly into the bloodstream. ■ The patient must have usable veins. ■ Cost of supplies and medications

ROUTE: PARENTERAL: INTRAMUSCULAR   The drug is injected into the muscle mass.

PREPARATION TYPES	ADVANTAGES	DISADVANTAGES
Primarily aqueous solutions (see intravenous route), although some preparations (e.g., penicillin) are suspensions	■ Rapid absorption, except for oily preparations or suspensions ■ Allows use of drugs that are not stable in solution. ■ Causes less pain (than do subcutaneous injections) from irritating drugs because they are deep in the muscle. ■ Allows administration of a larger volume than does subcutaneous administration. ■ Allows more rapid absorption than does subcutaneous or oral administration.	■ May cause irritation and local reactions. ■ Poses risk for tissue and nerve damage if site is improperly located. ■ Cannot be used where tissue is damaged (e.g., bruised) or peripheral circulation is decreased.

ROUTE: PARENTERAL: SUBCUTANEOUS   The drug is injected into the subcutaneous tissue under the skin

PREPARATION TYPES	ADVANTAGES	DISADVANTAGES
Primarily solutions—Drugs dissolved in a liquid carrier	■ Allows faster action than does oral administration. ■ Allows better absorption of lipid-soluble drugs than does intramuscular administration.	■ Only very small amounts can be given. ■ Absorption is relatively slow and often confined to the injected area.

ROUTE: PARENTERAL: INTRADERMAL   The drug is injected under the skin, into the dermis. Most commonly used for diagnostic testing or screening or for injecting local anesthetic.

ROUTE: PARENTERAL

Intraspinal—Injection of drug into the spinal canal

Intrathecal—Injection of drug into the subarachnoid space around the spinal cord

Epidural—Injection of drug between the vertebral spines into the extradural space.

Most commonly used for regional anesthesia.
For advantages and disadvantages, see Chapter 37.

decomposed by gastric secretions; the coating thus prevents the medication from being diluted before it reaches the intestines. In this way, the coating delays the action of the medication. It also decreases irritating effects of the medication on the stomach. **Timed-release (sustained-release)** medications are formulated to dissolve slowly, releasing small amounts for absorption over several hours.

To be absorbed, oral preparations must be water soluble and at least partially lipid soluble. *Liquids* (e.g., suspensions or solutions) are absorbed faster than tablets or capsules because the medications are already dissolved.

■ *Water-soluble drugs.* Drugs must be water soluble in order to dissolve in the *aqueous* (watery) contents of the GI tract.

■ *Lipid-soluble drugs.* Lipid solubility depends partly on the drug's chemical structure and partly on the environment at the site of absorption. Lipid-soluble drugs can penetrate lipid-rich cell membranes and enter the cells, whereas water-soluble drugs, such as penicillin, cannot penetrate these areas. That is why a highly fat-soluble drug, such as nitrous oxide, can cross the blood–brain barrier and effect sedation.

Which of your patients ("Meet Your Patient") is most likely to receive a water-soluble medication?

Effects of pH and Ionization

The **pH** (relative acidity or alkalinity) of the local environment also affects the absorption of a drug. The acid content of the stomach aids in transporting the medication across the mucous membranes, so *acidic* medications, such as aspirin, are more readily absorbed in the stomach than *basic* (alkaline) medications, such as sodium bicarbonate, which are readily absorbed in the more alkaline small intestine. For best absorption, should Mr. Pearson's ("Meet Your Patient") medications be acidic or alkaline preparations?

In solution, some of a drug's molecules are in **ionized** (electrically charged) form, and others are **nonionized** (neutral or noncharged). The ionized molecules are lipid insoluble and thus cannot pass easily through the phospholipid layer of cell membranes. Drug molecules can be converted easily from one form to the other, depending primarily on the pH of the environment. For example, when aspirin is dissolved in the stomach acid, most of its molecules remain nonionized, so they easily pass through the membranes of the gastric mucosa and enter the bloodstream. If the person ingests an antacid before taking aspirin, however, it will likely reduce the effects of the aspirin.

Blood Flow to the Area

Medications are absorbed rapidly in areas where blood flow to the tissue is greatest (e.g., oral mucous membranes). Areas with poor vascular supply (e.g., the skin, scarred areas) experience delayed absorption. Consider the following examples:

■ Excessive exercise draws blood away from the stomach and intestines to the muscles. Which route would promote absorption for a person who has just exercised heavily: oral or intramuscular (IM)? Why?

■ A person in shock has poor peripheral circulation. Which route would promote faster absorption: intramuscular or intravenous (IV)? Why?

For the first question, the IM route would be better for the person who has recently engaged in heavy activity.

This is because medication injected deep into the muscle where there is a rich blood supply would be absorbed more readily; while medication administered orally must first dissolve and be absorbed in the GI tract. For the second question, the IV route would be more efficient for the person with poor circulation because drugs act more rapidly, even in healthy people, when they are injected directly into the bloodstream and do not have to be absorbed.

KnowledgeCheck 23-3
■ Define *absorption*.
■ How are drugs absorbed?
■ What factors affect absorption?

 Go to Chapter 23, **Knowledge Check Response Sheet and Answers,** on the Student Resource Disk or DavisPlus at http://davisplus.fadavis.com/Wilkinson2

How Are Drugs Distributed Throughout the Body?

Distribution is the transportation of a drug in body fluids (usually the bloodstream) to the various tissues and organs of the body. Because blood goes to all parts of the body, theoretically a drug can produce effects (intended or unintended) anywhere. The rate of distribution depends on the adequacy of local blood flow in the **target area** (the site where the drug effects occur). It is also influenced by the permeability of capillaries to the drug's molecules as well as the protein-binding capacity of the drug. For a visual description,

 Go to Student Resources for pharmacokinetic animation, **Medication Absorption, Distribution, Metabolism, and Excretion,** on DavisPlus at http://davisplus.fadavis.com/Wilkinson2

Local Blood Flow

The blood supply of the target site affects distribution of a drug. For example, it is difficult to deliver a systemic medication to the skin and toes, where the blood vessels are very small. Circulation in the tissues is affected by a variety of factors. Factors that cause vasodilation in an area (e.g., application of warmth to an injection site, fever, and rest) increase circulation to area tissues. Factors that cause vasoconstriction (e.g., shock and chilling of the body) decrease circulation to the target tissue.

Membrane Permeability

Drug molecules must leave the blood and cross capillary membranes to reach their sites of action. Some capillary membranes act as barriers. The capillary networks in some organs consist of tightly packed endothelial cells that prevent some drugs from crossing them. For example, the **blood–brain barrier** allows distribution into the brain and cerebrospinal fluid of only those drugs that are (1) lipid soluble (e.g., anesthetics and barbiturates) and (2) not tightly bound to plasma proteins. Many antibiotics are only water soluble, and thus cannot be used to directly treat infections of the central nervous system. This barrier can be bypassed by injecting medications intrathecally (via the spinal canal) into the cerebrospinal fluid.

Protein-Binding Capacity

A drug's tendency to bind to plasma proteins in the blood also affects distribution. For a given amount of a drug, some molecules bind to plasma proteins, and the remainder will be "free." For example, nearly all acetaminophen (Tylenol) molecules are free in the bloodstream and are therefore pharmacologically active. By contrast, about 99% of the anticoagulant warfarin (Coumadin) is bound in the blood; its effects are produced by only the 1% of warfarin molecules that are free. Only free (unbound) drug molecules can produce pharmacological effects because only free molecules can be metabolized or excreted. A drug's tendency to bind to plasma proteins depends mostly on its chemical structure. Some medical conditions also affect protein binding. For example, malnourishment and liver disease reduce the amount of protein (serum albumin) available for binding.

KnowledgeCheck 23-4

- Define distribution.
- What factors affect distribution of drugs in the body?

 Go to Chapter 23, **Knowledge Check Response Sheet and Answers,** on the Student Resource Disk or DavisPlus at http://davisplus.fadavis.com/Wilkinson2

How Are Drugs Metabolized in the Body?

Metabolism (or **biotransformation**) is the chemical inactivation of a drug through its conversion into a more water-soluble compound or into metabolites that can be excreted from the body. Once a medication reaches its site of action, it is metabolized (changed into the inactive form) in preparation for excretion.

Metabolism takes place mainly in the liver, but medications can be detoxified also in the kidneys, blood plasma, intestinal mucosa, and lungs. If liver function is impaired (e.g., due to liver disease or aging), the drug will be eliminated more slowly, and toxic levels may accumulate. Disease states also affect drug metabolism. For example, patients with diabetes do not metabolize sugar effectively, so they should not take elixirs, which are high in sugar content.

Oral medications are absorbed from the GI tract and circulate through the liver before they reach the systemic circulation. Many oral medications can be almost completely inactivated in this way. This inactivation is known as the **first-pass effect**. For this reason, oral medications are formulated with a higher concentration of the drug than are parenteral medications. Alternatively, some medications can be given parenterally, allowing the drug to be distributed directly to target sites before it passes through the liver. For example, nitroglycerin undergoes this first-pass effect when taken orally; therefore, it is given sublingually or intravenously so that it bypasses the stomach and liver and reaches therapeutic levels in the blood.

KnowledgeCheck 23-5

- Define drug metabolism.
- Where are drugs metabolized?
- What factors affect drug metabolism?

 Go to Chapter 23, **Knowledge Check Response Sheet and Answers,** on the Student Resource Disk or DavisPlus at http://davisplus.fadavis.com/Wilkinson2

How Are Drugs Excreted from the Body?

A drug continues to act in the body until it is excreted. For **excretion** to occur, drug molecules must be removed from their sites of action and eliminated from the body. Drugs may be metabolized completely, partially, or not at all when they are excreted. The following are common organs of excretion.

Kidneys. The kidneys are the primary site of excretion. Adequate fluid intake facilitates renal excretion. If your patient has decreased renal function (e.g., as indicated by an elevated creatinine level), you should monitor for medication toxicity; if signs of toxicity are present, obtain a prescription for adjusted dosing.

Liver and GI Tract. Some drugs broken down by the liver are excreted into the GI tract and eliminated in the feces. Others (e.g., fat-soluble agents) are reabsorbed by the bloodstream, distributed to the target site, and returned to the liver. This is called **enterohepatic recirculation.** The kidneys later excrete these compounds. Anything that increases peristalsis (e.g., diarrhea, laxatives, enemas, chronic bowel disease, etc.) accelerates drug excretion via feces. Inactivity, poor diet, and decreased peristalsis delay excretion, increasing the effects of a drug.

Lungs. Most drugs removed by the lungs are not metabolized first. Gases and volatile liquids (e.g., general anesthetics) administered by inhalation usually are removed through exhalation. Other volatile substances, such as ethyl alcohol and paraldehyde, are highly soluble in blood and are excreted in limited amounts by the lungs. Strenuous exercise and deep breathing increase pulmonary blood flow and thereby promote excretion. By contrast, decreased cardiac output (as in shock) and hypoventilation (as can happen when a patient is in pain) prolong the period of time for drug elimination.

Exocrine Glands. Drug excretion through the **exocrine** (sweat and salivary) **glands** is limited. The elimination of metabolites in sweat is frequently responsible for such side effects as dermatitis. Drugs excreted in the saliva are usually swallowed and absorbed as other orally administered agents.

 Critical**Thinking** 23-4

You are notified of a patient being transferred from the ICU to your unit. The patient is 79-year-old Hattie Banks, admitted 2 days ago to the ICU for digoxin toxicity.

- What theoretical knowledge do you have about the metabolism and excretion of digoxin (Lanoxin)?
- What assessments should you be sure to make for Ms. Banks?

Concepts Relevant to Drug Effectiveness

In addition to the processes of absorption, distribution, metabolism, and excretion, you need to understand four other concepts related to a drug's effectiveness: (1) onset, peak, and duration of drug action; (2) therapeutic range; (3) bioavailability of the drug; and (4) concentration of the drug at target sites.

Onset, Peak, and Duration of Action

The **onset of action** is the time needed for drug concentration to reach a high enough blood level for its effects to appear. This is the **minimum effective concentration.** When the concentration of medication is highest in the blood, the medication has reached its **peak action.** The **duration of action** is that period of time in which the medication has a pharmacological effect (before it is metabolized and excreted) (Fig. 23-4). If the serum level of a medication falls below the minimum effective concentration, then the drug is not effective during that time. If the drug level exceeds the peak level, toxicity occurs.

 Critical**Thinking** 23-5

Refer to Table 23-1. James Bigler ("Meet Your Patient") is having right arm pain and needs relief quickly.

- Would it be better to give him oral acetaminophen with codeine (Tylenol #3) or an IM injection of a similar-strength medication? Why?
- Do you have enough information to be completely sure your choice of route will bring the quickest onset of action? Explain.

Therapeutic Range

When giving multi-dose medication (e.g., an antibiotic), the goal is to achieve a constant, therapeutic blood level. Because a fraction of the drug is constantly being excreted, repeated doses of the medication are given to achieve and maintain a constant therapeutic

Onset of action = 30 minutes
Peak effect = 1 hour
Duration of action = 2.0 hours

FIGURE 23-4 Once the drug is administered and absorption begins, blood levels begin to rise. When the *minimum effective concentration* is reached, drug effects begin (*onset of action*). *Maximum effect* occurs at peak blood level.

concentration. Even after absorption stops, distribution, metabolism, and excretion continue.

Therapeutic level is the concentration of a drug in the blood serum that produces the desired effect without toxicity.

Therapeutic range of a drug is a range of therapeutic concentrations. At onset of action, serum drug level is minimal.

Peak level occurs when the drug is at its highest concentration (when the rate of absorption is equal to the rate of elimination). After that, metabolic and excretory processes begin to remove the drug from the tissues and blood.

Trough level occurs when the drug is at its lowest concentration, right before the next dose is due.

A test called a *peak and trough level* helps to ensure the safety and effectiveness of certain drugs. The peak level must be measured when absorption is complete. This, of course, depends on all the factors that affect absorption. The trough level is typically measured about 30 minutes before the next dose of the drug is due. The drug's half-life and the time between doses affect the trough level. You will sometimes need to monitor serum drug levels so the primary care provider can adjust the dose and timing of a medication as needed. For a graphic illustration of peak, trough, and therapeutic levels,

 Go to Chapter 23, **Tables, Boxes, Figures: ESG Figure 23-1, Peak and Trough,** on the Student Resource Disk or DavisPlus at http://davisplus.fadavis.com/Wilkinson2

Biological Half-Life

A medication's **biological half-life** is the amount of time it takes for half of the drug to be eliminated. For example, tramadol (Ultram), a narcotic-like pain reliever, has a half-life of approximately 6 hours. This means if you take a 50-mg dose at 0800, by 1400 half of that dose (25 mg) will still be left in your body. In 12 hours, one-fourth of the initial dose (12.5 mg) will be left in your body. Because of their effects on metabolism and excretion, the following prolong half-life: liver and kidney disease, aging, absence of food, and slowed metabolic rate. Drug composition and distribution also affect half-life.

Critical Thinking 23-6

Rebecca Jones ("Meet Your Patients") received tramadol (Ultram) 50 mg for pain at 0800. The prescription allows the patient to have the drug every 6 hours. So at 1400, you give her another 50 mg. Ultram is metabolized in the liver and excreted mainly in the urine.

- When this medication reaches onset of action, about how much Ultram does Ms. Jones now have in her body?
- If the "normal" half-life of Ultram is 6 hours, you would expect Ms. Jones to still have about 25 mg of her first dose left in her body at the time of the second dose. Given her age, though, do you think she probably has more or less than 25 mg left at 6 hours? Why?

Concentration of Active Drug at Target Sites

The effectiveness of a medication depends ultimately on its concentration at the intended site. For example, a medication such as nitrofurantoin (Macrodantin) may be prescribed to treat a urinary tract infection. This drug is used because it is highly soluble in urine, and therefore tends to accumulate and concentrate in the bladder and kidneys, where the infection exists.

What Factors Affect Pharmacokinetics?

A drug's pharmacokinetics and therefore its effectiveness and safety, are affected by the following factors:

Age. Infants and young children need smaller doses because of their smaller body mass and immature body systems. Older adults may have declining liver and kidney function and are therefore at higher risk for drug toxicity. Table 23-2 summarizes life-span variations in pharmacokinetics.

Table 23-2 ➤ Drug Therapy Across the Life Span

PHARMACOKINETIC PROCESS	CHILDREN	OLDER ADULTS
Absorption	■ Exaggerated in infants as a result of lack of gastric acidity and shorter intestines ■ More complete topical absorption results from a larger body surface and thinner epidermis. ■ Enteral route is unpredictable. ■ Decreased muscle tone makes absorption of parenteral drugs unpredictable. ■ Gastric pH is higher, so that medications absorbed in acid environments are absorbed much more slowly.	■ Delayed but more complete ■ Gastric pH is less acidic because of decreased acid production in the stomach. ■ Decreased gastric pH delays absorption of medications absorbed in acid environments. ■ Because of decreased intestinal motility, drugs remain in the system longer, allowing for more absorption.
Distribution	■ Protein binding may be a problem. ■ Greater chance of toxicity because of low albumin levels. ■ Water content in the child's body is higher than in adults, so water-soluble drugs are less concentrated in the child and fat-soluble drugs are more highly concentrated.	■ Low albumin level could create a problem with plasma protein binding. ■ Increased risk of toxicity due to multiorgan slowdown. ■ Altered because of less lean mass ■ Less body water, greater body fat ■ Dehydration, poor nutrition, and electrolyte imbalances decrease absorption.
Metabolism	■ Metabolism may be altered because of immature liver. ■ Best to base dosage on body weight to avoid toxicity.	■ Presence of diseases may decrease metabolism of the drug. ■ Changes due to age, higher blood concentration, and less excretion cause greater chances of toxicity. ■ Some drugs interfere with the liver's ability to metabolize another drug.
Excretion	■ Excretion is delayed as a result of immature kidneys. ■ Repeat dosing may cause problems.	■ Decreased glomerular filtration rate inhibits excretion from the kidneys. ■ Diminished renal function inhibits excretion, thereby increasing the risk of toxicity.

Body Mass (Weight). The final concentration of a drug in the body depends on the patient's body mass. The average adult dose is based on the drug quantity that will produce a particular effect in 50% of people 18 to 65 years of age and weighing 150 lb. Obviously, a person who is much larger or smaller than this "average" requires an adjusted dose.

Sex. Women usually have lower muscle mass than men, a different hormone profile, and different fat and water distribution, which affect drug absorption.

Pregnancy. Most drugs are contraindicated during pregnancy because of their possible adverse effects on the embryo or fetus. Drugs known to cause developmental defects are called **teratogenic** drugs. Examples are alcohol and the anticonvulsant phenytoin (Dilantin).

Environment. Heat and cold affect peripheral circulation. A noisy environment may interfere with a person's response to antianxiety, sedative, or pain medications.

Route of Administration. The route of administration influences the amount of a drug absorbed into the circulatory system and the distribution to the sites of action.

Timing of Administration. The presence or absence of food in the GI tract affects an oral drug's pharmacokinetics. Biorhythms and cycles (e.g., drug-metabolizing enzyme rhythms, blood pressure cycles) also influence drug action.

Fluids. Insufficient fluid intake affects the absorption of solid dosage forms.

Pathological States. Intense pain decreases the effect of opioids; diseases causing circulatory, hepatic, or renal dysfunction interfere with pharmacokinetic processes.

Genetic Factors. Abnormal susceptibility to certain chemicals is genetically determined. Enzyme deficiencies and altered metabolism change a patient's responses to a drug. For example, blacks usually respond better to diuretics for blood pressure control than do other racial groups; and people of Asian descent metabolize some opioids at a slower rate. Use your critical thinking now. What important nursing intervention should you perform after you administer an opiate to an Asian patient?[1]

Psychological Factors. Some patients have the same response to a placebo—a pharmacologically inactive substance—as they do to the active drug. If a person has faith that a drug will help him, a *placebo effect* similar to the effect of an active drug may occur. Emotional states, such as anxiety, may cause resistance to tranquilizing drugs. Hostility toward or mistrust of medicine or health personnel can also interfere with a drug's effectiveness.

---

[1]How did you answer the question? If you said that you would need to observe closely for unexpected side effects, good thinking!

What Is Pharmacodynamics?

Pharmacodynamics is the study of *how* medications achieve their effects at various sites in the body—how specific drug molecules interact with target cells and how biological responses occur.

What Are Primary Effects?

Primary or **therapeutic effects** of medications are effects that are predicted, intended, and desired. The primary effects, in short, are the reason the drug was prescribed. All other consequences are **secondary effects** (unintended, nontherapeutic). Both primary and secondary effects are dose related, so increasing the dose increases the effects. Medications are given for the following effects:

- **Palliative effects** relieve the signs and symptoms of a disease but have no effect on the disease itself. For example, morphine sulfate may be given to a patient with cancer to manage pain, but it does not destroy cancer cells. The goal of palliative therapy is to make the patient as comfortable as possible when treatment options have been exhausted.
- **Supportive effects** support the integrity of body functions until other medications or treatments can become effective. For a patient with a bacterial infection, you may give acetaminophen (Tylenol) to control fever until blood levels of the prescribed antibiotic are effective in combating the infection causing the fever.
- **Substitutive effects** replace either body fluids or a chemical required by the body for improved functioning. You may, for example, administer insulin to a diabetic patient to replace the insulin no longer produced by the pancreas.
- **Chemotherapeutic effects** destroy disease-producing microorganisms or body cells. Two examples are (1) antibiotics, used to treat infections by killing or limiting the reproduction of certain bacteria and (2) antineoplastic drugs, used to treat cancer by limiting cell reproduction and destroying malignant cells.
- **Restorative effects** return the body to or maintain the body at optimal levels of health. For example, vitamin and mineral supplements are administered to many patients recovering from surgery.

KnowledgeCheck 23-6

- Name and define the four pharmacokinetic processes.
- How does absorption differ in children and older adults?
- What factors affect excretion?
- You are to administer the following drugs to Cyndi Early ("Meet Your Patient"): (1) insulin for her diabetes, administered subcutaneously and (2) morphine to relieve her pain, administered intravenously. For which primary effect is each of these drugs being given?

Go to Chapter 23, **Knowledge Check Response Sheet and Answers,** on the Student Resource Disk or DavisPlus at http://davisplus.fadavis.com/Wilkinson2

What Are Secondary Effects?

All medications can cause secondary effects (e.g., side effects, adverse reactions, allergic reactions), which can either be harmless or cause injury and which can sometimes be predicted.

Side Effects

Side effects are unintended, often predictable, physiological effects that are usually well tolerated by patients. They occur at the usual prescribed dose and may be immediate (e.g., dizziness) or delayed (e.g., constipation). For hospitalized patients, you will most often see side effects caused by analgesics, antibiotics, antipsychotics, and sedatives. The most common side effects are nausea, vomiting, diarrhea, dizziness, drowsiness, dry mouth, abdominal distention or distress, and constipation.

If side effects are significant, the medication may be discontinued. For example, lanoxin (Digoxin), which is given to regulate and strengthen the heartbeat, can cause cardiac irregularities, a side effect that can be life-threatening. Persistent or undesired side effects may require symptom management with laxatives, antidiarrheals, and antiemetics. For example, levofloxacin (Levaquin), an antibiotic, may cause diarrhea, which is treated with antidiarrheals (e.g., loperamide [Imodium]). Teach your patients what side effects to anticipate with medications and how to manage them.

Adverse Reactions

Adverse reactions are harmful, unintended, usually unpredicted reactions to a drug administered at the normal dosage. They are more severe than side effects and often require discontinuation of the drug.

- When adverse reactions are *dose related,* the undesired effects result from known pharmacological effects of the medication. For example, a diabetic patient treated with insulin may develop very low blood sugar if too much insulin is administered or he doesn't eat.
- Adverse reactions also occur because of *patient sensitivity,* meaning that the patient is unusually susceptible to the effects of the drug. Box 23-1 lists patients at high risk for adverse reactions.

The FDA defines **severe adverse reactions** as those that (1) are life-threatening, (2) require intervention to prevent permanent impairment or death; or (3) lead to congenital anomaly, disability, hospitalization, or death. Health professionals must document serious adverse reactions according to agency policy and report them to the FDA MedWatch program. To make a report, contact the FDA by calling 1-800-332-1088, or

 Go to the **FDA Medwatch** Web site at http://www.fda.gov/medwatch/

BOX 23-1 ■ Risk Factors for Adverse Drug Reactions

- Receiving treatment from two or more providers at the same time
- Concurrent illnesses (e.g., diabetes and renal failure)
- A change in the ability to absorb, metabolize, or excrete the drug
- Taking multiple prescription drugs in addition to over-the-counter preparations and herbal remedies and supplements. This is also called polypharmacy.
- Taking a drug inconsistently
- Confusion/cognitive impairment
- History of allergies
- History of previous adverse drug reactions
- Long-term use of a drug (may promote accumulation, leading to toxicity)
- Very old or very young age
- Obesity or extreme thinness
- Impaired hepatic and renal function
- Dehydration or rapid change in hydration status

Or contact the Institute for Safe Medication Practices (ISMP) to report errors, close calls, or hazardous conditions. ISMP guarantees the confidentiality and security of the information received. Contact ISMP by phone 800-FAIL-SAFE, by email **ismpinfo@ismp.org**.

 Go to https://www.ismp.org/orderforms/reporterrortoismp.asp

Toxic Reactions

Toxic reactions are dangerous, damaging effects to an organ or tissue. They are more severe than adverse reactions, sometimes even causing permanent damage or death. It may help to think of toxicity as poisoning. Antidotes are available for some medications; for example, naloxone (Narcan) is given for opiate toxicity. Toxicity may be caused by any of the following:

- *Overdosing* (administrating a dose that exceeds the prescribed amount). Examples are respiratory depression from excessive morphine and hypoglycemia from too much insulin)
- *Accumulation* of the drug in the tissues (related to long-term use or incomplete metabolism/excretion)
- *Abnormal sensitivity* or allergic response to the drug

Toxic reactions are usually localized, reversible, and immediate. However, they can be:

- Localized to a particular tissue or organ, or they can affect several organ systems.
- Reversible (e.g., tinnitus caused by aspirin) or permanent (e.g., hearing loss caused by aminoglycoside antibiotics).

- Evident soon after administration; although, some toxic reactions take months or even years to develop (e.g., drug-induced cancers).

CriticalThinking 23-7

- You have just looked up the antihypertensive drug, lisinopril (Zestril) and found the following side effects. What strategy could you use to help you remember all the side effects listed below?

  neutropenia, dizziness, headache, fatigue, depression, somnolence, paresthesia, hypotension, orthostasis, chest pain, nasal congestion, diarrhea, nausea, dyspepsia, impotence, rash, cough, muscle cramps, angioedema, lethargy, hypokalemia, decreased libido

- You have checked the medication record (MAR) for Margaret Marks ("Meet Your Patients") and prepared her next dose of antibiotic for intravenous administration. The MAR also indicates that she is receiving morphine for pain and that her last dose was given 1 hour ago. When you enter the room, you find her apparently sleeping. You are not able to awaken her to verify her identity. What do you suspect is happening, and how should you respond? (If you need information about antibiotics and morphine, look it up in an appropriate reference.)

Allergic Reactions

In an **allergic reaction,** the immune system identifies a medication as a foreign substance that should be neutralized or destroyed. The patient experiences no problems with the first dose of the medication, but it acts as an antigen, activating the formation of antibodies against the drug. When the drug is again administered, the antigen–antibody binding complex prompts an allergic reaction.

Allergic reactions range from minor to serious; however, even a small amount of a medication can cause a severe reaction. Urticaria (hives), pruritus (itching), edema of soft tissue and mucosa, and rhinitis (inflammation of the nasal mucosa) usually occur within minutes to 2 weeks after exposure and are considered mild. Such reactions often disappear after the medication is discontinued and the blood level of the drug falls. Medications most frequently implicated in allergic reactions are antibiotics, biological agents, and diagnostic agents. For a list of specific drugs, see Table 23-3, Medications Frequently Triggering Allergic Reactions.

An **anaphylactic reaction** is a life-threatening allergic reaction that occurs immediately after administration. The allergic response produces sudden constriction of bronchioles, edema of the larynx and pharynx, severe shortness of breath, wheezing, and severe hypotension (low blood pressure). Immediate treatment includes discontinuing the medication and giving epinephrine, IV fluids, steroids, and antihistamines. Respiratory support ranging from oxygen to intubation or ventilation may be required. A patient who is allergic to one drug may also be allergic to other medications in the same class. For example, many patients who are allergic to

Table 23-3 ➤ Medications Frequently Triggering Allergic Reactions

DRUG CLASSIFICATION	EXAMPLE DRUGS
Analgesics, Anesthetics, and Anti-inflammatory Agents	Codeine
	Morphine
	NSAIDs (ibuprofen, acetaminophen, naproxen)
	Indomethacin
	Aspirin
	Tranquilizers
	Local anesthetic agents, such as tetracaine, phenylbutazone, procaine, lidocaine, cocaine, benzocaine, general anesthetics
Antiseizure Drugs	Phenytoin
	Carbamazepine
Antibiotics	Cephalosporins
	Erythromycin
	Neomycin
	Penicillin
	Streptomycin
	Sulfonamides
	Tetracycline
	Vancomycin
Biological Agents	Allopurinol
	Antitoxins
	Corticotropin (ACTH)
	Enzymes
	Gamma globulin
	Insulin
	Vaccines
Diagnostic Agents	Iodinated media contrasts
	Intravenous pyelogram (IVP) dye
Other Drugs	Dextran
	Histamines
	Iodines
	Iron
	Phenothiazides
	Quinidine

penicillin are also allergic to cephalexin (Keflex), a synthetic penicillin.

Allergic reactions occur with 5% to 10% of all prescriptions, so always explore the patient's allergy history; use Allergy Alert bracelets and stickers; and document allergies in the patient's chart and care plan.

People with severe allergic reactions should wear a Medic Alert bracelet (Fig. 23-5) that identifies the person and the allergen, and carry epinephrine for emergency injection.

Critical Thinking 23-8

You are administering medications to your assigned patients ("Meet Your Patients"). What should you do in each of the following situations? Which patient should you attend to first? Explain your thinking.

- Ms. Jones has ibuprofen (Motrin) prescribed for her back pain. She tells you she cannot take this medication because it makes her feel nauseated.
- Mr. Bigler had an open reduction internal fixation of his arm performed yesterday and is receiving an antibiotic, cefazolin (Ancef), 500 mg IV every 8 hours. He has already received three doses of this medication, and you initiated his 0800 dose about 10 minutes ago. He tells you that he thinks his throat is closing shut.

Idiosyncratic Reactions

An **idiosyncratic** reaction is an unexpected, abnormal, or peculiar response to a medication. Idiosyncratic reactions may take the form of extreme sensitivity to a medication, lack of response, or a paradoxical (opposite of expected) response, such as agitation in response to a sedative. In children, for example, diphenhydramine (Benadryl) occasionally causes agitation or excitability instead of the expected drowsiness.

Cumulative Effect

A **cumulative effect** is the increased response to repeated doses of a drug that occurs when the rate of administration is greater than the rate of metabolism and excretion. This happens when (1) the body cannot metabolize a dose of the medication before the next dose is given, (2) excretion is slowed but absorption is normal or rapid, or (3) absorption is slowed. Unless the dose is

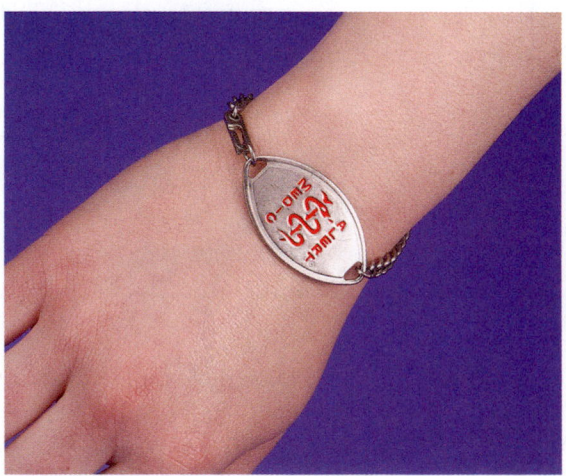

FIGURE 23-5 People with severe allergies to a medication should wear a Medic Alert bracelet.

changed, the medication accumulates in the system until a toxic level is reached. Opiates and barbiturates are known for their cumulative effects.

KnowledgeCheck 23-7

- Differentiate between primary and secondary effects of medications.
- List one adverse reaction for each of the following systems: blood, gastrointestinal, neurological, cardiovascular, hepatic, renal.
- What are some of the symptoms you will see in an anaphylactic reaction?
- What type of patient is most likely to experience an allergic reaction?

Go to Chapter 23, **Knowledge Check Response Sheet and Answers,** on the Student Resource Disk or DavisPlus at http://davisplus.fadavis.com/Wilkinson2

How Do Medications Interact?

When one drug alters or modifies the action of another, a **drug interaction** occurs. In an **antagonistic drug relationship,** one drug interferes with the actions of another and decreases the resultant drug effect—that is, the combined effect is less than that of one drug given alone. In a **synergistic drug relationship,** there is an additive effect; that is, the effect of both drugs together is greater than the individual effects. **Drug incompatibilities** occur when multiple drugs are mixed together, causing a chemical deterioration of one or both drugs. The result is an incompatible solution that should not be administered. You can usually recognize an incompatibility when the mixed solution takes on a changed appearance. However, you should always consult medication resources and compatibility charts *before* mixing medications. Then, after mixing, double-check the medication for changes in appearance.

As a nurse, you must be knowledgeable of drug interactions and monitor your patients for them. For a list of common drug-drug and drug-food interactions,

Go to Chapter 23, **Tables, Boxes, Figures: ESG Table 23-5, Drug-Drug and Food-Drug Interactions,** on the Student Resource Disk or DavisPlus at http://davisplus.fadavis.com/Wilkinson2

The more drugs a patient takes, the higher the risk of a drug interaction. Other variables influence drug interactions: intestinal absorption, competition for protein binding, drug metabolism, renal excretion, and alteration of electrolyte imbalance. Drugs may also interact with certain foods. For example,

High-fat foods and those low in fiber will delay stomach emptying and medication absorption by up to 2 hours.
Acidic citrus fruits and juices enhance absorption of iron. Some citrus fruits, such as grapefruit, interact with medication in an antagonistic manner.

Carbonated soft drinks can cause medications to dissolve faster, be neutralized, or experience a change in absorption rate in the stomach.

Dairy products taken with an antibiotic such as tetracycline, decrease the absorption of the drug in the stomach.

Foods containing tyramine (e.g., aged, dried, or fermented products), when consumed while taking monoamine oxidase (MAO) inhibitors, may produce a hypertensive crisis.

For a list of several medications that should be taken with food and those that should be taken on an empty stomach,

Go to Chapter 23, **Tables, Boxes, Figures: ESG Box 23-1,** on the Student Resource Disk or DavisPlus at http://davisplus.fadavis.com/Wilkinson2

KnowledgeCheck 23-8

- What type of interaction occurs when one drug interferes with the action of another?
- What interactions occur when one drug has an additive effect on another drug?
- What is drug incompatibility?

Go to Chapter 23, **Knowledge Check Response Sheet and Answers,** on the Student Resource Disk or DavisPlus at http://davisplus.fadavis.com/Wilkinson2

What Should I Know About Drug Abuse or Misuse?

You should be able to differentiate between tolerance and dependence. **Tolerance** is a decreasing response to repeated doses of a medication. The person then requires more of the drug to achieve the desired effect. In contrast, a person's reliance on, or need for, a drug constitutes **drug dependence.** Dependence leads to compulsive patterns of drug use wherein the user's lifestyle centers on procuring and taking the drug.

Drug misuse is the nonspecific, indiscriminate, or improper use of drugs, including alcohol, over-the-counter (OTC), and prescription drugs. In performing self-care, people frequently misuse laxatives, aspirin, acetaminophen, ibuprofen, cough and cold remedies, and sleep-inducing drugs. Older adults are especially prone to misuse of laxatives.

Drug abuse is the inappropriate intake of a substance by amount, type, or situation, continuously or periodically. For example, consuming alcohol at work is considered abuse, but having a glass of wine with dinner is not. Drug abuse may or may not lead to drug dependence. **Illicit drugs,** also known as street drugs, are drugs sold illegally. Many are prescription drugs (e.g., hydrocodone [Oxycontin or Vicodin]) sought for their mood-altering effects. Prescription drugs can be abused when taken for purposes other than medically intended.

How Do I Measure and Calculate Dosage?

Medications are not always available in the exact dosage the patient needs. Therefore, you must be proficient in calculating drug dosages to be sure your patients receive the correct amount of medication.

Medication Measurement Systems

Medications are usually prescribed and measured using the metric system; however, there are still a few medications dispensed using the apothecary and household systems, so you will need to learn how to work with all three systems. For a complete discussion of measurement systems and equivalents,

VOL 2 Go to Chapter 23, **Measuring and Calculating Dosage,** in Volume 2.

Metric System. The metric system is the preferred system. The metric system promotes accuracy by allowing for calculation of small drug dosages. A disadvantage of this system in the United States is that many people outside the healthcare system are not familiar with it.

Apothecary System. The British apothecary system of measurement has been in use in the United States since colonial times. Only a few medications (e.g., aspirin) are measured using this system because it is less convenient and less precise. Apothecary measurements are usually written using Roman numerals, but you may also see them in Arabic numerals. For example, *5 grains* might be written as *grains V* or *gr V.*

To avoid a dosage error, write out the intended unit of measurement (grains) so gr (grains) is not mistaken for gm (grams).

Household System. Because most people are familiar with the household system, it is easier to teach a patient about home medications using this system. However, nurses do not often use it because dosages measured in this system are less precise (e.g., teaspoons, ounces, cup) and can lead to medication dosing error.

Special Measurements: Units and Milliequivalents

Insulin, a drug used by diabetics to help control blood sugar, is measured in **units,** with 100 international units (U100) being the standard strength preparation. In this strength, 1 mL of the fluid medication contains 100 units of insulin. Heparin, an anticoagulant, and penicillin are also prescribed in units. Be aware that not all units are the same. For example, 1 mL of heparin does *not* contain 100 units of heparin. You must always read the container label to know the number of units per milliliter. The following is a medication prescription using units: "NPH insulin 14 units subcutaneously every morning."

Milliequivalents (mEq) indicate the strength of the ion concentration in a drug. A milliequivalent is the number of grams of a solid contained in one mL of a solution. Electrolytes, such as potassium chloride (KCl), are measured in mEq. The following are medication prescriptions using mEq:

KCl 20 mEq by mouth twice daily
D_5W 1000 mL with KCl 40 mEq every 8 hours

Note that units and mEq *cannot* be directly converted to the apothecary, metric, or household systems.

Calculating Dosages

You should be able to verify using dosage calculations accurately using several different methods and formulas. Inaccurate calculations result in incorrect dosages and could harm the patient. For expanded instructions on calculating dosages for adults and children,

 Go to Chapter 23, **Measuring and Calculating Dosage,** in Volume 2.

The Electronic Study Guide also contains several practice problems. To use them,

 Go to Chapter 23, **Practice Dosage Problems,** on the Student Resource Disk or DavisPlus at http://davisplus.fadavis.com/Wilkinson2

What Must I Know About Medication Prescriptions?

Prescriptions for medication are either entered into an electronic health record for automated dispensing or printed in the patient orders on the chart or prescription pad using the format below. Before administering any medication you must obtain a medication prescription from the care provider and verify that it is complete, correct, and completely legible. A complete medication prescription contains the following essential elements (Fig. 23-6):

- Patient's full name (some agencies and some states require the address of the patient)
- Name of the prescriber, including relevant credentials and legal registration number, such as the National Provider Identification (NPI) in the United States
- Address of the prescriber
- Date and time prescription was written
- Name of medication
- Dosage (including size, frequency, and number of doses)
- Route of administration
- Signature of prescriber

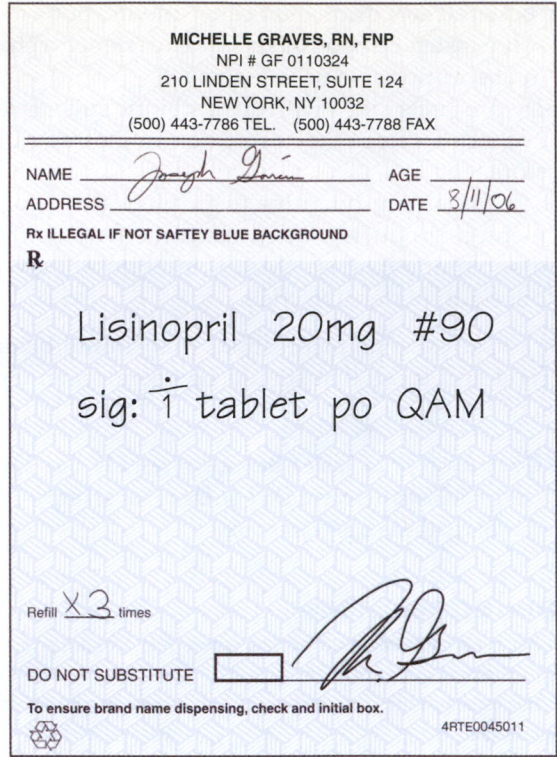

FIGURE 23-6 Example of a prescription.

To verify a medication prescription, ask yourself the following questions:

- Is the prescription legible enough for me to clearly read?
- Is the prescribed dose within the normally prescribed dosage range and comparable to previously prescribed dose?
- Is the prescribed route appropriate?
- Is the drug appropriate for the patient? (For example, you would question an antihypertensive drug to be prescribed for a patient with hypotension.)
- Is the patient allergic to the medication prescribed?
- Are the administration times appropriate? For example, is an antibiotic prescribed for every 6 hours when the drug formulary indicates it should be taken every 24 hours?
- What is the address and National Provider Identification (NPI) of the person prescribing?
- How many doses are there before the prescription needs to be refilled?
- How many refills are prescribed?

KnowledgeCheck 23-9

- What are the essential parts of a medication prescription?
- How does an inpatient prescription (order) differ from an outpatient prescription?

 Go to Chapter 23, **Knowledge Check Response Sheet and Answers,** on the Student Resource Disk or DavisPlus at http://davisplus.fadavis.com/Wilkinson2

What Abbreviations Are Used in Medication Prescriptions?

For a list of medication-related abbreviations you may see used when prescribing and documenting medications,

 Go to Chapter 23, **Tables, Medication-Related Abbreviations,** in Volume 2.

You should write out drug names in full. Abbreviations can be easily confused and many are not universally understood. However, you will see and use some abbreviations when administering and documenting medications (e.g., mL, mEq). Always do so carefully because some may be similar and confusing. Consult The Joint Commission's official Do Not Use list and know the acceptable abbreviations used in your facility. Also,

 Go to Chapter 23, **Tables, Institute for Safe Medication Practices: List of Error-Prone Abbreviations, Symbols, and Dose Designations,** in Volume 2.

Types of Medication Prescriptions

Common types of medication prescriptions are based on the duration, frequency, and/or urgency of the prescription.

- **Standard written prescriptions** apply without a renewal date until the prescriber writes a prescription to alter or discontinue the medication or indicates on the original prescription a specific stop date. For example, "Give furosemide 20 mg IVP twice a day for 5 days." This type of prescription should be renewed regularly.
- **Automatic stop dates** are protocols that hospitals use for discontinuing medications after a certain length of time. Most narcotic prescriptions are in effect only for 7 days. If the medication is needed after the automatic stop date, the care provider must write another prescription.
- **STAT** prescription means that a single dose of medication is to be given immediately and only once. The word *stat* or *now* should appear in the prescription, for example, "Give furosemide 20 mg IVP STAT," or "Give lorazepam 1 mg IV push now."
- **Single** prescription, or *one-time prescription*, indicates that the medication is to be given only once at a specified time. Preoperative medications, given before surgery or diagnostic procedures or treatments, are an example of a single prescription. For example:
    Versed 25 mg intramuscularly on call for when surgical staff requests premedication to be administered
    Tetanus toxoid 0.5 mL intramuscularly before discharge
- **Standing orders.** When a unit frequently provides care to a standard population of patients—for example, coronary care patients or knee replacement patients—the primary care provider may develop a set of *standing orders*. These are officially accepted sets of prescriptions to be applied routinely by nurses for the care of patients under certain conditions or under certain circumstances, such as drug allergies or sensitivities. They establish guidelines for treating a particular disease or set of symptoms. For example:

    Coronary care or intensive care units (CCUs or ICUs) may have standing orders for the administration of nitroglycerin for chest pain (e.g., "Give nitroglycerin 0.4 mg sublingually q3–5 min for chest pain, to a maximum of 3 doses in 15 min").

- Many postoperative patients receive a prescribed number of injectable analgesic medications for pain relief. So, for all the postoperative patients on a unit, standing orders would include, "ketorolac 30 mg IV push q12hr for 2 days."
- **prn prescription.** The care provider may prescribe a medication to be given whenever the patient requires (prn). A prn prescription requires the nurse to determine, in collaboration with the patient, when the medication is to be given. The prescription specifies (1) the condition for which the medication is to be given and (2) the minimum time intervals between doses. The medication cannot be given any more frequently than prescribed, even if symptoms persist. Pain medications, antiemetics (antinausea medications), and laxatives are usually given prn. For example:

    Morphine 10 mg intramuscularly q3–4hr prn incisional pain.
    Acetaminophen 650 mg PO q4hr prn for temp >101°F.

How Are Medication Prescriptions Communicated?

Medication prescriptions can be communicated in various ways. The nursing implications are slightly different for each. In general, prescribers either write or speak to communicate the intended prescription.

Written Prescriptions. You will find **written prescriptions** either hand written on a prescription form or preprinted standard medication orders and protocols. Some agencies accept medication orders or prescriptions transmitted electronically or via facsimile from the prescriber to the nurse, with the original copy provided later. Although this step may save time, the risk of errors is greater because faxed copies may be illegible.

Verbal Prescription. A prescriber may sometimes give a spoken prescription while present with the nurse. This is called a **verbal prescription.** When you receive a verbal prescription, you, as the RN, will write the prescription and sign it with the provider's name followed by your name and credentials. Medication names that sound the same can be confusing and lead to administering the wrong drug (Box 23-2). Repeat the prescription to the provider and spell the medication name to ensure accuracy. Avoid taking verbal prescriptions, and use them only in urgent situations because they increase the risk for miscommunication and errors.

Telephone Prescription. Prescribers may also give medication prescriptions by the telephone. You will not be surprised to know that we call these **telephone prescriptions**. Usually this will be in response to a call you have placed to report a change in the patient's condition or the results of laboratory or other tests. The provider usually must cosign verbal and telephone prescriptions within 24 hours.

What Steps Should I Take if I Think a Prescription Is Incorrect?

As a nurse, you are legally responsible for medications you administer. If you believe a prescription is incorrect, perform the following steps:

- Ask another nurse or physician to check the prescription.

- Look up the medication in a reliable resource (e.g., drug formulary) to verify spelling, usage, dosages, and routes.
- Contact the prescriber for clarifications, concerns, or questions.
- Do not assume you are correctly interpreting the prescription if you have any question at all.

Use your knowledge, common sense, and intuition when administering medications. To avoid errors, you must know and understand the procedures at your facility, be familiar with the medications you give, and always check the prescription. Each agency will have a policy specifying the procedure for checking medication prescriptions. For example, a unit clerk may copy the original prescription onto a medication administration record (MAR), but the nurse must check to be sure the transcription is correct.

 Critical**Thinking** 23-9

Find the errors in these medication prescriptions. Look the medications up in a drug formulary or nursing drug handbook to check dosages, spelling, and so on.

- Ancef 10 g q6hr IV
- Capatril 25 mg orally twice a day
- Digoxin 0.125 mg daily
- Lasix 400 mg by mouth
- NTG grain 1/150 prn chest pain
- Tylenol orally prn fever

Medication Errors

All medications are prescribed, prepared, and administered with the best intentions to improve patient health and comfort. However, medication errors occur with surprising frequency. A **medication error** is any preventable event that may cause or lead to inappropriate medication use or harm to a patient. Medication errors are among the most common adverse events that occur in hospitalized patients.

About one out of five drug doses administered by nurses are in error in some way. The most common errors are confusion caused by similar drug names, lack of knowledge of the drug (e.g., incorrect dosages, incorrect mixing), lack of information about the patient (e.g., allergies, lab results, medical condition). A fairly high percentage of medication errors involve anticoagulants (blood thinners), with nearly 3% or those resulting in patient harm or death (Joanna Briggs Institute, 2005). Box 23-3 describes several causes of medication errors by nurses.

How Can I Avoid Errors?

A variety of system-wide measures help to prevent medication errors in healthcare agencies. The Joint Commission recommends standardizing protocols for prescribing, administering, and documenting

BOX 23-2 ■ Medications With Similar-Sounding Names

Alprazolam	lorazepam
Baclofen	Bactroban
Cefzil, Keflin	Keflex
Celebrex	Celexa, Cerebyx
Cytoxan	Ciloxan
Demerol	dicumarol
Digoxin	digitoxin
Glyburide	glipizide
Humalog	Humulin R
Keflex	Kantrex
Lamictal	Lamisil
Lodine	Iodine
Morphine	meperidine
NovoLog	Humalog
NovoLog	Novalin R
Ophthalgan	Auralgan
Percocet	Percodan
Phenergan	Phenaphen
Procardia	Procardia XL
Quinine	quinidine
Ranitidine	amantadine
Serzone	Seroquel
Taxotere	Taxol
Zantac	Xanax
Zantac	Zyrtec
Zostrix	Zestril

BOX 23-3 ■ Why Do Medication Errors Occur?

The following are several factors associated with medication errors:

Lack of Knowledge or Information

- Lack of knowledge of the drug (e.g., incorrect dosages, incorrect mixing, overly rapid infusion, drug interaction, adverse effects, etc.) is the most common factor contributing to medication errors.
- Lack of information about the patient (e.g., allergies, other medications, lab results, medical condition for which the medication is contraindicated). This is the second most frequent cause of errors.
- A drug is given by the wrong route.

Faulty Communication

- The written prescription is unclear, illegible, or transcribed incorrectly, resulting in administering the wrong drug or dosage (e.g., confusion between drugs with similar names).
- The telephone prescription is taken incorrectly.
- Protocol is not understood or is violated.
- A drug prescription is written on the wrong patient's chart.
- The wrong dosage is prescribed (e.g., by misplacing a zero or decimal point).
- Abbreviations are misunderstood.
- Poor, or no, documentation can result in error. For example, a nurse administers a medication yet fails to record it immediately afterward. A second nurse checking the patient's chart thinks the drug has not been given so administers a dose. The patient receives a double dose.

Equipment Errors

- Wrong equipment is used to administer the drug.
- Equipment malfunctions or is not used properly.

Calculation and Measurement Errors

- An error in calculating the dosage is made so the patient receives the wrong dose.
- There is confusion in the unit of measurement; for example, a drug is prescribed based on kilograms and dispensed or administered based on pounds (and vice versa).

Other

- Medication is improperly handled or stored.
- The patient's identity is not checked, and the wrong patient receives the medication.
- Lighting is inadequate.
- The nurse is fatigued, distracted, or interrupted.

Sources: The Joanna Briggs Institute. (2005). Strategies to reduce medication errors with reference to older adults. *Best Practice,* 9(4), 1–6; Roy, V., Gupta, P., & Srivastava, S. (2005). Medication errors: Causes & prevention. *Health Administrator,* XIX(1), 60–64.

medication. Errors can be reduced in the home setting if the patient is prescribed the same dose at home as in the hospital.

To ensure patient safety you need to learn from your mistakes and the mistakes of others. You also need to think defensively. Ask "what if" and "why" questions: "What will happen if I don't do something or if I do something wrong? Why am I hanging this IV or giving this medication?" As a nurse, your critical thinking is the best defense to avoid errors and improve patient care and safety.

For guidelines to help individual nurses prevent medication errors,

 Go to **Clinical Insight 23-7: Guidelines for Avoiding Medication Errors,** in Volume 2.

Error-Prevention Technology

Computers can decrease errors by improving access to information and communication among health professionals. Some healthcare agencies provide nurses with laptops and PDAs, allowing them to tap into detailed information about diseases, similar-sounding drugs, interactions, and side effects. A variety of error-prevention technologies can reduce the likelihood of medication errors.

Use of Smart Technologies. So-called smart pumps, used at the point of care, can help you avoid programming the wrong dose into the pump. Drug protocols can be linked to a drug library with predefined dosing limits. If a nurse attempts to program outside that parameter, the pump halts or triggers an alarm. Smart infusion pumps also ensure the correct dose is delivered. Once programmed, the delivery rate does not change; if there is a blocked line, an alarm will sound. In contrast, when using a gravity IV, the drip rate can change (e.g., with patient movement) and you may not notice it immediately.

Computerized Prescriber Order Entry (CPOE). CPOE helps prevent errors in reading and transcribing orders, particularly when handwritten orders are illegible. Electronic prescribing systems are safer when combined with decision-support tools that automatically alert prescribers to possible interactions, allergies, and other potential problems.

Barcoding Medications. Barcode medication administration, especially when combined with CPOE, provides a nearly foolproof system for identifying the right patient and transfers data electronically, eliminating the error-prone paper transcription process. Barcoding at the unit-dose level helps prevent nurses from selecting an incorrect medication.

Automated Dispensing Units in the pharmacy minimize human handling, which can also reduce error.

Pediatric Considerations

Confusion between pounds and kilograms is a source of dosing error. The Joint Commission advises nurses to weigh patients in kilograms because it is the standard measurement for dosing pediatric prescriptions, medical records, and staff communication. Prescriptions for medication should be written with the dose per kilogram of body weight so that the intended dosage can be easily double-checked by nurses and pharmacists. When available, pediatric-specific medication formulations and concentrations are safer than medications dispensed for adults.

What Should I Do if I Commit a Medication Error?

As a nurse, you have a duty to do no harm. With that said, if an error were to occur, even though you might be anxious about having put your patient at risk, and might even be embarrassed to admit that you made a mistake or fear you could lose your job, you must immediately assess the patient's vital signs and physical status; report findings to the primary care provider; and notify the nurse manager of your unit. You must report the event surrounding the error for risk management. Check with your institution for agency-specific policy regarding incident reporting. For detailed guidelines about actions to take if you commit a medication error,

 Go to **Clinical Insight 23-8: Taking Action after a Medication Error,** in Volume 2.

Practical **Knowledge**
knowing how

Regardless of the type of medication or the route of administration, when administering a medication you should:

- Perform assessments relevant to the medication.
- Review the medication prescriptions and the medication administration record (MAR); clarify any differences.
- Consult with a reference for medications unfamiliar to you.
- Explain to the patient the actions and the side effects of the medication.
- Administer the medication using the "rights of medication." (See Ensuring Safe Medication Administration section.)
- Perform related interventions, for example:
  - Explain the importance of drinking fluids, timing of medication in relation to food consumption, and whether medication tablets or capsules may be crushed.
- Assess vital signs.
- Assess for contraindications and adverse effects.
- Evaluate and record the patient's response to the medication.

The rest of the chapter explains these activities to you. You should also

 Go to Chapter 23, **Medication Guidelines: Steps to Follow for All Medications (Regardless of Type or Route),** in Volume 2.

 Critical **Thinking** 23-10

Mr. Pearson ("Meet Your Patients") refuses to take his 1400 dose of antibiotic, stating that he had just taken it. What actions do you take to ensure sound decision-making and maintain patient safety?

ASSESSMENT

During your initial patient assessment, you will gather data that you need to administer medications safely. The following are highlights of medication-related assessments.

Before administration, assess:

- Vital signs
- Whether the patient's general condition is appropriate for the medication
- Your knowledge of the medication
- Biological factors that affect drug metabolism

 Go to Chapter 13, **Clinical Insight 13-1: Assessing for Biological Variations,** in Volume 2.

During administration, assess the patient's:

- Mental status
- Coordination
- Ability to self-administer the drug
- Swallowing (for oral medications)

After administration, assess:

- Effectiveness of the drug
- For side effects
- For signs of toxicity or adverse reactions

When taking a medication history, you should ask about the patient's history of illness, history of allergies, medications, attitudes toward medications, learning needs, and whether the patient (if a woman) is pregnant or breastfeeding. Also check relevant laboratory test results. For more discussion of the components to include in a medication history, and to print out a tool you can use for a full medications history and physical,

Go to Chapter 23, **Supplemental Materials: Components of a Medication History,** on the Student Resource Disk or DavisPlus at http://davisplus.fadavis.com/Wilkinson2

As with the nursing history, the physical examination allows you to identify potential problems and the need for adapting medication administration procedures. For example, you will assess relevant body systems to confirm the need for the drug and provide a baseline for evaluating the patient's responses to it. For oral medications, assess the patient's ability to swallow; for intramuscular medications, assess muscle mass. For more complete information about the physical examination related to medications,

 Go to Chapter 23, **Supplemental Materials: Physical Examination Related to Medications,** on the Student Resource Disk or DavisPlus at http://davisplus.fadavis.com/Wilkinson2

ANALYSIS/NURSING DIAGNOSIS

The following are some examples of nursing diagnoses associated with patient medications:

Deficient Knowledge related to lack of motivation to learn about medications
Ineffective Management of Therapeutic Regimen related to confusion
Risk for Aspiration related to Impaired Swallowing

For examples of other nursing diagnoses,

 Go to Chapter 23, **Standardized Language; Standardized Diagnoses, Outcomes, and Interventions Related to Medication Administration,** in Volume 2.

A few nursing diagnoses represent medication side effects; however, because a wide range of adverse effects is possible, no attempt was made to include them all. The following sections discuss Risk for Injury and Noncompliance.

Risk for Injury

Risk for Injury may be related to polypharmacy, misuse, overuse, or underuse of medications. Many people self-prescribe or rely on over-the-counter (OTC) medications for relief of symptoms such as insomnia, headaches, joint pains, and indigestion. They may continue taking them in combination with prescribed medications. This practice is **polypharmacy:** the ingestion of numerous medications in an attempt to treat many conditions simultaneously. Polypharmacy increases the potential for adverse reactions and dangerous drug and food interactions.

Older adults are especially prone to polypharmacy. They typically take several medications prescribed for chronic diseases, and many medicate for symptoms related to the aging process (e.g., constipation). The combination of polypharmacy, increased sensitivity to medications, and declining cognitive and sensory function can be especially dangerous.

Some patients misuse, overuse, underuse, or use drugs inconsistently. They may even use them when contraindicated. For example, when a person takes an antibiotic and then "feels better" after a few days of the medication, she may stop taking it or take it erratically as symptoms come and go. Such an inconsistent dosage schedule hinders the body's ability to achieve a blood level high enough to treat the infection or disease. Some drugs, for instance beta blockers, when taking inconsistently can be dangerous, even life-threatening.

Noncompliance

Noncompliance (nonadherence) is failure to follow the treatment plan (e.g., not taking a prescribed medication, or skipping doses). You cannot assume that the reason a patient may be noncompliant is because he hasn't been taught the importance of following the treatment plan. Prescription medications are expensive. Faced with choosing between food and pills, people on a limited budget or without health insurance often simply do not buy the more costly medications, or they may take only partial doses of maintenance medications (e.g., thyroid medications, oral hypoglycemics for diabetes). Some patients, particularly older adults, have visual and motor deficits that limit their ability to read labels and manipulate bottle caps, syringes, and so on. Other reasons for noncompliance include lack of symptoms, inability to tolerate side effects, forgetfulness, and impaired mental capacity. Always investigate the patient's reasons for nonadherence so you can take appropriate actions.

KnowledgeCheck 23-10

- What are the risks involved for patients who engage in polypharmacy?
- List at least three reasons for noncompliance with a medication regimen.

 Go to Chapter 23, **Knowledge Check Response Sheet and Answers,** on the Student Resource Disk or DavisPlus at http://davisplus.fadavis.com/Wilkinson2

PLANNING OUTCOMES/EVALUATION

NOC standardized outcomes depend on the specific nursing diagnoses you choose. For NOC outcomes for selected nursing diagnoses,

 Go to Chapter 23, **Standardized Language; Standardized Diagnoses, Outcomes, and Interventions Related to Medication Administration,** in Volume 2.

Individualized goals/outcome statements you might write for a client should be stated so their achievement reflects resolution of the problem (NANDA-I label). The following are some examples:

After explanation, and within 1 week, describes the expected actions and side effects of his medications.
Self-administers his medications in the correct amounts and on the prescribed schedule.
Describes possible interactions with other drugs; names the drugs to avoid taking with this medication.
After demonstration and practice, and within 1 week, correctly draws up and self-administers insulin.

Will consult the primary care provider before adding any new OTC or other medications or homeopathic/herbal preparations.

 PLANNING INTERVENTIONS/IMPLEMENTATION

NIC standardized interventions depend on the patient's nursing diagnoses, especially on the etiologies.

VOL 2 Go to Chapter 23, **Standardized Language; Standardized Diagnoses, Outcomes, and Interventions Related to Medication Administration,** in Volume 2.

Specific individualized nursing activities include preparing and administering medications. You will use specific, step-by-step procedures for these activities. However, only the general principles and the critical aspects of the procedures are presented in this volume.

Nursing interventions also include activities to address specific nursing diagnoses and, for all patients, the activities to ensure safe administration of medications presented in the remainder of this chapter.

Ensuring Safe Medication Administration

Medication mistakes are the most common type of healthcare error. Errors include giving the dose at the wrong time, omitting doses, giving the wrong dose, and giving the dose without authorization. To help prevent errors, perform "three checks" and "rights of medication" when giving medications.

VOL 2 Go to Chapter 23, **Medication Guidelines: Steps to Follow for All Medications (Regardless of Type or Route),** in Volume 2.

Three Checks

Check each medication three times:

1. *BEFORE you pour, mix, or draw up a medication,* check its label against the entry on the MAR. Be sure that the name, route, dose, and time match the MAR entry.
2. *AFTER you prepare the medication,* and before returning the container to the medication cart or discarding anything, check the label against the MAR entry again.
3. *AT THE BEDSIDE, check the medication again* before actually administering it.

Observing the "three checks" rule will help you to practice the "rights of medication."

Rights of Medication

Following the "**rights of medication**" means that you will give the (1) right medication to the (2) right patient in the (3) right dose using the (4) right route at the (5) right time with the (6) right documentation of the medication administration. This system helps you prevent medication errors.

Right Drug. Obviously, you must always administer the correct medication. That is one reason for reading each label three times (see the "three checks"). Be familiar with the drugs you administer. If you don't know, look it up. Always check the prescription, and think critically. Ask yourself if the medication prescription is suitable for the patient's condition. If not, question the prescriber.

Right Dose. The right dose is the dose prescribed for the particular patient. Be sure the dose is within the recommended range for the patient's age, weight, and condition. Perform the "three checks" of the container against the MAR. If the pharmacist has sent a dose different from the one prescribed, you may need to calculate how much of it to give. It is a good idea to have another nurse check your calculations, paying close attention to the decimal point.

Right Time. Check the prescription against the time to give the drug, and document the exact time of administration on the MAR. Never assume the patient received it as scheduled. Medications are designed to be given at specific times to maintain constant therapeutic blood levels.

Right Route. Recall that drug absorption is highly dependent on the route of administration. Perform the "three checks," and be sure that the drug is in the proper form for the route prescribed. Many medications are available in multiple forms; others are made for one specific route. The right route also includes **right site**. If an intramuscular injection is prescribed, be sure the site is appropriate considering the age of the patient (child, adult, elderly) and the medical condition.

Right Patient. Just before giving the medication, always double-check the patient's identification (ID) bracelet to ensure you have the correct patient. The Joint Commission National Patient Safety Goals recommend using two methods of patient identification (The Joint Commission, 2007); so, also ask the patient to state his name. It is best to say, "Please tell me your name," because patients with hearing impairment or confusion might respond "yes" incorrectly when asked, for example, "Are you Mary Smith?" Never skip this step, even if you are familiar with the patient. If you are busy and distracted, it is possible to enter the wrong room. Also, patients, especially when they are confused or emotionally disturbed, may move about. You may enter room 214 with a medication for Mr. Jones but discover an entirely different person in Mr. Jones's bed!

Suppose you are taking an oral tablet to a patient's room. He is in the bathroom and says, "Just leave it; I'll take it when I come out." What would you do? If you leave the tablet, how would you know whether he really took it? And what might happen if another confused patient (or even a visiting child) wandered into the room and took the tablet?

Right Documentation. Most nurses consider documentation the sixth right. After administering a medication, document it immediately on the patient's MAR, as in Figure 23-7. To see an electronic MAR, go to Chapter 16. Be sure to document the following information:

- Name of medication given
- Dose of medication given
- Route of administration and injection site for parenteral medications
- Date and time administered
- Your name or initials as administering nurse

Most MARs are preprinted with the patient's name, name of the medication, dosage, and route administered (e.g., intramuscular, oral, or intravenous). If so, you need only to write the time you actually gave the medication, initial each medication, and sign the form one time. As for all charting, write legibly in ink.

If for some reason you do not administer a prescribed medication, document that information on the MAR and write a nurse's note explaining why it was not given. Reasons may include patient refusal, NPO for surgery, tests, or procedures being performed. For example:

06/20/11 0800—Pt NPO for surgery this a.m. 0800 meds held as prescribed. —————— Janet King, RN

When giving a prn medication, in addition to recording on the MAR, you should write a nursing note documenting your assessment and the time the drug was given. Then, after allowing time for the medication to be absorbed and take effect, evaluate and document the patient's responses. For example:

06/20/11 0800—Pt reports abdominal pain at incision site rated as a #6 on a scale of 1–10. Active bowel sounds auscultated. Resp 16 breaths/minute, HR 88 beats/min, BP 130/84. Denies N/V. Morphine 10 mg given intramuscularly in right vastus lateralis (see MAR). ———————————————— Janet King, RN

06/20/11 0900—States pain relieved; "about 3" (scale of 1–10). Resp 14 breaths/min, HR 68 beats/min. BP 126/80. ———————————————— J. King, RN

You are responsible for documenting the client's responses to all medications, including therapeutic effects, side effects, and unexpected or adverse reactions.

In addition to the "rights" already discussed, patients also have the following rights about medications they receive:

Right Reason. This includes the right to not receive unnecessary medications. For example, a tranquilizer or sleeping pill should be given because the patient is

---

HOSPITAL MEDICATION ADMINISTRATION RECORD

<u>Codes For Injection Sites</u>

A - Left Anterior Thigh	H - Right Anterior Thigh
B - Left Deltoid	I - Right Deltoid
C - Left Gluteus Medius	J - Right Gluteus Medius
D - Left Lateral Thigh	K - Right Lateral Thigh
E - Left Ventral Gluteus	L - Right Ventral Gluteus
F - Left Lower Quadrant	M - Right Lower Quadrant
G - Left Upper Quadrant	N - Right Upper Quadrant

Mary Smith 086432

age 46   John Miller, M.D.

ALLERGIES: PCN, Sulfa				4.16.11	4.17.11	4.18.11
4.16.11		Lanoxin 0.25mg po Q D	0900	09 JW		
4.16.11		Rocephin 1 gm IV Q D	1200	1200 JW		
4.16.11		Zinacef 1 gm IV Q 8 hr	0800	08 JW		
			1600			
			2400			

SIGNATURE / SHIFT INDICATES	7-3	JW		
NURSE ADMINISTERING MEDICATIONS	3-11			
J Wilson, RN	11-7			

FIGURE 23-7 After administering a medication, immediately document the date, time, dose, route, and person administering the medication on the MAR.

very anxious or cannot sleep, not for the convenience of caregivers who are weary of his incessant demands.

Right to Know. This means that you tell the patient the name of the medication, why it is being given, its actions, and potential side effects.

Right to Refuse. The patient always has the right to refuse a medication regardless of her reasons and regardless of the consequences.

KnowledgeCheck 23-11

- What are the rights of medication?
- Give an example of each one.
- How many times, and when, should you check the medication against the MAR?

 Go to Chapter 23, **Knowledge Check Response Sheet and Answers,** on the Student Resource Disk or DavisPlus at http://davisplus.fadavis.com/Wilkinson2

FIGURE 23-8 When pouring a liquid medication, measure the dose while holding the calibrated cup at eye level.

Administering Oral Medications

The oral route is the one most commonly used for medications. Recall what you already know about oral medications: Where are they absorbed? What are their advantages and disadvantages? What assessments should you make? If you cannot answer these questions, review discussions of drug preparations and routes of administration, and review Table 23-1. For critical aspects of administering oral medications, see the Critical Aspects box for Procedures 23-1 through 23-18. To see procedural steps for administering various types of oral medications,

 VOL 2 Go to Chapter 23, **Procedure 23-1: Administering Oral Medications,** in Volume 2.

Pouring Liquid Medications

Liquid medications are frequently used for children and older adults. They usually come in multidose bottles, so you will need to pour individual doses into a disposable, calibrated cup, as in Figure 23-8. When pouring, hold the bottle so the liquid does not run over the label, making it difficult to read.

- Measure the dosage with the calibrated cup at eye level or draw up a liquid medication in a syringe.
- Read the dosage where the lowest part of the concave surface (meniscus) of the fluid is on the line.
- When you are finished, wipe the rim of the bottle with a clean tissue or paper towel before replacing the cap.

Buccal and Sublingual Medications

Buccal and sublingual medications, although placed in the mouth, are intended for absorption in the mucous membranes rather than in the GI tract. Some soluble forms of medications and enzyme preparations are ad-

ministered by this route and are rapidly absorbed, some within seconds. Buccal medications are held in the cheek; sublingual medications are held under the tongue.

Enteral (Nasogastric and Gastrostomy) Medications

For patients who cannot swallow or who have feeding tubes, you can give oral medications through nasogastric (NG), gastrostomy, or jejunal tubes. Observe the following precautions when administering enteral medications:

- Do not give hydrophilic medications, such as psyllium (Metamucil), through feeding tubes because they attract water and will solidify in the tube.
- Be sure to check that crushing is acceptable. Some tablets should not be crushed, because crushing changes aspects of their action. Never crush an enteric-coated or extended-release medication.
- Give medications separately, and flush with water between each. Some medications are less effective when given in combination with others.
- If the patient is receiving a continuous tube feeding, disconnect it before giving the medications; leave the tube clamped for a few minutes after administering the medication, according to agency protocol.
- If the enteral tube is connected to suction, you will usually discontinue the suction for 30 minutes after administration and keep the tube clamped to allow time for the drug to be absorbed.
- Document on the intake and output (I&O) record the amount of liquid medication and the water used for flushing.
- If the patient is on fluid restriction, use the smallest amount of water possible to dissolve tablets and flush the tube.

For other procedures related to enteral tubes,

 Go to Chapter 26, **Procedure 26–2: Inserting Nasogastric and Nasoenteric Tubes, Procedure 26-3: Administering Feedings Through Gastric and Enteric Tubes,** and **Procedure 26-4: Removing a Nasogastric or Nasoenteric Tube,** in Volume 2.

Special Situations

Some oral medications can discolor or damage tooth enamel. Mix these drugs with liquid, and have the patient drink it through a straw and drink water afterward. The following methods help to disguise the taste for medication with objectionable taste:

- Unless contraindicated, encourage the patient drink a liberal amount of flavored liquid (e.g., juice) or water to dilute the medication.
- Have the patient suck on ice chips for several minutes before taking the medication. Ice numbs the taste buds.
- Store the medication in the refrigerator, unless contraindicated. Especially if it is an oily liquid, the smell and taste is less objectionable when chilled.
- Use a syringe to place the medication on the back of the patient's tongue. There are fewer taste buds there.
- Some medications can be constituted with flavored additive to make the elixir more appealing, particularly for children.
- Regardless of method, offer oral hygiene immediately after giving the medication.
- Some patients have difficulty swallowing medications; they gag, or the pills become "stuck" in their throat. It may help to crush soluble tablets and place them in liquids or in a small amount of applesauce or pudding. Remember that some forms (e.g., time-released tablets) should *not* be crushed, so check your drug reference sources to be certain.
- Do not give oral medications to patients who:

    Cannot swallow fluids. The risk for aspiration is too great.
    Have nausea or vomiting; the medication would be lost in the emesis.
    Are NPO.
    Are not coherent or are comatose.

- In those situations obtain a medical prescription for an alternative route or, if the patient is NPO, permission to give the medication with small sips of water. To learn more about which medication to take with or without food.

 Go to **ESG Box 23-1, Oral Medications Taken with or Without Food,** on the Student Resource Disk or DavisPlus at http://davisplus.fadavis.com/Wilkinson2

KnowledgeCheck 23-12

- Describe two ways to ensure an accurate dosage when pouring liquid medications.

- What instructions should you give to a patient who is taking a sublingual medication?
- Explain the special steps required when administering enteral medications to a patient who is receiving continuous tube feedings.
- Describe three methods for disguising the taste of objectionable tasting drugs.
- For which patients are oral medications contraindicated?

 Go to Chapter 23, **Knowledge Check Response Sheet and Answers,** on the Student Resource Disk or DavisPlus at http://davisplus.fadavis.com/Wilkinson2

Medicating Children

Giving medication to young children might be difficult because they are not motivated by logic. They do not grasp the cause and effect of "Take this; it will make you feel better." If they do not like the taste, they simply will not swallow it. Another challenge is that before the age of 5 years, children may not be able to swallow tablets and capsules. For these reasons, most oral medications for children are prepared as sweetened and flavored liquids. Chewable tablets are also popular. For very young children and infants, you must take care to prevent choking and aspiration. Parents can often suggest the best methods for getting their child to take medicines. For other parents, you may need to teach techniques for administering medications at home (Self-Care: Teaching Parents About Medicating Children).

Medicating Older Adults

As you already know, because of physiological changes (e.g., diminished liver or renal function) associated with aging, older adults usually require smaller dosages of drugs. In addition, physical responses to some medications are unpredictable. You need to observe carefully for both therapeutic and undesired effects. Other issues include:

Difficulty Swallowing Medications. It may help to crush tablets or give drugs in liquid form. Gently massaging the area just below the chin may help to initiate swallowing. Consult an occupational or speech therapist for other strategies.

Reduced Thirst. As the desire to drink liquids decreases with age, the mouth often becomes drier. Some older adults find it difficult to take large pills or tablets.

Slow Reflexes and Reasoning Ability. You may need to allow more time to explain and administer medications to older adults. Keep the instructions simple.

Forgetting to Take the Medications. Impaired memory is more common with age, so clients need simple plans that they can follow at home. A written schedule or a med calendar might help, especially if you plan the drugs to be taken other than at mealtimes and bedtime. Many people take their medication, only to forget shortly thereafter that they did so. Advise the patient to

Self-Care

Teaching Parents About Medicating Children

1. Mark each bottle or syringe with medication using a different color of tape or adhesive label. That way each is clearly distinguishable, even though many medication bottles look alike.

2. You can reuse syringes for oral medications until the markings or tape begins to wear off or the plunger becomes difficult to move. Wash syringes with warm, soapy water, rinse well, and allow to air dry.

3. Take your time when giving medication, and find a quiet environment. Don't rush the process. It can be frustrating to struggle with a young child who is resisting taking a medication, especially if your time is limited.

4. Give the medication at the same time each day so it becomes a matter of routine. It is easier to remember when a pattern is established.

5. If the child is old enough to understand, warn him when a medication has an unpleasant taste (e.g., "John, this doesn't taste very good, but you can have a big drink of juice as soon as you swallow it."). You may lose his trust if you surprise him with a bad taste.

6. Give the child a frozen fruit bar or frozen flavored ice pop just before the medication. This helps to numb the taste buds to weaken the taste of the medication.

7. To mask bad-tasting medicines, you can crush tablets or empty the contents of a capsule and mix with soft foods, such as applesauce, hot cereal, or pudding. This is helpful for children who might aspirate liquids, as well. (*Caution:* Check with the prescriber before crushing a tablet or emptying a capsule. Some medications should not be crushed.)

8. Do not use essential foods in the child's diet (e.g., milk or orange juice) to mask the taste of medications. The child may later refuse a food he associates with the medicine.

9. Take care to prevent choking or aspiration. When giving liquids to infants and toddlers, hold the child in a sitting or semi-sitting position. Use a medicine dropper or syringe to place the medication between the gum and cheek. Apply gentle pressure; avoid giving too much medication too fast.

10. Always praise the child after she swallows the medication.

---

use a divided pill container or a small glass filled with the medications for each dosage time during the day. If the A.M. container is empty, the person will know he has taken the morning drugs.

Impaired Visual Acuity. For patients who cannot see well, write out the home medication schedule in large letters, or ask family members to help. Display the schedule or med calendar in a convenient and highly visible location.

Difficulty Opening Containers and Administering Medications. Because of pain or stiffness in the hands and fingers, and also because of decreased visual acuity, older adults often find it difficult to open containers or to administer their own insulin injections, inhalers, eye medications, and so on. Help them find solutions or assistance from family and friends. Avoid childproof, safety lids on containers. Older adults are allowed to sign a release with their pharmacy to have the childproof covers removed for easier handling.

Families with young children visiting the homes of older adults need to be alert to the risk of accidental ingestion of medication.

Lack of Understanding of the Purpose of Medication. Some older adults accept unquestioningly everything a physician says, but they may not understand what each drug is for. For example, suppose a patient's tranquilizer is not effective. The physician prescribes a new one, but the patient does not understand that he should stop taking the old one; so for a period of time, he takes both

medications. This type of situation can happen, too, when patients are being treated by more than one provider (e.g., a podiatrist and an internist may both prescribe a medication to treat toenail fungus).

Not Seeing the Need for the Medication. Some patients may think, "I don't feel any better when I take all this stuff," so they simply do not take it. In the hospital, they may refuse to take medications, or they may put the tablets in their mouths but spit them out when you leave the room. You should stay with the patient until you see that he has swallowed the medications.

To reduce medication-related problems for older adults, nurses need to alert the prescriber to impaired visual acuity, memory, dexterity to open medication containers, mobility, and swallowing.

Some action steps you can take as a nurse are listed in Box 23-4.

KnowledgeCheck 23-13

- What is the chief danger when administering oral medications to children?
- How can you help a person who has some difficulty swallowing oral medications?
- Keeping in mind that patients do have the right to refuse medications, how can you be sure that they are actually taking them and not spitting them out after you leave the room?

Go to Chapter 23, **Knowledge Check Response Sheet and Answers,** on the Student Resource Disk or DavisPlus at http://davisplus.fadavis.com/Wilkinson2

BOX 23-4 ■ Reducing Risk for Medication Errors for Older Adults

■ Be alert to unnecessary drug therapy. It is not unusual for prescribers to be reluctant to stop a medication or simply forget to do so. The likelihood of a poor outcome increases as the number of drugs prescribed increases.

■ Request the indication for use on all medication prescriptions.

■ Suggest primary care provider trials of nonpharmacologic interventions (such as warm massage and guided imagery) before prescribing medication for new symptoms.

■ Consider the "snowball effect" when symptoms occur as a side effect of prescribed medication, and the care provider then prescribes another drug to deal with the side effect. This results in yet another side effect, another drug, and so on. To interrupt this phenomenon, the prescriber can either discontinue the medication, reduce the dose, or substitute with one the patient tolerates better.

■ Verify that the newly prescribed medication does not have documented drug–drug interaction. Check that the prescribed dosage is correct within the desired range.

■ When titrating drug doses, start low and go slow. It's best to start with the lowest possible dose when starting a medication because adverse drug effects are dose-related and older adults tend to be more sensitive.

■ Assess urinary status. Many drugs are cleared through the renal system. Some have toxic effects on the kidneys, particularly for older adults.

■ Recommend safer drugs if the prescriber initiates medication associated with adverse outcomes for older adults. The benefit must exceed the risk to the patient (Zwicker and Fulmer, 2008).

Administering Topical Medications

Topical medications are applied directly to a body site or placed in body cavities by irrigation or instillation. They are usually used for their local effects (e.g., zinc oxide ointment to protect the skin against chafing and chapping associated with bowel and bladder incontinence), but some are absorbed through the skin and mucous membranes for their systemic effects (e.g., estrogen patches), depending on the drug preparation. Most must be applied to the skin two to three times per day for maximum effect.

Skin Applications: Lotions, Creams, and Ointments

To enhance absorption, cleanse the skin with soap and water and pat dry before applying lotions, creams, and ointments. If you warm the medication in your gloved hands, it will be more comfortable for the patient and make the preparation easier to apply. Use a cotton swab, tongue blade, or gloved finger to apply corticosteroid

creams and other topical medications so that your skin does not absorb them. The Critical Aspects box summarizes key points for applying skin medications, including powders and aerosols. For the step-by-step procedure,

 Go to Chapter 23, **Procedure 23-7A: Applying Medications, Lotions, Creams, and Ointment to the Skin,** in Volume 2.

Transdermal Medications

Designed to be absorbed through the skin, transdermal medications are prepared as patches made of a special membrane. Patches allow constant, controlled amounts of medications to be released over 24 hours or more, giving a prolonged systemic effect. Examples of drugs administered by patch are: nitroglycerin (used to control angina or chest pain), scopolamine (used to treat motion sickness), nicotine (used to control smoking urges), and fentanyl (used to treat chronic pain). Most patches are prepared with the correct dose already applied and should not be cut. Other gel patches can be cut and are self-adherent, for example, lidocaine and diclofenac. Be sure to check the package insert or ask a pharmacist about proper handling, application, and disposal of patches.

Wear gloves when applying transdermal patches (Fig. 23-9). Avoid placing the patch on areas where there are skin lesions. When removing and discarding patches, be aware that they may still contain medication. Wear gloves, fold the medicated side to the inside, and dispose of the patches where they are not accessible to children or pets. For guidelines,

 Go to Chapter 23, **Procedure 23-7D: Applying Transdermal Medications to the Skin,** in Volume 2.

Performing Irrigations and Instillations

Washing out a body cavity with a steady stream of fluid or water is called **irrigation.** Sterile water, saline, or antiseptic solutions are flushed into the eyes, ears, throat,

FIGURE 23-9 Patches allow constant, controlled amounts of medications to be released over a 24- to 72-hour period, giving a prolonged systemic effect. Wear gloves when removing and applying them.

vagina, rectum, or urinary tract to wash out the cavity. **Instillation** is the insertion of medication into a body cavity (e.g., eye drops) so the medication can be retained or absorbed through that body cavity. Some medications need to remain in the body cavity for a period of time for maximum absorption and effect.

Irrigations and instillations are performed to remove discharge or foreign bodies (e.g., from the eye or ear); to apply heat and cold to an area; to apply medications, such as antiseptics; and to prepare an area for surgery (e.g., an enema for cleansing the bowels). You will usually not use sterile technique unless there are breaks in the skin. Several types of syringes are used for irrigating and instilling medications and fluids. Each is calibrated to allow you to control the amount and speed of solution delivered into the cavity (Fig. 23-10).

Ophthalmic Medications

Ophthalmic ointments or solutions are used for their local effects, for example, to treat eye irritations, infections, and glaucoma or to lubricate the eye. During an eye examination, eye medications may also be used to anesthetize the eye, dilate the pupil, or temporarily stain the cornea to identify abraded areas. Eye irrigation may be performed to remove foreign bodies, secretions, or harmful chemicals.

Ophthalmic medications are packaged in small bottles or tubes that state, *"For ophthalmic use only."* Do not place any medication in the eye unless this statement appears on the container. The **cornea** (the transparent part of the sclera in front of the iris and pupil) is easily injured, so you should not place medications directly onto the eyeball. Take care to not touch the tip of the dropper or tube to the eye or conjunctiva; doing so may lead to bacterial growth on the container or damage the eye.

FIGURE 23-10 Syringes for administering enteral medications and performing irrigations and instillations. *A,* Asepto syringe: Plastic syringe with rubber bulb. *B,* Toomey (piston) syringe: Calibrated plastic syringe with removable tip that fits into the end of a tube (e.g., urinary catheter or enteral tube). For deep wound irrigation bladder irrigations, and administration of enteral medications. *C,* Rubber bulb syringe, for ear irrigations.

See Chapters 19 and 29 for information about the structure and function of the eyes. The Critical Aspects box summarizes key points in performing ophthalmic instillations. For the step-by-step procedure,

 Go to Chapter 23, **Procedure 23-2: Administering Ophthalmic Medications,** in Volume 2.

Otic Medications

Medications or solutions may be dropped into the ear to treat internal and external ear infections, to apply heat to the area, and to soften and remove earwax. Use solutions at room temperature because a solution that is too hot or too cold may cause vertigo, nausea, and pain. If the solution has been refrigerated, warm the solution by rubbing the bottle between your hands for a minute or two before use, especially for medication dispensed in a glass container. You will use clean technique when administering otic medications. However, if the tympanic membrane (eardrum) has been ruptured or if a surgical procedure has been done, you will use sterile technique to help prevent infection.

See Chapters 19 and 29 for information about the structure and function of the ear. The Critical Aspects box provides guidelines for performing otic instillations. For the complete procedure,

 Go to Chapter 23, **Procedure 23-3: Administering Otic Medications,** in Volume 2.

Nasal Medications

Clients usually self-administer nasal drops and sprays. The most common nasal medications are used to shrink swollen mucous membranes and to loosen secretions and provide drainage for treatment of nasal cavity or sinus infections. Because many nasal medications are available without prescription, caution the patient regarding overuse. Long-term use of decongestants may cause a **rebound effect;** that is, they will be effective immediately after administration, but the nasal congestion often recurs and even increases when the effects of the drug wear off. Frequent use of or swallowing excess decongestant can also cause systemic side effects, such as increased heart rate and increased blood pressure. These effects can be serious in children; saline drops are safer for them.

See Chapters 19 and 29 for information about the structure and function of the nose. The Critical Aspects box provides guidelines for performing nasal instillations. For the complete procedure,

 Go to Chapter 23, **Procedure 23-4: Administering Nasal Medications,** in Volume 2.

Vaginal Medications

Vaginal medications come in various forms: foams, jellies, liquids (douches), creams, tablets, and suppositories. They may be used for contraception; to destroy bacteria in the vagina before gynecological surgery; to reduce vaginal dryness related to menopause; to treat vaginal itching or infection; or to induce labor. Store suppositories in the refrigerator to keep them firm enough to insert. Insert them with a lubricated, gloved finger. After insertion, the body temperature causes the suppository to melt. Foams and jellies are inserted using an applicator or inserter. For optimal effect, have the patient remain supine for at least 20 minutes after insertion. Apply a clean perineal pad if there is heavy drainage or if the woman is ambulatory (the medication may melt and drain from the vagina by gravity).

A **douche** is a vaginal irrigation using low pressure. Vaginal irrigations are used to administer antimicrobial solutions to prevent infection (e.g., before surgery), to remove irritating discharge, and to apply heat or cold (e.g., to reduce inflammation). In the acute care setting, you will usually use sterile supplies. However, this is not usually necessary when the irrigation is self-administered at home because people usually have some resistance to the microorganisms in their daily environment.

✚ Teach women that douching is not necessary for ordinary female hygiene and that it may even be harmful because it disturbs the normal pH and healthy balance of microorganisms in the vagina.

The Critical Aspects box provides guidelines for administering vaginal medications. For the complete procedure,

 Go to Chapter 23, **Procedure 23-5: Administering Vaginal Medications,** in Volume 2.

Rectal Medications

Rectal suppositories and liquid instillations **(enemas)** are used to encourage bowel movements or to treat systemic complaints. For example, antiemetic suppositories are often used to treat nausea. Absorption is slow and erratic because of rectal contents, local drug irritation, and uncertainty of drug retention in the rectum. Other disadvantages include embarrassment to the patient and possible rectal pain if the patient has hemorrhoids. However, the rectal route may provide for higher blood levels of the medication than does the oral route because the venous blood from the rectum does not pass through the liver before entering the general circulation (review the discussion of the first-pass effect, as needed). Also, rectal administration may be preferred when a drug has an unacceptable taste or odor or when it is not safe to use the oral route, as with a patient who is vomiting or unconscious. As a rule, rectal medications are contraindicated when there is active rectal bleeding.

The Critical Aspects box provides guidelines for administering rectal medication. For the complete procedure,

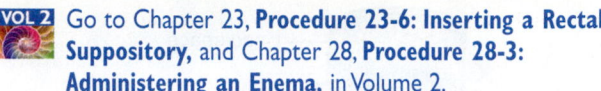 Go to Chapter 23, **Procedure 23-6: Inserting a Rectal Suppository,** and Chapter 28, **Procedure 28-3: Administering an Enema,** in Volume 2.

Administering Respiratory Inhalations

Nebulization is the production of a fine spray, fog, powder, or mist from a liquid drug. The patient inhales the medication mixture by breathing deeply through a mouthpiece attached to the nebulizer. The airways and alveoli are highly vascularized, and therefore, absorb inhaled medications rapidly.

Types of Nebulizers

The following are four types of devices for achieving nebulization:

- *Atomizers* disperse the medication in the form of large droplets.
- *Aerosol sprayers* suspend the droplets of medication in a gas (e.g., oxygen).
- *An ultrasonic (handheld) nebulizer* mixes a small volume of medication, usually less than 1 mL, with 3 mL of normal saline. The device forces air through the nebulizer and delivers medication and humidity as a fine mist. Because the particles are so small, the mist can be inhaled deep into the lungs.
- *A metered-dose inhaler (MDI)* (Fig. 23-11) is a type of nebulizer that delivers measured doses of a nebulized drug.

No matter which device is used, the smaller the droplets, the farther the medication can be inhaled into the respiratory tract.

Metered-Dose Inhalers

A Metered-Dose Inhaler (MDI) is a pressurized container prefilled with several doses of a drug and an eco-friendly substance, called hydrofluoroalkane, or HFA, for propelling the medication forward. The patient inhales while pushing the canister's pump to release a measured dose of medication through a mouthpiece (Fig. 23-11a). Sometimes an extender (spacer) is attached to the mouthpiece to enhance the delivery of medication into the respiratory tract (Fig. 23-11b). Medication is pumped into the extender instead of directly into the patient's mouth. The patient inhales the drug from the chamber.

A Dry Powder Inhaler (DPI) is similar to a MDI. The medication is activated by a pump rather than by inhalation. Each powdered dose is in a blister pack that is activated according to the manufacturer's instructions. Once the dose is loaded, the patient simply takes a deep breath. DPIs are not designed to be used with a spacer.

Patients frequently self-administer inhalations (most often bronchodilators or steroids) using an MDI. You may need to teach your patients how to use the device correctly (Fig. 23-12). Also,

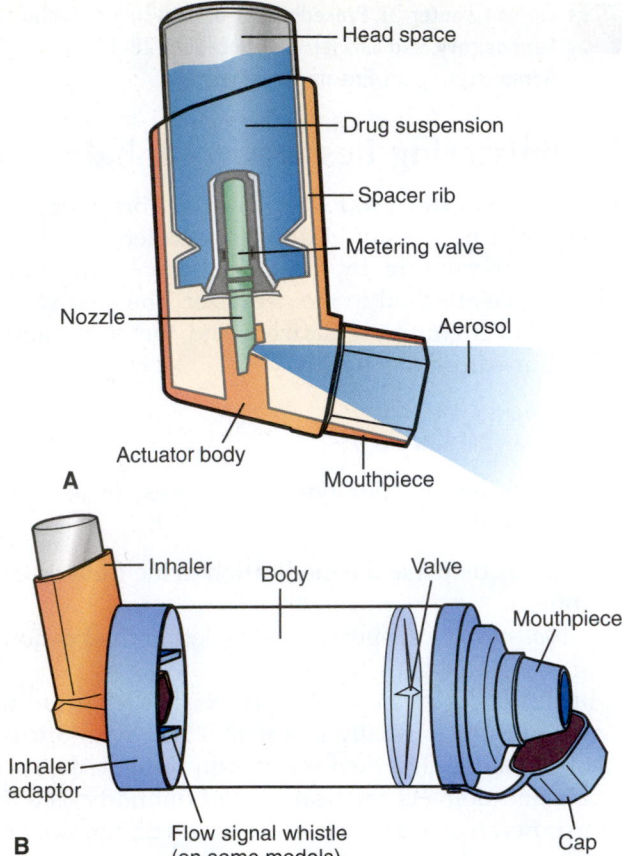

A

- Head space
- Drug suspension
- Spacer rib
- Metering valve
- Nozzle
- Aerosol
- Actuator body
- Mouthpiece

B

- Inhaler
- Body
- Valve
- Mouthpiece
- Inhaler adaptor
- Flow signal whistle (on some models)
- Cap

FIGURE 23-11 Inhalers. *A*, Metered-dose inhaler. *B*, Inhaler with a spacer.

FIGURE 23-12 Child using a metered dose inhaler with an extender.

Go to Chapter 23, **Procedure 23-8: Administering Metered-Dose Inhaler Medication**, in Volume 2.

The advantage of MDIs is that high doses of medication can be rapidly instilled in the lungs, producing local effects directly in the airway while avoiding systemic side effects. Disadvantages are the need for manual dexterity, which is often compromised in older adults and young children; skill in coordinating the inhalation of the medication and the pushing of the canister to administer the dose; and the ability to inhale and exhale deeply enough

to allow penetration of the medication in the more distal bronchioles. Keeping track of how many puffs have been used is problematic for some users, which can lead to a canister being unexpectedly empty when needed.

KnowledgeCheck 23-14

- Why should you use a cotton swab, tongue blade, or gloved finger to apply corticosteroid creams and other topical medications?
- Most of the following routes are used for both local and systemic effects. Which one is used only for medications intended for systemic absorption (that is, which one is not used for local effects): lotions, creams, ointments, transdermal patches, or irrigations?
- When administering eye drops, how can you prevent injury to the cornea?
- When should you use sterile technique when performing otic instillations?
- What are two of the undesired effects of self-administered nasal decongestants?
- What possible harm can result from vaginal douching?
- When is rectal instillation of a drug preferred over oral administration?
- When, as a rule, are rectal medications contraindicated?
- Define *nebulization*.
- What is the best way to determine if a metered-dose inhaler is empty?

Go to Chapter 23, **Knowledge Check Response Sheet and Answers,** on the Student Resource Disk or DavisPlus at http://davisplus.fadavis.com/Wilkinson2

Administering Parenteral Medications

Parenteral medications include those that are injected via the intradermal, subcutaneous, intramuscular, or intravenous routes. Parenteral injections are absorbed faster and more completely than drugs given by other routes; the results are more predictable; and the dosage can be measured more accurately. In addition, they can be used for patients who cannot take oral medications. However, injectable medications have some disadvantages:

- They penetrate the skin barrier, increasing the risk for infection if aseptic technique is not used.
- Tissue damage may result if the pH, osmotic pressure, or solubility of the medication is not appropriate to the tissue where the medication is given. For example, medications intended for injection into muscle may damage subcutaneous tissue.
- Preparation and administration must be performed accurately, because the onset of action is relatively rapid and the medications, once given, cannot be retrieved.

Preparing Injectable Medications

Injectable medications are those that are injected or infused into body tissues or into the bloodstream. When administering them, you must know about various kinds of needles and syringes. You will need to decide, based on each situation, what size and type of needle and syringe to use. For a summary of the sites and equipment used for parenteral administration,

 Go to Chapter 23, **Tables, Boxes, Figures: ESG Table 23-6, Parenteral Injections: Comparison of Sites and Equipment,** on the Student Resource Disk or DavisPlus at http://davisplus.fadavis.com/Wilkinson2

Needles

Needles are disposable, stainless steel sheaths that attach to a syringe. Figure 23-13 shows the parts of a needle. Needles are made in various lengths and gauges and with different bevel sizes.

Gauge refers to the inside diameter of the needle lumen. Needle gauges are numbered 14 through 30. The smaller the gauge, the larger the diameter (i.e., a 16-gauge needle has a larger diameter than a 20-gauge needle). Choose the gauge based on the patient's size and skin condition, the viscosity of medication used, and the speed of administration desired. Smaller needles (25- to 30-gauge) cause less pain and trauma to the tissue, so they are useful for patients who must have frequent or long-term injections (e.g., for insulin and heparin). Larger needles (14- to 18-gauge) are used for blood and more viscous medications, to mix intravenous (IV) medications, or for rapid infusion of IV medications.

Bevel is the slanted tip with a narrow slit. The slant of the tip creates an opening that will close quickly to prevent leakage of medication, blood, and serum. A long bevel tip is sharper and narrower and therefore causes less discomfort during injection. Long bevels are usually used for subcutaneous and intramuscular injections. Short bevels are used for intradermal or IV injections.

Needle length is the distance from the tip to the hub (bottom) of the needle. Common needle lengths range from ⅜ to 3 inches. Use a longer needle for intramuscular injections, and a shorter one for intradermal injections. Vary the length according to the thickness of the patient's muscle and adipose tissue. Although a 1½ inch needle is common for intramuscular injections, you would use a shorter one for a child or a very thin person.

Filter needles and **filter straws** are used to trap rubber or glass fragments when drawing up a medication from a vial or an ampule. You must replace the filter needle with a regular needle before injecting the medication into the patient or into the IV solution.

See also the Home Care box, Reusing Needles and Syringes.

Critical Thinking 23-11

- You are to give repeated intramuscular injections to a patient who is frail and has very little muscle mass (5 ft, 5 in. tall and weighing 96 lb). You are to give 1 mL of a thin, watery medication. You have these needle sizes available: 16-gauge, 20-gauge, 25-gauge. Which would you use, and why?
- For the same patient, you have needles available in 1 inch and 1½ inch lengths. Which would you use, and why?

Syringes

A syringe consists of a barrel, plunger, and syringe tip (Fig. 23-13). Because injections require strict sterile technique, you may touch the outside of the barrel and end of the plunger but not the inside of the barrel, hub, shaft of the plunger, or needle.

Syringes are usually made of plastic and are disposable. Some have the needle attached; others do not. The syringe tip, either **luer-lock** (twist on) or **non-luer-lock** (slip on), fits into the needle hub (Fig. 23-14). Syringes are made in various sizes, from 0.5 mL to 60 mL. The larger sizes are used for adding medications to IV solutions and for irrigating wounds. You will usually use a 2-mL or 3-mL syringe for intramuscular injections. Syringes larger than 5 mL are used for IV administration, instillations, and irrigations. Three syringes are shown in Figure 23-15. For interactive exercises to familiarize yourself with syringe markings,

 Go to **Animations: Syringe Exercises** in Student Resources on DavisPlus at http://davisplus.fadavis.com/Wilkinson2

Home Care

Reusing Needles and Syringes

Many people (e.g., those who have diabetes) must give themselves repeated injections, perhaps several each day. Supplies for home use are costly. Insurance may or may not cover the cost, or the person may not have insurance. Therefore, although manufacturers and health professionals recommend disposable syringes and needles be used only once, some people find it practical to reuse needles and syringes. Do not encourage this practice, but when clients feel they must reuse needles, teach them about potential risks and precautions to take.

VOL 2 Go to Chapter 23, **Clinical Insight 23-1: Reusing Needles and Syringes: Home Care,** in Volume 2.

FIGURE 23-13 Parts of a needle and syringe.

FIGURE 23-14 Syringe tips. *A*, Luer-lock (twist-on) tip. *B*, Non-luer-lock (slip-on) tip.

FIGURE 23-15 Syringe types. *A*, 100-unit insulin syringe marked in units. *B*, 1-mL tuberculin syringe marked in increments of 0.01 mL. *C*, 3-mL standard syringe marked in increments of 0.1 mL.

- **Standard syringes** are supplied in 3-, 5-, and 10-mL sizes. They are commonly supplied without needles or with 18-, 21-, 23-, or 25-gauge needles that are 0.5 to 3 inches long. They are calibrated and marked in 0.1-mL and 1- or 2-mL increments so that drugs can be measured accurately.
- **Tuberculin syringes** have a 1-mL capacity and are calibrated in 0.01-mL increments; they come with a small (usually 25- to 28-) gauge, short (½ to ⅝ in.) needle. Use tuberculin syringes to administer small, precise doses of medication (e.g., when medicating infants or children, for allergy tests, or when administering potentially dangerous medications, such as heparin).
- **Insulin syringes** are calibrated in units and are used to administer insulin. Insulin syringes are calibrated in 100 units per milliliter. They are made in 0.3-, 0.5-, or 1-mL sizes with very small-gauge needles (26- to 30-gauge).
- **Prefilled unit-dose systems** are reusable syringe holders that hold disposable, single-dose, prefilled medication cartridges. No medication preparation is necessary, but you must check each cartridge and dose carefully because all of the cartridges look alike. You simply insert the cartridge into the holder and lock it in place. After administering the medication, dispose of the cartridge; keep the holder for reuse.

FIGURE 23-16 (Left) Prefilled unit-dose system. (Right) Disposable, prefilled, self-contained system.

- **Disposable prefilled, self-contained systems** are available for hospitals, office practices, nursing homes, and self-administration. The injection plunger is attached to the medication barrel and twists in directly. This ready-to-use syringe reduces the risk of constituting or dosing errors. Because you do not need to remove the cartridge from the holder after using it, the risk of a needlestick injury is reduced (Fig. 23-16).

There are many new safety needle devices available today. Some common types include resheathing systems with sliding barrels that shield the needle. Syringes with retractable needles that spring back into the barrel of the syringe are protective against needlestick injury. Needles with attached covers reduce the risk of accidental puncture with contaminated needles. Wing-tipped needles are also available for clinical use.

 VOL 2 Go to Chapter 23, **Clinical Insight 23-2: Using Prefilled Unit-Dose Systems,** in Volume 2.

KnowledgeCheck 23-15
- What does the term *parenteral* mean?
- What are two disadvantages of the parenteral route?
- To maintain sterile technique, which part of a syringe must you *not* touch?
- You need to irrigate a wound. Which syringe size would you probably need: 0.5-mL, 3-mL, 5-mL, or 50-mL?
- Which syringe would you use for an intramuscular injection, as a rule: tuberculin, 50-mL, 5-mL, or 3-mL syringe?

 Go to Chapter 23, **Knowledge Check Response Sheet and Answers,** on the Student Resource Disk or DavisPlus at http://davisplus.fadavis.com/Wilkinson2

Drawing Up Medications from an Ampule

An **ampule** is a thin-walled, disposable glass container with a narrow neck that you must snap off to access the medication (Fig. 23-17). To prevent injuries, use an ampule opener to snap the glass. Each ampule holds a single dose of a liquid medication, usually 1 mL to 10 mL, but some hold 50 mL. Because glass fragments may be introduced into the medication, most agencies require you to use a filter needle or filter straw to draw up the medication. See the Critical Aspects box. Also,

 VOL 2 Go to Chapter 23, **Procedure 23-9A: Preparing and Drawing Up Medications from Ampules,** in Volume 2.

FIGURE 23-17 Safety device for opening glass ampules. (Courtesy of Medi-Dose®, Inc. EPS®, Inc., Ivyland, PA.)

Drawing Up Medications from a Vial

A **vial** is a single-dose or multidose plastic or glass container with a rubber stopper that reseals the top after each needle introduction. A plastic or metal cap covers the rubber stopper to protect it until it is used (Fig. 23-18). Because the vial is a closed system, you must inject air into it to withdraw the solution. Otherwise, a vacuum is created in the vial that makes withdrawal difficult. See the Critical Aspects box. Also,

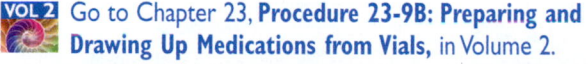

VOL 2 Go to Chapter 23, **Procedure 23-9B: Preparing and Drawing Up Medications from Vials,** in Volume 2.

Nurses traditionally wipe the rubber stopper with alcohol after removing the cap, even on a single-dose vial; however, there is conflicting scientific justification for this practice as an infection control measure. The practice does remove dust and rubber particles from the top of the vial; however, using a filter needle or straw achieves that purpose as well. You will need to follow the policy of the institution in which you work.

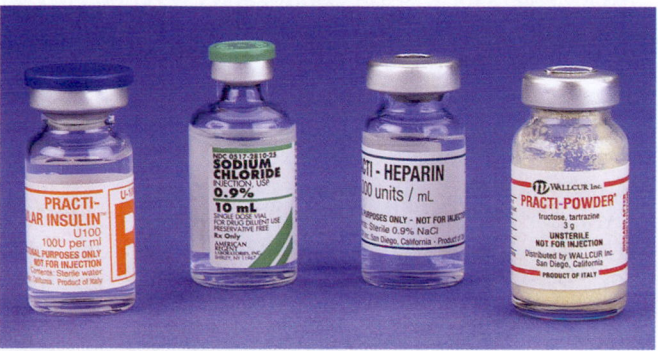

FIGURE 23-18 Vials containing medications.

Reconstituting Medications

Medications that are not stable in solution are dispensed as powders in vials. You must add a diluent or solvent to the powder to create a solution for injection. The diluent is usually sterile water or saline; however, each packaged vial includes the manufacturer's instructions for the amount and kind of solvent to add. For safety, use a plastic vial access cannula instead of a needle when possible. For guidelines,

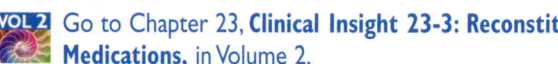

VOL 2 Go to Chapter 23, **Clinical Insight 23-3: Reconstituting Medications,** in Volume 2.

Mixing Medications in the Same Syringe

You can mix two medications in the same syringe (1) if they are compatible, (2) if the total dose is within accepted limits, and, obviously, (3) if they are both to be given by the same route. This technique allows for efficient use of supplies and allows the patient to receive fewer injections.

Medications are *compatible* if they can be mixed without affecting their constituents or actions. Package inserts and medication references usually include compatibility information.

✚ Always check the compatibility before mixing medications together. If the contents of the syringe become discolored, there are visible particles in the solution, or there is a change in consistency, do not administer the medications.

When mixing medications in one syringe, you must follow these principles:

1. Maintain sterile technique.
2. Do not contaminate one container with medication from the other container. You must use a separate needle to withdraw from each vial (exceptions: when both are single-dose vials, and in the case of different types of insulin).
3. Verify that the dosage of *each* medication is accurate before administering.
4. Draw the second drug up slowly and carefully. If you draw up too much of the second drug, you must discard the syringe and medication and begin again.
5. Ensure the total, final dosage is correct. Add the volumes of the 2 meds you drew up and ensure that the total is actually the amount you have in the syringe.

At each measurement step, either to expel or account for air in the syringe.

✚ Never reuse a needle or syringe for drawing up a later dose of medication. A single-use vial contains only one dose of medication. Even if you do not administer the entire dose, the vial should be used only once for one patient, using a sterile needle and sterile syringe.

See the Critical Aspects box for guidelines. For the complete steps,

 Go to Chapter 23, **Procedure 23-9C: Mixing Medications in One Syringe Using Two Vials,** in Volume 2.

Accounting for Needle "Dead Space"

Some nurses believe a small amount of the patient's medication remains in the needle when an injection is given. Therefore, in the past, some recommended adding 0.2 mL of air to the syringe after measuring a medication for IM injection. Nurses are not in agreement about the need for adding air and, unfortunately, there is scant research to settle the question. Theoretically, on injection the air clears the needle of medication, ensuring that the patient receives the entire dose. However, because syringes are calibrated to account for medication left in the needle, and because the medication left in the needle after injection is the same amount as before the injection, many believe that air should not be added. We recommend that you add air only in the following situations:

1. *When the medication is irritating to subcutaneous tissues,* add 0.2 mL of air after measuring the proper dose. The air drives the medication deep into the subcutaneous tissue; the air injected into the tissue creates an air lock above the medication, preventing it from tracking through subcutaneous tissue.
2. *When you change needles after drawing up the medication.* For example, when you draw up a dose using a filter needle, then replace it with a new needle, the new needle has air in it instead of medication. If you push the plunger until you see a drop of medication at the tip of the needle, you will see that you no longer have a complete dose in the syringe. Pulling in 0.2 mL air before changing the needle and then pushing the plunger until you see a drop of medication at the tip of the new needle will prevent the loss of medication with the needle change.

 Go to Chapter 23, **Clinical Insight 23-4: Measuring Dosage When Changing Needles,** in Volume 2.

Preventing Needlestick Injuries

Workplace injuries occur from needles and other "sharps," putting healthcare workers at risk for blood-borne diseases, such as hepatitis B, hepatitis C, and HIV (see Chapter 21). For this reason, special safety devices have been designed to reduce the risk of needlestick injuries through blunting, shielding, retracting needles, and needles with attached covers as in Figure 23-19a, b, and c. Figure 23-20 is a photo of a safety syringe with a guard that pulls forward to cover the needle immediately after it is withdrawn from the skin to reduce the risk of accidental punctures with contaminated needles. You then dispose of both needle and sheath in a "sharps" container. Needles with attached covers reduce the risk of accidental punctures with contaminated needles.

FIGURE 23-19 Needle safety features. *A,* Self-sheathing safety feature: Sliding needle shields attached to disposable syringes and vacuum tube holders. *B,* Syringe with retractable needle. *C,* Needles with covers.

FIGURE 23-20 Special safety syringe. *A,* Needle guard position before injection. *B,* Needle guard position after injection.

Wing-tipped needles are also available in many clinical settings.

The Centers for Disease Control and Prevention (CDC) and the Occupational Safety and Health Administration (OSHA) recommend the use of "needleless" systems. Most systems involve adapters that can be used with regular intravenous tubing and medication vials, permitting access through a valve system without a needle. Figure 23-21 shows three such devices.

Another needle-free system is the jet injection most often used for immunizations. The jet injectors drive liquid medication into the intradermal, subcutaneous, or intramuscular tissues by creating a narrow stream under high pressure that penetrates the skin. However,

FIGURE 23-21 Needleless systems. *A*, Lever-lock cannula. *B*, Threaded lock cannula. *C*, Blunt-tipped syringe for drawing up medication.

local reactions or injury, such as redness, bruising, and pain, occur more often with jet injectors than by use of a needle.

✚ Always dispose of needles, glass, and other "sharps" in clearly marked, usually red, puncture-proof containers (Fig. 23-22). Never force a needle into an already full container; you may be injured by sharps protruding from the top. Never put a needle or other sharp in a wastebasket, in your pocket, or at the patient's bedside.

For tips to prevent needlestick injury,

 Go to Chapter 21, **Clinical Insight 21-2: Preventing Needlestick Injuries,** in Volume 2.

Recapping Contaminated Needles

You should never recap a contaminated needle (e.g., after giving an injection); place it uncapped, needle pointing downward, directly into a sharps disposal container. However, you may occasionally find that you must recap a contaminated needle. The 1991 Bloodborne Pathogens Standard (last updated November, 2008) requires bending, recapping, or needle removal using a mechanical device or a one-handed technique. For step-by-step instructions,

VOL 2 Go to Chapter 23, **Procedure 23-10: Recapping Needles Using a One-Handed Technique,** in Volume 2.

FIGURE 23-22 Disposal system for sharp objects, such as needles and glass. The container must be clearly marked, usually red, and puncture-proof.

Recapping Sterile Needles

OSHA and the National Institute of Occupational Safety and Health (NIOSH) do not advise against recapping sterile needles (e.g., after drawing up a medication), except to recommend needleless systems and safety systems. We suggest that you not use the one-handed "scoop" technique to recap a sterile needle because the risk of contaminating it is high. Consider one of the other methods described in Procedure 23-10.

Administering Parenteral Injections

Parenteral techniques are invasive. They carry the potential for tissue trauma and provide a portal of entry for pathogens through the skin. Therefore, you must maintain strict aseptic (sterile) technique to minimize the risk of infection. When you choose a site for injection, consider the type of medication to be administered, the viscosity of the medication, the volume of the medication, the anatomical landmarks underlying injection sites, and the patient's situation (e.g., the condition of the tissues at the injection site, the accessibility of certain sites). Your injection technique is critical to patient safety. The following are examples of errors and their consequences:

- Injecting a large volume of medication into a small muscle causes pain and may damage the tissues.
- Injecting into the wrong tissue (e.g., giving an intramuscular medication too shallowly into the subcutaneous tissue) may (1) accelerate or delay the rate of absorption and (2) cause tissue injury and pain.
- Incorrectly locating an injection site may result in bone or nerve injury when you insert the needle.
- An unsteady needle and syringe while injecting the drug could lead to pain and tissue trauma.

- Forgetting to aspirate before injecting risks administration of medication into an artery or vein instead of the muscle. This could result in an adverse, even fatal, effect.

Minimizing Discomfort

The discomfort associated with an injection comes from three sources: the prick of the needle, the pressure of the volume of the drug in the tissues, and chemical irritation caused by some drugs. Fear and anxiety magnify discomfort. Use the following techniques to reduce discomfort:

- Use the smallest needle suited for the site and medication.
- Use two needles when drawing up medications: one to withdraw the medication from the container, and the second one for the injection. If the needle is not free of medication, it may irritate tissues as it is inserted.
- Do not administer too much solution into an injection site. If the total volume is more than the recommended amount, give it in two injections and at two sites.
- For intramuscular injections, help the patient to assume a position that reduces muscle tension.
- For intramuscular injections, use the Z-track technique (see Procedure 23-14B). This prevents leakage of the medication up through the needle track after the needle is withdrawn. The Z-track method is particularly useful when giving medications that irritate or discolor the subcutaneous tissue. It should also be used for elderly patients who have reduced muscle mass.
- Pull the skin taut, and insert the needle quickly to avoid pulling the tissues. Remove the needle quickly and at the same angle you inserted it.
- Steady the syringe with one hand while injecting the medication.
- Inject the medication slowly.
- Distract the patient from the procedure by talking to her.
- Apply gentle pressure (not massage) after injection unless contraindicated.
- Especially with children, acknowledge that they will feel some pain (e.g., "This may hurt a little bit."). If you deny or minimize the pain, the patient might lose trust in you and be even more anxious about future injections.
- After injecting a child, pat or hug him, speak softly to him, and perhaps play with him, so that he does not associate you only with pain.
- Other methods for decreasing pain can be cooling the skin (e.g., applying ice) or flicking or tapping over the injection area before injecting. Both send distracting signals to the brain so that when the needle comes, it can't process the stimulus as easily.

Developmental Considerations

Because older adults may experience muscle atrophy or have decreased muscle mass, you may need to use a shorter needle. Infants and children also require shorter,

thinner needles. Also, you should ask a parent or another caregiver to immobilize an infant or young child to prevent injury during the injection.

The preferred intramuscular site for infants is the vastus lateralis muscle, because there are no major nerves or blood vessels in the area and the gluteal muscles have not yet been developed by walking. For children who are walking, the site of choice is the ventrogluteal muscle because the muscle is more developed.

 Do not use the dorsogluteal site for patients of any age, including older children and adults.

Intradermal Injections

Intradermal injections are given into the **dermis,** or the layer of the skin located beneath the skin surface. The intradermal route is commonly used for allergy or tuberculosis (TB) testing. Most nurses use the patient's nondominant arm for TB screening and the dominant arm, chest, or upper back for all other tests (Fig. 23-23). Give only small amounts of medication by this route—about 0.1 mL. Use a 1-mL syringe and a short, small (26- to 28-gauge) needle, and insert at an angle of 5° to 15° (see Fig. 23-25).

 Do not apply pressure or massage the injection site, because the capillaries in the dermal tissue will quickly absorb the medication.

Refer to the Critical Aspects box for critical elements of intradermal injections. Also,

VOL 2 Go to Chapter 23, **Procedure 23-11: Administering Intradermal Medications,** in Volume 2.

Subcutaneous Injections

Subcutaneous (subQ) injections are given into the subcutaneous tissue, the layer of fat located below the dermis and above the muscle tissue. Absorption is slower than through the intramuscular route because subcutaneous tissue does not have as rich a blood supply as muscle. However, speed of absorption varies with the

FIGURE 23-23 Sites commonly used for intradermal injection.

Toward Evidence-Based Practice

Zaybak, A., & Khorshid, L. (2008). A study on the effect of the duration of subcutaneous heparin injection on bruising and pain. *Journal of Clinical Nursing, 17*(3), 378–385.

This study was done to learn whether there is a difference in bruising or pain when subcutaneous injections of heparin are given quickly or slowly. Researchers studied 50 patients who required treatment with heparin. Injections on the right abdomen were given over 10 seconds; on the left abdomen, over 30 seconds. Bruising occurred in almost two out of every three (64%) of those who received the rapid injection; however, fewer than half (42%) of the patients bruised after receiving slower injection. Also, the size of the bruising was smaller in the 30-second injection. Pain intensity and pain duration were statistically significantly lower for the slower injection than for the more rapid one.

Chan, H. (2001). Effects of injection duration on site-pain intensity and bruising associated with subcutaneous heparin. *Journal of Clinical Nursing, 25*(6), 882–892.

This study was done to examine the relationship between how quickly a subcutaneous injection is performed and the occurrence of bruising and pain at the injection site. The research involved 34 stroke patients receiving heparin. For each subject, two injection techniques were used: one injection 10 seconds in duration and the other 30 seconds. Results showed the 30-second duration injection technique resulted in statistically significantly less intense site-pain and fewer and smaller bruises. Researchers concluded that administering a subcutaneous heparin injection over longer duration reduces injection site-pain and bruising.

Ipp, M., Taddio, A., Sam, J., et al. (2007). Vaccine-related pain: Randomized controlled trial of two injection techniques. *Archives of Disease in Childhood, 92*(12), 1105–1108.

The aim of this study was to compare pain during immunization using a slow injection versus a rapid technique. One hundred and thirteen healthy infants 4 to 6 months of age receiving routine DPTaP-Hib immunization were studied. One group received the intramuscular dose using a technique with slow aspiration before injection, slow injection, and slow withdrawal. The technique used for infants in the other group involved no aspiration, rapid injection, and rapid withdrawal. Infants receiving the slower injection technique cried twice as often, cried longer, and took more time to have the vaccine injected. Researchers concluded that immunization using a rapid intramuscular injection technique is less painful than a slower technique and should be recommended for routine intramuscular immunization.

1. You are providing care to an older adult patient who is receiving heparin therapy via subcutaneous injection. Based on the preceding studies, would you give subcutaneous doses over 10 seconds or 30 seconds?

2. You are working in a pediatric clinic. You want to administer intramuscular medication and immunizations to children in as pain-free a way as possible. Would you give IM injection slowly or more rapidly? Why would you choose that technique?

3. Why do you think subcutaneous injection might be less painful and produce less bruising when given more slowly even though IM injection using the same technique might be more painful?

 Go to Chapter 23, **Toward Evidence–Based Practice Suggested Responses,** on the Student Resource Disk or DavisPlus at http://davisplus.fadavis.com/Wilkinson2

---

subcutaneous site selected. Sites on the abdomen and arms offer fastest absorption; those on the thigh and upper buttocks, the slowest absorption. Medication is absorbed more evenly from the abdomen than from the thighs and buttocks because it is less affected by activity.

Aspiration for blood return is not necessary for subcutaneous injection because of the shallow depth of the needle into the subcutaneous layer under the skin. The Critical Aspects box contains critical elements of the procedure. For the full procedure,

VOL 2 Go to Chapter 23, **Procedure 23-12: Administering Subcutaneous Medications,** in Volume 2.

Choosing a Subcutaneous Site
See Figure 23-24 for sites to use for subcutaneous injections. Avoid sites of abnormal subcutaneous tissue, such as areas lying beneath burns, birthmarks, inflamed tissue, or scars. Do not use sites with lesions or sites over bony prominences, large underlying vessels, or nerves. When using the abdominal site, do not inject any closer than 5 cm (2 inches) from the umbilicus. For repeated injections, each injection should be at least an inch apart. It is important to rotate sites for repeated injections. Using the same spot can cause scarring and hardening of fatty tissue that will interfere with the absorption of medication.

Choosing a Subcutaneous Needle
As a general rule, use a syringe with a short and small needle for subcutaneous injection—that is, long enough to penetrate beyond the skin into the fatty subcutaneous layer and yet not into the muscle. The needle length will vary depending on the amount of adipose the patient has and the type of injection that is needed (e.g., insulin, immunization, or other medication). For most subcutaneous

FIGURE 23-24 Sites used for subcutaneous injections.

injections, a ⅝-inch needle is preferred. However, shorter needles are more comfortable for some insulin users, for instance a 3/16- to 5/16-inch needle.

The **gauge**, or needle thickness, for subcutaneous injection should be small, typically 25- to 27-gauge; however, finer needles are often preferred by insulin users (e.g., 28- to 31-gauge). For children and persons with little or average subcutaneous fat, insert a standard length needle (⅝ inch) at a 45° angle; however, when using a shorter needle, inject at a 90° angle. Obese patients will need a longer needle (e.g., 1-inch) and a 90° angle for injection, and the nurse needs to spread the skin taut rather than pinching. See Figure 23-25.

The medication you are giving influences your choice of syringe. Recall there are special insulin syringes and that you will use a tuberculin syringe or prefilled cartridge when giving heparin.

◆ Inject only small amounts (0.5 to 1 mL) of water-soluble medication subcutaneously to avoid creating sterile abscesses (hardened, painful lumps under the skin).

Administering Insulin

Insulin must be administered subcutaneously or intravenously because it is a protein and would be destroyed in the gastrointestinal tract. Recall insulin is administered using a special insulin syringe. The pre-

scriber will specify the number of units rather than the number of milliliters or milligrams. Insulin vials contain 100 units/mL. Insulin may be prescribed in specific dosages at specific times or on the basis of the patient's blood glucose level before meals. The latter is a **sliding scale**, also called a correction scale. However, the sliding scale is controversial as many studies cite poor glycemic control and deleterious effects with its use. Sliding scale is used less now because basal insulin is available to stabilize blood sugar with fewer fluctuations, and because insulin pumps are in more common use. However, it can be useful when initiating insulin therapy and during times of physical stress such as illness, surgery, and trauma. Be sure to check with your institution regarding the sliding scale.

Categories of Insulin. Understanding the categories of insulin and how they are used for blood sugar control is essential for preventing errors and giving insulin safely.

- **Basal insulin** is given to cover the body's energy needs without taking the diet into account. Common basal insulins are NPH, insulin glargine (Lantus), and insulin detemir (Levemir).
- **Prandial** and **preprandial insulin** is given to prevent high blood sugar after eating a meal. Regular insulin is this type.
- **Correction insulin** is given to reduce an elevated blood sugar level to a normal range. This type of sliding scale blood sugar management is not the best way to manage diabetes because it achieves damage control more than damage prevention.

Appearance of Insulin. Regular (unmodified) insulin is rapid acting. It is a clear solution. If a vial of regular insulin is cloudy, you should discard it. Other types of insulin (e.g., Lente, insulin glargine, and neutral protamine hagedorn [NPH]) are cloudy because of the addition of proteins, which slow the absorption of the drug, giving the insulin an intermediate to long duration of action. As a rule, remember "clear before cloudy"; that is, draw up the regular (clear) insulin first, and then draw up the modified (cloudy) insulin. Actually, though, you will rarely need to mix insulins because stable premixed insulins are available.

FIGURE 23-25 Standard angles of insertion for intramuscular, subcutaneous, and intradermal injections.

Storing Insulin. The length of time insulin can be stored depends on whether it is refrigerated or stored at room temperature. Check the package insert to know how long the insulin will remain effective after the vial is opened.

 Go to Chapter 23, **Supplemental Materials, Insulin Administration,** on the Student Resource Disk or DavisPlus at http://davisplus.fadavis.com/Wilkinson2

 Go to Chapter 23, **Clinical Insight 23-5: Mixing Two Kinds of Insulin in One Syringe,** in Volume 2.

Insulin can be administered in a variety of ways.

- **Disposable syringes** for subcutaneous injection are the most common.
- **Automatic injectors** are used by some patients for subcutaneous dosing. By pressing a button on the device, the injector releases the needle into the skin, releasing the insulin dose.
- **Insulin pumps** are becoming more common as a way to maintain glycemic control because of the benefit of fine-tuning the dosing. The pump consists of a tube with a needle on the end of it that is taped to the abdomen, and a computerized device that is worn at the waist. Insulin is received continuously from the pump. A button is pressed at mealtime to release an extra insulin dose.
- **Insulin pen devices** contain a cartridge and disposable needles to deliver certain doses with each injection. Patients who use insulin pens do not have to draw up insulin from a vial.
- **Nondisposable syringes** (glass syringe and metal needle) may be used repeatedly if they are sterilized after each use.
- **Spray injectors** forcefully spray the insulin dose into the skin. This involves a wider area of skin than an injection would.

People with diabetes usually administer their own insulin injections. They should rotate injection sites to promote absorption and minimize tissue damage. Insulin is absorbed at different rates from different parts of the body. For hospitalized patients, you should document site rotation (usually on a diagram of the body) to prevent repeated use of the same site.

KnowledgeCheck 23-16

- List three errors in technique that can occur when giving parenteral injections. State their possible consequences.
- Describe at least four ways to minimize the discomfort of an injection.
- Name two reasons for giving an intradermal injection.
- As a rule, what gauge and length of needle would you use for a subcutaneous injection?
- Why should people rotate injection sites when they must have repeated injections over a long time?

 Go to Chapter 23, **Knowledge Check Response Sheet and Answers,** on the Student Resource Disk or DavisPlus at http://davisplus.fadavis.com/Wilkinson2

CriticalThinking 23-12

- What do intradermal and subcutaneous injections have in common?
- How are they different?

Administering Heparin

Heparin is a fast-acting medication that interrupts the blood clotting process. It may be used for patients at risk for harmful clot formation, for example, those who are immobile after major surgery, have undergone vascular surgery, or have problems related to blood clotting, such as cerebrovascular accident (stroke) or myocardial infarction (heart attack). Because heparin is absorbed poorly from the gastrointestinal tract, it is given intravenously or subcutaneously. If mistakenly given intramuscularly, it will cause hematoma and pain. The dosage is based on the patient's weight and results of blood coagulation studies, so always check laboratory values for coagulation studies before giving.

Give the injection deep into the subcutaneous tissue of the abdomen, at least 5 cm (2 inches) away from the umbilicus. Rotate sites. Because of the anticoagulant properties of heparin, you will need to modify your injection technique. Primarily, this means:

1. Add 0.2 mL of air after drawing up the correct dose.
2. Do not massage the site after the injection.
3. Never aspirate when giving heparin subcutaneously because this will increase bruising.
4. If injecting low molecular weight heparin (LMWH [Lovenox]), be sure to alternate between the left and right anterolateral and left and right posterolateral abdominal wall.
5. Inject the whole length of the subcutaneous needle into a skin fold held between the thumb and forefinger; the skin fold should be held throughout the injection.

For detailed guidelines,

 Go to Chapter 23, **Clinical Insight 23-6: Administering Anticoagulant Medication Subcutaneously,** in Volume 2.

Intramuscular Injections

Intramuscular injections (injections into muscle tissue) are absorbed faster than subcutaneous medications because of the rich blood supply in the muscles. Muscles can also tolerate more fluid—you can give as much as 3 or 4 mL of liquid in the large vastus lateralis and ventrogluteal muscles. The smaller the muscle, the less fluid it can tolerate. For example, you should usually give no more than 0.5 to 1 mL in the average deltoid muscle.

Aspiration is the technique of pulling back on the plunger of the syringe before injection to be sure the needle tip is not in a blood vessel. Conventional IM injection techniques call for you to aspirate before injecting medication; if there is no blood return, you are confident that the medication will not be injected into a blood vessel. However, because there are no large blood vessels at the sites used for most immunizations (i.e., deltoid for adults, anterolateral thigh for infants), the CDC

Advisory Committee on Immunization Practices (ACIP) does not require aspiration when giving immunizations to adults and children (Kroger, Atkinson, Marcuse, et al., 2006). As there is little strong evidence at this time to support the practice one way or the other, aspirating for blood is common and does not pose a risk to the patient. However, for children who have difficulty remaining still during the procedure and for those with anxiety regarding injection, a no aspiration technique reduces the difficulty of IM injection.

Choosing an Intramuscular Site

When selecting an IM site, you should look for a site that is:

- A safe distance from nerves, large blood vessels, and bones
- Free from injury, abscesses, tenderness, necrosis, abrasion, or other pathology
- Large enough to accommodate the volume of medication to be given

Muscles commonly used are the vastus lateralis, ventrogluteal, and deltoid. Because of their proximity to major nerves and vessels, the rectus femoris and dorsogluteal are no longer recommended sites (Greenway, 2004; Nicholl & Hesby, 2002). For a summary description of intramuscular injection sites, refer to the Critical Aspects box. For the complete procedure,

VOL 2 Go to Chapter 23, **Procedure 23-13: Locating Intramuscular Injection Sites,** in Volume 2.

Ventrogluteal Muscle—Site of Choice. Whenever possible, use the ventrogluteal site for intramuscular injections; it is the site of choice for adults and young children who are walking. The ventrogluteal site, located on the lateral hip, involves the gluteus medius and gluteus minimus muscles (Fig. 23-26). Because it is located away from major blood vessels and nerves, it is the safest and least painful site for intramuscular injections. Be aware though, that some medications and immunizations, such as those used to treat influenza/pneumonia, are normally given in the deltoid; be sure to check the package insert.

When learning to locate this site, many students notice that it feels "hard" when they palpate it. They worry the needle will hit the bone. In part, the muscle feels hard because there is little subcutaneous tissue over it. To reassure yourself it is safe, examine a skeleton model with the muscles attached. Notice the ilium is concave (curves in) and the muscle lies deep down in the "cup" it forms. If you are sure you have located the anterosuperior iliac spine and if you follow the procedure steps, you will not hit a bone. In fact, you are less likely to do so than if you use other sites. For guidelines in locating the ventrogluteal site, refer to the Critical Aspects box and Procedure 23-13 (in Volume 2).

Dorsogluteal Site. The dorsogluteal site consists of the gluteal muscles of the buttocks. ✚ Because of its close proximity to the sciatic nerve and superior gluteal artery, this site is not recommended for use. It is always

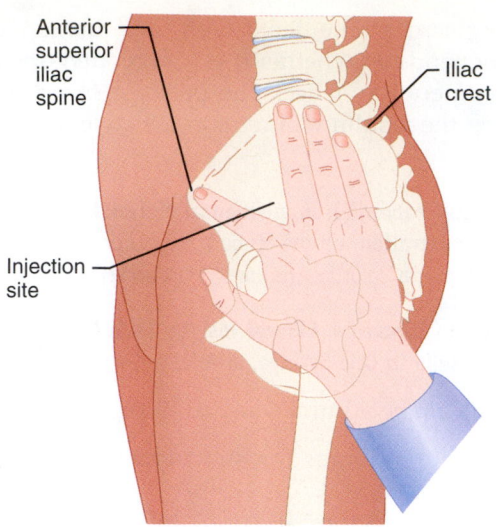

FIGURE 23-26 Locating the ventrogluteal site.

contraindicated for use in infants or children. Using this site increases the risk of injection into a major blood vessel, as well as damage to the sciatic nerve, which can cause permanent or partial paralysis of the leg involved. Furthermore, the site is difficult to identify accurately in older adults or people with flabby skin.

✚ Avoid using the dorsogluteal site for IM injections. Accidental injection of the sciatic nerve and superior gluteal artery can lead to complications.

You may observe some nurses continue to use the dorsogluteal site because they were taught to use it long ago and have not learned how to locate the ventrogluteal site. This gives you the opportunity to improve practice by demonstrating correct technique for locating the preferred site.

Deltoid Site. The deltoid site is located in the middle third of the upper arm (Fig. 23-27). The area has a small muscle mass with little subcutaneous tissue, so medications are absorbed rapidly. This muscle is easily accessible but is not well developed in many older adults; so, you should use it only for small amounts of up to to 1 mL or when other sites are inaccessible. Avoid using the deltoid site in infants; you can use it in children if you are sure the muscle mass is adequate, but the anterolateral thigh is preferred.

The deltoid is small and lies close to the radial nerve and brachial artery. When locating this site, do not merely roll up the sleeve; fully expose the entire upper arm and shoulder. Otherwise, you may miss the muscle mass and injure a nerve or blood vessel. For a guide to locating the deltoid site, see the Critical Aspects box and Procedure 23-12 (in Volume 2).

Vastus Lateralis Site. The vastus lateralis muscle, located in the anterolateral thigh (Fig. 23-28), is the preferred site for young infants, particularly before walking age (Centers for Disease Control, 2002) because it's usually the best developed and contains no large nerves

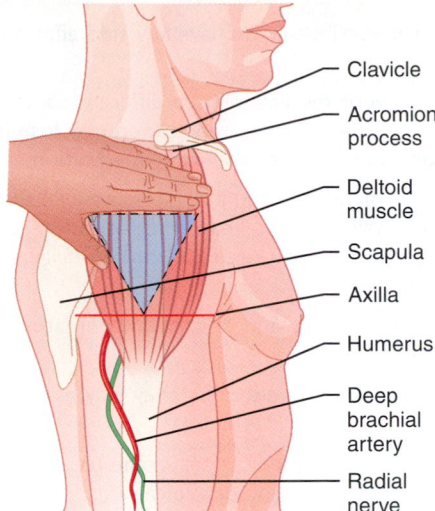

FIGURE 23-27 Locating the deltoid site.

Clavicle

Acromion process

Deltoid muscle

Scapula

Axilla

Humerus

Deep brachial artery

Radial nerve

Vastus Lateralis Site. The vastus lateralis muscle, located in the anterolateral thigh (Fig. 23-28), is the preferred site for young infants, particularly before walking age (Centers for Disease Control, 2002) because it's usually the best developed and contains no large nerves or blood vessels, minimizing the risk for injury. Its main advantage is that drugs are rapidly absorbed from this area. Moreover, it can accommodate a larger volume of medication than the deltoid, and it is not near any major blood vessels or nerves. For children and adults, a disadvantage is that the patient can see you administer the injection, and the psychological effect may create some discomfort. However, this is a convenient location for those who self-administer injections. Also, because this muscle is used in walking, an ambulatory patient may notice more residual soreness than in another site.

To relax this muscle for injection, have the patient sit or lie flat with his knee slightly flexed. For children and adult patients with small muscle mass, you should grasp ("pinch up") the body of the muscle during injection to be sure that the medication reaches muscle tissue and the needle does not penetrate to the underlying bone. For

FIGURE 23-28 Locating the vastus lateralis.

Rectus femoris

Vastus lateralis

guidelines in locating the vastus lateralis site, refer to the Critical Aspects box and Procedure 23-13 (in Volume 2).

Rectus Femoris Site. The rectus femoris site, located in the anterior thigh, is no longer recommended for infants and children, although you may rarely use it for adults when rapid absorption is needed or other sites are inaccessible. It is often used by patients who self-administer their intramuscular injections because it is easy for them to reach. A disadvantage is that it is usually painful. Use a shorter needle when injecting this site. For a guide to locating the rectus femoris site, refer to the Critical Aspects box and Procedure 23-13 (in Volume 2).

Choosing an Intramuscular Needle

Although a 1½-inch needle is considered "standard" for intramuscular injections, you should choose the needle gauge and length based on the site, the size of the muscle, the amount of medication to be given, and the amount of adipose tissue over the muscle. In the deltoid muscle, for example, you might use a 23- or 25-gauge, 1-inch needle. But if the solution is viscous, you would need a larger-bore needle (e.g., 20-gauge). For a very thin person, you could use a 1-inch needle, even when injecting into the larger muscles. For an obese person, you might need a needle as long as 3 inches to penetrate adipose tissue and reach the muscle (unfortunately, long needles may not be available in some settings). As a rule, the angle of insertion for an intramuscular injection is 90° (see Fig. 23-25). The Critical Aspects box presents the key elements for IM injections. For the complete steps,

Go to Chapter 23, **Procedure 23-14: Administering Intramuscular Injections,** in Volume 2.

✚ CDC (2007) recommends a 1-inch needle for all thigh intramuscular immunizations in infants ages 1 to 12 months, a 1- to 1¼-inch needle for all thigh intramuscular immunizations in toddlers ages 12 to 24 months, and a ⅝- to 1-inch needle for all deltoid intramuscular vaccinations in children ages 1 to 18 years.

Z-Track Technique

Procedure 23-14B describes the procedure for using the Z-track technique for intramuscular injections. This technique seals the needle track and prevents medication from leaking out of the muscle up through the needle track and into the subcutaneous tissues. You must use this technique for irritating medications, such as iron preparations. The Z-track method is also good for older adults with reduced muscle mass. It is recommended for all intramuscular injections, because it is less painful and helps to prevent irritation of subcutaneous tissues. For this technique, it is best to use the larger muscles: the ventrogluteal and vastus lateralis sites.

KnowledgeCheck 23-17
- Name three sites for giving IM injections.
- What is the preferred site for adults? Why?
- From which route is medication absorbed more rapidly: subcutaneous or intramuscular? Why?

Self-Care

Teaching Your Patient About Self-Medication

➤ Do not take medications prescribed to others, and do not share your medications with others.

➤ Keep a list of your medications, including doses and times taken. Take this list with you when you visit any primary care provider or an emergency department.

➤ If you take a variety of medications, post a list of them in a prominent place that is easy to get to in the event of an emergency.

➤ Wear a Medic Alert bracelet or necklace if you are a diabetic, take anticoagulants, or have allergies to any medication.

➤ When you are prescribed a new medication, ask why you are taking it, how long you should take it, what side effects you should expect, whether you should take it with food, and whether there are any special precautions.

➤ Be sure to read the label carefully on the bottle each time you take the medication so that you take the correct medication. Many pills look alike.

➤ Take only the amount and dose prescribed. If you have questions, call your prescriber.

➤ To measure liquids, use kitchen measuring spoons rather than tableware, which can vary in volume.

➤ Take the medication for the prescribed length of time to make certain you receive the full benefit of the drug. For example, some patients may take only part of an expensive antibiotic, hoping to "save it for later." If you do not take the full course of medication, the infection may recur. Antibiotic resistance may develop, leading to "superinfection," such as methicillin-resistant *Staphylococcus aureus* (MRSA).

➤ Notify your prescriber if you have any side effects or adverse reactions.

➤ Do not store your medication in a different container from the one it came in. The medication may lose its strength, or you may take the wrong medication.

➤ Store all your medications in a dry place out of the sunlight and away from the heat. If a medication requires a cold storage, be sure you return it to the refrigerator immediately after use.

➤ Check expiration dates, and discard any outdated medications.

➤ Do not take expired medications; they may have lost their strength.

➤ Do not place expired medications in the trash within the reach of children. Disposing of expired medications in the sink or toilet is not environmentally sound (e.g., they can appear in the community water supply). Some communities sponsor an "old medications discard day" or provide a place to discard them to avoid contamination. Some local pharmacies may offer medication disposal as a community service.

➤ Use childproof caps if children have access to your medications. If no children are in the home, replace with simple closure cap for elderly patients who might have difficulty opening the containers.

➤ Monitor your prescription amounts, and get refills before you run out. If you get medications by mail, be sure you send for them in plenty of time.

➤ If you become pregnant, notify your primary care provider as soon as possible so your medications can be discontinued or adjusted.

- For an "average" adult, what is the standard needle length for IM injections?
- Why is the dorsogluteal site *not* recommended?
- What are the disadvantages of the deltoid site?
- When using the vastus lateralis to give an intramuscular medication to a person with small muscle mass, how can you ensure the medication reaches muscle tissue and the needle does not penetrate to the underlying bone?

 Go to Chapter 23, **Knowledge Check Response Sheet and Answers,** on the Student Resource Disk or DavisPlus at http://davisplus.fadavis.com/Wilkinson2

Intravenous Medications

Intravenous (IV) medications are given through a catheter or cannula inserted into a vein. The onset of medication action takes place within seconds, so IV administration is especially useful in emergencies. However, because an IV drug begins to act immediately, there is no way for you to stop its action if an adverse reaction occurs (unless there is a known antidote). Review Table 23-1 for advantages and disadvantages of using the IV route.

IV medications may be administered by a variety of programmable electronic pumps and infusers. These are discussed in Chapter 36.

To prevent complications, when administering IV medications, you should:

- Use sterile technique.
- Administer the medication slowly.
- Be aware that in addition to the effects of the medicine, the volume of fluid infused has possible consequences.
- Observe the patient carefully for signs of adverse reactions.
- Have an antidote on hand if the drug has potentially serious side effects. Be aware, though, that many drugs do not have an antidote.
- If your patient shows signs of serious allergic reaction, you will need to prepare to support the patient's airway, deliver oxygen, and administer medication to reduce the reaction.
- Assess the patient before, during, and after giving the medication.
- Determine the drug is compatible with the fluid that is infusing; consult a pharmacist if necessary.
- Determine the drug is compatible with the plastic IV bag and tubing; you may occasionally need to use a glass IV bottle and special tubing.
- Observe the insertion site often; check to be sure the cannula is in the vein before administering a medication. Figure 23-29 provides an example of

FIGURE 23-29 Tissue and skin injury after intravenous medication leaks into an infiltrated site. (Used by permission of the National Extravasation Information Service (UK). www. extravasation.org.uk)

tissue damage that can occur when certain IV medications escape from the vein into surrounding tissues.

The following sections explain how to administer IV medications by (1) adding medication to the large-volume primary or maintenance fluids, (2) IV push or bolus, (3) intermittent infusion (piggyback or tandem setups), and (4) volume-control infusion sets. You will find the procedures for initiating and maintaining intravenous fluids and using intermittent injection ports in Chapter 36.

Adding Medications to Large-Volume (Primary) Infusions

The safest and easiest way to administer a drug intravenously is to mix it into a bag of fluid that is already infusing. This is often normal saline or lactated Ringer's solution or, sometimes, glucose. Vitamins, potassium chloride, oxytocin, and several blood pressure and cardiovascular drugs are commonly given this way. This method is useful when the drug can be infused continuously over a long period of time or when it must be given continuously to achieve the desired effect. The main disadvantage is the danger of infusing too much fluid, especially for children, older adults, and people with cardiac or renal disease. In some instances, the drug may be premixed with the IV fluid in the pharmacy. Or you may need to add a drug to a bag before you hang it or to one that is already infusing.

 A safe method for mixing medication from multi-dose IV vials while providing sterile air filtration is to use a **reconstitution device**—designed with a sharp, thin, piercing spike to minimize coring and permit easy penetration of rubber top vials. The luer-lock port maintains a secure closure between the device and the syringe. The hinged cap and the sheath over the spike help maintain sterility before use, minimize "touch" contamination, and ensure a closed system for disposal.

A safe method for adding medications to an IV container is to use a **transfer needle** or **cannula**—a

blunted plastic needle with a double beveled tip. One end is inserted into the powdered or liquid medication and the other end is inserted into a port of the IV bag. Solution is transferred from the IV bag into the medication vial, which you shake lightly to mix the medication. Then the medication is transferred back into the IV bag for administration.

Refer to Figure 23-30 and the Critical Aspects box. Also,

 Go to Chapter 23, **Procedure 23-15: Adding Medications to Intravenous Fluids,** in Volume 2.

IV Push Medications

IV push (bolus) medications are injected directly into the systemic circulation. Many drugs given by IV push have a package insert that contains specific guidelines for their administration rate (usually between 1 and 10 minutes). Read the package insert or ask the prescriber how fast the drug can be pushed. Even just a minute can seem like a very long time when you are pushing a medication, so don't guess—look at your watch! Take note that "IV push" does not mean the same thing as "give rapidly." If given too rapidly, IV drugs—particularly potassium—can be quite dangerous. Because you cannot retrieve the medication once it is injected, there is no margin for error.

Because many IV push medications can irritate tissues, you must confirm the IV cannula is in the vein before injecting the drug. If the medication is accidentally injected into tissues, sloughing, pain, and abscesses may occur (see Fig. 23-29). The medications may also be irritating to the lining of the vein, so evaluate the condition of the injection site frequently. Refer to the Critical Aspects box, and

Go to Chapter 23, **Procedure 23-16: Administering IV Push Medications,** in Volume 2.

Intermittent Infusion

Many medications, such as antibiotics, are administered intravenously by intermittent infusion. Intermittent infusions may be given through the port of a running IV

FIGURE 23-30 A reconstitution device is used to add medication from multidose IV vials while providing sterile air filtration. (Courtesy of Medi-Dose® Inc./ EPS® Inc., Ivyland, PA.)

line or, if the patient does not need the IV fluids, through an intermittent injection port, also called a saline or heparin lock (Fig. 23-31).

Most intermittent infusion medications are supplied in bags containing 50 to 250 mL of 5% dextrose in water (D_5W) or normal saline. The drug is given over a period of time, usually 30 to 60 minutes, and at regular intervals (e.g., every 6 hours). The small bag of diluted medication (the "secondary" bag) is attached to the primary IV infusion line for administration. There are two types of setups for intermittent infusion using a primary IV line:

1. A **tandem setup** is connected to the primary IV line at the lower (secondary) port (Fig. 23-32). The medi-

cation can be given intermittently or at the same time as the primary IV infusion—both bags can infuse at the same time.

2. With an **IV piggyback** setup the smaller (secondary) container is connected to the primary (continuous) infusion line at the upper (primary) port (Fig. 23-33). This setup allows for intermittent use only.

Traditionally, the secondary tubing was attached to the primary set tubing by inserting a needle into the port and taping it in place. However, most agencies now use needleless systems (see Fig. 23-21), which use a threaded or lever-type lock to make the connection. In addition to helping prevent needlestick injuries, a needleless system prevents contact contamination at the IV connection site. The Critical Aspects box provides guidelines for administering intermittent infusions. Also,

VOL 2 Go to Chapter 23, **Procedure 23-17: Administering Medications by Intermittent Infusion,** in Volume 2.

Volume-Control Infusion Sets

To effectively control the infusion of smaller amounts of solutions, particularly with pediatric patients, a volume-control infusion set (e.g., Buretrol, Soluset, Volutrol, or Pediatrol) may be used (Fig. 23-34). These are

FIGURE 23-31 Intermittent injection port.

FIGURE 23-32 Tandem (secondary) setup is attached to the primary (continuous infusion) IV line at the lower port, allowing for both intermittent and simultaneous infusion.

FIGURE 23-33 Piggyback setup is attached to the primary (continuous infusion) IV line at the upper port, allowing for intermittent infusion only.

FIGURE 23-34 Volume-control infusion set for intermittent infusion administration; used when the fluid volume is critical and must be carefully monitored.

are inserted into the central circulation via a peripheral vein and can remain in place for months. For short-term use, the nontunneled central catheter can be inserted into the jugular, subclavian, or femoral veins.

An **internal, or implantable, port** is a CVAD that can remain in place and be functional for years. Access is gained through the skin via a hollow port with a self-sealing silicone cap. These devices are inserted when long-term IV medication is needed or the medication is too irritating for a peripheral site. See Figure 23-35A for an example of a port for injecting medication into the subclavian vein.

Catheters for central venous delivery can be single- or multilumen (Fig. 23-35B). Although they are more convenient for administering different medications and fluid, some types of multilumen catheters have a higher infection rate than single-lumen catheters.

small fluid containers (100 to 150 mL) that are attached directly below the primary fluid container. The medication and the desired amount of IV fluid are added to the volume-control container and administered through the primary line. This system decreases the risk of overhydration because the amount of fluid that can infuse into the patient is limited to the amount that you place in the small container.

Central Venous Access Devices

Intravenous medication can be delivered through a central or peripheral vein. The most common reasons for a patient to have a central venous access device (CVAD) are:

- To give long-term IV therapy
- To provide total parenteral nutrition when the patient cannot eat normally
- To have blood drawn without the trauma and complications of repeated venipuncture
- When peripheral IV placement is difficult

External CVADs can be either tunneled or nontunneled. The *tunneled devices* are surgically implanted peripherally and tunneled to a central vein, typically the superior vena cava. *Nontunneled catheters* are inserted near the destination site. These catheters can be single- or multilumen. This category includes peripherally inserted central catheters (PICCs), which

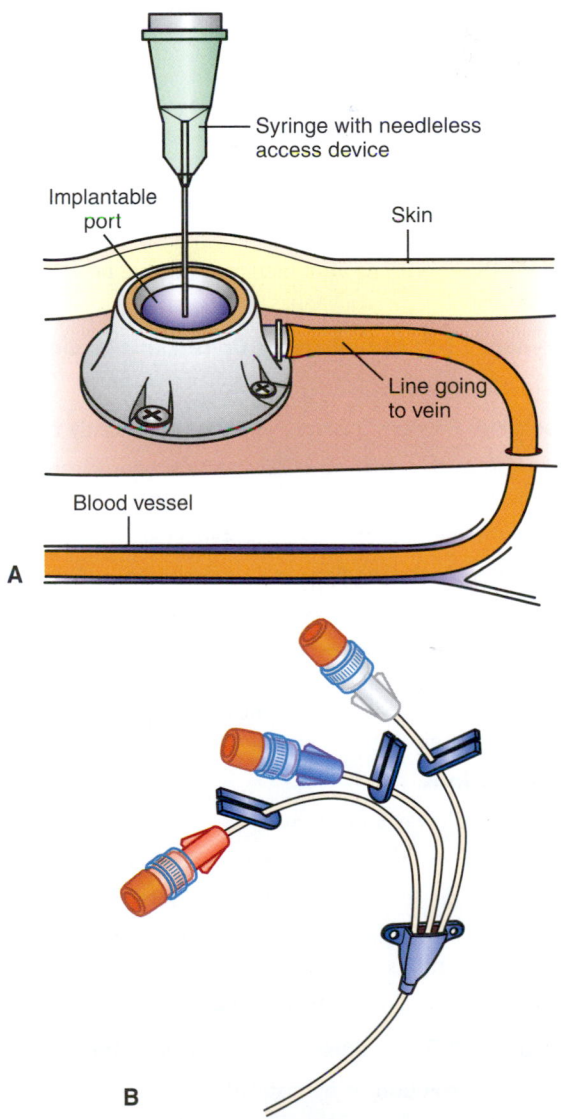

FIGURE 23-35 Central vascular access device: *A,* Implantable device. *B,* Multilumen catheter with blunt cannula, split septum, needleless access device.

VOL 2 For steps to follow in *all* procedures, refer to the Universal Steps for All Procedures found on the inside back cover of Volume 2. Go to full procedures in Volume 2 to practice and learn the procedure steps. Use these Critical Aspects later to help you review key points.

Procedure 23-1: Administering Oral Medication

➤ Observe the "three checks" and the "rights of medication": right patient, drug, dose, time, route, and documentation.

➤ Tablets and capsules: Pour the correct number into the medication cup.

➤ Liquids: Hold the plastic medication cup at eye level to measure the dose.

➤ Assist the patient to a high-Fowler's position, if possible.

➤ For enterically administered medications, check for correct placement of the nasogastric or gastric tube.

➤ Correctly administer the medication.

Powder: Mix with liquid, and give it to the patient to drink.

Lozenge: Instruct the patient not to chew or swallow it before dissolving it in his mouth.

Tablet or capsule: Place the tablet or medication cup in the patient's hand or mouth, and instruct the patient to swallow with sips of liquid.

Sublingual: Have the patient place the tablet under the tongue and hold it there until it is completely dissolved.

Buccal: Instruct the patient to place the tablet between the cheek and teeth and hold it there until it is completely dissolved.

➤ Stay with the patient until medications have been swallowed or dissolved.

Procedure 23-2: Administering Ophthalmic Medication

For instillations

➤ Use a high-Fowler's position, with the head slightly tilted back.

➤ Work from the inner to outer canthus when cleansing or instilling medication.

➤ Apply the medication into the conjunctival sac.

➤ Do not apply the medication to the cornea.

➤ Do not let the dropper or tube touch the eye.

➤ For eye drops, press gently against the same side of the nose for 1 to 2 minutes to close the lacrimal ducts. For an eye ointment, ask the patient to gently close the eyes for 2 to 3 minutes.

For irrigations

➤ Use a low-Fowler's position.

➤ Check the pH in the conjunctival sac, if indicated.

➤ Use a Morgan lens or IV tubing to irrigate the eyes.

➤ For direct-flow irrigation, irrigate from the inner canthus to the outer canthus.

➤ Irrigate for 20 minutes or until the desired pH is reached.

Procedure 23-3: Administering Otic Medication

➤ Warm the solution to be instilled.

➤ Assist the patient to a side-lying position, with the appropriate ear facing up.

➤ Straighten the ear canal. For an adult patient, pull the pinna up and back; for a child 3 years or younger, down and back.

➤ Instill the prescribed number of drops into the ear canal.

➤ Do not force the solution into the ear or occlude the ear canal with the dropper.

➤ Instruct the patient to remain on his side for 5 to 10 minutes.

Procedure 23-4: Administering Nasal Medication

➤ Determine head position: Consider the indication for the medication and the patient's ability to assume the position.

➤ Explain to the patient that the medication may cause some burning, tingling, or unusual taste.

➤ Position the patient with the head down and forward or supine with the head back.

➤ Place the tip of the sprayer into the right nostril, pointing the tip toward the outside of the nose (toward the outside corner of the right eye). Never point the tip toward the middle of the nose (the septum) or straight up (toward the sinus).

➤ Have the patient blow his nose, occlude one nostril, and exhale.

➤ Squirt the spray into the nose while patient inhales through his other nostril.

➤ Repeat for the other nostril.

➤ If the patient tastes the medicine, the head was not down or he did not inhale long enough. Advise him to put his head back down and sniff again without the medicine.

➤ If nose drops are used, ask the patient to stay in the same position for approximately 5 minutes.

Procedure 23-5: Administering Vaginal Medication

For instillation

➤ Position the patient in a dorsal recumbent or Sims' position.

➤ Inspect and cleanse the vaginal area before administering the medication.

➤ Use a water-soluble lubricant.

➤ Insert the suppository or applicator along the posterior vaginal wall about 8 cm (3 inches).

➤ Instruct the patient to maintain the position for 5 to 15 minutes after the medication is inserted.

For irrigation (douche)

➤ Warm the irrigation solution to approximately 105°F (40.6°C).

➤ Hang the irrigation solution approximately 30 to 60 cm (1 to 2 ft) above the level of the patient's vagina.

➤ Position the patient in a dorsal recumbent position on a waterproof pad and bedpan.

➤ Insert the nozzle approximately 7 to 8 cm (3 in.) into the vagina, and start the flow of irrigation solution.

Procedure 23-6: Inserting a Rectal Suppository

➤ Before inserting the suppository, assess for contraindications, such as rectal surgery, rectal bleeding, or cardiac disease.

➤ Position the patient in the Sims' position.

➤ Don gloves

➤ Lubricate the suppository.

➤ Insert the suppository past the internal sphincter about ½ to 1 inch in infants and 1 to 3 inches in adults. Never force the suppository during insertion.

➤ Instruct the patient to stay on his side for 5 to 10 minutes and retain (not expel) the suppository for about 30 minutes.

Procedure 23-7: Applying Medication to the Skin

➤ Wear gloves to avoid absorbing the medication through your own skin and to avoid cross-contamination.

➤ Before applying topical medication, cleanse the skin with soap and water.

➤ Do not apply medication to skin with open lesions, irritation, or known hypersensitivity.

➤ Avoid exposure to UV light/sunlight after applying medication.

➤ Assess for adverse skin reactions (e.g., hypersensitivity, redness, itching, or local irritation).

➤ Use gentle technique when applying topical medication to fragile skin, which is typical in older adults.

➤ Take care to not over-apply the medication.

Procedure 23-8: Administering Metered-Dose Inhaler (MDI) Medication

➤ Identify the number of remaining inhalations in the canister. The "float method" is no longer recommended for determining whether an MDI canister is empty.

➤ Assist the patient to a seated position.

➤ Shake the inhaler. Remove the mouthpiece cap of the inhaler and insert the mouthpiece into the spacer while holding the canister upright.

➤ Remove the cap from the spacer.

➤ Ask the patient to breathe out slowly and completely.

➤ If a patient is unable to use the metered-dose inhaler independently, time the use of the device with the patient's own respirations.

➤ Place the spacer's mouthpiece into the patient's mouth and ask him to seal his lips around the mouthpiece. Press down on the inhaler canister to discharge one puff of medication into the spacer.

➤ Ask the patient to slowly inhale, and then hold his breath for as long as possible.

➤ If a second puff is needed, wait at least 1 minute and repeat.

Procedure 23-9: Preparing, Drawing Up, and Mixing Medication

➤ Maintain sterile technique.

➤ Recap the needle or vial access device (VAD) using a needle safety device or the one-handed method.

➤ Change the needle, if indicated.

Procedure 23-9A: Drawing Up Medication from Ampules

➤ Tap the ampule to remove medication trapped in the top of the ampule or shake it with a quick snap of the wrist.

➤ Use an ampule opener to break the ampule neck. Or wrap gauze or an alcohol swab in its wrapper around the neck of the ampule, and snap the ampule away from you.

➤ Use a filter needle or filter straw to withdraw the medication.

➤ Withdraw all of the medication from the ampule by inverting or tipping the ampule.

➤ Remove the filter needle and replace it with an appropriate size needle.

➤ Dispose of the broken ampule and filter needle in a sharps container.

Procedure 23-9B: Drawing Up Medication from Vials

➤ Scrub the rubber top of the vial with an alcohol prep pad or chlorhexidine–alcohol product (for a multidose vial only).

➤ Draw air into the syringe equal to the amount of medication to be withdrawn.

➤ When inserting the needle or VAD through the rubber top of the vial, insert at a 45°- to 60° angle, bevel up. Puncture the rubber top at that angle, but immediately raise to 90° as you insert the needle.

➤ Keeping the needle above the fluid line, inject air into the vial before inverting the vial and withdrawing the medication.

➤ Remove bubbles from the syringe, hold the vial at eye level, and check that the dose is correct before removing the needle.

Procedures 23-9C, D, and E: Mixing Medication in One Syringe

➤ Make sure the medications are compatible.

➤ Before beginning, determine the total volume of all medications to be put in the syringe and whether that volume is appropriate for the administration site.

➤ Maintain the sterility of the needles and medication.

➤ Avoid contaminating a multidose vial with a second medication.

➤ Carefully expel air bubbles.

➤ Withdraw the second medication very carefully because the medications are mixed as you pull back the plunger; therefore, you must withdraw the exact amount. If there is any excess, you must discard the contents of the syringe and start over.

➤ When opening ampules, protect yourself from injury.

➤ Use a filter needle or straw to withdraw medication from ampules; change to a needle of the proper length and gauge for administering the medication.

➤ When drawing up from a single-dose vial and ampule, draw up from the vial first.

➤ Do not use prefilled cartridges unless they have a safety device; transfer the medication to a syringe with a safety device before administering.

Continued

➤ Always recap a sterile needle using a safety capping device or the one-handed scoop method.

Procedure 23-10: Recapping Needles Using One-Handed Technique

Procedure 23-10A: Recapping Contaminated Needles

➤ Recap a contaminated needle only if you cannot avoid it.

➤ Do not place your nondominant hand near the needle cap when recapping the needle or engaging the safety mechanism.

➤ If you are using a safety needle, engage the safety mechanism to cover the needle.

➤ Place the needle cap in a mechanical recapping device if one is available.

➤ If recapping devices are not available and you must recap the needle for your own and/or the patient's safety, use the one-handed scoop technique or one of the methods in Procedure 23-10B.

Procedure 23-10B: Recapping Sterile Needles

➤ Be sure to keep the needle and cap sterile.

➤ Do not place your nondominant hand near the needle cap when recapping the needle or engaging the safety mechanism.

➤ Use one of the following methods:

   ➤ Place the needle cap in a medication cup, and recap the needle.

   ➤ Place the cap on a clean surface so that the end of the needle cap protrudes over the edge of the counter or shelf, and scoop with the needle.

   ➤ Use a hard syringe cover: Stand it on end; insert the needle cap into the cover, and then insert the needle.

   ➤ Place the needle cap on a sterile surface, such as on open alcohol prep pad, and use the one-handed scoop technique. This is the least desirable method.

Procedure 23-11: Administering Intradermal Medication

➤ Have appropriate antidotes for certain injections readily available before beginning the procedure.

➤ Know the location of resuscitation equipment in case of a life-threatening adverse reaction.

➤ Maintain sterile technique and standard precautions.

➤ Use a 1-mL syringe and a 25- to 28-gauge, 1/4- to 5/8-inch needle.

➤ Be aware that an intradermal dose is small, usually about 0.01 to 0.2 mL.

➤ Administer the injection on the ventral surface of the forearm, upper back, or upper chest.

➤ Hold the syringe parallel to the skin at a 5° to 15° angle, with the bevel up.

➤ Stretch the skin taut to insert the needle.

➤ Do not aspirate.

➤ Inject slowly, and create a wheal or bleb.

➤ Do not wipe the site with alcohol, massage, or bandage the site.

Procedure 23-12: Administering Subcutaneous Medication

➤ Maintain sterile technique and standard precautions.

➤ Use a 1-mL syringe and a 25- to 27-gauge needle that is less than 1 inch long (usually 3/8 to 5/8 in.).

➤ A subcutaneous dose is typically no more than 1 mL.

➤ Most common injection sites: Use the outer aspects of the upper arms, abdomen, and anterior aspects of the thighs.

➤ Pinch the skin to inject, as a general rule.

➤ For an average-weight or thin patient, inject at a 45° angle. For an obese patient, inject at a 90° angle; as a general rule, use a longer needle and spread the skin taut instead of pinching.

➤ Aspiration is optional for most medications, but do not aspirate when injecting heparin or insulin.

➤ Do not massage the site.

Procedure 23-13: Locating Intramuscular Injection Sites

➤ Always palpate the landmarks and the muscle mass to ensure correct placement.

Procedure 23-13A: Locating the Ventrogluteal Site

➤ On adults, a triangle is formed between your fingers when you place your palm on the head of the trochanter, index finger on the anterior superior iliac spine, and middle finger on the iliac crest. This is the preferred site for adults and children older than 7 months.

Procedure 23-13B: Locating the Deltoid Site

➤ The injection site is an inverted triangle on the upper arm. The base is two to three fingerbreadths below the acromion process, and the tip is even with the top of the axilla. This is a good site in healthy adults for small-volume injection, especially when other sites aren't easily accessible because of drains or dressings.

Procedure 23-13C: Locating the Vastus Lateralis Site

➤ Midlateral thigh: On adults, one handbreadth below the head of the trochanter and one handbreadth above the knee. The site is the middle third of this area. This is the preferred site for infants who are not walking.

Procedure 23-13D: Locating the Rectus Femoris Site

➤ Middle third of the anterior thigh. Use this site only if no others are accessible. It is more painful than other sites.

Procedure 23-14: Administering Intramuscular Injections

➤ Maintain sterile technique and standard precautions.

➤ Use a 1- to 5-mL syringe and a 21- to 25-gauge, 1- to 3-inch needle (longer needle if the patient is obese).

Critical Aspects of Procedures 23-1 through 23-18

- The usual volume is no more than 3 mL per injection.
- Select an appropriate injection site, and identify the site using anatomical landmarks:
  - The ventrogluteal site is preferred except in special circumstances (e.g., for many adult immunizations).
  - The deltoid site is acceptable for IM doses of 1 mL or less.
- Aspirate before injecting. If blood appears, withdraw the needle, discard it, and start over.
- Inject at a 90° angle.
- Z-track technique is recommended. Mnemonic:

Deliver	**D**isplace
All	**A**spirate
Injections	**I**nject (wait 5–10 seconds)
With	**W**ithdraw
Responsibility	**R**elease

Procedure 23-15: Adding Medication to Intravenous Fluids

- Check the compatibility of the IV solution and medication.
- Refer to agency policy regarding maximum number of meds that can be added to one IV solution.
- Assess the patency of the IV site.
- Maintain the sterility of IV fluids and medication admixture.
- Affix the medication label to the bag, with the name and amount of medication, date and time administered, and your name or initials.

Procedure 23-16: Administering IV Push Medication

- Determine the type and amount of dilution needed for the medication.
- Determine the amount of time needed to administer the medication.
- Ensure the patency of the line before administration.

- Flush the line before and after administering the medication.
- Maintain sterility.

Procedure 23-17: Administering Medications Intermittent Infusion

- Ensure the compatibility of the IV solution and medication—both the solution in the primary IV system and in the secondary system.
- Assess the IV site and the patency of the line.
- Calculate the amount of medication to add to the solution.
- Use the correct amount and type of diluent solution.
- Use the correct rate of administration.
- Determine the correct primary line port in which to infuse the medication.
- Affix the correct label to the secondary bag identifying the infusate, patient name, start date and hour, discard date and hour, and your initials.

Procedure 23-18: Administering Medication Through a Central Venous Access Device

- First verify the medication can safely be administered through a central site.
- Scrub all surfaces of the catheter port, including the extension "tail," using an alcohol or chlorhexidine–alcohol combination product every time you enter the line.
- Flush the line before and after administering medication. Use saline, heparinized flush solution, or solution from the infusing IV line.
- Frequency for flushing varies from once every 8 hours to once weekly.
- For multilumen catheters, flush all lumens.
- Clamp the line between the IV infusion set and the medication port. Open the clamp after medication is administered.
- After administration, monitor and report suspected CVAD dislodgement, line-related infection, or other complications.

 Go to Chapter 23, **Resources for Caregivers and Health Professionals,** on the Student Resource Disk or DavisPlus at http://davisplus.fadavis.com/Wilkinson2

 Suggested Readings: Go to Chapter 23, **Reading More About Administering Medications,** on the Student Resource Disk or DavisPlus at http://davisplus.fadavis.com/Wilkinson2

 Bibliography: Go to Volume 2, Bibliography.

CHAPTER 24

Teaching Clients

Learning Outcomes

After completing this chapter, you should be able to:

➤ Present three factors contributing to the expanding role of teaching in professional nursing.

➤ Describe the concepts of teaching and learning.

➤ Name, define, and give one example of each of Bloom's three domains of learning.

➤ Discuss how each of the following factors can affect learning: motivation, readiness, physical condition, emotions, timing, active involvement, feedback, repetition, environment, scheduling of the teaching session, amount and complexity of the content, communication, special needs (e.g., learning disability), developmental stage, culture, and literacy.

➤ List at least six barriers to teaching and learning.

➤ Describe some strategies for motivating learners.

➤ Develop strategies for working with clients with cultural or learning differences.

➤ Describe the content of a learning assessment.

➤ Discuss correct and incorrect uses of the nursing diagnosis Deficient Knowledge.

➤ Develop teaching plans for clients.

➤ List four methods for evaluating the outcomes of teaching and learning.

➤ Document teaching content, methods, and patient responses to learning.

Meet Your Patients

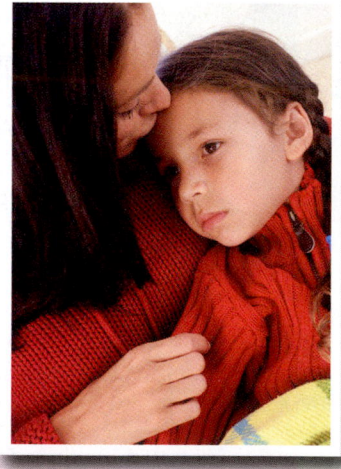

You are the student nurse assigned to Heather, a 20-year-old mother, and her 4-year-old preschooler. They have come to a family practice clinic for a well-child checkup. During the healthcare visit, you notice that the child speaks in one- or two-word phrases. The mother's tone to her daughter is impatient and she repeatedly tells her to "stop using that baby talk."

Heather says, "I don't know what I'm doing wrong. All her friends are taller and talking more. She was even small when she was born, so I suppose it's my fault."

Your assessment shows the child is below the 5th percentile for height and weight. What health teaching could you provide that might help resolve this problem? Your nursing instructor tells you to assess for teaching needs and provide anticipatory guidance to the mother. How would you begin to address Heather's learning needs without reinforcing her feelings of self-blame?

Your anticipatory guidance should include information about safety measures for a 4-year-old, nutrition for preschool-aged children, and expected growth and development. How can you evaluate whether or not the teaching has been effective and further promote Heather's retention of this new information?

By the time you finish working through this chapter, you should be able to answer these questions and provide teaching to meet the unique needs of other patients you encounter.

Theoretical **Knowledge** **knowing** why

Much of your work as a nurse will involve patient teaching. This has been true for well over 100 years—certainly since Florence Nightingale taught both nurses and patients about the value of good nutrition, fresh air, exercise, and personal hygiene (Nightingale, 1860/1992). Since that time, teaching has become progressively more important. The following are a few of the reasons why:

Patients Participate in Healthcare Decisions. Patients are taking responsibility for their own healthcare. Primary care providers expect patients to take an active role in making decisions about their health; patients and families need information so that they make *informed* decisions. You can help patients get answers to their questions, find resources, recognize problems, and develop self-care behaviors.

Hospital Stays are Brief. A great deal of complex care is being given in homes and the community. Patients are often sent home still needing medications, dressing changes, and skilled procedures, such as urinary catheterization. Nurses have a responsibility to teach family members how to provide care and to teach patients to care for themselves as they are able.

Healthcare is Expensive. Patient education can help to decrease the overall cost of healthcare. It does so by helping to increase patient compliance with medical and nursing regimens, which can shorten hospital stays and decrease frequency of medical treatments and admissions (Bastable, 2008).

As you may have guessed from the foregoing discussion, the basic purpose of teaching and learning is to provide information that will empower clients and families to (1) perform self-care, and (2) make informed decisions about their healthcare options. Like other interventions, you can use teaching to promote wellness, prevent or limit illness, restore health, adapt to changes in body function, and facilitate coping with stress, illness, and loss.

Who Are the Learners?

As a nurse, your learners are clients, families, and others who care for the client. You will often provide informal one-to-one teaching while performing other nursing interventions. For example, as you give a medication, you will teach about its therapeutic and side effects. Or you may do more formal teaching to groups of people. You might demonstrate a baby bath to a class of expectant parents.

You will find your learners wherever you work: hospital, an ambulatory setting, home care, or in the community. As a community health nurse, you would be more likely to teach large groups of people; for example,

you might teach a healthy lifestyles class to a group of teens.

As nurse, you will also be responsible for teaching healthcare workers whom you supervise. For example, you may instruct nursing assistive personnel when you observe an error in technique. Or you may help a new nurse learn how to use new equipment on the unit. Nurses in practice are also involved in clinical instruction of nursing students, new graduates, and other members of the healthcare team. Most of this teaching may be informal, although you might also present specific topics at unit meetings and conferences. For example, if there is a change in the agency's documentation system, you might teach a class to the nurses on your shift to learn the new system.

What Are My Teaching Responsibilities?

Teaching is a major component of clinical practice skills and is an independent nursing function. In many states, nurses' teaching role and responsibility is defined in the Nurse Practice Act.

The American Nurses Association (ANA). The *ANA Code of Ethics for Nurses with Interpretive Statements* (2001) purports that nurses are responsible for promoting and protecting health, safety, and rights of patients. Patient teaching is essential in fulfilling that responsibility.

ANA standards of practice (2010, in press), Standard 5B, states, "The registered nurse employs strategies to promote health and a safe environment." The following are the specific measurement criteria for that standard[1]:

- Provides health teaching that addresses such topics as healthy lifestyles, risk-reducing behaviors, developmental needs, activities of daily living, and preventive self-care.
- Uses health promotion and health teaching methods appropriate to the situation and the patient's values, beliefs, health practices, patient's developmental level, learning needs, readiness and ability to learn, language preference, spirituality, culture, and socioeconomic status.
- Seeks opportunities for feedback and evaluation of the effectiveness of the strategies used.

The Joint Commission. *The standards* require educators in healthcare organizations to consider the literacy, developmental and physical limitations, financial limitations, language barriers, culture, and religious practices of every patient. Teaching must also include any person who will be responsible for the patient's care (The Joint Commission, 2009).

---

[1]*Caveat*: This material is from the draft for public comment (ANA, 2010, in press); its wording may be changed somewhat in the final published version. For that version of the ANA Standards of Professional Nursing Practice, go to www.nursingworld.org.

The American Hospital Association (AHA). The AHA "*Patient Care Partnership*" (previously the "Patient's Bill of Rights") that describes in simple language the right of patients to receive high-quality care. Patient rights include a clean and safe environment; protection of privacy; complete and current information about their diagnosis, treatment, and prognosis; information communicated in ways they can understand; and the right to be informed of hospital policies and practices that relate to them (American Hospital Association [AHA], 2003).

What Are Some Basic Learning Concepts and Principles?

The educational process consists of both teaching and learning. **Teaching** is an interactive process that involves planning and implementing instructional activities to meet intended learner outcomes or providing activities that allow the learner to learn (Bastable, 2008). Teachers must have effective communication skills to (1) adequately convey information, (2) assess verbal and nonverbal feedback, and (3) accommodate various learning styles. In patient education, nurses can use teaching, counseling, and behavioral modification together to achieve effective client learning.

Learning is a change in behavior, knowledge, skills, or attitudes. It occurs as a result of planned or spontaneously occurring situations, events, or exposures. *Conscious, goal-oriented learning* is intended and deliberate. It involves motivation to learn. Learning can occur in a rote manner, informally by circumstance, by formal instruction, or by a combination of approaches. It is not enough for the teacher to give the person written or verbal information; information alone will not change behaviors. Box 24-1 summarizes some basic principles of learning and provides a quick check for planning teaching sessions. For information about learning theories,

Go to Chapter 24, **Supplemental Materials: Learning Theories,** on the Student Resource Disk or DavisPlus at http://davisplus.fadavis.com/Wilkinson2

KnowledgeCheck 24-1

- Identify at least three reasons why nurses have a responsibility to teach clients.
- Define *teaching*.
- Define *learning*.

Go to Chapter 24, **Knowledge Check Response Sheet and Answers,** on the Student Resource Disk or DavisPlus at http://davisplus.fadavis.com/Wilkinson2

Learning Occurs in Three Domains

People learn in three ways, or *domains:* cognitive, psychomotor, and affective (Bloom & Krathwohl, 1956). You should include each of these domains, involving think-

---

> ### BOX 24-1 ■ Five Rights of Teaching
>
> When you are making a teaching plan, you can use this as a checklist to ensure that you consider each of the five "rights" of teaching in the plan.
>
> **Right Time**
> - Is the learner ready, free of pain and anxiety, and motivated?
> - Have you and the learner a trusting relationship?
> - Have you set aside sufficient time for the teaching session?
>
> **Right Context**
> - Is the environment quiet, free of distractions, and private?
> - Is the environment soothing or stimulating, depending on the desired effect?
>
> **Right Goal**
> - Is the learner actively involved in planning the learning objectives?
> - Are you and your client both committed to reaching mutually set goals of learning that achieve the desired behavioral changes?
> - Are family or friends included in planning so that they can help follow through on behavioral changes?
> - Are the learning objectives realistic and valued by the client; do they reflect the client's lifestyle?
>
> **Right Content**
> - Is the content appropriate for the client's needs?
> - Is it new information or reinforcement of information that has already been provided?
> - Is the content presented at the learner's level?
> - Does the content relate to the learner's life experiences or is it otherwise relevant to the learner?
>
> **Right Method**
> - Do the teaching strategies fit the learning style of the learner?
> - Do the strategies fit the client's learning ability?
> - Are the teaching strategies varied?

ing, doing, and feeling/caring, when writing objectives and planning teaching and evaluation strategies, which are discussed later in this chapter. Table 24-1 provides examples of client learning in each of the domains. For a more detailed version of this table, which identifies levels of behavior associated with each domain,

Go to Chapter 24, **Tables, Boxes, Figures: ESG Table 24-1,** on the Student Resource Disk or DavisPlus at http://davisplus.fadavis.com/Wilkinson2

Cognitive Learning

Cognitive learning includes storing and recalling information in the brain. Ranging from simple to complex

Table 24-1 ➤ Bloom's Domains of Learning

DOMAIN AND LEVELS OF BEHAVIOR	EXAMPLES
Cognitive (thinking) Includes memorization, recall, comprehension, and ability to analyze, synthesize, apply, and evaluate ideas.	A client is able to report the names and doses of the three medications he is taking. A client explains the expected effect of the medication she has been prescribed. A client designs a planned schedule for dressing changes for a wound on her leg. A client describes how to distinguish between normal inflammation and signs of infection in a wound. A client recognizes the need for behavioral changes to decrease the chance of recurrence of infection.
Psychomotor (skills) Includes sensory awareness of cues involved in learning, as well as imitation and performance of skills and creation of new skills.	A client identifies that he needs to read directions before starting a project. A client brings personal equipment to a teaching session. A new mother follows the instructor who is demonstrating diapering of her newborn, imitating her movements. A new father is observed diapering his newborn after observing a demonstration. A client independently changes her complex dressing. The wound heals with no signs of infection. A client with limited vision creates a new approach to giving his daily injections.
Affective (feelings) Includes receiving and responding to new ideas, demonstrating commitment to or preference for new ideas, and integrating new ideas into a value system.	An adolescent makes eye contact with the nurse as she explains the admission process. A client asks questions about what to expect during a procedure he is to undergo. A parent of a child who has just been admitted to the hospital expresses commitment to staying with her child after the nurse explains the impact of hospitalization. A client who has overcome drug addiction chooses to present his story to high school groups.

Adapted from Bloom, B. S., Mesia, B. B., & Krathwohl, D. R. (1964). Taxonomy of educational objectives (Vol. 1: *The affective domain* and Vol. 2: *The cognitive domain*). New York: David McKay; Bloom B. S., & Krathwohl, D. R. (1956). Taxonomy of educational objectives: The classification of educational goals. *Handbook I: Cognitive domain.* New York: Longmans, Green.

processes, it encompasses six levels of behavior: memorization, recall, comprehension and analysis, synthesis, application, and evaluation of ideas (Table 24-1). Strategies and tools to support teaching cognitive-type content include lectures, reading materials, panel discussions, audiovisual materials, programmed instruction, computer-assisted instruction (CAI), and problem-based learning (e.g., case studies and care plans).

Psychomotor Learning

Psychomotor learning involves learning a skill that requires both mental and physical activity. It requires the learner to accept and value the skill (the affective domain) as well as know about the skill (the cognitive domain). Strategies and tools used to teach psychomotor skills include demonstration and return demonstration, simulation models, audiovisual materials (e.g., DVDs, streaming video), journaling and self-reflection, and printed materials (especially with photographs and illustrations).

Affective Learning

Affective learning involves changes in feelings, beliefs, attitudes, and values. It is considered the "feeling domain." Levels of affective behavior are shown in Table 24-1. Strategies and tools for promoting affective learning include role modeling, group work, panel discussion, role playing, mentoring, one-to-one counseling and discussion, audiovisual materials (e.g., DVDs, streaming video, interactive computer-based modules, movies), and printed materials.

Anderson and Krathwohl (2001) adapted Bloom's model describing learning using a more outcomes-based approach, including the following domains:

Remember
Understand
Apply
Analyze
Evaluate
Create

KnowledgeCheck 24-2

- What are the three domains of learning?
- What strategies and tools are used to promote learning within each of the three domains of learning?
- Give an example of each of the domains of learning.

  Go to Chapter 24, **Knowledge Check Response Sheet and Answers,** on the Student Resource Disk or DavisPlus at http://davisplus.fadavis.com/Wilkinson2

CriticalThinking 24-1

By now, you have probably already learned how to assess a patient's blood pressure (BP).

- Think about how you were taught to perform that *skill*. What would have been the best way for *you* to learn to take a BP? To read a book and look at the photos closely? To watch a DVD? To have someone tell you how to do it? To have someone demonstrate the skill? Perform the blood pressure measurement yourself? Some other way?
- Now think about the *principles* involved with BP (e.g., normal ranges, the physiological regulation of the BP). What, for you, would have been the best way to learn the principles? Read a book? Listen to a lecture? Physically obtain a BP reading for a patient? Work a case involving BP? Some other way?
- From your answers to the two preceding questions, what (if anything) can you conclude about different domains of learning and the kinds of activities to use in teaching and learning in each domain?

Many Factors Affect Client Learning

Learning is complex. Many factors can either enhance or interfere with it. An understanding of the following factors will help you to design effective teaching interventions and promote client learning.

Motivation

Motivation is desire from within. It is created by an idea, a physical need, an emotion, or some other kind of force. Without motivation, little learning can occur. Motivation is greatest when clients recognize the need for learning, believe it is possible to improve their health, and are interested in the information they are being given. Think about classes you have taken. Have you studied harder in some than in others? What motivated you? Was it because you were intrigued by the information, wanted to earn a good grade or the approval of the instructor, or had other incentives?

Motivation may be based on physical and social needs, the need for task mastery or success, and health beliefs. In your teaching, try to apply the following principles for motivating learners.

- Conveying your interest in and respect for the learner and the learning process helps to motivate the learner.
- Creating a warm, friendly environment can enhance social needs motivation, as can your enthusiasm.

- You can sometimes motivate clients by helping them identify a physical need. For example, Heather ("Meet Your Patient") may not be aware that her child is at risk for accidents and injury from home hazards. Helping her to understand the normal behavior of a 4-year-old may help her to see the need for child-proofing her home.
- The need for achievement and competence is related to task mastery and self-efficacy. When a person succeeds at a task, he is usually motivated to continue learning. Rewards and incentives can provide this type of motivation.
- The client will be motivated to learn only if she believes that health is important. For example, Heather may understand that a 4-year-old likes to explore and may recognize there are safety hazards in the home; however, she will not be motivated to learn safety measures if her attitude is that "it is no big deal."

Many of the following factors also provide motivation as well as contributing in other ways to learning.

Readiness

Readiness is the demonstration of behaviors that indicate the learner is both *motivated* and *able* to learn *at a specific time*. For instance, a client may not be "ready" for teaching right before scheduled diagnostic tests or invasive treatments because anxiety makes it difficult to focus on the material. In addition, readiness for learning includes the physical and emotional capacity to take in, process, and recall information.

Physical Condition

Physical factors (e.g., pain, strength, coordination, energy, senses, mobility) and intact cognition contribute to a patient's readiness to learn. You must consider them in your planning. For example:

- Pain interferes with the ability to concentrate on the material the nurse presents.
- The client needs adequate strength, coordination, energy, and mobility to demonstrate psychomotor learning.
- You will need to adapt your teaching and evaluation strategies to accommodate clients with impaired hearing or vision.

Emotions

Emotions are another aspect of readiness. Severe anxiety, stress, or emotional pain interfere with the ability to learn. In addition, the learning itself, and the idea that behaviors must be changed, can create anxiety. However, a mild level of anxiety can enhance learning by providing motivation. For example, a client newly diagnosed with diabetes may not be experiencing physical complications related to the disease, so he may not be interested in learning about diabetes. You may be able to motivate him (i.e., create some anxiety) by pointing out the potential and serious complications (e.g., blindness, kidney damage) of uncontrolled diabetes. Provoke mild anxiety carefully so the client does not interpret your words as a threat or excessive negativity.

Timing

You must present information at a time when the learner is open to learning. Timing is therefore related to readiness, and it is important in the following ways, as well.

- People retain information better when they have an opportunity to use it soon after it is presented. For example, a student reads about insulin in her textbook and takes a test on the content 2 weeks later. Another student reads the same information and during the 2 weeks also administers different types of insulin to several patients. The second student will have an advantage at test time.
- For some concepts, the learner might need more time to be able to absorb and apply information, especially when more complex thinking is required.

Active Involvement

Learning is more meaningful when the client is actively engaged in the planning and the learning activities. Learners retain 10% of what they read, but they retain 90% of what they speak and do (London, 1999). Passive listening is not typically as effective for processing and retaining information as activities involving more than one style of learning. For instance, a demonstration with a return demonstration and a patient education brochure is often a better way to teach patients how to perform a new skill. Demonstration is particularly effective for kinesthetic learners (which most adults are). Can you think of other examples of learning that involve multiple senses?

Feedback

Feedback is information about the learner's performance. For example, a test grade is feedback for students, conveying the message, "You need to work on that content some more," or "You have successfully mastered the lesson." Feedback in the clinical setting or skills lab might be, "You consistently maintained sterile technique." Positive feedback encourages learners and boosts morale when it comes to tackling difficult content or devoting the time and effort needed to get the most out of the educational process. This is especially critical when significant behavioral changes are required to be a successful learner. Patients, too, tend to respond well to positive interaction while learning. For example, the patient teaching experience reinforces the patient with a new ostomy who successfully changes her appliance or a patient with diabetes who learns to correctly draw up a mixed insulin dose. Sometimes you may need to act like a coach, encouraging the learner with frequent feedback and praise and suggesting alternatives. When teaching, you may sometimes need to point out errors, but do so in a positive way when you can. Be careful not to seem judgmental when clients are learning a new skill or are giving home care. Fear of failure or judgment can be a serious barrier to learning at what could be the patient's most teachable moment.

Repetition

The client is more likely to retain information and incorporate it into his life if the content is repeated. Each time the learner hears the information, the likelihood of retention increases. For example, often patients forget what medication is prescribed for certain conditions. Repeating the name of the drug can help patients better remember it. This is especially true for learning psychomotor skills. Do you remember the first time you counted a radial pulse? Even that simple skill may have been difficult at first. By now it is probably very easy for you.

 Critical**Thinking** 24-2

Use examples from your own experience, if you can. Do not use examples you have read in the preceding sections.

- Give an example to illustrate the importance of relevance in learning.
- Give an example to illustrate the importance of repetition in learning.
- Give an example to illustrate the importance of timing in learning.

Learning Environment

For most people, an ideal learning environment is private, quiet, physically and psychologically comfortable, and free from distractions. Have you ever tried to concentrate on a lecture right after lunch when you were sitting in a warm, stuffy room? Or when someone is talking or texting you via cell phone? However, keep in mind that some learners are best motivated and engaged when teaching occurs in a group situation. Social learners can be distracted from the task when alone in a quiet space.

When you are planning a teaching session, provide good lighting and comfortable seating that is conducive for conversations. Have your teaching materials ready at hand to avoid gaps in the teaching session. If you have an area that is set aside for teaching, try to use inspirational or motivational accessories (e.g., photographs, posters).

A quiet, private space is ideal for teaching, but sometimes there is none available. You can at least try to find a quiet corner, pull the bed curtain shut, close the door, or sit close to the client so that you can talk softly (Fig. 24-1). Make the best of what you have to work with.

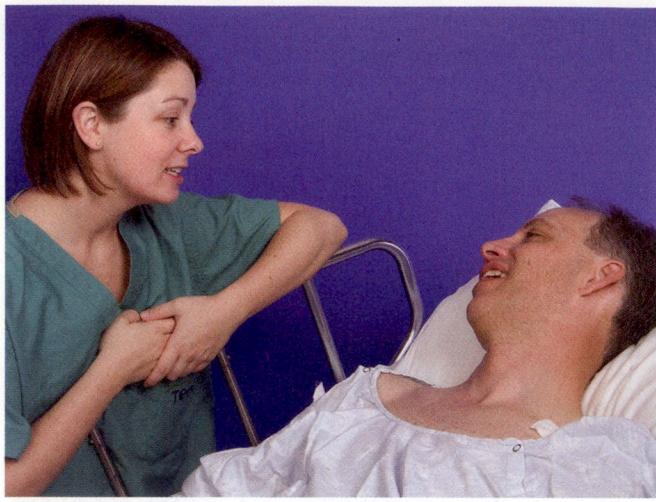

FIGURE 24-1 To provide privacy, sit or stand close to the patient so that you can talk privately.

Scheduling the Session

Plan for uninterrupted time to allow you to adequately assess and understand the client. The teaching time doesn't need to be long, just uninterrupted. Based on the client's condition (e.g., activity intolerance, attention span, fatigue, pain), shorter teaching sessions may be best for comprehension and retention. Finding suitable time to teach can be a challenge, but a moment can be a teaching session, as shown in Box 24-2.

Amount and Complexity of Content

The more complex or detailed the content, the more difficult it is for most people to learn and retain, as you probably know from your own learning experiences. For example, imagine teaching parents about the need for isolation precautions for their newborn who has just

BOX 24-2 ■ Teachable Moments

A student nurse walks into her patient's room. This week in class she has been studying patient teaching. Her instructor has informed the students that she expects them to incorporate teaching into each clinical day. But the student ponders, "I am way too busy to find time to teach. What am I going to do?" Later in the day, she asks the nurse who is co-assigned to her client for suggestions. The nurse questions the student: "Did you take the patient's blood pressure?" When the student answers that she did, the nurse says, "Did you explain why you were doing that and what the BP readings mean?" Again the student says, "Yes." The nurse asks, "When you gave your patient his medications, did you explain why you are giving each one and the common side effects?" The student says, "Yes," and a light dawns! The student begins to understand that almost every patient contact presents an opportunity for teaching and that teaching can be fit into a short time frame.

been diagnosed with a profound immune disorder. In comparison, teaching parents of a healthy newborn about the recommended immunization schedule would be far less challenging.

In addition, the greater the change, the greater the challenge for both teacher and client. For example, a client rehabilitating after a stroke who has to relearn using eating utensils, swallowing, and other basic tasks for daily hygiene and self-care will experience a more intense learning challenge than one who has to learn only a daily schedule for taking medications.

Communication

Communication is central to the teaching and learning process in which teachers and learners communicate information, perceptions, and feelings. Barriers to communication include pain, anxiety, fatigue, illness, hunger, dysfunctional relationships, language differences, vision and hearing impairment, cultural factors, and various environmental issues, such as noise and distraction. Attend carefully to verbal and nonverbal feedback that the client gives; it can tell you whether or not the learner is attentive and focusing on the learning activities. For more information about communication, see Chapter 18.

CriticalThinking 24-3

A client who has a brain injury needs to learn how to administer insulin. Another learner, who must learn to change a wound dressing, has attention-deficit/hyperactivity disorder (ADHD).

■ How do you think these clients' health status might affect:
  1. Their motivation to learn?
  2. Their ability to be actively involved in the learning?
■ What approaches or changes might you need to make in:
  1. The learning environment?
  2. The timing of the teaching session?
  3. The use of repetition?
  4. Your communication?
  5. The amount and complexity of content presented in a session?
  6. Your use of feedback?
  7. The amount of teacher support?

Special Populations

For clients who have special needs (e.g., those with learning disabilities, attention deficit disorder, mental illness, affective or communication disorders, mental illness, or brain injury) you must plan carefully to ensure that you use appropriate strategies to maximize learning. Consider a variety of teaching approaches— one size does not fit all. For example, you may need to use brief, frequent learning sessions or pay special attention to minimizing distracting stimuli in the environment. Or you may need to present information slowly, use repetition, and be satisfied with slower progress. The adaptations you make will depend on the nature of the special need, so if you are not familiar with the patient's condition, you must acquire theoretical knowledge of it. Include a family member, caregiver, or other significant person in the teaching to reinforce the learning and act as a safety net for implementing the information.

Developmental Stage

An understanding of intellectual development will help you to gear your teaching strategies and content to the level of the learner. When teaching psychomotor skills, you will need to assess the person's fine and gross motor development. For example, a young child may not have adequate fine motor skills to complete a skill such as tying shoes without assistance (Fig. 24-2). If you would like to review an extensive discussion of intellectual development, including Piaget's theory (1966),

 Go to Chapter 9, **Expanded Discussion,** on the Student Resource Disk or DavisPlus at http://davisplus.fadavis.com/ Wilkinson2

Stages of Cognitive Development

Piaget identified three stages of cognitive development that are especially important in client teaching in the cognitive domain:

- **The Preoperational Stage** (2 to 7 years old), in which the child begins to acquire language skills and find meaning through use of symbols and pictures.
- **The Stage of Concrete Operations** (7 to 11 years old), in which the child learns best by manipulating concrete, tangible objects and can classify objects in two or more ways (e.g., identify a shape as a triangle and also as green). Logical thinking begins, and the child can understand the relationship between numbers and the idea of reversibility. He also can begin to recognize and adapt to the perspective of others.
- **The Formal Operational Stage** (age 11 years or older), in which the person can use abstract thinking and deductive reasoning. The person can relate general

FIGURE 24-2 When teaching psychomotor skills, consider the person's gross and fine motor development.

concepts to specific situations, consider alternatives, begin to establish values, and try to find meaning in life. Not everyone reaches this stage, including some adults.

Always assess cognitive development. For clients who have not achieved the stage of formal operations, use examples instead of definitions; use concrete rather than abstract terms.

Teaching Older Adults

When teaching older adults, consider the numerous factors that can adversely affect the teaching. Possible barriers include vision and hearing impairments, illness, pain, reduced social interaction, reduced mobility, medication effects, sensory deficit, sociocultural factors, and a noisy or chaotic environment. Allow extra time for teaching, and stop occasionally for rest periods. Assess for sensory deficits (e.g., hearing and vision) and adapt your style according to any restrictions. Use large print for the visual aids, and repeat information as necessary. Refer to Table 24-2 for some principles that apply specifically to adult learners as well as tips for effectively teaching older adults.

Teaching Children

When you work with children, use strategies to gain trust, reduce their anxiety, promote cooperation, and enhance their emotional readiness to learn. For instance, for a child who needs surgery, schedule a tour of the hospital at least 1 week before the admission date, and introduce the child to staff members and other patients of the same age (if possible). Have the child practice breathing exercises or other aspects of tests or treatments that he will be involved in. With the parents' permission, provide the child with ice cream or other food, game, or material "reward," and give the child a coloring book or other item about the upcoming surgery to take home.

If you are teaching a child in the preoperational stage or an adult with limited intellectual development, you will need to simplify the content and use pictures and concrete examples. For example, there is little point in going into detail with a preschooler regarding the rationale for taking an antibiotic. Instead, tell the child that the medicine will keep her from getting sick; use pictures of a child drinking from a medicine cup, or provide a calendar that the child can mark each time she takes a dose. A reward system is often an effective way of improving compliance.

Cultural Factors

Awareness of norms, values communication, social structure, time orientation, and cultural identification are important in planning teaching (see Chapter 13 to review these concepts). If English is not the client's primary language, you may need to use an interpreter. The bottom line is that cultural sensitivity involves respect for clients' identity and needs, regardless of who they are, where they're from, how they speak,

Table 24-2 ➤ Incorporating Principles of Adult Learning into the Teaching of Older Adults

CHARACTERISTICS OF ADULT LEARNERS, PARTICULARLY OLDER ADULTS	TIPS FOR TEACHING OLDER ADULTS
Adults are independent and self-directed learners.	Help them to identify their own learning needs.
Adults must recognize the need to learn before they become willing to learn.	Explain why the information or new skill is important. Be sure to include materials with practical tips and realistic goals for learning.
Some older adults may be afraid of the learning process because of (1) fear of failure, (2) past unsatisfactory experiences with educational processes, (3) not having participated in formal education for many years, or (4) feeling that "being taught" is for children.	Present content in a nonthreatening environment, where there is no risk of judgment or embarrassment in front of peers. Offer feedback (evaluation) simply to improve important skills and not for the sake of a grade. Remember the intent of patient education is to improve clinical outcome. Privacy is often necessary.
Adults are more motivated to learn if they think they will be able to use the information or skills immediately.	Plan the teaching session at the time of greatest need. That is, hold the teaching session close to the time the patient will need the information or need to perform a new skill.
Adults prefer to be partners in the learning process—to have some control over what they learn and how they learn it.	Encourage learners to tell you first what they intend to gain from the educational session. You might spell out the goals of your session in advance and allow the learner to customize it.
Adults have previous life experiences that can enhance learning.	Relate new content to past experiences and knowledge and have learners use their experiences to solve problems. Encourage older adults to share life experiences.
Many adult learners do well when a hands-on approach is used. Older adults must practice a new skill, or rehearse new information, in order to learn it.	Offer active participation and opportunities for interaction with instructor and other learners. Demonstrations and practical tips are useful for adult learners, particularly older adults.
Many older adult learners need to review new information away from the initial learning environment in order to retain it. It might not be until later that information sinks in.	Use take-home materials, such as colorful posters, table tents, and tip sheets, and patient-friendly brochures to reinforce information.
Messages are best received when they are part of the real-life experience.	In the teacher role, model the message you are conveying to your audience. "Walk the walk" and not just "talk the talk."
Some older adults may feel threatened by the need to learn new information. They may feel, "I've gotten along just fine all these years without needing to know that; why should I learn it now?" Or they may believe that they are "too old to learn." These attitudes may be defenses to avoid failure or to resist change.	Work with the learner to establish the "need to know" at the onset of the program. Involve the learner in defining what he or she intends to gain from the educational session. Reassure the learner about the importance of the information and encourage the learner to tackle a little at a time.
Some older adults learn better when they are not overwhelmed with multiple needs, topics, or skills at one time.	Introduce only a few topics at a time. Usually tackling one to three new topics or skills is enough. Identify what is the most important information for your learner to walk away with. Define those topics and cover them well. Remember, slow and steady wins the race, especially when it comes to learning information that is essential to the patient's health.
Changes in visual distance, depth, acuity, and light perception occur with aging, thus diminishing the ability to take in information. Older adults experience increased sensitivity to glare and reduced color perception with aging. Processing of sensory information is also slower in the latter decades of life.	(1) Avoid colors such as blue, green, and lavender, because they are difficult for older adults to differentiate. (2) Remove physical barriers that could compromise the field of vision, such as projector position, tables, and so on. (3) In teaching materials, choose fonts that are bold, black, and a minimum size of 18-point. Fancy lettering is harder to decipher. (4) A nonglare background without a stylized pattern is easier to see and process than complex designs. (5) For those who cannot read or who have severe visual impairment, consider recording instructional material.
Reduced hearing acuity is common in older adults. Auditory perception for various tones and filtration of extraneous noise also diminish with age.	(1) Speak slowly, using a normal tone of voice. If you must speak more loudly than normal, be careful not to sound demeaning as though speaking to a child. You don't want learners to perceive annoyance in your tone. (2) Many older adults do some lip reading, although they may be unaware of it. You can facilitate lip reading by not distorting your facial features by exaggerated pronunciation. (3) Provide a quiet setting and decrease background noise. Close the door or windows if outside noise interferes with the teaching/learning experience.

Table 24-2 ➤ Incorporating Principles of Adult Learning into the Teaching of Older Adults—cont'd

CHARACTERISTICS OF ADULT LEARNERS, PARTICULARLY OLDER ADULTS	TIPS FOR TEACHING OLDER ADULTS
Older adult learners can be distracted and annoyed by cellular phones and other electronic devices.	Request phones, radios, or other electronic devices are turned off for the educational session. Turn your own phone off, as well!
Older adults may be socially less active and might perceive bias, ageism, or isolation.	As for any group of people, it is essential to honor cultural backgrounds, local customs and practices, and personal preferences.
Because of some short-term memory loss that occurs with aging, some older adults learn better when they have a source of supplemental information or support.	Reinforce your teaching with follow-up opportunities and connections to the community for information and support in grasping new information or acquiring a new skill.
Older individuals may bring family members or other caregivers to the teaching session to help interpret or remember information presented. Sometimes the extra people in the room can be noisy and distracting to the patient's learning situation.	If they are distracting, it may be helpful to ask others in the room to minimize other conversations, or in some circumstances, to leave the room for a time.
Older adult learners can be particularly affected by fatigue, illness, medication, pain, stress, and other personal factors.	Be sure to plan the teaching session when the patient is well rested, pain-free as possible, and comfortable.
Many older adults were raised in an era when learning occurred primarily through the reading, discussion, and retelling of stories. Technology was not as prevalent as today.	Use informal teaching sessions that include storytelling. Tie the patient's past experiences to what you are teaching. To elicit stories, you must be a patient and empathetic listener. Keep your stories short. Ask open-ended questions and be willing to wait for the answer. Convey your genuine interest in your learners before sharing personal stories. Allow more time for older adults, especially those with chronic illness, to tell their own stories.

how old they are, what religion they practice or not, whether disabled or not, how much wealth or poverty they experience, how much they weigh, how socially popular they are, or any other aspect that can lead to unfair treatment. Box 24-3 highlights key concepts of teaching with a culturally competent approach.

Health Literacy

Health literacy is the ability to understand basic health information and services needed to make appropriate healthcare decisions (*Healthy People 2020*, 2009). On the contrary, **health illiteracy** occurs when the language spoken is not the patient's preferred language (i.e., limited English proficiency). Or perhaps the format through which the information is communicated is not suited to the patient. For example, if the patient has a hearing impairment and discharge teaching is done verbally, then a communication gap can occur. A gap in health literacy results when a healthcare provider uses medical terminology that is unfamiliar or misunderstood by the patient, thus resulting in an unintended message or lack of meaningful information. Limited health literacy is more common among the medically underserved community, minority populations, and older adults. Patients with low health literacy might have difficulty taking medication as prescribed or managing complex or chronic health problems. They are not as likely to

understand the connection between risky behavior and health.

In light of the high number of people in the United States who cannot read and/or write English, reading literacy is yet another significant barrier interfering with the communication between patients and healthcare providers. These patients would not be as likely to communicate health history to the provider or complete lengthy forms for obtaining healthcare. Patients with limited reading proficiency in English might not be able to grasp information in health-related brochures or printed discharge instructions. To enhance understanding between you and your patients, refer to Box 24-4, which presents tips for promoting health literacy.

Barriers to Teaching and Learning

As you gain experience in teaching, you will learn to recognize the factors we have just discussed (e.g., timing, the environment) and to manipulate those that can be changed to enhance the teaching and learning experience. At the same time, take care to avoid factors that act as outright barriers to teaching/learning.

In a study about barriers influencing online learning for students, the highest rated problem revolved around the lack of social interactions when learning outside the traditional classroom. Poor learner motivation, time issues, and technical problems also contribute to student dissatisfaction with the online learning environment.

Teaching Plan

Client Data

Emily O'Connor is the APN in charge of the student health center on campus at State University. A research project by one of her nursing students last semester revealed that only 35% of women surveyed on campus performed monthly breast self-examination (BSE). Emily has decided to teach students and interested campus staff members about the importance of BSE and the proper technique. To reinforce the content information, Ms. O'Connor develops handouts with pictures and charts to make them more visually appealing. She also follows one of the first principles of adult motivation: Provide food, so people who are not a captive audience (as hospitalized patients are) will have an additional reason to attend.

Nursing Diagnosis

Deficient Knowledge (health behaviors) about BSE as evidenced by campus-wide survey results showing that only 35% of women performed monthly BSE.

NOC Outcome

Knowledge: Health Behavior (1805)

NIC Intervention

Teaching: Group (5604)

Teaching Environment

1. Provide an environment conducive to learning. Promote relaxation by making personal introductions and offering refreshments during break time.

Rationale: When adult learners are in an environment in which they feel comfortable, they are less distracted and more able to learn. Physical and emotional comfort of the participants is important for creating a positive atmosphere for adult learning. The environment influences a learner's interest level and actual motivation acquire new knowledge (Rankin & Stallings, 2004).

Overall Strategy / Approach

1. Focus on real-world problems.
2. Emphasize application of content to everyday life.
3. Relate content to life experience.
4. Explain how the education will solve a problem.
5. Involve learners in the educational process.
6. Use a variety of methodologies.

Rationale: Utilizes principles of adult learning. Using a variety of methodologies is important because different people learn in different ways.

Instructional Materials

1. Printed materials (brochures, fact sheets)

Rationale: Print materials at an appropriate reading level for the target audience allow participants to review information when it is convenient for them. In a study looking at the effectiveness of five different types of media (print paperback booklet, online booklet, spoken audio files, audio with text Web page, and Flash) for improving patient's learning, findings show that although participants preferred multimedia presentations, patients retained information using supplementary materials regardless of form the content was presented in (Bader & Strickman-Stein, 2003).

Teaching Plan (continued)

Instructional Materials

2. Videotape (DVD) of BSE

Rationale: In a study investigating the effectiveness of videotape for women learning to perform BSE, findings indicate use of an educational videotape increased the frequency of BSE among premenopausal women (Janda, Stanek, Newman, et al., 2002). Another study examining the effectiveness of using DVD to teach clinical skills to medical students found highly significant improvement in outcomes as compared to the group who received instruction through the traditional didactic method (Lee, Boyd, & Stuart, 2007).

3. Flash or other interactive multimedia (animation, narration, and text) on computer, to accompany PowerPoint slides.

Rationale: In one study, participants learning about lung cancer received instruction in five forms, and 71% ranked the Flash presentation as their preferred format for learning (Bader & Strickman-Stein, 2003). Women who participated in an interactive multimedia educational program about breast cancer perceived breast cancer to be a more personally important health issue, learned more and reported less anxiety about cancer screening than did women learning from written materials. It is no longer sufficient to ask the question of whether various forms of educational media are effective or not but rather look carefully at the quality of the media and software for meeting learners' needs. These researchers have clearly demonstrated that not all multimedia are created equal (Wiljer & Catton, 2003).

Learning Objective	Schedule/ Sequence	Content	Teaching Strategy
By the end of the first educational session, participants will be able to explain why BSE is important.	April 1–8	**1.** Determine date, time, and content of class to be held.	Advertise the educational session by using posters on campus, the campus newspaper, newsletter, and e-mail blasts.
	April 9 6:30–7:00 P.M.	**2.** Social hour. Dessert and beverages. Get acquainted.	
	7:00–7:30 P.M.	**3.** Identify risk factors for breast cancer.	Lecture with slides
		4. Discuss current treatments for breast cancer.	
		5. Describe how BSE helps with early diagnosis, enhancing chances for cure.	
	7:30–7:50 P.M.	**6.** Provide thorough instruction on BSE technique.	Videotaped demonstration of BSE
	7:50–8:00 P.M.	**7.** Promote awareness and incorporate reminders in follow-up contact with participants.	Questions and answers
	8:00–9:00 P.M.	**8.** Provide optional practice and/or online program on BSE.	Set up an online program on three computers for participants to use before and after the formal class hour.

Rationale: Content is based on the Health Belief Model, designed by the U.S. Public Health Service. It identifies four key factors that promote health-seeking behavior (adapted for this setting): (1) Person perceives she is at risk for disease (breast cancer). (2) Person perceives the disease is harmful and has serious consequences. (3) Person believes the suggested intervention is of value. (4) Person believes treatment (screening), effectiveness is worth overcoming barriers to treatment (screening) (Clarke-Tasker & Wade, 2002; Rankin, Stallings, & London, 2004; The Communication Initiative [TCI], 2003).

(continued on next page)

Teaching Plan (continued)

Evaluation

Eighteen women attended the session. When Ms. O'Connor began the educational session, participants were seated in chairs facing the front of the room, where the screen was set up for a PowerPoint presentation. She distributed the handout materials and provided a short introduction. Before she began teaching, two women asked questions about breast cancer and screening tests. Three women shared stories about friends and family members who had breast biopsies. One had a question about mammograms. During this discussion, the women turned their chairs to face each other and talked among themselves. When there was a lull in the discussion, one of the participants said she thought she had a lump and was too scared to do anything about it.

Ms. O'Connor realized that learning takes place when participants share stories with facilitation by the group leader. Teaching does not have to be led exclusively by the facilitator. Even though she had a teaching plan, she was flexible enough to modify the plan to meet participants' needs. She turned off the projector, turned on the lights, and, instead of lecturing, she shared information by answering questions and guiding the discussion.

During this process, Ms. O'Connor realized she had made assumptions about the participants' goals for this educational program and their educational needs. She learned that the women who attended came to the program with an understanding of risk factors for breast cancer; they knew that the disease is serious and that interventions are valuable. They wanted to talk about their fears, concerns, and questions; they wanted to separate myths from facts; and they wanted to learn proper technique and how they could remember to do monthly BSE.

After the session, Ms. O'Connor realized that she needed to revise her plan and hold a second session in a week or two. Her assumption that a lack of knowledge was responsible for the low number of women performing BSE was not confirmed by discussion with the women. She developed new goals for the second session:

1. By the end of the educational intervention, participants will:
   a. State that questions about breast cancer have been addressed.
   b. Share strategies for overcoming barriers to performing BSE.
   c. Identify the role anxiety plays as a barrier to BSE.
   d. List steps to follow if a lump or other abnormality is identified.
2. At the 1-year follow-up point, participants will report that they performed monthly BSE in 10 of the last 12 months.

References

Bader, J. L., & Strickman-Stein, N. (2003). Evaluation of new multimedia formats for cancer communications. *Journal of Medical Internet Research, 5*(3), e16.

Clarke-Tasker, V. A., & Wade, R. (2002, May–June). What we thought we knew: African American males' perception of prostate cancer and screening methods [electronic version]. *Association of Black Nursing Faculty Journal, 13*(3), 56–60.

Janda, M., Stanek, C., Newman, B., Obermair, A., & Trimmel, M. (2002). Impact of videotaped information on frequency and confidence of breast self-examination. *Breast Cancer Research and Treatment, 73*(1), 37–43.

Lee, J. C., Boyd, R., & Stuart, P. (2007). Randomized controlled trial of an instructional DVD for clinical skills teaching, *Emergency Medicine Australasia, 19(3)*, 241–245.

Rankin, S. H., Stallings, K. D., & London, F. (2004). *Patient education in health and illness.* Philadelphia: Lippincott Williams & Wilkins.

The Communication Initiative (TCI). (2003, July 29). *Health belief model.* Retrieved from http://www.comminit.com/ctheories/sid-8180.html

Wiljer, D., & Catton, P. (2003). Multimedia Formats for patient education and health communication: Does user preference matter? *Journal of Medical Internet Research, 5*(3), e19.

BOX 24-3 ■ Culturally Competent Teaching

- Inquire or observe interactions among family members to decide who is the decision maker and how decisions are made. Include the family in the planning and teaching.
- Assess for customs or taboos that may conflict with the information you plan to present.
- Observe verbal and nonverbal communication patterns.
- Assess whether the family is past, present, or future oriented.
- Determine if the patient and/or family prefers a same-sex nurse to teach a client about personal topics, such as birth control and sexually transmitted infections. Different cultures have different ideas about what is appropriate for discussion between men and women.
- Determine whether the client's values and wishes are in congruence or conflict with the family.
- Respect, accept, and validate the client's beliefs.
- Find sources of information that can help you learn about the culture and its healthcare practices.
- Admit unfamiliarity with the culture, but express willingness to learn.
- Find ways to incorporate the client's current healthcare practices and beliefs into the plan of care unless there is potential for harm.
- Speak slowly and clearly; avoid slurring syllables.
- Do not use slang expressions.
- Use short sentences and concrete rather than abstract words. Present only one idea in each sentence.
- Use pictures and other visual aids to help communicate your meaning.
- Provide teaching materials in the client's language. If you cannot read it, have it translated so that you can judge its appropriateness.
- Avoid using humor; jokes often do not translate well because of connotations, jargon, and culture-specific context.
- Obtain feedback carefully. Do not assume that a client who smiles, nods, and says yes really understands what you are teaching. The client may be embarrassed to ask questions or may feel that it will embarrass you.
- Encourage the client to ask questions; stop often to evaluate client understanding.

BOX 24-4 ■ Promoting Health Literacy with Patients

- Ask questions that involve "how" and "what" rather than "yes" and "no".
- Assist patients in completing forms and/or health histories as needed.
- Organize information so the most important material stands out and is repeated for emphasis and clarity.
- Avoid medical jargon and technical terms.
- Speak using simple words, short sentences, and structuring sentences with active rather than passive voice. For example, instead of saying, "The pill should be taken every 8 hours," say "Take the pill every 8 hours."
- Use as many drawings and photographs as possible to illustrate your statements.
- For those with Limited English Proficiency (LEP), provide information in primary language or seek an interpreter to translate.

BOX 24-5 ■ Barriers To Effective Teaching and Learning In The Healthcare Environment

Barriers for the Teacher
- Limited time
- Limited opportunity to prepare for teaching
- Lack of space and privacy
- Teaching not seen as a priority (either by the nurse or the organization)
- No third-party reimbursement for teaching
- Frustration with the amount of documentation needed
- Lack of coordination by various healthcare providers

Barriers for the Learner
- Personal stress
- Illness
- Physical condition
- Anxiety
- Low literacy
- A negative environmental influence
- Lack of time to learn
- Overwhelming amount of behavioral change needed
- Lack of support and ongoing positive reinforcement
- Lack of willingness to take responsibility
- The complexity of the healthcare system, which can lead to discouragement or abandonment
- Communication gap resulting from language barrier
- Teaching not adapted to the learner's preferences and learning style
- Provider who uses excessive jargon and technical terminology
- Lack of perceived need for the information taught

Access to the Internet can be problematic for some students (Muilenburg & Bergeb, 2005). When deciding whether online learning is best suited to your learners, consider students' technical and academic skills.

Transportation, class schedule, time, child care, didactic-style instruction are a few of the barriers for some students choosing traditional classroom education. The most common barriers to effective teaching and learning in the traditional and technology-based learning environments are identified in Boxes 24-5 and 24-6.

BOX 24-6 ■ Barriers to Technology-based Learning Environment

Technical

- Anxiety about use of technology
- Limited bandwidth or lack of adequate Internet access
- Lack of consistent platforms, browsers, software
- Difficulty with navigation throughout the site, including pages where required assignments are located
- Technical failure with hardware
- Insufficient training to use the delivery system
- Fear of incorrectly submitting required assignments or missing them altogether
- Unfamiliar with online learning technical tools

Instructional

- Online learning environment appeals to learners who perform well seated with visual instruction. Not all learners process and retain information in this manner.
- Might not be suited to learners with physical restriction for effective keyboard use, such as repetitive use syndrome or other disability involving motor activity of the upper extremities or visual impairment.
- Some instructors lack the skills to teach online.
- Some lower quality materials/instruction are used online.
- There might be lack of access to instructor/expert and other support services, such as tutor, technical service.
- Class size is not right for online learning.
- The student might not have sufficient time to commit to completing assignments and meeting expectations involved in online courses, which at times can be more demanding than traditional didactic-style classrooms.

- Clear expectations and instructions are even more important because the instructor isn't present for the student to ask questions.
- Lack of timely feedback from the instructor might occur.
- Frustration occurs when learners have difficulty contacting academic or administrative staff.
- Insufficient language, writing, reading, and communication, and typing skills for online learning interferes with effective learning.
- Learners must take on more responsibility for learning.
- Lack of sufficient academic advisors online can be a problem.

Social/Personal

- Lack of face-to-face contact with instructor and peers
- Reduced motivation to participate in the online learning program (procrastination, cannot get started)
- Shy or lacks confidence for online learning
- Fear family life will be disrupted
- Lacks support from family, friends, employer
- Online learning affecting personal time
- Online learning seems impersonal.
- Afraid of feeling isolated and too little student collaboration
- Significant interruptions during study at home/work

Adapted from Muilenburg, L.Y., & Bergeb, Z. L. (2005). Student barriers to online learning: A factor analytic study. *Distance Education,* 26(1), 1475–1498.

KnowledgeCheck 24-3

- List and define six factors that affect the learning process.
- What is one strategy you could use to motivate a client who seems uninterested in learning?
- What are some aspects of the environment that can enhance or interfere with learning?
- What two strategies might you use with a learner functioning with low cognitive ability?

  Go to Chapter 24, **Knowledge Check Response Sheet and Answers,** on the Student Resource Disk or DavisPlus at http://davisplus.fadavis.com/Wilkinson2

CriticalThinking 24-4

- List some actions you can take to avoid each of the teaching barriers.
- Give an example of each of the barriers to the learner. For "stress of illness," here is one example: A patient is frightened after having a heart attack, worried about the cost of the medical treatment, and worried about not being able to go to work, so he cannot concentrate on the material being presented to him.

Note: These questions may be difficult, depending on your knowledge base and experience. Work with others to answer the questions, as necessary.

Practical **Knowledge**
knowing how

The teaching process parallels the nursing process. You will assess learning needs and readiness, make educational diagnoses, write learning objectives, plan and implement teaching strategies, and evaluate client learning. Effective client teaching begins with assessment of learning needs.

■ ASSESSMENT

A learning assessment will help you to determine the right setting for the teaching, the necessary content to cover, learning goals, and teaching strategies. Your initial assessment consists of general information about the amount of time and resources available for your teaching. Also be clear about your intended audience. For example, with Heather ("Meet Your Patient") assess the following:

Learning Needs. To understand her own child's behaviors, Heather needs to learn about normal growth and development and nutritional needs of 4-year-olds. She will need safety and health instructions for the next year because her child may not return for another checkup until age 5.

Client's Knowledge Level. You need to identify Heather's current expectations of her preschooler as well as her understanding of how the child has developed up to this point. You should also find out what Heather knows about preschooler nutrition and language development.

Health Beliefs and Practices. Determine Heather's (and her daughter's) current healthcare practices as well as trust and investment in the healthcare system. For example, what kinds of meals does she offer the preschooler?

Physical Readiness. Is Heather able to sit and listen to the information presented? You may need to provide appropriate play materials for her preschooler so that she will require less attention from her. Some interruptions are likely, because 4-year-olds have short attention spans.

Emotional Readiness. In the case of Heather, emotional maturity is a factor in her readiness to learn. Heather has expressed concern that her child is so small, which offers you an opportunity to begin the teaching based on her interest in her child's progress and health. However, she may have trouble focusing on her responses to the care provider during the healthcare visit if her child is restless or if she has limited time for her appointment.

Ability to Learn. During the interview, you can begin to assess Heather's ability to learn, based on her responses to questions. You can also ask about her educational level.

Literacy Level. You might ask Heather to read a short statement or paragraph related to the topic you're teaching. Then ask questions to determine if Heather understood the printed information.

Neurosensory Factors. By observing Heather's interactions with her preschooler, you can assess her vision, hearing, and manual dexterity. Observe her response to visual and auditory clues that are given by her child or healthcare providers. Watching her manipulate a pen, pencil, or toy could help you determine manual dexterity.

Learning Styles. Ask Heather how she learns best. Understanding that she probably doesn't have extensive blocks of time or focused attention to read or listen, you might give her single-page handouts, videos, or pamphlets instead of books or more detailed booklets.

For guidelines and questions to ask when conducting a learning assessment,

VOL 2 Go to Chapter 24, **Assessment Guidelines and Tools, Learning Assessment Guidelines,** in Volume 2.

ANALYSIS/NURSING DIAGNOSIS

Deficient Knowledge is the most frequently used (and perhaps misused) nursing diagnosis for a teaching plan. It may be either a problem or the etiology of a problem.

Deficient Knowledge as the Primary Problem

You should use Deficient Knowledge only if you believe that the lack of knowledge is the *primary* problem. Use it to describe conditions in which the patient needs new, additional, or extensive knowledge. Identify the specific knowledge deficit as the problem, and follow with the etiology and related signs and symptoms. For example:

> Deficient Knowledge (diabetic foot care) related to lack of prior experience, as manifested by anxiety and many questions about foot care

Deficient Knowledge as the Etiology

Deficient Knowledge is probably most effectively used as the etiology of other nursing diagnoses, such as the following:

- Ineffective Health Maintenance related to (r/t) Deficient Knowledge of immunizations
- Risk for Impaired Parenting r/t Deficient Knowledge of child developmental stages and needs for stimulation
- Ineffective Therapeutic Regimen Management r/t Deficient Knowledge of the procedure for drawing up and injecting insulin
- Risk for Imbalanced Nutrition: Less Than Body Requirements r/t the pregnant woman's Deficient Knowledge about additional calories and nutrients needed during pregnancy and her fear of "getting fat"

Wellness Diagnoses

Teaching is the primary intervention for wellness diagnoses, such as Effective Breastfeeding, Health-Seeking Behaviors, Readiness for Enhanced Communication, and the more than 22 other NANDA-I labels beginning with the phrase "Readiness for Enhanced."

Incorrect Uses of Deficient Knowledge

Beware of routine or premature diagnosing. It is easy to see that a patient lacks information, label it as a Deficient Knowledge problem, and try to solve the problem by giving information—which may not be what the patient needs at all. Always look beyond the knowledge deficit to see what problematic *responses* it produces.

Do not use Deficient Knowledge routinely as a problem label for all patients. There are information needs associated with almost every medical and nursing diagnosis. However, you cannot assume a particular patient needs to be taught that information. For example, a person with a foot ulcer secondary to long-standing diabetes may already know more than you do about foot care. For most nursing diagnoses (e.g., Anxiety, Imbalanced Nutrition), you can merely write a nursing order to provide the informal teaching needed instead of writing a Deficient Knowledge diagnosis.

Do not use Deficient Knowledge for problems involving the client's *ability to learn*. To accurately describe such situations, use non-NANDA-I diagnoses such as:

- Impaired Ability to Learn r/t fear and anxiety
- Impaired Ability to Learn r/t delayed cognitive development
- Lack of Motivation to Learn r/t feelings of powerlessness

PLANNING OUTCOMES

Before making a teaching plan, educators contract with the learner for what they want to accomplish together. **Contractual agreements** are statements of understanding between teacher and learner about how to achieve mutually set goals. The contract usually describes the responsibilities of both teacher and learner, time frame for the teaching, content to be included, and expectations of all participants. Learning contracts increase commitment by the learner to reach the teaching and behavioral goals. They are usually informal.

Teaching goals are broad in scope and set down what is expected as the final outcome of the teaching and learning process. They should address all three domains of learning. In contrast, **learning objectives** are single, specific, one-dimensional behaviors that must be completed to accomplish the goal. They are short term and ideally are accomplished in one or two sessions. Similar to patient outcomes in the nursing process, learning objectives/goals should include an action verb, an activity that can be measured or observed, the circumstances of the learner's performance, and how learning will be measured. For example:

Goal: Client will demonstrate ability to perform newborn care in 3 days.
Learning Objectives: (1) Client changes infant's diaper, making sure that umbilical cord remains outside the diaper. (2) Client demonstrates bathing baby while maintaining newborn's axillary temperature of greater than 98.5°F (36.9°C).

See Table 24-3 for examples of active verbs for each domain of learning. See Chapter 5 for a review of goals and outcomes.

Critical**Thinking** 24-5

A client has just been diagnosed with diabetes mellitus. He must monitor and record his blood glucose three times a day. The two of you establish a goal that he will be able to perform glucose testing independently within 1 week. What objectives would you need to write to achieve this goal?

Table 24-3 ➤ Active Verbs for Domains of Learning		
COGNITIVE DOMAIN	**AFFECTIVE DOMAIN**	**PSYCHOMOTOR DOMAIN**
Compare	Cry	Adapt
Define	Choose	Apply
Describe	Defend	Arrange
Design	Discuss	Assemble
Differentiate	Display	Begin
Explain	Form (e.g., an opinion)	Change
Give examples	Express	Construct
Identify	Give	Create
List	Help	Demonstrate
Name	Initiate	Draw up (e.g., medication)
Plan	Justify	Inject (e.g., medication)
State	Relate	Manipulate
Summarize	Revise	Move
	Select	Organize
	Share	Show
	Smile	Start
	State a feeling	Take
	Use	Work
	Value	

NOC standardized outcomes for Deficient Knowledge depend on the content that needs to be taught. *Nursing Outcomes Classification (NOC)* (Moorhead, Johnson, & Maas, 2008) has identified 42 "Knowledge" outcomes for specific topics, for example, Knowledge: Diabetes Management and Knowledge: Infant Care.

VOL 2 Go to Chapter 24, **Standardized Language, NOC Outcomes for Health Knowledge,** in Volume 2.

If you use Deficient Knowledge as the etiology of another diagnosis (e.g., Imbalanced Nutrition) then you would use NOC outcomes linked to that diagnosis (e.g., Knowledge: Diet, or Nutritional Status).

Individualized goals/outcome statements you might write for a client with a diagnosis of Deficient Knowledge include examples such as the following:

- For Deficient Knowledge (Breastfeeding): After demonstration and teaching, mother will position infant correctly at breast.
- For Deficient Knowledge (Child Physical Safety): After demonstration and explanation, parents will fasten preschooler safely and securely in infant car seat.

- For Deficient Knowledge (Diabetes Management): After reading pamphlets, client will explain the relationship of carbohydrate intake and exercise to blood sugar.

As you can see, choice of outcome is directly related to the area in which the client lacks knowledge or information.

The outcomes you choose depend on whether you have used Deficient Knowledge in the problem clause or the etiology clause of the nursing diagnosis. For example, if your nursing diagnosis for Heather ("Meet Your Patient") were Deficient Knowledge (Preschooler Nutrition) related to lack of experience and family support; then one outcome might be, "Heather will plan nutritious meals for her child, based upon the MyPyramid." If, however, your diagnosis for the child were Risk for Impaired Nutrition: Less Than Body Requirements related to the mother's Deficient Knowledge about nutrition, then one outcome might be, "Preschooler will gain weight so that she is in at least the 10th percentile for weight by September of this year."

PLANNING INTERVENTIONS/IMPLEMENTATION

In Chapters 5 and 6, you learned about creating a nursing care plan. For clients and families with learning needs, you will create individualized teaching plans. The teaching plan is often one part of the client's complete nursing care plan. For an example see a sample nursing care plan at end of this chapter.

Creating Teaching Plans

The process of creating a teaching plan differs from that of creating a nursing care plan in two key ways: First, in a teaching plan, the interventions are actually teaching strategies. Second, when planning teaching, you will plan content, sequencing, and the types of instructional materials to be used. Let's apply these aspects of a teaching plan, using the example of Heather in the "Meet Your Patient" scenario. You have assessed the need for anticipatory guidance regarding safety for her 4-year-old. Your nursing diagnosis is Deficient Knowledge (safety for a 4-year-old) related to the mother's inexperience.

- *Teaching strategies* are the method used to present content. For Heather, they might include one-to-one instruction and printed information. (A description of various teaching strategies follows shortly.)
- The *content* of your teaching includes the information your learner must understand to reach the desired goal. It can include facts, skills, or emotions. For Heather, the content of your informal teaching might include the following:

  Poison control and prevention—Curiosity and lack of ability to understand danger puts the preschooler at greater risk.

  Accident prevention—This would include the need for car seats, increased supervision when exploring, and the use of a helmet when the child rides a tricycle.

  Risk of choking—Foods that are hard to swallow or chunky (e.g., hot dogs) are a concern for a 4-year-old.

  Need for immunizations and physical checkup during the next year.

- *Scheduling and sequencing* refer to how you organize the information, that is, in what order to present the topics. As a general rule, you should present simple before complex topics and nonthreatening topics before more controversial ones. You must also determine when the teaching session(s) should be scheduled based on the client's and teacher's needs. When extensive content is involved, it is best to schedule a teaching session in advance; the teacher and learner are then committed and prepared for the session. Using small amounts of time can be effective if teaching is brief and organized.

  In the example at the beginning of this chapter, you could teach Heather about poison control and accident prevention in the lobby while she and her preschooler are waiting for the child to be examined. During the child's examination, you could review immunizations and the need for an annual checkup. At the end of the examination, when discussing the child's nutrition, you might include a discussion of foods that are a choking hazard, such as a hot dog.

- *Instructional materials* are tools that are used to introduce information and reinforce learning. You might give Heather printed handouts about poison control (including the Poison Control Center [PCC] telephone number) and about accident prevention (e.g., how to properly install a child car seat). The child's immunization record would list current immunizations and the schedule for further immunizations may be printed on it. To involve the child, you might include a coloring book and stickers about one of the topics.

Selecting NIC Interventions

NIC standardized interventions related to patient learning depend on the nursing diagnoses you have identified. The *Nursing Interventions Classification (NIC)* (Bulechek, Butcher, & Dochterman, 2008) lists 30 patient education interventions from which to choose, depending on the content being taught. An example is Health Education and Teaching: Disease Process. To see the entire list,

VOL 2 Go to Chapter 24, **Standardized Language, NIC Interventions for Patient Education,** in Volume 2.

Selecting Specific Teaching Strategies

Several different types of teaching strategies are currently available. Before selecting one, consider the learner's differences, needs, learning style, and advantages and disadvantages of each method.

Lecture

Lecture is a traditional method in which one or more presenters orally share information while learners listen (Fig. 24-3). It can be enhanced by including discussion and question-and-answer periods for clarifying content and by use of computer-projected slide presentation, streaming video, flip charts, transparencies, posters, brochures, models, and other audiovisual formats. Teachers can engage learners with an attention-getting opening and by supporting teaching points with stories, quotes, images, analogies or metaphors, and humor.

- **Advantages.** A lecture is an efficient and cost-effective way to impart information, especially to large groups. The format is useful for conveying basic concepts and information that serves as the foundation for higher-level, critical thinking later. The presenter can use media-rich formats within the lecture in order to reach learners with auditory and visual learning styles. Lectures may be recorded for future use.
- **Limitations.** Does not allow for individualization of teaching. Didactic learning is a passive-learning technique that for most learners is not suited for optimal retention of information. The lecture may not be geared to the level of the learner. This type of instruction is not effective for teaching in the psychomotor or affective domains. Lectures can lead to oversaturation if too much information is presented in too short a time frame. Boredom is common. This format is not a good strategy for promoting critical thinking. There is little opportunity for assessment of learner comprehension.

Group Discussion

In a group discussion, several participants discuss topics, exchanging information and presenting their points of view. The teacher acts as a facilitator to achieve objectives shared with the group at the beginning of the session. Effective group discussion requires an atmosphere

FIGURE 24-3 The advantage of lecturing is that you can teach more than one person at a time.

of trust that encourages everyone to participate. Openness to new ideas and confidentiality of the content expressed are essential for participation. One type of group discussion is *brainstorming*, which is a process for generating multiple ideas for solving a problem. Participants suggest a maximum number of ideas and consider a wide array of creative ideas; then they analyze options, identify a best solution, and develop a plan of action.

- **Advantages.** Group discussion is learner-centered and effective for teaching in the affective and cognitive domains. Many students enjoy a learning environment with opportunities for interaction with peers. Social involvement can enhance content.
- **Limitations.** This method may be less effective with large groups. The teacher must be comfortable with less structure and with unpredictable learner responses. Managing group discussion requires good leadership skills of the instructor. Group discussion is not well suited for teaching in the psychomotor domain. The quality of group work can be negatively affected by "group think"—a force that stifles creativity by succumbing to the often subtle pressure of agreeing with the group even though affirmation doesn't reflect the learner's individual opinion. Brainstorming fails when participants are distracted or fail to contribute ideas because of fears of rejection or ridicule by peers. Some might even hold back with brainstorming when anticipating the ideas to be unpopular with the instructor. Individuals who dominate can be equally problematic when crowding out less confident participants. Those who are disruptive or intentionally sabotage the activity can interfere in successful group discussion.

Demonstration and Return Demonstration

In this method, the teacher explains and demonstrates a skill or task. The learner then demonstrates comprehension by returning the demonstration. Return demonstrations should be scheduled close to the initial teaching of the skill. This format allows for targeted questions and answers and practical matters, rather than theory. This method requires the demonstrator to have specialized expertise if highly technical tasks are involved.

- **Advantages.** Demonstration is most effective in teaching psychomotor skills (e.g., use of equipment, self-injection, dressing changes). It can be used in small groups if enough equipment is available. When the task or skill is performed correctly, return demonstration can increase self confidence.
- **Limitations.** It does not work well with large groups or for those who do not learn best by observing others. Demonstration may not be best suited for participants who learn at different rates; some might need repeated demonstration or slow enactment of steps, while others do not. The method is time-consuming and labor intensive. It involves preparation time to set up equipment. The space must be suitable for the demonstration format.

One-to-One Instruction and Mentoring

In one-to-one instruction, generally one teacher presents information to an individual learner. They mutually formulate objectives at the beginning of the session. Often the learner receives printed or audiovisual materials to reinforce the information presented. As a nurse, you will often use this method for patient teaching. Mentoring involves a more personal interaction between teacher and learner, involving not only the exchange of information but also role modeling and problem-solving. It offers an opportunity to directly observe and offer feedback on the learner's performance. Mentoring often involves learners in an authentic clinical setting.

- **Advantages.** One-on-one instruction gives the teacher the opportunity to establish a relationship with a learner; convey interest in his learning needs; and tailor the teaching to the learner's needs as the session proceeds. Mentoring allows reluctant learners to more readily ask questions. It enables the teacher to obtain frequent feedback so that material can be repeated and clarified as needed. The method is useful for teaching in all three domains: affective, psychomotor, and cognitive. It provides an opportunity for learners to build skills and problem-solve in situations with expert supervision, guidance, and feedback.
- **Limitations.** The method can be labor intensive and reaches the fewest numbers of learners. It may be overwhelming to learners because of the large quantity of information given in a short period of time, and therefore may not promote retention. One-on-one instruction tends to isolate the learner from others who may share the same learning needs and who could provide support. It can be hampered by personality conflicts. It relies heavily on the instructor, preceptor, or nurse being a good role model and having effective teaching skills.

Printed Materials

Printed materials may be available in the form of fact sheets, discharge instructions, printed pamphlets, or detailed booklets. Printed materials for children include storybooks, coloring books, and activity books with mazes and other games. To be sure the clients comprehend the information, you must provide an opportunity for them to ask questions after they have read the materials. You will usually use printed materials to supplement other teaching strategies.

When you are creating your own teaching materials, remember the tips for ensuring readability in the "Health Literacy" section of this chapter (see Box 24-4). Many standard word processing programs allow you to check the reading level of materials you create. However, keep in mind that health-related information often contains medical terminology, which tends to have more syllables. Reading levels computed based on the syllable count can falsely indicate a higher-grade for reading level than what is reflected predominantly in the document. Figure 24-4 is an example of a patient teaching fact sheet written at the level of grade 6.8.

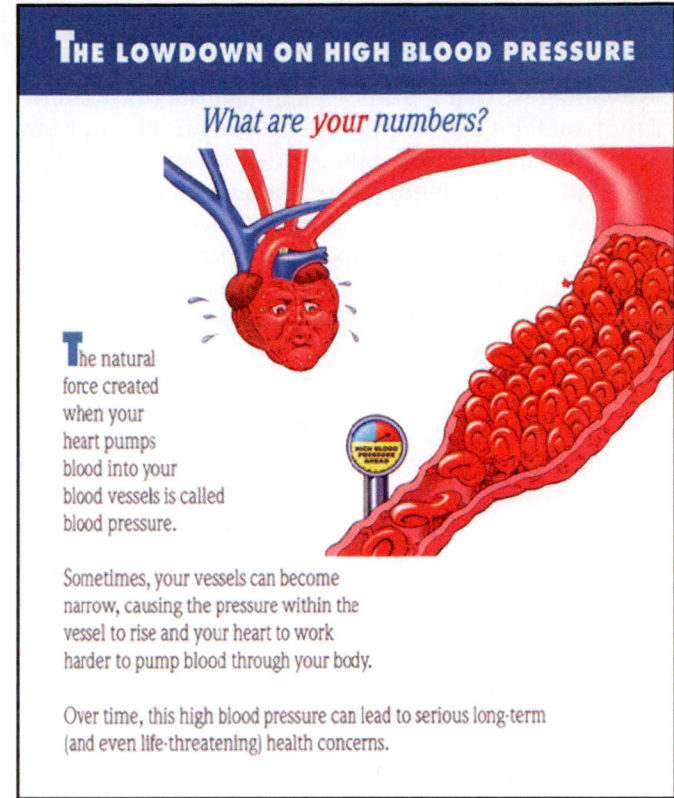

FIGURE 24-4 Reading level of this patient teaching aid is grade 6.8.

Provide your clients with a take-home summary of the main points you want them most to remember after the teaching session. Having something clients can put their hands on to refer to at a later time can be invaluable for reinforcing important information.

- **Advantages.** Printed materials allow for standardized information to be presented to each client, but with some room for individualization. Hard-copy documents are an excellent way to reinforce material taught in lecture, demonstration and return demonstration, or one-to-one instruction. Handouts allow the teacher to cover just the main ideas and high points while using the time more efficiently for face-to-face instruction. Printed materials are portable, so people can read the information when it is most convenient.
- **Limitations.** The method assumes literacy, motivation to read the content, organization to keep track of materials, and visual acuity to decipher the print. Materials must be written at a 5th grade reading level with words that most people understand.

Audiovisual Materials

Teachers often use materials that make use of visual illustrations and sound. Audiovisual materials may include streaming video or Flash format, computer animations, audio clips online or per CD/DVD, film, slides, or computer-generated material. They can be effective supplements to other methods if the teaching session is followed by a question-and-answer session, a discussion of the content, a test, or printed materials to expand understanding.

- **Advantages.** Using audiovisual materials is a stimulating method because it engages both sight and hearing, and can accommodate large groups.
- **Limitations.** The method is not as efficient as a lecture or reading in terms of the amount of content that can be covered. It can be expensive because it requires special hardware (e.g., projectors, screens) and media (e.g., videotapes), which must be replaced when they become outdated.

Simulation

Simulation creates an experience that is similar to actual nursing practice but without risks and consequences associated with learning new nursing skills using live patients. Simulation requires the learner to make decisions, solve problems, and review the effects of nursing actions. Simulations can occur through written case studies as well as human models, mannequins (Fig. 24-5), computer programs, and physical setups (e.g., practicing injections in the nursing lab). Technology allows students to learn and practice airway placement, external defibrillation, IV placement with replaceable skin and veins, injections, nasogastric tube insertion, and chest compressions. Students can check a pulse or blood pressure and assess lung, heart, and bowel sounds. Most simulators can cough, vomit, moan, and make other life-like vocal sounds. Optional features provide more specialized training, such as trauma care, resuscitation, and wound care. Pregnancy mannequins offer experience with simulated delivery. Infant and child simulators are available to teach age-specific interventions.

- **Advantages.** Simulation portrays realistic patient-based situations. Practicing through simulations can increase learner confidence. It also allows the teacher to evaluate effectiveness of the teaching and trouble-shoot areas of concern before a real-world situation arises. Simulation allows nurses to learn new skills without risk to patients. Simulators allow instructors to program the mannequin to test students over specific procedures and different scenarios and provide immediate feedback.

FIGURE 24-5 Simulation mannequins can offer realism and relevance to the educational experience.

- **Limitations.** Human patient simulators require special equipment. The instructor needs extensive preparation time and specialized training to use the equipment properly. Simulation models are expensive and technically complex. Only a small number of learners can participate at a time, which can create scheduling and logistical challenges. If commercially prepared cases are not available, the instructor must create the case, which is time consuming and requires special skill.

Role-Playing

Role-playing is used primarily with groups to achieve learning in the affective domain. Participants take on unrehearsed roles without a script to follow. The teacher must develop the situation so that participants can develop understanding of the roles they are given. Role-playing can involve a typical patient scenario the student is likely to encounter. One person enacts a specific patient role, acting as a "real patient," reacting differentially depending on the action of the learners. Learners are challenged to respond appropriately and might be evaluated by the instructor accordingly.

- **Advantages.** Similar to simulation, this is a safe method to rehearse real-life situations before being confronted with them. Role-playing is usually even less structured than simulation, although the two can be combined. This method works well for social learners who are stimulated by interaction with others.
- **Limitations.** Role-playing requires follow-up discussion to allow learners to express feelings, attitudes, and observations. Learners must be willing to participate either as observers or role-players. Some people may feel self-conscious when role-playing. Others might dominate and occupy more of the learning experience than less social or less prepared classmates.

Role Modeling

In role modeling, the instructor teaches by example, demonstrating the behaviors and/or attitudes that learners should adopt. Role modeling is even more effective when the teaching point corresponds with the role model's action. Role modeling is integral to mentoring relationships in which students or patients learn by seeing, hearing, and doing. Be aware that learning occurs unconsciously as well as intentionally. Therefore, you must consider what you are communicating. Role models must connect the learning to the objectives. Role modeling is more successful when the teaching point is made apparent to learners during the learning experience.

Many experienced pediatric nurses find that role modeling using a puppet or a child's own doll or stuffed animal can be helpful in reducing the child's anxiety and enhancing the child's learning. For instance, you can suggest that the child be "the nurse" and "feel Miss Bunny's pulse," or have a puppet "suggest" to a child, "When I get a shot, I say, 'Ouch!' real loud, and then it's all over!"

- **Advantages.** The method allows the learner to identify with the teacher. It can be a subtle but powerful method to increase motivation and ability to perform a desired behavior. It tends to generate high learner interest, and doesn't usually require additional preparation on the part of the role model.

- **Limitations.** Learners need to be aware and receptive to this type of teaching. A role model who does not effectively represent desired behaviors can send the wrong message.

Self-Instruction

Self-instruction is a method in which the learner studies independently using carefully designed materials. Self-study modules are developed with objectives and various types of materials, including workbooks, computer programs, videotapes, and audiotapes with worksheets. Because feedback (evaluation) is an essential part of the educational process, teachers need to be available for questions or feedback at certain points in the process.

- **Advantages.** Learners can work at their own pace and on their own time schedule. This convenience is appealing to many learners, particularly those with employment, marriage, and family life demands. Since transportation is not required, the expense and inconvenience of commuting to a traditional classroom setting are avoided.
- **Limitations.** Self-instruction requires literacy skills and motivation to pursue individualized instruction; it can be isolating for those who need frequent feedback and support from others. This method requires a great deal of time for the initial preparation of modules. Without access to an instructor, students might not know if they are on track and adequately understand the material.

Distance Learning

With distance learning, teacher and learner are not in the same physical location. Live or taped instructions are sent from the teacher to the learner. Two or more individuals or classrooms may be connected by video or teleconferencing. Computers offer individual and groups of learners access to information from distant locations, at different times, and in different formats. Distance learning is flexible to accommodate the needs of learners who cannot or choose not to participate in face-to-face instruction.

- **Advantages.** This method allows for teaching to remote or multiple sites at the same time, and can link many individuals separated by great distances. Current technology provides the opportunity for interactive teaching rather than a one-way process.
- **Limitations.** Distance learning requires good technological skills from the teacher, expensive equipment, and a great deal of time for preparation and organization.

Online Sources of Information

Learners can obtain extensive information and support geared toward the lay public as well as healthcare professionals via the Internet through listserves and credible Web sites (e.g., CDC, The Joanna Briggs Institute [Best Practice], Hartford Geriatric Nursing Initiative). Electronic learning platforms offer education through multimedia, search engines, electronic libraries, content portals, and social networking sites and blogs. Learners can connect with others in similar situations through listserves, which are online communities sharing a common focus or interest. Through listserve and other-threaded discussions, participants exchange information; express opinions; offer support; and inquire about topics of interest to the greater community; promote special interests; and network with others for personal or professional intent.

- **Advantages.** The Internet makes a vast amount of information readily available. The easily available health-related information makes it possible for consumers to participate in self-care and make informed decisions. Patients feel empowered when they have access to relevant and understandable information. They often cope better and experience less uncertainty when health information is available.
- **Limitations.** The teacher has little control over the quality of information learners access via the Internet. Before recommending particular Web sites to a patient, you need to read it yourself to be sure the information is accurate and the format and reading level are best suited to your patient. See Chapter 39 for information about evaluating materials you obtain from a Web site.

Computer-Assisted Instruction and Online Coursework

Computer-assisted instruction (CAI) involves the use of computer software or Web-based, learning management systems to present information and provide a virtual classroom experience. CAI may include video or audio clips that enhance learning. CAI typically incorporates functions such as:

Assessing the learner's capabilities with a pre-test
Presenting educational materials in a navigable form—may be multimedia, such as Flash or streaming video, audio, PDF, PowerPoint, or other interactive formats
Providing exercises, quizzes/tests to improve the learner's mastery of the content
Providing game-based drills to increase attention within the learning enjoyment
Assessing the learner's progress with a post-test
Documenting learners' scores and progress for later evaluation by the courseware instructor

- **Advantages.** This method allows learners to proceed at their own pace. Learners can access programs at a time that is convenient for them. CAI provides feedback while the learner progresses through the study module. Teachers and learners interact through electronic discussion pathways that are with instructor and/or peers. It provides interactive learning, which promoted retention of information.
- **Limitations.** Learners must have access to a computer, have adequate visual acuity and literacy skills, and have computer skills. Because this method is technology driven, and because personal support facilitates

learning, be sure to also plan occasional person-to-person contact with the learner.

Gaming

Gaming requires the learner to participate in activity that promotes learning through specialized techniques using competition, distraction, activity, and pleasure. Activities are structured with preset rules (e.g., a board game that allows players to move when they answer a question correctly). Choose games that are relevant to the teaching point with objectives clear to learners. The teacher serves as a facilitator who sets the ground rules, explains the process, and keeps the flow going. Games can be created by the teacher or purchased commercially.

- **Advantages.** Gaming can be used with individuals or groups and can make learning fun. It can be used to introduce new information or reinforce previous learning. Because it involves active learning, it enhances retention of information. Meeting the challenges of the game can build the learner's confidence in knowing and expressing the material.
- **Limitations.** Some participants may not enjoy the competitive atmosphere or may have physical or social impairments that preclude participation. Gaming can create disinterest for learners who are not competitive by nature. Some learners might reject the gaming approach when feeling insecure about gaming skills. Learners might be distracted from the teaching point if winning is overemphasized.

Concept Mapping

A concept map is a diagram used to represent a teaching point or ideas by using key word, symbols, images, or other code word or phrase. This spatial learning strategy visually portrays how key concepts are logically ordered. The relationship among concepts is shown with lines, arrows, and other graphic linkages. Concept maps can be used to construct care plans; summarize key points from lectures; organize papers before beginning the actual writing; outline review materials before a test; create a summary of reading assignments; and undertake a comprehensive review of the research literature. You can use concept maps as a patient teaching tool to simplify the content; however, learning is best when the learner constructs the map rather than viewing a map made by someone else.

- **Advantages.** Concept mapping promotes reflection and critical thinking. This method helps to identify patterns and structure within the content. It takes a large amount of information and summarizes the key aspects into a concise, visual format. Because concept mapping involves active learning, it discourages rote memorization.
- **Limitations.** Constructing a concept map might be difficult for learners with limited spatial reasoning ability. Some learners might not prefer this educational approach. Additionally, learners need to be taught how to create a concept map. For complete information about mind-mapping,

Go to Chapter 5, **Supplemental Materials: Mind-Mapping,** on the Student Resource Disk or DavisPlus at http://davisplus.fadavis.com/Wilkinson2

KnowledgeCheck 24-4

- True or false: When a patient has a learning disability, you should use a non-NANDA diagnosis (e.g., Impaired Ability to Learn) to describe the problem.
- True or false: Learning objectives are short-term and, ideally, should be accomplished in one or two teaching sessions.
- List and state the advantages and disadvantages of at least six teaching strategies.

Go to Chapter 24, **Knowledge Check Response Sheet and Answers,** on the Student Resource Disk or DavisPlus at http://davisplus.fadavis.com/Wilkinson2

▬ EVALUATION OF LEARNING

As with all nursing interventions, evaluation is central to the educational process—that is, patient learning is an outcome that is achieved or not. Evaluation of the effectiveness of the teaching plan is essential to improving the quality of instruction. You should evaluate the entire nursing process (as you may recall from Chapter 7). Was your assessment adequate, or did you fail to notice that the patient was physically uncomfortable and therefore not ready to learn? Was your nursing diagnosis accurate? Were your learning objectives realistic? When evaluating the teaching, consider the type of strategy you used, the timing of the teaching, the content, the amount of information, and the teaching materials. The client is your best source for feedback. He can tell you whether the materials and methods were helpful, or uninteresting, and so on.

The following methods are commonly used for outcomes evaluation (client learning).

- *Tests and written exercises* can be used to measure retention and progress toward meeting cognitive objectives. This method requires the learner to be actively involved and have adequate literacy skills.
- *Oral questions/interviews/questionnaires/checklists* allow clients to evaluate their own progress and determine future learning needs. You may obtain more information by talking with the client; however, you may obtain more honest responses by using written questions and providing for anonymous completion of the evaluations.
- *Direct observations of client performance* are anecdotal, descriptive notes that you make of the learner's performance. They will help you in providing feedback to the client either to reinforce accurate learning or to correct misinformation. Provide feedback as soon as possible after you observe performance.
- *Reports and client records.* Clients and/or families can keep records of performance and results. You can then evaluate the data and give feedback accordingly. Documentation of performance is best when following criteria or other clear expectations You can make plans for further teaching when you analyze the data and determine the learners' knowledge deficits.

Clients will not remember everything you teach them. That is normal. If you start to question your effectiveness as a teacher, think about one of the courses you took last semester. Did you score 100% on every test? How much of the material presented in that course do you remember now? Repetition, reinforcement, and practice are necessary for retention; and so is information made memorable.

Documentation of Teaching and Learning

As is true for all nursing interventions (as you learned in Chapter 16), it is important to record the responses of the client and family to teaching interventions. Documentation also provides legal evidence that teaching was done and communicates the information to other health professionals. Write objective statements about what was taught and the client skills and behaviors that demonstrate learning. For informal teaching that occurs during other care activities, you may simply record in the nursing notes. For planned teaching that is provided frequently for a particular population of clients, many agencies provide special documentation forms. For an example of a patient education record,

 Go to Chapter 24, **Tables, Boxes, Figures: ESG Figure 24-1,** on the Student Resource Disk or DavisPlus at http://davisplus.fadavis.com/Wilkinson2

Toward Evidence-Based Practice

| Caruana, E. (2007, August). Patient information (pre-operative): Knowledge retention. Evidence Summaries – Joanna Briggs Institute. Retrieved from ProQuest Nursing & Allied Health Source database at www.joannabriggs.edu.au/pdf/BPISEng_4_6.pdf. (Document ID: 1451740781).

Nineteen scientific trials were analyzed to determine which patient education strategies are most effective in promoting patient knowledge and the use of good technique for self-care activities after surgery. This analysis suggests patient education before surgery is useful for improving patients' knowledge of postoperative treatment and their ability to perform the care needed after surgery. Instruction is likely to be more effective if provided before admission. If done after admission, teaching in a group format is equally as effective as individual instruction. The researchers supported the use of educational pamphlets to inform patients and improve their skills.

| Palmer, M. H., Kowlowitz, V., Campbell, J., et al. (2008). Using clinical simulations in geriatric nursing continuing education. *Nursing Outlook, 56*(4), 159–166.

This study of 312 nurses attending a continuing education program to improve geriatric nursing competencies was conducted to determine whether simulation is effective for adult education. Three types of clinical simulations were studied, including unfolding cases, human patient simulator, and online case studies. Clinical simulations involving the human patient simulator were most highly rated of all types

of simulation, especially when it came to relevance of the experience to real-life scenarios (97.9% of participants strongly agreed or agreed). Most participants (97.5%) strongly agreed or agreed that human patient simulators helped to apply the information to clinical practice. Unfolding cases and online case studies were rated nearly as high, respectively. Nurse participants enjoyed the interactive nature of the human patient simulator experience. Further research is needed to demonstrate if the self-reported increase in skills levels actually means better patient care.

1. What important points does the first study pertaining to preoperative teaching make that you could use in your teaching?

2. In the first article discussing patient retention of information, why do you think group learning for postoperative care could be an effective approach for patient teaching after admission?

3. In the first article, why do you think a patient education pamphlet is important as a teaching aid before admission?

4. Based on the results of the second study, why do you think simulation might be an effective method of instruction?

5. Have you experienced simulation as part of your own nursing education? Was it beneficial to you for learning new information or nursing skills? Why or why not?

 Go to Chapter 24, **Toward Evidence-Based Practice Suggested Responses,** on the Student Resource Disk or DavisPlus at http://davisplus.fadavis.com/Wilkinson2

 Go to Chapter 24, **Resources for Caregivers and Health Professionals,** on the Student Resource Disk or DavisPlus at http://davisplus.fadavis.com/Wilkinson2

 Suggested Readings: Go to Chapter 24, **Reading More About Teaching Clients,** on the Student Resource Disk or DavisPlus at http://davisplus.fadavis.com/Wilkinson2

 Bibliography: Go to Volume 2, Bibliography.

How Nurses Support Physiological Functioning

CHAPTER 25

Stress & Adaptation

Learning Outcomes

After completing this chapter, you should be able to:

➤ Define stress.

➤ Explain the difference between adaptive and maladaptive coping strategies.

➤ Explain the relationship between stressors, responses, and adaptation.

➤ Describe physical changes occurring during the three stages of Selye's general adaptation syndrome (GAS).

➤ Explain how Selye's local adaptation syndrome (LAS) is different from the GAS.

➤ Discuss the inflammatory response: What triggers it, and what physiological changes occur?

➤ Explain how anxiety, fear, and anger relate to stress.

➤ Provide examples and definitions of specific ego defense mechanisms.

➤ Describe the effects of prolonged stress and unsuccessful adaptation on the various body systems.

➤ Briefly describe: hypochondriasis, somatization, somatoform pain disorder, and malingering.

➤ Compare and contrast crisis and burnout.

➤ State three ways in which you could assess for each of the following: (1) stressors and risk factors, (2) coping methods and adaptation, (3) physiological responses to stress, (4) emotional and behavioral responses to stresses, (5) cognitive responses to stress, and (6) adequacy of support systems.

➤ Describe several interventions or activities for preventing and managing stress.

Meet Your Patients

Gloria and her husband, John, live in a residential community from which John commutes to work in a nearby city. Gloria runs an accounting business from their home. They have two teenage boys, who are active in sports, church activities, Boy Scouts, and the school band. The boys need transportation to activities. Gloria and John teach Sunday school and are Boy Scout leaders. Gloria's mother needs knee replacement surgery and so cannot take care of Gloria's father, who has early-stage Alzheimer's disease. In addition to her own home responsibilities, Gloria must go to her parents' home to prepare meals and to provide care for them during the day. Gloria's sister comes at 8:00 P.M. to sleep in the parents' home during the night.

Theoretical **Knowledge** knowing why

Everyone experiences stress as a part of daily life, but we each perceive and respond to stress in our own unique way. Our responses are holistic—that is, physical, psychological, spiritual, and social. Stress has been directly linked to heart disease, stroke, injury, suicide, and homicide. Indirectly, it is also linked to cancer, chronic liver disease, chronic bronchitis, and emphysema (Quick, Saleh, Sime, et al., 2006).

As a nurse, you need to understand stress to help your clients cope effectively and adapt to the stressors of illness and caregiving. In addition, you will encounter many stressful situations in your career, so you must develop healthful ways of responding.

What Is Stress?

Stress is any disturbance in a person's normal balanced state. A **stressor** is a stimulus that the person perceives as a challenge or threat; it disturbs the person's equilibrium by initiating a physical or emotional response. When stress occurs, it produces voluntary and involuntary **coping responses** aimed at restoring equilibrium (balance, or homeostasis). The changes that take place as a result of stress and coping are called **adaptations.** We can also define adaptation as an ongoing effort to maintain external and internal equilibrium, or **homeostasis.**

Stress is not necessarily bad. It can keep you alert and motivate you to function at a higher performance level. For example, when you are preparing for an examination, your desire to succeed can create just enough anxiety to motivate you to study. On the other hand, if you become too anxious, you may be unable to focus on the task or think clearly.

Types of Stressors

The sources of stress are infinite; however, stressors are commonly categorized in the following ways:

Distress/Eustress. **Distress** threatens health, and **eustress** (literally "good stress") is protective. A passionate kiss can produce as strong a stress response as a slap in the face. On the Holmes–Rahe stress scale, for example, marriage and divorce receive similarly high scores. To see this scale,

 Go to Chapter 25, **Assessment Guidelines and Tools, The Holmes–Rahe Social Readjustment Scale,** in Volume 2.

External/Internal. Stressors may be **external** to the person, for example, death of a family member, a hurricane, or even something as simple as excessive heat in a room. Stressors may also be **internal,** for example,

diseases, anxiety, nervous anticipation of an event, or negative self-talk.

Developmental/Situational. **Developmental stressors** are those that can be predicted to occur at various stages of a person's life. For example, most young adults face the stress of leaving home and beginning a career, and many middle-aged adults must adjust to aging parents and accepting their own physical changes. In a sense, developmental stressors may be easier to cope with because they are expected and the person has some time to prepare for them. For theoretical knowledge about developmental stages, refer to the theories of Erikson and Havighurst in Chapter 9 of Volume 1. Also see Box 25-1 for examples of developmental stressors.

Situational stressors are unpredictable. For example, you cannot predict if you will experience an automobile accident, a natural disaster, or an illness. Situational stressors can occur at any life stage and can affect infants, children, and adults equally.

Physiological/Psychosocial. **Physiological stressors** are those that affect body structure or function. You can categorize them as follows; a few examples are given for each category.

Chemical—poison, medications, tobacco
Physical or mechanical—trauma, cold, joint overuse
Nutritional—vitamin deficiency, high-fat diet
Biological—viruses, bacteria
Genetic—inborn errors of metabolism
Lifestyle—obesity, sedentary lifestyle

Psychosocial stressors are external stressors that arise from work, family dynamics, living situation, social relationships, and other aspects of our daily lives. The Holmes–Rahe Scale in Volume 2 contains examples of psychosocial stressors.

KnowledgeCheck 25-1

Refer to the "Meet Your Patients" scenario.

- What are Gloria's stressors? Classify each of them as follows: (1) Are they physiological or psychosocial? (2) Are they developmental or situational?
- What are John's stressors?

 Go to Chapter 25, **Knowledge Check Response Sheet and Answers,** on the Student Resource Disk or DavisPlus at http://davisplus.fadavis.com/Wilkinson2

Models of Stress

Some theorists conceptualize stress as a complex, dynamic, and reciprocal transaction between person and environment. Other theorists view stress solely as a stimulus that causes psychological or physiological responses that in turn increase vulnerability to disease. This chapter uses the **response-based model** of Hans Selye (1974, 1976), and our distinction between *stressors* and *stress* stems from this model. Selye found that physical, emotional, psychological,

BOX 25-1 ■ Stressors Throughout the Life Span

The following are common developmental stressors. Of course not everyone will experience these stressors.

Childhood

School-age children may also experience stressors at school or among peers; however, children's stressors occur primarily in the home:

- Absence of parental figures
- Failure of parents to meet needs for safety, security, love, and belonging
- Failure of parents to meet basic physiological needs for oxygen, food, elimination, rest, and cleanliness

Adolescence

- Exposure to an expanded environment and a wider circle of friends and acceptance by peers
- Rapid changes in body appearance
- Need for academic achievement, sports performance, or demonstration of other talents
- Peer pressure
- Maintaining self-esteem while searching for identity
- Decisions about the future in the areas of school, work, and relationships
- Conflicts between standards for behavior and the sex drive
- Decisions about and involvement with alcohol and drugs

Young Adult

- Separation from family, starting college or a job
- Making the transition from youth to adult responsibilities
- Preparing for careers: graduation from college, learning a trade
- Establishing career goals and planning how to achieve success and career stability
- Financial stressors around relationships and providing a home for self or family
- Parenting children
- Conflicts between responsibilities for work and family or other relationships

Middle Age

- Concern with career achievement and continuing career challenges
- Continuation of child rearing; marriage of the children; grandparenting
- Changes in appearance and health due to aging
- Dealing with too many responsibilities: e.g., children, work, elderly parents, community activities
- Empty-nest syndrome when the children leave home
- Being "sandwiched" between caring for aging parents as well as children or grandchildren
- "Mid-life crisis" (wanting to escape from one's present life): The person regresses and unrealistically tries to recapture youth, for example, by buying a new sports car that is too small to hold the entire family, making a geographic move, taking an exotic vacation that strains the budget, engaging in an affair, daydreaming excessively about the ideal life in retirement, "partying" and overuse of alcohol and illicit drugs, engaging in "workaholic" behavior, or unhealthy "addiction" to cosmetic surgery. Any one of these behaviors does not necessarily signal mid-life crisis, but they are all examples of behaviors someone might use as an escape.

Older Adults

- Loss of family and friends due to illness or death, resulting in loneliness and isolation
- Changes in physical appearance and functional abilities, including mobility
- Major life changes (e.g., retirement, loss of life partner)
- Health problems (e.g., chronic diseases) with accompanying discomfort or pain
- The cost of healthcare
- Learning to live on a fixed, perhaps inadequate, income
- Adjusting to loss of independence
- Reduction in social status
- Substance and alcohol misuse and abuse is a problem for about 15% of adults older than the age of 50 (Substance Abuse and Mental Health Services Administration, 2007).

---

and spiritual stressors, or the anticipation of a stressor (as in anxiety), can initiate nonspecific physiological *responses*. Selye defined these responses as stress.

For more information about the transaction and stimulus models of stress,

 Go to Chapter 25, **Supplemental Materials: Models of Stress,** on the Student Resource Disk or DavisPlus at http://davisplus.fadavis.com/Wilkinson2

 Critical**Thinking** 25-1

- Make a list of your own stressors in the following areas: work, school, family, and living situation.
- What physiological stressors do you have?

How Do Coping and Adaptation Relate to Stress?

Coping strategies are the thinking processes and behaviors a person uses to manage stressors. Some examples are problem-solving, daydreaming, making changes in lifestyle (e.g., exercising more, eating less), sleeping, and consulting others for support or advice. Coping strategies can be adaptive or maladaptive.

Adaptive (effective) coping consists of making healthy choices that reduce the negative effects of stress (e.g., exercising to relieve tension, engaging in a favorite hobby). Sometimes the difference between effective and ineffective coping is in the degree to which a technique is used (for examples, see the section "Ego Defense Mechanisms" later in this chapter).

Maladaptive (ineffective) coping does not promote adaptation. Unhealthful coping choices include overeating, working too much, and substance abuse. Although a maladaptive behavior may temporarily relieve anxiety, it may have other harmful effects. For example, a person who smokes to relieve the tensions of a stressful work situation may experience an immediate decrease in anxiety. However, the person is doing nothing to change or adapt to the stressful situation, and, over time, is increasing her risk of respiratory disease.

Three Approaches to Coping Are Commonly Used

People use three approaches to cope with stress, at different times and in various combinations:

- *Altering the stressor.* In some situations, a person takes actions to remove or change the stressor. For example, Gloria ("Meet Your Patients") might remove one of her stressors by resigning her position as a Scout leader.
- *Adapting to the stressor.* It is not always possible to remove or change a stressor. Adapting involves changing one's thoughts or behaviors related to the stressor. Gloria cannot change the fact that her father needs ongoing care and her mother needs surgery, but as she gains experience as a caregiver, she may find easier, more efficient ways to care for her parents. This would give her a little more time to relax or attend to other responsibilities.
- *Avoiding the stressor.* Sometimes it is healthful to avoid a stressor. For example, you may find that being with a certain person is stressful for you, even though you have tried many times to change the dynamics of the relationship. In that case, it may be best to minimize or end your relationship with the person. In other situations, avoidance may be maladaptive. For example, a woman who discovers a lump in her breast becomes anxious that she may have cancer. She copes with her anxiety by putting it out of her mind and avoids seeking medical care. As a result, if the lump is cancerous, it would not be treated at an early stage.

The Outcome of Stress Is Either Adaptation or Disease

Stress results in either adaptation or disease. Successful adaptation allows for normal growth and development and effective responses to changes and challenges in daily life. The outcome depends on the balance between the strength of the stressors and the effectiveness of the person's coping methods (Fig. 25-1). In the following equation, **E** is the event (stressor), **R** is the person's response (which is determined in part by past experiences, perception of the stressor, and coping methods used), and **O** is the outcome.

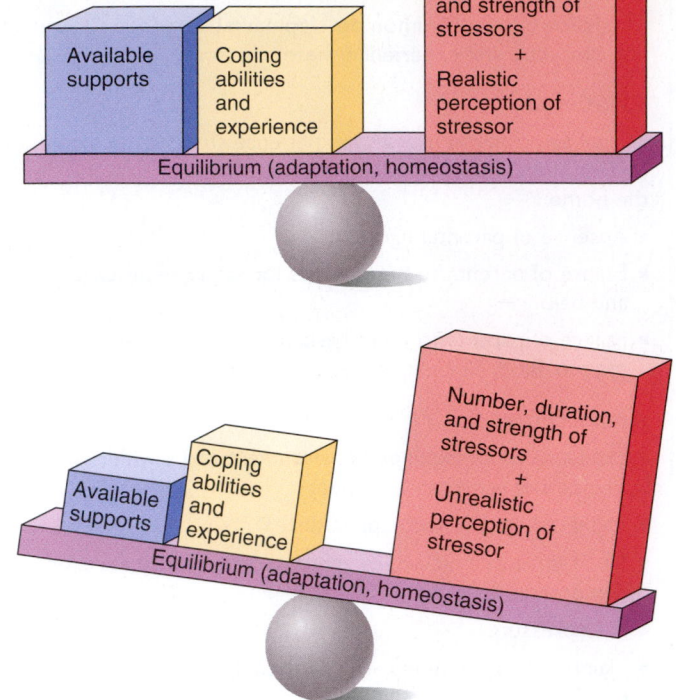

FIGURE 25-1 Adaptation occurs when a person has supports and coping abilities adequate to enable him to deal with the stressors. A realistic perception of the stressful event promotes adaptation, whereas an unrealistic perception makes adaptation more difficult.

E	+	R	=	0
stressful event		response (experience, perception, coping methods)		outcome (adaptation or disease)

Some events produce more stress than others. However, a person with good coping skills can usually adapt to a single stressful event, even a demanding one. But suppose several stressors occur in a short period of time. Gloria ("Meet Your Patients") has many stressors, so her coping abilities may be taxed to the limit. When there are many stressors or when stressors continue for a long period of time, adaptation is more likely to fail.

Personal Factors Influence Adaptation

Why do some people succumb to overwhelming stress while others adapt and thrive? Fortunately, successful adaptation does not depend entirely on being able to alter or avoid stressors. Various personal factors also influence the outcome:

Perception of the Stressor. A person's perception may be realistic or exaggerated. Suppose two women with similar coping skills and support systems both must have a mastectomy. Mrs. King thinks, "Yes, I am losing a part of my body, but I am more than just a breast. This will be a difficult adjustment, but I am so grateful to be alive." Mrs. Alan thinks, "I will be so ugly. My husband won't want to touch me. I won't be much of a woman now. This is the worst thing that could ever happen." Which woman do you think is more likely to adapt successfully to this change in her body?

Overall Health Status. On the one hand, stressors may actually cause a healthy person to engage in constructive adaptive behaviors that improve health. A person who has just discovered that he has hypertension may react by modifying his diet and exercising to lower his blood pressure and prevent complications. On the other hand, if a person with hypertension also has been coping for years with pain and immobility from arthritis, he may be too overwhelmed and exhausted to take any actions to lower his blood pressure.

Support System. A **support system** may include friends, family, counseling groups, church groups, or other like-minded people who share common interests. A good support system can help a person adapt to stress, provide emotional support, encourage expression of feelings, and help the person solve problems. It may also provide financial and other concrete types of support, such as a place to live, meal preparation, household help, child care, and transportation.

Hardiness. People who thrive despite overwhelming stressors tend to have a quality that has been termed **hardiness**. They maintain three key attitudes that help them weather adversity: commitment, control, and challenge. Commitment lets them seek to be involved with ongoing events, rather than feeling isolated. Control enables them to struggle and try to influence outcomes instead of becoming passive and feeling powerless. Challenge allows them to perceive stressful changes as opportunities for learning (Maddi, 1987, 2002).

Other Personal Factors. Age, developmental level, and life experiences (e.g., learning which coping methods have worked for you) all affect a person's response to stress. For example, infants and the very old may lack the physiological reserves to adapt to physical stressors, such as temperature extremes, dehydration, or illness.

Even with a positive attitude and good coping skills, excessive amounts of stress can lead to maladaptation and disease. Some people succumb to illness after experiencing only a few stressors, whereas others seem to adapt to multiple, intensely difficult stressors. Each person has a different ability to tolerate stress, but everyone has a breaking point at which stress becomes overwhelming.

KnowledgeCheck 25-2

- True or false: The difference between adaptive and maladaptive coping is that maladaptive coping does not relieve stress.
- In addition to avoiding the stressor, what are two other approaches to coping?
- (Complete the sentence.) The outcome of stress (adaptation or disease) depends on the balance among the strength, number, and duration of the stressors and _____.

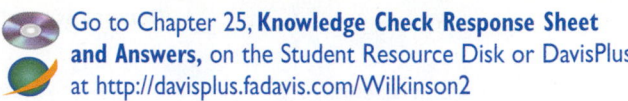

Go to Chapter 25, **Knowledge Check Response Sheet and Answers,** on the Student Resource Disk or DavisPlus at http://davisplus.fadavis.com/Wilkinson2

How Do People Respond to Stressors?

Although Selye's (1974, 1976) response-based model acknowledges physical, emotional, psychological, and spiritual *stressors*, his ideas about responses (*stress*) are primarily physiological. As you know, the body has various homeostatic mechanisms for regulating its internal environment to maintain homeostasis. In Selye's theory, physiological responses to stress are described by the general adaptation syndrome (GAS) and the local adaptation syndrome (LAS).

The General Adaptation Syndrome Includes Nonspecific, Systemic Responses

Would you be surprised to know that a near-miss automobile accident and kicking the winning field goal at a football game would both produce the same general body responses? It is true. Regardless of the specific stressor, the responses involve the whole body, especially the autonomic nervous system and the endocrine system. The **general adaptation syndrome (GAS)** is Selye's name for the group of nonspecific responses that all people share in the face of stressors. The GAS has three stages: (1) the initial alarm stage, (2) resistance (adaptation), and (3) the final stage of either recovery or exhaustion (Fig. 25-2).

Alarm Stage—"Fight or Flight"

Imagine yourself in this situation: It is dark. You are alone, walking to your car, when you hear footsteps behind you. You stop and look around and see no one. As you begin walking again, the footsteps return. You walk faster; the footsteps are faster. Stop reading, shut your eyes, and use your imagination. How do you feel? Pay attention to your physical and emotional reactions. If you are not feeling a response to this imaginary situation, think back to a time when something similar happened to you—when something frightened you.

Is your heart pounding?
Are you breathing fast?
Is there a flutter in your stomach?
What is the physical sensation in your muscles?
Do you feel frightened? What are your emotions?
Are you straining to hear the footsteps?
Do you want to run away, or are you "frozen"?
If someone were to walk into the room where you are studying right now, would it startle you?

This scenario should help you to imagine the experience of the alarm stage, during which the body prepares for *"fight or flight."* The alarm stage has two phases: shock and countershock. The **shock phase** begins when the cerebral cortex first perceives a stressor

FIGURE 25-2 The stages of Selye's general adaptation syndrome (GAS) are (1) *alarm* (also called "fight or flight"); (2) *resistance* (or adaptation), in which the body enacts physical and psychological adaptive mechanisms to maintain homeostasis; and (3) either *recovery* or *exhaustion* (which usually ends in disease or death).

and sends out messages to activate the endocrine and sympathetic nervous systems. Large amounts of epinephrine (adrenaline) and various other hormones prepare the body for fight or flight. The shock phase does not last long—usually less than 24 hours, and sometimes only a minute or two. In the **countershock phase,** all the changes produced in the shock phase are reversed, and the person becomes less able to deal with the immediate threat.

Endocrine System Responses

In response to a perceived stressor, the following endocrine responses occur:

1. The *hypothalamus* releases corticotropin-releasing hormone (CRH).
2. *CRH,* together with messages from the cerebral cortex, directs the pituitary gland to release adrenocorticotropic hormone (ACTH) and antidiuretic hormone (ADH).
3. *ACTH* stimulates the adrenal cortex to produce and secrete glucocorticoids (especially cortisol) and mineralocorticoids (especially aldosterone).

   - *Cortisol,* in general, has a glucose-sparing effect. It increases the use of fats and proteins for energy and conserves glucose for use by the brain. Cortisol also has an anti-inflammatory effect. See Figure 25-3 for the effects of cortisol during the alarm reaction of the GAS.
   - *Aldosterone* promotes fluid retention by causing the kidneys to reabsorb more sodium. In that way, it helps to increase fluid volume and maintain or increase blood pressure.

4. *ADH* also promotes fluid retention by increasing the reabsorption of water by kidney tubules. See Figure 25-4 for the effects of aldosterone and ADH.

5. *Endorphins,* secreted by the hypothalamus and posterior pituitary, act like opiates to produce a sense of well-being and reduce pain.
6. *Thyroid-stimulating hormone (TSH)* is secreted by the pituitary gland to increase the efficiency of cellular metabolism and fat conversion to energy for cell and muscle needs.

Sympathetic Nervous System Responses

The cerebral cortex also sends messages via the hypothalamus to stimulate the sympathetic nervous system. The sympathetic nervous system then stimulates

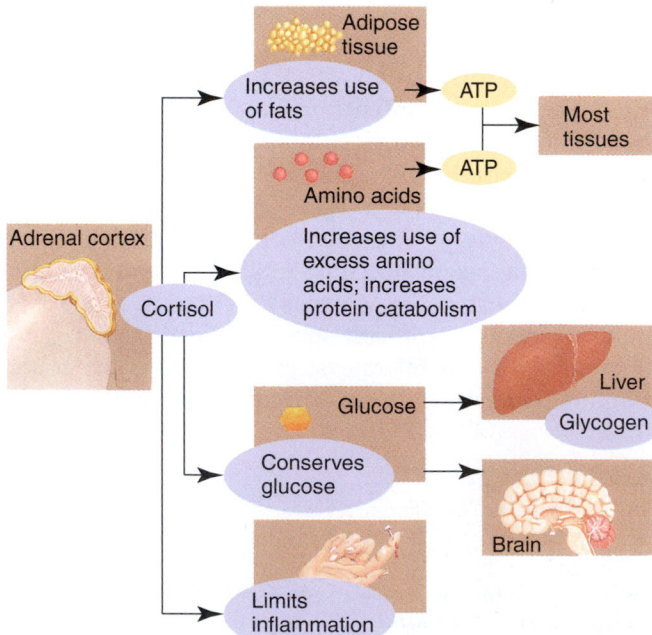

FIGURE 25-3 Functions of cortisol during the alarm stage of the GAS. (From Scanlon, V., & Sanders, T. (2007). *Essentials of anatomy and physiology* (5th ed.). Philadelphia: F. A. Davis, p. 241.)

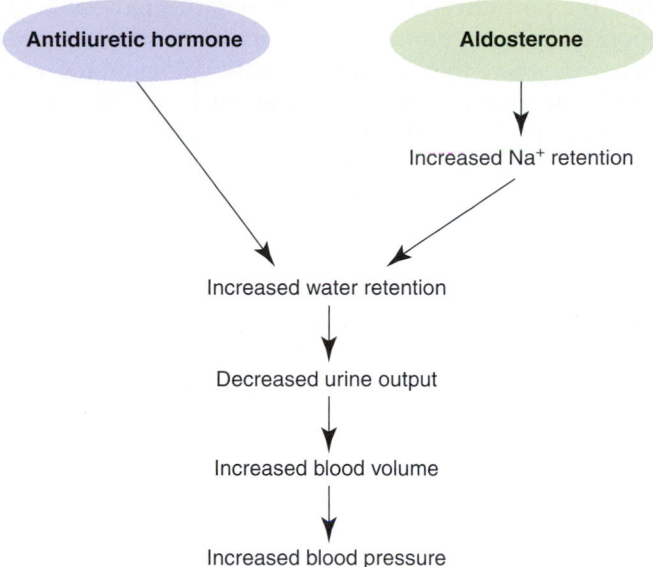

FIGURE 25-4 The release of ADH (from the posterior pituitary gland) and aldosterone (from the adrenal cortex) leads to sodium and water retention, increases blood volume, and increases blood pressure.

the adrenal glands to secrete adrenaline and norepinephrine, which increase mental alertness. This allows the person to assess the situation and aids in a decision to stand and fight or run away in flight. Adrenaline also increases the ability of the muscles to contract and causes the pupils to dilate, producing greater visual fields. See Figure 25-5 for the effects of adrenaline during the alarm reaction of the GAS.

Other Body System Responses in the Alarm Stage

The following are some body system responses that occur in the alarm stage as a result of endocrine and sympathetic nervous system activity. Refer to Figures 25-2 through 25-5 to see how these changes are produced.

- *Cardiovascular system.* The heart rate and contraction force increase. Peripheral and visceral vasoconstriction increases blood flow to vital organs (e.g., brain, lungs) and to muscles preparing for flight. Blood volume and blood pressure also increase, and the blood clots more readily.
- *Respiratory system.* The bronchioles dilate, thereby increasing the depth of respiration and tidal volume. This makes oxygen available for diffusion to muscle, brain, and cardiac cells.
- *Metabolism.* The metabolic rate increases. The liver converts more glycogen to glucose (*glycogenolysis*), making it available for energy. Except in the brain, the body uses less glucose for energy. The use of amino acids and the mobilization of fats for energy (*lipolysis*) increase.
- *Urinary system.* Blood flow to the kidneys decreases, and they retain more sodium and water. The kidneys secrete renin, which produces *angiotensin*. In turn, angiotensin constricts the arterioles and tends to increase blood pressure.

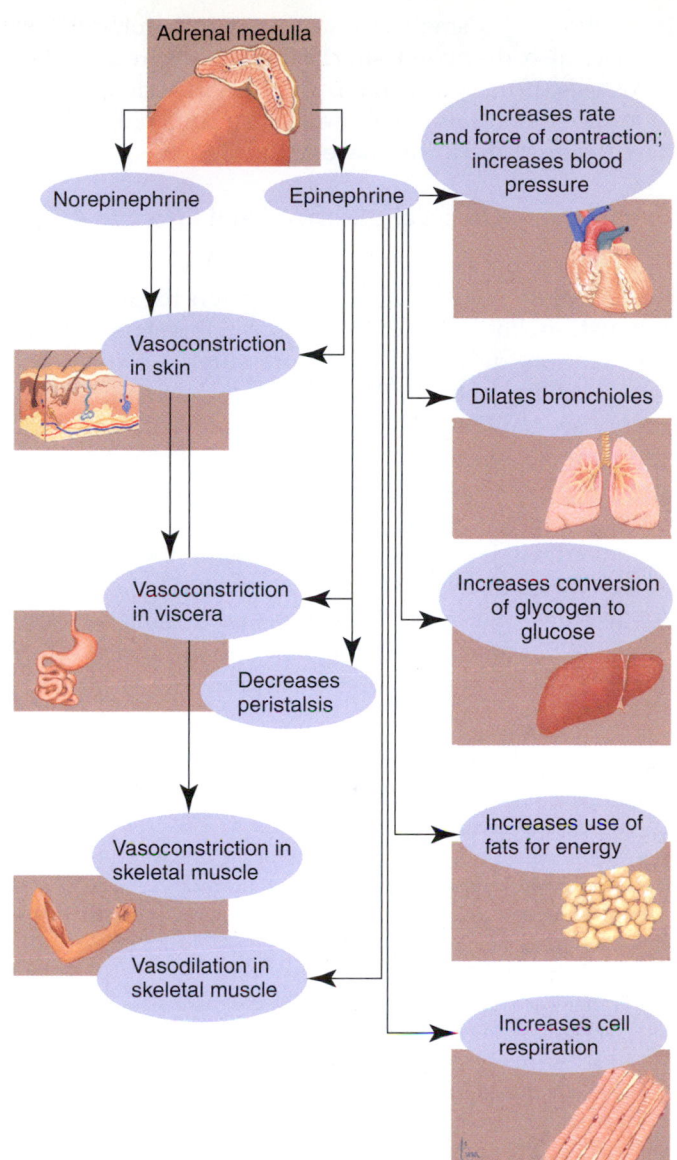

FIGURE 25-5 Functions of epinephrine and norepinephrine during the alarm stage of the GAS. (From Scanlon, V., & Sanders, T. (2007). *Essentials of anatomy and physiology* (5th ed.). Philadelphia: F. A. Davis, p. 239.)

- *Gastrointestinal system.* Peristalsis and secretions of digestive enzymes decrease. The blood glucose level increases to fuel the energy needed for fight or flight.
- *Musculoskeletal system.* Blood vessels dilate, increasing flow of blood (and thus oxygen and energy) to skeletal muscles.

Resistance Stage—Coping with the Stressor

During the second stage of the GAS, **resistance** (or *adaptation*), the body tries to cope, protect itself against the stressor, and maintain homeostasis. Stabilization involves the use of physiological and psychological coping mechanisms. Psychological defense mechanisms for coping are discussed shortly. Physical adaptations help the heart rate, blood pressure, cardiac output, respiratory function, and hormone levels return to normal. If the person adapts successfully or if the stress can be be confined to a small area (as in the inflammatory response, also discussed shortly), the body regains homeostasis. If the stress is too great (as in serious illness or severe blood loss), defense mechanisms fail, and the person enters the third phase of the GAS.

Exhaustion or Recovery Stage—Final Effort to Adapt

If stress continues and adaptive mechanisms become ineffective or are used up, a person enters the final stage, **exhaustion.** Physiological responses in this stage include vasodilation, decreased blood pressure, and increased pulse and respirations. Physical adaptive resources and energy are depleted. The body is unable to defend itself and cannot maintain resistance against the continuing stressors. Exhaustion usually ends in injury, illness, or death.

In contrast, if adaptation is successful, the final stage is **recovery.** For example, after a miscarriage, a couple participates in a support group and begins to focus more deeply on their relationship with each other. They are able gradually to resolve their grief.

KnowledgeCheck 25-3

- In general, what is the difference between the alarm stage and the resistance stage of the GAS?
- Name the gland that releases each of the following hormones in response to stress, and name each hormone's function: corticotropin-releasing hormone (CRH), antidiuretic hormone (ADH), adrenocorticotropic hormone (ACTH), aldosterone, cortisol, epinephrine, and norepinephrine.
- In the alarm stage of the GAS, what are the effects of the sympathetic nervous system on each of the following: heart, brain, glycogen stores, and skeletal muscle?
- What is the effect of Selye's resistance stage on the cardiovascular and respiratory systems? On hormone levels?

 Go to Chapter 25, **Knowledge Check Response Sheet and Answers,** on the Student Resource Disk or DavisPlus at http://davisplus.fadavis.com/Wilkinson2

The Local Adaptation Syndrome Involves a Specific Local Response

Whereas the GAS is a whole-body response to a stressor, the **local adaptation syndrome (LAS)** is a localized body response; that is, it involves only a specific body part, tissue, or organ. It is a short-term attempt to restore homeostasis. As a nurse, the two most common LAS responses you will deal with are the reflex pain response and the inflammatory response (others include blood clotting and pupil constriction in response to light).

Reflex Pain Response

When you perceive a painful stimulus, especially in one of your limbs, you immediately and unconsciously withdraw from the source of pain. If you've ever accidentally touched a hot stove, you certainly didn't stop to ponder, "Hmmm, I think I will withdraw my hand." You pulled your hand away before you could even think about it.

This is a protective **reflex** (an involuntary, predictable response). Pain receptors send sensory impulses to the spinal cord, where they synapse with the spinal motor neurons. The motor impulses travel back to the site of stimulation, causing the flexor muscles in the limb to contract. This is a local, rather than a whole-body, response.

Inflammatory Response

The **inflammatory response** is a local reaction to cell injury, either by pathogens or by physical, chemical, or other agents (Box 25-2). Regardless of the injuring agent (stressor), its mechanisms are the same, and they produce the classic symptoms of inflammation: pain, heat, swelling, redness, and loss of function. The inflammatory process includes a vascular response, a cellular response, formation of exudate, and healing.

Vascular Response. Immediately after injury, blood vessels at the site constrict (narrow) to control bleeding. After the injured cells release histamine, the vessels dilate, increasing blood flow to the area **(hyperemia).** Under the influence of kinins released by the dying cells, the capillaries become more permeable, allowing movement of fluid from capillaries into tissue spaces. The tissue becomes edematous. After leukocytes move into the area, localized blood flow again decreases, to keep them in the area to fight infection.

Cellular Response. Specialized white blood cells **(phagocytes)** migrate to the site of injury and engulf bacteria, other foreign material, and damaged cells and destroy them. Sometimes they form a "wall" around an invading pathogen. The accumulation of dead white cells, digested bacteria, and other cell debris in the presence of infection is called *pus.*

BOX 25-2 ■ Agents Causing Inflammatory Responses

The following agents stimulate the inflammatory response by causing cell injury:

- Autoimmune disorders
- Antigen–antibody responses
- Body substances (e.g., digestive enzymes leaking into the abdomen; accumulation of uric acid crystals in joints)
- Chemical injury (e.g., acid or alkali burns)
- Ischemia
- Neoplastic growth (i.e., cancer)
- Pathogens (e.g., bacteria, viruses)
- Physical agents:
    Heat or cold
    Radiation
    Electrothermal injury
    Mechanical trauma (e.g., abrasion, contusion, laceration, puncture, incision, fractures, sprains)

Exudate Formation. The fluid and white blood cells that move from the circulation to the site of injury are called **exudate.** The nature and quantity of exudate depend on the severity of injury and the tissues involved. For example, a surgical incision may ooze serosanguineous (clear or pinkish) exudate for a day or two.

Healing. Healing is the replacement of tissue by regeneration or repair. **Regeneration** is replacement of the damaged cells with identical or similar cells. However, not all cells can regenerate (e.g., some central nervous system neurons and cardiac muscle cells cannot regenerate). Most injuries heal by **repair,** wherein scar tissue replaces the original tissue. You will find a thorough discussion of wound healing in Chapter 34.

The inflammatory response is adaptive in that it protects the body from infection and promotes healing. However, chronic inflammation, as in arthritis, is itself a stressor.

Do not confuse inflammation with infection. Inflammation is a mechanism for eliminating invading pathogens; therefore, you always see inflammation when there is infection. However, inflammation is stimulated by trauma as well as by pathogens (as in the example of a sprained ankle); thus, it can occur when there is no infection.

KnowledgeCheck 25-4

- What are four characteristics of the local adaptation syndrome (LAS)?
- Name two LAS responses.
- What are the classic symptoms of the inflammatory process?

 Go to Chapter 25, **Knowledge Check Response Sheet and Answers,** on the Student Resource Disk or DavisPlus at http://davisplus.fadavis.com/Wilkinson2

Psychological Responses to Stress Include Feelings, Thoughts, and Behaviors

Health professionals understand most human health disorders to be *biopsychosocial* in nature (Alford, 2007). That is, they consist of interactions among biological, psychological, and social factors. Recall that stress responses are holistic. That means we respond and adapt to stress physically, mentally, and behaviorally, and many would add spiritually.

Psychological responses are both emotional and cognitive, and they include feelings, thoughts, and behaviors (Box 25-3). They may be fleeting, as in a flash of anger that is gone in seconds; or long-term, as in the avoidance of relationships by an adult whose needs for love and security were not met as a child.

As with physical responses, psychological responses can be adaptive or harmful. Consider this example case:

Case example: Both Mr. Laslow and Mr. Harvey have had heart attacks and are both anxious about the future. To relieve his anxiety, Mr. Laslow takes a prob-

BOX 25-3 ■ Psychological Responses To Stressors

Cognitive Responses

Difficulty concentrating

Poor judgment

Decrease in accuracy (e.g., in counting money)

Forgetfulness

Decreased problem-solving ability

Decreased attention to detail

Difficulty learning

Narrowing of focus

Preoccupation, daydreaming

Emotional Responses

Adjustment disorders

Anger

Anxiety

Depression

Fear

Feelings of inadequacy

Low self-esteem

Irritability

Lack of motivation

Lethargy

Behavioral Responses

Academic difficulties

Aggressiveness

Crying, emotional outbursts

Dependence

Nightmares

Poor job performance

Substance use and abuse

Sleeplessness (or sleeping too much)

Change in eating habits (e.g., loss of appetite, overeating)

Decrease in quality of job performance

Preoccupation (i.e., daydreaming)

Illnesses

Increased absenteeism from work or school

Increased number of accidents

Strained family or social relationships

Avoiding social situations or relationships

Rebellion, acting out

lem-solving approach, learning about diet, exercise, and lifestyle changes that he must make. Mr. Harvey uses denial; he cannot even accept that he has "really" had a heart attack. He says, "I'm not an invalid. I feel fine. I could follow all those rules and still get hit by a truck and die tomorrow." Both of these responses may relieve the person's anxiety. Which one do you think is more adaptive in the long term?

Common emotional responses to stress include anxiety, fear, anger, and depression.

Anxiety and Fear

As discussed in Chapter 11, **anxiety** is diffuse and not easily defined. NANDA International (2009, p. 242) defines it as a "vague, uneasy feeling of discomfort or dread accompanied by an autonomic response (the source often nonspecific or unknown to the individual); a feeling of apprehension caused by anticipation of danger. . ." Notice that the response is not to a danger but to the *anticipation* of danger—to imagining it. An anxious person worries; feels nervous, uneasy, and fearful; may be tearful; and often has physical symptoms, such as nausea, trembling, and sweating.

Fear is an emotion or feeling of apprehension (dread) from an identified danger, threat, or pain. The danger may be real or imagined. Anxiety and fear produce similar responses; however, some experts differentiate them as follows:

- Fear is a cognitive response, whereas anxiety is an emotional response.
- Fear is related to a present event, whereas anxiety is related to a future (or anticipated) event.
- The source of fear is easily identifiable, whereas the source of anxiety may not be identifiable.
- Fear can result from either a physical or a psychological event; anxiety results from psychological conflict rather than physical threat.

Mild to moderate anxiety may be adaptive because it motivates and mobilizes the person to action. However, severe anxiety consumes energy and interferes with the person's ability to focus on and respond to what is really happening. See Chapter 11 to refresh your theoretical knowledge of anxiety and fear, including levels of anxiety.

Anxiety and fear initiate the release of epinephrine, which stimulates the sympathetic nervous system and prepares the person for fight or flight. Therefore, living with anxiety can be physically, emotionally, and spiritually exhausting.

 Critical**Thinking** 25-2

Read the following two scenarios.

1. You are a student assigned to a 6-hour day in the clinical area. Each time you have a clinical day coming up, you feel anticipation and look forward to working in the clinical area. However, you do not know what to expect. You think: "What will my patients be like? How will the day go? Do I know enough to handle it? Do I need to practice any procedures?" It is hard to answer these questions until you are actually on the unit and see your patients.

2. Given the same situation, suppose that when you begin your clinical day, your clinical instructor tells you that he will be in the agency asking questions, supervising, evaluating your performance—and, perhaps from your perspective, making your life miserable.

In which situation are you most likely to feel fear rather than anxiety? Explain your reasoning.

Ego defense mechanisms are unconscious mental mechanisms that make a stressful situation more tolerable by decreasing the inner tension associated with the stressors. Just as the body responds physiologically to stressors, it has psychological responses that protect the person from anxiety and assist with adaptation. When used sparingly, and for mild to moderate anxiety, defense mechanisms can be helpful. When overused, however, they become habits that give us the false illusion that we are coping. If psychological defense mechanisms are inadequate to diminish the threat and restore equilibrium, the person may develop an anxiety disorder. Table 25-1 identifies some common psychological defense mechanisms.

Anger and Depression

Anger is a strong, uncomfortable feeling of animosity, hostility, extreme indignation, or displeasure. A person who cannot control stressors may become apprehensive (anxious about what may happen) and respond with anger. Thus, moderate anger is often a first protective response against anxiety. As anxiety increases and the person recognizes fear, he feels more threatened and may resort to bullying behavior to increase the personal feeling of power, control, and self-esteem.

Anger may be expressed in screaming or shouting, throwing things, or hitting, or more subtly with sarcastic, caustic remarks. Some people attempt to hide their emotions and soften their hurtful remarks, or make them more socially acceptable, through the use of humor and joking. When anger involves destructive behaviors such as physical or verbal abuse, it is called **hostility.** When expressed appropriately and clearly (i.e., verbally), anger can be adaptive, because it temporarily releases the person's feelings of tension. When the anger is out in the open, both parties can deal with it. Nevertheless, even verbal expressions of anger can be destructive if the anger continues after the person expresses it.

Depression is sometimes associated with unresolved anger and may result from stress. It is normal to feel depression in response to any loss or a traumatic event, but long-term depression is a reason for concern. Review Chapter 11 for information about anger and depression.

Knowledge Check 25-5

- In addition to ego defense mechanisms, name four common emotional responses to stress.
- Explain how mild to moderate anxiety can be adaptive.
- True or false: One difference between anxiety and fear is that the danger in anxiety may be imagined, whereas in fear the danger is real.
- What are ego defense mechanisms?

 Go to Chapter 25, **Knowledge Check Response Sheet and Answers,** on the Student Resource Disk or DavisPlus at http://davisplus.fadavis.com/Wilkinson2

Table 25-1 ➤ Psychological Defense Mechanisms

DEFENSE MECHANISM	EXAMPLES	EXAMPLES AND CONSEQUENCES OF OVERUSE
Avoidance—Unconsciously staying away from events or situations that might open feelings of aggression or anxiety	"I can't go to the class reunion tonight. I'm too tired; I have to sleep."	The person becomes socially isolated because of the tension he feels when around other people.
Compensation—Making up for a perceived inadequacy by developing or emphasizing some other desirable trait	A small boy who wants to be on the football team instead becomes a great singer.	Use of drugs or alcohol to gain courage to enter a social situation
Conversion—Emotional conflict is changed into physical symptoms that have no physical basis. The symptoms often disappear after the threat is over.	Feeling back pain when it is difficult to continue carrying the pressures of life; developing nausea that causes the person to miss a major exam	Laryngitis, inability to speak on the anniversary of father's death. Continued anxiety can lead to actual physical disorders, such as gastric ulcers.
Denial—Transforming reality by refusing to acknowledge thoughts, feeling, desires, or impulses. This is unconscious; the person is *not* consciously lying. Denial is usually the first defense learned.	A student refuses to acknowledge that he is barely passing anatomy, does not withdraw from the class, and is now failing a nursing course. An alcoholic states, "I can quit any time I want to."	Overuse can lead to repression and dissociative disorders (e.g., dual personalities, selective amnesia).
Displacement—"Kick the dog." Transferring emotions, ideas, or wishes from one original object or situation to a substitute inappropriate person or object that is perceived to be less powerful or threatening	Husband loses his job, goes home, and yells at his wife. (This mechanism is rarely adaptive.)	In extreme situations, this mechanism leads to verbal and physical abuse.
Dissociation—Painful events are separated or dissociated from the conscious mind.	A person who was sexually abused as a child describes the events as though they happened to a sibling.	May result in a dissociative disorder, such as multiple personality disorder.
Identification—A person takes on the ideas, personality, or characteristics of another person, especially someone that the person fears or respects.	Children play cowboy, police, fireman, or mommy.	Assumes mannerisms, wears clothing, and arranges hair and physical appearance to match those of the other person.
Intellectualization—Cognitive reasoning is used to block or avoid feelings about a painful incident.	When her husband dies, the wife relieves her pain by thinking, "It's better this way; he was in so much pain." A person says, "I think" rather than, "I feel."	"My husband loves me, so he doesn't like it when another man talks to me; that's why he beats me."
Minimization—Not acknowledging or accepting the significance of one's own behavior, making it less important	"It doesn't matter how much I drink. I never drive when I'm drinking."	Person engages in unhealthy or antisocial behavior; there is no motivation to change behavior
Projection—Blaming others. Attributing one's own personality traits, mistakes, emotions, motives, and thoughts to another; "finger pointing"	"The clinical instructor makes me nervous, so I cannot do well." "I forgot to bake cookies because you did not tell me that cookies were due at school today."	Person cannot see his own responsibility for a situation, so he cannot make adaptive behaviors. Person criticizes habits in others that are the same as one's own bad habits.
Rationalization—Use of a logical-sounding excuse to cover up or justify true ideas, actions, or feelings. An attempt to preserve self-respect or approval or to conceal a motive for some action by giving a socially acceptable reason. Similar to intellectualization, but uses faulty logic.	"It was God's will that this happened to me." "If I didn't have to work, I would be a better wife."	This mechanism can lead to self-deception.

Continued

Table 25-1 ➤ Psychological Defense Mechanisms—cont'd

DEFENSE MECHANISM	EXAMPLES	EXAMPLES AND CONSEQUENCES OF OVERUSE
Reaction formation—Similar to compensation, except the person develops the exact opposite trait. The person is aware of her feelings but acts in ways opposite to what she is really feeling.	"It's OK that you forgot my birthday" (when it really is not OK).	Overuse can cause failure to resolve internal conflicts.
Regression—Using behavior appropriate in an earlier stage of development to overcome feeling of insecurity in a present situation	Cooks and eats a comfort food (e.g., hot fudge sundae). A 60-year-old divorcee dresses and acts like a teenager.	Can interfere with perception of reality
Repression—Unconscious "burying" or "forgetting" of painful thoughts, feelings, memories, ideas; pushing them from a conscious to an unconscious level. It is a step deeper than denial.	Having no memory of sexual abuse by sibling or father An adolescent forgets to put out the trash because being "bossed" makes him angry, but he feels guilty if he consciously chooses not to do it.	Flashbacks, traumatic stress syndrome, and amnesia
Restitution (undoing)—Making amends for a behavior one thinks is unacceptable, to reduce guilt	Giving a treat to a child who has been punished for wrongdoing	May send double messages. Relieves the person of the responsibility for honesty about the situation
Sublimation—Unacceptable drives, traits, or behaviors (often sexual or aggressive) are unconsciously diverted to socially accepted traits.	Anger is expressed by aggression when playing sports. A person who chooses to not have children runs a day-care center.	The "acceptable" behavior might reinforce the negative tendencies, and the person may still show signs of the undesirable trait or behavior. For example, a person indulges in child pornography to obtain sexual gratification.

Adapted from Neeb, K. (2006). *Fundamentals of Mental Health Nursing* (3rd ed.). Philadelphia: F. A. Davis.

Spiritual Responses to Stress Are Multifaceted

Spiritual responses—as do all human responses—vary among individuals. Many people depend on a higher power or religious community for support when coping with stress. Some search for a larger meaning in the illness or other stressor. Others may view stress as a test, a punishment, or a challenge.

Often, a first response during the alarm stage is to pray or ask for help (e.g., healing, coping). Prayer, meditation, and religious affiliation can also help during the second stage (adaptation). In the final stage, spiritual resources may be exhausted, leaving the person feeling abandoned, helpless, and hopeless. If your own spiritual life is healthy, you will be better equipped to support patients who are experiencing spiritual challenges. For more information about spiritual responses to stress, see Chapter 14.

What Happens When Adaptation Fails?

Living with continual stress strains adaptive mechanisms. This strain can lead to exhaustion and disease, which in turn can lead to more stress. Once established, this type of positive feedback loop is difficult to break.

Three types of disorders that can develop when adaptation fails are stress-induced organic responses, somatoform disorders, and psychological disorders.

Stress-Induced Organic Responses

As a result of repeated central nervous system stimulation and elevation of certain hormones, continual stress brings about long-term changes in various body systems. People who use maladaptive coping strategies (e.g., overeating, substance abuse) create additional stress on the body, further contributing to disease.

Cardiovascular System. Continued secretion of epinephrine may cause cardiovascular disorders including angina, myocardial infarction, cardiomegaly, and congestive heart failure, all of which lead to decreased cardiac output. As cardiac output decreases, less oxygen circulates to meet cellular metabolic demands, and the body becomes fatigued. Prolonged secretion of epinephrine and renin result in vasoconstriction, causing hypertension. ADH, aldosterone, ACTH, and cortisol create electrolyte imbalance and retention of sodium and water, thus promoting peripheral edema.

Endocrine System. Continuing high levels of blood glucose and insulin can cause diabetes. Metabolic disorders of hyperthyroidism or hypothyroidism can result as persistent demands for thyroid hormone production cause a rebound failure of the gland. Even prenatal stress can cause adaptive changes in fetal endocrine and metabolic processes that impact later adult health (Sullivan, Hawes, Winchester, et al., 2008).

Immune System. Stress reduces the ability of the body's immune cells to differentiate between self and nonself. Thus, the immune cells begin to attack body tissues, producing autoimmune illness. Common autoimmune illnesses include rheumatoid arthritis, lupus, cancer, and allergies. Research has linked stress to suppression of the immune system and even to viral replication in HIV patients (e.g., Davidson, Kabat-Zinn, Schumacher, et al., 2003; Robinson, Mathews, & Witek-Janusek, 2000).

Gastrointestinal System. The gastrointestinal system may respond to central nervous system stimulation with constipation or diarrhea, gastroesophageal reflux, colitis, or irritable bowel syndrome. Continued secretion of hydrochloric acid produces gastric hyperacidity and erosion of the gastrointestinal tract.

Musculoskeletal System. Constant readiness for fight or flight produces muscle tension and pain in various body sites. Tension headache and temporomandibular joint pain result from prolonged muscle tension in the head, neck, and spine.

Respiratory System. Epinephrine and circulating hormones dilate the bronchial tubes and increase the rate of respiration. Hyperventilation can produce symptoms of alkalosis, including dizziness, tingling hands and feet, and anxiety. Distress in the respiratory system can exacerbate existing asthma, hay fever, and allergies.

Somatoform Disorders

Somatoform disorders are conditions characterized by the presence of physical symptoms with no known organic cause. They are believed to result from unconscious denial, repression, and displacement of anxiety. Certain people seem predisposed to somatoform disorders—for instance, those who suffer from personality disorders and major psychiatric illness, those who do not handle anxiety well, and those who are dependent, emotionally needy, frustrated, and resentful (Neeb, 2006). The physical symptoms allow the person to avoid a situation that, if confronted, would provoke extreme anxiety. The following are examples of somatoform disorders:

- **Hypochondriasis.** The person is preoccupied with the idea that he is or will become seriously ill. The person is abnormally concerned with his health and interprets his real or imagined symptoms unrealistically, fearing that they will get worse or become incurable. The person is not "faking it"; anxiety about his health may trigger the physical sensations.
- **Somatization.** In this disorder, anxiety and emotional turmoil are expressed in physical symptoms, loss of physical function, pain that changes location often,

and depression. The patient is unable to control the symptoms and behaviors, and complaints are vague or exaggerated.

- **Pain disorder.** Previously called *somatoform pain disorder*, this is emotional pain that manifests physically. Pain is the main focus of the person's life. The level of pain the person states is inconsistent with the physical condition—that is, the physical cause is either disproportionate to the pain or cannot be found at all. The pain does not change location.
- **Malingering.** Malingering is different from the other disorders because it is a *conscious* effort to escape unpleasant situations. The patient merely pretends to have the symptoms for personal or tangible gain (e.g., calling in sick because the person does not want to go to work).

KnowledgeCheck 25-6

- Name and describe three stress-induced organic or systemic responses to stress.
- Name and describe at least three somatoform disorders.

 Go to Chapter 25, **Knowledge Check Response Sheet and Answers,** on the Student Resource Disk or DavisPlus at http://davisplus.fadavis.com/Wilkinson2

Stress-Induced Psychological Responses

Even if coping mechanisms are effective initially, with long-term stress, exhaustion sets in, and the mechanisms begin to fail. The person may then try maladaptive ways to cope. As work and personal relationships deteriorate, the person loses self-esteem. Prolonged stress can eventually result in crisis and burnout (Fig. 25-6). More severe responses include psychiatric illnesses, such as anxiety disorders, clinical depression, and post-traumatic stress disorder (PTSD). Anxiety and depression were discussed in Chapter 11. We discuss crisis, burnout, and PTSD next.

Crisis

A **crisis** exists when (1) an event in a person's life drastically changes the person's routine and he perceives it as a threat to self, and (2) the person's usual coping methods are ineffective, resulting in high levels of anxiety and inability to function adequately. Such events are usually sudden and unexpected (e.g., serious illness or death of a loved one, serious financial losses, an automobile accident, rape, and natural disasters).

Keep in mind that each person has a different tolerance for stress and that an event that creates a crisis for one may be just a minor nuisance for another. Nevertheless, most experts agree that people experiencing crisis go through five phases (Neeb, 2006; Stuart & Sundeen, 2009).

1. *Precrisis.* In response to the event and the anxiety, the person uses her usual coping strategies. The person has no symptoms, denies any stress, and may even report a feeling of well-being.

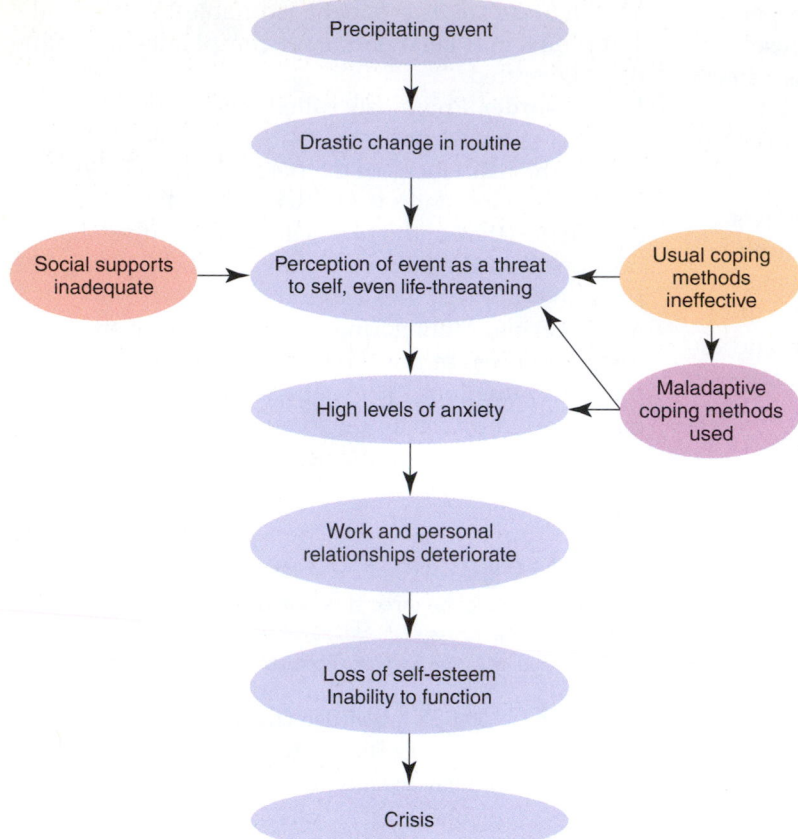

FIGURE 25-6 How a crisis develops.

2. *Impact.* If the usual strategies are not effective, anxiety and confusion increase. The person may have trouble organizing her personal life. The person may feel the stress but minimize its severity.

3. *Crisis.* The person experiences more anxiety and tries new ways of coping, such as withdrawal, rationalization, and projection (refer to Table 25-1). The person recognizes the problem but denies that it is out of control.

4. *Adaptive.* The person redefines the threat and perceives the crisis in a realistic way. She begins to think rationally and does some positive problem solving, regains some self-esteem, and is able to begin socializing again. Adaptation is more likely if the person can use effective coping strategies and if situational supports are available.

5. *Postcrisis.* The aftermath of a crisis may have both positive and negative effects on functioning. The person may have developed better ways of coping with stress. Or, she may be critical, hostile, and depressed, and she may use maladaptive strategies (e.g., overeating or substance abuse) to deal with what has happened.

People in crisis are at risk for physical and emotional harm, so intervention is essential (see "Crisis Intervention" later in the chapter).

 Critical**Thinking** 25-3

Suppose you are the charge nurse on a 30-bed surgical unit. In addition, you must assume care of three patients because

another nurse called in sick. It is a normal, busy day with seven postoperative patients and eight discharges. In addition, a patient went into cardiac arrhythmia and was transferred to the coronary care unit. Because the sick nurse was supposed to work a 12-hour shift and no replacement has been found, you are told you must stay and work 4 hours overtime. You had plans to have dinner with your spouse this evening because it is your anniversary. Now you will surely not be home before 8:00 P.M., and you will be exhausted.

- What would be the stressors for you in this situation?
- What thoughts and feelings would you have?
- What physical responses would you probably notice?
- What are some psychological responses that you would use to help you adapt and cope with this day?
- How would you probably react if the same thing were to happen on the following day?

Burnout

Burnout occurs when nurses and other professionals cannot cope effectively with the physical and emotional demands of the workplace. You will find examples of stressors specific to nursing in Box 25-4.

Excessive demands by an employer serve as a catalyst for burnout. In some situations, the nurse receives no respect and little support from the employer or coworkers. Filled with feelings of injustice for treatment received, the nurse may respond with anger and frustration, feel overwhelmed and helpless, and suffer low self-esteem and depression. Some nurses experience grief reactions, moral distress, and guilt feelings because the situation prevents them from performing as

BOX 25-4 ■ Stressors that Can Lead to Burnout

- Dealing with difficult personalities (e.g., patient, supervisors, physicians)
- Working 12-hour shifts with minimal breaks for food, water, or rest
- Frequent rotating shifts that upset the circadian rhythm of the body and lower the immune system response
- Mandatory overtime
- Being "floated" to an unfamiliar unit (e.g., a maternity nurse may be "floated" to an orthopedic unit)
- Workload: low staffing ratio (one nurse to many patients)
- Frustration with patients (e.g., who do not follow therapeutic routines)
- Need to constantly anticipate patients' needs and cope with the unexpected
- Feeling helpless against a patient's disease process or lack of healing
- Dealing with death and dying
- Lack of rewards (both intrinsic and extrinsic)
- Lack of participation in decision-making
- Inability to delegate responsibilities
- Organizational philosophy that conflicts with personal philosophy

well as they believe they should (Badger, 2008). The nurse who burns out may develop a physical illness or a negative attitude or may use maladaptive coping techniques such as smoking, substance abuse, or distancing from patients—"going through the motions" but not really interacting with patients in a meaningful way. Many nurses feeling empty and discontented in such situations give up and leave nursing. You will find suggestions for preventing burnout later in the chapter.

Post-Traumatic Stress Disorder

Post-traumatic stress disorder (PTSD) is a specific response to a violent, traumatizing event, such as an earthquake or other natural disaster, or to physical or emotional abuse, such as rape, torture, or war experience. The victim experiences anxiety and flashbacks that may last for months or years. Other symptoms include social withdrawal, feelings of low self-esteem, changes in existing relationships, difficulty forming new relationships, irritability and outbursts of anger for no obvious reason, depression, and chemical abuse or dependence.

Counseling and special intervention are needed to help the person cope with and recover from the impact of the traumatic event. Stress management has also been found to be effective (Bisson & Andrew, 2007).

Toward Evidence-Based Practice

Hall, L., Doran, D., & Pink, L. (2008). Outcomes of interventions to improve hospital nursing work environments. *The Journal of Nursing Administration, 38(1), 40–46.*

This study evaluated the effects of workplace change interventions on nurse and patient perceptions of work quality and work environment. The intervention was a workplace change designed to improve the availability of resources on patient care units (e.g., improving the linen supply, identifying basic equipment needs). The only statistically significant change after the intervention was that nurses had a more positive perception of work quality and the work environment. Based on data from patients, researchers speculate that nurses' satisfaction with work arrangements can influence patient care.

Hegge, M., & Larson, V. (2008). Stressors and coping strategies of students in accelerated baccalaureate nursing programs. *Nurse Educator, 33(1), 26–30.*

Students in six baccalaureate nursing programs reported their stress level, sources of stress, and coping strategies. Findings indicate that students experienced higher levels and more extended periods of stress than in prior life events. The most helpful coping categories, in order, included seeking social (emotional) support, turning to religion, trying to grow as a person, planning, and acceptance. Students recognized the stress of the nursing program, appraised it in light of previous experience, resolved to meet their academic goals, and used helpful coping strategies to promote positive learning outcomes.

Morgan, P., Fogel, J., Rose, L., et al. (2005). African American couples merging strengths to successfully cope with breast cancer. *Oncology Nursing Forum, 32(5), 979–987.*

This qualitative study examined the process of coping with breast cancer among African American couples. The couples described the importance of combining their strengths and working together as a couple to cope with a breast cancer diagnosis. Nurses should use this information to facilitate couples' working through a similar experience.

Recall the three approaches to coping and adaptation: Altering the stressor, adapting to the stressor, and avoiding the stressor.

1. In which study (or studies) is stress relieved by altering the stressor? Explain your thinking (e.g., what the stressor was, how it was altered).

2. Which study or studies report using support systems to help in adapting to a stressor? Explain your thinking (e.g., what the stressor was and what support system was used).

3. What ideas does each study give you for ways in which you might help Gloria and John ("Meet Your Patients")?

 Go to Chapter 25, **Toward Evidence-Based Practice Suggested Responses,** on the Student Resource Disk or DavisPlus at http://davisplus.fadavis.com/Wilkinson2

KnowledgeCheck 25-7

Define *crisis, burnout,* and *post-traumatic stress disorder.*

 Go to Chapter 25, **Knowledge Check Response Sheet and Answers,** on the Student Resource Disk or DavisPlus at http://davisplus.fadavis.com/Wilkinson2

Practical **Knowledge**
knowing how

People under stress may not be thinking clearly or able to communicate effectively; so it is important to intervene to relieve their immediate anxiety as much as possible, demonstrate empathy, and develop rapport before beginning an assessment. Focus the patient by asking short, direct questions and then proceeding to open-ended questions that will provide you with as much information as possible (see Chapter 18 if you need to review questioning techniques).

■ ASSESSMENT

Assessment should explore subjective and objective data about the person's stressors, risk factors, coping and adaptation, support systems, and stress responses (psychosocial and physiological).

Assess Stressors, Risk Factors, and Coping and Adaptation

Data about the patient's stressors and risk factors should help you to:

- Determine whether the client has a realistic or an exaggerated perception of the stressors
- Identify factors that increase risk for future stress
- Identify interventions to reduce current stress and to provide anticipatory guidance to prevent future stress

You might begin gathering these data by having the patient complete a stress inventory, such as the Holmes–Rahe Scale. Then follow up with questions such as those in "Assessment Guidelines and Tools" in Volume 2. You will also find questions to help you obtain information about patients' coping methods and adaptation in those guidelines.

 Go to Chapter 25, **Assessment Guidelines and Tools, the Holmes–Rahe Social Readjustment Scale** and **Assessing for Stress: Questions to Ask,** in Volume 2.

Assess Responses to Stress

When assessing responses to stress, recall that stress responses are holistic. Therefore, you will need to assess physiological, emotional, cognitive, and behavioral indicators of stress. For examples of questions to ask,

 Go to Chapter 25, **Assessment Guidelines and Tools, Assessing for Stress: Questions to Ask,** in Volume 2.

Assessing Physiological Responses. Because the GAS is nonspecific, you must obtain data from all body systems (for physical examination techniques, see Chapter 19). A check of vital signs for elevations in pulse, respiration, and blood pressure will indicate whether the fight-or-flight response is present. In your general survey, or overview, of the patient, you should note hygiene, grooming, facial expression, and ability to make eye contact. Box 25-5 summarizes physiological responses that indicate stress. If coping is successful, clinical signs and symptoms of stress may not be present.

Assessing Emotional and Behavioral Responses. Assess for the emotional and behavioral responses to stress that are described in Box 25-3. As the client answers questions, note posture, facial expression, body tension, and other nonverbal behaviors. Also note mood and affect. Does the client seem angry, anxious, or depressed? Check the client's records, and observe for and ask the client about destructive behaviors (e.g., drug abuse, anger). The client may or may not be aware that the feelings or behaviors are related to stress.

Assessing Cognitive Responses. You can assess the client's cognitive functioning as you assess other functional areas. See Box 25-3 to review examples of cognitive responses. Notice whether the person has difficulty focusing and responding to your questions. When you ask the client to describe and rate the intensity of the stressors, you can begin to assess whether he perceives the stressors realistically or in an exaggerated way. The

BOX 25-5 ■ Physiological Responses to Stressors

- Dilated pupils
- Muscle tension
- Stiff neck
- Headaches
- Nail biting
- Skin pallor
- Skin lesions (e.g., eczema)
- Diaphoresis, sweaty palms
- Dry mouth
- Nausea
- Weight or appetite changes
- Increased blood glucose
- Increased heart rate
- Cardiac dysrhythmias
- Hyperventilation
- Chest pain
- Water retention
- Increased urinary frequency or decreased urinary output
- Diarrhea or constipation
- Flatulence

client's responses concerning any coping strategies will give you an idea of his problem-solving abilities.

Assess Support Systems

Recall that support systems such as family, friends, and co-workers are important to the success of a client's coping strategies. Conversely, these people may be affected by the same stressors or by the client's responses to them. For these reasons, you should determine the supports available and their ability to assist the client—that is, do the significant others have the sensitivity and skills to be supportive? For examples of questions to ask,

 Go to Chapter 25, **Assessment Guidelines and Tools, Assessing for Stress: Questions to Ask,** in Volume 2.

 Critical**Thinking** 25-4

Review the scenario of Gloria and John ("Meet Your Patients"). How much does it really tell you about the clients' situation?

- Which aspect of stress do you have the most information about: their stressors, their coping methods and adaptation, their responses to stress, or their support systems?
- What facts do you have about either Gloria's or John's physiological responses to their multiple stressors? What can you infer their responses might be?
- What facts do you have about the clients' emotional and behavioral responses to their stressors?
- What information do you have about how well they are adapting to stress?
- What data do you have about their support systems? What information do you need?

ANALYSIS/NURSING DIAGNOSIS

Stress is nonspecific, so there is almost no limit to the number of nursing diagnoses that could be stress-induced. Your theoretical knowledge of the holistic nature of stress should lead you to identify diagnoses in the physical, behavioral, cognitive, emotional, interpersonal, and spiritual domains. The following are some examples.

Physical	Constipation r/t decreased peristalsis secondary to stress
Behavioral	Ineffective Therapeutic Regimen Management r/t use of denial as an ego defense mechanism to relieve anxiety
Cognitive	Impaired Short-Term Memory r/t overwhelming number and severity of stressors
Emotional	Anxiety r/t uncertainty about the future and ineffectiveness of usual coping mechanisms
Interpersonal	Impaired Parenting r/t maladaptive use of alcohol to cope with recent stress of divorce
Spiritual	Hopelessness r/t perceived lack of support and ability to change the present situation

For a more extensive list of stress-related nursing diagnoses,

 Go to Chapter 25, **Standardized Language, NANDA-I Nursing Diagnoses Associated with Stress,** in Volume 2.

It is important to correctly identify the etiology of the diagnosis so that you can choose interventions to remove or modify the stressor. For example, if you believe a patient's diarrhea is being caused by stress, you would intervene by modifying the stressor, helping the patient to perceive the stressor differently, and so on. If, instead, the diarrhea were being caused by a gastrointestinal virus, your interventions would not have been helpful.

Knowledge Check 25-8

- How might you identify and assess Gloria and John's stressors ("Meet Your Patients")?
- List three questions you could ask to find out how Gloria is coping and adapting to stress.
- List three questions you could ask to assess Gloria's physiological responses to stress. What observations might you also make?
- List three questions you could ask to assess Gloria's emotional and behavioral responses to stress.
- How might you determine whether stress is affecting Gloria's cognitive functioning?
- You know Gloria's sister is providing some support. How could you find out more about the extent of Gloria and John's support system?

 Go to Chapter 25, **Knowledge Check Response Sheet and Answers,** on the Student Resource Disk or DavisPlus at http://davisplus.fadavis.com/Wilkinson2

PLANNING OUTCOMES/EVALUATION

NOC standardized outcomes are outcomes that, if achieved, demonstrate resolution of the problem stated by the nursing diagnosis. For example, if you make a diagnosis of Anxiety related to client's perception that he will not be able to fulfill family responsibilities, you might use the NOC outcome, Anxiety Control. For a list of NOC outcomes to use for stress diagnoses,

 Go to Chapter 25, **Standardized Language, Standardized Outcomes and Interventions for Stress-Related Nursing Diagnosis,** in Volume 2.

Individualized goal or outcome statements are also specific to each nursing diagnosis. Broad, general goals for clients experiencing stress are to (1) reduce the strength and duration of the stressor, (2) relieve or remove responses to stress, and (3) use effective coping mechanisms. Examples of specific outcome statements you might write include the following:

- Reports (or physical exam reveals) reduction in physical symptoms of stress.
- Demonstrates less physical tension in facial expression and other muscle groups.

- Verbalizes increased feelings of control in the stressful situation.
- Uses problem-solving and anxiety-reducing techniques.
- Demonstrates relaxation and stress-reducing strategies.

PLANNING INTERVENTIONS/IMPLEMENTATION

NIC standardized interventions for stress may be linked to both the problem and the etiology of the nursing diagnosis. Using the preceding example of Anxiety related to the client's perception that he will not be able to fulfill family responsibilities, some interventions may focus on supporting the client's ability to fulfill family roles; others may focus on general techniques for relieving anxiety (e.g., aromatherapy, calming technique). For other stress-related NIC interventions,

 Go to Chapter 25, **Standardized Language, Standardized Outcomes and Interventions for Stress-Related Nursing Diagnoses,** in Volume 2.

Specific nursing activities will be individualized on the basis of the patient's needs and the etiologies of the nursing diagnoses. As you implement stress-reduction interventions, it is essential to consider compliance. Will the patient adhere to or cooperate with therapeutic suggestions? Does the person wish to use complementary or alternative care measures? How open is he to deviating from traditional Western therapies? Confer and collaborate with patients to determine what will fit most comfortably into their lifestyle. Those are the interventions that will be most effective.

Most stress-relieving interventions work by one or more of the following means:

- Removing or modifying the stressor(s)
- Supporting coping abilities (e.g., changing the person's perception of the stressor)
- Treating the person's responses to stress (e.g., symptoms such as anxiety or diarrhea)

As you read through the following interventions, see whether you can identify the rationale for the action. Look back at the list above as you need to.

Health Promotion Activities

People cannot always control the occurrence of a stressful event, and there are no high-tech treatments for coping with stress. However, a healthy lifestyle can prevent some stressors and improve the ability to cope with others. Chapter 41 provides an in-depth discussion of wellness promotion. The following suggestions are a brief guide to a healthy lifestyle.

Nutrition

Nutrition is important for maintaining physical homeostasis and resisting stress. For example, adequate nutrition is essential to maintain the integrity of the immune system; and proteins are needed for tissue building and healing. In addition, overweight and malnutrition are stressors that may lead to illness. See Chapter 26 if you need detailed information about nutrition. To summarize, you should advise clients to:

- Maintain a normal body weight.
- Limit the intake of fat (especially animal fat) to no more than 30% of daily calories.
- Limit the intake of sugar and salt.
- Eat more fish and poultry and less red meat.
- Eat smaller, more frequent meals to aid digestion.
- Consume 25 grams of fiber (fruits, vegetables, and whole grains) daily to promote bowel elimination.
- Consume no more than one or two alcoholic beverages per day.

Exercise

Regular exercise promotes physical homeostasis by improving muscle tone and controlling weight. It also improves the functioning of the heart and lungs and reduces the risk of cardiovascular disease. Exercise also improves emotional homeostasis by promoting relaxation and reducing tension. During exercise, the brain releases **endogenous opioids** (e.g., endorphins), which create a feeling of well-being. To achieve any health benefits, the client needs to exercise for at least 30 minutes at least 5 days of the week.

- Advise clients who are obese, chronically ill, or who have always been sedentary to consult a primary caregiver before beginning a new exercise program.
- Suggest that the client identify a variety of physical activities that he enjoys (e.g., swimming, bicycling, walking, sports) and, if possible, schedule regular sessions with one or more exercise "buddies." These strategies help the client adhere to the exercise routine.

Sleep and Rest

Sleep and rest restore energy levels, allow the body to repair itself, and promote mental relaxation. Most people need 7 or 8 hours of sleep a day; however, the amount of sleep varies among individuals. Stress, pain, and illness may interfere with the ability to sleep, so some clients may need help identifying and implementing techniques for relaxing and going to sleep (see Chapter 33 for more information on sleep, as needed).

Leisure Activities

Compared to exercise, which not everyone enjoys, leisure activities are any activities that provide joy and satisfaction. They may involve physical activity (after all, many people do enjoy exercising), or they may be sedentary activities, such as reading, painting, and even watching television. Leisure activities are a form of rest and, as such, are restorative.

Time Management

People who manage their time efficiently and organize their life routines feel more in control and, therefore, less stressed. If clients feel overwhelmed, you can help them to prioritize tasks and make "to do" lists. It is also important that they learn to delegate responsibilities and set boundaries on the use of time. For example, a working couple with three children may need to assign each child mealtime tasks, such as setting the table, drying the dishes, and so forth. Or they may need to limit the amount of time they spend cooking, reserving elaborate meals for weekends.

Time management also includes learning to say no. Out of a need to be liked or a strong sense of responsibility to others, people sometimes try to make everyone happy by agreeing to every request for assistance: from spouse, children, parents, friends, church, school, and the community. You can prompt clients to identify how much they can realistically accomplish—what is essential to do, and what would be "nice" to do.

Avoiding Maladaptive Behaviors

Some people use maladaptive behaviors as a response to stress. For others, the behaviors themselves become stressors. Advise clients to avoid the following unhealthful behaviors:

Consuming excess caffeine (e.g., coffee, tea, colas)
Abusing alcohol
Smoking or chewing tobacco
Using illegal street drugs
Abusing over-the-counter or nonprescribed medications, or using prescription medication in nonmedicinal ways
Avoiding social interaction

KnowledgeCheck 25-9

Name and discuss at least four aspects of a healthful lifestyle that can help prevent or relieve stress.

 Go to Chapter 25, **Knowledge Check Response Sheet and Answers,** on the Student Resource Disk or DavisPlus at http://davisplus.fadavis.com/Wilkinson2

Relieving Anxiety

Because anxiety is a common response to illness, medical tests, and treatments, you will use anxiety-relief interventions every day of your professional life. For example, when you tell patients what to expect before you perform a procedure or ask them to take deep breaths during a painful treatment, you lessen anxiety. If you have developed a therapeutic, trusting relationship, your very presence will help to ease the patient's anxiety. You will find specific interventions for anxiety in Chapter 11, and many of the interventions in the following sections provide anxiety relief as well (see also Complementary and Alternative Modalities (CAM): Using CAM for Stress Reduction).

Complementary & Alternative Modalities (CAM)

Using CAM for Stress Reduction

Bost, N., & Wallis, M. (2006). The effectiveness of a 15 minute weekly massage in reducing physical and psychological stress in nurses. *Australian Journal of Advanced Nursing, 23*(4), 28–33.

Thirty nurses received a 15-minute back massage once a week; the control group of 30 nurses received no therapy. Physiological stress was measured at weeks 1, 3, and 5 by urinary cortisol and blood pressure readings. Psychological stress levels were measured at weeks 1 and 5 with the State-Trait Anxiety Inventory (STAI). No significant difference in physiological measures was found between the two groups. However, anxiety decreased in the group receiving massage and increased in the control group. The difference was significant. Researchers concluded that massage therapy may be beneficial in reducing nurses' psychological stress.

Keegan, L. (2003). Therapies to reduce stress and anxiety. *Critical Care Nursing Clinics of North America, 15*(3), 321–327.

This article reports on the successful use of alternative and complementary therapies as adjunct therapies to help decrease stress for critical care patients. Therapies included in the report are aromatherapy, hydrotherapy, humor, imagery, massage, music, and relaxation.

Maville, J., Bowen, J., & Genham, G. (2008). Effect of healing touch on stress perception and biological correlates. *Holistic Nursing Practice, 22*(2), 103–110.

The researchers measured heart rate, blood pressure, muscle tension, skin conductance, and skin temperature in healthy adults before, during, and after healing touch treatment. All measures changed except for muscle tension. Results suggested that healing touch treatment is associated with both physiological and psychological relaxation and may be useful as an intervention for stress in healthy adults.

Pemberton, E., & Turpin, P. (2008). The effect of essential oils on work-related stress in intensive care unit nurses. *Holistic Nursing Practice, 22*(2), 97–102.

This small pilot study evaluated the effects of topical essential oils on nurses in intensive care unit settings. Nurses assessed their stress levels on a scale of 1 to 10. The nurses' perceived stress level decreased significantly in the intervention group. Researchers concluded that use of *L. angustifolia* and *S. sclaria* in sweet almond oil had a beneficial effect on work-related stress reduction.

Anger Management

Anger is a common response to stress. However, clients usually do not openly say, "I am angry." In fact, they may not even recognize that they are angry. Instead, they engage in angry behaviors. For example, they may become hypercritical of family members or caregivers, become verbally abusive, or become demanding. By now you have probably heard stories from nurses about the client who is "on the call light constantly." Unfortunately, such behaviors often provoke frustration or anger in others—even nurses. Be aware of how you are responding to stressed-out clients. Are you relieving your own stress, or are you relieving the client's stress? If you respond angrily to relieve your own stress, you may provoke further negative emotion in the client and even escalate the situation to the point of violence. Not only that, but anger also blocks communication and can lead to poor patient care and reduced patient satisfaction. For other tips on managing anger, refer to Box 21-8, Dealing With Violence, and

 Go to Chapter 25, **Clinical Insight 25-1: Dealing with Angry Patients,** in Volume 2.

Stress Management Techniques

It is important to teach your clients about relaxation and other stress management techniques. Most such techniques focus on discharging tension or simplifying one's life to modify stressors or control stress responses. **Relaxation** is a state of reduced physical and mental arousal. It is an important intervention because it reverses some stress responses. By elongating muscle fibers, relaxation reduces neural impulses sent to the brain and decreases the activity of the brain and other body systems. Blood pressure, heart rate, respiratory rate, and oxygen consumption decrease, while peripheral skin temperatures and brain alpha wave activity increase.

Many of the techniques in this section are complementary or alternative therapies that require special training, and which are discussed in detail in other chapters. For 12 weeks of daily suggestions for coping with stress,

 Go to Chapter 25, **Tables, Boxes, Figures: ESG Box 25-1,** on the Student Resource Disk or DavisPlus at http://davisplus.fadavis.com/Wilkinson2

- *Exercise* reduces stress because it releases tension held in muscles, improves muscle tone and posture, expresses emotions, and stimulates the secretion of endorphins, thus creating a feeling of well-being and relaxation.
- *Relaxation techniques* involve teaching the patient to relax individual muscle groups. **Progressive relaxation** in a quiet meditation state or lying in bed, relaxing and contracting muscle groups is much less traumatic and damaging to fragile joints and muscles than active exercise. Therefore, it may be used even by people who are not in good health. **Passive relaxation,** in which the person relaxes the muscle groups without first contracting them, is even less traumatic and requires even less energy.
- *Meditation* involves heightening one's attention or awareness. Regular meditation increases harmony among mind, body, and spirit, thereby reducing anxiety and giving the person control. See Chapter 40 for further information. For a script to lead a client through a guided meditation to reduce stress,

 Go to Chapter 25, **Tables, Boxes, Figures: ESG Box 25-2, Script for Visualization,** on the Student Resource Disk or DavisPlus at http://davisplus.fadavis.com/Wilkinson2

- *Visualization or imagery* techniques are often used to complement the effects of relaxation techniques. They are explained in Chapters 30 and 40.
- *Biofeedback* techniques use electronic instruments to measure neuromuscular and autonomic nervous system activity and provide information about those responses to the person. The immediate feedback helps the person become aware of and learn how to voluntarily control certain physiological responses, such as those produced by stress (Olson, 2003). Biofeedback practitioners require special training, and most are credentialed in biofeedback.
- *Acupuncture* involves insertion of a needle into "meridian points" to regulate the flow of energy or life force throughout the body. It can modify pain perception and restore normal physiological functions (e.g., decrease the heart rate). Special training is required to use this intervention (see Chapter 30).
- *Chiropractic adjustment* involves manual realignment of the vertebrae. Misalignment of the vertebrae is thought to lead to pain, loss of function, and illness. Realignment is performed to free energy, release muscle tension, and improve body function and health. Chiropractors undergo special education and training before they are qualified to perform adjustments. See Chapter 40 for more information.
- *Reiki and therapeutic touch* are focused on energy modulation. Healing energy is channeled through a practitioner's hands to improve well-being. See Chapters 30 and 40 for more information.
- *Massage,* through manipulation of the soft tissues, relaxes muscles, releases body tension, improves circulation, and allows energy and blood to flow through muscles and soft tissues more readily. See Chapters 30 and 40 for more information. For instructions on how to give a back rub,

 Go to Chapter 33, **Procedure 33–1: Giving a Back Massage,** in Volume 2.

- *Reflexology* is the application of pressure to specific points on the feet, hands, or ears, which are thought to correspond with certain organs of the body. The goal is to relieve blockage, promote the flow of energy, and reduce tension—thus, reflexology may be helpful in treating stress-related illnesses. Reflexology requires special training. See Chapter 40 for more information.

The following are simpler activities you can recommend to most clients to aid in relaxation and stress reduction:

- *Humor.* Reading and telling jokes, viewing funny movies or stand-up routines, and simply appreciating the humor of situations all help release tension and anger and increase coping abilities. Laughter releases endorphins and relieves feelings of stress (Fig. 25-7). It enhances respiration and circulation, oxygenates the blood, suppresses the stress-related hormones in the brain, and activates the immune system. Some medical centers have begun implementing in-house humor programs (Bennett & Lengacher, 2007; Cousins, 1979; du Pré, 1998; Johnson, 2002).
- *Listening to music.* Music soothes and relaxes when its vibrations are in harmony with body frequencies. Listening to tranquil music can also relax the mind.
- *Engaging in art activities.* Painting, working with clay, and engaging in other art activities help to express emotions and release endorphins.
- *Dance and sports,* like other forms of exercise, release pent-up physical tension and emotions. Steady-state exercises, such as running or swimming at a consistent pace, offer stress relief in a meditative manner through sustained deep breathing and movement. Physical activity can also enhance self-esteem and help people feel better by the simple act of accomplishing a personal goal.
- *Journal writing* helps the person to reflect on experiences and express emotions. The venting of emotion that can occur in journal writing often provides insights into causes of stress and ways to modify stressors.

FIGURE 25-7 Laughter releases endorphins and helps relieve stress.

Changing Perception of Stressors or Self

Recall that altering ones perception is one way to improve adaptation to stress. For clients who have an unrealistic perception of the stressor and can imagine only negative outcomes, a technique, called **cognitive restructuring,** may be helpful. With this technique, you help clients to recognize their negative focus and to restructure their thinking in more positive and realistic ways. For example, you might encourage a working mother with demanding family members to take a single positive step, such as saying no to someone at least once a day.

You can also help clients to identify positive aspects of themselves and their coping abilities. This promotes self-esteem and helps them to recognize and use the resources they have for coping with their stressors. **Positive self-talk** is another method for increasing self-esteem. Each time you hear negative self-talk, stop the client, and ask him to rephrase the statement so that it is positive.

Identifying and Using Support Systems

You can facilitate successful adaptation by helping clients to identify and contact people and groups who offer various supports (e.g., listening, encouragement, advice, problem solving, help with household tasks, financial support). Be aware of the groups available in your community (e.g., Weight Watchers, Alcoholics Anonymous, Parents Without Partners, Reach for Recovery). You may need to teach socialization skills to clients who are socially isolated so that they can begin to build a support system.

Reducing the Stress of Hospitalization

Illness and hospitalization are stressful for patients and their families. In addition to being sick, patients find themselves in unfamiliar surroundings, with little privacy, and a certain loss of control. Promote patient-centered care in the healthcare agency as much as you can. Involving patients and families actively in their care helps them adapt to the stressors of hospitalization. Teach patients what to expect from hospitalization, and give them a few tips to help plan ahead to minimize the stress they experience (Self-Care: Teaching Clients How to Reduce the Stress of Hospitalization).

Providing Spiritual Support

In addition to helping clients obtain spiritual support from church groups and clergy, you can help to strengthen the client spiritually. You may wish to:

- *Pray for or with clients,* if they desire, and if you are comfortable doing so. Prayer can help reduce their feelings of powerlessness and loneliness.
- *Help clients to define their values and set boundaries* that honor themselves and uphold those values.

Self-Care

Teaching Clients How to Reduce the Stress of Hospitalization

Share the following tips with clients, preferably before hospitalization.

➤ Bring what you need from home. Make a list of necessities and pack carefully before you go. For example, bring your own soap, toothpaste, lotion, pajamas, and slippers—or your favorite tea bags and sweetener. Having familiar things can make your stay more pleasant for you.

➤ If you will feel well enough, bring your computer, reading material, crossword puzzles, or whatever you like to do that can help prevent boredom and depression. You might want to bring a few family photos for your nightstand.

➤ Bring a notepad and pencils so that you can take notes about what your primary care providers tell you (e.g., about diagnostic tests, instructions for care, and so on).

➤ Do *not* bring jewelry, cash, credit cards, or other valuables.

➤ Do not bring clothing that is not washable or that is uncomfortable or tight.

➤ Do not allow family or friends to visit if they are ill.

➤ It helps to ask family or friends to stay at the bedside, particularly when the physician is "making rounds." They can advocate for you and help you feel confident that everything will go well. You may not feel well enough to ask for what you need, but a family member can do that for you.

➤ Your family members or friends can also help you interpret and remember information and instructions that you will receive from nurses, physicians, and other care providers. There may be 30 people in your room each day, and when you are ill or taking certain medications, it is hard to keep track of everything.

➤ Keep a bottle of hand sanitizer by your bed or insist visitors, including family members and care providers, use a hand hygiene product at the door when entering the room, just as you do.

➤ Know the name of your primary nurse (or nurses) on each shift, and ask as many questions as you need to.

➤ Even though some things seem to not make sense (e.g., taking your temperature at 3 A.M.), there is likely a medical reason for it. Try to be as patient and cheerful as possible.

■ Teach clients to silently recite an affirming mantra (e.g., on inhalation, say, "I am free." Exhale and say, "Stress, leave me.")

For other ways to provide spiritual support, see Chapter 14.

Crisis Intervention

As an entry-level nurse in acute and ambulatory care settings, you are more likely to see patients in the first three phases of crisis and not be present for the adaptive and postcrisis stages. The goals of crisis intervention at an entry level of practice include the following (Brammer & MacDonald, 2003; Neeb, 2006):

1. Assess the situation.
2. Ensure the patient's safety.
3. Defuse the situation.
4. Decrease the person's anxiety.
5. Determine the problem.
6. Decide on the type of help needed.
7. Return the person to precrisis level of functioning.

For further explanation,

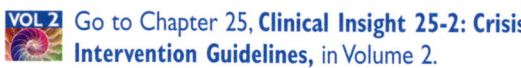 Go to Chapter 25, **Clinical Insight 25-2: Crisis Intervention Guidelines,** in Volume 2.

Crisis centers often rely on telephone counseling ("hotlines"). If telephone counseling is not adequate, or if observations of the home environment are needed, home visits may be necessary.

KnowledgeCheck 25-10

■ Describe at least five specific interventions for dealing with an angry person.

■ What is cognitive restructuring?
■ What is the purpose of positive self-talk?
■ List the seven steps of crisis intervention.
■ Why is relaxation an important stress intervention?

 Go to Chapter 25, **Knowledge Check Response Sheet and Answers,** on the Student Resource Disk or DavisPlus at http://davisplus.fadavis.com/Wilkinson2

Stress Management in the Workplace

You will need to pay attention to your feelings, your body, and your personal responses to stress. Do you notice that you are eating more than usual or have lost your appetite? Are you feeling edgy or impatient with family or co-workers, or not sleeping well? Check your body. Do you feel tired or often have headaches or gastrointestinal distress? Are the muscles in your face and shoulders tense? Do you often take work home with you? Are you unable to stop thinking about work, even when you are at home? Do concerns about finances or personal situations consume your thinking and create a sense of doom? If so, you probably need to start managing your stress. You can better manage workplace stress and avoid burnout by following the advice you give your patients. For some tips,

 Go to Chapter 25, **Tables, Boxes, Figures: ESG Box 25-1,** on the Student Resource Disk or DavisPlus at http://davisplus.fadavis.com/Wilkinson2

When stressors arise from the workplace, the following actions are especially important:

Examine your expectations. Have realistic expectations of yourself and others. Don't be overcritical; most people, including you, are doing the best they can.

Ask for help. Some nurses feel that they must know everything or be able to handle things, but asking for help does not indicate weakness. It can even make others feel good by giving them the opportunity to practice collegiality.

Support colleagues. Offer support to colleagues who need help with tasks or with their feelings. This adds to the overall good feeling on a unit and improves the efficiency of performing many tasks.

Be proactive about the things you can change and accept the things that you cannot change. Complaining and negative talk add to your own stress and that of others. Get involved in constructive efforts to change policies (e.g., regarding staffing, overtime, safety practices, and so on). If you cannot effect the changes, and if you cannot accept things as they are, you may need to think about leaving the organization rather than subjecting yourself to continual stress.

Join and support professional organizations that address workplace issues (e.g., the National Student Nurses Association [NSNA] and the ANA).

Strive for balance. Try to keep these six key points in balance in your life: family; financial responsibilities; health; social contributions; career, vocation, or education; and spirituality or faith. Work affects life, but your life also affects your work. Try to achieve control of the various aspects of your life by focusing on the most important items and tasks.

Obtain counseling for stress that exceeds your ability to cope.

Making Referrals

This chapter has presented many assessments and interventions for reducing stress. Remember, though, you are not yet an expert nurse and no one, not even an experienced nurse, is an expert in all areas. It is important not to "get in over your head" with clients who are under stress and showing maladaptive coping. You can help by recognizing your limitations and by referring the client to the appropriate professionals as needed (e.g., a spiritual leader, a counselor, a social worker, a practitioner of complementary therapies, a physician, a psychologist, or a psychiatrist).

 Critical**Thinking** 25-5

Sally is an RN seeking employment at a local nursing home. She left her previous employer because of stress and frustration with agency policy, for which the bottom line was financial gain rather than quality patient care. What can Sally do to help ensure that she will not experience the same problem in the new agency?

 Care**Planning** & **Mapping**Practice

For Care Planning/Care Mapping practice,

Go to Student Resources, **Care Planning & Care Mapping Practice,** at http://davisplus.fadavis.com/Wilkinson2

Go to Chapter 25, **Resources for Caregivers and Health Professionals,** on the Student Resource Disk or DavisPlus at http://davisplus.fadavis.com/Wilkinson2

Suggested Readings: Go to Chapter 25, **Reading More About Stress and Adaptation,** on the Student Resource Disk or DavisPlus at http://davisplus.fadavis.com/Wilkinson2

Bibliography: Go to Volume 2, Bibliography.

CHAPTER 26

Nutrition

Learning Outcomes

After completing this chapter, you should be able to:

➤ Identify the types, functions, metabolism, and major food sources of (1) the energy nutrients, (2) vitamins, (3) minerals, and (4) water.

➤ Differentiate among the various sources of nutritional information (e.g., USDA dietary guidelines, food guide pyramids, DRIs, Nutrition Facts labels).

➤ Calculate a client's basal metabolic rate.

➤ Identify the primary nutritional considerations for various developmental stages.

➤ Discuss how each of the following affects and is affected by nutritional status: lifestyle choices, vegetarianism, dieting for weight loss, culture and religion, disease processes, functional limitations, and special diets.

➤ Describe tools and techniques for gathering subjective data about nutritional status.

➤ Compare the effectiveness of various anthropometric measurements.

➤ Calculate the body mass index for a client.

➤ Explain the significance of body mass index.

➤ List at least five physical assessment findings that indicate nutritional imbalance.

➤ Identify laboratory values that are indicators of nutritional status.

➤ Discuss the need for and advisability of vitamin and mineral supplementation.

➤ Describe nursing interventions for patients with special needs: Impaired Swallowing, NPO, older adults, and Nausea.

➤ Describe techniques for assisting patients with meals.

➤ Identify and discuss six nursing interventions for Imbalanced Nutrition: Less Than Body Requirements and six interventions for Imbalanced Nutrition: More Than Body Requirements.

➤ Safely provide enteral and parenteral nutrition for patients.

Meet Your Patients

As part of a class assignment, you are to assist a local business with their wellness program. You will be completing health risk appraisals and gathering the following data on each of the employees: height, weight, medical and nutritional history, and lifestyle practices. Today you will screen two employees, and then each will have blood drawn for a complete blood count (CBC), comprehensive metabolic panel, and lipid panel:

- Isaac Schwartz, a 65-year-old accountant, works long hours. He describes a sedentary lifestyle, no tobacco use, infrequent alcohol use, no medical problems, and a nutritional history of skipping meals and daily consumption of restaurant food. You measure his height as 69 in. and weight as 245 lb.
- Sujing Lee, a 29-year-old project manager, regularly works 65 hours per week. Sujing is 30 weeks pregnant. She does not smoke or drink and has never been hospitalized or had surgery. She has gained a total of 25 lb since becoming pregnant. Her diet consists mainly of traditional Chinese food. She eats three meals a day and always brings lunch from home. Lately she has felt "tired all the time." At the screening, she weighs 126 lb and measures 63 in. tall.

At the end of your clinical day, you need to compile a report on the clients you have seen. How would you interpret the data on height, weight, and nutrition? What, if any, additional information do you need to help you evaluate their nutritional status? In this chapter, you will read about dietary recommendations, energy balance, and nutritional concerns across the lifespan. You will gain the theoretical knowledge to answer these questions, as well as practical knowledge about managing nutritional problems.

Theoretical **Knowledge** **knowing** why

Low-fat, sugar-free, reduced-calorie, low-sodium, calcium-enriched . . . these are just a few of the hundreds of claims you find on packaged foods. At home, a flood of TV and print media ads hypes nutritional supplements, weight-loss pills, and new diets, while the news carries conflicting reports on the benefits and dangers of phytochemicals, antioxidants, and *trans*-fatty acids. With so many options and so much advice available, it's no wonder that many people are confused about what to eat.

Nutrition is the study of food and how it affects the human body and influences health. Good nutrition is essential to wellness, and poor nutrition contributes to disease; so clients need accurate, current, and appropriate nutritional information. Before you can give effective individualized advice, you need to know about the nutrients found in foods, as well as how the body metabolizes food for energy. In this chapter you will also learn about principles of energy balance and factors that influence nutritional status.

What Are Some Reliable Sources of Nutrition Information?

Standards and guides provide credible nutrition information. **Standards** are a reference for nutrient intake thought to meet the nutritional needs of most healthy population groups. They list nutrient amounts in measurements, such as grams and milligrams, and are not intended to indicate individual requirements or therapeutic needs. **Food guides** are more practical tools that you can use to educate patients and families. They specify the number of servings of foods needed daily so nonprofessionals can use them in making healthful meal choices. In general, standards and guides provide recommendations to healthy individuals but they are not sensitive to the needs of people experiencing metabolic or other medical problems.

Dietary Reference Intakes

The National Academy of Sciences, in a collaborative effort by the United States and Canada, has established standards, the **Dietary Reference Intakes (DRIs),** to promote the consumption of healthful nutrient levels. For carbohydrates and lipids, the *acceptable macronutrient distribution range (AMDR)* is used. To view the DRIs and AMDRs for males and females in various age groups,

Go to Chapter 26, **Supplemental Materials, Dietary Reference Intakes: Vitamins; Dietary Reference Intakes: Electrolytes; Dietary Reference Intakes: Elements; and Dietary Reference Intakes: Macronutrients,** on the Student Resource Disk or DavisPlus at http://davisplus.fadavis.com/Wilkinson2

The DRIs are a revision of the older **Recommended Dietary Allowances (RDAs)** for vitamins and minerals, protein, and total kcal that are thought to meet the needs of about 98% of individuals in a group. For vitamins and minerals, the DRI tables include RDAs and **Adequate Intakes (AIs).** AIs are the intakes adequate to meet the needs of all individuals in a group. For files you can download,

 Go to "Browse by Subject," **U.S. Department of Agriculture, National Agricultural Library, Food and Nutrition Information Center,** a government Web site, at http://fnic.nal.usda.gov/nal_display/index.php?info_center=4&tax_level=1

Canada's Food Guide to Healthy Eating

Canada's Food Guide to Healthy Eating advises choosing a variety of foods from each of four groups, plus a small amount of unsaturated fat (ESG Fig. 26-1). People are advised to choose their total amount of food based on age, body size, activity level, gender, pregnancy, and lactation. To see this figure,

 Go to Chapter 26, **Tables, Boxes, Figures: ESG Figure 26-1,** on the Student Resource Disk or DavisPlus at http://davisplus.fadavis.com/Wilkinson2

USDA Dietary Guidelines

In 1980, the United States Department of Agriculture (USDA) developed dietary guidelines for Americans. The guidelines are revised every 5 years. Box 26-1 presents the 2005 guidelines to help people evaluate their food habits and work toward general improvement in their diet. The guidelines do not specify daily amounts of food and nutrients.

USDA Dietary Guidelines for Americans 2005. The U.S. Department of Agriculture intends this document to be a primary source of dietary health information for nutrition educators, policymakers, and healthcare providers. It is based on the latest scientific evidence and provides information about choosing a nutritious diet, maintaining healthy weight, achieving adequate exercise, and food safety to avoid food-borne illness. The dietary guidelines are updated every 5 years. You can access them at the USDA Dietary Guidelines Web site, at

 http://www.cnpp.usda.gov/dietaryguidelines.htm

Food Pyramids

MyPyramid is a food guide for use as a diet-teaching tool (Fig. 26-1). Based on USDA dietary guidelines, it visually illustrates healthful daily food choices. The width of each of the areas of the pyramid offers a clue as to the proportion of the intake you should get from that food group. An interactive Web site allows individuals to plan and track their food choices. For access to MyPyramid,

---

BOX 26-1 ■ Dietary Guidelines for Americans 2005—Key Points

- Consume a variety of nutrient-rich foods daily.
- Adopt a balanced eating pattern (e.g., the USDA Food Guide) to meet recommended intakes.
- Limit the intake of saturated fats, *trans*-fats, and cholesterol. Keep fat intake below 20% to 35% of total calories. Most fats should come from foods such as fish, nuts, and vegetable oils.
- Limit your intake of added sugars, salt, and alcohol. 1500 mg (1 teaspoon) per day is an adequate adult salt intake; 2300 mg is the recommended daily limit. However, most people in the United States consume far more than that, and more than half of U.S. groups are in high-risk groups that would benefit from a salt intake of no more than 1500 mg per day (Centers for Disease Control and Prevention [CDC], 2009).
- Achieve and maintain a healthy weight.
- Be physically active each day.
- Balance calorie intake with increase or decrease in activity.
- Choose a variety of fruits and vegetables each day.
- Choose fiber-rich fruit, vegetables, and whole grains often. At least half the grains should come from whole grains.
- Cook, chill, and store foods to keep them safe from microorganisms.
- Clean hands, food contact surfaces, and fruits and vegetables. Do not wash or rinse meat and poultry. (Also see Chapter 21 for food safety.)

Source: Abstracted from U.S. Department of Agriculture. (2005). *Dietary guidelines for Americans 2005.* Retrieved from http://www.health.gov/dietaryguidelines/; and CDC (2009). Application of lower sodium intake recommendations to Adults – United States, 1999–2006. *MMWR, 58*(11), 281–283. Retrieved from http://www.cdc.gov/mmwr/preview/mmwrhtml/mm5811a2.htm

---

 Go to the **MyPyramid** Web site at http://www.MyPyramid.gov

MyPyramid is also provided in Spanish, with the same foods as the English MyPyramid. For the Spanish version,

 Go to http://www.mypyramid.gov/sp-index.html

MyPyramid stresses the following concepts for healthy eating:

- *Activity.* The steps are a reminder of the importance of daily physical activity.
- *Moderation.* The wider base represents foods with little or no solid fats or added sugars. The narrower top area stands for foods with more solid fats and sugars, which you should eat less often.
- *Personalization.* The person on the steps of the pyramid symbolizes the need to individualize diet choices (one size does *not* fit all). To find the kinds and amounts of food you need to eat each day, based on personal factors, check the MyPyramid Web site.

MyPyramid
STEPS TO A HEALTHIER YOU
MyPyramid.gov

GRAINS	VEGETABLES	FRUITS	MILK	MEAT & BEANS
Make half your grains whole	Vary your veggies	Focus on fruits	Get your calcium-rich foods	Go lean with protein
Eat at least 3 oz. of whole-grain cereals, breads, crackers, rice, or pasta every day	Eat more dark-green veggies like broccoli, spinach, and other dark leafy greens	Eat a variety of fruit	Go low-fat or fat-free when you choose milk, yogurt, and other milk products	Choose low-fat or lean meats and poultry
1 oz. is about 1 slice of bread, about 1 cup of breakfast cereal, or 1/2 cup of cooked rice, cereal, or pasta	Eat more orange vegetables like carrots and sweetpotatoes	Choose fresh, frozen, canned, or dried fruit	If you don't or can't consume milk, choose lactose-free products or other calcium sources such as fortified foods and beverages	Bake it, broil it, or grill it
	Eat more dry beans and peas like pinto beans, kidney beans, lentils	Go easy on fruit juices		Vary your protein routine – choose more fish, beans, peas, nuts, and seeds

For a 2,000-calorie diet, you need the amounts below from each food group. To find the amounts that are right for you, go to MyPyramid.gov.

Eat 6 oz. every day	Eat 2 1/2 cups every day	Eat 2 cups every day	Get 3 cups every day; for kids aged 2 to 8, it's 2 cups	Eat 5 1/2 oz. every day

Find your balance between food and physical activity
- Be sure to stay within your daily calorie needs.
- Be physically active for at least 30 minutes most days of the week.
- About 60 minutes a day of physical activity may be needed to prevent weight gain.
- For sustaining weight loss, at least 60 to 90 minutes a day of physical activity may be required.
- Children and teenagers should be physically active for 60 minutes every day, or most days.

Know the limits on fats, sugars, and salt (sodium)
- Make most of your fat sources from fish, nuts, and vegetable oils.
- Limit solid fats like butter, margarine, shortening, and lard, as well as foods that contain these.
- Check the Nutrition Facts label to keep saturated fats, *trans* fats, and sodium low.
- Choose food and beverages low in added sugars. Added sugars contribute calories with few, if any, nutrients.

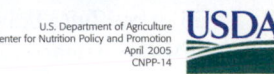

U.S. Department of Agriculture
Center for Nutrition Policy and Promotion
April 2005
CNPP-14

FIGURE 26-1 USDA MyPyramid: Steps to a Healthier You. (From U.S. Department of Agriculture, 2005.)

- *Proportionality.* Notice that the food group bands are of different widths. The widths are a general guide to how much food you should choose from each group. For example, the "Oils" group is a very thin area, and the "Grains" area is very large. This gives you a general idea that you should eat many more servings of grains than of oils.
- *Variety.* Six different colors represent the food groups. This illustrates the importance of variety in your diet; you need foods from all groups each day.
- *Gradual improvement.* The slogan "Steps to a Healthier You" suggests that you can benefit from taking even small steps to improve your diet and lifestyle.

MyPyramid does not specify number of servings per day; it specifies measurable amounts, such as ounces and cups. However, should you need information about serving sizes and nutrients provided by each food group when assisting patients with nutritional choices,

 Go to Chapter 26, **Clinical Insight 26-1: Serving Sizes for Daily Food Choices,** in Volume 2.

You can find several other food guide pyramids, as well. For a vegetarian diet pyramid, see Figure 26-2. For an alternative that has been proposed to that pyramid,

 Go to Chapter 26, **Reading More About Nutrition,** the article by **Messina, Melina, & Mangels (2003),** on the Student Resource Disk or DavisPlus at http://davisplus.fadavis.com/Wilkinson2

For Asian, Latin American, Vegetarian, and Mediterranean Diets, which include some of the traditional foods of those cultural groups,

 Go to the **Oldways Preservation and Exchange Trust** Web site at http://www.oldwayspt.org

For the Diabetes Food Pyramid,

 Go to the **American Diabetes Association** Web site at http://www.diabetes.org/food-and-fitness/food/planning-meals/diabetes-food-pyramid.html

The Diabetes Food Pyramid, unlike MyPyramid, groups foods based on their carbohydrate and protein content. For example, you will find potatoes and beans in the "breads, grains, and other starches" group instead of the "vegetables" group.

Food Guides for Older Adults

For an updated (2007) Modified MyPyramid for Older Adults,

 Go to the **Tufts University Friedman School of Nutrition Science and Policy** Web site at http://nutrition.tufts.edu/1197972031385/Nutrition-Page-nl2w_1198058402614.html

The Tufts University pyramid emphasizes nutrient-dense foods and stresses the importance of fluids by showing an entire row of glasses as the foundation of the pyramid. It shows packaged fruits and vegetables in addition to fresh because they are easier to prepare and have a longer shelf life. This is important to consider when it is difficult for an older adult to make frequent trips to the grocery store. The pyramid also emphasizes whole fruits and vegetables rather than juices. A flag at the top suggests that older adults may need to discuss with their health care providers nutrient supplements such as calcium, vitamin D, and vitamin B_{12}.

Nutrition Facts Label

You are probably familiar with the **Nutrition Facts label** shown in Figure 26-3, because the United States Food and Drug Administration (FDA) requires this label on all packaged foods sold in the United States. The Nutrition Facts panel contains important information about serving size, number of servings per package, total calories and calories from fat per serving, a list and amounts of the key nutrients in the food, and the *percent daily values* (% DV) for the nutrients listed on the panel. The % DV identifies the percentage that a serving of the food contributes to a consumer's overall intake of the nutrient listed.

If you need a more thorough, easy to understand, explanation of how to use Nutrition Facts labels,

 Go to Chapter 26, **Supplemental Materials, Nutrition Facts Panels – Food Labels,** on the Student Resource Disk or DavisPlus at http://davisplus.fadavis.com/Wilkinson2

KnowledgeCheck 26-1

- What are the DRIs?
- List the current USDA dietary guidelines for Americans.

 Go to Chapter 26, **Knowledge Check Response Sheet and Answers,** on the Student Resource Disk or DavisPlus at http://davisplus.fadavis.com/Wilkinson2

 CriticalThinking 26-1

How might you use the various sources of nutritional information to evaluate the nutritional status of the clients introduced in the "Meet Your Patients" scenario?

What Are the Energy Nutrients?

The cells and tissues of the body depend for their functioning on building blocks called **nutrients.** Any one food may contain a variety of nutrients; for instance, cheese contains carbohydrates, protein, lipids, sodium, vitamins, and minerals. Some nutrients, called *macronutrients,* supply the body with energy (kilocalories), whereas others, called *micronutrients,* help manufacture, repair, and maintain cells. In this section, we discuss the three classes of nutrients that provide the body with energy: carbohydrates, proteins, and lipids. Table 26-1 lists the sources of and requirements for macronutrients.

My Vegetarian Food Pyramid

Whole Grains | Vegetables | Fruits | Dairy | Proteins | Fats

Consult your dietitian or physician to determine the amount of water, iodized salt, calcium, vitamin D, and B12 to add to your daily diet.

Feel Good — Look Good Guidelines

Desire Drinks: Prioritize water instead of soda, alcohol, or sugary fruit drinks.

Engage Exercise: 10,000 steps for fitness or walking 90–120 minutes for weight loss.

Enjoy Eating: In a clean kitchen, wash all fresh fruits and vegetables in clean water to reduce harmful bacteria. Serve cold foods chilled and hot foods hot.

Pyramid Plan: Use the pyramid above as a guide for meal planning and shopping.

Plate Portions: Locate your daily calorie target below and read down that column to see how many servings from each Pyramid Food Group will best meet your calorie and nutrition requirements.

Choose Colors: Select the most intense colors of green, red, yellow, orange, brown, blue, and purple vegetables, fruits, and whole grains.

Welcome Whole: Favor natural, unprocessed foods and minimize processed foods high in sodium, sugar, cholesterol, refined flour, total fat, and trans-fat.

Value Variety: Daily select a variety of foods from all pyramid groups to get all essential nutrients.

Food Groups	Many Women and Older Adults 1600 Calories Daily	Children, Active Girls and Women 2000 Calories Daily	Boys and Active Men 2500 Calories Daily	Sample Serving Sizes
Go Whole Grains	5 Servings	6 Servings	8 Servings	• 1 slice whole grain bread • 1/2 cup cooked pasta, rice, or other grains • 1 cup dry cereal • 1/4 cup granola • 1 tortilla or chapatti • 1/2 bagel or muffin
Vary the Vegetables	4 Servings	5 Servings	6 Servings	• 1/2 cup cooked, canned, or frozen vegetable • 1 cup raw vegetable salad • 3/4 cup vegetable juice • unlimited fresh herbs and spices
Focus on Fruits	3 Servings	4 Servings	4 Servings	• 1 medium fresh fruit • 1 cup berries • 1/4 cup dried fruit • 1/2 cup cooked, canned, or frozen fruit • 3/4 cup unsweetened fruit juice
Delight in Dairy or Equivalents	3 Servings	3 Servings	3 Servings	• 1 cup low fat milk or fortified full fat soy beverage • 1 cup low fat yogurt or kefir • 1/2 cup low fat ricotta, cottage, or soy cheese • 1.5 ounces low fat fresh cheese
Protect with Proteins	3 Servings	3 Servings	4 Servings	• 1/2 cup meat analog, soy beans, or tofu • 2 grilled medium portabello mushrooms • 1/2 cup cooked, canned, or frozen legumes (beans or peas) • 1 egg or 2 egg whites • 1/4 cup almonds, pistachios, pumpkin or sunflower seeds
Find Healthy Fats	2 Servings	3 Servings	5 Servings	• 1 teaspoon vegetable oil or margarine • 1 tablespoon nut butter or mayonnaise • 1/4 cup avocado • 2 tablespoons nuts, sesame or ground flax seeds • 4 large olives
Select Few Sweets	Avoid unhealthy fats and minimize or eliminate refined sugars to lose weight.			• 1 tablespoon fruit preserves • 1/8 fruit pie • 1/2 cup ice milk or low fat ice cream • 1.5 ounce chocolate bar • 1 small nut and fruit cookie

FIGURE 26-2 A food guide pyramid for vegetarians. (*Source:* Vegetarian Diet Pyramid ©1998–2009. Mayo Foundation for Medical Education and Research (MFMER), with permission. Retrieved from http://www.mayoclinic.com/health/medical/IM02769)

FIGURE 26-3 A Nutrition Facts panel. (From U.S. Food and Drug Administration, 2004.)

The body requires a constant supply of energy. Physiological mechanisms constantly convert stores of more complex forms of chemical energy into usable energy, which is then carried to individual cells. The term **metabolism** encompasses all the ways in which the body changes and uses nutrients. Two types of metabolic reaction, anabolism and catabolism, occur continually and are adjusted according to the needs of the body. **Anabolism** involves the formation of larger molecules from smaller ones. For example, if protein is needed for tissue repair, amino acids are recombined to form proteins. This process requires energy. **Catabolism** involves the breakdown of larger molecules into smaller components. One of the results of this separation is the release of energy. Most metabolic reactions, including metabolism of nutrients, are catalyzed by enzymes; each is specific and catalyzes only one type of reaction.

Carbohydrates

Carbohydrates (CHOs) are the primary energy source for the body. **Simple carbohydrates,** commonly called *sugars,* are named according to the number of sugar

(or *saccharide*) units making up their chemical structure (Fig. 26-4). **Monosaccharides** (simple sugars) consist of a single unit; **disaccharides** are molecules made up of two saccharides. **Complex carbohydrates** consist of long chains of saccharides, called **polysaccharides. Dietary fiber,** a polysaccharide, is the indigestible "fibrous skeleton" of plant foods. Humans do not have the enzymes to digest fiber; thus, it provides no usable glucose. Carbohydrates perform several functions:

1. *Supply energy for muscle and organ function.* Carbohydrates, which are more easily and quickly digested than proteins and lipids, fuel strenuous short-term skeleton muscle activity and provide nearly all the energy for the brain. Humans store glucose in liver and skeletal muscle tissue as **glycogen.** Glycogen is converted back into glucose to meet energy needs. This process is called **glycogenolysis.** If carbohydrates are not available, proteins and lipids (fats) can also be used for energy.

2. *Spare protein.* If glycogen stores are low (for instance, in a person who is undernourished), physical activity

Table 26-1 ➤ Energy Nutrients

NUTRIENT	SOURCES	ENZYMES INVOLVED IN DIGESTION	REQUIREMENTS
Carbohydrates	*Simple sugars* occur mainly in corn syrup, honey, milk, table sugar, molasses, sugar cane, sugar beets, and fruits. *Complex carbohydrates* occur in vegetables, breads, cereals, pasta, grains, and legumes.	Salivary amylase (mouth) Ptyalin (mouth and stomach) Pancreatic amylopsin Intestinal: sucrase, lactase, maltase	There is debate about the amount of carbohydrate needed in the diet. Many popular diet plans alter carbohydrate intake: the Atkins diet is a low-carbohydrate plan, whereas the Pritikin and Ornish diets recommend high intake of complex carbohydrates. Body size and activity level affect the amount of carbohydrate used by the body. The 2002/2005 DRIs specify that adults should get 45%–65% of their calories from CHOs, or 130 grams per day (g/day).
Proteins	*Complete proteins* come mostly from animal sources: meat, poultry, fish, eggs, and milk products. *Incomplete proteins* are supplied by plant sources (e.g., grains, nuts, legumes, seeds, vegetables). They can be combined to make complete proteins.	Stomach: Pepsin Pancreas: Trypsin, chymotrypsin, carboxypeptidase Intestine: Aminopeptidase, dipeptidase	Protein needs depend on age, body size, and physical state. Needs are increased during growth periods, such as childhood and pregnancy. The average adult needs about 1 gram of protein per kilogram of body weight per day. The 2002/2005 DRIs specify that adults should get 10%–35% of their calories from protein, or 0.8 g/kg of body weight (46–56 g/day for an "average" person).
Lipids	*Saturated fats* occur in pork, beef, poultry, seafood, egg yolk, and dairy; coconut oil and palm oil. *Unsaturated fats (from plants)* occur in olives, olive oil, vegetable oils (peanut, soybean, cottonseed, corn, safflower), nuts, and avocados *Essential fatty acids (linoleic acid [omega-6] and alpha-linolenic acid [omega-3])* occur in polyunsaturated vegetable oils and in fatty fish (e.g., salmon). *Trans-fats* occur in hydrogenated oils, some margarines, packaged baked goods, and many processed foods	Lingual: Lipase Gastric: Lipase, tributyrinase, bile salts Pancreatic lipase (steapsin)	There is debate about the appropriate amount of fat in the diet. The American Heart Association recommends that people obtain <30% of their calories from fat; <7% of calories should come from saturated fats, and <1% from *trans*-fat. Clients with increased risk for heart disease may need stricter control. The 2002/2005 DRIs specify that adults should get 20%–35% of their calories from fat; children, 25%–40%.

Sources: Adapted from U.S. Department of Agriculture, Food and Nutrition Center (2002–2005). *Dietary Guidance. DRI Tables. Dietary Reference Intakes: Macronutrients.* National Academy of Sciences. Institute of Medicine. Food and Nutrition Board. Retrieved from http://fnic.nal.usda.gov/nal_display/index.php?info_center=4&tax_level=3&tax_subject=256&topic_id=1342&level3_id=5140; and American Heart Association (n.d[a].) Fat. AHA recommendation. Retrieved from http://www.americanheart.org/presenter.jhtml?identifier54582

causes the breakdown of body stores of protein (**gluconeogenesis**) and lipids (fats) to use for energy. But when proteins are used for energy, they are not available for their primary functions of tissue growth, maintenance, and repair. Fats are converted directly into an alternative fuel called **ketones;** ketones raise the acidity of the blood and can lead to acid–base imbalance. Fats are used for fuel in persons with diabetes, whose cells cannot use glucose for energy.

3. *Other physiological functions.* Carbohydrates enhance insulin secretion, increase satiety (feeling of fullness and satisfaction), and improve absorption of sodium and excretion of calcium. **Insulin** is a pancreatic hormone that promotes the movement of glucose into the cells for use.

Refer to Table 26-1: How many servings of carbohydrates did you eat yesterday? How many were simple carbohydrates? How many were complex carbohydrates?

FIGURE 26-4 Carbohydrates. Each hexagon represents a six-carbon simple sugar, such as glucose. *A,* A disaccharide, such as maltose. *B,* Cellulose, a polysaccharide. *C,* Starch, a polysaccharide. *D,* Glycogen, a polysaccharide.

Proteins

Proteins are complex molecules made up of *amino acids.* Every amino acid consists of a central carbon atom connected to a hydrogen atom, an acid, an *amine* (a region of the molecule containing nitrogen), and a side chain. Only the side chain varies from one amino acid to another (Fig. 26-5). Just 20 different amino acids are the building blocks of most of the proteins in the human body (Table 26-2). The **essential amino acids** are significant in our diets because the body cannot manufacture them. They must be supplied by food or nutritional supplements. In contrast, the body can synthesize the 10 **nonessential amino acids,** so we do not need to obtain them from food.

For protein synthesis to occur, every amino acid necessary to build that protein must be available. **Complete protein** foods contain all of the essential amino acids necessary for protein synthesis. These usually come from animal sources. **Incomplete protein** foods (e.g., nuts, grains) do not provide all of the essential amino acids. However, by combining two incomplete proteins, a complete protein can be made. For instance, peanut butter on whole-grain bread constitutes a complete

FIGURE 26-5 Amino acids. *A,* The structural formula of an amino acid. The "R" represents the variable portion of the molecule. *B,* A polypeptide. Several amino acids, represented by different shapes, are linked by peptide bonds.

protein. Protein complementing allows for a healthful vegetarian diet.

Refer to Table 26-1: How many servings of protein did you eat yesterday? How many were complete proteins? How many were incomplete proteins? Do you think that protein foods accounted for more than 10% of your food intake yesterday?

Protein Metabolism and Storage

Although protein digestion begins in the stomach, it occurs mostly in the small intestine, where enzymes break it down into amino acids (see Table 26-1). The body continually breaks down and resynthesizes protein into tissues, adjusting as needed to maintain overall protein balance. The body also maintains a balance between tissue protein and plasma protein. When amino acids are catabolized, the nitrogen-containing part is converted to ammonia (NH_3) and excreted in the urine as urea. Therefore, nitrogen balance reflects how well body tissues are being maintained.

Nitrogen balance occurs when intake and output of nitrogen are equal. A **positive nitrogen balance** exists when nitrogen intake exceeds output, making a pool of amino acids available for growth, pregnancy, and tissue maintenance and repair. **Negative nitrogen balance**

Table 26-2 ➤ Amino Acids		
TYPE	**DESCRIPTION**	**EXAMPLES**
Essential	Must be obtained from the diet; cannot be made in the body.	Arginine*, histidine, isoleucine, leucine, lysine, methionine, phenylalanine, threonine, tryptophan, and valine
Nonessential	Easily synthesized by the body.	Alanine, asparagine, aspartic acid, cysteine**, glutamic acid, glutamine, glycine, proline, serine, and tyrosine**

*Considered by some to be "semiessential" because it cannot be synthesized at a rate that will support growth. Therefore, it is essential for children, but not for most adults.
**Considered conditionally essential. That is, essential in some situations (e.g., in immaturity, during severe stress).
Sources: American Heart Association (n.d. [a]); Guyton & Hall (2000); Lutz & Przytulski (2006); Thompson & Manore (2008); U.S. Department of Agriculture, Food and Nutrition Center (2002–2005).

exists when nitrogen intake is lower than nitrogen loss. This occurs in illness, injury (e.g., burns), and malnutrition. Which patient ("Meet Your Patients") is probably in positive nitrogen balance?

Functions of Protein

Dietary proteins perform the following functions:

1. *Tissue building.* Protein is the structural material of every cell in the body. In fact, except for water, protein makes up the biggest part of the body. It is essential for growth, maintenance, and repair of body cells and tissues.
2. *Metabolism.* Proteins are essential for building body tissue. For example, proteins are precursors to digestive enzymes and hormones (e.g., thyroxine). **Enzymes** facilitate cellular reactions throughout the body. In addition, proteins combine with iron to form hemoglobin, the oxygen carrier in red blood cells.
3. *Immune system function.* **Lymphocytes** (specialized white blood cells) and antibodies (components of our immune system that defend against foreign invaders) are proteins.
4. *Fluid balance.* Because they attract water, proteins in cells and the bloodstream help regulate fluid balance.
5. *Acid–base balance.* Blood proteins function as buffers, helping to regulate acid-base balance.
6. *Secondary energy source.* As noted earlier, proteins can be broken down to provide energy when stores of the other energy nutrients are inadequate (Thompson & Manore, 2008).

Protein needs vary according to age, sex, weight, and health. Most North Americans eat more protein than they need, especially in the form of meat. There is no health benefit from eating more than the recommended amount of protein. In fact, there may be health risks in eating diets high in animal protein. Animal proteins are high in saturated fat, which increases the risk for certain cancers and coronary artery disease, and which has been associated with kidney stones and calcium loss through the urinary system.

Lipids

Lipids are organic (carbon-containing) substances that are insoluble in water. They are made up of carbon, hydrogen, and oxygen—the same basic elements that make up carbohydrates. The term *lipid* comes from *lipos,* the Greek word for "fat." Lipids that are solid at room temperature are called *fats,* whereas those that are liquid at room temperature are called *oils.* For example, butter is a fat even when it is melted, because it would be solid at room temperature. You will hear the terms (lipids and fats) used interchangeably.

People in developed countries typically eat a diet relatively high in fat. In the United States about 45% of

our total kcal comes from fat. Fat is an essential nutrient, but certain types, when overconsumed, can also be a health hazard.

Lipid metabolism occurs in the small intestine, where bile and pancreatic enzymes begin splitting the fatty acids from their glycerol backbone. Lipids are stored as adipose tissue. Because lipids are insoluble in water, and because blood is primarily water, lipid absorption requires a solvent carrier.

Types and Sources of Lipids

The three types of lipids found in foods are glycerides, sterols, and phospholipids (Box 26-2). **Glycerides** (also called **true fats**) consist of one molecule of glycerol attached to one, two, or three fatty acid chains (Fig. 26-6). *Glycerol* is an alcohol composed of three carbon atoms. *Fatty acids* are long chains of carbon and hydrogen atoms ending in an acid. Most glycerides found in foods are *triglycerides,* which are compounds consisting of a glycerol molecule attached to three fatty acids.

Sterols are lipids, but they are not made of fatty acids. They consist of rings of carbon and hydrogen. The most important sterol in the body is **cholesterol,** a waxlike substance needed for the formation of cell membranes, vitamin D, estrogen, and testosterone.

BOX 26-2 ■ Types of Lipids

Glycerol Molecules (bonded to) Fatty Acid Molecules

Glycerides		
Monoglycerides	1	1
Diglycerides	1	2
Triglycerides	1	3
Sterols	0	0
Phospholipids	1	2 + a phosphate group

FIGURE 26-6 Lipids. A, A triglyceride made of one glycerol and three fatty acids. B, The steroid cholesterol. The hexagons represent rings of carbon and hydrogen.

Cholesterol is synthesized in the liver, and it is also found in animal foods.

Phospholipids (which contain a phosphate group) are soluble in water. They are a key component of **lipoproteins,** which consist of phospholipids and a protein. Because they are water soluble, lipoproteins are the major transport vehicles for lipids in the bloodstream. By "wrapping" triglycerides with water-soluble phosphates and proteins, lipoproteins deliver these substances to body cells.

- **Low-density lipoproteins (LDLs)** transport cholesterol to body cells. Diets high in saturated fats increase LDLs circulating in the bloodstream and may result in fatty deposits on vessel walls, causing cardiovascular disease. As a result, LDL is often known as the "bad cholesterol."
- **High-density lipoproteins (HDLs)** remove cholesterol from the bloodstream, returning it to the liver, where it is used to produce bile; thus, a high blood level of HDL is considered protective against cardiovascular disease. It is often known as the "good cholesterol."

Saturated and Unsaturated Fatty Acids

Fatty acids are classified as saturated, unsaturated, or *trans* fats (Table 26-3). **Saturation** means that a substance is holding all that it is capable of holding (e.g., think of a wound dressing saturated with blood).

- An **unsaturated fatty acid** is one that is not completely filled with all the hydrogen it can hold. Therefore, it is lighter and less dense. Fats made up primarily of unsaturated fatty acids are called **unsaturated fats.** Molecules of **monounsaturated fats** have one unfilled spot where hydrogen is not attached. **Polyunsaturated fatty acids** contain two or more unfilled spots for hydrogen. At the spot(s) where the molecule does not have a hydrogen attached, it becomes kinked and does not pack together. This is why these fats are liquid at room temperature. Replacing saturated fats in the diet with mono- and polyunsaturated fats reduces the risk of heart disease and stroke. Dietary fat should mainly be polyunsaturated and unsaturated, from food sources, such as fish and nuts.
- **Saturated fatty acids** are those in which every carbon atom is fully bound to (or "saturated" with) hydrogen. The molecules pack tightly together at room temperature and are dense, solid, and heavy. A fat made up mostly of saturated fatty acids is called a **saturated fat.** Animal fats are the primary source of saturated fats in the North American diet; however, many processed foods contain saturated fats.
- *Trans*-**fatty acids** are saturated fats created when food manufacturers add hydrogen to polyunsaturated plant oils, such as corn oil, to break the double carbon bonds and straighten out the molecules. This process solidifies the fat and extends the shelf life of the food. *Trans*-fats are found in many margarines and other processed foods containing *hydrogenated vegetable oils.*

Saturated fats and *trans*-fats are the main dietary factors in increasing blood cholesterol levels. They raise LDL cholesterol levels. The FDA mandates that *trans*-fat content be listed on all food labels. Intake of saturated fats and *trans*-fats should be limited.

Refer to Table 26-3: How many servings of fat did you eat yesterday? How many were saturated fats; how many were unsaturated?

Essential and Nonessential Fatty Acids

A fatty acid is considered **essential** if (1) the body cannot manufacture it and (2) its absence creates a deficiency disease. The essential fatty acids, **linoleic acid (omega-6)** and **alpha-linolenic acid (omega-3)**, help protect against heart disease. Omega-6 fatty acid is found mainly in polyunsaturated vegetable oils, nuts, and seeds. Omega-3 fatty acid can be obtained in adequate amounts by eating fatty fish (e.g., tuna, shellfish) twice a week (American Heart Association, 2008).

Functions of Lipids

Lipids perform the following functions:

1. *Supply essential nutrients.* Food fats supply the essential fatty acids and aid in the absorption of fat-soluble vitamins.
2. *Energy source.* Although carbohydrates are the primary energy source during strenuous physical activity, our bodies burn fat for energy when we are engaging in sustained light activity, such as walking or mowing the lawn, and when we are at rest. The body also burns fat for energy when glycogen stores are exhausted.
3. *Flavor and satiety.* Lipids give food its creamy taste and texture and promote our sense of satiety (being "full"). Fats are digested more slowly than carbohydrates, so stomach emptying time is slower.
4. *Other functions of lipids.* Body fat provides insulation, protects vital organs, aids in thermoregulation, and enables accurate nerve-impulse transmission. In addition, lipids are a component of every cell membrane and are essential to cell metabolism.
5. *Cholesterol functions.* Cholesterol is a component of every cell in the body, where it lends suppleness and support. It is also an ingredient of bile, which helps digest fats, and serves as a precursor to all steroid hormones, including sex hormones. When lipid metabolism is "disordered," cholesterol contributes to atherosclerosis.

Critical Thinking 26-2

Review the information you collected on the two employees ("Meet Your Patients").

- What conclusions, if any, can you make about their intake of carbohydrates, protein, and fats?
- How might you gather additional data on their intake of the energy nutrients?

Table 26-3 ➤ Dietary Fats

TYPE OF FAT	SOURCES	EFFECT ON BLOOD CHOLESTEROL
Monounsaturated	Olives; olive oil, canola oil, peanut oil; cashews, almonds, peanuts, and most other nuts; avocados	Lowers LDL and raises HDL.
Polyunsaturated	Corn, soybean, safflower, sesame, sunflower, and cottonseed oils; fish, nuts, and seeds	Lowers LDL and raises HDL.
Saturated	Whole milk, butter, cheese, and ice cream; lard; red meat; chocolate; coconuts, coconut milk, and coconut oil; palm oils; cocoa butter	Raises LDL and HDL.
Trans-fats	Most margarines; vegetable shortening; partially hydrogenated vegetable oil; deep-fried chips; many fast foods (e.g., French fries, donuts); most commercial baked goods	Raises LDL.
Dietary Cholesterol	Foods from animals: meats, egg yolks, dairy products, organ meats (e.g., heart, liver), fish, and poultry	Raises cholesterol.

AMERICAN HEART ASSOCIATION RECOMMENDATIONS

Limit foods high in saturated fat, *trans*-fat, and/or cholesterol. Instead choose foods low in saturated fat, *trans*-fat and cholesterol. Here are some helpful tips (AHA, n.d.[a]):

- Limit intake of whole-milk dairy products, fatty meats, tropical oils, partially hydrogenated vegetable oils, and egg yolks.
- Include a variety of fruits and vegetables in the diet.
- Eat a variety of grain products; include whole grains.
- Eat fish, particularly fatty fish, at least twice a week.
- Include fat-free and low-fat milk products and legumes.
- Choose skinless poultry and lean meats.
- Choose fats and oils with 2 grams or less saturated fat per tablespoon (e.g., liquid and tub margarines, canola oil).

What Are the Micronutrients?

Vitamins and minerals are called **micronutrients** because they are required by the body in only very small amounts. Although they provide no energy, they are critical in regulating a variety of body functions.

Vitamins

Vitamins are organic substances that are necessary for metabolism or preventing a particular deficiency disease. Because the body cannot make vitamins, they must be supplied by the foods we eat. Vitamins are critical in building and maintaining body tissues, supporting our immune system so we can fight disease, and ensuring healthy vision. They also help our bodies to break down and use the energy found in carbohydrates, proteins, and lipids. Vitamins are especially critical during periods of rapid growth, pregnancy, lactation, and healing. Some evidence supports the claim that certain vitamins prevent chronic illness (Institute of Medicine, 2000; Jockers, 2007).

Table 26-4 summarizes information about vitamins, including specific functions and recommended dietary allowances (RDAs). RDAs represent the daily dietary intake that is adequate to meet the needs of about 98% of all healthy individuals in a group, such as men, women, or infants. The RDAs for some of the vitamins were established as long ago as 1997, and some researchers are suggesting the need to increase the requirements. The American Pediatric Society, for instance, now recommends that infants, children, and adolescents have a minimum daily intake of 400 international units (IU)[1], or 10 micrograms, of vitamin D—double the current adequate intake amount listed in Table 26-4 (Wagner & Greer, 2008). Other research suggests that the RDAs should be increased dramatically for both children and adults to help prevent various chronic diseases, such as hypertension and type 2 diabetes (Jockers, 2007).

Fat-Soluble Vitamins. The fat-soluble vitamins are A, D, E, and K. They are stored primarily in the liver and adipose tissues, although vitamin E is deposited in all body tissue. Because the body can store these vitamins, we do not need to consume them every day if we are consuming them in adequate amounts; however, diets extremely low in fat and disorders affecting fat digestion and absorption can lead to deficiency of fat-soluble vitamins. In contrast, because they are not readily excreted, excessive supplementation with the fat-soluble vitamins can lead to toxicity. Vitamin D is unique in that the body can synthesize it from a cholesterol compound in the skin when

---

[1]Although The Joint Commission includes the abbreviation *IU* on its "do not use" list, the abbreviation is nevertheless used in other settings (e.g., on vitamin labels).

Table 26-4 ➤ Vitamins: Adult Dietary Reference Intakes (DRIs)*

VITAMIN	FUNCTION	RDA†	SOURCES	EFFECTS OF DEFICIENCY	SYMPTOMS OF EXCESS
Fat-Soluble Vitamins					
A	Night and color vision Cellular growth and maturity Maintaining healthy skin and mucous membranes Growth of skeletal and soft tissues Reproduction	Women: 700 mcg/day Men: 900 mcg/day	Fish liver oil, liver, butter, cream, egg yolk, yellow fruit, green leafy vegetables, fortified milk	Night blindness, xerosis, xerophthalmia, keratomalacia, skin lesions	GI upset, headache, blurred vision, poor muscle coordination, fetal defects
D‡	Regulates blood calcium levels. Regulates rate of deposit and resorption of calcium in bone.	5 mcg/day (AI), to age 50 10 mcg/day (AI), ages 51–70 15 mcg/day (AI), after age 71	Fish liver oil, fish, fortified milk, sunlight exposure	Bone and muscle pain, weakness, softening of bone, fractures, rickets	Fatigue, weakness, loss of appetite, headache, mental confusion, mental retardation in infants
E	Antioxidant Protects red blood cells and muscle tissue cells	15 mg/day, age 14+	Vegetable oils, nuts, milk, eggs, muscle meats, fish, wheat and rice germ, green leafy vegetables	Hyporeflexia, ataxia, hemolytic anemia, myopathy	Insufficient blood clotting, impaired immune system
K	Synthesis of clotting factors Bone development	Women age 19+: 90 mcg/day (AI) Men age 19+: 120 mcg/day (AI)	Green leafy vegetables, liver (Intestinal bacteria synthesize a form of vitamin K, so deficiency is unlikely.)	Increased bleeding	Jaundice and hemolytic anemia in infants
Water-Soluble Vitamins					
Thiamin	Cellular metabolism (producing energy from glucose and storing energy as fat) Nervous system function Gastrointestinal system function Cardiovascular system function	Women: 1.1 mg/day Men: 1.2 mg/day	Whole grain, enriched cereal, beef, pork, liver, peas, beans, nuts	Peripheral neuritis, loss of muscle strength, depression, memory loss, anorexia, constipation, dyspnea, decreased alertness and reflexes, fatigue, irritability, beriberi	Unlikely; readily excreted
Riboflavin	Cellular metabolism Antioxidant Tissue health and growth	Women: 1.1 mg/day Men: 1.3 mg/day	Milk, cheese, eggs, green vegetables, whole grain, enriched grains, bread, organ meats, poultry, fish	Tissue inflammation and breakdown: Sore throat, stomatitis, swollen tongue, facial dermatitis, anemia; poor wound healing	Unlikely; readily excreted
Niacin	Cellular metabolism to produce energy	Women: 14 mg/day Men: 16 mg/day	Enriched breads and cereals, chicken, tuna, liver, peanuts, dairy products	Weakness, poor appetite, indigestion, dermatitis, diarrhea, headache, dizziness, insomnia. Chronic: CNS damage (confusion, neuritis, dementia), pellagra	Facial flushing, itching, nausea, liver damage

Table 26-4 ➤ Vitamins: Adult Dietary Reference Intakes (DRIs)*—cont'd

VITAMIN	FUNCTION	RDA†	SOURCES	EFFECTS OF DEFICIENCY	SYMPTOMS OF EXCESS
B₆ (Pyridoxine)	Protein (and some carbohydrate) metabolism RBC production Neurotransmitter synthesis	Men and women through age 50: 1.3 mg/day Women 50+: 1.5 mg/day Men 50+: 1.7 mg/day	Meats, poultry, fish, beans, nuts, seeds, dairy products, enriched cereals	Rash, stomatitis, seizure, peripheral neuritis, depression	Irreversible nerve damage (i.e., extremity numbness, walking difficulties)
Pantothenic acid	Cell metabolism of fat and cholesterol Amino acid activation Heme formation	All adults: 5 mg/day (AI)	Occurs widely in most foods. Best sources: Meats, whole grain cereals, legumes	Deficiency is unknown.	Unlikely; readily excreted
Folacin (folate, folic acid)	Cellular metabolism Neurotransmitter synthesis Cell division DNA synthesis Hemoglobin formation	400 mcg/day (folic acid); 600 mcg/day when pregnant Women capable of becoming pregnant should take a daily supplement of 400–800 mcg	Green leafy vegetables, asparagus, liver, yeast, eggs, beans, fruits, enriched cereals	Megaloblastic anemia, neural tube defects	Increased seizure activity, hives, respiratory distress, itching, rash
B₁₂ (cyanocobalamin)	Metabolic reactions Maintain myelin sheath Hemoglobin synthesis	2.4 mcg/day	Dairy products, meat, poultry, fish, liver, milk, cheese, eggs	Pernicious anemia, irreversible nerve damage, memory loss, dementia	Unlikely; readily excreted
C	Collagen synthesis "Cementing" substance for capillary walls Antioxidant Iron absorption Immune function	Women: 75 mg/day Men (age 19+): 90 mg/day Additional 35 mg/day for those who smoke	Citrus fruits, tomatoes, potatoes, green vegetables, cauliflower	Anemia, tissue bleeding, easy bone fracture, gingivitis, petechiae, poor wound healing, joint pain, scurvy	Stomach inflammation, diarrhea, oxalate kidney stones

Note: 1 mcg = 40 International Units.

*Values in the table are RDAs unless marked (AI). Dietary Reference Intakes (DRIs) represent:
- Recommended Dietary Allowances (RDAs)—Intake set to meet the needs of 97%–98% of individuals in a group.
- Adequate Intakes (AIs)—Believed to cover the needs of all individuals in the group.
- Upper Intake Levels (UIs)—The maximum daily intake likely to pose no risk of adverse effects.

†RDAs are usually less than adult values for infants and children, more for pregnant women, and highest for lactating women. RDAs for some vitamins (e.g., vitamin A) are higher for older adults and higher for men than for women.

‡The American Academy of Pediatrics recommends 10 mcg/day of vitamin D for infancy through adolescence (Wagner, Greer, & the Section on Breastfeeding and Committee on Nutrition, 2008). Other clinicians and researchers have suggested that the RDA for adults should be dramatically increased as well, to 20-25 mcg (800-1000 IU) for adults age 50 and older (Jockers, 2007).

 Go to Chapter 26, **Supplemental Materials, Dietary Reference Intakes: Vitamins,** on the Student Resource Disk or DavisPlus at http://davisplus.fadavis.com/Wilkinson2

Sources: Adapted from National Institutes of Health, Office of Dietary Supplements, National Institutes of Health. *Dietary Reference Intakes: Vitamins.* (Last modified 2008). Retrieved from http://ods.od.nih.gov/health_information/Dietary_Reference_Intakes.aspx. Complete reports are available at http://fnic.nal.usda.gov/nal_display/index.php?info_center=4&tax_level=3&tax_subject=256&topic_id=1342&level3_id=5140; summary tables are available at http://www.iom.edu/Object.File/Master/7/296/0.pdf; Lutz, C., & Przytulski, K. (2006). *Nutrition and diet therapy: Evidence-based applications* (4th ed.). Philadelphia: F.A. Davis.

we receive adequate exposure to sunlight. However, adequate exposure is difficult in winter months for anyone living at a latitude of 40° or more north or south of the equator (e.g., in Canada and the northern United States). Newest recommendations are that adults age 50 years and older should receive 20 to 25 mcg (800 to 1000 IU) of vitamin D per day.

Water-Soluble Vitamins. The water-soluble vitamins include vitamin C and the B-complex vitamins: thiamine, riboflavin, niacin, pyridoxine (vitamin B_6), folic acid, pantothenic acid, biotin, and cyanocobalamin (vitamin B_{12}). Because these vitamins are soluble in water, excess amounts are regularly excreted by the kidneys in the urine. Thus, toxicity is rare except in people with renal disease. However, because excess amounts are excreted, the body cannot store these vitamins; so they need to be consumed every day. Inadequate intake is much more likely to lead to deficiency in water-soluble vitamins than to deficiency in fat-soluble vitamins.

Minerals

Minerals are inorganic elements found in nature. They occur in foods either naturally or as additives, as well as in supplements. **Major minerals (macrominerals)** are minerals that the body needs in amounts of 100 mg/day or greater. **Trace minerals** are essential, but in a lower concentration. In the United States, calcium deficiency is one of the most common mineral deficiencies (Table 26-5).

Minerals assist in fluid regulation, nerve impulse transmission, and energy production; they are essential to the health of bones and blood and help rid the body of by-products of metabolism. Evidence also shows that minerals play key roles in disease prevention and treatment. For example:

1. Adequate *calcium* intake throughout the lifespan decreases the likelihood of osteoporosis (a condition marked by porous bones). The recommended daily intake of 1200 mg for adults aged 50 years and older is difficult to achieve by diet alone.
2. *Iron* deficiency causes anemia, the most common nutritional problem worldwide.
3. *Magnesium* may decrease the risk of hypertension and coronary artery disease in women.
4. *Sodium*, consumed in high amounts (>2500 mg/day), increases the risk for high blood pressure, heart attacks, and stroke.

Minerals are absorbed mostly in the small intestine. Salt and potassium are absorbed in the large intestine, however. If the body is deficient in a mineral, it absorbs more; if the body has enough, it absorbs less and excretes more in the feces. Minerals interact with other minerals, vitamins, and other substances to accomplish absorption and metabolism and perform their functions. For example, iron absorption is enhanced in the presence of vitamin C, and vitamin D deficiency inhibits calcium absorption.

Why Is Water an Essential Nutrient?

Water is made up of hydrogen and oxygen. Water makes up about half of total body weight (55% to 65% in men and 50% to 55% in women). Men have greater muscle mass; muscle contains a relatively large amount of water. Water is distributed in two body compartments. **Intracellular fluid** is the water contained within each living cell. It makes up about 40% of the total body weight. **Extracellular fluid** is external to the cell membrane (e.g., in the fluid portion of blood and lymph and in the gastrointestinal tract); it accounts for 20% of body weight. Water is critical to the body because its functions are essential to life:

1. *Solvent.* Water is the basic solvent for the body's chemical processes.
2. *Transport.* Circulating as a component of blood, water serves as a medium for transporting oxygen, nutrients, and metabolic wastes.
3. *Body structure and form.* Water "fills in the spaces" in body tissues (e.g., in muscle).
4. *Temperature.* Water helps maintain body temperature. When body temperature rises, evaporation of sweat helps cool the body.

The amount of water a person requires varies according to the environmental humidity and temperature, activity level, age, and metabolic needs. The average AI for adult women is about 2.7 liters of water per day and 3.7 liters for men. Eighty percent of those amounts should come from fluids. We also obtain water in the foods we eat (Lutz & Przytulski, 2006). What foods can you think of that are high in water content?

Overall fluid balance is maintained when fluid intake in liquids, foods, and metabolic reactions matches fluid output through urine, feces, respiration, and sweat. Fluid and electrolyte balance is discussed in Chapter 36.

KnowledgeCheck 26-2

- What is the body's most usable energy source?
- Which nutrient's primary function is growth and repair of tissue?
- Identify five functions of adipose tissue (body fat).
- Which type of vitamin requires daily consumption to maintain appropriate levels?
- What distinguishes a major mineral from a trace mineral?
- Identify at least four functions of water.

Go to Chapter 26, **Knowledge Check Response Sheet and Answers,** on the Student Resource Disk or DavisPlus at http://davisplus.fadavis.com/Wilkinson2

What Must I Know About Energy Balance?

The energy in carbohydrates, proteins, and lipids is measured in terms of **calories,** or, more precisely, **kilocalories (kcal).** A kcal is the amount of heat required to

Table 26-5 ➤ Minerals: Adult Dietary Reference Intakes*

MINERAL	FUNCTION	RDA†	SOURCES	EFFECTS OF DEFICIENCY	SYMPTOMS OF EXCESS
Macrominerals					
Calcium (Ca)	Bone and teeth formation, blood clotting, nerve conduction, muscle contraction, cellular metabolism, heart action	1000 mg/day (AI), ages 19–50 1200 mg/day (AI) ages 51+ 1300 mg/day (AI), ages 9–18	Dairy products, sardines, green leafy vegetables, broccoli, whole grains, egg yolks, legumes, nuts, fortified products	Bone loss, tetany, rickets, osteoporosis	Kidney stones, constipation, intestinal gas
Magnesium (Mg)	Aids thyroid hormone secretion, maintains normal basal metabolic rate, activates enzymes for carbohydrate and protein metabolism, nerve and muscle function, cardiac function	Men: 400 mg/day (AI), ages 19–30; 420 mg/day, age 31+ Women: 310 mg/day (AI), age 19+	Whole grains, nuts, legumes, green leafy vegetables, lima beans, broccoli, squash, potatoes	Tremor, spasm, convulsions, weakness, muscle pain, poor cardiac function	Weakness, nausea, malaise
Phosphorus (P)	Bone and tooth strength, overall metabolism, formation of enzymes, acid–base balance	700 mg/day (AI), age 19+	Dairy products, beef, pork, beans, sardines, eggs, chicken, wheat bran, chocolate	Bone loss, poor growth	Tetany, convulsions
Potassium (K)	Intracellular fluid control, acid–base balance, nerve transmission, muscle contraction, glycogen formation, protein synthesis, energy metabolism, blood pressure regulation	4.7 g/day (AI)	Unprocessed foods, especially fruits, any vegetables, meats, potatoes, avocados, legumes, milk, molasses, shellfish, dates, figs	Muscle weakness (including weakness of heart and respiratory muscles), weak pulse, fatigue, abdominal distention. (Rarely occurs as a result of inadequate dietary intake. More likely due to losses from prolonged vomiting, diarrhea, or some diuretic drugs.)	Cardiac dysrhythmias, cardiac arrest, weakness, abdominal cramps, diarrhea, anxiety, paresthesia
Sodium (Na)	Water balance, acid–base balance, muscle action, nerve transmission, convulsions	1.5 g/day (AI), ages 19–50; 1.3 g/day, age 51–70; 1.2 g/day, age 70+	Table salt (NaCl), milk, meat, eggs, baking soda, baking powder, celery, spinach, carrots, beets	Dizziness, abdominal cramping, nausea, vomiting, diarrhea, tachycardia, convulsions, coma. (Rarely occurs except in heavy exercise and sweating.)	Thirst, fever, dry and sticky tongue and mucous membranes, restlessness, irritability, convulsion
Trace Minerals					
Copper	Aids in iron metabolism, works with many enzymes in protein metabolism and hormone synthesis	900 mcg/day (AI)	Liver, seafood, cocoa, legumes, nuts, whole grains	Rarely occurs: anemia, low WBC count, poor growth	Vomiting, nervous system disorders

Continued

Table 26-5 ➤ Minerals: Adult Dietary Reference Intakes*—cont'd

MINERAL	FUNCTION	RDA†	SOURCES	EFFECTS OF DEFICIENCY	SYMPTOMS OF EXCESS
Fluoride	Increases resistance to dental caries	Women: 3 mg/day (AI) Men: 4 mg/day (AI)	Fluorinated water, toothpaste, dental treatment, seaweed, fish, tea	Increased dental caries	Stomach upset, staining of teeth, bone pain
Iodine	Synthesis of the thyroid hormone, thyroxine	150 mcg/day	Iodized salt, salt water fish, dairy products, enriched white bread	Goiter, poor infancy growth, cretinism, hypothyroidism	Skin lesions, thyroid malfunction
Iron	Synthesis of hemoglobin, general metabolism (e.g., of glucose), antibody production, drug detoxification in the liver	Women: 18 mg/day, ages 19–50; 8 mg/day, age 50+ Men age 19+: 8 mg/day	Meats, eggs, spinach, seafood, broccoli, peas, bran, enriched breads, fortified cereals	Small, pale RBCs, anemia	Hemochromatosis
Zinc	Cofactor for many enzymes involved in growth, insulin storage immunity, alcohol metabolism, sexual development and reproduction	Men: 8 mg/day Women: 11 mg/day	Primarily meats and seafood; also legumes, peas, and whole grains	Skin rash, diarrhea, decreased appetite, hair loss, poor growth and development, poor wound healing	Reduced copper absorption, diarrhea, cramps, depressed immune function

*Dietary Reference Intakes (DRIs) represent:
- Recommended Dietary Allowances (RDAs)—Intake set to meet the needs of 97%–98% of individuals in a group.
- Adequate Intakes (AIs)—Believed to cover the needs of all individuals in the group.
- Upper Intake Levels (UIs)—The maximum daily intake likely to pose no risk of adverse effects.

Values in table are RDAs unless marked (AI).

†RDAs are usually less than adult values for infants and children, more for pregnant women, and highest for lactating women. RDAs for some minerals are higher for older adults and different for men and women.

 Go to Chapter 26, **Supplemental Materials, Dietary Reference Intakes: Elements; Electrolytes;** and **Elements,** on the Student Resource Disk or DavisPlus at http://davisplus.fadavis.com/Wilkinson2

Sources: Lutz, C., & Przytulski, K. (2006). *Nutrition and diet therapy: Evidence-based applications* (4th ed.). Philadelphia: F. A. Davis; United States Department of Health and Human Services and U.S. Department of Agriculture. *Dietary guidelines for Americans,* 2005 (6th ed.). Washington, DC: U.S. Government Printing Office; U.S. Department of Agriculture (2005). Inside the pyramid. Retrieved from http://www.mypyramid.gov/pyramid/index.html; Shaw, A., Fulton, L., Davis, C., et al. (n.d.) *Using the Food Guide Pyramid: A resource for nutrition educators.* U.S. Department of Agriculture Food, Nutrition, and Consumer Services. Retrieved from http://www.cnpp.usda. gov/Publications/MyPyramid/OriginalFoodGuidePyramids/FGP/FGPResourceForEducators.pdf#xml=http://65.216.150.53/texis/search/pdfhi.txt?query=SERVING+SIZE&pr=MyPyramid&sufs=2&order=r&cq=&id=4592b7130

raise the temperature of 1 kg of water 1° centigrade. To maintain a stable weight, the number of kcal we consume must equal the number of kcal we burn. Any deviation results in weight loss or weight gain. Below is the amount of energy liberated from the metabolism of 1 gram of energy nutrients:

- Carbohydrates = 4 kcal/g
- Protein = 4 kcal/g
- Fat = 9 kcal/g

KnowledgeCheck 26-3

Imagine that you have just eaten a food consisting of 4 grams of protein, 18 grams of carbohydrate, and 1 gram of fat.
- What would your total kcal intake be?

- What percentage of your kcal is from carbohydrates? Protein? Fat?

 Go to Chapter 26, **Knowledge Check Response Sheet and Answers,** on the Student Resource Disk or DavisPlus at http://davisplus.fadavis.com/Wilkinson2

A diet of too few kcal is likely also to lack essential nutrients. People who are undernourished may experience weakened immunity, stunted growth, and hormonal disruption. Too many kcal cause obesity, which increases the risk for chronic diseases, such as diabetes, arteriosclerosis, hypertension, hyperlipidemia, and cancers. In determining total energy (kilocalorie) needs, consider two factors: the client's basal metabolic rate and the duration and intensity of daily physical activity.

What Is Basal Metabolic Rate?

The **basal metabolic rate (BMR)** is a measure of the energy used while at rest in a neutral temperature environment—the energy required for vital organs such as the heart, liver, and brain to function. *Direct measurement* of BMR requires use of a calorimeter: an insulated unit that measures temperature changes of water that are produced by exposure to a fasting individual at rest. Although it is very accurate, it is rarely used because most institutions do not have calorimeters and because the test requires a controlled environment and a 12-hour fast. Direct measurement of BMR is used primarily by researchers. *Indirect calculation* of BMR, sometimes called the resting energy expenditure (REE), includes the following:

- Measuring oxygen uptake per unit of time. This can be done in an exercise lab or with portable machines at the bedside. This is most often done for patients in intensive care units. Not all facilities have this capability.
- Serum thyroxine levels (a blood test).
- A formula for calculating BMR when precise measurement is not required (Box 26-3).

What Factors Affect Basal Metabolic Rate?

When interpreting test results, consider the following factors that influence BMR:

- *Body composition.* Lean body tissue has greater metabolic activity than fat and bones. This explains why women, who have on average more adipose tissue than men, also have lower BMRs.
- *Growth periods.* BMR increases during periods of growth, such as the first 5 years of life, adolescence, pregnancy, and lactation.
- *Body temperature.* The BMR increases 7% for each 1°F (0.83°C) rise in body temperature.
- *Environmental temperature.* Cold weather, especially temperatures below freezing, causes a slight rise in the BMR to generate body heat and maintain normal body temperature.

- *Disease processes.* Diseases involving increased cellular activity, such as cancer, anemia, cardiac failure, hypertension, and asthma, result in BMR elevation. For the same reason, systemic injury (e.g., severe burns, traumatic injury) increases BMR.
- *Prolonged physical exertion.* Metabolic demands are also elevated during prolonged physical exertion (e.g., chopping wood, running).

How Do I Calculate a Client's Total Energy Needs?

The amount of energy required varies according to the intensity of the activity (Table 26-6). A person's total daily energy requirement is the number of kcal necessary to replace those used for basic metabolism plus those used in physical activities. The following are simple estimates based on activity level and age:

- Sedentary women and older adults need 1600 kcal/day.
- Children, teenage girls, active women, and most men need 2200 kcal/day.
- Teenage boys, active men, and very active women need 2800 kcal/day.

However, these estimates have limited usefulness. For instance, is a woman who works a desk job but walks for 30 minutes a day sedentary, active, or somewhere in between? To calculate energy use more precisely, you need to know the person's age, weight, and physical activity, including the intensity and duration of the activity. See Table 26-7.

Heightened emotional states may also increase energy needs, not because they directly increase metabolic activity, but because they increase muscular activity in the form of muscle tension, restlessness, and agitated movements.

KnowledgeCheck 26-4

You have already calculated the expected BMR for Mr. Schwartz ("Meet Your Patients") for a 24-hour period.

- If Mr. Schwartz describes himself as working at a desk 8 to 10 hours per day, lawn mowing manually every other week during the summer, and playing an occasional game of golf, how would you classify his general activity level?
- After interviewing Mr. Schwartz, you estimate his average caloric intake to be approximately 3000 kcal per day. Determine whether his kcal intake is sufficient or insufficient to maintain his present activity level.

 Go to Chapter 26, **Knowledge Check Response Sheet and Answers,** on the Student Resource Disk or DavisPlus at http://davisplus.fadavis.com/Wilkinson2

What Are Some Body Weight Standards?

Weight standards have been established to correlate weight with good health and longevity and to help determine a client's ideal body weight. The **general ideal**

BOX 26-3 ■ Calculating Basal Metabolic Rate (BMR)

Women: 0.9 kcal/kg of body weight per hour

Men: 1.0 kcal/kg body weight per hour

Example: Isaac Schwartz ("Meet Your Patients") weighs 245 lb.

   1 kilogram = 2.2 pounds.

   Divide 245 by 2.2 to convert pounds to kilograms:

   $245 \div 2.2 = 111.3$

   Now complete the calculation:

   $1.0 \times 111.3 \times 24 \text{ hours} = 2671.2$

Table 26-6 ➤ Levels of Physical Activity: Energy Expended and Examples*

INTENSITY LEVEL	LIGHT	LIGHT TO MODERATE	MODERATE	HIGH
Energy Expended	120–150 kcal/hr	150–300 kcal/hr	300–420 kcal/hr	420–700+ kcal/hr
Examples of Activities	Dressing	Housework (e.g., sweeping)	Digging	Shoveling snow
	Showering	Light gardening	Mowing lawn (manually)	Walking 5 mph
	Shaving	Mowing lawn (motorized)	Walking 3½–4 mph	Climbing
	Rocking	Painting	Ballet	Bicycling 15–25 mph
	Writing	Walking 2–3 mph	Ballroom dancing	Cross-country skiing
	Typing	Bicycling 5½ mph	Golf (no cart)	Jogging 5 mph or 1 mile in 10 min
	Standing	Canoeing 2–3 mph	Tennis (doubles)	Swimming
				Aerobic dancing

*Precise energy use varies with body weight. For example, an individual weighing 200 lb burns about 740 calories per hour during aerobic dance, whereas an individual weighing 125 lb burns about 470 during the same activity.

weight guide uses a formula to determine a reasonable weight based on height:

Men: 106 lb (47.7 kg) for the first 5 ft (150 cm), then add 6 lb/in. (2.7 kg/2.5 cm)
Women: 100 lb (45 kg) for the first 5 ft (150 cm), then add 5 lb/in. (2.25 kg/2.5 cm)
Add 10% for large body frame; subtract 10% for small body frame.

Various **height–weight tables** have been developed over the years. The classic one was first released by the Metropolitan Life Insurance Company in 1943, last revised in 1983, and is no longer available. However, many other organizations and researchers have developed their own such tables, and controversy exists as to which is best. To see the World Health Organization (WHO) child growth standards (e.g., length and height-for-age, weight-for-age),

 Go to http://www.who.int/childgrowth/standards/Technical_report.pdf

Height–weight tables are based on statistical estimates and often include variations for age, sex, and body frame. Use standards and standardized tables with caution because they are based on limited samples and may create unrealistic expectations, especially at the low weight ranges. Consider the following example. You have two male clients; each weighs 200 lb. Mason is 72 in. tall, works out vigorously 5 days per week, and has 18% body fat. Travis is 72 in. tall, rarely exercises, and has 35% body fat. Which of these clients requires more kcal to maintain his present weight? Which of these clients is at lower risk for cardiovascular disease?

If you answered Mason, you are correct. Although both men have the same height and weight, Mason has more lean body mass. He will burn energy more rapidly and be able to eat more without gaining weight. Height–weight tables cannot replace a thorough assessment and analysis of body composition when attempting to determine a client's overall fitness.

Body composition analysis attempts to quantify lean body mass versus percentage body fat. Lean body mass includes muscle, bone, and connective tissue. Lean tissue weighs more than fat; thus, a person who engages in regular weight-bearing exercise and is physically fit may actually weigh more than an individual of similar appearance who is sedentary and unfit. Various methods to assess body composition, known as *anthropometric measurements,* are provided in the "Assessment" section later in the chapter.

Table 26-7 ➤ Energy Needs Based on Weight and Activity

For *each pound of body weight*, a person needs the following per day:

ACTIVITY LEVEL	UNDERWEIGHT	NORMAL WEIGHT	OVERWEIGHT
Sedentary	13 kcal	13 kcal	9–11 kcal
Moderately active	18 kcal	16 kcal	13 kcal
Active	18–23 kcal	18 kcal	16 kcal

CriticalThinking 26-3

Examine your dietary intake for the next 3 days to determine how balanced your diet is. Use the form on the Electronic Study Guide and record all intake.

Go to Chapter 26, **Critical Thinking Response Sheet (Volume 1),** on the Student Resource Disk or DavisPlus at http://davisplus.fadavis.com/Wilkinson2

- How does your diet compare to the USDA MyPyramid or Canada's Food Guide in terms of:
  a. Servings of bread, cereal, rice, and pasta?
  b. Servings of vegetables?
  c. Servings of fruits?
  d. Servings of milk, yogurt, and cheese?
  e. Servings of meat, poultry, fish, dry beans, eggs, and nuts?
  f. Servings of fats, oils, and sweets?
- From what you have learned from this activity, what habits could you change in patterns of eating in order to achieve optimal nutrition?

What Factors Affect Nutrition?

Several factors influence nutritional needs and choices. Some can be modified; some cannot. The most influential factors are development, knowledge, lifestyle, culture, disease processes, and functional limitations.

Developmental Stage

At specific developmental stages, nutritional needs and eating patterns vary according to physiological growth, activity level, metabolic processes, disease prevention, and other factors.

Infants to One Year

Humans grow most rapidly during the first year of life. Birth weight doubles by 5 months of age and triples during the first year, and length increases 50%. A baby 20 inches long at birth grows to about 30 inches by age 1 year. Nutritional needs per unit of body weight are greater than at any other time.

Calories and Protein. The infant needs adequate protein for tissue building and enough carbohydrates to furnish energy and "spare" the protein. The period from conception into the second year of life is most critical to brain development. For maximum brain growth, the baby needs optimal nutrition. Severe protein-calorie deficiency in the last trimester of pregnancy or the first 6 months of life may decrease the number of brain cells by 20%.

Vitamins and Minerals. Fetal iron stores are depleted at 4 to 6 months, so intake of iron becomes important. The infant needs calcium for bone growth and development of teeth, calcium and vitamin C for iron absorption, and vitamin D for calcium regulation.

Fluids. Compared to adults, infants have a higher metabolic rate. They also have greater water loss through the skin, which comprises a greater proportion of the body. These factors, along with immature kidneys, mean that infants need proportionately more fluid than adults. To meet nutritional and fluid needs, the infant requires 1.5 to 2 ounces of breast milk or formula per pound of body weight per day.

Infant Feedings. The only safe choices for meeting fluid and nutrient needs in the first months of life are breast milk and commercially prepared formulas. Breast milk is the ideal food for infants because it is matched to their nutritional requirements. It contains enzymes to digest fats, protein, and carbohydrates. In addition, it enhances maturation of the infant's immune system and provides passive immunity against a number of infections. Breastfed infants also may have a reduced exposure to foreign dietary antigens and a reduced risk of subsequent allergies (Friedman & Zeiger, 2005). They may also have less risk of developing diabetes mellitus later in life (Owen, Martin, Whincup, et al., 2007; Rosenbauer, Herzig, Kaiser, et al., 2007).

When breastfeeding is contraindicated or the mother chooses not to breastfeed, numerous commercial formulas are available. The most commonly used formula is modified cow's milk available in powder, liquid concentrate, or ready-to-use liquid. Other types include iron-fortified, soy, and hypoallergenic formulas. Potable (drinkable) water should be boiled for 1 minute and cooled before mixing with infant formula. Infant formulas should contain between 4 and 12 mg/L of iron (Kazal, 2002).

✚ Infants younger than 1 year old should not receive regular cow's milk because it may cause gastrointestinal bleeding and may place too much strain on the infant's kidneys. It also can contribute to iron-deficiency anemia.

✚ Honey and corn syrup should not be used as a source of carbohydrates in preparing infant formula. They are potential sources of botulism toxin, which can be fatal in children younger than 1 year old (Schlenker & Roth, 2006).

At 4 to 6 months, infants may be started on solid foods, beginning with iron-fortified infant rice cereal. They progress to eating table food by 1 year of age. If solid foods are begun too early, they may trigger allergies. Vitamin supplements may be prescribed for both breastfed and bottle-fed infants; iron supplements are usually prescribed at age 6 months. Fluoride might also be prescribed for infants without a fluoridated water supply.

Toddlers and Preschoolers

Toddlers grow more slowly in comparison to infants, and have fewer energy demands. Toddlers require about 900 to 1800 kcal and 1250 mL of fluid per day, depending on body weight. As the gastrointestinal system matures, they are able to eat most foods and adjust to the adult pattern of three meals a day. By age 3, most children have all of their deciduous teeth and can chew adult food.

✚ Food should be cut in small pieces to avoid choking in toddlers who sometimes are "too busy" to chew food sufficiently. Sometimes young children "chipmunk" their food and can later choke on it. Do not give food when the child is in a car seat or bouncy chair, where choking is more likely and can occur without a parent noticing.

Toddlers' diets are sometimes deficient in fat and meat. One- and 2-year-old children should drink reduced-fat (2%), or in some cases, whole milk to provide adequate fat for the still-growing brain. Deficiencies in iron, calcium, and vitamins A and C are also common during this period. Parents need to offer a variety of foods to provide these essential nutrients. This can be a challenge, because toddlers assert their autonomy and manipulate their parents by refusing foods. They may take a long time to eat or refuse to eat at all. Parents should not turn mealtime into a battle of wills or use foods to punish or reward; such reactions may affect the child's attitude toward food. To encourage the child to eat, you may offer parents the suggestions in the accompanying Home Care box.

Preschoolers are similar to toddlers in their growth and nutritional needs; however, their eating patterns typically improve. They begin to form responses to specific foods, such as refusing all green vegetables or drinking less milk. They often refuse casseroles and foods with sauces. They might also eat only one particular food for several days. Because they are active, preschoolers require nutritious between-meal snacks. Lifelong food habits are developed during this stage, so encourage families to widen the variety of foods offered to preschoolers and to investigate the diet provided by their child's day care or preschool. Between ages 2 and 5 fat should provide only about 30 percent of the child's intake.

Home Care

Tips for Encouraging Toddlers to Eat

➤ Keep only nutritious foods in the house to avoid battles over nutrient-poor snacks.

➤ Serve foods in a "child-friendly" way; for example, arrange tortillas, cheese, tomato slices, and beans in a smiling face.

➤ Allow the child to "graze" throughout the day on healthful foods rather than insisting that she sit for formal meals at the table.

➤ Avoid "combined" foods, such as casseroles and stews.

➤ Limit consumption of sweets and snack foods.

➤ Do not use dessert as a reward for eating other foods (e.g., "You can't have cookies until you eat your meat").

➤ Offer healthy foods that are easy to eat (e.g., "finger foods" or those easily chewed).

School-Age Children

In the school-age period, growth and body changes occur gradually. Permanent teeth erupt, and the digestive system matures. School-age children need about 2400 kcal and 1750 mL of fluid per day. An adequate supply of vitamins and minerals is critical because the body is still growing and preparing for the demands of adolescence.

Parental control over food intake declines because advertising influences the child's food choices. The child eats away from home and may buy junk food with his lunch money or choose less nutritious foods in the school cafeteria. Even if the child brings lunch from home, he may trade his food or not eat lunch at all. Parents should encourage their children to eat breakfast to provide nutrients and energy to fuel problem-solving skills, memory, and sports and playground activities. Poor eating habits may lead to obesity. Thirty-two percent of U.S. children are overweight; 16% are obese; and 11% are extremely obese (CDC, 2008). Leading causes of childhood obesity include the following:

- Routine consumption of high-fat, high-sugar fast foods, nutrient-poor foods, and high-calorie snacks and beverages (Sugared soft drinks are no longer a treat, but rather a staple of children's diets.)
- Loss of family mealtime
- Eating in front of a TV or computer
- Lack of regular physical activity to burn the kcal consumed

Adolescents

Adolescence is a time of dramatic growth and development of the reproductive system. Boys experience an increase in muscle tissue and bone length and density. At menstruation, girls experience fat deposition. The needs of the adolescent body for energy, vitamins, and minerals approach those of the infant. In particular, adolescents need protein, calcium, iron, and B and D vitamins. Boys, in particular, seem to eat constantly. Adolescents have active lifestyles and snack often, preferring ready-to-eat, eat-on-the-run foods, such as chips, pizza, cookies, and fast foods. Unfortunately, most such foods have little nutrient value. Adolescents are responsible for their own food decisions, so the best approach for parents is to keep only healthful snack foods (e.g., cheese, fruit, raw vegetables) in the home.

For girls, the need for nutrients conflicts with intense social pressure to be slim. About half of all teenage girls report that they are either dieting or that they need to be. Eating disorders are a concern in this group. Most people with eating disorders exhibit their first symptoms before age 20, some as early as age 10. The majority of eating disorder sufferers are female (National Association of Anorexia Nervosa and Associated Disorders, n.d.). Underweight and undernutrition are discussed more in the Practical Knowledge Section.

Adults

Young adults continue to require adequate amounts of protein, vitamins, and minerals, but not at the same levels as in adolescence. If adults continue unhealthful behaviors developed in earlier stages, repercussions will begin to show up in adulthood. Calcium, vitamin D, folic acid, and iron continue to be critical, especially in women, for bone and reproductive health. U.S. Preventive Services Task Force officials recommend that women capable of becoming pregnant should take a daily folic acid supplement of 0.4 mg to 0.8 mg (400 to 800 micrograms) to lower the risk for neural tube defects in the fetus (USPSTF, 2009).

The BMR of middle adults decreases, potentially causing weight gain if dietary intake and activity level are unchanged. Individuals may begin to experience chronic illnesses such as diabetes, hypertension, obesity, and hyperlipidemia, often as a result of heredity or poor lifestyle choices. Dietary modification and exercise are essential to control these diseases. Overweight and obesity are discussed more in the Practical Knowledge section. For dietary strategies for preventing cancer,

 Go to Chapter 26, **ESG Box 26-2, Dietary Strategies for Preventing Cancer,** on the Student Resource Disk or DavisPlus at http://davisplus.fadavis.com/Wilkinson2

Older Adults

Nutritional needs of older adults vary only slightly from middle adulthood. Lean body mass, physical activity, and BMR decrease, so older adults tend to need fewer kcal; but they still need the same or higher levels of nutrients. However, it is not unusual for older adults to lose interest in eating and for the thirst sensation to decrease.

Older adults with chronic diseases may need to adjust to therapeutic diets low in salt, simple sugars, or fat. Unfortunately, the ability to taste and smell diminishes with age, and many clients find these diets unappealing. Other sensory changes, such as diminished vision or hearing, limit mobility and interaction, making it more difficult to purchase and prepare food. Tooth loss and gum disease limit chewing ability, forcing many older adults to eat only soft food. Arthritic hands may have difficulty preparing and eating food, and when they are no longer able to drive, many older adults must rely on local markets, where food choices may be limited and expensive. Other physical problems that may affect nutrition include gastroesophageal reflux, decreased gastric secretions, decreased intestinal peristalsis, and glucose intolerance.

See Table 26-8 for dietary requirements for adults older than 70 years. Notice the main difference is that older adults require smaller quantities of most foods. In general, they require slightly more of the milk/yogurt/cheese group and slightly less of all other groups, especially the breads/cereal group. Older adults need complex

Table 26-8 ➤ Daily Food Requirements for Adults Older than Age 70

FOOD GROUP	ADULTS ≥ 70 YEARS
Supplement of calcium, vitamin D, and vitamin B_{12}	As prescribed. Not everyone needs supplements. People should consult their healthcare providers.
Fats, oils, and sweets	Use sparingly
Milk, yogurt, and cheese group	3 servings
Meat, poultry, fish, dry beans, eggs, and nut group	2 or more servings
Vegetable group	3 or more servings
Fruit group	2 or more servings
Bread, fortified cereals, rice, and pasta group	6 or more servings
Water equivalents	8 or more servings

Sources: Russell, R., Rasmussen, H., & Lichtenstein, A. (1999). Modified food guide pyramid for people over seventy years of age. *Journal of Nutrition,* 129(3), 751–753; and Modified MyPyramid for Older Adults (2007). Tufts University, Gerald J. & Dorothy R. Friedman School of Nutrition Science and Policy. Retrieved from http://nutrition.tufts.edu/1197972031385/Nutrition-Page-nl2w_1198058402614.html

carbohydrates (i.e., fiber) to maintain bowel function. They should be sure to drink at least eight glasses of water or other fluids (e.g., soups) per day and choose primarily green leafy vegetables and brightly colored fruits to help prevent constipation and dehydration. All of this, of course, assumes their medical condition allows.

Many older adults may need supplements of calcium, vitamin D, and vitamin B_{12}. For example: (1) As bone density decreases, calcium requirements increase, especially in women at risk for *osteoporosis;* and (2) low concentrations of vitamin B_{12} have been linked to cognitive decline in older adults (Clark, Birks, Nexo, et al., 2007).

With advancing age, older adults face many losses. As a result, depression and social isolation are common. Both negatively affect appetite. **Adult failure to thrive** is a complex disorder seen in many institutionalized older adults. It is characterized by weight loss, decreased activity and interaction, and increasing frailty.

Pregnant and Lactating Women

Nutritional requirements increase dramatically during pregnancy as the mother provides for the nutritional needs of the fetus. Folic acid intake is critical in the first trimester of pregnancy (the first 13 weeks) to prevent neural tube defects; a daily supplement of 0.6 to 0.8 mg is recommended during pregnancy. Adequate protein and calcium are important for growing muscle, brain, and bone tissues; iron is essential to maintain maternal and fetal blood supplies and stores during pregnancy. It is almost impossible to consume the recommended amount of dietary iron, so supplements are commonly prescribed, as are supplements of folic acid and calcium. Pregnant women need about 300 additional kcal/day in the second and third trimesters of pregnancy.

Women who are breastfeeding need 500 additional kcal per day. They continue to need additional protein and calcium, as well as increased fluid intake to make adequate amounts of breast milk. Needs vary based on the size of the baby and the frequency of breastfeeding. The quantity of the breast milk depends on an adequate supply of fluids and nutrients. However, the nutritional quality of the milk remains the same even if dietary intake is not adequate. For more information on nutrition in pregnancy and lactation, consult a maternal–newborn nursing textbook.

KnowledgeCheck 26-5

- Why is breast milk an ideal food source for infants?
- Why are an infant's nutritional needs per unit of body weight greater than at any other time?
- Why is it sometimes a challenge to meet the nutritional needs of toddlers?
- What is the challenge in meeting the nutritional needs of school-age children?
- Which age group experiences a growth spurt second only to that of infants?
- Why are energy (kcal) requirements less for older adults?

 Go to Chapter 26, **Knowledge Check Response Sheet and Answers,** on the Student Resource Disk or DavisPlus at http://davisplus.fadavis.com/Wilkinson2

 Critical**Thinking** 26-4

Make a list of all the food products you have seen advertised on television and in magazines. What implications does this have for the nutritional status of the public?

Lifestyle Choices

Nutrition-related lifestyle choices include the following:

Dietary Patterns. Obviously, consuming more kcal than are expended in activity results in weight gain; however, the type of food consumed is equally important to health. Whole foods, such as fresh fruits and vegetables, whole grains, and legumes, promote health, whereas foods high in simple sugars, saturated and trans fats, and sodium increase the risk for health problems.

Cooking Methods. Up to one-half of the water-soluble vitamin content (vitamins B and C) is lost in the cooking water of boiled vegetables. Keeping foods hot longer than 2 hours results in even further loss.

Oral Contraceptive Use. This method of family planning lowers the serum level of vitamin C and several B vitamins. Women with marginal nutrient intake may need vitamin supplements.

Using Food to Cope. If used often, poor coping patterns, such as reacting to stress by skipping meals, binge eating, or consuming too much of a single food (e.g., snack foods or chocolate) can result in poor nutrition.

Tobacco Smoking. Smokers use vitamin C faster than nonsmokers. Even children exposed to second-hand smoke tend to have lower plasma levels of ascorbate than unexposed children (Aghdassi, Royall, & Allard, 1999; Preston, 2003). If the person cannot quit smoking, a vitamin C supplement may help compensate.

Alcohol. Alcohol contributes to obesity. A 12-oz beer contains 150 calories; a juice-based cocktail contains about 160 calories. This can add many unnecessary calories to the regular diet. In addition, alcohol significantly decreases the rate of fat metabolism, contributing to obesity. Excessive alcohol use interferes with adequate nutrition by (1) replacing the food in the person's diet, (2) depressing the appetite, (3) decreasing the absorption of nutrients by its toxic effects on intestinal mucosa, and (4) impairing the storage of nutrients. People who use alcohol heavily need multivitamin supplements, especially B vitamins and folic acid.

Caffeine. The most common source of caffeine is coffee—the leading beverage in the United States. Over the years, research reports have claimed a variety of dangers and health benefits for caffeine. Recently a privately funded group (Schardt, 2008) published an analysis of nine scientific reports in which they state that many of our accepted beliefs about coffee are myths. They report coffee does not create risk for dehydration, heart disease, or cancer, and has little or no role in hypertension. Caffeine may be associated with bone loss; however, its negative effect can be offset by as little as 2 tablespoons of milk. In high doses, caffeine can sometimes cause anxiety and stomach upset. On the positive side, caffeine can enhance mood and mental and physical performance. It aids the ability to burn fat for fuel instead of carbohydrates, and has been linked to a lower risk of Parkinson's disease, type 2 diabetes, stroke, and dementia (Brody, 2008; Schardt, 2008). So it appears that while the evidence is still mixed, caffeinated beverages in moderation are not the villains we once thought.

Vegetarianism

All vegetarian diets exclude red meat and poultry, but beyond this distinction is a wide spectrum of diets. **Semi-vegetarians** are the most inclusive, allowing fish, eggs, and dairy products as well as plant-based foods. **Ovo-lacto vegetarians** are somewhat more strict; they eat eggs and dairy products, but not fish. **Lacto-vegetarians** consume only dairy and plant-based foods. **Vegans** eat only foods of plant origin, and a **fruitarian** diet includes only fruits, nuts, honey, and vegetable oils. Soy beans, soy milk, tofu, and processed protein products can be used by all but fruitarians to enhance the nutritional value of the diet.

People choose vegetarian diets for a number of reasons. As noted in Chapter 14, some religions prohibit consumption of animal flesh or foods of animal origin. Ethical considerations related to humane treatment of animals also cause some people to adopt a vegetarian diet. However, many people adopt a vegetarian diet simply as a health choice, noting the abundant research indicating that vegetarianism reduces the risk of disease and promotes wellness by limiting fat intake.

Although ovo-lacto vegetarians have no higher rate of nutrient deficiencies than the meat-eating population, they must choose foods carefully to include enough of the following nutrients:

- *Vitamin B$_{12}$* is found only in animal products, such as eggs and milk. Vegans must eat foods fortified with B$_{12}$ or take B$_{12}$ supplements. Long-standing B$_{12}$ deficiency can result in severe and irreversible neurological impairment.
- *Vitamin D* may be inadequately supplied by vegetarian diets, so vitamin D-fortified foods (e.g., soy and dairy milk are usually vitamin D fortified) should be included. Adequate sun exposure also helps to compensate for lack of dietary intake.
- *Calcium, iron, and zinc.* Vegans, fruitarians, and others who limit animal foods may need to supplement the diet with calcium, iron, and zinc. This is especially important for children and women who are pregnant or lactating.
  - (a) *Iron:* The iron from plant foods is not absorbed as well as that from animal sources. However, it is easier to absorb dietary iron when it is eaten with foods containing vitamin C, so eating fruit or vegetables containing vitamin C with meals *helps to compensate.*
  - (b) *Calcium:* Vegans, especially, may find it difficult to obtain enough dietary calcium. It is important to include fortified soy milk and calcium-rich vegetables (e.g., bok choy, broccoli, collards, Chinese cabbage, kale, mustard greens, okra, and fortified tomato juice). Calcium-fortified cereals are also available.
- *Protein* may be inadequate, especially in vegan children who do not care for the taste of soy milk, tofu, and other soy-based meat substitutes. For adults, a varied diet that meets normal nutrient and energy needs is also likely to supply adequate amounts of essential amino acids. Complementary proteins should be eaten throughout the day, but careful meal-by-meal balance of amino acids is usually not necessary. Review Table 26-1 and the discussion of complete and incomplete proteins earlier in the chapter.

In addition to following the information contained in the Vegetarian Food Pyramid (see Fig. 26-2), to ensure adequate nutrients it may be wise for vegetarians to consult a qualified nutrition professional, especially during periods of growth, breastfeeding, pregnancy, or recovery from illness. For recommended servings of vegetarian food groups,

Go to Chapter 26, **Tables, Boxes, Figures: ESG Table 26-1,** on the Student Resource Disk or DavisPlus at http://davisplus.fadavis.com/Wilkinson2

Dieting for Weight Loss

One popular Internet bookseller recently offered no fewer than 36,655 books on weight-loss diets! Many diets, including the *Dietary Approaches to Stop Hypertension* (DASH) diet, the American Heart Association diet, and others, are nutritionally sound, but many others are "fad diets," claiming to produce speedy, effortless, almost miraculous, weight loss. You can recognize fad diets by the following characteristics. They:

- Promise quick and dramatic weight loss, which is usually achieved only temporarily because it results from loss of body fluids.
- Limit the range of foods from which the dieter can select (e.g., only fruits and vegetables for the first week), leading to an imbalance in nutrients.
- Often recommend purchase of supplements and/or special packaged meals; in many cases, these are brands that they endorse or actually produce.
- Fail to include practical strategies that help dieters permanently change eating and activity patterns.

As soon as they achieve their weight-loss goal, fad dieters typically revert to former eating habits and regain the weight. In contrast, more moderate calorie-restriction diets, such as the American Heart Association diet:

- Describe food selection and preparation tips and other behavior modifications that can lead to slow, sustained weight loss.
- Promote a diet that includes a variety of food choices and a balance of nutrients.
- Encourage physical activity as a cornerstone of weight loss.
- Emphasize self-monitoring, cognitive strategies, and behavior modification.

Ethnic, Cultural, and Religious Practices

As described in Chapters 13 and 14, religion and culture can have a major impact on diet and lifestyle. The following are examples:

- Language barriers may make it difficult for a client to understand nutritional information. For those patients, simple visual aids may be useful.
- Ethnic/cultural food choices often reflect the foods that were plentiful in the region of origin (e.g., fish in coastal communities, coffee and cocoa beans in equatorial regions), as well as foods that were readily grown in the native soil (e.g., rice in warm wetlands, potatoes in colder climates).
- Other diet choices reflect a concern for food preservation: for instance, people from various geographic regions eat salted meats and dried fruits and cook with fiery spices to combat microbes.

- Certain religions may require fasting or abstaining from certain foods. For example, Roman Catholics fast on Ash Wednesday and Good Friday; kosher dietary laws prohibit eating pork and shellfish.
- The burden of childhood obesity is not spread equally across the U.S. population. For example, obesity has been increasing faster among Mexican American and African American children (National Center for Health Statistics, 2008a).
- Cultural beliefs, perceptions, and attitudes about weight issues may often not match those of health providers. For example, some parents may perceive their children as cute and healthy, even though their BMI indicates they are obese. A slim body is not the ideal in all cultures.

Traditional diets of many cultures are healthful and should not be discouraged; in fact, contemporary adaptations made to these diets may compromise their nutritional quality. Examples of adapted traditional diets are the Asian, Latin, and Mediterranean Diet Pyramids, mentioned earlier. The Mediterranean diet, which includes a glass of red wine and is rich in fish, fruits, vegetables, and nuts and low in dairy foods, saturated fats, and red meat, has been linked to decreased risk of death from all causes, including deaths due to cancer and cardiovascular disease in a U.S. population (Mitrou, Kipnis, Thiébaut, et al., 2007).

Disease Processes and Functional Limitations

Chronic diseases (e.g., diabetes mellitus, gastrointestinal disorders) can alter nutrient intake, digestion, absorption, use, and excretion. Any illness, especially when accompanied by fever, increases the need for protein, water, and kilocalories to meet the demands of increased metabolic rate. Traumatic injury (e.g., burns, surgery) requires extra protein and vitamin C for wound healing and tissue rebuilding. People with long-term insufficient calorie intake (e.g., patients with cancer) also suffer from **protein-calorie malnutrition,** which is characterized by weight loss and muscle and fat wasting. A variety of other physical and psychological disorders and/or their treatments can adversely affect a client's nutrition:

Appetite. A poor appetite results in decreased intake of food and therefore of nutrients. It is a common problem in alcoholism. Almost all oral medications have the potential to cause nausea or vomiting, thereby decreasing appetite. Examples of medications that often cause nausea include acetylsalicylic acid (aspirin), antibiotics, anticonvulsants, antidepressants, anti-inflammatory agents, antineoplastic agents (chemotherapy), asthma medications (especially theophylline), birth control pills, fluoride supplements, opioids, potassium chloride, and vitamin and mineral supplements. Some medications directly decrease appetite, for example, amphetamine and dextroamphetamine (Adderal), aspirin, diphenhydramine (e.g., Benadryl), and lithium carbonate (e.g., Lithobid).

Cognitive Function. A person with a developmental delay, severe mental illness, confusion, or memory loss may be unable to remember what, when, or whether she has eaten.

Ability to Obtain Food. Paralysis or hemiplegia (e.g., from a stroke) can cause functional limitations that affect mobility and, hence, the ability to shop for food. Social factors also limit the ability to gather or procure food. People with limited income may be forced to choose between buying food, medication, or household utilities. Homeless people and others in extreme poverty are often reduced to eating from trash cans and dumpsters or consuming nonfoods, such as paper, grass, and clay.

Ability to Prepare Food. Preparing food takes time and energy. A person with severe dyspnea from chronic obstructive pulmonary disease (COPD), for example, may not have the stamina to prepare a nutritious meal. Instead, she may eat prepared foods that are high in sodium content. Fatigue is also caused by advanced chronic disease, severe anemia, pregnancy, depression, or excess work.

Chewing. Decayed or missing teeth and ill-fitting dentures make chewing difficult. The person often resorts to eating only soft foods, many of which lack fiber.

Swallowing. Acute disorders affecting the throat, such as pharyngitis, make swallowing painful. Cancer of the larynx or esophageal strictures also make swallowing painful or difficult, and frequently leads to avoiding food.

Stomach Function. Heartburn, indigestion, and other stomach disorders are common. People may eat only bland foods or avoid certain foods to prevent the pain or burning that follow eating.

Peristalsis. Peristalsis is the wavelike action that propels food through the intestinal tract. Bowel inflammation or infection, diverticuli (outpouchings of the intestine), or tumors may increase peristalsis, thereby decreasing absorption of nutrients. In addition, high stress levels may either speed or slow transit time. If peristalsis is slow, the stomach may not empty properly (gastroparesis). This could lead to early satiety, nausea, or vomiting and affect nutrient intake. This is not unusual in patients with diabetes.

Intestinal Surface Area. The amount of intestinal surface area may be diminished either by surgery or disease, thereby decreasing absorption of nutrients. This may result in malnutrition despite the fact that the patient is consuming adequate calories and protein.

Enzyme Secretions. Liver, gallbladder, or pancreas problems affect the secretion of enzymes involved in digesting foods. Nearly 50 million Americans lack the enzyme (lactase) needed to digest milk. Up to 80% of African Americans, 80% to 100% of Native Americans, and 90% to 100% of Asian Americans are lactose intolerant (National Digestive Diseases Information Clearinghouse, 2006).

Medications. In addition to the direct effects of diseases and disorders, nutrition may be affected by the drugs and therapies used to treat them. For example, chemotherapy and radiation therapy may cause oral ulcers, intestinal bleeding, or diarrhea—which interfere with eating and absorbing nutrients from food. Certain drugs alter nutrient metabolism, and others increase or decrease nutrient excretion. Some drugs affect specific nutrients. For example, acetylsalicylic acid (aspirin) decreases folate levels and increases excretion of vitamin C; laxatives may cause calcium and potassium depletion; and thiazide diuretics decrease the absorption of vitamin B_{12}.

KnowledgeCheck 26-6

- List at least three nutrients that may be more difficult to supply through a vegetarian diet.
- When selecting a program for weight loss, what factors should a person consider?
- Why should you encourage clients from various cultures to follow their traditional diets?
- Describe the effects on nutrition of (1) smoking and (2) heavy alcohol use.

Go to Chapter 26, **Knowledge Check Response Sheet and Answers,** on the Student Resource Disk or DavisPlus at http://davisplus.fadavis.com/Wilkinson2

Special Diets

Many people must follow a modified diet to assist in managing their illness. In addition, all inpatients at healthcare facilities must have a diet prescribed by their primary care provider. The following are the most commonly prescribed modified diets.

Regular Diet

A regular diet, also called the "house diet," is appropriate for clients without special nutritional needs. This diet is a balanced meal plan that supplies 2000 kcal per day. Many facilities provide vegetarian and ethnic variations (Asian menu, kosher, and so on). Inpatients choose each meal from a list of menu choices.

Have you ever eaten "hospital food"? Or have you heard someone complain that "hospital food is bland and unimaginative"? There is some justification for that complaint. House diets must accommodate the varied tastes of all patients, so they are usually lightly seasoned. Selections are limited to avoid unpopular items (e.g., brussel sprouts) and restrict fatty, fried, or gassy foods, which many patients tolerate poorly. However, you should refrain from making negative comments to patients about the food.

NPO

NPO means no food or fluid (including water) by mouth. This may be ordered before surgery or an invasive procedure to limit the risk of aspiration. Common examples are "NPO after midnight," or "NPO 8 hours prior to procedure." Most well-nourished, well-hydrated patients easily tolerate short-term NPO status. However, no one can tolerate prolonged periods of NPO. Intravenous fluids may be given to provide hydration, and clients who must remain NPO for a lengthy period need enteral (through a stomach tube) or parenteral (IV) nutrition to prevent malnutrition.

Diets Modified by Consistency

Patients undergoing surgery, bowel procedures, or acute illness may, for a short period of time, need a diet modified by consistency. Patients with chronic health concerns that affect their ability to chew or swallow (e.g., Impaired Dentition and Impaired Swallowing) may need long-term changes in the consistency of their diet.

Clear Liquids. A clear liquid diet provides fluids to prevent dehydration, and supplies some simple carbohydrates to help meet energy needs. Items in a clear liquid diet include water, tea, coffee, broth, clear juice (usually apple, grape, or cranberry juice), popsicles, carbonated beverages, and gelatin. Clear liquids do not supply adequate calories, protein, and other nutrients, so timely progression to more nutritious diets is recommended. If clear liquids are required for more than 3 days, commercial clear liquid supplements are usually prescribed.

Full Liquids. A full liquid diet contains all the liquids included in the clear liquid diet plus any food items that are liquid at room temperature: soups, milk, milk shakes, puddings, custards, juices, some hot cereals, and yogurt. It is difficult to obtain a balanced diet on a full liquid plan, so it should be used for a short time only. If it is needed for a longer time, it should be planned by a professional dietitian. High-calorie, high-protein supplements are often added.

Mechanical Soft Diet. Mechanical soft diet is the diet of choice for people with chewing difficulties resulting from missing teeth, jaw problems, or extensive fatigue. A soft diet includes all items on the full liquid diet plus soft vegetables and fruits; chopped, ground, or shredded meat; and breads, pastries, eggs, and cheese. Many food items can be added to this diet by cooking them extensively or blending or grinding to alter their texture. This diet can supply a full range of nutrients but is quite low in fiber. As a result, constipation is a risk.

Pureed Diet. A pureed diet is a blended diet. Any food item may be eaten; however, the consistency must be altered by blending. Often liquids are added to the food to create a texture that may be scooped onto serving plates.

Diets Modified for Disease

Some health conditions require modification of dietary intake. The following are the most common diets:

- *Calorie-restricted.* For clients requiring weight reduction
- *Sodium-restricted.* For clients with blood pressure or fluid balance problems
- *Fat-restricted.* For clients with elevated cholesterol or triglyceride levels; may also be ordered for general weight loss.
- *Diabetic.* To manage calories and carbohydrate intake for clients with diabetes mellitus
- *Renal diet.* To manage electrolytes and fluid for clients with renal insufficiency
- *Protein-controlled diet.* To manage liver and kidney disease
- *Antigen-avoidance diets.* For clients allergic to or intolerant of certain foods, such as a gluten-free diet for clients with celiac disease
- *Calorie-protein push.* Used when there is a need to heal wounds, maintain or increase weight, or promote growth. If the person cannot consume enough kcal by adding fats and proteins to his regular diet, high–calorie, high-protein supplements may be used.

 Critical**Thinking** 26-5

Analyze the following diets. Which nutrients are missing or difficult to obtain from these diets?

- Clear liquid
- Full liquid

Practical Knowledge knowing how

Good nutrition not only is essential for health, but also is a key aspect of disease management. In the rest of this chapter, we look at assessing nutritional status and diagnosing and planning care for some nutrition problems. In addition, we discuss specifically the care of patients who are underweight/undernourished or overweight/obese.

Nursing Care to Meet Nutritional Needs

Nutrition is a basic human need. But more than a physical necessity, it also has emotional associations. We eat when we are hungry, but we also eat for pleasure because the food tastes good! Food has become a part of most social events and activities. A certain food may symbolize one's cultural or religious affiliation or even be a political statement (e.g., refusal to eat lettuce in support of migrant workers). It is wise to keep in mind that food has different meanings to different people. Personal beliefs, habits, and preferences are as important as nutritional knowledge in determining what a person eats.

 ASSESSMENT

The nutrition component of the overall health history provides information for identifying nutrition-related problems. It includes subjective data about the client's dietary history and related factors. For the components of a nutritional history,

VOL 2 Go to Chapter 26, **Assessment Guidelines and Tools, Nutritional History,** in Volume 2.

You can obtain a dietary history during any routine assessment. When you take a **dietary history,** whether you use a self-administered form or an interview, you collect general knowledge of the client's basic eating habits, food attitudes and preferences, cultural factors, and use of dietary supplements. A dietary history creates a picture of the client's food habits and eating behaviors.

Food Diaries

To collect detailed data on what the client is actually eating, ask him to keep a **food diary.** The following are three types of food diaries:

24-Hour Recall. A 24-hour recall requires the client to name all food eaten within a day. Simply ask questions such as "Yesterday, what did you eat for breakfast/lunch/dinner/snacks?" A 24-hour recall is simple, requires no equipment, and can be used as often as required. However, accuracy of the data may be questionable, because some people have difficulty remembering everything they ate the previous day, and any single day may be atypical. Sometimes, a family member can help the client recall intake more accurately.

Food Frequency Questionnaire. A food frequency questionnaire asks the client to identify the number of times per day, week, or month a particular food group is eaten (e.g., fruits, red meats). You can modify the questions according to the client's specific issues. Food frequency questionnaires provide a more global image of the client's nutritional intake than the 24-hour recall; however, accuracy is still a problem.

Food Record. A food record is the most accurate food diary. It provides information on the quantity as well as the types of foods eaten. You ask the client in advance to keep a record of measured and weighed amounts of all foods he eats in a 3-day period. From the detailed information collected, you can analyze the total kilocalories and nutrient content for the recorded period. Although the food record provides meaningful results, it requires a high level of cognitive and psychomotor functioning that not all clients have. It also requires commitment to the process for 3 days, which may be difficult for some people.

You may wish to remind some patients there are websites that can help them with journaling their diet and tracking nutritional intake, goals, and so on. For example,

Go to one of these three Web sites: http://www.fitday.com/fitness/Login.html?_a_Date=1247356800
http://www.nutrawatch.com/
http://www.fitwatch.com/

How Do I Screen Clients for Nutritional Problems?

Nutritional screening is performed to determine deficiencies or excesses in the diet. The Joint Commission requires a nutritional screening to be completed within 24 hours of inpatient admission (The Joint Commission, 2008). The degree of screening performed depends on the patient's condition or concerns. **Cursory screening** consists of evaluation of height, weight, and body mass index (BMI) coupled with a brief dietary history. Clients who are found to be at risk for nutritional problems should be further evaluated. It is especially important to assess nutritional status in elderly clients carefully to ensure that you detect marginal deficiencies before major problems occur.

- *The subjective global assessment.* This commonly used screening method makes use of information from the overall medical history and physical examination to evaluate a client's nutritional status.
- *The Nutrition Screening Initiative (NSI),* developed for older adults, identifies indicators of impaired nutritional status.
- *The Mini Nutritional Assessment,* also developed for older adults, can be used with clients of all ages.

To learn more about those screening methods and a tool to use in assessing nutritional status for clients with dementia,

 Go to Chapter 26, **Assessment: Screening for Nutritional Problems,** in Volume 2.

How Can I Assess Body Composition?

When assessing body composition (the proportion of fat in the body), you use **anthropometric measurements.** These are noninvasive physical examination techniques to determine body dimensions such as height and weight. Other examples are discussed in the following sections. Anthropometric measurements are used to assess growth rate in children; to indirectly assess adults' protein and fat stores; and to diagnose overweight, obesity, and underweight. To obtain accurate data, you must use standardized equipment and procedures and compare the data to existing reference standards for men and women.

Skinfold Measurements

Approximately half of body fat is located subcutaneously. Therefore, you will use measurement of

skinfold thickness to estimate a person's body fat content. Skinfold thickness reveals information about current nutritional status as well as long-term changes in fat stores. Use a caliper to obtain the most accurate measurement. The most reliable location is the triceps for children and women and the subscapular area in men. The combined measurements of triceps skinfold and mid-upper arm circumference yield a better estimate of muscle and fat areas than a single measurement. For instructions on taking skinfold measurements,

 Go to Chapter 26, **Clinical Insight 26-2: Skinfold Measurement,** in Volume 2.

Circumferences

Another method of estimating the percentage of body fat is to use girth, or circumference measurements. *Mid-upper arm circumference* is routinely measured as part of screening. For people who are obese, *abdominal circumference* is the preferred measurement. *The waist-to-hip ratio (WHR)* evaluates obesity by assessing abdominal fat. A WHR of greater than 1 in men and greater than 0.8 in women indicates obesity. A high level of abdominal fat is associated with increased risk for hypertension, diabetes, hyperlipidemia, and cardiovascular disease. For specific instructions on measuring mid-upper arm circumference and WHR,

 Go to Chapter 26, **Clinical Insight 26-3: Measuring Circumferences to Evaluate Body Composition,** in Volume 2.

Body Mass Index

Body mass index (BMI) can be precisely measured using scanning devices that measure *bioelectrical impedance*—the conduction of a harmless electrical charge through the client's body. Lean tissue readily conducts the charge, whereas adipose tissue does not. However, you will usually roughly estimate BMI by using the calculation formula in Box 26-4. You may also consult tables with precalculated values based on height and weight. For an example of a height–weight BMI table,

 Go to Chapter 19, **Procedure 19–1: Performing the General Survey,** in Volume 2.

You can also find BMI calculators on the Web. Two reliable examples are at:

 Centers for Disease Control and Prevention, at http://www.cdc.gov/healthyweight/assessing/bmi/adult_bmi/english_bmi_calculator/bmi_calculator.html and **National Heart Lung and Blood Institute,** at http://www.nhlbisupport.com/bmi/bmicalc.htm

The normal BMI for adults ranges from 18.5 to 24.9 (although this may vary slightly among professional organizations). The usefulness of BMI values is

BOX 26-4 ■ Calculating Body Mass Index (BMI)

BMI = weight in kilograms ÷ (height in meters)^2

Example:

Robert weighs 165 lb. Convert his weight to kilograms:

$$165 ÷ 2.2 = 75 \text{ kg}$$

He is 71 inches tall. Convert his height to meters.

$$1 \text{ meter} = 39.37 \text{ inches.}$$

Divide 71 inches by 39.37 inches; he is 1.8 meters tall (rounded off)

His BMI is 75 kg ÷ $(1.8)^2$ = 23

The normal BMI for adults ranges from 18.5 to 24.9.

Classification of Body Mass Index Values

Classification	BMI (kg/m^2)
Severely underweight	<16
Moderately underweight	16–16.99
Mild underweight	17–18.49
Underweight	<18.5
Healthy weight	18.5–24.9
Pre-obese	25.0–29.9
Class I obesity	30.0–34.9
Class II obesity	35.0–39.9
Class III obesity	40.0 or higher

Source: Adapted from National Heart Lung and Blood Institute (1998); and World Health Organization (2006).

limited for athletes because of their highly developed muscle mass, and for pregnant and postpartal women because their increased weight is normal. In addition, BMI values have not been specifically calculated for people older than age 65. Despite these limitations, BMI is useful in identifying underweight and obese individuals.

KnowledgeCheck 26-7

- What is the most accurate type of food diary?
- Compare and contrast four nutritional screening approaches: cursory screening, subjective global assessment, Mini Nutritional Assessment, and Nutrition Screening Initiative.
- Identify three nutritional risk factors.

 Go to Chapter 26, **Knowledge Check Response Sheet and Answers,** on the Student Resource Disk or DavisPlus at http://davisplus.fadavis.com/Wilkinson2

 Critical**Thinking** 26-6

1. Calculate your WHR.
2. Use Box 26-5 to calculate your BMI. Evaluate the result.
   - How useful are these data?
   - Do you feel you need to pursue a program of weight loss? Why or why not?

Imaging Techniques

Imaging techniques are not widely used to evaluate lean body mass because they are quite expensive to perform. Imaging methods include the following:

Dual-energy X-ray Absorptiometry (DEXA). DEXA is used to assess bone mineral content and density. Because lean tissue has different absorptive properties than adipose tissue, this technique shows promise for wider use because it is quick and noninvasive.

Computed Tomography (CT). CT scans measure volume rather than actual body tissue composition. They can provide information about the quantity of adipose tissue, particularly in body cavities.

Magnetic Resonance Imaging (MRI). MRI is an excellent noninvasive method for directly assessing body composition. The cost and availability of the machinery, however, make it impractical for day-to-day evaluation of clients.

Underwater Weighing

Hydrodensitometry, or underwater weighing, is another method of determining body composition. It requires total submersion of the patient in a tank of water. Because fat readily floats, the person's buoyancy will vary depending on his percentage of body fat. This method is considered the gold standard for body composition measures. However, clinical use of this method is limited because it is impractical to use with children, the elderly, or individuals who are severely ill.

KnowledgeCheck 26-8

- What are the most reliable locations for skinfold measurement?
- What are the implications of an increased WHR?

 Go to Chapter 26, **Knowledge Check Response Sheet and Answers,** on the Student Resource Disk or DavisPlus at http://davisplus.fadavis.com/Wilkinson2

What Physical Examination Findings Are Cues to Nutrient Imbalance?

You should correlate physical examination findings with other assessments, such as nutritional and medical history, dietary intake, anthropometric measurements, and laboratory results. Refer to Chapter 19 as needed for a review of physical examination techniques. For guidelines in performing a nutrition-focused physical examination,

VOL 2 Go to Chapter 26, **Assessment Guidelines and Tools, Focused Nutritional Assessment,** in Volume 2.

What Are the Signs of Severe Malnutrition?

Malnutrition is a condition of impaired development or function caused by a long-term deficiency, excess, or imbalance in energy and/or nutrient intake. Malnutrition caused by deficiency of protein in a diet that is primarily starches is called **kwashiorkor**. When protein sources in food are scarce and overall caloric intake is low, **marasmus** occurs, particularly in young children. Undernourished people are prone to infections. Symptoms of undernutrition due to insufficient food are reduced physical activity, weight loss, and reduced height, abdominal enlargement, and hair loss. Other diseases develop as a result of specific vitamin and mineral deficiency, such as beriberi (neurological deficits), scurvy (delayed wound healing and poor bone growth), and pellagra (diarrhea and dementia). See Tables 26-4 and 26-5 for specific signs of vitamin and mineral excesses and deficits.

Malnutrition is most common in underdeveloped nations and among children, older adults, and people with chronic illnesses such as cancer, HIV, and COPD. Others at risk for malnutrition include those with the following:

- Serum albumin level 3.5 g/dL or less
- Nausea or vomiting lasting 3 days or more
- Clear liquid diet or NPO for 3 days or longer
- Increased nutritional requirements (e.g., wound healing, burns)
- Recent, unplanned loss of 10% or more of patient's usual weight

To assess for malnutrition in children, compare weight, height, and head circumference to the standards (norms) for the child's age. In cases of severe malnutrition, abdominal circumference can signal worsening disease. Other indicators in children include the presence of iron deficiency anemia and, in adolescents, a delay of stages of sexual maturation.

KnowledgeCheck 26-9

- Identify at least 10 physical examination findings that would lead you to suspect nutritional problems.
- What factors would lead to poor wound healing?

 Go to Chapter 26, **Knowledge Check Response Sheet and Answers,** on the Student Resource Disk or DavisPlus at http://davisplus.fadavis.com/Wilkinson2

What Laboratory Values Indicate Nutritional Status?

Various laboratory or biochemical indicators provide information about nutritional status. These include blood glucose, serum protein level and associated indices, total lymphocyte count, and hemoglobin. To see the norms for these lab tests,

 Go to **Diagnostic Testing, Tests Reflecting Nutritional Status: Norms,** in Volume 2.

Blood Glucose

The blood glucose level indicates the amount of fuel available for cellular energy. A homeostatic mechanism regulates the concentration of glucose in the blood. Levels above the normal set point trigger the release of insulin, which causes the glucose to move into body cells and to be stored in the liver and muscles. A level falling below the normal set point triggers the release of glucagons, leading to the release of glucose from storage.

Hypoglycemia limits the fuel supply to the body, resulting in symptoms ranging from weakness to coma. Hypoglycemia is usually defined as blood glucose of less than 50 mg/dL, but some people may feel symptoms at higher levels. Often the cause is insufficient food intake, excessive physical exertion, or a disproportionate amount of hypoglycemic agents.

Hyperglycemia (blood glucose greater than 109 mg/dL fasting or greater than 126 mg/dL at random) may be a sign of diabetes mellitus, an endocrine problem, which may develop as a result of either insufficient insulin production or resistance to the existing supply of insulin. A high blood glucose level does not mean that there is more fuel available for cellular energy, though. A characteristic of diabetes is that although there is more than enough glucose in the blood, it cannot enter and be used by the cells. Repeated blood glucose measures are required before making a diagnosis of diabetes mellitus because glucose levels may be temporarily elevated as a result of excessive carbohydrate intake or emotional and physical stressors.

A temporary rise in blood sugar may produce weakness or fatigue. Prolonged elevations lead to weight loss, blurred vision, **ketosis** (incomplete metabolism of fat due to inability to use carbohydrates as fuel), renal failure, and **peripheral neuropathy** (damage to nerves due to prolonged exposure to high glucose levels).

Patients with diabetes usually monitor their own blood sugar levels, but you may need to do it for some. Usually this is done by a fingerstick to obtain capillary blood for testing. Some meters can use blood from alternative sites such as upper arm, forearm, base of thumb, or thigh. Other types of monitors are available. For example, one kind uses a disposable sensor placed just under the skin. The sensor communicates with a receiver that reads the levels. Another is a skin testing device, worn like a watch, that pulls tiny amounts of fluid from the skin without puncturing it. See the Critical Aspects box for a summary of the fingerstick procedure. For complete steps,

 Go to Chapter 26, **Procedure 26-1: Checking Fingerstick (Capillary) Blood Glucose Levels,** in Volume 2.

Serum Protein Levels and Indices

Protein molecules dissolve in blood to form plasma proteins. Tissue proteins are a combination of albumin and globulin, so serum protein levels are indicators of protein stores.

- **Albumin** is synthesized in the liver and constitutes 60% of total body protein. Low levels of albumin are associated with malnutrition, malabsorption, acute and chronic liver disease, and repeated loss of protein through burns, wounds, or other sources. The half-life of albumin is 18 to 21 days. As a result, there is a lag in detecting nutritional problems based on serum albumin. Albumin is also affected by fluid status and, therefore, is not an accurate measure in the patient with fluid imbalance. For example, a patient in positive fluid balance (taking in more than excreted) will have a falsely low albumin level.

- **Prealbumin** level fluctuates daily and is considered a better marker of acute change than albumin.
- **Transferrin** is a protein that binds with iron. Because it has a half-life of only 8 to 9 days, it allows for faster detection of protein depletion than does measuring albumin. Transferrin can be measured directly or indirectly (by a total iron-binding capacity test [TIBC]). It also reflects iron status. In a person with iron deficiency, the TIBC will be increased; in a person with anemia, the TIBC will be decreased.

Other markers are used to monitor protein metabolism:

- **Urea** is formed in the liver as an end product of protein metabolism and is excreted through the kidneys. As such, the serum blood urea nitrogen (BUN) level is an indicator of liver and kidney function. An elevated BUN level is seen with impaired kidney function, dehydration, excessive protein breakdown (often seen with diabetes mellitus, hyperthyroidism, or starvation) or excessive dietary protein intake. Low levels are seen with impaired liver function, fluid overload, and low protein intake.
- **Creatinine,** an end product of skeletal muscle metabolism, is excreted through the kidneys and is an excellent indicator of renal function. Increased levels may indicate impaired kidney function or loss of muscle mass.
- **Lymphocytes,** or white blood cells (WBC), are the body's first line of defense against microorganisms. For a detailed discussion of the role of WBCs in infection control, as well as a discussion on the types of WBCs and their normal values, see Chapter 20. A decrease in total lymphocytes, known as **leukopenia,** is associated with malnutrition, protein deficiency, alcoholism, bone marrow depression, and anemia.
- **Hemoglobin** is composed of **heme,** an iron-rich compound, and **globulin,** a serum protein. Adequate iron intake is required to produce heme. Therefore, a low hemoglobin may indicate inadequate iron intake or chronic blood loss. Globulin forms the backbone of hemoglobin as well as antibodies, glycoproteins, lipoproteins, clotting factors, and a variety of key enzymes. A decreased globulin level indicates insufficient protein intake or excessive protein loss.

May I Delegate Nutritional Assessments?

You may safely delegate to nursing assistive personnel (NAPs) the measurement of weight, height, and intake and output; other nursing staff (e.g., licensed practical/vocational nurses) can collect a nutritional history. However, the registered nurse (RN) is responsible for reviewing and interpreting these findings. When delegating these tasks, you must also tell the NAP or LPN how often the measurements are to be made. Review Chapter 7 for making delegation decisions.

KnowledgeCheck 26-10

- What are the likely causes of hyperglycemia?
- Why is it important to identify the serum albumin level?

  Go to Chapter 26, **Knowledge Check Response Sheet and Answers,** on the Student Resource Disk or DavisPlus at http://davisplus.fadavis.com/Wilkinson2

CriticalThinking 26-7

The Mini Nutritional Assessment (MNA®) in Volume 2 is completed for a 70-year-old woman and yields the following results:

Part I Screening = 8
Part II Assessment = 10

- What would her Malnutrition Indicator Score be, and what does this indicate?
- What type of physical assessment findings would support this score?
- What type of anthropometric findings would support this score?
- What type of laboratory values would support this score?

▮ ANALYSIS/NURSING DIAGNOSIS

For clients who have no symptoms of or risk factors for nutrition problems, use the diagnostic label Readiness for Enhanced Nutrition. NANDA-I defines this as "a pattern of nutrient intake that is sufficient for meeting metabolic needs and can be strengthened" (2009, p. 67).

Nutrition as the Problem

You can use the following NANDA-I labels to describe general nutrition problems:

- Adult Failure to Thrive
- Imbalanced Nutrition: Less Than Body Requirements
- Imbalanced Nutrition: More Than Body Requirements
- Risk for Imbalanced Nutrition: More Than Body Requirements
- Self-Care Deficit (Feeding)

As you have learned, nutrition problems have many causes. Etiologies for undernutrition include eating disorders, difficulties with chewing, swallowing, vomiting, alcoholism, food intolerances, metabolic disorders, digestive disorders, and absorption disorders. For overnutrition, etiologies include overeating, lack of exercise, and metabolic or endocrine disorders. The following nursing diagnoses may contribute to nutrition problems: Diarrhea, Health-Seeking Behaviors

(Nutrition), Impaired Swallowing, Nausea, Noncompliance (with prescribed diet), and Deficient Knowledge (nutrition).

The following is an example of a nutrition nursing diagnosis statement:

Imbalanced Nutrition: Less Than Body Requirements related to difficulty chewing and Impaired Swallowing

Nutrition as the Etiology

Nutritional problems can also be the etiology of problems in other functional areas, for example:

- Ineffective Breastfeeding r/t inadequate milk production 2° insufficient intake of calories and fluids
- Constipation r/t insufficient intake of fluids and fiber
- Diarrhea r/t excessive intake of alcohol and/or sugar
- Risk for Infection r/t inadequate intake of calories and protein
- Impaired (or Risk for Impaired) Skin Integrity r/t inadequate intake of protein and/or vitamin A
- Disturbed Sleep Pattern r/t excessive caffeine intake or to eating fatty and spicy foods near bedtime
- Impaired Social Interaction r/t low self-esteem 2° obesity

PLANNING OUTCOMES/EVALUATION

The overall *Healthy People 2020* nutrition goal for the United States population is to "promote health and reduce chronic disease associated with diet and weight" (U.S. Department of Health and Human Services, 2010). For specific objectives related to that goal,

 Go to Chapter 26, **Tables, Boxes, Figures: ESG Box 26-1,** on the Student Resource Disk or DavisPlus at http://davisplus.fadavis.com/Wilkinson2

The final *Healthy People 2020* goals should be available after this text is published. You should read the new nutrition goals and objectives

 At **Healthy People** home page at www.healthypeople.gov

NOC standardized outcomes directly linked to nutritional problems include the following: Nutritional Status, Nutritional Status: Food and Fluid Intake, Nutritional Status: Nutrient Intake, and Weight Control.

You would choose other NOC outcomes based on the patient's nursing diagnosis. For example, for Situational Low Self-Esteem related to obesity, you might use Self-Esteem; for Noncompliance (prescribed diet), you could use Adherence Behavior, Compliance Behavior, or Treatment Behavior: Illness/Injury.

Individualized goals/outcome statements you might write for a patient with nutrition-related problems include the following:

Loses 1 lb per week until ideal weight is attained.

Follows the prescribed modified diet that, at a minimum, meets the DRIs.

Eats a variety of foods that provide a balanced diet.

PLANNING INTERVENTIONS/IMPLEMENTATION

NIC standardized interventions directly linked to nutrition problems include the broad interventions of Nutrition Management, Nutrition Therapy, Nutritional Counseling, and Nutritional Monitoring. These interventions could probably be used for most nutrition problems, regardless of the etiologies. The other 13 interventions grouped under Nutritional Support address specific etiologies (e.g., Swallowing Therapy).

 Go to Chapter 26, **Standardized Language, NOC Outcomes and NIC Interventions Related to Nutrition,** in Volume 2.

Individualized nursing actions are determined by the patient's nursing diagnosis. They may include, for example, counseling regarding vitamin and mineral supplementation, teaching clients on a limited budget how to buy nutritious foods, supporting special nutritional needs, and assisting clients with meals. These are discussed in the rest of this chapter.

Vitamin and Mineral Supplementation

Do you take a vitamin tablet every day? Do you know anyone who takes megadoses of vitamin C to prevent a cold? Or zinc to cure one? Noncredentialed nutrition "experts" recommend, and sell, megadoses of the entire alphabet of vitamin and mineral supplements to prevent cancer and heart attacks, improve your sex life, prevent aging, and work other miracles. However, conservative health professionals may scoff at supplements, insisting that a nutritious diet supplies all the micronutrients you need. Somewhere in the middle, most likely, lies the truth. A growing body of research suggests that certain supplements provide health benefits. Remember, too, that RDAs are for "average" needs. Individual needs for micronutrients vary. During periods of increased nutrient demands, it may be difficult to get enough nutrients from diet alone.

NIC Intervention—Nutritional Counseling

When teaching clients about supplements, keep the following principles in mind:

1. Dietary supplements may be appropriate for people whose diet does not provide the recommended intake of specific vitamins. With a few exceptions, there is little evidence to suggest that people will be harmed by taking vitamin supplements in appropriate amounts (Agency for Healthcare Research and Quality, 2003).
2. Individual needs vary, and those needs should determine the specific nutrients and amounts used. For example:
   - Newborn infants are given a vitamin K injection to prevent hemorrhaging because they do not yet

have bacterial flora in the gut to synthesize enough vitamin K.

- Breastfed infants may need a vitamin D supplement (but not other vitamins) if the mother does not have an adequate diet or if the baby does not receive enough exposure to sunlight. Fetal iron stores are depleted at 4 to 6 months, so breastfed infants also need iron supplementation at that age.
- Vegetarians who eat little or no animal products may need a vitamin D supplement.
- Folic acid supplementation is recommended for people taking methotrexate (a drug used to treat certain types of cancer).
- All women who are capable of becoming pregnant should take a daily folic acid supplement of 400 to 800 micrograms, in addition to the naturally occurring folate they eat in foods. Pregnant women need at least 600 micrograms daily.
- Most adults older than 50 years should obtain vitamin B_{12} from fortified foods or supplements.
- Women age 50 and older should take calcium supplements to prevent osteoporosis; and there is growing evidence that men may need to do so, as well. Adults in the United States do not typically obtain adequate calcium from their diets (Barclay & Lie, 2008). Most calcium supplements come in combination with vitamin D to promote absorption of the calcium.
- People who do not eat dairy products need supplemental calcium.

3. Food is the best source of nutrients. Supplements do not replace the need to eat a nutritious diet. Vitamins need carbohydrate, protein, and fat to do their work. Specific supplements for certain individual situations are more effective if the person also has an adequate diet.
4. Read supplement labels carefully. They provide information about toxicity levels, dosage, and side effects.
5. Encourage patients to ask their primary care provider's advice before taking vitamins.
6. Advise patients to follow the dosages recommended in the DRIs or RDAs.
7. Be certain that any health claims made for a supplement are based on sound research.
8. The long-term effects of most nutritional supplements have yet to be fully researched.

The same principles apply with regard to mineral supplementation. Supplements of specific minerals may be needed during growth periods (i.e., pregnancy, lactation, and adolescence), but as a rule healthy adults eating balanced diets do not need supplements. People who require mineral supplementation include those who refuse dairy products (and therefore lack calcium), and those with clinical problems such as iron-deficiency anemia, zinc deficiency (e.g., in alcoholism and long-term low-calorie diets), and treatment with certain diuretics (e.g., for hypertension).

Nutritious Foods on a Limited Budget

Hunger and malnutrition are not unusual among the poor in the United States. When your clients cannot afford to buy food, you should teach them about available assistance and make appropriate referrals to programs such as the following:

SNAP (The Supplemental Nutrition Assistance Program) is the new name for the federal Food Stamp Program. For low-income households, this program issues coupons that can be used to buy food to cover the household's needs.

Commodity Supplemental Food Program. The federal government buys surplus food items to support certain agricultural products. These include both perishable and nonperishable commodities (e.g., peanut butter, cheese, green beans). The foods are made available to low-income pregnant and breastfeeding women, infants, children younger than 6 years old, and older adults at least 60 years old.

Women, Infants, and Children (WIC). This federal program provides free food to low-income women who are pregnant or breastfeeding and to children younger than age 5. Typical available foods are milk, eggs, cheese, cereals, juice, and infant formulas. They are intended to supplement the diet with protein, iron, and vitamins. They are not meant to supply all necessary food for the household.

National School Lunch and Breakfast Programs. These federally assisted programs subsidize schools that provide free or reduced-rate breakfasts and/or lunches to low-income children. All students, then, pay slightly less than the full cost of the meal. Lunches must supply about one-third of the child's RDA for energy and nutrients.

NIC Intervention—Teaching: Individual

You can help your clients to use their food dollars creatively by teaching them to follow the suggestions in the Self-Care box.

Supporting Special Nutritional Needs

Patients with special needs (e.g., patients with Impaired Swallowing, patients who are NPO, and older adults) require specific nutrition interventions.

Impaired Swallowing

The NANDA-I diagnosis Impaired Swallowing may be caused by mechanical obstruction (e.g., tumor), neuromuscular impairment (e.g., facial paralysis), stroke, cerebral palsy, or a host of other anatomical or physiological defects. Nutritional support for patients with Impaired Swallowing includes activities from the NIC intervention, Swallowing Therapy (Bulechek, Butcher, & Dochterman, 2008, pp. 707–708). For a list of these activities,

Teaching Your Patients to Buy Nutritious Foods on a Limited Budget

Plan ahead

➤ Look at the grocery advertisements in the paper or in their fliers, and plan meals around the sale items that are also the most nutrient-dense.

➤ Make a list of the foods you need. This will help you to control impulse buying and extra trips to the store.

➤ Avoid eating at fast-food restaurants. Meals are more expensive and less nutritious than those you can prepare at home.

➤ If transportation is not a problem, buy fresh foods at farmers' markets, at consumer co-ops, and from neighbors who have gardens.

Buy wisely

➤ Buy generic instead of more expensive and widely advertised brands.

➤ Watch for sales of nutrient-dense items. Stock up on and freeze them for later use if you do not need them right away.

➤ Buy in quantity—if it results in real savings and if you can use that amount of food before it spoils.

➤ Limit convenience foods (e.g., frozen dinners); they are expensive and often high in fat and sodium.

➤ Buy foods when they are in season; for example, fresh tomatoes are less expensive, and better tasting, in the summer than in the winter.

➤ Purchase oatmeal and cream of wheat instead of cold, sugared cereals. Buy in bulk rather than single-serving packages.

➤ Avoid shopping at convenience stores. Items are usually more expensive than in supermarkets.

➤ Buy inexpensive cuts of meat; avoid processed lunchmeats and hot dogs.

➤ Buy frozen concentrated fruit juices instead of juice in plastic jugs and cardboard boxes.

➤ Substitute dairy products, beans and lentils, and peanut butter for more expensive meat. Substitute powdered milk for whole milk.

➤ Read the Nutrition Facts panels on prepared foods to be sure you obtain the most nutrition for the money.

 Go to Chapter 26, **Clinical Insight 26-4: Interventions for Patients with Impaired Swallowing,** in Volume 2.

Patients Who Are NPO

Patients who cannot have oral food and fluids need comfort measures. Intravenous fluids for hydration may also include small amounts of glucose, but certainly not enough to meet bodily needs. Provide or assist the patient with oral hygiene. If allowed, provide ice chips, hard candy, chewing gum, or sips of water for rinsing the mouth. Advise family or visitors not to eat or drink around the patient, and try to schedule other activities for the patient at mealtimes. Remember, too, that remaining NPO for more than 3 days puts the patient at risk for malnutrition.

Patients Who Have Nausea

Nausea can cause vomiting and loss of appetite, leading to Impaired Nutrition. Nursing interventions include assessing for the cause of the nausea, and providing comfort and prevention measures. For other interventions,

 Go to **Clinical Insight 26-5: Interventions for Patients Who Have Nausea,** in Volume 2.

Older Adults

Nutritional problems of older adults are similar to those for adults of all ages, but the incidence of problems may be higher among older adults. The following interventions are appropriate for patients of any age who experience the problems.

Self-Care Deficit: Feeding. You will find interventions in the section "Assisting Patients with Meals," following.

Loss of Appetite; Diminished Sense of Smell and Taste. Refer to the section "Stimulating the Patient's Appetite," later in this chapter.

Decreased Income. Refer to the Self-Care box, Teaching Your Patients to Buy Nutritious Foods on a Limited Budget. In addition, for older adults in the United States, two types of food programs are available for you to recommend. Everyone older than age 60, regardless of income, can eat hot noon meals at a community center (under the Congregate Meals programs). Those who are ill or disabled can receive meals at home under the Home Delivered Meals Program. Socially needy persons (e.g., those who are homeless) are given priority. These programs are funded by public/private partnerships (e.g., Meals on Wheels).

Nutritional Deficiencies. Advise clients to eat nutrient-dense foods and to eat essential foods first. Because the sense of taste is decreased, older adults may prefer concentrated sweets; and because they may also have a poor appetite, once they eat sweets they may not be hungry enough to eat other foods.

Gastroesophageal Reflux. Advise clients to not eat just before bedtime and to elevate the head of the bed 30 to 40 degrees. It is also important to avoid overeating, avoid bending over, and take their prescribed medications. They should also avoid fruit juices, fatty foods, chocolate, alcohol, and smoking; all of these stimulate reflux. If overweight, the client with reflux should lose weight.

Decreased Gastric Secretions. People with this problem should eat regularly scheduled meals, chew their food thoroughly, and take prescribed medications. They should be certain to eat foods rich in vitamin D to ensure calcium absorption.

Dry Mouth. This is an age-associated change. Advise clients to avoid caffeine; alcohol; tobacco; and dry, bulky, spicy, salty, or highly acidic foods. Offer sugarless hard candy or chewing gum to stimulate salivation (unless the patient has dementia). Use lip moisturizer and encourage frequent sips of water.

Glucose Intolerance. Obviously, patients with glucose intolerance should avoid concentrated, refined sugars (e.g., candy, ice cream, desserts), unless they have been told to use it to treat hypoglycemia. Complex carbohydrates (e.g., whole-grain cereals, vegetables) are better tolerated. Smaller, more frequent meals may also be necessary.

Decreased Intestinal Peristalsis. To prevent constipation, advise patients to eat a diet high in fiber, including a minimum of five servings of fresh fruits and vegetables every day (prunes and prune juice are often effective); exercise regularly; drink at least eight glasses of water or other fluids per day; and eat meals on a regular schedule.

Avoiding Dementia. At least one study suggests that dementia, especially Alzheimer's disease, is less common among people who eat fruits and vegetables daily, eat fish once a week, and use fats rich in omega-3 fatty acids (e.g., walnut and soy oil) (Barberger-Gateau, Raffaitin, Letenneur, et al., 2007). Of course, this doesn't prove that diet can prevent dementia. It merely suggests there may be a connection. Either way, clients can benefit from this dietary advice.

Nothing by Mouth (NPO) Orders. When older adults must be NPO for tests or procedures, schedule them early in the day to decrease the length of time the patient must be NPO. If testing must be late in the day, ask the primary care provider whether the patient can have an early breakfast.

Assisting Patients with Meals

Some patients are at risk for nutritional deficits as a result of a Self-Care Deficit (Feeding), which may be caused by loss of cognitive, musculoskeletal, or neuromuscular function; weakness; pain; or environmental barriers. Elderly patients, especially, are at risk for undernutrition or malnourishment in inpatient settings.

You should institute special nutrition interventions in patients who have one of the following:

- An involuntary weight loss of more than 5% in 30 days or 10% in 180 days.
- Leaving more than one-fourth of their food in the past 7 days or two-thirds of meals (based on a 2000-kcal diet).
- A body mass index (BMI) of 19 or less.

NIC Interventions for this situation are Feeding and Self-Care Assistance: Feeding. Important nursing actions include assisting patients with meals. Other nursing activities include the following:

- Assess for functional deficits that contribute to Self-Care Deficit or Imbalanced Nutrition.
- Monitor intake for nutritional adequacy. Some patients may need liquid oral supplements of protein and calories.
- Collaborate with occupational and physical therapists in planning care.
- See that the patient has protein- and energy-enriched meals.
- Provide mid-afternoon snacks.
- Ensure the nutrition prescribed is actually implemented. Assign someone to be responsible for assisting the patient with meals as necessary. Include this in your instructions to NAPs and other assistive personnel.
- Refer the patient and family to an agency that can help them obtain a home health aide.

For guidelines more specific to assisting with meals, including care of patients with dementia,

 Go to Chapter 26, **Clinical Insight 26-6: Assisting Patients with Meals,** in Volume 2.

What Are Overweight and Obesity?

The BMI is commonly used to define weight status. A client with a BMI greater than 25 but less than 30 is considered **overweight** (or pre-obese). **Obesity** is a BMI of 30 or higher. Something like 32% of noninstitutionalized adults are obese (National Center for Health Statistics, 2008b). Obesity and overweight together affect two-thirds of our adult population, and are associated with several chronic diseases. Therefore, major health agencies consider obesity to be a national epidemic and have issued guidelines encouraging weight reduction. As a nurse you can assist your clients to achieve and maintain a healthy weight.

Obesity in Older Adults

Older adults are a part of the obesity epidemic. The proportion of obese older adults has doubled in the past 30 years. Nevertheless, most older adults lead active and healthy lives and are not obese. Obesity is more prevalent in adults younger than age 70 and becomes less prevalent after that. Still, more than 15% of older adults are obese (Newman, 2009).

As we age we tend to exercise less, but our eating patterns do not usually change. In addition, aging is associated with hormonal changes and slowing metabolism that cause accumulation of fat (e.g., decreased growth hormone and serum testosterone). Many of the chronic problems associated with aging are made worse by obesity (e.g., respiratory problems, arthritis, cardiovascular disease, cancer, and diabetes).

Interventions are the same as for other groups: dietary modification, exercise, and use of community supports. Older adults may require more assistance improving physical function so they can exercise more. To avoid injuries, exercise should start at low intensity and progress gradually over several months.

ANALYSIS/NURSING DIAGNOSIS

NANDA-I diagnoses define overweight and obesity in the following ways:

- *Imbalanced Nutrition: More Than Body Requirements* is used when a person consumes nutrients in excess of metabolic needs. The defining characteristics are (1) triceps skinfold greater than 15 mm in men and 25 mm in women, or (2) weight 20% over ideal for height and frame.
- *Risk for Imbalanced Nutrition: More Than Body Requirements* identifies the potential for an individual to experience intake of nutrients in excess of metabolic needs.

Etiologies of those NANDA diagnoses include the following:

- Consuming more kcal than needed for activity, gender, height, and weight
- Reducing activity level without modifying food intake
- Genetic predisposition to obesity. For example, low BMR and excess adipose tissue distribution are common in certain ethnic groups.
- Ineffective coping mechanisms—for instance, the use of binge eating to reduce anxiety or relieve boredom
- Cultural influences—some cultural norms encourage excess weight, particularly as an indication of wealth.
- Decreased levels of thyroid hormone can lower BMR, causing weight gain.
- Ineffective Health Maintenance—for example, high-fat diet, inactivity, and avoidance of health assistance
- Impaired Physical Mobility, which limits physical activity and decreases energy expenditure

Being overweight may lead to the development of other nursing diagnoses. Excess weight, and especially obesity, makes activity more difficult; therefore, over time, the person becomes more sedentary, and the body becomes deconditioned (weakened). The following are examples:

- Activity Intolerance r/t deconditioned state secondary to long-term sedentary lifestyle
- Decreased Cardiac Output r/t prolonged deconditioned state
- Constipation r/t inadequate physical activity
- Risk for Injury (and/or Risk for Falls) r/t deconditioned state and generalized weakness
- Social Isolation r/t poor self-image secondary to excess weight

PLANNING OUTCOMES/EVALUATION

A part of your nursing role will be to work with clients to help achieve the Healthy People 2020 nutrition goals. To review them,

Go to Chapter 26, **ESG Box 26-1, Nutrition Objectives from *Healthy People 2020,*** on the Student Resource Disk or DavisPlus at http://davisplus.fadavis.com/Wilkinson2

For *NOC standardized outcomes* for evaluating weight:

Go to Chapter 26, **Standardized Language, NOC Outcomes, and NIC Interventions for Overweight/Obesity and Underweight/Malnutrition,** in Volume 2.

Individualized goals/outcome statements include the following examples:

States pertinent factors contributing to weight gain.
Designs dietary modifications to meet individual long-term goal of weight control.
Accomplishes desired weight loss in a reasonable time frame (1 to 2 lb/week).
Incorporates appropriate physical activities requiring energy expenditure into daily life.

PLANNING INTERVENTIONS/IMPLEMENTATION

For the *NIC standardized interventions* for overweight and obese clients,

Go to Chapter 26, **Standardized Language, NOC Outcomes, and NIC Interventions for Overweight/Obesity and Underweight/Malnutrition,** in Volume 2.

Individualized nursing activities include the following:

- ***Weigh the client weekly under the same conditions.*** Weekly weights allow the client to monitor his progress and can motivate him to follow the weight-loss regimen.
- ***Suggest keeping a food diary for a number of days.*** Research suggests that this can double diet weight loss. Analyzing the diary will provide valuable information on intake and circumstances that trigger eating. It may help to identify behavioral or coping issues. Keep in mind that many patients eat less than usual when they are keeping a food diary (Hollis, Gullion, Stevens, et al., 2008).
- ***Educate the client about a healthy diet.*** Lifestyle changes must be ongoing to maintain weight loss. For the client, the first step is to learn about a balanced diet and food quality.
- ***Encourage the client to eat more fresh fruits and vegetables and fewer fatty foods and sugar-sweetened beverages.***
- ***Discuss fat substitutes,*** which are available to improve flavor and texture of low-fat foods while reducing total dietary fat. Recall that fats contain 9 kcal per gram, so reducing fat intake is an important part of most weight-loss diets. Fat substitutes are not absorbed; therefore, they contribute few kcal. The American Heart Association (n.d.[b]) states that fat substitutes, used

appropriately, can provide flexibility in diet planning. Although the USDA (FDA) considers fat substitutes to be safe, long-term benefits and risks are not yet known. In addition, it is not unusual for people to experience diarrhea and stomach cramps when using fat substitutes.

■ *Encourage the client to commit to regular exercise.* Increased physical activity will not only use up excess stores of fat but also increase the body's resting metabolic rate. Individuals should begin gradually with low-impact activities, such as walking for 20 minutes at least four times a week. The American College of Sports Medicine (ACSM) recommends 150 to 250 minutes of exercise per week to prevent weight gain. More than 250 minutes per week are needed to bring about significant weight loss—that is, 50 minutes on 5 days of the week or 40 minutes on 6 days of the week (ACSM, 2009). Although increased physical activity aids in weight control, advise your client to set realistic expectations for what exercise can achieve. A recent study concludes that overeating, more than a lack of exercise, is to blame for the American obesity epidemic (Swinburn, Sacks, Lo, et al., 2009).

■ *Be encouraging and nonjudgmental,* especially when there are setbacks.

■ *Provide weight loss tips* such as those in Self-Care: Teaching Weight Loss Tips.

■ *For children, recommend the 5-2-1-0 program* (Marion County Children's Alliance, 2008). Children should have:

    5 – Servings of fruits and vegetables each day.
    2 – Hours or less of "screen" time per day.
    1 – Hour of physical activity per day.
    0 – Servings of sweetened beverages.

■ *For children and adolescents,* weight loss is more effective when it involves the child, the parents, and the community in limiting soda and junk food consumption and limiting hours spent watching television and playing video games. Children can be taught to make "best choices" regarding activities and the foods they eat (Speroni, Early, & Atherton, 2007). To learn more about obesity in adolescents and children,

Go to Chapter 26, **Reading More About Nutrition,** on the Student Resource Disk or DavisPlus at http://davisplus. fadavis.com/Wilkinson2

Care**Planning** & **Mapping**Practice

For Care Planning/Care Mapping Practice,

Go to Student Resources, **Care Planning & Care Mapping Practice,** at http://davisplus.fadavis.com/Wilkinson2

What Are Underweight and Undernutrition?

A BMI of less than 18.5 is considered underweight (see Box 26-4). For patients in long-term care settings, parameters include one of the following:

1. Involuntary weight loss of more than 5% in 30 days or 10% in 180 days

2. Leaving more than one-quarter of food in the past 7 days or two-thirds of meals based on a 2000-kcal diet

3. A BMI of 19 or less

For hospitalized patients with serious illness, increased mortality is associated with a BMI of 21 or less (National Guideline Clearinghouse, 2005a).

A person becomes underweight when he consumes fewer kcal than needed based on his activity, sex, height, and weight. Consuming too few kcal may result in serious undernutrition; that is, insufficient intake of protein, fat, vitamins, and minerals. The causes of underweight status may be psychological, social, economic, or physiological (e.g., hospitalization, self-care deficits, illness, eating disorders). A person can also be malnourished with regard to specific nutrients without being underweight.

Eating disorders are a growing problem in North America. **Anorexia nervosa** is a psychiatric disorder characterized by self-starvation. **Bulimia nervosa** refers to binge eating (eating an excessive amount of food in a short period of time) followed by self-induced vomiting or laxative abuse to purge food. Although all segments of society are affected, eating disorders are more common in women, and most report the onset of illness before the age of 20. About half of teenage girls either are or think they should be on a diet.

Both anorexia and bulimia can result in hair loss, low blood pressure, generalized weakness, amenorrhea, and cold intolerance. Serious medical complications include osteoporosis and increased risk for fractures; brain damage; decreased resistance to infection; cardiac, renal, liver, and metabolic disorders; and even death. You will need to recognize the early warning signs of eating disorders, such as the behavior changes described in Box 26-5.

■ ANALYSIS/NURSING DIAGNOSIS

Imbalanced Nutrition: Less Than Body Requirements may be the patient's problem, or it may be the etiology of other nursing diagnoses. The following are examples. For other useful nursing diagnoses and etiologies, see Table 26-9.

Imbalanced Nutrition: Less Than Body Requirements r/t Impaired Swallowing 2° pain with swallowing
Risk for Disproportionate Growth r/t Imbalanced Nutrition: Less Than Body Requirements 2° anorexia nervosa

■ PLANNING OUTCOMES/EVALUATION

The NOC standardized outcome for assessing weight is Weight Control. If it becomes necessary to monitor nutritional status, you could use the labels of Nutritional Status: Food and Fluid Intake and Nutritional Status: Nutrient Intake.

Self-Care

Teaching Weight Loss Tips

Getting Ready

Make a commitment.
- Promise yourself; promise others. "I will do this."

Set realistic goals.
- Aim to lose 1 to 2 lb/week. To do this you need to burn 500 to 1000 calories more than you consume. Losing weight faster usually means losing water weight or muscle tissue rather than fat.
- Set "process" rather than "outcome" goals. For example, "I will exercise every day" instead of "I will lose 10 pounds this month." Changing your habits (your "processes") is the key to weight loss.
- Write your goals, your plan for achieving them, and your start date. This makes it reality, not just a thought.
- Review your goals each week. Readjust them as needed. If you are exercising more than you thought, adjust your goal upward, for example.

Plan for setbacks.
- Identify situations that might trigger eating or interfere with exercise; plan specific actions you will take to overcome them.

Beginning New Behaviors

Eat healthier foods.
- Eat more fruits and vegetables.
- Limit fatty foods and sugar-sweetened beverages.

Get active and stay active.
- If you have not been exercising, start slowly.
- Work up to at least 250 minutes per week to lose weight and maintain the loss.

Get adequate sleep.
- For most people, this is 7 to 8 hours a night.
- New research suggests that sleep deprivation can affect levels of the appetite-regulating hormones leptin and ghrelin.
- Sleep loss can affect the type of food you crave. When you are tired you are less able to cope with stress and emotional triggers for eating, and more likely to crave comfort foods such as chocolate and ice cream.

"Sticking with It"

Keep a food diary.
- This can double your weight loss.

Decide what and when to eat.
- Decide what foods you will eat as well as when you will eat. For example, "I will eat only at the table, 3 meals and 2 snacks daily."
- Make a conscious effort to take small bites and eat slowly.
- Serve your food on small plates.

Shop wisely.
- Shop for food on a full stomach.
- Read food labels when purchasing food (for information about calorie and fat content).

Find ways to exercise.
- Lay out your exercise clothing ahead of time (e.g., at night if you exercise in the morning).
- Use the stairs instead of the elevator; park in the back of the parking lot, as far from the door as possible.
- Walk or bike to work when possible.

Get emotional support.
- Family members can help by not offering you desserts. Weight-loss support groups let you know you are not alone. An exercise partner can help keep you motivated.

Recognize that lifestyle changes must be permanent.

Remember: Healthy eating, physical activity, and sleep are necessities, not luxuries!

Individualized goals/outcome statements include the following:

Progressively gains weight toward desired goal.
Verbalizes willingness to follow diet.
Body mass and weight are within normal limits.
Laboratory values (e.g., albumin, complete blood count [CBC]) are within normal limits.
Recognizes factors contributing to underweight.

PLANNING INTERVENTIONS/IMPLEMENTATION

For the *NIC standardized interventions* for undernutrition,

 Go to Chapter 26, **Standardized Language, NOC Outcomes and NIC Interventions for Overweight/Obesity and Underweight/Malnutrition,** in Volume 2.

BOX 26-5 ■ Early Warning Signs of an Eating Disorder

Food Behaviors

- Deliberate self-starvation with weight loss
- Continuous dieting
- Skips meals.
- Takes only tiny portions.
- Will not eat in front of others.
- Always has an excuse not to eat.
- Usually has a diet soda or coffee in hand.
- Eats only food that is low in fat.

Physical Signs

- Excessive facial or body hair (because of inadequate protein in the diet)
- Hair loss
- Abnormal weight loss
- Sensitivity to cold
- Absent or irregular menstruation

Appearance and Body Image Behaviors

- Wears baggy clothes.
- Complains of being fat.
- Obsesses about clothing size.
- Spends lots of time inspecting self in the mirror.

Exercise Behaviors

- Exercises excessively and compulsively.
- May tire easily.
- Pushes self beyond normal expectations.

Social Behaviors

- Tries to please everyone and withdraws if unsuccessful.
- Tries to care for everyone but self.
- Tries to control what and where family eats.
- Relationships tend to be superficial or dependent.

Emotional Behaviors

- Intense fear of gaining weight

Table 26-9 ➤ Nursing Diagnoses Associated with Undernutrition

IMBALANCED NUTRITION AS THE PROBLEM

NANDA-I Label	Use when:
Imbalanced Nutrition: Less Than Body Requirements	Intake of nutrients is insufficient to meet metabolic needs.
Risk for Imbalanced Nutrition: Less Than Body Requirements (This is not a NANDA-I label.)	Clients are at risk for insufficient intake of nutrients to meet metabolic needs.
Adult Failure to Thrive	There is progressive functional deterioration of a physical and cognitive nature. The person has no appetite, is apathetic, and consumes < 75% of normal requirements at each or most meals.
Some Etiologies of Imbalanced Nutrition	
Impaired Dentition	Dental caries, dental fractures, or missing teeth affect the ability to chew food.
Impaired Swallowing	Intake is decreased because the client has pain with swallowing or chokes and/or coughs with swallowing attempts.
Impaired Oral Mucous Membrane	A condition such as stomatitis or ulcers limits intake because of pain or altered sense of taste.
Diarrhea	Frequent, loose, liquid stools prevent absorption of nutrients.
Chronic Confusion	Cognitive decline creates problems with reasoning and responding appropriately to stimuli. The person may forget to eat or forget how to prepare and eat food.
Other Diagnoses that May Result from Undernutrition	
Risk for Delayed Development	There is a 25% or more delay in the development of cognitive, language, or motor skills due to poor nutritional intake.
Risk for Infection	A client is in a debilitated state due to inadequate nutrition.
Risk for Impaired Skin Integrity	Inadequate intake of food and fluids and excessive weight loss create skin fragility and slow healing.

Individualized nursing activities for clients who are underweight or undernourished include the following:

- **Assess for recent changes in physiological status as underlying cause of weight loss or undernourishment** (e.g., pain, fatigue, illness, and immobility).
- **Offer high-calorie and high-protein (nutrient-dense) foods.** Serve these foods when the person is most likely to be hungry. Avoid food with little nutritional value; when intake is limited, it is essential that it not be wasted on empty calories.
- **Consult with a dietitian** about strategies to increase the nutritional content of foods.
- **Weigh the client regularly under the same conditions.** Weigh the client one to two times per week if nutritional status is severely jeopardized to assess the effectiveness of the therapeutic plan.
- **Offer high-protein supplements.** Offer nutritious high-protein supplements between meals to increase intake of protein and kcal. It may be easier for the client to drink a small amount of a supplement than to eat enough food to supply the equivalent nutrients.
- **Suggest community resources** (e.g., Meals on Wheels for clients with Adult Failure to Thrive). Additional assistance may be needed to improve access to food.
- **For eating disorders, see that the client is referred for appropriate counseling** (e.g., dietitian, mental health professional).

The following sections discuss more fully nursing interventions for improving the appetite, as well as alternative feeding methods.

Stimulating the Patient's Appetite

Illness, with its accompanying pain, anxiety, and medications, often causes appetite loss. This is especially true for institutionalized patients, who have little control over food choices and preparation. You will need to make an effort to see that hospitalized patients eat the food that is served. It is not enough merely to order meals and deliver the trays. The following measures may help improve appetite and intake, and subsequently, nutritional status:

- **Offer frequent, small meals.** This helps prevent gastric distention and improves appetite by keeping the patient from being overwhelmed with a large amount of food.
- **Suggest smokers refrain for 1 hour before a meal.**
- **Restrict liquid intake with meals** to prevent gastric distention or feeling full before the patient consumes sufficient nutrients.
- **Keep the patient's environment neat and clean** and free of unpleasant sights, odors, and medical equipment. These often trigger loss of appetite. For example, remove bedpans, urinals, and the emesis basin from the room before mealtimes.
- **Order a late food tray or warm the food** if the patient is not in his room during mealtime.
- Provide or assist with **frequent oral hygiene.**
- **Provide a pleasant eating environment.**

- **Serve foods attractively;** vary textures, colors, and flavors; arrange the tray so the person can easily reach the food.
- **Position the person comfortably** for mealtime.
- **Find out what the person likes to eat,** and encourage family and friends to bring foods from home.
- **Control pain around the clock,** and avoid painful treatments before meals.
- **If the patient receives a nutritional supplement, delay the meal for at least an hour afterward.**
- **Encourage meals with friends** for those who live alone, or meals at a senior center.
- **Provide nutrient-dense foods** (e.g., add ice cream to appropriate beverages and foods).
- **Arrange for a home health aide** to shop and prepare meals for those who are unable to leave home for groceries, or arrange for Meals-on-Wheels.

Providing Enteral Nutrition

If a patient cannot meet his nutritional needs through an enhanced diet and measures to stimulate the appetite, you may need to use an alternative feeding method. Feeding can occur through the intestinal tract as enteral nutrition, or intravenously as parenteral nutrition. **Enteral nutrition** (tube feeding) refers to the delivery of liquid nutrition into the upper intestinal tract via a tube. Tube feeding may be used in addition to or instead of oral intake. It is the preferred method of feeding for a patient who has a functioning intestinal tract but needs nutritional support (e.g., patients with high metabolic needs, such as those with trauma, burns, or severe malnutrition; neurological disorders that affect swallowing; anorexia nervosa; prematurity; failure to thrive; or specific bowel diseases). Tube feeding may be a short- or long-term therapy.

Enteral feedings are preferred to parenteral (i.e., intravenous) nutrition because they have a lower incidence of sepsis and maintain intestinal structure and function (Kaushik, Pietraszewski, Holst, et al., 2005). However, there are a number of risks associated with enteral feedings. If enteral formula is aspirated into the lungs, it can lead to infection, pneumonia, abscess formation, adult respiratory distress syndrome (ARDS), and in some cases death. The high glucose content of enteral formulas provides a medium for bacterial growth. Other complications include diarrhea, nausea and vomiting, nasopharyngeal trauma, alterations in drug absorption and metabolism, and various metabolic disturbances.

There have been some instances where enteral feedings have been mistakenly connected to intravascular (IV) lines and feeding solutions have been infused into veins. These events, termed "tubing misconnections," are potentially fatal to the patient. An enteral device manufacturer and a professional organization dedicated to improving patient care by advancing the science and practice of nutrition support therapy have cooperated to develop the "BE A. L. E. R. T." Safety Campaign© to increase the safety of patients on enteral nutrition (see Box 26-6).

✚ BOX 26-6 ■ Be A.L.E.R.T©

To reduce errors and help ensure safe enteral nutrition, use the following mnemonic:

A   **Aseptic** technique---------------------------------- When preparing and delivering enteral formula, practice good hand hygiene; wear gloves when handling feeding tube; avoid touching can tops, container openings, spike and spike port.

L   **Label** enteral equipment-------------------------- with patient name and room number, formula name and rate, date and time of initiation, and nurse initials.

E   **Elevate** the head of the bed---------------------- a minimum of 30 degrees for feedings whenever clinically possible; may mitigate risk of reflux and aspiration of gastric content.

R   **Right** patient, **Right** formula, **Right** tube------- Match formula to patient's feeding order; verify **enteral** tubing set connects formula container to feeding tube.

T   **Trace** all lines and tubing back to patient------- Avoid misconnections – trace all lines from origin to patient; only enteral-to-enteral connections.

Sources: © 2009 Nestlé HealthCare Nutrition, Inc. The BE A. L. E. R. T.© poster is a joint effort of the American Society for Parenteral and Enteral Nutrition (A.S.P.E.N.) and Nestlé HealthCare Nutrition, Inc. Retrieved from http://www.nutritioncare.org/WorkArea/showcontent. aspx?id52968; A.S.P.E.N. (2009). Special report: Enteral nutrition practice recommendations. *Journal of Parenteral and Enteral Nutrition,* Retrieved from http://www.nutritioncare.org/wcontent.aspx?id52078.

Administer feedings at room temperature, and be sure to check the expiration date of any feedings before starting an infusion. In this volume, the Critical Aspects box summarizes a procedure for enteral feedings. For complete instructions,

 VOL 2 Go to Chapter 26, **Procedure 26-3: Administering Feedings Through Gastric and Enteric Tubes,** in Volume 2.

Patients may receive enteral or parenteral nutrition in the home as well as in inpatient settings. The box, Home Care: Home Nutritional Support, reviews teaching related to alternative feeding methods in the home. You should review these topics with the patient or caregiver.

Types of Enteric Tubes

Enteric tubes are available in various materials, lengths, diameters, and types. Choose the type of tube you need based on the intended use and the length of time you anticipate it will be left in place. This chapter focuses on the use of enteric tubes as a route for feeding; however, they are inserted for other reasons, as well:

- Lavage of the stomach (e.g., when there is disease, surgery, or bleeding in the GI tract, and in cases of poisoning or medication overdose)
- Collecting a specimen of stomach contents for laboratory tests
- To prevent nausea, vomiting, and gastric distention postoperatively.

Home Nutritional Support

Home Care

Clients frequently administer enteral and parenteral nutrition at home. To assist the client or caregiver with the management of home nutritional therapy, teach the following aspects.

➤ *Formula.* Review the type of formula the patient should receive. Enteral or IV solutions are clearly marked with their contents. Emphasize that the caregiver double-check that the correct solution is being used and that the expiration date and time have not been reached before administering any feeding.

➤ *Administration.* Carefully review how to administer the feeding. Emphasize the need for hand washing before hanging the infusion. After a period of time, the client may be able to tolerate delivering 1 to 3 L of enteral feeding at night. The rate must be increased at the beginning and decreased when ending the delivery. If parenteral nutrition is administered at home, be sure that the client or caregiver is aware of proper technique.

➤ *Access device.* Review the care required for the access device, including site care, dressing changes, and flushing.

➤ *Storage.* Stored enteral and parenteral nutrition must be refrigerated to prevent bacterial contamination.

➤ *Monitoring.* Instruct the client or caregiver to report a rise in temperature, weight loss, change in bowel movements, decrease in urine output, or change in condition.

➤ *Follow-up.* Arrange for the client to be weighed and assessed regularly to monitor the adequacy of the feedings. Often clients weigh at home and report to the primary care provider's office or the nutrition support team for ongoing monitoring of progress and review of lab work.

These are complicated therapies to manage at home. These patients will typically go home with a referral for a home care nurse to assist in the transition from hospital to home and follow-up with nutritional support service.

When a nasogastric (or orogastric) tube is placed so the stomach can be emptied (lavage), larger bore, tubes made of polyvinyl chloride (PVC), are used. These are called **Salem sump tubes** (Fig. 26-7). A Salem sump tube has a lumen for drainage and one to allow air to enter the stomach. The air port (pigtail) is usually blue. A **Levin tube**, also used for drainage, has a single lumen, with holes in the tip and along the sides.

Selecting a Feeding Tube

Short-term (<6 weeks) enteral feedings are usually delivered through a nasogastric (NG) or a nasoenteric (NE) tube. As a nurse, you may be asked to place a small-bore, **nasogastric,** or a **nasojenunal (NJ) feeding tube**. The tube is inserted through one naris, passed through the nasopharynx into the esophagus, and finally into the stomach. Placing the tube through the mouth is an option (oropharyngeal), but this method is more likely to trigger gagging or unconscious chewing on the tube. The Critical Aspects box in this volume provides a summary of a procedure for inserting nasogastric and nasoenteric tubes. For the entire procedure,

VOL 2 Go to Chapter 26, **Procedure 26-2: Inserting Nasogastric and Nasoenteric Tubes,** in Volume 2.

A **nasoenteric (NE) tube** is longer than an NG tube, extending through the nose down into the duodenum or jejunum (if it extends into the jejunum, it is called an NJ tube). A small, flexible tube is preferred for feeding. An NE tube may be used instead of an NG tube for patients at risk for aspiration. This includes patients who have a decreased level of consciousness, absent or diminished gag reflex, or severe gastroesophageal reflux.

The **lumen** (inside diameter) of a feeding tube is measured using the **French (Fr) scale:** The larger the lumen, the larger the diameter. Most feeding tubes for adults are 8 to 12 Fr and 90 to 108 cm (36 to 43 in.) long. Each Fr unit is about 0.33 mm, so a 12 Fr tube is about 4 mm in diameter. Large-bore (>12 Fr) NG tubes, such as the Salem sump (Fig. 26-7), are occasionally used for feeding, but are converted to a smaller tube within the first 2 days. They are less flexible, less comfortable, and are more commonly used if it is necessary to empty (lavage) the stomach. Figure 26-8 shows two types of feeding tubes.

For long-term feedings, a **gastrostomy tube (G-tube), percutaneous endoscopic gastrostomy tube (PEG)** (Fig. 26-9), **jejunostomy tube (J-tube, PEJ),** or **gastrostomy button (G-button)** (Fig. 26-10), is preferred. These are placed surgically or laparoscopically through the skin and the abdominal wall into the stomach or jejunum. They can also be placed endoscopically. The surgical incision is sometimes sutured tightly around the tube to hold it in place and prevent leakage. You must use surgical asepsis to care for a new incision. A gastrostomy tube can be converted to a **G-button** once healing has taken place. Historically, a PEG or PEJ was reserved for clients needing long-term nutritional support. However, that trend is changing. Patient comfort and improved technology leading to ease of insertion have made PEG or PEJ an option even for short-term use. The G-tubes and G-buttons, which can be capped off flush with the abdominal wall when not in use, are the most comfortable of all for long-term use.

FIGURE 26-7 A large-bore, polyvinyl-chloride (PVC) Salem sump tube used for gastric lavage.

FIGURE 26-8 *A,* A double-lumen, weighted (Dobhoff) feeding tube. *B,* A nonweighted (kangaroo) feeding tube.

FIGURE 26-9 A percutaneous gastrostomy (PEG) tube for feeding.

Checking Feeding Tube Placement

NG and NE feeding tubes are placed without direct visualization. As a result, there is risk of placing the tube into the respiratory tract. Therefore, you must check the location of the tip of the feeding tube before each enteral feeding or once per shift for continuous feedings. Failure to verify placement could be disastrous because it may result in infusion of formula into the lungs.

⊕ Radiographic verification is the most reliable method for confirming tube placement, and must be performed before the first feeding is administered. All feeding tubes contain markings that can be detected by radiographic films. Radiography reliably confirms initial tube placement; however, it is too expensive and time-consuming to use for ongoing verification of placement. Reliable bedside assessment is necessary because even when the tube is initially placed correctly in the stomach (or intestine), it may later move upward. No other method to verify the tube location

FIGURE 26-10 A gastrostomy button (G-button) in place for feeding.

is as reliable as radiographic verification, so it is recommended that you use the pH of the aspirate in combination with other methods for bedside verification. If in doubt, obtain a radiograph to determine tube location.

Bedside methods include the following—again, it is best to use a combination of these:

Measuring the pH (acidity) of the aspirate. This is currently the most reliable method for verifying tube placement at the bedside. The lower the pH, the more likely the tube is in the stomach. The outcome of pH testing is useful only if the fluid is acidic, indicating gastric placement. If the fluid is alkaline, it might be because the gastric contents are alkaline, or because the tip of tube is in the small intestine or the lung. Because of the frequency of such situations, even this method should be used in combination with other verification methods (Clarke, 2008; Guedon, 2000; May, 2007; Schmieding, Waldman, & Desaulles, 1997).

Aspirating stomach contents and inspecting for color and curdling.

Measuring the residual volume of the aspirate and observing for unexpected changes in the volume. A dramatic increase in the residual volume may indicate that a small bowel tube has moved into the stomach.

Injecting air into the feeding tube (the "whoosh test"). If the tube is in the stomach, injecting 5 to 30 mL of air produces a gurgling sound audible by listening with a stethoscope over the stomach. This is the least reliable method for checking placement of an NG or NE tube.

Measuring the tube that extends outside of the body. At the time it is placed, the feeding tube should be marked where it exits the body (e.g., the abdominal wall, the naris). If there is a change in the length of the external portion of the tube, it may have moved out of the original placement site.

Other repeated observations and assessments. The following assessments must be made repeatedly over time to be at all useful for confirming tube placement. They include:

- Observing for respiratory distress
- Determining whether the patient can speak

Other bedside verification methods. Capnometry and additional tests of gastric juices may also serve as measures to verify the tube is correctly placed.

- **Capnometry** tests for carbon dioxide (CO_2). The presence of CO_2 with the placement of an NG or NE tube would indicate that the tube has been placed in the respiratory tract. This method is not yet in wide use, and is best used only at the time the tube is placed. Figure 26-11 is a CO_2 detector.
- Measuring bilirubin, trypsin, and pepsin in the aspirate provides a positive determination that the

FIGURE 26-11 A carbon dioxide detector for checking gastric tube placement.

tube is placed in the stomach. Test devices for these three gastric components are not yet commercially available (Elpern, Killeen, Talla, et al., 2007; Peter & Gill, 2009).

 No longer recommended: Adding dye to enteral feedings as a method for identifying aspiration of gastric contents is not recommended because it has been associated with several adverse effects, including gastric bacterial colonization, diarrhea, systemic dye absorption, and death (AACCN, 2005b).

Remember, you should not rely on any one of these methods alone. Always use them in combination. For more information and guidelines for checking enteral tube placement,

VOL 2 Go to Chapter 26, **Clinical Insight 26-7: Checking Feeding Tube Placement,** in Volume 2.

KnowledgeCheck 26-11

- When is enteral nutrition the preferred alternative feeding?
- Identify and describe the types of enteral nutrition tubes.
- List four tube placement verification techniques.

 Go to Chapter 26, **Knowledge Check Response Sheet and Answers,** on the Student Resource Disk or DavisPlus at http://davisplus.fadavis.com/Wilkinson2

Administering Enteral Feedings

In a few institutions, enteral feeding formulas are blended in the kitchen, but most use one of the many commercially prepared products. The type of product selected depends on the patient's health condition. Products vary in nutritional components and caloric concentration (Box 26-7).

Feeding Schedules

Continuous feedings provide a constant flow of formula and an even distribution of nutrition throughout the day. For example, an infusion of 50 mL/hr for 24 hours of a 1 kcal/mL formula provides 1200 kcal per day. Continuous infusions are usually administered via small-bore NG, NJ, PEG, or PEJ tubes, or G-buttons, to patients in debilitated states who require intensive nutritional support. Feedings may be interrupted for periodic instillation of medications or flushing with water.

- **Pump-controlled infusions** are recommended for jejunal feedings and for gastrostomy feedings given by continuous infusion to decrease gastroesophageal reflux (American Gastrointestinal Association, 1995). A feeding pump ensures a steady flow rate.
- **Gravity feedings** can also be used, but the rate of delivery is not precise, and they increase the risk of gastroesophageal reflux, diarrhea, and aspiration. You regulate the drip rate by adjusting a clamp on the tubing, much the same as adjusting an IV rate.

BOX 26-7 ■ Types of Enteral Feeding Solutions

- **Basic feeding formulas** are used for clients who have no significant nutritional deficits but are unable to eat or drink sufficiently. They provide 1 kcal/mL of solution, and meet the needs of most clients. A standard formula contains 12%–20% of kcal from protein, 45%–60% of kcal from carbohydrates, and 30%–40% of kcal from fats. They also contain vitamins and minerals. They are usually lactose-free and contain complex forms of carbohydrates, fats, and proteins. Therefore, they require digestion and absorption.

- **High-protein formulas** are for clients who have a substantial need for protein, such as those with burns, open wounds, or malnutrition.

- **Elemental formulas** do not contain complex proteins; instead, they contain amino acids or peptides. They are reserved for patients with severe small bowel absorptive dysfunction. These formulas are fiber-free and highly osmotic. Their use is controversial.

- **Diabetic formulas** are for clients who require tube feedings to meet nutritional needs but have type 1 or type 2 diabetes mellitus. These formulas control carbohydrate intake.

- **Renal formulas** are for clients who require tube feedings to meet nutritional needs but have renal failure or renal insufficiency as a comorbidity. These formulas limit potassium, sodium, and nitrogen intake.

- **Pulmonary formulas** provide 55% of the calories as fat so that less CO_2 is produced per unit of oxygen consumed. They are used, for example, for patients with lung disease.

- **Fiber-containing formulas.** Because fiber has a potential protective effect for multiple disease states, including diverticulosis, colon cancer, diabetes, and heart disease, fiber-containing formulas may be used for patients in long-term care facilities or patients who require enteral feedings for a prolonged period of time.

Cyclic feedings are administered regularly; however, the infusion time is less than 24 hours per day. Nocturnal feedings are a form of cyclic feedings. The patient is able to eat meals and participate in activities throughout the day but receives an infusion of enteral formula at night while at rest. Another variant is a 20-hour infusion. A 4-hour break allows time for the feeding pump to be disconnected for hygiene and other activities.

Intermittent feedings are given to supplement oral intake or for patients who want greater mobility to take part in activities, such as physical therapy. Feedings are given on a regular or periodic basis several times a day, usually over 30 to 60 minutes. An example of a prescription for a *regular feeding* is, "Give 250 to 500 mL of enteral nutrition every 4 to 6 hours." *Periodic feedings* are often based on oral intake and are considered to be more physiologically similar to normal eating patterns. Consider the following periodic feeding prescription:

If the client consumes 90% to 100% of the ordered diet, give no additional feeding.

>75% but <90%, give 100 mL of formula after each meal.

>50% but <75%, give 200 mL of formula after each meal.

>25% but <50%, give 300 mL of formula after each meal.

0 to 25% of the ordered diet, give 400 mL of formula.

Intermittent feedings are sometimes given by **bolus,** if the patient can tolerate this method. In this method, you use a syringe to deliver 300 to 400 mL of formula through the tube over a 5- to 10-minute period. This is the easiest method to teach family members for home care, and it frees the patient from mechanical devices that limit activity. But because the fluid is given more rapidly by this method, it increases the risk for respiratory aspiration and for stomach distention. You can use it only with gastric tubes, never with intestinal tubes.

Open and Closed Feeding Systems

An **open system** is exposed to the environment. One example is to open cans of formula and use a syringe to inject the formula into the tube; alternatively, you can pour it into a reservoir (e.g., a plastic bag). You should flush and clean the system after each delivery. Most agencies require that an open-system feeding not hang for more than 4 hours.

A **closed system** is a prefilled system (e.g., a bag or a bottle) that functions much like IV fluid. The nurse spikes the container with tubing that is attached to the feeding pump or run through a manually controlled drip chamber. Closed systems decrease the risk of contamination. A prefilled closed-system container can safely hang for 24 to 48 hours if you use sterile technique. You can measure out the specified amount in the drip chamber, allowing the remainder of the container to be used later in the day.

Monitoring Patients Receiving Enteral Nutrition

For patients receiving enteral nutrition, you will need to monitor tube placement, skin condition, laboratory values (especially blood glucose, BUN, and electrolytes), feeding residual, and gastrointestinal status. This will allow you to detect complications that affect metabolism or fluid and electrolyte balance and to assess responses to enteral feeding. Feedings may need to be increased or decreased depending on the patient's changing clinical condition. For guidelines,

 Go to Chapter 26, **Clinical Insight 26-8: Monitoring Patients Receiving Enteral Nutrition,** in Volume 2.

 Go to Chapter 26, **Clinical Insight 26-9: Preventing Infection in Patients Receiving Enteral Feedings,** in Volume 2.

Removing Feeding Tubes

When a patient's condition has stabilized and she no longer requires enteral nutrition, the feeding tube may be removed. A PEG tube is usually clamped if feedings are no longer required. The Critical Aspects box at the end of the chapter summarizes a procedure for removing a feeding tube. For a complete set of steps to follow,

 Go to Chapter 26, **Procedure 26-4: Removing a Nasogastric or Nasoenteric Tube,** in Volume 2.

Critical Thinking 26-8

Your client has dementia and is frequently agitated. She has been progressively losing weight. An interdisciplinary team recommended enteral nutrition due to poor oral intake; however, the client has repeatedly pulled out her NG tube and had an episode of aspiration pneumonia last month. What recommendations might you consider at the next meeting?

Providing Parenteral Nutrition

Parenteral nutrition (PN) is the delivery of nutrition intravenously into a large, central vein. This is the preferred method of feeding for clients who cannot be nourished through the gastrointestinal tract. Some clients (e.g., those with shortened small bowel secondary to injury or disease) who are able to meet some of their nutritional needs may use PN in addition to some oral intake to meet caloric and nutrient needs. Others, such as clients who are severely malnourished, have extensive burns or trauma, or have conditions that require resting the gastrointestinal system, are nourished entirely by PN.

PN solutions usually contain a 10% to 70% concentration of dextrose in water (but usually not more than 20%)

along with amino acids, and can provide 20 to 30 kcal per kilogram per day, depending on the patient's calculated energy need. Note though, that the most common concentrations of glucose provide only 200 kcal per liter. PN also contains vitamins, minerals, and trace elements. Standard PN formulas are available at many healthcare facilities; however, PN can be modified to meet individual needs.

The type of venous access device used to administer PN will depend on the components of the PN and the anticipated duration of PN. Because PN solutions are hypertonic, they should be administered in a large, high-flow vein through a central venous access catheter. The subclavian vein has been the site of choice; however, the jugular vein is preferred for tunneled catheters and implanted ports. Peripherally inserted central catheter (PICC) lines are also used for PN. Whatever the insertion site, all PN catheters must have chest x-ray confirmation that the tip is in the lower portion of the superior vena cava adjacent to the right atrium (see Fig. 26-12) before beginning the first infusion. High blood flow through that vessel causes rapid dilution of the concentrated PN and thereby prevents vessel damage. Some types of PN solutions may be infused via a peripheral vein, but this is not usual.

Lipid emulsions contain essential fatty acids, triglycerides, and supplemental kcal. They are administered weekly for patients who rely on PN to prevent essential fatty acid deficiency. They also add calories to the PN mixture so that lower glucose concentrations can be used, thus reducing the risk of glucose fluctuations. Most IV fats are supplied by safflower or soybean oil. They provide 1.1 to 3 kcal/mL.

You may administer lipids at the same time as the PN, through a peripheral line or by Y-connector tubing

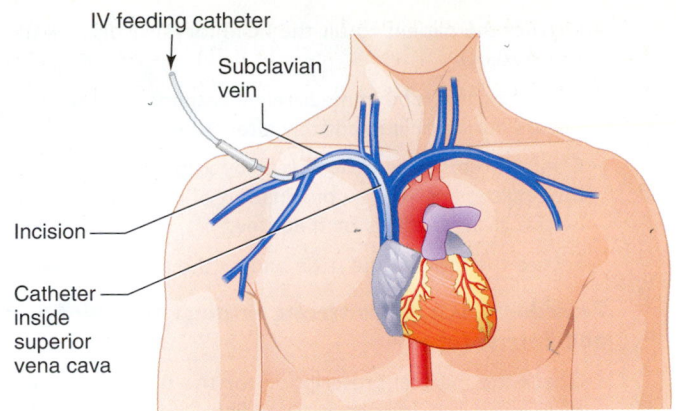

FIGURE 26-12 The subclavian vein is the site of choice for parenteral nutrition.

through a central line. Lipids are also sometimes added to the PN solution (this is called a 3-in-1 admixture), and administered over a 24-hour period. The Critical Aspects box summarizes procedures for administering parenteral nutrition and lipid emulsions. For the complete procedures,

 Go to Chapter 26, **Procedure 26-5: Administering Parenteral Nutrition,** and **Procedure 26-6, Administering Lipids,** in Volume 2.

To learn about monitoring and maintenance of patients receiving parenteral nutrition,

 Go to Chapter 26, **Clinical Insight 26-10: Monitoring and Maintaining Patients Receiving Parenteral Nutrition,** in Volume 2.

VOL 2 For steps to follow in *all* procedures, refer to the Universal Steps for All Procedures found on the inside back cover of Volume 2. Go to the full procedures in Volume 2 to practice and learn the procedure steps. Use these Critical Aspects later to help you review key points.

Critical Aspects of Procedures 26-1 through 26-6

Procedure 26-1: Checking Fingerstick (Capillary) Blood Glucose Levels

➤ Have the patient wash hands with warm soap and water. Dry well with a clean towel.

➤ Don procedure gloves.

➤ Cleanse the patient's finger with an alcohol prep pad if agency policy requires.

➤ Prepare the lancet and meter and obtain a clean test strip that is correct for the meter.

➤ Stick the side of the fingertip.

➤ Wipe off the first drop of blood; then place the second drop on the test strip.

➤ At the indicated time, read the glucose level on the digital display. (Follow the manufacturer's instructions.)

Procedure 26-2: Inserting Nasogastric and Nasoenteric Tubes

➤ Place the patient in a sitting or high-Fowler's position.

➤ Measure the length of the tube:

NG tubes: Measure from the tip of the nose to earlobe and from earlobe to the xiphoid process.

Nasoenteric tubes: Add 8 to 10 cm (3 to 4 in.) to the NG measurement, as directed.

➤ Lubricate the tube with a water-soluble lubricant.

➤ Ask the patient to hyperextend the neck and breathe through the mouth.

➤ Insert the tube gently through the nostril; advance the tube as the patient swallows.

Continued

- ➤ Instruct the patient to tilt the head forward, drink water, and swallow.
- ➤ Withdraw the tube immediately if respiratory distress occurs during or immediately after insertion.
- ➤ Confirm tube placement initially by x-ray. Always reconfirm tube placement with a combination of bedside methods before giving feedings or medicine.
- ➤ Secure the tube to the nose and to the patient's gown.

Procedure 26-3: Administering Feedings Through Gastric and Enteric Tubes

- ➤ Check the medical prescription for the type of formula, rate, route, and frequency of feeding.
- ➤ Check the chart to make sure a confirmation x-ray of tube placement was performed.
- ➤ Confirm tube placement at the bedside before administering the feeding.
- ➤ Elevate the head of the bed at least 30 to 45 degrees while administering the feedings and for an hour after administration.
- ➤ Check residual volume before feeding for intermittent feedings.

  For continuous feeding: Check the gastric residual volume at least once every shift. If residual is 10% greater than the formula flow rate for 1 hour (or alternatively, a total of 150 mL), hold the feeding for 1 hour and recheck. Notify the physician if the residual is still not within normal limits.

  For gastrostomy and percutaneous endoscopic gastrostomy (PEG) tubes and gastrostomy buttons (G-buttons): Check residual volume every 4 hours.

  For jejunostomy tubes: Residual volumes are not checked.

- ➤ Flush tubing with 30 mL of water before and after feeding (every 4 hours for continuous feedings), and before and after medication administration. Some closed continuous feeding systems run sterile water tandem with the tube feeding; you can program the pump to deliver flushes according to the feeding protocol.
- ➤ Change the tube feeding administration set and other supplies a minimum of every 24 hours.
- ➤ Continuous feedings should be infused by pump.

Procedure 26-4: Removing a Nasogastric or Nasoenteric Tube

- ➤ Verify the primary provider's prescription for removal of nasogastric or nasoenteric tube.
- ➤ Assist the patient to a sitting or high-Fowler's position.
- ➤ Clear the tube of secretions by injecting 10 mL of air through the main lumen.
- ➤ Ask the patient to hold his breath, and gently, but quickly, withdraw the tube.
- ➤ Discard the equipment.
- ➤ Provide or assist with care of nose and mouth.

Procedure 26-5: Administering Parenteral Nutrition (PN)

- ➤ Perform pre-procedure assessments: Check patient record (e.g., to confirm CVC tip placement), check blood glucose, and assess patency of the line.
- ➤ Position the patient supine.
- ➤ Examine the PN solution for leaks, cloudiness, and particles. If the solution contains lipids, also look for a brown layer, oil droplets, or oil on the surface. Have a co-worker verify.
- ➤ Identify the patient, using two identifiers; have identification verified by a second staff member.
- ➤ Compare the bag to the patient's ID band and with the original prescription.
- ➤ Observe meticulous sterile technique in the appropriate steps of the procedure. During all steps, observe careful aseptic (clean) technique. Or follow agency policy.
- ➤ Use a filter.
- ➤ Attach the new administration set to the new bag.
- ➤ Prime the tubing (either now or after placing in the pump).
- ➤ Place the tubing in the infusion pump; set the rate.
- ➤ Clamp the catheter and the old administration set.
- ➤ Remove gloves, perform hand hygiene, and don clean gloves.
- ➤ Observe meticulous sterile technique in the appropriate steps of the procedure. During all steps, observe careful aseptic (clean) technique.
- ➤ Scrub all surfaces of the needleless connector and Luer locking threads with an antiseptic pad.
- ➤ Determine patency of the IV line.
- ➤ Trace the tubing back to the patient, attach the new infusion tubing to the designated PN lumen (usually the largest one), and secure the Luer-lock connection. Have the patient perform the Valsalva maneuver when connecting the tubing for the new infusion.
- ➤ Start the infusion.
- ➤ Label tubing.

Procedure 26-6: Administering Lipids

- ➤ Lipids require a special administration set.
- ➤ Position the patient supine.
- ➤ Be certain lipids are not cold.
- ➤ Examine the bottle for a layer of froth or separation into fat globules or layers.
- ➤ Complete the infusion within 20 hours.
- ➤ Use new tubing for each bottle of lipids.
- ➤ If infusing simultaneously with PN, use a separate port below the PN filter.
- ➤ Take vital signs before infusing, then every 10 minutes for 30 minutes, and observe for side effects.
- ➤ Begin the infusion slowly. If no reactions occur after 30 minutes, adjust to the prescribed rate.

Toward Evidence-Based Practice

Scarmeas, N., Luchsinger, J., Mayeux, R., et al. (2007). Mediterranean diet and Alzheimer disease mortality. *Neurology, 69,* 1084–1093.

A Mediterranean diet (MeDi) consists of an average nine servings of fruits and vegetables daily, whole grains, fish once or twice a week, and up to 5 ounces of red wine daily. It limits red meat and avoids *trans*-fats and saturated fats, using instead olive oil for its antioxidant effect and canola oil and nuts to provide omega-3 fatty acids.

Researchers followed 192 community-based individuals diagnosed with Alzheimer's disease (AD) for 4.4 years. 85 of the AD patients died during that period. Researchers concluded that adherence to the MeDi may reduce not only risk for AD but also subsequent disease course: Higher adherence to the MeDi is associated with lower mortality in AD.

Barberger-Gateau, P., Raffaitin, C., Letenneur, L., et al. (2007). Dietary patterns and risk of dementia. *Neurology, 69,* 191–193.

This study included 8085 nondemented participants ages 65 and older in three cities in France. An independent committee validated 281 cases of dementia (including 183 AD). Daily consumption of fruits and vegetables was associated with a decreased risk of all-cause dementia; weekly consumption of fish was associated with a reduced risk of AD, but only among people carrying a high-risk AD gene; regular use of omega-3–rich oils was associated with a decreased risk for all-cause dementia. Researchers concluded that frequent consumption of fruits and vegetables, fish, and omega-3 rich oils may decrease the risk of dementia and AD, especially among those who do not carry the high-risk AD gene.

Vogiatzoglou, A., Refsum, H., Johnston, C., et al. (2008). Vitamin B$_{12}$ status and rate of brain volume loss in community-dwelling elderly. *Neurology, 71*(11), 826–832.

This was a 5-year study of 107 community-dwelling elders aged 61 to 87 years with no cognitive impairment at the beginning of the study. They were assessed yearly by magnetic resonance imaging (MRI) scans, cognitive tests, and blood studies. The decrease in brain volume over the 5-year period was greater for those with lower vitamin B$_{12}$ levels. Researchers concluded that low vitamin B$_{12}$ status should be further researched as a cause of brain atrophy and likely cognitive impairment in the elderly.

1. Suppose you are a manager in a long-term care facility that specializes in treating residents with AD. You are planning nutritional interventions for these residents. Which of these three studies is best suited to your patients, and why?

2. How was the cognitive status of the subjects different in all three studies?

3. Based on the third study, for which group would vitamin B$_{12}$ supplementation be most likely to be of benefit? Explain your thinking.
   a. People who have AD and want to extend their life expectancy
   b. Older adults who wish to prevent getting AD
   c. Older adults who want to avoid cognitive impairment from brain changes other than AD.

 Go to Chapter 26, **Toward Evidence-Based Practice Suggested Responses,** on the Student Resource Disk or DavisPlus at http://davisplus.fadavis.com/Wilkinson2

 Go to Chapter 26, **Resources for Caregivers and Health Professionals,** on the Student Resource Disk or DavisPlus at http://davisplus.fadavis.com/Wilkinson2

 Suggested Readings: Go to Chapter 26, **Reading More About Nutrition,** on the Student Resource Disk or DavisPlus at http://davisplus.fadavis.com/Wilkinson2

 Bibliography: Go to Volume 2, Bibliography.

CHAPTER 27

Urinary Elimination

Learning Outcomes

After completing this chapter, you should be able to:

➤ Describe the normal structure and function of the organs in the urinary system.

➤ Describe the processes of urine formation and elimination.

➤ Discuss factors that affect urinary elimination.

➤ Describe the contents of a nursing assessment and physical examination focused on urinary elimination.

➤ Accurately measure urine output.

➤ Describe procedures for collecting various types of urine specimens.

➤ List and describe diagnostic tests used in identification of urinary elimination problems.

➤ Discuss common elimination problems: urinary tract infection, urinary retention, and urinary incontinence.

➤ Identify nursing diagnoses associated with altered urinary elimination.

➤ Describe nursing interventions that promote normal urination.

➤ Provide care for clients experiencing urinary problems.

➤ Perform urinary catheterizations following accepted procedures.

➤ Discuss nursing care appropriate for clients who have a urinary diversion.

Meet Your Patient

During your assigned clinical experience at University Hospital, the RN asks you to complete the admission process for Marlena, a 55-year-old woman who is complaining of frequent, painful urination. As you interview her, Marlena becomes embarrassed. "I really don't enjoy talking about this," she admits. Then, she asks to use the bathroom. You ask her to give you a midstream clean-catch urine sample while she is in the restroom. When she returns, she gives you a small specimen of pink-colored, strong-smelling urine. "I feel like I have strong urge to go and then I hardly have any urine. It's a little bloody and burns like crazy during my stream," she reports.

You close the door and interview Marlena in private about her usual urination pattern and current symptoms. Your calm approach and straightforward manner put her at ease. She confides that she is sexually active and that her symptoms began after spending the weekend with her new partner. You take her vital signs: oral temperature 99.4°F (37.4°C), radial pulse 88 beats/min, respiratory rate 20 breaths/min, and blood pressure 108/72 mm Hg.

After you report your assessment data to the RN, the emergency department (ED) physician asks you to perform a dipstick urinalysis on the urine sample and to send the urine sample to the lab for culture and sensitivity. He asks you: "Well, what do you think we need to do next?" How would you answer his question?

As you gain theoretical and practical knowledge in this chapter, we will return to this case study to discuss how you might answer the physician's question and support Marlena's recovery. You will also have the opportunity to examine your feelings about giving care that patients may regard as personal or even embarrassing.

Theoretical Knowledge
knowing why

A variety of factors, including personal hygiene, age, nutrition, stress, sexual activity, and medications, play a role in urinary health. That's why it is vitally important that you take a holistic approach to patients who have altered urinary elimination patterns. Such an approach requires theoretical knowledge of normal urinary system physiology, factors that influence urinary elimination, and common alterations in urinary function.

How Does the Urinary System Work?

To understand problems affecting the urinary system, you'll need to first understand how the urinary system functions in a healthy individual. The organs of the urinary system include the kidneys, ureters, bladder, and urethra (Fig. 27-1).

The Kidneys Filter and Regulate

The kidneys filter metabolic wastes, toxins, excess ions, and water from the bloodstream and excrete them as urine. If kidney function is impaired, these substances reach toxic levels and damage body cells. The kidneys also help to regulate blood volume, blood pressure, electrolyte levels, and acid–base balance by

selectively reabsorbing water and other substances. Secondary functions of the kidneys are to produce erythropoietin, secrete the enzyme renin, and activate vitamin D_3 (calcitriol). The kidneys are located against the posterior abdominal wall behind the peritoneum (they are **retroperitoneal**). The average kidney weighs about 5 ounces and is the shape of a kidney bean (see Fig. 27-1).

The outer layer, or **cortex,** of the kidney is composed of millions of microscopic functional units, called *nephrons* (Fig. 27-2). The inner layer, or **medulla,** consists of 8 to 10 wedge-shaped cones, called the *renal pyramids*. The renal pyramids are made up of bundles of collecting tubules. The innermost area is the **renal pelvis.** Funnel-shaped extensions known as **calyces** (singular: **calyx**) enclose the central portion of each renal pyramid and direct urine into the renal pelvis.

The Nephrons Form Urine

The **nephron** is the basic structural and functional unit of the kidney (see Fig. 27-2). There are about 1 million nephrons in each kidney. Each nephron consists of:

- A double-walled hollow capsule, the **Bowman's capsule,** enclosing a **glomerulus,** a knotty ball of capillaries
- A series of filtrating tubules
- A collecting duct

Together, these structures act as a microscopic filter, controlling the excretion and retention of fluids and solutes according to the body's moment-by-moment needs. Urine is formed by filtration, reabsorption, and secretion, as discussed next.

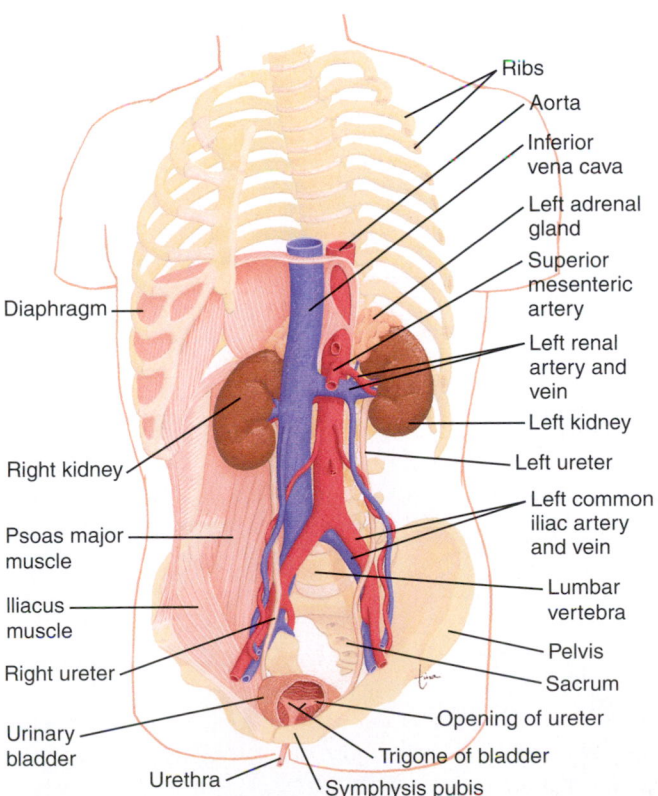

FIGURE 27-1 The organs of the urinary system include the kidneys, ureters, bladder, and urethra.

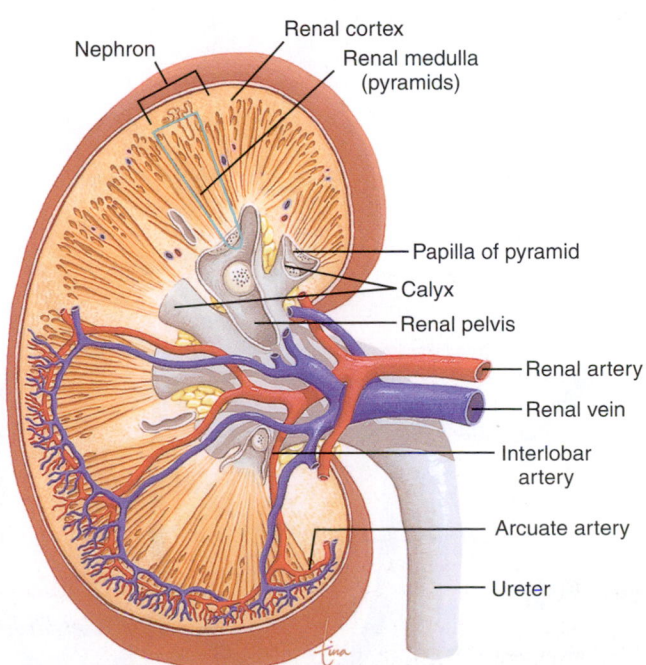

FIGURE 27-2 A cross-section of the kidney, showing the renal cortex, medulla, pyramids, and calyces.

For a detailed view of a nephron,

 Go to Chapter 27, **Tables, Boxes, Figures: ESG Figure 27-1,** on the Student Resource Disk or DavisPlus at http://davisplus.fadavis.com/Wilkinson2

Glomerular Filtration

Figure 27-3 summarizes the process of urine formation. The first step, **filtration,** occurs in the glomeruli. The renal arteries bring blood to the kidneys and into the glomeruli. Blood pressure forces plasma, dissolved substances, and small proteins out of the porous glomeruli into Bowman's capsule to form a liquid called **filtrate.** The **glomerular filtration rate** is the amount of filtrate formed by the kidneys per minute.

Unless the glomerular capillaries are inflamed or damaged, large molecules, such as blood cells and blood proteins, are too large to filter across their walls. Glomerular filtrate resembles blood plasma, except that it contains much less protein and no blood cells.

To see an animated explanation of the processes of osmosis, diffusion, filtration, and active transport,

 Go to **Animations: Osmosis, Diffusion, Filtration, and Active Transport** on DavisPlus at http://davisplus.fadavis.com/Wilkinson2

Tubular Reabsorption

The filtrate moves from Bowman's capsule into a highly twisted tubule (*proximal convoluted tubule,* Fig. 27-3). As the filtrate journeys through the tubule, 99% is reabsorbed into the peritubular capillaries. Approximately 1% of filtrate returns, as urine, to the *collecting tubule,* which transports it into the ureters. Wastes and toxins that remain in the blood after filtration are actively transported into the filtrate (reabsorbed) in the *distal* and *collecting tubules.* Water and sodium are reabsorbed in these structures when antidiuretic hormone (ADH) and aldosterone are secreted. For an animated explanation of urine formation and elimination,

 Go to **Animations: Formation and Elimination of Urine** on DavisPlus at http://davisplus.fadavis.com/Wilkinson2

When the amount of fluid in the body decreases (e.g., because of low intake or blood loss), the posterior pituitary gland secretes more ADH. This causes the distal and collecting tubules to reabsorb more water into the blood. At the same time, the adrenal cortex secretes more aldosterone, which increases the reabsorption of sodium, and water follows sodium back into the blood. ADH and aldosterone thus have the effect of maintaining normal blood volume and blood pressure.

FIGURE 27-3 A schematic representation of the formation of urine.

When the amount of water in the body increases (e.g., as in ingestion of excessive fluids), ADH is suppressed and the opposite effect occurs. Urine becomes dilute and water continues to be eliminated until its concentration returns to normal (Scanlon & Sanders, 2007).

Tubular Secretion

Some substances are actively secreted from the blood in the peritubular capillaries into the renal filtrate. For example, metabolic waste products, such as ammonia and creatinine, and some medications are secreted into the filtrate and then eliminated in urine. In addition, the kidneys help maintain the normal pH of blood by secreting hydrogen ions (H^+).

 Critical**Thinking** 27-1

If a client is suffering from impaired kidney function, what signs and symptoms might you expect to see?

The Ureters Transport Urine

The remaining organs of the urinary system transport or store the urine once it is formed. From the collecting tubules, urine travels into the renal pelvis and enters the ureter. Each kidney has one ureter, approximately 26 to 30 cm (10 to 12 in.) long and 1.25 cm (0.5 in.) in diameter (see Fig. 27-1). The ureters contract in peristaltic waves to move urine toward the bladder. At the opening between the ureter and the bladder is a flap of mucous membrane that acts as a one-way valve, allowing urine to enter the bladder but preventing backflow (**reflux**) into the ureter.

The Urinary Bladder Stores Urine

The urinary bladder (see Fig. 27-1) is a sac-like organ that receives urine from the ureters and stores it until discharged from the body. The wall of the bladder consists of four layers:

- An innermost mucous membrane seals off the remaining layers from exposure to urine.
- A layer of connective tissue supports the mucous membrane.
- Three layers of longitudinal and circular smooth muscle fibers are collectively called the **detrusor muscle.**
- An outermost layer of fibrous connective tissue covers the detrusor layer.

When the bladder is empty, it shrivels and its elastic wall becomes heavily folded. As it receives newly formed urine, it expands and the wall becomes smooth. An average, normal bladder can store 500 mL (one pint) of urine, but it may distend when needed to a capacity twice that amount. You cannot palpate an empty bladder, but a full or distended bladder extends upward to form a pear shape that you can feel in the suprapubic region.

The Urethra Transports Urine

The urethra transports urine from the bladder to the body's exterior. In women, the urethra is about 3 to 4 cm (1.5 in.) long and is anchored to the anterior wall of the vagina by connective tissue; it opens at the **urinary meatus** between the clitoris and vaginal opening. Because the female urethra is so short, women are especially prone to urinary tract infection from microorganisms residing in the vagina and rectum. In men, the urethra extends about 20 cm (8 in.) from the bladder to the urinary meatus at the distal end of the penis. As it leaves the bladder, the male urethra passes through a surrounding gland known as the **prostate.** In addition to urine, the male urethra also carries semen.

The mucous membrane of the urethra (in both men and women) is continuous with the bladder and the ureters. Therefore, infection in the urethra can easily spread through the bladder and up into the kidneys.

Knowledge Check 27-1

- Identify the major structures of the urinary system.
- What are the functions of the kidneys?
- Briefly describe how urine is formed.
- What role do the ureters, bladder, and urethra play in urinary elimination?

 Go to Chapter 27, **Knowledge Check Response Sheet and Answers,** on the Student Resource Disk or DavisPlus at http://davisplus.fadavis.com/Wilkinson2

How Does Urinary Elimination Occur?

Where the bladder connects to the urethra is a thickening of smooth muscle, called the **internal urethral sphincter.** When closed, the internal sphincter keeps urine in the bladder from entering the urethra. When the bladder contains 200 to 450 mL of urine (50 to 200 mL in children), the distention activates stretch receptors in the bladder wall. The stretch receptors send sensory impulses to the *voiding reflex center* in the spinal cord, triggering motor impulses that cause the detrusor muscle to contract and the internal sphincter to relax. The internal urethral sphincter is not under voluntary control.

Voiding (also called **urination** or **micturition**) occurs when contraction of the detrusor muscle pushes stored urine through the relaxed internal urethral sphincter into the urethra. This triggers the conscious urge to void. However, voiding may be voluntarily delayed by inhibiting release of a second, **external urethral sphincter.** When the person is ready to urinate, the brain signals the external sphincter to relax, and urine flows through the urethra. Further contraction of the detrusor muscle normally forces out any urine remaining in the bladder. After the detrusor muscle relaxes, the bladder begins to fill with urine again.

As you can see, voiding and control of urination require that, in addition to normal functioning of the bladder and urethra, the brain, spinal cord, and nerves supplying the bladder and urethra be intact. The person must be aware of the need to urinate and able to respond by either inhibiting the reflex or by going to the toilet.

Normal Urination Patterns

The kidneys produce urine at a rate of about 50 to 60 mL per hour, or 1500 mL per day. However, output may fluctuate by 1000 mL to 2000 mL depending on various factors discussed in the next section. Most people void about five or six times per day, even eight times is normal—typically after awakening, after each meal, and just before bedtime. When fluid intake is increased, urination will be more frequent. Sometimes frequent urination is a sign of other medical problems, such as diabetes or urinary tract infection.

Characteristics of Normal Urine

Specific gravity is a measure of dissolved solutes in a solution. As the concentration of the urine solutes increases, specific gravity increases. The specific gravity of distilled water is 1.000 because there are no dissolved solutes. The normal specific gravity range for urine is 1.002 to 1.028. As fluid intake increases, urine becomes dilute and lighter in color to almost clear as it approaches a specific gravity of 1.000. In contrast, if fluid intake is low or there have been fluid losses, as with diarrhea or vomiting, the urine darkens as the specific gravity rises. Characteristics of urine are discussed in depth later in this chapter. Also,

 Go to Chapter 27, **Procedure 27-3: Bedside Urine Testing: Measuring Specific Gravity** in Volume 2.

 Critical**Thinking** 27-2

- How does Marlena's ("Meet Your Patient") urinary elimination pattern differ from normal?
- What would you expect to find if you measured her specific gravity?
- Marlena's symptoms suggest a urinary tract infection. How might this be related to the fact that she is sexually active?

What Factors Affect Urinary Elimination?

Given the complex structure and physiology of the urinary organs, it isn't surprising that many variables affect their function.

Developmental Factors

Developmental factors affect urine volume and frequency and control of voiding.

Infants and Children

A newborn's kidneys produce 15 to 60 mL of urine per kilogram of body weight per day. Newborns do not concentrate urine well and, therefore, may void up to 25 times during the first 24 hours of life. The normal specific gravity of their urine is 1.008. Over the first weeks of life, the urine gradually becomes more concentrated, and the well-hydrated infant produces eight to ten wet diapers a day. Infants do not have voluntary control of voiding because neuromuscular functioning is immature.

The timing of toilet training is highly variable and is influenced by family and culture (e.g., the presence of older children who can act as role models). In the United States, most parents begin toilet training when their child is between 18 and 36 months of age. This timing can vary widely. Before toilet training can occur, toddlers must be able to control the external urethral sphincter, sense the urge to void, communicate their need to use the toilet, and remove their clothing. Toddlers usually stay dry in the daytime before they can go without a diaper all night.

Occasional wetting (**enuresis**) is entirely normal in children, even in the early school years, especially when the child is intensely involved in a game, test, or other absorbing activity. Such events should be accepted calmly and not punished.

- **Nocturnal enuresis,** or night-time bedwetting, occurs in 15% to 25% of 5-year-old children. By the age of 12 years, 8% of boys and 4% of girls still wet the bed.
- **Primary nocturnal enuresis** is bedwetting in a child who has not achieved consistent dryness at night.
- **Secondary enuresis** occurs in a child who has had at least 6 months of nighttime dryness (Thiedke, 2003).

Older Adults

Renal blood flow progressively decreases with aging, primarily because of changes to the micro blood vessels to the kidney. This decline in glomerular filtration is the most important functional deficit caused by aging (*Merck Manual of Geriatrics*, 2000 [updated 2006]).

The size and functioning of the kidneys begin to decrease at about age 50, and by age 80 only about two-thirds of the functioning nephrons remain. This results in a decline in filtration rate, which affects the ability to dilute and concentrate urine, but does not normally create problems unless an illness alters fluid balance. For example, when older adults lose fluids and electrolytes through vomiting and diarrhea, it is difficult for their kidneys to maintain acid–base and electrolyte balances. Chronic diseases such as arteriosclerosis, common in older adults, can reduce blood flow and impair renal function. Decreased kidney function places older adults at risk for drug toxicity, as well.

The potential volume of the bladder decreases because of a loss of elasticity in the bladder wall; thus, older adults need to urinate more frequently, especially during the night (**nocturnal frequency**). Loss of elasticity and muscle tone also decreases the ability of the bladder to empty completely. Retention of urine after voiding then increases the risk for bladder infections. In women, childbearing may have weakened the pelvic muscles, which can lead to leakage of urine. In older men, the prostate gland may be enlarged, causing urinary frequency and hesitancy. Most older men have some degree of difficulty starting urination or reduced force of the urinary stream, and may experience dribbling.

Personal, Sociocultural, and Environmental Factors

Many people put off voiding while they are working, watching TV, or busy with other tasks. Delaying urination promotes urinary stasis and can lead to bladder infections. Other situations can inhibit voiding, as well, such as the following:

Anxiety. A person who is anxious and tense cannot relax the abdominal and perineal muscles and the external urethral sphincter. It is then difficult to void.

Lack of Time. Most people find it difficult to void when they feel rushed; therefore, when helping patients to void, make sure you have scheduled enough time for them to relax fully.

Lack of Privacy. Many people require privacy for voiding and if they are in a restaurant or other unfamiliar environment, they may be embarrassed even to ask for directions to a bathroom. Some hospitalized clients may also avoid asking for assistance to the bathroom.

Loss of Dignity. In Chapter 10, we talked about the loss of dignity that hospitalized patients experience. Patients who need assistance with toileting may be especially vulnerable to such feelings, especially if they require catheterization or a bedpan. It is important, therefore, to acknowledge such feelings and encourage the patient to participate in other aspects of self-care, such as bathing and dressing.

Cultural Influences. Some patients will state personal, cultural, or religious requirements for toileting assistance to be provided by a person of the same gender, or they will wait until a visit from a family member before acknowledging their need for help with voiding.

Nutrition, Hydration, and Activity Level

Substances that contain caffeine, such as coffee, tea, cola, and chocolate, act as diuretics and increase urine production. Consuming large amounts of alcohol impairs the release of antidiuretic hormone (ADH), resulting in increased production of urine. In contrast, a diet high in salt causes water retention and decreases urine production.

The kidneys also "spare" water when a person is dehydrated, such as after heavy exercise or when fluid intake is inadequate. This causes the urine to be concentrated and low in volume. During prolonged periods of physical activity, especially in hot weather, the body loses sodium and other electrolytes rapidly through sweat; for this reason, electrolyte replacement beverages may be more beneficial than plain water in helping to prevent dehydration for prolonged or vigorous-intensity activity (Thompson & Manore, 2008). For most adults, pale to clear urine indicates adequate hydration.

KnowledgeCheck 27-2
- What quantity of urine in the bladder will stimulate the urge to void?
- Identify at least three methods for determining whether hydration is adequate and urine output is within normal limits.

 Go to Chapter 27, **Knowledge Check Response Sheet and Answers,** on the Student Resource Disk or DavisPlus at http://davisplus.fadavis.com/Wilkinson2

Medications

Various medications affect urination. *Phenazopyridine hydrochloride (Pyridium),* a bladder analgesic, turns the urine a deep orange-red color. *Diuretics,* sometimes called "water pills," treat blood pressure, fluid retention, and edema by increasing elimination of urine.

Diuretics are classified as thiazide, potassium-sparing, or loop-acting diuretics (Box 27-1). In contrast, a number of medications have a side effect of urinary retention. They inhibit the free flow of urine due to *anticholinergic effects* (e.g., medications given to relieve bladder spasms). See Box 27-2 for a listing of the most common medications associated with urinary retention.

BOX 27-1 ■ Diuretics

Thiazide diuretics are used to treat high blood pressure by reducing the amount of sodium and water in the body. They also dilate blood vessels, thereby lowering blood pressure.

Potassium-sparing diuretics reduce the amount of water in the body. Unlike other diuretic medicines, these medicines do not cause potassium loss.

Loop-acting diuretics cause the kidneys to excrete more urine by reabsorbing less water. This reduces the amount of water in the body and lowers blood pressure.

Medications that have significant interactions with diuretics include: Digoxin, antihypertensives, lithium, certain antidepressants (especially when taking thiazide or loop-acting diuretics), and the immunosuppressant cyclosporine, especially when the patient is taking a potassium-sparing diuretic.

Common side effects of diuretics include weakness, muscle cramps, skin rash, increased sensitivity to sunlight (with thiazide diuretics), dizziness, lightheadedness, joint pain.

BOX 27-2 ■ Medications Associated with Urinary Retention

Class	Examples
Antihistamines loratadine	Chlorpheniramine (Chlor-Trimeton), (Claritin)
Tricyclic antidepressants	Amitriptyline (Elavil), desipramine (Norpramin)
MAO inhibitors	Phenelzine (Nardil), tranylcypromine (Parnate)
Antispasmodics	Dicyclomine (Bentyl)
Antiparkinsonism medications	Benztropine mesylate (Cogentin), levodopa
Beta-adrenergic blockers	Propranolol (Inderal), nadolol (Corgard)

Still other medications are **nephrotoxic** (damaging to the kidneys). These include some antibiotics, such as gentamicin (Garamycin) and amphotericin B (Amphotec, a fungicide), and high doses or long-term use of aspirin and ibuprofen.

Surgery and Anesthesia

Surgery can have various effects on the urinary tract.

Reproductive and Urinary Tract Surgeries can affect urine solutes, normal urine characteristics, and the ability to pass urine normally. Manipulation of the urinary tract frequently leads to trauma, bleeding, or the introduction of bacteria into a normally sterile tract. Swelling after diagnostic or invasive procedures and childbirth may cause urinary retention.

Surgery in the Pubic Area, Vagina, or Rectum is associated with a high incidence of trauma to the urinary organs, lower abdominal swelling, loss of pelvic muscle control, and increased pressure on the kidneys, ureters, or bladder. Surgery on the reproductive organs, such as hysterectomy in women or transurethral resection of the prostate in men, usually requires the use of an indwelling catheter (tube) for draining the bladder postoperatively. The urine may be red or pink-tinged after any invasive urinary tract surgery or procedure.

Anesthetic Agents can decrease blood pressure and glomerular filtration, thus decreasing urine formation. Spinal anesthesia decreases the patient's awareness of the need to void, which may lead to bladder distention.

Pathological Conditions

Disorders of the urinary system that affect urinary elimination include the following:

Infection or inflammation of the bladder, ureters, or kidneys

Renal calculi (kidney stones) or tumors, which obstruct the normal flow of urine

In older men, **hypertrophy** (excessive growth) of the prostate gland due to benign or cancerous lesions, which interferes with flow of urine from the bladder into the urethra

Diseases involving other systems can indirectly affect urinary function. For example:

- *Cardiovascular and metabolic disorders* decrease blood flow through the glomeruli and thus impair filtration and urine production.
- Any condition that affects *nervous system* control of the urinary system organs will impair urinary elimination. After a stroke or spinal cord injury, for example, some patients may lose bladder control.
- *Neurogenic bladder* occurs as a result of impaired neurological function. The person cannot perceive bladder fullness or control the urinary sphincters. The bladder becomes flaccid or spastic, causing frequent involuntary loss of urine.
- *Systemic infection*, especially when accompanied by a high fever, causes the kidneys to reabsorb and retain water.
- *Immobility and impaired communication* may interfere with the ability to get to the bathroom in time or to communicate the need for assistance. This may result in urination in inappropriate settings or at inappropriate times.
- *Cognitive changes* that alter perception of the urge to void or severe psychiatric conditions involving altered perception or ability to manage activities of daily living may lead to **incontinence**, which is involuntary loss of urine.

KnowledgeCheck 27-3

- What common medications increase the amount of urine voided?
- What types of medications are associated with urinary retention?
- What types of conditions or surgeries are associated with a high incidence of altered urination?

 Go to Chapter 27, **Knowledge Check Response Sheet and Answers,** on the Student Resource Disk or DavisPlus at http://davisplus.fadavis.com/Wilkinson2

Practical Knowledge knowing how

As a nurse, you will monitor and assist clients with urinary elimination, teach them about body functions, and work collaboratively with the healthcare team to facilitate normal urinary function. In the remainder of the chapter, we discuss these activities.

■ ASSESSMENT

To assess urinary elimination, you will use data from the nursing history, physical examination, and diagnostic and laboratory reports.

Nursing History

Because urination patterns vary among individuals, you will need a nursing history to determine what is normal for a particular person. As you interview the client, pay attention to her reaction to your questions. Many people are embarrassed about discussing urination. Tailor your assessment to the client's needs, and use language that makes her comfortable. For a set of interview questions,

 Go to Chapter 27, **Assessment Guidelines and Tools, Urinary Elimination History Questions,** in Volume 2.

For clients with a urinary diversion, you should also gather data on the client's usual care of the stoma, use of appliances, and adjustment to the ostomy.

Physical Assessment

Physical assessment for urinary elimination includes examination of the kidneys, bladder, urethra, and skin surrounding the genitals, as appropriate. For a complete discussion of physical examination of the genitourinary system,

 Go to Chapter 19, **Procedure 19-17: Assessing the Male Genitourinary System,** and **Procedure 19–18: Assessing the Female Genitourinary System,** in Volume 2.

KnowledgeCheck 27-4

- What should you discuss with your client when performing a nursing history focused on urinary elimination?
- What are the key elements of a physical assessment for a client with urination problems?

 Go to Chapter 27, **Knowledge Check Response Sheet and Answers,** on the Student Resource Disk or DavisPlus at http://davisplus.fadavis.com/Wilkinson2

 CriticalThinking 27-3

In the "Meet Your Patient" scenario, some assessment findings were given for Marlena. If you performed the preceding urinary tract assessments, what findings might you expect?

Assessing the Urine

In addition to observations already mentioned, assessment of the urine includes measuring urine output and conducting a variety of bedside tests.

Measuring Intake and Output

Measuring urine output is part of a comprehensive plan to monitor a client's fluid status. Recall that the kidneys produce urine at a rate of approximately 50 to 60 mL per hour, or 1500 mL per day. However, urinary output fluctuates depending on the quantity of fluids the patient drinks and on other factors, such as the ability of the heart to circulate the blood, adequate kidney functioning, and the ability of the patient to void the urine. Urine output might be low if the person is sweating excessively or has significant vomiting and diarrhea. High fever can contribute to reduced urine output.

You must know both the intake and the output (I&O), as well as relevant physical condition, to interpret the meaning of the patient data. For example, if urine output is low, you cannot assume the patient's kidneys are not working properly. If his intake is also low, he may be dehydrated. But what does it mean if his intake is high and his output low? Yes, this could mean his kidneys are not working well. However, it could also mean that his kidneys are producing urine but that he has urinary retention because of something that is obstructing flow.

To measure fluid intake, record all fluids the patient drinks or receives intravenously. Include the following items as fluid intake: oral fluids, semiliquid foods, ice chips, IV fluids, tube feedings, and irrigations instilled and not withdrawn immediately. Fluid output includes the following items: urine output, gastrointestinal fluid loss (e.g., emesis), liquid feces, and drainage (e.g., from suction devices or wounds). Explain to the client, family members, and all caregivers that I&O are being monitored. Posting a sign at the bedside or on the door to the room is a helpful reminder. When possible, have the client assist you with monitoring.

You will usually total the I&O at the end of each shift, as well as for each 24-hour period. In intensive care units, you may measure I&O hourly. Most healthcare facilities have standardized I&O forms. I&O may be recorded on a separate form or be part of a flowsheet.

 Go to Chapter 16, **Forms: Nursing Assessment Flow Sheet,** in Volume 2.

For more discussion of intake and output, go to Chapters 16 and 36. See Figure 16-2 for an example of a form to document the I&O. Also,

 Go to Chapter 16, **Charting Forms, Intake & Output Sheet,** in Volume 2.

Observe universal precautions when handling urine to prevent exposure to body fluids. Always wear disposable procedure gloves, and avoid splashing the urine and contaminating your uniform. The method you use to measure urine is dictated in part by the amount of help the client needs with urination.

Voided Urine

Many ambulatory clients need no assistance with urination. Be sure to inform them you are monitoring their intake and output (I&O), and explain how they can help. Place a specimen "hat" (collection container) under the toilet seat to collect urine, or have male clients void into a urinal. Periodically measure the output and empty the urine into the toilet. For clients who can assist with recording the I&O, provide a bedside clipboard.

For the client with mobility problems, use a bedpan or urinal to collect urine output. Use a fracture pan for clients with a fracture of the pelvis, lower back, or legs or for clients who have casts, splints, or braces on their legs. Male clients may void into a urinal while remaining in bed.

 Go to Chapter 28, **Procedure 28–2: Placing and Removing a Bedpan,** in Volume 2.

For complete instructions for measuring urine output from a bedpan or urinal,

 Go to **Chapter 27, Procedure 27-1A: Measuring Urine Output from a Bedpan or Urinal,** in Volume 2.

Urine from a Catheter

An **indwelling urinary catheter**, also known as a Foley or a retention catheter, is a flexible tube that is inserted through the urethra into the bladder. It is held in place by a balloon that is inflated in the bladder above the detrusor muscle (Fig. 27-4). Catheter insertion and ongoing care are discussed in the "Planning Interventions/Implementation" section of this chapter.

You will usually measure urine output from the indwelling catheter at the end of each shift unless otherwise prescribed. Clients who require close monitoring of I&O will have a special collection bag with a measuring chamber. Often this is used to assess hourly urine output.

For complete instructions for measuring urine from a catheter,

 Go to Chapter 27, **Procedure 27-1B: Measuring Urine from an Indwelling Catheter,** in Volume 2.

Obtaining Samples for Urine Studies

Many disorders of the urinary system can be assessed by examining urine. You will perform some of these tests at the bedside. For others, you will collect a specimen that is analyzed in the lab. The various types of urine samples are discussed in the text that follows.

FIGURE 27-4 An indwelling catheter may be used for patients who are unable to void because of inflammation or disease or who require continual observation of urine flow.

Freshly Voided Specimen

To collect a freshly voided sample, collect the urine in the same manner as when you are measuring intake and output. Pour the urine into a specimen container labeled with the patient's name, the date, and the time of collection. Many facilities require packaging the container in a moisture-proof specimen-handling bag. Follow agency policy on additional packaging. Transport the specimen to the lab as soon as possible (according to agency policies). If there is a delay in getting the specimen to the lab, most agencies recommend refrigeration.

 Go to Chapter 27, **Procedure 27-1 and 27-2: Measuring Voided Urine and Obtaining a Urine Specimen for Testing,** in Volume 2.

For infants and very young children, you will apply a special collection device over the genitals to collect the specimen. While wearing procedure gloves, cleanse the genital area and allow the skin to dry. Remove the covering over the adhesive strips on the collection bag, and apply the bag over the genitals. When the child urinates, remove the collection bag and place the entire bag in a specimen container.

Clean-Catch Specimen

Many diagnostic tests require a clean-catch urine specimen. The client must cleanse the genitalia before voiding and collect the sample in midstream because the initial flow of urine may contain organisms from the urethral meatus, distal urethra, and perineum. A midstream sample is free of these contaminants. The Critical Aspects box in this chapter summarizes key steps in collecting a clean-catch sample. For the complete procedure,

 Go to Chapter 27, **Procedure 27-2A: Collecting a Clean-Catch Urine Specimen,** in Volume 2.

Sterile Urine Specimen

A sterile urine specimen aids in determining the presence of a urinary tract infection. You can obtain a sterile urine specimen by inserting a catheter into the bladder or by withdrawing a sample from an indwelling catheter. Do not take the specimen from the collection bag because that urine may be several hours old.

✚ Never disconnect the catheter from the drainage tube to obtain a sample. Interrupting the system creates a portal of entry for pathogens, thereby increasing the risk of contamination. Figure 27-5 illustrates how to obtain a sterile specimen from an indwelling catheter. For a discussion of the steps involved,

 Go to Chapter 27, **Procedure 27-2B: Obtaining a Sterile Urine Specimen from a Catheter,** in Volume 2.

24-Hour Urine Collection

A 24-hour urine collection, may be prescribed to evaluate some renal disorders by showing kidney function at different times of the day and night. You

FIGURE 27-5 Inserting a sterile needleless access device and syringe into the specimen port to obtain a sterile specimen from an indwelling catheter.

must use a large container and preserve all urine voided in the 24-hour time period. Occasionally you will be asked to store each voiding in a separate container. To begin collecting, have the patient void and record the time. Discard this first voiding, but save all urine for the next 24 hours. Be sure to inform the patient and all staff about the collection. Post signs in prominent locations, such as the client's bathroom or entry door, to remind staff of the ongoing test and alert them to not discard urine. Also,

Go to Chapter 27, **Procedure 27-2C: Collecting a 24-Hour Urine Specimen,** in Volume 2.

Routine Urinalysis

A routine urinalysis (UA) is one of the most commonly prescribed laboratory tests. It is used as an overall screening test as well as an aid to diagnosing renal, hepatic, and other diseases. Urinalysis requires a freshly voided sample.

Urinalysis techniques include "dipstick" testing and/or microscopic analysis. Dipstick testing is commonly performed at the bedside; microscopic examination is done in the lab. Box 27-3 contains several terms used to describe urine characteristics and quantity. For the expected findings and common variants of urinalysis,

Go to Chapter 27, **Diagnostic Testing, Urinalysis,** in Volume 2.

Bedside Testing (Dipstick)

Dipstick testing can determine pH and specific gravity and the presence of protein, glucose, ketones, and occult blood in the urine. Commercially prepared kits contain a reagent designed to detect a specific substance (e.g., glucose). The reagent may be a paper test strip, a fluid, or a tablet. When contacted by the urine, a chemical reaction causes a color change that you compare to a color chart (Fig. 27-6). You will need good lighting to evaluate the test strip results. Read

---

BOX 27-3 ■ Terms Associated with Urination

Acute renal failure (ARF): An acute rise in the serum creatinine level of 25% or more. May be caused by inadequate blood flow to the kidney, injury to the kidney glomeruli or tubules, or obstruction of kidney outflow.

Anuria: The absence of urine, often associated with kidney failure or congestive heart failure. This term is used when urine output is less than 100 mL in 24 hours.

Dysuria: Painful or difficult urination. May be associated with infection or partial obstruction of the urinary tract as well as medications that trigger urinary retention.

End-stage renal disease (ESRD): A chronic rise in serum creatinine levels associated with loss of kidney function that must be treated with dialysis or transplantation. Also known as chronic renal failure (CRF).

Enuresis: Involuntary loss of urine

Frequency: The need to urinate at short intervals

Hematuria: Blood in the urine. May be due to trauma, kidney stones, infection, or menstruation.

Micturition: To start the stream of urine; to urinate; release urine from the bladder

Nephropathy: A broad term meaning disease of the kidney

Nephrotoxic: A substance that damages kidney tissue. Some antibiotics (gentamicin, tobramycin, and amikacin), nonsteroidal anti-inflammatory drugs, lead, and contrast media have the potential to be nephrotoxic.

Nocturia: Frequent urination after going to bed. May be caused by excessive fluid intake as well as a variety of urinary tract and cardiovascular problems.

Nocturnal enuresis: Involuntary loss of urine while asleep

Oliguria: Urine output of less than 400 mL in 24 hours. For pediatric patients, oliguria is < 0.5–1.0 mL/kg per hour.

Pessary: An incontinence device that is inserted into the vagina to reduce organ prolapse or pressure on the bladder

Polyuria: Excessive urination. May be caused by excessive hydration, diabetes mellitus, diabetes insipidus, or kidney disease.

Proteinuria: The presence of protein in the urine. May be a sign of infection or kidney disease.

Pyuria: Pus in the urine. May be caused by lesions or infection in the urinary tract.

Urgency: A sudden, almost uncontrollable need to urinate.

---

the kit label to be certain that you are using the correct reagent and that the kit is not past the expiration date. Follow the manufacturer's directions regarding the amount of urine needed and the time needed for the reagent to develop. For guidelines for dipstick testing,

FIGURE 27-6 Commercial testing kits contain a reagent for a specific substance. A chemical reaction with the urine causes a color change that you interpret using a color chart.

Go to Chapter 27, **Procedure 27-3A: Dipstick Testing of Urine,** in Volume 2.

You may delegate bedside urine testing to nursing assistive personnel (NAP) if you know that they have the knowledge and skill to perform the procedure. Ask the NAP to report the test results to you and to save the urine sample in case you should need to repeat the test.

Specific Gravity

Specific gravity, an indicator of urine concentration, can be measured with a reagent strip. However, when you need to be precise and accurate, you should use a refractometer. Specific gravity is usually tested in the laboratory, but it is a nursing responsibility in some settings. For guidelines when testing urine specific gravity,

Go to Chapter 27, **Procedure 27-3B: Measuring Specific Gravity of Urine,** in Volume 2.

A **refractometer** (Fig. 27-7) measures the extent to which a beam of light changes direction when it passes through the urine (the *refractive index*). If the concentration of solids is high, the light is refracted more. The method is quick and easy to perform and requires only a few drops of urine. A refractometer is more precise, requires a much smaller specimen, is more compact, and poses less risk of spills and exposure to body fluids than does a urinometer, which for the most part is no longer used.

KnowledgeCheck 27-5

- Explain how to collect a clean-catch urine specimen.
- You are caring for a patient on a hospital unit from 0700 to 1200. Based on the following information, calculate the I&O and comment on your findings.
  Receiving IV fluid at 125 mL/hr
  0800 breakfast—4 oz juice, toast, scrambled eggs, 8 oz coffee

FIGURE 27-7 A refractometer indicates urine concentration by measuring the extent to which a beam of light is refracted ("bent") when passed through the urine. (Courtesy of Atago USA, Inc.)

0930—3 oz water
0700 to 1200—wound drainage: 360 mL
0700 to 1200—urine output per indwelling catheter: 180 mL

Go to Chapter 27, **Knowledge Check Response Sheet and Answers,** on the Student Resource Disk or DavisPlus at http://davisplus.fadavis.com/Wilkinson2

Critical**Thinking** 27-4

- Why do you think the first voided urine is discarded at the start of a 24-hour urine collection?
- Below are the dipstick findings you obtained on the clean-catch specimen from Marlena ("Meet Your Patient").

Urinalysis	Result
pH	8.0
Specific gravity	1.030
Protein	Negative
Glucose	Negative
RBCs	Trace
Nitrite	11
WBCs	12
Bilirubin	Negative
Ketones	Negative
Urobilinogen	Negative

a. Identify the abnormal findings.
b. What would you expect the findings of her urine culture and sensitivity to demonstrate?

Blood Studies

Blood urea nitrogen (BUN) and creatinine levels are commonly measured to assess renal function and hydration. For normal ranges,

Go to Chapter 27, **Diagnostic Testing, Blood Studies: BUN and Creatinine,** in Volume 2.

Common Diagnostic Procedures

A variety of diagnostic procedures may be performed on the urinary tract. These procedures are conducted in the operating room, procedures suite, or radiology department. Typically nurses are responsible for preparing the client for the procedure, assisting with specimen collection, delivering aftercare, and sometimes assisting the physician. For a discussion of urinary system studies and the nursing responsibilities associated with them,

 Go to Chapter 27, **Diagnostic Testing, Studies of the Urinary System,** in Volume 2.

ANALYSIS/NURSING DIAGNOSIS

Urinary elimination problems are described by several nursing and medical diagnoses. NANDA-I diagnoses specific to urinary elimination include the following:

> Impaired Urinary Elimination
> Urinary Incontinence (Functional, Reflex, Stress, Urge)
> Risk for Urge Urinary Incontinence
> Urinary Retention
> Overflow Urinary Incontinence
> Readiness for Enhanced Urinary Elimination
> Risk for Infection (Urinary Tract)
> Risk for Ineffective Renal Perfusion

Urinary problems may also be the etiology of other nursing diagnoses, such as the following:

> Anxiety related to urinary urgency and recent episode of incontinence
> Disturbed Body Image secondary to new urostomy
> Acute Pain related to bladder spasms and urinary tract infection
> Social Isolation related to frequent periods of incontinence
> Risk for Imbalanced Fluid Volume
> Ineffective Self Health Management

Common urinary elimination problems, including urinary tract infection, retention, incontinence, and urinary diversions are discussed at length in the remainder of this section.

Urinary Tract Infections

Normally urine is free of bacteria, viruses, and fungi. A urinary tract infection (UTI) occurs when microorganisms, usually *Escherichia coli (E. coli),* which normally lives harmlessly in the colon, enter the urethra and begin to multiply, overwhelming the normal flora. An infection limited to the urethra is called **urethritis. Cystitis** occurs when bacteria travel up the urethra into the bladder, causing a bladder infection. If not treated promptly, the infection may progress superiorly (upward) to the ureters or kidneys (**pyelonephritis**).

Several biological safeguards are in place in the urinary system to prevent UTIs. One-way valves at the junction of the ureters and bladder help prevent urine from backing up toward the kidneys. In addition, the flow of urine during urination helps wash bacteria out of the body. In men, the prostate gland produces secretions that slow bacterial growth. But despite these safeguards, infections still occur.

Risk Factors for Urinary Tract Infection

People who are more prone to UTIs include the following:

- *Sexually active women.* During sexual activity, perineal pathogens may enter the urethra. Because a woman's urethra is short, pathogens, particularly *E. coli,* can gain rapid access to the bladder.
- *Women who use spermicidal contraceptive gel.* Spermicides reduce normal flora in the vagina, allowing pathogens to multiply unrestricted.
- *Older women.* The loss of estrogen associated with menopause leads to drying of the mucosa in the vagina and urethra and a decrease in protective normal flora.
- *Pregnant women.* Some pregnant women are more prone to UTI because of hormonal changes and because of pressure of the uterus on the bladder.
- *Men with an enlarged prostate.* An enlarged prostate may develop as a result of aging or cancerous changes. Pressure from the prostate creates difficulty emptying the bladder, resulting in stagnant urine, which provides an excellent medium for the growth of bacteria.
- *People with kidney stones.* Kidney stones (*renal calculi*) obstruct the flow of urine, creating stagnation, and irritate the urinary tract as they are passed.
- *Anyone who has an indwelling catheter.* Indwelling catheters pose several risks:

  > Failing to maintain a closed drainage system increases the risk for infection by allowing bacteria to enter the catheter; the catheter provides a pathway for bacteria to migrate up into the urinary system (Wong, 2005, Wound, Ostomy, and Continence Nurses Society, 2008).
  > The catheter irritates the mucosal lining of the urethra, which then creates a portal of entry for microbes. The longer the catheter is indwelling the higher the risk of developing UTI.
  > The urine collection bag is a reservoir for microorganisms.

- *People who have diabetes mellitus.* Glucose in the urine provides nutrients for bacteria to multiply.
- *Immunocompromised patients.* Susceptible hosts (e.g., neonates, elderly, those receiving immunosuppressive drugs, people with weakened immune systems) are less able to maintain a healthy balance of microbes in the urinary tract.
- *People who have a history of UTIs.* Anyone with a previous UTI is more likely to experience a recurrence. This is

thought to be related to the absence of certain antigens against bacteria that attach to the lining of the urethra (National Kidney and Urologic Diseases Information Clearinghouse, 2005).

Recognizing and Treating Urinary Tract Infections

The presence of bacteria in a symptomatic patient is used in the medical diagnosis of UTI. To assist in the diagnosis of UTI, assess for the signs and symptoms in Box 27-4. You will also need to collect a midstream, clean-catch, urine specimen.

Antibiotics are used to treat UTI. The length and type of treatment depends on the location and severity of infection. In general, a bladder infection may be treated with oral antibiotics for 1 to 5 days. In contrast, pyelonephritis (kidney infection) may require IV antibiotics for several days followed by a course of oral antibiotics. Preventive antibiotic treatment is not recommended for people requiring long-term urinary catheterization (Wooten, Bradley, Cardenas, et al., 2010; Lo, Nicholle, Classen, et al., 2008; Wound, Ostomy and Continence Nurses Society, 2008). Drug resistance develops easily; therefore, antibiotics are reserved for symptomatic infections (Wilde & Getliffe, 2006).

 CriticalThinking 27-5

As you may have concluded, Marlena ("Meet Your Patient") has a UTI. What additional history questions would you like to ask Marlena?

Urinary Retention

Urinary retention is an inability to empty the bladder completely. Etiologies include obstruction, inflammation and swelling, neurological problems, medications, and anxiety.

Obstruction. Among men, an enlarged prostate is the most common cause of obstruction in the lower urinary tract. Other obstructions include stones lodged in the urethra, strictures or scars from previous injury, tumors or blood clots in the urinary system, and fecal impaction. Impacted stool distends the rectum and causes forward pressure on the urethra, interfering with the flow of urine out of the bladder.

Inflammation and Swelling. Obstruction may also occur as a result of inflammation and swelling, for example, from infection or surgery in the pelvic region. Swelling narrows the diameter of the urethra so that urine cannot flow freely.

Neurological Problems. Recall that voiding requires that the brain, spinal cord, and nerves supplying the bladder and urethra must be intact. Conditions that affect innervation of the bladder include spinal cord tumors or injury, herniated disk, and viral infections involving perineal nerves (e.g., genital herpes).

Medications. Anesthesia and other medications can also cause temporary problems with urination.

Anxiety. Painful urination may produce anxiety and lead to voluntary withholding of urination.

Urinary Incontinence

Urinary incontinence (UI) is a lack of voluntary control over urination. Urinary incontinence will affect about two-thirds of older adults, to at least some degree. Incontinence is associated with skin impairment, obesity, UTIs, self-rated poor health, reduced mobility, depression, and increased caregiver burden. It can lead to social isolation and increased caregiver burden (Dowling-Castronovo & Bradway, 2003; updated 2008, January).

The total number of people affected by incontinence is presumed to be greater than current estimates because healthcare providers often fail to ask specific questions about it or people are embarrassed to admit to experiencing leakage of urine. Incontinence affects people of all ages and social and economic levels. It affects both sexes, but women are twice as likely as men to have this condition. Risk factors for incontinence also include older age, neurological disease (e.g., stroke), obesity, sedentary lifestyle, depression, and diabetes.

Although incontinence is common, it is not a normal change that occurs with aging. This myth is pervasive and often leads older adults to avoid seeking treatment. Many people do not mention leakage of urine to healthcare providers because they are embarrassed, believe nothing can be done, or believe it is an inevitable condition of older age. Unfortunately, these views may lead to restriction of activities and ultimately to loneliness, depression, and isolation (Dowling-Castronovo & Bradway, 2003; updated 2008, January).

In men, UI is most often related to benign prostatic hyperplasia (enlarged prostate) or to prostatectomy. In women, it is often related to childbirth, specifically to vaginal delivery. Incidence is even higher among those who required episiotomy or forceps- or vacuum-assisted birth. Other risk factors for UI are perimenopausal status, high body mass index, diabetes, and current cigarette smoking.

BOX 27-4 ■ Signs and Symptoms of Urinary Tract Infection

Urinary frequency	Bladder spasms
Urgency	Edema
Foul-smelling urine	Chills
Pyuria	Fever
Dysuria	Back pain
Hematuria	Nausea and vomiting

Types of Urinary Incontinence

The Agency for Healthcare Research and Quality guidelines (Dowling-Castronovo & Bradway, 2008) identified the following seven types of UI:

- **Urge incontinence** is the involuntary loss of larger amounts of urine accompanied by a strong urge to void. It is often referred to as **overactive bladder**.
- **Stress incontinence** is an involuntary loss of small amounts of urine with increased intra-abdominal pressure. NANDA-I specifies "loss of less than 50 mL of urine" in the absence of an overactive bladder (2009, p. 94). Etiological factors include pregnancy, childbirth, obesity, chronic constipation, and straining at stool. Activities that produce leakage of urine also include exercise, laughing, sneezing, coughing, and lifting.
- **Mixed incontinence** is a combination of urge and stress incontinence.
- **Overflow incontinence** is the loss of urine in combination with a distended bladder. Causes of Overflow Incontinence include fecal impaction, neurological disorders, and enlarged prostate (NANDA-I, 2009).
- **Functional incontinence** is the untimely loss of urine when no urinary or neurological cause is involved. This type of incontinence occurs because of physical disability, immobility, pain, external obstacles, or problems in thinking or communicating that prevent a person from reaching a toilet. NANDA-I (2009, p. 91) defines Functional Incontinence as the "inability of [a] usually continent person to reach the toilet in time to avoid unintentional loss of urine." Etiologies include confusion, disorientation, or mobility problems.
- **Transient incontinence** is a short-term incontinence that is expected to resolve spontaneously. Causes include UTI and medications, especially diuretics.
- **Unconscious (reflex) incontinence** is loss of urine when the person does not realize the bladder is full and has no urge to void. Central nervous system disorders and multisystem problems are common causes. NANDA-I defines Reflex Urinary Incontinence as the "involuntary loss of urine at somewhat predictable intervals when a specific bladder volume is reached" (2009, p. 93). Tissue damage from radiation, cystitis, bladder inflammation, or radical pelvic surgery can also trigger reflex incontinence.

The following are other types of incontinence.

- **Enuresis,** which tends to be familial, is involuntary urination after about 5 to 6 years of age, when control is usually established. Enuresis is *primary* if bladder training was never achieved and *secondary* if control was established and then lost. Enuresis has been associated with stress (e.g., marital discord), UTI, allergies, abnormal electroencephalographic patterns, sleep disorders, hearty laughing, and small bladder capacity; however, the cause is not always apparent.
- **Nocturnal enuresis** (bedwetting) can persist until age 10 or later. If one parent had nighttime bedwetting as a child, there is a high chance the child will also experience it. Most often children outgrow the condition. Only a small percentage of the secondary type is caused by a medical condition, such as UTI, urinary obstruction, diabetes, pressure on the bladder from extreme constipation, or neurological disorders of the spinal cord.

Treatments for Urinary Incontinence

The first-line treatment for urinary incontinence is using behavioral interventions, such as timed voiding and Kegel exercises. Pelvic floor training should include at least eight contractions, three times a day. Pelvic muscle training should be continued for at least 3 months before moving to more aggressive treatment. Patients should also reduce caffeine intake, as this irritates the bladder. People with body mass index (BMI) greater than 27 who suffer urinary incontinence may consider losing weight to control symptoms.

The following medical and surgical treatments may be used to manage UI:

Medications. Medications include topical estrogen for women who have UI associated with urogenital atrophy, and anticholinergic drugs such as oxybutynin (Ditropan) and tolterodine (Detrol), which inhibit involuntary bladder contractions.

Devices. Indwelling intravaginal (e.g., pessary) or intraurethral devices to manage urinary incontinence are not to be used routinely, but instead reserved to prevent occasional leakage, for example, during exercise.

Sacral Nerve Stimulation might be recommended for the treatment of certain types of urinary incontinence in women who have not responded to conservative treatment.

Surgical Treatment, such as bladder suspension and prostate resection, relieve the pressure of other pelvic organs against the bladder.

Do not use absorbent products, hand-held urinals, and other toileting aids to routinely manage urinary incontinence, unless used to supplement other therapy.

For more information about helping patients to manage urinary incontinence,

VOL 2 Go to Chapter 27, **Clinical Insight 27-2: Caring for Patients with Urinary Incontinence,** in Volume 2.

Conditions Requiring Urinary Diversions

A **urinary diversion,** or **urostomy,** is a surgically created opening for elimination of urine. Urostomies are used to treat patients who have conditions such as birth defects, cancer, trauma, or disease of the urinary system. A patient with a urinary diversion does not eliminate urine via the urethra. Instead, urine bypasses the bladder and is expelled through the **stoma** or **ostomy.** The patient no longer has voluntary control of urination. Urine constantly flows through the stoma and is collected in a pouch that the patient wears. Risks associated with urinary diversions are primarily infection and permanent kidney damage, which can occur from hydronephrosis (distention of the kidneys with urine, which results from obstruction of the ureter).

The following are three types of urinary diversions:

A Cutaneous Ureterostomy reroutes the ureter(s) directly to the surface of the abdomen, forming a small stoma. It may be unilateral or bilateral. This procedure has limited use because it provides a pathway for pathogens on the skin to directly enter the kidney. The stomas are small and difficult to fit with a collection appliance.

An Ileal Conduit **(also known as a Bricker's loop or ileal loop)** is the most common type of urinary diversion (Fig. 27-8). A small piece of ileum is removed with blood and nerve supply intact. The remainder of the ileum is reconnected to prevent disruption of flow through the bowel. The free segment of ileum is sutured closed at one end, and the other end is brought out to the abdominal wall to create a stoma. The result is a small pouch into which the ureters are implanted. Urine, along with mucus from the ileum, drains continuously from the stoma. This procedure is preferable to a cutaneous ureterostomy because the mucous membrane lining the ileum protects the kidneys from ascending infection. In addition, the ileum creates a stoma that is easier to fit with an appliance.

A Continent Urostomy, also known as an **ileal bladder conduit,** or **Kock pouch** (Fig. 27-9), is a variation of the ileal conduit. Urine drains from the ureters into a surgically created ileal pouch. The stoma created on the abdomen contains a nipple valve to keep urine from leaking. Rather than having urine flow constantly, the patient with an ileal bladder conduit inserts a catheter into the stoma to drain urine through the valve. A second valve prevents reflux of urine back into the kidneys.

Critical**Thinking** 27-6

What types of challenges or problems do you think a patient with a urinary diversion might experience?

FIGURE 27-8 An ileal conduit is the most common urinary diversion.

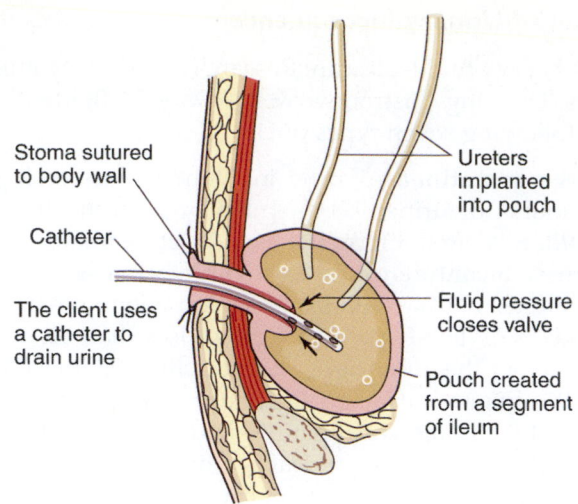

FIGURE 27-9 A continent urostomy allows the client to manage urine without the need to wear an ostomy appliance.

▬ PLANNING OUTCOMES/EVALUATION

The general goal related to urinary elimination is that patients will comfortably void approximately 1500 mL of light yellow urine in 24 hours. Because normal urine elimination patterns vary, the frequency and amount of urine are based on the individual's pattern, food and fluid intake, medications, and other factors.

NOC standardized outcomes for urinary problems, regardless of the specific problem, are the following: Kidney Function, Urinary Continence, Urinary Elimination, and Tissue Integrity: Skin & Mucous Membranes (because urinary elimination problems often place the patient at Risk for Impaired Skin Integrity).

Individualized goals/outcome statements you might use to evaluate the effectiveness of interventions for urinary problems include the following:

- Will resume his normal urination pattern by (date).
- Will discuss his feelings about his urostomy.
- Will have no visible blood in urine after 2 days on antibiotics.
- Responds to the urge to void in a timely manner.
- After voiding, states he feels he has emptied his bladder completely.
- Postvoiding residual volume is <150 mL.

▬ PLANNING INTERVENTIONS/IMPLEMENTATION

For *NIC standardized interventions* for patients with urinary elimination nursing diagnoses,

 Go to Chapter 27, **Standardized Language, NIC Interventions for Urinary Problems,** in Volume 2.

You should select nursing activities to meet individual needs and address problem etiologies. *Specific nursing activities* for patients with elimination problems fall into the following categories: promoting normal urination, preventing urinary tract infection, managing

urinary retention, managing urinary incontinence, and caring for patients who have urinary diversions. The rest of this chapter discusses those activities.

Promoting Normal Urination

As a nurse, you should have a repertoire of independent nursing activities for promoting normal urination. These include providing privacy, positioning, scheduling elimination, providing and monitoring fluid and nutrition, and assisting with hygiene.

Provide Privacy

Although urination is a normal physiological process, most people consider it a private matter. Taking a matter-of-fact approach confirms to patients that you are comfortable with this aspect of care. Provide privacy when discussing or providing care related to urination. Excuse visitors from the room, draw the dividing curtains in shared rooms, and close the door to the room. Whenever possible, give the patient time alone to void. Do not, for example, hover outside the bathroom door asking, "Are you OK?" or "Are you finished?" However, if the client is weak and frail, you may need to remain with him.

Assist with Positioning

Most men stand to void and may have difficulty voiding in other positions. Whenever possible, assist the patient to the bathroom to use the toilet and allow him to assume his preferred position. Alternatively, provide a bedside commode or urinal for the patient to use. To place a urinal, position the patient in a semi-Fowler's position with the legs slightly spread. Place the urinal on the bed between the patient's legs, and insert his penis in the urinal.

Women generally find an upright seated or squatting position to be the most comfortable position for voiding. If a female patient must remain in bed, provide a bedpan. Place her in a semi-Fowler's position to urinate unless contraindicated. Raise the siderails or provide an overhead trapeze so that the patient will have grip holds to maneuver herself onto and off the bedpan. If the patient is very weak, you may need an assistant to help you position her on the bedpan, and you may need to stay with her to help her maintain her position on the bedpan. For the steps involved,

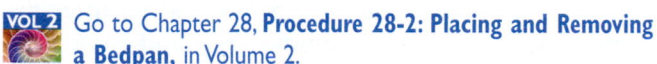 Go to Chapter 28, **Procedure 28-2: Placing and Removing a Bedpan,** in Volume 2.

The Critical Aspects box in Chapter 28 of this volume summarizes that procedure.

Facilitate Toileting Routines

Most patients void on awakening, after meals or drinking a large volume of fluid, before bedtime, or during the night for some. Identify your patient's pattern, and

stick to it as much as possible. If you anticipate a change in the pattern for elimination, inform the patient. For example, if the patient is to receive a diuretic, explain that he will need to urinate more often. Similarly, if the patient is scheduled for a diagnostic procedure or activity, inform him ahead of time so that he may void before the activity begins.

Provide assistance to all patients who have mobility problems and those who use the bedpan. Discuss with all NAP the need to offer assistance so that patients experience minimal delays.

Promote Adequate Fluids and Nutrition

Adequate hydration promotes urinary tract function and flushes the system of waste products. Unfortunately, many people do not meet the recommended intake. Water is the preferred fluid because soda, coffee, and tea often contain caffeine or additives that may cause diuresis. However, the amount of fluid is more important than the type. If the patient will not or cannot drink water, provide the fluid he prefers. Most people should drink eight to ten 8-ounce glasses of fluid daily unless health problems limit the fluid. See Box 27-5 for strategies to increase your patient's fluid intake.

Assist with Hygiene

Urine is irritating to the skin. Therefore, perineal cleansing is an integral part of toileting hygiene. Many ill patients are unable to do this for themselves, so you would need to provide perineal care. If the patient can ambulate to the bathroom, you merely need to assist with her

---

BOX 27-5 ■ Strategies to Increase Patients' Fluid Intake

- For patients with limited mobility, keep water or other liquids in easy reach.
- You may need to remind young children or patients with cognitive or psychiatric disorders to drink fluids.
- For patients who have increased fluid needs, provide goals for intake, and frequently remind them to drink.
- Many foods have a high fluid content. If the patient requires additional fluid for hydration, consider adding soup and watery foods, such as watermelon, to the diet. In contrast, if the patient requires fluid restriction, you will have to account for these foods into the fluid balance.
- Try offering liquids with a straw. Patients tend to drink more this way.
- Chilled drinks might be more appealing, particularly if the patient's mouth is dry. Offer beverages with ice if they are to be served cold.
- Provide good mouth care. Patients will often drink more readily if their mouth feels fresh.

usual cleansing routines. You may assist the patient by pouring warm soapy water over the genitals while she is seated on the toilet, the bedside commode, or on the bedpan. Be sure to rinse with warm water because soap may be drying to the genital mucosa. Also offer a moist washcloth or towelette for washing hands after toileting. For further information,

 Go to Chapter 22, **Procedure 22-4: Providing Perineal Care,** in Volume 2.

KnowledgeCheck 27-6

- Identify activities that promote normal urination patterns.
- Write at least two nursing diagnostic statements that would be appropriate for Marlena in the "Meet Your Patient" scenario.

Go to Chapter 27, **Knowledge Check Response Sheet and Answers,** on the Student Resource Disk or DavisPlus at http://davisplus.fadavis.com/Wilkinson2

Teaching Prevention of Urinary Tract Infection

An important part of UTI treatment is prevention of future infection. The accompanying Self-Care box presents the teaching points that you should include in your sessions with patients at risk for UTI or recovering from a UTI.

Self-Care

Teaching Your Client About Preventing UTI

➤ Drink at least 8 to 10 eight-ounce glasses of water per day to keep urine dilute and to flush bacteria from the urinary tract. The Institute of Medicine (IOM, 2004) recommends even more, particularly with heat exposure or prolonged exercise. Water is best. Some reports claim a benefit to drinking cranberry juice but this practice is controversial (Kiel & Nashelsky, 2003).

➤ Urinate when you first feel the urge. Do not make a habit of postponing urination because bacteria can multiply in stagnant urine.

➤ Always wipe from front to back after urination or defecation.

➤ Wear cotton underwear because nylon or other synthetic fabrics prevent evaporation of moisture. Also avoid tight-fitting clothing in the groin area. Bacteria and other microorganisms grow well in a warm, moist environment.

➤ Urinate after having intercourse to flush away bacteria that might have entered the urethra.

➤ If you have a history of UTI, avoid using a diaphragm, spermicidal contraceptive gel, or unlubricated or spermicidal condoms.

➤ If you have a history of UTI, avoid bubble baths and baking-soda baths.

➤ Promptly report any symptoms of UTI to your healthcare provider.

Managing Urinary Retention

Clients with a mechanical obstruction to urine flow are treated by surgical removal or repair of the obstruction (e.g., resection of the prostate gland, removal of bladder calculi). For clients who have loss of bladder tone, collaboratively, you may (1) administer cholinergic medications, such as bethanechol chloride (Urecholine), which promote bladder emptying by stimulating contraction of the detrusor muscle; (2) use **Credé's maneuver** (apply manual pressure over the bladder to promote emptying); or (3) perform urinary catheterization. When caring for patients with urinary retention, nurses may do the following:

- Monitor intake and output.
- Assess for risk factors for urinary retention (e.g., prostatic hypertrophy, pelvic surgery and medications with anticholinergic side effects, such as diazepam [Valium], some antidepressants, and diphenhydramine [Benadryl]).
- Inspect and palpate for bladder distention.
- Apply heat to the lower abdomen to relax the muscles near where the bladder lies.
- Run water nearby, or place the patient's hands in warm water.
- Pour water over the perineum, or assist the patient to take a warm sitz bath.
- Measure postvoiding residual urine (see the section that follows).
- Advise the patient to contact a medical professional:
  If not previously evaluated for urinary hesitancy, dribbling, or weak urine stream
  For fever, vomiting, side or back pain, shaking chills, or passing little urine for 1 to 2 days
  For blood in the urine, cloudy urine, frequent or urgent need to urinate, or a discharge from the penis or vagina

Urinary Catheterization

Catheterization is the introduction of a pliable tube (catheter) into the bladder to allow drainage of urine. Urinary catherization is performed to:

- Obtain a sterile urine specimen.
- Drain the bladder for surgical or diagnostic purposes or when emptying is incomplete after urination.
- Prevent or treat bladder overdistention and urinary retention (e.g., after surgery) when other measures fail.
- Measure urine that remains in the bladder after the patient voids. This is commonly referred to as *postvoid residual volume* and is measured as part of the diagnostic workup for a patient with urinary retention or incontinence.
- Protect excoriated skin from contact with urine.
- Reduce the need for unnecessary movement of patients who are near death.

Indwelling urinary catheterization is associated with complications of bacteriuria and urinary tract infection. A catheter provides a connection between the external environment and a normally sterile system. In addition, when the patient has an indwelling catheter, microorganisms are no longer flushed from the urethra through voiding. In fact, an indwelling urinary catheter is the most common cause of nosocomial infections. To reduce the risk of bacterial contamination, observe strict sterile technique when inserting and caring for a urinary catheter and maintain a closed system (Lo, Nicholle, Classen, et al., 2008).

Catheterization can injure the urethra if the catheter is too large, is forced through strictures, or is inserted at an incorrect angle. For male patients, when inserting a catheter you must elevate the penis so that it is perpendicular to the body; this straightens the normally curved urethra, helping to prevent trauma. Catheters must be well lubricated on insertion to prevent damaging the delicate mucosa of the urethra.

Patients with spinal cord injuries or neurological disorders use intermittent catheterization to drain the bladder and limit the risk of infection. Many actually perform **intermittent self-catheterization,** although caregivers may assist. Although you will use sterile technique for catheterization, most patients who self-catheterize use clean technique. In spite of this difference, intermittent catheterization carries a substantially lower risk of infection than does an indwelling catheter (Pilloni, Krhut, Mair, et al., 2005; Ord, Lunn, & Reynard, 2003). To teach patients the procedure for self-catheterization,

 Go to Chapter 27 **Clinical Insight 27-4: Teaching Clients About Clean, Intermittent Self-Catheterization,** in Volume 2.

Types of Urinary Catheters

There are a variety of catheter types and materials to choose from, depending on whether the patient requires catheterization for long-term or short-term use, has product sensitivity, or is at increased risk for infection.

- *Silver-alloy* coated catheters were found to reduce infection rates significantly when catheters remained in place for less than 7 days, although they were less effective when used for longer than 1 week (Grabe, Bishop, & Bjerklund-Johansen, 2008; Schumm & Lam, 2008). Silver-coated catheters are not routinely used for short-term catheterization (Lo, Nicholle, Classen, et al., 2008) because they are more costly than standard catheters; however, using standard catheters may be a false economy if the patient acquires an infection.
- *Teflon-bonded latex* is used for short- to medium-term use (< 28 days) because the coating reduces friction and tissue irritation during insertion and while the catheter remains in place.
- *Polyvinyl chloride* (PVC) catheters are designed for long-term use (up to 6 weeks) because they soften and conform to the urethra.
- For even longer periods of use (e.g., up to 3 months), *silicone or hydrogel-coated* catheters may be used because these types help prevent encrustation around the urinary meatus and reduce friction with insertion, removal, and while in place. They are recommended by the International Continence Society (ICS) as well as manufacturers for long-term use (Wilde & Getliffe, 2006).

Toward Evidence-Based Practice

Kessler, T. M., Ryu, G. R., & Burkhard, F. C. (2008). Clean intermittent self-catheterization: A burden for the patient? *Neurourology and Urodynamics, 27*(8). Retrieved from http://www3.interscience.wiley.com/journal/121385630/abstract. DOI 10.1002/nau.20610

The aim of this study was to assess patients' perceptions of clean intermittent self-catheterization (CISC) for voiding dysfunction. This study suggests CISC is an easy and painless procedure that did not interfere with daily activities. CISC does not appear to be a burden for the patient and can be a worthwhile approach for patients in the outpatient setting to manage dysfunctional urinary elimination.

1. As a nurse providing home care to a patient with urinary retention, you teach her how to perform clean intermittent self-catheterization (CISC). What information might you convey to maximize the client's receptiveness to performing the procedure?

2. What suggestions might you make for the client performing CISC so that the procedure does not interfere with daily living?

Sublett, C. M. (2008). Adding to the evidence base: A review of two qualitative studies. *Urologic Nursing, 28*(2), 130–131.

Two qualitative studies compared women with urinary incontinence (UI) and healthcare-seeking behavior. Nurses and other practitioners need to be consistently informed that women are choosing to live with UI for many reasons, including lack of knowledge of resources for UI or the fear that providers may not pay attention to them or take their concerns seriously.

3. As nurse providing care to older adult women, what should you do in your practice to help women with urinary incontinence?

 Go to Chapter 27, **Toward Evidence-Based Practice Suggested Responses,** on the Student Resource Disk or DavisPlus at http://davisplus.fadavis.com/Wilkinson2

- Some catheters have a *lubricant and/or antimicrobial coating* to help prevent infection.

➕ Always check for latex or Teflon and iodine allergies before performing a catheterization.

Catheters are sized by the *diameter* of the lumen; the larger the number, the larger the lumen. For example, 8 and 10 French (Fr) catheters are used for children; they are smaller in diameter than the 14 and 16 Fr catheters typically used for adults. Men usually need a larger size (e.g., 18 Fr) than women. Catheters also come in different *lengths*: a 22-cm catheter is appropriate for women, whereas for men you will need a 40-cm catheter.

Straight Catheter. **A straight catheter** is a single-lumen tube that is inserted for immediate drainage of the bladder (e.g., to obtain a sterile urine specimen, to measure postvoid residual volume, or to relieve temporary bladder distention). After the bladder is empty or the sample obtained, the catheter is removed and the patient resumes voiding independently.

Indwelling Catheter. An **indwelling catheter,** also known as a *Foley* or *retention catheter,* is used for continuous bladder drainage (e.g., when the bladder must be kept empty or when continuous urine measurement is needed). It is usually a double-lumen tube: one lumen is used for urine drainage, and the second lumen is used to inflate a balloon near the tip of the catheter. The inflated balloon holds the catheter in place at the neck of the bladder. The balloon is sized according to the volume of fluid used to inflate it. For most patients you will use a 5-mL balloon; for children 3-mL; and for achieving hemostasis after a prostatectomy, a 30-mL balloon. A triple-lumen indwelling catheter is used when the patient requires intermittent or continuous bladder irrigation. Figure 27-10 illustrates the different types of catheters.

Suprapubic Catheter. **A suprapubic catheter** is used for continuous urine drainage when the urethra must be bypassed (e.g., after gynecological surgery or where there is prostatic obstruction). A suprapubic catheter is inserted through an incision above the symphysis pubis (Fig. 27-11). It is often sutured in place but may

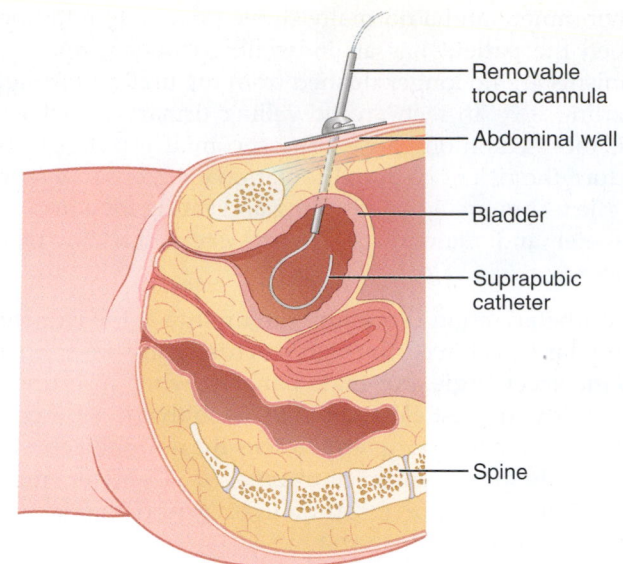

FIGURE 27-11 A suprapubic catheter drains urine from a surgically created opening into the bladder, bypassing the urethra.

occasionally be a double-lumen catheter held in place by a balloon.

Supplies for Urinary Catheterization

The supplies used for inserting an indwelling catheter are usually prepackaged (Fig. 27-12). Included in the kit are sterile gloves, swabs or cotton balls, a solution for cleansing the urethral meatus, sterile lubricant, a sterile indwelling catheter, a syringe filled with sterile water to inflate the retention balloon, drainage tubing, and a drainage collection bag. Kits contain the most common catheter sizes, usually 12, 14, or 16 Fr. Pediatric kits contain 8 or 10 Fr catheters. The smallest diameter catheter possible that provides proper drainage is recommended to minimize urethral trauma (Lo, Nichole, Classen, et al., 2008). Many facilities also have prepackaged kits for straight (single-lumen) catheterization. Instead of a drainage collection bag, these have a drainage basin for collecting urine. Both types of kits may also contain a sterile urine cup for collecting a sterile specimen.

FIGURE 27-10 Types of catheters. *A,* A single-lumen catheter is used to obtain a urine sample or immediately drain the bladder. *B,* A double-lumen catheter is the most commonly used indwelling catheter. *C,* A triple-lumen catheter is inserted when the patient requires irrigation of the bladder.

Catheter tip   Cross section   Urine drainage
A

Catheter tip   Inflated balloon   Cross section   Balloon inflation   Urine drainage
B

Catheter tip   Inflated balloon   Cross section   Irrigation   Balloon inflation   Urine drainage
C

FIGURE 27-12 Supplies for catheter insertion usually come in a prepackaged kit. *A,* Straight catheter kit. *B,* Indwelling catheter kit.

Knowledge Check 27-7

- Describe the difference between a catheter used for straight catheterization and one used for ongoing drainage.
- Why is intermittent catheterization preferred for patients who must be catheterized over lengthy periods of time?

Go to Chapter 27, **Knowledge Check Response Sheet and Answers,** on the Student Resource Disk or DavisPlus at http://davisplus.fadavis.com/Wilkinson2

Urinary Catheter Insertion

To insert a urinary catheter, you will need to gather the appropriate supplies and prepare the patient. Explain to the patient the reason for the catheter insertion, the expected length of time the catheter will be needed, and the sensations he is likely to have. Most patients experience a sensation of pressure and some discomfort (but not pain) when a catheter is inserted. Explain that

when the catheter is inserted it may feel as though he is voiding, but the urine is going into the tube, not on the bed. If there is swelling or bleeding in the urinary tract, insertion may be painful.

Many patients feel embarrassed during this procedure. A professional approach, along with draping and other privacy measures, helps relieve discomfort or distress. As you are draping the patient, offer to answer any further questions he may have.

Use a dorsal recumbent position and supine position for men and women. For female patients, make sure to lower the knee gatch of the bed so that you can easily visualize the urinary meatus. You may need to place a firm cushion under the patient's buttocks to prevent her sinking into a soft mattress and obscuring visibility of the meatus. For women who are unable to assume a dorsal recumbent position, consider Sims' or a lateral position (Fig. 27-13).

The Critical Aspects box provides an overview of urinary catheterization. For the complete procedure,

Go to Chapter 27, **Procedure 27-4: Inserting a Urinary Catheter,** in Volume 2.

Caring for the Patient with an Indwelling Catheter

The following are nursing goals when providing care for a patient with an indwelling catheter:

Prevent Urinary Tract Infection. An indwelling catheter is connected to a drainage tube and collection bag,

FIGURE 27-13 *A, B,* For women who cannot assume a dorsal recumbent position, you can use the side-lying position and lift the superior buttock to expose the urethral meatus.

VOL 2 For steps to follow in *all* procedures, refer to the Universal Steps for All Procedures found on the inside back cover of Volume 2. Go to the full procedures in Volume 2 to practice and learn the procedure steps. Use these Critical Aspects later to help you review key points.

Procedure 27-1: Measuring Urine

➤ Don clean procedure gloves.

➤ Record the amount of urine on the input and output (I&O) flow sheets.

Procedure 27-1A: Measuring Urine Output from a Bedpan or Urinal

➤ Place the bedpan or urinal in the proper position and encourage your patient to begin voiding. Instruct the patient to press the call light button when finished or remain close by.

➤ Pour the urine from the bedpan or urinal into a graduated measuring device. Place on a flat, even surface and read the amount at eye level.

Procedure 27-1B: Measuring Urine from an Indwelling Catheter

➤ Open the drainage spout and allow urine to drain into the measuring device, being careful to avoid touching the spout to the inside of the container.

➤ Pour the urine from the bedpan or urinal into a graduated measuring device. Place on a flat even surface and read the amount at eye level.

Procedure 27-2: Obtaining a Urine Specimen for Testing

➤ Don clean procedure gloves.

Procedure 27-2A: Collecting a Clean-Catch Urine Specimen

➤ Wash the perineum or the end of the penis first with soap and water, then with an antiseptic solution. (For women, wash from front to back; for men, use a circular motion from urethra outward.)

➤ Ask the patient to begin voiding. After the stream begins, collect a 30- to 60-mL specimen.

➤ Maintain sterility: Do not touch the inside of the container or the container lid. Avoid getting toilet paper, feces, pubic hair, or anything else in the urine sample.

➤ Pour the urine into a specimen container that is labeled with the patient's name, the date, and the time of collection.

➤ Place a lid on the container, label the container with the patient's name, the date and time of collection.

➤ Follow agency policy on additional packaging. (Many facilities require packaging the container in a specimen handling bag.)

➤ Transport the specimen to the lab as soon as possible. If there is a delay in getting the specimen to the lab, most facilities recommend refrigeration.

Procedure 27-2B: Obtaining a Sterile Urine Specimen from a Catheter

➤ Empty the drainage tube of urine.

➤ Don clean gloves, and swab the specimen port with an antiseptic swab.

➤ Insert the needleless access device (or needle if the port will not accommodate a needleless device) with a 20- or 30-mL syringe into the specimen port, and aspirate to withdraw the amount of urine you need.

➤ Transfer the specimen into a sterile specimen container.

➤ Maintain sterility: Do not touch the needleless access device or the inside of the container, or the container lid.

➤ Transport the specimen to the lab as soon as possible.

➤ Label the specimen container with the correct patient identification and transport it to the lab in a timely manner.

Procedure 27-2C: Collecting a 24-Hour Urine Specimen

➤ Ask the patient to void. Record the time. Discard this first voiding.

➤ Collect all urine voided during the next 24 hours.

➤ Apply a label on the storage container, identifying the patient's name, date, and time the test ended. Transport it to the lab after the collection is complete. Otherwise, place the urine in a refrigerator designated for specimen storage.

Procedure 27-3: Testing Urine at the Bedside

➤ Follow the manufacturer's directions carefully regarding the amount of urine needed.

Procedure 27-3A: Dipstick Testing of Urine

➤ Read the kit label to be certain that you are using the correct reagent and that the kit has not passed the expiration date.

➤ To ensure accuracy, the reagent strip should be read at the exact time indicated on the label. You will need adequate lighting to evaluate the results.

➤ Dipstick testing is considered a preliminary test for screening.

Procedure 27-3B: Measuring Specific Gravity of Urine

➤ Before use, be sure the equipment is calibrated to 1.000 according to the manufacturer's instructions.

➤ Use fresh urine; if you cannot perform the test within 1 hour, refrigerate the specimen.

➤ Place a drop of urine on the glass plate and close the flap.

➤ Hold the refractometer up to the light when looking through the eyepiece.

➤ Read the specific gravity by looking for the point where the contrast line between the dark and light fields crosses the scale.

➤ Clean the instrument when finished.

Procedure 27-4: Inserting a Urinary Catheter

➤ Allow adequate time for these procedures: Experienced nurses need at least 15 minutes. You will need more time if problems arise—and even more if you are a novice.

➤ Take an extra pair of sterile gloves and an extra sterile catheter into the room.

➤ Be sure that you have good lighting.

➤ Work on the right side of the bed if you are right-handed and on the left side if you are left-handed.

➤ Drape the patient for privacy.

➤ Perform perineal care before the procedure; wash your hands; open the kit.

➤ Don sterile gloves and maintain sterile technique while manipulating the supplies in the kit and performing the procedure.

➤ Once you have touched the patient with your nondominant hand, do not remove that hand from the patient.

➤ For indwelling urinary catheterization, pretesting the balloon by inflating it before insertion is not necessary, especially with silicone catheters. The practice can cause the balloon to form cuffs. Cuffing can cause harm to the patient's urethra.

➤ Lubricate the catheter tip before insertion.

➤ Insert the catheter 5 to 7.5 cm (2 to 3 in.) for women, 17 to 22.5 cm (7 to 9 in.) for men, until urine flows.

➤ Drain the bladder; collect needed samples; measure urine; and connect the drainage bag as needed or remove it if catheterization is intermittent.

Procedure 27-5: Applying an External (Condom) Catheter

➤ Application of a condom (external) catheter is a clean procedure.

➤ Clean and dry the penis before catheter application.

➤ When applying the condom, stabilize the penis with your nondominant hand.

➤ Leave a gap of 2.5 to 5 cm (1 to 2 in.) between the condom and the tip of the penis to prevent skin irritation.

➤ Use only the tape supplied in the application kit to secure the catheter.

➤ For condom catheters that contain adhesive material on the inside of the condom, grasp the penis and gently compress the condom onto the shaft.

➤ Be certain that the tubing from the end of the catheter to the bedside drainage (or leg) bag is free from kinks.

Procedure 27-6: Removing an Indwelling Catheter

➤ Use clean technique. Wash hands before and after removing the catheter. Wear clean procedure gloves.

➤ Be sure to remove the tape securing the catheter to the patient.

➤ Obtain a sterile specimen if needed.

➤ Deflate the balloon completely by aspirating the fluid.

➤ Check the balloon size on the valve port to verify that all fluid has been removed.

➤ If you cannot aspirate all the fluid, do not pull on the catheter. Report to the charge nurse or the primary care provider before continuing.

➤ Observe the first few voidings after the catheter is removed.

Procedure 27-7: Irrigating the Bladder or Catheter

Procedure 27-7A: Intermittent Bladder Irrigation

➤ Establish a sterile field under the specimen removal port or the irrigation port on a three-way catheter.

➤ Because of the risk of infection, never disconnect the drainage tubing from the catheter.

➤ Use a sterile irrigation solution, warmed to room temperature.

➤ Instill the irrigation solution slowly.

➤ Repeat the process as necessary.

Procedure 27-7B: Continuous Bladder Irrigation

➤ Drape the patient, exposing only the irrigation port of the catheter.

➤ Using aseptic technique, attach the connecting tubing to the irrigation solution container.

➤ Prime the tubing.

➤ Don clean procedure gloves.

➤ Pinch the irrigation port of the catheter and connect the irrigation tubing to the port.

➤ Regulate the flow of the irrigant.

➤ Monitor for urine output.

---

which constitute a closed system. This means that it cannot be opened at any point. This minimizes the chance for pathogens to enter the system and infect the urinary tract. UTIs are the most common healthcare-associated infection. More than one-third of all UTIs are associated with indwelling urinary catheters.

Maintain Free Flow of Urine. Free flow of urine prevents backflow of urine into the bladder, which can cause bladder distention and injury. Stasis of urine also provides a medium for growth of microorganisms.

Prevent Transmission of Infection. When providing catheter care, observe universal precautions.

Promote Normal Urine Production. Adequate urine production flushes pathogens out of the bladder, provides natural irrigation of the tubing, and prevents stasis of urine.

Maintain Skin and Mucosal Integrity. Secure the tubing to the leg to prevent traction on the bladder. Provide hygiene care so that the perineal skin and mucosa do not become irritated by feces encrustation of the catheter.

For a comprehensive list of nursing activities to help you meet the preceding goals,

 Go to Chapter 27, **Clinical Insight 27-1: Caring for a Patient with an Indwelling Catheter,** in Volume 2.

Bladder Irrigation

You may perform an irrigation to maintain patency of a urinary catheter, to wash out the bladder (e.g., remove blood clots in the bladder after surgery), or to instill medications into the bladder. An *intermittent irrigation* is most commonly used for medication instillation, whereas a *continuous irrigation* is used to maintain patency when blood, clots, or debris is anticipated. Routine intermittent irrigations (e.g., every shift, every week) are sometimes prescribed to ensure patency; however, these should be avoided and irrigation done only as necessary.

A client requiring a continuous irrigation should have a triple-lumen catheter in place: one lumen for injecting water into the balloon when the catheter is inserted, another for the irrigating solution to flow into the bladder, and a third for the solution and urine to flow out of the bladder. A double-lumen catheter system may need to be opened for irrigation and, therefore, creates a high risk for infection. Although "open" irrigation was used in the past, it is no longer recommended. The Critical Aspects box provides overviews of bladder irrigation procedures. For complete procedures,

 Go to Chapter 27, **Procedure 27-7A: Intermittent Bladder or Catheter Irrigation,** and **Procedure 27-7B: Continuous Bladder Irrigation,** in Volume 2.

Removing an Indwelling Catheter

Removing a urinary catheter is a simple task, but you must monitor patients carefully afterward. Gather the necessary supplies, and tell the patient what you are about to do, what she will feel, and that you will need to monitor her urination after removal. Explain that this procedure is usually painless.

Ask the patient to notify you the first time she voids. The catheter may have caused some edema of the urethra, which can interfere with voiding at first. Therefore, you must assess regularly for bladder distention until normal voiding is reestablished. The same is true for patients who have had rectal, perineal, or lower abdominal surgery, which also creates perineal edema.

If a catheter is in place for several weeks and the urine has been draining continuously, the bladder does not stretch and contract as it does in normal voiding. Therefore, the muscle loses tone and the patient may require bladder retraining. Agencies have differing procedures for this; however, one method is to begin clamping the catheter for certain periods of time (e.g., 1 to 4 hours) to allow the bladder to fill, and then releasing the clamp to allow urine to drain from the bladder. This should

stimulate the bladder muscle and improve tone. However, there is limited evidence to support a practice guideline for clamping the catheter before discontinuing it (Griffith & Fernandez, 2007, updated 2009).

For hospitalized patients who have had a urinary catheter for a short time, it may be a good idea to time catheter removal for late at night instead of in the morning. A review of research found that when this was done, patients (on average) held urine in the bladder for a longer period of time before voiding in the morning. This led to larger volume for the first void after the catheter was discontinued. Patients with late night catheter removal were discharged sooner and without having to have the urinary catheter reinserted for urine retention (Griffith & Fernandez, 2007, updated 2009).

For guidelines to follow when removing a retention catheter,

 Go to Chapter 27, **Procedure 27-6: Removing an Indwelling Catheter,** in Volume 2.

After removing the catheter, note and record the time and amount of the first voiding and the appearance of the urine. Compare the patient's intake to output for the next 8 to 12 hours, and palpate the bladder for distention.

KnowledgeCheck 27-8

- What actions should you take before inserting a catheter?
- When caring for a client with an indwelling catheter, you notice sandy particles around the urethral meatus. What should you do?
- How often should the urine collection bag be emptied?

 Go to Chapter 27, **Knowledge Check Response Sheet and Answers,** on the Student Resource Disk or DavisPlus at http://davisplus.fadavis.com/Wilkinson2

CriticalThinking 27-7

You are caring for a patient who had an indwelling catheter removed 12 hours ago. The patient has not voided. What action should you take?

Managing Urinary Incontinence

Because urinary incontinence is so prevalent, you are likely to be called on to deal with this problem in your practice. Most incontinence is managed with skin care and behavioral interventions, but medications are sometimes used (see the box, Home Care: Managing Incontinence).

For a comprehensive list of nursing interventions for managing urinary incontinence,

 Go to Chapter 27, **Clinical Insight 27-2: Caring for Patients with Urinary Incontinence,** in Volume 2.

Perineal Skin Care

Normal urine is acidic. When it remains in contact with the skin, it becomes alkaline, causing dermatitis and

Home Care

Managing Incontinence

➤ Routinely ask clients and families about incontinence. Patients and families often do not raise the issue. Be direct and ask about continence using simple questions in a way that wouldn't embarrass the patient, such as "Do you wear a pad to keep your clothes dry?" "Do you ever wet your clothing?"

➤ If you determine that the client is incontinent, ask follow-up questions to identify the type of incontinence. For example: "Do you sometimes not make it to the toilet in time?" "Do you ever dribble urine when you sneeze or cough?"

➤ Ask where the toilet is and whether the patient can get there easily.

➤ Encourage use of a bladder diary for at least 3 to 7 days, covering routine day-to-day activities as well as atypical situations.

➤ Advise patients to contact a healthcare provider if:

   ➤ They have not been previously evaluated for this problem.

   ➤ The urinary stream is weak.

   ➤ There is burning, fever, chills, pain, or passing little urine for 1 to 2 days.

   ➤ Urine is cloudy, unusually foul-smelling.

   ➤ Discharge occurs from the penis or vagina.

➤ Place a commode near where the patient spends most of his time.

➤ In a two-story house with a toilet on only one floor, place a commode on the other floor in the room where the patient spends most of his time. With a written prescription, Medicare/Medicaid may reimburse this expense.

➤ For some patients, a commode should be placed by the bedside on a large, absorbent, washable mat (to absorb any urine that leaks).

➤ Advise women who have a body mass index (BMI) > 27 to lose weight.

➤ Because many home caregivers are middle-aged or older women, they may have continence problems of their own. Teach them pelvic muscle exercises and the best techniques for lifting and turning the patient in bed. For more information,

 Go to Chapter 27, **Clinical Insight 27-2: Caring for Patients with Urinary Incontinence,** in Volume 2.

---

skin excoriation. It is essential to keep the skin, clothing, and bedding clean and dry, especially after any leakage of urine. Barrier creams may be used for irritated skin; antifungals may be prescribed (e.g., nystatin [Mycostatin]) to prevent or eliminate fungus growth. You may use absorbent products as an adjunct to other control measures, especially for those with intractable UI.

Behavioral Interventions

Nurses have taken the lead in investigating incontinence and treatment options. Aggressive nursing intervention can help to improve patients' quality of life, capacity for physical activity, and self-esteem. It can also help to reduce the cost of healthcare.

Recent guidelines outline five categories of nonpharmacological treatment options nurses commonly provide independently: lifestyle modification, bladder training, pelvic floor muscle rehabilitation, anti-incontinence devices, and supportive interventions (Wyman, 2003). These therapies have been proven to be effective for most patients. They are summarized in the following paragraphs. For detailed guidelines,

 Go to Chapter 27, **Clinical Insight 27-2: Caring for Patients with Urinary Incontinence,** in Volume 2.

Lifestyle Modification. Lifestyle modifications involve dietary changes, increased fluid intake, smoking cessation, avoidance of caffeine, preventing constipation, and physical activity that does not include high-impact exercise. Weight reduction by as little as 5% to 10% alleviates incontinence symptoms and improves the

quality of life. Fluid restriction is recommended only if daily fluid intake is greater than 3000 mL (Finnish Medical Society, 2008).

Bladder Training. The goal of bladder training is to enable the patient to hold increasingly greater volumes of urine in the bladder and to increase the interval between voidings. This involves patient teaching, scheduled voiding, and self-monitoring using a voiding diary. In addition to teaching the mechanisms of urination, teach distraction and relaxation strategies to help inhibit the urge to void. Other techniques include deep breathing and guided imagery.

Scheduled Voiding. This is a form of bladder training involving timed voiding and habit retraining. The client must be mentally and physically capable of self-toileting. Initially the patient may be scheduled to attempt voiding every 2 hours or even more often. As a pattern develops and the person gains greater control, the length of time between voiding may be increased. Scheduled voiding is usually combined with other techniques, including lifestyle adjustments and pelvic muscle exercises.

Pelvic Floor Muscle Rehabilitation. Pelvic floor muscle exercises (PFME) are a mainstay of UI treatment for women. PFME strengthen perineal muscles and help to prevent and treat stress, urge, and mixed UI. **Kegel exercises** are the most commonly used method for preventing and reversing incontinence in women for the first year after giving birth. This approach may also prevent or reduce urinary incontinence in older women and in men undergoing prostate surgery. Cure rates of UI, based on patient diaries, range from 16% to 27%, and improvement rates vary from 48% to 80.7% with PFME alone. To be successful, the patient must do the exercises correctly and practice them daily. A period of 6 to 12 months may be required before treatment is effective.

Vaginal Weight Training. Vaginal weight training is another form of PFME. However, this method has not been shown to produce better outcomes than Kegel exercises (Gamiero, Gamiero, Gamiero, et al., 2010).

Biofeedback. Biofeedback has been advocated by some women as an adjunct to PFME. Electrodes attached to the skin on the perineum provide feedback to the patient about the perineal contraction.

Supportive Interventions. Supportive interventions focus on helping the patient reach the toilet, urinate independently, and perform toileting self-care. Examples include bedside commodes and gait and strength training. When continence cannot be achieved, absorbent products with waterproof coverings are available. Under no circumstances should you refer to these as "diapers." To do so is disrespectful of the patient's dignity.

 Critical**Thinking** 27-8

How do you feel about instructing patients about pelvic floor muscle exercises? Do you think a woman should always provide this instruction? Explain your thinking.

Anti-incontinence Devices

Anti-incontinence devices are designed to reduce the incidence of UI or provide a pathway for urine flow. They include the following:

- An *incontinence pessary,* or intravaginal support device. This is inserted into the vagina to reduce pelvic organ prolapse or pressure on the bladder. This helps to support the bladder neck and prevent UI.
- An *external occlusive device* that is removed before voiding. For women, a urethral meatus covering is used. For men, a penis clamp is a reusable, soft spongy rubber device used to control stress incontinence or dribbling urine, common with enlarged prostate.
- An *internal urethral meatus plug,* which may be used by men and women. This is a disposable, single-use device, typically used for activities that cause stress incontinence.
- A *valved catheter* that allows urine to be drained on a schedule.
- An *indwelling urethral catheter*. This is used as a last resort to control the flow of urine and protect the perineal skin.
- A *bed alarm,* which will waken the patient if incontinence occurs.

- An *external collection device*. Condom catheters, also known as uro-sheaths, are most commonly used for men who have adequate bladder emptying and intact genital skin. To learn how to apply a condom catheter,

 Go to Chapter 27, **Procedure 27-5: Applying an External (Condom) Catheter,** in Volume 2. Also see the Critical Aspects box for a summary of the procedure.

When anti-incontinence devices are used, it is important to observe for vaginal or urinary tract infection, blood in the urine, and vaginal erosion.

Pharmacological and Surgical Interventions

Although it is not the treatment of choice, some forms of incontinence may respond to pharmacological treatment. Estrogen may be prescribed for postmenopausal women when incontinence is secondary to atrophic vaginitis. For urge incontinence, medication may be used to relax the detrusor muscle and increase bladder capacity (e.g., anticholinergics, smooth-muscle relaxants, calcium-channel blockers, and antidepressants). For stress incontinence, drugs may be given to improve urethral sphincter muscle functioning (e.g., the decongestant phenylpropanolamine [Triaminic]).

When incontinence is caused by cystocele, rectocele, or an enlarged prostate gland, surgical techniques may be appropriate (e.g., bladder neck suspension to create a normal angle between the bladder and urethra, and prostatectomy).

Managing Enuresis

Occasional wetting (called *enuresis*) is entirely normal in children even in the early school years, especially when the child is intensely involved in a game, test, or another absorbing activity, or when restricted from using the toilet. Parents should accept such events calmly and not punish the child (see the box, Home Care: Managing Enuresis in Children).

Children, especially older ones, can be embarrassed by *nocturnal enuresis,* or bedwetting, not to mention the inconvenience it poses. Young children may feel anxious about using the bathroom in a clinic, hospital, or any unfamiliar environment. They may be especially anxious about using a bedpan. Also, be aware that the stress of an illness or hospitalization may cause a child to regress in his ability to toilet independently. You may need to schedule regular trips to the bathroom and to watch for nonverbal cues that the child needs to void.

 Critical**Thinking** 27-9

What treatment options for incontinence have you seen used in your clinical experience? What options do you believe should be used more frequently? Less frequently? Explain your thinking.

Caring for a Patient with a Urinary Diversion

A patient with a urinary diversion requires physical and psychological care. Initially you will care for the ostomy. However, the goal is for the patient to become comfortable with his changed body and to assume self-care.

Patients experience a variety of reactions to the stoma. Patients with continent ostomies are usually more comfortable with their stoma because of the control it offers while avoiding the embarrassment, odor, and inconvenience of UI. Your attitude and willingness to discuss the body changes associated with an ostomy will help your patient begin his adjustment. In many communities, the local ostomy association has counselors available to visit patients, discuss the psychological changes associated with a urinary diversion, and help them with physical care of the stoma. Most counselors are adept because they too have ostomies. They are able to share practical and personal information with patients based on their own experience with similar challenges.

Nursing care of a patient with a urinary diversion should begin with a thorough assessment. A healthy stoma ranges in color from deep pink to brick red, regardless of skin color, and is shiny and moist at all times. A pale, dusky, or black stoma often indicates inadequate blood supply. Immediately document and report such findings to the surgeon. Assess the skin surrounding the stoma for signs of irritation, such as redness, tenderness, skin breakdown, and drainage. A moisture-proof skin barrier is usually placed around the stoma to protect surrounding skin. More extensive discussion about stoma care is covered in Chapter 28.

VOL 2 Go to Chapter 28, **Procedure 28-6: Changing an Ostomy Appliance,** in Volume 2.

Home Care

Managing Enuresis in Children

➤ Reassure parents that in most cases, loving acceptance and passage of time provide the cure.

➤ Cover the mattress with plastic.

➤ Limit fluid intake in the evening.

➤ Wake the child to urinate just before the parents go to sleep.

➤ Use a bed alarm that wakens the child when wetting occurs. Over time, this conditioning may be effective; however, once the alarm is removed, the child may relapse into enuresis.

➤ If bedwetting persists into the school-age years, the child should receive a thorough medical evaluation to rule out underlying disease processes.

➤ Parents should plan to bathe the child in the morning rather than at bedtime to minimize urine odor.

➤ Medication can be effective for managing nocturnal enuresis for children younger than age 10. Medication is helpful when the child is not sleeping at home.

For guidelines for caring for a patient with a urinary diversion,

 Go to Chapter 27, **Clinical Insight 27-3: Caring for Patients with Urinary Diversions,** in Volume 2.

 Go to Chapter 27, **Resources for Caregivers and Health Professionals,** on the Student Resource Disk or DavisPlus at http://davisplus.fadavis.com/Wilkinson2

 Suggested Readings: Go to Chapter 27, **Reading More About Urinary Elimination,** on the Student Resource Disk or DavisPlus at http://davisplus.fadavis.com/Wilkinson2

 Bibliography: Go to Volume 2, Bibliography.

Nursing Care Plan

Client Data

Desmond Washington, a 69-year-old man, comes to the clinic 4 weeks after having a prostatectomy for prostate cancer. He was discharged from the hospital on postoperative day 4 and went home with an indwelling urinary catheter. The catheter was removed at his last visit, 9 days after surgery.

Mr. Washington is meticulously groomed. He is friendly, greeting other patients in the clinic and chatting with the clinic personnel. When his nurse brings him to an exam room and asks how he feels, he says, "I saw the sun come up today. I appreciate that more now. The good Lord has given me a new lease on life, and I intend to use it!" His nurse continues, "That's great, Mr. Washington. How have you been doing since the catheter was removed?" Mr. Washington's smile fades. He lowers his voice and says, "You know, I think that's the worst part of this whole thing. I hate wearing these diapers—they make me feel, well, like an old man. I'm certainly not ready for this."

The nurse continues, "Do you have *any* control of your urine?" Mr. Washington explains, "I may go for hours and stay dry, and then it seems for no reason, I wet myself. Take yesterday, for example. I was sitting on the sofa watching the ball game when someone came to the door. I got up to answer the door, and all of a sudden, I felt wet. I didn't even have anything to drink so I could make it through the afternoon and stay dry. And if I cough? Forget it. Can something be done so I can hold my urine again?"

Nursing Diagnosis

Stress Urinary Incontinence related to disruption of the urinary sphincter and related pelvic muscles by surgery as evidenced by client report of involuntary loss of urine with increased intra-abdominal pressure.

NOC Outcomes	Individualized Goals/Expected Outcomes
Urinary Continence (0502) Urinary Elimination (0503)	*By the next visit, Mr. Washington will:* 1. Describe three things he can do that will help regain urinary continence. 2. Explain three interventions to cope with leaked urine. 3. Report that he is drinking adequate amounts of fluids during the day.

Nursing Care Plan (continued)

Nursing Interventions and Activities	Rationale

NIC Interventions

Urinary Elimination Management (0590)
Urinary Incontinence Care (0610)

Nursing Activities

1. Obtain midstream voided urine specimen for urinalysis.

   Urinary tract infection can cause or worsen incontinence (Nazarko, 2008; Urinary Continence Guideline Panel [UCGP], 1992; Wilde & Getliffe, 2006).

2. Identify factors that contribute to Mr. Washington's incontinence by using an incontinence diary.

   Identifying activities or other factors that cause loss of urine control can guide specific interventions. A diary facilitates monitoring over time and can identify patterns that could otherwise be missed (National Institute for Health and Clinical Excellence [NICE], 2006).

3. Teach pelvic floor muscle exercises (PFME).

   PFME strengthen pelvic muscles and enhance sphincter control. They have been shown to increase urinary continence without side effects in men who have undergone prostatectomy (National Collaborating Centre for Women's and Children's Health, 2006; NICE, 2006; Sampselle, Wyman, & Thomas, 2006; van Kempen, De Weerdt, & van Poppel, 2000).

4. Use biofeedback when needed in conjunction with PFME training to help Mr. Washington isolate pelvic floor muscles.

   Biofeedback allows clients to receive auditory or visual (or both) cues when the proper muscles are contracted, so they learn what the proper muscle contraction feels like. Biofeedback also allows the nurse or therapist to objectively measure strength of contractions (Burgio, Goode, Urban, et al., 2007; Hunter, Moore, Cody, et al., 2004; UCGP, 1992).

5. Teach timed voiding. Have Mr. Washington void on a schedule of every 2 hours.

   Voiding on a schedule of every 2 hours can reduce the amount of urine in the bladder, thus reducing the likelihood of leakage with activities of daily living (National Collaborating Centre for Women's and Children's Health, 2006; NICE, 2006; Sampselle, Wyman, Thomas, 2006; UCGP, 1992).

6. Explain the need to drink adequate fluids and *not* limit fluids in an effort to prevent incontinence. Help Mr. Washington identify ways to drink a minimum of 1500 mL/day.

   Adequate fluid intake is important to maintain dilute urine, which is less irritating to the bladder; to maintain systemic hydration; and to reduce the risk for constipation, which can contribute to urinary incontinence (Dowling-Castronovo & Bradway, 2003; IOM, 2004; UCGP, 1992).

7. Assist the client in selecting appropriate absorbent products that collect urine strictly for temporary management while continence management is ongoing.

   Proper absorbent garments and pads can collect and trap urine, keep skin clean and dry, reduce odor, and minimize the risk of soiling accidents (NICE, 2006; UCGP, 1992).

(continued on next page)

Nursing Care Plan (continued)

Nursing Interventions and Activities	Rationale

Nursing Activities

8. Help the client develop a personal hygiene routine that will maintain skin integrity.

   Proper hygiene will reduce the risk of skin irritation and infection. Use warm (not hot) water, and pat (don't scrub) the perineal area. A barrier cream will repel fluid and protect the skin from urine.

9. Offer referral to a support group.

   Support groups provide a sense of community and enhance problem-solving skills of members. Mr. Washington may feel less embarrassment when he discovers that others share his problems.

10. Explain that urinary incontinence is common after prostatectomy, but that it may be only temporary.

    Urinary incontinence can be a troubling complication of prostatectomy for many men. Fortunately, it usually resolves with active management within 6 to 12 months of surgery (Burgio, Goode, Urban, et al., 2007).

Nursing Care Plan (continued)

There are many treatment recommendations that are not supported by research. Anecdotally, they may work for some clients. These include reducing caffeine consumption; eliminating bladder irritants, such as artificial sweeteners, spicy foods, and citrus from the diet; losing weight; and quitting smoking. In addition, it is important for nurses to understand the pathophysiology of urinary incontinence differs between men and women and that interventions that are successful in women may or may not be equally successful in men.

Evaluation

At the end of the visit, Mr. Washington said, "I didn't know there were things I could do about the leaking urine. Before surgery, all I cared about was getting rid of the cancer. I don't need a support group for me but maybe I'll lead one!" Mr. Washington had been placing folded paper towels in his underwear to collect urine because he thought absorbent products were too expensive, but with guidance from his nurse, he identified products he could afford. He liked that they would not be visible through his clothing.

At Mr. Washington's next visit, the nurse will review the initial collaborative goals and stated outcomes and perform a client assessment to determine whether the goals were reached in the stated time frame.

Mr. Washington currently has a positive attitude and is focused on "beating" his cancer first and on managing complications of surgery second. As time passes, incontinence may persist and may become more frustrating for him once he is fully recovered from surgery. Mr. Washington initially declined referral to a support group, but he may be more interested in joining one in the future for help dealing with long-term consequences of prostatectomy.

References

Burgio, K. L., Goode, P., Urban, M., et al. (2007). Postoperative biofeedback assisted behavioral training to decrease prostatectomy incontinence: A randomized, controlled trial. *Journal of Urology, 175*(1), 196–210.

Dowling-Castronovo, A., & Bradway, C. (2003). Urinary incontinence. In M. Mezey, T. Fulmer, I. Abraham, & D. A. Zwicker (Eds.), *Geriatric nursing protocols for best practice* (pp. 83–98). New York: Springer.

Hunter, K. F., Moore, K. N., Cody, D. J., & Glazener, C. M. (2007). Conservative management for postprostatectomy urinary incontinence (Cochrane Review). In *The Cochrane Library*. Chichester, UK: John Wiley & Sons.

National Collaborating Centre for Women's and Children's Health. (2006, October). Urinary incontinence: The management of urinary incontinence in women. London (UK): *Royal College of Obstetricians and Gynaecologists* (RCOG, 221). In National Guideline Clearinghouse Summary. Retrieved on May 12, 2009, from http://www.guideline.gov/summary/summary.aspx?view_id=1&doc_id=9926

National Institute for Health and Clinical Excellence (NICE). (2006). Urinary incontinence. The management of urinary incontinence in women. Quick reference guide. National Collaborating Centre for Women's and Children's Health, Retrieved on May 12, 2009, from http://www.nice.org.uk/nicemedia/pdf/word/CG40quickrefguide1006.pdf

Nazarko, L. (2008). Reducing the risk of catheter-related urinary tract infection. *British Journal of Nursing, 17*(16), 1002–1010.

Urinary Continence Guideline Panel (UCGP). (1992). Urinary incontinence in adults. Rockville, MD: Agency for Healthcare Policy and Research, Public Health Service, U.S. Department of Health and Human Services.

VanKampen, M., DeWeerdt, W., VanPoppel, H., DeRidder, D., Feys, H., & Baert, L. (2000, January 8). Effect of pelvic-floor re-education on duration and degree of incontinence after radical prostatectomy: A randomised controlled trial. *The Lancet, 355*, 98–102.

Wilde, M. H. & Getliffe, K. (2006). Urinary catheter care for older adults. *Annals of Long-term Care: Clinical Care and Aging, 8*(14), Retrieved on May 11, 2009, from http://www.annalsoflongtermcare.com/article/6051.

Care Map

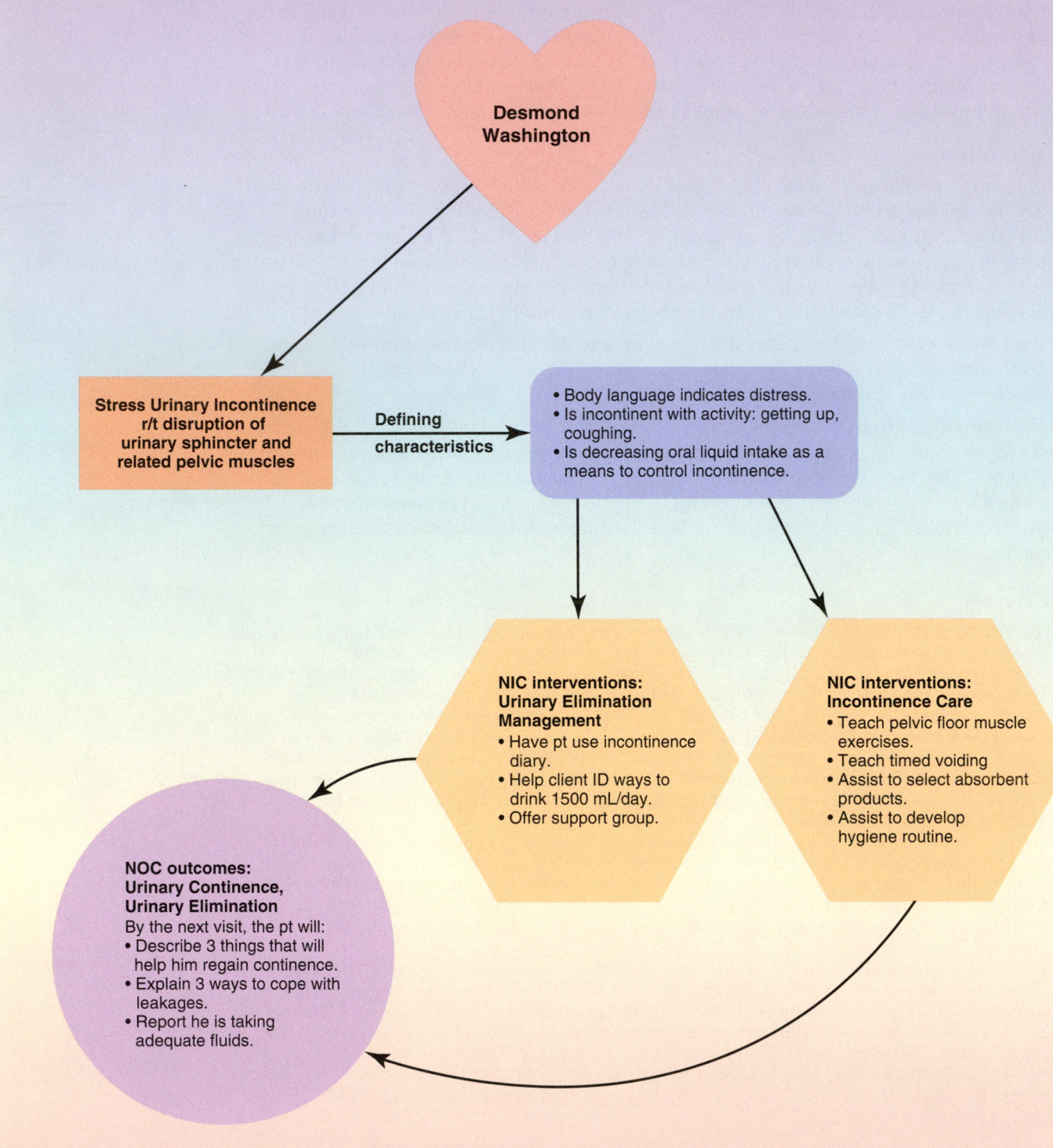

Desmond Washington

Stress Urinary Incontinence r/t disruption of urinary sphincter and related pelvic muscles

Defining characteristics

- Body language indicates distress.
- Is incontinent with activity: getting up, coughing.
- Is decreasing oral liquid intake as a means to control incontinence.

NIC interventions: Urinary Elimination Management
- Have pt use incontinence diary.
- Help client ID ways to drink 1500 mL/day.
- Offer support group.

NIC interventions: Incontinence Care
- Teach pelvic floor muscle exercises.
- Teach timed voiding
- Assist to select absorbent products.
- Assist to develop hygiene routine.

NOC outcomes: Urinary Continence, Urinary Elimination
By the next visit, the pt will:
- Describe 3 things that will help him regain continence.
- Explain 3 ways to cope with leakages.
- Report he is taking adequate fluids.

Key:
- Nursing diagnosis
- Defining characteristics
- NIC interventions and nursing activities
- NOC outcomes

CHAPTER 28

Bowel Elimination

Learning Outcomes

After completing this chapter, you should be able to:

➤ Identify the basic structures and functions of the gastrointestinal system.

➤ Discuss factors that affect bowel elimination.

➤ Describe normal bowel elimination.

➤ Differentiate among the various types of bowel diversions.

➤ Discuss common bowel elimination problems.

➤ Identify appropriate nursing history questions to assess bowel elimination problems.

➤ Perform a physical examination focused on bowel elimination.

➤ List and describe diagnostic tests used to identify bowel elimination problems.

➤ State nursing diagnoses associated with altered bowel elimination.

➤ Describe nursing interventions that promote normal bowel elimination.

➤ Provide care for clients experiencing alterations in bowel elimination.

➤ Discuss nursing care associated with the use of bowel diversions.

Meet Your Patients

You are assigned to care for Mrs. Zeno, a frail 96-year-old woman who broke her hip last month after a fall at home. Mrs. Zeno was hospitalized for surgical repair of her hip and is now in a skilled nursing facility (SNF) for rehabilitation. The nursing assistive personnel (NAP) informs you that Mrs. Zeno has eaten poorly for the past week, eating less than half of the food on her meal trays and refusing the protein supplements that were added to her diet. Mrs. Zeno tells you she would like to go home: "I have my routine and the foods I like. I think I'd be better there." As you review the chart in preparation for clinical, you note that she has not had a bowel movement (BM) for 3 days. Her last BM was small and very hard.

What additional assessments should you perform? What, if anything, is of concern about her bowel pattern?

What actions should you take with Mrs. Zeno?

In this chapter, we discuss bowel function and common disorders associated with bowel elimination. You will gain theoretical and practical knowledge to help you answer those questions and provide care for clients with bowel elimination concerns.

Theoretical **Knowledge**
knowing why

Bowel elimination is a normal process by which we eliminate waste products from our bodies. To understand bowel elimination, you will need knowledge of the anatomy and physiology of the gastrointestinal tract.

What Are the Anatomical Structures of the Gastrointestinal Tract?

The gastrointestinal (GI) tract is a smooth-muscle tube approximately 5 m (15 ft) long, running through the body from the mouth to the anus. Its major functions are to digest and absorb the nutrients present in food and to eliminate food waste products as feces (Fig. 28-1). Feces consist primarily of bacteria, insoluble fiber, and other material that was not absorbed during passage through the GI tract. The structures of the GI tract are the mouth, esophagus, stomach, small intestine, large intestine, rectum, and anus.

The Mouth

Mechanical digestion begins in the mouth with **mastication,** or chewing. Food is torn into small pieces, mashed, moistened with saliva, and formed into a bolus that is then swallowed into the esophagus. The mouth contains glands that secrete enzymes, such as ptyalin and salivary amylase, which begin the digestion of carbohydrates.

The Esophagus

The bolus of food travels through the esophagus to the stomach. The esophagus is a tube of smooth muscle, which alternately contracts and relaxes in waves of **peristalsis** to push the bolus toward the stomach. The bolus travels the length of the esophagus (about 25 cm, or 10 in.) in about 15 seconds. The *cardiac sphincter* (also called the *gastroesophageal sphincter*) relaxes to allow food to pass into the stomach. When the cardiac sphincter is constricted, it prevents acidic stomach contents from flowing back into the esophagus.

The Stomach

The stomach is a distensible sac that extends from the esophagus to the small intestine. The stomach stores food while it churns and mixes it, providing further mechanical breakdown. Chemical digestion continues in the stomach, which secretes hydrochloric acid (HCl), a protein-digesting enzyme called *pepsin,* and *gastric lipase,* an enzyme that begins the digestion of lipids. The stomach lining also secretes a mucous coating that protects the stomach from being corroded by HCl. Food

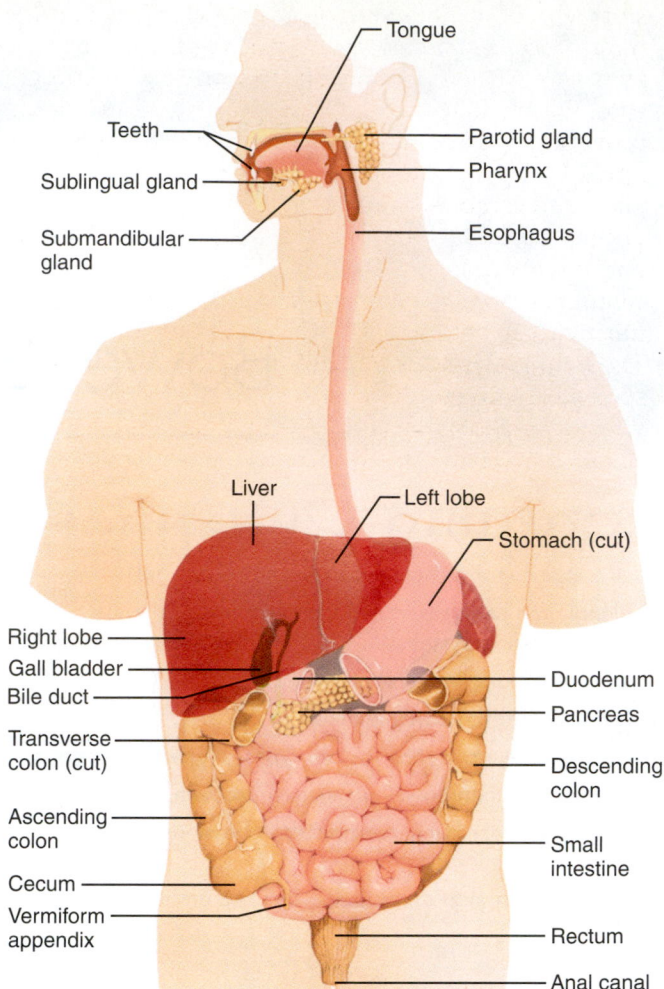

FIGURE 28-1 The gastrointestinal tract extends from the mouth to the anus. The major functions of the GI system are to digest and absorb the nutrients in food and to eliminate food waste products as feces. (*Source:* Scanlon, V., & Sanders, T. (2007). *Essentials of anatomy and physiology* (5th ed., p. 371). Philadelphia: F. A. Davis. Used with permission.)

remains in the stomach an average of 4 hours. Food leaves the stomach as a liquid, called **chyme.**

The Small Intestine

The small intestine is a folded, twisted, and coiled tube that connects the stomach and the large intestine. About 2.5 cm (1 in.) in diameter and approximately 6 m (20 ft) long if fully extended, it occupies most of the abdominal cavity. Most digestion and absorption of food occurs in the small intestine, with the aid of enzymes from the pancreas and bile from the gallbladder. Chyme travels slowly, by peristalsis, through the small intestine; peristalsis halts periodically to allow for absorption. The small intestine consists of three segments: the duodenum, jejunum, and ileum.

- The **duodenum** is the first section of the small intestine. It is a C-shaped tube that branches off from the stomach, about 30 to 60 cm (1 to 2 ft) long. The duodenum processes chyme by mixing it and adding enzymes. The bile duct and main pancreatic duct both enter the small intestine at the level of the duodenum, providing bile from the liver and gallbladder to digest lipids and pancreatic enzymes to digest lipids, proteins, and carbohydrates.

■ The **jejunum** is the coiled midsection of the small intestine. It is about 1.8 to 2.4 m (6 to 8 ft) long and forms the connection between the duodenum and ileum. Its major function is to absorb carbohydrates and proteins.

■ The **ileum** joins the small and large intestine. It is responsible for absorption of fats; bile salts; and some vitamins, minerals, and water. However, nutrients are absorbed mainly in the duodenum and jejunum.

As mentioned previously, the total length of the small intestine, if it were stretched out, is approximately 6 m (20 ft), but in the body it is much shorter because it is folded to provide a vast surface area for absorption. The inner wall of the small intestine is covered by millions of tiny fingerlike projections called **villi** (Fig. 28-2). The villi are covered with even tinier projections, called **microvilli**. The combination of folds, villi, and microvilli increases the surface area of the small intestine greatly, facilitating absorption of nutrients.

The Large Intestine

The **large intestine,** also known as the **colon,** is larger in diameter than the small intestine (6.3 cm, or 2.5 in.) but shorter in length—about 1.5 to 1.8 m (5 to 6 ft). It extends from the ileum of the small intestine to the anus. It contains seven segments: the cecum, ascending colon, transverse colon, descending colon, sigmoid colon, rectum, and anus (Fig. 28-3).

Undigested food entering the first portion of the large intestine, the **cecum,** consists mostly of cellulose and water. The connection of the ileum to the cecum is controlled by the **ileocecal valve.** Under most conditions, the valve prevents backflow of chyme from the colon into the small intestine. The **appendix** is a small, fingerlike appendage off the cecum. It is believed to be a **vestigial organ**—one whose significance has diminished over time—however, it is lined with lymphatic tissue and may play a role in immune function.

The next three segments, the **ascending, transverse,** and **descending colon,** ring the small intestine. The **sigmoid colon** is a final, small segment of bowel that twists medially and downward to connect with the rectum and anus.

The colon secretes mucus, which facilitates smooth passage of stool, and absorbs water, some vitamins, and minerals. Approximately 80% of the fluid that enters the colon is reabsorbed along its passage. Normal flora in the colon aid in the digestive process. These bacteria are

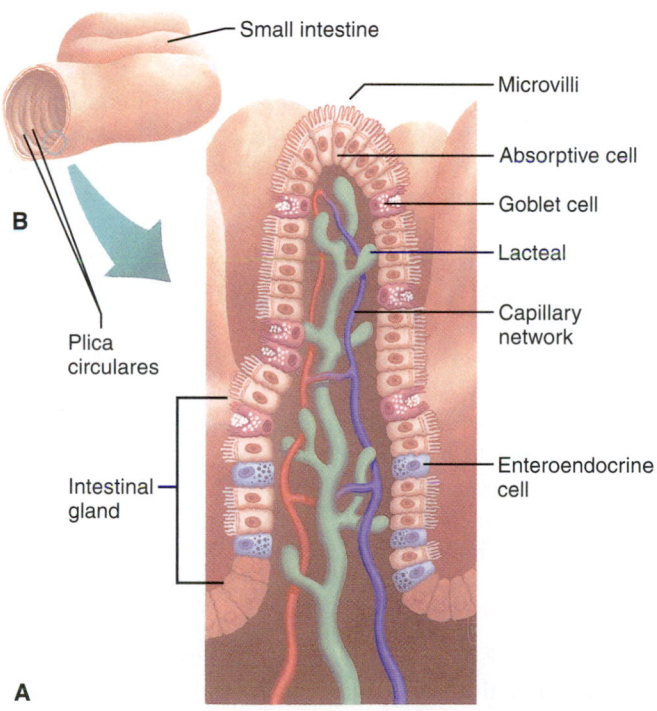

FIGURE 28-2 The small intestine is highly folded, providing a vast surface area for absorption of nutrients. The microvilli form a brush border, which is the site of most nutrient absorption. *A,* Section through the small intestine showing the plica circulares (circular folds) of the mucosa and submucosa. *B,* Microscopic view of a villus showing the internal structure. (*Source:* Scanlon, V., & Sanders, T. (2007). *Essentials of anatomy and physiology* (5th ed., p. 383). Philadelphia: F. A. Davis. Used with permission.)

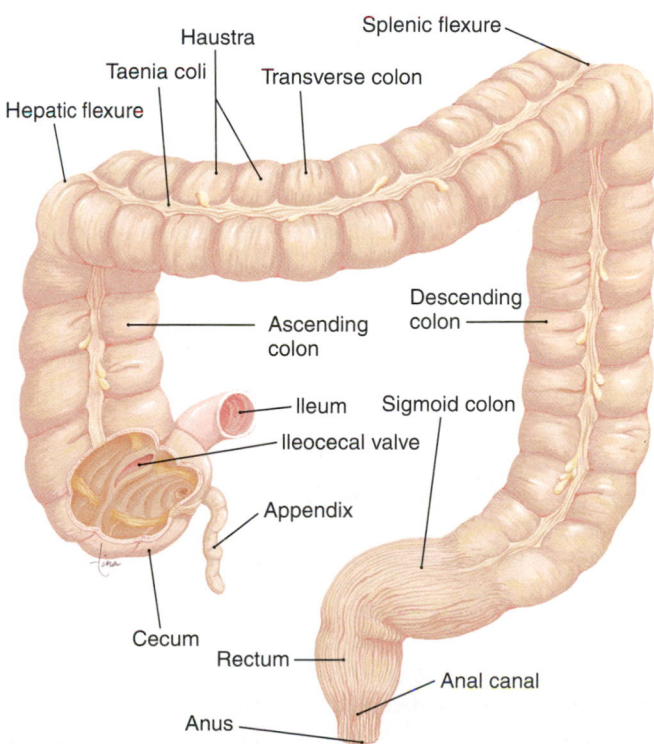

FIGURE 28-3 The large intestine shown in anterior view. The term *flexure* means a turn or bend. (*Source:* Scanlon, V., & Sanders, T. (2007). *Essentials of anatomy and physiology* (5th ed., p. 385). Philadelphia: F. A. Davis. Used with permission.)

responsible for producing vitamin K and several of the B vitamins.

The large intestine has two sets of muscles that give it a puckered appearance. Longitudinal muscles, known as **taenia coli,** run lengthwise along the colon surface. Tension in these muscles gathers up the colon into pouched segments known as **haustra** all along its length (see Fig. 28-3). In addition, the colon wall contains circular muscles that, together with the taenia coli, cause the colon to expand and contract in length and width to achieve haustral churning, peristalsis, and mass peristalsis.

- **Haustral churning** moves digestive contents around within each haustra. This action promotes reabsorption of water.
- **Peristalsis** continues throughout the length of the large intestine, where it propels intestinal contents toward the rectum and anus.
- **Mass peristalsis** is a powerful contraction along a lengthy segment of bowel. It is facilitated by the **gastrocolic reflex,** which is triggered by food entering the stomach and small intestine. Mass movements usually occur only one to three times each day, and they are responsible for most of the propulsion of the contents in the transverse and sigmoid colon.

The Rectum and Anus

The **rectum** is approximately 15 cm (6 in.) long and is continuous with the **anus,** the last 2.5 cm (1 in.) of the colon. A highly vascular folded tube, the rectum is free of waste products until just before defecation.

The anus has two ringlike muscles that function as sphincters. The **internal sphincter** involuntarily relaxes and opens when stool is present in the rectum. The **external sphincter** is under voluntary control. Voluntary relaxation of the external sphincter allows stool to be expelled from the body (Fig. 28-4). The anus is highly vascular. Chronic pressure on the veins within the anal canal, as with prolonged sitting or retained feces, can cause **hemorrhoids** (distended blood vessels within or protruding from the anus).

KnowledgeCheck 28-1

- What are the major functions of the small intestine and large intestine?
- How do the rectum and anus control elimination of feces from the body?

 Go to Chapter 28, **Knowledge Check Response Sheet and Answers,** on the Student Resource Disk or DavisPlus at http://davisplus.fadavis.com/Wilkinson2

 Critical**Thinking** 28-1

Based on your knowledge that hemorrhoids are dilated blood vessels in the anal canal, what symptoms would you expect a patient with hemorrhoids to exhibit?

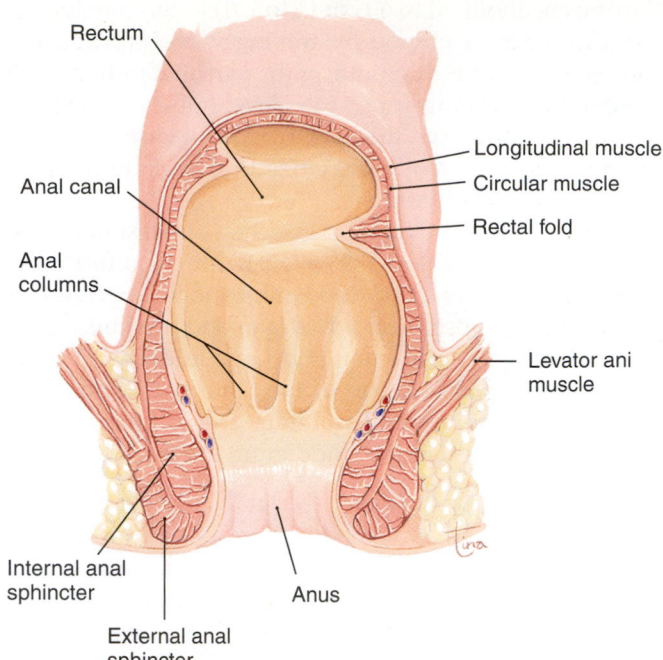

FIGURE 28-4 Internal and external anal sphincters shown in a frontal section through the lower rectum and anal canal. (*Source:* From Scanlon, V., & Sanders, T. (2007). *Essentials of anatomy and physiology* (5th ed., p. 387). Philadelphia: F. A. Davis. Used with permission.)

How Does the Bowel Eliminate Waste?

As you have learned, reabsorption of water from chyme in the large intestine produces a semisolid mass known as **feces.** Feces are a mixture of fiber and undigested food, shed epithelial cells, inorganic material (e.g., calcium and phosphates), bacteria, and water. Small amounts of fat may be present. Feces are usually brown in color because **bile salts,** which aid in the digestion of fat, are excreted in the feces. Bile is normally golden yellow, but the action of bacteria in the GI tract changes the color to brown. Bacteria are also responsible for the odor of feces.

Flatus, or gas, is formed in the digestive process. Some is swallowed air that accompanies the intake of food. A small portion diffuses from blood into the GI tract. However, most of the gas is created by bacterial fermentation in the colon. Flatus is a mixture of nitrogen, carbon dioxide, hydrogen, methane, and hydrogen sulfide.

The Process of Defecation

The process by which the bowel eliminates waste is called **defecation.** When fecal material reaches the rectum and causes it to distend, (a) stretch receptors are stimulated to start contraction of the sigmoid colon and rectal muscles, and (b) the internal anal sphincter relaxes. At the same time, sensory impulses transmitted to the central nervous system (CNS) produce a conscious urge to defecate. We respond to this signal by voluntarily contracting our diaphragmatic and abdominal muscles to increase downward pressure, while at the same time relaxing the external anal sphincter. These actions allow feces to be propelled through the anus. If we ignore the signal to defecate, the reflexive contractions ease for a few minutes, until mass peristalsis occurs again.

A person can increase the pressure to expel feces by contracting the abdominal muscles (straining) while maintaining a closed airway (e.g., holding the breath). This is called the **Valsalva maneuver.** Although it assists with the passage of stool, you should caution clients with heart disease, glaucoma, increased intracranial pressure, or a new surgical wound to avoid the Valsalva maneuver because it increases pressure within the abdominal cavity, raises blood pressure, and is associated with an increased risk for cardiac arrhythmias.

Normal Defecation Patterns

Grocery stores, pharmacies, and even convenience stores may have half an aisle or more of products devoted to bowel function. Some products promote bowel movements (BMs), and others treat diarrhea. All claim to return the consumer to "regularity." The sheer volume of products suggests that bowel function problems are common. Nevertheless, many people avoid the topic of bowel elimination—it is not typically something they chat about with their neighbors. As a result, many patients have unanswered questions about their bowel function and may turn to you for information.

Part of the confusion about bowel function is that there is a wide range of "normal." The frequency of BMs may range from several times per day to once a week. As long as the person passes stools without excessive urgency (needing to rush to the toilet), with minimal effort and no straining, without blood loss, and without the use of laxatives, you can regard bowel function as normal.

Normally stool is approximately 75% water and 25% solid when expelled. This combination yields a soft, formed semisolid. If passage through the colon is slowed, more water is reabsorbed from the feces. The stool becomes dry and hard, requiring more effort to pass. If transit time through the colon is faster than normal, less water is reabsorbed, and stools are watery.

Critical**Thinking** 28-2

- Based on your knowledge of normal bowel function, how would you describe Mrs. Zeno's ("Meet Your Patient") bowel function? Is it normal or abnormal?
- What additional information, if any, do you need to know to answer this question?

What Factors Affect Bowel Elimination?

There is a wide range of acceptable frequency for BMs. Each person develops a pattern that is based on several factors, discussed in the sections immediately following.

Developmental Stage

Bowel elimination patterns change throughout the life span.

Infants. During the first few days of life, the term newborn passes meconium through the anus. **Meconium** is green-black, tarry, and sticky and is formed by swallowed mucous, hair, and amniotic fluid. It has no odor. Stools transition to a yellow-green color over the next few days. After that, the appearance of the feces depends largely on the type of feeding the infant receives. Breastfed babies pass golden yellow stools, whereas formula-fed babies pass tan stools. Initially babies defecate frequently, usually after each feeding—especially when they are breastfeeding. The stools tend to be watery while the large intestine is still immature. Gradually normal flora develop in the colon, and stools become firmer and less frequent.

Children. The ability to control defecation typically develops at about 2 to 3 years of age. Toilet training requires neural and muscular control as well as conscious effort. The child must be aware of the urge to defecate, be able to maintain closure of the external anal sphincter while getting to the toilet, and be able to remove clothing. When toddlers become engrossed in play, they sometimes ignore the need to move their bowels, and soiling is common. As children mature, they gradually learn to gain more control over defecation. In fact, school-age children and adolescents often delay defecation until they have come home or have completed an activity.

Adults. The bowel pattern set in childhood normally continues into late adulthood if the client consumes adequate fiber and fluid and engages in regular physical activity. However, peristalsis, intestinal smooth muscle tone, perineal muscle tone, and sphincter control normally decrease with aging. These physiological processes can contribute to bowel elimination problems among older adults, especially if they decrease their activity and fiber intake.

Personal and Sociocultural Factors

Privacy is important to most people, as is sufficient time to have a bowel movement without feeling the need to hurry. Clients working in fast-paced jobs may have difficulty even consciously recognizing the need to defecate, and some habitually ignore the need, promoting bowel dysfunction. Parents and caregivers of infants and toddlers may postpone their own toileting needs because of fear of leaving the children alone. Some clients are acutely embarrassed by the thought that anyone might realize they are having a bowel movement and will wait until they are entirely alone before even entering the bathroom.

Have you ever heard the following phrase: "He puts his stress in his gut"? Stress has a major influence on motility of the GI tract. It may cause diarrhea or constipation, and it is a primary risk factor in the development of *irritable bowel syndrome*, a disorder associated with bloating, pain, and altered bowel function.

Nutrition, Hydration, and Activity Level

Nutrition, hydration, and activity all relate to bowel function.

Foods and Fiber. As noted earlier, regular intake of food promotes peristalsis. People who eat on a regular schedule are likely to develop a regular pattern of defecation. Irregular eating creates irregular bowel elimination. Adequate intake of high-fiber promotes peristalsis and defecation by increasing bulk. Bulky foods absorb fluids and increase stool mass. The increased mass stretches bowel walls, initiating peristalsis and the defecation reflex. Most people should have at least five servings of high-fiber foods each day. Examples are fresh fruits and berries; dried fruits; vegetables (especially raw); whole-grain cereal products; flaxseed; popcorn; and dried beans, peas, and legumes.

Other foods have specific effects in the bowel. For example, the active bacteria in yogurt stimulate peristalsis, while at the same time promoting healing of intestinal infections. Low-fiber foods, such as pasta and other simple carbohydrates and lean meats, slow peristalsis. Foods like broccoli, onions, and beans lead to excess gas in many people. Spicy foods may also cause gas, as well as more frequent bowel movements.

Dietary Supplements. Dietary supplements can also affect bowel function. For example, calcium supplements cause constipation in many clients, whereas magnesium loosens stools. Supplemental vitamin C softens stools and, in high doses, may cause diarrhea in sensitive clients.

Fluids. A minimum of six to eight 8-ounce glasses (1500 to 2000 mL) of fluid per day is required to promote healthful bowel function. Inadequate fluid intake or excessive fluid loss, as in diarrhea or vomiting, slows peristalsis and leads to dry, hard stools that are difficult to pass (Wilson, 2005). Excessive fluid intake (especially beverages with high sugar content) may lead to rapid passage through the colon and soft or watery stools. Different types of fluids have varying effects on sensitive individuals. For instance, consuming large amounts of milk may cause constipation in some people. Coffee promotes peristalsis in many clients and may even cause loose stools in sensitive clients.

Activity. Physical activity seems to stimulate peristalsis and bowel elimination. In addition, sedentary people are likely to have weaker abdominal muscles. Clients with health concerns that limit activity (e.g., shortness of breath, pain, or required bed rest) often experience constipation.

Medications

Many medications may affect peristalsis. All oral medicines have the potential to affect the function of the GI tract. Examples include the following:

- *Antacids,* often used for heartburn, neutralize stomach acid but may slow peristalsis.

- *Aspirin and other nonsteroidal anti-inflammatory drugs (NSAIDs),* such as naproxen and ibuprofen, irritate the stomach. Repeated use can lead to ulceration of the stomach or duodenum.

- *Antibiotics* given to combat infection decrease the normal flora in the colon. The result is often diarrhea. Bacterial populations can be maintained with supplements of probiotics (e.g., acidophilus) or daily consumption of yogurt.

- *Iron,* a common mineral supplement, is available as an over-the-counter (OTC) medication and is often prescribed for the treatment of anemia. Iron has an astringent effect on the bowel and is notorious for causing constipation and changing stool color to black. It also causes nausea when taken when there is no food in the stomach.

- *Pain medications,* particularly opioids (narcotics), slow peristalsis and are associated with a high incidence of constipation.

- *Antimotility drugs,* such as diphenoxylate (Lomotil), may be used to treat diarrhea. They work by slowing peristalsis.

- *Laxatives* are used to treat constipation. In general, laxatives work by stimulating peristalsis (see Box 28-1). They come in many forms and are frequently abused by people who self-medicate with OTC drugs. They may become dependent on them, requiring ever-increasing dosages until the intestine fails to work properly.

Box 28-2 lists medications commonly associated with constipation.

Surgery and Procedures

Clients undergoing anesthesia and surgery often experience sluggish bowel elimination. The delay in bowel elimination may be caused by a variety of circumstances:

Anesthesia. General anesthesia (which renders the patient unconscious) and analgesics (administered preoperatively and postoperatively for pain) slow bowel motility. Spinal anesthesia and epidural anesthesia are less likely to cause this effect.

Stress. Regardless of the type of anesthesia, most clients find surgery a stressful event. As you may recall from Chapter 25, if stress activates the general adaptation syndrome (GAS), autonomic nervous system and endocrine responses ensue. Among those responses is a slowing of peristalsis.

Manipulation of the Bowel During Surgery. Abdominal or pelvic surgery in which the bowel is manipulated may result in a **paralytic ileus,** a cessation of bowel peristalsis. Although peristalsis halts, the bowel continues to produce secretions. Without peristalsis, secretions remain stagnant, causing distention and discomfort. To decrease the complications of paralytic ileus, patients who have

BOX 28-1 ■ Types of Laxatives

- ***Stool softeners*** enable moisture and fat to penetrate the stool, thereby softening it and making it easier to pass. Example: docusate sodium. Effectiveness of stool softeners in relieving chronic constipation is being questioned, but they are still in use.

- ***Osmotic laxatives*** work by drawing water into the bowel from surrounding tissue, resulting in bowel distention. Examples: polyethylene glycol, lactulose

- ***Lubricant laxatives*** coat the stool and the GI tract with a thin waterproof layer. Mineral oil is an example. Because the lubricant coats the entire GI tract, it may interfere with the absorption of nutrients. ✚ Mineral oil is potentially dangerous in debilitated patients. Inhaled droplets can lead to a form of pneumonia.

- ***Stimulant laxatives*** are bowel irritants. They irritate the intestinal wall, stimulating intense peristalsis. Examples: senna, bisacodyl, castor oil

- ***Bulking agents*** are high in fiber. They must be combined with sufficient fluid intake to be effective. The fiber attracts fluid into the colon, and the increased bulk of the stool stimulates the urge to evacuate. These are considered the safest form of laxative, but may interfere with absorption of some medicines. They are the drug of choice for chronic constipation. Examples: Metamucil, Citrucel, psyllium, FiberCon

- ***Chloride channel activators*** increase intestinal fluid and motility to help stool pass.

- ***Combination laxatives*** are laxatives that contain more than one type of laxative ingredient. The most common type is a combination stimulant laxative and stool softener.

BOX 28-2 ■ Medications Associated with Constipation

Antacids containing aluminum hydroxide or calcium carbonate

Anticholinergic drugs (e.g., belladonna)

Anticonvulsant drugs (e.g., phenytoin)

Antidiarrheals (e.g., loperamide)

Antihistamines (e.g., diphenhydramine)

Antiparkinsonian drugs (e.g., amantadine hydrochloride)

Antipsychotic drugs (e.g., chlorpromazine)

Calcium channel blockers (e.g., verapamil hydrochloride)

Calcium supplements

Diuretics (e.g., furosemide)

Iron supplements

Lithium

Nonsteroidal anti-inflammatory drugs (e.g., ibuprofen)

Opioids (e.g., morphine, codeine)

Sympathomimetics (e.g., ephedrine)

Tricyclic antidepressants (e.g., nortriptyline)

had bowel surgery typically have a nasogastric (NG) tube with low constant or intermittent suction. The NG tube removes secretions until peristalsis returns. To review insertion of an NG tube or management of a patient with an NG tube,

 Go to Chapter 26, **Procedure 26-2: Inserting Nasogastric and Nasoenteric Tubes,** in Volume 2.

Decreased Mobility. After surgery, patients often experience discomfort that affects mobility. This further hinders GI motility and increases the risk for constipation.

Perineal Surgery. Patients who have had surgical interventions involving the perineal region (e.g., an episiotomy after childbirth) may fear pain or that their sutures will "tear" or "break" during bowel elimination, and therefore they resist the urge to evacuate their bowel.

Anal Sphincter Surgery. Patients who have had surgery that disrupts the anal sphincter may experience uncontrolled drainage after surgery.

Pregnancy

In early pregnancy, many women experience fluid loss due to "morning sickness"—periods of nausea and vomiting which, despite the name, may occur at any time of day. As the pregnancy progresses, the growing uterus crowds and displaces the intestines, and the increased level of progesterone slows intestinal motility. As a result, pregnant women often experience constipation, decreased appetite, and irregular food intake. In addition, the increasing pressure of the uterus and the increased blood volume of normal pregnancy increase the woman's risk for hemorrhoids.

 Critical**Thinking** 28-3

- Review the case of Mrs. Zeno ("Meet Your Patient"). What factors may be affecting her bowel elimination?
- What additional information do you need?

Pathological Conditions

Several disorders affect bowel function. Among them are neurological disorders that affect innervation of the lower GI tract, cognitive conditions that limit the ability to sense the urge to defecate, pain or immobility that leads to sluggish peristalsis, and pathological conditions of the GI tract. Constipation and diarrhea are discussed in the "Nursing Diagnosis" section of the chapter. Other common disorders are food allergies, food intolerances, and diverticulosis.

Food Allergies. The National Institute of Allergy and Infectious Diseases (NIAID) characterizes a **food allergy** as a true immune system reaction prompted by the presence in the body of an allergenic food (NIAID, 2001). Some common food allergens include dairy products, egg whites, shellfish, gluten, peanuts and other nuts, citrus fruits, and soy. Immune responses to foods manifest as a variety of symptoms ranging from a mild rash to anaphylactic shock. Common GI symptoms suggesting food allergy include constipation, diarrhea, a red, blistering rash around the anus, abdominal discomfort, bloating, excessive gas, and intestinal bleeding (Chapman, Bernstein, Lee, et al., 2006).

Food Intolerances. In contrast to a food allergy, a **food intolerance** is specifically linked to the GI system. It produces such symptoms as GI discomfort, pain, gas, bloating, diarrhea, or constipation after the person consumes the food. An example is *lactose intolerance,* a deficiency of the enzyme lactase, which is responsible for the breakdown of milk sugar (lactose). Such symptoms can mimic those of a food allergy, but food intolerances are not caused by immune responses.

Diverticulosis. When the colon must repeatedly move highly compacted fecal material, over time the longitudinal and circular muscles enlarge. This increases force on the mucosal tissues, causing them to "balloon" out between the muscles and to form pouches in which fecal matter becomes trapped. The development of these saclike outpouchings of mucosa through the muscle layers of the colon wall is a condition called **diverticulosis.** In some cases, the pouches become infected, a condition called **diverticulitis,** and antibiotics or surgery is required. People whose diets are low in fiber or consist mainly of refined foods are especially at risk for diverticulosis. Obesity and red meat intake are also risk factors (Korzenik, 2008).

KnowledgeCheck 28-2

- What is a normal defecation pattern?
- Identify the factors that affect bowel elimination.

 Go to Chapter 28, **Knowledge Check Response Sheet and Answers,** on the Student Resource Disk or DavisPlus at http://davisplus.fadavis.com/Wilkinson2

Bowel Diversions

A **bowel diversion** is a surgically created opening for elimination of digestive waste products. The procedure is performed for clients with a variety of conditions, including cancer, ulcerations, trauma, or inadequate blood supply. A client with a bowel diversion does not eliminate via the anus. Instead, the **effluent** (output, fecal material) is expelled through a surgically created opening in the abdominal wall, called a **stoma** or **ostomy.** The effluent may range from liquid to solid, depending on the part of the bowel that is being diverted. A bowel diversion close to the ileocecal valve (between the small and large intestine) will have a constant flow of liquid effluent. In contrast, a bowel diversion close to the rectum will have effluent that resembles feces (Fig. 28-5).

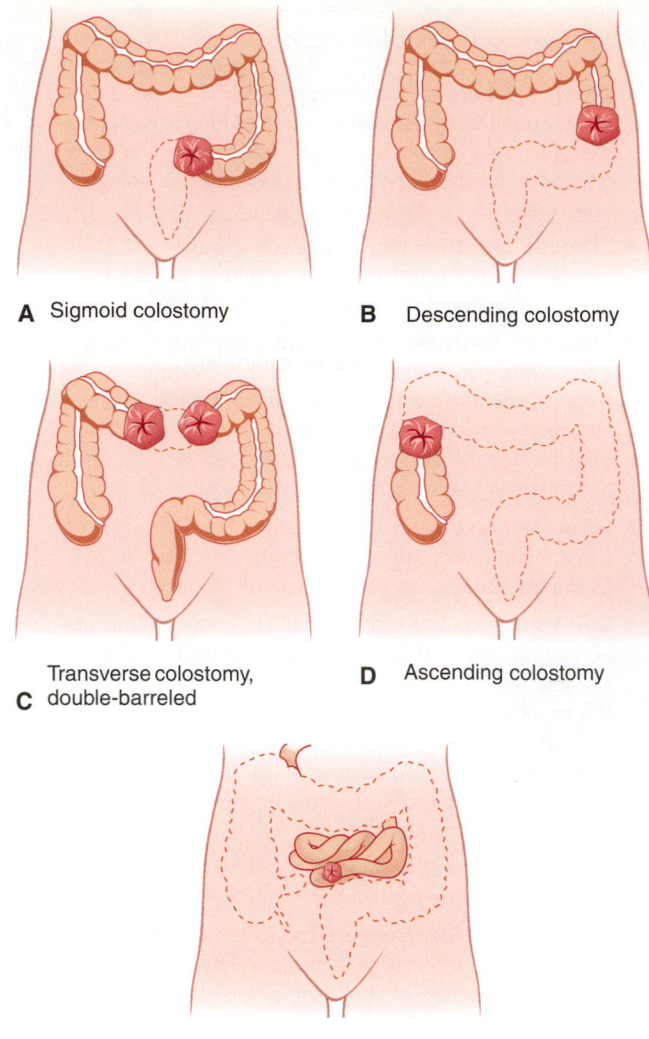

A Sigmoid colostomy   **B** Descending colostomy

C Transverse colostomy, double-barreled   **D** Ascending colostomy

E Ileostomy

FIGURE 28-5 *A–E,* Location of various bowel diversion ostomies. Shaded areas indicate sections of the bowel that are removed or being "rested." The closer the colostomy is to the ascending colon ("higher"), the more liquid and continuous the drainage will be.

Bowel diversions may be temporary or permanent. *Temporary bowel diversions* are common after surgical interventions for benign conditions of the bowel. They allow healing of the distal portion of the bowel. Once adequate healing has occurred, surgical **reanastomosis** (reconnection) of the bowel is performed, and the patient once again has BMs from the anus. *Permanent bowel diversions* are performed if the bowel is necrotic (dead) or cannot be salvaged because of severe disease or trauma.

Ileostomy

An **ileostomy** brings a portion of the ileum through a surgical opening in the abdomen, bypassing the large intestine entirely. Drainage at this level is liquid and continuous. The patient must wear an ostomy appliance at all times to collect the drainage. Two variations of an ileostomy are designed to control drainage more effectively and to cause less body image disturbance. However, many clients are not candidates for these procedures because of their underlying disease.

- A **Kock pouch,** or continent ileostomy, creates an internal pouch, or reservoir, to collect ileal drainage (Fig. 28-6A). To drain the pouch, the patient inserts a tube through the external stoma into the pouch several times per day. This alternative avoids continuous drainage and allows the patient to be free of an ostomy appliance.
- A **total colectomy with ileoanal reservoir** is a surgical procedure in which the colon is removed, a pouch is created from the ileum, and the ileum is connected to the rectum (Fig. 28-6B). The patient evacuates the bowel on the commode in the usual manner. Although this procedure should result in continence of bowel elimination, the feces will still be liquid.

Colostomy

A **colostomy** is a surgical procedure that brings a portion of the colon through a surgical opening in the abdomen. The location of the colostomy determines the consistency of the feces eliminated, as well as the need to wear an ostomy appliance (see Fig. 28-5). The closer the colostomy is to the ascending colon, the more liquid and continuous the drainage will be. In contrast, a colostomy close to the sigmoid colon will produce solid feces. Colostomies near the rectum, such as sigmoid colostomies, can often be controlled by diet and irrigation. As a result, the client may not need to wear an ostomy appliance to collect drainage.

A colostomy created in the transverse colon is usually temporary and may be either a double-barreled or loop colostomy.

- A **double-barreled colostomy** (see Fig. 28-5C) has two separate stomas that externalize the bowel on both sides of the portion that has been removed. The proximal stoma is the functioning end that drains fecal material. The distal stoma may drain mucus and is sometimes called a mucous fistula.
- A **loop colostomy** (Fig. 28-7) consists of a segment of bowel brought out to the abdominal wall. The posterior wall of the bowel remains intact, but a plastic rod is wedged under the bowel to keep it from slipping back into the abdomen. The anterior wall is incised, and the mucosal surface is left visible and open to air. It, too, has a functioning proximal end and limited drainage from the distal end.

You may also be interested in seeing an animation about colostomies at

Go to Student Resources, **Animations: Colostomy,** on DavisPlus at http://davisplus.fadavis.com/Wilkinson2

KnowledgeCheck 28-3

- What changes in bowel elimination are associated with constipation? With diarrhea?
- Why are bowel diversions performed?
- What determines the nature of the effluent from a bowel diversion?

Go to Chapter 28, **Knowledge Check Response Sheet and Answers,** on the Student Resource Disk or DavisPlus at http://davisplus.fadavis.com/Wilkinson2

FIGURE 28-6 Ileostomy variations. A, Continent ileostomy (Kock pouch). B, Ileoanal reservoir.

FIGURE 28-7 A loop colostomy.

Practical **Knowledge**
knowing how

As a nurse, you will monitor and assist clients with bowel elimination, teach about bowel function, and work collaboratively with the healthcare team to facilitate normal bowel function in well and ill clients. In the remainder of the chapter, we discuss these activities.

▌ ASSESSMENT

To assess bowel elimination, you must obtain a nursing history, perform a physical examination focused on elimination, and review diagnostic and laboratory data associated with bowel function and elimination.

Focused Nursing History

Because bowel patterns vary, you will need a nursing history to determine what is normal for each client. As you interview clients, pay attention to their reactions to your questions. Many people are embarrassed by discussion about bowel function. Tailor your assessment to the client's needs, and use language that makes the client comfortable. The following items should be part of your assessment:

- Normal bowel pattern
- Appearance of stool
- Changes in bowel habits or stool appearance
- History of elimination problems
- Use of bowel elimination aids, including diet, exercise, medications, and remedies

For a list of questions that you may use to assess each of these areas,

 Go to Chapter 28, **Assessment Guidelines and Tools, Focused Assessment: Bowel Elimination,** in Volume 2.

For clients with a bowel diversion, you will also gather data on the client's usual care of the stoma, use of appliances, and adjustment to the ostomy. Table 28-1 describes characteristics of normal and abnormal stool.

Focused Physical Assessment

Physical assessment for bowel elimination includes examination of the abdomen, rectum, and anus. Observe the size, shape, and contour of the abdomen, and listen to bowel sounds. You might also palpate the anus and rectum for the presence of stool or masses. When auscultated:

- *Normal bowel sounds* are high-pitched, with approximately 5 to 15 gurgles every minute.
- *Hyperactive bowel sounds* are very high-pitched and more frequent than normal. They may occur with

small bowel obstruction and inflammatory disorders and may produce diarrhea.

- *Hypoactive bowel sounds* are low-pitched, infrequent, and quiet. A decrease in bowel sounds indicates decreased peristalsis, which can result in constipation.
- *Absent bowel sounds.* If after listening for 3 to 5 minutes you hear no bowel sounds, you can describe them as *absent*. Absent bowel sounds indicate a lack of intestinal activity, which may occur after abdominal surgery and indicate a paralytic ileus.

For complete details about a focused assessment of bowel function,

 Go to Chapter 28, **Assessment Guidelines and Tools, Focused Assessment: Bowel Elimination,** in Volume 2. Also go to Chapter 19, **Procedure 19-14: Assessment of the Abdomen** and **Procedure 19-19: Assessment of the Rectum and Anus,** in Volume 2.

Knowledge Check 28-4

- What should you discuss with your client when performing a nursing history focused on bowel elimination?
- Describe the physical assessment you would perform for a client with constipation.

 Go to Chapter 28, **Knowledge Check Response Sheet and Answers,** on the Student Resource Disk or DavisPlus at http://davisplus.fadavis.com/Wilkinson2

Diagnostic Tests

Several diagnostic tests may be performed to assess for bowel elimination problems (e.g., to screen for colorectal cancer, to diagnose diverticulosis). They may be classified as direct or indirect visualization studies. **Indirect visualization studies** are radiographic views of the lower GI tract. The simplest of the tests is an abdominal flat plate, an anterior to posterior (AP) x-ray view of the abdomen used to detect gallstones, fecal impaction, and distended bowel.

Direct visualization studies are used for diagnostic and treatment purposes. They are invasive procedures and are conducted by a gastroenterologist, who inserts various instruments (e.g., *endoscopes*) to examine the interior of the GI tract. The nurse's role during these studies is to prepare the patient for the test, function as an assistant, and provide aftercare. You might need to assist the patient to the appropriate position, monitor the patient's tolerance of the procedure, provide pain medication or sedation to keep the patient comfortable during the exam, and provide reassurance to the patient as the test proceeds. For a description of the most common visualization tests,

 Go to Chapter 28, **Diagnostic Testing, Direct Visualization Studies of the Gastrointestinal Tract, and Indirect Visualization Studies of the Gastrointestinal Tract** in Volume 2.

Table 28-1 ➤ Normal Characteristics of Feces and Variations

FREQUENCY

Normal	Number of BMs per day varies.
	Infants:
	Bottle-fed, 1–3 per day
	Breastfed, 4–6 per day
	Adults: Daily or 2–3 per week
Variations	Hypermotility:
	Infants: More than 6 stools per day
	Adults: More than 3 stools per day
	Hypomotility:
	Infants: Fewer than every 1 or 2 days
	Adults: Fewer than once a week

COLOR

Normal	*Infants*: Yellow
	Adults: Brown
Variations	Bile pigment gives feces its brown color. Infant stools are yellow because of their rapid passage.
	White or clay-colored stool may indicate absence of bile (e.g., as in bile duct obstruction) or use of some antacids.
	Light brown stool may indicate diet high in milk products and low in meat.
	Pale, fatty stool may indicate malabsorption of fat.
	Black, tarry stool (**melena**) may indicate use of iron medications or upper GI bleeding; eating large quantities of red meat, spinach, and dark green vegetables may cause feces to be almost black.
	Red stool may indicate bleeding in lower intestinal tract or hemorrhoids.
	Stool darkens the longer it is left standing after defecation.

QUANTITY

Normal	*Adults*: About 150 g per day
Variations	Quantity varies with amount of food eaten, from 100 to 400 g per day.

SHAPE

Normal	Approximately the diameter of the rectum: about 2.5 cm (1 in.) in diameter; tubular shape
Variations	Narrow, pencil-shaped stool may indicate intestinal obstruction or constriction, or rapid peristalsis.
	Small, marble-shaped stool may indicate slow peristalsis, with longer time in the large intestine.

CONSISTENCY

Normal	Formed, soft, moist
Variations	Consistency is related to gastric motility and is affected by food and fluid intake.
	Hard stool indicates constipation. The more time spent in the large intestine, the more water is reabsorbed, and the harder the stool. May also indicate dehydration.
	Liquid stool may indicate diarrhea; rapid peristalsis (e.g., from infection).

ODOR

Normal	Pungent; affected by foods eaten
Variations	Normal odor is created by putrefaction and fermentation in the lower GI tract. Odor is also influenced by the pH of the stool, which is normally neutral or slightly alkaline.
	Strong, foul odors may indicate blood in the stool, especially in the upper GI tract, or infection.

*All information about infant stool patterns applies after passage of meconium.

For nursing care before, during, and after each of these tests,

Go to Chapter 28, **ESG Box 28-1, Diagnostic Testing, Direct Visualization Studies of the Gastrointestinal Tract,** and **ESG Box 28-2, Indirect Visualization Studies of the Gastrointestinal Tract** on the Student Resource Disk or DavisPlus at http://davisplus.fadavis.com/Wilkinson2

 Critical**Thinking** 28-4

A client asks you why he must perform a bowel prep with a strong laxative before having a colonoscopy. How might you reply?

Laboratory Studies of Stool

Stool specimens may be analyzed to detect blood, infection, or parasitic infestation. The client must void first and then defecate into a clean, dry bedpan, bedside commode, or a special container (half hat) placed under the toilet seat. A small sample is obtained and sent to the laboratory for analysis or analyzed at the bedside. To obtain a specimen from an infant or young child, you will collect freshly passed feces from a diaper.

Handling Stool Specimens

 Wear clean gloves when you handle the container or manipulate stool specimens. Use tongue blades to transfer the stool specimen to the container provided by the lab. Do not contaminate the outside of the specimen container. In most cases you will need approximately 2.5 cm (1 in.) of formed stool or 20 to 30 mL of liquid stool. If blood, mucus, or purulent material is present, be sure to include this with the sample. Transport the specimen to the laboratory as soon as possible. If that is not possible, consult the laboratory for appropriate storage. Usually you will need to refrigerate the specimen until it can be received in the lab.

Testing for Fecal Occult Blood

You may be called on to assess stool for the presence of blood. Blood may be visible to the eye or **occult** (hidden). You can perform the test for occult blood at the bedside, although some institutions require that it be done in the laboratory. The test is called a *guaiac test* or *fecal occult blood test*. It requires use of a special reagent that detects the presence of **peroxidase,** an enzyme present in hemoglobin. Only a small smear of stool is required. For home testing, remind patients to wash their hands before and after collecting stool. The Critical Aspects box in this chapter presents highlights. For the complete procedure,

Go to Chapter 28, **Procedure 28-1: Testing Stool for Occult Blood,** in Volume 2.

The patient should restrict certain types of foods and medications for 3 days before stool testing:

- Red meat, chicken, fish, horseradish, and some raw fruits and vegetables, such as radishes, may result in a false-positive reading.

- Bleeding gums can also produce a positive result of blood in the stool.
- Ingestion of a large amount of vitamin C can produce a false-negative result (Allison, 2005; American College of Physicians, 1997).
- Some drugs can cause GI bleeding, even if microscopic (e.g., anticoagulants, aspirin and other NSAIDs, colchicines, iron supplements in large doses, and corticosteroids). The patient should avoid these and oxidizing drugs (e.g., iodine, bromides, and boric acid) for the 7 days before testing to avoid results that could be misinterpreted (Atkins, 2008).
- The test should not be done if a woman is having her menstrual period or if the person has bleeding hemorrhoids or hematuria. Complying with these restrictions may not always be possible in clinical settings, though.

Colorectal cancer is the third most common cancer in both women and men. Screening can detect colorectal polyps so they can be removed before becoming cancerous. Annual guaiac-based fecal occult blood testing is recommended for all patients 50 to 75 years of age and older as one method of screening for colorectal cancer (some guidelines suggest every 2 years). The recommended age for annual testing drops to 45 and older for blacks, as they are at higher risk (National Guideline Clearinghouse, n.d., updated 2009). Some suggest the cut-off age to stop screening should be age 80, or an expected remaining life span of less than 8 to 10 years. Based on 2005 data, fewer than half of adults aged 50 and older were screened for cancer at the recommended intervals (American Cancer Society, 2009a).

Assessing for Pinworms

Pinworms (an intestinal parasite) are small, white, threadlike worms that live in the cecum. They come to the anal area to deposit eggs during the night and migrate back up through the rectum during the day. In assessing a child, you can spread the buttocks while the child is sleeping and examine the anus to see whether any pinworms are visible to the naked eye. You can test for the presence of the eggs with tape. In the morning, as soon as the patient awakens, press clear cellophane tape against the anal opening. Remove the tape immediately, and place it adhesive side down on a slide. You may also need to do perianal swabs for microscopic study. You may also check at night by using a flashlight. The test may need to be repeated on consecutive days. For guidelines,

 Go to Chapter 28, **Clinical Insight 28-1: Testing for Pinworms,** in Volume 2.

 Critical**Thinking** 28-5

You are reviewing a client's chart and note that the client was tested for fecal occult blood. The results are as follows:

3/10 negative for occult blood

3/11 no BM
3/12 no BM
3/13 no BM
3/14 positive for occult blood
3/15 negative for occult blood
3/16 negative for occult blood

What can you conclude? What questions do these findings raise?

ANALYSIS/NURSING DIAGNOSIS

Common nursing diagnoses related to bowel elimination include the following:

- *Bowel Incontinence* is a change in normal bowel habits characterized by involuntary passage of stool. It is more common among women and older adults. Other risk factors include neurological diseases, stroke, sphincter damage, and inflammatory bowel disease.
- *Constipation.* Because frequency of bowel elimination varies, constipation is usually defined as a decrease in the frequency of bowel movements resulting in the passage of hard, dry stool. Constipation can be a temporary problem wherein symptoms resolve in a short time. Nearly everyone experiences constipation at some point. *Chronic constipation* typically lasts 3 months or longer and may persist for years. Unrelieved constipation may eventually result in a **fecal impaction,** in which dry, hard stools lodged in the rectum cannot be passed.
- *Risk for Constipation* is an appropriate diagnosis for clients at increased risk because of bedrest, medications such as opioids, or surgery. Use this diagnosis for a client with a condition or taking medications known to decrease peristalsis.
- *Perceived Constipation* is an appropriate diagnosis for a client who makes a self-diagnosis of constipation and uses laxatives, suppositories, or enemas to ensure a daily bowel movement.
- *Diarrhea* is the passage of loose, unformed, or watery stools.
- *Dysfunctional Gastrointestinal Motility* is a broad label that encompasses increased, decreased, ineffective, or absent peristaltic activity within the GI system. If you use this label, you need to specify whether the GI motility is increased, decreased, and so on (e.g., Dysfunctional GI Motility: Increased).
- *Toileting Self-Care Deficit* is impaired ability to perform or complete own toileting activities.

For definitions and defining characteristics of these diagnoses, consult a nursing diagnosis handbook or

 Go to Chapter 28, **Standardized Language, Nursing Diagnoses Associated with Bowel Elimination,** in Volume 2.

Bowel elimination problems may also form the etiology of other nursing diagnoses and collaborative problems. Examples include the following:

- Social isolation r/t embarrassment secondary to bowel incontinence

- Potential Complication: Electrolyte imbalance secondary to diarrhea. Older adults, very young children, and infants are at especially high risk.
- Impaired Skin Integrity r/t irritating effects of feces secondary to diarrhea
- Anxiety r/t perceived need for a daily bowel movement
- Disturbed Body Image r/t bowel diversion

CriticalThinking 28-6

- What data do you have about Mrs. Zeno's ("Meet Your Patient") bowel function?
- What else would you like to know about her bowel function? What other symptoms often accompany these cues?
- Which NANDA-I nursing diagnosis best describes this cue cluster?
- In addition to this nursing diagnosis, what other data in the scenario might also be contributing to her infrequent BMs?
- From the scenario data, how would you describe the etiology of Mrs. Zeno's problem?
- What questions do you still have about the etiology?

PLANNING OUTCOMES/EVALUATION

The general bowel elimination goal is that the patient will have soft, formed bowel movements regularly.

For *associated NOC standardized outcomes* for bowel elimination diagnoses,

 Go to Chapter 28, **Standardized Language, Selected Standardized Outcomes and Interventions for Bowel Elimination Diagnoses,** in Volume 2.

When bowel elimination is the etiology, choose outcomes linked to the problem side of the diagnosis. For example, for Impaired Skin Integrity r/t irritating effects of diarrhea stool, the NOC outcomes might fall within Tissue Integrity: Skin and Mucous Membranes.

Individualized goals/outcome statements depend on the nursing diagnosis. Because normal bowel elimination patterns are individualized, regularity is based on the individual's pattern. Examples include the following:

Will resume his normal bowel pattern by (date).
Will discuss his feelings about his colostomy.

PLANNING INTERVENTIONS/IMPLEMENTATION

Bowel elimination is a normal physiological function. It is important for you to convey an attitude of acceptance and display professionalism when providing care for patients with bowel elimination problems.

For *NIC standardized interventions and activities* for patients with bowel elimination problems,

 Go to Chapter 28, **Standardized Language, Selected Standardized Outcomes and Interventions for Bowel Elimination Diagnoses,** in Volume 2.

Specific nursing activities to promote normal bowel function and relieve elimination problems are found in the next section.

Promoting Normal or Regular Defecation

Promoting regular defecation entails a number of independent nursing activities. These include providing privacy, positioning, timing, providing hydration and nutrition, promoting exercise, and teaching clients when they should seek medical assistance.

Provide Privacy

Try this exercise. Imagine that your class assignment for today is to stand in front of the classroom and describe to the class your normal pattern of defecation, including frequency, appearance, and other characteristics of the stool. How would you feel about that? Would you do it?

Although defecation is a normal physiological function, most patients consider it a very private matter. Provide privacy for your patient when discussing or providing care related to bowel elimination. Taking a matter-of-fact approach confirms to patients that you are comfortable with this aspect of care. When assisting a patient with bowel elimination, excuse visitors from the room, draw the dividing curtains in shared rooms, and close the door. Many patients are embarrassed by the odor of bowel movements and therefore may ignore the urge to defecate. Using an aromatic spray or other odor-reducing product may help to reduce embarrassment.

Assist with Positioning

An upright seated or squatting position is the most comfortable for defecation and decreases the need to strain. When possible, assist the patient to the bathroom to use the toilet. An alternative is to place a bedside commode next to the bed for patients who are unable to ambulate to the bathroom. A patient who must remain in bed should assume a semi-Fowler's position to use the bedpan. Patients who are unable to assume this position because of surgery, trauma, or other medical conditions must use supine or side-lying positions. These positions are unnatural for bowel elimination and place the patient at risk for constipation.

Raise the siderails or provide an overhead trapeze so that the patient can grip them to maneuver on and off the bedpan. If the patient is very weak, you may need an assistant to help you position him on the bedpan. In addition, you may need to stay with the person while he uses the bedpan to help him maintain his position. The Critical Aspects box in this chapter provides highlights of this procedure. For the complete procedure,

VOL 2 Go to Chapter 28, **Procedure 28-2: Placing and Removing a Bedpan,** in Volume 2.

Consider the Timing of Defecation

Recall that food entering the duodenum triggers mass peristalsis. As a result, the urge to defecate often occurs after meals. Advise patients not to ignore this urge, because doing so may result in constipation. For patients who are ambulatory, allow some free time after meals to use the restroom. For those who cannot toilet independently, assist them to ambulate to the bathroom or using the bedpan. Discuss with nursing assistive personnel (NAP) the need to offer assistance without waiting to be asked, so patients experience minimal delays.

Support Healthful Intake of Food and Fluids

Unfortunately, a typical American diet is low in fiber, often as low as 5 to 8 grams per day. Teach clients the importance of a balanced diet in promoting soft, formed, regular bowel movements. Encourage a daily intake of 25 to 30 grams of fiber to provide bulk, attract water into the stool, and promote peristalsis. The diet should be rich in fresh fruits and vegetables, whole-grain foods, legumes, and water, yet low in simple sugars, fats, carbonated beverages, and processed foods.

Without adequate fluid intake, a high-fiber diet can actually cause constipation. Recommend a minimum intake of 1500 mL of fluid per day to keep stool soft and aid in production of mucus to lubricate the colon. Ideally, a person should drink eight to ten 8-ounce glasses of fluid daily (2000 to 2400 mL). Water is the preferred fluid because soda, coffee, and tea often contain caffeine or additives that promote diuresis. However, because the diuretic effect of these fluids is minimal, they are acceptable for clients who simply will not drink enough plain water.

Also keep in mind that adding fiber does not help to relieve opioid-induced constipation unless the patient's current intake is deficient. In fact, excessive fiber might put the patient at risk for bowel obstruction due to the opioid-induced decreased peristalsis, delayed gastric emptying, and prolonged intestinal transit time of the feces (Müller-Lissner, Kamm, Scarpignato, et al., 2005; Yuan, 2005).

Encourage Exercise

Physical activity increases peristalsis and promotes defecation. Encourage patients to exercise three to five times per week and to engage in daily walking or light activity. Assist hospitalized or institutionalized patients to ambulate as soon as their condition permits. Even limited activity, such as getting out of bed or walking 10 feet, decreases the risk for constipation.

Provide range-of-motion (ROM) exercises for patients who must remain on bedrest. Even passive ROM (the joints are moved through ROM by the nurse) promotes peristalsis. Chapter 31 provides additional information about activity and ROM exercises, if you need it.

For clients who can assist with exercise, the following exercises promote abdominal and perineal strength:

- *Thigh strengthening.* Have the client slowly bring one knee up to his chest, briefly hold it, then lower the leg to the bed. Repeat this pattern alternating legs. Encourage the client to perform this exercise several times per hour while he is awake.
- *Abdominal tightening.* Have the client tighten and hold the abdominal muscles for a count of five and then

relax. This core exercise works the abdominal muscles used during defecation.

Teach Clients When to See a Primary Care Provider

Obviously many GI symptoms are normal and do not require treatment. For example, everyone has excessive flatus and abdominal distention at some time—perhaps as a result of a high-fat, high-sugar meal. And it is common for bowel movements to occasionally become a little irregular. However, clients need to know when a symptom may be signaling a more serious condition.

Teach clients to see their primary care provider for the following if a symptom lasts longer than 3 weeks or is disabling:

- Blood in the stool (unless they have hemorrhoids and this is not an unusual occurrence for them)
- Severe stomach pain
- Change in bowel habits
- Unintended weight loss
- Constipation is not relieved after trying fiber, fluids, and exercise

KnowledgeCheck 28-5

Identify at least five independent nursing actions that you can take to encourage regular elimination in a well client.

  Go to Chapter 28, **Knowledge Check Response Sheet and Answers,** on the Student Resource Disk or DavisPlus at http://davisplus.fadavis.com/Wilkinson2

CriticalThinking 28-7

How could you facilitate regular bowel elimination for Mrs. Zeno ("Meet Your Patient")? What information do you need?

Managing Diarrhea

Diarrhea may occur as a result of contaminated food, a viral infection, or dietary change, or as a side effect of a medication. Patients with diarrhea are at risk for fluid and electrolyte imbalance. Water and potassium loss are the primary concerns. Infants, young children, and the frail elderly are most vulnerable and may require hospitalization and intravenous fluid replacement therapy. Ideally, oral liquids replace the lost fluid and potassium.

Nursing interventions focus on treating the diarrhea itself, as well as its associated problems (cramping, fluid and electrolyte imbalances, and Impaired Skin Integrity):

Preventive Interventions

Diarrhea can be prevented in the following ways:

- Teach hand hygiene. Teach patients to wash their hands often. This helps prevent diarrhea caused by viruses and other pathogens.
- Provide information about foods that can cause diarrhea. Highly spiced foods, high-fat foods, greasy snacks, or large quantities of raw fruits and vegetables may cause diarrhea in some patients. Tell patients to keep track of foods that trigger diarrhea and to eat them in moderation.

Monitoring Interventions

During the diarrhea episode, assess and monitor the following:

- Monitor stools. Assess frequency, amount, color, and consistency of stools to determine the severity of the diarrhea.
- Monitor fluid balance. Monitor intake and output, body weight, and vital signs to assess hydration. Also assess skin turgor and moistness of mucous membranes.
- Monitor electrolyte status. Check serum electrolyte levels to detect imbalances.
- Monitor skin integrity. Assess the perineal area for alterations in skin integrity. Clients with diarrhea may experience perianal irritation and excoriation.

Treatment Interventions

Treatments include medications, diet modification, and attention to fluid balance and skin integrity. Opiates (e.g., paregoric) and opiate derivatives (e.g., loperamide) are the primary antidiarrheal drugs prescribed. Although they slow peristalsis and inhibit diarrhea, they may cause drowsiness; advise patients, especially older adults, to use them with caution. Pepto-Bismol (bismuth subsalicylate) is a readily available OTC medication that is useful for traveler's diarrhea because it has antimicrobial and antisecretory properties.

Antidiarrheal medications are not recommended for acute diarrhea. In many cases, diarrhea is a response to infection or unusual foods and serves as a mechanism to rid the body of the pathogens or troublesome food. Although antidiarrheal medications are available without a prescription, caution patients to avoid using them unless instructed by their healthcare provider. Medication is usually reserved for use with chronic diarrhea—diarrhea that has persisted for more than 1 month—which is often due to a disease state.

During the acute episode, the patient may need to modify his diet to control the diarrhea. You will need to promote skin integrity and fluid balance with interventions such as the following:

- Provide assistance with hygiene to protect the skin.
- Teach the patient about, or provide, a clear liquid diet, including electrolyte replacement fluids, (e.g., Pedialyte or sports drinks that have been diluted by 50% or more). Clear broth and gelatin are also good choices.
- Encourage your patient to sip liquids or take ice chips or popsicles often to replace the losses.
- Reduce the amount of fiber in your client's diet by cutting back servings of whole grain bread and fresh fruits and vegetables.
- Limit foods containing caffeine, such as coffee, strong tea, and colas.

- Avoid a sudden large intake of fluid or food when resuming a normal diet, because this may trigger mass peristalsis.
- Several medications, especially antibiotics, may cause diarrhea. A change in medications may be required. Plain yogurt and other probiotic foods consumed daily may help to prevent this response to antibiotics.
- Breastfed infants with acute diarrhea should be continued on breast milk without any need for interruption. In fact, breastfeeding not only has a well-known protective effect against the development of enteritis, but it also promotes faster recovery and provides improved nutrition.
- Advise a BRAT diet if a child with diarrhea has an appetite. A BRAT diet consists of bananas, (white) rice, applesauce, and toast. These are easy to digest, provide calories for energy without gastric irritation, and help offset potassium loss. Although developed for pediatric use, the BRAT diet is sometimes used for adults.

Managing Constipation

Many of the nursing strategies to prevent and treat constipation are identical to the activities that promote regular bowel elimination.

Short-Term Constipation is usually caused by the person's lifestyle. Clients most likely to experience constipation are those who (1) have decreased activity or are on bedrest, (2) are receiving opioids or other medications that slow peristalsis, and (3) have decreased fluid and fiber intake. The following are some interventions:

- Increase the intake of high-fiber foods if intake is inadequate (normal adult RDA/AI is 25 to 38 grams, depending on age and sex).
- Increase fluid intake.
- Increase physical activity.
- Provide privacy for using the toilet.
- Assist the patient to a seated or squatting position whenever possible. A semi-Fowler's position is preferred for a client on bedrest.
- Allow the patient uninterrupted time to use the toilet, especially after meals, when mass peristalsis occurs.
- Assess for complications such as impaction and hemorrhoids.

Chronic Constipation. Chronic constipation may be associated with physiological factors such as dysfunctional intestinal motility, nervous system problems, and dysfunctional anorectal musculature. Chronic constipation causes significant psychological distress and decreased quality of life for many clients, and it may result in complications, which include intestinal impaction, anal fissures, hemorrhoids, volvulus, intestinal obstruction, rectal ulcers, fecal seepage, and bowel perforation. Lifestyle changes and nonprescription medications do not usually adequately treat chronic constipation.

Medications. When lifestyle modifications are ineffective in preventing and treating constipation, medications may be given (Box 28-1). Bulking agents are actually fiber in a nonfood source. They are the preferred medications for treating constipation. Many laxatives are readily available without prescription and are used by clients to treat actual or perceived constipation. Habitual laxative use, except for bulking agents, may cause reliance on medications for bowel elimination and, ironically, may lead to further constipation. See Self-Care: Teaching Your Patient About Laxative Use for key points to discuss with patients about managing constipation.

Older Adults should be screened for risk factors, including a history of polypharmacy and taking laxatives. Other risk factors include impaired cognitive status, inadequate fluid intake, inadequate dietary fiber, reduced mobility, lack of privacy for toileting, and reliance on others for assistance. These are the same as risk factors for all ages, but they are more likely for older adults. Prevention measures are the same for all ages. However, for those unable to walk or who are restricted to bed, exercises such as trunk rotation, pelvic tilt, and leg lifts may be helpful. For older adults, osmotic laxatives (e.g., polyethylene glycol [PEG] and lactulose) and bulking agents have been found to be beneficial (The Joanna Briggs Institute, 2008).

Self-Care

Teaching Your Patient About Laxative Use

Discuss the following topics with clients who have concerns about the frequency of their bowel movements or ask about laxatives.

1. The frequency of BMs may range from several times per day to once per week. As long as stools are passed without excessive urgency, with minimal effort and no straining, and without the use of laxatives, bowel function may be regarded as normal.

2. To maintain normal bowel function:
   - Eat a well-balanced diet that includes five servings of whole grains, fresh fruits, and vegetables.
   - Drink eight to ten glasses of fluid per day.
   - Engage in daily exercise to stimulate peristalsis.
   - Set aside uninterrupted time after breakfast or dinner for using the toilet.
   - Do not ignore the urge to defecate.
   - Whenever there is a significant or prolonged change in bowel habits, report this to your healthcare provider.

3. If you are experiencing constipation, choose bulking agents, such as Metamucil or psyllium, to treat the problem rather than other over-the-counter laxatives. Be sure to drink plenty of water when using bulking agents.

Managing Fecal Impaction

Fecal impaction is the presence of a hardened fecal mass in the rectum. The impaction often blocks the passage of normal stool and sets up a vicious cycle of furthering hardening. Liquid stool may leak, seeping around the hardened mass, and the patient may report feelings of fullness, bloating, constipation, diminished appetite, and a change in bowel habits. You can detect fecal impaction by digital examination of the rectum. To treat a fecal impaction, you will use enemas or digital removal of stool. Once the impaction has been removed, establish a bowel regimen to prevent recurrence of impactions. You will learn more about digital removal of stool in a later section.

Administering Enemas

An **enema** is the introduction of solution into the rectum to soften feces, distend the colon, and stimulate peristalsis and evacuation of feces. Some enema solutions are chosen because they irritate the mucosa of the rectum and sigmoid colon and assist with forceful evacuation of stool. The Critical Aspects box summarizes the procedure for various types of enemas. To learn the procedure,

 Go to Chapter 28, **Procedure 28-3: Administering an Enema,** in Volume 2.

Enemas may be classified as cleansing, retention, or return-flow. The primary care provider generally orders the specific type to administer to a patient.

Cleansing Enemas

Cleansing enemas promote removal of feces from the colon. They may be used to:

- Treat severe constipation or impaction.
- Clear the colon in preparation for visualization procedures, such as colonoscopy.
- Empty the colon when starting a bowel training program.

Historically, cleansing enemas were used before surgical procedures and childbirth to prevent the escape of feces. That use is rare now; they are used only before surgeries of the lower GI tract and for some pelvic surgeries.

Cleansing enema solutions include hypotonic solutions and hypertonic solutions. With *hypotonic solutions* (saline, tap water, and soap) you introduce a large volume (500 to 1000 mL for adults, 100 to 250 mL for infants) of fluid into the rectum. The volume causes intestinal distention and leads to rapid evacuation of stool. Large-volume solutions may be contraindicated in patients who have weakened intestinal walls.

In contrast, *hypertonic solutions* are usually smaller in volume (70 to 120 mL, or 2.5 to 4 oz, for adults). The

hypertonic solution attracts water into the colon, causing distention and stimulating peristalsis and defecation (Table 28-2). ✚ Hypertonic solutions may be contraindicated for patients who tend to retain sodium or water (e.g., those with renal failure and congestive heart failure).

A cleansing enema may be given "high" or "low." A "low" enema is given by standard procedure. A "high" enema attempts to clear as much of the large intestine as possible. With a "high" enema, the client receives initial instillation of the fluid in the left lateral position. The client then moves to the dorsal recumbent position and then the right lateral position for the remainder of the instillation. This turning process allows the fluid to follow the shape of the large intestine.

Retention Enemas

Retention enemas introduce a solution into the colon that is meant to be retained for a prolonged period. Consequently the volume is small, usually 90 to 120 mL (3 to 4 oz). The following are the most common forms of retention enemas.

Oil-Retention Enemas. Oil-retention enemas instill 90 to 120 mL of oil into the rectum to soften stool and lubricate the rectum. This type of enema may be used to assist a client to pass hard stool or before digital removal of stool. It may also be used in conjunction with a cleansing enema—at least 1 hour before the cleansing enema.

Carminative Enemas. Carminative enema is a procedure in which 60 to 180 mL (2 to 6 oz) of solution are instilled into the rectum to help expel flatus and relieve bloating and distention. This procedure is used after abdominal or pelvic surgery when peristalsis is slow to return and the client experiences pressure from gas. Solutions may be commercially prepared or prepared on the unit. A common carminative enema is the "MGW" enema; a mixture of magnesium sulfate, glycerin, and water in a ratio of 1:2:3 (e.g., 15 mL of magnesium sulfate, 30 mL of glycerin, and 45 mL of water).

Medicated Enemas. Medicated enemas may be used to instill antibiotics to treat infections in the rectum or anus or to introduce anthelminthic agents for treatment of intestinal worms and parasites.

Nutritive Enemas. Nutritive enemas administer fluid and nutrition through the rectum for patients who are dehydrated and frail. They are most commonly used in hospice care as a means to provide hydration for dying patients.

Return-Flow Enemas

A return-flow enema, known as a *Harris flush,* may be ordered to help a patient expel flatus and relieve abdominal distention. For adults, approximately

Table 28-2 ▶ Solutions Commonly Used in Enemas

SOLUTION	EXAMPLES	ACTION	TIME UNTIL BM	ADVERSE EFFECTS
Hypotonic	500–1000 mL of tap water	Large volume distends the colon, thereby stimulating peristalsis; water also softens stool.	15 minutes	Fluid and electrolyte imbalance, especially water intoxication, is possible if enema is not expelled.
Isotonic	500–1000 mL of normal saline (0.9% NaCl solution)	Large volume distends the colon, thereby stimulating peristalsis; some softening of stool also occurs.	15 minutes	Fluid and electrolyte imbalance, especially sodium retention
Hypertonic	120–180 mL of sodium phosphate (e.g., Fleets); available as a commercially prepared solution	Attracts water into the colon, thereby causing distention.	Rapid acting: 5–10 minutes	Sodium retention
Oil	90–120 mL of mineral oil, cottonseed oil, or olive oil; available as a commercially prepared solution	Softens the feces, lubricates the rectum.	Varies widely. An oil-retention enema is often given 1–3 hours before a cleansing enema is administered.	
Soapsuds	Pure Castile soap is added to tap water or saline.	Intestinal irritation stimulates peristalsis.	Varies.	Only pure Castile soap is safe. Other soaps and detergents can cause bowel inflammation.
Carminative	For example 1:2:3 "MGW" solution (e.g., 30 mL magnesium, 60 mL glycerin, and 90 mL water)	Provides relief from abdominal distention caused by flatus.		

100 to 200 mL (3 to 7 oz) of tap water or saline is instilled into the rectum. The rectal tube and solution container are then lowered below the level of the rectum to encourage return flow of the solution. This process is repeated several times, or until distention is relieved. If the solution becomes thick, discard it and begin again with new solution.

Guidelines for Administering an Enema

Before administering an enema, explain the purpose of the enema and what the patient can expect. For example, the patient will probably experience some cramping with a large-volume enema. Reassure the patient that you will be immediately available to help her to the restroom or onto the bedpan.

Responses to an enema are governed by the height of the solution container, the speed of flow, the concentration of the solution, and the resistance of the rectum. Hypotonic and isotonic solutions are easier to retain. Hypertonic solutions irritate the intestinal mucosa and cause a rapid evacuation. Muscle tone and history of constipation or other bowel disorders determine the resistance of the rectum. A client with a long

history of constipation is more likely to be able to tolerate a large-volume enema, because the rectum and colon have become distended over time.

The higher the solution container, the greater the effect of gravity and the faster the solution flows into the bowel. As a rule, place the solution container no higher than 30 cm (12 in.) above the rectum (7.5 cm, or 3 in., for children). This allows for a steady flow of solution that is easily tolerated. Rapid instillation will cause rapid distention of the bowel and intense cramping. Slower instillation is more comfortable for the client and allows him to retain the fluid for a period of time to soften the stool.

KnowledgeCheck 28-6

- Identify the types of enemas available for use.
- How do hypotonic and isotonic enemas differ from hypertonic enemas?
- What actions can you take to make the patient more comfortable when he receives an enema?

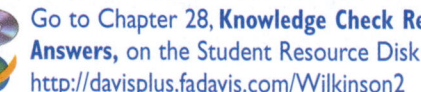 Go to Chapter 28, **Knowledge Check Response Sheet and Answers,** on the Student Resource Disk or DavisPlus at http://davisplus.fadavis.com/Wilkinson2

Digital Removal of Stool

If fecal impaction does not respond to use of stool softeners and enemas, you will need to digitally remove feces from the rectum. Digital removal is accomplished by breaking up the hardened mass into pieces and manually extracting the pieces. You may administer an oil-retention enema at least 30 minutes before digital removal to soften the stool and decrease the patient's discomfort during the procedure.

✚ Aside from discomfort, the pressure generated in the rectum may stimulate the vagus nerve, slowing the heart rate. For that reason, you must have a prescription from the primary care provider. The Critical Aspects box in this chapter summarizes the procedure. For complete steps,

 Go to Chapter 28, **Procedure 28-4: Removing Stool Digitally,** in Volume 2.

 Critical**Thinking** 28-8

Mrs. Zeno ("Meet Your Patient") begins to pass liquid stool. What actions should you take? Explain your reasoning.

Critical Aspects of Procedures 28-1 through 28-8

VOL 2 For steps to follow in *all* procedures, refer to the Universal Steps for All Procedures found on the inside back cover of Volume 2. Go to the full procedures in Volume 2 to practice and learn the procedure steps. Use these Critical Aspects later to help you review key points.

Procedure 28-1: Testing Stool for Occult Blood

➤ According to colorectal screening guidelines, all persons age 50 or older should be screened every 1 to 2 years for occult (hidden) blood in the stool. The 2008 NGC and the 2007 American Cancer Society recommendations suggest annual screening. High-risk groups require initial screening at a younger age.

➤ Patients should avoid foods that may alter the accuracy of the test for 3 days before collecting the stool specimen.

➤ Review the patient's medications. If the patient is taking salicylates, NSAIDs, iron, anticoagulants, or colchicines, consult with the physician.

➤ Take care that the sample is not contaminated by urine or menstrual blood.

➤ Test two small stool samples from separate areas of the large sample.

➤ Following the manufacturer's directions, place the correct number and size of drops of developer solution into the "windows" of the opposite side on the Hemoccult slide.

➤ Record a positive result if the slide windows turn blue.

Procedure 28-2: Placing and Removing a Bedpan

➤ Determine whether the patient will need to use a regular bedpan or a fracture pan.

➤ Don clean procedure gloves.

➤ Help the patient to achieve a position on the bedpan that will be most helpful in facilitating urinary or bowel elimination. Place the patient in a semi-Fowler's position whenever possible. Modify the position based on the patient's condition.

➤ Provide toilet tissue, clean washcloths, and towels for the patient to perform personal hygiene when elimination is complete. Assist if the patient cannot perform these tasks independently.

Procedure 28-3: Administering an Enema

➤ Generously lubricate and gently insert the rectal tube.

➤ Instill warm solution at a slow rate.

➤ For best results:
  ➤ Be sure patient is properly positioned.
  ➤ Instruct her to retain the solution for 3 to 15 minutes, depending on the type of enema.
  ➤ Assist the patient in a sitting or squatting position to promote defecation.

➤ Before leaving the bedside, implement fall prevention measures that are appropriate for your patient.

➤ Use nursing judgment to modify the procedure based on the patient's mobility and ability to follow your instructions.

Procedure 28-4: Removing Stool Digitally

➤ Be aware that this procedure is both painful and embarrassing to your patient.

➤ Trim and file your fingernails so they do not extend over the ends of your fingertips.

➤ Obtain baseline vital signs, and determine whether the patient has a history of cardiac problems or other contraindications.

➤ Determine whether the procedure will be accompanied by suppository insertion or enema administration.

➤ Use only one or two gloved fingers, and remove stool in small pieces.

➤ Allow the patient periods of rest, and monitor for signs of vagal nerve stimulation.

➤ Teach the patient lifestyle changes necessary to prevent stool retention.

Procedure 28-5: Inserting a Rectal Tube

➤ A rectal tube may be used to facilitate the passage of gas for clients experiencing intestinal distention.

➤ Position the patient on his left side.

➤ Lubricate the tip of the tube; insert 10 to 12.5 cm (4 to 5 in.).

➤ Attach the collecting device to the end of the tube.

➤ Leave the tube in place for 15 to 20 minutes.

Continued

➤ Assist the patient to move about in bed; the knee–chest position is ideal if tolerated.

Procedure 28-6: Changing an Ostomy Appliance

➤ Change the pouch every 3 to 5 days, as a general rule.

➤ Empty the old pouch before removing it, if possible.

➤ Remove the wafer or pouch, pulling down from the top with one hand while holding counter-tension with the other.

➤ Assess the stoma and the peristomal skin area (e.g., for discoloration, swelling, redness, irritation, excoriation, bleeding).

➤ Use a measuring guide to determine the size of the stoma.

➤ Trace the size of the opening onto the back of the wafer, and cut the wafer opening about 2 to 3 mm ($^{1}/_{16}$ to $^{1}/_{8}$ in.) larger.

➤ Apply the new wafer with gentle pressure.

Note: Some pouches come with the wafer attached, some without. These instructions assume that the wafer is attached.

Procedure 28-7: Irrigating a Colostomy

➤ Consult with the ostomy nurse and/or physician to see if colostomy irrigation is appropriate for your patient.

➤ Determine the patient's normal bowel pattern before surgery.

➤ Prime the tubing before irrigation, using 500 to 1000 mL, preferably 1000 mL, of warm tap water.

➤ Position the patient in front of or on the toilet or bedside commode. If the patient is immobile, place her in left side-lying (Sims') position, and use a bedpan.

➤ Prepare the new appliance before removing the existing one.

➤ Examine the stoma and peristomal skin.

➤ Lubricate the cone at the end of the tubing and insert it gently.

➤ Allow approximately 30 minutes for evacuation.

➤ Remove the sleeve, and rinse, dry, and store it.

Procedure 28-8: Placing Fecal Drainage Devices

Procedure 28-8A: Applying an External Fecal Collection System

➤ Select the fecal management system appropriate for the patient.

➤ Obtain assistance as needed.

➤ Place the patient side-lying.

➤ Cleanse and dry the perineal area; clip hair as needed.

➤ Spread the buttocks and apply the device; avoid gaps and creases.

➤ Hang the drainage bag lower than the patient.

Procedure 28-8B: Inserting an Indwelling Fecal Drainage Device

➤ Select the fecal management system appropriate for the patient.

➤ Obtain assistance as needed.

➤ Place the patient left side-lying.

➤ Remove any indwelling device.

➤ Cleanse and dry the perineal area; clip hair as needed.

➤ Prepare the device according to instructions (e.g., remove residual air from the balloon).

➤ Lubricate the balloon generously with water-soluble lubricant.

➤ Spread the buttocks and gently insert the balloon end of the catheter.

➤ Inflate the device with water or saline.

➤ Remove the syringe from the inflation port; gently tug the catheter.

➤ Position the tubing, avoiding kinks; position the collection bag lower than the patient.

Managing Flatulence

Recall that flatus is a natural by-product of digestion. When gas is excessive or leads to complaints of abdominal distention, cramping, or discomfort, it is known as **flatulence.** Some people develop flatulence after eating gas-producing foods, such as beans, cabbage, cauliflower, onions, or highly spiced foods. For others, flatulence occurs when fiber intake is increased. Clients with irritable bowel syndrome experience a cluster of symptoms that include flatulence. Constipation is often accompanied by flatulence because digestive by-products undergo prolonged fermentation in the colon. Use the following interventions to help clients manage flatulence:

■ Teach clients to be aware of and avoid foods that trigger flatulence.

■ Teach clients to follow self-care strategies (identified earlier) for maintaining regular bowel movements.

■ Encourage patients who have had surgery with gaseous anesthesia to ambulate and perform bed exercises to stimulate peristalsis and the passage of gas.

■ In severe cases, you may need to insert a rectal tube to aid in the elimination of flatus. For a summary, see the Critical Aspects box. To learn the entire procedure,

VOL 2 Go to Chapter 28, **Procedure 28-5: Inserting a Rectal Tube,** in Volume 2.

Managing Bowel Incontinence

Bowel incontinence (or *fecal incontinence*) is the inability to control the discharge of feces and flatulence. One study suggests that one-third of critically ill patients have fecal incontinence, and it is a leading cause of admission to long-term care facilities in the United States (Beltz, 2006; Landefeld, Bowers, Feld, et al.,

2008). Physiological conditions causing bowel incontinence include conditions that affect innervation of the rectum and anus, uncontrolled diarrhea, impaction resulting in leakage of stool, and cognitive changes that alter perception of the urge to defecate. Patients who have severe psychiatric problems may be incontinent because of altered perception or inability to manage activities of daily living. Bowel incontinence is also created by functional limitations—for example, when a client recognizes the need to have a BM but cannot get to the toilet independently or in time to defecate in the toilet. Illnesses that limit mobility often lead to incontinence.

Clients with persistent bowel incontinence require special nursing care to prevent Impaired Skin Integrity because of the moisture and the activity of enzymes in the stool. In addition, bowel incontinence may be embarrassing. As clients worry about future episodes, anxiety escalates. Refer to the Nursing Care Plan and Care Map for a patient with fecal incontinence at the end of this chapter. In general, nursing interventions include the following:

- Monitor the pattern of BMs.
- Provide the bedpan or assist the patient to the bathroom at regular intervals and at times BMs are most likely to occur.
- Change clothing and/or bed linens as soon as possible to prevent skin irritation and embarrassment.
- Provide prompt hygiene care after any episodes of incontinence.
- Monitor skin for evidence of breakdown. Use moisture-barrier cream if redness or irritation is noted. Consider use of a fecal incontinence pouch for skin protection (discussed in a following section).
- Review diet, fluid intake, activity, and medicines. Work with the primary care provider to alter the above factors to encourage regular bowel movements.
- Consider a bowel training program.
- Use containment or indwelling methods to prevent fecal drainage from soiling clothing. Research on patient outcomes of most of these methods is limited.

Absorbent Products

You may use absorbent products to prevent fecal drainage from soiling clothing and linens. Products are available to fit different needs. For small quantities of stool, a long, rectangular pad or a belted absorbent shield can be placed inside clothing. For larger quantities, adult incontinence garments are used. They may pull on like underwear or fasten like a diaper. Moisture-resistant pads placed under the patient help to protect bed linens. When using absorbent products, remember these important points:

- Never refer to incontinence pads as "diapers" when caring for adults or children who have been toilet-trained. This inappropriate reference may cause embarrassment and lower the patient's self-esteem.

- Never place the plastic side of the pad next to the patient's body. This holds moisture next to the skin, which leads to irritation and breakdown.
- Use state-of-the-art skin protection products, such as perineal cleansers and skin barrier products.
- Change the pad as soon as possible after defecation. Keep the skin scrupulously clean.

External Fecal Collection Devices

You may apply an external fecal incontinence pouch to protect perianal skin or to collect large fecal samples. The pouch collects fecal drainage, keeping feces away from the skin. This is a common approach for clients with uncontrolled diarrhea. A variety of pouch systems may be used. Most frequently, a moisture-proof barrier is applied around the anus, and a plastic pouch is secured to the barrier (Fig. 28-8). The equipment may be the same as that used for patients with an ostomy. (Ostomy care is discussed later in the chapter.)

External collection systems can prevent skin breakdown, minimize odor, track output accurately, and enhance patient comfort. However, they are not typically used for patients who are ambulatory, agitated, or active in bed because the device may be dislodged, causing skin breakdown. External systems cannot be used effectively when the patient has Impaired Skin Integrity because they will not seal tightly.

You will need to assess the system regularly to ensure that it has not become dislodged, that no leaks have occurred, and to empty contents. Empty the fecal pouch when it is one-third to one-half full to prevent the pouch from getting too heavy. Pay close attention to

FIGURE 28-8 A fecal incontinence pouch. A skin barrier is applied around the anus and a plastic pouch is secured to the barrier. (Courtesy of Hollister Incorporated, Libertyville, IL.)

the perianal skin as you perform your assessment. You may need to use moisture-barrier cream on the surrounding skin. You will usually change the fecal pouch at least every 72 hours and whenever there is evidence of leakage.

The Critical Aspects box summarizes a procedure for placing both external and internal fecal drainage devices. To learn the procedure,

VOL 2 Go to **Procedure 28-8: Placing Fecal Drainage Devices,** in Volume 2.

Indwelling Fecal Drainage Devices

Indwelling fecal drainage devices are used to collect liquid stool from bedbound, immobilized ill patients. They consist of a soft, latex-free catheter and a collection bag (Fig. 28-9). The tube is inserted and a balloon on the end is filled with saline or water. Internal devices protect perianal skin, protect caregivers from potentially infectious stool, and are thought to decrease urinary tract infections. They are FDA approved, but only for 29 consecutive days, and not for pediatric patients. Other contraindications include patients who have severe hemorrhoids; recent bowel, rectal, or anal surgery or injury; rectal or anal tumors; or stricture or stenosis.

You must follow the manufacturer's recommendations carefully for insertion and maintenance. When the bag is filled, empty or replace it, depending on the type.

FIGURE 28-9 An indwelling fecal drainage device. (Courtesy of Hollister Incorporated, Libertyville, IL.)

You must also monitor to confirm placement and may need to irrigate the device.

Bowel Training

A bowel training program assists the patient to have regular, soft, formed stools. It is appropriate for clients who have chronic constipation, impaction, or bowel incontinence. Elements of a bowel training program include the following:

- Plan the program with the patient and caregiver.
- Gradually increase fiber in the diet while monitoring consistency of the stool.
- Increase fluid intake to at least eight glasses of water per day, if not contraindicated.
- Initiate a designated uninterrupted time for defecation: usually after meals, especially in the morning.
- Provide privacy for the patient during the designated time.
- Develop a staged treatment plan if constipation develops. Usually, additional fiber is added as a first measure. A stool softener is next, followed by a suppository such as bisacodyl (Dulcolax).
- Regularly modify the plan based on the patient's response.

KnowledgeCheck 28-7

- What are the major patient care concerns associated with bowel incontinence?
- What are the elements of a bowel training program?

 Go to Chapter 28, **Knowledge Check Response Sheet and Answers,** on the Student Resource Disk or DavisPlus at http://davisplus.fadavis.com/Wilkinson2

Caring for Patients with Bowel Diversions

Patients experience a variety of reactions to a bowel diversion, and each person has unique physical and psychological needs. Initially you will care for the ostomy, but the goal is for the patient to assume self-care.

Ongoing Assessments

Part of your role, as always, is to assess and monitor. You should begin care with a thorough assessment of the stoma. A healthy stoma (Fig. 28-10) ranges in color from deep pink to brick red, regardless of the patient's skin color, and is shiny and moist. Pallor or a dusky blue color indicates ischemia, and a brown-black color indicates necrosis.

Immediately after surgery, the stoma will be swollen and enlarged. As the inflammation subsides and healing occurs, the stoma will shrink. By 6 to 8 weeks, it will be at its permanent size. Stoma size varies according to the size of the person and the part of the bowel that was externalized (see Fig. 28-5). An ileostomy stoma is generally smaller than a colostomy stoma. The stoma will

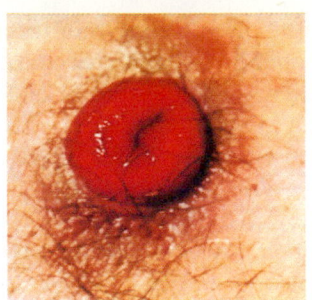

FIGURE 28-10 A healthy stoma is deep pink to brick red and is shiny and moist.

protrude above the level of the abdomen by approximately 1.3 to 2.5 cm (0.5 to 1 in.).

Output from an ileostomy stoma is liquid and contains digestive enzymes. An ostomy lower in the GI tract will have more solid output and fewer enzymes. The presence of enzymes in the effluent increases the likelihood of skin breakdown. Assess the skin surrounding a stoma for signs of irritation, such as redness, tenderness, skin breakdown, and/or drainage. You will usually need to place a moisture-proof skin barrier around the stoma to protect surrounding skin. The Critical Aspects box provides a summary of ostomy care. For a full description of the care of an ostomy appliance, including changing and emptying,

 Go to Chapter 28, **Procedure 28-6: Changing an Ostomy Appliance,** in Volume 2.

Helping Patients Adapt to the Diversion

Patients experience a variety of reactions to a bowel diversion, and each person has unique needs. Initially you will care for the ostomy, but the goal is to have the patient assume self-care and a normal life. The first step in that direction is for the patient to adjust to the presence of an ostomy. If the patient has been sick before the surgery and the ostomy leads to less pain or discomfort, the transition may be easier. Similarly, patients with continent ostomies may adapt more easily to their stoma.

With the exception of a temporary double-barreled colostomy, ostomy care is a lifelong task. Patients must learn about appliances, stoma care, and ongoing management of the ostomy. Some nurses receive additional education in enterostomal therapy and specialize in care of ostomy patients. In many hospitals and large communities, you can find an enterostomal therapist to assist patients with their ongoing care and to provide consultation on ostomy appliances.

The following interventions will promote physical and psychological adaptation:

- Be available to discuss the patient's reaction to the stoma. Your attitude and willingness to discuss the

Toward Evidence-Based Practice

Baldwin, C., Grant, M., Wendel, C., et al. (2008). Influence of intestinal stoma on spiritual quality of life of U.S. veterans. *Journal of Holistic Nursing, 26*(3), 185–194. Retrieved from http://jhn.sagepub.com/cgi/content/abstract/26/3/185

A survey was used to obtain spiritual quality-of-life (QOL) data from male veterans with intestinal ostomies. Researchers used both statistical and qualitative analysis data to explore differences among those with high QOL scores and those with lower QOL scores. Those in the high QOL group expressed more feelings of hope and meaning in life in their narratives. Both the high and low QOL groups reported odor and noise from the ostomy as problematic to church attendance. However, the high QOL group indicated that positive support from church members or clergy was helpful, whereas the low QOL group did not. The high QOL group also reported receiving support through praying, meditating, and attending church or temple.

Simmons, K., Smith, J., Bobb, K-A, et al. (2007). Adjustment to colostomy: Stoma acceptance, stoma care self-efficacy and interpersonal relationships. *Journal of Advanced Nursing, 60*(6), 627–635.

Researchers collected data from 51 patients with colostomies. They used questionnaires to measure

acceptance of the stoma, relationship with others, and stoma self-care efficacy 6 months after surgery. Results indicated that these three variables, along with location of the stoma, were strongly associated with adjustment. They concluded that routine care for stoma patients should address psychosocial concerns, with more emphasis on dispelling negative thoughts and encouraging social interaction.

1. Based on these studies, write three nursing interventions that you would use to help a patient accept and adapt to a stoma.

2. Suppose you wanted to know whether those interventions would be effective for patients with other medical conditions. For example, would the interventions that help clients adapt to a stoma help other clients to adapt to a different issue? Think of at least two health conditions for which you might want to perform the two studies just described. Explain your thinking.

 Go to Chapter 28, **Toward Evidence-Based Practice Suggested Responses,** on the Student Resource Disk or DavisPlus at http://davisplus.fadavis.com/Wilkinson2

patient's body changes will help your patient begin adapting.

- Show acceptance when working with the patient and the stoma.
- Provide adequate ventilation and odor control when assessing the stoma or ostomy appliance.
- Provide ample time to explain stoma care and use of ostomy appliances. For most patients, this is a lifelong task; therefore, patient teaching is essential.

- Teach the client about diet modifications. Ostomy patients no longer have sphincter control, so they may need to modify their diet. Box 28-3 discusses the effects of some foods on a patient with an ostomy.
- Encourage patients to return to their usual activities as much as possible.
- Refer the patient to the local ostomy association, if one is available. In many communities the local ostomy association has counselors available to visit patients,

---

BOX 28-3 ■ Dietary Changes Associated with an Ostomy

Note: These are only suggestions. Each person must, by trial and error, discover what works best for him.

General Guidelines for Patients

- Initially you may be asked to follow a bland, low-residue or soft diet for a month or two, to prevent obstructions and GI upsets. Advance the diet by adding one new food at a time.
- Eat three or more meals daily at regular times.
- People with ostomies may require additional fluid to compensate for the loss of the large intestine.
- Avoid chewing gum, as it may cause you to swallow air, causing a noisy stoma.
- Avoid foods that cause gas, odor, blockage, or loose stools. Eventually introduce them into your diet one at a time and be aware of their effects.
- Chew your food well to avoid blockage of the stoma.
- Avoid excessive weight gain.

Foods that May Cause Gas or Odor

Alcoholic beverages	Dairy products
Asparagus	Eggs
Beans	Fish
Beer	Garlic
Broccoli	Melons
Brussels sprouts	Nuts
Cabbage	Onions
Carbonated beverages	Peanut butter
Cauliflower	Peas
Cod liver oil	Radishes
Cucumbers	

Foods that May Help Control Gas or Odor

Buttermilk
Cranberry juice
Parsley
Yogurt

High-Fiber Foods that May Cause Blockage

You can eat some of these foods (e.g., mushrooms, shrimp) if you cut them into small pieces and chew them very thoroughly. As long as blockage does not occur, these foods should not necessarily be avoided, but used carefully.

- Foods with seeds (e.g., raspberries)
- Foods with tough skins (e.g., corn, dried fruits, pears, tomatoes)
- Mushrooms
- Nuts, popcorn
- Raw or minimally cooked fruits and vegetables (e.g., coleslaw, Chinese stir-fried vegetables, oranges, apple skins)
- Shrimp, lobster
- Stringy foods (e.g., celery, coconut, spinach, bean sprouts, green beans, orange pulp)

Foods that May Cause Loose Stools

Alcoholic beverages	Large meals
Baked beans	Licorice
Beer	Milk
Bran cereals	Onions
Cabbage, cooked	Prunes
Caffeine	Raisins
Chocolate	Raw fruits
Fresh fruit	Raw vegetables
Fried foods	Whole grains
Highly seasoned foods	

Note: Never restrict fluids in an effort to control diarrhea.

Foods that May Alleviate Diarrhea

Applesauce
Bananas
Cheese
Creamy peanut butter
Starchy foods (e.g., boiled rice, bread, potatoes)

Sources: United Ostomy Associations of America (2005). *Ostomates food reference chart.* Retrieved from http://www.uoaa.org/ostomy_info/pubs/uoa_diet_nutrition_en.pdf; Lutz, C., & Przytulski, K. (2006). *Nutrition and diet therapy: Evidence-based applications* (4th ed.). Philadelphia: F. A. Davis.

discuss the psychological changes associated with a bowel diversion, and help them with physical care of the stoma. Most of the counselors are skillful because they, too, have ostomies. They are able to share practical and personal information based on their own experience with similar challenges. To find the local chapter consult your phone book, or

 Go to the **United Ostomy Associations of America** Web site at http://www.uoaa.org

Caring for the Ostomy

In addition to helping the patient adapt, other nursing interventions include the following:

- Pay close attention to the skin surrounding the stoma. Skin breakdown may lead to infection, pain, and leakage. Use recommended barrier creams and skin care products.
- Monitor the amount and type of drainage from the stoma.
- ✚ Immediately report to the surgeon a stoma that is pale, dusky, or black in color; dry; or with sloughing tissues. These are signs of inadequate blood supply to the portion of intestine that has been externalized.
- Perform colostomy irrigation as needed.

Colostomy Irrigation may be indicated as an occasional intervention for constipation or in a select population of patients. Consult with the ostomy nurse and/or physician to see if colostomy irrigation is appropriate for your patient. A stoma above the descending colon usually has liquid output that cannot be controlled. Therefore, it is not irrigated. Patients with an ostomy in the descending or sigmoid colon may use colostomy irrigation as a means to control bowel evacuation and possibly eliminate the need to wear an ostomy pouch.

Colostomy irrigation is similar to an enema. The nurse or patient inserts a flexible tube into the stoma and instills irrigation fluid (traditional enema solutions). The patient may use a special plastic sleeve over the stoma or an ostomy appliance to direct the output into the toilet. After evacuation of the bowel, the client may wear a small covering over the stoma instead of a pouch. When illness occurs, it may be difficult to control the output, so the patient will use an ostomy appliance. The Critical Aspects box contains a summary. For the complete procedure,

 Go to Chapter 28, **Procedure 28-7: Irrigating a Colostomy,** in Volume 2.

KnowledgeCheck 28-8

- How can you help a patient adapt psychologically to living with a bowel diversion?
- What does a healthy stoma look like?
- Why is skin care around a stoma so important?

 Go to Chapter 28, **Knowledge Check Response Sheet and Answers,** on the Student Resource Disk or DavisPlus at http://davisplus.fadavis.com/Wilkinson2

 Go to Chapter 28, **Resources for Caregivers and Health Professionals,** on the Student Resource Disk or DavisPlus at http://davisplus.fadavis.com/Wilkinson2

 Suggested Readings: Go to Chapter 28, **Reading More About Bowel Elimination,** on the Student Resource Disk or DavisPlus at http://davisplus.fadavis.com/Wilkinson2

 Bibliography: Go to Volume 2, Bibliography.

Nursing Care Plan

Client Data

Olivia Grimaldi, 59 years old, is admitted to the orthopedic unit after having a total knee replacement. She is receiving intravenous opioid analgesics for pain. Mrs. Grimaldi's nurse sits down to talk and complete the nursing admission assessment. The conversation turns to a discussion of bowel habits.

Nurse: Mrs. Grimaldi, we pay special attention to bowel elimination because many people on this unit have problems. How often do you have a bowel movement?

Mrs. G: Not as often as I'd like. I used to be very regular, but lately everything is all mixed up.

Nurse: What has changed? Tell me what's going on.

Mrs. G: Oh, it's so embarrassing. I haven't told anyone about this.

Nurse: When did this problem start?

Mrs. G: Everything started going bad when I fell and landed on this knee a few months ago. Nothing was broken, but the pain has been just awful. I knew I had arthritis, but I never felt anything like this. I couldn't sleep, the pain was so bad. The doctor put me on some pain pills—narcotics—and they helped, but I got so constipated. I started using laxatives to go to the bathroom, but I kept needing to use more and more. Sometimes I would take a laxative and then I would have to get to the bathroom quickly. I had a couple accidents because I couldn't get to the toilet quickly enough.

Nurse: I think this is something we'll be able to help you with, Mrs. Grimaldi.

The nurse discovers that Mrs. Grimaldi drinks about 32 to 40 ounces of fluid each day and has used several stimulant laxatives and enemas to relieve her constipation. Her mobility has been significantly impaired for the past 2 months.

Nursing Diagnosis

Bowel Incontinence related to overdistention of the rectum secondary to chronic constipation, as evidenced by client report of constipation when taking opioids and subsequent fecal incontinence with the use of laxatives.

NOC Outcomes   Individualized Goals/Expected Outcomes

Bowel Continence (0500)
Bowel Elimination (0501)

By discharge, Mrs. Grimaldi will:
1. Be free from fecal impaction.
2. Begin to establish a regular pattern of stool evacuation.
3. Describe four actions she can take to reduce the risk of constipation.

Within 1 month, Mrs. Grimaldi will:
1. Control stool passage without any episodes of fecal incontinence.

Nursing Care Plan (continued)

Nursing Interventions and Activities

NIC Interventions

Bowel Management (0430)
Bowel Training (0440)

Nursing Activities

1. Conduct a comprehensive assessment of all factors related to fecal incontinence and impaired bowel elimination.

2. During physical examination, inspect the perianal skin for possible causes of fecal incontinence or skin irritation resulting from exposure to liquid stool.

3. Inquire about Mrs. Grimaldi's access to the bathroom and toileting facilities at home and work. Provide regular toileting assistance as long as the client needs it during her hospitalization.

4. Work with Mrs. Grimaldi to establish a bowel reeducation program, starting with bowel cleansing.

5. Ensure that Mrs. Grimaldi drinks 30 mL/kg of fluids per day and gradually increase dietary fiber with bran or with bulking agents. Mrs. Grimaldi is drinking only about 1200 mL of fluid per day. If she weighs 125 lb (56.7 kg), she would need to drink at least 1700 mL of fluid per day.

6. Teach Mrs. Grimaldi about how her body works to produce stool; ways to gently signal the body to defecate; the importance of responding to the urge to defecate; and how immobility, medications, and dehydration can cause constipation.

Rationale

Fecal incontinence has multiple possible causes. The best nursing interventions are those based on client assessment (Norton & Chelvanayagam, 2000). Constipation is attributed to immobility, weak straining ability, use of constipating drugs, neurological disorders, lack of dietary fiber, and poor fluid intake (Scarlett, 2004; Schnelle & Leung, 2004).

Congenital abnormalities and hemorrhoids can lead to incontinence. Skin tags can make cleansing difficult and lead to minor soiling that is difficult to distinguish from actual fecal incontinence (Norton & Chelvanayagam, 2000).

A lack of convenient access to the toilet can precipitate fecal incontinence (Schnelle & Leung, 2004).

Cleansing is indicated for rectal impaction or palpable stool in the descending or sigmoid colon. Cleansing with manual disimpaction, laxatives, and/or enema removes any potential blockages to stool elimination (Scarlett, 2004; Schnelle & Leung, 2004).

Increasing fluid intake may help to normalize stool consistency in clients with constipation who do not have adequate fluid intake (Müller-Lissner, Kamm, Scarpignato, et al., 2005). Increasing dietary fiber improves stool consistency and reduces fecal incontinence (Shakil, Church, & Rao, 2008); however, unless the diet is lacking in fiber, adding fiber does not necessarily alleviate constipation.

Bulk should be added to the diet slowly to reduce the risk of bloating, gas, or diarrhea. Dosing of bulking agents can be increased weekly until desired results are achieved; the results are more important than the amount of fiber ingested.

Gaining knowledge about bodily functions allows clients to be active participants in their care. Addressing causes of constipation can reduce the risk of recurrence (Schnelle & Leung, 2004).

(continued on next page)

Nursing Care Plan (continued)

Evaluation

Review initial outcomes and goals. Reassess daily progress toward stated discharge goals.

The day before Mrs. Grimaldi's discharge, she had no palpable stool on physical exam, and she no longer needed the intravenous analgesics; her PCA pump was discontinued. She was drinking approximately 20 mL/kg per day of fluids, she had begun taking 2 tablespoons of psyllium dissolved in water every morning, and she had a bowel movement each of the previous 2 days with stool of normal consistency for the first time in more than a month. She was able to state the actions she would take at home: continue the bulk supplements, try to increase her fluid intake to 30 mL/kg per day, use nonconstipating analgesics, and increase her mobility each day. The nurse charted that the goals were met.

References

Bulechek, F., Butcher, H., & Dochterman, J. (2008). *Nursing interventions classification (NIC)*. (5th ed.). St. Louis, MO: C. V. Mosby.

Gallagher, P., O'Mahony, D., & Quigley, E. (2008). Management of chronic constipation in the elderly. *Drugs & Aging, 25*(10), 807–822.

Ginsberg, D., Phillips, S., Wallace, J., et al. (2007). Evaluating and managing constipation in the elderly. *Urologic Nursing, 27*(3), 191–200.

Moorhead, S., Johnson, M., Maas, M., et al. (Eds.). (2008). *Nursing outcomes classification (NOC)* (4th ed.). St. Louis, MO: C. V. Mosby.

Müeller-Lissner, S., Kamm, M., Scarpignato, C., et al. (2005). Myths and misconceptions about chronic constipation. *American Journal of Gastroenterology, 100,* 232–242.

Norton, C., & Chelvanayagam, S. (2000). A nursing assessment tool for adults with fecal incontinence. *Journal of Wound, Ostomy and Continence Nursing, 27,* 279–291.

Norton, W. (2008). An overview of bowel incontinence: What can go wrong? *The Exceptional Parent, 38*(9), 67–70.

Scarlett, Y. (2004). Medical management of fecal incontinence. *Gastroenterology, 126,* S55–S63.

Schnelle, J. F., & Leung, F. W. (2004). Urinary and fecal incontinence in nursing homes. *Gastroenterology, 126* (1 Suppl 2), S41–S47.

Shakil, A., Church, R., & Rao, S. (2008). Gastrointestinal complications of diabetes. *American Family Physician, 77*(12), 1697–1703.

Care Map

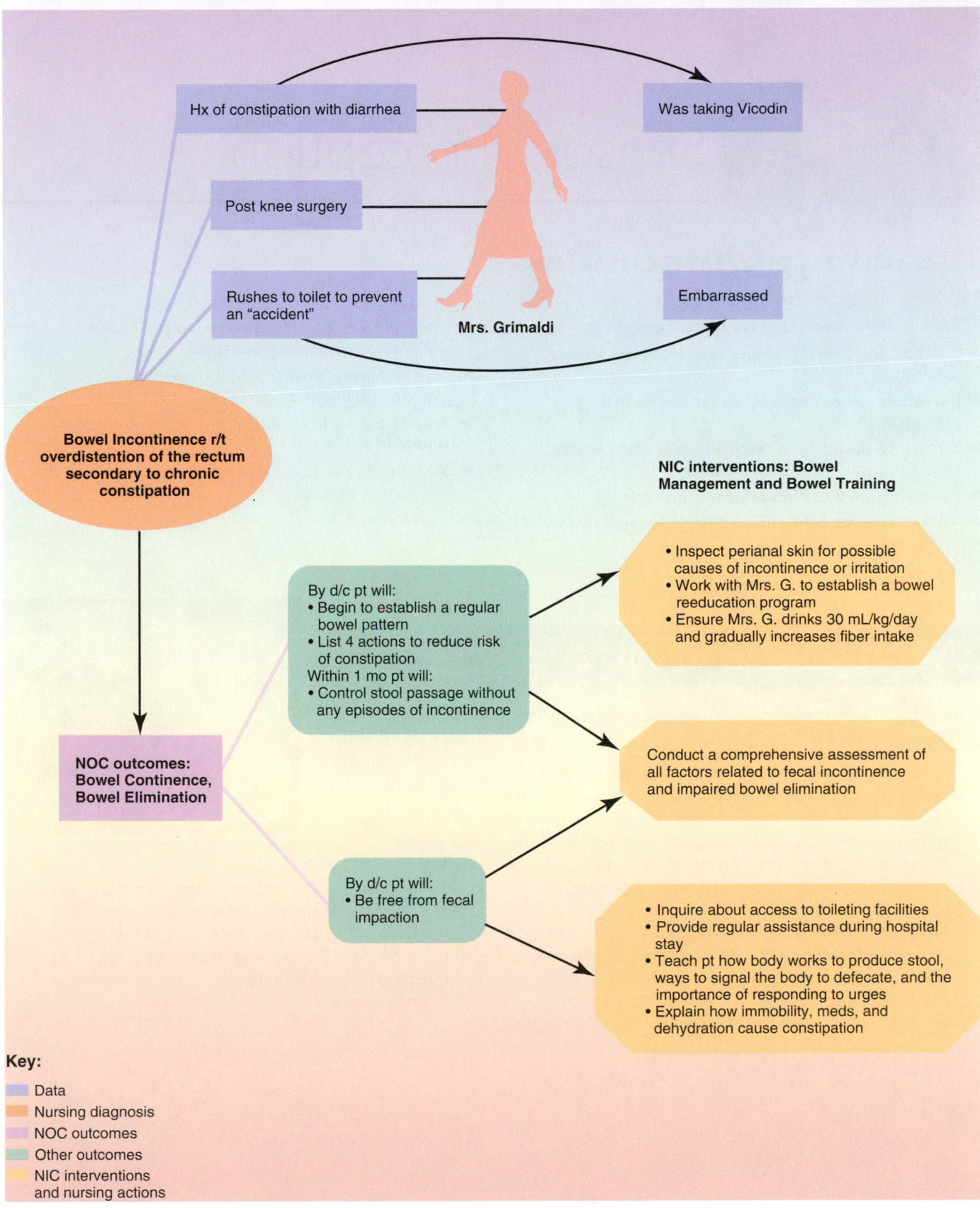

Hx of constipation with diarrhea

Post knee surgery

Rushes to toilet to prevent an "accident"

Mrs. Grimaldi

Was taking Vicodin

Embarrassed

Bowel Incontinence r/t overdistention of the rectum secondary to chronic constipation

NOC outcomes: Bowel Continence, Bowel Elimination

By d/c pt will:
• Begin to establish a regular bowel pattern
• List 4 actions to reduce risk of constipation
Within 1 mo pt will:
• Control stool passage without any episodes of incontinence

By d/c pt will:
• Be free from fecal impaction

NIC interventions: Bowel Management and Bowel Training

• Inspect perianal skin for possible causes of incontinence or irritation
• Work with Mrs. G. to establish a bowel reeducation program
• Ensure Mrs. G. drinks 30 mL/kg/day and gradually increases fiber intake

Conduct a comprehensive assessment of all factors related to fecal incontinence and impaired bowel elimination

• Inquire about access to toileting facilities
• Provide regular assistance during hospital stay
• Teach pt how body works to produce stool, ways to signal the body to defecate, and the importance of responding to urges
• Explain how immobility, meds, and dehydration cause constipation

Key:
- Data
- Nursing diagnosis
- NOC outcomes
- Other outcomes
- NIC interventions and nursing actions

CHAPTER 29

Sensory Perception

Learning Outcomes

After completing this chapter, you should be able to:

➤ Identify the components of the sensory experience.

➤ Compare and contrast sensory deprivation and sensory overload.

➤ List factors placing clients at risk for altered sensory perception.

➤ Discuss the hazards of sensory deficits in vision, hearing, taste, smell, touch, and proprioception.

➤ Identify factors that affect sensory stimulation.

➤ Assess clients for signs and symptoms of altered sensory perception.

➤ State nursing diagnoses and outcomes appropriate for clients with problems of sensory perception.

➤ Describe nursing interventions to prevent sensory deprivation and sensory overload.

➤ Describe nursing interventions for clients with sensory deficits.

➤ Discuss strategies to enhance communication with clients with sensory deficits.

Meet Your Patients

At a clinical post-conference, your instructor presents the following cases:

■ Joshua is a 28-year-old patient in the intensive care unit (ICU). He had a car accident 3 weeks ago and has had several surgeries to repair a fractured femur, ruptured spleen, and intracranial bleeding. He was ventilated mechanically for 10 days and has had numerous invasive procedures. The nurses report that he is very confused and has been hallucinating.

■ Richard is a 90-year-old man who has been a resident at a skilled nursing facility for 10 years. He has no visitors, never leaves his room, has no television or radio in the room, and no longer speaks. He does not respond to verbal or tactile stimulation. He lies in bed in a fetal position.

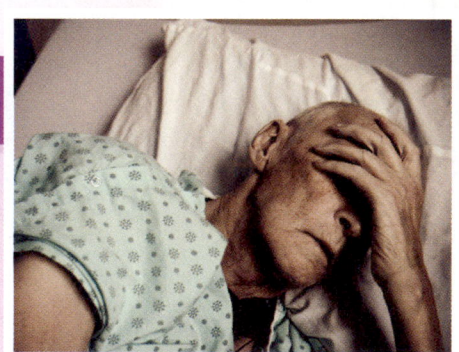

When staff members try to move him, he moans and howls.

Your instructor asks you to consider how these patients are similar and how their care might overlap. It seems hard to imagine that these patients could have much in common. What similarities can you see? What differences? As you read this chapter, follow these cases and other examples illustrating the effects of altered sensory or perceptual function.

Theoretical **Knowledge**
knowing why

We experience the world through our senses. Vision, hearing, smell, taste, touch, and our sense of our body in space all help us to interpret and interact with our environment in a meaningful way. To grow, develop, and function, we must be able to sense and respond to sensory input.

Many patients who are being treated for one condition also have a preexisting sensory deficit (e.g., a diabetic client whom you are teaching self-injection may also be blind). Others develop alterations in sensory function as a result of their illness or of medications they are taking. The Joint Commission (2008) requires that you address the communication needs of patients with vision, speech, hearing, language, and cognitive impairments. This chapter will help you provide care for such patients.

Components of the Sensory Experience

Our senses give us information about our environment and what is happening inside our bodies. The purpose of sensation is to allow the body to respond to changing situations and maintain homeostasis. A sensory experience involves four components in the nervous system: stimulus, reception, perception, and an arousal mechanism. A **stimulus** may be a sight, sound, taste, touch, pain, or anything that stimulates a nerve receptor. The brain must receive and process it to make it meaningful.

Reception

Reception is the process of receiving stimuli from nerve endings in the skin and inside the body. A receptor converts a stimulus to a nerve impulse and transmits the impulse along sensory neurons to the central nervous system (CNS). Some receptors remain activated for as long as the stimulus is applied. However, most receptors *adapt* to stimuli; that is, their response declines with time. Adaptation explains why, over time, you become unaware of an unpleasant smell or the persistent hum of an air conditioner.

Receptors usually respond to only one type of stimulus. For example, taste buds in the mouth detect sweet, sour, salty, or bitter, whereas receptors in the retina detect light rays. The following are examples of the many types of sensory receptors in the body:

- *Mechanoreceptors* in the skin and hair follicles detect touch, pressure, and vibration.
- *Hair cells* are receptors for hearing. Located in the cochlea of the ear, they detect sound waves. In the vestibular apparatus of the ear, receptors for equilibrium and balance also detect acceleration of the body and position of the head.

- *Thermoreceptors* in the skin detect variations in temperature.
- *Proprioceptors* in the skin, muscles, tendons, ligaments, and joint capsules coordinate input to enable us to sense the position of our body in space (proprioception).
- *Photoreceptors* located in the retina of the eyes detect visible light.
- *Chemoreceptors* for taste are located in our taste buds. *Olfactory receptors* (chemoreceptors for smell) are located in the epithelium of the nasal cavity.

Perception

Perception is the ability to interpret the impulses transmitted from the receptors and give meaning to the stimuli. After the receptors generate nerve impulses, the impulses travel along neural pathways to the spinal cord and brain. They are then relayed to specialized locations in the brain where perception of the stimuli occurs (Fig. 29-1). For example, vision is perceived in the occipital lobes, hearing in the temporal lobes, and touch in the somatosensory area. Perception requires functioning of the sensory receptors, the reticular activating system, neural pathways, and brain.

Perception occurs when the person becomes aware of the stimulus and receives the information. It would not be possible to process all the stimuli that constantly bombard us. The brain discards about 99% of all sensory information as irrelevant and unimportant. For example, you are usually unaware of your clothing touching your body. However, if you focus on it, you can feel it.

Perception of a stimulus is affected by several factors:

- *Location* of the receptors and pathway activated
- *Number* of receptors activated
- *Frequency* of action potentials generated (which varies according to the intensity of the stimulus)
- *Changes* in location, number, and frequency

Past experiences, knowledge, and attitude also influence perception.

Arousal Mechanism

For the central nervous system to perceive, interpret, and react to incoming stimuli, it must be active. The **reticular activating system (RAS),** located in the brain stem, controls consciousness and alertness. The neurons of the RAS make connections between the spinal cord, cerebellum, thalamus, and cerebral cortex, relaying visual, auditory, and other stimuli that help keep us awake, attentive, and observant. Without such stimuli, the CNS becomes lethargic, and the person may lose consciousness. Anesthesia, sedatives, opioids, and some other drugs depress the RAS, as does a darkened, quiet environment. Not surprisingly, as you will learn in Chapter 33, sleep is regulated by the RAS.

Frontal lobe

Premotor area

Motor area

General sensory area

Sensory association area

Parietal lobe

Occipital lobe

Visual association area

Visual area

Motor speech area

Auditory association area

Auditory area

Temporal lobe

FIGURE 29-1 Special sensory areas of the brain receive and interpret stimuli from the sensory receptors. (*Source:* Scanlon, V., & Sanders, T. (2007). *Essentials of anatomy and physiology* (5th ed.). Philadelphia: F. A. Davis. Used with permission.)

The level of stimuli needed to maintain arousal varies: Some people feel optimally alert in bright, noisy, fast-paced environments, whereas others prefer much lower levels of stimulation. As discussed earlier, the brain adapts to constant stimuli, such as a ticking clock. Thus, to maintain arousal, some variation in stimuli is required, such as different pieces of music or an ever-changing view.

Responding to Sensations

Once a stimulus is perceived, the brain either discards it, stores it in memory, or sends impulses along motor pathways to various parts of the body (e.g., the muscles, the heart, and so on), bringing about a response. Humans respond to sensations when they are alert and receptive to stimulation. For example, a fatigued new mother may wake up to the soft cry of her infant yet sleep through the persistent ringing of the doorbell. The response to a stimulus is based on the following factors:

Intensity. An intense stimulus excites more receptors, leading to a greater response. For example, a bright, glaring light can cause you to respond by squinting and shielding your eyes, whereas a dim light may cause little reaction.

Contrast. Contrast is also stimulating. Imagine being outside in cold, windy weather. If you enter an un-heated garage, you instantly feel warmer because the building blocks the wind. If you then go inside a room with a blazing fireplace, you will need to take off layers of clothing rapidly because the contrast in temperature will make you feel hot.

Adaptation. Often we take stimuli for granted. Have you ever taken a vacation to a remote place? Suddenly you notice the stars, quiet surroundings, and the smell of the flowers. At home, you fail to notice these things because they have become familiar to you. But in a different setting, they become noticeable. Now recall your first clinical experience. Did you notice the noise and activity on the unit? Nurses become accustomed to the noise, lights, activity, and even alarms and are able to "tune them out." Unfortunately, these stimuli are all new to patients, so they notice them and may have difficulty resting.

Previous Experience. Prior experience with a stimulus affects ongoing responses to the same stimulus. Have you ever seen a patient scrunch her eyes, grit her teeth, or turn away from an injection before you are even ready to give it? This may mean that she has memory of a prior negative experience with injections.

KnowledgeCheck 29-1

- What is the difference between reception and perception?
- What are the four components of a sensory experience?
- What is the role of the reticular activating system in the sensory experience?

 Go to Chapter 29, **Knowledge Check Response Sheet and Answers,** on the Student Resource Disk or DavisPlus at http://davisplus.fadavis.com/Wilkinson2

Factors Affecting Sensory Function

Among the many factors affecting sensory function are developmental stage, culture, health status, medications, stress level, personality, and lifestyle.

Developmental Variations

People have differing sensory perceptual abilities at different stages of life. In addition, the need for and use of sensory stimulation differs throughout life.

Infants

Newborns can track objects and respond to light, but their vision is far less acute than that of older children and adults. Newborn hearing is especially acute at low frequencies. Newborns can also discriminate between different tastes, and they prefer sweet over sour. They react to odors and seem to be able to discriminate between the smell of their own mother's breast milk and that of another woman. The sense of touch is keenly present at birth; the face, hands, and soles of the feet are the most sensitive (Polan & Taylor, 2007).

Infants require sensory stimulation to grow and develop normally. Tactile stimulation through cuddling, feeding, and soothing creates a bond between infant and caregiver, provides comfort and pleasure, and teaches the infant about the external environment. Exposure to voices, music, and ambient noise develops the auditory nervous system. By 1 year of age, the child can discriminate between different sounds and often recognizes the source. Lights, colors, and contrast allow the infant to observe the world in which she lives and stimulate continued development.

Children and Adolescents

In *early childhood*, visual acuity improves; full depth perception is achieved during the preschool period. Hearing is usually fully developed in young children; however, they may experience reversible hearing loss as a result of frequent ear infections and cerumen impaction. In contrast to toddlers, who often lose their balance when walking, older children are sure and steady on their feet. During the *school-age years* and *adolescence*, children experience increasing social interaction and formal education. They are developmentally driven toward peers, and these experiences provide a wealth of sensory stimulation.

Adults and Older Adults

By *early adulthood*, senses are at their peak, unless they are affected by illness or injury. As the adult ages, all of the senses are affected. Table 29-1 describes sensory changes associated with aging. *Older adults* experience a generalized decrease in the number of nerve conduction fibers, resulting in slower reflexes and delayed response to stimuli. Structural changes occur in the aging eye and

Table 29-1 ➤ Sensory Function Changes with Aging	
SENSE	**CHANGES ASSOCIATED WITH AGING**
Vision	All structures of the eyes undergo changes:
	The vitreous humor becomes thinner, and "floaters" appear in the visual field.
	The lens becomes discolored and opaque; the pupil becomes smaller. Therefore, less light reaches the retina, limiting vision.
	The lens becomes less flexible and less able to focus on near objects.
	The ciliary body contracts and the lens thickens, bringing loss of visual acuity, decreased ability to accommodate to distance and sudden changes in illumination, and decreased night vision.
	Decreased peripheral vision
	Decreased tear production
Hearing	Cerumen is drier and more solid, creating hearing loss.
	Scarring (e.g., from previous inflammation over the life span)
	Hearing changes commonly include presbycusis (hearing loss of high-frequency tones) and decreased speech discrimination.
Taste	Taste buds atrophy and decrease in number, decreasing the ability to perceive tastes, especially sweetness.
	Dry mouth may alter the sense of taste.
Smell	Atrophy and loss of olfactory neurons decreases the ability to perceive smell (which may also alter the sense of taste).
Touch	Loss of sensory nerve fibers and changes in the cerebral cortex decrease the ability to perceive light touch, pain, and temperature variations.
Kinesthesia	Kinesthetic changes include a decrease in muscle fibers and diminished conduction speed of nerve fibers, resulting in slowed reaction time, decreased speed and power of muscle contractions, and impaired balance. These place older adults at increased risk for falling.

ear; for example, cerumen (wax) accumulation in the ear canal and impaction are more common in older adults. Sensory decline with aging may cause withdrawal, depression, social isolation, and hallucinations. Keep in mind that aging is not the only cause of sensory deficits in older adults, though.

Culture

Culture affects the nature, type, and amount of interaction and stimulation that people feel comfortable with. People of different cultural backgrounds tend to prefer differing amounts of eye contact, personal space, and physical touch. Compare the day-to-day experience of an older adult living in a remote farming community to someone living in an extended family home in the center of a large city. The amount of stimulation perceived as normal would be very different for each of these people.

Assess your clients' cultural needs to see how they impact their sensory–perceptual status. For example, you may think your hospitalized patient needs quiet time alone to rest. However, if he is accustomed to being surrounded by a large family, he may actually rest better in the midst of what seems like chaos to you. Also, use touch advisedly. For some people it is comforting; for others, it may be offensive.

Illness and Medications

Many illnesses affect sensory reception and perception. Neurological disorders, such as multiple sclerosis, slow the transmission of nerve impulses. Diseases that affect circulation (e.g., atherosclerosis) may impair function of the sensory receptors and the brain, thereby altering perception and response. Some diseases affect specific sensory organs. For example, diabetic retinopathy is the leading case of blindness among adults ages 20 to 74. Hypertension, too, can damage the retina of the eyes.

Several **medications** affect sensory function. For example, aspirin and furosemide (Lasix) become ototoxic if taken for a long period of time and impair function of the auditory nerve. CNS depressants, such as opioid analgesics and sedatives, blunt reception and perception of stimuli.

Stress

Have you ever been under a great deal of stress? How did it feel? When you are under stress, do you find yourself looking for or avoiding stimuli? Obviously, stress provides added stimulation. As a result, a person who is bored may add stress. By setting a goal, such as running a marathon, the person undertakes a series of activities to reach that goal. In that regard, stress provides sensory stimulation at a time when the person may have been experiencing deprivation.

However, stress can cause too much stimulation. Physical illness, pain, hospitalization, tests, and surgery are all stressors that can lead to sensory overload—more stimuli than the person can handle. Jason ("Meet Your Patients") has been under tremendous physical and emotional stress as a result of his injuries and surgeries. His situation is one in which you might want to limit unnecessary stimuli (e.g., noise, lights, too many visitors).

Personality and Lifestyle

Are you the kind of person who likes to have people around all the time? Do you thrive on noise and action? Or are you the kind of person who loves to curl up with a book and a cup of tea? Clients, too, vary in their personalities and lifestyles. Some people, by nature, like excitement, change, and stimulation; others prefer a more predictable and quiet life. Clients are at risk for sensory alterations if their previous level of stimuli does not match their current level. Health problems, a change of environment, or loss of a partner can each create changes in stimuli.

KnowledgeCheck 29-2

- List five major factors that affect sensory function.
- Compare and contrast the sensory changes in childhood with those in older adulthood.

 Go to Chapter 29, **Knowledge Check Response Sheet and Answers,** on the Student Resource Disk or DavisPlus at http://davisplus.fadavis.com/Wilkinson2

Sensory Alterations

Humans are constantly striving to achieve **sensoristasis,** a state of optimum arousal. Sensory alterations occur when the body experiences meaningless or limited stimulation (sensory deprivation), excessive stimulation (sensory overload), or sensory deficits.

Sensory Deprivation

Sensory deprivation is a state of RAS depression caused by a lack of meaningful stimuli. When environmental stimuli are deficient, the remaining stimuli, such as distant noises, minor pain, and cold extremities, can become overly noticeable or distorted, filling in the "sensory gap" and causing the patient a level of distress that is out of proportion to the intensity of the stimulus. Sensory deprivation can be caused by environmental conditions or by interference with the reception or perception of stimuli. Clinical manifestations include problems with perception, cognition, and emotion (Box 29-1).

The following situations increase the risk for sensory deprivation:

- Impaired sensory reception (e.g., neurological injury, dementia, depression, sleep deprivation, sensory losses, and CNS depressant medications)
- Inability to transmit or process stimuli (e.g., nerve or brain injury)

BOX 29-1 ■ Signs of Sensory Deprivation and Sensory Overload

Sensory Deprivation	Sensory Overload
Irritability	Irritability
Confusion	Confusion
Reduced attention span	Reduced attention span
Decreased problem-solving ability	Decreased problem-solving ability
Drowsiness	Drowsiness (due to insomnia)
Depression	Muscle tension
Preoccupation with somatic complaints (e.g., heart palpitations)	Anxiety
Delusions (misinterpretations of external stimuli)	Inability to concentrate
Hallucinations (seeing, hearing, feeling, tasting, or smelling something that is not there)	Decreased ability to perform tasks
	Restlessness
	Disorientation

- Restricted mobility
- Sensory deficits (e.g., vision, hearing)
- A nonstimulating, monotonous environment. Examples include children in orphanages; people in prison; homebound disabled and older people; patients in nursing homes and other institutions; and hospitalized patients in isolation, seclusion, or private rooms.
- Being from a different culture and unable to interpret received cues

As you might expect, interventions for sensory deprivation focus on providing stimuli and supporting sensory perceptual function. They are discussed in more detail in the "Practical Knowledge" section of this chapter.

Sensory Overload

Sensory overload develops when either environmental or internal stimuli—or a combination of both—exceed a higher level than the patient's sensory system can effectively process. This sometimes occurs in patients who, because of neurological or psychiatric disorders, are unable to adapt to continuing, nonmeaningful stimuli. Some clinical manifestations of sensory overload are similar to those of sensory deprivation (see Box 29-1).

Hospitalized patients often experience sensory overload due to a combination of physical discomfort, anxiety, separation from loved ones, and the experience of being in the unfamiliar hospital environment. Medications that stimulate the CNS may also contribute to overload, as will substances, such as caffeine and over-the-counter weight-loss pills. In addition, physical conditions that activate the CNS (e.g., hyperthyroidism) contribute to sensory overload.

Patients at risk for sensory overload are those in an environment with excessive stimuli or more stimuli than is usual for that person. For example, a patient who lives alone might experience sensory overload on a busy medical–surgical unit.

KnowledgeCheck 29-3

- How does sensory deprivation occur?
- Identify five signs of sensory deprivation.
- How does sensory overload occur?
- Identify five signs of sensory overload.

 Go to Chapter 29, **Knowledge Check Response Sheet and Answers,** on the Student Resource Disk or DavisPlus at http://davisplus.fadavis.com/Wilkinson2

 Critical**Thinking** 29-1

Review the stories of Joshua and Richard ("Meet Your Patients"). How are these patients similar? What factors may have contributed to each patient's current concerns?

Sensory Deficits

Sensory deficits may stem from impaired reception, perception, or both. Of the six basic sensory deficits discussed here, impaired vision and hearing are the ones you are most likely to encounter in nursing practice. Drawing on your personal experience, think how many people you know who wear glasses or contact lenses or who wear a hearing aid. How many do you know whose vision or hearing is not completely corrected by such aids? You can see that sensory deficits are common.

A sudden onset of a deficit is unnerving and may lead to disorientation and anxiety. Gradual changes allow the person to adapt, often without even realizing the extent of it. The patient who has progressively lost hearing may, over time, keep turning up the sound on his radio and telephone and not realize that others find the sound blaring. When there is a deficit in one sense, the other senses may become sharper to compensate (e.g., a person who is blind may develop more acute hearing). Six sensory deficits are discussed in the following sections.

Impaired Vision

Vision occurs when light rays that focus on the retina trigger a nerve impulse that is transmitted to the visual area of the brain in the occipital region. Visual deficits may result from trauma or disease of the eye, microvascular problems, or CNS disorders. Common causes of visual deficits include age-related changes, refractive errors, orbital trauma, cataracts, glaucoma, diabetic or hypertensive retinopathy, macular degeneration, or loss of visual fields after a stroke (Box 29-2). Changes in vision affect all aspects of daily living and may severely limit mobility and interaction.

Impaired Hearing

Hearing occurs when sound waves entering the ear canal are converted to vibrations and transferred from the middle ear to the inner ear. Vibrations cause the hair cells in the cochlea to bend, generating impulses that are carried by cranial nerve VIII to the brain. The auditory area in the brain is located in the temporal lobes. The auditory area interprets the sound and allows you to determine the direction from which the noise is coming. See Chapter 19, Figure 19-5, for an illustration of the structures of the ear.

Hearing deficits may result from injury or disease in structures of the ear, the nerves, or the brain (Box 29-3). Inability to hear decreases the ability to communicate and thus hampers social interaction. It may interfere with a patient's ability to understand instructions from healthcare professionals and create a safety hazard due to inability to hear warnings.

BOX 29-2 ■ Common Visual Deficits

- **Myopia,** or nearsightedness, means that the patient is able to see close objects well but not distant objects. For example, a person with 20/200 vision can see an object from 20 feet away that a person with normal sight could see from a distance of 200 feet.

- **Hyperopia,** or farsightedness, implies that the eye sees distant objects well. A person with hyperopia may have 20/10 vision—he can see an object from 20 feet that a normal eye can see from 10 feet; however, near vision is impaired.

- **Presbyopia** is a change in vision associated with aging. The lens becomes less elastic and less able to accommodate to near objects. If you're older than 40 years of age, there's a good chance you may be experiencing this problem.

- **Astigmatism** is caused by an irregular curvature of the cornea or lens that scatters light rays and blurs the image on the retina. The person has blurred vision with distortion.

- **Cataracts** are a clouding of the lens, resulting in blurred vision, sensitivity to glare, and image distortion.

- **Glaucoma** is a type of vision loss caused by increased pressure in the anterior cavity of the eyeball that distorts the shape of the cornea and shifts the position of the lens, resulting in loss of peripheral vision. It can eventually lead to blindness.

- **Macular degeneration** is the loss of central vision due to damage to the *macula lutea,* the central portion of the retina. The leading cause of visual impairment in U.S. residents older than age 50, it is characterized by slow, progressive loss of central and near vision. It is usually present in both eyes.

- **Strabismus** (crossed eyes), in which one eye deviates from a fixed image, can cause permanent vision loss.

BOX 29-3 ■ Common Hearing Deficits

- **Conduction deafness** results when one of the structures that transmits vibrations is affected. It may be a temporary or permanent condition caused by infection of the middle ear, a punctured tympanic membrane, or arthritis of the auditory bones. A hearing aid may be helpful for conduction deafness.

- **Nerve deafness** occurs when there is damage to cranial nerve VIII or the receptors in the cochlea. It may result from ototoxic medications (e.g., gentamicin) or viral infections that affect cranial nerve VIII. Chronic exposure to loud noise may also lead to nerve and receptor impairment.

- **Presbycusis** is a progressive sensorineural loss associated with aging. It results from deterioration of the hair cells in the cochlea. Presbycusis leads to diminished ability to hear high-pitched sounds and to distinguish sounds in a noisy environment. Hearing aids may be of no value in sensorineural hearing loss.

- **Central deafness** results from damage to the auditory areas in the temporal lobes. Tumor, trauma, meningitis, or CVA (cerebrovascular accident, i.e., stroke) in the temporal lobe may cause this.

- **Tinnitus** is a term used to describe ringing in the ears. Most tinnitus comes from damage to the microscopic endings of the nerve in the inner ear, for example, trauma, turbulent blood flow, hypertension, ear infection, medications, otosclerosis, or arthritic changes of the bones of the ear.

- **Impacted cerumen** is a condition in which earwax becomes tightly packed in the ear canal, blocking the canal. Patients with impacted cerumen may experience a feeling of fullness or pain, decreased hearing, or tinnitus.

- **Otosclerosis** is a hardening of the bones of the middle ear, especially the stapes. The stapes becomes fixed, leading to poor sound transmission to the inner ear. The cause of this disorder is unknown.

- **Otitis media** is a middle ear infection. It is a common childhood illness that may be caused by viruses or bacteria.

Impaired Taste

Taste imparts flavor and interest to food. Taste deficits may decrease the pleasure associated with eating; weight loss and malnutrition may result. Taste depends on the functioning of the taste buds on the tongue and, to a lesser extent, on the soft palate. Four types of taste buds exist: sweet, sour, salty, and bitter. A proposed fifth taste bud, glutamate, can detect savory flavors. The buds for sweet and salty tastes are primarily on the tip of the tongue; for sour taste, on the two lateral sides of the tongue; and for bitter taste, primarily on the posterior tongue and the soft palate (Fig. 29-2). When stimulated, taste buds generate nerve impulses that travel along the facial and glossopharyngeal nerves (cranial nerves VII and IX, respectively) to the taste area in the parietal–temporal cortex. Foods stimulate different combinations of taste buds. That stimulation, together with the sense of smell, produces the vast number of tastes we can perceive.

Impaired taste most commonly results from **xerostomia** (excessively dry mouth), which may be caused by medications, decreased saliva production, inadequate fluid intake, poor nutrition, or poor oral hygiene. In addition, loss of the sense of smell commonly causes loss of taste. Other causes of taste deficits include the common cold; infections of the nose, sinuses, mouth, or salivary glands; smoking; vitamin B_{12} or zinc deficiency; and injury to the mouth, nose, or head (Box 29-4).

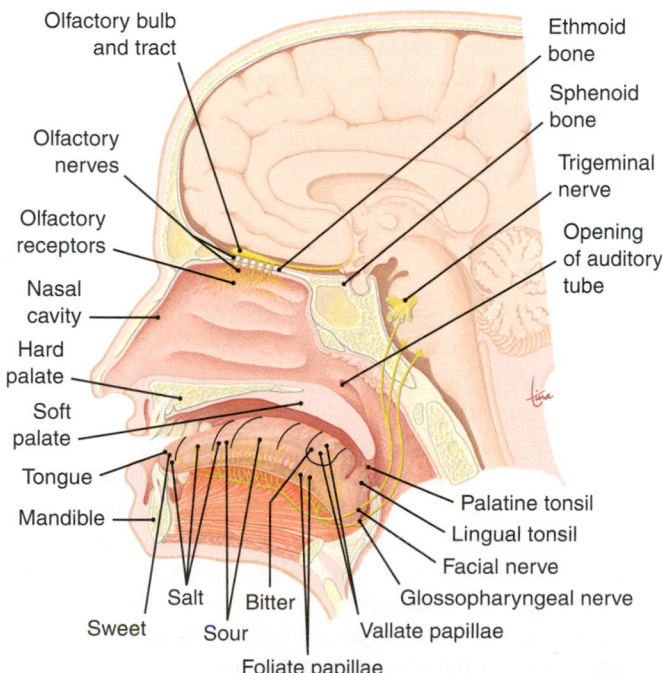

FIGURE 29-2 Structures concerned with the sense of smell and taste. (*Source:* Scanlon, V., & Sanders, T. (2007). *Essentials of anatomy and physiology* (5th ed., p. 201). Philadelphia: F. A. Davis. Used with permission.)

BOX 29-4 ■ Medications that Cause Taste Disturbance

Numerous medications affect the sense of taste. A study by Zervakis and Schiffman (2004) found that most prescription medications are foul-tasting and may have a profound effect on the sense of taste. In a test of 62 prescription medications, "bitter, sour, and metallic" described all the medications. Medications with the highest incidence of taste disturbance include the following:

- Antibiotics
- Anticonvulsants, such as phenytoin (Dilantin) and carbamazepine (Tegretol)
- Antihistamines and decongestants
- Antihypertensive and cardiac medications
- Chemotherapy agents
- Lithium carbonate (Lithobid)
- Antipsychotics
- Antidepressants
- Statins
- Muscle relaxants

Impaired Smell

The sense of smell is triggered when chemoreceptors in the upper nasal cavities detect vaporized chemicals. Chemoreceptors generate impulses carried by the olfactory nerve (cranial nerve I) into the olfactory area in the temporal lobes (see Fig. 29-2). Vaporized molecules can be detected from a distance, so the sense of smell can serve as an early warning system for detection of smoke and noxious chemicals.

The sense of smell is vital to the sense of taste. Recall the last time you had a cold or nasal congestion. When the sense of smell is lost **(anosmia)**, food does not taste the same. Patients who are unable to smell food lose their appetite, and nutritional deficits may result. Permanent anosmia may develop after cranial nerve damage, a tumor, or atherosclerosis. It may also be inherited and nonpathological. Zinc deficiency, heavy smoking, cocaine use, rhinitis, and sinusitis can cause reversible anosmia.

Nurses may make therapeutic use of a patient's sense of smell. **Aromatherapy,** the use of odors for therapeutic effect, has become one of the most widely practiced complementary therapies among nurses in the United States. See the box, Complementary and Alternative Modalities (CAM): Essential Oils. Also see Chapter 40 for more information about aromatherapy. Olfaction has been shown to play a role in memory, mood, and safety. See Toward Evidence-Based Practice for a discussion of current research on smell, memory, and mood.

Complementary & Alternative Modalities (CAM)

Essential Oils

Aromatherapy is the use of naturally extracted aromatic essences from plants to balance, harmonize, and promote the health of body, mind, and spirit. It is a natural, noninvasive treatment system designed to affect the whole person, not just the symptom or disease. Although scientific evidence is weak and preliminary, essential oils are thought to work by promoting the body's natural ability to balance, regulate, heal, and maintain itself. The following are some essential oils frequently used in aromatherapy. Note that some may be used topically in certain situations (e.g., minor burns). Beginning research supports the following; however, the evidence base is not strong.

- **Eucalyptus,** *Eucalyptus globulus* **or** *Eucalyptus radiata.* Helpful in treating respiratory problems, such as coughs, colds, and asthma. Used to treat burns, wounds, and insect bites. Also helps to boost the immune system and relieve muscle tension.

- **Ylang Ylang,** *Cananga odorata.* Helps one to relax, and can reduce muscle tension. Good antidepressant. Used for anxiety, hypertension, and stress.

- **Geranium,** *Pelargonium graveolens.* Helps to balance hormones in women, good for balancing the skin. Can be both relaxing and uplifting, as well as antidepressant. Used for acne and oily skin.

- **Peppermint,** *Mentha piperita.* Used in treating headaches, sinusitis, vertigo, muscle aches, asthma, digestive disorders such as slow digestion, indigestion, nausea, and flatulence.

- **Lavender,** *Lavandula angustifolia.* Relaxing, and also useful in treating wounds, burns, and skin care. Also used for asthma, itching, labor pains, colic, and dysmenorrhea.

- **Lemon,** *Citrus limon.* Uplifting, yet relaxing. Helpful in treating wounds and infections, and for house cleaning and deodorizing. Sometimes used for athlete's foot, colds, and warts.

- **Clary sage,** *Salvia sclarea.* Natural pain killer, helpful in treating amenorrhea and muscular aches and pains. Relaxing, and can help with insomnia. Also helpful in balancing hormones. Used to treat sore throat, stress, and exhaustion.

- **Tea tree,** *Melaleuca alternifolia.* A natural antifungal oil, good for treating all sorts of fungal infections including vaginal yeast infections, "jock itch," athlete's foot, and ringworm. Used for insect bites, itching, and migraine. Also helps to boost the immune system.

- **Roman chamomile,** *Anthemus nobilis.* Relaxing, and can help with sleeplessness and anxiety. Also good for muscle aches, arthritis, and tension. Useful in treating wounds and infection. Used for insomnia, nausea, PMS, and earache.

- **Rosemary,** *Rosmarinus officinalis.* Uplifting and promotes mental stimulation. Also stimulating to the immune, circulatory, and digestive systems. Good for muscle aches and tension.

Impaired Tactile Perception

Touch is crucial to growth and development. It provides pleasure, warns us of injury, and transmits information about the external environment. The dermis of the skin contains receptors for the cutaneous sensations of light touch, pressure, heat, cold, and pain. Information from these receptors is transmitted to the sensory areas in the parietal lobes. The number of cutaneous receptors determines the sensitivity of an area and the amount of space devoted to that region in the sensory cortex area. The hands and face have the most receptors and therefore the largest area in the sensory cortex.

A person's ability to perceive touch is often measured in terms of *two-point discrimination,* that is, the ability to perceive as distinct two close but separate points pressed against the skin. On the lips and fingertips, a person can normally distinguish between points less than 4 mm apart, whereas on the torso, normal two-point discrimination is greater than 2 cm.

Loss of tactile sensitivity can be caused by a cerebrovascular accident (stroke), brain or spinal tumor or injury, or peripheral nerve damage caused by diabetes, Guillain-Barré syndrome, or chronic alcoholism.

 Critical**Thinking** 29-2

- Why do you think a person with impaired tactile perception is at risk for injury?
- Speculate as to the possible nature of injuries that might occur.

Impaired Kinesthetic Sense

Kinesthesia, or muscle sense, is a complex process involving **proprioceptors** that detect stretch in muscles to create a mental picture of how the body is positioned. Conscious muscle sense is perceived in the parietal lobes. Unconscious muscle sense occurs in the cerebellum, which coordinates movement.

Problems of the inner ear commonly impair kinesthesia. The vestibular apparatus of the inner ear has hair cells that detect rotation or acceleration of the body. Because the vestibular cell nuclei also receive input from neurons involved in vision, a mismatch between the position or acceleration of the head and the visual field can result in motion sickness. This is why it is not advisable to read a book while riding in a car traveling on a winding road.

Parkinson's disease, other neurological disorders, tumors, cerebrovascular accident, and even certain

Toward Evidence-Based Practice

Jirovetz, L., Buchbauer, G., Stoilova, I., et al. (2006). Chemical composition and antioxidant properties of clove leaf essential oil. *Journal of Agricultural and Food Chemistry, 54*(17), 6303–6307.

These researchers studied the chemical properties of clove leaf essential oil in laboratory experiments. They found it to have antioxidant properties.

Sonboli, A., Babakhani, B., & Mehrabian, A. (2006). Antimicrobial activity of six constituents of essential oil from *Salvia. Zeitschrift fur Naturforschung, 61*(3-4), 160–164.

Using bioassay research, this laboratory found that *Salvia* has some antimicrobial activity, the degree of which varies among different species of the herb.

Kyle, G. (2005). Evaluating the effectiveness of aromatherapy in reducing levels of anxiety in palliative care patients: Results of a pilot study. *Complementary Therapies in Clinical Practice, 12*(2), 148–155.

This pilot study evaluated the effectiveness of aromatherapy massage with a sweet almond carrier oil as compared to two different types of sandalwood in reducing anxiety in patients receiving palliative care. No firm conclusions could be drawn, but the results seemed to support the notion that sandalwood oil is effective in reducing anxiety.

McCaffrey, R., Thomas, D., & Kinzelman, A. (2009). The effects of lavender and rosemary essential oils on test-taking anxiety among graduate nursing students. *Holistic Nursing Practice, 23*(2), 88.

Researchers studied the use of rosemary and lavender essential oil sachets on test-taking stress in graduate nursing students. The intervention reduced stress as measured by scores on a test anxiety measure, personal statements, and pulse rates.

Jayasekara, R. (2008). Dementia: Wandering. *Evidence Summaries – Joanna Briggs Institute.* Retrieved from http://www.guideline.gov/summary/summary.aspx?ss=15&doc_id=12992&nbr=6688

One finding of this systematic review of 11 studies suggested that there is no robust evidence to recommend aromatherapy as an intervention to reduce wandering in patients with dementia.

Several of these studies provide beginning support for the usefulness of a specific oil for a specific purpose. For each of the following questions, (a) state whether one of the studies can answer the question for you; (b) if it can, give the answer; and (c) if it cannot, say why.

1. Is there research support that aromatherapy with clove leaf essential oil may help prevent aging because of its antioxidant properties?

2. What essential oil is thought to have antimicrobial properties?

3. What would be a good way to deliver rosemary and lavender essential oils for the purpose of reducing stress?

4. Is there research to support that sandalwood oils help to reduce stress?

 Go to Chapter 29, **Toward Evidence-Based Practice Suggested Responses,** on the Student Resource Disk or DavisPlus at http://davisplus.fadavis.com/Wilkinson2

---

medications can impair kinesthesia. Kinesthetic deficits place the patient at risk for balance and coordination problems and falls. Box 29-5 highlights activities that enhance proprioception.

Seizures

A **seizure** is the abrupt onset of disturbance in electrical activity in the brain—a group of neurons fires abnormally. This results in motor symptoms, such as rhythmic jerking of the limbs. Symptoms and the duration of the seizure vary, depending on the area of the brain affected. In addition to motor symptoms, the person may have a decreased level of consciousness or a loss of consciousness. This places the patient at high risk for injury from falls.

BOX 29-5 ■ Activities to Enhance Proprioception

Kinesthesia, or muscle sense, is enhanced by activities that tone muscles and increase coordination. These activities are helpful for individuals of any age. Examples include the following:

- Rhythmic movement (e.g., T'ai chi, dance, yoga)
- Aerobic activities, such as walking, running, or bicycling
- Strength training, such as weight-bearing exercise or use of light weights
- Flexibility activities, such as stretching
- Balance conditioning with eyes open and closed (e.g., standing on one foot)
- Putting joints through full range of motion, especially rotational movements

Seizures are not uncommon. Incidence is highest for those younger than age 10 or older than age 65. Males are more likely to have seizures than females, especially children. Each year, 200,000 new cases of epilepsy are diagnosed. Most seizures last less than three or four minutes. In 7 out of 10 people with seizures, no identifiable cause can be found. Among adults, the most common cause is a tumor or head trauma. The most common reason for seizures in a person with epilepsy is failure to take prescribed antiseizure medication. Other common triggers are ingesting substances, sleep deprivation, stress, illness, and hormone fluctuations. Half of the people newly diagnosed with a seizure disorder will have generalized seizures. Three-quarters of children with seizures outgrow the events (Epilepsy Foundation, 2009).

You need to take measures to protect patients who are at risk for seizures. Pad the head, foot, and siderails of the bed and place oral suction at the bedside. If a seizure occurs, you may need to perform suctioning after the episode to prevent aspiration of oral secretions. Do not attempt to open the mouth and insert a padded tongue depressor. This can result in airway obstruction by pushing the tongue back into the pharynx. When anxious, the first responder also could break teeth trying to insert the depressor. For guidelines,

VOL 2 Go to Chapter 29, **Clinical Insight 29-1: Seizure Precautions,** in Volume 2.

KnowledgeCheck 29-4

- Discuss the difference between myopia and hyperopia.
- What is the difference between conduction deafness and nerve deafness?
- Identify three factors that may impair the sense of taste.
- How is the sense of smell triggered?
- What areas of the body have the greatest number of tactile receptors?
- What type of health concerns may be generated by kinesthetic deficits?

 Go to Chapter 29, **Knowledge Check Response Sheet and Answers,** on the Student Resource Disk or DavisPlus at http://davisplus.fadavis.com/Wilkinson2

 CriticalThinking 29-3

Imagine that you are experiencing sensory deficits. Which deficits would you find most challenging?

Practical **Knowledge** knowing how

As a nurse, you should always consider your client's sensory perceptual status. Sensory deficits, excess, and overload influence a person's safety and quality of life and may be especially troublesome for those in inpatient facilities.

ASSESSMENT

Assessment of sensory perception includes a history and physical exam to gather data about the following items (see Chapter 19):

- Factors affecting sensory perception
- Mental status
- Level of consciousness
- Recent changes in sensory stimulation
- Use of sensory aids
- The client's environment
- The support network
- Focused examination of vision, hearing, taste, smell, touch, and balance

In your nursing interview, you will assess the client's usual and current state of sensory function, as well as gather a history of sensory problems and use of sensory aids. In addition to interviewing the client and family, assess the environment and client situation for factors that may alter sensory function. This section provides a brief overview of each of those items.

Physical assessment of sensory function requires assessment of the six senses. For guidelines,

 Go to Chapter 19, **Procedure 19-16: Assessing the Sensory Neurological System, Procedure 19-6: Assessing the Eyes,** and **Procedure 19-7: Assessing the Ears and Hearing,** in Volume 2.

For a bedside assessment that you can use to easily assess sensory function,

 Go to Chapter 29, **Assessment Guidelines and Tools, Bedside Assessment of Sensory Function,** in Volume 2.

Assess Changes in Sensory Function

To assess changes in sensory function, you will need to obtain a history of the client's usual sensory function as well as information about the client's current status. For a list of questions you can use for this purpose,

 Go to Chapter 29, **Assessment Guidelines and Tools, Nursing History: Sensory Perceptual Status,** in Volume 2.

Assess Risk Factors for Impaired Sensory Perception

You should perform a comprehensive assessment for any client at increased risk for sensory alterations: older adults, clients with limited mobility, clients who are bedbound or homebound, clients in intensive care units, and clients with known sensory deficits, especially if the change has been acute. Routinely assess developmental level, health status, medications, stress and coping mechanisms, personality, and lifestyle related to sensory alterations.

Assess Mental Status

Sensory alterations may trigger changes in mental status, and altered mental status can interfere with sensory perception. A check of mental status includes assessment of behavior, appearance, response to stimuli, speech, memory, and judgment. Normal findings include an ability to express and explain realistic thoughts with clear speech, follow directions, listen, answer questions, and recall significant past events.

You can assess many of those factors as you interact with the client. For example, if you have asked the client the questions covered in the previous section, you have already formed an impression about his appearance, speech, ability to express himself, and other facets of mental status. In addition, you must specifically assess the client's level of orientation. Chapter 19 presents additional discussion of mental status screening and orientation.

Assess Level of Consciousness

Level of consciousness (LOC) is one indicator of cerebral function. It includes arousal (from alert to deeply comatose) and orientation (to time, place, person, and situation). An alert client will respond to auditory stimuli. If the client does not respond, progress to tactile and then painful stimuli (refer to Chapter 19). Remember, however, that if your client does not speak your language he may not respond to questions or commands. The Glasgow Coma Scale is commonly used to assess LOC. It assesses eye, motor, and verbal responses. The FOUR (Full Outline of Un-Responsiveness) scale adds to that, brain stem reflexes and respirations. To use the Glasgow Coma Scale or the FOUR Scale for assessing level of consciousness,

VOL 2 Go to Chapter 19, **Procedure 19-16: Assessing the Sensory Neurological System,** in Volume 2.

If you are not using a coma scale, document your findings specifically and objectively in your nursing notes. Be sure to assess whether the patient is alert, confused, lethargic, obtunded, stuporous, or comatose. For explanations of those states and observations to make,

VOL 2 Go to Chapter 29, **Assessment Guidelines and Tools, Nursing History: Sensory Perceptual Status** (section, **"Assess Mental Status"),** in Volume 2.

Assess Use of Sensory Aids

Sensory aids are devices that assist with sensory function. They include glasses, contact lenses, hearing aids, canes, and walkers. For sample interview questions,

VOL 2 Go to Chapter 29, **Assessment Guidelines and Tools, Nursing History: Sensory Perceptual Status,** in Volume 2.

Assess the Environment

The environment is an important source of stimulation. Consider how different the environment is for Joshua and Richard ("Meet Your Patients"). Joshua is in a crowded space with lights and noise 24 hours per day. He has had a number of invasive procedures and is most likely receiving pain medication. In contrast, Richard is in a quiet room with little exposure to light, noise, or touch. As Joshua's and Richard's situations demonstrate, a healthcare environment can have too many or too few stimuli. As part of your assessment, assess how the client is responding to the conditions of the environment.

Compare Your Data About the Patient's Personality and Lifestyle with the Current Environmental Situation. In healthcare facilities, patients are subjected to lights, noises, and odors that cause them anxiety. They may hear others who are crying out in pain. For most, this environment is very different from anything they are used to. A patient from a small family and a quiet environment may become overwhelmed and develop sensory overload in a hospital setting. Even a client used to a rapid-paced lifestyle may experience overload if he also feels pain, nausea, dizziness, or other symptoms of illness. In contrast, a client used to an active life may find the hospital setting boring.

Assess the Effect of the Environment on Sensory Deficits. For example, for a patient with age-related hearing changes, the background noise of the healthcare environment may make it difficult to hear voices. A patient with visual deficits or impaired balance will often modify his home environment to allow optimal function; however, when the patient is in an institution, these aids are no longer present. To assist the patient, you must determine which environmental factors make his deficits worse and which help to compensate.

Assess the Support Network

For a client with a sensory deficit, his support network may serve as a buffer or a hindrance. For example, an older adult with macular degeneration has progressive loss of vision. If he lives alone, the effect of the visual loss will be quite different than if he lived with an extended family. Support persons may help the client to adapt to deficits by assuming chores that the client can no longer perform or by providing comfort to the client so he is less distressed by the sensory losses.

A support network can also be influential when clients are experiencing sensory deprivation or overload. Recall that Richard ("Meet Your Patients") has no visitors. What influence do you think frequent visits by family members would have on Richard? If you say that Richard would receive more stimulation and may have less sensory deprivation, you are correct. Family members can also help clients who are confused from sensory alterations by reorienting and calming the client.

KnowledgeCheck 29-5

- Identify six areas you should assess for a client with known or suspected sensory alterations.
- What factors must be evaluated when it is known that a client uses a sensory aid?
- Identify at least two ways that you can assess vision and hearing deficits at the bedside.

 Go to Chapter 29, **Knowledge Check Response Sheet and Answers,** on the Student Resource Disk or DavisPlus at http://davisplus.fadavis.com/Wilkinson2

 Critical**Thinking** 29-4

How would you assess Joshua and Richard ("Meet Your Patients") for sensory alterations? You may need to review the "Meet Your Patients" scenario at the beginning of this chapter to answer this question.

ANALYSIS/NURSING DIAGNOSIS

NANDA International (2009) identifies the following diagnostic labels for use with sensory-perceptual problems. For definitions,

 Go to Chapter 29, **Standardized Language, Selected NOC Outcomes and NIC Interventions for Sensory Perceptual Nursing Diagnoses,** in Volume 2.

Disturbed Sensory Perception (specify): Visual, auditory, kinesthetic, gustatory, tactile, olfactory
Acute Confusion
Chronic Confusion
Impaired Environmental Interpretation Syndrome
Impaired Memory
Risk for Peripheral Neurovascular Dysfunction
Unilateral Neglect

Disturbed Sensory Perception may also be the etiology of other nursing diagnoses. Examples include the following:

Risk for Falls r/t visual impairment
Risk for Injury r/t reduced tactile sensation
Self-Care Deficit: Total, r/t kinesthetic impairment
Deficient Diversional Activity r/t reluctance to be in social situations because of hearing impairment
Imbalanced Nutrition: Less Than Body Requirements r/t loss of appetite secondary to impaired taste
Social isolation r/t embarrassment about Impaired Memory

PLANNING OUTCOMES/EVALUATION

For *NOC standardized outcomes* associated with sensory perception diagnoses,

 Go to Chapter 29, **Standardized Language, Selected NOC Outcomes and NIC Interventions for Sensory Perceptual Nursing Diagnoses,** in Volume 2.

Individualized goals/outcomes statements you might write for a client with Disturbed Sensory Perception include the following:

- Compensates for visual impairment by maximizing the use of touch and hearing.
- Verbalizes the importance of eating nutritious foods, despite the fact they "taste funny."
- Demonstrates proper use of her hearing aid.
- Participates in at least one unit activity daily.

As always, use the goals and outcomes you write to evaluate the client's responses to nursing interventions. The outcomes focus your data collection; comparing the new data against the outcomes allows you to determine patient progress.

PLANNING INTERVENTIONS/IMPLEMENTATION

For *NIC standardized interventions* associated with sensory perception nursing diagnoses,

 Go to Chapter 29, **Standardized Language, Selected NOC Outcomes and NIC Interventions for Sensory Perceptual Nursing Diagnoses,** in Volume 2.

Specific nursing activities to address sensory perception problems are based on the nursing diagnosis chosen, especially on its etiology. Common nursing activities are discussed in the following sections.

Promoting Optimal Sensory Function

Optimal sensory function requires periodic health screening along with early identification and treatment of health problems. Comprehensive healthcare is the ideal approach, because sensory problems are often related to other health disorders. For example, to protect his vision, a client with hypertension needs to have periodic eye examinations and to control his blood pressure. See the Self-Care box for information to teach your clients about self-care to promote their vision and hearing. For additional information on health promotion and health screening, see Chapter 41.

Preventing Sensory Deprivation

If your assessment indicates the client is at risk for sensory deprivation, include that information in the nursing care plan, along with specific strategies for prevention. Be sure to communicate this information to nursing assistive personnel (NAPs) so they can participate in this aspect of care.

To prevent sensory deprivation, you will need to (a) provide stimulation and (b) support the patient's ability to perceive and interpret stimuli. Ideally you will

Self-Care

Teaching Your Client About Sensory Perceptual Health

Vision

➤ Have regular eye examinations.

➤ Infants and preschoolers should be screened at their routine office visits.

➤ Young adults should have a complete eye exam at least three times between the ages of 20 and 39.

➤ Have a baseline screening at age 40, and based on that information, the ophthalmologist will determine how frequently your eyes need to be re-examined.

➤ Those age 65 and older should have a complete eye exam every 1 to 2 years to check for cataracts and other eye conditions (The Foundation of the American Academy of Ophthalmology, 2007).

➤ Have more frequent eye exams, regardless of your age, if you are at risk for eye disease. For example, if you: (1) take steroids; (2) are of African ancestry; (3) have a family history of eye disease, diabetes, or high blood pressure; (4) or if you have any symptoms. Your ophthalmologist will recommend how often you should have an exam.

➤ Call your healthcare provider for prompt examination if you have eye pain, discharge, a change in vision, or bleeding.

➤ Have your prescriptions for glasses or contact lenses reviewed at each screening and updated if needed.

➤ Be sure that visual screening is done at your child's elementary school. If not, consult your pediatrician or other care provider.

➤ Work with your primary healthcare provider to control conditions such as hypertension and diabetes.

➤ If you are pregnant, obtain early and adequate prenatal care to prevent the danger of premature birth and exposure of the newborn to high-volume oxygen.

➤ Keep sharp or pointed tools (e.g., scissors) out of reach of infants, toddlers, and preschoolers.

➤ Teach children to walk carefully, tool point downward, when carrying pointed tools or other objects.

➤ Teach children to stay away from projectile activities, such as lawn-mowing.

➤ Keep the child away from firearms and fireworks.

➤ Insist that your child use eye protection when playing sports such as tennis or baseball.

➤ Insist that children wear helmets when skating or riding bicycles and that teenagers wear helmets when riding motorcycles.

➤ For children who wear glasses, be sure the lenses are made of shatterproof safety glass.

Hearing

➤ Auditory screening is often performed in elementary school; however, most adults do not have their hearing screened regularly. If you work in an area with a high noise level, you should have your hearing checked regularly. Early detection may prevent hearing loss.

➤ If you are pregnant:

➤ Obtain early prenatal care.

➤ Avoid ototoxic drugs.

➤ Be sure you are tested for syphilis and rubella (German measles).

➤ Avoid anyone you suspect may have rubella.

➤ Children with frequent ear infections require evaluation to determine whether hearing loss has occurred.

➤ Middle and older adults may begin to experience difficulty distinguishing voices in a crowd or hearing the television or radio. These are indications of hearing loss and should be evaluated; you may need a hearing aid.

➤ Hearing loss is not a "natural part of aging."

Taste

Dental health is an important aspect of maintaining taste. Decayed teeth, gum disease, and other disorders of the mouth may affect the ability to taste. Have your teeth cleaned and examined at least yearly. You may need additional dental work to promote oral health.

use the following as preventive actions. However, you will use these same activities in care for patients who have been diagnosed with sensory deprivation.

Visual Stimulation. For visual stimulation, help the patient with glasses to apply them whenever she is not sleeping. Make sure eyeglasses are clean and in good repair. This will allow the patient to receive available stimuli. Put artwork on the walls, furnish colorful pajamas and robes, and place pictures or flowers where the patient can see them. Unless the patient objects, open curtains during the daytime to allow sunlight to enter the room. Avoid keeping the patient in a dark room, except to promote sleep.

Auditory Stimulation. To stimulate hearing, help the patient with a hearing aid to apply it whenever she is not sleeping. Check that the hearing aid has working batteries and the sound is set at the appropriate level. When possible, move the patient to a quiet area to avoid background noise when communicating.

Olfactory Stimulation. Stimulate the sense of smell with fruits and flowers, or even aromatherapy. Pleasant smells may also stimulate appetite.

Tactile Stimulation. Use touch carefully in your patient-care activities. You may want to hold a patient's hand while talking or provide a back rub with morning and bedtime care. Gentle hand massage is sometimes effective in calming agitated patients. However, people do respond differently to being touched, so adjust the amount of touch you provide according to the patient's reaction.

Audiovisual Media. A television or radio in the room may provide meaningful stimulation. Teach NAPs to choose appropriate music and programs for the patient. Inappropriate choices (e.g., cartoons with laugh tracks) offer meaningless stimulation and may lead to sensory deprivation.

Social Interaction. Social interaction is a type of stimulus. The following are some social interaction measures:

- Make regular contact with the patient. Introduce yourself, and address the patient by name.
- Provide continuity of care by assigning the same personnel whenever possible.
- Encourage patients to have some form of social interaction. For example, urge long-term care patients to take part in scheduled activities. Assist acute-care patients out of bed for meals or visits from family and friends. Advise staff members to visit at intervals or encourage patients to leave their rooms. Children may play video games with others online.
- Avoid isolating the patient when at all possible. Ensure that any patient in isolation receives adequate stimulation from nurses, family members, or assistive personnel.

Minimizing Anxiety and Confusion. Minimize anxiety and confusion so the patient can accurately perceive stimuli. For example:

- Explain all procedures and care. This will decrease anxiety and help orient confused clients.
- Hang a calendar in the room, along with a schedule of activities.
- A large clock on the wall is also helpful.
- Encourage family members to bring in familiar objects from home.
- If the patient is disoriented, provide information at each visit. For example, "Good morning, Mr. Booker. My name is Elsa. I am the nurse taking care of you this morning. It is a few minutes after eight in the morning. I'm going to take your blood pressure and get you ready for breakfast."

Facilitating Communication. Develop alternative methods of communication when interacting with clients with aphasia, or who speak another language, or who have difficulty hearing. Communication boards, a magic slate, pictures, or writing may be helpful. You might also hang a message board in the room and ask family members to post photos, cards, or notes. Computers are useful if the patient has one; and telephone texting might also be used.

Pet Therapy. Consider using pet therapy. Many facilities have resident pets or can arrange to have pets visit.

A singing bird may delight a resident who cannot be out of bed. In long-term care facilities, resident cats often favor bedbound clients for their frequent naps. Pet therapy can increase socialization, lower blood pressure, and decrease loneliness and pain (Braun, Stangler, Narveson, et al., 2009; Hooker, Freeman, & Stewart, 2002).

Collaboration. Collaborate with other healthcare team members in caring for clients with sensory deprivation. Music therapy, activities, physical therapy, speech therapy, nutritional therapy, and occupational therapy may all be valuable in the care of the client. Carefully monitor the use of sedating medications that may contribute to sensory deprivation.

Self-Stimulation. Finally, when they are able, teach patients to provide their own stimulation by counting, singing, reading, playing computer video games, or reciting poetry.

Critical Thinking 29-5

Which of the strategies to treat sensory deprivation would be most appropriate for Richard ("Meet Your Patients")?

Preventing Sensory Overload

Sensory overload is sometimes an unfortunate outcome of hospitalization. To prevent or treat sensory overload, consider the following strategies. Oddly, some of the interventions are the same as those for preventing sensory deprivation.

Control Visual Stimuli. Minimize unnecessary light. Instruct NAPs to be aware of appropriate light levels, especially at night. Use a flashlight instead of turning on room lights, for example.

Control Auditory Stimuli. Minimize unnecessary noise. Instruct NAPs to be aware of appropriate noise and light levels, especially at night. Speak in a moderate tone of voice, using a calm and confident manner. Do not speak about the client to others in his presence, even when he seems unresponsive. Consider the use of earplugs for the client.

Control Olfactory Stimuli. Reduce noxious odors by promptly emptying commodes and bedpans, removing meal trays, using deodorant sprays, and keeping wounds covered.

Use Radio and TV Appropriately. Choose programs to meet the client's interests. Do not leave the TV or radio on 24 hours a day.

Minimize Stress. Stressors create internal stimuli such as anxiety. Observe for the client's reaction to environmental stimuli. Remove annoying or bothersome stimuli if possible.

- Introduce yourself when meeting the client and address him by name. Provide a calm presence; for example, do not hurry with care or speak rapidly.

- If possible, provide a private room and limit visitors. Reduce unessential tasks by other health team members.
- Control pain and nausea with ordered medications.
- Teach clients about stress reduction techniques.
- Provide relaxing music that promotes visualization and deep-breathing techniques.

Promote Adequate Sleep and Rest. Establish a schedule for care that allows for uninterrupted periods of sleep and rest. Besides preventing interruptions during rest periods, a schedule will provide the client with advance notice of what to expect during the day. Instruct NAPs on the importance of allowing the client adequate rest and the need to avoid interruptions.

 Critical**Thinking** 29-6

Review the scenario of Joshua, the young ICU patient with sensory overload ("Meet Your Patients").

- Which strategies to prevent sensory overload would be most appropriate for an ICU patient?
- Which would be least likely to be successful or not feasible based on the setting?

Provide a rationale for your choices. You may need to visit an ICU or talk with classmates who have been to an ICU to answer this question.

Caring for Clients with Sensory Deficits

Recall that in addition to sensory deprivation and sensory overload, many clients have sensory deficits. The Joint Commission (2008) requires that you address the communication needs of patients with vision, speech, hearing, language, and cognitive impairments. Regardless of the primary medical diagnosis, you may need to modify your approach to the client or alter the environment. The specific interventions depend on the type of deficit (i.e., visual, hearing, olfactory, taste, tactile, kinesthetic, and altered mental status). Describe the sensory deficits on the nursing care plan, along with strategies to deal with them. For example, if the patient recovering from an abdominal surgery has no vision in his left eye, nursing orders should specify to approach the patient from the right.

Interventions for Visual Deficits

Visual deficits range from minor problems requiring corrective lenses to complete blindness. Surgical procedures of the eye may cause temporary visual problems. Problems that limit movement of the head may limit peripheral vision but have no effect on central vision. To provide care for the client with visual deficits, you will need to describe fully the scope of the deficit on the care plan. For the client with sight, your interventions focus on enhancing vision.

- Make sure eyeglasses are clean, in good repair, and of the proper prescription. Place them within easy reach or help the client put them on if necessary.

- Offer a magnifying lens or large-print books and magazines for clients with presbyopia.
- Provide enough light, but avoid glare: (1) use soft, diffuse lighting; (2) provide sunglasses, visors, or hats with brims when the client is outdoors.
- For information on caring for contact lenses, see Chapter 22, and

 Go to Chapter 22, **Procedure 22–12,** in Volume 2.

For clients with severely limited vision:

- Be sure that all staff are aware of the client's limited vision.
- Provide an uncluttered environment, and do not rearrange furniture.
- Place the call bell, phone, and self-care items within easy reach.
- Consider books on tape or Braille for the client's enjoyment.
- Keep the bed in a low position.
- When helping the client walk, ask which side she prefers to have you on. Offer her your arm and allow her to grasp it.
- If the client refuses an offer of help, don't insist.
- For safety measures, see Home Care: Sensory Deficits—Safety and Health Measures.
- If a visually impaired client uses a guide dog do not distract the dog. A guide dog in a harness is working and should be approached only with the owner's permission.

To learn about communicating with visually impaired clients,

 Go to Chapter 29, **Clinical Insight 29-2,** in Volume 2.

Interventions for Hearing Deficits

A hearing impairment can limit communication and place the client at risk for social isolation. In addition, clients with impaired hearing are unable to receive warnings. This places them at risk for injury (e.g., they may not hear a fire alarm). Your nursing interventions should focus on supporting auditory function, improving communication, and creating a safer environment.

Support Auditory Function
See that hearing aids are functioning properly. If the client has a hearing aid, check to make sure that it is working, the batteries are functional, and the sound is adjusted to a comfortable level. Encourage your client to wear her hearing aid as much as possible. A significant number of people with hearing impairment do not wear hearing aids. To review care of a hearing aid,

 Go to Chapter 22, **Procedure 22-16,** in Volume 2.

Inspect ear canals for cerumen impaction, a common cause of conduction hearing loss. Regular inspection will detect this problem. See Critical Aspects of

Sensory Deficits—Safety and Health Measures

Home Care

To promote safety and health, instruct clients on the following points:

Visual Deficits

➤ Do not use throw or area rugs on any floors.

➤ Keep spaces uncluttered.

➤ Orient the client to new surroundings, for example, "The couch is directly ahead 3 feet. There is a table next to it."

➤ Do not rearrange furniture.

➤ Keep the bed in a low position.

➤ Clients with significant visual impairment should be evaluated for the ability to drive. Many people resist giving up driving privileges, because this severely limits their lifestyle. However, poor vision places the driver, passengers, pedestrians, and other drivers at risk for harm.

Hearing Deficits

➤ Install blinking lights that alert the person to an incoming call or the ring of a doorbell.

➤ Install blinking alarm clocks, burglar alarms, and smoke detectors.

Olfactory Deficits

➤ Have gas appliances regularly inspected and maintained to prevent gas leaks.

➤ Check smoke detectors and replace batteries regularly.

➤ If you cannot detect food spoilage by smell or taste, date foods and inspect them for any evidence of spoilage. Spoilage usually causes changes in the color and consistency of canned, fresh, or leftover foods.

Gustatory Deficits

➤ Perform frequent oral hygiene to encourage appetite and enhance the sense of taste.

➤ Enhance the meal experience by concentrating on the visual appeal of the meal, the plates, and the dinner table.

➤ Avoid bland, overcooked food. Use spices liberally unless they are contraindicated.

➤ Vary food texture, color, and temperature to provide more interest.

Tactile Deficits

➤ Use a bath thermometer to monitor water temperature and prevent burns.

➤ Change position frequently to relieve pressure on bony prominences.

➤ Use properly fitting shoes and socks.

➤ Immediately report any signs of circulatory impairment (e.g., declining motor function, cool temperature, gray-blue coloration).

➤ Inspect daily for open areas, cuts, abrasions, or areas of redness.

Procedure 29-1 for key information on otic irrigation. For the complete steps,

VOL 2 Go to Chapter 29, **Procedure 29-1: Performing Otic Irrigation,** in Volume 2.

Other support measures include closed-caption television, which allows the client to read the dialogue and continue to enjoy his favorite shows or stay current with the news. For telephones, the client might want to consider sound amplification or conversion to text-telephone service. Finally, some clients may also be candidates for hearing aid dog service.

Adapt and Improve Communication

For a client with hearing impairment, provide written instructions to ensure that she understands the teaching and instructions. For additional suggestions for communicating with hearing-impaired persons,

VOL 2 Go to Chapter 29, **Clinical Insight 29-3: Communicating with Hearing-Impaired Clients,** in Volume 2.

Promote Safety

Suggest that your client modify the home environment. For example, install blinking lights that alert the person to an incoming phone call or the ring of a doorbell. Blinking alarm clocks, burglar alarms, and smoke detectors are also available. Also refer to the accompanying Home Care box. For institutionalized patients, keep

Critical Aspects of Procedure 29-1

VOL 2 For steps to follow in *all* procedures, refer to the Universal Steps for All Procedures found on the inside back cover of Volume 2. Go to the full procedures in Volume 2 to practice and learn the procedure steps. Use these Critical Aspects later to help you review key points.

Procedure 29-1: Otic Irrigation

➤ Warm the irrigating solution to body temperature.

➤ Assist the patient into a sitting or lying position, with the head tilted slightly toward the affected ear.

➤ Straighten the ear canal by pulling up and back on the pinna. For a young child, pull down and back to straighten the canal.

➤ Instruct the patient to notify you if he experiences any pain or dizziness during the irrigation.

➤ Place the tip of the nozzle (or syringe) into the entrance of the ear canal, and direct the stream of irrigating solution gently along the top of the ear canal toward the back of the client's head.

➤ Continue irrigating until the canal is clean.

➤ Perform an otoscopic examination.

➤ Place a cotton ball loosely in the outer ear.

➤ If cerumen is very hard, you may repeat the procedure later after the solution has had time to soften the cerumen.

background noise to a minimum, and keep a call bell within easy reach of the patient.

KnowledgeCheck 29-6

- Identify three safety measures that may be used with clients with visual impairment.
- Identify three safety measures that may be used with clients with hearing impairment.

 Go to Chapter 29, **Knowledge Check Response Sheet and Answers,** on the Student Resource Disk or DavisPlus at http://davisplus.fadavis.com/Wilkinson2

Interventions for Olfactory Deficits

An impaired sense of smell diminishes taste and denies the client the pleasure of enjoying food. This often leads to weight loss. Home safety issues are also a concern for the client who cannot smell. Measures to protect the client with olfactory impairment are found in the Home Care box, Sensory Deficits—Safety and Health Measures.

Interventions for Gustatory Deficits

Many people find great pleasure from the different tastes of food. Without the gustatory sense, a client may eat less and be at risk for nutritional deficits and weight loss. If the client has lost weight, be sure to check the fit of any dentures or dental appliances. Weight changes may affect their fit and make it even harder to eat.

For hospitalized clients, provide frequent oral hygiene. Assess for sores or open areas in the mouth. These require prompt treatment because they may become infected and further damage the sense of taste. Teach clients to eat foods separately or drink water between bites to distinguish the taste of the food more readily. Seasonings, salt substitutes, spices, or lemon may improve the taste of foods and encourage the client's appetite (see Home Care box).

Interventions for Tactile Deficits

Patients with peripheral vascular disease, spinal cord injury, diabetes, cerebrovascular accident, trauma, or fractures are at risk for diminished tactile sensation. They may not notice a cut or wound in an area with limited sensation. For institutionalized patients, inspect the affected area daily and teach the patient to continue this practice at home. Look for open areas, cuts, abrasions, or areas of erythema. Any of these findings requires care. Also see the Home Care box.

If the patient consents, you can stimulate the sense of touch by brushing his hair, giving a back rub, or touching him when giving care. You may need to use firm pressure for him to feel the touch. Frequent turning and positioning may also help. In contrast to tactile deficit, some patients are overly sensitive to touch. In those instances, you must minimize irritating stimuli:

Use a bed cradle, and keep bed linens loose to keep them off the skin as much as possible.

Although traditionally we have thought of touch as a caring and healing intervention, there is actually not a lot of empirical evidence that supports its use as a nursing intervention. Furthermore, there are wide differences in how touch is perceived among both patients and nurses. Although many patients are comforted by touch, others are not. Use touch carefully, observing the patient's reaction, until research evidence provides clear guidelines for practice (Gleeson & Timmins, 2005, 2009).

Interventions for Confused Clients

Confusion interferes with the ability to interpret stimuli accurately. It can be temporary or permanent. Confusion is an aspect of both delirium and dementia. **Delirium** is an acute, reversible state of confusion caused by medications and a variety of physiological processes, such as hypoxia, metabolic disturbances, infection, or sensory alterations. It may be accompanied by changes in the level of consciousness. In contrast, **dementia** is a chronic and progressive deterioration in mental function caused by physical changes in the brain and is not associated with changing levels of consciousness.

Your nursing care should promote orientation, use simple communication, decrease anxiety, keep the patient safe, and provide continuity of care. Notice that some of the following interventions are the same as for preventing sensory deficit.

Promote Orientation. Introduce yourself and state the client's name each time you meet with him. Wear a readable (large, plain type) name tag to reinforce your introduction. Also identify the day, date, and time as you interact. Provide visual clues to time, such as opening the drapes during the day and closing them at night, and placing calendars and clocks where they are easy to see. Also place personal objects, photos, and mementos in the immediate environment, and discuss them with the client. Encourage the patient to participate in familiar activities, such as bathing.

Simplify Your Communications. The patient cannot interpret stimuli accurately and may not understand what you say. Take an unhurried approach, allowing adequate time for the client to answer any questions you raise. Face the client and speak calmly, simply, and directly. Provide simple explanations for all care and treatments. Use short sentences with few words: "It's bath time," rather than, "Let's go have a bath and get you all nice and clean for visitors." Do not offer too many choices because this confuses the confused patient.

Decrease Anxiety. People with dementia are often anxious, worried, and fearful. Find ways to make the person feel more secure and comfortable before you focus on the content of your conversations.

- Gently hold or pat the patient's hand.
- Realize that the person is probably distressed and is doing the best he can. Be affectionate, reassuring, and calm, even when things make no sense.
- Try to respond to the person's feelings instead of the content of his words. This helps to reassure her. For example, if a woman is constantly searching for her husband, don't say, "Your husband is not here." Rather, say, "You must miss your husband," or "Tell me about your husband."
- If the person has difficulty finding the right word, supply it for him unless it upsets him. This helps control his frustration.
- If you do not understand what the patient is trying to say, ask him to point to it or describe it (e.g., "What does a zishmer look like?").
- Consider using alternative therapy, such as music therapy.

Provide for Safety. Recognize that the client's decision-making may be poor. Maintain a safe environment. For example, store medications away from the patient's reach, keep doors and windows closed securely, and use bed or chair monitors to prevent wandering.

Provide Continuity of Care when Possible. It helps to establish a routine for care and assign the same caregivers each day.

KnowledgeCheck 29-7

- What are the major concerns associated with loss of smell and taste?
- What safety measures should be taught to a client with tactile impairment?
- How can you best assist a client who is confused?

 Go to Chapter 29, **Knowledge Check Response Sheet and Answers,** on the Student Resource Disk or DavisPlus at http://davisplus.fadavis.com/Wilkinson2

Interventions for Unconscious Clients

The unconscious client is unable to interact with you but requires reality orientation nevertheless. In addition to some of the preceding suggestions, you should include the patient's support persons in the care. Teach them the necessary strategies. You can usually incorporate more touch into the plan of care.

Safety measures are a priority for unconscious patients. Keep the bed in low position when you are not at the bedside, and keep the siderails up. If the patient's blink reflex is absent or her eyes do not close totally, you may need to give frequent eye care to keep secretions from collecting along the lid margins. The eyes may be patched to prevent corneal drying, and lubricating eye drops may be ordered. Oral care is also important because the unconscious patient can have no oral fluids.

CriticalThinking 29-7

What types of interventions would be most appropriate for Joshua and Richard ("Meet Your Patients")—that is, interventions for sensory deficits, sensory deprivation, sensory overload, or confusion?

CarePlanning & MappingPractice

For Care Planning/Care Mapping practice,

 Go to Student Resources, **Care Planning & Care Mapping Practice,** at http://davisplus.fadavis.com/Wilkinson2

 Go to Chapter 29, **Resources for Caregivers and Health Professionals,** on the Student Resource Disk or DavisPlus at http://davisplus.fadavis.com/Wilkinson2

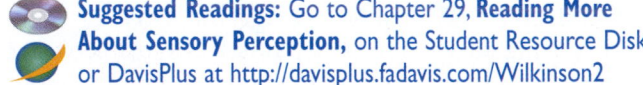 **Suggested Readings:** Go to Chapter 29, **Reading More About Sensory Perception,** on the Student Resource Disk or DavisPlus at http://davisplus.fadavis.com/Wilkinson2

 Bibliography: Go to Volume 2, Bibliography.

CHAPTER 30

Pain Management

Learning Outcomes

After completing this chapter, you should be able to:

➤ Define pain.

➤ Classify pain according to origin, cause, duration, and quality.

➤ Describe the physiological changes that occur with pain.

➤ Discuss two physiological mechanisms involved in pain modulation.

➤ Discuss factors that influence pain.

➤ Identify the effect of unrelieved pain on each of the body systems.

➤ Discuss nonpharmacological pain relief measures.

➤ Describe pharmacological measures, including nonopioid analgesics, opioid analgesics, and adjuvant analgesics.

➤ Describe chemical and surgical pain relief measures.

➤ Explain why pain should be considered the fifth vital sign.

➤ Identify the steps involved in creating a pain management program for a client.

➤ Write an individualized goal for a client with a nursing diagnosis of Acute Pain.

➤ Write an individualized goal for a client with a nursing diagnosis of Chronic Pain.

➤ Explain how to use a patient-controlled analgesia (PCA) system.

➤ Describe a method for evaluating a pain management program.

Meet Your Patient

As a special experience, your instructor has arranged for you to spend a half-day in the intensive care unit (ICU). As you enter the ICU, you are a little apprehensive. Your patient today is a 23-year-old Asian woman who was in an automobile accident yesterday and sustained chest and abdominal injuries. You walk into the room with your clinical instructor to meet your patient, Ms. Eunice Chu Ling. She was taken to the operating room during the night to have her spleen removed. She is intubated (has an endotracheal tube in her airway that is connected to a ventilator), has an intravenous line running, and a chest tube on the left side that is draining bloody fluid. Her parents and siblings are in the room sitting rigidly in the chairs, smiling at you. Ms. Chu Ling is awake and grimacing. You want to ask her if is she is in pain, but she cannot speak.

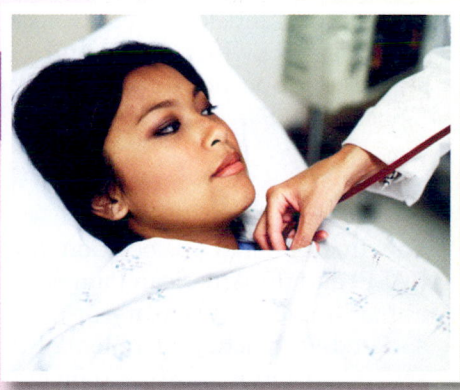

Theoretical **Knowledge** **knowing** why

Many of us enter nursing to relieve suffering and promote healing. Pain is one of the most distressing symptoms we deal with, yet it is the most frequent reason people seek medical attention (American Academy of Pain Management, 2008). Nurses are often considered the gatekeepers of pain management; thus, it is crucial that you gain solid theoretical knowledge of what pain is and why it occurs. The prevalence of pain will continue to grow as people are treated for diseases that were previously fatal. Most of the top 10 causes of death, such as heart disease, cancer, and chronic lower respiratory diseases, are associated with pain. The following are some facts about the incidence of pain:

- More than 1 in 4 American adults experience pain lasting more than 24 hours.
- 1 in 6 American adults live in chronic pain (American Academy of Pain Management, 2008).
- About ¼ to ½ of community-dwelling older adults report pain that interferes with normal functioning
- An estimated 1 in 5 adults experiences pain or physical discomfort that disrupts sleep a few nights a week or more.
- In spite of measures to relieve pain, ½ to ¾ of hospitalized patients die in moderate to severe pain.
- Non-Hispanic white adults reported pain more often than adults of other races. Women and men reported pain at about the same frequency.
- The most commonly reported types of pain are severe headaches and lower back, neck, and facial ache or pain. People with arthritis and joint issues account for a large proportion of pain sufferers (American Pain Society, 2007).

What Is Pain?

The International Association for the Study of Pain (IASP) and the American Pain Society (APS) define pain as "an unpleasant sensory or emotional experience associated with actual or potential tissue damage, or described in terms of such damage" (APS, 1994, p. 16; Mersky & Bogduk, 1994, p. 971). Although this definition provides an excellent foundation for our discussion of pain, as a nurse, you will also need to understand the holistic dimensions of the pain experience.

Pain can cause sleep loss, irritability, cognitive impairment, functional impairment, and immobility, and thus it can be destructive to the patient and family. Although we usually think of pain in this negative context, pain is also protective, warning us of potential injury to the body. Recall the last time you touched a hot object with your bare hand. Undoubtedly, you quickly pulled your hand away when you felt discomfort. Without the ability to sense pain, you might have been burned. Pain can also prompt us to change our actions: After we have been sitting at the computer for a while, muscle pain may prompt us to get up and stretch or go out for a walk; or the gastrointestinal discomfort we experience after overeating may remind us to eat more moderately in the future.

Pain is a multidimensional experience, affecting and being affected by nearly every other aspect of life. For instance, severe back pain can affect a patient's job performance, engagement in social activities, sexual intimacy, sleep and rest, ability to exercise, and ability to perform activities of daily living. These factors, in turn, can affect the intensity of the patient's pain, as well as his response to pain.

Margo McCaffery, a nursing expert on pain, describes pain as "whatever the person says it is, and existing whenever the person says it does" (1989, p. 17). In other words, pain is a subjective experience. Unlike a pulse or blood pressure, you cannot measure pain objectively. In addition, your expectations of your patients' pain will be influenced by your own values, ideals, and life experiences. However, as McCaffery's definition indicates, you will need to put aside your personal beliefs about pain and focus on the *patient's* experience.

You will be able to manage pain more effectively if you can classify the type of pain the patient is experiencing. But remember that patients often experience more than one kind of pain (Institute for Clinical Systems Improvement, 2008). Pain can be classified by the origin of pain, cause, duration, and quality of pain.

Origin of Pain

The origin of pain refers to the site where pain is felt, and not necessarily the source of pain.

Cutaneous or **superficial pain** arises in the skin or the subcutaneous tissue. If you have ever touched a hot object or received a paper cut, you have experienced superficial pain. Although the injury is superficial, it may cause significant short-term pain.

Visceral pain is caused by the stimulation of deep internal pain receptors. It is most often experienced in the abdominal cavity, cranium, or thorax. Visceral pain may vary from local, achy discomfort to more widespread, intermittent, and crampy pain. The description of the quality and extent of the pain often serves as a strong clue to the cause. Menstrual cramps, labor pain, gastrointestinal infections, bowel disorders, and organ cancers all produce visceral pain.

Deep somatic pain originates in the ligaments, tendons, nerves, blood vessels, and bones. Deep somatic pain is more diffuse than cutaneous pain and tends to last longer. A fracture or sprain, arthritis, and bone cancer can cause deep somatic pain.

Radiating pain starts at the origin but extends to other locations. For instance, the pain of a severe sore throat may extend to the ears and head. Or the pain of an episode of gastroesophageal reflux ("heartburn") may radiate outward from the sternum to involve the entire upper thorax.

Referred pain occurs in an area that is distant from the original site. For example, the pain from a heart attack may be experienced down the left arm, through the back, or into the jaw. See Figure 30-1 for other examples of referred pain.

Phantom pain is pain that is perceived to originate from an area that has been surgically removed. Patients with amputated limbs may still perceive that the limb exists and experience burning, itching, and deep pain in that area.

Psychogenic pain refers to pain that is believed to arise from the mind. The patient perceives the pain despite the fact that no physical cause can be identified. Psychogenic pain can be just as severe as pain from a physical cause. See the discussion of somatoform pain disorder in Chapter 25, if you would like more information.

Cause of Pain

Physical pain is either nociceptive or neuropathic. These two types of pain differ in the way they affect the patient as well as in how they are treated.

Nociceptive pain is the most common type of pain experienced. It occurs when pain receptors, which are called **nociceptors,** respond to stimuli that are potentially damaging, for example, as a result of noxious thermal, chemical, or mechanical types of injury. Nociceptive pain may occur as a result of trauma, surgery, or inflammation. It is most commonly described as aching. Two types of nociceptive pain are visceral pain (i.e., pain originating from internal organs) and somatic pain (i.e., pain originating from the skin, muscles, bones, or connective tissue).

Neuropathic pain is a complex and often chronic pain that arises when injury to one or more nerves results in repeated transmission of pain signals even in the absence of painful stimuli. The nerve injury may originate from any of a variety of conditions, such as poorly controlled diabetes, a stroke, a tumor, alcoholism, amputation, or a viral infection (e.g., shingles or HIV/AIDS). Some medications, such as chemotherapeutic agents, can trigger nerve injuries that may cause neuropathic pain even after the medication is discontinued. Neuropathic pain is described as burning, numbness, itching, and "pins and needles" prickling pain.

Duration of Pain

Acute pain has a short duration and is generally rapid in onset. It varies in intensity and may last up to 6 months (American Pain Society, n.d.). This type of pain is most frequently associated with injury or surgery. It is protective in that it indicates potential or actual tissue damage. Although acute pain may absorb a patient's physical and emotional energy for a short time, it is helpful for the patient to know that it will generally disappear as the tissues heal.

Chronic pain is pain that has lasted 6 months or longer and often interferes with daily activities. It can be related to a progressive disorder, or it can occur when there is no current tissue injury, as in neuropathic pain. Patients with chronic pain may experience periods of remission and exacerbation. Unlike acute pain, chronic pain is often viewed as insignificant and may lead to withdrawal, depression, anger, frustration, and dependence. Next to incurability, chronic pain is the most feared aspect of contracting cancer or other progressive diseases.

Intractable pain is both chronic and highly resistant to relief. This type of pain is especially frustrating for the patient and care provider. It should be approached with multiple methods of pain relief.

Quality of Pain

The words patients use to describe the quality of their pain help care providers to determine the probable cause and most effective treatment. Patients may describe pain quality with a variety of adjectives, such as *sharp* or *dull, aching, throbbing, stabbing, burning, ripping, searing,* or *tingling.* They may refer to its periodicity as *episodic, intermittent,* or *constant.* Patients also use a variety of terms to convey the intensity of their pain, such as *mild, distracting, moderate, severe,* or *intolerable.*

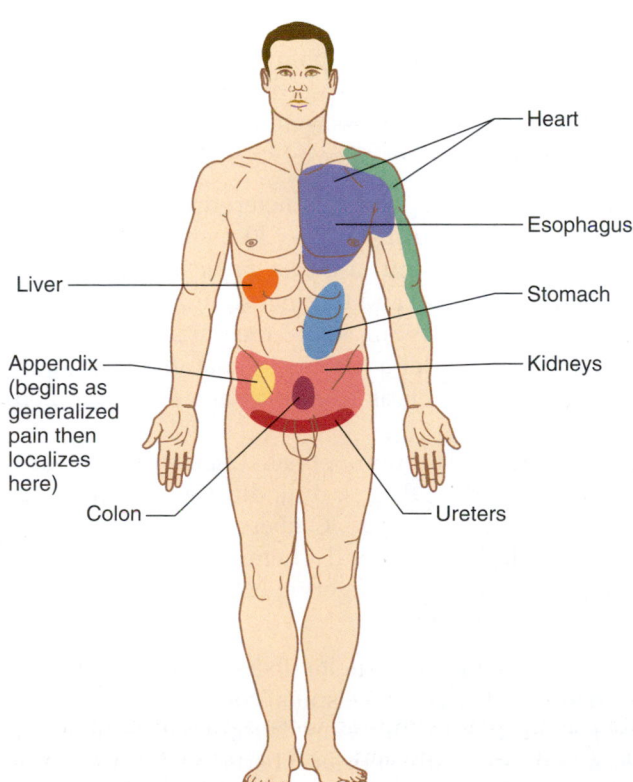

FIGURE 30-1 Most common areas of referred pain.

KnowledgeCheck 30-1

How would you classify the pain that the following patients are experiencing?

- A patient with metastatic cancer
- A patient with back pain that was the result of an automobile injury a year ago
- A patient who had bowel surgery yesterday
- A patient with a fractured leg
- A patient who just had his leg amputated but feels as though the leg is still there
- You just received a paper cut while turning the pages of a book.

  Go to Chapter 30, **Knowledge Check Response Sheet and Answers,** on the Student Resource Disk or DavisPlus at http://davisplus.fadavis.com/Wilkinson2

CriticalThinking 30-1

How would you expect a patient with neuropathic pain to appear?

What Happens When Someone Has Pain?

Review the story of Eunice Chu Ling in the "Meet Your Patient" scenario. Eunice had been in an auto accident that caused severe injuries. She has had surgery and requires monitoring and invasive devices, such as a ventilator and IV line. She is awake but cannot speak. However, through the maze of equipment you can see that she is grimacing. Consider these aspects of Eunice's experience as we explore the physiology of pain.

Transduction

Pain-sensitive nociceptors are found in the skin, subcutaneous tissue, joints, walls of the arteries, and most internal organs. The skin has the highest density of nociceptors, and the internal organs the least. Eunice's injuries, surgery, and procedures have stimulated nociceptors throughout her body. In a process called **transduction,** nociceptors become activated by the perception of potentially damaging mechanical, thermal, and chemical stimuli.

Mechanical stimuli are external forces that result in pressure or friction against the body. Eunice's injuries are predominantly of this type. They involve stretching of tissue in joints and body cavities related to bleeding and swelling, and compression of body tissues caused by the force of the accident. Other types of mechanical stimuli are surgical incisions, friction or skin shearing that occurs from sliding down in bed, or pressure from a mechanical device, such as a cast or brace.

Thermal stimuli result from exposure to extreme heat or cold. If you've ever touched a hot object and rapidly pulled away or suffered an earache when outdoors on a cold day without a hat, you have experienced pain from thermal stimuli.

Chemical stimuli can be internal or external. Lemon juice or any acidic substance on an open area in the skin causes sharp, sudden pain. This is an example of pain from *external* chemical stimuli. In contrast, the chest pain experienced during a myocardial infarction (heart attack) is caused by *internal* chemical stimuli; specifically, the chemical changes that result from tissue ischemia. Another example of a chemical source is ingestion of lead-based paint chipping from a deteriorating residence built before the 1940s. The lead poisoning (also called plumbism) produces neurological damage, headache, and other multisystem effects.

In the "Meet Your Patient" scenario, the physical cues that Eunice may be in pain include bruising, swelling, surgical incisions, and her tubes and IV. However, you will not always see physical, external cues when tissue injuries are present. This is especially true of injuries caused by internal chemical stimuli. This is one reason you need to believe the patient's report of pain.

Tissue damage prompts the release of substances such as bradykinin, histamine, and prostaglandins, which activate nociceptors in the surrounding tissues. Bradykinin is also a powerful vasodilator that triggers a release of inflammatory chemicals that cause the injured area to become red, swollen, and tender. Inflammation is the most frequent cause of pain.

Transmission

Peripheral nerves carry the pain message to the dorsal horn of the spinal cord in a process known as **transmission** (Fig. 30-2). Pain messages are conducted to the spinal cord along either of two types of fibers:

- **A-delta fibers** are large-diameter myelinated fibers that transmit impulses at 6 to 30 meters per second. These fibers transmit *fast pain impulses* from acute, focused mechanical and thermal stimuli. For instance, when you bump your knee, the initial sharp pain is carried by A-delta fibers. Pleasurable stimuli to skin receptors, such as from massage, also stimulate A-delta fibers.
- **C fibers** are smaller unmyelinated fibers that transmit *slow pain impulses*, that is, dull, diffuse pain impulses that travel at a slow rate. C fibers conduct pain from mechanical, thermal, and chemical stimuli. If you bump your knee, the lingering ache in the tissue will be carried by C fibers.

At the dorsal horn, A-delta fibers synapse with long fiber neurons that cross the spinal cord and transmit the message directly to the brain. In contrast, C fiber impulses synapse with shorter fiber neurons that pass through several synapses before reaching the brain. Communication of pain impulses across any of these

FIGURE 30-2 After nociceptors are activated, pain is transmitted along A-delta fibers or C fibers to the dorsal horn of the spinal cord. From there, the pain message is sent to the brain for perception.

synapses requires chemicals, called neurotransmitters, one of the most important of which is *substance P.* Once transmitted, some pain messages enter the reticular formation of the brain stem. However, most pain impulses are transmitted to the thalamus of the brain. An integrating center, the thalamus directs the impulses to three regions of the brain: (1) the somatosensory cortex perceives and interprets physical sensations; (2) the limbic system is involved in emotional reactions to stimuli; and (3) the frontal cortex is involved in thought and reason. The person now perceives pain.

Pain Perception

Perception involves the recognition and definition of pain in the frontal cortex. The point at which the brain recognizes and defines a stimulus as pain is called the **pain threshold.** The number and intensity of stimuli necessary to produce pain, as well as the duration and characteristics of the pain produced, vary from patient to patient. Although the pain threshold usually remains fairly constant for an individual over time, repeated experience with pain can reduce a patient's threshold.

Pain tolerance is the duration or intensity of pain that a person is willing to endure. This varies not only from person to person but also for the same person in different situations. For example, a mother donating a kidney to her child may not report a great deal of post-operative pain. Yet if this same person had a kidney removed because it was cancerous, her pain tolerance

may be completely different. Extreme sensitivity to pain is called **hyperalgesia.**

Pain Modulation

A process called **modulation** changes the perception of pain by either facilitating or inhibiting pain signals. Two mechanisms allow for modulation of pain: the endogenous analgesia system and the gate-control mechanism.

The Endogenous Analgesia System

In the **endogenous analgesia system,** neurons in the brain stem activate descending nerve fibers that conduct impulses back to the spinal cord. These impulses trigger the release of endogenous opioids and other substances to block the continuing pain impulses and provide pain relief. *Endogenous opioids* are naturally occurring analgesic neurotransmitters that inhibit the transmission of pain impulses and the release of substance P. The three neurotransmitters are enkephalins, dynorphins, and beta endorphins. Endogenous opioids bind to opiate receptor sites in the central and peripheral nervous system at four receptor sites, designated as mu (μ), kappa (κ), delta (δ), and sigma (σ). These sites are also involved in reception when patients take pain medicines. Each of the receptor sites has a different affinity for various medications. In addition, nonpharmacological measures, such as exercise, meditation, visualization, and music therapy, can prompt the release of endogenous opioids.

The Gate-Control Theory

Pain impulses can also be modulated at the spinal level. The **gate-control theory of pain modulation** describes the mechanism of pain sensation, based on the idea that the perception of pain does not occur by direct stimulation of only nociceptors (pain-producing fiber). Instead, pain is perceived by the interplay between two different kinds of fibers—those that produce pain and those that inhibit pain.

As slow-pain impulses travel along C (small) fibers from the periphery to the brain, they encounter a "gate" that either allows or blocks the transmission of pain sensation to the brain. If the source of stimulation is non-painful, the gate would be blocked to feeling pain. Likewise, noxious stimulation keeps the gate open to pain. Imagine that you've just hit your arm against a hard surface. Almost without thinking, you reach down and rub the area. Your massage stimulates skin receptors. These send sensory impulses along fast A-delta (large) fibers, which quickly excite inhibitory neurons at the "gate." These neurons in turn block some of the pain signals being carried along the slower C fibers (Fig. 30-3). Another application of the Gate Control Theory is use of a Sitz bath after childbirth to produce relief from pain at the perineum. The warm water and gentle pressure block the gate to the perception of pain in the brain. The Gate Control

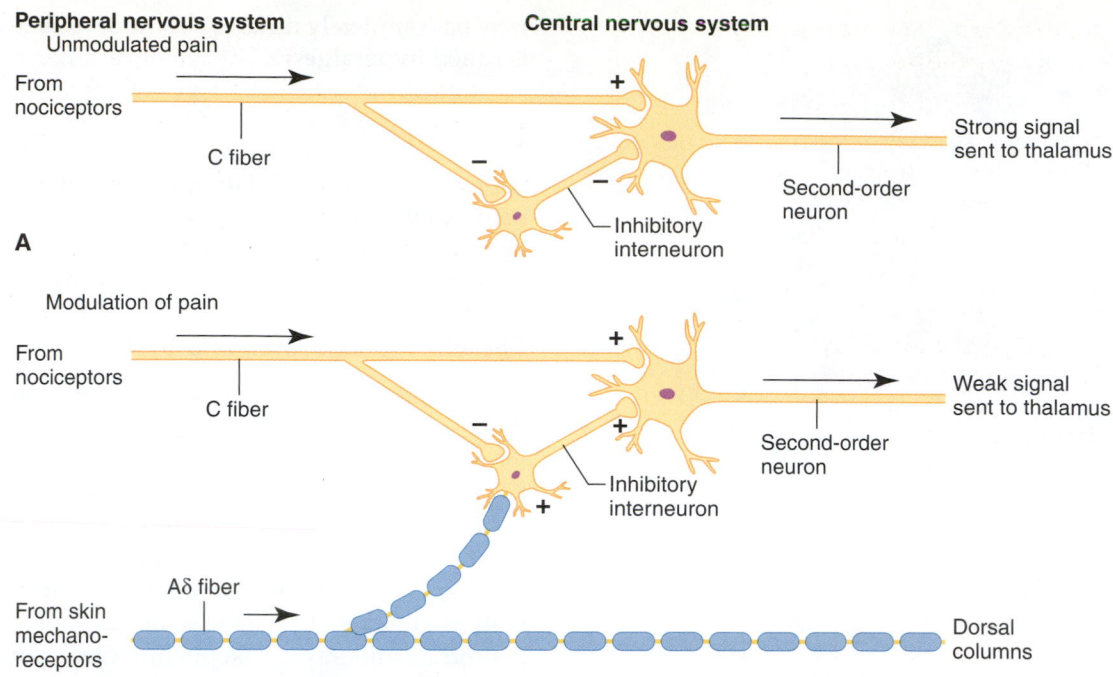

FIGURE 30-3 The gate-control theory of pain modulation. *A,* Normally, C fibers carrying slow-pain signals block inhibitory interneurons and transmit their signals across the synapse unimpeded. *B,* A-delta fibers carrying pleasurable signals (e.g., from touch) excite inhibitory interneurons, which then block the transmission of slow-pain signals (+ equals transmission, − equals no transmission).

Theory is the basis for development and use of the transcutaneous electrical nerve stimulation (TENS) as a pain relief measure.

Descending impulses from the brain, including impulses related to mood or emotion, are also thought to open or close the gate. For this reason, medications for depression are sometimes used for patients with chronic pain. Nonmedication therapies, such as meditation, exercise, relaxation techniques, and laughter, may also compete with C fiber impulses and block the gate. These strategies are discussed later in this chapter. In summary, on a purely physiological basis, pain is simply transduction, transmission, perception, and modulation. However, as we discuss next, our experience of pain involves far more than these four processes.

KnowledgeCheck 30-2

- What must occur to generate pain?
- What are the four physiological steps involved in the pain process?

  Go to Chapter 30, **Knowledge Check Response Sheet and Answers,** on the Student Resource Disk or DavisPlus at http://davisplus.fadavis.com/Wilkinson2

CriticalThinking 30-2

Based on what you have learned about pain modulation, what nursing interventions might help Eunice ("Meet Your Patient") be more comfortable?

What Factors Influence Pain?

Think back to the last time you experienced significant pain. Was it obvious to others that you were in pain? Were you demonstrative? Quiet? Withdrawn? Did you moan or cry out? Now recall Eunice Chu Ling's reaction. What accounts for these different responses to pain?

Pain is universal, yet each person experiences and responds to pain differently. This uniqueness gives you a hint about its nature: Pain is a complex phenomenon that influences and is influenced by emotions, age, sociocultural factors, and communication and cognitive impairments.

Emotions

The most common emotions associated with pain are fear, guilt, anger, helplessness, and loneliness. In Meet Your Patient, imagine how Eunice Chu Ling must be feeling. How might her feelings affect and be affected by her pain?

Fear. Undoubtedly, Eunice is experiencing fear. She was involved a serious accident and can't even ask questions about what is going on. In addition, she may be feeling any of a variety of specific fears. Some patients fear that their pain means their illness or injury is life-threatening. Others fear their pain will eventually become intolerable. Many fear that if they ask for pain medication, they will be judged as weak. Still others fear that if they accept pain medication, they will become addicted to it. When such fears remain unresolved, they can prolong or increase the patient's pain.

Confusion and Helplessness. In addition to fear, Eunice is also probably experiencing confusion and helplessness. Depending on her role in the accident, she may also feel angry or guilty. Fortunately, family members have come to visit, but when they leave and she is by herself, Eunice may experience loneliness or even a sense of abandonment.

Anger and Depression. As you learned in Chapter 11, anxiety and depression are common in people who are ill or hospitalized. Anxiety is most often associated with acute pain, but the anticipation of pain may also trigger anxiety. Waiting for surgery or a procedure that you know will be painful offers plenty of time to think about the unpleasantness and to become anxious. In contrast, depression is most often linked with chronic pain, especially intractable pain.

Previous Pain Experience. Emotional responses to pain are affected by previous pain experiences. Often patients who have had numerous painful experiences are more anxious about the prospect of experiencing pain and are more sensitive to pain. This is especially troublesome for children and adults who require a series of surgeries or painful treatments for their medical conditions. Conversely, patients who have had effective pain relief in the past are usually less anxious and are more confident they will achieve satisfactory pain relief.

You can easily see that people in pain do not experience one single emotional reaction to the experience. Instead, a flood of feelings may overwhelm them, and these emotions in turn may escalate their pain. Often patients get in a vicious cycle: illness and pain trigger emotional reactions, and the emotional reactions exacerbate the pain.

Rarely is pain purely physical or emotional. Instead, it is usually a combination of both. Interventions to relieve pain may relieve feelings of fear and helplessness, and interventions addressing these emotions, such as reflective listening and gentle touch, often aid in pain relief.

Critical Thinking 30-3

Imagine being in a situation similar to that of Eunice Chu Ling. What emotions might you experience?

Developmental Stage

The behavior people exhibit when they have pain is strongly influenced by their stage of development.

Infants and Children

Newborns have the same sensitivity to pain as older infants and children, and preterm infants may have a greater sensitivity (McCaffery & Pasero, 1999). The most common kind of pain that children experience is acute pain resulting from injury, illness, or necessary medical procedures. Infants and small children usually respond to pain by crying loudly. However, in premature and term newborns, the experience of pain does not always evoke detectable behavioral response. Indicators of pain in neonates might be as subtle as skin mottling, grimacing, twitching, crying, poor feeding, increased or decreased activity, averting gaze, temperature fluctuation, elevated blood pressure, and decreased oxygen saturation. As a result, even though an infant has a low pain score based on behavioral assessment tools, he may not be pain free (Slater, Cantarella, Franck, et al., 2008).

Research suggests that infants' and children's memories of painful experiences can influence later behavior. For example, in a study of pain experienced with routine vaccinations, it was found that boys who had been circumcised and not received anesthesia cried longer and had higher pain scores after the injections than those who had not been circumcised (Taddio, Katz, Hersich, et al., 1997).

Older Adults

Pain occurs in approximately one-half to three-quarters or more of the geriatric population. Estimates are that as many as 45% to 80% of nursing home residents have significant pain that is undertreated. These older adults may be unable to report pain because of cognitive impairment. Often their discomfort is evident only in nonverbal cues, such as grimacing, rapid blinking, withdrawal, labored breathing, altered gait, or decreased activity. Some older patients respond to pain in atypical ways, such as mental confusion or collapse (American Geriatrics Society (AGS), 2002; Flaherty, 2007). Undertreated pain often leads to other problems that diminish the quality of life, such as social isolation, depression, sleep disturbances, and mobility-related problems.

Sociocultural Factors

We learn behaviors associated with pain through interaction with family and social support groups. Beliefs about the value of expressing pain or minimizing it are often tied to culture. As you care for clients of various backgrounds, you may notice patterns of behavior. For example, some patients may gain comfort from crying or moaning when they are in pain, whereas some cultures may value silence and brave endurance of pain. Be careful, however, not to assume that patients will react according to responses you have seen in others of the same ethnic or cultural group, because each patient is unique. For example, do you respond to pain in exactly the same way as your parents and siblings?

The family and friends patients in pain may also have culturally determined responses to the experience. From the "Meet Your Patient" scenario, recall how Eunice Chu Ling's family is responding. Although you may think it odd that they are smiling, they may be doing so because they want to make a favorable connection with you, the nurse, because you will be responsible for providing care to Eunice. As a nurse, you will be caring for many people in pain and will see a wide variety of responses. Avoid reaching hasty conclusions about the meaning of those responses.

Nursing has its own culture. Most nurses respond compassionately to those in pain. However, if you fail to recognize that pain is a unique multidimensional experience, you may misjudge a patient's reaction to injury, surgery, or other discomforts. Disparities exist in the treatment of chronic pain among people of different racial backgrounds. Clinicians should strive to provide culturally competent care and adequate pain control to every patient.

Communication and Cognitive Impairments

One of your greatest challenges as a nurse will be caring for patients in pain who have impaired cognition or communication (e.g., patients who have suffered stroke or dementia, who are intubated, or have limited command of the local language). Although people with dementia might not appear to be experiencing pain, there is no evidence they have less pain than do other older adults. Cognitively-impaired adults are not less sensitive to pain but may rather fail to interpret sensations as painful. Or they might not be able to effectively communicate their pain to others. Also even though those with dementia may not be able to recall their pain, they nonetheless still experience it (American Geriatrics Society, 2002). These patients are at risk for underassessment of pain and inadequate pain relief (Horgas, 2007). You will need to consider their behavioral cues as a form of self-report.

Common nonverbal cues of pain include decreased activity, grimacing, frowning, crying, moaning, and irritability. Less obvious indicators you may see in cognitively impaired patients include the following:

- Facial expressions (e.g., a sad or frightened expression, rapid eye blinking)
- Vocalizations (e.g., noisy breathing, profanity, verbally abusive language)
- Changes in physical activity (e.g., fidgeting, increased pacing or rocking, disruptive behavior)
- Changes in routines (e.g., refusing food, difficulty sleeping)
- Mental status changes (e.g., increased confusion)
- Physiological cues include elevated blood pressure, respiration, and pulse.
- Be aware, however, that the absence of these cues does not automatically mean that pain is absent.

KnowledgeCheck 30-3
- What are the most common emotional responses to pain?
- What factors influence behavioral responses to pain?

 Go to Chapter 30, **Knowledge Check Response Sheet and Answers,** on the Student Resource Disk or DavisPlus at http://davisplus.fadavis.com/Wilkinson2

 CriticalThinking 30-4

Eunice Chu Ling is unable to communicate verbally because of her intubation. She is grimacing in pain. After you medicate her for pain, how would you determine whether her pain has been relieved?

How Does the Body React to Pain?

Our bodily reactions to pain are influenced primarily by the stage of the pain experience, as well as the intensity, duration, and quality of the pain. Pain triggers a variety of changes in the body. The onset of acute pain activates the sympathetic nervous system. As discussed in Chapter 25, this fight-or-flight (stress) response is protective. It minimizes blood loss, maintains perfusion to vital organs, prevents and fights infections, and promotes healing.

If the pain continues, the body adapts, and the parasympathetic nervous system takes over. However, the pain receptors continue to transmit the pain message so that the person remains aware of the tissue damage. Again, this is largely protective; for example, the pain you feel for several days after you sprain your ankle reminds you to stay off it until it is fully healed.

The severity and duration of the pain significantly affect how the person continues to respond to it. Often the person is able to ignore mild pain, but pain that is severe and unrelieved can consume thoughts and change daily living patterns. Box 30-1 identifies common pain responses.

Unrelieved Pain

Unrelieved pain can produce harmful effects in various body systems.

Endocrine System. Ongoing pain triggers excessive release of hormones, including adrenocorticotropic hormone (ACTH), cortisol, antidiuretic hormone (ADH), growth hormone (GH), catecholamines, and glucagon. Insulin and testosterone levels decrease. These hormone shifts activate carbohydrate, protein, and fat catabolism (breakdown), hyperglycemia, and poor glucose use. The inflammatory process, combined with these endocrine and metabolic changes, can result in weight loss, tachycardia, fever, increased respiratory rate, and even death.

Cardiovascular System. Unrelieved pain leads to hypercoagulation and an increase in heart rate, blood pressure, cardiac workload, and oxygen demand. The combination of hypercoagulation and increased cardiac workload may lead to unstable angina (chest pain), intracoronary thrombosis (clot formation in the vessels that supply the heart), and myocardial ischemia and infarction (heart attack).

Musculoskeletal System. Unrelieved pain causes impaired muscle function, fatigue, and immobility.

BOX 30-1 ■ Common Pain Responses

Physiological (Involuntary) Responses
Sympathetic Responses (Acute Pain)
Increased systolic blood pressure

Increased heart rate and force of contraction

Increased respiratory rate

Dilated blood vessels to the brain, increased alertness

Dilated pupils

Rapid speech

Parasympathetic Responses (Deep or Prolonged Pain)
Decreased systolic blood pressure, possible syncope

Decreased pulse rate

Changeable breathing patterns

Withdrawal

Constricted pupils

Slow, monotonous speech

Behavioral Responses (Voluntary)
Withdrawing from painful stimuli

Moaning

Facial grimacing

Crying

Agitation

Guarding the painful area

Psychological (Affective) Responses
Anxiety

Depression

Anger

Fear

Exhaustion

Hopelessness

Irritability

Poorly controlled pain can prevent the patient from performing activities of daily living and engaging in physical therapy.

Respiratory System. Patients in pain tend to breathe shallowly—to limit thoracic and abdominal movement in an effort to reduce pain. This is called **splinting**. Splinting reduces tidal volume (air exchanged with each breath) and increases inspiratory and expiratory pressures. These changes can lead to pneumonia and atelectasis as well as underventilation (retained carbon dioxide, also called hypercarbia) and respiratory acidosis.

Genitourinary System. Unrelieved pain causes release of excessive amounts of catecholamines, aldosterone, ADH, cortisol, angiotensin II, and prostaglandins. These hormones lead to decreased urinary output, urinary retention, fluid overload, hypokalemia, hypertension, and increased cardiac output.

Gastrointestinal (GI) System. In response to pain, intestinal secretions and smooth muscle tone increase, and gastric emptying and motility decrease.

KnowledgeCheck 30-4
- What are the effects of untreated pain on each of the body systems?
- How might untreated pain affect the progress of a patient recovering from major illness?

 Go to Chapter 30, **Knowledge Check Response Sheet and Answers,** on the Student Resource Disk or DavisPlus at http://davisplus.fadavis.com/Wilkinson2

Practical Knowledge
knowing how

As we discussed earlier, a person's *pain threshold* is the point at which that person perceives a stimulus as painful, whereas *pain tolerance* is the amount of pain a person is willing to endure. Both differ greatly from person to person. You should regularly assess for pain and accept the patient's report of pain. Increases in pain may indicate change in condition or a need for more aggressive pain management.

ASSESSMENT

The patient self-report is the most reliable indicator of pain, including those with mild cognitive impairment (Institute for Clinical Systems Improvement, 2008; National Institutes of Health [NIH], National Institute on Drug Abuse, 2005, revised). Self-report is especially important for patients with chronic pain. When pain is ongoing, the autonomic nervous system eventually adapts, so physiological and behavioral signs become less evident (Schneider, 2006–2007).

To treat pain effectively, you must first understand the patient's perception of pain. To do this, begin with a pain history. Each agency will have different assessment forms for this history. For a list of questions that are typically asked,

 Go to Chapter 30, **Assessment Guidelines and Tools, Taking a Pain History,** in Volume 2.

Pain, the Fifth Vital Sign

To raise awareness of pain and emphasize pain relief, the American Pain Society recommends assessing for pain as the fifth vital sign. This means that you should ask patients to rate their pain intensity whenever you take a full set of vital signs (Berdine, 2002; Molony, Kobayashi, Holleran, et al., 2005; Pasero, 1997). By simply raising the question with each vital signs check, you will prompt your clients to report pain more often. Also, teach nursing assistive personnel (NAP) to ask patients about their pain when taking vital signs and to report their findings to you. Box 30-2 provides the clinical approach to pain assessment recommended by the Agency for Health Care Policy and Research (AHCPR). Perform pain assessments routinely, but not limited to:

- On admission to a healthcare facility
- Before and after each potentially painful procedure or treatment
- When the patient is at rest, as well as when involved in a nursing activity
- Before you implement a pain management intervention, such as administering an analgesic drug, and 30 minutes after the intervention
- With each check of vital signs, if the pain is an actual or potential problem
- When the patient complains of pain

Assessing Pain in Children

You can assess pain in children through self-report, behavioral observation, or physiological measures. Be sure to consult the parents about the child's stress signals and reaction to pain. With children, use art and play as a way to assess the child's understanding of pain and the pain management plan. Choose age-appropriate toys to engage the child in acting out feelings. Sometimes this indirect method is more effective than directly asking the child. Remember, most children are fearful about injections and may deny pain if they think that describing their pain will lead to an injection. You can also use a pain-rating scale consisting of simple illustrations of faces. For an example,

 Go to Chapter 30, **Assessment Guidelines and Tools, Using Pain Scales,** in Volume 2.

<table>
<tr><td>

BOX 30-2 ■ Recommended Clinical Approach to Pain Assessment—Agency for Healthcare Policy and Research

Ask about pain regularly. **A**ssess pain systematically.

Believe the patient and family in their reports of pain and what relieves it.

Choose pain control options appropriate for the patient, family, and setting.

Deliver interventions in a timely, logical, coordinated fashion.

Empower patients and their families.

Enable patients to control their course to the greatest extent possible.

Source: Agency for Healthcare Policy and Research, Public Health Service, U.S. Department of Health and Human Services. (1994). AHCPR Publication no. 94-0592. Rockville, MD: Author.

</td></tr>
</table>

Culturally Competent Assessments

Three words—*pain, hurt,* and *ache*—seem to be used across many cultures to describe pain (American Geriatrics Society, 2002). You might also use descriptions of *burning, itching,* and *cramping* when asking patients about their pain experience. For this reason, many pain assessment tools can be successfully translated into various languages. If you work in an area where there are many non–English-speaking patients, you may benefit from pain assessment tools that have been translated into the languages you are most likely to encounter. To see pain translated into common languages,

 Go to Chapter 30, **Tables, Boxes, Figures: ESG Box 30-1, Pain in a Sample of Languages,** on the Student Resource Disk or DavisPlus at http://davisplus.fadavis.com/Wilkinson2

Difficult-to-Assess Patients

Patients who are under anesthesia or those receiving pancuronium bromide (Pavulon) are difficult to assess for pain. Those with brain injury may mimic pain-like behavior. Patients with Alzheimer's disease with severe cognitive and expressive deficits are also a challenge for assessing the extent of pain. It may not be possible to elicit a reliable self-report for pain, and their behavioral cues might not be reflective of the pain experience either.

When using a pain scale for cognitively impaired patients, you must allow sufficient time for the patient to respond. Although there are many pain assessment tools, the Pain Assessment in Advanced Dementia (PAINAD) Scale is a five-item, observational tool, specifically geared to older adults with dementia. The areas for rating include breathing, negative vocalization, facial expression, body language, and consolability. Lower scores indicate less pain. To see this tool,

 Go to Chapter 30, **ESG Table 30-3, Pain Assessment in Advanced Dementia (PAINAD) Scale,** on the Student Resource Disk or DavisPlus at http://davisplus.fadavis.com/Wilkinson2

You need to judge the intensity and quality of pain based on patient history and current environment. Does the patient have an underlying painful condition? What is the likely source of pain? Are there physical signs that indicate the patient has increased pain with movement, turning, or other motions? Nonverbal signs of pain become important cues for such patients.

How Do I Assess for Nonverbal Signs of Pain?

In addition to the patient's verbal report of pain, you must recognize other responses that may signal pain (see Box 30-1). Pay attention to the patient's physical signs and symptoms. Is the blood pressure or pulse elevated? Does the client appear ashen? These are signs of sympathetic nervous system stimulation. You will see these signs if the pain is acute. If the pain is unresolved or chronic, the blood pressure and pulse may be lower than normal, and the patient may report feeling faint. These are signs of parasympathetic nervous system stimulation. For guidelines to help you assess for nonverbal signs of pain,

 Go to Chapter 30, **Clinical Insight 30-2: Guidelines for Assessing Nonverbal Signs of Pain,** in Volume 2.

How Do I Use Pain Scales?

To help you assess the intensity of the pain as well as any changes in the pain, you can choose from among a variety of pain scales. Select a pain scale by considering the patient's age, level of education, language skills, eyesight, and developmental level. Keep in mind that when using a simple pain intensity scale, children can communicate the quality of pain before they are developmentally capable of indicating the intensity (O'Rourke, 2004). Once you choose a particular pain scale for a patient, use it consistently to prevent confusion and allow for comparison. To see some pain scales you might use,

 Go to Chapter 30, **Assessment Guidelines and Tools, Using Pain Scales,** in Volume 2.

KnowledgeCheck 30-5

- How often should you assess the patient for pain, if pain is a potential problem for the patient?
- What are some of the common pain scales used?
- Who should determine if the patient is in pain?

 Go to Chapter 30, **Knowledge Check Response Sheet and Answers,** on the Student Resource Disk or DavisPlus at http://davisplus.fadavis.com/Wilkinson2

 CriticalThinking 30-5

What pain rating scale would you use to assess Eunice ("Meet Your Patient")? Why?

ANALYSIS/NURSING DIAGNOSIS

For nursing diagnoses, NOC outcomes, and NIC interventions associated with Pain,

 Go to Chapter 30, **Standardized Language,** in Volume 2.

When writing a pain nursing diagnosis, specify the location of the pain and any etiological or precipitating factors that you are aware of. Also identify any knowledge deficits, fear of addiction, or any other fears or beliefs that may interfere with effective pain management. Focusing on the specific nature of pain enables you to choose the most useful interventions. For example: Acute Pain (headache) related to changes of position and secondary to increased intracranial pressure. The following NANDA-I labels are commonly used when pain is the focus of the problem:

- *Acute Pain.* Pain with an anticipated or actual duration of < 6 months.

- *Chronic Pain.* Pain with an anticipated or actual duration of > 6 months.

Notice that NANDA-I uses only duration, not speed of onset or severity, to differentiate between Acute Pain and Chronic Pain.

Pain affects many areas of functioning. Therefore, it is often the etiology of other nursing diagnoses, as you can see in the Standardized Language section of Volume 2.

PLANNING OUTCOMES

The overall objective when working with a client in pain is to prevent pain whenever possible or, if it is present, to reduce or eliminate pain.

Individualized goals/outcome statements you might write for a client with pain include the following:

- By day 2 post-op, will require only oral analgesics.
- Within 15 minutes of PCA injection, reports pain is < 3 on a 0–10 scale.
- Reports that chronic pain does not prevent her from performing activities of daily living.
- Pain Control: Uses pain diary (4: Often demonstrated) (NOC)

Use the goals set in the planning outcomes phase to evaluate the pain relief obtained from nursing and medical interventions.

PLANNING INTERVENTIONS/IMPLEMENTATION

When planning care, remember that each situation is unique. For example, one terminally ill patient may request complete relief of pain even if this leads to heavy sedation. Another patient with the same diagnosis and prognosis may prefer that the pain be decreased to a just manageable level so he can interact with his family or complete any unfinished business. The patient and family must be part of the pain management program. Generally, the most effective and least invasive method of pain control is preferable. Remember to include nonpharmacological interventions.

Although overall care of the patient depends on the cause of the pain, whether pain is acute or chronic, and on the patient's unique situation, there are nursing interventions and activities that address pain, regardless of its cause.

Specific nursing activities (including focused assessments) for clients with Acute Pain and Chronic Pain include the following:

- Actively listen to the patient's reports of pain.
- Support the patient in maintaining an active role in treatment by including her as part of the pain management team.
- Provide prescribed analgesics promptly.
- Assess for response to analgesics and nonpharmacological measures, including level of sedation. Make

assessments approximately 30 to 60 minutes after the administration of an oral medicine. Injectable medications work more quickly, so adjust the assessment time accordingly.

- Alter the treatment if the pain is not adequately relieved.
- Provide interventions to manage the side effects of medications.
- Reduce anxiety and fear by offering explanations about care and medications, by allowing the patient to be in control of his pain management, and by providing positive encouragement.
- Consult with the healthcare team about complex pain management issues.
- Delegate appropriate pain management strategies to nursing assistive personnel (NAP).

See Box 30-3 for a list of strategies that may be delegated to NAP.

Nonpharmacological Pain Relief Measures

Integrating complementary therapies into a pain management plan can help ease chronic pain and reduce the need for drug therapy (Hart, 2008). According to the 2002 National Health Interview Survey (NHIS), one-third of adults used some form of complementary alternative medicine (CAM) when confronted with pain or stress (Barnes, Bloom, & Nahin, 2008). Nonpharmacological therapies offer an alternative for people with mild pain who do not wish to take potent drugs for pain relief. For many patients, they are satisfying and empowering. However, they should be used as an adjunct to pharmacological therapies for patients with moderate to severe pain.

BOX 30-3 ■ Pain Management Tasks that May Be Delegated to Nursing Assistive Personnel

Nursing assistive personnel (NAP) may assist you in caring for patients with pain. However, you may never delegate the responsibility to assess the patient's pain, monitor the patient's response to pain management strategies, or evaluate the pain management plan. The following tasks may be delegated:

- Repositioning, using pillows for support
- Back rub or massage
- Providing darkness and quiet in the room for sleep
- Straightening sheets
- Mouth care
- Soft music of the patient's preference
- Using distraction (talking or setting up a favorite game for the patient)

Cutaneous Stimulation

Cutaneous stimulation (stimulation of the skin) is a method of pain relief based on the gate-control theory of pain. As we discussed earlier, skin stimulation sends impulses along the large sensory fibers, which in turn excite inhibitory interneurons in the spinal cord to "close the gate." This process diminishes the patient's perception of pain. Cutaneous stimulation works best on pain that is localized and not diffuse.

TENS Units. A **transcutaneous electrical nerve stimulator (TENS)** is a battery-powered device about the size of a pager that is worn externally. TENS units consist of electrode pads, connecting wire, and the stimulator. The pads are directly applied to the painful area. Once activated, the unit stimulates A-delta sensory fibers. A TENS unit can be worn intermittently or for long periods of time, depending on the patient's pain.

PENS Units. **Percutaneous electrical stimulation (PENS)** combines a TENS unit with percutaneously placed (through the skin) needle probes to stimulate peripheral sensory nerves. PENS is effective in short-term management of acute and chronic pain. PENS therapy in some patients promotes physical activity, increases the sense of well-being, reduces the use of nonopioid medication, and improves sleep.

Spinal Cord Stimulator. Chronic neurologic pain may be treated by a surgically implanted **spinal cord stimulator (SCS)**. The SCS produces a tingly sensation that interferes with the perception of pain.

Acupuncture. Application of extremely fine needles to specific sites in the body to relieve pain is called **acupuncture**. It is believed to stimulate the endogenous analgesia system. Acupuncture is well documented to provide relief from dental pain and has been used extensively after surgery and chemotherapy to treat nausea. Of all the complementary therapeutic approaches, acupuncture enjoys the most credibility in the medical community (Hart, 2008). There have been some reports in which acupuncture has led to lightheadedness, which may be a concern for patients who are at risk for falls. Assess these patients carefully after the treatment.

Acupressure. Similar to the ancient art of acupuncture, from which it evolved, **acupressure** stimulates specific sites in the body. However, instead of needles, fingertips provide firm, gentle pressure over the various pressure points. This process may have a calming effect through the release of endorphins. Patients can be readily taught key points to stimulate so that they can self-administer acupressure at any time.

Massage. Massage has been shown to be effective in reducing pain (Cassileth, Trevissan, & Jyothirmai, 2007). By providing cutaneous stimulation and relaxing the muscles, **massage** helps to reduce pain. **Effleurage**, or the use of slow, long, guiding strokes, is used for obstetrical patients during labor and as back rubs for postsurgical patients. Massage requires little effort from the patient and may improve sleep. For most patients, superficial massage is soothing and relaxing, both mentally and physically. However, some patients do not like to be touched, and you should always obtain verbal permission for a massage.

Application of Heat and Cold. The application of cold causes vasoconstriction and can help prevent swelling and bleeding. Cold can be especially effective in reducing the amount of pain that occurs during procedures. Apply a cold pack to the site before and after a procedure to reduce pain. Heat promotes circulation, which speeds healing. Use caution with these methods, however, because the skin may be injured by extremes of either hot or cold. Also, because the addition of moisture to heat or cold amplifies the intensity of the treatment, take extra precautions when applying moist heat or cold.

 To safely use heat and cold:

- Avoid direct contact with the heating or cooling device. Cover the hot or cold pack with a washcloth, towel, or fitted sleeve.
- Apply heat or cold intermittently, for no more than 15 minutes at a time, to avoid tissue injury.
- Check the skin frequently for extreme redness, blistering, cyanosis (blue color), or blanching (white color).
- If any of these occur, discontinue the treatment immediately and notify the provider.

Contralateral Stimulation. Why does a patient experiencing pain in the right arm experience some relief when lotion is applied and rubbed into the left arm? The principle involved is called **contralateral stimulation**—stimulating the skin in an area opposite to the painful site. Stimulation may be in the form of scratching, rubbing, or applying heat or cold. This intervention is especially helpful if the affected area is painful to touch, under bandages, or in a cast. It has provided some relief to patients who have phantom pain after an amputation.

Immobilization

Immobilizing a painful body part (e.g., with splints) may offer some relief. It is particularly helpful with arthritic joints. When this is done, however, you must remember to remove the splints at regular intervals so that the patient can exercise the area to strengthen the site and prevent further injury. Patients in severe pain have the tendency to immobilize a painful area by limiting its use.

Cognitive–Behavioral Interventions

Cognitive–behavioral therapy attempts to alter patterns of negative thoughts and to encourage more adaptive thoughts, emotions, and actions. It is used to decrease depression and anxiety, both of which play a role in

pain. Cognitive therapy helps patients to deal with their pain by fostering a sense of control over their illness and decreasing feelings of helplessness. Be sure to obtain the patient's permission before using these methods, because psychological or spiritual distress may occur if she considers them inconsistent with her belief system. Because they are complementary therapies, several of these interventions are discussed in more detail in Chapter 40.

Distraction

Distraction is a method of drawing the patient's attention away from the pain and focusing on something other than the pain. It is based on the belief that the brain can process only so much information at one time. When distraction works, the patient has only a peripheral awareness of pain. You may have responded to this strategy in the past. Have you ever had a headache or muscle pain go away when you became busy with other activities?

Distraction can be visual, tactile, intellectual, or auditory. The usefulness of the different methods varies among patients. For some patients, *visual* tactics, such as watching a football game on TV, serve as effective distraction. Others may respond better to *tactile* distraction such as massage, hugging a favorite toy, holding a loved one, or stroking a pet. Examples of *intellectual* distraction include becoming engrossed in a crossword puzzle or playing a challenging game. *Auditory* distraction in the form of music therapy has been shown to reduce anxiety during childbirth and appears to improve mood and pain tolerance. Music should not be limited to adults; it can be used for infants and children as well. Distraction is useful with all ages, but it should not be used in place of analgesics.

Although distraction can be used for severe pain, it is most effective for mild to moderate pain and for brief periods of time (e.g., for a short procedure such as an injection or infusion). Some patients experience an increase in pain and may become fatigued and irritable when they are no longer distracted.

Relaxation Techniques

Relaxation techniques reduce pain in a variety of medical conditions, especially in chronic pain. In **sequential muscle relaxation (SMR),** or progressive relaxation, the person sits comfortably and tenses a group of muscles for 15 seconds and then relaxes the muscle while breathing out. After a brief rest, this sequence is repeated using another set of muscles. Patients often start at the facial muscles and work downward to the feet.

Guided Imagery

Guided imagery uses auditory and imaginary processes to affect emotions and help calm and relax. Acute and chronic pain, physical and psychological, may respond to guided imagery; however, it is more effective for chronic pain. Audio media featuring guided imagery can help patients use their imagination to create images of temporary escape that will elicit a sense of well-being (Lewandowski, Good, & Draucker, 2005). For a script for a guided imagery session,

 Go to Chapter 25, **Supplemental Materials,** on the Student Resource Disk or DavisPlus at http://davisplus.fadavis.com/ Wilkinson2

Hypnosis

Hypnosis involves the induction of a deeply relaxed state. Once the person is in this state, the hypnotist offers therapeutic suggestions to provide relief of symptoms. For example, the hypnotist may suggest to a patient with arthritis that the pain can be turned down, like the volume of a radio. Special training in hypnotherapy is required.

Therapeutic Touch

Therapeutic touch (TT) was developed by nurses and derived from the ancient practice of laying on of hands. Despite its name, therapeutic touch does not require physical contact. It focuses on the use of the hands to direct energy fields surrounding the body. Although research studies on its effect are not consistent, some patients become relaxed and require less pain medication after a session of therapeutic touch.

Humor

Humor has positive effects on a patient's physical and emotional health. For most people, laughter is positive and indicates mental well-being. Humor may boost the immune system as well. It is especially helpful when used before a painful procedure because it lessens anxiety and serves as a form of distraction. Some institutions have humor carts and even humor rooms containing humorous videos, books, and playful items, such as bubbles, fingerpaints, and puppets. Humor is helpful for both children and adults, but it must always be in good taste and age-appropriate. Involve the patient in choosing the humor material, because what one person considers very funny another person may not.

Expressive Writing

Expressive writing can help reduce chronic pain. Some recommend structured writing sessions in which the patient describes stressful events for a specified period of time over consecutive days. This type of therapy is best when done in conjunction with a knowledgeable practitioner to provide direction and support (Hart, 2008). Others benefit from frequent journaling in an informal way, expressing feelings, fears, or what comes to mind.

Critical**Thinking** 30-6

What has been your experience with using nonpharmacological pain relief measures to manage your own pain? How would you incorporate these methods into your nursing practice?

Toward Evidence-Based Practice

> **Lewandowski, C. S., Good, M., & Draucker, C. B. (2005). Changes in the meaning of pain with the use of guided imagery.** *Pain Management Nursing, 6*(2), 58–67.

In a sample of 44 people experiencing chronic pain in the home setting, participants in the treatment group learned the guided imagery technique to reduce pain. Of the 210 verbal descriptions of pain reported by participants who used guided imagery and those who did not use the technique, six categories emerged from the data: pain is never-ending, pain is relative, pain is explainable, pain is torment, pain is restrictive, and pain is changeable. Before introducing the imagery technique, pain was described most often as never-ending in both groups. However, this phrase was not expressed by participants after using guided imagery.

> **Smith, C. A., Collins, C. T., Cyna, A. M., et al. (2006). Complementary and alternative therapies for pain management in labour. Cochrane Database of Systematic Reviews Issue 4.** Retrieved from http://www.cochrane.org/reviews/en/ab003521.html

Some women experience labor and childbirth without using drugs and turn to alternatives to manage pain. Alternative methods include acupuncture, mind–body techniques, massage, reflexology, herbal medicines or homoeopathy, hypnosis, and music. Researchers found evidence that acupuncture and hypnosis may help relieve pain during labor. More research is needed on these and other complementary therapies.

---

1. For patients using alternative therapies, such as guided imagery, acupuncture, and hypnosis to manage pain in various situations, why do you think these techniques might be effective?

2. When teaching alternative therapies for managing pain, how might you best prepare the setting in order to maximize the effectiveness of the technique?

3. Can you think of reasons why patients might resist trying alternative methods for managing chronic pain? What would you do to encourage patients who seem to oppose the idea of practicing nonpharmacological pain management?

 Go to **Chapter 30, Toward Evidence-Based Practice Suggested Responses,** on the Student Resource Disk or DavisPlus at http://davisplus.fadavis.com/Wilkinson2

Pharmacological Pain Relief Measures

Analgesics are classified into three groups: nonopioids, opioids, and adjuvants. Many health practitioners use the World Health Organization's (WHO) three-step ladder to assist in the selection and titration of an analgesic (Fig. 30-4). Each step in the ladder represents severity of pain, by which the analgesic selection is determined. Choice of treatment is based on the level of pain the patient is experiencing. Patients in severe pain should start at the third step. Titration is accomplished according to the patient's response. Monitoring should be regular and continuous. If the patient's pain is not controlled, adjust by moving up the pain ladder. To apply the ladder correctly, you need to know the interactions and side effects of all the drugs recommended on each step.

Around-the-Clock Dosing. Administer analgesics at regular times throughout the day if the patient has pain that lasts throughout the day. First, determine the dosage that relieves pain at the patient's desired level, then observe how long the first dose lasts. Administer the next dose before the last dose wears off. This around-the-clock (ATC) dosing prevents the patient from experiencing severe pain several times a day and is believed to be better than prn (as needed) dosing for pain. Explain to the patient that ATC dosing will keep pain at an acceptable level throughout the day and allow the patient to function at an optimal level.

Nonopioid Analgesics

Nonopioid analgesics include a variety of medications that relieve mild to moderate pain. Many also reduce inflammation and fever. Several of these medications, including acetaminophen (Tylenol), aspirin, and ibuprofen (Advil, Motrin), are available over the counter. All may be used for acute and chronic pain. Most have an onset of action within 1 hour. Box 30-4 features a number of commonly used nonopioid analgesics.

The analgesic properties of acetaminophen and aspirin are often underestimated. Research indicates that 650 mg of aspirin or acetaminophen may relieve as much pain as 50 mg of oral meperidine or 3 to 5 mg of oxycodone, both of which are narcotic analgesics.

Nonopioid analgesics are often compounded with opioids. This allows for a lower dose of opioid to be administered and reduces the incidence of side effects.

Nonsteroidal Anti-Inflammatory Drugs

The largest group of nonopioid analgesics is made up of nonsteroidal anti-inflammatory drugs (NSAIDs). These include aspirin and ibuprofen, as well as several others. NSAIDs act primarily in the peripheral tissues by interfering with the production of prostaglandins. Prostaglandins sensitize pain receptors and are involved with inflammation. One of the most common side effects of NSAIDs is gastric irritation. Taking the medication with food, lowering the dose, or using enteric-coated pills can reduce the incidence of this side effect. Some of the newer NSAIDs are less irritating to the GI tract, so they markedly decrease gastric irritation and bleeding. However, they are expensive and available only by prescription. NSAIDs should be used with caution in patients with impaired blood clotting, renal disease, and gastrointestinal bleeding or ulcers.

Aspirin is a unique NSAID. In addition to reducing inflammation, fever, and pain, it can inhibit platelet aggregation (clumping), the first step in clot formation. Myocardial infarction (heart attack), stroke, and thrombophlebitis (a clot in the peripheral veins) are all associated with platelet aggregation. Because of this property, low-dose aspirin (usually 81 mg) is prescribed to decrease risk of these disorders. Regular use of aspirin prolongs

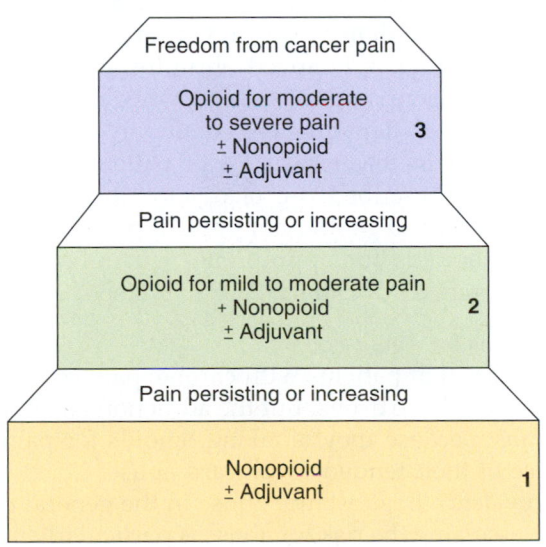

PAIN

FIGURE 30-4 The WHO three-step analgesic ladder. (World Health Organization [WHO, 1990]. Cancer pain relief and palliative care: Report of a WHO expert committee. WHO Technical Report series, No. 804. Geneva, Switzerland: Author. Used with permission.)

BOX 30-4 ■ Commonly Used Nonopioid Analgesics

Chemical Name	Brand Name
Acetaminophen	Tylenol
Acetylsalicylic acid (aspirin)	Excedrin, Bayer, others
Celecoxib	Celebrex
Diclofenac	Voltaren, Cataflam
Etodolac	Lodine
Ibuprofen	Motrin, Advil, others
Indomethacin	Indocin
Ketoprofen	Oruvail
Nabumetone	Relafen
Naproxen	Naprosyn, Aleve, Anaprox

clotting time, so teach patients who use aspirin that they will bruise easily and will bleed more if cut.

Combining two nonsteroidal anti-inflammatory drugs (NSAIDs) is not recommended because it increases the risks of side effects and may not be more effective. However, taking a small daily dose of aspirin to prevent myocardial infarction does not seem to increase the side effects for patients taking other NSAIDs.

Acetaminophen

Unlike most nonopioid analgesics, acetaminophen has very little anti-inflammatory effect. Instead it has analgesic and fever-reducing properties. It has fewer side effects and is probably the safest of the nonopioids. It does not affect platelet function, rarely causes gastrointestinal problems, and can be used in patients who are allergic to aspirin or other NSAIDs. However, even in recommended doses (up to a maximum of 4000 mg daily), it can cause severe hepatotoxicity (liver toxicity) in patients who consume alcohol and in patients with liver disease.

KnowledgeCheck 30-6

- How do NSAIDs induce pain relief?
- What is the main side effect of NSAIDs?
- In which patients are NSAIDs contraindicated?

Go to Chapter 30, **Knowledge Check Response Sheet and Answers,** on the Student Resource Disk or DavisPlus at http://davisplus.fadavis.com/Wilkinson2

Opioid Analgesics

Opioids are natural and synthetic compounds that relieve pain, although they vary in potency. To some degree opioids work by finding pain receptor sites to bind with and block the pain impulse. Keep in mind that the process of achieving analgesia is more complex than this. Opiate receptors include mu, delta, kappa, and sigma receptors; however, mu receptors are most effective in relieving pain.

- **Mu agonists** stimulate mu receptors and are used for acute, chronic, and cancer pain. They include codeine, morphine, hydromorphine (Dilaudid), fentanyl, methadone, and oxycodone. These are excellent medications for **breakthrough pain**—pain that "breaks through" relief provided by analgesics. Breakthrough analgesia refers to a rescue or extra dose. Drugs used for breakthrough pain should have a rapid onset and short duration. Whenever possible, use the same drug as that given for ongoing pain relief. There is no maximum daily dose limit and no "ceiling" to the level of analgesia from these drugs. You can steadily increase the dose to relieve pain.
- **Agonist-antagonists** are another group of opioids. These medications stimulate some opioid receptors but block others. Commonly used medications include mixed agonist-antagonists, such as pentazocine (Talwin) and nalbuphine (Nubain), and partial agonists, such as buprenorphine (Buprenex). These medications are appropriate for moderate to severe acute pain. Agonist-antagonists should not be given to patients taking mu agonists (e.g., morphine) because they may act as antagonists at the mu receptor sites and reduce or reverse the analgesia from the mu agonist.

Opioid Effectiveness

The effectiveness of opioids for pain relief can vary depending on individual differences in metabolism. Some are classified as poor, intermediate, extensive, and ultrarapid metabolizers. Body size has little to do with appropriate opioid dosing (D'Arcey, 2008b). For instance, a large person weighing near 300 pounds may not receive the same therapeutic effect with the same dosing as what is needed to effectively treat a 90 pound, frail, older adult.

Opioids are most effective for certain types of pain. For instance, visceral pain, which is more generalized, is most responsive to opioid treatment, whereas pain of neurological origin tends to be resistant to opioids, requiring that they be given as an adjunct to other therapies (Institute for Clinical Systems Improvement, 2008).

Patient Misconceptions About Opioids

Some people may be concerned about using opioids because they fear respiratory depression, drug tolerance, drug dependence, and addiction. Respiratory depression can be treated with naloxone (Narcan), an opioid antagonist.

- **Tolerance** to opioids can occur, but increasing the dose or changing the route of administration can correct that problem. There is no ceiling on the analgesic effects of opioids. Because of the problem of cross-tolerance, opioid rotation and new opioid compounds are used to produce better pain relief (D'Arcey, 2008b).
- **Physical dependence** leads to withdrawal symptoms when the drug is removed abruptly; it can be prevented by decreasing the dose slowly over time.
- **Psychological dependence,** commonly called *addiction,* occurs in fewer than 1% of patients even after long-term prescribed use of opioids for pain. Thus, fear of addiction should not prevent patients from receiving opioids for appropriate pain relief (Pasero, Manworren, & McCaffery, 2008; Patterson, 2008).

Screening for Abuse Potential

Be aware that patients with chronic pain *can* become addicted or abuse drugs. But the addiction is not necessarily *just* because they're taking opioids for pain, but because of their tendencies toward abuse. Considering the prevalence of substance abuse in the general population, assessing the risk for abuse is particularly important for the patient with chronic, nonmalignant pain.

Healthcare professionals often fail to recognize substance abuse unless they actively screen for it. Although you may be uncomfortable asking questions about alcohol and illicit drug use, gathering a reliable substance use history is important to provide a foundation for good pain management. This history should include information on the pattern and amount of alcohol intake because patients whose tolerance for alcohol is high may require a higher dose of opioids. Screening should be an integral part of chronic pain management using a validated risk assessment tools, such as the following:

- The **Opioid Risk Tool (ORT).** This is a five-question, yes/no self-report designed to predict a patient's tendency for aberrant behaviors when prescribed opioid analgesia.
- The **Screener and Opioid Assessment for Patients with Pain (SOAPP).** This is a longer, highly reliable tool that may be more appropriate for high-risk populations or when the clinician has time for a thorough assessment.

You can't rely on the normalcy of behavior to indicate opioid abuse. Random drug screening will show opioid use even when aberrant behavior is not evident (Schneider, 2006–2007). To use the Opioid Risk Tool,

 Go to Chapter 30, **Tables, Boxes, Figures: ESG Table 30-1, Using the Opioid Risk Tool,** on the Student Resource Disk or DavisPlus at http://davisplus.fadavis.com/Wilkinson2

Side Effects of Opioids

Most opioids share the same general side effects. The most common are nausea, vomiting, constipation, and drowsiness. Some side effects, such as drowsiness and nausea, improve after a few doses. Large doses may lead to respiratory depression and hypotension. Always assess the patient for level of alertness and respiratory status before you administer the drug. Excessive sedation will precede respiratory depression. Other side effects of opioids include difficulty with urination, dry mouth, sweating, tachycardia, palpitations, constipation, bradycardia, rashes, urticaria (hives), or pruritus (itching).

You should look up in a drug guide the specific opioid you will be administering for side effects of that particular drug. See Box 30-5 for strategies to prevent common side effects.

BOX 30-5 ■ Preventing and Treating Side Effects from Opioids

Before deciding to add another medication to treat a side effect, consider changing the dose or frequency of the current opioid or changing to another opioid.

Side Effect: Constipation

- Add more fruits, vegetables, and fiber to the diet. Keep in mind, though, this does not help relieve opioid-induced constipation unless the patient's current fiber intake is deficient. Excessive fiber might even put the patient at risk for bowel obstruction due to the opioid-induced decreased peristalsis (refer to Chapter 28, as needed).
- Increase exercise routine. Even walking short distances will help.
- Increase oral fluid intake to eight 8-ounce glasses of water per day.
- If needed, administer stool softeners.
- If the above are not effective, administer a mild laxative.
- If constipation continues, soften stool with glycerin suppository and follow up with a soapsuds enema.

Side Effect: Nausea and Vomiting

- Reduce opioid dose by combining nonopioid or adjuvant drugs.
- Teach patients that nausea will usually subside after several doses.
- Premedicate or medicate consecutively with an antiemetic. Be aware this may increase sedation, depending on the antiemetic chosen.
- Teach relaxation techniques.

Side Effect: Pruritus

- Reduce opioid dose by combining with nonopioid or adjuvant drugs.
- Use cool packs, lotion, or topical anesthetics.

- Administer antihistamines, such as diphenhydramine (Benadryl). Be aware that this may increase sedation.
- Teach the patient that he can generally expect to develop a tolerance to pruritus.
- Use distraction techniques, which frequently work well.

Side Effect: Respiratory Depression

- Assess the patient's respiratory status *before* administering the opioid and frequently afterward.
- Reduce the opioid dose by combining with nonopioid or adjuvant drugs.
- Reduce the opioid dose by 25% when you observe signs of oversedation.
- If the patient is not responsive or is only minimally responsive, stop the opioid and administer an antagonist, such as naloxone (Narcan). After dosing with a narcotic antidote, reassess the patient for respiratory depression. Naloxone is metabolized more quickly than opioids and therefore, repeat dosing might be needed.

Side Effect: Drowsiness

- Assess the patient to ensure that the drowsiness is due to opioid administration and not from another cause.
- Teach the patient that drowsiness will generally subside after a few days as she develops tolerance.
- If analgesia is adequate, reduce the opioid by 25%.
- Discontinue all other nonessential CNS depressant medications.
- During the daytime, offer simple stimulants, such as caffeine.
- Offer a lower dose more frequently to decrease peak concentration.
- Consider another opioid or route of administration.

■ *Paradoxical reactions.* For some individuals, opioids may lead to a paradoxical increase in pain despite receiving increasing doses of opioids (Institute for Clinical Systems Improvement, 2008).

■ *Sedation.* Most patients experience some degree of sedation at the beginning of opioid therapy or when the dose is increased. Monitor postoperative patients who receive opioids for sedation and respiratory depression every 1 to 2 hours during the first 12 to 24 hours after surgery. For an example of a sedation scale,

 Go to Chapter 30, **Assessment Guidelines and Tools, Sedation Rating Scale,** in Volume 2.

KnowledgeCheck 30-7

■ What are the most common side effects of opioids?
■ Identify at least three things that you should monitor when administering opioids.
■ What is the risk of addiction to opioids for patients with acute pain?

 Go to Chapter 30, **Knowledge Check Response Sheet and Answers,** on the Student Resource Disk or DavisPlus at http://davisplus.fadavis.com/Wilkinson2

Equianalgesia

Equianalgesia refers to the approximately equal analgesia that a variety of opioids will provide. Equianalgesic dose calculations provide a starting point when changing from one opioid to another or from one route of administration to another. For example, a parenteral dose of 5 mg of morphine is equivalent to

60 mg of parenteral codeine or 100 mg of oral codeine in terms of the analgesic effect it produces. As another example, 5 mg of parenteral morphine is the equivalent of 15 mg of oral morphine. These doses are approximate and vary according to the number of doses, the variety of opioids the patient has received, and the needs of the patient. To see a table of equianalgesic dosages among opioids,

 Go to Chapter 30, **Tables, Boxes, Figures: ESG Table 30-5, Equianalgesic Doses of Commonly Used Opioid Analgesics,** on the Student Resource Disk or DavisPlus at http://davisplus.fadavis.com/Wilkinson2

Routes of Administration for Opioid Analgesics

Use the safest and least invasive route to administer opioids. See Box 30-6 for an overview of opioid administration routes.

Patient-Controlled Analgesia (PCA). PCA pumps are an effective and safe way to deliver opioids by IV, epidural, or subcutaneous routes. They provide excellent pain relief and give the patient a sense of control over the pain. The system consists of a programmable infusion pump, a syringe, IV tubing, and a trigger that the patient presses to self-administer a dose. The success of the pump depends on programming a dose that can be administered frequently enough to manage the patient's pain effectively. Some providers order a low continuous rate of infusion as a base that can be supplemented with patient-initiated doses. Most PCA pumps can be programmed with 1- or 4-hour maximum medication limits. If the patient reaches the limit set, the pump will automatically trigger a "lockout" even if the patient keeps pressing the button. Patients need to be educated about this lockout feature; they may not activate the pump enough because they fear overdosing.

If you are educating the patient on the use of the PCA pump in the postoperative period, make sure the patient is alert enough to understand the directions and has been given a hearing aid or glasses, if needed, before you offer your explanation. Because of the potential to overdose the patient, only nurses who are trained in PCAs should set up the pump and the program. As a safeguard, another nurse should double-check the setup before patient use. Encourage patients to administer a dose before potentially painful activities, such as walking or physical therapy. PCA pumps are contraindicated in patients who have limited ability to understand directions. The accompanying Critical Aspects box summarizes the key points involved in use of the PCA. For detailed instruction on use of a PCA pump,

 Go to Chapter 30, **Procedure 30-1: Setting Up and Managing a Patient-Controlled Analgesia by Pump,** in Volume 2.

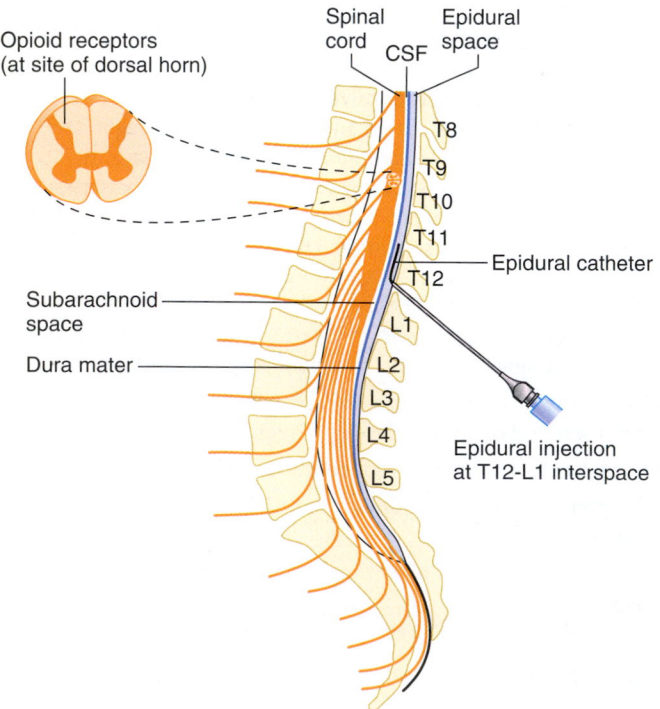

FIGURE 30-5 Placement of an epidural needle and catheter.

Opioid receptors (at site of dorsal horn)

Spinal cord
Epidural space
CSF
T8
T9
T10
T11
T12
Epidural catheter

Subarachnoid space
Dura mater
L1
L2
L3
L4
L5
Epidural injection at T12-L1 interspace

BOX 30-6 ■ Opioid Administration Routes

Oral

The oral route is convenient, safe, and generally produces steady analgesic levels. It is the preferred route of administration unless rapid onset of analgesia is desired. Use the oral route to provide relief for mild to severe pain. It includes medications that are swallowed but also includes sublingual, transmucosal, buccal, and gingival routes. Oral patient-controlled analgesia (oral PCA) is being used in some hospitals to eliminate the delay between the patient's request for medication and the nurse's administration of it.

Nasal

The intranasal route of administration of drugs has been used for centuries. A rich supply of blood in this area provides the drug easy access to systemic circulation. The mixed agonist–antagonist opioid butorphanol and the mu agonist sufentanil can be administered intranasally. One drawback to this route is that it may cause burning or stinging.

Transdermal

The transdermal route delivers a continuous release of drug for up to 72 hours. It is a convenient alternative for a patient who requires constant opioid treatment for pain. Fentanyl (Duragesic) is commonly given as a transdermal patch. Use it with care on patients who are febrile, because their increased temperature will increase absorption of the drug. This route is effective for ongoing pain relief but does not provide immediate relief. Inform the patient and family about safe storage and proper disposal of transdermal patches. Proper dating and removing patches after the dose is complete can prevent confusion and dosing errors.

Rectal

Suppositories are an excellent alternative to the oral route, especially in infants and young children. This route is effective when the patient is vomiting, has a gastrointestinal obstruction, or is at risk for aspiration if oral medications are used. The rectal route may be contraindicated in patients with neutropenia or thrombopenia because of the potential to cause rectal bleeding while inserting the suppository.

Subcutaneous

The subcutaneous route may be used for intermittent injections and continuous administration of opioids. Continuous subcutaneous infusion (CSCI) of opioids is gaining popularity. CSCI is appropriate for people who cannot tolerate oral opioids or who have dose-limiting side effects from oral administration (e.g., nausea) and who also have limited venous access. Absorption and distribution vary based on the placement site chosen. Hydromorphine and morphine are the drugs most commonly used. Frequently, CSCI of opioids is used for chronic cancer pain and in palliative care. It is better absorbed, is safer, and provides more continuous relief than the intramuscular (IM) route. Small portable medication pumps allow the patient to be mobile. However, some patients find this method painful and time-consuming. You will need to teach patients and their families how to use the pumps, needles, syringes, and other equipment. Because of the small volume of drug (2 to 3 mL per hour) that can be absorbed, two sites may be needed if higher doses are required.

Intramuscular (IM)

IM injections are painful, the onset of action is slow, and absorption is unreliable. Consequently, this is not the preferred route of administration of pain medication. With repeated administration, sterile abscesses and fibrotic tissue can result. Nevertheless, the IM route is often used for short-term pain relief postoperatively. This route should be avoided in children because they often refuse pain medication to avoid having an injection.

Intravenous (IV)

The IV route produces immediate pain relief and is desirable for acute or escalating pain. It is most commonly used for short-term therapy and for hospitalized patients who can be monitored. It is, however, also used in the home care setting for patients with cancer and other pain who are unable to tolerate oral opioids. Methods of IV delivery include continuous infusions, bolus, and patient-controlled analgesia (PCA). Patients on a continuous infusion can deliver a bolus for breakthrough pain or procedures such as wound care. Drawbacks to this route include the need for venous access and the need to maintain a patent line. Patients who previously used oral opioids may find the IV equipment cumbersome but they typically report less pain and fewer side effects than with the oral route.

Intra-articular

A pain pump is implanted into a joint during arthroscopic surgery as a measure to control postsurgical pain. A pain pump provides relief to patients by delivering continuous infusion of local anesthetic directly to the surgical site.

Intraspinal and Epidural Analgesics

Intraspinal analgesia requires placement of a catheter in the subarachnoid space (for intrathecal analgesia) or the epidural space by an anesthesiologist or a certified registered nurse anesthetist (CRNA). The epidural space is generally preferred because it poses less risk of complications although they can occur, such as dural puncture, infection, hematoma, and nerve damage (see Fig. 30-5). Placement of the catheter, as well as the type and concentration of medication, determines the area affected by the medication. Higher doses are needed for epidural than for intrathecal administration.

The most commonly used opioids for epidural administration are morphine sulfate (Duramorph), fentanyl citrate (Sublimaze), and hydromorphone (Dilaudid, Palladone). Local anesthetics are frequently combined with the opioids to reduce the total amount of drug necessary to produce analgesia. For nursing care activities associated with caring for a client with an epidural catheter for pain management,

 Go to Chapter 30, **Clinical Insight 30-1: Caring for a Patient with an Epidural Catheter,** in Volume 2.

For steps to follow in *all* procedures, refer to the Universal Steps for All Procedures found on the inside back cover of Volume 2. Go to the full procedures in Volume 2 to practice and learn the procedure steps. Use these Critical Aspects later to help you review key points.

Procedure 30-1: Setting Up and Managing Patient-Controlled Analgesia by Pump

➤ Determine the patient's baseline vital signs, cognitive status, physical mobility, and pain level.

➤ Review the physician prescription for PCA, including the initial bolus (loading) dose, the basal rate, the demand dose, the lockout interval between each dose, and the 1-hour or 4-hour lockout dose limit.

➤ Determine if the patient has an allergy to prescribed medication.

➤ Verify PCA with two nurses before initiating PCA, discontinuing it, change of shift, and when wasting the remainder of medication.

➤ Insert the medication cartridge/syringe into the pump, prime the connecting tubing, and lock the pump.

➤ Set the pump for the loading dose (if prescribed), basal rate, demand dose, lockout interval, and the 1-hour or 4-hour lockout dose limit.

➤ Connect the tubing into the patient's maintenance IV line.

➤ Start infusing the medication (loading, then basal, dose).

➤ Place the button that controls dosing within reach of the patient.

➤ Change tubing per facility protocol.

 ## Critical**Thinking** 30-7

- What routes of opioid administration have you seen in your clinical rotation?
- What types of pain relief and side effects have you observed?
- What routes of administration would you like to see? Why?

Adjuvant Analgesics

Adjuvant analgesics may be used as a primary therapy for mild pain or in conjunction with opioids for moderate to severe pain. Drugs in this category include anticonvulsants, antidepressants, local anesthetics, topical agents, psychostimulants, muscle relaxants, neuroleptics, corticosteroids, and others. **Adjuvant analgesics** reduce the amount of opioid the patient requires. They are especially useful if the patient experiences significant side effects from escalating doses of opioids. Adjuvant analgesics are frequently used in managing neuropathic pain, in which they may be the primary treatment or may be used in conjunction with opioids.

Chemical Pain Relief Measures

Nerve blocks and **epidural injection** are types of regional anesthesia. An anesthetic agent is injected into or around the nerve that supplies sensation to a specific part of the body. Most nerve blocks affect a network of nerves called a *plexus.* Nerve blocks may be used for short-term pain relief after surgical procedures or for long-term management of chronic pain.

Local anesthesia is the injection of local anesthetics into body tissues. Short-acting agents, such as lidocaine, and long-acting agents, such as marcaine, may be used. Local anesthetics are injected into subcutaneous tissue for minor surgical procedures. They may also be injected into joints and muscle for pain relief. Pumps are commonly used to administer local anesthetics at surgical sites for postoperative pain relief.

Topical anesthesia involves applying an agent that contains cocaine, lidocaine, or benzocaine directly to the skin, mucous membranes, wounds, or burns. Topical anesthesia is quickly absorbed and provides pain relief for mild to moderate pain. Many topical anesthetic agents are available over the counter. Sunburn relief agents, gel products for tooth and gum pain, and first aid sprays are forms of topical anesthetics.

Radiofrequency Ablation Therapy

Radiofrequency ablation therapy uses electromagnetic waves that travel at the speed of light to target nerves that carry pain impulses. This procedure is used to provide longer term pain relief than that provided by injections of steroids or pain relievers and nerve blocks.

Surgical Interruption of Pain Conduction Pathways

Surgical interruption of pain conduction pathways results in permanent destruction of nerve pathways and is used as a last resort for intractable pain. The various options depend on the type and location of pain.

- **Cordotomy** interrupts pain and temperature sensation below the tract that is severed. This is most frequently done for leg and trunk pain.
- **Rhizotomy** interrupts the anterior or posterior nerve route that is located between the ganglion and the cord. Anterior interruption is generally used to stop spastic movements that accompany paraplegia, and posterior interruption eliminates pain in the area innervated. This procedure may be safely performed at any level along the spine but is most often used for head and neck pain produced by cancer.
- **Neurectomy** is used to eliminate intractable localized pain. The pathways of peripheral or cranial nerves are interrupted to block pain transmission.
- **Sympathectomy** severs the paths to the sympathetic division of the autonomic nervous system. The outcomes of this procedure are improvement in vascular blood supply and the elimination of vasospasm. It is used to treat the pain from vascular disorders, such as Raynaud's disease.

Surgical therapies disrupting pain pathways are not widely used due to advances in oral and transdermal opioid therapies.

KnowledgeCheck 30-8

- Identify three types of chemical pain relief measures.
- What type of patient might be suitable for surgical interruption of a pain pathway?

 Go to Chapter 30, **Knowledge Check Response Sheet and Answers,** on the Student Resource Disk or DavisPlus at http://davisplus.fadavis.com/Wilkinson2

Misconceptions that Interfere with Pain Management

Pain is invisible to others but it exists when the patient says it does. It exists even when there are no sure-fire signs of pain or an apparent cause.

Patients, caregivers, and clinicians sometimes have beliefs about pain or pain management strategies that interfere with the treatment plan. For instance, one older patient may fear that severe pain is a sign of weakness and try to endure it. Others might perceive pain as a part of the normal physical declines that accompany aging instead of an acute situation that requires treatment. An athlete might believe no pain, no gain when actually pain can signal a problem. A "grin and bear it" approach for dealing with minor pain, such as an occasional headache or muscle soreness, is one thing but putting up with chronic pain can reduce quality of life. Or a family member may worry that pain medication may make the patient nonfunctional. Others might fear addiction to pain medication even though non-narcotic analgesics are not addictive.

The beliefs of healthcare providers can also interfere with pain management. For example, nurses and other caregivers sometimes doubt the patient's report of pain because:

- Most people don't have pain from that particular illness or procedure.
- There is no obvious, physical cause for the pain.

- They are concerned about drug-seeking behavior and patient addiction.

As you care for patients in pain, remain open to the patient's description of pain, and work with the patient and caregivers to provide pain control. Table 30-1 highlights some of the most common misconceptions about pain.

Managing Pain in Older Patients

Pain, particularly persistent pain, is common among older adults, especially those suffering from degenerative spine conditions, arthritis, nightly leg pain, or pain as a result of cancer. Pain management among older patients is especially difficult. Most older adults have at least one chronic condition and take multiple medications. Adding analgesics to an already complex medication regimen increases the likelihood of drug interactions. In addition, drug distribution is altered in older patients because of changes in blood flow to the organs, protein binding, and the difference in body composition. Older adults are at great risk for undertreatment of pain because they and their caregivers may be reluctant to administer analgesics for fear of producing confusion, excessive sedation, drug interactions, and respiratory depression.

Another problem for sufficiently treating pain in older adults is that pain is often unrecognized because of dementia, coexisting medical conditions, sensory impairment, or inability to verbally communicate the quality or intensity of pain. Poor pain management can result in falls, poor sleep, delayed healing, reduced activity, prolonged hospitalization, anxiety, and poor quality of life (Horgas, 2007). At the same time, there is a risk of overtreatment due to the higher peak effect and longer duration of pain relief that they experience as a result of changes associated with aging (AGS, Panel on Persistent Pain in Older Persons, 2002).

Table 30-1 ➤ Common Misconceptions Among Patients and Caregivers About Pain

FALLACY	TRUTH
The caregiver is more objective than the patient about the amount of pain experienced.	The patient's report is the "gold standard," and the patient is the authority.
You should wait until the pain is severe before taking medication.	You should take pain medication early and on a regular basis if pain is severe.
There is a significant danger of addiction to pain medications.	Patients in pain rarely become addicted to their pain medications.
Pain is a normal component of aging.	Pain is a symptom that something is wrong and should be treated.
Complaining of pain will label the person as a "bad patient."	The patient should report pain so that it can be treated.
Patients should have severe pain only if they have major surgery.	Even minor surgery and injury can produce severe pain.
Patients will have visible physical or behavioral signs if they are really in pain.	Even when patients are in severe pain, they may not exhibit physical or behavioral signs.

Persistent pain is not a normal part of aging and should not be ignored. For updated recommendations from the American Geriatrics Society (AGS) Panel on Pharmacological Management of Persistent Pain in Older Persons,

 Go to Chapter 30, **ESG Table 30-2, AGS Panel on Pharmacological Management of Persistent Pain in Older Persons,** on the Student Resource Disk or DavisPlus at http://davisplus.fadavis.com/Wilkinson2

There is a major change in the 2009 AGS guidelines for managing persistent pain in older adults. Original guidelines recommended seniors use over-the-counter or prescription anti-inflammatory drugs (NSAIDs), such as aspirin or ibuprofen, before being prescribed an opioid drug. However, in light of increased cardiovascular risk and gastrointestinal toxicity in this population, the AGS Panel now recommends all patients with moderate to severe pain or diminished quality of life due to pain should be considered for opioid therapy. Acetaminophen should be considered for treatment of persistent pain, particularly musculoskeletal pain, in light of its effectiveness and safety. The guidelines also provide recommendations about the use of adjuvant therapy for older persons with recurring pain.

 Critical**Thinking** 30-8

- Which groups of patients are most at risk for inadequate pain management?
- What can you do to assist each group?
- How do past pain experiences affect present pain experience?

Managing Pain in Patients with Substance Abuse or Active Addiction

It is important to differentiate between physical dependence, which is expected and treatable, and addiction. **Addiction** is a state of psychological dependence in which a person uses a drug compulsively and will engage in self-destructive behavior to obtain the drug. Many studies have shown that the properly managed, short-term medical use of opioid analgesic drugs is safe and rarely causes addiction with the exception of those with a personal or family history of drug abuse or mental illness (NIH, National Institute on Drug Abuse, 2005).

Although addiction related to the therapeutic use of opioids is uncommon, substance abuse is a common problem within our society and is a problem among individuals from all backgrounds. Behaviors that may indicate substance abuse or addiction include the following:

- Repeated requests for injections of an opioid or atypical high dosing when pain should normally be diminishing with recovery from an injury or surgery

- Refusal to try oral medication for pain relief
- "Doctor shopping"—moving from provider to provider in an effort to obtain multiple prescriptions for the drug(s) they abuse
- "Pharmacy shopping"—using multiple pharmacies to dispense controlled substances

If you observe these signs, assess the patient carefully because the signs may also indicate untreated withdrawal or increased pain due to complications. When dealing with clients with active addiction, try to assume a nonjudgmental approach.

Healthcare providers have long wrestled with the dilemma of how to adequately relieve the suffering of chronic pain while avoiding the potential for the patient to become addicted to the pain medication. Although it is important to recognize opioid addiction, you must be careful not to undertreat pain in patients whom you know or suspect to abuse substances. As a nurse, you will be in a position to help maintain the balance between providing adequate pain relief and protecting against inappropriate drug use.

 Critical**Thinking** 30-9

You are preparing to give your patient a bath. When you remove his bath equipment from under the bedside table, you find illicit drugs mixed in with the patient's bath equipment. What would you do?

Pain Relief from Placebos

A **placebo** is defined as "any medication or procedure, including surgery, that produces an effect in a patient because of its implicit or explicit intent, not because of its specific physical or chemical properties" (McCaffery & Pasero, 1999, p. 36). Placebos contain inactive substances that do not chemically provide analgesia. Clearly, placebos can relieve pain for some patients. How they do so is not well understood. Theories include operant conditioning, faith, anxiety reduction, and endorphin release. Although use of placebos may be appropriate in clinical trials, they are not suitable for pain management for the following reasons:

- If the patient responds to a placebo, it does not mean that the patient did not have pain. In classic studies done in the 1950s, 36% of patients demonstrated adequate pain relief from a placebo injection the day after abdominal surgery (Evans, 1974). However, there is no way to determine in advance which patients will experience pain relief; therefore, you risk inadequately treating the patient.
- Even in the same patient, placebos may relieve pain at one time and not at another.
- Ethically, the most important reason for not using placebos is that their use involves deceit. If discovered, and it frequently is, the patient's trust in healthcare professionals will be diminished, if not destroyed.

Teaching the Patient and Family About Pain

Patients and caregivers tend to cope more effectively when they are well informed. Because pain can interfere with a patient's learning, be sure to include the patient's family in your teaching. If the patient is discharged from the facility with a prescription for opioids, the family should be taught how to monitor for excessive sedation and to call the healthcare provider if the patient is not receiving adequate pain relief. The following topics should be discussed with the patient and family:

- The cause of the pain, if it is known
- The normal duration of the pain, if known (e.g., postoperative pain generally decreases every day as tissues heal)
- How to use the selected pain scale; ask for a demonstration of use
- The overall pain management plan
- Information about the analgesic prescribed—dose, interval, and route of administration
- If opioids are prescribed, explanation that the risk of addiction is extremely low
- Nonpharmacological ways to treat pain
- Side effects to observe for
- The need to alter the treatment plan if relief is not achieved
- How to contact the healthcare team regarding side effects, missed doses, change in condition, or ineffective pain management

Documentation

Thoroughly document the pain management plan and the patient's responses. Documentation may be narrative, in either nursing or interdisciplinary notes, or recorded on a pain management flowsheet. Although documentation varies from facility to facility, it typically reflects the entire spectrum of the nursing process:

- The expected outcome for pain management
- The patient's pain level at the present time
- The patient's response to any intervention for pain
- Any adverse reactions that may have resulted from the analgesic
- Planned interventions to improve the pain relief if needed

Typically, pain management flowsheets contain a column for time, pain ratings, and analgesic used, including dose and route, vital signs, and side effects. Pain management flowsheets are tailored to the patient population, the type of pain being monitored, and the clinical setting. For example, the pain flowsheet for a patient on an IV PCA pump will be more complex than a pain flowsheet for a patient on oral medications at home. Documentation is important because typically pain recall is poor and patients often underestimate their pain after the fact. If pain is not adequately documented, there is no way to prove that it was accurately assessed. For an example of a pain flow sheet,

 Go to Chapter 30, **Tables, Boxes, Figures: ESG Figure 30-4, Pain Flow Sheet,** on the Student Resource Disk or DavisPlus at http://davisplus.fadavis.com/Wilkinson2

▌ EVALUATION

Evaluation is critical to a pain management program. Compare your findings with the expected outcomes to determine whether the pain management strategy is effective. Questions to ask include the following:

- Are the patient's pain scores consistently at or better than the desired level? Are they improving?
- Is the patient's behavior, mobility, range of motion, mood, and affect consistent with pain relief?
- What is the quality of the patient's life, according to the patient's standards?

In addition to evaluating the extent to which the pain was relieved, you need to determine which interventions were or were not effective, as well as any adverse reactions to these interventions. Close examination of the patient's pain diary should provide most of the data you need for evaluation.

It is important to reassess the patient's pain regularly. An increase in pain may be a sign of inadequate pain management, but it may also be a sign of developing complications. Before implementing a change in the treatment plan, you should determine whether the pain management plan was carried out correctly. If the decision of the healthcare team is to make a change, remember to evaluate again the effect of this change. Do not assume your intervention will provide adequate pain relief.

Nursing Process in Action

Mary Jean Thompson, 30 years old, was admitted to the hospital with severe abdominal pain and underwent an appendectomy yesterday. The physician has prescribed hydromorphone (Dilaudid) 2 mg tablet PO q4-6 hr prn for pain. Ms. Thompson doesn't like the idea of taking pain medication and waits until she rates her pain a 9 or 10 on a scale of 0 to 10 before requesting an injection. Even after the medication, her pain never drops below a 7 on a scale of 0 to 10 and she is unwilling to turn or ambulate due to the pain.

When you perform your assessment, she tells you she does not want to be sedated. "I hate that groggy,

Pain Management: Nursing Care

Nursing Diagnosis: Acute Pain (surgical incision) related to possible inadequate analgesia (drug and dosing) because of reluctance to have IM injection, as manifested by not requesting medication until her pain is at a score of 9

EXPECTED OUTCOMES	NURSING INTERVENTIONS	RATIONALE
On a scale of 0–10, the patient will verbalize pain relief at a score of 3 or below while in bed and 4 or below while ambulating at all times.	Assess and document the patient's verbal and nonverbal expressions of pain relief with each check of vital signs, with every procedure and ambulation, and when the patient is at rest.	Assessment is necessary to determine the effectiveness of the prescribed medications. Assessment and documentation are legal responsibilities for the nurse as well.
	Discuss with the prescriber the need to modify prescriptions if pain relief measures are ineffective. Recommend PCA.	Ineffective pain management will cause the patient increased stress and can lead to further complications because the patient will be unwilling to move.
	When you obtain new pain orders for a PCA morphine pump, educate the patient about the pump.	A patient using PCA requires instruction about safe use of the pump.
	Provide nonpharmacological interventions, such as a back rub or other techniques described in this chapter, before rest or sleep, with any exacerbation of pain, and after painful procedures such as ambulation.	Nonpharmacological interventions are synergistic and enhance the relief the opioid gives.
The patient will demonstrate pain relief by participating in ambulation and turning within 24 hours.	Teach the patient to press the PCA pump before activities.	Peak blood levels enable the patient to ambulate, cough and deep-breathe, and perform activities of daily living.

drugged feeling. I'm willing to have some pain to avoid that." After you discuss the importance of pain management to aid in healing and ability to participate in activities and therapy, Ms. Thompson states that she would like to have a pain score of 3 to 4 today.

 Go to Chapter 30, **Resources for Caregivers and Health Professionals,** on the Student Resource Disk or DavisPlus at http://davisplus.fadavis.com/Wilkinson2

 Suggested Readings: Go to Chapter 30, **Reading More About Pain Management,** on the Student Resource Disk or DavisPlus at http://davisplus.fadavis.com/Wilkinson2

 Bibliography: Go to Volume 2, Bibliography.

Care Map

Data (blue box):
- Severe pain; appendectomy
- Dislikes use of IM opioid analgesics
- After med, still rates pain as 7 (0–10 scale); wants 3–4
- Not turning/ambulating
- Dislikes sedation

Mary Jean Thompson

Nursing diagnosis: Acute pain r/t surgical incision and possible inadequate analgesia

Outcomes:

On a scale of 0–10, pt will state relief at 3 in bed and 4 with ambulation.

Pt will demonstrate pain relief by ambulating and turning within 24 hr.

Nursing activities:

Provide nonpharmacological interventions. (e.g., backrubs)

Assess/document pain relief with VS, procedures, and ambulation.

Collaborate with prescriber to obtain PCA order.

Educate pt in use of narcotic PCA.

Teach patient to bolus PCA before activity.

Key:
- Data
- Nursing diagnosis
- Outcomes
- Nursing activities

CHAPTER 31

Activity & Exercise

Learning Outcomes

After completing this chapter, you should be able to:

➤ Discuss the physiology of movement.

➤ Use proper body mechanics when providing patient care.

➤ Describe the five types of exercise discussed in this chapter.

➤ Compare the effects of exercise and immobility on the body.

➤ Describe the physical activity recommended for health promotion, cardiovascular fitness, and maintenance of healthy weight.

➤ Discuss factors that affect body alignment and activity.

➤ Identify patients who are at risk for immobility concerns or activity intolerance.

➤ Develop a plan of care for patients with decreased activity tolerance.

➤ Implement care related to a patient's mobility problems.

Meet Your Patients

You are attending a health promotion series at the local hospital in order to fulfill the requirement in your state for continuing nursing education. For the next 4 weeks, the topic is exercise. In the group, you meet the following people:

▪ Phillip Flanders is a 40-year-old accountant. He works long hours in an office setting doing work that is sedentary and requires concentration. Although he is not physically active, he often feels tired. He does not exercise regularly. Many of his friends have suggested that he begin some kind of exercise program to improve his energy and health. Phillip would like to learn how to get started with an over-all fitness program that works with his work and family life. Before getting started, he makes an appointment with his primary care provider for a thorough health evaluation.

▪ Peter Phan is 28 years old and is a marathon runner and triathlete. On average, he runs 35 miles per week and cycles at least twice per week. Peter has had plantar fas-ciitis in the past that was painful and caused him to miss exercise. Peter would like to learn what he can do to prevent other injuries.

▪ Helen Jillian is 72 years old. She has hypertension and high choles-terol levels for which she takes four medications. She is 5 ft 1 in. tall and weighs 290 lb. Recently, she began having chest pain when starting a brisk walk. Her physician prescribed nitroglycerin for the chest pain, and after a thorough cardiac evaluation told her to enroll in this class and the CardioFit program at the hospital. She does not understand why she is being asked to do these things because activity seems to trigger her chest pain.

In this chapter, you will find answers to each of these patient questions about activity and exercise. In addition, you will learn more about assisting patients with mobility problems.

Theoretical **Knowledge**
knowing why

Before the rise of civilization, humans kept active just meeting their daily needs. Men hunted for game, and women gathered roots, fruits, and other edible plants. Survival depended on physical activity, such as changing locations to find suitable food sources or escape a dangerous situation. Later, the shift to an agricultural society reduced the need for most people to hunt and gather food. Farming was hard work that kept people active all day long. Today, with modern grocery distribution systems, people expend little to no energy to obtain food.

In addition, there are many other occupations where people spend many hours at a desk or a computer screen. Even popular leisure activities, such as watching television, sending e-mail, or playing video games, are sedentary.

To get enough exercise, most people need to make a conscious effort to build exercise and activity into their lives. Although fitness equipment and health clubs are popular among some groups of people, the overall level of fitness in the United States is declining. Nearly half of people ages 12 to 21 do not engage in regular, vigorous activity. And, more than 60% of adults do not achieve the recommended amount of physical exercise coupled with increasing the activity in everyday living.

Unfortunately, these standard guidelines tend to overlook the 30% of the population now considered obese. The American College of Sports Medicine (ACSM) recommends 150 to 250 minutes of exercise per week to prevent weight gain and chronic illness. More than 250 minutes per week are needed to bring about significant weight loss—that is, 50 minutes on 5 days of the week or 40 minutes on 6 days of the week (ACSM, 2009). Moderate activity (e.g., brisk walking) or 35 minutes per day of vigorous activity (e.g., running or cycling) over the long term is needed to maintain weight loss (Binks & Housle, 2009). Of course exercise alone does not guarantee weight maintenance or loss. You must also eat a sensible, nutritious diet.

Physiology of Movement

Activity and exercise require body movement **(mobility).** Mobility depends on the successful interaction among the skeleton, the muscles, and the nervous system.

Skeletal System

The skeletal system includes bones, cartilage, ligaments, and tendons. The skeleton forms the framework of the body, protects the internal organs, produces blood cells, and stores mineral salts (e.g., calcium) and fat.

Bones consist of a hard outer shell with a spongy interior (Fig. 31-1). There are 206 bones in the human

FIGURE 31-1 Bone is complex living tissue.

- Proximal epiphysis
- Diaphysis
- Distal epiphysis
- Marrow
- Yellow bone marrow
- Marrow (medullary) cavity
- Periosteum
- Compact bone
- Spongy bone
- Haversian system
- Haversian canal
- Concentric rings of osteocytes
- Venule
- Arteriole
- Canaliculi
- Osteocyte
- Fibrous layer
- Osteogenic layer (osteoblasts)
- Periosteum

body. Some bones are long (such as the femur and humerus), some short (phalanges and metacarpals), some flat (sternum and cranial bones), and some are irregularly shaped (vertebrae and tarsal bones). The short, flat, and irregular bones contain red bone marrow that produces red blood cells.

Bones feel strong and tough, so it is easy to forget that they are composed of living tissue that is constantly building and remodeling. **Osteoclasts** are specialized cells that function as housekeepers in the bone by breaking down old or damaged tissue. **Osteoblasts** repair damaged bone and build new bone to keep the skeleton strong. A delicate balance exists between the actions of the osteoblasts and the osteoclasts.

When two bones come close together **(articulate),** a joint is formed. Body movement occurs at the joints. Joints are classified based on the amount of movement they permit:

- **Synarthroses** are immovable joints (e.g., the sutures between the cranial bones). In youth, these joints have some flexibility to allow growth, but they gradually become rigid.
- **Amphiarthroses** allow for limited movement. Examples are the joints between the vertebrae and pubic bones.
- **Diarthroses,** or **synovial joints,** are freely movable because of the amount of space between the articulating bones. Synovial joints are filled with **synovial fluid,** and the joint surfaces of the articulating bones are covered with smooth **articular cartilage** (connective tissue found in the joints and skeleton). The synovial fluid and articular cartilage prevent friction as the bones move. Table 31-1 identifies the types of movable joints in the body.

Cartilage, ligaments, and tendons serve as the interface between the skeleton and the muscles. Ligaments are fibrous tissues that connect most movable joints. Ligaments are flexible to allow freedom of movement, but strong and tough so they do not yield under force of movement. Tendons are fibrous connective tissues that attach muscles to the bone. Muscles span a joint and attach by tendons to two different bones.

Muscles

Muscles comprise 40% to 50% of body weight. When they contract, they cause movement. The type of movement depends on the type of muscle: skeletal, smooth, or cardiac.

- **Skeletal muscle** moves the skeleton.
- **Smooth muscle,** occurring in the digestive tract and other hollow structures, such as the bladder and blood vessels, produces movement of food through the digestive tract, urine through the urinary tract, and blood through the circulatory system.
- **Cardiac muscle** is a unique form of muscle that has the ability to contract spontaneously. It is responsible for the beating of the heart.

Muscles attach to bone at two points: (1) at the *point of origin,* to the more stationary bone, and (2) at the *point of insertion,* to the more movable bone. The "belly" (thickest part) of the muscle lies between these two points. When a skeletal muscle contracts, it shortens, thus causing one bone to move at the joint. Muscles work in pairs. For example, the biceps brachii contracts to flex the forearm (bend the elbow joint). When the biceps contracts, the opposing muscle, the triceps brachii, relaxes. Similarly, contraction of the triceps is associated with relaxation of the biceps (Fig. 31-2).

Nervous System

The nervous system controls the movement of the musculoskeletal system. Motor nerves are either autonomic or somatic. The **autonomic nervous system** consists of

Table 31-1 ➤ Types of Synovial Joints		
TYPE	**DESCRIPTION**	**EXAMPLES**
Ball-and-socket	A rounded head (ball) fits into a cuplike structure (socket) to allow movement in all planes in addition to rotation.	Shoulder and hip joints
Condyloid	An oval-shaped bone fits into an elliptical cavity to allow movement in two planes at right angles to each other.	Wrist
Gliding	Two flat plane surfaces move past each other.	Intervertebral joints
Hinge	A convex surface fits into a cavity, allowing flexion and extension.	Knee and elbow
Pivot	The joint is formed by a ringlike object that turns on a pivot. Motion is limited to rotation.	The atlas and axis of the first vertebrae and base of the skull
Saddle	One bone surface is concave in one direction and convex in the other. The other surface has the opposite construction so that the bones fit together. Movement is possible in two planes at right angles to each other.	Carpal–metacarpal joint of the thumb

FIGURE 31-2 Antagonistic muscles. *A,* Extension of the forearm. *B,* Flexion of the forearm.

A   *Extension*   **B**   *Flexion*

the sympathetic and parasympathetic nervous systems, which innervate involuntary muscles, such as the heart, blood vessels, and glands. The **somatic nervous system** innervates the voluntary skeletal muscles.

When you make a conscious decision to bend your elbow, the thought originates in the motor area of your cerebral cortex. The upper motor efferent nerves communicate with the lower motor neurons that conduct impulses to the muscles. When the muscle receives sufficient stimuli, it contracts the biceps as the triceps relaxes and moves the elbow. Movement also occurs through reflex mechanisms. Common reflexes include the knee-jerk reflex and corneal reflex. Reflexes are discussed at length in Chapter 19.

A muscle contraction, whether conscious or reflexive, stimulates afferent nerves that convey information to the cerebral cortex and the cerebellum. This information helps control and coordinate movements.

KnowledgeCheck 31-1

- Name three purposes of the skeletal system.
- Define the following movements: abduction, adduction, flexion, extension, circumduction, internal rotation, supination, and pronation.
- Identify three types of muscle.
- How do the muscles and the nerves interact?

Go to Chapter 31, **Knowledge Check Response Sheet and Answers,** on the Student Resource Disk or DavisPlus at http://davisplus.fadavis.com/Wilkinson2

Body Mechanics

Body mechanics is a term used to describe the way we move our bodies and includes four components: body alignment, balance, coordination, and joint mobility. You should always use good body mechanics and teach them to patients as part of your health promotion and disease prevention efforts. In addition to discussing those components, we will also present some guidelines to use when teaching your patients about safe movement and lifting.

The following are terms used to describe problems with muscle mass, strength, or mobility:

Body Alignment

Body alignment, or posture, is an important aspect of body mechanics. Proper posture places the spine in a neutral (resting) position. There are four natural curves to the spine (Fig. 31-3). Proper posture maintains these natural curves because it allows movement to occur with less stress and fatigue; the bones are aligned, and the muscles, joints, and ligaments can work at peak efficiency. Good posture contributes to the normal functioning of the nervous system and improves feelings of well-being (Self-Care: Tips to Maintain Proper Posture). Most posture problems result from a combination of the following:

Accidents, injuries, and falls
Careless sitting, standing, or sleeping habits
Excessive weight
Foot problems or improper shoes
Negative self-image
Occupational stress

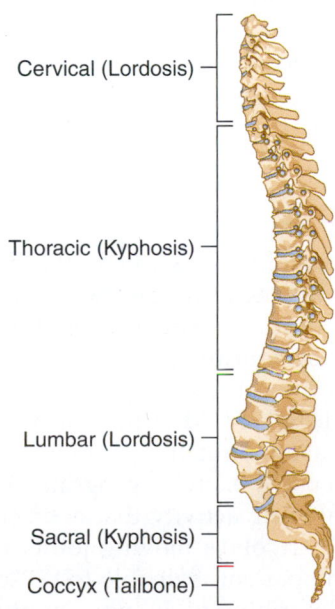

Lateral (side) spinal column

Cervical (Lordosis)

Thoracic (Kyphosis)

Lumbar (Lordosis)

Sacral (Kyphosis)

Coccyx (Tailbone)

FIGURE 31-3 There are four natural curves to the spine.

Poor sleep support (mattress)
Poorly designed work space
Visual difficulties
Weak muscles or muscle imbalance

Balance

The body achieves balance when it is in alignment. For your body to be balanced, your line of gravity must pass through your center of gravity, and your center of gravity must be close to your base of support. The **line of gravity** is an imaginary vertical line drawn from the top of the head through the center of gravity. The **center of gravity** is the point around which mass is distributed. In the human body, the center of gravity is below the umbilicus at the top of the pelvis. The **base of support** is what holds the body up. The feet provide the base of support.

To avoid injury when moving objects, place your center of gravity closest to your base of support and stand with your head erect, buttocks pulled in, abdominal muscles tight, chest high, shoulders pulled back, and feet wide (Fig. 31-4). Use a wide stance, with feet apart and one foot forward when standing for a long period of time. The broader the base of support, the lower the center of gravity, and the easier it is to maintain balance.

Coordination

Smooth movement requires coordination between the nervous system and the musculoskeletal system. Voluntary movement is initiated in the cerebral cortex. However, the cerebellum coordinates movements. As you may recall, *proprioception*—the awareness of posture, movement, and position sense—is largely controlled by the cerebellum. The basal ganglia, located deep in the cerebrum, assists with coordination of movement. Damage to the motor cortex, cerebellum, or basal ganglia affects coordination of movement. For example, a stroke affecting the motor cortex alters gait and changes posture.

Joint Mobility

Joint movement allows us to sit, stand, bend, walk, and perform other activities. **Range of motion (ROM)** is the maximum movement possible at a joint. **Active range of motion** (AROM) is defined as the movement of the joint through the entire ROM by the individual. Full ROM is part of being physically fit; for that reason, stretching exercises are included in a comprehensive exercise program. **Passive ROM** (PROM) is a nursing activity that is discussed later in this chapter. It involves moving joints through their ROM when the patient is unable to do so for himself. Other terms describing body movement are shown in Volume 2.

Tips to Maintain Proper Posture

➤ Avoid standing in one position for a lengthy period. If you cannot change positions, elevate one foot on a stool or box, and alternate foot placement frequently.

➤ Do not lock your knees when standing upright.

➤ Keep your stomach muscles tight to support your back.

➤ Do not bend forward at the waist or neck when you are working in a low position.

➤ When you are seated at your desk, work at a comfortable height.

➤ Do not wear high-heeled or platform shoes for long periods of time.

➤ Do not slump when you sit.

➤ Sit close to your work.

➤ Use a chair that supports your back in a slightly arched position.

➤ Sit with your feet flat on the floor and your knees below your hips.

➤ Sleep on a mattress that is firm but not extremely hard.

 Go to **Tables, Range of Motion at the Joints** in Volume 2

To see animations of joints and range of motion,

 Go to **Animations: Range of Motion Animations** on DavisPlus at http://davisplus.fadavis.com/Wilkinson2

FIGURE 31-4 A, With a wide stance, the center of gravity (x) is closer to the base of support. B, With a narrow stance, the body is less stable.

Body Mechanics Guidelines

Principles of body mechanics are the rules that allow you to move your body while reducing the risk for injury. Historically, nurses have used body mechanics guidelines as the cornerstone of safe practice for moving and lifting patients. However, patient characteristics and condition (e.g., obesity), as well as the patient care environment, make it difficult to rely on body mechanics alone to prevent injury (Nelson, Fragala, & Menzel, 2003). There is no reason to "prove yourself" by transferring without the use of an assistive device (e.g., lift, transfer board, or other staff). The American Nurses Association, in 2004, launched a national campaign titled "Handle with Care" to reduce the risk of back and musculoskeletal injuries among nurses. This campaign emphasizes the use of assistive devices to decrease the risk of injury and recommends virtually no manual lifting. Even though increasingly more assistive devices are becoming available in clinical facilities, to avoid injury it is essential to continue to use good body mechanics as you move and lift patients. For guidelines to help you assess patients' transfer abilities and use good body mechanics,

 Go to Chapter 31, **Clinical Insight 31-1: Applying Principles of Body Mechanics,** in Volume 2.

KnowledgeCheck 31-2

- Identify the four components of body mechanics.
- Give at least five guidelines for good body mechanics.

 Go to Chapter 31, **Knowledge Check Response Sheet and Answers,** on the Student Resource Disk or DavisPlus at http://davisplus.fadavis.com/Wilkinson2

 CriticalThinking 31-1

While you are attending the health promotion class, Helen Jillian ("Meet Your Patients") develops chest pain and must be assisted to a wheelchair for transport to the emergency department.

- Based on what you know about body mechanics, how would you be able to assist Ms. Jillian?
- What additional information do you need to know?

Exercise

Physical activity refers to bodily movement and energy expenditure involving contraction of the skeletal muscles above basal level. Bodily movement can be grouped into two basic categories:

- **Baseline activity** refers to the light-intensity activities of daily living, such as standing, walking slowly, and lifting lightweight objects.
- **Health-enhancing physical activity** is more than baseline to produce health-enhancing benefits (U.S. Department of Health and Human Services, 2008).

Types of Exercise

Exercise may be classified according to the type of muscle contraction it involves and according to whether it uses oxygen for energy.

Isometric exercises involve muscle contraction without motion. They are usually performed against an immovable surface or object, for example, pressing the hand against a wall. The muscles of the arm contract, but the wall does not move. Each position is held for 6 to 8 seconds and repeated 5 to 10 times. Isometric training is effective for developing total strength of a particular muscle or group of muscles. It is often used for rehabilitation because the exact area of muscle weakness can be isolated and strengthening can be administered at the proper joint angle. This kind of training requires no special equipment, and there is little chance of injury. Patients who are bed-bound can use this form of exercise to maintain or regain muscle strength.

Isotonic exercise involves movement of the joint during the muscle contraction. A classic example of an isotonic exercise is weight training with free weights. As the weight is moved throughout the ROM, the muscle shortens and lengthens. Calisthenics, such as chin-ups, push-ups, and sit-ups, all of which use body weight as the resistance force, are also isotonic exercises.

Isokinetic exercise is performed with specialized apparatuses that provide variable resistance to movement. Isokinetic exercise combines the best features of both isometrics and weight training by providing resistance at a constant, preset speed while the muscle moves through the full ROM. Specialized machines available at health clubs and physical therapy departments are used for this form of exercise.

Aerobic exercise acquires energy from metabolic pathways that use oxygen—the amount of oxygen taken into the body meets or exceeds the amount of oxygen required to perform the activity. Aerobic exercise uses large muscle groups, can be maintained continuously, and is rhythmic in nature. It increases the heart and respiratory rates, thereby providing exercise for the cardiovascular system while simultaneously exercising the skeletal muscles. Jogging, brisk walking, and cycling are common forms of aerobic exercise.

Anaerobic exercise occurs when the amount of oxygen taken into the body does not meet the amount of oxygen required to perform the activity. Therefore, the muscles must obtain energy from metabolic pathways that do not use oxygen. Rapid, intense exercise, such as lifting heavy objects or sprinting, are examples of anaerobic exercise.

Exercise Program Guidelines

A well-rounded exercise program focuses on flexibility, resistance training, and aerobic conditioning. Factors when designing or evaluating an exercise program include the following:

Flexibility Training. Stretching before exercise helps warm up the muscles and prevents injury during exercise. Stretching after exercise cools the muscles and limits post-exercise stiffness. As we get older, joints and muscles become stiffer. A regular flexibility program helps maintain mobility as aging occurs.

Resistance Training. Movement against resistance increases muscular strength and endurance. Perhaps the most common type of resistance training is weight lifting. When a person is exercising for strength, the goal is to increase the amount of resistance with each exercise (i.e., lift more weight). When a person is exercising for endurance, the goal is to increase the number of repetitions with each exercise (i.e., lift the weight more times).

Aerobic Conditioning. Fitness and body composition are improved by aerobic conditioning. Components of aerobic conditioning include intensity, duration, frequency, and mode. Intensity is how hard one is exercising. Box 31-1 describes three common tests used to evaluate exercise intensity.

Amount of Exercise. Duration is the amount of time one is exercising. To achieve and maintain healthy level of fitness, the U.S. Department of Health and Human Services (USDHHS) recommends 2.5 hours/week (150 minutes/week) or more of moderate-intensity physical activity coupled with increasing the activity every day (USDHHS, 2008). The **frequency** of exercise should be 3 to 5 days per week, although the more often and the longer duration the better. The **mode** of exercise is the type of activity. Aerobic (endurance) and muscle-strengthening (resistance) physical activities both promote better health. See Box 31-2.

Many people become discouraged because they don't see immediate results from their efforts. However, subtle changes occur long before the person sees changes in weight or shape. Some tips to help develop an exercise program are included in Self-Care: Teaching Clients How to Set Up an Exercise Program.

Benefits of Regular Exercise

Regular physical activity each week, sustained for months and years, can produce long-term health benefits. Strong evidence links regular physical activity with a lower risk for early death, heart disease, stroke, type 2 diabetes, hypertension, hyperlipidemia, metabolic syndrome, colon and breast cancers, and depression. Regular physical activity also promotes weight loss and maintenance of normal weight when combined with diet, better heart and lung function, muscular fitness, fall prevention, and improved memory and mental clarity in older adults. Weight-bearing exercise reduces loss of bone density in adults and older adults (Jitramontree, 2007; USDHHS, 2008). Resistance training does not lead to weight loss; instead, it may increase loss of fat mass and improve muscle tone and strength (ACSM, 2009).

Exercise is associated with an overall decrease in mortality in men and women of all ages and an overall improvement in quality of life for people in all ethnic groups and across the lifespan. People with disabilities also benefit from physical activity (USDHHS, 2008). Box 31-3 presents numerous other benefits of regular exercise.

BOX 31-1 ■ Tests for Determining Exercise Intensity

Target Heart Rate Method

In the target heart rate method, the target heart rate (THR) is calculated from an estimate of maximum heart rate. The estimated maximum heart rate is calculated using the following formula:

$$\text{Maximum heart rate} = 220 - \text{age}$$

The THR is calculated as a percentage of the maximum heart rate. Most persons can exercise at 60% to 80% of the maximum heart rate.

For example, consider a 50-year-old woman. Her maximum heart rate is 170 beats/min. To exercise at 75% intensity, her target heart rate is 128 beats/min.

$$\text{Maximum heart rate} = 220 - 50 = 170$$
$$\text{THR} = 0.75 \times 170 = 128$$

The person's heart rate during exercise should be 128 beats per minute, excluding warm-up and cool-down.

Talk Test

The talk test evaluates exercise intensity based on the person's ability to talk while exercising. Short phrases interspersed with breaths or feeling like you can "just respond" is considered an appropriate level of exercise. If you are too short of breath to answer, the level of intensity is too high. An ability to carry on a conversation indicates that you are not exercising hard enough.

Borg Rate of Perceived Exertion Scale®

The Rate of Perceived Exertion (RPE) scale is very easy to use. The person who is exercising selects the rating based on how difficult the exercise feels at that time. The exerciser selects one of eight categories that best describes the intensity of activity. RPE ratings range from *No Exertion at All* to *Extremely Hard*. *Extremely Hard* is associated with exercise that corresponds to almost 100% of maximum heart rate. *Somewhat Hard* corresponds with 75% of maximum heart rate; this is the level you should encourage for most individuals.

Sources: Borg, G. (1998). *Borg's perceived exertion and pain scales.* Stockholm, Sweden: Human Kinetics; Foster, C. (2004). "Talk test" measures exercise intensity. *Medicine & Science in Sports & Exercise,* 36(9), 1632–1636.

BOX 31-2 ■ U.S. Department of Health and Human Services 2008 Physical Activity Guidelines for Americans

Children and Adolescents

- Engage in at least 1 hour of physical activity daily.
- Physical activity should be enjoyable. A variety of activities will improve adherence.
- Most activity should be aerobic, either moderate- or vigorous-intensity.
- At least 3 days/week, children and teens should participate in vigorous-intensity exercise as well as muscle- and bone-strengthening physical activity.

Adults and Older Adults

- To gain substantial health benefits, get at least 150 minutes per week of moderate-intensity or 75 minutes a week of vigorous-intensity aerobic physical activity, or an equivalent combination of moderate- and vigorous-intensity aerobic activity. More frequent exercise (i.e., 300 minutes/week) is even more beneficial.
- Engage in aerobic activity throughout the week in episodes of at least 10 minutes. Longer periods of time provide additional benefits.
- For additional health benefits, perform moderate or high-intensity muscle and bone-strengthening activities on 2 or more days per week.

Specific to Older Adults

- Older adults unable to perform 150 minutes of moderate-intensity aerobic activity per week should be as physically active as abilities and conditions allow.
- Include exercises that maintain or improve balance and core strength.

Adults, Children, and Adolescents with Disabilities

- Be as physically active as abilities allow with guidance from their healthcare provider.

Healthy Pregnant and Postpartum Women

- Consult with the healthcare provider regarding activity level throughout pregnancy. If the pregnancy or postpartum recovery is uncomplicated, then those who regularly engage in vigorous-intensity aerobic activity or in high amounts of activity can continue with this regimen.
- If not already engaged in vigorous-intensity physical activity, get at least 150 minutes of moderate-intensity aerobic activity per week, preferably spread throughout the week after consulting with healthcare provider.

Adapted from U.S. Department of Health and Human Services. (2008). 2008 physical activity guidelines for Americans. Retrieved from www.health.gov/paguidelines

Toward Evidence-Based Practice

Frimel, T. N., Sinacore, D. R., & Villareal, D. T. (2008, July). **Exercise attenuates the weight-loss induced reduction in muscle mass in frail obese older adults.** *Medicine & Science in Sport & Exercise, 40*(7), 12-19.

The goal of this study was to assess the effect of adding exercise to a low-calorie diet on changes in lean mass and strength in frail, obese older adults who were voluntarily losing weight. Researchers found when exercise is added to weight-reducing diet, less muscle mass is lost as compared to diet alone. In adults ages 65 years and older, regular exercise that incorporates resistance training, combined with a diet for weight loss for 6 months, reduces the amount of lean muscle mass lost and increased strength.

Simoes, E. J., Kobau, R., & Waterman, B., et al. (2006, December). **Associations of physical activity and body mass index with activities of daily living in older adults.** *Journal of Community Health, 31*(6), 453-467.

This study was done to find out more about physical activity and the effect on body mass index (BMI) and activities of daily living (ADLs) and instrumental ADLs. Physically active individuals were less likely than inactive people to be dependent with ADLs/IADLs. Researchers supported a strategy to improve the quality of life for older adults by improving physical activity.

Maddalozzo, G. F., & Snow, C. M. (2000). **High intensity resistance training: Effects on bone in older men and women.** *Calcified Tissue International, 66*, 399–404.

This classic study revealed that a high-intensity resistance exercise improves bone mineral density, lean mass, and muscle strength. It is important to emphasize careful progression in order to prevent overtraining and possible injuries. Older adults should include resistance training within their lifestyles.

1. Based on these three studies, what benefits can you think of for older adults that support starting a community-based physical fitness program?

2. You are in charge of an outpatient healthy lifestyle program for adults 65 years and older. The program is geared for obese, sedentary older adults who want to lose weight and improve physical fitness. Based on the Maddalozzo and Snow study, how would you design the program?

 Go to Chapter 31, **Toward Evidence-Based Practice Suggested Responses,** on the Student Resource Disk or DavisPlus at http://davisplus.fadavis.com/Wilkinson2

Teaching Clients How to Set Up an Exercise Program

If you are older than 40, smoke or drink, are sedentary, are overweight, or have a chronic health condition, have a medical evaluation before starting an exercise program.

Getting Started

➤ Choose a variety of exercises that you enjoy and feel comfortable doing, such as walking, biking, dancing, or a team sport.

➤ Find allies. Exercising with someone else can make it more fun. If you choose to exercise by yourself, pick a friend with whom you can discuss your exercise progress.

➤ Vary your routine. You may be less likely to get bored or injured.

➤ Choose a comfortable time of day.

➤ Don't get discouraged. It can take weeks or months before you notice some of the changes from exercise.

➤ Forget "no pain, no gain." Although a little soreness is normal after you first start exercising, pain isn't. Stop if you hurt.

➤ Make exercise fun. Find fun things to do, such as taking a walk through the park or watching your favorite show while riding a stationary bike.

➤ Sign a contract committing yourself to exercise.

➤ Find an accountability partner. A fitness program is not only more enjoyable when shared with someone else but also is more successful with others for whom you are accountable.

➤ Keep a daily log of your activities.

➤ Think about joining a health club. The cost gives some people an incentive to exercise regularly.

Exercise Tips

➤ Warm up your muscles for 5 to 10 minutes before your main session of aerobic exercise.

➤ Maintain your exercise intensity for 30 to 45 minutes.

➤ Gradually decrease the intensity of your workout (cool down) and then stretch for 5 to 10 minutes at the end of your workout.

➤ Accumulate physical activity throughout the day. For example:

  ➤ Take the stairs instead of the elevator.

  ➤ Go for a walk during your coffee break or lunch.

  ➤ Walk all or part of the way to work.

  ➤ Park your car at the far end of the parking lot.

➤ Wear good, shock-absorbing footwear. Shoes that do not support your feet will cause stress on leg bones and the back and, over time, lead to injury.

➤ Alternate easy and hard exercise days, or alternate modes of exercise (e.g., alternate running, swimming, and biking).

➤ Take a day off periodically. The body needs a chance to rest and allow bones, joints, and muscles to rest and repair.

➤ To avoid becoming dehydrated, drink at least 8 ounces of fluid before the exercise, and then pause regularly during the exercise for more. If you are thirsty after the exercise session, drink until you feel satiated. Water is still the best liquid to drink during and after exercise. However, you can't rely on feeling thirsty as a reminder to replace fluid lost through sweating; one of nature's dirty tricks is that exercise suppresses thirst.

Risks Associated with Exercise

Armed with theoretical knowledge, you should be able to teach your clients realistically about the risks associated with exercise and thereby help them to exercise safely. Risks include cardiac injury, musculoskeletal injury, dehydration, hypoglycemia, and temperature regulation problems. Keep in mind that the benefits of exercise far outweigh the risks.

Cardiac Injury. Fear of triggering a cardiac event prevents some people from exercising. However, exercise itself is rarely life-threatening, especially when compared with the alternative (*not* exercising). Before starting an exercise program or significantly increasing the intensity of normal work-outs, seasoned athletes as well as rank beginners should be screened for underlying health problems, such as high blood pressure, thickened heart muscle (cardiac hypertrophy), electrical abnormalities, and blood vessel abnormalities. In people without underlying heart disease, recreational drug use is an important cause of sudden cardiac arrest, whether during exercise or at rest.

Musculoskeletal Injury. High-impact exercises, such as running or aerobic dance, may pose a risk for injuries to bones, joints, and muscles. However, you can prevent most such injuries by gradually increasing the activity level or varying activities. Walking is an exercise that most people can do without injury. Injury can also occur from lifting weights. Free weights can cause injury if the person lifts too much weight or uses poor body mechanics when lifting. Working with a fitness trainer to learn correct form and appropriate weights markedly decreases the risk of injury. In addition, exercise machines provide some degree of control and are less likely to cause injury.

Dehydration. It is possible to become dehydrated with prolonged exercise, with warm temperatures, or as a result of health problems or medications. During an

BOX 31-3 ■ Benefits of Regular Exercise

Cardiovascular System

- Improves pumping action of the heart.
- Decreases heart rate and blood pressure.
- Improves circulation by increasing the number of capillaries.
- Improves venous return to the heart.
- Increases high-density lipoprotein (HDL).
- Decreases low-density lipoprotein (LDL) and total cholesterol.
- Decreases risk of thrombophlebitis.

Respiratory System

- Improves pulmonary circulation.
- Improves gas exchange at the alveolar–capillary membrane.
- Dilates bronchioles to increase ventilation.

Musculoskeletal System

- Improves skeletal development in children.
- Increases muscle strength.
- Improves flexibility.
- Increases coordination.
- Helps maintain joint structure and function; reduces risk of osteoarthritis.
- Improves bone mineral density.
- Improves bone mass with aging; reduces risk of osteoporosis.
- Reduces risk of falls and helps older adults maintain an independent lifestyle.

Nervous System

- Speeds nerve impulse transmission.

Endocrine System

- Increases sensitivity to insulin at the receptor sites.
- Increases efficiency of metabolic processes.
- Improves temperature regulation.
- Facilitates weight management.

Gastrointestinal System

- Improves appetite.
- Improves abdominal muscle tone.
- Decreases risk of colon cancer.

Urinary System

- Increases efficiency of kidney function.

Integumentary System

- Improves skin tone as a result of improved circulation.

Immune System

- Reduces susceptibility to minor viral illnesses.

Mental Health

- Boosts energy level.
- Release endorphins, which assist with pain control and stress management.
- Improves self-esteem and body image.
- Provides a nonpharmacological way to relieve symptoms of anxiety and depression.
- Leads to positive outlook and sense of optimism.
- Promotes clearer thinking and improved memory in older adults.
- Enhances feelings of well being and diminishes depressive symptoms.
- Relieves some stress.
- Can be a source of social interaction.

Overall Health

- Burns calories to achieve and maintain healthy body weight.
- Leads to reduced abdominal obesity.
- Improves overall stamina.
- Reduces fatigue.
- Increases time spent in stage IV and REM sleep.

---

intense exercise period, the body can lose 2 liters of fluid for every hour of exercise. It is important to drink water before, during, and after the exercise period. Water is still the best choice during and after exercise. Some sports drinks have glucose and electrolytes for replacement and quick energy and can be used for endurance activities or prolonged, intense activity.

Temperature Regulation Problems. **Hyperthermia** can occur when the person exercises in a hot climate. Hyperthermia is often accompanied by dehydration. **Heat exhaustion** is a potentially life-threatening event. Signs of heat exhaustion include lightheadedness, nausea, headache, fatigue, hyperventilation, loss of concentration, and abdominal cramps. Body temperature rises,

but the skin is clammy and cold. In contrast, **hypothermia** can occur when the person does not wear proper clothing or is exposed to cool water for an extended period of time. Hypothermia is characterized by fatigue, confusion, and lack of coordination.

Advise clients to follow the tips in the Self-Care box to exercise safely and help prevent injury.

KnowledgeCheck 31-3

- Identify and describe four types of exercise.
- State the components of an exercise program

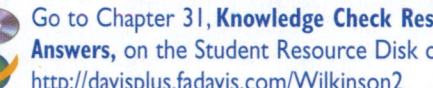 Go to Chapter 31, **Knowledge Check Response Sheet and Answers,** on the Student Resource Disk or DavisPlus at http://davisplus.fadavis.com/Wilkinson2

Teaching Your Older Adult Patient About Increasing Physical Activity and Exercise

What are the Benefits of Physical Activity for an Older Adult?

➤ Improves and maintains strength so you can stay as independent as possible.

➤ Maintains balance and prevents falls.

➤ Gives you more energy to do the things you want to do.

➤ Helps you to sleep better and feel more rested.

➤ Perks up your mood and helps reduce depression.

➤ Prevents or delays some diseases like diabetes, heart disease, and cancer.

What Kind of Physical Activity Should I Do?

➤ Get at least 30 minutes of *endurance* activity almost every day. Exercise that makes you breathe hard builds strength and staying power.

➤ Incorporate *resistance* into your exercise. That means, use some kind of weight or isometric activity to build strength. Remember you can do more and are less likely to fall when your muscles are strong.

➤ Do things to work on your *balance* (e.g., standing on one foot). This can help to prevent falls.

➤ Daily stretching will help you be more *flexible* and prevent injury.

Who Should Exercise?

Almost anyone can do some type of physical activity, but before starting a new exercise program check with your healthcare provider if you experience:

➤ Any change in your health in the past 6 months

➤ Shortness of breath or dizziness

➤ Chest pain or pressure, or fluttering heart

➤ Joint pain or swelling

➤ Unexplained weight loss

➤ An infection with fever

➤ Eye problems

➤ Blood clot

➤ Hernia

➤ Recent hip surgery or joint injury

Source: Adapted from The National Institutes of Health, National Institute on Aging. (2006, October) [Updated 2009, February]. Exercise and physical activity: Getting fit for life. Retrieved from http://www.nia.nih.gov/HealthInformation/Publications/exercise.htm

Critical Thinking 31-2

■ How would you address Helen Jillian's ("Meet Your Patients") concerns about the risks associated with her engaging in an exercise program?

■ Peter Phan ("Meet Your Patients") has experienced a number of injuries as a result of his exercise. Based on your knowledge of exercise, what questions would you like to ask Peter about his exercise program?

Factors Affecting Mobility and Activity

Factors influencing activity and exercise include developmental stage, nutrition, lifestyle, attitudes, external factors, diseases, and physical abnormalities. These factors are discussed in the next sections.

Developmental Stage

Neuromuscular development is related to age. A newborn can move his extremities and turn his head from side to side, but he is unable to get from place to place. As the child matures, motor skills and coordination develop. In spite of that, children in the United States are becoming more sedentary, and the incidence of obesity continues to rise. Twenty-four percent of young adults are obese and 28% more are overweight. Using 2005-2006 data, the Centers for Disease Control and Prevention (CDC) reported the following:

■ Obesity rates for young adults tripled compared to the 1971–1974 data.

■ Only 36% of young adults get regular physical activity in their spare time.

■ Only 26% of young adults were doing strength training at least twice per week, which is a minimum recommendation for adults of all ages (CDC, 2009).

Healthy People 2020 goals recommend older adults also need to increase physical activity (see Self-Care: Teaching Your Older Adult Patient About Increasing Physical Activity and Exercise).

The expected physiological changes associated with growing older make it harder to start or maintain an exercise program. The result is increased risk for chronic health problems. For a discussion of neuromuscular development across the life span and associated nursing considerations as it affects activity and exercise,

Go to Chapter 31, **Tables, Boxes, Figures: ESG Table 31-1, The Influence of Developmental Stage on Activity and Exercise,** on the Student Resource Disk or DavisPlus at http://davisplus.fadavis.com/Wilkinson2

Nutrition

In the United States, obesity is a major health problem. Obesity often leads to numerous health problems, which indirectly reduces activity and can in turn contribute to further obesity. For example, joint injuries and osteoarthritis are more prevalent with obesity, which in turn reduces a person's physical activity. Unhealthy eating patterns, such as large portions, consumption of convenience foods, and a diet high in saturated fat and simple carbohydrates, play a major role in the obesity problem. Although the obese person has plenty of calories available to expend on exercise, movement becomes more difficult as body size increases.

In contrast, people with chronic disease may be in negative nitrogen balance—that is, they do not have adequate protein stores available to maintain or repair body tissue. They experience muscle wasting and fatigue, which lead to decreased activity levels.

Lifestyle

Over the last century, manual labor has declined and work environments have become increasingly sedentary. As a result, individuals need to look toward leisure time for exercise and fitness activities. This requires "making time" for exercise. Personal values about exercise and fitness determine when, or whether, exercise becomes part of a person's routine.

Some people enjoy exercise. Others see it as pure drudgery or as "something I have to do." A person's culture and support system define what exercise the person is likely to accept. For example, swimming requires wearing a bathing suit. People raised in a culture that values modesty may not choose swimming as a form of exercise. Walking, which allows the person to dress in modest clothing, would be a preferred form of exercise.

Stress

How is your stress level? You may want to turn back to Chapter 25 in Volume 2 and evaluate your stress using the questionnaire provided there. A high stress level can produce fatigue. Although you may view exercise as one more thing you don't have time for, exercise is energizing and can be used to relieve stress. For example, taking a brisk 20-minute walk during a study break may allow you to continue working for several more hours. You can also use this technique when caring for patients. Hospitalized patients and family members often experience a great deal of stress. Helping the patient take a walk to the courtyard, or instructing family members how to handle the wheelchair so they can take a walk around the block, often will help lessen some of the strain.

Environmental Factors

Environmental factors affecting exercise include weather, pollution, neighborhood conditions, finances, and support systems. Weather has a strong influence on activity level. Cold, damp weather encourages people to stay inside, whereas warm, sunny weather makes it fun to go outside and exercise. Encourage patients to choose a variety of activities that they enjoy so they can exercise regardless of the weather. When air quality is poor, encourage indoor activities to reduce exposure to allergens and pollutants.

Neighborhood conditions, such as crime or lack of parks, influence attitudes about outside activities. Mall walking is an example of a successful way to incorporate exercise into daily patterns when neighborhood conditions do not encourage activity. Lack of money may make it difficult to join a gym and engage in some sports (e.g., skiing, golfing). However, many activities, such as walking or playing basketball or tennis in the community park, are inexpensive.

The support system is perhaps the most influential external factor. Family and friends who encourage activity are likely to help you find ways to exercise. Those who are themselves sedentary may not encourage you to be more active or lose weight.

Diseases and Abnormalities

Diseases and abnormalities in various body systems can negatively influence body alignment, balance, coordination, and joint mobility. In the next sections, we describe some disorders that affect activity and exercise.

Abnormalities of the Musculoskeletal System

The following are common congenital abnormalities that affect appearance, motor function, and mobility:

- **Syndactylism** is the fusion of two or more fingers or toes. Most cases involving the hands are treated surgically at an early age to limit the effect on fine-motor development.
- **Developmental dysplasia of the hip (DDH)** is a congenital abnormality of the development of the femur, acetabulum, or both that shows as hip dislocation.
- **Foot deformities,** such as club foot (talipes equinovarus), occur in about 4% of all newborns. Serial casts or surgery may be used to correct the defect and preserve function.
- **Scoliosis** is a lateral curvature of the spine. Scoliosis can result from congenital bone disorders, neuromuscular impairment, or trauma, but approximately two-thirds of cases have no known cause and are termed idiopathic scoliosis. Idiopathic scoliosis is classified as infantile, juvenile, or adolescent depending on the age at onset.

Nursing responsibilities for all of these disorders include early detection and referral for additional treatment, parent counseling, and careful attention to positioning and transfers.

Diseases Related to Bone Formation or Metabolism

Bone formation abnormalities may be congenital, related to dietary deficiencies, or the result of bone disease.

- **Osteogenesis imperfecta (OI)** is a congenital disorder of bone and connective tissue that is characterized by brittle bones that fracture easily. Infants with OI are often born with fractures and continue to fracture with minimal trauma or even spontaneously. Prompt recognition and treatment of fractures helps prevent deformities.

- **Achondroplasia,** or dwarfism, occurs when the bones ossify (harden) prematurely.
- **Paget's disease** is a metabolic bone disease in which increased bone loss results in pain, pathological fractures, and deformities. This disorder usually affects the skull, vertebrae, femur, and pelvis.
- **Vitamin D and calcium** are needed to form and maintain bone. Deficiencies lead to porous bones. In children, prolonged deficiencies can cause the long bones of the legs to become bowed, retard growth, and lead to frequent fractures.

Nursing responsibilities for patients with bone formation abnormalities include collaborative treatments, providing comfort, lifting and transferring patients safely, and patient education to promote mobility. Education should include teaching patients to consume a balanced diet that meets the minimum recommendations for vitamins and minerals.

Diseases Affecting Joint Mobility

Diseases of the joints may be degenerative or inflammatory. The most prevalent type of degenerative joint disease is **osteoarthritis (OA)**. OA involves a loss of articular cartilage in the joint, with pain and stiffness as the primary symptoms. Patients may also have decreased ROM and **crepitus,** a creaking or grating sound, with joint motion. Symptoms are aggravated by weight bearing and joint use and are relieved by resting the affected joints. OA is more common in women, older adults, and people who are overweight.

Rheumatoid arthritis (RA) is a systemic autoimmune disease involving chronic inflammation of the joints and surrounding connective tissue. RA causes joint pain, deformity, and loss of function; patients may also experience fever, fatigue, weakness, and weight loss. RA occurs most frequently in the fingers, wrists, elbows, ankles, and knees. RA occurs in 1% to 2% of the population, with a greater incidence in women. The illness usually begins in mid-life, but persons in any age group can be affected. Swann (2007) identified the most frequently affected age group as those in the 30- to 50-year-old range. Unlike OA, RA does not improve with rest. Pain is most intense when the person arises from bed. Pain and joint deformities may so severely affect mobility that patients cannot care for themselves.

Ankylosing spondylitis is a chronic inflammatory joint disease characterized by stiffening and fusion of the spine and sacroiliac joints. The inflammation occurs where the ligaments, tendons, and joint capsule insert into the bone. The disease usually develops in young adults, equally in men and women. Signs and symptoms include low back pain and stiffness and decreased ROM of the spine. The convex lumbar curve is lost, and the upper spine curve increases, causing kyphosis (see Chapter 19 for review).

Gout is an inflammatory response to high levels of uric acid. Crystals form in the synovial fluid, and small white nodules, or *tophi*, form in the subcutaneous tissues. Gout produces painful joints and severely limits activity during acute flare-ups.

Nursing activity for patients with joint mobility problems focuses on assisting with movement, providing comfort, and teaching about medications. If mobility is severely restricted, you will also assist patients with activities of daily living (ADLs).

Problems Affecting Bone Integrity

Osteoporosis is a decrease in total bone density, which occurs when osteoclast activity outpaces that of the osteoblasts. The internal structure of the bone diminishes, and the bone collapses in on itself. Normally bone mass continues to increase up to the third decade of life. After age 30, bone loss begins. Women experience a rapid decline in bone mass at menopause. In men, a gradual loss continues. As bones become porous, they become weak, leading to vertebral collapse or fractures of the long bones of the arms and legs. Fractures may occur spontaneously or with very slight trauma.

The best treatment for osteoporosis is prevention. Teach adolescents to eat a diet high in calcium, fluoride, and other minerals, and to start an exercise program they can continue throughout their lives. Advise older women that weight-bearing exercise can help decrease the rate of bone loss, and advise them to ask their provider about medications to reduce bone mineral loss.

The National Osteoporosis Foundation (2010) recommends calcium intake for adults age 50 and older to be 1200 mg/day and vitamin D 800 to 1000 IV/day to prevent bone loss, urge people of all ages, but particularly postmenopausal women, to avoid smoking because tobacco reduces the absorption of calcium in the intestine. In addition, more than two drinks of alcohol per day decreases the matrix of the bone and reduces the body's ability to absorb calcium (National Guideline Clearinghouse, 2010).

Osteomyelitis (infection of the bone) may develop after bone injury or surgery. It can be difficult and expensive to treat and can leave the patient with permanent disability. Bone contains microscopic channels that are impermeable to most of the natural defenses of the body. Once bacteria enter these channels, they multiply rapidly.

Bone tumors may also affect form and function. Tumors in the bone cause considerable pain and severely limit activity. Nursing responsibilities for patients with osteomyelitis or bone tumors include collaborative treatments, patient education about the treatment plan, and providing comfort.

Trauma

Trauma can affect the entire musculoskeletal system. One of the most significant forms of trauma is a **fracture,** or a break in the bone. Signs and symptoms of a fracture include tenderness at the site, loss of function, deformity of the area, and swelling of the surrounding tissues. However, x-ray is required for definitive diagnosis. Fractures are classified according to the extent of damage. The type and severity of fracture determine whether casting, traction, or surgical repair is necessary. For a classification and description of several types of fractures,

Go to Chapter 31, **Supplemental Materials: Fractures,** and to **Tables, Boxes, Figures: ESG Figure 31-2, Types of Fractures,** on the Student Resource Disk or DavisPlus at http://davisplus.fadavis.com/Wilkinson2

For information about nursing care for patients with a fracture,

Go to Chapter 31, **Clinical Insight 31-7: Caring for Patients with Casts and Traction,** in Volume 2.

Sprains and strains are more common than fractures. A **sprain** is a stretch injury of a ligament that causes the ligament to tear. A partial tear can usually heal with rest, but a complete tear often requires surgery to stabilize the joint. A **strain** is an injury to muscle caused by excessive stress on the muscle. Both strains and sprains cause pain at the site of injury, swelling, and loss of function. As you can see, the signs and symptoms are the same as those of a fracture. As a result, x-ray studies are used to distinguish these injuries. Initial treatment of fractures, sprains, and strains include rest, ice, compression, and elevation.

Stretching and tearing injuries to the meniscus (knee cap), lateral knee ligaments, and Achilles' tendon are also fairly common. Magnetic resonance imaging (MRI) studies are done to determine the extent of injury. Rest and ice are necessary, but often surgical repair is needed to achieve full healing.

Disorders of the Central Nervous System

Any disorder that affects the motor centers of the brain or the transmission of nerve impulses will affect mobility. Cerebrovascular accident (stroke), head or spinal cord injury, multiple sclerosis (a disorder affecting nerve transmission), and myasthenia gravis (a disease caused by antibodies to the acetylcholine receptors at the neuromuscular junction) are examples. Progressive degenerative disorders of the neurological system also affect mobility and coordination. For example, Parkinson's disease is a progressive degeneration of the basal ganglia. It produces tremor, rigidity, and difficulty coordinating movement.

Diseases of Other Body Systems

Diseases affecting other body systems may affect mobility and activity tolerance, as in the following examples:

- *Respiratory disorders.* Any disorder that affects oxygenation limits exercise tolerance. Chronic obstructive pulmonary disease, asthma, and pneumonia are associated with shortness of breath, which becomes worse with increased activity. Consequently, patients limit their activity.
- *Circulatory disorders* affect mobility. Impaired arterial circulation limits oxygen delivery to the tissue. As activity increases, skeletal muscle pain develops. Impaired venous circulation causes leg swelling and discomfort, which are relieved by elevating the legs. As a result, patients may become relatively sedentary to relieve the pain and discomfort.
- *Fatigue* also affects activity level. Acute illnesses, such as influenza, produce fatigue during the acute illness and limit activity for short periods of time. Disorders that produce long-standing fatigue include anemia, anorexia nervosa, cancer, depression, and grief.
- *Bed rest* is part of the treatment for a variety of disorders. For example, a woman with a high-risk pregnancy may be placed on bed rest. For patients on bed rest, the goal is to prevent additional problems caused by immobility, such as pressure injury, constipation, joint contracture, muscle weakness, balance problems, deep vein thrombosis, pooling of secretions, orthostatic hypotension, and various other hazards.

KnowledgeCheck 31-4

- In which age groups are you more likely to see health concerns that affect mobility?
- What types of disorders limit activity or mobility?
- What are the signs and symptoms of a fracture?
- What is the difference between a strain and a sprain?

Go to Chapter 31, **Knowledge Check Response Sheet and Answers,** on the Student Resource Disk or DavisPlus at http://davisplus.fadavis.com/Wilkinson2

CriticalThinking 31-3

- Your teenage daughter complains when you ask her to take a calcium supplement and encourage her to exercise. What information should you provide so she understands why these measures are important?
- Phillip Flanders ("Meet Your Patients") has never been involved in a regular exercise program. Phil works as an accountant, and most of his friends are work associates. Phil's siblings are overweight and do not exercise. Both of his parents died of heart disease. Many of Phil's friends have suggested that he begin exercising to improve his energy and health. What recommendations can you make to Phil to make it more likely that he will start and continue an exercise routine?

Hazards of Immobility

Most people take their mobility for granted until illness, disease, or trauma affects their ability to move. Even short periods of immobility may be difficult. If you've ever had the flu or an illness that sent you to bed, you know that it can take several days to return to your pre-illness state, especially for older adults and people with underlying chronic illness. Severe illness associated with prolonged immobilization causes physiological changes in almost every body system, along with psychological changes. Some changes are reversible, but others are not. These changes are discussed below.

Effect of Immobility on Muscles and Bones

Even a couple of days in bed can leave you feeling tired and weak, because the musculoskeletal system is one of the first systems affected by immobility. Inactivity causes significant wasting of the gastrocnemius, soleus, and leg muscles that control flexion and extension of the hip, knee, and ankle. Confinement to bed leads to 7% to 10% loss of muscle strength (atrophy) per week. Immobility also causes the joints to become stiff. The strongest muscles, usually the flexors, pull the joints in their direction, leading to **contractures,** or joint **ankylosis** (fusion of the joints).

Immobility affects parathyroid function, calcium metabolism, and therefore bone formation. The result of these changes is osteoporosis, calcium depletion in the joints, and **renal calculi** (kidney stones) due to increased excretion of calcium. These changes place the patient at risk for pathological fractures with minimal trauma.

Effects of Immobility on the Lungs

Immobility decreases the strength of all muscles, including those involved in chest wall expansion, which also affects ventilation. When a patient is in bed, the depth of respirations decreases, and secretions pool in the airways. The ability to effectively cough and expectorate secretions diminishes as muscle tone of the abdomen and chest decrease. As a result, pooled secretions block air passages and alveoli, decrease oxygen and carbon dioxide exchange, and often lead to atelectasis, (collapse of air sacs), or pneumonia. Even a sedentary lifestyle affects the capacity to increase ventilation in response to exercise (see Chapter 35 if you want more information about ventilation).

Effect of Immobility on the Heart and Vessels

Immobility increases the workload of the heart and promotes venous stasis. When you are active, the skeletal muscles of the legs help pump blood back to the heart. Recall that the veins are thin-walled vessels with valves. Muscle activity propels blood toward the right side of the heart, and the valves prevent backflow of blood. To compensate for immobility, heart rate and stroke volume increase to maintain blood pressure. But with immobility, cardiac reserves are lessened, which means the heart is less able to respond to demands above baseline. Without muscle activity, the force of gravity causes blood to pool in the periphery, which leads to edema. Fluid in the tissue (e.g., heels or sacrum) is more prone to pressure injury.

In addition to venous pooling, immobility leads to compression and injury of the small vessels in the legs and decreased clearance of coagulation factors, causing blood to clot faster. These three changes—stasis, activation of clotting, and vessel injury—make up what is known as **Virchow's triad,** a trilogy of symptoms associated with a greater chance of thrombus formation, such as deep vein thrombosis (DVT).

An immobile person is also more prone to **orthostatic hypotension.** Prolonged bedrest inactivates the baroreceptors involved with constriction and dilation of the blood vessels. As a result, when a person who has been immobilized changes position, he is less able to maintain his blood pressure. The patient complains of feeling dizzy and light-headed and may be unable to support his own weight.

Effects of Immobility on Metabolism

Inactivity increases the level of serum lactic acid and decreases adenosine triphosphate (ATP) concentrations. As ATP concentrations decrease, so do the body's energy reserves. In response, metabolic rate drops, protein and glycogen synthesis decrease, and fat stores increase. Together, these effects cause glucose intolerance and reduced muscle mass.

Immobility also triggers the release of epinephrine, norepinephrine, thyroid hormones, adrenocorticotropic hormone (ACTH) from the pituitary gland, and aldosterone from the kidneys. These changes in hormones are the same as occur in the stress response; so, as you can see, immobility can be a stressor in itself.

Effects of Immobility on the Integument

External pressure from lying in one position compresses capillaries in the skin, obstructing skin circulation. Lack of circulation causes tissue ischemia and possible necrosis (death). Nursing interventions include frequent turning and skin care to prevent wounds, known as pressure ulcers, from forming (see Chapter 34 as needed).

Effects of Immobility on the Gastrointestinal System

Immobility slows peristalsis, which leads to constipation, gas, and difficulty evacuating stool from the rectum. In extreme circumstances, a **paralytic ileus** (cessation of peristalsis) may occur. When peristalsis slows, appetite diminishes and food also is digested slowly. The net effect is usually decreased calorie intake and inability to meet the protein demands of the body. Body muscle is broken down as a fuel source, causing further wasting.

Effects of Immobility on the Genitourinary System

Being supine inhibits drainage of urine from the renal pelvis and bladder. Urine becomes stagnant, which creates an ideal environment for infection and kidney stone formation. Immobility triggers a rise in calcium levels, which also contributes to stone formation. Diminished muscle tone leads to a decrease in bladder tone, and many patients have difficulty voiding in a bedpan or urinal.

Psychological Effects of Immobility

Prolonged immobility, whether in the hospital or at home, leads to isolation and mood changes. In the 1960s, the effects of immobility were studied among astronauts. Early space travel placed solo astronauts in cumbersome suits strapped in recumbent positions. Along with the many physical effects of immobility, researchers found noticeable psychological changes. These healthy men showed signs of depression, anxiety, hostility, sleep disturbances, and changes in their ability to perform self-care activities. Patients who are in bed for long periods of time can suffer all these problems, as well as disorientation, apathy, and altered body concept. Other notable psychological effects of immobility/bed rest included a diminished ability to concentrate, recall sequential events, problem-solve, and perform self-care. For tips on preventing complications of bedrest, see Box 31-4.

KnowledgeCheck 31-5

- Identify the effects of immobility on the cardiovascular, musculoskeletal and integumentary systems.
- Why might immobility be referred to as a stressor?
- What are three effects of immobility on the GI system?
- What changes in mood might be seen with immobility?

 Go to Chapter 31, **Knowledge Check Response Sheet and Answers,** on the Student Resource Disk or DavisPlus at http://davisplus.fadavis.com/Wilkinson2

BOX 31-4 ■ Preventing Complications of Bedrest

- Position the patient to allow for lung expansion and prevent atelectasis and pneumonia.
- Provide a healthy diet to prevent loss of muscle mass.
- Prevent orthostatic hypotension by having the patient sit on edge of bed before the first time out of bed.
- Turn the patient every 2 hours to prevent pressure on the skin and minimize edema.

Practical Knowledge knowing how

As you have seen in the preceding sections, immobility can result in serious health consequences. In the remainder of the chapter, we discuss nursing activities to promote activity and exercise and eliminate the hazards of immobility.

■ ASSESSMENT

Perform an assessment focused on mobility and exercise for any patient who has musculoskeletal concerns, is obese, has limited mobility, or is confined to bed or home. As always, you will validate the nursing history data with physical examination. Box 31-5 defines a variety of terms used to describe problems with muscle mass, strength, or mobility. To help you with focused mobility assessments in the home, see the home care box, Home Assessment for a Patient with Mobility Concerns.

Focused Nursing History

A nursing history focused on activity and exercise addresses usual activity, fitness goals, mobility problems, underlying health problems, lifestyle, and external factors. For suggested questions for assessing activity and exercise,

 Go to Chapter 31, **Assessment Guidelines and Tools, Suggested History Questions for Assessing Activity and Exercise,** in Volume 2.

When caring for patients with very limited activity, assessing the ability to perform ADLs or instrumental

---

BOX 31-5 ■ Terms Used to Describe Problems with Muscle Mass, Strength, or Mobility

Atrophy is a decrease in the size of muscle tissue due to lack of use or loss of innervation.

Clonus is spasmodic contraction of opposing muscles resulting in tremorous movement.

Flaccidity is a decrease or absence of muscle tone.

Hemiplegia is paralysis of one side of the body.

Hypertrophy is an increase in the size or bulk of a muscle or organ.

Paraplegia is paralysis of the lower portion of the trunk and both legs.

Paresis is partial or incomplete paralysis.

Paresthesia is numbness, tingling, or burning due to injury of the nerve(s) innervating the affected area.

Quadriplegia is paralysis of all four extremities.

Spasticity is a motor disorder characterized by increased muscle tone, exaggerated tendon jerks, and clonus.

Tremor is involuntary quivering movement of a body part.

Home Assessment for a Patient with Mobility Concerns

Assess the Environment

➤ Are there stairs or other obstacles that the patient must negotiate?

➤ What aspects of the home environment assist with patient care?

➤ What aspects of the home environment hinder patient care?

➤ What is the patient's history of falls or other mobility concerns?

➤ Would the patient benefit from assistive equipment (e.g., hospital bed, walker)?

➤ Can the patient negotiate the distance between the bedroom, bathroom, and kitchen?

Assess the Family or Caregivers' Abilities and Needs

➤ Who is providing care?

➤ Is the available care sufficient to meet the patient's needs?

➤ Are additional support persons available to assist with care?

➤ Can the caregiver safely move the patient in bed or assist the patient out of bed?

➤ What are the health concerns or physical limitations of the caregivers?

➤ What is the backup plan if the family or caregiver can no longer meet the patient's needs?

Assess Resources

➤ What community resources are available to the patient or caregiver (e.g., Meals on Wheels, physical therapy, Visiting Nurses Association)?

➤ Are the patient and caregiver willing to use community resources?

➤ What services are provided by the patient's insurance?

➤ Can the patient or family afford private services? If so, what services are they interested in?

activities of daily living (IADLs) may be more appropriate. Recall that ADLs focus on hygiene, feeding, toileting, and transfer out of bed. In contrast, IADLs focus on tasks that are instrumental in helping a patient maintain independent living status. Assessment tools for ADLs and IADLs were presented in Chapter 3.

Focused Physical Assessment

Important data to include in a physical assessment related to activity and exercise include vital signs, height, weight, body mass index, body alignment, joint function, gait, muscle strength, and activity tolerance. This section summarizes a few of these components. For a

focused activity and exercise assessment that includes all the components,

 Go to Chapter 31, **Assessment Guidelines and Tools, Focused Physical Assessments for Activity and Exercise,** in Volume 2.

Before beginning the exam, be fully aware of the patient's mobility status and any restrictions in movement, pain, injury, or otherwise. As you move through the exam, observe for pain, inflammation and mobility limitations in all areas. For a thorough discussion of physical assessment of the musculoskeletal system, see Chapter 19. For an illustration of joint range or motion,

 Go to Chapter 31, **Clinical Insight 31-3: Performing Passive Range-of-Motion Exercises,** in Volume 2.

The Functional Independence Measure

Also known as the FIM Scale, the functional independence measure is used to measure multiple areas of a patient's care needs, such as ADLs, mobility, problem solving, memory, and others. On admission, patients are scored for baseline and then serially until discharge and later in the outpatient or home setting to monitor improvement.

Gait

The way a person moves communicates a great deal about his general state of health, mood, and risk for falls. You might want to assess abnormal gaits in patients with injury, neurological issues, or with the following characteristics:

- **Antalgic gait**—limp to avoid pain when bearing weight on the affected side
- **Propulsive gait**—a stooped, rigid posture, with the head and neck bent forward; movement forward is by small, shuffling steps with involuntary acceleration; also known as festinating gait; common in Parkinson's disease
- **Scissors gait**—legs flexed slightly at the hips and knees with the thighs crossing in a scissors-like movement; common with cerebral palsy, stroke, or spinal tumor
- **Spastic gait**—a stiff, foot-dragging walk caused by one-sided, long-term, muscle contraction; seen with cerebral palsy, head trauma, or brain tumor
- **Steppage gait**—an exaggerated motion of lifting the leg to avoid scraping the toes of a foot with foot drop (foot appears floppy with the toes pointing down); seen with Guillain-Barré syndrome
- **Waddling gait**—a distinctive rolling motion in which the opposite hip drops; seen in patients with muscular dystrophy or developmental dysplasia of the hip; characteristic gait in late pregnancy.

To see illustrations of these gaits,

 Go to Chapter 19, **Abnormal Atlas, Abnormal Gaits,** in Volume 2.

Activity Tolerance

To promote the benefits of physical activity, people need to pace themselves during exercise, especially those who have been inactive. Health professionals can teach people to rate the perceived level of exertion and monitor target heart rate. Target heart rate requires a pulse check during exercises and staying within 50% to 85% of the maximum heart rate. To figure this out, take 220 and then subtract the person's age and then multiply times 0.5 to 0.85.

For more information about optimal target heart rates during exercise, see Box 31-1 or

 Go to the American Heart Association Web site. **Target Heart Rates** are available at http://www.americanheart.org/presenter.jhtml?identifier=4736

KnowledgeCheck 31-6

- Describe a focused assessment for a patient experiencing mobility concerns.
- Identify the assessment methods (inspection, palpation, percussion, and auscultation) used when performing a physical examination focused on mobility concerns.

 Go to Chapter 31, **Knowledge Check Response Sheet and Answers,** on the Student Resource Disk or DavisPlus at http://davisplus.fadavis.com/Wilkinson2

 CriticalThinking 31-4

Review the "Meet Your Patients" scenario. Which, if any, of the class participants requires a physical examination focused on mobility concerns? Explain your reasoning.

ANALYSIS/NURSING DIAGNOSIS

Nursing diagnoses that specifically describe activity and exercise problems include the following:

- *Activity Intolerance* is a state in which a patient has insufficient physical or psychological energy to carry out daily activities.
- *Impaired Physical Mobility* is limitation of independent purposeful movement of the body. Impaired Physical Mobility is a broad, general diagnosis. Use the following, more descriptive diagnoses when the patient has specific deficits: Impaired Bed Mobility, Impaired Walking, Impaired Wheelchair Mobility, and Impaired Transfer Ability.
- *Risk for Disuse Syndrome* exists when a patient's prescribed or unavoidable inactivity creates the risk for deterioration of other body systems.
- *Sedentary Lifestyle* is a habit of life that is characterized by a low physical activity level.

Mobility problems may also be the etiology of other diagnoses. The following are examples:

- Acute Pain r/t musculoskeletal injury.
- Ineffective Health Maintenance r/t prescribed bedrest.

- Risk for Injury r/t unsteady gait.
- Self-Care Deficit (Bathing/Hygiene, Feeding, Dressing/Grooming, Toileting) r/t Impaired Physical Mobility
- Delayed Surgical Recovery

For further information about mobility diagnoses,

 Go to Chapter 31, **Standardized Language, NANDA-I Diagnoses for Activity and Exercise Problems,** in Volume 2.

PLANNING OUTCOMES/EVALUATION

For *associated NOC standardized outcomes* for mobility diagnoses,

 Go to Chapter 31, **Standardized Language, Selected NOC Outcomes for Energy Maintenance and Mobility,** in Volume 2.

Individualized goals/outcome statements depend on the nursing diagnosis used. Because activity and exercise abilities are individualized, goals must consider the patient's current condition, expected condition changes, lifestyle, and values. Examples:

Will independently transfer to the wheelchair by [date].
Will discuss his feelings about his activity restrictions by [date].

PLANNING INTERVENTIONS/IMPLEMENTATION

Because attitudes about fitness and activity vary widely, mobility is often a difficult topic. Some people are devastated by activity limitations caused by disease or treatment. Others are able to accept these changes. For these reasons, it is important for you to convey an attitude of acceptance about the patient's current activity level and provide care that helps the patient achieve his optimal level of function.

For *NIC standardized interventions and activities* for patients with mobility problems,

 Go to Chapter 31, **Standardized Language, Selected NIC Interventions for Activity and Exercise Management and Immobility Management,** in Volume 2.

Specific nursing activities to promote exercise and mobility include promoting exercise, preventing injury from exercise, positioning patients, moving patients in bed, transferring patients out of bed, performing ROM exercises, and assisting with ambulation.

Promoting Exercise

Nurses are in a perfect role to encourage and educate people of all ages to be active for healthy living. Here are some common steps to help people attain and maintain fitness. Also see the Self-Care box, Teaching Clients to Set Up an Exercise Program.

- *Personalize the benefits of regular physical activity.* In other words, find out what motivates your patient. For instance, your patient might want to lose weight and improve his physical appearance. Yet another patient might be interested in improving the quality of sleep or overcoming periods of low energy during the day.
- *Set personal goals for physical activity.* Simple, realistic goals tend to be best. Be sure to define them so they are specific and measurable.
- *Include a variety of activities to keep the patient from feeling bored.*
- *Remind your patient to recognize and appreciate success.*
- *Suggest strategies to achieve the patient's goals.* For instance, you might suggest a fitness program that is fun and entertaining. You can also inform your patient about ways to avoid joint injury or falls.
- *Provide encouragement.* Sometimes just the right approach is a positive, enthusiastic one. You might offer praise for taking steps toward health and fitness. Support from spouse, family members, friends, and coworkers can improve compliance and consistency.
- *Promote physical exercise as an enjoyable activity.*
- *Discuss barriers to regular activity and elicit ways to overcome those obstacles.*

People give various reasons for failing to develop a regular exercise program. See Box 31-6 for suggestions on dealing with such objections.

Preventing Injury from Exercise

As previously discussed, the benefits of exercise outweigh any associated risks. Advise clients to follow the tips in the self-care boxes: Teaching Clients How to Set Up an Exercise Program and Teaching Your Patient How to Prevent Back Injuries. Also re-read the theoretical knowledge in the section, Risks Associated with Exercise, if you need a review.

Positioning Patients

Healthy people regularly shift position to maintain comfort. However, many patients are unable to move without assistance. They require a change of position at least every 2 hours to prevent skin breakdown, muscle discomfort, damage to superficial nerves and blood vessels, and contractures. Immobile people are more prone to pressure injury as a result of reduced circulation, impaired oxygen exchange to the tissues, and edema.

A firm mattress provides support to the patient's body and makes it easier to turn the patient (because he does not sink down into the mattress). Most hospital mattresses are firm. However, when you provide

---

BOX 31-6 ■ Suggestions for Overcoming Objections to Exercise

Objection	Suggestion
"I hate to exercise."	Pick several activities that you enjoy.
"I burn out on exercise."	Plan ahead and build in rest days and varied activities.
"I am self-conscious about going to the gym and don't have the motivation to exercise by myself."	Find a friend to exercise with, or develop a reward system for yourself if you continue to exercise.
"I am too busy with work or family."	Develop a routine that you can do at lunchtime, or exercise with your family.
"I find exercise boring."	Change your routine frequently.
"Exercise hurts."	Make sure to exercise at your target heart rate, and plan a rest day after every weightlifting session.
"I don't have time."	Schedule your exercise time. If need be, schedule several short 10- to 15-minute sessions throughout the day.
"I have pain about all the time."	Take pain medication an hour or so before starting physical activity. If fatigue is the problem, try to arrange schedule to keep a balance of rest and activity as well as avoid stimulants (e.g., caffeine or nicotine) that might interfere with the quality of sleep.
"I have difficulty getting around sometimes."	Stretch adequately before starting exercise, but not to overstretch joints. Also, you will need to walk on smooth, even surfaces.
"I am diabetic and have trouble with my feet. My vision is not very good, either."	Be sure shoes fit properly and the area is well-lit.

Teaching Your Patient How to Prevent Back Injuries

➤ Poor posture is one of the main causes of back pain. Make a conscious effort to maintain good posture at all times.

➤ Use a firm mattress that provides adequate support.

➤ Sit with your knees slightly lower than your hips.

➤ If you must stand for a long period of time, flex your hip and raise one foot on a stool or object 6 to 8 inches off the ground. Periodically switch legs.

➤ Wear comfortable, low-heeled shoes. Avoid high heels as much as possible.

➤ Avoid restrictive clothing that inhibits your ability to use good body mechanics.

➤ Follow principles of body mechanics at all times (e.g., use wide base of support, and do not lift with your back).

➤ Exercise regularly to maintain your optimal weight and strengthen the muscles of your body.

➤ Include abdominal exercises in your routine. Strong abdominal muscles help support the back.

➤ Avoid lifting excessive weight.

➤ Avoid exercises or movements that cause spinal flexion (e.g., toe-touches, sit-ups with knees extended), excessive flexion of the neck (e.g., abdominal crunches with neck curved to chest), or spinal rotation (twisting).

home care, you will find mattresses of various types and conditions. To provide additional support, you can place a piece of plywood under a sagging mattress.

A clean, dry bed also makes it easier to turn the patient and decreases the risk of skin maceration or pressure ulcer formation. Bedding should provide coverage and warmth but not be tucked in so tightly as to restrict movement.

✚ To protect yourself from back injury as you move patients, avoid manual lifting as much as possible. Use assistive equipment and devices, as recommended by the ANA (2005), and always make sure you have adequate help. The amount of help you need depends on the size of the patient, the level of assistance the patient can offer, your size and strength, and the equipment or lines attached to the patient.

Positioning Devices

Devices used to maintain body alignment, prevent contractures, and promote comfort are briefly discussed in the next sections. For guidelines for using common positioning devices, including hip abduction pillows,

 Go to Chapter 31, **Clinical Insight 31-2: Using Common Positioning Devices,** in Volume 2.

Adjustable Beds

An adjustable bed, often referred to as a hospital bed, assumes a variety of positions. You can elevate or lower the head of the bed, and elevate the foot of the bed. Often the bed breaks, or "gatches," at the knee to keep the patient from sliding down when the head is elevated. You can also adjust the height of the bed. You should raise the bed to waist height when providing care so that you can use proper body mechanics; place the bed in its lowest position before helping a patient get out of bed or if the patient is at risk for falling.

Several types of specialized beds are used in treating and preventing pressure ulcers. These include alternating, low air loss, immersion (air-fluidized), and oscillating beds. The mattresses may be composed of air, water, or gel. Special beds are discussed further in Chapter 34. A circular bed and Stryker frame are used in the care of patients with severe mobility restrictions. Both can rotate a patient from supine to prone. With the advent of low-pressure specialized beds, these latter two types of beds are now in limited use.

Pillows

Pillows are the most common devices used to assist with positioning, provide support, and elevate body parts. They help position a patient by molding to the body and expanding the weight-bearing area. You will need a variety of sizes to position patients who are unconscious, paralyzed, frail, or who have had surgery. To obtain the right size or type (e.g., abductor pillows), or if pillows are not available, you can use folded blankets or towels. Foam wedge pillows are useful for elevating the upper body when an adjustable bed is not available and for abducting the hips after hip surgery.

Siderails

Most hospital beds are equipped with siderails. The rails may run the full length of each side of the bed or consist of an upper or lower rail on each side.

✚ Siderails are designed to ensure patient safety. They serve as a reminder that the patient should call for assistance before getting out of bed and provide a grip for the patient who is able to reposition himself in bed. Although siderails are designed to protect patients, they can be a source of injury. Patients can get tangled in the railing or fall between the bed and rail, and confused patients may injure themselves trying to climb over the rails.

Siderails may also be considered a form of restraint, so follow your agency's policy for use and be sure to discuss their purpose with patients and family. See Chapter 21 if you need to review restraint use.

Trapeze Bar

A trapeze bar is a triangular-shaped device that is attached to an overhead bed frame (Fig. 31-5). The patient can use the base of the triangle as a grip bar to move up in bed, turn, and pull up in preparation for getting out of bed or getting on and off the bedpan. Patients can use the trapeze to move about in bed and to exercise their upper extremities. Frail patients may not be able to use a trapeze bar because of the amount of effort it requires.

Footboard

When a person is supine, the toes tend to point downward toward the bed (*footdrop*), and the feet are in plantar flexion. Able-bodied persons usually shift position throughout the night, so the foot and leg muscles are periodically contracted and relaxed. In contrast, the patient who is unable to move independently will experience a shortening of the gastrocnemius muscle and may have difficulty walking again if prolonged plantar flexion occurs. A footboard is a device placed at the end of the bed to prevent foot drop and outward hip rotation, but it does not relieve heel pressure (Fig. 31-6). For the footboard to be effective, the heels must be touching it. Each time you turn the patient, you may need to reposition the footboard to ensure proper position.

Other Positioning Devices

The following are other positioning devices used in the clinical setting.

- *Trochanter rolls* are made from tightly rolled towels, bath blankets, or foam pads. They are placed snugly adjacent to the hips and thighs to prevent external rotation of the hips. To learn how to make them,

FIGURE 31-5 A trapeze bar provides a grip for the patient to reposition herself independently.

FIGURE 31-6 A footboard is placed at the end of the bed to prevent foot drop.

 Go to Chapter 31, **Clinical Insight 31-2: Using Common Positioning Devices,** in Volume 2.

- *Hand and wrist splints* may be manufactured or fashioned from rolled wash cloths. Often splints are custom made for patients. The purpose of splints is to hold the wrist and hand in natural position and prevent claw-hand deformities.
- *Hand rolls* prevent hand contractures. Some are commercially made. Otherwise, you can make a hand roll from a tightly rolled washcloth.
- *Hip abduction pillows* prevent internal hip rotation and hip adduction when the patient is in a supine position. These wedge-shaped pieces of spongy material are used after femoral fracture, hip fracture, or surgery. Lateral indentations and straps that wrap around the patient's thighs hold the patient in the correct position.
- *Boots* made of spongy rubber with heel cutouts and ankle cushioning prevent footdrop, skin breakdown, and external hip rotation.

   If any part of the boot is made of a latex product, be sure the patient does not have a latex allergy before applying.

- *Foot cradles* are metal or plastic devices that are secured at the foot of the bed to hold bedding up off the toes and feet, allowing for free movement.
- *High-top sneakers* may be used to prevent heel drop, but they do not reduce heel pressure. They do help in positioning hips and pelvis to prevent hip rotation.
- *Sandbags* are small fabric bags filled with sand. They are used in the same manner as pillows and trochanter rolls; however, they provide firmer support.

Positioning Techniques

In the next section we briefly describe the various ways to position patients. Table 31-2 illustrates these positions; identifies potential problems associated with them; and offers solutions to prevent the problems. The positions are also described and illustrated in Chapter 19, Table 19-1.

Fowler's Positions

Fowler's position is a semisitting position, in which the head of the bed is elevated 45° to 60°. This position promotes respiratory function by lowering the diaphragm and allowing the greatest chest expansion. It is also an ideal position for some patients with cardiac dysfunction. Common variations include **semi-Fowler's position,** in which the head of the bed is elevated only 30° and **high-Fowler's position,** in which the head is elevated 90°.

In the **orthopneic position,** the head of the bed is elevated 90° and an overbed table with a pillow on top is positioned in front of the patient (Fig. 31-7). Have the patient lean forward, resting his arms and head on the pillow. This position is helpful for a patient with shortness of breath.

Lateral Positions

The **lateral position** is a side-lying position with the top hip and knee flexed and placed in front of the rest of the body. The lateral position creates pressure on the lower scapula, ilium, and trochanter but relieves pressure from the heels and sacrum. The **lateral recumbent position** is side-lying with legs in a straight line (see Table 19-1). The **oblique position** is an alternative to the lateral position that places less pressure on the trochanter. The patient turns on the side with the top hip and knee flexed; however, the top leg is placed behind the body (Fig. 31-8).

Prone Position

In the **prone position,** the patient lies on his abdomen with his head turned to one side. This is the only position that allows full extension of the hips and knees. It also allows secretions to drain freely from the mouth and

---

Table 31-2 ▶ Positioning a Bed-Bound Patient

POSITION	POTENTIAL PROBLEM	SOLUTION
Fowler's 	Hyperextension of the neck	Use a small pillow under the head and neck.
	Posterior flexion of the lumbar curvature	Use a firm mattress.
		Position the patient so that the angle of elevation begins at the hip.
	Dislocation of the shoulders	Position a pillow under the forearms to prevent pull on the shoulders.
	Flexion contracture of the wrist and edema of the hands	Support the hands on pillows in alignment with the forearms.
	Flexion contracture of the fingers and abduction of the thumbs	Use hand splints if appropriate, or provide a large roll in the palm of the hand.
	External rotation of the legs	Place sandbags or rolls alongside the trochanters and upper thighs.
	Hyperextension of the knees	Place a small pillow under the lower legs from the ankles to below the knees. Do this for short periods only; avoid pressure on the popliteal area.
	Foot drop	Use a footboard or high-top sneakers to hold the feet in dorsiflexion.
Lateral 	Lateral flexion of the neck	Place a pillow under the head and neck to provide alignment.
	Internal rotation and adduction of the upper shoulder and limited respirations	Place a pillow under the upper arm, and comfortably flex the lower arm.
	Internal rotation and adduction of the femur	Support the upper leg from groin to foot with pillows.
	Twisting of the spine	Align the shoulders with the hips.
	Flexion of the cervical spine	Place a pillow under the head and neck to provide alignment, unless drainage from the mouth is desired.

Continued

Table 31-2 ➤ Positioning a Bed-Bound Patient—cont'd

POSITION	POTENTIAL PROBLEM	SOLUTION
Prone	Hyperextension of the lumbar curvature, pressure on the breasts in women or genitals in men, impaired respirations	Place a small pillow under the abdomen.
	Foot drop	Move the patient down in bed so the feet extend over the edge of the mattress, or place a small pillow under the shins so that the toes do not touch the bed.
	Lateral flexion of the neck	Place a pillow under the head and neck to provide alignment, unless drainage from the mouth is desired.
Sims'	Internal rotation and adduction of the upper shoulder and limited respirations	Place a pillow under the upper arm, and comfortably flex the arm at the elbow.
	Pressure on the shoulder and axilla of the inferior arm	Position the lower arm behind and away from the back.
	Internal rotation and adduction of the femur	Support the upper leg from groin to foot with pillows.
	Twisting of the spine	Align the shoulders with the hips.
	Foot drop	Support the feet in dorsiflexion with sandbags.
	Hyperextension of the neck	Place a pillow under the head and neck to provide alignment.
Supine	Internal rotation of the shoulders and extension of the elbows	Position the upper arms next to the body. Place pillows under the forearms, and position the wrists in slight pronation.
	Flexion of fingers and abduction of the thumbs	Use hand splints if appropriate, or provide a large roll in the palm of the hand.
	Flexion of the lumbar curvature and hips	Provide a firm mattress, or place a small pillow under the lumbar curvature.
	External rotation of the legs	Place sandbags or rolls alongside the trochanters and upper thighs.
	Hyperextension of the knees	Place a small pillow under the lower legs from the ankles to below the knees.
	Foot drop	Use a footboard or high-top sneakers to hold the feet in dorsiflexion.

thus is helpful for an unconscious patient. However, this is the most difficult position to move an unconscious or frail patient into, because it requires the greatest amount of manipulation to position the patient appropriately. The prone position creates a significant lordosis (inward curving of the spine in the lower back) and rotation of the neck. Therefore, it should not be used for patients with cervical or lumbar spine problems. You should not use the prone position for patients with cardiac or respiratory difficulty because it inhibits chest wall expansion and, therefore, oxygenation. As a rule, you can use this position only for short periods of time.

Sims' Position

Sims' position is a semiprone position. The lower arm is positioned behind the patient, and the upper arm

FIGURE 31-7 The orthopneic position is ideal for a patient with shortness of breath.

FIGURE 31-8 The oblique position is a modified lateral position that places less pressure on the trochanter.

is flexed. The upper leg is more flexed than the lower leg. Sims' position facilitates drainage from the mouth and limits pressure on the trochanter and sacrum. This is an ideal position for administering an enema or a perineal procedure.

Supine Position

In the **supine position,** also known as the **dorsal recumbent position,** the patient lies on his back with head and shoulders elevated on a small pillow. The spine is aligned and the arms and hands comfortably rest at the side.

KnowledgeCheck 31-7

- Describe the following positions: Fowler's, lateral, prone, Sims', and supine.
- What is the advantage of the oblique position versus the lateral position?
- Identify and describe six positioning devices.
- What are three uses for siderails?

 Go to Chapter 31, **Knowledge Check Response Sheet and Answers,** on the Student Resource Disk or DavisPlus at http://davisplus.fadavis.com/Wilkinson2

CriticalThinking 31-5

You are providing care for a young man who is recovering from Guillain-Barré syndrome, which produces a reversible paralysis after viral illness. He has been healthy until this present illness. How would you position this patient? Explain your reasoning.

Moving Patients in Bed

To position patients, you must be adept at moving and lifting them in bed. This involves positioning the patient in the length of the bed, as well as turning with as little friction and shearing on the skin as possible.

Moving Up in Bed

Frail patients slide down in bed because of gravity and their inability to correct their position. Elevating the head of the bed accentuates the slide and places the patient in an awkward position. If the patient is light in weight or able to provide assistance, you will be able to move her independently (Critical Aspects of Procedures 31-1 through 31-3). For complete instructions,

 Go to Chapter 31, **Procedure 31-1A: Moving a Patient Up in Bed,** in Volume 2.

Turning in Bed

Turn patients at least every 2 hours to protect their skin and prevent other complications of immobility. For efficient use of time, try to time turning to coincide with moving the patient up in bed. Use pillows and other positioning devices to help the patient maintain the new position (see Critical Aspects box for a summary). For a complete description,

 Go to Chapter 31, **Procedure 31-1B: Turning a Patient in Bed,** in Volume 2.

Logrolling

Logrolling is a special turning technique used when the patient's spine must be kept in straight alignment. You will need at least two nurses for this procedure, more if the patient is large. Logrolling moves the patient's body as a unit. One nurse is positioned at the level of the patient's head. The other staff members are distributed along the length of the patient. All must move the patient in unison (see Critical Aspects box for a summary). For a complete description,

 Go to Chapter 31, **Procedure 31-1C: Logrolling a Patient,** in Volume 2.

Friction-Reducing Devices

You can use one of a variety of friction-reducing devices when moving a patient in bed. **Transfer roller sheets** are thin, low-friction fabric sheets that may be placed beneath the draw sheet to facilitate moving the patient in bed (Fig. 31-9). A **scoot sheet** is also a thin, low-friction fabric sheet that is often positioned under the draw sheet of the patient, but it is attached to a mechanical crank (Fig. 31-10). By turning the crank, a single person can move a patient up in bed. Transfer roller sheets are relatively inexpensive and are widely available on clinical units. If one is not available, you can improvise by placing a large, clean, unused plastic bag under the draw sheet to help you move the patient. The plastic bag reduces drag and facilitates movement. However, unlike the thin fabric of transfer sheets, plastic allows moisture to pool under the patient. Consequently, you should not leave a bag in place under the draw sheet.

Transferring Patients Out of Bed

Stretchers and wheelchairs are used to transport patients between units and to tests or procedures. A stretcher is usually reserved for the patient who is weak, sedated, or has a condition that does not permit transfer by wheelchair. A wheelchair may be used for transport or as part of an activity program. In addition, you may transfer

VOL 2 For steps to follow in *all* procedures, refer to the Universal Steps for All Procedures found on the inside back cover of Volume 2. Go to the full procedures in Volume 2 to practice and learn the procedure steps. Use these Critical Aspects later to help you review key points.

Procedure 31-1A: Moving a Patient Up in Bed

➤ Use a friction-reducing device to move the patient if the patient can assist with movement. Use a full body sling if the patient cannot assist.

➤ Remove the pillow. Have the patient flex her neck, fold her arms across her chest, and place her feet flat on the bed.

➤ Position a nurse on either side of the patient.

➤ Use a wide base of support.

➤ Have the patient, on the count of 3, push off with his heels as you shift your weight forward.

Procedure 31-1B: Turning a Patient in Bed

➤ Use a friction-reducing device and draw sheet to move the patient. Position at least one nurse on each side of the bed.

➤ Place the patient's near leg and arm (e.g., the left arm and leg when turning to the right) across his body, and abduct and externally rotate the far shoulder.

➤ Each nurse places one arm at the level of the patient's shoulders and the other at the level of the patient's hips. Each nurse shifts her weight as both simultaneously roll the patient in the intended direction.

Procedure 31-1C: Logrolling a Patient

➤ Move the patient as a unit to the opposite side of the bed; raise the siderail on that side.

➤ Move to the side of the bed that the patient will be turning toward; lower the siderail.

➤ Each staff member evenly distributes his arms across the patient's length. One nurse is responsible for moving the head and neck as a unit.

➤ Shift your weight backward as you roll the patient toward you.

Procedure 31-2A: Transferring Patient from Bed to Stretcher

➤ Move the patient to the side of the bed where the stretcher will be placed.

➤ Position the stretcher next to the bed, and lock it in place.

➤ Keep the destination device (i.e., bed to stretcher or visa versa) situated a little lower than the surface the patient is on.

➤ Using the draw sheet, roll the patient away from the stretcher.

➤ Place the transfer board against the patient's back halfway between the bed and stretcher. Position a friction-reducing device over the transfer board. Turn the patient to his back and onto the transfer board with the draw sheet.

➤ On a count of three, use the draw sheet to slide the patient across the transfer board onto the stretcher.

Procedure 31-2B: Dangling a Patient at the Side of the Bed

➤ Place the patient in a supine position, and raise the head of the bed to 90°.

➤ Apply a gait transfer belt, and place the bed in a low position.

➤ Stand facing the patient with a wide base of support. Place your foot closest to the head of the bed forward of the other foot.

➤ Position your hands on each side of the gait transfer belt.

➤ Rock onto your back foot as you move the patient into a sitting position, and pivot to bring the patient's legs over the side of the bed.

➤ Stay with the patient as he dangles.

Procedure 31-2C: Transferring a Patient from Bed to Chair

➤ Ask the patient to wear nonskid footwear.

➤ Place the bed in the low position, and lock the wheels.

➤ Assist the patient to dangle at the side of the bed (see Procedure 31-2B).

➤ Brace your feet and knees against the patient. Bend your hips at the knees, and hold onto the transfer belt.

➤ If two nurses are available to assist with the transfer, one nurse should be on each side of the patient.

➤ Instruct the patient to place her arms around you between your shoulders and waist. Ask the patient to stand as you move to an upright position by straightening your legs and hips.

➤ Instruct the patient to pivot and turn with you toward the chair.

➤ Ask the patient to flex her hips and knees as she lowers herself to the chair. Guide her motion while maintaining a firm hold on her.

➤ If the chair is a wheelchair, lock the wheels.

Procedure 31-3: Assisting with Ambulation

➤ Ask the patient to wear nonskid footwear.

➤ Place the bed in low position, and lock the wheels.

➤ Assist the patient to dangle at the side of the bed (see Procedure 31-2B).

➤ If two nurses are available, each nurse should stand facing the patient on opposite sides of the patient.

➤ Brace your feet and knees against the patient. Bend your hips at the knees, and hold onto the transfer belt. Pay attention to any known weakness.

➤ Instruct the patient to place her arms around you between your shoulders and waist (the location depends on the height of the patient and the nurses). Ask the patient to stand as you move to an upright position by straightening your legs and hips.

➤ Allow the patient to steady herself for a moment.

➤ One nurse: Stand at the patient's side, placing both hands on the transfer belt. If the patient has weakness on one side, position yourself on the weaker side.

➤ Two nurses: One nurse stands on each of the patient's sides, grasping hold of the transfer belt.

➤ Slowly guide the patient forward. Observe for signs of fatigue or dizziness.

➤ If the patient must transport an IV pole, allow the patient to hold onto the pole on the side where you are standing. Assist the patient to advance the pole as you ambulate together.

FIGURE 31-9 A transfer roller sheet reduces friction and facilitates movement.

FIGURE 31-10 A scoot sheet allows a single person to move a patient up in bed.

patients to a stationary chair to increase their general activity level (see Critical Aspects box for a summary). For complete procedural steps,

 Go to Chapter 31, **Procedure 31-2A: Transferring a Patient from Bed to Stretcher, Procedure 31-2B: Dangling a Patient at the Side of the Bed,** and **Procedure 31-2C: Transferring a Patient from Bed to Chair,** in Volume 2.

Transfer Board

A **transfer board** is a wood or plastic device designed to assist with moving patients. Using a transfer board reduces your risk of injury and promotes a smooth transfer. Place the board under the patient on the side to which he will be moved. It is best to use a draw sheet to slide the patient across the board (Fig. 31-11). Transfer boards are also used by patients with long-standing mobility problems to increase their independence.

FIGURE 31-11 Transfer boards are used by patients with chronic mobility problems to increase their independence.

Mechanical Lift

A **mechanical lift** is a hydraulic device used to transfer patients. Place a fabric sling under the patient, and attach chains or straps from the sling to the lifting device (Fig. 31-12A). A mechanical lift is especially useful when providing care for obese and immobile patients. Lifts are often used in home care because they allow one person to transfer the patient safely. Most lifts position patients in a seated position and thus are ideal for assisting the patient into a chair. Others suspend the patient in a supine position; they may be used to transfer the patient from bed to stretcher or to suspend the patient while the bed is made. Many such lifts include scales that weigh the patient while he is suspended in the sling. Some mechanical lifts are mounted on the ceiling to reduce caregiver back injuries and increase patient safety (see Fig. 31-12B).

Standing assist devices are mechanical lifts that help the patient move from a sitting to a standing position or support a patient in the standing position. A sling is positioned around the back and under the arms of the patient (Fig. 31-13). Specialized chairs and wheelchairs are also available. Each has a mechanical lift in the seat that rises to assist the patient to a standing position. Mechanical lift devices reduce the risk of back and musculoskeletal injury.

Transfer Belt

A **transfer belt** is a heavy belt several inches wide that is used to facilitate transfer or provide a secure mechanism to hold the patient when ambulating. Apply the belt around the patient's abdomen, close to the patient's center of gravity. The belt may have external grip holds, or you may grip the entire belt with your hand (Fig. 31-14).

FIGURE 31-12 *A,* A mechanical lift is useful when providing care to patients with impaired mobility. *B,* A ceiling mounted mechanical lift is used to support patients in the standing position.

The fit should not be overly tight or cause the patient discomfort. You should be able to easily place your hand under the belt. Do not place it over the rib cage, as this could compromise breathing. Do not use a transfer belt around the patient's hip. This could cause unsteadiness and lead to a patient fall. You would not use a transfer belt after abdominal surgery or with other abdominal wound, colostomy, or internal organ contusion or other injury.

KnowledgeCheck 31-8

- What criteria determine whether your patient should be logrolled when he is repositioned?
- How often should you turn and reposition a patient?
- Identify the most appropriate device for the following activities:
    Transferring an obese patient from a bed to a stretcher
    Assisting an immobile patient to a recliner chair
    Helping a weak patient from bed to chair

 Go to Chapter 31, **Knowledge Check Response Sheet and Answers,** on the Student Resource Disk or DavisPlus at http://davisplus.fadavis.com/Wilkinson2

Performing Range-of-Motion Exercises

Patients with limited mobility are at risk for developing complications of disuse, such as muscle atrophy and contractures. ROM exercises limit the complications of immobility. **Active range of motion (AROM)** occurs when the patient independently moves his joints through flexion, extension, abduction, adduction, and circular rotation. Patients recovering from illness, injury, or surgery often perform this exercise as a rehabilitation procedure. Performing ADLs exercises most joints. **Passive range of motion (PROM)** is movement of the joints through their range of motion by another person. Both AROM and PROM improve joint mobility, increase circulation to the area exercised, and help maintain function. However, AROM also improves muscle strength and tone, as well as respiratory and cardiac function. For an explanation of how to perform PROM,

VOL 2 Go to Chapter 31, **Clinical Insight 31-3: Performing Passive Range-of-Motion Exercises,** in Volume 2.

FIGURE 31-13 A mechanical lift with a sling chair is used to safely transfer an immobile patient into a wheelchair.

Continuous passive motion, also called CPM, is a device that is used to gently flex and extend the knee joint. The CPM machine is often used after knee replacement or other knee procedures to allow the joint to improve range of motion, eliminate the problem of stiffness, and prevent the development of adhesions, which can limit motion further.

Assisting with Ambulation

Prolonged bedrest is no longer the standard of care. However, as a nurse, you will provide care to patients whose illnesses and injuries curtail their ability to walk and be active. Assisting patients with ambulation includes physical conditioning to prepare the patient for ambulation, as well as assisting the patient to walk.

Physical Conditioning

Patients who have been confined to bed for more than a week or who have sustained major injury require conditioning before they are able to resume walking. The following conditioning exercises are summarized here; they are explained in detail,

 Go to Chapter 31, **Clinical Insight 31-4: Assisting with Physical Conditioning Exercises to Prepare for Walking,** in Volume 2.

Quadriceps and Gluteal Drills. The quadriceps muscle group and the gluteal muscles are the largest muscles of the body. Patients who are confined to bed can perform isometric exercises to prepare them for walking.

Arm Exercises. Patients use the biceps and triceps muscles when getting out of bed and for crutch walking. Exercises to help prepare the patient for ambulation

FIGURE 31-14 A transfer belt is placed close to the patient's center of gravity. It may have external grip holds to facilitate transfer or provide a secure mechanism to hold the patient when ambulating.

include using a trapeze bar, and doing "push-ups" off the mattress or a chair. ✚ Be mindful of any cardiac or musculoskeletal precautions that restrict arm movement, weight bearing on the hands and wrists, or other upper body injury. If lymphedema is present in the upper extremities, do not encourage arm exercises or use of the trapeze, unless directed by the primary care provider.

Dangling. Use this position to prepare the patient to get up in a chair, to stand, or to ambulate.

✚ Patients who have been confined to bed frequently become lightheaded or develop orthostatic hypotension when first getting up. Dangling allows the patient to experience being upright with limited risk of falling.

Some common approaches used for orthostatic problems include antiembolism stockings with compression wraps to prevent pooling of venous blood. Sometimes abdominal binders are used for this purpose as well. Medication is available to control orthostatic hypotension. Patients with spinal cord injury experiencing autonomic dysfunctions need a high-back reclining wheelchair so the back of the chair can be lowered (and someone might even have to lift up their legs for a few minutes) until blood pressure stabilizes. Tilt-table therapies are also used.

Daily Activities. Moving around in bed and performing activities of daily living (e.g., brushing one's hair) exercise many of the muscle groups needed for ambulation. Getting up into a chair accustoms the patient to an upright posture and is an important predictor of success with ambulation.

Assisting the Patient to Walk

Before getting the patient out of bed, assess his readiness to walk. Also obtain the appropriate equipment and assistance. Move floor rugs and loose objects from the path of the patient and caregiver. Be sure the floor is not slippery. When possible, use a transfer belt. Have a chair or additional assistance available on the first few attempts at ambulation.

If the patient becomes faint or begins to fall, do not attempt to hold him up by yourself. Instead, protect the patient as you guide him to a seated or lying position. Create a wide base of support, and project forward the hip closest to the patient. Help the patient slide down your leg as you call for help (Fig. 31-15). Protect the patient's head as his body descends.

The Critical Aspects box summarizes ambulation with one-nurse assist and with two-nurse assist. For the complete procedures,

 Go to Chapter 31, **Procedure 31-3A: Assisting with Ambulation (One Nurse),** and **Procedure 31-3B: Assisting with Ambulation (Two Nurses),** in Volume 2.

Assisting Older Adults. When assisting older adults to ambulate, find out how much assistance, if any, the patient typically requires and modify support as needed. Consider the following nursing interventions.

- Observe constantly during ambulation for weakness and fatigue. Plan for periods of rest during ambulation, if needed. The older adult might become fatigued more quickly and recover more slowly from the physical demands of walking, especially if a heart or lung condition is present.
- Move the patient gradually to a sitting position and allow him to dangle at the bedside before coming to a standing position. Observe for dizziness or light-headedness.

FIGURE 31-15 If the patient begins to fall, the nurse guides the patient gently to the floor or to a chair.

- Assess for falls risk factors. For example, some medications cause dizziness or lethargy; and patients with neurological or cognitive disorders, such as Parkinson's or Alzheimer's disease, have a greater potential for falls. For more information about assessing a patient's risk for a fall see Chapter 21.
- To reduce the risk for falling in the home, recommend family place nonskid strips on stairs or other smooth flooring.
- Assistive devices, such as walkers, canes, and transfer belts, can be useful for older adults who require more support.
- Be cautious when using a transfer belt for the patient with osteoporosis or back pain. Too much pressure from the belt can cause injury or pain.

Knowledge Check 31-9

- Identify four principles to be followed when performing PROM.
- Describe activities that can promote a patient's readiness for ambulation.
- What action should you take if a patient begins to fall when ambulating?

Go to Chapter 31, **Knowledge Check Response Sheet and Answers,** on the Student Resource Disk or DavisPlus at http://davisplus.fadavis.com/Wilkinson2

Mechanical Aids for Walking

A variety of aids is available to promote stability and independence when walking. Some aids are intended for short-term use; others will be incorporated into the patient's lifestyle. Some patients consider the use of aids a sign of weakness or inconvenience. As a result, they avoid using the aid and increase their risk of falls. However, most people dread loss of independence, so you can promote the use of walking aids by stressing their importance in helping the person maintain independence. For instructions on sizing canes, walkers, and crutches,

 Go to Chapter 31, **Clinical Insight 31-5: Sizing Walking Aids,** in Volume 2.

For instructions on teaching patients to use these aids,

 Go to Chapter 31, **Clinical Insight 31-6: Teaching Patients to Use Canes, Walkers, and Crutches,** in Volume 2.

Canes

The following are three basic types of canes used (Fig. 31-16):

- *Single-ended cane with a half-circle handle.* This is ideal for the patient who needs minimal support and is able to negotiate stairs.
- *Single-ended cane with a straight handle.* This is ideal for the patient with hand weakness who has good balance.
- *Multiprong canes.* A multiprong cane usually has three or four prongs, and all types have a straight handle. These canes provide a wide base of support and are useful for patients with balance problems.

Walkers

A walker is a lightweight metal frame device with four legs that provides a wide base of support as a patient ambulates. Various forms of walkers are available. Some models have wheels that allow the walker to be rolled forward; others have a seat that allows the

patient to rest periodically (Fig. 31-17B). These walkers are best for patients whose mobility problems are related to fatigue or shortness of breath rather than gait instability.

Braces

Braces support joints and muscles that cannot independently support the body's weight. They are most commonly used in the lower extremities. Physical medicine specialists usually fit the brace. Nursing responsibilities include assisting the patient into and out of the brace and monitoring the condition of the skin under the brace.

Crutches

Crutches are commonly used for rehabilitation of an injured lower extremity. The purpose of using crutches is to limit or eliminate weight bearing on the leg(s) by forcing the user to rely on strength in the arms and shoulders for support. Two forms of crutches are available.

The *forearm support crutch* is more likely to be used by a patient with permanent limitations. It is usually constructed of lightweight aluminum with a hand hold and a forearm support (Fig. 31-18A).

Axillary crutches are for both short- and long-term use (Fig. 31-18B). Properly fitted axillary crutches support the body weight in the hands and arms, not the axilla. For guidelines on how to measure a patient for an axillary crutch,

 Go to Chapter 31, **Clinical Insight 31-5: Sizing Walking Aids,** in Volume 2.

Crutch walking taxes the arms and hands and may cause discomfort to the axillae, arms, and palms where the patient is bearing weight. There are five crutch gaits: two-point gait, three-point gait, four-point gait, swing-to gait, and swing-through gait. Two-point and four-point gait are used for partial weight bearing, whereas

FIGURE 31-16 Three types of canes.

FIGURE 31-17 Walkers. *A*, The basic walker is picked up and advanced as the patient steps ahead. *B*, Some walkers have wheels and seats that allow the patient to rest periodically.

FIGURE 31-18 Crutches. *A,* Forearm support crutches. *B,* Axillary crutches.

three-point gait is used when weight bearing must be avoided. Swing-to and swing-through are used when weight-bearing is permitted.

✚ Navigating stairs with crutches can be quite dangerous. When possible, have the patient practice this technique before discharge.

For basic gaits and guidelines for teaching patients to use crutches,

Go to Chapter 31, **Clinical Insight 31-6: Teaching Clients to Use Canes, Walkers, and Crutches,** in Volume 2.

To see animations of crutch gaits,

 Go to **Animations: 5 Types of Crutch Gaits** on DavisPlus at http://davisplus.fadavis.com/Wilkinson2

KnowledgeCheck 31-10

- What type of cane should a patient with significant balance problems use?
- When are forearm support crutches used?
- Identify five crutch gaits.

 Go to Chapter 31, **Knowledge Check Response Sheet and Answers,** on the Student Resource Disk or DavisPlus at http://davisplus.fadavis.com/Wilkinson2

CriticalThinking 31-6

Discuss crutch walking with your peers and family. What instruction would facilitate the best understanding of proper crutch-walking technique?

CarePlanning & Mapping Practice

For a nursing care plan for Impaired Physical Mobility,

 Go to Chapter 31, **Nursing Care Plan, Impaired Physical Mobility,** on the Student Resource Disk or DavisPlus at http://davisplus.fadavis.com/Wilkinson2

 Go to Chapter 31, **Resources for Caregivers and Health Professionals,** on the Student Resource Disk or DavisPlus at http://davisplus.fadavis.com/Wilkinson2

 Suggested Readings: Go to Chapter 31, **Reading More About Activity and Exercise,** on the Student Resource Disk or DavisPlus at http://davisplus.fadavis.com/Wilkinson2

 Bibliography: Go to Volume 2, Bibliography.

CHAPTER 32

Sexual Health

Learning Outcomes

After completing this chapter, you should be able to:

➤ Identify the female and male reproductive organs.

➤ Describe the physical, emotional, social, and spiritual aspects of human sexuality.

➤ Explain how gender, gender identity, and sexual orientation contribute to expression of sexuality throughout the life cycle.

➤ Differentiate between typical and atypical forms of sexual expression.

➤ Explore physical and psychological issues that affect sexuality and sexual functioning.

➤ Complete a sexual history as part of a comprehensive nursing assessment.

➤ State nursing diagnoses to describe sexuality problems.

➤ Explain how sexual health is challenged by high-risk sexual behaviors, sexually transmitted infections (STIs), menstrual problems, infertility, negative intimate relationships, sexual harassment, rape, and disorders of the sexual response cycle.

➤ Provide nursing interventions that enhance sexual well-being.

➤ Discuss strategies to increase your personal comfort and confidence in providing holistic nursing care.

➤ Describe approaches for dealing with inappropriate sexual behavior from patients or in the work environment.

Meet Your Patients

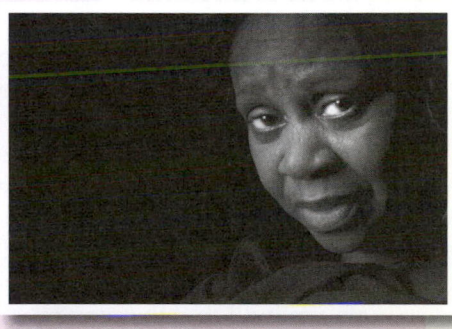

Two days after undergoing a fine-needle aspiration to evaluate a small breast mass, Jocelyn Carter's surgeon informed her that the mass was malignant. He recommended a mastectomy (removal of the breast). Today, she arrives alone at the surgery registration area. You ask how she is feeling, and she tells you that the last week has been a whirlwind of activity. "I had to arrange child care, cancel a business trip, and organize the house so that I could take a few days off to have the surgery. My husband is working overseas this fall, so he couldn't be here to help me. Honestly, I don't know how I'm feeling. I haven't had time to think about it." A few minutes later, as she waits in the surgery holding area, she begins to cry.

You hold her hand and ask whether she would like to talk. She asks you, "Do you think my husband will still want me? I'm afraid he will be turned off when he looks at me."

Gabriel Thomas comes to the outpatient clinic complaining of a throbbing headache over the last 3 days. He explains that he has tried several over-the-counter medicines and has had no relief. You check his blood pressure, and measure the reading at 240/130 mm Hg.

(continued on next page)

Meet Your Patients (continued)

When you ask whether he has ever been treated for high blood pressure, he replies, "Are you another one of these people trying to get me to take drugs that will ruin my sex life?"

Frank Thanee, who has heart disease, had a mitral valve replacement 3 days ago. He has been transferred to the cardiology floor for an additional day of hospitalization. His partner, Greg, has spent the last 3 days at the hospital and has just left to check on the apartment and feed their cat. Frank confides that he is worried about his parents' expected visit. "I've never been able to tell them about Greg. They wouldn't be able to understand it, never mind approve. I don't know how to handle this. What do you think I should do?"

Although each of these clients has a different medical diagnosis, all are experiencing a concern related to

sexuality. In this chapter, we explore the relationship between health and sexuality, as well as the nurse's role in promoting sexual health.

Theoretical **Knowledge**
knowing why

When a baby is born, the first question the parents ask is, "Is it a boy or a girl?" In fact, many parents want to know the gender of their baby at the first sonogram, early in the pregnancy. For most parents, this eagerness reflects the fact that their baby's gender will influence their choice of name, clothing, toys, nursery decor, and even the ways they handle and communicate with their infant. Hopes and dreams of future parent–child relationships (e.g., mother-daughter) often begin to form even during the first months of pregnancy. Such is the power of gender.

However, sexuality encompasses much more than gender. It includes how we perceive ourselves, how we relate to others, and how we express ourselves as sexual beings. Like many people, you may have been socialized to avoid talking openly about sexuality. As a nurse, though, you will find that you must discuss a variety of issues that are vital for clients' optimal wellness. Some of these discussions may include sexual concerns, dysfunctions, infections, or behaviors. As you gain theoretical knowledge and reflect on the issues of human sexuality, you will be challenged to confront your own biases related to sexuality and to set those aside as you work with your clients. You must meet this challenge to address your clients' sexual health needs in a comfortable and competent manner.

Sexual and Reproductive Anatomy and Physiology

The reproductive system plays a role in human life that extends far beyond its basic function of producing children. It influences body image, sexual desire, and sense of sexual identity. The first step in exploring human sexuality is to understand the basics of reproductive anatomy and physiology. (For more information to supplement the brief review that follows, consult an anatomy, physiology, or women's health text.)

Female Reproductive Organs

The female reproductive system consists of a pair of ovaries and fallopian tubes, the uterus, vagina, and external genital tissues (Fig. 32-1). **Ova** (eggs) are produced in the ovaries and travel through the fallopian tubes to the uterus. If fertilization occurs, the embryo embeds in the wall of the uterus for further development.

The **vagina** is a muscular tube that receives sperm during sexual intercourse, allows the exit of menstrual flow if fertilization does not occur, and serves as a birth canal at the end of pregnancy.

The external genitalia and the mons pubis are a source of pleasurable sensations. The **mons pubis** is a pad of fatty tissue over the symphysis pubis. It is covered with coarse hair and contains sensitive nerve endings. The external genitalia, or **vulva,** consist of the clitoris, labia majora, labia minora, Bartholin's glands, urinary meatus, and vaginal introitus. The **clitoris** contains erectile tissue, blood vessels, and nerves. It is extremely sensitive and reacts to pleasurable stimuli. The **labia majora** protect external genital organs, such as the clitoris. The **labia minora**, also engorge and become sensitive to during sexual stimulation.

The breasts play an important role in female sexual arousal; in fact, some women can be brought to orgasm solely by caressing the breasts and nipples. The mammary glands, enclosed within the breasts, are also part of the reproductive system. Their role is to produce milk after the birth of an infant.

FIGURE 32-1 The female reproductive system.

The Menstrual Cycle

The menstrual cycle governs reproductive ability. The menstrual cycle consists of three phases (Fig. 32-2):

Menstrual Phase. Menstruation usually lasts 3 to 7 days, averaging 5 days. During this phase, the uterus sheds the endometrial lining and several ovarian follicles develop. Follicle-stimulating hormone (FSH) from the anterior pituitary begins to increase during this phase, leading to a rise in estrogen levels.

Follicular Phase. This phase begins on the first day of menstrual bleeding and is associated with growth of ovarian follicles and regrowth of the endometrium of the uterus. This phase ends with **ovulation,** or release of the ovum from the mature follicle, around day 13 or 14 of the menstrual cycle. Luteinizing hormone (LH) levels from the anterior pituitary rise, as does the estrogen level.

Ovulatory Phase. Lasting about 16 to 36 hours, a surge in LH and FSH occurs. The follicle then ruptures and the egg is released for fertilization. Estrogen peaks and progesterone rises, which stimulates growth of the endometrium.

Luteal Phase. If fertilization occurs, the endometrium thickens to support an embryo. The pregnancy hormone, called chorionic gonadotropin, is produced; pregnancy tests are based on detecting levels of this hormone. If fertilization does not occur, progesterone levels drop, and menses begins.

Male Reproductive Organs

The male reproductive system consists of the testes and a series of ducts and glands that transport sperm. Sperm are produced in the testes and transported through the epididymis, ductus deferens, ejaculatory duct, and urethra (Fig. 32-3). Along the path, the reproductive glands (seminal vesicles, prostate, and bulbourethral glands) add secretions that mix with the sperm to produce semen.

The penis functions in the urinary system to transport urine from the bladder to the outside of the body. It has important functions in the reproductive system as well. Within the penis are three sections of erectile tissue: the corpus cavernosum and sections of corpus spongiosum above and below the urethra. During sexual arousal these erectile tissues fill with blood, making the penis erect. **Ejaculation** (the expulsion of semen) is brought about by peristalsis of the reproductive ducts and contraction of the prostate and muscles of the pelvic floor. With each ejaculation, approximately 100 million sperm cells are expelled in 2 to 4 mL of semen.

KnowledgeCheck 32-1

- Identify the major structures of the female reproductive system.
- Summarize the phases of the menstrual cycle.
- Identify the major structures of the male reproductive system.

 Go to Chapter 32, **Knowledge Check Response Sheet and Answers,** on the Student Resource Disk or DavisPlus at http://davisplus.fadavis.com/Wilkinson2

Sexuality

What do you think of when you see the term *sexuality*? A recent Internet search on the term *sexuality* turned up a hodgepodge of results, including scientific, pornographic, and product-oriented sites. The

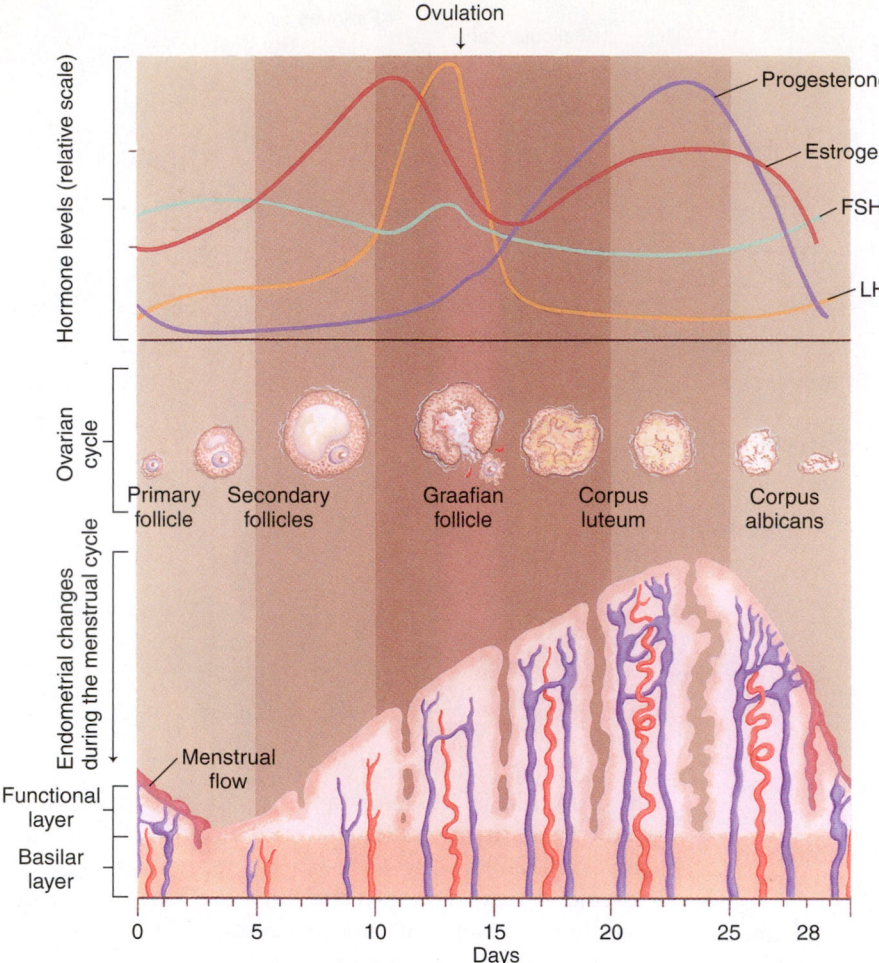

FIGURE 32-2 The menstrual cycle. Hormone levels and endometrial thickness throughout the cycle are shown.

World Health Organization (WHO) describes **sexuality** as a "central aspect of being human throughout life and encompasses sex, gender identities and roles, sexual orientation, eroticism, pleasure, intimacy and reproduction" (WHO, 2002). **Sexual identity** is a person's perception of his or her gender, gender identity, gender role, and sexual orientation. All of these are also a part of the person's overall self-concept (see Chapter 11 to review self-concept).

What Is Gender?

People often think of *sexuality* as a synonym for *sex*. This is inaccurate. In fact, even the word *sex* has multiple meanings. For example, *sex* is used to describe intimate pleasurable activity (e.g., "We had sex yesterday") or to indicate whether an individual is male or female (e.g., "What sex is your baby?"). In this chapter, we use the term **gender** to indicate biological sex status (male or female) and follow the World Health Organization's definition of sexuality.

Gender is determined at the moment of conception, when an ovum is fertilized by a sperm. The ovum always provides an X chromosome, whereas the sperm may contribute either a second X chromosome, which results in a female offspring, or a Y chromosome, resulting in a male offspring (Fig. 32-4).

Gender Roles

Gender roles are the societal norms for gender-appropriate behavior. During the 1950s, the media portrayed the father-in-a-suit who went off to work to support his family. Mother, in her apron, spent the day cooking, cleaning, and caring for her perfect children and devoted husband. Even then, many Americans did not identify with this stereotype, and today it may seem laughable. But many of these values remain embedded in our culture. Consider your class structure. How many of your classmates are female? How many are male? Nursing and teaching were among the first professions women assumed outside the home, and they are still predominantly female. In contrast, most auto mechanics, plumbers, and politicians are men.

Historically in North America, most people expected men to be strong and to control their feelings, and women to be gentle and to express their feelings. Boys received positive reinforcement for "masculine" behaviors, such as competitiveness, and may have endured teasing if they showed passivity. In girls, "feminine" behaviors, such as cooperation, were reinforced, whereas assertiveness was often labeled aggression. But in the past 40 or 50 years, many people have defied such stereotypes. Women now commonly perform jobs formerly thought to be "for men only,"

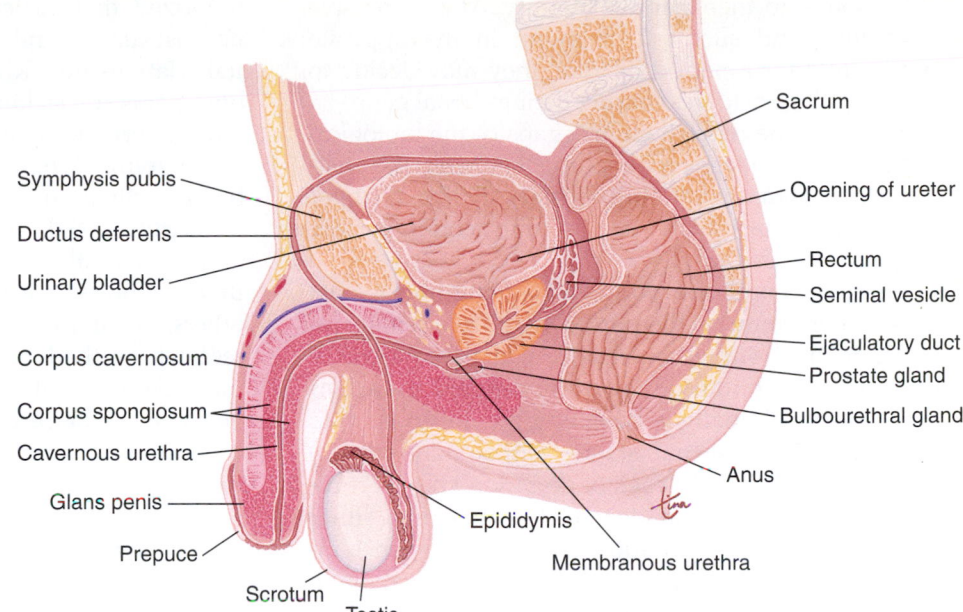

FIGURE 32-3 The male reproductive system.

and men are entering predominantly female professions. Our society's expectations regarding gender roles have changed and expanded.

Today, many parents encourage some **androgyny** in their children. The word *androgyny* is a combination of the Greek words for male, *andro,* and female, *gyn.* By one of its definitions, *androgyny* refers to a blending of traditional masculine and feminine roles. It means that everyone has some skills, traits, and behaviors that may be classified as "masculine" and some that may be "feminine." Androgyny is a positive trait in that it gives an individual greater adaptability in life situations.

FIGURE 32-4 The woman provides the X chromosome, and the man may contribute either a second X chromosome, which results in a female offspring, or a Y chromosome, resulting in a male offspring.

Critical Thinking 32-1

- Provide at least three examples of nonconformity to traditional gender role expectations.
- As a parent, how might you encourage androgyny in your children, if you wished to do so?

Gender Identity

Gender identity, one component of sexual identity, is the image we have about ourselves as a man or woman. It is an internal experience: whether we "feel like" a woman or a man. Usually a little girl sees herself growing up to be a woman, and a young boy sees his future as a man. However, some children form a gender identity that is not the same as their biological gender.

Transgendered (or "differently gendered") is a broad term used to describe people whose gender identity differs in some way from their apparent biological gender. For example, some people think of themselves as female even though they have male genitalia. Longitudinal studies have shown that transgendered persons may be transsexual, intersexed, or cross-dressing; and heterosexual, homosexual, or bisexual (Zucker, 2000).

- **Transsexuals** are people who identify with the opposite gender from their biology—for example, a person with the physical appearance and reproductive organs of a woman who "feels" and perceives herself to be a man. It is common for transsexuals to express dissatisfaction with their gender at an early age. They may insist that they will grow up to be the opposite gender. Their preference for dress and play is more typical of those of the other gender.
- **Preoperative transsexuals** are adults who alter their physical appearance through dress, make-up, and/or the use of hormones so that their external appearance

corresponds to their gender identity. After extensive counseling and successfully living in the opposite gender role for a period of time, they may decide to undergo surgery to reconstruct their external genitalia and remove the reproductive organs of the biological birth gender. After sex reassignment surgery, the **postoperative transsexual individual** legally changes gender. For the transsexual or transgender person, single rooms are best.

- **Intersexed** people are born with ambiguous sexual organs. For example, the person may have female internal organs (ovaries, a uterus), but an external penis. Previously, such individuals were referred to as **hermaphrodites.** Initially, a developing embryo is in an **undifferentiated sexual state**—neither male nor female. At about the 7th week of gestation, the sex chromosomes direct the gonads to differentiate into either testes or ovaries. A mutation of any of the genes involved in sexual differentiation or an alteration in hormonal secretion may result in gender alterations. Parents must then face the difficult decision whether to assign a sex and have the child undergo surgery to change the physical appearance or to delay assignment and allow the child to choose at a later time.

- A **cross-dresser** (or **transvestite**) is a person who occasionally or frequently wears the clothing characteristic of the opposite sex, particularly the undergarments, as a form of sexual expression. Often the person carries out this behavior in secret. Cross-dressers may be heterosexual, homosexual, or bisexual (see the next section, "What Is Sexual Orientation?"). The majority of research on transvestites has focused on men who choose to dress as women, but women also cross-dress.

KnowledgeCheck 32-2

- How is gender determined?
- Distinguish gender, gender role, and gender identity.
- What is androgyny?

  Go to Chapter 32, **Knowledge Check Response Sheet and Answers,** on the Student Resource Disk or DavisPlus at http://davisplus.fadavis.com/Wilkinson2

CriticalThinking 32-2

Do you believe that androgyny is a positive attribute? Explain your thinking.

What Is Sexual Orientation?

Sexual orientation refers to the general tendency of a person to feel sexually attracted to people of a certain gender. Because most people in North America are thought to be **heterosexual** (sexually attracted to members of the opposite sex), heterosexuality is the predominant cultural expectation. However, in the mid-20th century, the research of Alfred C. Kinsey indicated that a population's sexual orientation falls on a bell curve, with the majority of people experiencing at least some attraction to people of the same gender. Kinsey theorized that society influences people to sublimate homosexual feelings and choose exclusively heterosexual relationships. Kinsey's work, which was faulted by opponents for lacking objectivity, was followed by the work of Fritz Klein, who described sexual orientation as an ongoing dynamic process, with people's gender-based inclinations changing over time.

In truth, we do not fully understand what makes up sexual orientation or how it develops. Some theories hold that it evolves as a result of early learning experiences; others, that it is biologically determined. With increasing research on the biological aspects of sexual orientation, more professionals are concluding that people come to "recognize" the object of their sexual desire rather than "choose" or "prefer" it. Therefore, "sexual orientation" is probably a more accurate term than "sexual preference."

Heterosexuality

As just mentioned, **heterosexuals** are people who are sexually and emotionally attracted to members of the opposite sex. This segment of the population may be referred to as *straight*. Many major religious traditions reinforce heterosexual behaviors and gender roles. Although some heterosexuals have had same-gender sexual thoughts or limited experiences during childhood, adolescence, or adulthood, they still consider themselves heterosexual and have relationships with people of the opposite gender.

Homosexuality

The focus of sexual attraction for **homosexuals** is a person of the same gender. Homosexuals may be referred to as gay men and lesbian women. According to a CNN exit poll, approximately 4% of the voting population in the 2008 United States presidential election identified themselves as gay, lesbian, or bisexual. Accurate prevalence statistics are difficult to obtain because most of the studies listed below rely on self-report data. Because homosexuality is not an aspect of the dominant culture and is prohibited by some religions, there has been significant discrimination against homosexuals. It can be difficult for gays and lesbians to share this aspect of their lives with employers, colleagues, family, and friends, much less with researchers and pollsters. Some homosexuals openly acknowledge to both self and others that they are gay; others do not and hide their sexual preference from family, friends, employers, and people in their communities. Of note, the *Diagnostic and Statistical Manual of Mental Disorders IV* of the American Psychiatric Association (2000) does not classify homosexuality as a psychiatric disorder.

Bisexuality

A person who is **bisexual** is sexually and emotionally attracted to both males and females. This group is perhaps least understood and least accepted by both the heterosexual and homosexual communities. They are less likely to be found in long-term monogamous relationships and often experience feelings of isolation. However, some bisexuals maintain stable and satisfying marriages because of their sustained sexual attraction to and amiable relationship with their spouse and the importance they place on parenting. Compatibility within the marriage depends on the partner's acceptance of the bisexual spouse's sexual orientation and sexual relationships outside the marriage, if any.

KnowledgeCheck 32-3

- What are the majority and minority sexual orientations in our culture?
- What is meant by transgender?

  Go to Chapter 32, **Knowledge Check Response Sheet and Answers,** on the Student Resource Disk or DavisPlus at http://davisplus.fadavis.com/Wilkinson2

 CriticalThinking 32-3

- What sexual orientations are you comfortable working with?
- Would you have difficulty working with a transsexual or other transgendered client?

How Does Sexuality Develop?

We are sexual beings from birth to death. Expression of our sexuality evolves through the life span. For additional discussion on sexuality and developmental stages,

Go to Chapter 9, **Expanded Discussion,** on the Student Resource Disk or DavisPlus at http://davisplus.fadavis.com/Wilkinson2

Birth Through Preschool

Beginning at the moment of birth, parents, caregivers, and others respond to the infant with preconceived thoughts of what that gender role entails. The first 2 years of life can be highly sensual; as infants are nursed, stroked, bathed, and massaged, they develop their first attachment experience through bonding with the parent or other caregiver (Fig. 32-5). It is not unusual for

FIGURE 32-5 Parent-infant attachment occurs through daily contact and care through activities such as feeding, bathing, and holding.

children in this age group to touch their genitals and enjoy being nude. This behavior is part of their exploration of their bodies and is a normal part of child development. By age 3, most children recognize gender differences and know the names of body parts. Toddlers are interested in their bodies and curious to see the genitals of others.

By age 5, children mimic adults by holding hands or hugging. Adults, who find these actions amusing or endearing, frequently reinforce such behaviors. Young children also may practice getting married, playing house, or playing doctor. It is not unusual for preschool children to masturbate and ask questions about "where babies come from." Parents should give factual answers without offering explanations beyond what the child asks.

School Age Through Puberty

The school-age child strongly identifies with the same-sex parent and has mostly same-sex friends. Through interaction at home, school, and other activities, children gain awareness of gender roles and emerging gender identity.

From age 8 to 12, the child is in transition between childhood and puberty. Secondary sex characteristics become apparent. In females, breast buds form, and pubic hair appears. For a significant number of girls, **menarche** (beginning of menstruation) occurs. Boys become more muscular, the voice deepens, hair in facial and axillae develop, and the genitals begin to increase in size. The first attraction, either heterosexual or homosexual, may occur during this stage, and the child may begin to masturbate more frequently, but privately. For information on the Tanner stages of sexual development in boys and girls,

 Go to Chapter 19, **Procedures 19-17 and 19-18,** in Volume 2.

Many school-age children are curious about sexual activity, reproduction, and sex roles, and they may ask explicit questions. Parents and nurses should answer with facts and follow up with age-appropriate printed material. By age 10 to 12, parents should begin teaching children basic information about approaching body changes, menstruation, sexual intercourse, and reproduction.

Adolescents

Adolescence is a time of heightened sexual interest and activity. There are two reasons for this: (1) the hormonal changes accompanying puberty and (2) the culture's emphasis on sex. Masturbation is common. It is a safe and comforting sexual activity that has neither interpersonal nor disease risks. However, some adolescents may encounter parental, cultural, or religious disapproval of masturbation.

Sexual exploration usually begins with kissing, moves on to fondling, and can lead to genital contact. This progression may occur over a period of years, or there may be an early initiation of oral, vaginal, or anal intercourse. Although about 75% of adolescents are sexually active by their late teen years, the teen pregnancy rate is slowly dropping (Alan Guttmacher Institute, 2002, updated December 2006; U.S. Department of Health and Human Services [USDHHS], 2006, updated October 2008). However, the incidence of oral sex is increasing in early adolescence. Many teens believe that this behavior allows them to maintain their virginity and incorrectly assume that it carries no health risks.

Sexuality education in the home and school dispels myths and prepares teens for adult roles. To make informed choices as they move toward adulthood, adolescents need information about body changes, interpersonal relationships, **contraception** (birth control), and preventing **sexually transmitted infections (STIs)**. To review physical changes of adolescence, see Chapters 9, Expanded, and 19.

Young Adults

Not so many years ago it was generally assumed that young adults would abstain from sexual intercourse until marriage, when the husband and wife could become sexually active and start a family. Today, marriage is often delayed, and young adults engage more openly in premarital sex. Many young adults practice **serial monogamy,** in which the partners are mutually faithful but make no lifelong commitment. When the relationship ends, each partner usually enters another monogamous relationship.

During early adulthood, people define their sexual identity and resolve issues related to their sexual orientation. As a part of sexual maturity, they develop an intimate relationship in which there is both communication and respect. Many people find a life partner during this period and make long-term plans, which often include parenting. However, some adults continue to struggle with their sexual identity, sexual orientation, or ability to form or commit to intimate relationships.

Young adults often wonder whether their sexual behaviors and responses are normal (e.g., "How often do most people have intercourse?" "Do other women have an orgasm every time they have sex?"). Many still need information about birth control, prevention of STIs, and relationship and communication issues.

Middle Adults

Many adults in the middle years experience life changes that may enhance physical and emotional intimacy. The children have left the home, college and weddings are paid for, careers are settled or winding down, and concerns about pregnancy are gone. However, this may also be a time when physical changes and chronic diseases emerge to affect sexual patterns.

Women transition through **menopause** (cessation of menstruation), a process that varies widely. Some are relieved that the prospect of childbearing has ended; others may mourn the loss of the ability to give birth. Normal physiological changes that result from decreased

levels of estrogen and progesterone include decreased vaginal secretions and vaginal wall thinning. These changes may result in painful intercourse and decrease a woman's desire for sexual activity. Some women also experience hot flashes, sleep disturbances, and mood changes.

Men, as a result of the aging process or health conditions (e.g., type 2 diabetes or hypertension), may experience erectile difficulty. They may perceive this problem as a threat to their masculinity and sexual attractiveness, and their self-image may suffer. Men also experience a decrease in the sex hormone testosterone. Sexual desire and the ability to achieve and maintain erection may decrease gradually, but many men remain fertile into old age.

It is important to recognize that middle adults may have sexual concerns that should be addressed. This may be difficult for young nurses, because patients of this age may remind them of their parents. It can be a challenge to view them as individuals who engage in and enjoy sexual relations.

Aging Adults

Most older adults are sexually active and regard sexuality as an important part of life, according to national data from the National Social Life, Health, and Aging Project (NSHAP). Sexual activity does decline with age, yet a substantial number of men and women engage in vaginal intercourse, oral sex, and masturbation even in their 80s and 90s (Lindau, Schuman, Laumann, et al., 2007). Sexual problems are more likely to result from failing physical health and medication side effects than from age alone. For example, as noted earlier, men with diabetes are more likely to have difficulty achieving and maintaining an erection. Other obstacles for sexual expression are lack of a partner (especially for women) and lack of privacy (e.g., for those who live with family members or in a long-term care facility).

As a result of age-related changes, postmenopausal women report less sexual stimulation and reduced desire, so they tend to need more foreplay and direct clitoral stimulation for sexual enjoyment. They may have fewer orgasms or orgasms that are weaker in intensity. Nevertheless, some women "rediscover" sexual desire after menopause. Poorer health has been associated with a lower likelihood of masturbation among older women (Laumann, Paik, Glasser, et al., 2006). Many older women complain of loss of vaginal lubrication. Some have pain during intercourse, usually caused by vaginal thinning and dryness. You can help your patients by suggesting water-soluble lubricants to counteract vaginal dryness and enhance pleasurable sensations during sexual activity.

Some men report erectile difficulty and need more time and more direct genital stimulation to achieve erection. It may take longer to ejaculate, and the orgasmic contractions may be less intense. When penetration is not possible (e.g., because of male erectile dysfunction), many couples find satisfaction with alternate forms of sexual stimulation and expression.

Older adults frequently experience sexual problems, but may hesitate to discuss them with healthcare providers unless encouraged to do so. But if you bring up the subject and people feel comfortable, then they are eager for advice. In the past, many healthcare providers have hesitated to offer sexual counseling, out of fear that such intimate discussion might offend their patients. However, people with problems are eager for advice (American Geriatric Society Foundation for Health in Aging, n.d.). Even terminally ill people have sexual needs (e.g., reassurance from sexual partner or sexual stimulation) or sexual problems (e.g., lack of closeness).

You can help aging clients to understand that sexual feelings do not necessarily disappear with age, and sexual expression need not stop (Fig. 32-6). Suggest alternatives to intercourse when illness or disability interfere. For example, sexual expression may include hugging, caressing, oral sex, and mutual manual stimulation. In addition, you may suggest ways to adapt coital positions to accommodate bodily changes, for example, when a partner is obese or has joint immobility.

KnowledgeCheck 32-4

- Why is it important to consider sexuality throughout the life cycle?
- What are the two major contributing factors to adolescents' heightened sexual interest and activity?
- What aspects of human sexuality are associated with young and middle adulthood?
- What challenges to sexuality may be found in the aging adult?

 Go to Chapter 32, **Knowledge Check Response Sheet and Answers,** on the Student Resource Disk or DavisPlus at http://davisplus.fadavis.com/Wilkinson2

FIGURE 32-6 Healthy older adults maintain sexual intimacy.

What Factors Affect Sexuality?

Culture, religion, lifestyle, sexual knowledge, and physical health all influence our attitudes toward sexuality, sexual behaviors, and intimate relationships. This knowledge can help you to provide nonjudgmental, holistic care to people who have a wide range of values, lifestyles, and states of well-being.

Culture

Culture influences our ideas about gender role, gender identity, marriage, sexual expression, and social responsibilities. However, it is not unusual for people to be ethnocentric—that is, to see their own culture and sexual behaviors as the norm for all. Because the United States is a multicultural country, beliefs and practices related to human sexuality vary widely. Consider the following examples of cultural influences.

- Victorian-era and later Puritan legacies have influenced many European-Americans, some of whom consider sex to be "not nice," particularly if engaging in certain sexual activities or positions.
- Blacks are influenced by the dominant Anglo-Saxon culture as well as by their African heritage, history in America, and current economic and social situation. Marriage rates for blacks are lower than for other ethnic groups, in part because of an unequal gender ratio (84 males per 100 females), as well as cultural acceptance of single parenting (Hyde & DeLamater, 2008).
- Many Latinos have strong ties to the Roman Catholic Church and a tradition of rigidly defined gender roles. The norm in Hispanic culture is for the male to be given more freedom as a child, but he is expected to be a virile, responsible provider for his family as an adult. In contrast, the female is typically raised to be more passive and obedient throughout her life.
- Asian Americans and Muslim Americans tend to be the most sexually conservative of the major U.S. cultural groups.

Culture determines what is acceptable and what is not. In some societies, **polygamy** (marriage to more than one partner) may be acceptable. Another culture may permit or prohibit sexual play among children. Many cultures have special rites of passage at puberty, such as the Jewish bar mitzvah for boys and bat mitzvah for girls, or the Native American vision quest.

Generally, you should honor cultural practices unless they are harmful. An example of a harmful practice is female genital mutilation (formerly known as **female circumcision**), which is illegal in most countries but is still performed among certain tribes. In this procedure, the labia majora, labia minora, and clitoris are excised, and/or the vagina is sutured closed **(infibulation).** Infibulation may be done to ensure that the girl remains a virgin, whereas clitoral excision is meant to reduce sexual desire and ensure that the woman remains faithful to her husband. In addition to its psychosocial consequences, the procedure carries a high risk of infection and can cause the development of scar tissue that makes vaginal birth impossible. In 1997, the World Health Organization issued a statement to abolish the practice of female genital mutilation. A new statement with expanded United Nations support was released in 2008 to advocate abandonment of this practice (WHO, 2008). Domestically, the U.S. Congress passed a law in 1996 making female genital mutilation for girls younger than 18 a federal offense.

Religion

Religion also has a powerful influence on sexuality. Religious practices restricting premarital sex, birth control, homosexuality, abortion, extramarital relationships, and masturbation are common. Some religions have rules about body coverings, modesty, and restricting opposite gender healthcare providers. Even education about the structure and function of the human body is governed by some religions. The "sexual revolution" that began in the 1960s has led to permissive sexual values in the wider North American society. When these values conflict with a person's traditional religious values, anxiety and sexual dysfunction may result. To review the influence of religion on health, see Chapter 14.

CriticalThinking 32-4

How have religion and culture influenced your views on sexuality?

Lifestyle

Life experiences encompass our interactions with others and the environment. Family, socioeconomic status, employment factors, and interpersonal relationships shape our lifestyle, although they do not fully determine it. Consider the following examples:

- Having a beloved brother reveal to you that he is gay might alter your perception of homosexuality. Similarly, being raised by a lesbian couple might affect your view of gender roles.
- Growing up in a low-income neighborhood in which prostitution is a visible and accepted part of the environment might influence your views on what is acceptable sexual behavior.
- Dedication to a high-stress job or the demands of raising young children might leave you too exhausted to desire sex with your spouse, whereas retirement might bring time to develop your range of intimate expression.
- Being in an abusive relationship would affect how you feel about yourself and might cause you to avoid intimacy in the future.

Lessons learned through day-to-day experience create powerful impressions on our views and often modify cultural and religious influences.

Sexual Knowledge

Although sexuality and family life are part of the curriculum in many public schools, you cannot assume that young adults have adequate sexual knowledge. Community values play a large role in determining how sexuality is viewed and taught. Thus, even if a state mandates sex education, a particular school may limit discussion on reproduction, STIs, birth control, intimacy, exploitive relationships, domestic abuse, or rape, believing that these topics are best addressed by the family or church. In addition, many children are home-schooled or taught in private or church-affiliated schools that do not allocate any class time to sex education. Even in schools with a comprehensive curriculum, parents have the right to exclude their child from sex education classes. Do not let your clients' age, level of education, or life experiences lead you to make assumptions about their knowledge of sexuality. For example:

- A married person may not be sexually active.
- A woman with several children may not know what is involved in a pelvic exam or how conception occurs.
- A highly educated person may be uninformed regarding his body structure and function.

It is difficult for most people to admit to a professional that they lack knowledge. Therefore, you must assess each client's knowledge and understanding of sexual terms. At times you may need to use the vernacular or "street" terminology to be understood. You can then introduce medically specific terminology.

KnowledgeCheck 32-5

- What sexual knowledge would you expect an adult male with children to have?
- What sexual knowledge would you expect a nursing student to have?

Go to Chapter 32, **Knowledge Check Response Sheet and Answers,** on the Student Resource Disk or DavisPlus at http://davisplus.fadavis.com/Wilkinson2

Health and Illness

Sexuality involves body, mind, and spirit; so, it is not surprising that health status affects sexuality. For example, healthful nutrition and physical exercise are commonly reported to increase satisfaction in sexual relationships, whereas overweight and inactivity can undermine one's own feelings of attractiveness or one's attraction for one's partner. The importance of sexuality is readily apparent in the clinical setting. For example, the clients in the "Meet Your Patients" scenarios all expressed concerns related to their sexuality.

Physical Illness

Diseases, injuries, and medical treatments may demand lifestyle changes in multiple areas, including sexual functioning.

- *Heart disease or respiratory disease* may cause people to restrict sexual activity because of fatigue, dyspnea, or fear of overstressing the heart.
- *Diabetes mellitus* leads to neurological changes that may cause male erectile dysfunction; women may experience vaginal dryness and loss of orgasmic ability. In addition, vaginal yeast infections are common with diabetes, causing itching and painful intercourse.
- *Cancer* may be accompanied by body image changes, fatigue, treatments that create nausea, and fear of death—all of which lead to feeling unattractive and a reduced desire for sexual activity.
- *Spinal cord injury* may make it impossible for the person to feel physical stimulation. Depending on the level of the injury, the person may or may not experience psychogenic or reflexogenic genital arousal. Some men may be able to achieve erection and ejaculation and are fertile; others may have no genital response.
- *Surgeries,* in addition to causing pain in the early postoperative period, may alter a person's body image. At the least, surgery leaves a physical scar. At worst, it removes a body part or creates other disfigurement. When the surgery involves body parts important to sexual functioning (e.g., a breast, a testicle), the effect is even more likely to be negative. Because some people feel ugly after such procedures and worry about their partner's reactions to their appearance, they may avoid having sex. Two very common surgeries are hysterectomy and prostatectomy:

    Hysterectomy (surgical removal of a uterus) may enhance the sexual experience if it relieves pain and bleeding that were present before surgery. In contrast, some women report difficulty becoming aroused or having less intense orgasm after hysterectomy. These problems may be related to trauma to nerves in the pelvic area, to the absence of uterine contractions during orgasm, or to anxiety because so much of the woman's gender identity had been tied to childbearing.

    Prostatectomy (removal of the prostate gland, usually to treat prostate cancer) may be accompanied by erectile and other sexual dysfunction.

If a person becomes disabled while in a marriage or other committed relationship, the strain can threaten the partnership. In contrast, a person who is single or has a life-long disability may experience difficulty establishing an intimate relationship because of physical limitations, social isolation, poor self-image, or discrimination. Even when people lose interest in sexual intercourse, a need for intimacy still exists. Communication about sexual needs and desires may be difficult for couples, but as a nurse, you can support and facilitate it. Rehabilitation programs ideally offer holistic services and facilitate discussion regarding sexuality and relationship issues.

Psychiatric Disorders

Psychiatric disorders can lead to interpersonal disruptions and difficulty with sexual expression.

- A depressed person experiences significant loss of interest in activities that previously brought pleasure. Thus it is common for people with depression to avoid engaging in interpersonal activities, including sex.
- Conversely, a person with hypomania or mania may be preoccupied with pleasurable activities and increased sexual activity, as well as verbalization and acting out. Both extremes are disruptive to a relationship.
- For a person with psychosis, interpersonal relationships and sexual patterns are disrupted by lack of contact with reality or frank delusions.

Counseling for the couple is important when symptoms are controlled. During times of acute illness, support for the partner is vital.

Medications

Many medications used to treat health problems have unwelcome sexual side effects. Gabriel Thomas ("Meet Your Patients") clearly illustrates the concern some clients have about commonly prescribed medications. Table 32-1 lists a number of medications and their effects on sexual function.

Medications may be prescribed to enhance sexual function, particularly for men experiencing erectile dysfunction (ED), for example, those with diabetes mellitus or who are taking beta-adrenergic blocking agents to treat high blood pressure. Three oral drugs are available for impotence: sildenafil, vardenafil, or tadalafil. These drugs generally work within 1 hour of administration, but have no effect without sexual stimulation. They increase blood flow to the corpus cavernosum of the penis.

KnowledgeCheck 32-6

- Identify four factors associated with physical illness that may affect sexuality or sexual functioning.
- What determines our sexual attitudes?

 Go to Chapter 32, **Knowledge Check Response Sheet and Answers,** on the Student Resource Disk or DavisPlus at http://davisplus.fadavis.com/Wilkinson2

Sexual Health

The World Health Organization defines **sexual health** as a state of physical, emotional, mental, and social well-being related to sexuality; it is not merely the absence of disease, dysfunction, or infirmity. Sexual health requires a positive and respectful approach to sexuality and sexual relationships, as well as the openness and opportunity to have pleasurable and safe sexual experiences, free of coercion, discrimination, and violence. For sexual health to be attained and maintained, the sexual rights of all persons must be respected, protected, and fulfilled (WHO, 2002). To promote sexual health effectively, you will need theoretical knowledge about sexual responses, modes of sexual expression, and problems affecting sexuality.

Table 32-1 ➤ Effects of Drugs on Sexual Function

MEDICATION	POSSIBLE EFFECT
Alcohol	In limited quantities, alcohol may enhance desire and function. However, heavy or chronic use may lead to decreased libido, orgasmic dysfunction, and erectile dysfunction.
Antianxiety agents	Decreased libido, delayed ejaculation
Anticonvulsants	Decreased libido, prolonged painful erections, difficulty achieving orgasm
Antidepressants	Decreased libido, difficulty achieving orgasm
	Bupropion (Wellbutrin) and trazodone (Desyrel) are least likely to cause sexual side effects.
Antihistamines	Decreased libido, decreased vaginal lubrication
Antihypertensives	Decreased libido, erectile dysfunction, delayed ejaculation
	Calcium channel blockers are least likely to cause sexual difficulties.
Chemotherapy	Fatigue, decreased libido
Opioids	Decreased libido, erectile dysfunction
Stimulants (cocaine, methamphetamines)	Initially stimulants cause increased intensity of the sexual encounter; however, with continued use, sexual dysfunction develops.

Critical Thinking 32-5

Examine your own beliefs about sexuality. Identify areas of concern you have regarding sexuality. How do you think this will affect your ability to assist patients with sexual health concerns?

What Is the Sexual Response Cycle?

The **sexual response cycle** is the sequence of physiological events that occur when a person becomes sexually aroused. Based on research conducted in the 1950s, William Masters and Virginia Johnson identified a four-stage sexual response: excitement, plateau, orgasm, and resolution (Fig. 32-7). A growing body of research has called into question this four-stage model.

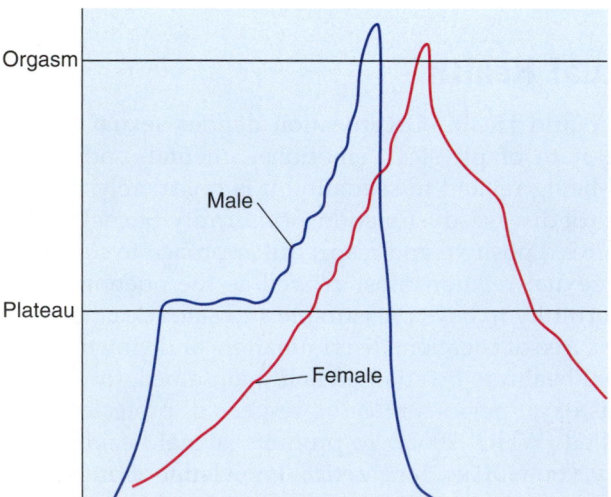

FIGURE 32-7 The sexual response cycle.

One suggested alteration of the original Masters and Johnson model is to add a stage of desire, which in some people precedes and in some people follows excitement (Basson, 2001).

Although it is most intense in the genitals, sexual response is a total body response, involving many physiological changes (e.g., increased heart rate, flushing). The emotional and mental aspects of sexual activity are equally important to the person's satisfaction. The body has many **erogenous zones** (areas that cause sexual arousal when stimulated): the genitals, the skin, lips, ears, breasts, buttocks, and thighs. Box 32-1 shows normal physiological changes in sexual response that occur with aging.

Desire

Desire is a stage of varying length characterized by an interest in sexual intimacy. Desire occurs in the mind and is communicated either verbally or through body language. This communication may be subtle and easily misread. In different cultures, behaviors meant to communicate desire may vary along gender lines. **Libido** is an individual's typical level of desire. In many people, desire is readily aroused by erotic stimuli, such as sights, sounds, and fantasies. However, recent research indicates that a majority of women and a minority of men do not experience desire until after they have become aroused; in these people, physical excitement prompts the desire for sex (Basson, 2001).

Although desire depends on both psychic stimulation and local sexual stimulation, it does increase in proportion to the level of the sex hormones (e.g., a man with low testosterone is not as interested in sex). For

Toward Evidence-Based Practice

Relatively little is known about the sexual behaviors of older people, and the relationship between quality of life and sexuality in older adults has not been fully explored.

Lindau, S. T., Schumm, P., Laumann, E. O., et al. (2007). A study of sexuality and health among older adults in the United States. *New England Journal of Medicine, 357(8),* 762–774.

This study was conducted to explore the sexual behaviors and sexual function of older people. In a sample of 3005 U.S. adults 57 to 85 years of age, researchers found that sexual activity declined with age. Women were significantly less likely than men at all ages to report sexual activity. Of those who were sexually active, about half of both men and women reported at least one sexual problem. The most common complaints among women were low desire, difficulty reaching climax, and difficulty with vaginal lubrication. Men reported erectile difficulty. Men and women who rated their health as poor were less likely to be sexually active. Sexual problems are frequent among older adults, but these problems are infrequently discussed with healthcare providers.

Kleinplatz, P. J. (2008). Sexuality and older people. *BMJ, 337,* a239.

Much of the literature on sexuality in older adults focuses on sexual problems, leaving healthcare providers with the impression that older adults have either dismal or nonexistent sex lives. Little research is available as it pertains to normal sexuality in older adults. This study reports sexual satisfaction is increasing among older adults, especially in women, even if sexual dysfunctions are present. Some dysfunctions, such as erectile dysfunction and female lack of orgasm, are decreasing, whereas sexual problems, such as ejaculatory dysfunction in men, have increased over the past 30 years.

Beckman, N., Waern, M., & Gustafson, D. (2008). Secular trends in self reported sexual activity and satisfaction in Swedish 70 year olds: Cross sectional survey of four populations, 1971–2001. *BMJ, 337,* A279.

Researchers studied trends in sexual behavior among 70-year-olds. They interviewed four samples of Swedish people over a 30-year period and found the 70-year-olds born more recently reported higher satisfaction with sexuality, fewer sexual dysfunctions, and more positive attitudes in sexuality in later life than those who were interviewed earlier in the century. Overall, self-reported quantity and quality of sexual experiences among 70-year-olds improved over time. At the same time, a relatively large proportion of participants had stopped having intercourse. However, most elderly people consider sexual activity and associated feelings a natural part of later life.

Penhollow, T. M., Young, M., & Denny, G. (2009, January/February). Predictors of quality of life, sexual intercourse, and sexual satisfaction in older adults. *American Journal of Health Education, 40,* 1, 13–22.

This study attempted to find out what aspects of sexuality have the greatest influence on sexual intercourse, sexual satisfaction, and overall quality of life in residents of a large active retirement community. Sexual self-confidence was found to be the single most important predictor of sexual intercourse and sexual satisfaction and (for women) quality of life. Cultural (sexual acceptance, sexual priority), psychological (sexual desire, sexual self-confidence, and control), and social factors (satisfaction in relationship and social life) help to explain sexual satisfaction beyond the physical health.

1. What trend in the research about sexuality in older adults do you see?

2. In the Penhollow et al. study, what was the single most important factor influencing sexual satisfaction and quality of life, other than physical health? What do you think nurses can do to promote it?

3. Based on these studies, how do you think nurses can affect the quality of sexuality in older adults?

 Go to Chapter 32, **Toward Evidence-Based Practice Suggested Responses,** on the Student Resource Disk or DavisPlus at http://davisplus.fadavis.com/Wilkinson2

---

women, desire reaches a peak each month near the time of ovulation, when estrogen levels are high.

What is considered "sexual" or "attractive" can vary greatly, because societal, cultural, and personal values influence the range of stimuli that provoke sexual desire. Desire may last only moments or be ongoing for years. Transient sexual thoughts are fleeting moments of desire that might be triggered by exposure to sexually explicit media or erotic thoughts, words or actions. Love and desire do not have to occur within a sexual relationship; this kind of example of desire can last for years.

Excitement

Excitement is the body's physical response to desire. During excitement the following bodily changes occur: Heart rate, blood pressure, and respiratory rate

BOX 32-1 ■ Normal Physiological Changes in Sexual Response that Occur with Aging

Sexual Response Stage	Changes in Women	Changes in Men
Desire	Decreased libido	Decreased libido
Excitement and plateau	Delayed nipple erection	Delayed nipple erection
	Reduced labial separation and swelling	Delayed and less-firm erection
	Reduced vaginal expansion	Longer excitement stage
	Reduced lubrication	Decreased preejaculatory emissions
	Decreased elevation of the uterus	Reduced muscle tension
	Reduced muscle tension	Reduced lifting of the scrotum and testes
	Reduced vaginal tone (in those who have had multiple vaginal deliveries); results in less stimulation during intercourse	Shorter phase of impending orgasm
		May require more direct stimulation to achieve and maintain an erection
Orgasm	Reduced spread of sexual flush	Shorter ejaculation time
		Fewer ejaculatory contractions
		Reduced volume of ejaculate
Resolution	No cervical dilation	More rapid loss of erection
		Longer refractory period
		Nipple erection lasts longer after orgasm

Sources: Stanley, M., et al. (2005). *Gerontological nursing: Promoting successful aging with older adults.* Philadelphia: F. A. Davis; Kennedy-Malone, L., Fletcher, K., & Plank, L. (2004). *Management guidelines for nurse practitioners working with older adults.* Philadelphia: F. A. Davis; Running, A., & Berndt, A. (2003). *Management guidelines for nurse practitioners working in family practice.* Philadelphia: F. A. Davis; EngenderHealth. (2007). Sexual response and aging. *Sexuality and sexual health: An online minicourse.* Retrieved from http://www.engenderhealth.org/res/onc/sexuality/.

increase; muscles tense **(myotonia);** nipples become erect; and genital and pelvic blood supply increases **(vasocongestion).** In women, vasocongestion leads to vaginal lubrication, swelling of the breasts, rise of the uterus, and swelling of the labia and clitoris. In men, erection begins as the penis increases in length and diameter. The testes rise closer to the body, and the scrotum thickens.

Excitement may lead to further sexual activity, but this is not inevitable. For both sexes, the person may lose and regain initial physical excitement many times without advancing to the next stage. Excitement may be communicated verbally or through body language.

Plateau

If stimulation continues, the person reaches the **plateau** phase. Plateau is associated with continued increases in pulse, respiratory rate, blood pressure, and muscle tension. Some people flush around the face, neck, and chest in this phase. In women, the areolae become firmer, the clitoris retracts into the clitoral hood, Bartholin's glands lubricate, and the lower vagina swells and narrows. With a male partner, the vagina tightens around the man's penis, increasing his sexual stimulation. In men, the ridge of the glans penis becomes more prominent, pre-ejaculate (two or three drops of fluid) is emitted, and the testes rise closer to the body. The person may achieve, lose, and regain the plateau phase several times without experiencing orgasm.

Orgasm

Orgasm occurs at the peak of the plateau phase. At the moment of orgasm, the sexual tension that has been building is released. The heart rate, respiratory rate, and blood pressure reach their peak, and there is loss of voluntary muscle tone.

- *In women,* spinal cord reflexes cause powerful rhythmic contractions of the vagina, uterus, anus, and pelvic floor muscles; feelings of warmth spread through the pelvic area. The cervical canal dilates, allowing easy transport of the sperm to the uterus. Orgasm may last for a few seconds or up to nearly a minute.
- *In men,* spinal cord reflexes cause the urethra, anus, and pelvic floor muscles to contract. Thrusting movements of the pelvis and penis occur, followed by **ejaculation** (the expelling of semen through the urethra). For men, orgasm usually lasts no more than 30 seconds.

The intensity of orgasm varies among individuals and in each individual from one sexual experience to another. Orgasm may involve intense spasm associated with intense focus on the sexual pleasure, or it may be signaled by as little as a sigh or subtle relaxation.

Resolution

Resolution is the period of time following orgasm. The muscles relax, and the body returns to its pre-excitement state. Immediately after orgasm, men experience a **refractory period,** during which they cannot achieve an erection. The duration of this period varies among individuals and increases with age. Women experience no refractory period—they can either enter the resolution stage or return to the excitement or plateau stage immediately following orgasm.

KnowledgeCheck 32-7

Identify the phase of the sexual response cycle described.

- This phase is reached if there is ongoing stimulation. This stage may be achieved, lost, and regained several times without the occurrence of orgasm.
- This stage occurs in the mind and may be communicated between potential sexual partners either verbally or through body language.
- This phase is associated with the release of sexual tension.

  Go to Chapter 32, **Knowledge Check Response Sheet and Answers,** on the Student Resource Disk or DavisPlus at http://davisplus.fadavis.com/Wilkinson2

CriticalThinking 32-6

Critique the theory of Masters and Johnson, as represented in the preceding discussion of the sexual response cycle. How would you respond to the statement that the theory does not adequately address variation among individuals and even within an individual's sexual response?

What Are Some Forms of Sexual Expression?

People express their sexuality and gain sexual satisfaction in many different ways. There is a range of behaviors that are socially acceptable and therefore considered "normal" by most people in our society. These are discussed in the next few sections. Keep in mind that people vary in what they consider to be "normal," as well as in their modes of sexual expression.

Developing Intimate Relationships

Developing intimate relationships involves a willingness to take risks and offer trust. Intimacy involves openness, mutual respect, caring, commitment, protection, honesty, and devotion. Although we often think of intimate relationships as sexual, they are not necessarily so. Furthermore, in our society, many sexual relationships occur without intimacy.

Fantasies and Erotic Dreams

Most men and women have sexual fantasies. They may be related to past experiences, dreams, desire, or stories heard, seen, or read. Sexual fantasies serve to increase self-esteem and sexual arousal and serve as an outlet to explore sexual desires. Fantasies may occur without sexual activity, during masturbation, or during intercourse. People in long-term monogamous relationships may fantasize to bring variety and excitement into a routine sexual encounter. Erotic dreams are also common among both men and women. Nocturnal orgasm may or may not occur.

Masturbation

Masturbation is self-stimulation of the genitals. Although there are many techniques, men typically hold and stroke the shaft of the penis, and women typically stimulate the clitoris manually. Young children touch their genitals as a part of body exploration, but they quickly learn either that touching certain areas is not acceptable or that it should be done in private. Adolescents, particularly males, may masturbate frequently. Adults may masturbate for sexual release when a partner is not available or for variety in a partnered relationship. Sex therapists often recommend masturbation as a means to resolve orgasm difficulties in women and ejaculatory problems in men.

Religious and social taboos discouraging masturbation are common. Some people mistakenly believe that masturbation is harmful, causing acne, warts, blindness, or insanity. More commonly masturbation is considered a "dirty," shameful, or perverted act. Although most people masturbate at some point in life, most do not talk about it openly in our society. For example, in 1994, U.S. Surgeon General Joycelyn Elder was removed from her position for advocating masturbation and suggesting, at an AIDS conference, that it should perhaps be taught as a method of safe sex (Frankel, 1994).

Shared Touching

An alternative to sexual intercourse may be mutual masturbation, or shared touching. This is particularly appealing to individuals who seek to maintain virginity, wish to decrease the risk of sexually transmitted infection, or have mobility or other physical problems that make intercourse difficult. Mutual masturbation is recognized as a form of safer sex because body fluids are not likely to be exchanged. This behavior can be satisfying because it allows for a significant level of sexual intimacy and allows participants to experience orgasm.

Sexual Intercourse

Sexual intercourse and **coitus** are terms used to describe penile penetration of the vagina. People use a variety of positions for intercourse, depending on preference, mobility, cultural and religious influences, the relationship, and other personal beliefs. For some women, manual stimulation of the clitoris is also necessary to achieve orgasm. Partners typically do not reach orgasm at the same time, despite the romantic preoccupation with this phenomenon.

Unprotected coitus may lead to conception, so the couple should use some method of contraception if they want to avoid pregnancy. Because it involves exchange of body fluids, sexual intercourse may also lead to the transmission of infections. Using a lubricated latex condom decreases this risk but is not a foolproof measure to prevent sexually transmitted disease.

Oral–Genital Stimulation

Both heterosexual and homosexual couples practice oral–genital stimulation (oral sex). Couples in committed relationships may engage in it for sexual variety or as foreplay. Others may engage in oral sex because it provides intimacy yet cannot result in pregnancy, and many believe that it does not affect their virginity status. For the latter reasons, oral sex has become more prevalent among adolescents. Oral-genital contact may, however, lead to STIs.

When a woman is the recipient of oral stimulation to her genitals, the practice is called **cunnilingus. Fellatio** is stimulation of the male genitals by a partner's mouth. Although swallowing semen is not a health issue, it may be a matter of personal preference whether the recipient ejaculates in his partner's mouth. If the couple is not in a long-term monogamous relationship, dental dams, plastic wrap, or latex condoms should be used to prevent the transmission of STIs.

Anal Stimulation or Anal Intercourse

Both homosexual and heterosexual couples engage in oral–anal stimulation (called **anilingus**). Objects for sexual stimulation, or the partner's finger, tongue, and mouth, may be used to stimulate the anus. **Anal intercourse** (also termed *sodomy*) is the insertion of the penis into the partner's rectum. When a couple engages in anal intercourse, lubrication is essential to lessen the chance of tiny tears to the rectal mucosa or damage to the anal sphincter. Unless the couple is in a long-term monogamous relationship, they should use a lubricated latex condom to lessen the chance of STIs. The condom must be changed before vaginal penetration to avoid the transfer of *Escherichia coli* bacteria from the rectum to the vagina. Couples should follow the same precaution when using objects for sexual pleasure.

Celibacy

Celibacy is a state in which an individual refrains from sexual activity. Traditionally, a celibate is a person who remains unmarried, often for religious reasons, and sublimates sexual desire through prayer, meditation, and service. However, some people choose to remain celibate out of fear of or lack of desire for intimate relationships. Childhood sexual trauma, for example, may lead an adult to choose celibacy. Some people are celibate

because a developmental or physical disability limits their opportunities for meeting prospective partners, limits their privacy, or interferes with their ability to communicate or act on their desires. Some celibate people simply have a low libido and focus their energies elsewhere. Married couples may be happily celibate. Others might be celibate after the loss of a relationship, whether through separation, divorce, or death, often feeling a considerable void.

Alternative Forms of Sexual Expression

The *Diagnostic and Statistical Manual of Mental Disorders IV* (American Psychiatric Association, 2000) describes eight categories of sexual deviation or **paraphilias:** exhibitionism, fetishism, frotteurism, pedophilia, sexual masochism, sexual sadism, transvestic fetishism, and voyeurism. Whereas some people experience guilt, shame, and depression about their paraphilia, others are distressed only by the societal disapproval, restrictions, and possible criminal charges associated with their mode of expression. If you need more information about paraphilias,

Go to Chapter 32, **Supplemental Materials: Alternative Forms of Sexual Expression,** on the Student Resource Disk or DavisPlus at http://davisplus.fadavis.com/Wilkinson2

There are some important things you can teach parents and other caregivers to do to reduce children's risk of sexual violence, predators, or other unhealthy exposure (Self-Care: Teaching Children About Predators).

KnowledgeCheck 32-8

- What are aspects of an intimate relationship?
- Identify solitary types of sexual expression and those that may be conducted with a partner.

Go to Chapter 32, **Knowledge Check Response Sheet and Answers,** on the Student Resource Disk or DavisPlus at http://davisplus.fadavis.com/Wilkinson2

What Problems Affect Sexuality?

Sexual well-being is a complex mesh of physical, emotional, cognitive, social, and spiritual components. Therefore, it is not surprising that many people experience challenges to their sexual health. Difficulties can arise in loving, healthy relationships as well as in dysfunctional couplings. Sexual dysfunction may be temporary and situational, or it may be long-standing.

Sexually Transmitted Infections

An STI is one that spreads through direct sexual contact. STIs are not transmitted by casual contact, such as touching, coughing, shaking hands, or sharing a glass with someone. They are spread by direct contact with an open wound or with body fluids, such as semen, vaginal secretions, or blood that contains pathogens.

Self-Care

Teaching Children About Predators

Set the Stage for Open Discussion

➤ Talk openly and directly with your child about her own development and sexuality. This establishes trust and makes it easier for the child to come to you when she has questions.

➤ Be open to your child's questions. Acting embarrassed discourages further conversation.

➤ Assure your child that she won't get in trouble for "tattling" on someone who asks her to keep a secret about sexual encounters.

➤ Make discussion a natural part of growing up—don't save it "for later."

Know What's Going On

➤ Be involved in your child's everyday life and ask questions—that is, where he is, who he's with, what he's doing.

➤ Know the other adults your child is around. Go to your child's activities and get to know the adults involved.

➤ Know what he watches on TV or media games.

➤ Locate computers in a central area in the home where you can monitor Internet use.

➤ Install a parental control to limit access to and monitor Web sites where your child could be exposed to sexual content or predators.

➤ Know if sexual predators live near you. Check out the sexual predators registry in your area.

Just Say No

➤ Teach your child about body parts that are private and should not be touched or looked at by others—except for medical reasons.

➤ Teach your child to firmly say "no" and get away if someone tries to touch or look at her in a way that makes her feel uncomfortable.

➤ Urge your child to tell you or another trusted adult if someone tries to touch or look at private areas or if the person tries to show the child his or her own private body parts.

➤ Place limits on Internet use.

➤ Teach children not to disclose personal information in public settings or on the Internet, even social networking sites.

An STI may be caused by bacteria, viruses, fungi, or parasites.

STIs are among the most common infectious diseases in the United States today. More than 20 different STIs have been identified, and they affect millions of men and women each year. **Reportable** (or **notifiable**) **diseases** are diseases that have a significant effect on public health. When healthcare providers diagnose a reportable disease, laws require it be reported to the CDC. Examples include the following:

- *Chlamydia trachomatis*. In 2007, over 1.1 million cases of sexually transmitted *Chlamydia trachomatis* infection were reported to CDC. This is the largest number of cases ever reported to CDC for any condition (CDC, 2007b).
- *Gonorrhea*. The incidence of gonorrhea has been declining for the past 20 years, and has now reached a plateau at about 350,000 new cases per year.
- *Syphilis*, although less common, is important because of the serious neurological complications it can lead to.

Nearly two-thirds of all STIs occur in people younger than 25 years. However, at least one in ten newly diagnosed cases of HIV occurs in a person older than 50 years.

Many STIs have few or no initial symptoms, allowing a person to be infected and transmit the infection without knowing it. For example, up to 90% of women infected with gonorrhea or chlamydia have no symptoms. To find out whether a patient has an STI, you must obtain a culture, that is, a swab of secretions from the genitals. In a man, the swab is put into the urethral opening.

In a woman, the swab is obtained from secretions near the cervix. A culture of the throat or rectum is obtained if the person has had oral or anal sex.

Many STIs can be treated fairly easily with antibiotics; however, if left untreated, they may cause serious problems. In women, the pathogens can travel up through the uterus into the fallopian tubes and cause pelvic inflammatory disease (PID). Untreated PID may cause sterility. One STI, human papillomavirus infection (HPV), causes genital warts and cervical and other genital cancers.

The best ways to prevent STIs are to be abstinent or to participate only in a committed, mutually monogamous sexual relationship with someone who has never had an STI and has never shared needles. Risk for an STI increases if a person has unprotected sex or has more than one sex partner. The more sex partners, the greater the risk. Other risk factors include alcohol and drug use, sexual activity at an early age, intercourse with a new partner, prior history of an STI, failure to utilize latex barriers with sexual contact, genital piercings, intercourse between men, intercourse with someone who has recently been in prison, sexual assault, sexual abuse, and failure to comply with prescribed treatment for an STI (Davidson, 2004).

To read about various STIs, their symptoms, treatment, and effect on sexual functioning, fertility, and childbearing,

 Go to Chapter 32, **Tables, Boxes, Figures: ESG Table 32-1, Common Sexually Transmitted Infections (STIs),** on the Student Resource Disk or DavisPlus at http://davisplus. fadavis.com/Wilkinson2

Dysmenorrhea

Dysmenorrhea is painful menstruation caused by strong uterine contractions that cause ischemia of the uterus. It is most common among adolescents and women experiencing perimenopause. The patient may experience cramping, lower abdominal pain, back and upper thigh pain, headache, vomiting, and diarrhea. Treatments include bedrest, application of heat to the back and abdomen, and analgesics such as aspirin and other nonsteroidal anti-inflammatory drugs (NSAIDs), for example, ibuprofen or naproxen.

Premenstrual Syndrome

Premenstrual syndrome (PMS) is characterized by physical and emotional changes occurring 3 to 14 days before the onset of the woman's menstrual period. Physical symptoms include headaches, constipation, breast tenderness, and weight gain associated with bloating, abdominal swelling, or swelling of the hands and feet. Some women feel as though they are on an emotional roller coaster, with periods of depression, anxiety, irritability, tension, and an inability to concentrate. Some women have difficulty maintaining social interactions at work or school because of severe emotional symptoms. Client teaching for PMS is discussed later in this chapter.

Women experiencing more severe form of menstrual cycle dysfunction (**premenstrual dysphoric disorder [PMDD]**) become seriously depressed for a week or more before their periods. In contrast, PMS is shorter, usually milder, and involves more physical symptoms. A woman can suffer from both PMS and PMDD at the same time, or may have one and not the other.

KnowledgeCheck 32-9

- Identify three methods to decrease the transmission of STIs.
- What are physical and emotional symptoms of premenstrual syndrome (PMS)?

Go to Chapter 32, **Knowledge Check Response Sheet and Answers,** on the Student Resource Disk or DavisPlus at http://davisplus.fadavis.com/Wilkinson2

Negative Intimate Relationships

Many couples are happy, and their sexual relationship becomes even more satisfying as they mature. However, some intimate relationships are not mutually satisfying, even when they do not involve neglect, or physical or emotional abuse. Couples may be involved in a celibate or loveless union for financial security, social status, for "the sake of the children," or because of cultural or religious restrictions regarding divorce. In reality, many couples' situation may be somewhere in between—sometimes satisfying and other times less so, depending on a wide variety of factors, ranging from stress, physical and mental illness, hormones, fatigue, distractions, low self-esteem, financial pressure, to name but a few. The most negative relationships involve *domestic violence* (also called *intimate partner violence*), which may include physical and/or emotional intimidation, assault, and rape.

Although either gender partner may be a victim of domestic violence, most often a man is the perpetrator. The anger, domination, and physical violence of the partner leads to fear, intimidation, and submission in the victim. Often victims come to believe they deserve the abuse and thus may hesitate to admit the cause of their injuries, even in the hospital setting. Many abused women are either emotionally or financially dependent on their partner and believe they have no options except to stay in the relationship.

Sexual Harassment

Sexual harassment occurs when a person in power makes unwanted sexual advances that implicitly or explicitly relate to the victim's employment, academic status, or success. "Advances" can take the form of sexual comments or behaviors (such as touching). Because of the power imbalance, the victim may keep silent and suffer physically and psychologically. Sexual assault includes contact with or without penetration, and touching sexual or intimate parts, and any unwanted sexual activity in situations of intoxication, coercion, or misconception.

Sexual harassment may take two forms: (1) In *quid pro quo* cases, the employer makes the employee feel that she must engage in unwelcome sexual advances to maintain employment; (2) In *hostile environment* cases, the sexual advances are more subtle, but persistent, and create an intimidating environment.

Rape

Although rape is actually a crime of violence rather than of sex, we discuss it here because it often involves the sexual organs and usually has negative effects on the victim's sexuality. **Rape** is nonconsensual vaginal, anal, or oral penetration. It occurs through force, by the threat of bodily harm, or when the victim is incapable of giving consent. In all 50 states, laws consider rape within a marriage is a crime.

Victims of rape range from infants to older adults and may be either gender, although girls and young women are more than 13 times more likely than males to be victims (American Academy of Pediatrics, Committee on Adolescents, 2001). Forced oral assault, multiple assailants, and weapons are more likely involved with male victims. In two-thirds of cases, the victim knows or is related to the assailant, especially when the victim is a young child (Rennison & Rand, 2008). People with developmental disabilities, especially mental retardation, are at double the risk for sexual assault than the general population.

Gang rape occurs when more than one person sexually assaults a victim. Group rape usually occurs when drugs and alcohol are involved. **Statutory rape** is sexual activity between an adult and a person under the "age of consent" (this ranges from 14 to 18 years of age, depending on state regulations). This charge may be filed even when the sex is consensual. **Date rape** is rape by an acquaintance when the assault occurs during an agreed-on social encounter. Although date rape is not a lesser violation, our society tends to blame the woman when date rape occurs.

Many rapes go unreported. An assault that involves significant physical injury is most likely to become known to the authorities because the victim requires medical attention. After a rape or other forms of sexual assault, care is more likely to be delayed, particularly for teens, if alcohol or drugs are involved. Other reasons for not reporting rape include fear of the assailant, fear of consequences to the assailant, knowledge of the low conviction rate for rapists, the desire to avoid a trial, shame and embarrassment, past sexual history, self-blame, wanting to "move on," and the wish to deny the event and its possible consequences.

If you follow accounts of rape charges and trials in the media, you can easily understand how victims may conclude that reporting a rape does not ensure justice will be served. In addition to psychological and physiological trauma, the rape victim is at risk for STIs and pregnancy. Three-quarters or more of sexually assaulted teens experience post-traumatic stress disorder. Referral to a local sexual assault support group is critical. A *sexual assault nurse examiner (SANE)* is a registered nurse who has received special training in the immediate care of sexual assault victims. For nursing interventions,

VOL 2 Go to Chapter 32, **Clinical Insight 32-1: Providing Care after Sexual Assault,** in Volume 2.

Sexual Response Cycle Disorders

A variety of disorders may occur throughout the sexual response cycle. These disorders affect desire, arousal, excitement, and orgasm.

Low Libido

A significant decrease in or absence of both sexual fantasies and sexual activity characterizes decreased sexual desire, or **low libido (hypoactive sexual desire).** Low libido may affect both men and women. It can be transient or long term. The person may experience low libido only with one particular partner, or the lack of desire can extend to all sexual activity. Persons with low libido may reluctantly engage in sexual encounters or avoid all sexual contact. However, once sexual activity has been initiated, the person is usually able to achieve orgasm.

Factors contributing to hypoactive sexual desire include sexual trauma, a negative attitude toward sex, negative relationships, and biological factors, including

hormone deficiencies, perimenopause, and side effects of various medications. Low sexual desire, in both men and women, in some cases may respond positively to testosterone administration.

Arousal Disorders

In women, arousal disorders manifest as minimal or absent pelvic congestion and vaginal lubrication even though desire may be present. Hormonal changes, the aging process, tampons, and medications, including antihistamines, also cause vaginal dryness. Vaginal dryness may result in **dyspareunia,** or painful intercourse, which further decreases sexual desire. A water-based lubricant or saliva helps to resolve vaginal dryness. Other causes of female dyspareunia include vaginal or urinary tract infections, pelvic inflammatory disease, and endometriosis.

A rare disorder affecting desire and arousal is vaginismus. **Vaginismus** is characterized by intense involuntary contractions of the perineal muscles, which close the vaginal opening and prevent penile penetration. Vaginismus may be associated with negative attitudes toward sex or a history of sexual abuse or trauma. Physiological disorders may also be the cause.

Sexual arousal disorders in men manifest as **erectile dysfunction (ED),** formerly known as *impotence.* Men with ED have persistent or recurring inability either to achieve or to maintain an erection sufficient for satisfactory sexual performance. Overall, testosterone plays a minor role in erectile function and a major role in libido (desire). The most common cause of ED is diseases of the blood vessels, such as hypertension or high cholesterol. ED may also result from underlying neurological (e.g., spinal cord injury, Parkinson's disease, stroke) or endocrine problems (diabetes). Common psychological problems that contribute to ED include performance anxiety, childhood sexual abuse, relationship issues, or mental illness. Some medications can also cause ED, such as antihistamines, antidepressants, antipsychotics, and antihypertensives.

Dyspareunia in men most commonly results from urinary tract infection or **phimosis,** a condition in which the foreskin of the penis is too tight. **Balanitis,** inflammation of the penis, is another cause of dyspareunia in men.

Orgasmic Disorders

Orgasmic disorder is a delay in or absence of orgasm after a normal sexual excitement phase. Once a woman has had orgasms, it is uncommon for her to lose that ability unless there has been a sexual trauma, poor sexual communication, a conflicted sexual relationship, a mood disorder, a medical condition, or direct physiological effects from a drug. Orgasmic disorder is more prevalent in younger women who have not had adequate sexual experience to learn how to reach orgasm. It is not unusual for a woman to require manual clitoral stimulation to reach orgasm; not all women can achieve orgasm through intercourse alone.

Men, too, can experience orgasmic disorders. Some cannot achieve orgasm during intercourse but are able to reach orgasm through masturbation or manual or oral stimulation by their partner.

In **premature ejaculation,** the male reaches orgasm and ejaculates before, at the time of, or shortly after penetration. The disappointment of both partners may lead to issues with self-esteem, sexual avoidance, and ED. There are sexual techniques as well as medications that help to delay ejaculation.

Retrograde ejaculation occurs when the semen empties into the bladder instead of being ejaculated through the urethra. Normally this cannot occur because the internal bladder sphincter closes in the orgasmic phase. However, some medications, prostate surgery, and spinal cord injuries may lead to retrograde ejaculation, resulting in sterility.

KnowledgeCheck 32-10

- Identify three forms of sexual victimization.
- In which phases of the sexual response cycle can sexual dysfunction occur?

 Go to Chapter 32, **Knowledge Check Response Sheet and Answers,** on the Student Resource Disk or DavisPlus at http://davisplus.fadavis.com/Wilkinson2

Practical **Knowledge** knowing how

Although you understand the importance of comprehensive client assessment, you may find it difficult to gather information related to sexuality. Students, and some nurses, may be shy, or may be concerned that the client will be embarrassed to talk about sexual topics. These matters are personal and private, and they can threaten a person's self-esteem. But including sexuality as a routine part of your nursing assessment reinforces the concept that sexuality is an integral part of life. It also provides an opportunity for much-needed patient teaching. Many patients will not raise the topic of sexuality, so if you do not mention it, you may not meet patient needs.

▮▮ ASSESSMENT

The extent to which you will assess a client's sexual health status varies. For example, for a woman with a suspected STI, you would perform a comprehensive health assessment in addition to a focused sexual health assessment. Similarly, clients with illnesses that affect their sexual functioning should receive a full assessment. Jocelyn Carter ("Meet Your Patients") is an example. Recall that chronic illness has a profound effect on sexual functioning. Frank Thanee and Gabriel Thomas ("Meet Your Patients") have chronic health problems that have created concerns related to their

sexuality. A focused sexual health assessment is needed in the following situations:

Pregnancy, infertility workup, request for birth control
Menstrual cycle irregularities or problems
Annual health visit
Unusual discharge from or change in genital organs
Urination problems
As part of a comprehensive physical examination
A known sexual problem (e.g., dyspareunia)
Illness that may affect sexual function (e.g., arthritis)
Medications

Sexual History

Most healthcare facilities use a standard nursing assessment form. Some address sexuality in a comprehensive manner, but most have only a few superficial questions or nothing at all. You will need to be sensitive to your client's verbal and nonverbal cues to identify and explore relevant issues that are not on the form. For topics to include in a sexual history and for suggestions for questions to ask,

 Go to Chapter 32, **Assessment Guidelines and Tools: Sexual History Questions,** in Volume 2.

Tips for Taking a Sexual History

When you are asking personal questions, be sure to provide privacy. It is not usually enough merely to pull the curtains around the bed. At some point, you will probably want to talk with both the client and partner. Nevertheless, you should be aware that clients may prefer to be alone when you take a sexual history. It is one thing to discuss blood pressure in the presence of family, but quite another to discuss sexual health issues, which may threaten the very core of a relationship. For example, a wife is not likely to discuss domestic violence with her abusing husband at her side. An 18-year-old man will probably not admit to having sex with another man when his father is present. An adolescent daughter may not want to discuss her STI in front of her mother.

For other suggestions,

 Go to Chapter 32, **Clinical Insight 32-2: Taking a Sexual History,** in Volume 2.

Focused Physical Examination

Sexual health assessment includes a physical examination focused on the reproductive system. For detailed instructions about performing these examinations,

 Go to Chapter 19, **Procedure 19-17: Assessing the Male Genitourinary System,** and **Procedure 19-18: Assessing the Female Genitourinary System,** in Volume 2.

If there is reason to suspect that a client has an STI, you should obtain cultures of any discharge or lesions. Other laboratory tests may be ordered as well.

KnowledgeCheck 32-11

What techniques can you use to increase comfort and communication during a sexual history assessment?

 Go to Chapter 32, **Knowledge Check Response Sheet and Answers,** on the Student Resource Disk or DavisPlus at http://davisplus.fadavis.com/Wilkinson2

 ## CriticalThinking 32-7

Review the three case scenarios in the "Meet Your Patients" discussion. Consider the following questions:

- Would you be comfortable caring for and responding to each of these clients?
- What topics, if any, that have been raised by these clients would be difficult for you to handle?
- How would you answer each of the client's questions?

ANALYSIS/NURSING DIAGNOSIS

NANDA-I has two nursing diagnoses for describing sexual problems. Use a diagnosis of:

- *Ineffective Sexuality Patterns* when the patient expresses concerns about his own sexuality. Examples of such concerns might include conflict about sexual orientation, values conflicts, fear of acquiring an STI, lack of knowledge about how to adapt sexual techniques to altered body function, lack of privacy, not having a partner, or impaired relationship with the partner.
- *Sexual Dysfunction* when there is an actual change in sexual function that the patient views as unsatisfying, unrewarding, or inadequate. This includes sexual response cycle disorders, such as low libido, arousal disorders, orgasmic disorders, vaginismus, premature ejaculation, and erectile dysfunction.

There is much overlap between these two NANDA-I diagnoses; however, Sexual Dysfunction is the more specific diagnosis for physiological problems and for concerns about sexual performance. Thus, it is best to use Sexual Dysfunction when the patient has one or more of the following defining characteristics:

Changes in achieving sexual satisfaction
Change of interest in self or others
Inability to achieve sexual satisfaction
Verbalization of a sexual problem
Actual or perceived limitations imposed by disease or therapy
Changes in ability to achieve perceived sex role
Seeking confirmation of desirability

If these defining characteristics do not seem to "fit" the patient, then use the more general diagnosis, Ineffective Sexuality Patterns (concern about one's sexuality). The only defining characteristic needed to make that diagnosis is that the patient reports difficulties, limitations, or changes in sexual behaviors or activities. Jocelyn Carter ("Meet Your Patients"), for example, is not actually experiencing problems with sexual satisfaction or performance. She is expressing a broader concern about her sexuality—about her future desirability as a sex partner. Therefore, the better diagnosis for her is Ineffective Sexuality Patterns. The same is true for Gabriel Thomas, who is expressing fear that he may have sexual problems in the future.

You could diagnose Sexual Dysfunction for Frank Thanee because he is experiencing a values conflict. He is expressing concerns, not about his sexual identity, performance, or satisfaction, but about how his homosexuality will affect his parents.

Etiologies of Sexuality Diagnoses

Several other nursing diagnoses may be the cause of sexuality problems. The following are the more common ones:

- *Activity Intolerance* and *Fatigue* may result from cardiac or respiratory disease, cancer, immune dysfunction, chronic pain, and morbid obesity. People with such conditions must alter their lifestyle, including sexual activity, to conserve energy. Lack of energy may decrease the person's interest in sex, or it may require a change in the mode of sexual expression.
- *Impaired Physical Mobility* (e.g., as occurs with arthritis, spinal cord injuries, or cerebral palsy) may affect a person's ability to interact, meet potential partners, and perform sexually (e.g., assume certain positions, make certain movements).
- *Fear* that sexual activity may be dangerous can inhibit desire and the ability to perform. This may occur, for example, after heart surgery. This diagnosis may also apply to the client's partner. A partner may be afraid that sexual activity will hurt the client after surgery, or hurt a pregnant partner or the baby.
- *Chronic Pain* may directly affect interpersonal relationships, interest in sex, or comfort during sexual intimacy. It may cause fatigue, indirectly affecting sexuality.
- *Chronic Low Self-Esteem* may result from chronic health problems and their consequences (e.g., loss of employment, inability to perform parenting roles). Sexual expression may also become a challenge, yet the intimacy and reassurance that accompanies sexual encounters can be vital to self-esteem and a sense of wholeness.
- *Self-Care Deficits.* For clients who need assistance with activities of daily living (ADLs), for example with toileting, family or caretakers often find it difficult to accept and facilitate sexual relationships. When a person with a physical disability lives in a residential facility, lack of opportunity and privacy may interfere with sexual expression (Fig. 32-8).
- *Delayed Development.* Relationship challenges also exist for people who are developmentally disabled. Those with very low cognitive functioning are unable to seek out or understand sexual relationships. Unfortunately, this makes them vulnerable to sexual abuse.

FIGURE 32-8 Adults with physical restrictions or those living within group settings, such as skilled nursing care, can maintain sexual relationships.

At a higher level of functioning, adolescents and adults have, as would be expected, a physical desire for sexual activity and often an accompanying desire for a loving, intimate relationship. Sex education is vital for these individuals to help them understand body structure and function, relationship issues, and ways to avoid exploitation and abuse.

Sexuality Problems as Etiologies of Other Diagnoses

Sexuality problems can be the etiology of other nursing diagnoses, for example:

- *Disturbed Body Image* related to change in appearance secondary to orchiectomy (removal of a testicle)
- *Pain (during coitus)* related to inadequate vaginal lubrication secondary to aging
- *Fear* related to sexual abuse by father
- *Rape-Trauma Syndrome* (Note that you do not need an etiology for this nursing diagnosis. It is self-explanatory, as are most syndrome diagnoses.)

Critical**Thinking** 32-8

Give a specific example (patient situation) for each of the defining characteristics of Sexual Dysfunction given in the preceding section.

PLANNING OUTCOMES/EVALUATION

For *NOC standardized outcomes* associated with Ineffective Sexuality Patterns and Sexual Dysfunction,

 Go to Chapter 32, **Standardized Language, Examples of NOC Outcomes for Sexuality Problems,** in Volume 2.

Individualized client outcomes and goals, as always, depend on the nursing diagnosis you identify. For Sexual Dysfunction and Ineffective Sexuality Patterns, you might write the following desired outcomes:

- Expresses comfort with sexual orientation.
- Describes plans for resolving values conflicts about extramarital sex (e.g., will talk to his minister).
- Describes techniques for preventing STIs.
- Reports using a condom for all sexual activities involving exchange of body fluids.

The following are examples of outcomes that apply specifically to Sexual Dysfunction:

- Communicates sexual needs and preferences to partner.
- Maintains penile erection through orgasm.
- Describes ways to adapt positions for intercourse to accommodate painful knee joints.

PLANNING INTERVENTIONS/IMPLEMENTATION

For *NIC standardized interventions* and selected nursing activities for sexuality,

 Go to Chapter 32, **Standardized Language, Examples of NIC Interventions and Nursing Activities for Sexuality Problems,** in Volume 2.

Specific nursing activities for sexuality problems depend on the etiology of the problem and on the goals selected. Broadly speaking, nursing interventions center around teaching about sexual health and self-care, counseling for altered sexual functioning, and dealing with inappropriate sexual behavior. Those interventions are discussed in the following sections.

You will find a nursing care plan and care map for Ineffective Sexuality Problems on the following pages.

Teaching About Sexual Health

Before you begin teaching, take the time to get to know your client and find out what she already knows about sexuality. Rapport and trust are essential to encourage clients to speak openly with you about sensitive or embarrassing topics. The time you take putting the client at ease is well spent. If the client is comfortable, she is more likely to retain what you teach and to feel free to questions. Offer to include the partner in the discussion if the client wishes. See Chapter 24 for a review of teaching and learning.

As part of teaching focused on sexuality, you should discuss prevention of STIs with all clients and discuss contraception with clients who are heterosexual or bisexual. Other common topics are presented in the next sections.

Body Function and Reproduction

A person's age, experience, and educational level do not ensure knowledge of sexual functioning. Before you begin any teaching, explore your client's knowledge base by asking open-ended questions such as "What questions do you have about sex?"

Visual aids (e.g., a diagram of reproductive system anatomy) are helpful. For example, for pregnant clients you could use drawings and charts illustrating fetal development. Most agencies provide handouts and brochures so that clients can review information at home.

As part of your general discussion on sexuality and bodily function, you may wish to discuss common myths and misconceptions about sex. Below are several statements about sex—all false—that provide a good starting point for discussion.

- You can't get pregnant the first time you have sex.
- You can't get pregnant if you're using a condom.
- You can tell the size of a man's penis by the size of his feet.
- You always have symptoms if you have an STI.
- People over 70 don't have sex.
- A vaginal orgasm is better than a clitoral orgasm.
- If the relationship is good, the man and woman will achieve simultaneous orgasm.
- It is not healthful to have intercourse during menstruation.
- The only normal position for intercourse is face to face. Anything else is deviant or at least "not nice."
- Only "dirty" people have STIs. You will not get an STI if your partner has good hygiene habits.
- If a person does not have an orgasm, they do not really love their partner.

Douching

Teach women that douching is unnecessary and is associated with significant risks. It can wash away the lactobacilli that clean the vagina and protect it from infection. Women who douche are at increased risk for some STIs and for pelvic inflammatory disease (Iannacchione, 2004). Furthermore, douching is essentially useless as a method of contraception. Some women douche because they notice an odor. Reassure them that this is normal during certain times of their menstrual cycle. If the odor doesn't disappear after washing, they should see their healthcare provider.

Menstruation

Many women require information about self-care to dispel myths about menstruation. For example, it is not dangerous to engage in sexual activity during menstruation. The bloody fluid is from the uterus, not the vagina, so intercourse will not harm the vagina. Actually, some women enjoy sex more during menstruation because the increased vascularity and lubrication in the pelvic region increases their pleasurable sensations, and orgasm may relieve their menstrual cramps. Some men, too, enjoy the warm, wet sensations. If the flow is very heavy, the woman can place a towel under her buttocks to protect the bed linens. Some women use a diaphragm to keep the flow from entering the vagina during sexual activity.

To prevent odor, the woman should use good perineal hygiene, bathe or shower every day, and change pads or tampons frequently. Advise women to follow the manufacturer's directions for reducing the risk for toxic shock syndrome. Deodorized pads and tampons are not very effective and can cause irritation to the vulva and vagina.

For mild cramping occurring before or during menses, aspirin and other NSAIDs, such as ibuprofen or naproxen, are effective and can be taken unless contraindicated for other reasons. These drugs inhibit uterine contractions as well as having analgesic properties. A heating pad or warm bath may be comforting; lying supine also keeps the abdomen warm.

Premenstrual Syndrome

For women with PMS, you may suggest a variety of nonpharmacological treatments: getting adequate sleep; eating small, frequent meals; reducing sugar, caffeine, alcohol, and salt in the diet; taking vitamin and mineral supplements; and exercising. Selective serotonin reuptake-inhibiting drugs (SSRIs) such as fluoxetine (Prozac) and sertraline (Zoloft) are increasingly being used as a front-line therapy for managing symptoms of PMS.

Menopause

Hormone replacement therapy (HRT) remains the most effective treatment to relieve symptoms of menopause, such as itching, dryness, discomfort with intercourse, hot flashes, sleep disturbances, and other symptoms. HRT can either increase or decrease risk of heart disease, depending on when hormone therapy is started; how long women remain on it; and individual differences. HRT can help prevent loss of bone density in menopausal women, which leads to fewer hip fractures among users. Also beneficial is the reduced risk of colorectal cancer. However, because of the risks associated with long-term use in a small number of women (e.g., heart disease, blood clots, breast and ovarian cancer, and dementia), consumers and healthcare providers alike have become more conservative in using HRT, reserving treatment for short-term use. Counsel women to discuss the risks and benefits of HRT with their primary care provider, and inform them that there are some natural remedies and bioidentical therapies that may provide symptom relief (Complementary and Alternative Modalities: CAM for Menopause Symptoms).

CAM for Perimenopausal Symptoms

Help, including hormone therapy, is available for menopause symptoms. In addition to finding a primary care provider with whom to discuss their symptoms, advise women to:

➤ Eat a balanced diet, low in fat and rich in calcium.

➤ Use supplemental vitamins, if necessary.

➤ Take supplemental calcium and magnesium.

➤ Get adequate sleep.

➤ Exercise daily.

➤ Avoid tobacco use.

➤ Limit alcohol and caffeine.

➤ Drink plenty of water to counteract the drying effect of low estrogen levels.

➤ Use soy products (e.g., soy milk, tofu, and soy flour), which are rich in phytoestrogens that are converted during digestion to very weak estrogens.

➤ Try the herbal remedies red clover and black cohosh.

➤ Use natural progesterone cream, which is made from a yam root. Women usually apply a small amount of the cream for 12 days out of each month.

Self-Examination

Breast self-examination and testicular self-examination are vital aspects of sexual health. Any change in how the breasts normally look and feel should be immediately provided to the healthcare provider. Although there is controversy about whether to advise routine breast self-examination, the American Cancer Society (2010) recommends it as an option for women in their 20s. Women should have yearly mammograms to screen for breast cancer after age 40. These guidelines represent an extensive review of the health literature and input from an expert advisory group. However, some researchers have not demonstrated clear benefit for performing breast self-exam in detecting cancer. For more information and for details about the assessments, see Chapters 9, 19, and 41.

Preventing Sexually Transmitted Infections

STIs are a worldwide health concern, and education is a key component of prevention. The only absolutely safe sex is total avoidance of sexual activity with a partner. However, most adults do not choose abstinence. The next safest sex occurs within a long-term, mutually monogamous relationship. Other safer sex practices involve the consistent, correct use of a condom and limiting the number of sexual partners. For information about the use of male and female condoms,

 Go to Chapter 32, **Clinical Insight 32-3: Teaching Your Client to Use a Condom,** in Volume 2.

Teach your clients the proper use of condoms and encourage them to discuss sexual feelings, activity, and safety with their partners. If people are not comfortable talking about birth control, STIs, and safer sex with a potential partner, they need to consider whether it is wise to begin a sexual relationship. Planned Parenthood advocates the following behaviors for safer sex:

■ Be honest about current sexual practices and sexual history, as well as sexual health concerns.
■ Avoid the exchange of body fluids, including semen, blood, and vaginal secretions, by correctly and consistently using latex barriers.
■ Avoid contact with genital sores or growths.
■ Have routine checkups for infection.
■ Consult a healthcare provider for diagnosis and treatment of symptoms such as abnormal discharge from the vagina, penis, or rectum; a burning sensation with urination; sores in the genital area; or painful intercourse.
■ Accept responsibility for your actions.

Also advise clients to choose a healthcare provider with whom they can comfortably discuss these issues. Freedom to speak frankly and openly about their sexual health concerns is important to their health. Assure them that testing, examination, and treatment for STIs are always confidential.

Contraception

For clients who are heterosexual or bisexual, your sexual health teaching may include methods for preventing unwanted pregnancies. Several fertility control and family planning strategies are available, each with advantages and disadvantages. For information on several fertility control methods,

VOL 2 Go to Chapter 32, **Tables, Fertility Control Methods,** in Volume 2.

Counseling for Sexual Problems

The PLISSIT model was developed as a guideline for counseling for sexual problems (Annon, 1974). Basic nursing education does not prepare you to provide sex therapy. However, the first three PLISSIT steps have been successfully adapted to address sexual knowledge deficits, which you are qualified to treat. The acronym PLISSIT represents the following:

*P*ermission. Permission means that you communicate an open, accepting attitude so that the client feels free to ask open-ended questions and express concerns and feelings and to engage in sexual behaviors with a consenting partner. For example, you might state, "Many women experience decreased vaginal lubrication after menopause. Tell me how well you have been lubricating."

Limited Information. Supplying limited information may include teaching about normal sexual functioning, expected changes in sexual functioning, medication side effects, and medical and surgical impacts on sexuality. For example, you might say, "Some women experience decreased vaginal lubrication because of decreased levels of certain hormones."

Specific Suggestions. You might make specific suggestions for self-care, as presented in this chapter. For example: "You might consider using a water-soluble lubricant."

Intensive Therapy. If these interventions do not relieve the client's concerns, you should refer the client to someone with specialized knowledge of sexual health. For example: "You might consider discussing this with your gynecologist."

Dealing with Inappropriate Sexual Behavior

Nursing involves intimate contact. We see people disrobed, literally touch bodies, and discuss private topics. In most cases, patients recognize this as professional behavior associated with providing health care. Occasionally they may respond inappropriately. For example, a client may make sexually suggestive comments, request sexually related care that is not required (e.g., ask you to bathe his genitalia when he can do it adequately himself), disrobe or expose body parts that are not involved in the care delivered, or touch or grab you as you provide care. The following are the most common reasons for sexually inappropriate behaviors:

- Confusion
- Neurological disorders, especially those involving the frontal lobe
- Psychiatric problems resulting in poor impulse control
- Misinterpretation of nursing care
- Need to have power or control over others, especially when the client feels powerless in other aspects of his life
- Worries about sexual functioning
- Unrealistic view of nursing based on sexual stereotypes

If you believe a client is demonstrating inappropriate sexual behaviors, immediately tell the client that the behavior is inappropriate. Do not express anger, but use clear statements, such as, "I don't like your comments. They are inappropriate. Please stop." Next, let the client know what behavior you expect. Be direct with your comments. If the client is exposing himself, let him know what you expect him to wear ("I expect you to keep your pajama bottoms on"). If the client is attempting to touch you, tell him, "Don't touch me." Refocus the client's attention to the care you are delivering ("Hold still now, while I tape your IV"). If you are extremely uncomfortable or the client persists in the comments or actions, leave the room and report the incident to your instructor or the nurse assigned to the client. Your instructor may need to change your assignment. You may also wish to consider discussing the situation with the client while another person is in the room.

Sexual harassment is a unique form of inappropriate sexual behavior (refer to "Sexual Harassment" in the "Theoretical Knowledge" section). If you believe you are being sexually harassed, you should confront your harasser and clearly state your concerns. If you feel unable to confront your harasser (e.g., if the harasser is a teacher or supervisor), keep a written record of the events, and report your concerns to the worksite or school official in charge of personnel. By law, all worksites and educational environments must have a written procedure for handling cases of sexual harassment. It will tell you how to file a grievance, what forms you need to use, to whom the incident is reported, and details of the procedure for a hearing and resolution. For further information, see Chapter 45.

Putting It All Together

Consider the three patients discussed in the "Meet Your Patients" scenario. Each situation illustrates how important sexual identity is to the sense of self.

- Jocelyn Carter is having a breast removed secondary to cancer. However, her question focuses not on the threat from cancer, but on how this surgery will affect her relationship with her husband.
- Gabriel Thomas has extremely high blood pressure, yet he is concerned that medications will impair his sexual abilities.
- Frank Thanee is recovering from open heart surgery but is focused on explaining to his visiting family his long-term relationship with a man.

The full-spectrum nursing model can help you to find the best approach when dealing with sexual health. We have used the three patients in "Meet Your Patients" to illustrate how this works.

Thinking

Theoretical Knowledge. You will need theoretical knowledge about sexuality, the effect of health concerns on sexual function and expression, and treatment of sexual health problems. Many myths and taboos surround the subject of sexuality; so it is important that you remain objective and current regarding these topics. A sound knowledge base enables you to teach and respond sensitively to all your clients. What knowledge do you already have that would enable you to address Gabriel Thomas's concerns? What knowledge do you still need?

Critical Thinking. Mr. Thomas has a markedly elevated blood pressure but is concerned about the effects of medications on his sexual function. To help him, you will need to focus on what he is experiencing and

Nursing Care Plan

Client Data

Emilio Juarez is a 50-year-old man hospitalized for cardiac monitoring after an acute myocardial infarction (MI; heart attack). He has no history of diabetes or hypertension. Mr. Juarez owns a computer software company and is active in the community (president of the Chamber of Commerce).

After dinner, Mr. Juarez's nurse sits down to teach Emilio and his wife, Luz, about the medications he will be taking. She also begins to talk to them about a cardiac rehabilitation program. Mr. Juarez asks, "What do you mean by 'activity restriction'? Do I have to stop doing all the things I did before?" The nurse asks, "What things are you thinking about?" Mr. Juarez hesitates, then says, "Oh, like working in the yard, going up the stairs, and, you know, personal things." Mrs. Juarez immediately says, "There is no need to talk about that now. The most important thing is for my Emilio to feel better and get home—there is plenty of time for other things later." The nurse tells the couple that many couples are anxious about resuming sexual activity after a heart attack and says, "I'd like to give you some information about that and answer any questions you might have."

Nursing Diagnosis

Ineffective Sexuality Patterns related to lack of knowledge about post-MI sexual activity and reluctance to ask questions, as evidenced by Mrs. Juarez's comment, "There is no need to talk about that now."

NOC Outcomes	Individualized Goals / Expected Outcomes
Sexual Identity (1207) Sexual Functioning (0119) Body Image (1200)	*By discharge, Mr. Juarez will:* 1. Be able to identify two resources he can use to learn more about sexual activity after myocardial infarction. 2. Commit to attending the cardiac rehabilitation classes offered at the hospital. *During and by the end of the cardiac rehabilitation program, Mr. Juarez will:* 1. Identify stressors in his life related to sexual activity. 2. Report a desire to resume sexual activity to pre-MI levels. 3. Resume previous sexual activity.

(continued on next page)

NIC Interventions/Activities	Rationale
NIC Interventions Sexual counseling (5248) Body image enhancement (5220) Anxiety reduction (5820) **Nursing Activities** 1. Initiate discussions about sexual activity after MI, beginning with general, nonthreatening statements.	Clients and significant others are often too embarrassed to ask about sexual matters. The client's perception of his sexuality impacts personal and social behavior outside the bedroom (Steinke, 2002; Steinke & Patterson-Midgley, 1996). Patients should be reassured that after recovery from an MI, sexual activity presents no great risk of another MI (Cooper et al., 2007).
2. Allow Mr. Juarez to control the discussion of sexual matters.	The subject of sexual activity should be raised with patients within the context of cardiac rehabilitation (Cooper et al., 2007; Miner, 2006). This shows respect for the client's privacy and his sexual being. Controlling what issues are discussed and when enhances self-esteem (Steinke, 2000).
3. Listen carefully to Mr. Juarez's verbal and nonverbal expression of concerns.	Anxiety interferes with patients' return to sexual activity after an acute cardiovascular event (Moser, 2009). Some men may overtly express disinterest in discussing sexual matters; others avoid the topic by joking, avoiding eye contact, or brushing off concerns as not pressing. Commonly, men avoid verbalizing feelings in this area because of the personal nature and threats to masculine identity. Although depressive symptoms are more common in women after an MI and contribute to higher rates of rehospitalization, men also show depression (Moser, 2009; Parashar et al., 2008).
4. Seek consultation from other members of the healthcare team as needed.	When nurses are uncomfortable talking about sexual matters and do not initiate the conversation, the client may think sexual activity is prohibited after MI. If the nurse is personally uncomfortable discussing these matters, it is imperative to consult with other members of the team who can meet the client's needs (Steinke, 2000; Steinke & Patterson-Midgley, 1996).
5. Include Mrs. Juarez in counseling as much as possible, with Mr. Juarez's consent.	Marriage and close interpersonal relationships allow each member to support the other and alleviate negative effects of stress. The client's ability to adapt physically and emotionally after MI depends on the spouse's ability to cope with situational stressors (Beach et al., 1992).

(continued on next page)

Nursing Care Plan (continued)

NIC Interventions/Activities	Rationale

Nursing Activities

6. Be clear about exploring Mr. and Mrs. Juarez's specific concerns, and correct any misinformation.

Anxiety about sexual activity after MI often arises from misconceptions. Fewer than 1% of MIs and 5% of angina attacks occur during sexual activity (Miner, 2006; Salamon, 2008). There is no evidence suggesting that sexual activity poses a risk for sudden death (Cooper et al., 2007). Regular exercise, such as in a cardiac rehab program, reduces the risk of MI from sexual activity (DeBusk et al., 2000; Muller, 2000). For some cardiac patients, sexual problems begin before a heart attack. Erectile dysfunction, the consistent inability to sustain an erection, affects more than 50% of men older than 60 and is a recognized symptom of cardiovascular disease. The typical period of maximum risk (which is still very low) is within 4 weeks of the MI (DeBusk et al., 2000). Exercise training after acute MI improves cardiovascular efficiency and reduces myocardial oxygen demand during customary activities, including sexual activity (Miner, 2006). Erectogenic drugs, when used correctly, do not increase overall cardiovascular risk in patients after an MI (Cooper et al., 2007).

7. Discuss the risks of using drugs for erectile dysfunction together with nitrates.

An unsafe drop in blood pressure can occur when erectile dysfunction medication is taken with nitrates (Cooper et al., 2007; Miner, 2004). Men should be taught to contact their prescribers if they experience an erection lasting more than 4 hours or if a change in vision occurs.

(continued on next page)

Nursing Care Plan (continued)

Evaluation

After Mrs. Juarez left for the evening, the nurse returned to bring Mr. Juarez a medication. He said, "Thanks for bringing that up and for leaving the booklet. I love my wife, and I was worried. I sure didn't want to have another heart attack. She was embarrassed to let on that it is important to her, but we will be sure to make use of the rehab program." The nurse followed up later by giving the Juarezes a videotape that discusses sexual issues, which they can take home and watch in privacy and comfort when they are ready to do so.

References

Beach, E. K., Maloney, B. H., Plocica, A. R., et al. (1992). The spouse: A factor in recovery after acute myocardial infarction. *Heart & Lung, 21*(1), 30–38.

Cooper, A., Skinner, J., Nherera, L., et al. (2007). *Clinical guidelines and evidence review for post myocardial infarction: Secondary prevention in primary care and secondary care for patients following a myocardial infarction (full NICE guideline).* National Collaborating Centre for Primary Care and Royal College of General Practitioners. www.nice.org.uk (Accessed February 17, 2009).

DeBusk, R., Drory, Y., Goldstein, I., et al. (2000). Management of sexual dysfunction in patients with cardiovascular disease: Recommendations of the Princeton consensus panel. *American Journal of Cardiology, 86*(2), 175–181.

Friedman, S. (2000). Cardiac disease, anxiety and sexual functioning. *American Journal of Cardiology, 86 (Supplement)* (2A), 46F–50F.

Miner, M. M. (2006). Sexual activity after myocardial infarction: When to resume the use of erectogenic drugs. *Current Sexual Health Reports, 3*(1), 30–34.

Moser, D. K. (2007). The rust of life: Impact of anxiety on cardiac patients. *American Journal of Critical Care, 16*(4), 361–369.

Muller, J. E. (2000). Triggering of cardiac events by sexual activity: Findings from a case-crossover analysis. *American Journal of Cardiology, 86 (Supplement)* (2A), 14F–18F.

Parashar, S., Rumsfeld, J. S., Reid, K. J., et al. (2008). Impact of depression on sex differences in outcome after myocardial infarction. *Circulation: Cardiovascular Quality and Outcomes, 2*, 33–40.

Salaman, M. (2008). Sex after a heart attack—for men: Be careful with performance enhancing drugs. About.com: Heart Disease. Retreived from http://heartdisease.about.com/lw/Health-Medicine/Conditions-and-diseases/Sex-after-a-Heart-Attack-for-Men.htm.

Steinke, E. E. (2000). Sexual counseling after myocardial infarction. *American Journal of Nursing, 100*(12), 38–43.

Steinke, E. E. (2002). A videotape intervention for sexual counseling after myocardial infarction. *Heart & Lung, 31*(5), 348–354.

Steinke, E. E., & Patterson-Midgley, P. (1996). Sexual counseling of MI patients: Nurses' comfort, responsibility, and practice. *Dimensions of Critical Care Nursing, 15*(4), 216–223.

Care Map

Status post MI

Mr. & Mrs. Juarez

- Lack knowledge of post-MI activity in relation to sexual activity
- Refer to sexual activity as "personal"

By discharge, Mr. J will:
- Identify two resources he can use to learn more about sexual activity post MI.
- Commit to attending cardiac rehab classes.

During and by the end of cardiac rehab, he will:
- Identify stressors r/t sexual activity.
- Report a desire to resume sexual activity to pre-MI levels.
- Resume previous sexual activity.

NOC outcomes:
Sexual Identity,
Sexual Functioning

Ineffective Sexuality Patterns r/t lack of knowledge about post-MI sexual activity and reluctance to ask questions

NIC interventions:
Sexual Counseling

NIC interventions:
Body Image,
Anxiety Reduction

- Start discussions about sexual activity with general, nonthreatening information.
- Use input from other team members.
- Include spouse in talks.
- Discuss dangers of medications for erectile dysfunction.

- Allow Mr. J to control discussion of sexual matters.
- Listen carefully to concerns, jokes, and nonverbal communication.
- Correct any misinformation.

Key:
- Data
- Nursing diagnosis
- NOC outcomes
- Other outcomes
- NIC interventions
- Nursing actions

critically examine his concerns in light of what is known about hypertension and its treatment. You will need to prioritize your concerns about Mr. Thomas, balancing the need to control his blood pressure with his sexual needs, and consider the consequences of various approaches. You might, for example, discuss alternative forms of sexual expression.

Doing

Practical Knowledge. When dealing with sexuality, communication skills are essential practical knowledge. Your verbal and nonverbal skills demonstrate to patients your comfort with sensitive topics. Consider the situation of Jocelyn Carter. Suppose you responded to Jocelyn's question by telling her, "That's the least of your worries." How do you think she would feel? Now consider what might happen if you responded, "You must be worried about your sexual relationship. Tell me a little more about what you're feeling."

Nursing Process. Gabriel Thomas has a markedly elevated blood pressure but is concerned about the effects of medications on his sexual function. To help him, you will need to assess his knowledge and concerns, clearly identify his problems (elevated blood pressure and Ineffective Sexuality Pattern) and use the nursing process to develop a plan of care that is acceptable to him. When working with patients with sexual health concerns, tailor your approach to each individual's needs, just as you do in all areas of health.

Caring

Self-knowledge. To help patients identify and resolve sexual health concerns, you will need to examine your own beliefs and values. The self-knowledge gained from examining your own views on sexuality will help you to be open to your patients' sexual concerns. What are your beliefs about sex and sexuality? Are you uncomfortable around people whose sexual orientation is different from yours? Imagine how you would feel if Frank Thanee asked you for help.

 Go to Chapter 32, **Resources for Caregivers and Health Professionals,** on the Student Resource Disk or DavisPlus at http://davisplus.fadavis.com/Wilkinson2

 Suggested Readings: Go to Chapter 32, **Reading More About Sexual Health,** on the Student Resource Disk or DavisPlus at http://davisplus.fadavis.com/Wilkinson2

 Bibliography: Go to Volume 2, Bibliography.

CHAPTER 33

Sleep & Rest

Learning Outcomes

After completing this chapter, you should be able to:

➤ Explain why rest and sleep are important.

➤ Describe the functions and physiology of sleep.

➤ Explain circadian rhythms and how they relate to sleep.

➤ Identify factors that influence rest and sleep.

➤ Describe nursing implications for age-related differences in the sleep cycle.

➤ Identify at least five common sleep disorders.

➤ Perform a comprehensive sleep assessment using appropriate interview questions, a sleep diary, and a sleep history.

➤ Formulate nursing diagnoses that identify sleep problems that may be treated through specific nursing interventions.

➤ Plan, implement, and evaluate nursing care related to specific nursing diagnoses addressing sleep problems.

Meet Your Patients

You are a nurse working on a surgical unit. Today you are meeting with Anne for preoperative teaching. She is scheduled for a complete hysterectomy next Monday. She has a secondary diagnosis of fibromyalgia, a chronic disorder characterized by widespread muscle pain and nonrestorative sleep.

Anne is a 49-year-old married woman with three children. She works full time and manages the family with her husband. She says, "I'm a little nervous about the surgery, but I know I need it. But I haven't been sleeping well because of thinking about it." Anne tells you that she has actually had trouble sleeping for the last 20 years. "I take an Ambien pill, 10 mg, every night to help me sleep. Will I be able to get that in the hospital? I really can't sleep at all without it," explains Anne.

As you continue the interview, Anne explains that she suffered from physical and emotional abuse as a young woman and has had sleep problems ever since. She has been to counseling, but that did not improve her sleep.

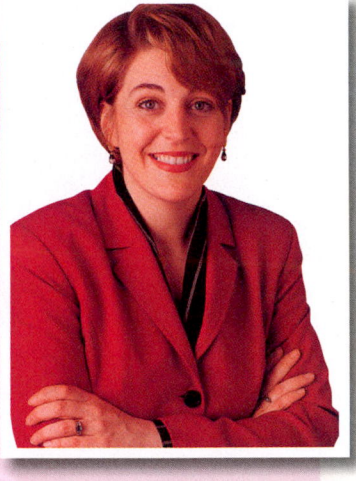

Recently her sleep has been even more troublesome. Aside from her upcoming surgery, she has been coping with the recent death of her father. After meeting with Anne, you realize that sleep-promoting measures will be an important part of her nursing care while she is in the hospital.

What clues in Anne's situation would cause you to suspect that she will have difficulty sleeping while in the hospital? What characteristics of the hospital environment might interfere with Anne's sleep? You may not have enough theoretical knowledge and experience to feel confident about your answers to these questions, but use your present knowledge base and your life experiences to think about them.

Theoretical Knowledge
knowing why

Have you felt tired after waking up from a night's sleep? Have you ever been tired, but not sleepy, and, after relaxing a while, felt your normal energy return? How do you think sleep and rest are different? How are they alike?

Rest is a condition in which the body is inactive or engaging in mild activity, after which the person feels refreshed. A person at rest is calm, at ease, relaxed, and free of anxiety and stress (Fig. 33-1). People rest by doing things that they find calming and relaxing (e.g., reading, listening to music, surfing the Internet, watching television, doing needlework, praying or meditating, gardening, playing golf, walking, and camping).

Sleep is a cyclically occurring state of decreased motor activity and perception (Germann & Stanfield, 2008) (Fig. 33-2). Body functions slow, and metabolism falls by 20% to 30%, so the body conserves energy. Sleep is characterized by altered consciousness: a sleeping person is unaware of the environment and responds selectively to external stimuli. For example, an alarm clock, bright light, or other meaningful stimuli usually awaken a sleeper, but everyday background noises and soft light do not.

Although necessary and beneficial, rest without sleep is inadequate. At rest, the body is disturbed by all exterior stimuli, whereas in sleep it is screened from them by altered consciousness. Thus, sleep restores the body; rest alone cannot do this.

Why Do We Need to Sleep?

We spend more time sleeping than in any other single activity: about 8 hours a day, or 2688 hours a year—nearly one-third of our lives! So why is sleep so important? Before you try to answer, think back to the last time you slept poorly. Remember the mental fogginess, the physical fatigue, the feeling of slight nausea? Poor quality or insufficient length of sleep for even one night can reduce mental performance, and long periods of

FIGURE 33-1 Woman receiving Hospice care resting comfortably.

FIGURE 33-2 Boy sleeping in hospital setting.

sleep deprivation can result in stress-related illnesses and injuries (e.g., from an automobile accident). The reason is that sleep and rest are essential for physical, mental, and spiritual well-being.

Theorists do not agree on all of the functions of sleep, but studies have shown that adequate sleep restores energy. Despite the fact that some regions of the brain are more active during sleep than when we are awake, total energy output is reduced during sleep, giving the body time for restoration and repair. Research also indicates that sleep strengthens the immune system (Cohen, Doyle, Alper, et al., 2009; Ranjbaran, Keefer, Stepanski, et al., 2007) and helps the body to fight infection. Sleep may also improve learning and adaptation, giving the individual a chance to mentally repeat and rehearse facts and situations before they are encountered in wakeful life. Some evidence suggests that sleep and dreaming may facilitate the storage of long-term memory (Germann & Stanfield, 2008), perhaps by assisting the brain in reorganizing and storing information. Sleep also appears to reduce stress and anxiety, improving our ability to cope and concentrate on activities of daily living.

Sleep/rest and illness are interrelated (Fig. 33-3). Illness and injury increase the need to sleep and at the

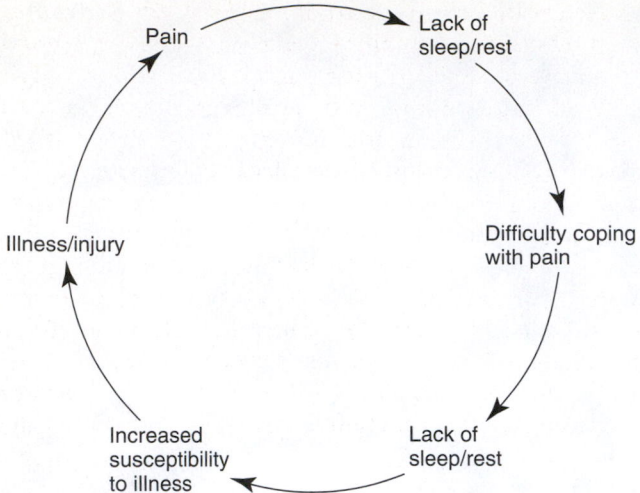

FIGURE 33-3 Relationship between sleep/rest and illness. Lack of sleep and rest increases susceptibility to illness. Likewise, the pain and stress of illness disturbs sleep.

same time make it difficult to sleep. In turn, lack of sleep increases the susceptibility to illness by compromising the immune system. People who are ill or injured need more sleep than usual to restore energy needed for tissue repair and healing. However, they often have difficulty resting because of pain and other symptoms of their illness.

Because sleep enhances wellness and speeds recovery from illness, promoting sleep is an important independent nursing intervention. In this chapter, you will learn how to recognize signs of sleep disturbance, as well as factors that interfere with patients' sleep, and specific measures to facilitate sleep for each client.

For further discussion of sleep theories,

 Go to Chapter 33, **Supplemental Materials: Theories of Sleep,** on the Student Resource Disk or DavisPlus at http:// davisplus.fadavis.com/Wilkinson2

KnowledgeCheck 33-1

- Compare and contrast sleep and rest. How are they different? Alike?
- Why is promoting sleep an important nursing intervention?

 Go to Chapter 33, **Knowledge Check Response Sheet and Answers,** on the Student Resource Disk or DavisPlus at http://davisplus.fadavis.com/Wilkinson2

 Critical**Thinking** 33-1

What effect do you think surgery will have on Anne's sleep ("Meet Your Patient")? Why?

How Much Sleep Do We Need?

Sleep needs vary widely among individuals. Even though the accepted standard has been 8 hours per night for adults, there is really no universal amount or pattern of sleep that is best suited for all people. In spite

of individual variations, however, different sleep patterns are characteristic of different age groups.

Infants have an overall greater total sleep time than any other age group. Newborns sleep as much as 16 to 20 hours a day, in periods ranging from one to several hours. Sleep time gradually decreases over the next few months, but throughout the first year of life, a minimum of 14 hours of sleep per day is recommended (Tuller, 2004). Most infants sleep several hours during one overnight period, with a morning and afternoon nap each day.

After the first year of life, sleep duration gradually lessens (Table 33-1). In most adults, sleep of 7 to 8 hours is fully restorative; however, there are wide individual variations. In some cultures, total sleep time is divided into an overnight sleep period and a midafternoon nap.

Older adults spend significantly less time sleeping but need more rest than younger adults. Usually older adults rest or nap during the day, go to bed early, and get up early. They take longer to fall asleep, and their arousal periods during sleep are longer and more frequent. Frequent waking is commonly due to physical discomfort, anxiety, and nocturia (Polan & Taylor, 2007). If sleep is interrupted, the person needs to sleep longer to feel restored. If the older adult does not increase the total time in bed, she may experience fatigue, irritability, and impaired cognition.

Critical**Thinking** 33-2

- How much sleep might Anne ("Meet Your Patient") need in a normal night?
- How will a good night of sleep benefit Anne while she is in the hospital?
- If you were preparing for an important test, would it be better to stay up all night studying, or should you try to get a good night of sleep?
- How many hours of sleep do *you* need to feel rested and function well the next day? Compare notes with family members, friends, and classmates. Do they all need the same amount of sleep as you?

Table 33-1 ➤ Average Sleep Requirements	
AGE GROUP	**HOURS PER DAY**
Newborns (birth–4 weeks)	16–20
Infants (4 weeks–1 year)	14–16
Toddlers (1–3 years)	12–14
Preschoolers (3–6 years)	11–13
Middle and late childhood (6–12 years)	10–11
Adolescents (12–18 years)	8–9
Young adults (18–40 years)	7–8
Middle-age adults (40–65 years)	7
Older adults (65 years and older)	5–7

Physiology of Sleep

Our environment plays a role in the physiology of our sleep, so we begin with an exploration of circadian rhythms, by which the body maintains synchronicity with nature. **Synchrony** occurs when things happen at the same time, or work or develop on the same time scale as something else.

How Do Circadian Rhythms Influence Sleep?

Biorhythms are "biological clocks" that are controlled within the body and synchronized with environmental factors (e.g., gravity, electromagnetic forces, light, and darkness). Biorhythms influence many physical and mental functions. For example, body temperature is typically lowest when the person wakes up in the morning, and female menstruation follows an approximately 28-day cycle, like the lunar cycle on which our calendar months are based.

A **circadian rhythm** is a biorhythm based on the day–night pattern in a 24-hour cycle. The term comes from the Latin words circa, meaning "about" and dies, meaning "day"—once a day. A person's circadian rhythm is regulated by a cluster of cells in the hypothalamus of the brain stem that respond to changing levels of light. Circadian rhythm affects our overall level of functioning; most people have a higher energy level in the daytime and less energy at night. However, some people are more alert and active in the morning, whereas others function at a higher level in the afternoon or evening.

Do you feel sleepy at about the same time each night? Do you often awaken before the alarm clock goes off? If so, that's because the timing of sleep and waking is also influenced by your circadian biorhythm. Sleep quality is best when the time at which you go to sleep and wake up is in synchrony with your circadian rhythm. For this reason, people who work evening and night shifts (e.g., healthcare workers, police officers) can suffer significant sleep deprivation until their bodies adjust to the new pattern. Changing time zones can also disrupt sleep–wake cycles and can thus be troublesome for people who travel frequently. Hospitalization can also interfere with a patient's circadian rhythm. Noises, lights, waking the patient for vital signs or medications, altered normal bedtime rituals, absence or presence of family members, recent losses, or fear of the unknown may compromise the patient's quality of sleep and the ability to fall and stay asleep.

 Critical**Thinking** 33-3

What may upset Anne's circadian rhythm?

How Is Sleep Regulated?

What makes us fall asleep? What happens in the brain during sleep? The mechanisms of sleep are complex and poorly understood, but we know that sleep is controlled by centers in the lower part of the brain, which produce sleep by actively inhibiting wakefulness. As just noted, a major factor in regulating sleep is the amount of light received through the eyes. The increasing light of a dawning sky signals the hypothalamus (Fig. 33-4) to induce gradual arousal from sleep. Another collection of nerve cell bodies within the brain stem, called the **reticular formation,** is responsible for maintaining wakefulness. The reticular formation is activated by stimuli from the cerebral cortex. Together, these reticular and cortical neurons are called the **reticular activating system (RAS).** Neurotransmitters associated with excitatory and inhibitory sleep mechanisms include catecholamines, acetylcholine, serotonin, histamine, and prostaglandins. L-Tryptophan and adenosine promote feelings of sleepiness.

An **electroencephalogram (EEG)** is used to record the electrical activity of the neurons in the brain. Electrical impulses are transmitted from the brain through electrodes attached to the scalp. These impulses create five different wave patterns, or *brain waves*. Figure 33-5 shows examples of different types of brain waves during sleep:

- **Alpha waves** are high-frequency, medium-amplitude, irregular waves. These occur in the drowsy stage.
- **Beta waves** are high-frequency, low-amplitude, irregular waves. These occur during periods of wakefulness.
- **Spindles** or **K-complexes** are peaked, irregular waveforms that occur in the earlier phases of NREM sleep.
- **Theta waves** are high-amplitude waves that are common in children but rare in adults. These occur with delta waves when transitioning to a deeper sleep stage.
- **Delta waves** are low-frequency, high-amplitude, regular waves common in deep sleep.

FIGURE 33-4 The reticular activating system works to regulate sleep and wakefulness.

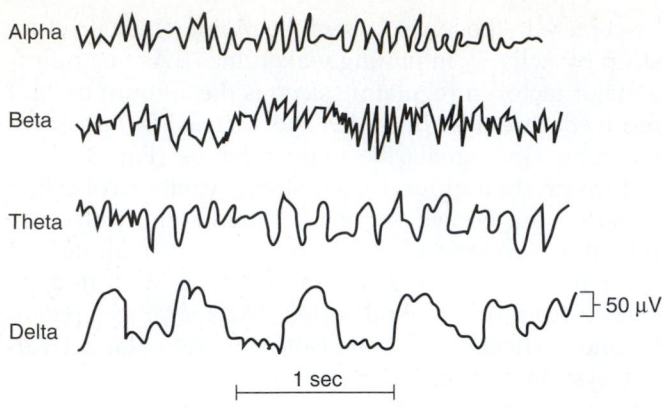

FIGURE 33-5 Four different types of brain waves.

The EEG of a waking person differs greatly from that of a sleeping person. In general, the greater the brain activity, the more rapid the brain waves on the EEG. While the person is awake, brain waves are very rapid, irregular, and low in amplitude, mostly alpha and beta waves. Many neurons are firing at different intervals, at different times, and with different strengths. When a person is relaxed without intense stimulation of the senses, the EEG records mostly alpha activity. During sleep, alpha waves disappear. They are replaced by slower, higher amplitude delta waves.

What Are the Stages of Sleep?

There are two distinct types of sleep:

- **NREM** (non–rapid eye movement) sleep is generally the restful phase of sleep where physiological function is slow.
- In **REM** (rapid eye movement) sleep, the brain is highly active, with brain waves similar to those that occur when a person is awake and alert.

The sleep cycle is typically 90 to 120 minutes. Cycling between REM and NREM sleep produces restorative rest. Five stages of sleep (four NREM stages and the REM stage) have been identified, based on brain activity and other physiological characteristics (Table 33-2).

NREM Sleep

NREM sleep is also called *slow-wave sleep (SWS)* because it is characterized by the presence of delta waves. NREM is divided into four stages, each deeper than the one preceding it. The parasympathetic branch of the autonomic nervous system becomes progressively more dominant during each stage of NREM sleep. During this phase, muscles relax, body temperature lowers, and heart rate, respirations, and blood pressure decrease.

Stage I is a light sleep from which the sleeper can easily be awakened. The person is relaxed; breathing is regular and deep; the eyelids slowly open and close, and the eyes roll from side to side. The person feels drowsy, the eyelids feel heavy, and suddenly without awareness the person falls asleep. Within 5 to 10 minutes, sleep progresses to stage II. Stage I accounts for about 5% of our total sleep during the night. Brain activity consists of alpha waves, with occasional low-frequency theta waves (McCance & Heuther, 2005).

Stage II is also light sleep. Brain activity slows, characterized by sleep spindles. The eyes are still, and body processes begin to slow down (e.g., temperature, pulse, and blood pressure decrease). There are spontaneous periods of muscle tone mixed with periods of muscle relaxation. Stage II usually lasts for 10 to 15 minutes.

Stage III is a deeper sleep. Progressively more delta and slow-wave activity begins to occur in this stage. The person is difficult to rouse, slow eye movement stops, skeletal muscles are very relaxed, and snoring may occur. This stage may last 5 to 15 minutes. A young adult spends about 8% of sleep time in Stage III.

Stage IV is the deepest sleep. In this stage, the delta waves are highest in amplitude, slowest in frequency, and highly synchronized. The body, mind, and muscles are very relaxed. It is difficult to awaken someone in stage IV slow-wave sleep, and if she is awakened, the person may appear confused and react slowly. Some dreaming may occur in stage IV, but dreams are less vivid than those that occur in REM sleep. Stage IV sleep appears to be especially important for restorative processes such as protein synthesis, cell division, and tissue renewal. During this stage, the body releases human growth hormone, which is essential for repair and renewal of brain and other cells (McCance & Huether, 2005). A young adult spends about 11% of sleep time in stage IV.

REM Sleep (Stage V)

About 90 minutes after the onset of sleep and after the deep sleep of stage IV, the brain becomes highly active, and the brain waves resemble those of a person who is fully awake. This is REM sleep, so called because of its characteristic rapid eye movements, which can often be detected even though the sleeper's eyelids are closed. Metabolism, temperature, pulse, heart rate, and blood pressure increase, but muscle activity and deep tendon reflexes are depressed. Because most people awakened during REM sleep report that they have been dreaming, this loss of muscle tone is thought to be a protective response that prevents the person from acting out the dreams. People are difficult to rouse during REM sleep; however, more spontaneous awakenings occur during this stage than any other. For this reason, REM sleep is also called *paradoxical sleep* (Germann & Stanfield, 2008). When sleepers are successfully awakened during this stage, they are usually alert and can react normally; in contrast, sleepers who are awakened during stages III or IV of slow-wave (NREM) sleep take a few moments to wake up and react.

Table 33-2 ▶ Characteristics of Stages of Sleep

STAGE	TYPICAL DURATION	CHARACTERISTICS
I	5–10 minutes	Transition between wakefulness and sleep
		Light sleep; can be awakened easily
		Relaxed but aware of surroundings
		Groggy, heavy lidded
		Regular, deep breathing; eyelids open and close slowly.
		Accounts for about 5% of total sleep.
		Dreams are usually not remembered.
II	10–15 minutes	Light sleep
		Easily roused
		Temperature, heart rate, and blood pressure decrease slightly.
		Accounts for about 50% of total sleep
III	5–15 minutes	Deep sleep
		Difficult to rouse
		Parasympathetic nervous system predominates: temperature, pulse, respirations, and blood pressure slow even more
		Skeletal muscles are very relaxed.
		Snoring may occur.
		Accounts for about 8% of total sleep.
IV	20–50 minutes	The deepest sleep
		Difficult to awaken
		Body, mind, and muscles are very relaxed.
		Parasympathetic nervous system still predominates; heart rate and respirations are slow and regular; temperature and blood pressure are low.
		If roused, may be confused.
		Accounts for about 11% of total sleep.
REM (V)	5–30 minutes (usually at least 20–30)	Paradoxical sleep
		Less restful than NREM sleep
		Eyes move rapidly.
		Small muscles twitch.
		Metabolism, temperature, pulse, and blood pressure increase.
		Pulse may be rapid and irregular.
		Apnea may occur.
		Gastric secretions increase.
		Large muscle activity and deep-tendon reflexes are depressed.
		Dreaming occurs.
		If awakened, will react normally.
		Accounts for about 25% of total sleep.

REM sleep is essential for mental and emotional restoration. Loss of REM sleep impairs memory and learning. A person who is deprived of REM sleep for several nights will usually experience *REM rebound;* that is, the person will spend a greater amount of time in REM sleep on successive nights, keeping the total amount of REM sleep constant over time.

Sleep Cycles

Sleep is cyclic. The NREM/REM sleep cycle repeats four to six times throughout the night, depending on the total amount of time spent sleeping (Fig. 33-6). Each cycle lasts approximately 100 minutes. The first REM period may last only about 20 minutes, but with each

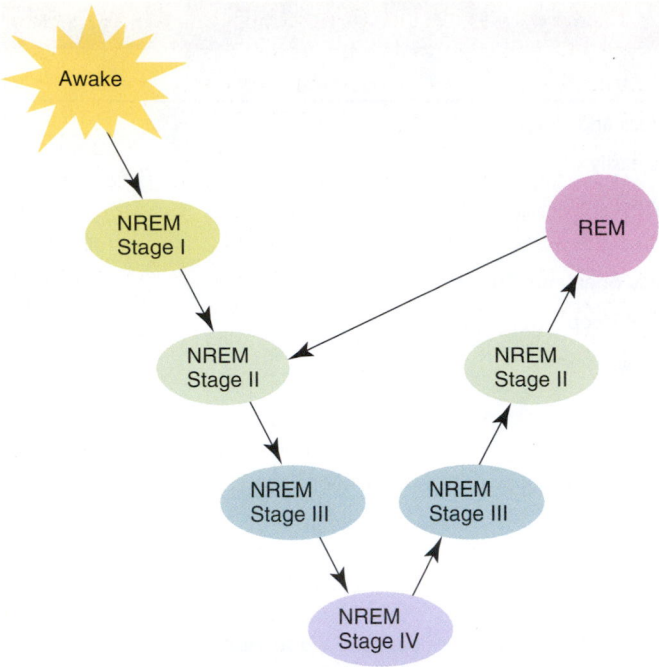

FIGURE 33-6 The normal adult sleep cycle. All but NREM stage I are repeated four or more times a night.

cycle, the REM period lengthens until, in the last cycle of a typical 8-hour sleep period, REM may last as long as 60 minutes. The amount of time spent in each sleep stage varies over the life span.

KnowledgeCheck 33-2

- List the five stages of sleep.
- Describe the progression of a typical sleep cycle for a young adult.
- Describe the physiological activity characteristic of each stage of sleep.
- What is the stage that must be "made up" if not enough time is spent in it?

 Go to Chapter 33, **Knowledge Check Response Sheet and Answers,** on the Student Resource Disk or DavisPlus at http://davisplus.fadavis.com/Wilkinson2

 Critical**Thinking** 33-4

- Anne's ("Meet Your Patient") physician has prescribed zolpidem (Ambien) for her. Ambien is a sedative/hypnotic (nonbarbiturate) used in the short-term treatment of insomnia. Why do you think the doctor prescribed a sleeping medication even though Anne is physiologically and psychologically dependent on the medication?
- Anne will undoubtedly receive narcotic analgesics after surgery. How do you think they will affect her sleep?

What Factors Affect Sleep?

People vary not only in the amount of sleep they need, but also in their sleep patterns. Some people are refreshed after napping for 15 or 20 minutes; others feel groggy after napping; others cannot nap at all. Many people routinely waken several times a night and do not report being tired, whereas others report fatigue and loss of mental clarity if their sleep is even minimally interrupted. In short, **sleep quality** has both subjective and objective components. It is related to (1) the total amount of sleep, (2) how well the person slept, and (3) whether the person obtained the needed amounts of NREM and REM. Several factors affect the amount and quality of sleep.

Age

Age is an important factor affecting the duration of sleep (see Table 33-1). But sleep *patterns* are also affected by age. For example, newborns and young children experience prolonged REM sleep periods; young adults spend about 25% of their sleep in REM sleep; and older adults typically enter REM sleep quicker and spend more time in this active phase of sleep.

Children and Adolescents

A survey by the National Sleep Foundation found that two out of three young children experience sleep-related problems a few times a week. The problems included trouble falling asleep, frequent awakenings, nightmares, and heavy snoring (Tuller, 2004). Environmental stimuli, such as the sounds and lights of older family members' activities, may make it difficult for a young child to sleep, or the child may have difficulty "winding down" after hectic activities in the late afternoon and early evening hours. Toddlers and preschoolers may be frightened to go to bed because of imaginary figures or intruders, or they may waken frequently at night because of bad dreams, the need to use the bathroom, illness, heavy snoring, tossing off the bedclothes, or falling out of bed. Some have difficulty self-calming enough to achieve a restful state before falling asleep. Some school-age children may suffer significant sleep disturbances because of anxiety or depression. Others might have more temporary sleep difficulty related to isolated situations, stress, excitement, or social concerns, such as anticipating a school event or sports competition.

The growth spurt that occurs during adolescence increases the need for sleep (Polan & Taylor, 2007). At the same time, teenagers may not sleep well because of increased demands at school; staying up late to watch television, texting or other social networking, or study; dating or staying out late with friends; or the effect of alcohol or drugs. Some teens consume large amounts of caffeinated colas and other beverages that can delay or disturb sleep.

Young Adults

College students may pull "all-nighters" to cram for exams or experience insomnia because of worries about grades or future career choices. Young adults may drive themselves too hard to succeed, prompting late nights at work or sleep loss due to hectic travel schedules or work-related stress. Others might not obtain enough sleep because of social choices and personal entertainment choices during the night. Others might work the evening or night shift.

Sleep for parents of young children is often interrupted. Breastfeeding mothers typically need to feed their infants one or more times each night until the infant begins solid foods. Parents of toddlers often wake to care for a child who is having a nightmare, is ill, or needs to use the bathroom. The National Sleep Foundation survey found that some parents lose as many as 200 hours of sleep a year because of their children's poor sleeping patterns (Tuller, 2004).

Middle-Aged and Older Adults

Middle-aged adults may experience insomnia because of the depression, anxiety, and tension that result from the stress of career demands, the need to care for a parent, marital discord, worry about teenaged children, or financial problems. The lack of sleep compounds the problem, leading to reduced ability to cope, and again to lack of sleep. As a physiological example, menopausal women may be awakened by hormonal fluctuations.

Older adults may feel displaced in the workforce and worry about their impending retirement. Many suffer sleep disturbances because of nocturia, the side effects of medications, and discomfort or pain. In addition, the levels of melatonin, the natural hormone that controls sleep, decline in the latter decades of life.

Lifestyle Factors

Lifestyle factors influencing sleep include work, exercise, nutrition, and use of medications and drugs. As noted earlier, a person who changes work shifts frequently may find it difficult to sleep at the right time. Moreover, people who cross time zones frequently because of travel may experience difficulty falling asleep, early wakening, or daytime fatigue.

Exercise. If it occurs at least 2 hours before bedtime, exercise promotes sleep. Fatigue from a normal physically active day is thought to promote a restful night's sleep. However, the more tired a person is, the shorter the first period of REM sleep.

Diet. Foods can either promote or interfere with sleep. A meal high in saturated fat near bedtime may interfere with sleep. Dietary L-tryptophan, an amino acid found in milk and cheese, may help to induce sleep, although some studies indicate that the protein in these foods actually increases alertness and concentration. Carbohydrates seem to promote relaxation through their effects on brain serotonin levels. In general, satiation induces sleep, whereas many people, especially infants and children, have difficulty falling asleep when they are hungry.

Nicotine and Caffeine. Central nervous system stimulants, such as nicotine and caffeine, interfere with sleep. Smokers tend to have more difficulty falling asleep and are more easily roused than nonsmokers. People who stop smoking often experience temporary sleep disturbances during the withdrawal period. Caffeine blocks adenosine and thereby inhibits sleep. However, individuals vary greatly in their sensitivity to caffeine. Some people can consume coffee throughout the day and evening and suffer no loss of sleep, whereas others cannot consume even small amounts of caffeine early in the day without suffering insomnia later.

Alcohol. Consumption of alcohol, especially if heavy, may hasten the onset of sleep; however, it disrupts REM and slow wave sleep and may cause spontaneous awakenings with difficulty returning to sleep. In addition, in some people heavy alcohol can prompt vivid dreams during REM sleep. Because alcohol is a diuretic, it can interrupt sleep by inducing nocturia.

Medications. Many of the medications people take cause either sleeplessness or excessive grogginess and sedation. Medications to induce sleep (i.e., *hypnotics*) tend to increase the amount of sleep while decreasing the quality. Zolpidem tartrate (Ambien) promotes normal REM sleep and appears to influence sleep quality less than do other hypnotics. Amphetamines, tranquilizers, and antidepressants reduce the amount of REM sleep; barbiturates, in addition, interfere with NREM sleep. Opioids, such as morphine, suppress REM sleep and cause frequent awakening. Beta-blockers are reported to cause insomnia and nightmares.

Illness

Illness increases the need for sleep and rest. At the same time, its associated mental and physical distress can cause sleep problems. Fear of the unknown outcome of an illness and role changes associated with hospitalization can cause anxiety. Disease symptoms, such as fever, pain, nausea, and respiratory conditions (e.g., shortness of breath, dyspnea, sinus congestion), can also interfere with sleep. Specific disease conditions altering the quality of sleep are allergies, hyperthyroidism, and Parkinson's disease.

Anxiety increases gastric secretions, intestinal motility, heart rate, and respirations, all of which contribute to a restless night. Anxiety also stimulates the sympathetic nervous system, increasing the level of norepinephrine. This decreases stage IV and REM sleep and leads to more awakenings. Depression may be associated either with almost constant sleeping or with insomnia.

Environmental Factors

Environmental factors can promote or inhibit sleep. Some people need a cool room, whereas others need warmth. Some prefer heavy blankets, and others like to sleep with just a light sheet. Noise can also inhibit sleep, but a person can become habituated to noise over time and be less affected by it. Some people routinely fall asleep to music or while listening to a radio or television. Often loud noises are needed to awaken a person in NREM stages III and IV and REM sleep.

Any change in the usual environmental stimuli can affect sleep. For example, a patient used to falling asleep next to his wife may have trouble sleeping alone in a hospital bed. Equipment noise, the muffled sounds of a busy medical–surgical unit, or the labored breathing or snoring of a roommate also can interfere with the patient's ability to sleep.

When people who are accustomed to sleeping in a dark room are hospitalized, they may have trouble falling asleep because of light outside their window or filtering into the room from the hallway. However, light can be therapeutic for some patients suffering from sleep problems. Exposure to bright light can alter circadian rhythms in some adults. However, light therapy has not been shown to be effective in older adults with dementia living in skilled nursing facilities (Haesler, 2004).

KnowledgeCheck 33-3

- For each of the following patients, propose at least two factors that might affect sleep:

    A newborn in the NICU
    A preschooler being treated for pneumonia
    An adolescent with cancer
    A breastfeeding mother of a newborn
    An elderly man who has fractured his hip

- Identify at least three types of environmental stimuli that can disturb sleep.

 Go to Chapter 33, **Knowledge Check Response Sheet and Answers,** on the Student Resource Disk or DavisPlus at http://davisplus.fadavis.com/Wilkinson2

What Are Some Common Sleep Disorders?

Sleep disorders are classified by their signs and symptoms. The more common disorders fall into two groups:

- **Dyssomnias**—Sleep disorders characterized by insomnia or excessive sleepiness. They include insomnia, sleep–wake schedule (circadian) disorders, sleep apnea, restless leg syndrome, hypersomnia, and narcolepsy.
- **Parasomnias**—Patterns of waking behavior that appear during sleep (e.g., sleepwalking)

Insomnia

Insomnia is the inability to fall asleep, remain asleep, or go back to sleep. Insomnia may be *transient/short term* (less than a month) or *chronic* (longer than a month).

People with insomnia usually report an insufficient quantity and quality of sleep and wake without feeling refreshed, even though they are often observed to sleep more than they perceive that they do. Most people are distressed by the daytime consequences of insomnia, which include symptoms of excessive daytime sleepiness, poor concentration, fatigue, lethargy, and irritability.

Insomnia is the most common sleep disorder. Two out of three people say they have insomnia at least once a week (National Sleep Foundation, 2008). It is more prevalent in women and in adults older than 60 years. Recent evidence suggests a link between neuroendocrine activity insomnia and depression, linking abnormal hypothalamic–pituitary–adrenal gland activity with insomnia and mood disorders (Roth, Roehrs, & Pies, 2007). Insomnia may occur as a result of illness, depression, anxiety disorders, acute stress, substance abuse, side effects of medications (e.g., steroids, central adrenergic blockers, bronchodilating agents), or inadequate sleep hygiene (e.g., watching TV in bed, drinking caffeine-containing beverages before bedtime). It may also be the presenting symptom of other primary sleep disorders, such as restless leg syndrome.

Primary care providers can diagnose and manage most cases of insomnia. Once underlying medical or psychiatric conditions have been identified and treated, a combination of behavioral and pharmacological therapy may be effective. The use of medication to induce sleep is controversial because some types can become habit-forming, become less effective when taken continuously, and can have serious side effects. However, sedative–hypnotic treatment is justified in short-term insomnia to avoid the negative effects of insomnia on mood and performance. Short-term aggressive treatment may prevent the development of chronic insomnia.

Sleep–Wake Schedule (Circadian) Disorders

Abnormalities in sleep–wake schedules may be caused by rapid time-zone changes (jet lag), shift work, or a change in total sleep time from day to day. Symptoms include decreased vigilance, decreased ability to perform psychomotor tasks, and short sleep episodes (*microsleeps*) that the person is not aware of. People suffering jet lag need several days to adjust their sleep–wake schedule.

Restless Leg Syndrome (RLS)

Restless leg syndrome (RLS) is a disorder of the central nervous system characterized by an uncontrollable movement of the legs while resting or before sleep onset. It tends to run in families. Children and young adults experience this condition, but it is especially common in older adults, and is sometimes associated with low levels of iron (Ball & Caivano, 2008; Hening, 2007) and use of some antidepressants. Symptoms include unpleasant creeping,

Toward Evidence-Based Practice

Kazuo, E., Pickering, T. J., Phil, D., et al. (2008). Short sleep duration as an independent predictor of cardiovascular events in Japanese patients with hypertension. *Archives of Internal Medicine, 168,* 2225–2231.

Researchers found out that short duration of sleep is a predictor of future cardiovascular events in patients with hypertension. Healthcare providers should ask patients with high blood pressure about how many uninterrupted hours of sleep they get.

Ong, J. C., Stepanski, E. J., & Gramling, S. E. (2009, February 15). Pain coping strategies for tension-type headache: Possible implications for insomnia. *Journal of Clinical Sleep Medicine, 5(1),* 52–56.

Study participants reported sleep problems as a trigger of headaches, stress as a trigger of headache, and going to sleep as a strategy for dealing with pain. Study findings suggest too much or too little sleep can lead to headaches; and people with headaches often take naps to deal with headache pain. Chronic insomnia can occur from napping during the day.

1. Sleep deprivation produces detrimental effects for many people, especially for those with high blood pressure and those experiencing stress. In what other ways do you think sleep deprivation creates problems for the physical body?

2. Considering the findings of the Kazuo, Pickering, Phil, et al., study, what else would you want to know about your patient with high blood pressure?

3. On one hand, sleep can be a way for people with headaches to deal with the pain. On the other hand, too much sleep, such as daytime naps, can wreak havoc on getting a good, restful sleep at night. How would you use the Ong, Stepanski, and Gramling study to guide patients who are dealing with the pain of a migraine?

 Go to Chapter 33, **Toward Evidence-Based Practice Suggested Responses,** on the Student Resource Disk or DavisPlus at http://davisplus.fadavis.com/Wilkinson2

---

crawling, itching, or tingling sensations in the legs. Symptoms are relieved only by moving the legs, which prevents the person from relaxing and falling asleep. If RLS is severe, treatment may include neuroleptic agents and medication used to treat Parkinson's disease (Birath & Martin, 2009). People with RLS should avoid stimulants (e.g., caffeine). Other self-care measures include walking, massaging, stretching, heat or cold compresses, medication, vibration, and acupressure.

Sleep Deprivation

Sleep Deprivation is a NANDA-I nursing diagnosis. It is not actually a sleep disorder, but rather a result of prolonged sleep disturbances (e.g., insomnia and parasomnias). It can result from NREM or REM deprivation, or both. Signs and symptoms of sleep deprivation include daytime drowsiness, impaired cognitive functioning, restlessness, perceptual disorders, slowed reaction time, irritability, somatic (body) complaints (e.g., hand tremors), and a general feeling of malaise. Functional imaging studies contrasting sleep-deprived and well rested brains reveal the importance of adequate sleep for memory and learning (Chee & Chuah, 2008). If sleep deprivation is severe and prolonged, delusions, paranoia, and other psychotic behavior may occur. Studies of sleep-deprived adults revealed changes in the levels of certain immunoglobulins and other markers of the immune system (Ranjbaran, Keefer, & Stepanski, 2007; Hui, Hua, Diandong, et al., 2007), which means going without sleep can weaken the body's protection against infection.

Illness and hospital care are common causes of sleep deprivation, especially for patients in critical care units (CCUs). In this environment, lights are on most of the time, and equipment noise, frequent treatments, and assessments all combine with the client's fragile physical condition to create sleep deprivation. Likewise, healthcare providers who work long and late hours or rotating day–night shifts experience serious fatigue that can lead to medical error and patient injury or death (Lockley, Barger, Ayas, et al., 2007).

Hypersomnia

Hypersomnia is excessive sleeping, especially in the daytime. People with excessive daytime sleepiness doze, nap, or fall asleep at times and in situations when they need or wish to be awake and alert. The sleep disorders that commonly cause hypersomnia are obstructive sleep apnea and narcolepsy. Hypersomnia may also be caused by disorders of the central nervous system, kidney, or liver or by metabolic disorders (e.g., diabetic acidosis and hypothyroidism). It can also be a symptom of depression.

Sleep Apnea

Sleep apnea is a periodic interruption in breathing during sleep—an absence of air flow through the nose or mouth during sleep. Typically the soft tissue of the pharynx and soft palate collapse and obstruct the airway. Episodes may occur several or a hundred times a night and may last for as long as 1 minute or longer

(American Sleep Apnea Association, 2008). During periods of apnea, the oxygen level in the blood drops, and the carbon dioxide level rises, causing the person to wake up. This may result in cardiac dysrhythmias (irregularities) and increases in pulse and blood pressure. Many people with sleep apnea complain of fatigue and morning headache; however, some may experience mild sleep apnea without any symptoms.

To diagnose sleep apnea, a sleep study consisting of an electroencephalogram (EEG), monitoring of arterial oxygen saturation, and an electrocardiogram (ECG) is recommended. Treatment depends on the type of apnea involved. Untreated sleep apnea is associated with polycythemia, hypertension, angina, coronary artery disease, right-sided heart failure, stroke, impotence, depression, personality changes, and mood swings.

The two main types of sleep apnea have different etiologies. **Mixed apnea** is a combination of the two main types. **Obstructive sleep apnea (OSA)** is caused by airway occlusion (usually by the tongue or palate) during sleep, but the person continues to try to breathe. The person is not aware of waking. Sleeping partners often report that the person snores, snorts, grunts, or thrashes about during sleep. Airway occlusion may be due to a collapse of the hypopharynx or from other structural abnormalities (e.g., enlarged tonsils, adenoids, a deviated nasal septum, or thyroid enlargement). Although most often males over age 40, particularly if overweight, are affected by sleep apnea, the condition occurs in females of any age and weight. Treatment of OSA might involve surgery to remove any obstruction within the airway or applying CPAP (continuous positive airway pressure) treatment. This is a device that delivers oxygen using forced air pressure and keeps the airways open when apnea occurs. Patients with OSA should avoid alcohol and smoking and lose excess weight (American Sleep Apnea Association, 2008; Marshall, Glazier, & Grunstein, 2008).

Central sleep apnea (CSA) is a complete suspension of breathing resulting from a dysfunction in central respiratory control. Only about 10% of sleep apnea is central in origin. People with CSA tend to awaken during sleep and, therefore, experience daytime sleepiness.

Snoring

Snoring is a hallmark sign of obstructive sleep apnea, but it does not necessarily indicate OSA. Even so, snoring can significantly reduce the quality of sleep for the bed partner. Snoring results when the muscles at the back of the mouth relax during sleep, obstruct the airway, and vibrate with each breath. Obstruction is usually more pronounced when the person sleeps on his back. Many treatments have been invented to open the air passages, such as nose tapes or even surgery. Saline sprays, nose drops, and cortisone sprays are also used—all with mixed success.

Narcolepsy

Narcolepsy is a chronic disorder caused by the brain's inability to regulate sleep–wake cycles normally. At various times, the person with narcolepsy experiences a sudden, uncontrollable urge to sleep lasting from seconds to minutes, even though the person sleeps well at night. The person cannot avoid the sleep episodes but awakens easily. Narcolepsy is characterized by sleepiness, slurred speech, slackening of the facial muscles, a feeling of impending weakness of the knees, paralysis, and hallucinations. Performance is impaired during these micro-sleep episodes. Sleep episodes can come on suddenly, even while the person is having a conversation. If they occur while the person is driving, working, or even operating machinery, they can be dangerous. People with narcolepsy will awaken from episodes of unavoidable sleep feeling refreshed (National Institute of Neurological Disorders and Stroke [NINDS], 2009). Some have other symptoms, such as **cataplexy,** a sudden loss of muscle tone usually triggered by an emotional event (e.g., laughter, surprise, or anger), but most only have hypersomnia.

Narcolepsy affects up to 1 in every 2,000 Americans, males about as often as females (NINDS, 2009). It is thought to be caused by a genetic defect of the central nervous system in which REM sleep cannot be controlled. Each micro-sleep episode begins in the REM stage instead of progressing through the NREM stages first. People with narcolepsy do not tolerate irregular sleep–wake patterns, such as shift work, and have difficulty staying awake with passive activity, such as watching television. The condition is controlled by central nervous system stimulants, such as methylphenidate (Ritalin), with little evidence of tolerance, dependence, or abuse.

Other individuals might suffer pseudo-narcolepsy, which is characterized by involuntary episodes of sleep but are related by acute or chronic sleep deprivation. In this case, when the person is well rested, the episodes resolve.

KnowledgeCheck 33-4

- What is the most common dyssomnia?
- What factors in the hospital may contribute to sleep deprivation in patients?
- What are the clinical signs of sleep deprivation?
- Why are sleeping pills not recommended for chronic insomnia?
- Why is snoring significant?

 Go to Chapter 33, **Knowledge Check Response Sheet and Answers,** on the Student Resource Disk or DavisPlus at http://davisplus.fadavis.com/Wilkinson2

 Critical**Thinking** 33-5

Compare and contrast insomnia and hypersomnia. How are they different? How are they alike?

Parasomnias

The parasomnias include sleepwalking, sleeptalking, bruxism, night terrors, REM sleep behavior disorders, and nocturnal enuresis.

Sleepwalking

Sleepwalking (somnambulism) occurs during stages III and IV of NREM sleep, usually 1 to 2 hours after the person falls asleep. The sleeper leaves the bed and walks about, with little awareness of surroundings. He may perform what appear to be conscious motor activities (e.g., brush his teeth, make coffee), but he does not wake up. The person is not aware of sleepwalking and has no memory of the event on awakening. The event may last 3 to 4 minutes or longer. Children sleepwalk more than adults do. If the child does not outgrow the condition or serious safety risks exist, drugs may be given to suppress stage IV sleep. Stress, fatigue, and some drugs can trigger sleepwalking.

Sleeptalking

Sleeptalking occurs during NREM sleep, just before the REM stage. It does not usually interfere with the person's rest but may be disturbing to a bed partner.

Bruxism

Bruxism, grinding and clenching of the teeth, usually occurs during stage II NREM sleep. It can eventually erode tooth enamel and loosen the teeth. The noise can also disturb the bed partner's sleep.

Night Terrors

Night terrors are sudden arousals in which the person (often a child) is physically active, often hallucinatory, and expresses a strong emotion such as terror. Children experiencing night terrors typically cry or scream in fear, thrash about, and resist all attempts by their parents or other caregivers to hold or console them. The child appears to be fully awake, but she is not; in fact, children in the midst of night terrors are extremely difficult to awaken. Episodes may last from 10 to 30 minutes. However, the child typically returns to sleep without awakening, and in the morning has no memory of the event (Cohen, 2004). Unlike *nightmares* (unpleasant, frightening dreams), which occur during REM sleep, night terrors occur during stage IV (deep NREM) sleep.

REM Sleep Behavior Disorders

REM sleep behavior disorders are associated with REM (or dreaming period) sleep, in which the sleeper violently acts out the dream. People have actually injured themselves or others without waking.

Nocturnal Enuresis

Nocturnal enuresis (bedwetting) is nighttime incontinence past the stage at which toilet training has been well established (Polan & Taylor, 2007). It has incorrectly been associated with dreaming; however, most incidents occur during NREM sleep, during the first third of the night when the child is difficult to rouse. It may be distressing to the child and family because of the importance society places on continence, the inconvenience of keeping bed linens clean, and the misconception that the child is bedwetting to act out against parents. Because the great majority of children outgrow enuresis, the best strategy is patience (McCance & Huether, 2005). If the problem persists, the child should have a full medical evaluation.

Secondary Sleep Disorders

Secondary sleep disorders occur when a disease causes alterations in sleep stages or in quantity and quality of sleep. The following are the most common causes:

Depression. Depressed people may spend a great deal of time in bed. However, in general, they have difficulty falling asleep, experience less slow-wave (deep) sleep, spend less time in REM sleep, awaken early, and have less total sleep time.

Hyperthyroidism or Hypothyroidism. An increase in thyroid secretion causes an increase in stage III and IV sleep; hypothyroidism causes a decrease in those stages. Hyperthyroidism increases metabolic rate, making it difficult for the person to fall asleep.

Pain. Both acute and chronic pain interfere with sleep. Chronic pain affects both the quality and quantity of sleep. It inhibits sleep, increases arousals during sleep, and causes longer waking intervals during the night.

Airway Passage Obstruction or CNS Dysfunction, Which Cause Sleep Apnea. These conditions were discussed under "Sleep Apnea."

Disorders that Are Provoked by Sleep

Sleep-provoked disorders are those that occur when signs and symptoms of the disease appear or become worse during sleep. Diseases affected by sleep include the following (McCance & Huether, 2005):

Coronary Artery Disease. During REM sleep, dreams may increase heart rate and provoke angina and ECG changes.

Asthma. People with asthma may experience bronchospasm during REM sleep. In adults, asthma attacks frequently occur during the night as the esophageal sphincter relaxes and reflux results. In children, they occur mostly during the final two-thirds of the night, when there is less stage IV sleep.

Chronic Obstructive Pulmonary Disease (COPD). Persons with COPD experience lowered oxygen tension and increased carbon dioxide retention during sleep, especially during REM sleep, when neuromuscular control is normally depressed. This can result in pulmonary spasm and transient pulmonary hypertension.

Diabetes. Blood glucose levels vary during sleep. When diabetes is uncontrolled, it may profoundly affect the blood sugar level during sleep, when the person is not alert enough to deal with it. Therefore, patients with uncontrolled diabetes may need to have blood glucose levels monitored during sleep.

Gastric and Intestinal Ulcers. During REM sleep, people with duodenal ulcers secrete up to 20 times more gastric acid than do people who do not have duodenal ulcers. Peptic ulcers also contribute to increased acid, often producing nocturnal epigastric pain and sleep loss.

KnowledgeCheck 33-5

- List and define at least three parasomnias.
- Describe ways in which depression can affect sleep.
- List two sleep-provoked disorders, and explain how the sleep stage affects the disease.

 Go to Chapter 33, **Knowledge Check Response Sheet and Answers,** on the Student Resource Disk or DavisPlus at http://davisplus.fadavis.com/Wilkinson2

Practical **Knowledge** **knowing** how

ASSESSMENT

It is important to assess usual sleep patterns and rituals for all patients who are being admitted to the hospital or seeking help for a sleep problem. A brief assessment for all patients should include questions about the following:

- Usual sleeping pattern
- Sleeping environment
- Bedtime routines/rituals
- Sleep aids
- Sleep changes or problems

For a list of questions you can use to obtain this information,

 Go to Chapter 33, **Assessment Guidelines and Tools, Questions for a Sleep History,** in Volume 2.

If the person reports experiencing satisfactory sleep, that is an adequate assessment, and you merely need to support her usual sleep patterns and rituals. When you suspect a sleep problem, you will perform a more in-depth assessment, such as a detailed sleep history or sleep diary.

A **sleep history** includes in-depth questions about the person's usual times for sleep, any preparation, preferences and routines, quality of sleep, napping habits (if any), and whether she wakes early and cannot return to sleep.

A **sleep diary** provides very specific information on your patient's patterns of sleep. This allows you to identify trends in sleep/wakefulness and associate behaviors interfering with sleep. You will usually tell the patient to keep the diary for 14 days; remind him that it is important to be diligent in maintaining it.

For examples of a sleep history and a sleep diary,

 Go to Chapter 33, **Assessment Guidelines and Tools, Questions for a Sleep History** and **Sleep Diary,** in Volume 2.

To find the National Sleep Foundation Sleepiness Diary online,

Go to Chapter 33, **Resources for Caregivers and Healthcare Professionals,** on the Student Resource Disk or DavisPlus at http://davisplus.fadavis.com/Wilkinson2

A **sleep study** is most useful in detecting sleep apnea and other sleep disorders, such as narcolepsy, night terrors, and periodic limb movement disorder. One of the most common sleep studies performed in a sleep lab is polysomnography, which records brain activity, eye movement, oxygen and carbon dioxide levels, vital signs, and body movements during the sleep phases.

ANALYSIS/NURSING DIAGNOSIS

It is important to determine whether lack of sleep is a problem, is a symptom of a problem, or is contributing to (etiology of) a different problem. For health promotion applications, use the NANDA-I diagnosis Readiness for Enhanced Sleep when a client has no particular sleep problem but wishes to move to a higher level of functioning in the area of sleep.

Sleep as the Problem

When you wish to focus on interventions to promote sleep, use the diagnoses Disturbed Sleep Pattern or Sleep Deprivation on the problem side of the nursing diagnosis.

Use *Sleep Deprivation* as the nursing diagnosis when the patient's amount, consistency, or quality of sleep is decreased over prolonged periods of time. Defining characteristics of Sleep Deprivation are more severe than those for Disturbed Sleep Pattern, so nursing activities may focus as much on relieving symptoms (e.g., confusion, paranoia) as on sleep promotion.

Use *Disturbed Sleep Pattern* as the diagnosis when assessment data points to a time-limited sleep problem due to external factors (e.g., inability to sleep in the unfamiliar hospital environment). The problem should be one that can be treated by nursing therapy. Add modifying words to specify the type of sleep problem, as in the examples. This will help you to focus goals appropriately.

- Disturbed Sleep Pattern (difficulty falling asleep) related to worries about family

- Disturbed Sleep Pattern (difficulty falling and remaining asleep) related to noise of hospital environment and need for scheduled treatments
- Disturbed Sleep Pattern (premature awakening) related to sleeping aid dependence and lack of knowledge of nonpharmacological aids for insomnia
- Disturbed Sleep Pattern (excessive daytime sleeping) related to effects of biological aging and depression
- Disturbed Sleep Pattern (altered sleep–wake patterns) related to frequent rotations of shift and overtime

Use *Insomnia* for patients who have a disruption in the amount of quality of sleep to the extent that it impairs functioning. Use *Readiness for Enhanced Sleep* for clients who are sleeping well enough to obtain adequate rest and desired functioning, but whose sleeping can be improved in quality.

Carefully describe the etiologies for sleep problems, because they determine your interventions.

 Critical**Thinking** 33-6

In the following nursing diagnoses, how do you think your interventions would be different for each diagnosis?
Disturbed Sleep Pattern related to:

- Changes in bedtime routines
- Exercising within 2 hours before sleep
- Drinking caffeinated beverages, eating chocolate, and drinking alcohol
- Emotional or physical pain
- Drug dependence or withdrawal
- Physical illness

Sleep Pattern as an Etiology

Disturbed Sleep Pattern and Sleep Deprivation affect many areas of functioning, so they often are the etiology of other nursing diagnoses, as in these examples:

- Risk for Injury or Falls related to sleepwalking (or REM sleep behavior disorder or narcolepsy)
- Fatigue (or Activity Intolerance) related to chronic insufficient quality or quantity of sleep (e.g., secondary to insomnia)
- Ineffective Coping related to decreased cognitive functioning and awareness, secondary to lack of sleep
- Disturbed Thought Processes related to decreased cognitive functioning, secondary to lack of sleep
- Anxiety (or Fear) related to fear of death from sleep apnea

Sleep Pattern as a Symptom

Difficulty sleeping may be one of the symptoms of another problem. For example, a client may have Spiritual Distress related to challenges to belief system *as manifested by nightmares, sleep disturbances, and verbalization of inner conflict about beliefs.* In this instance, you would focus on interventions for Spiritual Distress, assuming that the sleep pattern would improve as the Spiritual

Distress is resolved. Other nursing diagnoses that may cause sleep loss include Anxiety, Chronic Sorrow, Death Anxiety, Decisional Conflict, Complicated Grieving, Diarrhea, Impaired Gas Exchange, Nausea, Pain, and Relocation Stress Syndrome.

KnowledgeCheck 33-6

- For a chronic, long-term sleep problem, would you use a diagnosis of Sleep Pattern Disturbance, Sleep Deprivation, or Readiness for Enhanced Sleep?
- Name at least two nursing diagnoses that might have a sleep problem as the etiology.
- Name at least one nursing diagnosis that might have a sleep problem as the defining characteristic.

 Go to Chapter 33, **Knowledge Check Response Sheet and Answers,** on the Student Resource Disk or DavisPlus at http://davisplus.fadavis.com/Wilkinson2

PLANNING OUTCOMES/EVALUATION

NOC standardized outcomes linked to the NANDA-I sleep labels are as follows:

- For Disturbed Sleep Pattern: Rest, Sleep, and Personal Well-Being
- For Sleep Deprivation: Rest, Sleep, and Symptom Severity
- For the Insomnia diagnosis, linkages have not yet been established.

When sleep disturbances are the etiology of another nursing diagnosis, you will need to use the NOC outcomes associated with that diagnosis. For example:

Nursing diagnosis: Anxiety related to Sleep Deprivation
NOC outcomes for Anxiety: Anxiety Control, Coping

Individualized goals/outcome statements you might use to evaluate the success of interventions to promote sleep include the following:

- Verbalizes feeling rested or feeling less fatigue.
- Falls asleep within 30 minutes; sleeps 6 hours without awakening.
- Maintains a sleep–wake pattern that provides sufficient energy for the day's tasks.
- Demonstrates self-care behaviors that provide a healthy balance between rest and activity.
- Identifies stress-relieving rituals that enable falling asleep more easily.
- Demonstrates decreased signs of sleep deprivation.
- Verbalizes feeling less fatigued and more in control of life activities.

PLANNING INTERVENTIONS/IMPLEMENTATION

NIC standardized interventions for Sleep Deprivation and Sleep Pattern Disturbance include the following: Coping Enhancement, Energy Management, Environmental Management: Comfort, Simple Relaxation Therapy, and Sleep Enhancement. Linkages have not yet been established for Insomnia.

Specific nursing activities for clients with sleep problems are described in the next sections.

For a care plan and care map for Sleep Pattern Disturbance,

 Go to Chapter 33, **Care Plan and Care Map,** on the Student Resource Disk or DavisPlus at http://davisplus. fadavis.com/Wilkinson2

Schedule Nursing Care to Avoid Interrupting Sleep

Use nursing judgment to decide when a procedure must be done and when it is more important for your patient to sleep. Healthcare routines usually allow time for rest periods. In addition, you may consider the following:

- Some patients need to rest after a procedure or after meals.

VOL 2 For steps to follow in *all* procedures, refer to the Universal Steps for All Procedures found on the inside back cover of Volume 2. Go to the full procedures in Volume 2 to practice and learn the procedure steps. Use these Critical Aspects later to help you review key points.

Procedure 33-1: Giving a Back Massage

➤ Warm the lotion.

➤ Raise the bed to working height.

➤ Position the patient comfortably on her side or prone.

➤ Place lotion on your hands.

➤ Rub down the length and then up the sides of the back.

➤ Never rub directly over the spine.

➤ Apply gentle thumb pressure on either side of the spine at the midback, pushing outward for about 2.5 cm (1 in.) along the trapezius muscle.

➤ Always apply pressure away from the spine, not toward it.

➤ Go to the spots that felt the tightest or that the patient states are tight. Work in small circles, using gentle thumb pressure.

➤ Gently shake the scapula.

➤ Apply horizontal strokes across the scapula, using your thumb.

➤ Apply pressure in circles using the heels of your hands down both sides of the spine.

➤ Apply horizontal strokes using the heels of your hands across the latissimus dorsi muscle.

➤ Gently rub your hands up either side of the spine from the base of the back to the base of the neck, and then down the sides of the back.

Critical Aspects of Procedure 33-1

- If the person looks sleepy, give a prescribed sleeping pill early to avoid waking him later in the evening.
- You can often alter routines; for example, you can allow the patient to sleep as long as he can in the morning and bring his breakfast later.
- Cluster care to avoid unnecessary interruptions in sleep. Unless the patient is critically ill, do not wake him for morning vital signs if he is sleeping.
- Keep the noise level to a minimum. Be aware that activities, conversation, and equipment, even outside the patient's room, can disrupt sleep.

Create a Restful Environment

Many people find it difficult to sleep in a strange bed, even a comfortable one. Hospital beds are not noted for their luxury, but you can help make them more comfortable.

- Be sure the bed linens are tight on the bottom and loose on top to allow movement.
- Keep linens clean, dry, and free of irritants. Perspiration on the hospital gown or linens can lead to chill.
- Good body alignment also facilitates relaxation. Use extra pillows, a blanket from home, or any other item that may help the patient rest.
- Keep the room dark and quiet, unless the patient prefers a light.
- As much as possible, control the temperature of the room and provide good ventilation.

Promote Comfort

Pain, itching, and nausea may all be deterrents to rest and sleep in an ill person. Be sure to offer pain medications at their scheduled times, and before the patient's sleep time. Other comfort measures include providing a restful environment (see the preceding intervention) and offering fluids, cool cloths, or a massage or back rub. For detailed instructions for back massage,

 Go to Chapter 33, **Procedure 33-1: Giving a Back Massage,** in Volume 2.

Also see the accompanying Critical Aspects box for the critical aspects of this procedure.

Support Bedtime Rituals and Routines

Most people have some kind of a routine before bed, be it reading, watching TV, drinking warm milk, or praying or meditating, to allow them to prepare for sleep. For children, a favorite doll, blanket, bedtime story, as well as brushing their teeth and hair, may enhance sleepiness. Be sure to include any routines or rituals in the nursing plan of care to ensure continuity. Advise patients who smoke not to smoke after the evening meal.

Offer Appropriate Bedtime Snacks or Beverages

Complex carbohydrates (e.g., bread, cereal) seem to help most people sleep. A small amount of protein (e.g., milk, cheese) with the snack reduces the sugar boost and keeps blood glucose more stable. The dietary amino acid L-tryptophan promotes sleep. Advise the client to avoid alcohol, especially in the evening. Although it may induce sleepiness at first, alcohol interferes with the deep sleep cycle. The client should also avoid taking caffeine-containing foods and beverages (e.g., tea, coffee, chocolate, colas) after the evening meal. Advise the client to drink plenty of fluids during the day but to restrict fluids close to bedtime. Nicotine is a stimulant and should be avoided.

Promote Relaxation

You will base your choice of relaxation strategies on your repertoire of techniques and on patient preference. Relaxation strategies may include a massage, a warm bath, or one of the following:

- *Guided imagery* can be used to help your patient move in his mind to a safe place, where relaxation is possible. You may ask the patient what type of place will soothe him and "guide" him there through visualization. See Chapter 25 if you need to review.

- *Progressive muscle relaxation*, relaxing each muscle independently and progressing from head to toe, may help to promote sleep.
- *Music therapy* has been shown to be effective in promoting relaxation. Some patients respond well and can put away their troubles while listening to music, whereas others may find music irritating. Slow, quiet music or a recording of forest or ocean sounds may be soothing.

You may wish to refer to Chapter 40 for more details about relaxation strategies.

Maintain Patient Safety

A person who sleepwalks needs protection from injury, because the risk of falling is great (e.g., stairs). Intravenous infusions, catheters, and nasogastric tubes can produce injury if they are pulled out of the body when the person gets out of bed. Guide sleepwalkers back to bed, and remember that they startle easily, so be gentle and quiet.

Teach About Sleep Hygiene

Most people with sleep problems manage them at home by creating a restful environment, relaxing, avoiding distractions, and trying various sleep strategies without using sleep-inducing medication. Refer to the Self-Care box when teaching clients self-care for sleep (Self-Care: Teaching Your Client About Sleep Hygiene).

Self-Care

Teaching Your Client About Sleep Hygiene

➤ Follow a regular routine for bedtime and morning awakenings.

➤ Go to bed each night at the same time, even on days you are off work.

➤ If you cannot fall asleep in 30 minutes, get up and do something nonstimulating. When you feel sleepy, go back to bed.

➤ Use relaxation methods to promote sleep; read a book, pray, or meditate.

➤ Avoid going to bed angry.

➤ Don't depend on sleeping aids; be aware of the potential dangers of sleeping medications.

➤ Use your bedroom only for sleep; do not turn your bedroom into the family room.

➤ Avoid caffeine, alcohol, smoking, and heavy meals before going to sleep. Remember beverages and foods, such as black tea, chocolate, and cola, contain caffeine. Alcohol interferes with the transition to deeper phases of sleep.

➤ Eat a small amount of carbohydrates (e.g., crackers, cereal, or bread) before bed; they aid in sleeping.

➤ Use aromatherapy to relax.

➤ If you take prescription drugs, ask your prescriber or pharmacist about the side effects.

➤ Use earplugs to block out noise.

➤ Walk or exercise in the early evening at least one hour before going to sleep; doing so will raise your body temperature and tire your muscles. Even 15 minutes a day of exercise will give your body the activity and oxygen it needs to help you relax more and sleep better.

➤ Take a warm bath just before going to sleep. This will raise your body temperature and relax you to help you fall asleep more easily.

➤ Avoid naps during the day, unless you are an older adult who takes short "power naps." Daytime napping can lead to nighttime insomnia.

➤ Don't try to "catch up" on sleep. Rise at your regular time, even if you went to bed later than usual.

➤ Try to keep your bedroom as dark as possible. An illuminated bedroom clock is a source of light that can be distracting when trying to fall asleep. Either replace the clock or block the light with something.

➤ Close your eyes and visualize something peaceful when trying to fall asleep. Imaging your favorite, relaxing place where you find comfort or familiarity can relax you and help you get to sleep.

➤ Try progressive relaxation to fall asleep. Follow recorded instructions directing you in a sequence of relaxing certain muscle groups.

Administer and Teach About Medications to Produce Sleep

When considering sleep medications, it is important for the patient to understand the options, be aware of potential side effects, and know what questions to ask. Some medications are habit-forming; others may have unpleasant side effects. As a general rule, they are not recommended for long-term use. Others are considered safe and indicated for longer-term use. Some natural or homeopathic aids can lead to rest and sleep. The most common side effects of sleep medicines include dizziness, lightheadedness, daytime drowsiness, diarrhea, and difficulty with coordination.

Prescription Sleep Medications

You should be familiar with the various prescription and nonprescription sleep medications your patients may be taking.

Non-Benzodiazepines. This is the newest class of sedative/hypnotics (sleep medicines). These have a short half-life, which means that they are eliminated from the body quickly and do not cause "hangover" (daytime sleepiness). They are also selective, which means they target specific receptors that are thought to be associated with sleep rather than depressing the entire central nervous system. Examples are zolpidem tartrate (Ambien) and zaleplon (Sonata). Long-term effects of these medications are not yet known.

Benzodiazepines. This class of sedative/hypnotics includes both long-acting and short-acting drugs. Long-acting medications linger in the body and potentially cause daytime drowsiness. Many benzodiazepines were originally formulated to treat anxiety. Examples are diazepam (Valium), alprazolam (Xanax), flurazepam (Dalmane), lorazepam (Ativan), and triazolam (Halcion).

Barbiturates. These sedative/hypnotics and anticonvulsants are rarely prescribed for insomnia because of the risk of addiction, abuse, and overdose. Examples are amobarbital (Amytal), pentobarbital (Nembutal), and secobarbital (Seconal).

Tricyclic Antidepressants. At times, primary care providers prescribe antidepressants to promote sleep. Although none of these medicines is specifically FDA-approved for this purpose they have shown clinical benefit for some people with insomnia. Examples are amitriptyline (Elavil), doxepin (Sinequan), imipramine (Tofranil), and nortriptyline (Aventyl, Pamelor).

Nonprescription Sleep Medications

Nonprescription sleep medications usually contain an antihistamine, which may induce drowsiness that lasts into the next day. It is important to check the ingredient label of any over-the-counter (OTC) medication to see whether it contains an antihistamine. Advise clients that OTC sleep medications can interact with other medicines they may be taking, so they should consult their prescriber or pharmacist before using them. An example is diphenhydramine hydrochloride (Benadryl). Other nonprescription sleep aids include the following:

- *Melatonin.* This is widely sold as a sleep aid but remains controversial in medical circles. Melatonin is a natural hormone produced by the pineal gland.
- *Herbal sleep aids.* Herbal remedies for sleep problems include chamomile tea, valerian root, hops, lavender, and passionflower. Like melatonin, these herbal remedies have not undergone extensive testing for benefits and safety.

KnowledgeCheck 33-7

- What is the classification of zolpidem (Ambien)? Why is it an especially desirable medication for sleep?
- What are two other classes of medications that are sometimes prescribed for sleep?
- Describe three independent nursing interventions to promote sleep.
- Why should people contact their prescriber before taking nonprescription sleep aids?

 Go to Chapter 33, **Knowledge Check Response Sheet and Answers,** on the Student Resource Disk or DavisPlus at http://davisplus.fadavis.com/Wilkinson2

Putting It All Together

Anne ("Meet Your Patient") has arrived back on the surgical unit after her surgery. She has a urinary catheter, oxygen mask, IV line, and morphine by PCA for pain control. She is nauseated from the anesthesia and moaning in pain. Her husband, Eric, and their three children are there to greet her, and they are worried. Anne looks dreadful! "With all this equipment, and her moaning, is she going to be OK?" Eric asks. He tells you that Anne didn't sleep at all the night before surgery. "She was nervous and didn't want to take a sleeping pill because we were supposed to be at the hospital by 5:30 A.M.," he explains.

You perform an initial assessment. Anne's vital signs are as follows: BP, 118/74 mm Hg; pulse, 88 beats/min and regular; respirations, 26 per minute; and T, 99.48°F. Her lungs are clear, the dressing is dry and intact, and the urinary catheter shows a small amount of light yellow urine draining from the bladder. The oxygen mask is partially off. You check Anne's oxygen saturation. It is 99%. The notes from the operating and recovery rooms indicate that Anne has not received anything for pain in more than 90 minutes. The PCA is connected, but the pump supplies analgesia only when the patient triggers the device. Anne has been groggy and does not understand or remember that she must push the button to obtain pain medication. You trigger a bolus of morphine and show Anne and the family how the PCA works. You realize that she is sedated and may not remember what you have taught her, but Eric assures you that they will be staying for the day and will reinforce your instruction.

Several minutes later Anne is calm. Her respirations have slowed to 20 breaths/min, and she is lightly snoring. Eric sighs in relief. "I guess she'll sleep for awhile now," he says. You explain that she will sleep with the pain medication, but it will not be as restful as good-quality sleep. "With the morphine she will wake frequently and not get much REM sleep—that's a type of sleep we all require for health," you explain.

You were able to gather data preoperatively from Anne about her sleep habits and routines. You are also aware that Anne has had chronic sleep problems. In the nursing care plan, you have written the diagnosis Disturbed Sleep Pattern related to pain, dependence on Ambien, anxiety and other stresses of surgery and the recent loss of father, and unfamiliar environment; and secondary to fibromyalgia. You tell Eric that you would like him to bring from home Anne's pillow, toothbrush, and face cream because she has indicated that these are all part of her usual bedtime ritual.

When Eric volunteers that Anne sometimes listens to music before bedtime, you suggest that he also bring her favorite MP3 player.

At dinner time, Eric and the kids go home and gather Anne's belongings. When they return, she is more alert and comfortable. She tells them she feels exhausted, but not in pain. When you make your rounds, you explain that you would like to keep her usual bedtime routine and that she will be getting Ambien this evening. She is visibly relieved by your comments.

This scenario demonstrates full-spectrum nursing and shows how a nurse can make a difference for patients and their families by recognizing the need for sleep and providing appropriate interventions.

 Go to Chapter 33, **Resources for Caregivers and Health Professionals,** on the Student Resource Disk or DavisPlus at http://davisplus.fadavis.com/Wilkinson2

 Suggested Readings: Go to Chapter 33, **Reading More About Sleep and Rest,** on the Student Resource Disk or DavisPlus at http://davisplus.fadavis.com/Wilkinson2

 Bibliography: Go to Volume 2, Bibliography.

CHAPTER 34

Skin Integrity & Wound Healing

Learning Outcomes

After completing this chapter, you should be able to:

➤ Discuss the factors that affect skin integrity.

➤ Identify wounds based on accepted classification schemes.

➤ Describe the three phases of wound healing.

➤ Distinguish primary intention healing, secondary intention healing, and tertiary intention healing.

➤ Describe three types of wound drainage.

➤ Review the major complications of wound healing.

➤ Explain the factors involved in the development of pressure ulcers.

➤ Use the Braden scale to assess risk for pressure ulcers.

➤ Assess and categorize pressure ulcers based on the pressure ulcer staging system.

➤ Provide nursing care that limits the risk of pressure ulcer development.

➤ Differentiate the kinds of chronic wounds.

➤ Accurately chart assessment of a wound.

➤ Demonstrate appropriate technique for irrigating a wound.

➤ Describe care of a wound with a drain.

➤ Differentiate the five forms of wound débridement.

➤ Discuss the different kinds of tissue found in wounds.

➤ Discuss when and how to use absorbent, alginate, collagen, gauze dressings, transparent films, hydrocolloids, hydrogels, and foam and antimicrobial dressings.

➤ Describe guidelines to follow when applying heat or cold therapy.

➤ Demonstrate bandage and binder application.

Meet Your Patient

William Harmon is a 78-year-old man who fell 3 days ago. His fall resulted in a fractured left hip. He was admitted to the hospital and underwent an open reduction and internal fixation (ORIF) of the left hip. Today is his second postoperative day. He is still bed bound and is unable to roll or pull himself up in bed.

Mr. Harmon's weight on admission was 140 lb (63.64 kg). His height is 73 in. His family reports that he has been steadily losing weight. He expresses little interest in eating and says he has been depressed since his wife died last year.

While performing your assessment of Mr. Harmon, you notice that a large dressing covers the left hip incision. You loosen the dressing and see the staples are intact at the incision site and there is a minimal amount of serosanguineous drainage on the bandage. As you turn him in bed, you see a 10 cm by 6 cm reddened area on his coccyx and a 2 cm by 3 cm purple bruise-like area on his left heel. William now has three wounds, an intentional surgical wound and two pressure ulcers that have resulted from his impaired mobility. How will you care for each of these wounds? What factors contributed to each of the wounds, and how will you promote healing?

Theoretical **Knowledge** **knowing** why

The integumentary system consists of the skin, hair, nails, sweat glands, and the subcutaneous tissue below the skin. The skin is the largest organ of the body. The major functions of the skin include protection of the internal organs, unique identification of an individual, thermoregulation, metabolism of nutrients and metabolic waste products, and sensation.

What Factors Affect Skin Integrity?

It is important first to understand the structure of the skin (Fig. 34-1). The **epidermis** is the outer portion of the skin. The epidermis is made up of four or five layers, of which the most important are the inner and outer layers. The outermost layer of the epidermis, the **stratum corneum,** is composed of numerous thicknesses of dead cells. Functioning as a barrier, it restricts water loss and prevents fluids, pathogens, and chemicals from entering the body.

The innermost layer of the epidermis, the **stratum germinativum,** continually produces new cells, pushing the older cells toward the skin surface. Keratinocytes, melanocytes, and Langerhans cells are located in the epidermal layer. The **keratinocytes** are protein-containing cells that give the skin strength and elasticity. Deeper in the epidermis are **melanocytes,** which produce **melanin,** a pigment that gives skin its color and provides protection from ultraviolet light. **Langerhans cells** are mobile. Their function is to phagocytize (engulf) foreign material and trigger an immune response.

The **dermis** lies below the epidermis and above the subcutaneous tissue. It is made of irregular fibrous connective tissue that provides strength and elasticity to the skin and is generously supplied with blood vessels. Within the dermis are sweat glands, sebaceous (oil) glands, ceruminous (wax) glands, hair and nail follicles, sensory receptors, elastin, and collagen.

The **subcutaneous layer** is composed primarily of connective and adipose tissue. It provides insulation, protection, and a reserve of calories in the event of severe malnutrition. This layer varies in thickness in different body sites. Sex hormones, genetics, age, and nutrition also influence the distribution of subcutaneous tissue.

For optimal function, all layers of the skin must be intact. Breaks in the skin increase the risk of infection. Surgery and injuries may result in a loss of skin integrity. In the following sections you will learn about factors that influence the ability to maintain intact skin and heal wounds (e.g., age).

Age-Related Variations

Age affects the condition and structure of the skin. Infants, for example, are born with varying amounts of *vernix caseosa,* a creamy substance that protects their skin. Their skin is thinner and more permeable than that of adults, which predisposes infants to skin breakdown (e.g., diaper rash). The subcutaneous layer (brown fat) and sweat glands are not fully developed, especially for preterm infants. As a result, in the first few weeks of life thermoregulation is inadequate, and the infant must be swaddled to maintain body heat.

The skin of infants and young children feels smooth because of less exposure to the environment. As children are exposed to sun and other elements, skin texture

FIGURE 34-1 The structure of the skin.

becomes coarser. Sex hormones released during puberty increase sebaceous and sweat gland activity, which leads to perspiration odor and sometimes acne. In women, high estrogen levels may contribute to the softening of connective tissue and cause striae and darkening of the skin, particularly on the face, areolae, nipples, vulva, and umbilicus, particularly in people with dark skin.

As adults age, the activity of the sebaceous and sweat glands diminishes, resulting in drier skin. **Xerosis** (itchy, red, dry, scaly, cracked, or fissured skin) is a problem for up to 85% of older adults and can be a threat to the integrity of their skin. Along with loss of lean body mass, the subcutaneous tissue layer thins, giving the individual a sharp, angular appearance. Excess weight can offset this change of appearance, though. The strong bond between the epidermal and dermal layer decreases as the dermal layer loses elasticity as a result of changes in its collagen fibers. These changes make the skin prone to breakdown and prolong wound-healing time. Regeneration of healthy skin takes at least twice as long in an 80-year-old as in a 30-year-old. In addition, many older adults have chronic diseases that interfere with healing. Diabetes, for instance, predisposes to infection, and liver dysfunction interferes with synthesis of blood-clotting factors.

Impaired Mobility

A healthy person moves and shifts position unconsciously when he senses pressure or discomfort. However, many people are unable to move independently. For them, immobility causes an increase in pressure and may lead to skin breakdown. Impaired mobility is caused by conditions that require complete bedrest or that seriously limit activity. Examples are paralysis, extreme fatigue, high-risk pregnancy, sedation, altered levels of consciousness, casts, traction, and altered sensory perception.

KnowledgeCheck 34-1

- Identify the major functions of the skin.
- What is the function of the stratum corneum, the outermost layer of the skin?
- What is the function of the subcutaneous layer?
- What effect does aging have on skin?
- What effect does immobility have on skin?

 Go to Chapter 34, **Knowledge Check Response Sheet and Answers,** on the Student Resource Disk or DavisPlus at http://davisplus.fadavis.com/Wilkinson2

Nutrition and Hydration

Skin condition reflects overall nutritional status, while at the same time, nutritional intake affects the skin. Adequate intake of protein, cholesterol, calories, fluid, vitamin C, and minerals is essential to maintaining skin integrity.

Protein. Healthy skin depends on adequate protein levels. Protein is necessary to maintain the skin, repair minor defects, and preserve intravascular volume. As protein levels decline from excess loss or inadequate intake, minor defects cannot be repaired, fluid leaks from the vascular compartment of dependent areas, and edema (excess fluid in the tissues) develops. Edema decreases skin elasticity and interferes with the diffusion of oxygen to the cells. Therefore, the skin becomes prone to breakdown.

Cholesterol. Abnormally low cholesterol levels predispose patients to skin breakdown and inhibit wound healing. Patients on low-fat tube feedings may experience deficiencies in cholesterol, fatty acids, and linoleic acid. Together, these fats aid in providing fuel for wound healing and maintain a waterproof barrier in the stratum corneum.

Calorie Intake. If calorie intake is inadequate, the body uses proteins for energy (catabolism); they are then unavailable for building and maintenance functions (anabolism) (see Chapter 26 as needed). When undernutrition is prolonged, the person experiences weight loss, loss of subcutaneous tissue, and muscle atrophy. As a result, padding between the skin and the bones decreases, predisposing the skin to pressure ulcers.

Ascorbic Acid. Vitamin C, or ascorbic acid, is involved in the formation and maintenance of collagen, so a deficiency can delay wound healing. Zinc and copper are also involved in collagen formation, and deficiencies of either may impair healing.

Hydration. Skin turgor depends on hydration. Poor skin turgor may occur as a result of dehydration, whereas edema may result from overhydration. For further discussion on fluid requirements, see Chapter 36.

Diminished Sensation or Cognition

Clients with peripheral vascular disease, spinal cord injury, diabetes, cerebrovascular accident, trauma, or fractures often have diminished tactile sense, and they are therefore more prone to skin breakdown. If you've ever touched a hot surface and quickly pulled back your hand, you know the importance of tactile sensation. A client with diminished sensation is less able to sense a hot surface and would likely suffer a burn. If a client experiences a cut or wound in an area with limited sensation, it may go unnoticed and therefore untreated. The client with diminished sensation is also unable to feel pressure in an affected area. As a result, he may not shift position to relieve pressure over bony prominences or be aware that shoes or clothing are constricting.

Clients with impaired cognition (i.e., Alzheimer's disease, dementia, altered level of consciousness) are at higher risk to have skin breakdown because they are not aware of the need to reposition. Cognitive impairment can be subtle and difficult to recognize. Talk to your patient's family or caregiver and review past medical records so that the plan of care can be adjusted.

Impaired Circulation

The vascular system brings oxygen-rich blood to the tissues and removes metabolic waste products. Any form of circulatory impairment interferes with tissue metabolism. Impaired arterial circulation restricts activity, produces pain, and leads to muscle atrophy and development of thin tissue that is prone to ischemia and necrosis. Impaired venous circulation results in engorged tissues with high levels of metabolic waste products that are prone to edema, ulceration, and breakdown. Both forms of circulatory impairment delay wound healing. In fact, circulatory impairment is one of the main causes of chronic wounds.

Medications

Side effects and idiosyncratic reactions to medications can affect skin integrity and wound healing. Any medication that causes pruritus (itching), dermatoses (rashes), photosensitivity, alopecia, or pigmentation changes can result in changes that impair skin integrity or delay healing. The following are examples:

- *Blood pressure medications* decrease the amount of pressure required to occlude blood flow to an area, creating a risk for ischemia.
- *Anti-inflammatory medications*, such as over-the-counter nonsteroidal anti-inflammatory drugs (NSAIDs) and steroids, inhibit wound healing. Examples are ibuprofen (Motrin) and prednisone (Deltasone), respectively.
- *Anticoagulants* (e.g., heparin, warfarin [Coumadin]) can lead to extravasation of blood into subcutaneous tissue. As a result, even minimal pressure or injury can cause a hematoma.
- *Chemotherapeutic agents* delay wound healing because of their cellular toxicity.
- *Certain antibiotics, psychotherapeutic drugs,* and *chemotherapy agents* for cancer increase sensitivity to sunlight, increasing the risk for sunburn.
- *Several herbal products,* such as those containing lavender and tea tree oil, cleanse the skin but also have a drying effect.

Moisture on the Skin

Exposure to moisture leads to **maceration** (softening of the skin) and increases the likelihood of skin breakdown. Incontinence and fever are the most common sources of moisture. Bowel incontinence is particularly troublesome because feces contain digestive enzymes and microorganisms that can readily lead to **excoriation** (denuding) of superficial skin layers, placing such a patient at risk for **moisture-associated skin damage (MASD)**, **dermatitis** (inflammation of the skin), pressure ulcers, and infection.

Fever

Fever is a risk factor for skin breakdown for two reasons. First, it leads to sweating, which can cause maceration. Second, it increases the metabolic rate, thereby raising the tissue demand for oxygen. An increased demand for oxygen is difficult to meet if there is any circulatory impairment or tissue compression secondary to pressure.

Contamination or Infection

Contamination of a wound refers to the presence of microorganisms in the wound. All chronic wounds are contaminated. As bacteria begin to increase in number, a wound is said to be **colonized**, though the microorganisms are causing no harm. Wounds are colonized from the surrounding skin and local skin organisms, the external environment, and internal sources, usually from the mucous membranes of the gastrointestinal system. A wound becomes **critically colonized** when the bacteria begin to overwhelm the body's defenses. Critical colonization may be detected by subtle signs, such as an increase in drainage, or by more pronounced signs such as a new foul odor, a change in color of the wound bed, new tunneling of the wound, or absent or friable granulation tissue. An **infection** implies the microorganisms are causing harm by releasing toxins, invading body tissues, and increasing the metabolic demand of the tissue. Infection of the skin makes it more vulnerable to breakdown and impedes healing of open wounds. If not stopped, bacteria can then gain access to the systemic circulation.

Lifestyle

Some lifestyle habits affect skin integrity:

- *Tanning* exposes the skin to ultraviolet radiation, thereby increasing the risk for skin cancer.
- *Hygiene habits* that involve either excessive or insufficient skin hygiene are not healthy for skin integrity. Frequent bathing and use of soap remove skin oils and may lead to drying, which jeopardizes the skin's barrier function. Infrequent cleansing of the skin contributes to excessive oiliness, clogged sebaceous glands, and inadequate removal of microbes on the skin, which can infect a wound or lesion.
- *Regular exercise* improves circulation, which is necessary for maintaining skin integrity and wound healing.
- *A nutritious diet* helps maintain skin integrity, as already discussed.

- *Smoking* compromises the oxygen supply to the tissues, making skin more prone to breakdown and delaying wound healing. It also interferes with vitamin C absorption, which is needed for collagen formation.
- *Body piercings and tattoos* present a risk for infection and scarring. Complications, which occur in about 20% of piercings, include local infections, sepsis, endocarditis, hepatitis, and toxic shock syndrome. Intraoral and perioral piercings can result in gingivitis, damage to teeth and gums, and choking. Advise patients to become informed about the procedure and about aftercare and to find reputable piercers.

KnowledgeCheck 34-2

- Identify the factors that affect skin integrity.
- What nutritional components are essential to maintain skin?

  Go to Chapter 34, **Knowledge Check Response Sheet and Answers,** on the Student Resource Disk or DavisPlus at http://davisplus.fadavis.com/Wilkinson2

CriticalThinking 34-1

- Review the case of William Harmon ("Meet Your Patient"). What risks, if any, does William have for skin breakdown or delayed healing?
- What additional information do you need to know to fully evaluate his risk?
- What risks do you have for impaired skin integrity? What actions can you take to protect your skin?

Wounds

Wounds are a disruption in the normal integrity of the skin. Wounds may be intentional, such as a surgical wound, or unintentional, such as a cut or a pressure ulcer. As a nurse, you will be responsible for monitoring skin integrity and providing skin and wound care.

Types of Wounds

Wounds are classified according to length of time the wound has existed, as well as the condition of the wound (e.g., contamination, severity).

Skin Integrity. The simplest wound classification system is based on the integrity of the skin. If there are no breaks in the skin, the wound is described as **closed.** *Contusions* (bruises) or tissue swelling from fractures are common closed wounds. A wound is considered **open** if there is a break in the skin or mucous membranes. Open wounds include abrasions, lacerations, puncture wounds, and surgical incisions. A compound fracture may also lead to an open wound caused by the projection of bone through the skin. Several open and closed wounds are described in Table 34-1.

Length of Time for Healing. The length of time for wound healing varies according to the skin integrity and the factors affecting it, discussed in the previous section. **Acute wounds** are expected to be of short

Table 34-1 ➤ Types of Wounds

TYPE	DESCRIPTION
Abrasion	A scrape of the superficial layers of the skin; usually unintentional but may be performed intentionally for cosmetic purposes to smooth skin surfaces
Abscess	A localized collection of pus due to invasion from a pyogenic bacterium or other pathogen; must be opened and drained to heal
Contusion	A closed wound caused by blunt trauma. May be referred to as a bruise or ecchymotic area.
Crushing	A wound caused by force leading to compression or disruption of tissues. Often associated with fracture. Usually there is minimal or no break in the skin.
Incision	An open, intentional wound caused by a sharp instrument
Laceration	The skin or mucous membranes are torn open, resulting in a wound with jagged margins.
Penetrating	An open wound in which the agent causing the wound lodges in body tissue.
Puncture	An open wound caused by a sharp object. Often there is collapse of tissue around the entry point, making this wound prone to infection.
Tunnel	A wound with an entrance and exit site

duration. In a healthy person, these wounds heal spontaneously without complications through the three phases of wound healing (inflammation, proliferation, and maturation). Wounds that exceed the expected length of recovery are classified as **chronic wounds.** The natural healing progression has been interrupted or stalled because of infection, continued trauma, ischemia, or edema. Chronic wounds include pressure, arterial, venous, and diabetic ulcers. These wounds are frequently colonized with several types of bacteria, and healing is slow because of the underlying disease process. Unless the wound is properly diagnosed and the underlying disease process treated, a chronic wound may linger for months or years (Table 34-2).

Level of Contamination. **Clean wounds** are uninfected wounds with minimal inflammation. They may be open or closed and do not involve the gastrointestinal, respiratory, or genitourinary tracts (these systems frequently harbor bacteria). There is very little risk of infection for a clean wound. **Clean-contaminated wounds** are surgical incisions that enter the gastrointestinal, respiratory, or genitourinary tracts. There is an increased risk of infection for these wounds, but there is no obvious infection.

Contaminated wounds include open, traumatic wounds or surgical incisions in which a major break in asepsis occurred. The risk of infection is high for these wounds. Wounds are considered **infected** when bacteria

Table 34-2 ➤ Chronic Wounds

TYPE	ETIOLOGY	CHARACTERISTICS
Pressure Ulcers	Caused by pressure, resulting in tissue ischemia and injury	Appearance depends on the stage or tissue layers involved. Pressure ulcers tend to be located over bony prominences. Can cause serious tissue damage.
Arterial Ulcers	Caused by inadequate circulation of oxygenated blood to the tissue, which leads to tissue ischemia and damage	Ulcer appears "punched out," small and round with smooth borders. The wound base is usually pale with or without necrotic tissue. They tend to occur over the distal part of the leg, especially the ankles, toes, side of the foot, and shin. The surrounding skin appears shiny, thin, and dry and is cool to touch. Often there is loss of hair in the surrounding area. The area has delayed capillary refill time, and patients may complain of pain that worsens with increased activity. Arterial ulcers are most common in lower extremities but can occur anywhere. This type of ulcer can lead to serious injury and even death.
Venous Stasis Ulcers	Caused by incompetent venous valves, deep vein obstruction, or inadequate calf muscle function, resulting in venous pooling, edema, and impaired microcirculation of the skin	Located usually around the inner ankle, or in the lower part of the calf. Surrounding skin is reddened or brown and edematous. Wounds are usually shallow, with irregular wound margins. The wound bed appears "ruddy" or "beefy" red and granular. Drainage may be moderate to heavy depending on amount of edema. Pain usually occurs with leg dependence and dressing changes.

counts in the wound tissues are above 100,000 organisms per gram of tissue. However, the presence of *beta-hemolytic streptococci*, in any number, is considered an infection. Signs of wound infection include erythema and swelling around the wound, fever, foul odor, severe or increasing pain, large amount of drainage, or warmth of the surrounding soft tissue.

Depth of the Wound. **Superficial wounds** involve only the epidermal layer of the skin. The injury is usually the result of friction, shearing, or burning. **Partial-thickness wounds** extend through the epidermis but not through the dermis. **Full-thickness wounds** extend into the subcutaneous tissue and beyond (National Pressure Ulcer Advisory Panel [NPUAP], 2007c). The descriptor **penetrating** is sometimes added to indicate that the wound involves internal organs. Wound depth is a major determinant of healing time: The deeper the wound, the longer the healing time.

KnowledgeCheck 34-3

- Explain the difference between an acute and a chronic wound.
- Describe the wound categorization system based on the level of contamination.
- How does wound depth affect healing?

 Go to Chapter 34, **Knowledge Check Response Sheet and Answers,** on the Student Resource Disk or DavisPlus at http://davisplus.fadavis.com/Wilkinson2

Wound Healing Process

All wounds heal through a physiological process in which epithelial, endothelial, and inflammatory cells, platelets, and fibroblasts migrate into the wound to bring about tissue repair and regeneration. The process is essentially the same regardless of the type of injury or the type of tissues involved. Wounds may heal by regeneration or by primary, secondary, or tertiary intention.

Types of Healing

Regenerative/Epithelial Healing. When a wound affects only the epidermis and dermis, **regenerative/epithelial healing** takes place. No scar forms, and the new (regenerated) epithelial and dermal cells form new skin that cannot be distinguished from the intact skin. Partial-thickness wounds heal by regeneration.

Primary Intention Healing. When a wound involves minimal or no tissue loss and has edges that are well approximated (closed), primary (first) intention healing takes place (Fig. 34-2A). Little scarring is expected. A clean surgical incision heals by this method.

Secondary Intention Healing. Healing by **secondary (second) intention** occurs when a wound (1) involves extensive tissue loss, which prevents wound edges from approximating, or (2) should not be closed (e.g., because

it is infected). Because the wound is left open, it heals from the inner layer to the surface by filling in with beefy red **granulation tissue** (a form of connective tissue with an abundant blood supply) (Fig. 34-2B). Epithelial tissue may appear in the wound as small pink or pearl-like areas. Do not mistake this as a sign of infection. Wounds that heal by secondary intention heal more slowly, are more prone to infection, and develop more scar tissue. Pressure ulcers (discussed later) and infected wounds are examples.

Tertiary Intention Healing. A wound heals by **tertiary (third) healing**, also called *delayed primary closure*, occurs when two surfaces of granulation tissue are brought together (Fig. 34-2C). This technique may be used when the wound is clean-contaminated or contaminated. Initially the wound is allowed to heal by secondary intention. When there is no evidence of edema, infection, or foreign matter, the wound edges are closed by bringing together the granulating tissue and suturing the surface. Such wounds require strict aseptic technique during all dressing changes because they are prone to infection. Tertiary intention healing creates less scarring than does secondary, but more than primary intention healing.

Phases of Healing

Wound healing occurs in three stages: inflammatory, proliferative, and maturation (Fig. 34-3).

The Inflammatory Phase—Cleansing. The inflammatory (cleansing) phase lasts from 1 to 5 days and consists of two major processes: hemostasis and inflammation.

- *Hemostasis.* At the time of injury, tissue and capillaries are destroyed, causing blood and plasma to leak into the wound. Area vessels constrict to limit blood loss. Platelets are activated and aggregate (clump together) to slow bleeding. At the same time, the clotting mechanism is activated to form a blood clot.
- *Inflammation.* The inflammatory reaction is characterized by edema, erythema, pain, temperature elevation, and migration of white blood cells into the wound tissues. Within 24 hours, macrophages begin engulfing bacteria (**phagocytosis**) and clearing debris. In conjunction with plasma proteins and fibrin, they form a scab at the surface of the wound, which seals the wound and helps prevent microbial invasion.

The Proliferative Phase—Granulation. The proliferative (also called regeneration) phase occurs from days 5 to 21. Cells develop to fill the wound defect and resurface the skin. **Fibroblasts** (connective tissue cells) migrate to the wound where they form **collagen,** a protein substance that adds strength to the healing wound. New blood and lymph vessels sprout from the existing capillaries at the edge of the wound. The result is the formation of granulation tissue, a beefy red tissue that

Primary intention

A Clean wound   Sutured early   Results in hairline scar

Secondary intention

B Wound gaping and irregular   Granulation occurring   Epithelium fills in scar

Tertiary intention

C Wound not sutured   Granulation partially fills in wound   Granulating tissue sutured together

FIGURE 34-2 *A,* In a wound with minimal tissue loss, the edges may be sutured together, resulting in rapid healing and minimal scarring. *B,* A wound that heals by secondary intention heals from the inner layer to the surface. Healing takes longer, and there is scarring. *C,* A wound that heals by tertiary intention is initially healed by secondary intention and later sutured.

bleeds readily and is easily damaged. As the clot or scab is dissolved, epithelial cells begin to grow into the wound from surrounding healthy tissue and seal over the wound (**epithelialization**).

The Maturation Phase—Epithelialization. The maturation phase (or remodeling) is the final phase of the healing process. It begins in the second or third week and continues even after the wound has closed. Over the next 3 to 6 months, the initial collagen fibers that were laid in the wound bed during the proliferative phase are broken down and remodeled into an organized structure (e.g., scar tissue), increasing the tensile strength of the wound. A wound that has healed by primary intention leaves little scarring. Even so, a scar is only 80% as strong as the original tissue.

KnowledgeCheck 34-4

Identify the type of wound healing (primary, secondary, or tertiary intention):
- A wound that heals from inner layer to the surface

- A wound with approximated edges
- A wound that heals by approximating two surfaces of granulation tissue
- A wound that is sutured and has minimal or no tissue loss

 Go to Chapter 34, **Knowledge Check Response Sheet and Answers,** on the Student Resource Disk or DavisPlus at http://davisplus.fadavis.com/Wilkinson2

Wound Closures

Wounds that heal by primary and tertiary intention may be closed in a number of ways. Adhesive strips, sutures, staples, surgical glue, negative-pressure closure, and compression are the current choices.

Adhesive Strips. In the following situations, adhesive strips (e.g., Steri-Strips) are used:

- Closing superficial low-tension wounds, such as skin tears or lacerations
- Closing the skin on a wound that has been closed subcutaneously

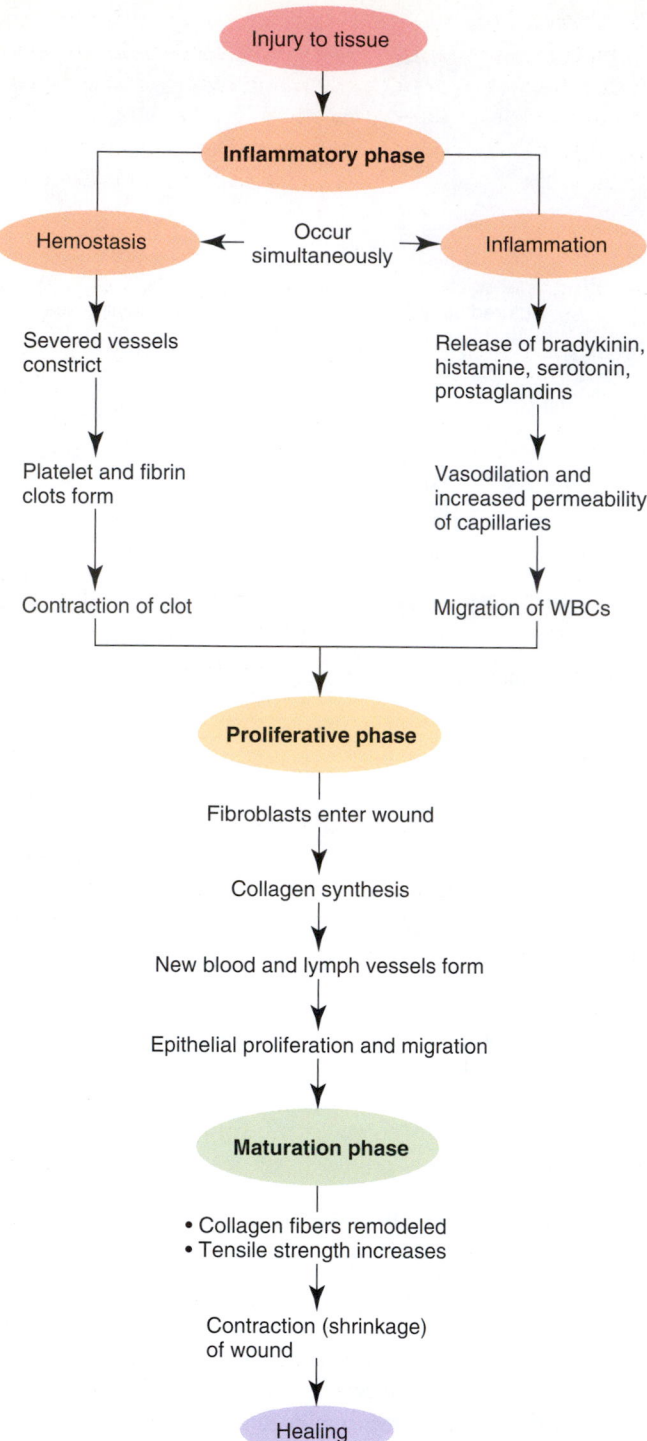

FIGURE 34-3 Stages in the wound healing process.

- Giving additional support to a wound after sutures or staples have been removed.

Adhesive strips are often kept in place until they begin to separate from the skin on their own. For instructions on applying Steri-Strips,

Go to Chapter 34, **Procedure 34-10: Placing Skin Closures,** in Volume 2.

Sutures. The traditional wound closures are sutures ("stitches"). Suturing leads to small puncture wounds along the track of the laceration or incision. Several types of suture materials are available.

- *Absorbent sutures* are used deep in the tissues, for example, to close an organ or **anastomose** (connect) tissue. Because they are made of material that will gradually dissolve, there is no need to remove absorbent sutures.
- *Nonabsorbent sutures* are placed in superficial tissues and require removal, often by a nurse. For instructions on removing sutures and staples,

Go to Chapter 34, **Procedure 34-13: Removing Sutures and Staples,** in Volume 2.

Surgical Staples. Made of lightweight titanium, surgical staples provide a fast, easy way to close an incision. They are also associated with a lower risk of infection and tissue reaction than sutures. The downside of staples is some wound edges are more difficult to align. The most common sites for wound stapling are arms, legs, abdomen, back, scalp, or bowel. Wounds on the hands, feet, neck, or face should not be stapled.

Surgical Glue. This is a relatively new method for wound closure. It is safe for use in clean, low-tension wounds. It is an ideal wound closure method for skin tears.

Negative Pressure Wound Therapy. Negative pressure wound therapy promotes healing by secondary and tertiary intention. Using a specialized pump, negative pressure is placed on a wound packed with foam or gauze dressings to create a vacuum. The subatmospheric pressure improves wound healing by reducing edema from swollen tissues; promoting granulation tissue formation; and removing exudate and infectious material. Negative pressure promotes granulation tissue formation by "stretching" cells and stimulating blood vessel growth and wound perfusion.

Advanced Wound Treatments

Collaborative treatments are necessary for wounds that will not heal despite aggressive care. Such treatments include the following:

- **Surgical options**, such as extensive débridement, skin grafts, secondary closure of the wound, and flap techniques (partially detached tissue placed over a wound) are used for complicated wounds.
- **Hyperbaric oxygen therapy** is the administration of 100% oxygen under pressure to a wound site. HBOT increases oxygen concentration in the tissue, stimulates the growth of new blood vessels, and enhances white blood cell (WBC) action.
- **Platelet-derived growth factor** augments the inflammatory phase of wound healing and accelerates collagen formation in the wound.

Types of Wound Drainage

Drainage is the flow of fluids from a wound or cavity. It is often referred to as **exudate**—fluid that oozes as a result of inflammation. Exudate may take several forms.

Serous Exudate. Clean wounds typically drain serous exudate. It is watery in consistency and contains very little cellular matter. Serous exudate consists of *serum,* the straw-colored fluid that separates out of blood when a clot is formed.

Sanguineous Exudate. You will often see sanguineous exudate with deep wounds or wounds in highly vascular areas. Sanguineous exudate is bloody drainage. It indicates damage to capillaries. Fresh bleeding produces bright red drainage, whereas older, dried blood is a dark, red-brown color.

Serosanguineous Drainage. In new wounds, you will most commonly see serosanguineous drainage, a combination of bloody and serous drainage.

Purulent Exudate. The thick, often malodorous, drainage that is seen in infected wounds is called **purulent exudate**. It contains pus, a protein-rich fluid filled with WBCs, bacteria, and cellular debris. It is commonly caused by infection from **pyogenic** (pus-forming) bacteria, such as streptococci or staphylococci. Normally, pus is yellow in color, although it may take on a blue-green color if the bacterium *Pseudomonas aeruginosa* is present.

Purosanguineous Exudate. Red-tinged pus is called **purosanguineous exudate**. It indicates that small vessels in the wound area have ruptured.

Complications of Wound Healing

Recall that wounds heal by moving through the phases of inflammation, proliferation, and maturation. At times, this process is interrupted by complications. The most common complications are hemorrhage, infection, dehiscence, evisceration, and fistulas.

Hemorrhage

Whenever a capillary network is interrupted or a blood vessel is severed, bleeding occurs. **Hemostasis** (cessation of bleeding) usually occurs within minutes of the injury. Hemostasis is delayed, however, when large vessels are injured, a clotting disorder exists, or the client is on anticoagulant therapy. If bleeding begins again after initial hemostasis, something is probably wrong. Possible causes include a slipped suture, erosion of a blood vessel, a dislodged clot, or infection. Bleeding may be internal or external. The risk of hemorrhage is greatest in the first 24 to 48 hours following surgery or injury.

Internal Bleeding. Swelling of the affected body part, pain, and changes in vital signs (i.e., decreased blood pressure, elevated pulse) may indicate internal bleeding.

By *internal bleeding,* in this chapter, we are referring to a **hematoma,** a red-blue collection of blood under the skin, which forms as a result of bleeding that cannot escape to the surface. The amount of blood in a hematoma varies. A large hematoma causes pressure on surrounding tissues. If the hematoma is located near a major artery or vein, it may impede blood flow.

External Hemorrhage. Compared to internal bleeding, external hemorrhage is easier to recognize. You will see bloody drainage on the dressings and in the wound drainage devices. When there is a brisk hemorrhage, blood often pools underneath the client as the dressings become saturated. To be sure that you recognize the full extent of the bleeding, remember to look underneath the patient.

Infection

Microorganisms can be introduced to a wound during an injury, during surgery, or after surgery. Suspect infection if a wound fails to heal. Localized swelling, redness, heat, pain, fever (temperatures higher than 38°C [100.4°F]), foul-smelling or purulent drainage, or a change in the color of the drainage may also indicate infection. The symptoms are likely to occur in a contaminated or traumatic wound within 2 to 3 days. In a clean surgical wound, you will usually not see signs and symptoms of an infection until the fourth or fifth postoperative day. Incisions that begin draining within 5 to 7 days of surgery are at risk for dehiscing.

Dehiscence

Rupture (separation) of one or more layers of a wound is called **dehiscence** (Fig. 34-4). Wound dehiscence is most likely to occur in the inflammatory phase of healing, before large amounts of collagen have been deposited in the wound to strengthen it. The most common causes of dehiscence are poor nutritional status, inadequate closure of the muscles, or wound infection. Obese clients are also more likely to experience dehiscence because fatty tissue does not heal readily and the patient's mass increases the strain on the suture line.

Dehiscence is usually associated with abdominal wounds. Patients often report feeling a pop or tear, especially with sudden straining from coughing, vomiting, or changing positions in bed. Usually there is an immediate increase in serosanguineous drainage. Nursing interventions include maintaining bedrest with head of bed elevated at 20° and the knees flexed. To prevent evisceration, a binder may be applied and activity modified. The physician should be notified of the dehiscence and may visit the patient to examine the wound.

Evisceration

Evisceration is total separation of the layers of a wound in which internal viscera protrude through the incision

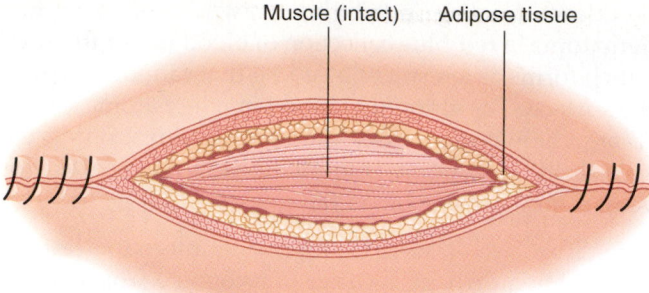

FIGURE 34-4 Dehiscence is separation of one or more layers of a wound. It is most common in the inflammatory phase of healing.

(Fig. 34-5). This is a rare complication and is a surgical emergency. Immediately cover the wound with sterile towels or dressings soaked in sterile saline solution to prevent the organs from drying out and becoming contaminated with environmental bacteria. Have the patient stay in bed with knees bent to minimize strain on the incision. Notify the surgeon and ready the patient for a surgical procedure (see Chapter 37 for perioperative care).

Fistulas

A **fistula** is an abnormal passage connecting two body cavities or a cavity and the skin. Fistulas often result from infection. An abscess forms, which breaks down surrounding tissue and creates the abnormal passageway. Chronic drainage from the fistula may lead to skin breakdown and delayed wound healing. The most common sites where fistulas form are the gastrointestinal and genitourinary tracts. Figure 34-6 illustrates a fistula between the rectum and vagina.

KnowledgeCheck 34-5

- Describe four types of wound closures.
- Identify five types of wound complications.
- Describe three signs of internal hemorrhage.
- Differentiate between dehiscence and evisceration.

 Go to Chapter 34, **Knowledge Check Response Sheet and Answers,** on the Student Resource Disk or DavisPlus at http://davisplus.fadavis.com/Wilkinson2

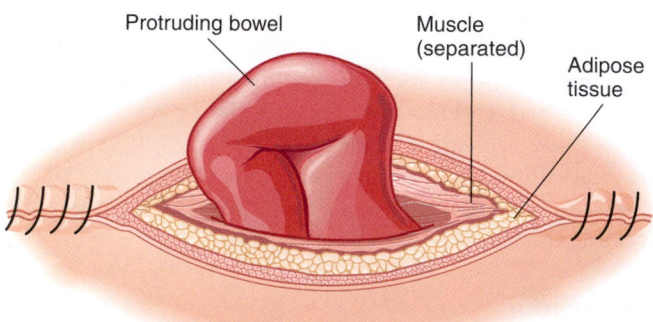

FIGURE 34-5 Evisceration is total separation of the layers of a wound with internal viscera protruding through the incision.

Fistula between rectum
and vagina (enterovaginal)

FIGURE 34-6 A fistula is an abnormal passage connecting two body cavities or a cavity and the skin. Fistulas are most common in the gastrointestinal and genitourinary tracts.

CriticalThinking 34-2

Recall the case of Mr. Harmon ("Meet Your Patient"). What form of wound healing (primary, secondary, or tertiary) is he undergoing? How long would you expect it to take before his wounds heal?

Chronic Wounds

A chronic wound is one that has not healed within the proper time frame. It has not moved through the repair process in an orderly fashion (inflammation, proliferation, maturation). Wounds that do not heal within 2 to 4 weeks may be considered chronic.

Pressure Ulcers

A pressure ulcer is a type of chronic wound. We discuss it separately because vigilant nursing care can prevent pressure ulcers. In the event pressure ulcers do form, nurses play a major role in their treatment. An estimated 1 million people in the United States have pressure ulcers: about 15% of hospital patients, 10% of home care patients, and 20% of long-term care patients (Ayello & Lyder, 2008; Black, Baharestani, Cuddigan, et al., 2007a). Unless the pressure injury is present on admission (POA), in most circumstances, Medicare will decline payment for treatment for that ulcer. Costs in lives can be high as well, with reported mortality rates of 70% for older adults within 6 months of an occurrence of a pressure ulcer (Brown, 2003).

How Do Pressure Ulcers Develop?

Pressure ulcers (formerly called *decubitus ulcers, pressure sores,* and *bedsores*) are localized areas of injury to the skin, and possibly the underlying tissue, usually over a bony prominence. They are caused by unrelieved pressure, or pressure in combination with shearing forces, which compromises blood flow to an area, resulting in *ischemia* (inadequate blood supply) in the underlying tissue (NPUAP, 2007e). Tissue ischemia leads to tissue anoxia (lack of oxygen) and cell death.

The key variables in ischemia are time and pressure. Small amounts of pressure over an extended period of time or a large amount of pressure for a short period of time results in tissue ischemia. Pressure ulcers can occur in as little time as 2 hours, though they may take as long as 5 days for the full extent of tissue damage to be known.

When ischemia first occurs, the skin over the area is pale and cool. When you relieve the pressure (e.g., by turning the patient), vasodilation occurs, and extra blood rushes to the area to compensate for the ischemic period. The area flushes bright red (**reactive hyperemia**). If the redness does not disappear quickly, tissue damage has occurred. The redness should last about half as long as the duration of the ischemia. For example, if the tissue was compressed for an hour, reactive hyperemia should not last more than about 30 minutes.

Although time and pressure are the key variables, several other factors predict the likelihood of pressure ulcer formation (Fig. 34-7). Some factors are intrinsic and some are extrinsic.

Intrinsic Factors. Certain intrinsic (internal) factors alter skin and tissue integrity or oxygen delivery capabilities, decreasing the amount of force required to create a pressure ulcer. Examples include immobility and impaired sensation, as occur with spinal cord injuries, stroke, or coma; poor nutrition; edema; aging; low arteriolar pressure; and fever. Septicemia is one of the most common principal reasons for hospitalization among patients with secondary pressure ulcers (Russo, Steiner, & Spector, 2008). The previous section, "What Factors Affect Skin Integrity?" discussed a variety of intrinsic factors.

Poor nutrition or dehydration can weaken the skin and lead to pressure ulcers. Adequate intake of calories, protein, vitamin C, and zinc is necessary to prevent pressure ulcers and promote healing of injured tissue (ICSI, 2007).

Extrinsic Factors. The following extrinsic (external) factors contribute to the development of pressure ulcers.

- ***Friction*** damages the outer protective epidermal layer, decreasing the amount of pressure needed to develop skin lesions (Black, Baharestani, Cuddigan, et al., 2007a).
- *Shearing* occurs when the epidermal layer slides over the dermis, causing damage to the vascular bed. It most commonly occurs when the head of the bed is elevated and the patient slides downward, causing shear to develop in the sacral area. When shearing occurs, the amount of pressure needed to occlude circulation is cut in half.
- *Moisture,* especially in the form of urine or feces, macerates the skin and also decreases the amount of pressure required to produce ulceration.
- Pressure ulcers most commonly develop over ***bony prominences,*** but can occur under casts, splints, or other assistive devices. Skin is compressed between the bone and the hard surface of the bed or chair, reducing blood flow to the area. When the patient is supine, these pressure points are the occiput, scapulae, elbows, sacrum, and heels. Figure 34-8A–D illustrates the pressure points in the supine, lateral, prone, and sitting positions.
- Wounds caused by ***trauma*** have a greater risk of infections and slower healing (Institute for Clinical Systems Improvement, 2008).

How Are Pressure Ulcers Staged?

Pressure ulcers are classified by the degree of tissue involvement (Table 34-3). The National Pressure Ulcer Advisory Panel developed a standardized staging system (European Pressure Ulcer Advisory Panel [EPUAP] and National Pressure Ulcer Advisory Panel [NPUAP], 2009). Only wounds that are caused by pressure should be "staged" (NPUAP, 2007e). Other classification systems exist to describe other chronic wounds, such as diabetic foot ulcers and venous stasis ulcers.

Reverse staging does not occur as an ulcer heals. The healing process cannot cause a stage IV pressure ulcer to become a stage III. Pressure ulcers become progressively more shallow by filling with granulation tissue, but lost muscle, subcutaneous fat, and dermis are not replaced. Therefore, reverse staging does not accurately characterize what is physiologically occurring in the ulcer. Instead, pressure ulcers maintain their original

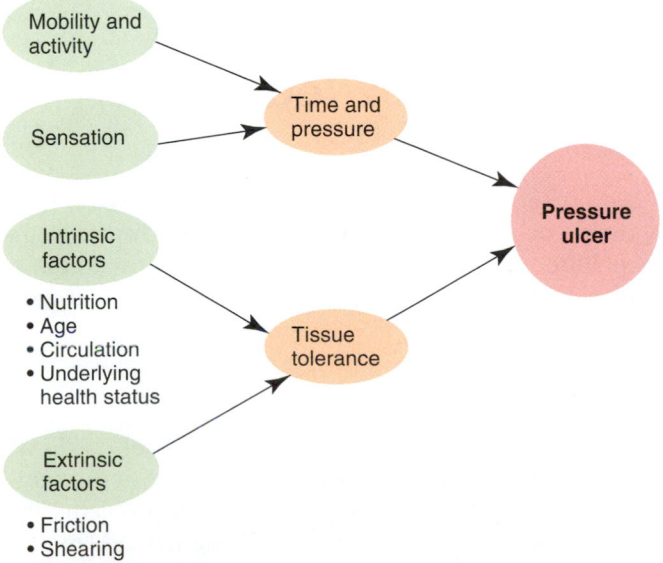

FIGURE 34-7 Several factors contribute to the development of pressure ulcers.

A

Vertebrae
(spinal processes)

Sacrum   Pelvis
           (ischial tuberosity)

Heels
(calcaneus)

B

Side of head Ear   Shoulder   Illium   Greater   Knee   Malleolus
(parietal and   (acromial   trochanter (medial   (medial
temporal bones)   process)   and lateral and
                                                    condyles)   lateral)

C

Back of head   Scapulae   Elbows   Sacrum   Heels
(occipital bone)   (olecranon   (calcaneus)
                          process)

D

Cheek and ear Shoulder Breasts   Genitalia Knees   Toes
(zygomatic   (acromial (women)   (men)   (patellas) (phalanges)
bone)   process)

FIGURE 34-8 *A–D,* Most commonly, pressure ulcers develop over the bony prominences. *A,* Sitting. *B,* Lateral. *C,* Supine. *D,* Prone. (Adapted from AHRQ Clinical Practice Guidelines.)

staging classification throughout the healing process, but they are described as *healing* (e.g., "stage IV ulcer: healing" or "stage I ulcer: healing").

Other Types of Ulcers

This chapter focuses primarily on pressure ulcers. However, not all lower extremity ulcers are related to pressure.

Venous Stasis Ulcers. Open lesions caused by venous stasis are called **venous stasis ulcers.** They are caused by venous stasis that results from damage to valves in

the veins (e.g., from deep vein thrombosis). They occur usually between the inside ankle and the knee, not necessarily over a bony prominence.

Diabetic Foot Ulcers. Diabetes causes narrowing of arteries, decreasing oxygenation to the feet and resulting in delayed healing and tissue necrosis. Because people with diabetes lose protective sensation, they may walk on sores, continuously damaging the tissues. Diabetic foot ulcers, often painless, occur mainly on the plantar surface of the foot, the ball of the foot, or top and bottom of the toes.

Arterial Ulcers. When a non–pressure-related blockage of arterial blood to an area (e.g., by a clot or stenosis of the arterioles), causes tissue necrosis the result is called an **arterial ulcers.** Arterial ulcer usually occur over the lower leg, ankle, or bony areas of the foot. The wound bed tends to be dry and pale, with little drainage.

For more detailed information about these three types of ulcers,

 Go to Chapter 34, **Supplemental Materials,** on the Student Resource Disk or DavisPlus at http://davisplus.fadavis.com/Wilkinson2

KnowledgeCheck 34-6
- What stage pressure ulcer does Mr. Harmon ("Meet Your Patient") have?
- What factors have contributed to its development?

 Go to Chapter 34, **Knowledge Check Response Sheet and Answers,** on the Student Resource Disk or DavisPlus at http://davisplus.fadavis.com/Wilkinson2

 CriticalThinking 34-3

Based on your knowledge of the factors that have contributed to Mr. Harmon's pressure ulcer development, what actions may lead to healing of the pressure ulcer? *Note:* To answer this question, you do not need to know about wound care (e.g., irrigation) for a pressure ulcer.

Practical **Knowledge** knowing *how*

As a nurse, you will care for many patients who have wounds or who are at risk for skin breakdown. In the remainder of the chapter, we will discuss how to maintain skin integrity, prevent pressure ulcers, and treat wounds.

▌ ASSESSMENT

The National Pressure Ulcer Advisory Panel (NPUAP) recommends nurses perform a comprehensive wound assessment while identifying other health problems and their impact on wound healing. Existing wounds require additional assessment. A thorough skin assessment

Table 34-3 ➤ Staging Pressure Ulcers

STAGE	CLINICAL FINDINGS	DISCUSSION
Suspected Deep Tissue Injury	An area of skin that is intact but discolored. It might be purplish or deep red, painful, boggy, or have a blister.	Occurs due to damage of underlying soft tissue from pressure or shear. Findings can be subtle enough that often DTI is not recognized until after severe tissue damage has occurred. May heal or evolve further and become covered by thin eschar, rapidly exposing additional layers of tissue even with optimal treatment. In darker pigmented individuals, discoloration might go undetected.
Stage I Pressure Ulcer	Localized area of intact skin with nonblanchable redness, usually over a bony prominence. The area may be painful, firm, soft, or warmer or cooler as compared to adjacent tissue. Discoloration will remain for >30 minutes after pressure is relieved.	Dark skin may not have visible blanching; its color may differ from that of the surrounding area. Therefore, Stage I may be difficult to detect.
Stage II Pressure Ulcer	Involves partial-thickness loss of dermis. Stage II pressure ulcers are open but shallow and with a red pink wound bed. There is no slough. May also be an intact or open/ruptured serum-filled blister; or a shiny or dry shallow ulcer without slough or bruising.	Do not use this stage to describe skin tears, tape burns, perineal dermatitis, maceration, or excoriation. Do not mistake moisture-associated skin damage or fungal infections for Stage II pressure ulcer. Stage II ulcers do not involve sloughing or bruising.

Continued

Table 34-3 ➤ Staging Pressure Ulcers—cont'd

STAGE	CLINICAL FINDINGS	DISCUSSION
Stage III Pressure Ulcer Stage III	A deep crater characterized by full-thickness skin loss with damage or necrosis of subcutaneous tissue. May extend down to, but not through, underlying fascia. Undermining (deeper-level damage under boggy superficial layers) of adjacent tissue may be present. Bone/tendon is not visible or directly palpable.	Some stage III pressure ulcers can be extremely deep when located in an area with significant adipose layers.
Stage IV Pressure Ulcer Stage IV	Involves full-thickness skin loss with extensive destruction, tissue necrosis, or damage to muscle, bone, or support structures. Exposed bone/tendon is visible or directly palpable. Slough or eschar may be present. Undermining and sinus tracts (blind tracts underneath the epidermis) are common.	The depth of a stage IV pressure ulcer varies by location. They can be shallow on the bridge of the nose, ear, occiput, and malleolus because these areas do not have subcutaneous tissue. Stage IV ulcers can extend into muscle and supporting structures (e.g., fascia, tendon, or joint capsule). Often require a full year to heal. Even once healed, the site remains at risk for future injury because the scar is not as strong as the original tissue.
Unstageable Pressure Ulcer	Involves full-thickness skin loss. The base of the wound is obscured by *slough* (tan, yellow, gray, green, or brown necrotic tissue) or *eschar* (tan, black, or brown leathery necrotic tissue).	Until enough slough and/or eschar is removed to expose the base of the wound, the true depth, and therefore stage, cannot be determined. *Stable eschar* is dry, adherent, and intact without erythema or fluctuance. Do not remove stable eschar, as it serves as "the body's natural cover."

includes a nursing history, physical examination, and diagnostic testing. For a list of competencies for nurses treating pressure ulcers (NPUAP, 2001),

 Go to Chapter 34, **ESG Box 34-2, Competencies for Registered Nurses Treating Pressure Ulcers,** on the Student Resource Disk or DavisPlus at http://davisplus. fadavis.com/Wilkinson2

Focused Nursing History

To assess wound healing ability and the risk for skin breakdown, you will need to gather data on factors that affect skin integrity (discussed previously): age, mobility, nutrition, hydration, sensation, circulation, medications, moisture, lifestyle, underlying health and disease status, and the presence of microorganisms. The psychosocial issues related to coping with chronic wounds also need to be considered. For instance, with care and compassion you will assess how patients cope with the pain of a chronic wound, handle the loss of control and independence, adapt to changes in body image, deal with the financial burden of caring for complex wounds, and adjust to the social isolation that comes with impaired mobility and chronic illness. For history questions to help you assess these factors,

 Go to Chapter 34, **Assessment Guidelines and Tools, History Questions for Skin and Wound Assessment,** in Volume 2.

For example, patients with poor circulation, such as those with diabetes, atherosclerosis, or low blood pressure, are at risk for tissue injury. Patients who use tobacco or are anemic have reduced oxygen supply in the blood, predisposing them to pressure ulcers. Those who have limited mobility or reduced sensation because of nerve damage, head injury or stroke, spinal cord injury, or diabetes, experience a loss of protective sensations to reposition themselves (Institute for Clinical Systems Improvement, 2008).

Pressure Ulcer Risk Assessment Measures

Patients may have multiple risk factors for skin problems. A comprehensive risk assessment tool enables you to evaluate the cumulative risk. Among the most commonly used tools are the Braden and Norton scales. To see these scales,

 Go to Chapter 34, **Assessment Guidelines and Tools, Braden Scale for Predicting Pressure Sore Risk,** and **Norton Scale for Assessing Risk of Pressure Ulcers,** in Volume 2.

The Braden Scale for predicting pressure sore risk is used to identify persons at risk for developing pressure ulcers. The Braden scale evaluates six major risk factors: sensory perception, moisture, activity, mobility, nutrition, and friction and sheer. The final score reflects the patient's risk; the lower the score, the more likely the patient will develop a pressure ulcer. A score of 18 or less for hospitalized patients indicates risk. Interventions should be based on the individual risk factors, as well as the total score. You should use this scale to assess the patient on admission to the facility and again in 48 to 72 hours. Studies have shown the second score to be more predictive, probably related to increased awareness of the patient's status. The Braden Q is a modified scale used in children.

The Norton Scale assesses risk based on the patient's physical condition, mental state, activity, mobility, and incontinence. A low score indicates a high risk. Some have suggested that the Norton scale should be modified by adding categories for skin appearance, medication, and nutrition.

 Critical**Thinking** 34-4

Review the Braden scale. Apply this risk assessment scale to Mr. Harmon ("Meet Your Patient").

■ What additional information, if any, do you need to complete these assessments?
■ Calculate a Braden score based on Mr. Harmon's risk factors, if he had also been incontinent of urine twice that day.

Focused Physical Examination

Physical assessment of skin integrity focuses on the two following areas:

Inspecting the Skin. Inspect all areas of the body routinely. Evaluate the skin for color, integrity, temperature, texture, turgor, mobility, moisture, lesions, and hair distribution. Check pressure points for erythema, tenderness, or edema. Assess all bony prominences of individuals "at risk" for skin breakdown routinely (Wound, Ostomy and Continence Nurses Society, 2007). Include skin under special garments, such as shoes, heel elevators, and antiembolism stockings. Also assess vulnerable pressure points for bed- or chair-bound patients. See Chapter 19 if you need more details on skin assessment.

Assessing Mobility and Activity Level. As you know, activity level and mobility affect skin integrity. See Chapter 19 if you need to review assessment of the musculoskeletal system. See Chapter 31 if you need additional information on activity and mobility.

Assessing Treated Wounds

All wounds require a focused assessment. Assessment frequency depends on the condition of the wound, the work setting, the patient's overall condition and underlying disease process, the type of wound, and the type of treatment used for the wound. If you are providing wound care, you will assess the wound with every treatment. For a wound assessment summary,

 Go to Chapter 34, **Assessment Guidelines and Tools, Physical Assessment: Wound Assessment,** in Volume 2.

Assessment parameters include the following:

Location. Describe the wound location in anatomical terms. For example, describe an incision from cardiac surgery as a midsternal incision extending from the manubrium to the xiphoid process. An accurate description of the location is important because:

- *Location influences the rate of healing.* Wounds in highly vascular regions, such as the scalp or hands, heal more rapidly than wounds in less vascular regions, such as the abdomen or a heel.
- *Location affects movement.* Wounds that can be readily stabilized heal more rapidly than those in areas that are affected by the constant stress of movement.
- *Location can give you clues to the wound etiology.* A wound over a bony prominence could be related to pressure, whereas one on the bottom of the foot could be a diabetic foot ulcer.

Type of Wound. Is it an acute wound? If the wound is sutured, examine the closure. Are the wound edges approximated (together)? Is there tension on any aspect of the wound? Are the stitches intact? Or is this a chronic wound?

Size. Measure the length and width of the wound in centimeters. It is important that nurses using a ruler measure a wound the same way. The NPUAP recommends using a head-to-toe orientation, the longest length head to toe, and the widest width side to side, perpendicular (90° angle) to length, encompassing the entire wound (NPUAP, 2007a). Use serial photographs showing the wound's dimensions, especially if the wound has an irregular border, to document the baseline and wound healing (EPUAP and NPUAP, 2009). To measure wound depth, gently insert a sterile cotton-tip applicator into the deepest part of the wound. Measure the applicator from skin level to the tip.

Undermining or Tunneling. Assess the wound edges for any undermining or tunneling. Pay close attention to any tissue that appears to have a separation either in tissue type or plane, as frequently tunnels may be found. Measure the depth and location of any undermining or tunneling using the face of a clock as a guide. If the top of the wound is 12:00 and the bottom of the wound is 6:00, for example, record "2 cm of undermining is present from 1:00 to 4:00" or "6 cm tunnel exists at the center of the wound tracking in the 3:00 direction."

Periwound. Examine the skin surrounding the wound. Skin discoloration may indicate a hematoma or additional injury to the surrounding tissue. Look for maceration, undermining, crepitus, blistering, erythema, and epiboly, slough, and eschar.

Maceration is caused by excessive moisture from pooled drainage on intact skin for periods of time or a moist dressing is inappropriately applied, left on too long, or overlaps onto healthy skin. The skin may appear as pale and wrinkled or "pruned," which may flake and peel.

Undermining will produce a boggy feel around the wound.

Crepitus is gas trapped under the skin. If you palpate the surrounding skin and feel a crackling sensation, this is crepitus. Crepitus may be due to air leaking from the lung in a chest wound or may indicate the presence of gas-producing bacteria.

Erythema, swelling, or other signs of irritation indicate that the surrounding tissue is in jeopardy.

Epiboly is closed or rolled wound edges. Examine wound edges for epithelial tissue and contraction. Epiboly may indicate that epithelial cells have moved down and rolled under the wound edges. Once the cells reach the wound bed, they will stall wound healing.

Slough is usually soft, stringy, and pale yellow or gray.

Eschar is thick, hard, and black or brown.

Percentage and Type of Tissue in Wound Base. Assessment of the types of tissue and their amounts can give you an idea of the severity of the wound, needed treatment options, and/or healing of the wound. Table 34-4 outlines different types of tissue you might see in a

Table 34-4 ➤ Types of Tissue in the Wound Bed		
TYPE OF TISSUE	**DESCRIPTION**	**NURSING GOAL**
Slough (Moist, devitalized tissue)	Soft, moist, devitalized (necrotic) tissue; may be white, yellow, tan; may be stringy, loose, or adherent to bed.	Débride the wound.
Eschar	Necrotic tissue; dry, thick, leathery; may be black, brown, or gray depending on moisture level.	Débride the wound.
Granulation Tissue	Pink to red moist tissue; made of new blood vessels, connective tissue, and fibroblasts; surface is granular or pebble-like.	Cleanse, protect.
Clean, Nongranulating	Absence of granulation tissue, but bed is pink, shiny, and smooth	Cleanse, protect.
Epithelial	Regenerating epidermis; may appear pink or pearly white as it crosses the wound bed; may begin as a ring around the wound or from epithelial cells lining hair follicles.	Cleanse, protect.

wound bed. Viable (living) tissue must be distinguished from nonviable tissue. Many wounds may have different types of tissue at the same time. Describe each type with percentages. For example, "80% of the wound bed contains granulation tissue, and 20% remains necrotic." Granulation tissue is evidence of healing. A pale color or dry texture may indicate a delay in healing. Necrotic tissue of any type will delay wound healing and should be removed. The exception is stable eschar on a heel that is firmly attached to the healthy wound edges without signs of infection.

Drainage. Determine whether exudate is present. If so, describe the amount, color, consistency, and odor. Compare changes in the exudate to the patient's previous status.

- *Amount.* Describe the amount as none, light, moderate, or heavy. Drainage amounts vary according to the type of wound (i.e., venous stasis ulcers usually produce more drainage than arterial ulcers).
- *Drains.* If a drain is present, measure the amount of fluid in the collection container.
- *Color.* Describe the color or consistency as serous or clear, serosanguineous, sanguineous, purulent, or seropurulent.
- *Odor.* Describe odor as absent, faint, moderate, or strong. Clean the wound of all exudate or foreign material before assessing for odor because odor characteristics vary depending on the wound moisture, organisms, amount of nonviable tissue or types of dressings used. Odor may indicate fistula formation or bacterial contamination. For example, if a patient has an abdominal wound that was odorless but begins to smell of bile or feces, you should carefully assess for presence of a fistula.

Wound and Tissue Pain. Routinely ask your patients about pain or discomfort related to the wound or wound care (European Pressure Ulcer Advisory Panel [EPUAP] and National Pressure Ulcer Advisory Panel [NPUAP], 2009). You will need to develop a pain management plan if the patient is uncomfortable. Always take seriously the patient's complaint of pain, especially if there is a sudden increase. Pain is often an early symptom of infection. In the immunocompromised patient, pain may be the only symptom of infection (Branom, 2002).

Nutritional Status. Screen and assess nutritional status for each patient with a pressure ulcer at admission. A referral to the dietitian for early assessment of and intervention may be necessary if nutritional problems are present. Sufficient calories are needed for wound healing, which may involve adding oral supplemental meals, or even enteral or parenteral nutrition (EPUAP and NPUAP, 2009).

Assessing Untreated Wounds

For an untreated wound, make the same assessments as for a treated wound. Also, make additional assessments that allow you to determine the immediate treatment needed. For example, assess for bleeding. If bleeding is profuse, apply direct pressure to the site. If bleeding continues after you apply pressure for 5 minutes or if blood is spurting from the wound, call the provider immediately. Severe pain, numbness, or loss of movement below the wound also requires immediate, comprehensive evaluation. For a description of the assessment process for an untreated wound,

VOL 2 Go to Chapter 34, **Assessment Guidelines and Tools, Physical Examination: Assessing an Untreated Wound,** in Volume 2.

Also determine whether the patient needs a tetanus immunization. Tetanus-prone wounds include compound fractures, gunshot wounds, crush injuries, burns, punctures, foreign object injuries, wounds contaminated with soil, and wounds neglected for more than 24 hours. An immunization should be given if:

- The last immunization was 10 years ago or longer (Immunization Action Coalition, 2007 [reviewed by the Centers for Disease Control and Prevention (CDC), 2009]).
- The wound is contaminated with dirt or debris, and the most recent tetanus immunization was given more than 5 years ago.
- It is uncertain when the patient last received an immunization.

Evaluating Pressure Ulcer Healing

In addition to the Braden and Norton risk assessments previously described, the AHRQ and NPUAP recommend use of the *PUSH tool* to evaluate pressure ulcers (NPUAP, 2002). The tool provides a comprehensive means of reporting the progression of a pressure ulcer. Surface area, exudate, and type of wound tissue are scored and totaled. As the ulcer heals, the total score falls. To see the PUSH tool,

VOL 2 Go to Chapter 34, **Assessment Guidelines and Tools, The PUSH Tool for Evaluation of Pressure Ulcers,** in Volume 2.

Laboratory Data

You should integrate laboratory data with your history and physical assessment findings. The most common laboratory assessments performed on clients with wounds or risk for skin breakdown are protein levels, complete blood count, erythrocyte sedimentation rate, glucose, thyroid and iron levels, coagulation studies, and wound cultures. To learn more about these tests and see the normal ranges,

VOL 2 Go to Chapter 34, **Diagnostic Testing: Tests for Assessing Wounds,** in Volume 2.

Wound cultures may be ordered to determine the types of bacteria present in the wound. Local or systemic signs of infection, suddenly elevated glucose levels, pain in a neuropathic extremity, or lack of healing after 2 weeks in a clean wound may indicate the need for a wound culture. Cultures may be obtained by swab, aspiration, or tissue biopsy.

Swabbing. The most common and most noninvasive method to obtain a culture is with a swab. Swab specimens have been shown to be acceptably accurate in representing bacteria counts biopsied from wound tissue (Gardner, Frantz, Saltzman, et al., 2006; Bill, Ratliff, Donovan, et al., 2001). The Wound, Ostomy and Continence Nurses Society (2007) recommends using swab cultures as a reasonable alternative to biopsy in the clinical setting. The Critical Aspects Box summarizes swabbing. For the full procedure,

 Go to Chapter 34, **Procedure 34-1: Obtaining a Wound Culture by Swab,** in Volume 2.

Needle Aspiration. Specifically trained providers may perform needle aspiration of a wound. This involves insertion of a needle in the tissue to aspirate tissue fluid. Organisms present in the tissue fluid can then be detected. Needle aspiration is an invasive procedure, with the risk of inadvertent needle damage to tissue and underlying structures. The Critical Aspects box summarizes needle aspiration. For the full procedure,

 Go to Chapter 34, **Procedure 34-2: Obtaining a Needle Aspiration Culture from a Wound,** in Volume 2.

Tissue Biopsy. The most accurate method for culturing a chronic wound is *tissue biopsy*. It has long been considered the "gold standard." Tissue is removed from the wound edge by a specially trained provider. However, many facilities do not have the equipment needed to process tissue samples. This is an invasive procedure, causes pain, and disrupts the wound bed, sometimes delaying healing. Biopsy also creates a risk of sepsis.

KnowledgeCheck 34-7

- What should be included in a wound assessment?
- What is the preferred method of wound culture that may be performed by a registered nurse?
- Identify three types of laboratory data that may be associated with a delay in wound healing.

 Go to Chapter 34, **Knowledge Check Response Sheet and Answers,** on the Student Resource Disk or DavisPlus at http://davisplus.fadavis.com/Wilkinson2

What Assessments Can I Delegate?

Initial assessment of a wound, as well as ongoing evaluation of a wound that requires treatment, must be done by the registered nurse. You may delegate to nursing assistive personnel (NAP) inspection of the skin for evidence of skin breakdown. Instruct the NAP to notify you of redness, tissue warmth, or drainage. You may

also delegate turning and position changes to the NAP. Turning and movement prevent tissue damage from ischemia, thereby preventing pressure ulcers.

■ ANALYSIS/NURSING DIAGNOSIS

The following nursing diagnoses are appropriate for patients who are at risk for skin breakdown or for patients who have wounds.

- *Risk for Impaired Skin Integrity* is appropriate for patients who have one or more risk factors for skin breakdown (e.g., immobility, incontinence, extremes of age, impaired circulation, impaired sensation, undernutrition, emaciation). NANDA International (2009) recommends that you use a risk assessment tool (e.g., Norton or Braden Scale) to identify these patients.
- *Impaired Skin Integrity* is appropriate for patients who have experienced damage to the epidermis or dermis, for example, patients who have superficial wounds or stage I or II pressure ulcers.
- *Impaired Tissue Integrity* is appropriate for patients with wounds that extend into the subcutaneous tissue, muscle, or bone. Use this diagnosis for patients with deep wounds or stage III or IV pressure ulcers.
- *Risk for Impaired Tissue Integrity* is appropriate for clients with Impaired Skin Integrity who are at risk for delayed healing. For example, Mr. Harmon ("Meet Your Patient") has a stage I pressure ulcer but is at risk for further progression of the ulcer because of his age, nutritional state, and the presence of another wound. Note that this is not a NANDA-I diagnosis; however, it is useful in the situation described.

Skin problems and wounds can be the etiology for other nursing diagnoses, for example:

- *Risk for Infection* is an appropriate diagnosis if the patient has a traumatic wound or is immunosuppressed, undernourished, or immobile.
- *Pain* is a diagnosis that may be used for patients who are experiencing discomfort from the wound or from the treatments required to heal the wound.
- *Disturbed Body Image* should be used if the patient is experiencing distress about the wound. Consider this diagnosis even if the patient is expected to make a complete recovery. Some patients experience extreme distress about wounds. You will certainly want to consider this diagnosis if the patient experiences an injury that is expected to result in disfigurement.

■ PLANNING OUTCOMES/EVALUATION

For associated NOC standardized outcomes for skin and tissue integrity diagnoses,

 Go to Chapter 34, **Standardized Language, Selected Standardized Outcomes and Interventions for Skin and Wound Diagnoses,** in Volume 2.

Individualized goals/outcome statements should address the need to maintain intact skin or heal the wound. For patients who have a diagnosis of Risk for Impaired Skin Integrity, you might write a goal such as the following:

Maintains intact skin throughout treatment, as evidenced by good skin turgor with no erythema, edema, or breaks in the skin.

For patients who have a wound (actual Impaired Skin Integrity or Impaired Tissue Integrity), you might write a goal such as the following:

Wound will heal by May 1, as evidenced by a progressive decrease in the size of the wound, a decrease in drainage from the wound, improvement in the condition of the surrounding skin, and no evidence of infection (erythema, purulent drainage, or odor).

▌ PLANNING INTERVENTIONS/IMPLEMENTATION

For NIC standardized interventions for skin and tissue integrity problems,

 Go to Chapter 34, **Standardized Language, Selected Standardized Outcomes and Interventions for Skin and Wound Diagnoses,** in Volume 2.

Specific nursing activities directed at maintaining skin integrity or healing wounds focus on preventing and treating pressure ulcers and other chronic wounds, providing wound care, and applying heat and cold therapies. In the next section, we discuss these nursing therapeutic measures.

What Are Some Nursing Measures to Prevent and Heal Pressure Ulcers?

Pressure ulcers are extremely difficult and time-consuming to treat. As a result, prevention is the most important nursing intervention. Healthy People 2020 proposed two public health objectives focused on pressure-related skin injury: 1) to reduce the proportion of nursing home residents with a current diagnosis of pressure ulcers, and 2) to reduce the rate of pressure ulcer-related hospitalizations among older adults 2020 (U. S. Department of Health and Human Services, 2010). The Institute for Healthcare Improvement (IHI) has made preventing pressure ulcers one of twelve goals in its 5 Million Lives Campaign. IHI recommended the six crucial elements in preventing pressure ulcers discussed in the following sections.

Conduct a Pressure Ulcer Admission Assessment for All Patients

Most agencies use a standardized risk assessment, such as the Braden and Norton scales, to assess the risk of pressure ulcers (see the previous section, "Pressure Ulcer Risk Assessment Measures"). You should use these scales to assess the patient on admission to any type of facility (hospital, nursing home or with home health care). Risk factors not found on those scales will place your patient at even higher risk. Examples include age, fever, hypotension, and poor dietary intake.

Reassess Risk for All Patients Daily

Reassess your hospitalized patient for risk daily because his condition can change frequently and rapidly. Any time your patient's condition changes or he is transferred to another unit, reassess his risk. Monitor a nursing home resident weekly for the first 4 weeks, then quarterly or whenever the patient's condition changes or deteriorates. Reassess home patients with every visit (Wound, Ostomy and Continence Nurses Society, 2007).

Once a patient is identified as being at risk for developing pressure ulcers, prevention programs or strategies can be implemented. Inform all members of the healthcare team (i.e., physical therapists, transporters, physicians, dietitians). Using visual cues, like stickers on charts or dots on ID bands, can help remind staff.

Inspect Skin Daily

Skin care begins with regular inspection of the skin—at least daily for patients at risk—and usually every 8 to 12 hours for institutionalized patients. You must have adequate light to detect subtle, early skin changes. Use a pen light to inspect bony prominences if direct sunlight is not available. Be sure to check pressure points for erythema, tenderness, or edema. Instruct family members and caregivers about the importance of early detection of skin problems. In obese patients, skin damage can occur under breasts, abdominal folds, or anywhere skin contacts skin.

Manage Moisture

Excess moisture creates a risk for skin breakdown. Use the following nursing actions to help you manage moisture:

Incontinence Care. Provide skin care regularly soon after each incontinence episode. Apply incontinence or moisture barrier cream to protect perineal skin from urine and stool. Keep these products readily available for use by all staff members. Use undergarments or products that will wick moisture away from the skin.

Bathing. Soaps and bathing techniques can contribute to skin breakdown, so be careful to keep the skin clean and intact. Diaphoretic (sweaty) patients may need frequent bathing as sweat can be irritating to sensitive or injury-prone skin. Older adults most likely will not need daily bathing due to decreased oil and sweat production. Use warm water; hot water dries the skin. Gently bathe fragile skin, using a minimum of force and friction, as washcloths can be abrasive. Use a mild cleansing soap only as needed and not routinely; and be sure to rinse thoroughly and gently pat the skin dry. Soaps are drying to the skin because they remove oils from the skin and may interfere with the ability of the skin to hold water.

Lotion and Massage. If the patient's skin is dry, apply a moisturizing lotion using a gentle massaging motion to promote circulation and wound healing. ✚ Do not massage over bony prominences, which can irritate the area and lead to tissue injury.

Linens. Keep the linen soft, clean, dry, and free from wrinkles by changing it frequently. Moisture and wrinkles in the sheets can damage skin integrity.

Optimize Nutrition and Hydration

Nutrition is vital to skin integrity. Patients with rapid weight loss, high metabolic demands, limited intake, or decreased serum albumin are particularly at risk for pressure ulcer development. Monitor hydration status and offer water (if appropriate) whenever you reposition the patient.

Carefully review the diet ordered for at-risk patients, and assess what the patient is eating. The diet may need to be modified to achieve adequate calorie and protein intake. Protein requirements may be as high as 2 grams per kilogram of body weight in a malnourished individual with a wound, so high-protein supplements may be necessary.

Consider the consistency of the diet as well. A soft diet may be helpful for a patient who is frail or is missing teeth. Tube feeding or parenteral nutrition may be prescribed to supplement oral intake if the patient is unable to consume adequate quantities of calories and protein. You may need to make a dietary referral.

Minimize Pressure

Most patients who are at risk for pressure ulcers have mobility problems. As a result, you must provide frequent position changes. This is one of the most important interventions for preventing pressure ulcers. You may delegate turning and position changes to the NAP. Turning and movement prevent tissue damage from ischemia, thereby preventing pressure ulcers.

Turning and Repositioning. Reposition the patient at least every 2 hours (Armstrong, Ayello, Capitulo, et al., 2008; Bergstrom, Bennett, Carlson, et al., 1994b; Buss, Halfens, & Abu-Saad, 2002). However, patients with very fragile skin or little subcutaneous tissue might need to be repositioned more frequently. At-risk individuals who are chair bound should be repositioned every hour or taught to shift their weight every 15 minutes. Place a turning schedule at the bedside so that all caregivers can participate in the prevention strategy. For an example of a patient turning schedule,

Go to Chapter 34, **Tables, Boxes, Figures: ESG Box 34-1, Scheduled Position Changes,** on the Student Resource Disk or DavisPlus at http://davisplus.fadavis.com/Wilkinson2

Use the "rule of 30" to guide your positioning:

✚ Elevate the head of the bed 30° or less, and when the patient is on her side, position the patient at a 30° angle to avoid direct pressure on the trochanter. If the head of the bed is elevated more than 30°, limit the time in this position to minimize pressure and shear.

✚ To protect skin during turning or repositioning, use lift devices or draw sheets, heel and elbow protectors, or sleeves and stockings. Never drag a patient when pulling her up in bed.

Support Surfaces. Numerous support surfaces are available for preventing and treating pressure ulcers. They do so by redistributing pressure and controlling moisture to prevent bacterial growth on the skin (microclimate between the skin and the surface of the bed). Support surfaces include specialty mattresses, integrated bed systems, mattress replacements, and overlays. These products may consist of air, gel, foam, or water, and are available in various sizes and shapes for beds, chairs, exam tables, and operating room tables (Fig. 34-9). Any patient at risk should be placed on a pressure-redistributing device. Of course, use of support surfaces should not be the only prevention measure, but should be coupled with effective turning and positioning schedules.

Protect heels by using products that completely raise the heels off the bed. Pillows may not be enough to redistribute the weight of your patient's foot and donut-type devices should not be used. Pressure redistributing devices are made for chairs and wheelchairs too. Figure 34-10 is a decision-making tree developed by AHRQ to guide selection of appropriate support surfaces (Bergstrom, Bennett, Carlson, et al., 1994b).

What Are Adjunctive Wound Care Therapies?

The use of adjunctive therapies is the fastest growing area in pressure-related wound management. Nurses apply adjunctive therapies that include negative pressure wound therapy, electrical stimulation, hyperbaric oxygen, radiant heat, tissue growth factors, ultrasound, bioengineered skin equivalents, and surgical options.

FIGURE 34-9 An egg crate mattress is a nonpowered foam mattress overlay used to redistribute pressure.

Management of tissue loads

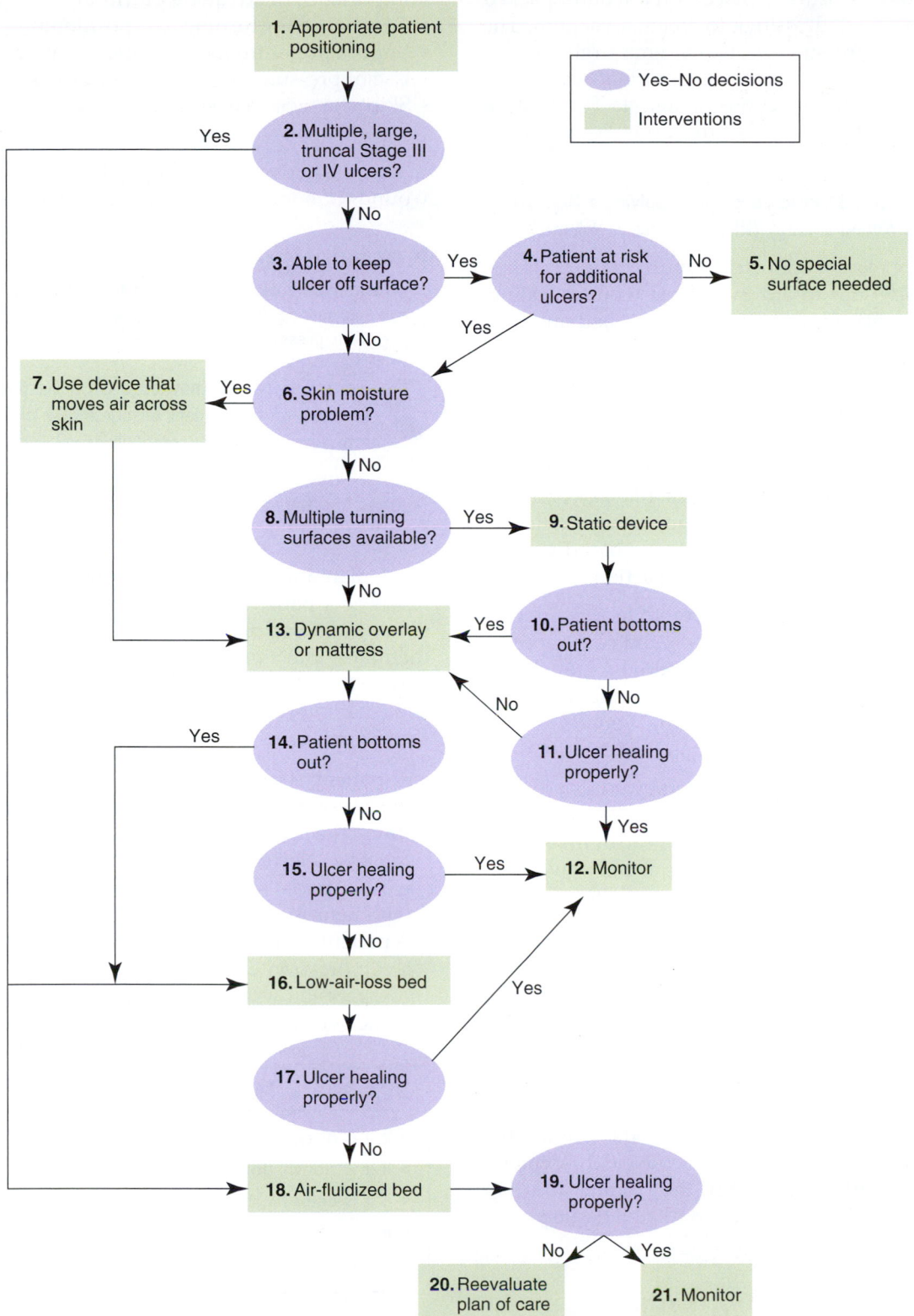

FIGURE 34-10 A decision-making tree to guide selection of appropriate support surfaces. (*Source:* Agency for Healthcare Quality and Research. (1994). *Clinical practice guidelines: Pressure ulcer treatment.* Rockville, MD: Author.)

Negative Pressure Wound Therapy. Using a specialized pump, negative pressure is placed on a wound packed with foam or gauze dressings to create a vacuum. The subatmospheric pressure reduces edema from swollen tissues, promotes granulation tissue formation, and removes exudate and infectious material. The Critical Aspects box summarizes this procedure. For complete guidelines,

 Go to Chapter 34, **Procedure 34-7: Applying a Negative Pressure Wound Therapy (NPWT) Device,** in Volume 2.

Electrical Stimulation. Electrical currents are transferred across tissues to aid in chronic wound healing. Electrodes are placed around the wound bed and connected to a machine that produces an electrical impulse. This therapy stimulates cellular growth through development of fibroblasts, new collagen, and increased blood flow and tissue oxygenation.

Hyperbaric Oxygen Therapy. Hyperbaric oxygen therapy (HBOT) is the administration of 100% oxygen under pressure. HBOT increases oxygen concentration in the tissue, stimulates the growth of new blood vessels, and enhances white blood cell (WBC) action.

Tissue Growth Factors. Tissue growth factors are proteins that occur naturally in the body and cause specific cells to grow and replicate. Platelet-derived growth factor has been used in chronic wound healing. It is indicated for diabetic and other nonhealing wounds that are clean of necrotic tissue and have good vascularity.

Ultrasound. Another adjunctive therapy used in chronic wound healing, is ultrasound. Sound waves are emitted by a control unit and hand-held sound head or transducer. Vibrations from the transducer create sound waves that pass into the tissue, causing it to vibrate and heat up. This stimulates movement of fluid within and between cells and aids in débridement and increased cell metabolism.

Bioengineered Skin Substitutes. This is a group of substances that aid in the temporary or permanent closure of wounds. Substitutes may be actual human epidermis or dermis, animal cells, or synthetic material. They can be used to treat partial- and full-thickness wounds.

Surgical Options. Complicated wounds require the use of surgical options, such as extensive débridement, skin grafts, secondary closure of the wound, and **flap techniques** (partially detached and rotated tissue placed over a wound to fill in the deficit).

What Patient and Family Teaching Do I Need to Do?

Teaching the at-risk patient and family about pressure ulcer prevention is a key prevention strategy. Include the following topics in your teaching:

- Characteristics of healthy skin
- Appearance of skin that has experienced unrelieved pressure
- Skin care and hygiene

- Protection of the skin and prevention of pressure ulcers
- Importance of adequate nutrition
- Techniques for turning and positioning
- Importance of frequent position changes
- Use of pressure-redistributing devices
- Skin changes that should be reported to healthcare professionals

Box 34-1 gives you simple tips for taking care of wounds at home that you can teach families.

KnowledgeCheck 34-8

- Identify the major interventions for preventing pressure ulcers.
- What nursing diagnosis is most appropriate for a patient at risk for pressure ulcer development?

 Go to Chapter 34, **Knowledge Check Response Sheet and Answers,** on the Student Resource Disk or DavisPlus at http://davisplus.fadavis.com/Wilkinson2

What Wound Care Competencies Do I Need?

Care planning to meet the complex, individualized needs of a patient with a chronic wound involves the entire multidisciplinary team (e.g., physical therapists, dietitians, infection control specialist, wound specialist, and so forth). Your wound assessment will guide your choice of interventions, which depend on the nature of the wound. Consider these two examples:

- A patient with a diabetic foot ulcer must have all the pressure taken off that area because every step traumatizes healing tissues. The appropriate dressing must be selected; in addition, this patient will need to wear a special shoe that is especially made for patients with neuropathy.
- A patient with a venous stasis ulcer will need to wear a compression garment (hose, stocking or multilayer compression wrap). These apply continuous pressure to the veins, which helps venous return and allows the

---

BOX 34-1 ■ Tips For Initial Wound Care

- If it is dirty, clean it.
- If it is slough, don't fluff.
- If it is deep, fill it.
- If it is open, cover it.
- If it is dry, moisten it.
- If it is wet, absorb it.

Reprinted with permission. Institute for Clinical Systems Improvement (ICSI), 8009 34th Avenue South, Suite 1200, Bloomington, MN 55425.
Institute for Clinical Systems Improvement (ICSI). (2008, January 28). Pressure ulcer treatment. Health care protocol. Bloomington (MN): Institute for Clinical Systems Improvement (ICSI); Retrieved on August 25, 2009, from http://www.guideline.gov/summary/summary.aspx?view_id=1&doc_id=13698

ulcer to heal. See Chapter 37 if you need more information about compression stockings.

Wound care is more than placing a dressing into a wound. It incorporates all of the strategies for preventing that wound, as well as treating it. ESG Box 34-2 lists the competencies of registered nurses for treating pressure ulcers (NPUAP, 2001). These interventions can also be used in treating other types of acute and chronic wounds.

 Go to Chapter 34, **ESG Box 34-2, Competencies of Registered Nurses for Treating Pressure Ulcers,** on the Student Resource Disk or DavisPlus at http://davisplus.fadavis.com/Wilkinson2

Cleansing Wounds

Wounds are cleansed to remove exudate, slough, foreign materials, and microorganisms. Cleansing also helps to promote healthy tissue healing. Historically, antiseptic solutions, such as Dakin's, acetic acid, hydrogen peroxide, povidone-iodine, and alcohol, were used to cleanse all types of wounds. However, research shows that these antiseptic solutions can damage granulating tissue and should not be used on healing tissue. Antiseptic solutions should be reserved for wounds that won't heal or those in which the bacterial burden is more harmful than the solution itself.

Because normal saline is physiological, it is safe and it will not harm injured or healing tissue. It will adequately cleanse most wounds if a sufficient amount is used to thoroughly flush the wound. Drinkable tap water is as effective as saline to cleanse a wound (Fernandez & Griffith, 2008). Liquid or foam skin cleansers that are pH balanced may be used to cleanse periwound skin or incontinence effluent. They are not for use in wounds. The thing to remember is to use universal precautions to minimize the risk of cross-contamination.

Always clean a wound initially and with each dressing change. To cleanse a wound, gently pat the surface with gauze soaked with saline or other prescribed wound cleanser. If there is granulation tissue, be careful not to disrupt it. Wound irrigation is a gentle technique. Some wounds do require vigorous cleansing though (see Table 34-4).

Irrigating Wounds

Nurses commonly use irrigation (**lavage**) to cleanse wounds gently by flushing. To remove debris from a wound, you must introduce the irrigation solution with a mild amount of force. Ideal irrigation pressures range from 4 pounds per square inch (psi) to 15 psi. To remove material adhering to the wound bed use a 35-mL syringe attached to a 19-gauge angiocatheter deliver the solution at approximately 8 psi (Institute for Clinical Systems Improvement, 2008; Branom, 2002; Campton-Johnston & Wilson, 2001). Pressures above 15 psi increase the risk of driving bacteria into the tissues, as well as causing mechanical damage.

Some agencies use a piston syringe for irrigation. Do not use a bulb syringe; it increases the risk of aspirating the drainage. Commercial irrigation systems are also available. Closely evaluate the amount of pressure they deliver before you use these devices.

There is a risk of splattering with this technique, so you must use gowns, masks, and goggles. Sterile technique is used for acute surgical wounds, wounds that have recently undergone sharp débridement, or when prescribed by the physician. The majority of wound irrigation uses clean technique. The Critical Aspects box provides a summary of the procedure. For the complete steps,

 Go to Chapter 34, **Procedure 34-3: Performing a Sterile Wound Irrigation,** in Volume 2.

Toward Evidence-Based Practice

Fernandez, R., & Griffiths, R. Water for wound cleansing. *Cochrane Database of Systematic Reviews,* Issue 1. Art. No.: CD003861. DOI: 10.1002/14651858.CD003861.pub2. Retrieved on June 11, 2009, from http://www.cochrane.org/reviews/en/ab003861.html.

Use of saline versus tap water for cleansing wounds is debated. Normal saline is traditionally preferred because it cleanses without interfering with the normal healing process. Yet, tap water is used commonly in the community for cleaning wounds and for care of chronic wounds because it is generally free of pathogens, yet easily accessible and inexpensive. Researchers wanted to know if rates of infection and healing differ depending on whether tap water or normal sterile saline is used to clean acute and chronic wounds. They analyzed findings from 24 clinical studies. Results showed no

differences in the rates of infections among acute and chronic wounds in adults and children cleansed with tap water as compared to those washed with saline.

1. What trend in the research about cleansing wounds do you see as compared to previous times?

2. If study findings indicate little difference in wound infection when tap water is used for cleansing, then what would you recommend to those using tap water in the community?

3. What implications does using tap water for cleaning wounds have when sending patients home after surgery?

 Go to Chapter 34, **Toward Evidence-Based Practice Suggested Responses,** on the Student Resource Disk or DavisPlus at http://davisplus.fadavis.com/Wilkinson2

Caring for Wounds with Drainage Devices

A variety of drains may be inserted into wounds to allow fluid and exudate to exit. Drains prevent excessive pressure from building up in the tissues. Drains are usually placed during a surgical procedure. Some are sutured into place, whereas others are simply placed into the cavity.

Types of Drains

A *Penrose drain* is a flexible latex tube that is placed in the wound bed but usually not sutured into place. A clip or pin may be attached to keep it from slipping further into the wound. You may be asked to advance the drain by gradually removing it from the wound bed. For example, the surgeon may prescribe "Advance the Penrose drain 6 mm (¼ inch) per day." Each day you pull the drain out of the wound 6 mm (¼ inch) until the drain is finally removed. The Critical Aspects box summarizes this procedure. For complete guidelines,

 Go to Chapter 34, **Procedure 34-14: Shortening a Wound Drain,** in Volume 2.

Some drains are attached to a collection device. Examples include Hemovac, Jackson-Pratt, and Davol drains (Fig. 34-11a). The surgeon may order a device to be "placed to suction." This means you will compress the device to create suction and facilitate removal of drainage (Fig. 34-11b). The Critical Aspects box summarizes this procedure. For complete guidelines,

 Go to Chapter 34, **Procedure 34-15: Emptying a Closed-Wound Drainage System,** in Volume 2.

If a specific pressure is to be applied, some drains can be connected to wall suction. The provider will prescribe the amount of suction. For example, a surgeon may order: "Place Hemovac to 20 mm Hg suction at all times."

FIGURE 34-11B Compress the bulb of the Jackson–Pratt drain to create suction and remove wound drainage.

Nursing Activities for Maintaining Drains

You are responsible for monitoring wound drains. The surgeon will describe the number and type of drains present. Describe drain placement according to the position on the clock face. Consider the patient's head to be at the 12 o'clock position. Some patients have more than one drainage device in a wound. Label the drains numerically with a marker or by placing tape on the collection apparatus so that each caregiver provides consistent care.

When removing dressings or irrigating wounds, take care to avoid dislodging any drains. Remember, many drains are not sutured in place. Monitor the amount and character of the drainage and the condition of the collection apparatus. Record this information in your nursing notes as well as on the I&O record.

Report to the surgeon any change in the amount or character of the drainage. If you suspect a drain is occluded, check the drain line from the insertion site to the collection device. Remove any kinks in the tubing. If this does not correct the problem, notify the provider of the blockage.

You need to empty the collection apparatus at a designated volume to maintain suction. As the device fills, suction pressure decreases. If there is significant drainage, you may need to empty the device several times during your shift.

KnowledgeCheck 34-9

- Identify goals for wound care before applying a dressing to a wound.
- What solutions are used to cleanse a wound?
- How can you control the amount of force applied for wound irrigation?
- Identify three nursing responsibilities when caring for a client with a wound drain.

 Go to Chapter 34, **Knowledge Check Response Sheet and Answers,** on the Student Resource Disk or DavisPlus at http://davisplus.fadavis.com/Wilkinson2

FIGURE 34-11A *Left,* Penrose drain. *Center,* Jackson-Pratt device. *Right,* Hemovac drainage system.

CriticalThinking 34-5

- Describe the percentage and type of tissue found in Mr. Harmon's wounds.
- What are the goals of treatment with both of Mr. Harmon's wounds?

Debriding a Wound

Débridement is the removal of devitalized tissue or foreign material from a wound. It also helps remove cells that are alive but not functioning (**senescent**) from the wound bed and edges. Removal of necrotic tissue, exudate, and infective material helps stimulate wound healing and prepare the wound bed for advanced therapies or biological agents. There are five types of débridement: sharp or surgical, mechanical, enzymatic, autolytic, and biotherapy or maggot débridement.

Sharp Débridement

Sharp débridement is the use of a sharp instrument, such as scalpel or scissors, to remove devitalized tissue. This method provides an immediate improvement of the wound bed and preserves granulation tissue. However, it requires specialized training. A physician, nurse, or physical therapist may perform this procedure at the bedside. If a wound requires extensive débridement, it may be performed in the operating room. Many stage IV ulcers extend into the bone, so a bone biopsy is often performed at the same time. The biopsy will detect **osteomyelitis**, extension of the infection into the bone.

Mechanical Débridement

Mechanical débridement may be performed via lavage (discussed in a preceding section), the use of wet-to-dry dressings, or hydrotherapy (whirlpool).

Wet-to-Dry Dressings. **Nonselective débridement** can be achieved with wet-to-dry dressings; that is, the dressings remove not only debris, but granulation tissue, from the wound. Coarse gauze moistened with normal saline is packed into the wound, allowed to dry, and then removed. The wound may require several dressing changes per day. This form of débridement was common once, but has declined in use because it removes granulation tissue and causes pain. If you must use this method, medicate the patient beforehand with opioid analgesics. Rewetting the gauze aids in its removal and decreases the pain, but it may eliminate the débriding action of the dressing change.

Hydrotherapy or Whirlpool Treatments. **Hydrotherapy or whirlpool treatments** also provide nonselective débridement. This is a vigorous form of débridement reserved for wounds with a large amount of nonviable tissue. Usually this treatment is performed in the physical therapy department once or twice per day. The wound is placed in a whirlpool containing tepid water for a prescribed amount of time (usually 5 to 15 minutes). Do not expose the wound directly to the water jets.

Whirlpool treatments increase the risk for periwound maceration, contamination by waterborne infections, and cross-contamination. Therefore, strict adherence to infection control measures is essential. Use hydrotherapy with caution in patients with venous stasis ulcers because it leads to vasodilation, which may increase edema and congestion. Persons with diabetic neuropathies are at increased risk for burns because of a decrease in sensory abilities.

Enzymatic Débridement

Enzymatic débridement uses proteolytic agents to break down necrotic tissue without affecting viable tissue in the wound. To use an enzymatic product, clean the wound with normal saline, apply a thin layer of the cream, and cover with a moisture-retaining dressing. This may be done once or twice daily, depending on the product. Apply the product only to devitalized tissue because it might cause some local irritation.

Autolysis

Autolysis is the use of an occlusive, moisture-retaining dressing and the body's own enzymes and defense mechanisms to break down necrotic tissue. This process takes more time than the other techniques, but it is tolerated better. The procedure involves applying the dressing and observing the fluid that collects under it (wound fluid may be tan in color). The dressing is normally changed every 72 hours. At that time, the wound is cleansed before a new dressing is applied. Observe the wound closely and regularly for signs of infection, such as an increase in pain or a foul odor. Autolysis is contraindicated in the presence of infection or immunosuppression.

Biotherapy or Maggot Débridement Therapy

Maggot débridement therapy is the use of medical-grade larvae of the greenbottle fly to dissolve dead and infected tissue from wounds. The larvae secrete enzymes that liquify dead tissue and create an alkaline environment. The enzymes are neutralized when they come in contact with normal tissue, so healthy tissue is unharmed. The larvae also digest bacteria from the wound. This therapy is effective and simple to use, though containing the larvae within the dressing can be problematic. Larvae are usually changed every 48 to 72 hours and disposed of as biohazardous medical waste.

Providing Moist Wound Healing

More than 65% of the human body is composed of water. The skin maintains this level of moisture by allowing water vapor to escape into the air around us in small amounts. With loss of or damage to the skin, body cells can dehydrate and die. A physiological wound environment is one that maintains the right amount of moisture for cells to flourish. Therefore, in the absence of skin, wound dressings must function as a barrier to water vapor loss. The type of dressing used on a wound depends on the characteristics of the wound and the goals of treatment. The dressing of choice should:

- Prevent drying of the wound bed.
- Absorb drainage.
- Keep the surrounding tissue dry and intact.
- Protect from contamination and infection.
- Aid in hemostasis.
- Débride the wound.
- Eliminate dead space.
- Prevent heat loss.
- Splint the wound site.
- Provide comfort to the patient.
- Control odor.

When choosing a dressing, ask yourself this question: Will it achieve the purposes listed above (e.g., can it be removed without damaging fragile skin or the wound itself?). Also consider how long it should stay in place and how often it needs to be changed.

The goal of all wound care is to heal the wound in the most rapid and comfortable manner, protect it from further injury and infection, and minimize scarring when possible. There is no single "recipe" for healing a wound. Each wound must be treated individually based on the patient history and assessment. Many wound materials are available, and new products are continually introduced. The "newest" dressing is not necessarily the best for the wound. You will need to become familiar with the different categories of dressings and how they are made. Each category has many different brands, so you must make your choice based on what the wound needs and not the manufacturer's brand name. Perform ongoing reassessment of your dressing choice every time you assess the wound. Modify dressings and wound treatments as the wound evolves.

KnowledgeCheck 34-10

- What should you consider when choosing a dressing?
- Describe the five types of wound débridement.
- Identify the purposes of a wound dressing.

 Go to Chapter 34, **Knowledge Check Response Sheet and Answers,** on the Student Resource Disk or DavisPlus at http://davisplus.fadavis.com/Wilkinson2

Primary dressings are ones that are placed in the wound bed and actually touch the wound. A **secondary dressing** is one that covers or holds a primary dressing in place. Many dressings can act as both, touching the wound bed and securing themselves to the wound with some type of adhesive (Table 34-5).

Absorption Dressings

Absorption dressings are made from highly absorptive layers of fibers such as cellulose, cotton, or rayon, and may or may not have an adhesive border.

Use—Appropriate for wounds with moderate to large amounts of exudate. Can be used as a primary

or secondary dressing to manage drainage from partial- or full-thickness wounds.

Cautions—Do not use to pack undermining wounds. Do not use if the wound is not draining.

Alginate Dressings

Alginates are fibers derived from brown seaweed and kelp. They are available in pad or rope form. Alginates are highly absorbent (20 to 40 times their weight).

Use—Should be reserved for wounds with large amounts of exudate. Ideal for wounds that have depth, tracts, tunneling, or undermining.

Technique—When the alginate comes in contact with exudate, a nonadhesive gel is created. You must irrigate this gel from the wound before placing the next dressing.

Cautions—Alginate dressings are extremely absorptive and will adhere to the wound bed if there is no drainage.

Antimicrobial Dressings

Antimicrobial dressings are topical antifungal and antibiotic agents that are available as ointments, impregnated gauzes, pads, gels, foams, hydrocolloids, and alginates. Silver and cadexomer iodine are two common ingredients in these dressings. The amount of drainage that can be absorbed depends on the type of dressing or delivery system that is combined with the antimicrobial agent.

Use—Can be used on partial- or full-thickness wounds, malodorous wounds with little to large amounts of drainage, or highly contaminated or infected wounds.

Purposes—To control or decrease the amount of bacteria in a wound, which helps to decrease exudate and prevent infection.

Collagen Dressings

Collagen is the most abundant protein in the body. Collagen dressings are made from bovine (cow) or porcine (pig) sources and made into sheets, pads, powders and gels.

Use—Use with partial or full thickness wounds, and contaminated or infected wounds.

Purposes—Collagen dressings stimulate wounds to produce collagen fibers and granulation tissue in the wound bed. Some collagen dressings are absorptive and help maintain a moist wound bed.

Advantages—These dressings do not stick to the wound bed and are easy to apply and remove.

Gauze Dressings

The simplest and most widely used dressings are gauze. Gauze is available in a variety of forms and textures (Fig. 34-12). Gauze is made of woven and nonwoven

Table 34-5 ➤ Types of Wound Dressings

TYPES OF DRESSINGS	USES	SIZE OF WOUND
Absorbent dressings	Highly absorbent	Large
Alginates	Absorbency Promote a moist environment Facilitate autolytic débridement	Large
Antimicrobials	Reduce and prevent infection Promote collagen deposition	Large
Collagens	Absorbency Promote a moist environment	Minimal to large
Foams	Absorbency Insulation Promote a moist environment Used under compression	Minimal to large
Gauze	Absorbency Packing Cleansing Protection	Large
Hydrocolloids	Promote a moist environment Provide a protective layer against friction/caustic agents Promote autolysis Used under compression	Light to moderate
Hydrogels	Promote a moist environment Rehydrate the wound bed Promote autolysis	Minimal
Transparent films	Promote a moist environment Occlusive with oxygen permeability Promote autolysis	Minimal to none

fibers of cotton, rayon, polyester, or a combination of these. Some gauze dressings are impregnated with antimicrobial agents, medications, or moisture, and others contain petrolatum to keep the wound moist. Gauze can be used in combination with **amorphous hydrogels**, saline, or medications. It may be packed as sterile or nonsterile, in bulk or in smaller packages.

Use—Gauze dressings can be used for packing large wounds, cavities, or tracts, deep or dirty wounds, or heavily draining wounds.

Disadvantages—Gauze dressings have, in the past, been considered the standard of care in advanced wound management. However, they have proven to be labor intensive and less cost effective than other advanced dressings, even though their initial cost of purchase may be less. Gauze dressings have the following disadvantages:

■ Gauze can stick to wound tissue (as with wet-to-dry débridement) and remove new, regenerated cells with each dressing change. Granulation tissue can grow into the material and be damaged with the gauze removal.

■ Gauze dressings do not ensure a moist wound environment, as they allow for fluid evaporation.

■ Many times gauze is applied incorrectly, as it must be fluffed to avoid pressure or overpacking of a wound.

■ The dressing change interval is dependent on the amount of fluid saturation of the gauze. If fluid wicks to the outer layer of the dressing, it must be changed more frequently. Frequent dressing changes disrupt the wound bed and cause the wound to become hypothermic (cold), which physiologically impairs cell growth.

The Critical Aspects box summarizes procedures for applying dry dressings and wet-to-damp (moist-to-moist) dressings. For complete steps,

VOL 2 Go to Chapter 34, **Procedure 34-4: Removing and Applying Dry Dressings,** and **Procedure 34-5: Removing and Applying Wet-to-Damp Dressings,** in Volume 2.

FIGURE 34-12 Gauze dressings are available in a variety of shapes and forms.

Foam Dressings

Foam dressings are made from semipermeable hydrophilic foam that forms an impermeable barrier over the wound. They are made into wafers, rolls, and pillows; have film coverings; and are adhesive or nonadhesive. They may be used in combination with other dressing materials, like alginates or films.

Use—Foams can absorb minimal to heavy exudates.
Purposes—They provide a moist environment and thermal insulation. The nonadhesive form protects friable periwound skin.
Techniques—When applying a foam dressing choose one that is approximately 2 to 3 cm (1 to 1½ in.) larger than the wound. The dressing may be changed up to three times a week.
Advantages—Conformable; can be shaped around body contours. They do not stick to the wound bed.
Cautions—Do not use with wounds that have tunneling or tracts. Foam is not recommended for dry, desiccated wounds. If the dressing becomes saturated, it may macerate periwound skin.

Hydrocolloid Dressings

Hydrocolloids are wafers, pastes, or powders that contain *hydrophilic* (water-loving) particles.

Use—When applied to a wound, the hydrophilic particles interact with exudate to form a gel that keeps the wound moist. The dressing forms a protective layer against friction and bacteria. This type of dressing is ideal for wounds with minimal drainage, such as partial-thickness wounds or stage II pressure ulcers. Hydrocolloid pastes or granules may be used to fill shallow cavities around stomas to create an even surface on which to place the ostomy appliance.

Advantages

- Wafers easily mold to the shape of the body, making them useful for difficult areas, such as heels or between buttocks.
- The protective layer also decreases pain.
- Hydrocolloids promote autolytic débridement.

Techniques

- Choose a dressing that is 3 to 4 cm (1½ to 2 in.) larger than the wound. Do not cut the wafer to fit into the wound. An edge is needed to stick to dry, intact skin.
- As a rule, hydrocolloid dressings do not need to be changed frequently. On a wound with minimal drainage, the dressing may remain in place for up to 7 days. Change the dressing if it begins to leak, develops an odor, or begins to separate from the skin.
- A secondary dressing is not required.
- When an exudate comes in contact with the hydrocolloid material, it can produce an odor that might be confused with a malodorous wound. Clean the wound bed first before determining if it is malodorous.

The Critical Aspects box highlights the procedure for applying a hydrocolloid dressing. For the complete steps,

 Go to Chapter 34, **Procedure 34-9: Applying a Hydrating Dressing and Hydrocolloid or Hydrogel,** in Volume 2.

 Cautions

- Not the dressing of choice for wounds that require frequent dressing changes (e.g., because it has moderate drainage or slough).
- Because hydrocolloid dressings are opaque, you cannot see the wound while they are in place.
- They are not recommended for wounds surrounded by friable skin because they can be difficult to remove.
- Their adhesive qualities can damage sensitive tissue.
- They should not be used on infected wounds because their occlusive nature (they are impermeable to oxygen, moisture, and bacteria) may facilitate the growth of anaerobic bacteria.
- They should not be used on wounds with tunneling or tracts because these wounds must be packed and allowed to drain. The wound should be shallow enough that the hydrocolloid touches the wound bed.

Hydrogels

Hydrogels are sheets, granules, or gels with a high water content, creating a jelly-like consistency that does not adhere to the wound bed.

Uses—Their soft, cooling texture promotes patient comfort. Hydrogels enhance epithelialization by providing moisture to the wound bed. They may also be used to soften slough or eschar in necrotic wounds, and they can be used in infected wounds.
Techniques—Because they are not adhesive, you will need to apply a secondary dressing over the hydrogel to maintain the moisture level in the wound and hold the product in place.
Cautions—Hydrogels have limited absorptive capabilities, so they are not practical for wounds with significant exudate. Their high moisture content can easily macerate periwound skin.

Skin Sealants and Moisture Barriers

Skin sealants are made from liquid transparent copolymer that can be wiped or sprayed on skin to protect it from wound exudate and moisture, friction, and skin stripping from adhesives. **Moisture barrier ointments** are petrolatum, dimethicone, or zinc-based products that can be applied to skin to protect it from exudate, moisture, urine, and feces. Both are simple and fast to use, and if needed, should be used with each dressing change.

> *Uses*—Skin sealants and moisture barrier ointments provide a barrier of protection over vulnerable skin from the effects of moisture and mechanical and chemical skin injury.
>
> *Cautions*—Ointments impair the adhesion of wound dressings or tapes.

Transparent Film Dressings

Transparent (thin film) dressings (Fig. 34-13) are clear and semipermeable. They allow exchange of air and water vapor between the wound and the environment while preventing external bacterial contamination.

> *Uses*—Transparent dressings are nonabsorbent, so they keep the wound moist. They are useful for wounds with minimal or no drainage. They are often used to dress IV sites.
>
> *Advantages*—The transparent dressing allows you to view the wound without removing or disturbing the dressing. Because they are thin and flexible, transparent films can be placed over joints without inhibiting movement.
>
> *Cautions*—If used over wounds that are draining, the tissues will become macerated. Transparent dressings adhere to the skin, so you should not use them on friable skin.

The Critical Aspects box highlights key steps in applying transparent films. For the complete procedure,

VOL 2 Go to Chapter 34, **Procedure 34-8: Applying a Transparent Film Dressing,** in Volume 2.

FIGURE 34-13 IV sites are commonly dressed with transparent film dressings.

KnowledgeCheck 34-11
- Differentiate among the different categories of dressings.
- What types of dressings may be used for wounds with a large amount of exudate?
- What form of dressing is appropriate for a wound with an eschar that needs to be eliminated?

Go to Chapter 34, **Knowledge Check Response Sheet and Answers,** on the Student Resource Disk or DavisPlus at http://davisplus.fadavis.com/Wilkinson2

Securing Dressings

What you will use to secure a dressing depends on wound size, location, amount of drainage, frequency of dressing changes, patient's activity level, and type of dressings used. Tape, ties, bandages, secondary dressings, and binders are among the choices. Tape is most commonly used. Tape is available in several forms:

Adhesive Tape provides stability to a dressing. It is tough and durable and can be used if you need to apply pressure to a wound. It leaves a residue on the skin and can cause trauma to surrounding intact skin when it is removed. However, commercial adhesive removers are available to remove the residue.

Foam Tape readily molds to the contours of the body and is ideal for dressings over joints.

Nonallergenic Tape and Paper Tape are best for sensitive skin. Ask patients whether they have any history of tape allergies or irritation, and use a tape that the patient has tolerated well in the past.

To tape a dressing, place strips of tape at the ends of the dressing, and space them evenly over the remainder of the dressing (Fig. 34-14A–C). The Critical Aspects box

FIGURE 34-14 *A*, Place strips of tape at the ends of the dressing and space them evenly over the remainder of the dressing. *B*, Choose a tape width appropriate for the size of the dressing. Use strips that are sufficiently long to secure the dressing in place. *C*, When taping over a joint, place the tape at a right angle to the direction in which the joint moves.

summarizes a procedure for taping dressings. To see the complete procedure,

 Go to Chapter 34, **Procedure 34-4: Taping a Dressing,** in Volume 2.

If a dressing requires frequent changes, you can use **Montgomery straps** with ties to secure the dressing (Fig. 34-15). Montgomery straps decrease the amount of pulling and irritation of skin around a wound. Apply the adhesive part of the straps to the skin at the ends of the dressing and at evenly spaced intervals. Lace the cloth ties between the straps to secure the dressing. Change the ties whenever they become soiled. Keep the straps in place until they begin to loosen from the skin.

Consider using thin hydrocolloids, low-adhesion foam dressings, or skin sealants under tape to also help prevent skin tears. For the fragile skin of older adults or infants, use porous tapes and avoid unnecessary tape use.

Controlling Infection

A wound provides a portal of entry or exit for microorganisms. When caring for patients with closed wounds, follow CDC Standard Precautions. For patients with open or draining wounds, follow CDC Tier Two: Contact Level Precautions in addition to Standard Precautions. See Chapter 20, and also,

 Go to Chapter 20, **Clinical Insight 20-4: Following Transmission-Based Precautions,** in Volume 2.

Observe the following guidelines:

Asepsis Measures. If the patient has an infection, place her in a private room or in a room with a patient who has an active infection caused by the same organism and no other infections. Follow any additional specific precautions for the microorganism identified. Most important, wash your hands frequently.

Use clean gloves when caring for the patient with a wound. Remove gloves, and wash your hands before coming in contact with another patient. Change your

FIGURE 34-15 Montgomery straps with ties may be used to secure a dressing that requires frequent changing.

gloves after removing a soiled dressing, before applying a clean dressing.

If a patient has multiple wounds, treat the least contaminated wound first, then progress to the most contaminated. Wash your hands and change gloves between each wound.

Sharp Débridement. Use sterile instruments for sharp débridement. Monitor the patient for signs and symptoms of sepsis (fever, tachycardia, hypotension, altered level of consciousness) after sharp débridement.

Dressings and Supplies. Use clean dressings when treating a chronic wound. Acute wounds may require sterile dressings. An immunocompromised patient may require sterile dressings even if the wound is chronic. Carefully dispose of contaminated dressings in biohazard waste receptacles.

Store patient dressing supplies in a clean and dry area. Do not share supplies among more than one patient. Access only the number of supplies you need for the dressing change. Do not touch the supply of dressings with gloves that have come in contact with the wound. Discard unused dressings if they become contaminated.

 Critical**Thinking** 34-6

What would be the best method to secure dressings for Mr. Harmon ("Meet Your Patient")?

How Are Wounds Supported and Immobilized?

Binders and bandages are used to hold a dressing in place, apply pressure to a wound to impede hemorrhage, and support and immobilize an injured area, thereby promoting healing and comfort. Before applying a bandage or binder, determine the intended purpose of the application and assess the part being bandaged.

Binders

Binders may be used to keep a wound closed when there is danger of dehiscence, or to immobilize a body part to aid in the healing process. They are typically used on large areas of the body and are designed for a specific body part. They may be made of cloth or elasticized material and fasten with straps, pins, or Velcro. The most common binders are the following:

- A *triangular arm binder or sling* is used to support the upper extremities. Because commercial slings are readily available, you will use the triangular sling infrequently.
- A *T-binder* is used to secure dressings or pads in the perineal area.
- An *abdominal binder* is used to provide support to the abdomen. It is often ordered when there is an open abdominal wound that is healing by secondary intention. The binder decreases the risk of dehiscence. Abdominal binders may be straight or multitailed.

To learn a procedure for applying binders, see the Critical Aspects box, and

VOL 2 Go to Chapter 34, **Procedure 34-11: Applying Binders,** in Volume 2.

Bandages

A bandage is a cloth, gauze, or elastic covering that is wrapped in place. With the exception of a sling, most bandages come in rolls and in various widths, commonly 1.5 to 7.5 cm (0.5 to 3 in.). Use a narrow width on small body parts, such as a finger, and wider bandages on arms and legs.

Cloth Bandages are most commonly used as slings to immobilize an upper extremity or to hold large abdominal dressings in place.

Gauze is the most frequently used type of bandage. It is available in many sizes and forms and readily conforms to the shape of the body. It may also be impregnated with medications for application to the skin or with plaster of Paris, which, when dried, hardens to form a cast.

Elastic bandages are used to apply pressure and give support (e.g., to improve venous circulation in the legs). Ace bandages are the most common form of elasticized bandage.

A rolled bandage is a continuous strip of material (gauze, stretchable gauze, or elastic webbing) that you unroll as you apply it to a body part. To apply a roller bandage, hold the free end in place with one hand, and use the other hand to pass the roll around the body part. Exert equal tension on each pass (or turn). Each turn should overlap the last one-half to two-thirds the width of the bandage, except for the circular turn. There are five basic turns for roller bandaging. To learn how to apply rolled bandages, see the Critical Aspects box for a summary, and

VOL 2 Go to Chapter 34, **Procedure 34-12: Applying Bandages,** in Volume 2.

How Should I Use Heat and Cold Therapy?

Local application of heat or cold has been used for therapeutic purposes for centuries. Temperature-sensitive nerve endings respond readily to temperatures between 59° and 113°F (15° and 45°C). Response to heat or cold depends on the area being treated, the nature of the injury, duration of the treatment, age, physical condition, and the condition of the skin. Monitor the patient especially carefully in the following situations:

Extremes of Age. The very young and the very old are the least tolerant of heat and cold therapies.

Sensory Impairment. Patients with sensory impairment are at increased risk for injury related to use of heat and cold therapy because they may not perceive temperature changes, burns, or ischemia.

Highly Vascular Areas. Highly vascular areas, such as the fingers, hand, face, and perineum, are very sensitive to temperature changes and thus are at high risk for injury from heat and cold.

Application to a Large Area. Application of cold or heat to a large body surface area decreases the patient's tolerance of the treatment. Application to a small area is best tolerated.

Injured Skin or Wounds. Intact skin tolerates heat and cold therapy better than skin that has been injured or has open wounds.

Safety Measures

✚ For patient safety, observe the following precautions when applying heat and cold:

- Avoid direct contact with the heating or cooling device. Cover the hot or cold pack with a washcloth, towel, or fitted sleeve.
- Apply hot or cold intermittently, leaving it on for no more than 15 minutes at a time in an area. This precaution helps prevent tissue injury (e.g., burns, impaired circulation). It also makes the therapy more effective by preventing *rebound phenomenon:* At the time the heat or cold reaches maximum therapeutic effect, the opposite effect begins.
- Check the skin frequently for extreme redness, blistering, cyanosis (blueness), or blanching. When heat or cold is first applied, the thermal receptors react strongly, and the person feels the temperature intensely. Over about 15 minutes, the receptors adapt to the new temperature, and the person notices it less. Caution clients not to change the temperature when this occurs because doing so can cause tissue injury.

Applying Heat Therapy

Local application of heat is used to relieve stiffness and discomfort associated with musculoskeletal problems. It may also be used for patients with wounds. Heat increases blood flow to an area through the mechanisms of vasodilatation, increased capillary permeability, and reduced blood viscosity. Increased blood flow brings oxygen and white blood cells to the wound and aids in the healing process. Heat promotes the delivery of nutrients and removal of waste products from the tissue, promotes relaxation, and decreases stiffness and muscle tension.

✚ When heat is applied to a large area of the body, vasodilatation may cause a drop in blood pressure and a feeling of faintness. Warn patients to be alert for this effect if they will be administering heat at home.

For steps to follow in *all* procedures, refer to the Universal Steps for All Procedures found on the inside back cover of Volume 2. Go to the full procedures in Volume 2 to practice and learn the procedure steps. Use these Critical Aspects later to help you review key points.

Procedure 34-1: Obtaining a Wound Culture by Swab

➤ Position the patient for easy access to the wound and in a manner that will allow the irrigation solution to flow freely from the wound with the assistance of gravity.

➤ Don protective equipment: Gown, face shield, and procedure gloves.

➤ Remove the soiled dressing, and dispose of gloves and dressing.

➤ Don clean gloves and fill a 35-mL syringe, with attached 19-gauge angiocatheter, with 0.9% (normal) saline solution.

➤ Holding the angiocatheter tip 2 cm from the wound bed, gently irrigate the wound (superior to inferior).

➤ Press the culture swab against an area of red granulating tissue, and rotate.

➤ Reinsert the swab into the culturette tube, label the tube, and transport it to the lab.

Procedure 34-2: Obtaining a Needle Aspiration Culture from a Wound

➤ Administer pain medication 30 minutes before the procedure, if necessary.

➤ Cleanse the wound with saline-moistened gauze, wiping from the center of the wound toward the edge.

➤ Draw up 1 mL of 0.9% (normal) saline for injection into a 22-gauge needle attached to a 3-mL syringe.

➤ Insert the needle 1 to 2 mm into the wound bed, and inject 1 mL of normal saline.

➤ Aspirate 1 mL of fluid from the wound bed.

➤ Express the fluid into the culture tube.

➤ Label the culture tube, and transport it to the lab.

➤ Apply a clean dressing to the wound as ordered.

Procedure 34-3: Performing a Sterile Wound Irrigation

➤ Administer pain medication 30 minutes before the procedure, if necessary.

➤ Position the patient for easy access to the wound and in a manner that will allow the irrigation solution to flow freely from the wound with the assistance of gravity.

➤ Don protective equipment: gown, face shield, and clean gloves.

➤ Remove the soiled dressing, and dispose of gloves.

➤ Set up a sterile field with a sterile irrigation kit or a 35-mL syringe and a 19-gauge angiocatheter with needle removed, dressing supplies, and irrigation solution.

➤ Wearing sterile gloves, fill either the syringe and angiocatheter or the piston-tip syringe with irrigation solution.

➤ Holding the syringe 2 cm (¾ to 1 in.) from the wound bed, gently irrigate the wound with a back-and-forth motion, moving from the superior aspect to the inferior aspect.

➤ Dry the tissue surrounding the wound with sterile gauze.

➤ Apply a new dressing as ordered.

➤ Dispose of used equipment and soiled dressings in a biohazard container.

➤ Reposition the patient.

Procedure 34-4: Taping a Dressing

➤ Place the patient in a comfortable position that provides easy access to the wound.

➤ Ensure the skin surrounding the dressing is clean and dry.

➤ Choose a tape that is appropriate for the dressing.

➤ Place the tape parallel to the incision.

➤ Tear strips that extend ½ inch beyond the dressing.

➤ Apply tape without pulling or stretching.

➤ Smooth tape in place by gently stroking the surface to maximize adhesion.

Procedure 34-5: Removing and Applying Dry Dressings

➤ Administer pain medication 30 minutes before the procedure, if necessary.

➤ Place the patient in a comfortable position that provides easy access to the wound.

➤ Wearing clean gloves, remove the soiled dressing and discard it in a biohazard receptacle.

➤ Change gloves and cleanse the wound with saline-moistened gauze.

➤ Assess the wound for location, appearance, odor, and drainage.

➤ Apply a dry dressing.

➤ Secure the dressing with tape.

Procedure 34-6: Removing and Applying Wet-to-Damp Dressings

➤ Assess for pain, and medicate 30 minutes before the procedure, if necessary.

➤ Place the patient in a comfortable position that provides easy access to the wound.

➤ Wearing clean gloves, remove the soiled dressing and discard it in a biohazard receptacle.

➤ Change gloves and cleanse the wound with saline-moistened gauze.

➤ Assess the wound for location, appearance, odor, and drainage.

➤ Don clean gloves and apply a single layer of moist, fine-mesh gauze to the wound. Be sure to place gauze in all depressions of the wound.

➤ Apply a secondary moist layer over the first layer. Repeat this process until the wound is filled with moistened sterile gauze.

➤ Cover the moistened gauze with an absorbent, surgical pad.

➤ Secure the dressing with tape or Montgomery straps.

Procedure 34-7: Applying a Negative Pressure Wound Therapy (NPWT) Device

➤ Administer an analgesic if needed.

➤ Select an appropriate dressing, per NPWT unit, to fill the entire wound cavity.

➤ Obtain a suction pump unit as ordered.

➤ Prepare a sterile field for supplies.

➤ Don sterile gloves for new surgical wounds; or clean gloves for chronic wounds.

➤ Irrigate the wound.

➤ Apply appropriate dressing per NPWT unit.

Procedure 34-7A: Open Pore Reticulated Polyurethane Foam (i.e., Vacuum Assisted Closure (VAC) Therapy)

➤ Cut the foam to fill the wound cavity.

➤ Do not place foam into blind/unexplored tunnels.

➤ Do not allow the foam dressing to overlap onto healthy skin.

Procedure 34-7B: Gauze Dressing Application (i.e., Chariker–Jeter Method)

➤ Measure the length of the drain.

➤ Moisten the gauze.

➤ "Sandwich" the drain in the moistened gauze and place in the wound base.

➤ Tuck the gauze into any undermining areas to ensure contact with the wound bed.

➤ Apply a strip or dollop of ostomy paste 1 cm from wound edge and secure the drain as needed.

For Both Types of Dressing

➤ Connect tubing attached to the dressing to the evacuation tubing going to the collection system.

➤ Position the tubing and connector away from bony prominences and skin creases.

➤ Ensure the clamps are open on all tubing.

➤ Turn on the pump and set to prescribed settings.

➤ Listen for audible leaks and observe for dressing collapse.

➤ Change the canister once a week or sooner if it fills.

Procedure 34-8: Applying a Transparent Film Dressing

➤ Place the patient in a comfortable position that provides easy access to the wound.

➤ Remove the soiled dressing, if necessary.

➤ Cleanse the surrounding skin and wound.

➤ Assess the condition of the wound.

➤ Apply the transparent film dressing to the wound by removing the center backing and holding the dressing firmly by the edges.

➤ Remove the edge liners.

Procedure 34-9: Applying a Hydrating Dressing (Hydrocolloid or Hydrogel)

➤ Place the patient in a comfortable position.

➤ Remove the soiled dressing, if necessary.

➤ Cleanse the wound, if necessary.

➤ Assess the wound, or other area where hydrocolloid dressing will be applied, for size, location, appearance, exudate, odor, and signs and symptoms of infection.

➤ Clip the area around the wound if necessary.

➤ Apply the hydrating dressing.

Procedure 34-10: Placing Skin Closures

➤ Place the patient in a comfortable position that provides easy access to the wound.

➤ Cleanse the surrounding skin and wound.

➤ Assess the wound and determine the size and type of skin closure needed.

➤ Peel the skin closure from the card at a 90° angle.

➤ Place closures across the wound without tension starting at the middle of the wound.

➤ Place closures 1/8 in. (3 mm) apart along the entire wound.

Procedure 34-11: Applying Binders

➤ Choose a binder of the correct type and size for the intended purpose.

➤ Make sure the binder is positioned properly to provide support but not compromise circulation or impair breathing.

➤ Pad any pressure areas or skin abrasions.

➤ *Abdominal binder*: Remove every 2 hours, and assess the underlying skin and dressings. Fasten from the bottom up.

➤ *Triangular strap binder*: Position the patient's arm across the chest with elbow flexed slightly. Place one end of the triangle over the shoulder of the uninjured arm, and allow the triangle to fall open so that the elbow of the injured arm is at the apex of the triangle.

➤ *T-binders*: They come in 2 basic types—those for females have a perineal strap; those for males have a split in the perineal strap.

Procedure 34-12: Applying Bandages

➤ Bandage the body part in its natural position.

➤ Work from distal to proximal position.

➤ Choose a bandage of the proper width.

➤ Clean the wound (if present).

➤ Apply primary dressing as prescribed.

➤ Apply the bandage as needed to secure the primary dressing.

Procedure 34-13: Removing Sutures and Staples

Procedure 34-13A: Suture Removal

➤ Place the patient in a comfortable position that provides easy access to the wound.

➤ Use the forceps to pick up one end of the suture. Slide the small scissors around the suture, and cut near the skin.

➤ With the forceps, gently pull the suture in the direction of the knotted side to remove it.

Continued

Procedure 34-13B: Staple Removal

➤ Position the staple remover so that the lower jaw is on the bottom.

➤ Place both tips of the lower jaw of the staple remover underneath the staple.

➤ Lift slightly on the staple ensuring that it stays perpendicular to the skin.

➤ Gently squeeze the handles together and lift the staple straight up.

➤ Place the removed staples on a piece of gauze.

➤ Dispose of the removed staples in the sharps container.

➤ Apply dressing if needed.

Procedure 34-14: Shortening a Wound Drain

➤ Before shortening a wound drain, make sure it is secured tightly.

➤ Firmly grasp the full width of the drain at the level of the skin and pull it out by the prescribed amount (e.g., 6 mm, [¼ in.]).

➤ Insert a sterile safety pin through the drain at the level of the skin.

➤ Hold the drain tightly, and insert the pin above your fingers.

➤ Using sterile scissors, cut the drain a little above the safety pin.

Procedure 34-15: Emptying a Closed-Wound Drainage System

➤ Don personal protective equipment as needed, including nonsterile procedure gloves, gown, and eyewear.

➤ Properly dispose of contaminated items into designated biohazard waste receptacles.

➤ Measure drainage and report excess volume to the primary care provider.

Moist Heat

The addition of moisture to heat amplifies the intensity of the treatment. Moist heat can be applied in several forms. The form used depends on the skin condition.

- *Washcloth or towel.* If heat is being applied for relaxation and the skin is intact, you can soak a washcloth or towel in warm water and wring out the excess moisture before applying to the skin.
- *Gauze compress.* If there are any open areas, you will need to use a gauze compress (usually sterile).
- *Soaks and baths* also provide moist heat. A **soak** involves immersion of the affected area. Soaking helps cleanse a wound and remove encrusted material. A **bath** is a modification of a soak in which a special tub or chair may be used. The most commonly used bath is a sitz bath (Fig. 34-16). A **sitz bath** soaks the patient's perineal area. Disposable sitz baths are often used to help prevent infection.

Dry Heat

Dry heat may be applied by several methods: electric heating pads, disposable hot packs, or hot water bags.

- *Electric heating pad*s have the advantage of providing a constant temperature, but the risk of burns is high. Caution patients to place the pad over the body area and never to lie on the pad.
- *Aquathermia pads* (Fig. 34-17) may also be used for dry heat application. Aquapads are plastic or vinyl pads that circulate water in the interior of the pad to create a constant temperature.
- *Disposable hot packs and hot water bags or bottles* are also available. Hot water bags are common in home use, but not in healthcare agencies because of the danger of burns from improper use.

For guidelines (including water temperatures) for applying moist and dry heat,

 Go to Chapter 34, **Clinical Insight 34-1: Applying Local Heat Therapy,** in Volume 2.

FIGURE 34-16 A sitz bath soaks the patient's perineal area.

FIGURE 34-17 Aquapads circulate water in the interior of the pad to create a constant temperature.

Applying Cold Therapy

The application of moist or dry cold causes vasoconstriction and decreases capillary permeability. It produces local anesthesia, reduces cell metabolism, increases blood viscosity, and decreases muscle tension. It also slows bacterial growth. Applications of cold are used to prevent or limit edema and reduce inflammation, pain, oxygen requirements, and bleeding. Cold therapy is often used to treat fevers and sports injuries (e.g., sprains, strains, fractures, and contusions), and to prevent swelling after surgery (e.g., an ice bag may be applied to the perineum after childbirth; an ice collar may be applied to the throat after a tonsillectomy). Cold applications have the following side effects:

- *Elevated blood pressure.* Because cold causes vasoconstriction, it may increase the patient's blood pressure.
- *Shivering.* Prolonged cold may cause shivering, a normal response as the body attempts to produce heat.
- *Tissue damage.* Prolonged exposure to cold may cause tissue damage due to impaired circulation.

For guidelines in applying cold therapy,

 Go to Chapter 34, **Clinical Insight 34-2: Application of Local Cold Therapy,** in Volume 2.

KnowledgeCheck 34-12

- What is the effect of adding moisture to heat or cold treatments?
- For how long should heat or cold be applied to an area?
- What precautions should you take before using heat or cold therapy?

 Go to Chapter 34, **Knowledge Check Response Sheet and Answers,** on the Student Resource Disk or DavisPlus at http://davisplus.fadavis.com/Wilkinson2

CarePlanning & MappingPractice

For a care plan and care map for Impaired Skin Integrity,

 Go to Chapter 34, **Care Plan** and **Care Map,** on the Student Resource Disk or DavisPlus at http://davisplus.fadavis.com/Wilkinson2

 Go to Chapter 34, **Resources for Caregivers and Health Professionals,** on the Student Resource Disk or DavisPlus at http://davisplus.fadavis.com/Wilkinson2

 Suggested Readings: Go to Chapter 34, **Reading More About Skin Integrity and Wound Healing,** on the Student Resource Disk or DavisPlus at http://davisplus.fadavis.com/Wilkinson2

 Bibliography: Go to Volume 2, Bibliography.

CHAPTER 35

Oxygenation

Learning Outcomes

After completing this chapter, you should be able to:

➤ Describe the structure and function of the respiratory and cardiovascular systems.

➤ Identify individual, environmental, and pathological factors that influence oxygenation.

➤ Assess oxygenation, breathing, circulation, and gas exchange.

➤ Interpret diagnostic testing related to oxygenation, breathing, circulation, and gas exchange.

➤ Develop nursing diagnoses related to oxygenation, breathing, circulation, and gas exchange.

➤ Plan outcomes and interventions for maintaining and improving oxygenation.

➤ Safely and correctly perform common nursing procedures related to oxygenation, breathing, perfusion, and gas exchange.

➤ Evaluate adequacy of oxygenation, breathing, perfusion, and gas exchange, and modify nursing activities appropriately based on outcomes.

➤ Describe a procedure for safe oxygen administration.

➤ Describe measures for mobilizing airway secretions.

➤ Implement measures for promoting optimal respiratory function (e.g., positioning)

➤ Explain how to suction the upper and lower airways.

➤ Provide care for patients requiring artificial airways.

➤ Provide care for patients requiring mechanical ventilation.

➤ Provide care for patients requiring chest tubes.

➤ Provide measures to promote peripheral circulation.

➤ Recognize medications used to enhance pulmonary and cardiovascular function.

➤ Use identified outcomes to evaluate care for patients with oxygenation and circulation problems.

Meet Your Patients

You are scheduled for a clinical placement in a pulmonary clinic. Your assignment is to (1) perform a focused assessment related to breathing and oxygenation, (2) perform common therapeutic interventions related to breathing and oxygenation, (3) identify desired outcomes and evaluate achievement of those outcomes, and (4) plan for follow-up and home care needs. In the course of your clinical day, you care for the following clients:

■ Mary is a 4-year-old girl with a history of asthma. Her mother, Ms. Green, has brought her in because of an "asthma attack." Mary is sitting in her mother's lap and breathing rapidly through an open mouth. Her cough sounds congested and wheezy. The nurse practitioner has ordered a nebulized treatment containing albuterol (Proventil) and ipratropium bromide (Atrovent).

■ Mr. Chu is a 78-year-old man complaining of cough, sore throat, fatigue, and weakness. His temperature is 100.4°F (38°C), pulse is 90 beats/min, respirations are 26 per minute, and blood pressure (BP) is 166/82 mm Hg.

■ William is a 19-year-old male who has had a sudden onset of right-sided chest pain and shortness of breath. His chest

(continued on next page)

Meet Your Patients (continued)

x-ray revealed a right pneumothorax, and he is currently receiving 35% oxygen by face mask while waiting for an ambulance to transport him to the hospital for further evaluation.

■ Ms. Saunders is a 45-year-old homemaker. She says she has been extremely tired, easily becomes short of breath, and is unable to complete her chores without frequent rest breaks. She is pale and moves slowly. Her vital signs are as follows: temperature 98.4°F (36.7°C); pulse, 86 beats/min; respirations 24 per minute and unlabored; BP 136/78 mm

Hg; and pulse oximetry 98% on room air. She is now waiting for her lab results, which include a complete blood count (CBC).

Each of these patients is experiencing an oxygenation problem. This chapter describes a variety of assessment techniques and interventions to support breathing, oxygenation, circulation, and gas exchange for patients such as these.

The concept **oxygenation** refers to how well the cells, tissues, and organs of the body are supplied with oxygen. The pulmonary, cardiovascular, musculoskeletal, and neurological systems work together to achieve oxygenation. The musculoskeletal and neurological systems regulate the movement of air into and out of the lungs. The lungs oxygenate the blood, and the heart circulates the blood throughout the body and back to the lungs. In this chapter, we present the pulmonary and cardiovascular systems separately to make your learning easier, but remember: the two systems work together. Changes in one system create changes in the other.

Part I. The Pulmonary System

Part I of this chapter describes the structures and functions of the pulmonary system and explains how breathing is controlled. You will also learn how to assess and support respiratory functioning.

Theoretical **Knowledge** **knowing** why

The pulmonary system has two major components: the *airway* and the *lungs.* The following presents a brief review of the anatomy and physiology of the pulmonary system (the airway and the lungs). For more in-depth information, consult anatomy and physiology texts, or

 Go to Chapter 35, **Supplemental Materials, Structures of the Pulmonary System,** on the Student Resource Disk or DavisPlus at http://davisplus.fadavis.com/Wilkinson2

The Airway

The airway consists of the nasal passages, mouth, pharynx, larynx, trachea, bronchi, and bronchioles (Fig. 35-1). Air flows through these structures into and out of the lungs. In addition, the airway structures do the following:

■ *Moisten the air*—A moist mucous membrane lining adds water to inhaled air.

■ *Warm the air*—Blood flowing through the vascular airway walls transfers body heat to the inhaled air.

■ *Filter the air*—(1) Specialized cells in the lining of the airways secrete sticky mucus to trap foreign particles. (2) **Cilia,** tiny hairlike projections from the walls of the airways, move rhythmically to sweep trapped debris up and out of the airway.

■ The **upper airway,** located above the larynx, includes the nasal passages, mouth, and pharynx. The *pharynx* (throat) contains the openings to the esophagus and trachea. The *trachea* lies just in front of the esophagus. The *epiglottis,* a small flap of tissue superior to the larynx, closes off the trachea during swallowing so that food and fluids do not enter the lower airway. The epiglottis opens during breathing to allow air to move through the airway.

■ The **lower airway,** located below the larynx, includes the trachea, bronchi, and bronchioles. The lower airway is considered sterile. The **trachea,** sometimes called the "windpipe," extends from the larynx to where it divides to form the right and left mainstem bronchi. As the airways branch and become smaller, they have progressively thinner and less cartilage, until it disappears completely in the smaller bronchioles. The walls of the bronchi and bronchioles contain layers of smooth muscles. Spasm of these muscles **(bronchospasm)** narrows the airway and obstructs airflow.

The Lungs

The *lungs* are soft, spongy, cone-shaped organs. They are separated by the **mediastinum,** which contains the heart and great vessels. The right lung has three lobes; the left lung has two lobes. The upper portion of each lung, the *apex,* extends upward above the clavicle. The lower portion of each lung, the *base,* rests on the diaphragm. Knowing the location of lung tissue beneath the chest wall helps you to perform a complete and accurate assessment of the lungs.

The lungs are composed of millions of **alveoli**—tiny air sacs with thin walls surrounded by a fine network of

FIGURE 35-1 An anterior view of the respiratory system. The upper airway lies above the larynx. The lower airway, located below the larynx, is considered sterile.

capillaries. Gases (oxygen and carbon dioxide) easily pass back and forth between the alveoli and capillaries. Alveoli are composed of two types of cells (Fig. 35-2).

- *Type I alveolar cells* are the gas exchange cells.
- *Type II alveolar cells* produce **surfactant,** a lipoprotein that lowers the surface tension within alveoli to allow them to inflate during breathing.

KnowledgeCheck 35-1

- What happens to inhaled air in the airways? How does this occur?
- In which structures of the lung does gas exchange take place?
- What does surfactant do for alveoli?

  Go to Chapter 35, **Knowledge Check Response Sheet and Answers,** on the Student Resource Disk or DavisPlus at http://davisplus.fadavis.com/Wilkinson2

CriticalThinking 35-1

You are assigned to care for an adult patient who has a medical condition with which you are not familiar. You look it up and find that the condition causes a dramatic loss of surfactant. Based on your knowledge of the function of surfactant, what problems are this patient at high risk for developing?

What Are the Functions of the Pulmonary System?

Two major processes occur in the pulmonary system: ventilation and respiration. **Ventilation** is the movement of air into and out of the lungs through the act of breathing. **Respiration** is the exchange of the gases oxygen and carbon dioxide in the lungs.

Pulmonary Ventilation

Oxygenation of the blood, and ultimately of organs and tissues, depends on adequate ventilation. Ventilation must move enough air through the lungs to make adequate oxygen available to the alveoli.

How Does Ventilation Occur?

Ventilation is accomplished through cycles of inhalation and exhalation. **Inhalation** is caused by expansion of the chest cavity and lungs, which creates negative pressure inside the lungs; this causes air to be drawn in through the nose or mouth and airways. The *diaphragm* is the major muscle of breathing. When it contracts with each inhalation, the chest cavity is pulled downward,

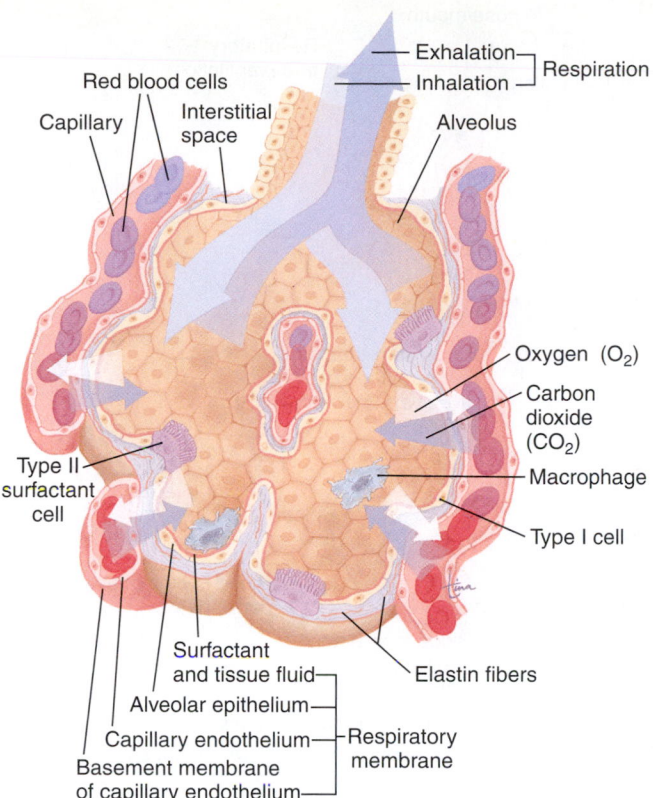

FIGURE 35-2 Alveolar structure showing type I and type II cells. Type I alveolar cells are the gas exchange cells. Type II alveolar cells produce surfactant.

FIGURE 35-3 A, During inhalation, the diaphragm contracts, pulling the chest cavity and lung bases downward; the intercostal muscles pull the rib cage up and outward. B, In exhalation, the diaphragm relaxes, the lung bases move upward, and the ribs and intercostal muscles move down and in, resulting in lung compression.

pulling the lung bases downward with it. *Intercostal muscles,* the small muscles around the ribs, also contract on inhalation and pull the ribs outward, slightly expanding the chest cavity and lungs. The pleural membrane covering the lungs adheres ("sticks") to the pleural membrane lining the chest cavity, so the lungs expand. Lung expansion creates negative pressure and draws air in through the only opening to the outside, the trachea. See Figure 35-3A.

Exhalation occurs when the diaphragm and intercostal muscles relax, allowing the chest and lungs to return to their normal resting size. See Figure 35-3B. The reduction in size causes the pressure inside the chest and lungs to rise above atmospheric pressure, so air flows out of the lungs. Exhalation requires no energy or effort.

What Factors Affect the Adequacy of Ventilation?

The adequacy of ventilation is affected by the rate and depth of respirations, lung compliance and elasticity, and airway resistance.

- **Respiratory rate and depth** are almost self-explanatory: **Rate** is how fast you breathe and **depth** is how much your lungs expand to take in air. These processes affect oxygen and carbon dioxide levels in the blood.
- **Hyperventilation** occurs when a person breathes fast and deeply to move a large amount of air through the lungs, causing too much carbon dioxide to be removed by the alveoli. Mild hyperventilation can occur in response to **hypoxemia** (a low level of oxygen in the blood). When blood oxygen is low, ventilation increases to draw additional air (and oxygen) into the lungs. However, as ventilation increases, carbon dioxide levels fall. Severe hyperventilation is usually triggered by medications, central nervous system abnormalities, high altitude, heat, exercise, panic, fear, or anxiety.
- **Hypoventilation** occurs when a decreased rate or shallow breathing moves only a small amount of air into and out of the lungs. Hypoventilation predisposes to the development of hypoxemia because less air (carrying oxygen) reaches the alveoli. The concern is that hypoxemia will lead to **hypoxia** (an oxygen deficiency in the body tissues).
- **Lung compliance** refers to the ease of lung inflation. Normally the lungs inflate easily because of their stretchy elastin fibers, low water content, and low alveolar surface tension. Lung compliance is reduced by conditions that cause elastin fibers to be replaced with scar tissue (collagen), increased lung water (edema), or loss of surfactant.
- **Lung elasticity** (or elastic recoil) refers to the tendency of the elastin fibers to return to their original position away from the chest wall after being stretched (think of stretching a rubber band, then letting go of it). Alveoli that have been overstretched, as with emphysema, lose their elastic recoil over time. This loss of elasticity allows the lungs to inflate easily but inhibits deflation, leaving stale air trapped in the alveoli.
- **Airway resistance** is the resistance to airflow within the airways. The larger the diameter of the airway, the more easily air moves through it. Normally, airway resistance is very low, so it takes little effort to move large volumes of air into and out of the lungs.

However, even small decreases in airway diameter (as might occur with secretions in the airway or mild bronchospasm) markedly increase airway resistance. Mary, the little girl with asthma in "Meet Your Patients," is undoubtedly experiencing airway resistance.

To see an animated demonstration of the physiology of ventilation,

 Go to **Animations: Physiology of Ventilation,** on DavisPlus at http://davisplus.fadavis.com/Wilkinson2

KnowledgeCheck 35-2

- What is the difference between ventilation and respiration?
- Describe how the diaphragm, accessory muscles, and pressure changes within the lungs create inhalation and exhalation.
- How does hypoventilation affect risk for hypoxemia and hypoxia?

 Go to Chapter 35, **Knowledge Check Response Sheet and Answers,** on the Student Resource Disk or DavisPlus at http://davisplus.fadavis.com/Wilkinson2

Respiration (Gas Exchange)

Respiration refers to gas exchange, that is, the oxygenation of blood and elimination of carbon dioxide in the lungs. Although nurses commonly use the term *respirations* to mean "breaths" in an assessment of vital signs, strictly speaking this is not accurate: you cannot measure gas exchange by counting breaths per minute. Gas exchange occurs at two equally essential levels: (1) at the alveolar–capillary membrane in the lungs (external), and (2) at the capillary–cellular membrane in body tissues (internal).

External respiration (alveolar–capillary gas exchange) occurs in the alveoli of the lungs. Oxygen (O_2) diffuses across the alveolar–capillary membrane into the blood of the pulmonary capillaries; carbon dioxide (CO_2) diffuses out of the blood and into the alveoli to be exhaled (Fig. 35-4). The rate of diffusion depends on the thickness of the membrane and the total surface of lung tissue available for gas exchange. Examples of conditions that slow diffusion are pleural effusion (fluid in the lungs), pneumothorax (lung collapse), and asthma (bronchospasms). If blood is not adequately oxygenated in the alveoli, **hypoxemia** (low blood-oxygen levels) occurs. Getting oxygen into the blood as it flows through the lungs is only the first step in oxygenation.

Internal respiration (capillary–tissue gas exchange) occurs in body organs and tissues. Oxygen diffuses from the blood through the capillary–cellular membrane into the tissue cells, where it is used for metabolism. From the cells, CO_2, a waste product of cellular metabolism, diffuses through the capillary–cellular membrane into the blood, from where it is transported to the lungs and exhaled. Tissue oxygenation requires both adequate external respiration and adequate peripheral circulation.

FIGURE 35-4 External respiration occurs at the alveolar–capillary membrane. Internal respiration occurs at the tissue–capillary membrane.

Limitations in either function may lead to **hypoxia** (oxygen deficiency in body tissues). In addition, if tissue cells are using more oxygen for metabolism than normal (e.g., during a high fever), hypoxia will occur unless more oxygen is made available to the tissues.

 ## CriticalThinking 35-2

William ("Meet Your Patients") has a right pneumothorax. Which of the two factors affecting the rate of gas diffusion is causing William to be hypoxemic? If you do not know what a pneumothorax is, look it up.

How Is Breathing Controlled?

The respiratory centers in the brain stem control breathing using feedback from chemoreceptors and lung receptors. **Chemoreceptors** located in the medulla of the brainstem, the carotid arteries, and the aorta detect changes in blood pH, O_2, and CO_2 levels, and they send messages back to the central respiratory center in the brain stem. In response, the respiratory center increases or decreases ventilation to maintain normal blood levels of pH, O_2 (Po_2), and CO_2 (Pco_2). Normally the blood CO_2 level provides the primary stimulus to breathe. High CO_2 levels stimulate breathing to eliminate the excess CO_2. A secondary, though important, drive to breathe is hypoxemia. Low blood O_2 levels stimulate breathing to get more oxygen into the lungs.

In addition, **lung receptors**, located in the lung and chest wall, are sensitive to breathing patterns, lung expansion, lung compliance, airway resistance, and respiratory irritants. The respiratory center uses feedback from the lung receptors to adjust ventilation. For example, if the lung receptors sense respiratory irritants such as dust, cold air, or tobacco smoke, the respiratory center triggers airway constriction and a more rapid, shallow pattern of breathing.

Voluntary control from the **motor cortex** can override the involuntary respiratory centers, but only temporarily. Voluntary control of breathing allows a person to continue breathing while doing activities such as talking, singing, swallowing, whistling, and blowing.

For a brief overview of the nervous system,

 Go to Chapter 35, **Supplemental Materials, The Nervous System,** on the Student Resource Disk or DavisPlus at http://davisplus.fadavis.com/Wilkinson2

KnowledgeCheck 35-3

- Describe two ways in which breathing is controlled.
- The level of which gas (oxygen or carbon dioxide) is the primary stimulant for breathing?

 Go to Chapter 35, **Knowledge Check Response Sheet and Answers,** on the Student Resource Disk or DavisPlus at http://davisplus.fadavis.com/Wilkinson2

 CriticalThinking 35-3

Ms. Saunders ("Meet Your Patients") has adequate blood oxygen levels, based on a pulse oximeter reading of 98%. Can you conclude that organ and tissue oxygenation are adequate? Explain your thinking.

What Factors Influence Pulmonary Function?

Factors that influence pulmonary function include developmental stage, the environment, individual and lifestyle factors, medications, and pathophysiological states.

Developmental Stage

Normal development influences lung, heart, and circulatory function, all of which affect oxygenation. Developmental factors have less effect on function in young and middle adults than in older adults.

Infants

Premature infants (less than 35 weeks' gestation) do not have a fully developed alveolar surfactant system. Surfactant is the substance that keeps air sacs inflated for effective respiration. Therefore, premature infants are at high risk for **respiratory distress syndrome** (RDS). RDS is characterized by widespread **atelectasis** (collapse of alveoli). The premature infant also has immature pulmonary circulation. Together with hypoventilation, this leads to hypercarbia (high CO_2 blood levels) and hypoxemia.

Infants born at term are also at risk for oxygenation problems (e.g., infection and airway obstruction) for the following reasons:

- Because the newborn's lower airway structures are immature and small, an infectious agent can spread rapidly.
- The infant's airways are quite narrow in diameter and, therefore, easily obstructed by edema, mucus, or a foreign body, such as meconium passed at birth.
- The central nervous system for preterm, and even some term, infants is immature, leading to periodic breathing patterns and apnea.
- The immune system of infants in the first few months of life is immature. Although at birth, infants enjoy the benefit of some maternal immunoglobulin circulating in their system; this protection is limited and not sufficient for fighting certain infections.
- By 6 months of age, infants can grasp small objects and put them in their mouths. This new skill, combined with small airway diameter, puts them at risk for choking on small objects.

Toddlers

As the toddler's respiratory and immune systems mature, his risk for frequent and serious infections diminishes. However, the incidence of *upper respiratory infections* (URIs) remains high because (1) the tonsils and adenoids are relatively large, predisposing to tonsillitis and (2) many children are exposed to new infectious agents in preschool and day care. Most children recover from URIs without difficulty. Toddlers actively explore the environment and often put objects in their mouths, which puts them at risk for other respiratory problems, for example:

- *Acquiring and transmitting infections* through toys and other objects
- *Airway obstruction* from aspiration of small objects (e.g., candy, buttons, coins, peanuts, grapes, and so on). The toddler's airway is still relatively short and small and may be easily obstructed.
- *Drowning* in very small amounts of water around the home (e.g., in a bucket of water or toilet bowl)

Preschool and School-Age Children

Preschool and school-age children have developed mature lungs, heart, and circulatory systems that can adapt to moderate stress and change. Healthy children typically have bouts of tonsillitis or URIs, which usually resolve without difficulty. Viral infections, such as croup and pneumonia, are common, especially in preschoolers and younger school-age children. Exercise-induced asthma is also a problem. Unfortunately, a few children as young as middle-school age begin social habits, such as tobacco use, that can have long-term adverse effects on oxygenation in both the pulmonary and cardiovascular systems.

Adolescents

In adolescence, the lungs develop adult characteristics. The average adolescent is developmentally at little risk for lung diseases. Some may, however, be developing behaviors and habits, such as tobacco use, that can create risk throughout life. As do adults, young people often begin smoking for social reasons (e.g., peer pressure, advertising, desire to feel cool), but nicotine addiction perpetuates the habit. Adolescents make fewer routine healthcare visits than do younger children, and as a result, many do not receive the recommended influenza vaccines. Exercise-induced asthma is still a problem in this age group.

Young, Middle, and Older Adults

Unhealthful practices (e.g., smoking and a lack of aerobic exercise) of adolescence often continue into adulthood. Half the adults who smoke were regular smokers by their 18th birthdays (American Lung Association, 2009a; CDC/NCHS, 2008).

Changes in the respiratory system that begin in middle-age and increase in older adulthood may become significant when the person experiences stressors such as infection, surgery, anesthesia, and emotional problems. The number of cells and the efficiency of the organs decline in a subtle and progressive way as a person ages. Keep in mind, though, that endurance training and regular exercise minimize the rate of these changes. In fact, an older person who is physically conditioned by regular exercise may have better lung function than a younger adult who is not well conditioned.

Older adults tend to experience the following changes:

- *Reduced lung expansion and less alveolar inflation*, especially in the bases of the lungs. This is because (1) costal cartilage begins to calcify, reducing chest wall movement during breathing; (2) the lungs have less recoil ability; and (3) the alveoli lose elasticity.
- *Difficulty expelling mucus or foreign material* due to a less effective cough reflex, drier mucus, and fewer cilia in the airways.
- *Diminished ability to increase ventilation* when oxygenation demands increase (e.g., with exercise). As diaphragm strength decreases, vital capacity is reduced; so exhalation becomes less efficient, causing progressive air-trapping.
- *Declining immune response*, especially cell-mediated immunity, T-cell activity, and the inflammatory response
- *Gastroesophageal reflux disease* is more common in older adults, creating a risk for aspirating stomach contents into the lungs. This may result in an inflammatory response.

All of these changes put older adults at risk for respiratory infections. Upper respiratory infections that would be mild and short-lived in a younger person may quickly lead to pneumonia in an older adult. In addition, chemoreceptors that control breathing respond more slowly to increased O_2 demand or rising levels of CO_2, making hypoxemia more likely.

Environment

Environmental factors, such as stress, allergic reactions, altitude, and temperature, affect oxygenation.

Stress

The stress response stimulates the release of catecholamines from the sympathetic nervous system. This results in increased tendency of blood to clot (e.g., as in pulmonary embolus). It also suppresses the immune system and inflammatory response. A chronically suppressed immune and inflammatory response increases the risk for all infections, including respiratory. For additional information on the effects of stress, see Chapter 25.

Allergic Reactions

An **allergy** is a hypersensitivity, or over-response, to an antigen. Pulmonary allergens include such things as dust, dust mites, cockroach particles, pollen, molds, newsprint, tobacco smoke, animal dander, and sometimes foods.

Hay Fever. Hay fever is an allergic reaction affecting the eyes, nose, and/or sinuses. It causes the release of *histamine,* which is largely responsible for accumulation of nasal fluid, swollen nasal membranes, nasal congestion; and itchy, swollen, watery eyes. Antihistamines are effective in combating hay fever.

Asthma. Asthma is an allergic reaction occurring in the bronchioles of the lungs. *Slow reacting substance of anaphylaxis* is released, which causes bronchoconstriction and lower airway edema and spasms, making breathing difficult and ineffective. Because histamine is not a major factor in causing the asthmatic reaction, antihistamines have little effect in the treatment of asthma. Asthma is the most common serious chronic disease of childhood, and it can be life-threatening.

Air Quality

Air pollution triggers respiratory problems (e.g., lung cancer, carbon monoxide poisoning) that interfere with oxygenation. Even healthy people may experience headache, coughing, and other symptoms when exposed to air pollution. People with existing respiratory disease may become unable to function. Some sources of air pollution are natural (e.g., forest fires), but the most common and damaging sources result from human activities (e.g., automobile exhaust emissions). Indoor air pollutants include carbon monoxide, nitrogen oxides, radon, and suspended particles (e.g., dust, mold spores, aerosols, and tobacco smoke). Pollutants are most harmful to infants, toddlers, older adults, and people with heart or lung disease. For more information about air quality,

Go to Chapter 35, **Supplemental Materials: Air Quality Affects Oxygenation,** on the Student Resource Disk or DavisPlus at http://davisplus.fadavis.com/Wilkinson2

Altitude

Atmospheric pressure falls from 760 mm Hg at sea level to 523 mm Hg at 10,000 feet. Oxygen pressure falls proportionally, leading to decreased oxygen diffusion from alveoli into capillaries (impaired gas exchange). Low oxygen levels at high altitudes can cause hypoxemia and hypoxia. If a person is suddenly exposed to low oxygen levels, arterial chemoreceptors stimulate ventilation, making more oxygen available in the alveoli and at the tissue level. Over the long term, people who live at high altitudes undergo physiological changes that facilitate oxygenation. Changes include increase in the following:

- Ventilation, which brings more oxygen into the lungs
- Production of red blood cells (RBCs), which aids in the transport of oxygen to organs and tissues
- Lung volume and pulmonary vasculature, which results in increased surface area for alveolar–capillary gas exchange
- Vascularity of body tissues, which allows for improved oxygen delivery to the tissues
- Production of hemoglobin, which readily binds with oxygen so that the tissue cells can use oxygen even when oxygen pressure is low in the environment.

Lifestyle

Lifestyle factors that affect oxygenation include pregnancy, occupational exposure to hazards, nutrition, obesity, exercise, smoking, and substance abuse.

Pregnancy

During pregnancy, oxygen demand increases dramatically. Maternal metabolism increases by approximately 15% during the last half of pregnancy, increasing the demand for O_2. At the same time, the enlarging uterus pushes upward against the diaphragm, limiting its downward movement. In response, the maternal respiratory rate increases in order to increase *minute ventilation* (amount of air moved into and out of the lungs in 1 minute) (Guyton & Hall, 2006).

Occupational Hazards

Occupational hazards may affect pulmonary function by irritating airways or causing cancer. Toxic agents may be categorized as follows:

- *Chemicals and their fumes* irritate the sensitive membranous lining of the lungs and airways and may lead to lung cancer or leukemia. Even common household cleaners can emit toxic fumes.

- *Products of combustion* (e.g., carbon monoxide) are known causes of lung cancer and chronic lung disease.
- *Microorganisms*, such as viruses, fungi, and mold may lead to infections and precipitate asthma.
- *Fine particles* (e.g., coal dust and asbestos) suspended in the air can be inhaled into the smallest airways, causing irritation and toxic reactions, including cancer.

Nutrition

The body needs an appropriate balance of proteins, carbohydrates, fats, and other nutrients for proper immune function. A healthy diet builds resistance to disease and infection, promotes normal cellular function and tissue repair, and maintains a healthy weight. Poor nutrition, especially in those with pulmonary disorders, can lead to loss of ventilatory muscle strength, making breathing more difficult.

Obesity

Obesity is a body mass index (BMI) above 30. Obesity causes multiple health problems, many of which affect pulmonary function. The following are two examples:

- *Respiratory infections.* Excess abdominal fat presses upward on the diaphragm, preventing full chest expansion, leading to hypoventilation and dyspnea on exertion. The risk for respiratory infection then increases because lower lung lobes are poorly ventilated and secretions not removed effectively.
- *Sleep apnea.* When the person lies down, chest expansion is limited even more. Excess neck girth and fat deposits in the upper airway often lead to obstructive sleep apnea, a condition characterized by daytime sleepiness, loud snoring, and periods of apnea lasting 10 to 120 seconds (Porth, 2008).

Exercise

Exercise increases metabolic demands. The body responds by increasing the heart rate and the rate and depth of breathing. Lack of exercise has the opposite effect. A sedentary lifestyle reduces the capacity to increase ventilation in response to exercise.

Smoking

Tobacco smoke contains tiny particles of tar and approximately 200 known toxic chemicals, more than 60 of which are known to cause cancer. *Mainstream smoke* (inhaled directly from the cigarette and then exhaled) and *sidestream smoke* (released from the burning tip of a cigarette into the air) are two types of *second-hand smoke.* Both are harmful to everyone in the environment, especially children, older adults, and people with allergies or lung disorders. Sidestream smoke has been found to have higher concentrations of harmful compounds than mainstream smoke, thus posing a significant health risk to nonsmokers (Schick & Glantz, 2005).

Tobacco smoke constricts bronchioles, increases fluid secretion into the airways, causes inflammation and swelling of the bronchial lining, and paralyzes cilia. These effects lead to reduced airflow and increased production of secretions that are not easily removed from the airways. Lung inflammation stimulates the release of enzymes that break down elastin and other alveolar wall components. Continued smoking leads to chronic bronchitis, obstruction of bronchioles and alveolar walls, and emphysema. Cigarette smoking is estimated to be the cause of more than 80% of cases of lung cancer. The longer a person smokes and the more cigarettes he smokes, the greater the risk for cancer and other chronic lung diseases (American Lung Association, 2008a). Roughly one in every five American adults smokes. However, once a person stops smoking, the body begins to repair the damage. In the first few days, the person will cough more as the cilia begin to clear the airways. Then the coughing subsides, and breathing becomes easier. Even long-time smokers can benefit from smoking cessation (Box 35-1).

Substance Abuse

People abuse various kinds of substances, including prescription medications. Excess use or overdose of respiratory depressants such as opioids, sedatives, antianxiety agents, and hypnotics can cause death due to hypoventilation, apnea, and respiratory failure. Over-the-counter medications and other legally available products, such as alcohol, caffeine, glue, and aerosols and other inhalants, also have abuse potential and can be lethal. Large amounts of alcohol, for example, depress respiratory and vasomotor centers of the brain. Illicit drugs, including stimulants (e.g., amphetamines, cocaine), hallucinogens (e.g., LSD, PCP), and marijuana also have adverse effects on the respiratory system. And of course, an overdose of these substances can depress respirations and increase the risk for aspiration.

KnowledgeCheck 35-4

- What are the major risks to oxygenation related to developmental factors?
- What environmental and lifestyle factors that influence ventilation can be avoided or minimized?

 Go to Chapter 35, **Knowledge Check Response Sheet and Answers,** on the Student Resource Disk or DavisPlus at http://davisplus.fadavis.com/Wilkinson2

 CriticalThinking 35-4

Review the "Meet Your Patients" scenario at the beginning of this chapter.

- Which patient(s) may be experiencing developmental, environmental, or lifestyle-related problems with oxygenation?
- Identify any additional information you need to know to answer this question.

Medications

Many drugs can interfere with pulmonary function by depressing respirations. Respiratory depressants generally act by depressing central nervous system (CNS) control of breathing or by weakening the muscles of breathing. They include general anesthetics, opioids (e.g., morphine), antianxiety drugs (e.g., diazepam [Valium]), sedative-hypnotics (e.g., barbiturates), neuromuscular blocking agents, and magnesium sulfate. Drugs that block beta-2 adrenergic receptors (e.g., used to lower the blood pressure) have little effect on healthy lungs but can lead to serious bronchiole constriction in people with asthma.

Medications are also used to improve respiratory function. Some examples are bronchodilators, anti-inflammatory agents such as corticosteroids, cough suppressants, expectorants, and decongestants.

For a more extensive discussion of individual medications that either interfere with or improve respiratory function,

 Go to Chapter 35, **Supplemental Materials: Medications that Can Interfere with Oxygenation and Medications Used to Improve Oxygenation,** on the Student Resource Disk or DavisPlus at http://davisplus.fadavis.com/Wilkinson2

Pathophysiological Conditions

Poor exchange of oxygen and carbon dioxide at the alveolar–capillary membrane or the tissue level may be life threatening. The pathophysiological conditions relevant to oxygenation can be classified into these groups: problems with gas exchange, respiratory infections,

---

BOX 35-1 ■ Health Effects of Smoking Cessation

- Life expectancy increases.
- Blood pressure and heart rate decrease.
- Circulation to the extremities improves within 2 hours.
- Carbon dioxide levels in the blood begin to drop within 4 hours.
- Oxygen levels in the blood begin to improve within 8 hours.
- Digestion improves.
- Coughing, congestion, and shortness of breath decrease.
- Overall energy increases.
- Lungs increase ability to clean themselves, thereby reducing the risk of infection.
- Risk of heart attack decreases and returns to that of a nonsmoker in 1 year.
- Risk of lung and other cancers, stroke, and chronic obstructive lung disease decreases.

pulmonary system abnormalities, pulmonary circulation abnormalities, central nervous system abnormalities, and neuromuscular abnormalities. Because it is difficult to separate pulmonary and cardiovascular causes and effects, both are included in the discussion of alterations in gas exchange that follows.

Problems with Gas Exchange

Poor exchange of oxygen and carbon dioxide in the lungs changes the levels of O_2 and CO_2 in the blood (Box 35-2). Unchecked, it affects oxygenation in tissues and organs. To determine adequacy of tissue oxygenation, you must assess both circulation and tissue/

BOX 35-2 ■ Problems with Gas Exchange

Hypoxemia—Low arterial blood oxygen levels.

Etiology: Poor oxygen diffusion across the alveolar–capillary membrane into the blood (ineffective external respiration) due to lung or pulmonary circulation disorders. Hypoventilation predisposes to the development of hypoxemia and may lead to hypoxia.

Comments: Even if the blood is adequately oxygenated, hypoxia may still occur in the organs and tissues because of poor circulation.

Hypoxia—Inadequate oxygenation of organs and tissues.

Etiology: Either hypoxemia or circulatory disorders

Comments: The effects of hypoxia depend on the organs affected. For example, hypoxic central nervous system tissue causes abnormal brain functioning (e.g., altered level of consciousness), whereas hypoxic renal tissue causes abnormal kidney functioning (e.g., poor urine output), and hypoxic limb tissue results in abnormal muscle functioning (e.g., muscle weakness and pain with exercise).

Hypercarbia (hypercapnia)—An excess of dissolved CO_2 in the blood.

Etiology: Hypoventilation is caused by abnormalities affecting the lungs or chest cavity or by neuromuscular abnormalities that interfere with normal breathing. Hypercarbia can occur suddenly, as in acute airway obstruction or drug overdose, or chronically, as in chronic lung disease.

Comments: Very high blood levels of CO_2 have an anesthetic effect on the nervous system and can lead to somnolence progressing to coma and death, a syndrome known as carbon dioxide narcosis.

Hypocarbia (hypocapnia)—A low level of dissolved CO_2 in the blood. In most cases (except high altitude), blood O_2 levels remain normal.

Etiology: Hyperventilation

Comments: Severe hypocarbia stimulates the nervous system, leading to muscle twitching or spasm (especially in the hands and feet) and numbness and tingling in the face and lips.

---

organ function. Poor peripheral circulation is characterized by weak or absent pulses; mottling (skin marbling); pale, ashen, or cyanotic skin and mucous membranes; and cool skin temperature. You can assess tissue oxygenation indirectly by determining whether organs are functioning normally.

Alterations in gas exchange are caused by a number of disorders that affect the structure, function, and regulation of the pulmonary and cardiovascular systems. The next section highlights pulmonary disorders. For a thorough description of these diseases and pathological conditions, consult a medical–surgical nursing text, or

 Go to Chapter 35, **Supplemental Materials: Pathophysiological Conditions That Influence Gas Exchange,** on the Student Resource Disk or DavisPlus at http://davisplus.fadavis.com/Wilkinson2

KnowledgeCheck 35-5

- What are some indirect indicators of tissue oxygenation?
- How are hyperventilation and hypoventilation related to carbon dioxide levels?
- What are the effects of carbon dioxide levels on the nervous system?

 Go to Chapter 35, **Knowledge Check Response Sheet and Answers,** on the Student Resource Disk or DavisPlus at http://davisplus.fadavis.com/Wilkinson2

 CriticalThinking 35-5

You are assessing a very anxious young man who looks frightened and is complaining of trouble breathing. His respiratory rate is 32 and deep. He states his fingers and hands are numb.

- What is the most likely cause?
- What blood levels would help you clarify what is going on?

Respiratory Infections

How many people do you know who have had "the flu" in the past year? A common cold? Respiratory infections are among the most common causes of short-term disability in the United States. Upper respiratory infections (URIs) and influenza are both caused by viruses. Both begin with similar symptoms. It is important to distinguish between them because antiviral medications are available for the flu. Diagnosis can be difficult because there are other conditions that start with cold-like symptoms (e.g., whooping cough, croup, allergies, measles, and pneumonia).

- *URI* symptoms include stuffy nose, sore throat, cough, sneezing, tearing, and a mild fever. Colds are more common in children, and tend to decline with age. They are rarely dangerous to healthy adults and children.
- *Influenza* is highly infectious and usually more severe than the common cold and may involve the lower airways. In addition to cold-like symptoms, the person

may experience headache, fatigue, weakness, exhaustion, and high fever. Most flu fatalities occur in children younger than age 2 and older adults, especially the frail elderly.

■ *Lower respiratory tract infections* (acute bronchitis, respiratory syncytial virus [RSV], pneumonia, and tuberculosis) occur more often, and are more severe, in children, older adults, and people with impaired immunity or lung function.

Pulmonary System Abnormalities

The following is a brief discussion of various pulmonary abnormalities that can lead to alterations in gas exchange.

Structural Abnormalities. Structural abnormalities include anything that restricts or limits the free movement of the chest wall (e.g., fractured ribs, kyphosis), interruptions in the chest cavity that inhibit inflation of the lungs (e.g., pneumothorax), or a collection of fluid (blood, lymph, pus) in the pleural space that inhibits lung expansion.

Airway Inflammation and Obstruction. Allergic reactions (e.g., asthma) or irritation from smoke or other irritants may cause airway inflammation. Obstruction may be mechanical, as with a foreign object or bolus of food, or due to spasm (e.g., laryngospasm). Swollen tonsils and a swollen epiglottis may also cause obstruction.

Alveolar–Capillary Membrane Disorders. These disorders are characterized by a change in the consistency of the lung tissue, especially at the alveolar level. The alveoli become stiff and difficult to ventilate, and gas exchange is impaired. Pulmonary edema, acute respiratory distress syndrome (ARDS), and pulmonary fibrosis are examples.

Atelectasis. Anything that reduces ventilation (e.g., tumor, obstructed airway) can cause **atelectasis**, or alveolar collapse.

Pulmonary Circulation Abnormalities

For gas exchange to occur in the alveoli, there must be adequate blood flow through the pulmonary circulation. The most common causes of impaired pulmonary circulation are pulmonary embolus and pulmonary hypertension. A **pulmonary embolus** is obstruction of pulmonary arterial circulation by a foreign substance (e.g., a blood clot, air, or fat).

Pulmonary hypertension is elevated pressure within the pulmonary arterial system. Normally this is a low-pressure system with thin-walled, compliant vessels. High pressure in the pulmonary circulation increases the workload of the heart. Over time, this causes right-sided heart failure, with a reduced amount of blood pumped into the pulmonary circulation. You will learn about the difference between right-sided

and left-sided heart failure in a medical-surgical nursing course. However, if you need some information about it now,

Go to Chapter 35, **Tables, Boxes, Figures: ESG Table 35-3,** on the Student Resource Disk or DavisPlus at http://davisplus.fadavis.com/Wilkinson2

Central Nervous System Abnormalities

Any condition that causes injury to the central nervous system (CNS) or alters CNS function can interfere with the regulation of breathing. Trauma and stroke (cerebrovascular accident) are the most commonly seen CNS problems in adults. Spinal cord injuries interfere with nerve transmission between the brain and the area below the level of the injury and may, for example, limit diaphragm function. Immature breathing patterns, such as apnea or periodic breathing, are common in preterm and term infants.

Neuromuscular Abnormalities

Neuromuscular abnormalities can affect gas exchange by interfering with the regulation of breathing or by limiting movement of the muscles involved with breathing. Any condition that alters CNS function can interfere with the regulation of breathing. Trauma, stroke, and medications are the most common causes. Neuromuscular disorders that affect the nerves involved in breathing can also depress respiratory function (e.g., Guillain-Barré syndrome, amyotrophic lateral sclerosis, and myasthenia gravis).

KnowledgeCheck 35-6

■ Identify four pathophysiological conditions that affect pulmonary function. How are they similar? How are they different?
■ What types of injuries are most likely to cause oxygenation problems?

Go to Chapter 35, **Knowledge Check Response Sheet and Answers,** on the Student Resource Disk or DavisPlus at http://davisplus.fadavis.com/Wilkinson2

CriticalThinking 35-6

You are the nursing supervisor on the night shift in a small community hospital. At the beginning of the shift, you have only one critical care bed available. During your shift, you receive calls for assistance on the following patients:

■ Patient A has burns on her face, scalp, and chest and is coughing up sputum with black streaks.
■ Patient B has pneumonia but has suddenly become confused.
■ Patient C is short of breath and complaining that he can't breathe. His skin is cool and moist, and he is coughing up clear sputum with small bubbles in it.

Which patient would you admit to the critical care bed? Why?

Practical **Knowledge**
knowing how

Nursing care to support pulmonary functioning is directed at assessing for and maximizing the effectiveness of ventilation and gas exchange. In this part of the chapter, we discuss these nursing activities. In Chapter 17, the section entitled "Respirations" provides information about assessing respirations. Also,

 Go to Chapter 17, **Procedure 17-5: Assessing Respirations,** in Volume 2.

ASSESSMENT

Although this section focuses on respiratory assessments, evaluation of overall oxygenation includes a history and physical examination to assess lung, heart, and circulatory function. The order in which you collect data and the priorities of assessment vary with the patient's condition and the purpose of the assessment. For example, for someone in obvious respiratory distress, the immediate assessment focus is to ask simple questions about current symptoms while performing a quick examination to determine adequacy of breathing, circulation, and oxygenation. In contrast, assessment for risk of respiratory disease in a healthy person might include more extensive questions about occupation, smoking habits, and living environment; a medical history; and an extensive physical examination. For a focused respiratory assessment, you will need to identify risk factors, perform a physical examination, and be familiar with certain diagnostic tests.

Assessing for Risk Factors

A health history related to pulmonary function includes questions about the presence of risk factors that affect lung and airway function. Topics to assess include the following:

- Demographic data
- Health history
- Respiratory history
- Cardiovascular history
- Environmental history
- Lifestyle

For a detailed list of interview questions for each of these topics,

 Go to Chapter 35, **Assessment Guidelines and Tools, Focused Assessment: Oxygenation,** in Volume 2.

All patients, not just those with oxygenation problems, should be asked if they use tobacco and should have their tobacco-use status documented on a regular basis.

Physical Examination

You will use all four examination techniques to assess respiratory function:

- *Inspect* to observe respiratory patterns, signs of respiratory distress, chest structures and movement, skin and mucous membrane color, presence or absence of edema, sputum characteristics, and overall general appearance. Refer to Chapter 19 to review the details of inspecting the skin and mucous membranes. Also

 Go to **Procedure 19-2: Assessing the Skin,** and **Procedure 19-12: Assessing the Chest and Lungs,** in Volume 2.

- *Palpate* pulses, skin temperature, heart pulsations through the chest wall, and areas of tenderness.
- *Percuss* over the lung fields to screen for areas of consolidation or excess air pockets in the lungs.
- *Auscultate* breath sounds, heart sounds, and vascular sounds. For a step-by-step discussion of how to assess the chest and lungs,

 Go to Chapter 19, **Procedure 19-12: Assessing the Chest and Lungs,** and **Procedure 19-13: Assessing the Heart and Vascular System,** in Volume 2.

Assess breathing patterns, cough and associated symptoms, and respiratory effort, as follows. You may also need to monitor oxygenation and ventilation with pulse oximetry and capnography.

Breathing Patterns

Assess for normal and altered breathing patterns. They include the following: eupnea, tachypnea, bradypnea, apnea or periodic breathing, Kussmaul's breathing, Biot's breathing, and Cheyne–Stokes respirations. These patterns are defined in Table 17-4. Also,

 Go to Chapter 35, **Clinical Insight 35-1: Assessing Breathing Patterns,** in Volume 2.

Recall that pain alters the rate and depth of respirations. Often patients in pain breathe shallowly and are at risk for atelectasis. Regularly assess all patients for pain. Once you have medicated the patient, reassess breath sounds, and encourage the patient to breathe deeply and cough.

Respiratory Effort/Dyspnea

A healthy person breathes effortlessly. A patient experiencing shortness of breath or dyspnea requires a thorough assessment. However, you must take care not to increase his respiratory effort. Use closed questions the patient can answer with yes, no, or only a few words. Ask whether the shortness of breath began suddenly or gradually, how severe it is right now, and whether it is getting better or worse. At the same time, observe for or ask about the signs of increased respiratory effort discussed below. Note that these signs are most easily visible in infants and small children.

- **Nasal flaring**—The visible enlargement of the nostrils with inhalation. It helps reduce resistance to airflow in the nose and keep the nasal passages open to take in more air.
- **Retractions**—The visible "sinking in" of intercostal, supraclavicular, and subcostal tissue, caused by excessive negative pressures generated in the chest to try to increase the depth of inhalation
- **Use of accessory muscles** during inspiration—The patient may use the intercostals, abdominal muscles, and muscles of the neck and shoulders when there is an increased demand for oxygen or problems with ventilation.
- **Grunting**—Caused by involuntary muscle contraction during expiration to help keep alveoli open and enhance gas exchange
- **Body positioning** to facilitate respirations—The patient usually finds an upright posture the most comfortable. In the upright position, gravity pulls the abdominal organs down and allows the diaphragm more room to contract. Most patients with dyspnea cannot tolerate lying down. **Orthopnea** is the term used to describe difficulty breathing when lying down. Ask how the patient usually sleeps. Some patients may report sleeping in a recliner or chair.
- **Paroxysmal nocturnal dyspnea**—Sudden awakening due to shortness of breath that begins during sleep. The patient feels panic and extreme dyspnea and must sit upright to ease breathing.
- **Conversational dyspnea**—The inability to speak complete sentences without stopping to breathe. The more frequently the patient pauses when speaking, the more severe the dyspnea.
- **Stridor**—A high-pitched, harsh, crowing, inspiratory sound caused by partial obstruction of the larynx or trachea. You can hear it without a stethoscope. Partial airway obstruction can easily become complete airway obstruction. Therefore, the patient with stridor needs immediate care.
- **Wheezing**—A musical sound produced by air passing through partially obstructed small airways. It is often heard in patients with asthma and lung congestion.
- **Diminished or absent breath sounds**—In a patient experiencing dyspnea these are signs of worsening ventilation and oxygenation. Oxygen therapy and measures to restore adequate ventilation may be required.

Cough

Everyone coughs from time to time to remove small amounts of mucus and debris from the airways. Coughing is a normal protective response to known respiratory irritants (e.g., cigarette smoke, irritating fumes, dust particles) or when food or fluid accidentally gets into the airways. A cough becomes significant if it persists, is recurring, or is productive. A persistent or recurring cough

may indicate ongoing or recurring airway irritation. Advise patients to obtain medical evaluation for a cough that lasts more than 3 weeks and cannot be explained.

Assess the Cough. Is it dry, productive, or hacking? When does the cough occur and how long has the patient been coughing? What makes it worse? What seems to help it? What has been used to treat the cough, and what were the effects?

Assess for Other Clinical Findings Associated with a Cough. This helps determine its cause. A cough associated with nasal congestion, sneezing, or watery eyes or nose discharge is most likely due to allergies and may be successfully treated with over-the-counter remedies. A cough occurring with fever, chest congestion, noisy breath sounds, and sputum production is more likely to be due to an upper respiratory tract infection, which may require antibiotics. A cough associated with dyspnea, chest tightness, and wheezing may be due to an airway obstruction disorder such as asthma, which requires corticosteroids and bronchodilating medications.

Assess Sputum Appearance, Color, and Odor. A cough is described as productive if it raises sputum (mucus and debris) up from the airways. Sputum appearance and odor provide valuable *clues* about the cause and significance of a cough (see Box 35-3).

Assess Sputum Amount. The amount of sputum can vary from a teaspoon to pints. In general, sputum production increases with the severity of the underlying condition. However, limited sputum production does not always indicate the problem is minor, because excess

---

BOX 35-3 ■ Significance of Sputum Appearance and Odor

Color/Appearance	Significance
White or clear	Usually present in viral infections (e.g., common cold, viral bronchitis), often requiring only supportive care
Yellow or green	A sign of infection
Black	Caused by coal dust, smoke, or soot inhalation
Rust colored	Associated with pneumococcal pneumonia, tuberculosis, and possibly the presence of blood
Hemoptysis	The coughing up of blood or bloody sputum. It may range from small streaks of blood to large amounts of frank blood.
Pink and frothy	Associated with pulmonary edema

Foul-smelling sputum usually indicates bacterial infection (e.g., pneumonia, lung abscess).

mucus and debris may be trapped in the airways and the patient is unable to cough it up and out of the body.

Assess Sputum Timing. Sputum production ranges from constant to once per day. Tobacco smokers often have a "morning cough," which helps clear their airways of mucus and debris accumulated overnight. They may not realize this is a result of long-term lung irritation and damage and is not a normal occurrence for everyone. In contrast, someone with an upper respiratory tract infection is more likely to produce sputum throughout the day.

Obtain Sputum Samples. Laboratory examination of sputum is a valuable diagnostic tool. Sputum samples are examined microscopically and cultured in the lab to identify organisms and test for sensitivity to different anti-infective agents. You may be responsible for collecting sputum specimens. For a summary of this procedure, see the Critical Aspects box. For the complete steps,

 Go to Chapter 35, **Procedure 35-1: Collecting a Sputum Specimen,** in Volume 2.

KnowledgeCheck 35-7

- What areas should you include in a nursing history for a patient with oxygenation concerns who is undergoing a comprehensive assessment?
- When is a cough significant? What aspects of a cough should be assessed?
- Identify at least five signs that you may observe in a patient experiencing dyspnea.
- A patient has a respiratory rate of 30 breaths/min that is rhythmic and moderate in depth. What term would you use to describe this breathing pattern?

 Go to Chapter 35, **Knowledge Check Response Sheet and Answers,** on the Student Resource Disk or DavisPlus at http://davisplus.fadavis.com/Wilkinson2

CriticalThinking 35-7

Review the patients presented in the "Meet Your Patients" scenario.

- Which patients are experiencing respiratory distress? Identify the signs of distress in these patients.
- Which patients require a comprehensive assessment, and which patients will need a rapid assessment and immediate treatment because of the severity of their symptoms?

Diagnostic Testing

Diagnostic testing helps clinicians identify the causes of impaired oxygenation and monitor patient responses to treatment. You will need to assist with and be familiar with the results of the tests of respiratory function. We discuss several of these tests in the next sections. For others,

 Go to Chapter 35, **Diagnostic Testing: Tests Related to Oxygenation,** in Volume 2.

Skin Testing

Tuberculin skin testing is widely used to detect exposure and antibody formation to the tubercle bacillus. Annual screening is recommended for low-income populations, residents in congregate living conditions (e.g., dormitories, correctional facilities), immigrants from countries with a high prevalence of TB, and healthcare workers. For the skin test to be effective, you must administer the antigen intradermally, not subcutaneously. Read the test site 48 to 72 hours after administration. To review a procedure for administering intradermal injections,

 Go to Chapter 23, **Procedure 23-11: Administering Intradermal Medications,** in Volume 2.

A positive skin test is defined as an area of induration (hardness) at the test site. The size of the induration that indicates a positive result depends on risk factors. Patients with positive TB skin tests must undergo further testing (chest x-ray study and sputum cultures) to determine whether they have merely been exposed to disease or whether they have active disease. For guidelines for interpreting test results,

 Go to Chapter 35, **Diagnostic Testing: Reading a Tuberculin Skin Result,** in Volume 2.

Allergy testing uses skin testing to identify antigens that may cause hypersensitivity reactions in susceptible individuals. Testing is performed by scratching antigen samples onto the skin. The area is then observed for allergic skin reactions. Skin testing is performed in facilities with resuscitation equipment and personnel trained in its use, because life-threatening airway obstruction sometimes occurs in response to the allergens.

Pulse Oximetry

Pulse oximetry is a noninvasive estimate of arterial blood oxygen saturation (SaO_2). SaO_2 reflects the percentage of hemoglobin molecules carrying oxygen. The normal value is 95% to 100%. Values below 94% are considered abnormal in healthy people and should be investigated to determine the cause. Pulse oximetry works by measuring light absorption by hemoglobin in the circulating red blood cells. Because well-oxygenated hemoglobin and deoxygenated hemoglobin absorb light differently, the oximeter is able to detect this difference and calculate the percentage of oxygenated hemoglobin.

Pulse oximetry is simple to perform, provides a rapid reading, and can be used intermittently or continuously (Fig. 35-5). A probe is placed on a part of the body where capillary blood flow is near the surface (e.g., a nail bed, earlobe, nose, or forehead). Be aware that factors such as movement, acrylic fingernails, nail polish, or cold extremities can interfere with the accuracy of the readings. The Critical Aspects box summarizes the use of pulse oximetry, including actions to take to obtain accurate readings.

FIGURE 35-5 Pulse oximetry is a noninvasive estimate of arterial blood oxygen saturation (Sao_2). It uses a light-emitting diode (LED) probe to measure light absorption by hemoglobin in the circulating red blood cells.

For the complete procedure,

 Go to Chapter 35, **Procedure 35-2: Monitoring Pulse Oximetry (Arterial Oxygen Saturation),** in Volume 2. Also, go to Chapter 35, **Clinical Insight 35-2: Tips for Obtaining Accurate Pulse Oximetry Readings,** in Volume 2.

Capnography

Capnography measures the carbon dioxide (CO_2) in inhaled and exhaled air. As a beam of infrared light passes through a sample of respiratory gases, more or less of it is absorbed depending on the amount of CO_2 that is present. The device displays the results digitally and prints out a graph showing CO_2 at various times in the breathing cycle. Capnography is often used with pulse oximetry. It provides information about ventilation because it shows accumulation or depletion of CO_2, whereas pulse oximetry reflects only oxygenation of the blood. Capnography is a more reliable indicator of respiratory depression than pulse oximetry. Some situations in which capnography is used are:

- When a patient is receiving opioids
- During general anesthesia
- For critical care patients
- In obstructive sleep apnea
- Monitoring some infants with respiratory distress
- For adjusting parameter settings in mechanically ventilated patients
- For validating endotracheal tube (ET) placement (if an ET tube is placed correctly, little or no CO_2 will be present)

Capnography directly measures ventilation, and indirectly measures the partial pressure of CO_2 in the arterial blood. Normally the difference between arterial blood and expired CO_2 is very small.

Although they do measure carbon dioxide, **CO_2 detectors** are different from capnography. They use chemically treated paper that changes color when exposed to CO_2. They do not give exact readings, but can measure only a range of values.

Spirometry

The process of ventilation can be studied clinically through **spirometry,** a measure of air that moves into and out of the lungs. To describe the events of pulmonary ventilation, the air in the lungs is divided into four volumes and four capacities. Normal lung volumes and capacities vary with body size, age, and exercise. Volumes and capacities are higher in men, in large people, and in athletes. For a summary of this information,

 Go to **Diagnostic Testing Boxes, Lung Volumes and Capacities,** in Volume 2.

 Critical**Thinking** 35-8

You hear a pulse oximeter alarm sound in a nearby patient room and find it reading 75%.

- What observations should you make?
- What actions should you take?

Arterial Blood Gases

Arterial blood gas (ABG) analysis measures the levels of oxygen and carbon dioxide in arterial blood. As the name suggests, an artery (usually the brachial, radial, or femoral) is used to obtain the blood sample. Arteries are located deep under the skin and alongside nerves, making needle insertion painful. The blood sample may be obtained by arterial puncture or by withdrawal from an arterial line. Nurses in critical care units routinely draw ABGs and monitor patients with invasive arterial monitoring; however, you may care for patients on medical–surgical units, or even outpatients, who will undergo periodic ABG evaluation. ABG analysis measures pH, partial pressure of oxygen (Po_2), partial pressure of carbon dioxide (Pco_2), saturation of oxygen (Sao_2), and bicarbonate (HCO_3) level. Here, we discuss only Po_2 and Pco_2. For a more thorough discussion of arterial blood gas values, see Chapter 36.

Measuring Arterial Blood Oxygen

Three values are important when assessing the degree to which the tissues are receiving oxygen:

- **Hemoglobin** is the iron-containing pigment of red blood cells that, as *oxyhemoglobin,* carries oxygen in the blood.
- **Po_2 (partial pressure of oxygen)** is the amount of oxygen available to combine with hemoglobin to make oxyhemoglobin.
- **Sao_2 (saturation of oxygen)** reflects oxygen that is actually bound to hemoglobin.

At sea level, the normal Po_2 range in arterial blood is 80 to 100 mm Hg. After tissues have extracted oxygen from arterial blood and the blood enters the veins to return to the heart, the venous blood P_{O_2} has fallen to around 40 mm Hg. The Sa_{O_2}, along with the P_{O_2} and hemoglobin level, indicates the degree to which the tissues are receiving oxygen. Small changes in Sa_{O_2} are associated with large changes in P_{O_2}. For blood gas values,

 Go to Chapter 35, **Diagnostic Testing: Arterial Blood Gas Values: Evaluating Adequacy of Oxygenation,** in Volume 2.

To fully interpret P_{O_2} and Sa_{O_2} values, you need to know the percentage of oxygen in the air the patient is inhaling. This is known as the **fraction of inspired oxygen,** or F_{IO_2}. At sea level, atmospheric air (commonly known as *room air*) is 21% oxygen ($F_{IO_2} = 21\%$). The norms quoted for P_{O_2} and Sa_{O_2} are based on an F_{IO_2} of 21%. If a healthy patient receives 100% oxygen for a few minutes, the arterial P_{O_2} would rise to 500 to 600 mm Hg, and the Sa_{O_2} would remain at 100%. The reason is that the Sa_{O_2} measures the oxygen *bound to hemoglobin*—and of course the hemoglobin cannot be "filled" with oxygen to more than 100% capacity. When gas exchange is impaired as a result of disease or injury, P_{O_2} and Sa_{O_2} levels fall. However, they can be kept at normal levels if supplemental oxygen is given.

Measuring Arterial Blood Carbon Dioxide

The **partial pressure of carbon dioxide (P_{CO_2})** is a measure of the CO_2 dissolved in the blood. Normal arterial P_{CO_2} is 35 to 45 mm Hg. Carbon dioxide readily diffuses across the alveolar–capillary membrane in the lungs even in the face of obstacles such as alveolar fluid or thickened membranes. As a result, P_{CO_2} levels remain normal until a severe disorder interferes with all gas exchange. Once in the alveoli, the amount of carbon dioxide exhaled from the lungs is directly influenced by how well air is moving into and out of the lungs (ventilation).

- **Hypocarbia**. When a person hyperventilates, he exhales large amounts of CO_2, causing arterial P_{CO_2} values to fall. Hyperventilation brings more oxygen into the lungs, so unless it is triggered by hypoxemia, oxygen levels (P_{O_2}) usually remain normal.
- **Hypercarbia**. Conversely, in hypoventilation less CO_2 moves into the alveoli for exhalation, leaving more CO_2 in the arterial blood. This causes P_{CO_2} values to rise. High P_{CO_2} levels (hypercarbia) have an anesthetic effect on the nervous system and can be toxic. Hypoventilation severe enough to cause hypercarbia is usually associated with hypoxemia because not enough oxygen is inhaled.

For additional information on interpreting arterial blood gases, see Chapter 36, "Interpreting ABGs" and Table 36-6 in Volume 1. Also

 Go to Chapter 36, **Clinical Insight 36-2: Interpreting Arterial Blood Gases,** in Volume 2.

KnowledgeCheck 35-8

- What does a pulse oximetry reading tell you?
- What is the relationship between arterial P_{O_2} and Sa_{O_2} levels?
- Identify normal P_{O_2}, Sa_{O_2}, and P_{CO_2} levels.
- What effect does ventilation have on arterial P_{CO_2}?
- How is P_{CO_2} related to oxygenation?

 Go to Chapter 35, **Knowledge Check Response Sheet and Answers,** on the Student Resource Disk or DavisPlus at http://davisplus.fadavis.com/Wilkinson2

 Critical**Thinking** 35-9

You are caring for two patients, both of whom have a P_{O_2} of 95 mm Hg and Sa_{O_2} of 99%. Do they have similar lung function? Explain your answer.

Peak Flow Monitoring

Peak expiratory flow rate (PEFR) measures the amount of air that can be exhaled with forcible effort. Patients with asthma use PEFR monitoring to detect subtle changes in their condition, often before symptoms occur. A peak flow meter is used to monitor these changes (Fig. 35-6). Peak flow is expressed in liters per minute. Patients with asthma are often asked to measure their peak flow daily and with the onset of any symptoms. Treatment protocols describe the use and frequency of medications based on individualized peak flow rates. The home care box: Home Use of a Peak Flow Meter describes self-monitoring.

ANALYSIS/NURSING DIAGNOSIS

Alterations in pulmonary function may be nursing diagnoses, etiologies of other problems, or merely symptoms of other problems. In analyzing the assessment data, you must determine which. For example, suppose a patient is breathing shallowly and slowly. The pulmonary problem might be one of the following:

- **A nursing diagnosis**: *Ineffective Breathing Pattern (hypoventilation)* related to pain secondary to rib fractures. In this case, you would provide pain relief; the desired outcome is that the patient will have effective (normal) ventilation.
- **An etiology**: Ineffective Tissue Perfusion (Cerebral) *related to Ineffective Breathing Pattern (hypoventilation),* as manifested by slurred speech and drowsiness. In this case, you would address the etiology by administering oxygen; the desired outcome would be effective cerebral perfusion, evidenced by normal speech and alertness. Activity Intolerance is another example of a problem with pulmonary function as an etiology.
- **A symptom**: Ineffective Tissue Perfusion (Cerebral) related to edema from head trauma, *as manifested by Ineffective Breathing Pattern (hypoventilation).* In this situation, you would, of course, support ventilation (the symptom) until the problem subsides. However,

Scale (LPM)

Piston

Red indicator

Spring

Opening

Mouthpiece

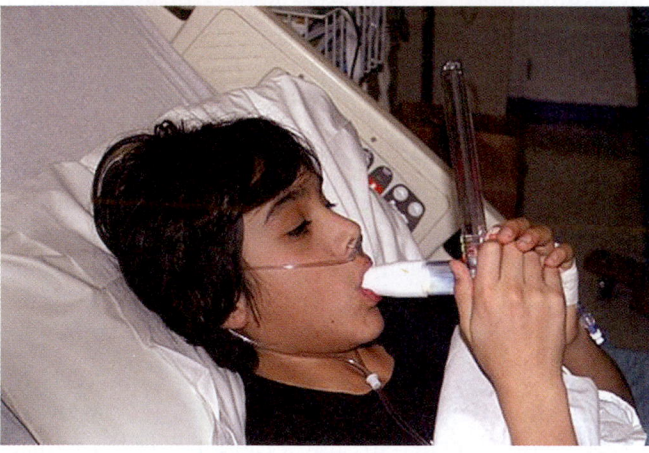

FIGURE 35-6 A patient with asthma using a peak flow meter to monitor peak expiratory flow rate (PEFR).

Home Care

Home Use of a Peak Flow Meter

People with asthma are often asked to monitor their peak flow readings at home and to compare their current readings to their baseline "personal best."

➤ Teach patients that to get an accurate reading, they need to take a deep breath and forcefully exhale.

➤ Teach patients to take a series of three readings and record the highest reading.

➤ Teach patients to maintain or adjust their medication according to their highest reading. They should follow the color-coded treatment protocols prescribed by their physician. These are individualized for each patient. Notice that these correspond to the color-coded markers on their peak flow meter.

Green = All clear: Baseline peak flow—Peak flow is within 80% to 100% of personal best baseline.

Treatment protocol calls for routine medication use.

Yellow = Caution: Peak flow is 50% to 80% of usual or "normal" rate. Said another way, there is a 20% to 50% reduction in peak flow—This reading signals the onset of airway changes.

Treatment protocols usually specify an increase in the dosage of maintenance medications, use of rescue therapies (e.g., fast-acting bronchodilators), or a call to the healthcare provider. These measures are designed to reverse acute exacerbations before they become severe.

Red = Medical alert: Peak flow is less than 50% of personal best baseline. Severe reduction in peak flow.

Treatment protocols usually specify immediate treatment with rescue medications and to seek emergency treatment if symptoms do not improve.

Adapted from American Lung Association (2008). Asthma & Allergy: Peak flow meters. Retrieved from http://www.lungusa.org/site/pp.asp?c=dvLUK9O0E&b=22586.

the primary interventions would be directed toward the edema and head trauma. Once these etiologies were corrected, the hypoventilation would disappear. The goal would be effective cerebral perfusion, evidenced by normal breathing pattern.

Problems of Ventilation and Gas Exchange

Five NANDA-I diagnoses directly describe problems with ventilation and gas exchange. Use these diagnoses when they are the central problem and you intend to use interventions to eliminate the cause of the problem.

- *Ineffective Airway Clearance* is the inability to maintain a clear airway.
- *Ineffective Breathing Pattern* is used to describe inadequate ventilation, such as hypoventilation, hyperventilation, tachypnea, or bradypnea.
- *Impaired Gas Exchange* is the appropriate diagnosis if the patient is ventilating adequately but diffusion of gases across the alveolar–capillary membrane is impaired.
- *Impaired Spontaneous Ventilation* describes a condition in which a patient, as a result of decreased energy reserves, is unable to maintain breathing adequate to support life.
- *Dysfunctional Ventilatory Weaning Response* represents a specific situation in which a patient who is being mechanically ventilated cannot adjust to lower levels of ventilator support, prolonging the ventilatory weaning process.

- *Risk for Aspiration* should be used when there is a risk for secretions, solids, or fluids entering into tracheobronchial passages (e.g., for patients who have had head or neck surgery or who have a reduced level of consciousness).

For further discussion of these diagnoses,

 Go to Chapter 35, **Standardized Language, Nursing Diagnoses Associated with Impaired Ventilation and Gas Exchange,** in Volume 2.

PLANNING OUTCOMES/EVALUATION

NOC standardized outcomes appropriate for patients with pulmonary function problems include the following:

Mechanical Ventilation Weaning Response: Adult
Respiratory Status: Airway Patency
Respiratory Status: Gas Exchange
Respiratory Status: Ventilation
Vital Signs.

For examples of NOC outcomes and NIC interventions for selected oxygenation nursing diagnoses,

 Go to Chapter 35, **Standardized Language, Examples of NOC Outcomes and NIC Interventions Linked to Oxygenation Diagnoses,** in Volume 2.

These provide a general care planning guide. Depending on individual patient needs, other NOC outcomes or NIC interventions may also be appropriate.

Individualized goals/outcome statements depend on the nursing diagnosis you identify. For diagnoses related to gas exchange, the following are examples of goals you might write:

Expectorates secretions effectively
No dyspnea or shortness of breath
Lungs clear; no adventitious sounds present
Respiratory rate and rhythm within normal limits for patient

Table 35-1 ➤ Respiratory Medications that Promote Ventilation and Oxygenation

CLASS	ACTION	EXAMPLES AND COMMENTS
Bronchodilators	▪ Relax the smooth muscles lining the airways. ▪ Can be administered as oral or inhaled medicines.	Beta-2 adrenergic agonists Anticholinergics Methylxanthine
Respiratory Anti-inflammatory Agents	▪ Combat inflammation in the airways. ▪ Important in treating and controlling respiratory conditions characterized by hypersensitive airways and airway inflammation (e.g., asthma).	Corticosteroids Cromolyn Leukotriene modifiers
Nasal Decongestants	▪ Relieve stuffy, blocked nasal passages by constricting local blood vessels through stimulation of alpha-1 adrenergic nerve receptors in the vessels. ▪ Although the desired effect is on the nasal mucosa, these medications can have systemic adrenergic effects causing elevated blood pressure, tachycardia, and palpitations, especially in those with a history of cardiovascular conditions.	Ephedrine Pseudoephedrine Phenylephrine
Antihistamines	▪ Prevent the effects of histamine release. ▪ Used to treat upper respiratory and nasal allergy symptoms.	diphenhydramine (Benadryl) chlorpheniramine (Chlor-Trimeton) brompheniramine (Dimetane) loratadine (Claritin) fexofenadine (Allegra) cetirizine (Zyrtec)
Cough Preparations	▪ *Antitussives* (cough suppressants) reduce the frequency of an involuntary, hacking, nonproductive cough. ▪ *Expectorants* help make coughing more productive. ▪ The goal is to reduce the frequency of dry, unproductive coughing while making voluntary coughing more productive.	These agents are often found mixed together in one preparation to achieve both desirable effects with one medication.

■ PLANNING INTERVENTIONS/IMPLEMENTATION

NIC standardized interventions related to oxygenation are found in the Respiratory Management category. Respiratory Management interventions focus on maintaining a patent airway and promoting gas exchange. They include Airway Management, Airway Suction, Cough Enhancement, Oxygen Therapy, and Respiratory Monitoring.

Specific nursing interventions for patients with oxygenation problems address ventilation, gas exchange, and circulation. These interventions, which include health promotion, prevention, and treatment activities, are discussed in the sections that follow.

Administering Respiratory Medications

Respiratory medications promote ventilation and oxygenation by their effects on the respiratory system itself. The major types of respiratory medicines include bronchodilators, corticosteroids, cough preparations, decongestants, antihistamines, and mucolytics. Some need a prescription; others do not. See Table 35-1.

✚ Do not give over-the-counter cough and cold medicines to children younger than the age of 4 years. There is a risk of serious and even life-threatening side effects. Safety and effectiveness for children ages 5 through 11 years is still in question. See Self-Care: Cough and Cold Medicines: Tips for Parents.

See the accompanying CAM box for some common cold remedies.

Promoting Optimal Respiratory Function

Deep, regular breathing promotes ventilation and optimizes gas exchange. Other interventions to promote optimal function include preventing upper respiratory infections, performing immunizations, supporting smoking cessation, preventing and treating pneumonia,

---

Complementary & Alternative Modalities (CAM)

Common Cold Remedies

➤ Cold care products containing *Pelargonium sidoides*, an extract of the South African geranium, may reduce the intensity of the common cold. However, more evidence is needed (Herbal solution hastens. . . , 2008). In the United States, Zucol products are one example.

✚ Honey is more effective than dextromethorphan in children with nocturnal cough (Paul, Beiler, McMonagle, et al., 2007). However, avoid giving honey to children younger than the age of 1 year because it is a reservoir of *Clostridium botulinum* spores, and may cause botulism in infants.

➤ Vitamin C in daily doses of 200 mg or more has not been found to prevent colds, but it did reduce the length and severity of symptoms. Be aware that in amounts of 2,000 mg, it may cause diarrhea and gas (Hemilä, Chalker, Treacy, et al., 2007).

➤ A Cochrane Review found there is no evidence that Echinacea preparations are effective for preventing and treating the common cold (Linde, Barrett, Bauer, et al., 2006).

➤ Although lab studies are preliminary, elderberry (*Sambucus nigra*), a herb, has been found to help combat viruses, specifically influenza. It is thought to strengthen the immune system and keep the flu virus from adhering to cells.

---

positioning, incentive spirometry, and preventing aspiration.

Prevent Upper Respiratory Infections

Upper respiratory infections (URIs) may be viral or bacterial. Teach clients that viral infections usually last about 10 to 21 days and are self-limiting. URIs may, however, lead to other respiratory diseases and seriously

---

Self-Care

Cough and Cold Medicines: Tips for Parents

➤ Do not give children medicines labeled for adults only.

➤ Do not give over-the-counter (OTC) cough and cold remedies to children younger than age 4 years. There is a risk of serious and even life-threatening side effects.

➤ Read labels! Some labels are marked "Do not use for children under age 4."

➤ The safety and effectiveness of OTC cough and cold remedies for children ages 2 through 11 years is still in question. It is not certain they are safe, and they may not be effective.

➤ Choose medications with safety caps. Close caps tightly and store out of sight and reach of children.

➤ Do not give more than one medicine with the same active ingredient. Check the "active ingredients" on the label. Your

child could be harmed by getting too much of the ingredient.

➤ Carefully follow the directions on the label for how to use the medicine. Overuse or misuse can cause serious side effects (e.g., drowsiness, breathing problems, and seizures).

➤ Measure carefully. Do not use household spoons because they come in different sizes.

➤ Understand that OTC medicines do not cure the cold or cough. They only treat symptoms such as runny nose, congestion, fever, and aches. They do not shorten the length of time your child is sick.

Source: Centers for Disease Control and Prevention (2008b); U.S. Food and Drug Administration (2008).

compromised oxygenation in children, older adults, and people who have other illnesses. Therefore, it is important to teach clients measures for preventing URIs. For teaching tips, see Self-Care: Teaching Clients How to Prevent URIs, in Chapter 41.

The overuse of antibiotics to treat URIs has contributed to the current crisis of antimicrobial resistance. Teach clients that antibiotics should be used only as prescribed for diagnosed bacterial infections. This includes taking the full course of prescribed antibiotics, even if symptoms are no longer present. Antibiotics are not without risks, and they are not effective for treating the common cold anyway. Advise clients not to pressure clinicians for a prescription, nor to take any antibiotics left over from previous prescriptions or from others who might offer to share antibiotics.

Prevent Influenza

The most effective strategy for preventing influenza is annual vaccination. Vaccines are developed annually to closely match the major known strains of the virus that have evolved. Immunizations given to healthy young adults are 70% to 90% effective. Though less effective in preventing the disease in older adults, immunization decreases the severity of the disease, the development of secondary complications, and the incidence of death (Fiore, Shay, Broder, et al., 2008).

Other prevention measures are to avoid exposure to the virus. That is, avoid contact with or proximity to people who are sick, if possible; and use recommended hand hygiene measures.

Infection rates are highest among children. Rates of serious illness and death are highest among older adults, children younger than age 2 years, and people with certain medical conditions. Therefore, for most types of influenza the Centers for Disease Control and Prevention (CDC) recommends that the following people should receive influenza immunization annually:

- Children ages 6 months to 18 years
- Adults age 50 years and older
- Women who will be pregnant during the influenza season
- People with certain medical conditions (e.g., chronic pulmonary diseases, diabetes mellitus)
- People with compromised immune systems
- Healthcare personnel
- Persons at risk for medical complications
- Persons who live with or care for persons at high risk for influenza
- Residents in nursing homes and chronic-care and other congregate living facilities (e.g., correctional institutions, college dormitories)

Prevent Pneumonia

Pneumonia is a leading cause of infectious death in the United States, with a mortality rate of approximately 50% in people older than age 65. Therefore, people who are most susceptible should be immunized against pneumonia. Historically this vaccine was thought to convey lifetime immunity, but recent data illustrate that this may not be so. As a result, the vaccine is recommended annually for high-risk groups, including the following (CDC, 2009):

- Adults 65 years old or older
- Children < 5 years old
- Adults of any age who:
  - Have chronic illnesses (e.g., those with heart disease, diabetes, pulmonary disease, alcoholism, HIV infection)
  - Smoke cigarettes
  - Have lowered resistance to infection

CDC recommended immunization schedules change periodically. To be certain you have the most current information, always check the CDC Web site at

 http://www.cdc.gov/vaccines/recs/schedules/

Healthcare-Associated Pneumonia tends to be more complicated and to have a higher mortality rate than community-acquired pneumonia. Guidelines for preventing healthcare-associated pneumonia include following standard precautions for hand hygiene and gloving.

Wear gloves for handling respiratory secretions or objects contaminated with respiratory secretions of all patients. Change gloves and decontaminate hands:

- Between contacts with different patients
- After handling respiratory secretions or contaminated objects and before contact with another patient, object, or environmental surface
- Between contacts with a contaminated body site and the respiratory tract or respiratory device on the same patient (Tablan, Anderson, Besser, et al., 2004)

Support Smoking Cessation

Nurses can provide effective support to patients who want to quit smoking. When nurses offer smoking cessation advice, smokers are more likely to quit as compared to smokers who do not have such advice from nurses (Rice & Stead, 2008). *All* patients should be asked if they use tobacco. Furthermore, a systematic review of evidence indicates that their tobacco-use status should be documented regularly (e.g., by chart stickers or computer prompts) (National Guideline Clearinghouse, 2008). The U.S. Public Health Service guidelines suggest the "5A's" model for treating tobacco dependence (Box 35-4) (Fiore, Jaén, Baker, et al., 2008).

Motivational counseling includes discussion about the connection between tobacco use and current health status, the risks of continued tobacco use, the rewards of quitting, anticipated barriers to quitting, and strategies for addressing barriers. It may also be important to refer the person to a tobacco cessation program.

BOX 35-4 ■ The 5A's for Treating Tobacco Dependence

Ask about tobacco use and document tobacco use status for every patient at every visit.

Advise to quit. Use a clear, strong, personalized approach to urge the patient to quit.

Assess willingness to make a quit attempt at this time.

Assist in a quit attempt. If the patient is willing, refer for counseling and medication. If the patient is not willing to quit at this time, provide interventions designed to increase future quit attempts.

Arrange follow-up. If the patient is willing to quit, make follow-up contacts beginning the first week after the quit date. If the patient is not willing to quit at this time, address tobacco dependence and willingness to quit at the next clinic (or other) visit.

Adapted from Fiore, M., Jaén, C., Baker, T., et al. (2008). Treating tobacco use and dependence: 2008 update. Clinical Practice Guideline. Rockville, MD: U.S. Department of Health and Human Services. Public Health Service.

Most smokers are not able to quit "cold turkey." Combining medication and counseling is more effective than either used alone. Encourage patients to contact their primary care provider for nicotine replacement therapy or other medications (e.g., antidepressants, clonidine) to treat tobacco dependence. For pregnant women, smokeless tobacco users, light smokers, and adolescents, medications may be contraindicated or may lack evidence of effectiveness (National Guideline Clearinghouse, 2008).

Box 35-1 highlights some of the benefits of smoking cessation. Share these and smoking cessation tips with patients (Self-Care: Smoking Cessation Tips).

Position for Maximum Ventilation

Position affects ventilation. An upright or elevated position pulls abdominal organs down, allowing maximum diaphragm excursion and lung expansion.

- If the patient is short of breath, provide an overbed table to lean forward on. Patients with impaired respiratory function adopt a tripod position to allow maximum expansion. They may need to rest their arms on an overbed table.
- When the patient is lying on her side, provide pillows to support the upper arm.
- Assist with frequent position changes to keep all areas of the lungs well ventilated, and ambulate as often as possible without creating fatigue.

Assist with Incentive Spirometry

Incentive spirometers are designed to encourage patients to take deep breaths by reaching a goal-directed volume of air. Incentive spirometry is usually reserved for patients at risk for developing atelectasis or pneumonia, for example, patients who have had abdominal, chest, or pelvic surgery, patients on prolonged bedrest, or patients with a history of respiratory

---

Self-Care

Smoking Cessation Tips

➤ Identify several personal reasons to quit smoking, such as: "I'll live longer and be able to spend more time with my children and grandchildren," or "My father died of lung cancer. He really suffered. I have no desire to experience that."

➤ Make a list of things you enjoy doing. Choose one of these items as a reward for not smoking.

➤ Before smoking, ask yourself, "What can I do instead of smoking this cigarette?"

➤ Identify friends who do not smoke, and plan to spend time with them.

➤ Have carrot sticks, celery, gum, or sunflower seeds available to chew instead of smoking a cigarette. These also help you cope with the increased hunger you may feel.

➤ Learn several relaxation techniques, such as meditation or visualization, to help you through the stress of quitting.

➤ Use positive affirmations daily. "I can successfully quit smoking. I am no longer a smoker."

➤ Tell several supportive people of your plan to quit. Ask them to help you be successful.

➤ Plan a time to quit. Choose a time that will not require many additional demands on you.

➤ Talk with friends and co-workers who have successfully quit smoking.

➤ Save the money you would have spent on cigarettes. Treat yourself to an activity or event with the money you have saved.

➤ Tell your healthcare providers that you would like to quit smoking.

➤ When you feel a craving to smoke, breathe deeply, find something to distract yourself, or call a supportive person.

➤ To help cope with irritability, use relaxation exercises or deep breathing; take a hot bath; or do something else you enjoy.

➤ Participate in a structured smoking cessation program, if possible.

➤ Consider asking your healthcare provider about nicotine-replacement therapy, for instance, gum or patches.

problems. Incentive spirometers offer various visual cues (such as elevation of a ball or piston) to show patients whether they are inhaling deeply enough. As an RN, you can delegate incentive spirometry coaching to licensed practical nurses (LPNs) and qualified nursing assistive personnel (NAPs). However, you are responsible for ensuring that incentive spirometry is carried out correctly and at required frequencies. You must also evaluate patient responses, airway clearance, and ventilation. See Figure 37-6 and Self-Care: Teaching Your Patient About Incentive Spirometry, in Chapter 37.

Take Aspiration Precautions

Aspiration is a risk for patients with a decreased level of consciousness, diminished gag or cough reflex, or difficulty with swallowing. You should keep a suction setup available for routine and emergency use. Preventing aspiration requires you to have practical knowledge about positioning, enteral and oral feedings, and administering medications. For guidelines to use with at-risk patients,

 Go to Chapter 35, **Clinical Insight 35-3: Guidelines for Preventing Aspiration,** in Volume 2.

Many of the guidelines involve basic care and can be delegated to qualified LPNs and NAP. The RN is responsible for monitoring for aspiration. Record in the nursing notes any preventive measures taken.

KnowledgeCheck 35-9

Identify at least three nursing interventions to promote optimal respiratory function in a hospitalized patient with chronic lung disease.

 Go to Chapter 35, **Knowledge Check Response Sheet and Answers,** on the Student Resource Disk or DavisPlus at http://davisplus.fadavis.com/Wilkinson2

CriticalThinking 35-10

- Review the "Meet Your Patients" scenario. For which of these patients should you recommend annual flu or pneumonia immunizations? Why?
- A 24-year-old nursing student has no previous hospitalizations or known chronic health problems, takes no medications, and has no current respiratory symptoms. On routine purified protein derivative, or PPD, testing (tuberculin skin testing), the student has an area of induration measuring 5 mm. How would you interpret these results?

Mobilizing Secretions

Coughing promotes deep inhalation and forceful expulsion of secretions. Interventions that help enhance coughing and mobilize secretions include deep breathing, coughing exercises, and hydration.

Teach Deep Breathing and Coughing

Deep breathing promotes ventilation and gas exchange. Coughing after deep breathing mobilizes secretions, which keeps airways and alveoli open and provides greater surface area for gas exchange. For information about teaching patients to deep-breathe,

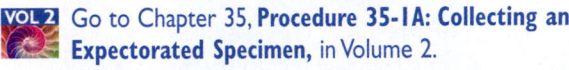 Go to Chapter 35, **Procedure 35-1A: Collecting an Expectorated Specimen,** in Volume 2.

Alter this procedure for patients with chronic lung disease. Have the patient exhale through pursed lips and cough throughout expiration in several short bursts to avoid high expiratory pressures, which collapse diseased airways.

Maintain Hydration

The following activities are important to keep pulmonary secretions thin and mobile:

- *Maintain systemic hydration.* Encourage oral fluid intake as much as possible. Supplement oral intake by intravenous fluid administration if the patient cannot ingest adequate amounts of fluid. For guidelines to use in teaching patients to maintain hydration, refer to the Self-Care box: Teaching Patients to Prevent Fluid and Electrolyte Imbalances in Chapter 36.
- *Humidify inhaled air.* You can accomplish this with humidification devices or nebulizers. A **nebulizer** is a device that turns liquids into an aerosol mist that can be inhaled directly into the lungs. Nebulizers are often used to deliver medications to the lungs, but they can also be used to deliver moisture to the airways and lungs. See "Administering Respiratory Inhalations" in Chapter 23, and Figures 23–11 and 23-12. Also,

 Go to Chapter 35, **Clinical Insight 35-4: Oxygen Therapy Safety Precautions,** in Volume 2.

Humidifiers are also used to keep secretions thin and mobile. A **humidifier** is a device that delivers small water droplets from a reservoir. Small humidifiers filled with sterile distilled water are attached to oxygen delivery systems to moisten the dry oxygen.

Perform Chest Physiotherapy

Chest physiotherapy moves secretions to the large, central airways for expectoration or suctioning (Fig. 35-7). It involves postural drainage, chest percussion, and chest vibration. In many institutions, respiratory therapists routinely perform chest physiotherapy. However, these procedures are briefly discussed below and in the Critical Aspects box. For detailed discussion,

 Go to Chapter 35, **Procedure 35-4: Performing Percussion, Vibration, and Postural Drainage,** in Volume 2.

FIGURE 35-7 Patient receiving chest physiotherapy.

- *Postural drainage* is the use of positioning to promote drainage from the lungs. Check chest x-ray results to see what segments of the lungs are affected. With this information, you can plan how to position your patient. Postural drainage uses gravity to drain the lungs, so you will place the affected area in an uppermost position so that secretions will drain down toward the large, central airways. For example, if the patient has pneumonia of the right lower lobe, you would place her on her left side and elevate the foot of the bed. This position allows the right lower lobe to drain.
- *Chest percussion and chest vibration* are used in conjunction with postural drainage. Have the patient assume the desired position for 10 to 15 minutes. Then percuss and vibrate to loosen and mobilize the secretions. **Chest percussion** is the rhythmic clapping of the chest wall using cupped hands. **Chest vibration** is the vibration of the chest wall with the palms of the hands. Vibration is a gentle procedure, so you can use it in frail patients who cannot tolerate percussion. If one is available, you can use a vibrating machine instead of the palms of your hands.

Critical**Thinking** 35-11

Your patient has pneumonia in the right lower lobe. She is mildly dyspneic with any activity. Strategize how you would perform chest physiotherapy on this patient. What activities would you consider to make this procedure more tolerable for the patient?

Providing Oxygen Therapy

Oxygen therapy provides oxygen at concentrations greater than the level found in room air. Room air contains only about 21% oxygen. Because oxygen is a medication, it requires a medical prescription for dosage (concentration) and route. Many agencies have protocols with standing orders for oxygen administration in an emergency. Oxygen is supplied in several different ways.

- *Wall outlets* connected to a large central tank of oxygen are usually provided in healthcare facilities (Fig. 35-8).
- *Compressed O_2 in portable tanks* may also be available (Fig. 35-9).
- *Liquid oxygen units* are often used for home oxygen therapy (Fig. 35-10).
- *Oxygen concentrator.* An oxygen concentrator removes nitrogen from room air and concentrates O_2. It requires a battery pack or electrical outlet for power. Oxygen concentrators can deliver flow up to 4 liters per minute (L/min) to create an FIO_2 of approximately 36%. Concentrations are higher at lower flow rates (e.g., an FIO_2 of 95% at 1 L/min). These devices eliminate the need for buying oxygen cylinders, relieving clients' anxiety about running out of oxygen. However, they are expensive, noisy, and not portable; moreover, the client must still have backup oxygen in case of a power failure.

An oxygen flow meter must be connected to the oxygen source to control the flow rate of oxygen from its source to the patient. Flow meters are set in liters per minute.

Various devices (e.g., mask, cannula) are used to deliver oxygen to a patient. They differ in the amount of oxygen they can deliver and the degree to which they enclose the patient. Low-flow devices are the nasal cannula, simple face masks, and rebreather masks. High-flow devices include Venturi masks, aerosol face masks, face tents, and tracheostomy collars—all capable

FIGURE 35-8 Healthcare facilities usually have oxygen available through wall outlets connected to a large central tank of oxygen.

FIGURE 35-9 Portable oxygen tanks come in a variety of sizes.

of reaching up to 100% oxygen concentration (Stich & Cassella, 2009).

The Critical Aspects box summarizes how to set up and apply oxygen therapy. For the complete procedure and to see the various types of masks,

 VOL 2 Go to Chapter 35, **Procedure 35-5: Administering Oxygen,** in Volume 2.

Oxygen administration is a nursing responsibility. NAP may assist in maintaining oxygen use (e.g., adjusting the

FIGURE 35-10 Liquid oxygen units are small and portable. They are ideal for home use.

face mask), but you are responsible for monitoring the patient's response to therapy.

Transtracheal Oxygen Delivery

A **tracheostomy** is a surgical opening into the trachea through the neck. It may be permanent or temporary. When a patient has a tracheostomy, inhaled air bypasses the upper airway, which normally warms and moistens air before it reaches the lower airway. Oxygen may be delivered through the tracheostomy via a collar or an adapter. A **transtracheal catheter** is a catheter placed into the tracheostomy to deliver O_2 directly into the trachea. Because oxygen cannot be humidified through this device, it is rarely used.

Oxygen Hazards

The following risks are associated with oxygen therapy:

- *Oxygen toxicity can develop* when O_2 concentrations of more than 50% are administered for longer than 48 to 72 hours. Prolonged use of high O_2 concentrations reduces surfactant production, which leads to alveolar collapse and reduced lung elasticity.
- *Oxygen supports combustion,* although it does not burn. High concentrations of oxygen will turn a small spark or fire into a large fire. Fire prevention precautions must be used near oxygen delivery systems.
- *Oxygen tanks contain oxygen under pressure.* If the tank ruptures or falls, compressed oxygen shoots forcefully from the tank, turning it into an unguided missile. Oxygen tanks have been known to hurtle through walls when ruptured. They must be handled carefully, and secured well, to prevent this hazard.

 VOL 2 Go to Chapter 35, **Clinical Insight 35-4: Oxygen Therapy Safety Precautions,** in Volume 2.

KnowledgeCheck 35-10

- Why is oxygen humidified?
- Which oxygen delivery method is appropriate for the following patients?
  A patient prescribed to receive 2 L/min of oxygen
  A patient who complains of being claustrophobic and requires low-flow humidified oxygen
  A patient with chronic obstructive pulmonary disease (COPD) with an order for oxygen at an F_{IO_2} of 24%
  A patient who wants to avoid intubation but requires an F_{IO_2} of 100%

Go to Chapter 35, **Knowledge Check Response Sheet and Answers,** on the Student Resource Disk or DavisPlus at http://davisplus.fadavis.com/Wilkinson2

Using Artificial Airways

Artificial airways provide an open airway for patients who have or who are at risk for airway obstruction. The most common artificial airways are discussed in the following sections.

Pharyngeal Airways

Pharyngeal airways provide an open air passage by holding the tongue away from the back of the pharynx. When artificial airways are properly placed, air can flow around and through them, and suction catheters can be passed through them.

Oropharyngeal airways should be used only in unconscious patients because they are likely to trigger gagging, vomiting, or laryngospasm in responsive patients with intact airway reflexes. They are C-shaped, hard plastic devices available in infant, pediatric, and adult sizes. To select the appropriate size, hold the airway next to the patient's face. The length of the airway should extend from the front of the teeth to the end of the jawline (Fig. 35-11). If it is *too short,* it will not keep the tongue pulled forward; if it is *too long,* it may push the epiglottis against the laryngeal opening and completely obstruct the airway. To learn how to insert an oropharyngeal airway,

 Go to Chapter 35, **Procedure 35-13: Inserting an Oropharyngeal Airway,** in Volume 2.

Nasopharyngeal airways are flexible rubber tubes that are inserted through a nostril into the pharynx. Patients who are semiconscious can tolerate nasal airways because they do not stimulate the gag reflex. Nasopharyngeal airways are available in a variety of pediatric and adult sizes. Generally, the larger the internal diameter, the longer the tube. To select the appropriate size, hold the airway next to the patient's face. The length of the airway should extend from the nares to the end of the jawline (Fig. 35-12). To learn about inserting a nasopharyngeal airway,

 Go to Chapter 35, **Procedure 35-14: Inserting a Nasopharyngeal Airway,** in Volume 2.

Endotracheal Airways

Patients who cannot breathe effectively because of airway obstruction or respiratory or cardiac failure need an airway inserted directly into the trachea. **Endotracheal**

FIGURE 35-11 Oropharyngeal airway in place.

FIGURE 35-12 A nasopharyngeal airway in proper position.

airways are pliable tubes inserted into the trachea through the following routes:

Orotracheal tube—the mouth
Nasotracheal tube—the nose
Tracheostomy tube—an opening directly into the trachea

There are several types of tracheostomy tubes, made of various materials. They may be cuffed or uncuffed and may have a single or double lumen. A cuffed tube is used for patients who are being ventilated or who have difficulty swallowing. For self-care at home, a tube with an inner cannula is preferred because the inner tube can be removed and cleaned to avoid tube occlusion, primarily due to accumulation of secretions in the airway.

Because tracheostomy tubes bypass the upper airway, the patient inhales air directly into the lower airway without humidification, filtering, or warming. For this reason, devices that warm and humidify inhaled air are used with endotracheal airways. Figure 35-13A illustrates the parts of an endotracheal airway. Figure 35-13B shows the placement of an orotracheal tube. Nursing responsibilities related to endotracheal airways are to assist in their insertion, maintain stabilization, and provide routine suctioning and management.

Assisting with Endotracheal Airway Insertion

Insertion of endotracheal airways is within the scope of practice of certain specially trained nurses (e.g., nurse anesthetist). As a general-practice nurse, you will assist with insertion by gathering equipment and preparing the patient. On most units, you will find intubation equipment in the resuscitation cart. You will need an oxygen source and a bag (e.g., Ambu or nonrebreather bag) to inflate the lungs; and also a laryngoscope, endotracheal tubes of various sizes, water-soluble lubricant, a syringe to inflate the cuff, and tape to secure the tube in place. Keep suction at the bedside to clear the mouth and airway if secretions are obstructing your view of the cords. If a tracheostomy is performed to create the direct opening into the trachea, you will also need a surgical tray.

FIGURE 35-13 *A*, An endotracheal tube. *B*, Placement of an orotracheal tube.

Intubation must often be done quickly, in response to a temporary decline in the patient's respiratory function during a procedure. Remain calm, and explain to the patient that the airway will enable him to breathe effectively. Once the airway is in place, listen to breath sounds to establish that both lungs are ventilated. Reassess breath sounds periodically. After the airway is inserted, record the type and size, as well as the patient's response to the procedure. A portable chest x-ray will be prescribed to confirm correct placement.

Managing Endotracheal and Tracheostomy Tubes

Managing endotracheal and tracheostomy tubes generally requires the expertise of a respiratory therapist or an RN, but you can delegate this activity to specially trained and skilled LPNs, especially in critical care areas. Once the ostomy is well healed, the airway will not collapse if the tracheostomy tube is dislodged; so a NAP, or even the patient, can reinsert it if necessary. Many patients with permanent tracheostomies perform self-care at home.

Evidence is still mixed about whether to use sterile or clean gloves when performing endotracheal care. Sterile technique is usually used for new tracheostomies. Some have this as policy, and others use sterile technique only for patients who have increased susceptibility to infection. However, for healed tracheostomies, and in many institutions for all tracheostomies, the trend is toward a modified sterile technique. Clean technique is the usual method in the home setting. Anyone who is not a family member and anyone concerned about acquiring an infection should wear nonsterile procedure gloves, even in the home setting. The following are the different levels of asepsis currently in use for tracheostomy care:

- **Sterile technique** is the use of a sterile suction catheter and other supplies with sterile gloves.
- **Modified sterile technique** is use of a sterile suction catheter and supplies, but with nonsterile procedure gloves.
- **Clean technique** is use of a clean catheter and clean hands or nonsterile gloves. The portion of the catheter that will be inserted in the tracheostomy tube is protected to avoid contact with unclean surfaces.

You should follow the procedure used in your healthcare organization or school. The Critical Aspects box summarizes the care for patients with a tracheostomy. To learn the procedure and guidelines for tracheostomy care, respectively,

VOL 2 Go to Chapter 35, **Procedure 35-6: Performing Tracheostomy Care,** and **Clinical Insight 35-5: Caring for Patients with Endotracheal Airways,** in Volume 2.

KnowledgeCheck 35-11

- In what circumstances would you use an oropharyngeal airway? A nasopharyngeal airway?
- What facts should you record if a patient is intubated?
- Describe seven interventions associated with caring for a patient with an endotracheal tube.

Go to Chapter 35, **Knowledge Check Response Sheet and Answers,** on the Student Resource Disk or DavisPlus at http://davisplus.fadavis.com/Wilkinson2

Suctioning Airways

Airways are suctioned to remove secretions and maintain patency. Signs that indicate the need for suctioning include agitation, gurgling sounds during respiration, restlessness, labored respirations, decreased oxygen saturation (Sao_2), increased heart and respiratory rates, and adventitious breath sounds on auscultation. Although suctioning helps remove secretions, it also removes air from the airways and causes the patient's O_2 levels to fall. As a result, suctioning must be done quickly and is often accompanied by supplemental oxygen. Suctioning can also irritate mucous membranes if done too frequently.

Suction catheters may be open tipped or "whistle tipped" (Fig. 35-14*A* and *B*). Most suction catheters have a port on the side, over which you place your thumb to control the suction. A Yankauer tube (Fig. 35-14*C*) is a rigid device for suctioning the oral cavity.

You will need to collaborate with respiratory therapists in managing a patient's airway. Both respiratory therapists and nurses are responsible for suctioning and trach care. The respiratory therapist and the nurse should keep each other informed of changes in the patient's

FIGURE 35-14 *A,* Whistle-tipped suction catheter. *B,* Open-tipped suction catheter. *C,* Yankauer (oral) suction tube.

condition. Airway suctioning is usually performed by RNs and LPNs, but not by NAP. NAP may use a Yankauer tube to suction the oral cavity as part of maintaining hygiene and preventing aspiration of oral secretions.

Suctioning the Upper Airway

Pharyngeal suctioning is performed to prevent oral and nasal secretions from entering the lower airway when the patient is too weak to cough up secretions. Suctioning the pharynx triggers a cough, which helps loosen and mobilize secretions. The patient's condition determines whether you suction the pharynx through the mouth or nose. Most patients find oropharyngeal suctioning more comfortable than the nasal approach. However, if the patient is unable to cooperate and automatically bites down when anything is placed in his mouth or if the jaw is wired, use a nasal approach. To suction the pharynx you must first estimate the distance to which you will advance the catheter. Use a gentle approach and do not force the catheter to advance. The Critical Aspects box summarizes this procedure. For the complete steps,

 Go to Chapter 35, **Procedure 35-10: Performing Upper Airway Suctioning,** in Volume 2.

If an oropharyngeal or nasopharyngeal airway is in place, follow the same procedure, but insert the suction catheter through the nasal airway or alongside the oral airway.

Suctioning the Lower Airway

In tracheal suctioning, a catheter is passed beyond the pharynx into the trachea to remove secretions from the lower airways. The trachea may be suctioned through

the mouth, nose, or an endotracheal airway. In the healthcare setting, deep tracheal suctioning is a sterile procedure.

Orotracheal or Nasotracheal (NT) Approach. When suctioning through the nose or mouth, insert the catheter into the pharynx, and advance it into the trachea during inspiration. This prevents the catheter from entering the esophagus and causing the patient to gag or vomit. When the suction catheter enters the trachea, it will stimulate coughing. Except in an emergency, NT suctioning should be done through a nasopharyngeal airway. The Critical Aspects box provides highlights of this procedure. For the complete steps,

 Go to Chapter 35, **Procedure 35-9: Performing Orotracheal and Nasotracheal Suctioning,** in Volume 2.

Endotracheal or Tracheostomy Approach. An endotracheal or tracheostomy tube provides a direct path into the trachea. To suction, insert the catheter through the artificial airway into the trachea. You do not need to insert the catheter as far into a tracheostomy tube, because you are bypassing the long upper airway. Before suctioning, make sure the airway is secured so it is not dislodged by the coughing or suctioning. The Critical Aspects box further describes this procedure. For the complete steps,

 Go to Chapter 35, **Procedure 35-8: Performing Tracheostomy or Endotracheal Suctioning,** in Volume 2.

KnowledgeCheck 35-12

- Describe the difference between pharyngeal and tracheal suctioning.
- How can you ensure that the suction catheter enters the trachea and not the esophagus?

 Go to Chapter 35, **Knowledge Check Response Sheet and Answers,** on the Student Resource Disk or DavisPlus at http://davisplus.fadavis.com/Wilkinson2

Caring for a Patient Requiring Mechanical Ventilation

A **mechanical ventilator** is a machine that assists a patient to breathe. Usually the patient is intubated before he is placed on the ventilator. An endotracheal tube or a tracheostomy tube is connected by oxygen tubing to the ventilator. Before initiating ventilation, be certain that the healthcare team is aware of advance directives and consults with family members. Many patients do not wish to be mechanically ventilated if it might be a permanent intervention.

Negative pressure ventilators consist of shells that fit externally around the chest. Negative pressure generated inside the shell pulls the chest outward and forces the patient to inhale air, similar to normal breathing. These ventilators are rarely used for acutely ill patients, but they are occasionally used for chronic conditions, for example, in patients with muscle weakness from neuromuscular disease.

Positive pressure ventilators, the most widely used type, require the patient to have an artificial airway (Fig. 35-15). Positive pressure ventilation carries risks, including *barotrauma* (injury to the airways due to pressure changes) and drop in cardiac output as the positive pressure in the chest decreases venous return to the heart.

To care for a patient receiving mechanical ventilation (also called positive pressure ventilation), you need a thorough understanding of the ventilator, its settings, and how to troubleshoot problems. You will need to be familiar with the types of ventilators in use. In the event of a malfunction, if the repair is not readily obvious, manually ventilate the patient with an Ambu bag (resuscitation bag) connected to supplemental oxygen while a colleague troubleshoots the problem.

Patients receiving mechanical ventilation are usually cared for by RNs. In critical care settings, specially trained LPNs may provide care, but the RN is responsible for ensuring that procedures are implemented safely and effectively. RNs also provide ongoing assessment of the patient's ventilatory and oxygenation status. Mechanical ventilation is indicated for acute or chronic respiratory failure, and may be a short- or long-term therapy. Patients requiring long-term ventilation are often cared for at home or in specialized long-term care units, where LPNs and family members often provide care.

The Critical Aspects box describes care of the patient on a mechanical ventilator, including ventilator terminology you will hear used. For the complete procedure,

VOL 2 Go to Chapter 35, **Procedure 35-11: Caring for Patients Requiring Mechanical Ventilation,** in Volume 2.

Patients being mechanically ventilated, even for a short period, are at high risk for developing *ventilator-associated pneumonia (VAP)*. VAP is associated with high mortality rates. Procedure 35-11 includes guidelines for nursing interventions to help prevent VAP.

Caring for a Patient Requiring Chest Tubes

Normally there is negative pressure in the pleural space and only a thin layer of fluid between the membranes. Accumulation of fluid and blood in the pleural space (**hemothorax**) interferes with lung expansion, ventilation, and gas exchange. Air in the pleural space (**pneumothorax**) creates positive pressure, causing lung tissue to collapse. Chest tubes remove air or fluid from the pleural space to make room for the lungs to fully expand. A chest-drainage system is composed of a chest tube inserted into the pleural space and a drainage collection system. The system usually is attached to some form of suction. To see diagrams of different types of pneumothorax,

 Go to Chapter 35, **Tables, Boxes, Figures: ESG Figure 35-3, ESG Figure 35-4,** and **ESG Figure 35-5,** on the Student Resource Disk or DavisPlus at http://davisplus.fadavis.com/Wilkinson2

The purpose of a chest-drainage system is to remove air or fluid from the pleural space without allowing it to re-enter. This is accomplished by means of a valve in the line or by a water-sealed compartment. Flow of air and fluid must be in one direction: from the patient to the collection system. Think of the chest tube as an extension of the pleural space. To provide negative pressure within the chest tube, the open end of the tube is placed under water. With each exhalation, air is expelled through the chest tube into the water, but no air is drawn in during inhalation (Fig. 35-16). Once all air is expelled from the pleural space, negative pressure is reestablished and the lung can fully expand. When the lung tissue is reexpanded, the chest tube can be safely removed.

Types of Drainage Systems

Various chest drainage systems are available, including the older, reusable glass, three-bottle, water-seal system. However, you will most often use a disposable system. These are more compact and lightweight. Disposable systems may be water-seal or dry-seal, and may or may not use suction.

Water-Seal Systems

Water-seal systems can consist of one, two or three chambers (or bottles, in the traditional glass bottle system).

One-Chamber Device. A one-chamber device is the simplest chest drainage system. The chest tube connects to one drainage chamber, which serves as both a collector and a water seal. This system can handle only small volumes of fluid or air (e.g., from **empyema**, a collection of pus in the pleural space). As fluid drains through the chest tube, it raises the fluid level in the chamber,

FIGURE 35-15 A patient on a ventilator via tracheosotomy.

Attached to suction

Suction chamber

Water seal chamber

Atmospheric air

Attached to chest tube

Drainage collection chamber

FIGURE 35-16 A disposable chest drainage system.

making it harder for the patient to exhale. It is important that the device not be tipped over because the vent tube would no longer be below water and air would enter the pleural space.

Two-Chamber System. A two-chamber system has one chamber that connects directly with the chest tube and serves as a collection bottle. The second chamber serves as the water seal; it maintains negative pressure as air flows through it. Because the chest drainage never enters the water-seal chamber, you can measure the amount of drainage more accurately. The two-chamber system can handle large amounts of fluid drainage, but its design can still contribute to labored breathing.

Three-Chamber System. This system adds a third chamber, which connects to the water-seal chamber and placed to suction (see Fig. 35-16). This creates controlled negative pressure within the system. The suction control chamber has three vent tubes: one connected to suction, one connected to the water seal chamber, and a long middle tube with one end open to air at the top. The amount of sterile water in the suction chamber determines the maximum suction possible within the system. For adults you will usually fill the suction chamber to the 15- or 20-cm water level. Suction pressure is expressed in centimeters of water.

Adjusting the suction regulator does not increase the amount of suction. Instead, it simply draws more air in from the atmosphere and causes more bubbling within the bottle. This is a safety feature that prevents excessive negative pressure from being created in the system. For

proper functioning, adjust the suction regulator to create gentle bubbling in the suction control bottle.

Dry-Seal Systems

Dry-seal systems are fairly new. They are a one-piece device with three chambers: fluid collection, dry seal, and dry suction control. They do not use water in the suction chamber, relying instead on a mechanical automatic control valve (ACV) and an air leak monitor. The valve allows air to pass out of the patient and prevents it from returning to the patient—even if the system is knocked over. Pressure is set by adjusting the rotary suction dial. The ACV keeps the pressure constant by adjusting to changes in air leaks and fluctuations in the suction source.

Portable Systems

Portable or mobile systems consist of a single, dry-seal chamber attached to the patient's chest tube (Fig. 35-17). It drains by gravity, but can be connected to wall suction. Portable systems improve ambulation and reduce the risk of deep vein thrombosis and pulmonary embolism. They are thought to decrease the length of time a patient must stay in the hospital. The collection chamber holds a maximum of 500 mL, so portable systems are not practical for patients whose drainage is more than 500 mL daily.

The Critical Aspects box summarizes how to set up disposable chest drainage system. For the complete procedure,

VOL 2 Go to Chapter 35, **Procedure 35-12: Setting Disposable Chest Drainage Systems,** in Volume 2.

Preventing Complications of Chest Drainage

Drainage is usually greatest when the chest tube is initially inserted and decreases as the lung reexpands.

FIGURE 35-17 A one-chamber, dry-seal, portable chest drainage system.

Care of a patient with a chest drainage system involves four broad nursing interventions:

- Monitor breathing, gas exchange, and chest drainage.
- Maintain an intact, properly functioning drainage system.
- Promote lung reexpansion.
- Monitor for complications and intervene promptly.

> ✚ Do not clamp chest tubes. Doing so can rapidly lead to a **tension pneumothorax**—a life-threatening complication. It occurs when positive pressure builds up in the pleural space and pushes the lungs, great vessels, and heart toward the other side of the chest. Clamp chest tubes only for changing the drainage system. Limit the clamp time, and monitor the patient's respiratory status constantly until the clamp is removed.

For guidelines to help you manage care for patients with chest tubes,

 VOL 2 Go to Chapter 35, **Clinical Insight 35-6: Managing Chest Tubes,** in Volume 2.

KnowledgeCheck 35-13

- What is the purpose of mechanical ventilation?
- Why is a chest tube inserted?
- What is the advantage of a three-chamber system (compared to a one-chamber or two-chamber system)?
- How does a portable chest drainage system compare to a water-seal drainage system?

 Go to Chapter 35, **Knowledge Check Response Sheet and Answers,** on the Student Resource Disk or DavisPlus at http://davisplus.fadavis.com/Wilkinson2

Part II. The Cardiovascular System

The first step in oxygenation is getting oxygen into the blood as it flows through the lungs. In the second step, the cardiovascular system transports oxygenated blood to the tissues. **Perfusion** refers to the circulation of blood to all body regions. Limitations in either function (i.e., oxygenating the blood and perfusion) may lead to **hypoxia** (oxygen deficiency in body tissues). In addition, if tissue cells are using more oxygen for metabolism than normal (e.g., during a high fever), hypoxia will occur unless more oxygen is made available to the tissues.

Theoretical **Knowledge** **knowing** why

This section discusses the structures, functions, regulation, and factors affecting the cardiovascular system.

What Are the Structures of the Cardiovascular System?

The structures of the cardiovascular system are the heart, the systemic and pulmonary blood vessels, and the coronary arteries.

The Heart

The heart is a four-chambered muscular organ encased in the **pericardium** (a sac of connective tissue) located inside the chest cavity. The two thin-walled **atria** receive

---

Critical Aspects of Procedures 35-1 through 35-14

VOL 2 For steps to follow in *all* procedures, refer to the Universal Steps for All Procedures found on the inside back cover of Volume 2. Go to the full procedures in Volume 2 to practice and learn the procedure steps. Use these Critical Aspects later to help you review key points.

Procedure 35-1: Collecting a Sputum Specimen

Procedure 35-1A: Collecting an Expectorated Specimen

➤ Use a high- or semi-Fowler's position.

➤ Caution the patient not to touch the inside of the sterile container or lid.

➤ Instruct the patient to breathe deeply for three or four breaths, cough forcefully, then expectorate in the container.

➤ Label the specimen container with the patient's name, test name, and collection date and time.

➤ Place the specimen in a plastic bag with a biohazard label. Follow agency policy.

➤ Send the specimen to the laboratory immediately. If specimen transport is delayed, consult the lab; refrigeration may be required.

Procedure 35-1B: Obtaining a Specimen by Suction

➤ Position in a high- or semi-Fowler's position.

➤ Don protective eyewear.

➤ Attach the suction tubing to the male adapter of the inline sputum specimen container.

➤ Don sterile gloves.

➤ Attach the sterile suction catheter to the rubber tubing on the inline sputum specimen container.

➤ Lubricate the suction catheter with sterile saline solution.

➤ Insert the tip of the suction catheter through the nasopharynx, endotracheal tube, or tracheostomy tube. Advance into the trachea.

➤ When the patient begins coughing, apply suction for 5 to 10 seconds to collect the specimen.

Continued

(Procedure 35-1B, continued)

➤ If an adequate specimen is not obtained, allow the patient to rest for 1 minute, and then repeat the procedure. Administer oxygen at this time, if indicated.

➤ When an adequate specimen is collected, discontinue suction, and gently remove the suction catheter.

➤ Label the specimen container.

➤ Place the specimen in a plastic bag with a biohazard label.

➤ Send the specimen to the laboratory immediately. If specimen transport is delayed, consult the lab; refrigeration may be required.

Procedure 35-2: Monitoring Pulse Oximetry (Arterial Oxygen Saturation)

➤ Choose a sensor that is appropriate for the patient's age, size, and weight and for the desired location.

➤ Attach the probe sensor to the site. Photodetector and light-emitting diodes on the probe sensor should face each other.

➤ Connect the sensor probe to the oximeter, and turn it on.

➤ Read the SaO_2 measurement on the digital display when it reaches a constant value.

➤ Set and turn on the alarm limits for SaO_2 and pulse rate, according to the manufacturer's instructions, patient condition, and agency policy if continuous monitoring is necessary.

➤ When monitoring is no longer needed, remove the probe sensor, and turn off the oximeter.

Procedure 35-3: Performing Cardiac Monitoring

➤ Identify electrode sites based on the monitoring system and the patient's anatomy.

➤ With an alcohol pad, clean the areas for electrode placement; allow to dry.

➤ Connect lead wires to electrodes.

➤ Apply the electrodes, pressing firmly.

➤ If the patient's chest is very hairy, shave the small areas for the electrodes.

➤ Check the ECG tracing on the monitor. If necessary, adjust the gain to increase the waveform size.

➤ Set the upper and lower heart rate alarm limits and turn them on.

➤ Obtain a rhythm strip by pressing the "record" button.

Procedure 35-4: Performing Percussion, Vibration, and Postural Drainage

➤ Help the patient assume the appropriate position based on the lung field that requires drainage.

➤ Keep the patient in the desired position for 10 to 15 minutes.

➤ Using cupped hands, perform percussion over the affected lung area for 1 to 3 minutes while the patient is in the desired drainage position.

➤ Next, perform vibration.

➤ Assist the patient to sit up. Ask him to cough at the end of a deep inspiration to clear the airways of secretions.

➤ Repeat postural drainage, percussion, and vibration for each lung field that requires treatment. The entire treatment should not exceed 60 minutes.

➤ Provide mouth care.

Procedure 35-5: Administering Oxygen

➤ Attach the flow meter to the oxygen source.

➤ Assemble and apply the oxygen equipment according to the device prescribed (nasal cannula, face mask, or face tent).

➤ Turn on the oxygen using the flow meter, and adjust according to the prescribed flow rate.

➤ Double check that the oxygen equipment is set up correctly and functioning properly.

➤ Assess the patient's respiratory status before you leave the bedside.

Procedure 35-6: Performing Tracheostomy Care

➤ Position the patient in a semi-Fowler's position.

➤ Don gown, eye protection, and sterile gloves.

➤ Suction the tracheostomy.

➤ Remove soiled dressing; remove gloves; wash hands.

➤ Set up sterile field and prepare the equipment, keeping supplies sterile.

➤ Don sterile gloves (procedure gloves for modified sterile technique).

➤ Remove the oxygen source, if the patient is receiving supplemental oxygen, and attach to outer cannula if possible. If not possible, clean and return the inner cannula before proceeding.

➤ Remove the inner cannula with your nondominant hand, and dispose of it (if it is a disposable cannula) or clean it (if it is a reusable cannula).

➤ Clean the stoma under the faceplate with the cotton-tipped applicators saturated with normal saline solution (or tap water for modified sterile technique).

➤ Clean the top surface of the faceplate and the skin around it with the gauze pads and cotton-tipped applicators saturated with normal saline solution. (You may use wash cloth and tap water for modified sterile technique.)

➤ Dry the skin around the faceplate and stoma with dry sterile gauze.

➤ With the help of an assistant, remove soiled tracheostomy ties.

➤ Ask the patient to flex his neck, and apply new tracheostomy ties.

➤ Insert a precut, sterile tracheostomy dressing under the faceplate and new ties.

Procedure 35-7: Performing Tracheostomy or Endotracheal Suctioning (Open System)

➤ Suction only when necessary.

➤ Use a suction catheter that is no more than half the internal diameter of the airway tube.

➤ Position the patient in a semi-Fowler's position.

➤ Adjust the suction regulator according to agency policy, using the lowest possible suction pressure.

> ➤ Adults: 100 to 150 mm Hg

> ➤ Children: 100 to 120 mm Hg

> ➤ Infants: 50 to 95 mm Hg

➤ Don sterile gloves. (Dominant hand is sterile; nondominant is unsterile.)

➤ Using your dominant hand, attach the suction catheter to the connecting tubing.

➤ Hyperoxygenate the patient.

➤ Insert the catheter gently, without suction.

➤ Advance the suction catheter, gently aiming downward, no further than the carina tracheae (or a maximum of 6 inches).

  Do not force the catheter.

  Do not apply suction as you enter the airway.

➤ Apply continuous suction as you withdraw the catheter. Apply suction for no longer than 15 seconds.

➤ Avoid saline lavage during suctioning.

➤ Repeat suctioning as needed, allowing intervals of at least 30 seconds between suctioning. Hyperoxygenate the patient between each pass.

➤ Replace the oxygen source when finished.

➤ Provide mouth care.

➤ Reposition the patient.

Procedure 35-8: Performing Tracheostomy or Endotracheal Suctioning (Inline System)

➤ Position the patient in a semi-Fowler's position unless contraindicated.

➤ Adjust the suction regulator according to guidelines or agency policy.

➤ Hyperoxygenate the patient according to agency policy.

➤ Insert the suction catheter gently, with suction off.

➤ Advance the suction catheter gently, aiming downward, no further than the carina trachea (premeasure). Do not force the catheter.

➤ Do not apply suction as you enter the airway.

➤ Apply continuous suction as you withdraw the catheter, but for no longer than 15 seconds.

➤ Avoid saline lavage during suctioning.

➤ Repeat suctioning as needed, allowing intervals of at least 30 seconds between suctioning. Make sure to hyperoxygenate the patient between each pass.

➤ Withdraw suction catheter completely into the sleeve, until you see the indicator line.

➤ Use normal saline to clear secretions from the catheter.

➤ Lock the suction regulator port.

➤ Provide mouth care.

➤ Reposition the patient.

Procedure 35-9: Performing Orotracheal and Nasotracheal Suctioning (Open System)

➤ Position the patient in a semi-Fowler's position.

➤ Adjust suction pressure according to guidelines or agency policy (typically 100 to 150 mm Hg for adults, 100 to 120 mm Hg for children, and 80 to 100 mm Hg for infants, and 60-80 for neonates).

➤ Prepare the suction equipment. For the nasotracheal (NT) approach open the water-soluble lubricant.

➤ Don sterile glove(s).

➤ Use protective eye equipment and gown.

➤ Pick up the suction catheter with your dominant hand, and attach it to the connection tubing.

➤ Approximate the depth the suction catheter should be inserted.

➤ Preoxygenate, if indicated.

➤ Lubricate (for NT approach) and insert the catheter, and advance it to the pharynx as the patient inhales.

➤ Advance the catheter to the predetermined distance as the patient inhales.

➤ Apply suction (no longer than 15 seconds) while you withdraw the catheter, using a continuous rotating motion.

➤ Withdraw the catheter and clear it with sterile saline.

➤ Repeat lubrication and suctioning as needed, allowing intervals of at least 30 seconds between suctioning.

➤ Replace the oxygen source.

➤ Coil the suction catheter in your dominant hand. Pull the sterile glove off over the coiled catheter. Discard in a biohazard receptacle.

➤ Make sure new suction supplies are readily available for future suctioning.

➤ Provide mouth care.

Procedure 35-10: Performing Upper Airway Suctioning

➤ Position the patient in a semi-Fowler's position.

  Oropharyngeal: Patient's face turned toward you

  Nasopharyngeal: Neck hyperextended

➤ Adjust suction regulator according to agency policy (typically 100 to 120 mm Hg for adults, 95 to 110 mm Hg for children, and 50 to 95 mm Hg for infants).

➤ If using the nasal approach, open the water-soluble lubricant.

➤ Don procedure gloves.

Continued

➤ Using your dominant hand, attach the suction catheter to the connection tubing.

➤ Approximate the depth the suction catheter should be inserted.

➤ Remove the oxygen delivery device, if necessary.

➤ If the oxygen saturation is <94%, or if the patient is in distress, administer supplemental oxygen before, during, and after suctioning.

➤ Lubricate and insert the suction catheter.

➤ Gently advance the catheter the premeasured distance into the pharynx.

➤ Engage the suction and apply it while you withdraw the catheter, using a continuous rotating motion.

➤ Clear the catheter with sterile saline.

➤ Lubricate the catheter, and repeat suctioning as needed, allowing 20-second intervals between suctioning.

Procedure 35-11: Caring for Patients Requiring Mechanical Ventilation

➤ Prepare the resuscitation bag; keep it at the bedside.

➤ Wear protective eye covering and gown.

➤ Respiratory therapists are responsible for setting up mechanical ventilation in most agencies. If you must assume the responsibility, refer to the manufacturer's instructions.

  ➤ Verify ventilator settings with the medical prescription.

  ➤ Make sure the ventilator alarm limits are set appropriately.

  ➤ Don gloves.

  ➤ Attach the ventilator tubing to the endotracheal tube or tracheostomy tube.

  ➤ Secure the ventilator tubing.

  ➤ Attach capnography device, if available.

  ➤ Prepare the inline suctioning equipment.

After the initial ventilator setup:

➤ Check arterial blood gases and respiratory assessment about 30 minutes after setup.

➤ Maintain the patient in a semirecumbent position (head of bed at 30° to 45°).

➤ Check the ventilator tubing frequently for condensation.

  Drain the condensate into a collection device, or briefly disconnect the patient from the ventilator and empty the tubing into a waste receptacle, according to agency policy.

  Never drain the condensate into the humidifier.

➤ Provide the patient with an alternative form of communication.

➤ Check ventilator and humidifier settings regularly.

➤ Check the inline thermometer.

➤ Give sedatives or antianxiety drugs as needed.

➤ Reposition the patient regularly (every 1 to 2 hours), being careful not to pull on the ventilator tubing.

➤ Moisten the lips with a cool, damp cloth and water-based lubricant.

➤ Provide frequent antiseptic oral care.

➤ Ensure the call light is always within reach; and answer the call light and respond to ventilator alarms promptly.

➤ Monitor tracheostomy tube for proper cuff inflation.

➤ Monitor for gastric distention.

Procedure 35-12: Setting Up Disposable Chest Drainage Systems

➤ Obtain and prepare the prescribed drainage system.

➤ Position the patient according to the indicated insertion site.

➤ Set up the sterile field and supplies you will need for dressing the insertion site.

➤ Don mask, gown, and sterile gloves.

➤ As soon as the chest tube is inserted, attach it to the drainage system.

➤ Turn on wall (or other) suction source (usually −80 mm H_2O).

➤ Set the prescribed suction level on the chest drainage unit (CDU).

➤ Don a clean pair of sterile gloves.

➤ Using sterile technique, wrap petroleum gauze around the chest tube at the insertion site, and dress the site with two precut sterile drain dressings covered by a large drainage dressing.

➤ Apply an occlusive dressing over the insertion site (e.g., with 2-in. silk tape); cover the dressing completely. Date, time, and initial the dressing.

➤ Using the spiral taping technique, wrap 1-inch silk tape around the connections. Wrap from top to bottom and bottom to top. (Or use locking connections, if furnished with the CDU.)

➤ With an 8-inch-long piece of 2-inch tape, secure the top end of the drainage tube to the chest tube dressing.

➤ Make sure the tubing lies with no kinks and no dependent areas, in a straight line to the CDU.

➤ Prepare the patient for a portable chest x-ray exam.

➤ Keep emergency supplies at the bedside in the event of tube dislodgement or system failure.

➤ Maintain the chest tube and drainage system by preventing kinks, ensuring patency of the air vent, and keeping the system below the level of the chest tube.

➤ Keep the head of the bed always elevated to at least 30°.

Procedure 35-13: Inserting an Oropharyngeal Airway

➤ You will need a variety of sizes of airway, procedure gloves, tongue blade, suction equipment, and possibly a handheld resuscitation bag and oxygen source.

Critical Aspects of Procedures 35-1 through 35-14

➤ Measured on the outside of the cheek, the airway should extend from the front teeth to the end of the jaw line.

➤ Clear the mouth of debris and secretions. Suction if needed.

➤ Position patient in supine or semi-Fowler's position, neck hyperextended.

➤ Hold the tongue down with a tongue blade, as needed, and insert the airway in the upside-down position.

➤ Rotate the airway 180° and continue inserting until the front flange is flush with the lips.

➤ Keep the patient's head slightly tilted and chin elevated.

➤ Verify airway patency by auscultating breath sounds.

➤ Do not tape the airway in place.

➤ Keep suction available at the bedside.

➤ Suction the oropharynx as needed.

Procedure 35-14: Inserting a Nasopharyngeal Airway

➤ You will need a correctly sized nasopharyngeal airway, procedure gloves, tongue blade, water soluble lubricant, suction equipment, and possibly a handheld resuscitation bag and oxygen source.

➤ Measured on the outside of the cheek, the airway should extend from the tip of the nose to the earlobe. It should be slightly smaller than the nares.

➤ Position patient in a supine or semi-Fowler's position, neck hyperextended.

➤ Lubricate the airway with water-soluble lubricant.

➤ Advance the airway through the naris until the outer flange rests on the nostril. Do not force.

➤ Visually inspect the top of the posterior pharynx; only the tip of the tube should be visible.

➤ Use your finger to check for air exchange at the naris.

➤ Auscultate the lungs bilaterally.

➤ Keep suction available at the bedside.

➤ Suction as needed.

blood into the heart, and the two thick-walled **ventricles** pump blood out of the heart. Valves between the heart chambers open widely to allow blood to flow easily and without turbulence from one chamber to another, and the valves close tightly to prevent backflow of blood. The **base,** or broadest side of the heart, which houses the atria, faces upward. The **apex,** or tip of the heart, which houses the ventricles, faces downward (Fig. 35-18).

A strong, efficient heartbeat keeps blood flowing through the vascular system. Deoxygenated blood from organs and tissues flows through the venous system into the right side of the heart and then into the pulmonary circulation. At the alveolar–capillary membrane, external gas exchange occurs. The newly oxygenated blood then flows from the lungs into the left side of the heart and out into the arterial circulation.

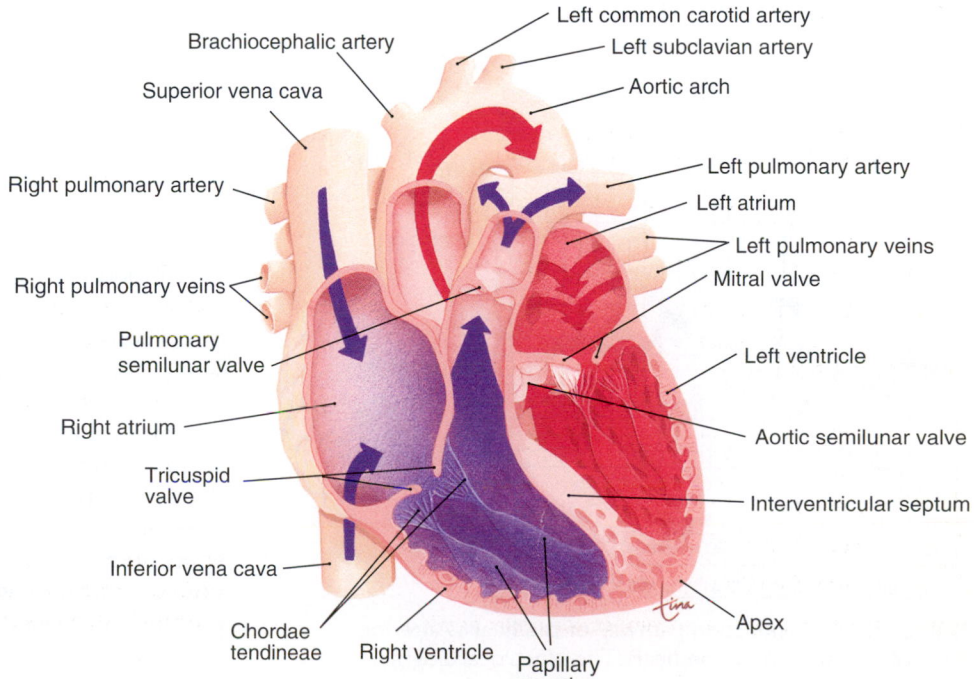

FIGURE 35-18 The atria receive blood into the heart; the ventricles pump blood out of the heart. Valves between the chambers allow blood to flow in one direction from one chamber to another without backflow.

The Cardiac Cycle

The **cardiac cycle** is the sequence of mechanical events that occurs during a single heartbeat. Very simply, it is the simultaneous contraction of the two atria, followed a fraction of a second later by the simultaneous contraction of the ventricles. The electrical activity of the myocardium regulates the cardiac cycle (Fig. 35-19).

Electrical Conduction

The heart contains specialized areas of nerve tissue that initiate electrical impulses.

- The **sinoatrial (SA) node** acts as the pacemaker. Located in the right atrium, it initiates an impulse that triggers each heartbeat. The impulse travels rapidly down the atrial conduction system so that both atria contract as a unit.
- At the **atrioventricular (AV) node**, there is a slight delay. From the AV node, impulses pass into the left and right *bundles of His* and into the *Purkinje fibers* to the ventricles.

In this way, myocardial fibers are electrically stimulated almost simultaneously to create a unified cardiac muscle contraction strong enough to pump blood out of a heart chamber. If there are defects in this electrical system, impulses travel more slowly through the heart and some areas contract before others. This can lead to ineffective heart pumping and decreased cardiac output.

Normally, the SA node is in charge and initiates a rate of 60 to 100 beats/min, depending on the body's oxygen needs. If the SA node fails, the AV node can take over as the pacemaker, but it generally triggers a slower heart rate. If both the SA and AV nodes fail, the conduction fibers can initiate impulses. Ventricular conduction generates a very slow rate, usually less than 40 beats/min; however, this can be life-saving if no other node or fiber is initiating an impulse.

FIGURE 35-19 Conduction pathway of the heart. Anterior view of the interior of the heart. The electrocardiogram tracing is one of a normal heartbeat. See text for description.

Systemic and Pulmonary Blood Vessels

The vascular system is composed of three types of vessels: arteries, veins, and capillaries. All vessels are lined with a smooth endothelial layer that promotes nonturbulent blood flow and prevents platelets from sticking to the sides of the walls and beginning a clot.

- **Arteries** have thick, elastic walls that allow them to stretch during cardiac contraction **(systole)** and to recoil when the heart relaxes **(diastole).**
- **Arterioles** are smaller branches of arteries. They are primarily smooth muscle and thinner than arteries. Under control by the sympathetic nervous system, the arterioles constrict or dilate to vary the amount of blood flowing into capillaries and help maintain blood pressure.
- **Capillaries** are microscopic vessels, created as arterioles branch into smaller and smaller vessels. Because they are only one cell thick, capillaries facilitate the exchange of gases, nutrients, and wastes between the tissue cells and the blood. Billions of capillaries provide blood flow to every cell in the body. Capillaries connect the arterial and venous systems and carry blood from arterioles to venules.
- The **venous system** returns the deoxygenated blood to the heart. **Veins** and **venules** have thin, muscular, but inelastic walls that collapse easily. These walls contract or relax in response to feedback from the sympathetic nervous system: When blood volume is low, the veins contract to provide a smaller space for smaller volume of blood; when blood volume is high, veins relax and enlarge to accommodate increased volume of blood. Think of the venous system as a holding tank for fluctuations in blood volume.

For illustrations of the systemic arteries and veins,

Go to Chapter 35, **Tables, Boxes, Figures: ESG Figure 35-1** and **ESG Figure 35-2,** on the Student Resource Disk or DavisPlus at http://davisplus.fadavis.com/Wilkinson2

To see an animated illustration of the circulatory system,

Go to **Animations, Cardiovascular/Pulmonary Animations: Blood Flow** on DavisPlus at http://davisplus.fadavis.com/Wilkinson2

The Coronary Arteries

The heart has its own blood supply through the coronary arteries (Fig. 35-20). The coronary sinus (not shown), located just above the aortic valve, fills with blood during diastole. From the coronary sinus, blood flows into the two main coronary arteries, which branch into several sections to supply the heart muscle with blood. The coronary arteries are the only arteries in the body that fill during diastole. To see an animated illustration of the coronary circulation,

Go to **Animations, Cardiovascular/Pulmonary Animations: Blood Flow Through the Heart** on DavisPlus at http://davisplus.fadavis.com/Wilkinson2

KnowledgeCheck 35-14

- Describe oxygenation and perfusion.
- Trace the path of normal electrical impulses in the heart.
- How do the walls of arteries, veins, and capillaries differ?
- What is the importance of diastole to perfusion of the heart?

FIGURE 35-20 Coronary vessels in anterior view. The pulmonary artery has been cut to show the left coronary artery emerging from the ascending aorta.

Labels: Aorta; Left coronary artery; Anterior interventricular branch; Great cardiac vein; Right coronary artery and vein

Go to Chapter 35, **Knowledge Check Response Sheet and Answers,** on the Student Resource Disk or DavisPlus at http://davisplus.fadavis.com/Wilkinson2

CriticalThinking 35-12

Your patient has a condition that has caused the mitral valve to become stiff with only a narrow opening for blood flow. What type of problems related to oxygenation would you anticipate in this patient?

How Are Oxygen and Carbon Dioxide Transported?

The cardiovascular system circulates oxygenated blood to organs and tissues and returns deoxygenated blood to the heart. Maintaining this blood flow requires:

- Adequate cardiac output
- Adequate circulation
- Effective regulation of cardiovascular function

A full 97% of blood oxygen is bound to hemoglobin, the iron-containing protein in red blood cells; only 3% is in a dissolved state. At the tissue level, O_2 leaves the hemoglobin, becomes dissolved in the blood, and passes through the capillary membrane into the tissues. Only the dissolved form of O_2 can pass through capillary membranes. Hemoglobin thereby serves as a reservoir for oxygen until it is needed in the dissolved state.

Carbon dioxide is a waste product of normal aerobic tissue metabolism. Carbon dioxide can be carried in the blood in three ways: about 7% of CO_2 is dissolved in plasma, 23% attaches to hemoglobin, and 70% is converted into bicarbonate ions. However, CO_2 diffuses through cellular and alveolar–capillary membranes only in its dissolved state. The CO_2 bound to hemoglobin eventually detaches and becomes dissolved in the plasma for diffusion into the alveoli of the lungs. The bicarbonate ions in the plasma are converted back to CO_2, which becomes dissolved, diffuses into the alveoli, and is exhaled.

To see an animated explanation of CO_2 and O_2 transport,

Go to **Animations, Cardiovascular/Pulmonary Animations: CO$_2$/O$_2$ Transport** on DavisPlus at http://davisplus.fadavis.com/Wilkinson2

How Is Cardiovascular Function Regulated?

Cardiovascular function is regulated by the autonomic nervous system (ANS) and by control centers in the brain stem.

Autonomic Nervous System

The autonomic nervous system regulates cardiovascular function through its influence on cardiac rate and muscle contractility, as well as vascular tone.

The Heart. Through branches at the thoracic level of the spinal cord, *sympathetic fibers* stimulate the heart to beat faster and contract more strongly. *Parasympathetic fibers* innervate the heart through the vagus nerve. Parasympathetic stimulation results in a slowed heart rate, but it does not influence myocardial contractility.

The Vascular System. All blood vessels are innervated by *sympathetic fibers* that maintain them in a constant baseline state of partial contraction (**tone**). Vascular tone maintains blood pressure and blood flow even when a person is resting or asleep. Sympathetic stimulation above and beyond baseline tone varies in response to body needs. Increased sympathetic stimulation causes constriction of some vessels (e.g., skin, gastrointestinal tract, and kidneys) and dilatation of other vessels (skeletal muscle). This shunts blood flow to the skeletal muscles for a fight-or-flight response. The *parasympathetic nervous system* has no significant control over blood vessels.

For more complete information, consult an anatomy and physiology text. For a brief overview of the nervous system,

 Go to Chapter 35, **Supplemental Materials: The Nervous System,** on the Student Resource Disk or DavisPlus at http://davisplus.fadavis.com/Wilkinson2

Brain Stem Centers

The brain stem centers integrate feedback from baroreceptors and chemoreceptors in the body to regulate cardiac function and blood pressure. The *vasomotor center* controls sympathetic stimulation of the heart and vascular system. The *cardioinhibitory center* controls parasympathetic slowing of the heart rate.

Baroreceptors. Baroreceptors located in the walls of the heart and blood vessels are sensitive to pressure changes. The aortic arch and carotid artery baroreceptors are particularly important in the regulation of heart rate and vascular tone. When baroreceptors sense even a small drop in pressure, they send messages to the brain stem centers to stimulate the sympathetic nervous system to increase heart rate and induce vasoconstriction. This mechanism allows us to change positions and maintain blood pressure.

Chemoreceptors. Chemoreceptors located in the aortic arch and the carotid arteries are sensitive to changes in blood pH, oxygen levels, and carbon dioxide levels. Their main function is to regulate ventilation, but they also send information to the vasomotor center in response to lack of oxygen. The vasomotor center responds by activating sympathetic stimulation.

If you would like further review of nervous regulation of the heart,

 Go to Chapter 35, **Tables, Boxes, Figures: ESG Figure 35-6,** on the Student Resource Disk or DavisPlus at http:// davisplus.fadavis.com/Wilkinson2

 KnowledgeCheck 35-15

- How are oxygen and carbon dioxide transported in the blood?
- How is the cardiovascular system regulated?
- Does poor peripheral perfusion increase the risk for hypoxemia?

 Go to Chapter 35, **Knowledge Check Response Sheet and Answers,** on the Student Resource Disk or DavisPlus at http://davisplus.fadavis.com/Wilkinson2

Critical**Thinking** 35-13

The second person you meet at the pulmonary clinic is Mary, a 4-year-old girl with a history of asthma ("Meet Your Patients"). She is receiving a nebulized treatment containing Proventil (albuterol) and Atrovent (ipratropium bromide). These medications stimulate the sympathetic nervous system.

- What cardiovascular side effects can you anticipate?
- How might these side effects affect oxygenation?
- What do you need to know about the patient's history to safely administer the drugs?

What Factors Influence Cardiovascular Function?

Similar to respiratory function, cardiovascular function is influenced by developmental stage, environment, lifestyle, substance abuse, medications, and pathophysiological conditions.

Developmental Stage

Normal development influences heart and circulatory function. Developmental factors exert more of an influence on older adults than on young and middle adults.

Preschool and School-Age Children

Preschool and school-age children have body systems mature enough to adapt to moderate stress and change, including the heart and circulatory systems. However, children as young as school age sometimes begin social habits, such as tobacco use, that can have long-term adverse effects on the cardiovascular system.

Adolescents

In adolescence, the heart and blood components develop adult characteristics. The average adolescent is developmentally at little risk for heart or circulatory disorders, although some athletes can be at risk for collapse and sudden cardiac dysrhythmia that is familial. New guidelines for health professionals performing sports assessments call for thorough investigation of the family history for fainting, collapse, or sudden death.

Some adolescents adopt behaviors and habits that can create risk throughout life. For instance, about half the adults who use tobacco were regular smokers by their 18th birthdays, and 20% of students in high schools report they have smoked cigarettes on one or more of the 30 days preceding the survey (American Lung Association, 2009a; CDC/NCHS, 2008). The U.S. incidence of childhood obesity is also rising to epidemic incidence in the United States. As a result, some adolescents exhibit signs of cardiovascular disease (e.g., high blood levels of lipids and cholesterol, a known factor in the development of high blood pressure, heart disease, and blockages in the arteries of the heart).

Young and Middle Adults

Lifestyle in young and middle adulthood can create cardiac risk factors. Some adults become "too busy" to prepare and eat nourishing foods, or more often simply prefer the taste of high-fat, high-sugar foods. A sedentary lifestyle, lack of aerobic exercise, and tobacco use also contribute to cardiovascular disorders in this group. Crack cocaine and methamphetamine abuse can lead to sudden cardiac failure. Family history of cardiovascular disease is yet another risk factor for this age group.

Older Adults

In general, the number of cells and the efficiency of the organs decline gradually as a person ages. Keep in mind, though, that endurance training and regular exercise slow the rate of these changes. In fact, an older person who is physically conditioned by regular exercise may have better heart and circulatory function than a younger adult who is not well conditioned.

Cardiac efficiency gradually declines as the heart muscle loses contractile strength and heart valves become thicker and more rigid. The peripheral vessels become less elastic, which creates more resistance to ejection of blood from the heart. As a result of these changes, the heart becomes less able to respond to increased oxygen demands, and it needs longer recovery times after responding. For example, in response to exercise, an older adult's heart rate does not increase as much as a younger person's, but it does remain elevated longer. Thus, older adults have lower exercise tolerance, need more rest after exercise, and are more prone to orthostatic hypotension.

Environment

Environmental factors, such as stress, allergic reactions, altitude, and temperature, affect cardiovascular function. These factors are discussed in the text that follows.

Stress

The stress response stimulates:

- *Release of catecholamines* from the sympathetic nervous system. This results in increased heart rate and contractility, vasoconstriction, and increased tendency of blood to clot.

- *Suppression of the immune and inflammatory responses,* which decreases resistance to infection
- *Release of cortisol* from the adrenal cortex, which results in altered glucose, fat, and protein metabolism

Sustained stimulation of the sympathetic nervous system can lead to cardiovascular disease. In addition, a chronically suppressed immune and inflammatory response increases the risk for all infections. For additional information on the effects of stress, see Chapter 25.

Allergic Reactions and Air Quality

An **allergy** is a hypersensitivity, or over-response, to an antigen. Inflammatory substances released during an allergic response (e.g., histamine, protease) cause the following cardiovascular events:

- Blood vessels dilate in areas affected (which increases blood flow to the areas).
- Eosinophils and neutrophils are attracted to the reaction site.
- Local tissues are damaged by protease.
- Capillaries become more permeable, resulting in fluid leak into tissues.
- Local (e.g., vascular) smooth muscle cells contract.

Altitude

Oxygen pressure falls proportionally with increased altitude (to review, refer to Part I, The Pulmonary System, "Altitude,") making more oxygen available in the alveoli and at the tissue level. Over the long term, people who live at high altitudes undergo physiological changes that facilitate oxygenation. Among the cardiopulmonary changes are the following:

- Increased production of red blood cells (RBCs)
- Increased vascularity of body tissues
- Increased ability of tissue cells to use oxygen even when atmospheric oxygen pressure is low

Heat and Cold

Heat generally causes vasodilatation, which increases cardiac output and oxygenation. However, heat also increases metabolism. As a result, people are naturally more sedentary in hot weather.

Cold slows cell metabolism, reducing O_2 demand. It also causes vasoconstriction, and slows the heart rate. Induced hypothermia is used in some surgical procedures. As another example, victims of cold-water near-drowning have been revived after long periods of time, in part because of the reduced O_2 demands associated with hypothermia. Prolonged exposure to cold causes frostbite, loss of hypothalamic temperature regulation, and death.

Lifestyle

Lifestyle factors that affect cardiovascular function include pregnancy, nutrition, obesity, exercise, tobacco use, and substance abuse.

Pregnancy

During pregnancy, oxygen demand increases dramatically, due to the needs of the fetus and an approximate 15% increase in maternal metabolism during the last half of pregnancy. To compensate, the mother's blood volume increases by 30%. The woman requires additional iron to produce this blood as well as to meet fetal requirements. Failure to meet these iron demands can result in maternal anemia, reducing tissue oxygenation to the mother and fetus.

Nutrition

The body needs an appropriate balance of proteins, carbohydrates, fats, and other nutrients for proper immune function, resistance to disease and infection, normal cellular function and tissue repair, and maintenance of a healthy weight. A diet high in saturated fat predisposes to the development of atherosclerosis, coronary artery disease, and hypertension, all of which can compromise circulation and oxygenation. A low-fat, low-cholesterol, low-sodium diet is considered "heart healthy." Vitamins, minerals (especially iron), and protein are important to prevent anemia, which reduces blood-oxygen–carrying capacity. Green tea consumption has been associated with reduced mortality due to cardiovascular disease (Kuriyama, Shimazu, Ohmori, et al., 2007).

Obesity

Obesity is a body mass index (BMI) above 30 (see Chapter 26). Obesity causes multiple health problems, many of which affect the heart and circulation. Obesity increases the risk of developing atherosclerosis and hypertension. Excess fat stores in and around the heart itself reduce its effectiveness as a pump. At the same time, the workload of the heart is increased by the need to perfuse the excess body tissues.

Exercise

Exercise improves blood circulation and delivery of oxygen to tissues and cells. It also increases metabolic demands. The body responds by increasing the heart rate and the rate and depth of breathing. Like skeletal muscles, the heart muscle is strengthened with regular aerobic exercise. As the heart becomes stronger, it becomes a more efficient pump. As a result, resting heart rate is slower because a higher heart rate is not required to maintain cardiac output. Lack of exercise has the opposite effect. A sedentary lifestyle reduces the efficiency of the heart and the capacity to increase ventilation in response to exercise.

Tobacco Use

Tobacco use is a major risk factor in several chronic cardiovascular conditions: stroke, peripheral arterial disease, aortic aneurysm, and heart disease. Smoking is implicated in atherosclerosis (fatty buildups in the arteries), hypertension, and decreased HDL (good) cholesterol—all of which lead to coronary heart disease and heart attack. Other factors contribute to coronary heart disease (e.g., obesity, diabetes, physical inactivity). However, cigarette smoking is such a significant risk factor that the U.S. Surgeon General has called it the leading preventable cause of disease and deaths in the United States. Cigar and pipe smoking are also implicated, but not to the extent of cigarettes (American Heart Association, 2009a).

Substance Abuse

Substances that people abuse include over-the-counter and prescription medications, commonly available commercial products, and illegal substances. Large amounts of alcohol depress respiratory, cardiac, and vasomotor centers of the brain. Chronic alcohol abuse causes fatty infiltration of the heart muscle, thrombi in the coronary arteries, heart enlargement, and dysrhythmias, all of which can ultimately lead to heart failure. Illicit drugs, including stimulants (e.g., methamphetamine, cocaine), hallucinogens [e.g., LSD (acid), mescaline (buttons)], and cannabinoids (e.g., marijuana) also have adverse effects on the cardiovascular system. For example, cocaine has been linked to myocardial dysfunction, dysrhythmias, endocarditis, and aortic dissection.

Medications

Many drugs can interfere with oxygenation by depressing cardiovascular function. For a more complete discussion of medications,

 Go to Chapter 35, **Supplemental Materials: Medications that Can Interfere with Oxygenation** and **Medications Used to Improve Oxygenation, Cardiovascular Medications,** on the Student Resource Disk or DavisPlus at http://davisplus.fadavis.com/Wilkinson2

Cardiovascular depressants are used therapeutically to slow the heart rate or reduce the force of myocardial contraction. This may reduce cardiac output and impair tissue oxygenation. The following are the most commonly used cardiovascular depressants:

- *Beta-adrenergic blocking agents* (e.g., bisoprolol fumarate [Zebeta]) are used therapeutically to reduce the work load of the heart, to control abnormal heart rhythms (dysrhythmias), and to control hypertension. Drugs that block beta-1 receptors slow the heart rate and decrease the strength of myocardial contraction.
- *Calcium channel blocking agents* (e.g., nifedipine [Procardia]) block the flow of calcium into cells of the heart and blood vessels. They decrease blood pressure and the strength of myocardial contraction, slow the heart rate, and dilate the arteries and arterioles.

KnowledgeCheck 35-16

- What changes occur in the cardiovascular system with aging?
- How does smoking affect the cardiovascular system?

 Go to Chapter 35, **Knowledge Check Response Sheet and Answers,** on the Student Resource Disk or DavisPlus at http://davisplus.fadavis.com/Wilkinson2

Pathophysiological Conditions

Alterations in oxygen and carbon dioxide levels at the alveolar–capillary membrane or the tissue level may be life threatening. The following common alterations were discussed in the section, "Problems with Gas Exchange":

Hypoxemia—Low arterial blood oxygen levels
Hypoxia—Poor oxygenation of organs and tissues. It may be due to hypoxemia or circulatory disorders.
Hypercarbia—An excess of dissolved CO_2 in the blood due to hypoventilation
Hypocarbia—A low level of dissolved CO_2 in the blood due to hyperventilation

Cardiovascular Abnormalities

Alterations in gas exchange are caused by a number of disorders that affect the structure, function, and regulation of the cardiovascular system. Cardiovascular abnormalities interfere with the flow of oxygenated blood to organs and tissues. Major abnormalities are as follows:

- **Heart failure** occurs when the heart becomes an inefficient pump and is unable to meet the body's demands. Blood is oxygenated when it passes through the lungs, but it is not well circulated to the organs and tissues. Impaired circulation leads to systemic and pulmonary edema, which further impairs gas exchange.
- **Cardiomyopathy** is a heart muscle disorder that results in heart enlargement and impaired cardiac contractility.
- **Cardiac ischemia** occurs when oxygen requirements of the heart are unmet. Prolonged ischemia leads to myocardial infarction (MI) as parts of the heart *necrose* (die) from inadequate oxygen. **Angina pectoris** is transient chest pain due to myocardial ischemia. The tissue becomes injured but does not necrose.
- **Coronary artery disease**, a leading cause of cardiac ischemia, is a condition in which plaque builds up inside the coronary arteries. Plaque narrows the arteries, reducing blood flow to the heart muscle and making it more likely that clots will form and block the arteries. If you are interested in seeing animated explanations of plaque buildup and coronary artery disease, respectively,

 Go to **Animations: Atherosclerosis,** and **Coronary Artery Disease,** on DavisPlus at http://davisplus.fadavis.com/Wilkinson2

- **Dysrhythmias** (alterations in heart rate or rhythm) can lower cardiac output and decrease tissue oxygenation.
- **Heart valve abnormalities** create turbulent flow, leading to a decrease in cardiac output and compromised tissue oxygenation. Often there is an audible murmur. The valves most commonly affected are the mitral and aortic valves.

If you are interested in a more extensive discussion of cardiovascular abnormalities,

 Go to Chapter 35, **Supplemental Materials, Cardiovascular Abnormalities,** on the Student Resource Disk or DavisPlus at http://davisplus.fadavis.com/Wilkinson2

Peripheral Vascular Abnormalities

Disorders of peripheral blood vessels impair blood flow to and from organs and tissues. Arterial abnormalities disrupt flow of oxygenated blood to tissues. When arterial blood flow is compromised, signs and symptoms include pallor, pain, weak or absent pulses, poor capillary refill, cool skin, and tissue dysfunction. Venous abnormalities disrupt blood return to the heart. Clinical signs of compromised venous blood flow include edema, brown skin discoloration, and tissue dysfunction (e.g., stasis ulcers). If you are interested in a more extensive discussion of peripheral vascular abnormalities,

 Go to Chapter 35, **Supplemental Materials, Peripheral Vascular Abnormalities,** on the Student Resource Disk or DavisPlus at http://davisplus.fadavis.com/Wilkinson2

Oxygen Transport Abnormalities

Even if the heart is functioning well and arterial blood flow is intact, tissues can become hypoxic if the blood is unable to carry adequate amounts of oxygen. The most common causes are anemia and carbon monoxide poisoning. **Anemia** is an abnormally low level of red blood cells, hemoglobin, or both. **Carbon monoxide** is a colorless, odorless gas produced by the combustion of flammable materials and fuels. When inhaled, carbon monoxide binds tightly to hemoglobin at the oxygen receptor sites, making it impossible for hemoglobin to carry oxygen. If you are interested in a more extensive discussion of oxygen transport abnormalities,

 Go to Chapter 35, **Supplemental Materials, Oxygen Transport Abnormalities,** on the Student Resource Disk or DavisPlus at http://davisplus.fadavis.com/Wilkinson2

KnowledgeCheck 35-17

- What changes occur in the cardiovascular system with aging?
- How does smoking affect the cardiovascular system?

 Go to Chapter 35, **Knowledge Check Response Sheet and Answers,** on the Student Resource Disk or DavisPlus at http://davisplus.fadavis.com/Wilkinson2

Practical **Knowledge**
knowing how

Nursing care for patients with cardiovascular problems is directed at assessing for and maximizing the effectiveness of the heart and circulatory system.

■ ASSESSMENT

Although this section focuses on cardiovascular assessments, evaluation of overall oxygenation status includes a history and examination that gathers information about lung, heart, and circulatory function. The patient's condition and the purpose of the assessment determine your priorities for assessment and the order in which you gather information. For example, for someone with a cardiac emergency, the immediate assessment focus would be to ask simple questions about current symptoms while performing a quick examination to determine adequacy of breathing, circulation, and oxygenation. In contrast, the assessment for risk of coronary artery disease in a healthy individual might include more extensive questions about occupation and smoking habits, a medical history, and an extensive physical examination.

You will need information about the patient's past and present cardiovascular signs and symptoms, risk factors, medications, activity level, tolerance of activity, and lifestyle factors that affect cardiovascular functioning.

Assessing for Risk Factors

A health history related to cardiovascular functioning includes questions about the presence of risk factors that affect the heart, and peripheral vascular function. Topics to assess include the following:

- Demographic data
- Health history
- Family history
- Respiratory history
- Cardiovascular history
- Environmental history
- Lifestyle

You should also assess the patient's level of anxiety. Patients with cardiac or respiratory problems are almost certain to be anxious, and anxiety interferes with achieving good outcomes for these patients. Pay close attention to verbal cues because heart rate and blood pressure changes may not be useful in assessing acutely ill patients for anxiety (Moser, 2007). For a detailed list of interview questions for each of these topics,

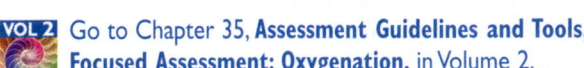 Go to Chapter 35, **Assessment Guidelines and Tools, Focused Assessment: Oxygenation,** in Volume 2.

Physical Examination

Assessment of heart and peripheral vessels includes inspection, palpation, and auscultation (and occasionally percussion). Use inspection to observe for signs of distress (e.g., chest pain), skin and mucous membrane color, presence or absence of edema, and overall general appearance. Palpate pulses, skin temperature, edema, heart pulsations through the chest wall, and areas of tenderness. Auscultate heart sounds, vascular sounds, and blood pressure. Auscultate the lungs because adventitious sounds, such as rales, may signal decreased cardiac output. For a step-by-step discussion of how to assess the heart and vascular system,

 Go to Chapter 19, **Procedure 19-13: Assessing the Heart and Vascular System,** in Volume 2.

Assess Pain

If a patient has chest pain, evaluate it immediately because chest pain is the most common heart attack symptom. Ask the patient to describe the pain, its location, duration, frequency, and radiation. Chest pain may also be caused by musculoskeletal or respiratory conditions, for example, a fractured rib or pleuritis (inflammation in the pleural space). You can differentiate cardiac pain because it is usually in the center or on the left side of the chest and radiates to the left arm, at least in men. The pain typically lasts several minutes; it may go away and come back. Some women have milder chest pain, sometimes none at all. They are thought to be more likely than men are to experience other symptoms, such as jaw or back pain, nausea, fatigue, and shortness of breath. Cardiac pain typically does not change with inhalation or exhalation. Ask the client to rate the pain on a scale of 0 to 10, with 0 representing no pain and 10 representing the worst possible pain. See Chapter 30 for pain assessment, as needed.

Patients experiencing chest pain are likely to be fearful—most people are aware that chest pain may signal a heart attack. You need to work quickly but calmly to instill confidence in the patient. If the person is experiencing a cardiac event, anxiety and stress can make it worse by increasing oxygen consumption, thereby extending hypoxic damage to the heart.

Assess Fatigue

Fatigue is a subjective experience. The patient feels tired and lacks endurance. Fatigue is a common symptom of various oxygenation problems, including anemia and heart failure. Ask your patient to rate his fatigue on a 0 to 10 scale, as you do for pain.

Assess Dyspnea

Dyspnea (shortness of breath) was discussed earlier in the chapter in relation to respiratory conditions. Recall that dyspnea is a sign of hypoxia, which can be associated with cardiovascular diseases and anemia, as well as with respiratory problems. As with pain, dyspnea provokes anxiety.

Assess Peripheral Circulation

Even if the lungs and heart are functioning well, pathology in the arteries and veins can interfere with tissue perfusion. Palpate the peripheral pulses, assess skin color and temperature, and note the distribution of hair on the extremities. Weak pulses, cool feet, lack of hair, and shiny skin on lower legs and feet usually accompany peripheral vascular disease. Look for skin ulcers that often accompany severe venous or arterial disease. Check for edema of the feet and ankles; this is one symptom of heart failure.

KnowledgeCheck 35-18

Why would you auscultate the lungs as a part of your assessment of cardiac function?

 Go to Chapter 35, **Knowledge Check Response Sheet and Answers,** on the Student Resource Disk or DavisPlus at http://davisplus.fadavis.com/Wilkinson2

 Critical**Thinking** 35-14

Why might it be more difficult to recognize a heart attack in a woman than in a man?

Diagnostic Testing

Diagnostic testing helps clinicians identify the causes of cardiovascular symptoms and monitor patient responses to treatment. We discuss several of these tests in the next sections. For others,

 Go to Chapter 35, **Diagnostic Testing: Tests Related to Oxygenation,** in Volume 2.

Tests of Blood Oxygenation

Pulse oximetry, capnography, and arterial blood gases were discussed in the Diagnostic Testing section in Part I of this chapter. You should understand, though, that results from all of those tests are pertinent to cardiac conditions. Remember: The heart and lungs work together to provide oxygenation; a problem in one creates a problem in the other. The Critical Aspects box explains the use of pulse oximetry. For the complete procedure,

 Go to Chapter 35, **Procedure 35-2: Monitoring Pulse Oximetry (Arterial Oxygen Saturation),** and **Clinical Insight 35-2: Tips for Obtaining Accurate Pulse Oximetry Readings,** in Volume 2.

To review (and use in clinical assignments) arterial blood gas values and other tests of blood oxygenation, respectively,

 Go to Chapter 35, **Diagnostic Testing: Arterial Blood Gas Values: Evaluating Adequacy of Oxygenation,** and **Diagnostic Testing: Tests Related to Oxygenation,** in Volume 2.

Cardiac Monitoring

Cardiac monitoring is the continuous monitoring of the **electrocardiogram (ECG),** a rendering of the electrical activity of the heart. Three to five electrodes placed on the skin of the chest display a waveform on a monitor screen or printout (Fig. 35-21). The ECG illustrates electrical activity, but not mechanical activity. In other words, the ECG reflects what the nerves are telling the heart muscle to do, but *not* what the heart muscle is actually doing in response.

The purposes of cardiac monitoring are to:

- Identify the patient's baseline rhythm and rate.
- Recognize significant changes in the baseline rhythm and rate.
- Recognize lethal dysrhythmias that require immediate intervention.

The ECG reading illustrates the complete cardiac cycle. Each part of the ECG complex has been given a letter to identify it: **P, Q, R, S,** and **T** (see Fig. 35-19).

- The **P wave** represents the firing of the SA node and conduction of the impulse through the atria. In the healthy heart, this leads to atrial contraction.
- The **QRS complex** represents *ventricular depolarization* and leads to ventricular contraction.
- The **T wave** represents the return of the ventricles to an electrical resting state so they can be stimulated

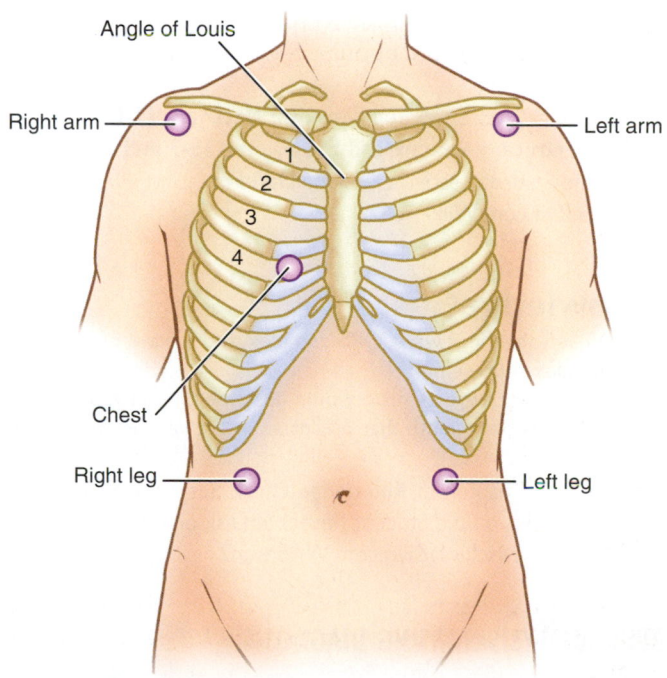

FIGURE 35-21 Electrodes placed for continuous cardiac monitoring.

again (*ventricular repolarization*). The atria also repolarize, but they do so during the time of ventricular depolarization; thus, they are obscured by the QRS complex and cannot be seen on the ECG complex.

Dysrhythmias are abnormal heart rhythms. Dysrhythmias can be broadly categorized according to rhythm as follows:

Tachydysrhythmias—Rates > 100 beats/min
Bradydysrhythmias—Rates < 60 beats/min
Ectopy—extra beats

Within each or those categories, dysrhythmias can be further classified by their site of origin:

Supraventricular—Above the ventricles
Junctional—Within the AV node
Ventricular—In the ventricles

Note that a tachy- or bradydysrhythmia depends on the patient's baseline heart rate. Some people have a low resting heart rate (less than 60 beats/min) without distress. Keep this in mind before assuming that the heart rate is abnormal.

All dysrhythmias have the potential to decrease cardiac output, resulting in hypotension and tissue hypoxia. Skill in identifying cardiac rhythms (both normal and abnormal) requires study and experience and is beyond the scope of this chapter. However, the Critical Aspects box highlights activities involved with the care of a patient requiring a cardiac monitor. For the complete procedure,

 Go to Chapter 35, **Procedure 35-3: Performing Cardiac Monitoring,** in Volume 2.

In contrast to cardiac monitoring, *electrocardiography* uses 12 "leads" (views of the heart). These are done by specially trained nurses or technicians. If you are interested in reading more about 12-lead ECGs,

 Go to Chapter 35, **Supplemental Materials, 12-Lead Electrocardiography,** and **ESG Figures 35-7 and 35-8,** on the Student Resource Disk or DavisPlus at http://davisplus.fadavis.com/Wilkinson2

KnowledgeCheck 35-19

- What does the P wave, QRS complex, and T wave of an ECG complex represent?
- What kind of dysrhythmia would describe a heart rate of 140 beats per minute that originates in the ventricles?

 Go to Chapter 35, **Knowledge Check Response Sheet and Answers,** on the Student Resource Disk or DavisPlus at http://davisplus.fadavis.com/Wilkinson2

ANALYSIS/NURSING DIAGNOSIS

Several nursing diagnoses address impaired circulation and tissue or organ hypoxia. They are briefly discussed below. For additional information,

 Go to Chapter 35, **Standardized Language, Nursing Diagnoses Associated with Impaired Circulation,** in Volume 2.

- *Decreased Cardiac Output* is the appropriate diagnosis when the heart is unable to pump adequate amounts of blood to meet the metabolic demands of the body. Definitive interventions for this problem are collaborative.
- *Ineffective Tissue Perfusion (Renal, Cerebral, Cardiopulmonary, Gastrointestinal, or Peripheral)* is appropriate for a patient experiencing poor perfusion to an organ or tissue, specifically, for a patient experiencing organ dysfunction rather than the overall effects of poor circulation that are evident with decreased cardiac output.
- *Risk for Shock* should be used for patients who have inadequate blood flow to body tissues that may lead to life-threatening cellular dysfunction (e.g., patients with sepsis and hypovolemia).

Cardiovascular functioning can also be the etiology of other nursing diagnoses, such as the following examples:

- Risk for Activity Intolerance related to decreased oxygen-carrying capacity of the blood secondary to anemia
- Acute Pain secondary to myocardial ischemia
- Anxiety related to shortness of breath
- Death Anxiety related to diagnosis of myocardial infarction (heart attack)
- Ineffective Coping related to hospitalization for oxygenation impairment

■ PLANNING OUTCOMES/EVALUATION

NOC standardized outcomes and evaluation criteria related to cardiovascular status are included in the Cardiopulmonary class of NOC Domain II: Physiologic Health. They include the following: Blood Loss Severity, Cardiac Pump Effectiveness, Circulation Status, Tissue Perfusion (Abdominal Organs, Cardiac, Peripheral, Pulmonary), and Vital Signs.

Individualized goals/outcome statements depend on the nursing diagnosis you identify. For diagnoses related to cardiac function or circulation, the following are examples of goals you might write:

- No dyspnea or shortness of breath
- Heart rate in expected range
- Peripheral pulses strong and equal bilaterally
- Brisk capillary refill
- Normal skin color (no pallor or cyanosis)

■ PLANNING INTERVENTIONS/IMPLEMENTATION

NIC standardized interventions related to the cardiovascular system are found in NIC Domain 2: Physiological Interventions: Complex, in the subcategory of Tissue Perfusion Management. Tissue Perfusion Management focuses on optimizing circulation. For examples of NOC outcomes and NIC interventions for selected oxygenation nursing diagnoses,

 Go to Chapter 35, **Standardized Language, Examples of NOC Outcomes and NIC Interventions Linked to Oxygenation Diagnoses,** in Volume 2.

These provide a general care planning guide. Depending on individual patient needs, other NOC outcomes or NIC interventions may also be appropriate.

Specific nursing interventions for patients with cardiovascular problems focus on relieving anxiety, promoting circulation, administering medications, and performing cardiopulmonary resuscitation (CPR).

Manage Anxiety

Almost everyone who experiences dyspnea or chest pain becomes anxious—some, extremely so. It is important to reduce anxiety because anxiety activates the sympathetic nervous system and triggers the stress response. Hormone changes occur, including the release of aldosterone, which promotes fluid retention and increases blood pressure. The heart rate and contraction force increase; peripheral and visceral vessels constrict, and the blood clots more readily. All of these make a cardiac or vascular condition more serious.

Prioritize your interventions. You will, of course, need to intervene first to prevent life-threatening situations. But try not to appear rushed, and speak calmly and quietly to the patient and to those around you. Do not leave the patient alone. Provide clear factual information and keep the patient and family informed about treatments being given. Many patients are reassured by the presence of a family member. If you need a review of detailed information about assessments and interventions for anxious patients, go to Chapter 11.

Promote Circulation

Adequate circulation ensures that oxygenated blood reaches tissues and organs and that venous blood returns to the heart. Two important nursing interventions are to promote venous return and prevent clot formation.

Promote Venous Return

Measures that promote venous return increase the flow of blood back to the vena cava and the right side of the heart.

- Elevate the patient's legs above the level of the heart. Gravity promotes venous return from the feet and legs.
- Flexion of the hips, legs, and knees constricts the veins and slows venous blood flow. If one is available, have the patient sit in a recliner that elevates the legs rather than sitting upright in a chair with legs elevated on a stool.
- Teach patients to avoid sitting with the legs crossed; this interferes with blood flow.
- Encourage and support early and frequent ambulation (e.g., after surgery). Contraction of the muscles in the legs moves blood upward against gravity.
- Encourage or provide range-of-motion (ROM) exercises, which increase venous blood flow through rhythmic massaging of the veins by the active muscles (see Chapter 31 to review ROM).
- Apply compression devices. *Antiembolism stockings (TED hose)* are elastic stockings that compress superficial leg veins and promote venous return. *Sequential compression devices (SCDs),* also called *pneumatic compression devices,* are cuffs that surround the legs and alternately inflate and deflate to promote venous return to the heart. Antiembolism stockings and SCDs are frequently used in perioperative patients to promote venous return and prevent clot formation. See Chapter 37 for further discussion and instructions on how to apply these stockings and appropriate follow-up care.

 Go to Chapter 37, **Procedure 37-2: Applying Antiembolism Stockings,** in Volume 2.

Prevent Clot Formation

A **thrombus** is a stationary clot adhering to the wall of a vessel. An **embolus** is a clot that travels in the bloodstream. Clots can form after injury to vessels, or in response to hypercoagulability. Of course, all the strategies to promote venous return also help prevent clot formation.

- Turn patients frequently; teach patients to change positions frequently. This prevents vessel injury from prolonged pressure in one position.
- Use scrupulous sterile technique when inserting or handling intravenous lines. This prevents infection that can damage the vessel lumens.
- Be sure intravenous medications are adequately diluted. This prevents chemical irritation of veins during IV medication therapy.
- Promote adequate hydration (i.e., monitor intake and output, assess hydration, manage fluid intake, teach patients to drink plenty of fluids). Unless contraindicated, adult fluid intake should be approximately 2000 mL per day to keep urine output around 1500 mL per day. Adequate hydration keeps respiratory secretions thin but also keeps the blood from becoming viscous ("thick"). Viscous blood clots more readily.
- Promote smoking cessation. Nicotine increases the risk for thrombus formation because of its constricting effects on vessel walls.
- Patients at particularly high risk for thrombus formation may receive anticoagulant therapy to help prevent abnormal clot formation.

Toward Evidence-Based Practice

Wood, S., & Nghiem, H. (2007). Raw garlic and garlic supplements offer no effect on lipids. *Archives of Internal Medicine, 167,* 125–126, 346–353.

Researchers randomly divided 192 adults with low-density lipoprotein (LDL) cholesterol concentrations of 130 to 190 mg/dL into four groups. One group received treatment with raw garlic, another with powdered garlic supplement, another with garlic extract, and another with placebo. None of the forms of garlic used had statistically or clinically significant effects on LDL cholesterol or other plasma lipids.

Jenkins, D., Kendall, C., Faulkner, D., et al. (2008). Long-term effects of a plant-based dietary portfolio of cholesterol-lowering foods on blood pressure. *European Journal of Clinical Nutrition, 62,* 781–788.

The intent of this study was to determine the effect of a cholesterol-lowering diet on blood pressure. Sixty-six subjects who had high blood lipid levels and hypertension were followed for 1 year. They consumed a diet of plant-based, cholesterol-lowering foods. Those who complied with almond intake advice experienced significant reduction in blood pressure; the rest did not.

Sesso, H., Buring, J., Christen, W., et al. (2008). Vitamins E and C in the prevention of cardiovascular disease in men. *JAMA, 300*(18). Retrieved from http://jama.ama-assn.org/cgi/content/full/300/18/2123.

This 10-year longitudinal research evaluated 14,641 men at low risk of cardiovascular disease to determine whether long-term vitamin E or vitamin C supplementation decreases the risk of major cardiovascular events among men. They concluded that there was no support for the use of these supplements for prevention of cardiovascular disease in middle-aged and older men.

Spangler, L., Newton, K., Grothaus, L., et al. (2007). The effects of black cohosh therapies on lipids, fibrinogen, glucose and insulin. *Maturitas, 57*(2), 195–204.

Black cohosh is an herb commonly used to treat menopausal symptoms. The researchers randomly assigned 351 peri- or postmenopausal women, 45 to 55 years old, either black cohosh, a multibotanical including black cohosh, a multibotanical plus soy diet counseling, estrogen, or placebo. Baseline blood lipids levels were established at the beginning of the study. At the end of 3 months, there were no differences among the herbal groups and placebo in total cholesterol, LDL, HDL, or triglycerides.

Use the information provided above as you answer the following questions:

1. If you had several risk factors for cardiovascular disease, specifically coronary artery disease, which of the following might help lower your risk? Explain your thinking.
   a. Taking a garlic supplement and cooking with garlic
   b. Eating a handful of almonds every day
   c. Taking vitamin E and vitamin C supplements daily
   d. Taking black cohosh every day

2. A male client says, "I've heard that black cohosh will help lower my cholesterol. Is that true?" Based on the Spangler study, how would you answer: Yes, no, I don't know? Explain your thinking.

 Go to Chapter 35, **Toward Evidence-Based Practice Suggested Responses,** on the Student Resource Disk or DavisPlus at http://davisplus.fadavis.com/Wilkinson2

Administer Medications

Cardiovascular medications are used to enhance cardiac output, thus providing increased blood flow and oxygenation to organs and tissues. They include vasodilators, beta-adrenergic blocking agents, diuretics, and positive inotropes.

- *Vasodilators* cause vessel dilatation, which eases the work of the heart. Drugs that dilate arterioles decrease the resistance against which the heart pumps (afterload). Drugs that dilate veins decrease venous return to the heart (preload). Vasodilators can cause hypotension, especially when the person rises from a sitting or lying position. Patients should be warned of this effect. You will need to monitor the patient's blood pressure and observe for symptoms of hypotension. Vasodilating agents include angiotensin-converting enzyme (ACE) inhibitors, angiotensin II receptor blockers, and nitrates.

- *Beta-adrenergic agents* block stimulation of beta receptors, which are located primarily in the heart, lungs, and blood vessels. Beta-1 selective agents are used to treat angina, acute myocardial infarction, and congestive heart failure (CHF). They decrease heart rate, slow conduction through the AV node, and decrease myocardial oxygen demand by reducing myocardial contractility.

- *Diuretics* increase removal of sodium and water from the body by increasing urine output. In patients with CHF, diuretics are used to reduce the volume of circulating blood and prevent accumulation of fluid in the pulmonary circulation.

- *Positive inotropes* increase cardiac contractility. They are used therapeutically to make the heart a more effective pump. The goal is to improve pumping effectiveness without creating excess heart work and oxygen demand. The two main classes of positive inotropes are cardiac glycosides and phosphodiesterase inhibitors.

Performing Cardiopulmonary Resuscitation

All of the previously discussed interventions, and those in Part I, are designed to promote circulation, ventilation, and gas exchange. However, the patient's condition can rapidly deteriorate. You must be prepared to perform *cardiopulmonary resuscitation (CPR)* in the event your patient experiences a respiratory, cardiac, or cardiopulmonary arrest. **Cardiac arrest** is the cessation of heart function. Signs of cardiac arrest are pale, cool, grayish skin; absence of femoral or carotid pulses; apnea; and pupil dilation. In the event of cardiac arrest, you have only 4 to 6 minutes before the brain is damaged by lack of oxygen. **Respiratory (pulmonary) arrest** is cessation of breathing. It can be caused by a blocked airway or occur after a cardiac arrest; it may be sudden or preceded by increasingly labored breathing.

CPR procedures are regularly updated as new knowledge is gained. The American Heart Association provides training sessions for healthcare professionals to become certified in CPR. This is a prerequisite for employment and clinical practice. We recommend you obtain CPR training from certified professionals. However, if you are already trained and just want to review the procedure,

 Go to Chapter 35, **ESG Procedure 35-1: Performing Cardiopulmonary Resuscitation, One- and Two-Person,** on the Student Resource Disk or DavisPlus at http://davisplus. fadavis.com/Wilkinson2

Key points of the most recent guidelines *for trained professionals* include the following:

- Focus on effective, uninterrupted chest compressions. Push hard, push fast in the center of the chest. About 100 compressions per minute
- 30 compressions to 2 breaths—for all victims except newborns

- Give breath over 1 second and make the chest rise visibly (Sayre, Berg, Cave, et al., 2008).

In-Hospital Arrests

All agencies have procedures (called a "Code Blue" in many agencies) for announcing cardiac or respiratory arrest, and there is usually an emergency alert system in the patient rooms in acute care facilities. Activating the alert system (e.g., by pulling down a handle) summons a code team, trained in CPR. However, you will probably need to begin CPR before they arrive. Begin CPR immediately after activating the alert, and use an automatic external defibrillator (AED) or manual defibrillator as soon as one is available. For a manual defibrillator, use a dose of 2 J/kg for the first shock and a dose of 4 J/kg for the second and subsequent shocks. Before beginning CPR, you are responsible for knowing whether your patient has an advance directive stating whether or not he would want CPR.

"Hands-Only™" CPR

The American Heart Association recommends different responses for laypersons, first responders, and CPR-trained professionals. The goal of these changes is to make it easier to learn, remember, and perform CPR. Referred to as "Hands-Only™" CPR, the method is recommended for people who see an adult collapse suddenly in the community. It has only two steps:

1. Call 911, or send someone to make the call.
2. Push hard and fast in the center of the victim's chest.

See Self-Care: Teaching Your Client Hands-Only™ CPR for a more detailed description of CPR that you can teach to lay persons.

Self-Care

Teaching Your Client Hands-Only™ CPR, for a Single Rescuer, Adult Victim

Witnessed Collapse

If you see an adult suddenly collapse in an "out-of-hospital" setting:

1. Call 911 (or send someone to do that).
2. Push hard and fast in the center of the chest (100 pumps per minute)
3. Continue until help arrives.

Unwitnessed Collapse

For an unwitnessed collapse of an adult victim:

1. Establish unresponsiveness (ask "Are you OK?")
2. Call 911 (or send someone to do it).
3. Obtain an AED, if possible.
4. Start traditional CPR, if you know how, while waiting for the AED.

Traditional CPR

1. When the AED arrives, turn it on for rhythm analysis.
2. After turning on the AED, open the airway (tilt the head, lift the chin).
3. Check for breathing.
4. Give two rescue breaths (each 1 second long). Look for chest movement, listen for breathing, and feel for air coming from the mouth or nose.
5. Administer one shock and wait for the AED to tell you what to do next.
6. When the AED says to continue CPR, start alternating 30 compressions with 2 breaths. Continue until help arrives. Stop only to check the AED for rhythm.

Remember: The most important action is to deliver uninterrupted, hard and fast chest compressions.

Source: American Heart Association (2008).

Rescuers should use Hands-Only™ CPR only for adults they observe to suddenly collapse. They should use CPR that combines breaths and compressions for:

Adults found already unconscious and not breathing normally

Victims of drowning or collapse due to breathing problems

All infants and children

KnowledgeCheck 35-20

- Identify three strategies that prevent clot formation.
- How do diuretics affect oxygenation?

 Go to Chapter 35, **Knowledge Check Response Sheet and Answers,** on the Student Resource Disk or DavisPlus at http://davisplus.fadavis.com/Wilkinson2

 Go to Chapter 35, **Resources for Caregivers and Health Professionals,** on the Student Resource Disk or DavisPlus at http://davisplus.fadavis.com/Wilkinson2

 Suggested Readings: Go to Chapter 35, **Reading More About Oxygenation,** on the Student Resource Disk or DavisPlus at http://davisplus.fadavis.com/Wilkinson2

 Bibliography: Go to Volume 2, Bibliography.

CHAPTER 36

Fluids, Electrolytes, & Acid–Base Balance

Learning Outcomes

After completing this chapter, you should be able to:

➤ Identify the fluid compartments within the body.

➤ Describe the location and function of the major electrolytes of the body.

➤ Differentiate among active and passive transport, osmosis, diffusion, and filtration.

➤ Describe the body mechanisms for maintaining fluid and electrolyte balance.

➤ Summarize the major fluid and electrolyte balance disorders.

➤ Describe respiratory and metabolic acidosis and alkalosis.

➤ Describe compensatory mechanisms for acid-base imbalances.

➤ Provide nursing interventions for clients with fluid, electrolyte, and acid-base imbalances.

Meet Your Patients

Your instructor has assigned you to care for Jackson LaGuardia, a 60-year-old man with end-stage renal disease. You have arrived at the hospital to review his chart so you can provide care the following day. When you arrive on the unit, the charge nurse informs you that Mr. LaGuardia is still in the emergency department (ED) while waiting to be admitted to the medical-surgical unit. You go to the ED to review his chart and gather data.

In the ED, you introduce yourself and explain your purpose. The charge nurse tells you that five members of the LaGuardia family have all come to the ED complaining of nausea, vomiting, and diarrhea related to severe gastroenteritis, a viral intestinal disorder. The family members include the following:

8-month-old Jason, grandson of Jackson
26-year-old Susanna, Jackson's daughter and Jason's mother

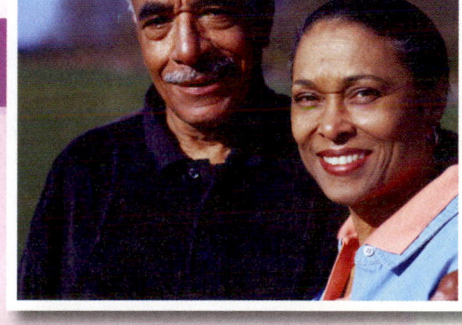

60-year-old Jackson
58-year-old Gemma, Jackson's wife
82-year-old Martha, Jackson's mother

Jason, Jackson, and Martha are being admitted to the hospital. However, Susanna and Gemma have been asked to follow up tomorrow in the urgent care clinic. As you prepare for your clinical day, you think, "If they all have the same disorder, why are only three family members being admitted? What makes these patients different?" In this chapter, we follow the LaGuardias and answer these questions.

Theoretical **Knowledge**
knowing why

In a healthy state, the fluid and chemical state of our bodies is in balance. However, illness can disturb this balance and threaten our existence. In this chapter, we examine how fluid, electrolyte, and acid–base balances are maintained, as well as what happens when there are disturbances in each of these areas.

Body Fluids

Body fluid is primarily water, with various dissolved substances. Gases, such as carbon dioxide and oxygen, readily dissolve in body fluids. In fact, body fluids transport gases throughout the body. Solid substances, called **solutes,** also dissolve in body fluids. Many solutes are **electrolytes**—substances (e.g., sodium, potassium) that develop an electrical charge when dissolved in water. Other solutes are nonelectrolytes. **Nonelectrolytes** (e.g., glucose, urea) do not conduct electricity. Body fluids perform several important functions:

- Maintain blood volume.
- Regulate body temperature.
- Transport material to and from cells.
- Serve as a medium for cellular metabolism.
- Assist with digestion of food.
- Serve as a medium for excreting waste.

Fluid makes up approximately 60% of an average adult's body weight. However, total body water content varies with the number of fat cells, age, and sex. Women have less body fluid than men because they have proportionately more body fat. An obese person has less fluid than a person of lean build. Body water progressively decreases with age. Table 36-1 demonstrates the distribution of fluid based on age and gender.

Table 36-1 ➤ Total Body Fluid in Relation to Sex and Age	
AGE	**TOTAL BODY FLUID (PERCENTAGE OF BODY WEIGHT)**
Full-term newborn	70–80%
1 year old	64%
Young adult	Men: 60%
	Women: 50%–55%
Middle adult	Men: 55%
	Women: 45%–50%
Older adult	Men: 50%
	Women: 45%

What Are the Body Fluids Compartments?

Most body fluid is contained within two compartments. **Intracellular fluid (ICF)** is contained within the cells. Essential for cell function and metabolism, it accounts for approximately 40% of body weight. **Extracellular fluid (ECF)** is outside the cells. ECF carries water, electrolytes, nutrients, and oxygen to the cells and removes the waste products of cellular metabolism. ECF accounts for 20% of body weight. ECF exists in three main locations in the body:

- *Interstitial fluid* lies in the spaces between the body cells. Excess fluid within the interstitial space is called edema.
- *Intravascular fluid* is the plasma within the blood. Its main function is to transport blood cells.
- *Transcellular fluid* includes specialized fluids, such as cerebrospinal, pleural, peritoneal, and synovial fluid; and digestive juices.

Figure 36-1 illustrates the distribution of body fluids. In times of illness, fluid may move into an area that makes it physiologically unavailable, such as the peritoneal space (a condition called *ascites*), the pericardial space (a condition called *pericardial effusion*), or the *vesicles* (blisters) produced by a burn wound. This type of fluid movement is known as **third spacing** because fluid is literally trapped in a third compartment—not within interstitial (cells) and not within intravascular spaces (blood vessels).

What Electrolytes Are Present in Body Fluids?

In addition to water, body fluid is composed of oxygen, carbon dioxide, dissolved nutrients, metabolic waste products, and electrolytes. Electrolytes that carry a positive charge are called **cations.** They include sodium (Na^+), potassium (K^+), calcium (Ca^{2+}), and magnesium (Mg^{2+}). Electrolytes that carry a negative charge are called **anions.** Examples are chloride (Cl^-), bicarbonate (HCO_3^-), phosphate (HPO_4^{2-}), and sulfate (SO_4^{2-}). Electrolytes are measured in milliequivalents per liter (mEq/L) of water or milligrams per 100 mL (mg/100 mL or mg/dL). Note that 1 dL, or deciliter, equals 100 mL. *Milliequivalent* is a measure of chemical combining power, whereas *milligram* is a weight measure.

The composition of body fluids varies between compartments:

- **In the ICF,** the major cations are potassium and magnesium. The major anion is phosphate. Other electrolytes are present, but to a lesser degree.
- **In the ECF,** the major electrolytes are sodium, chloride, and bicarbonate. Albumin is also present in the ECF, mostly in the intravascular fluid. Gastric and intestinal secretions (transcellular fluids) also contain electrolytes.

FIGURE 36-1 Normal distribution of body fluids. Transcellular fluid includes specialized fluids such as cerebrospinal and peritoneal fluid and digestive juices.

Severe electrolyte imbalances can occur if electrolytes move into a compartment they do not normally occupy or if they are lost in excess amounts from the body through perspiration, wounds, injury, or illness.

 KnowledgeCheck 36-1

- Define *solute, electrolyte, intracellular fluid, extracellular fluid, cation,* and *anion.*
- Identify the major electrolytes in the ICF and ECF.

 Go to Chapter 36, **Knowledge Check Response Sheet and Answers,** on the Student Resource Disk or DavisPlus at http://davisplus.fadavis.com/Wilkinson2

CriticalThinking 36-1

- Based on the information presented in the "Meet Your Patients" scenario, rank the members of the LaGuardia family based on total body water content.
- Does this information help you understand which family members were admitted to the hospital?

How Do Fluids and Electrolytes Move in the Body?

The selectively permeable membranes of cells and capillaries separate ICF and ECF (see Fig. 36-1). Fluid and electrolytes move across these membranes by passive and active mechanisms. In **active transport,** movement of fluid and solutes requires energy. **Passive transport** requires no energy. The three passive transport systems are osmosis, diffusion, and filtration. To see an animated illustration of these three systems,

 Go to **Animations: Osmosis, Diffusion, Filtration, and Active Transport** on DavisPlus at http://davisplus.fadavis. com/Wilkinson2

Osmosis

Osmosis involves movement of water (or other pure solute) across a membrane from an area of a less concentrated solution to an area of more concentrated solution. Water moves across the membrane to dilute the higher concentration of solutes (Fig. 36-2). Recall that a solute is a substance dissolved in body fluid. Solutes may be crystalloids or colloids. **Crystalloids** are solutes that readily dissolve (e.g., electrolytes). **Colloids** are larger molecules that do not dissolve readily (e.g., proteins).

The concentration of solutes providing pressure in body fluid is called **osmolality. Osmols** refers to the number of particles of solute per kilogram of water and

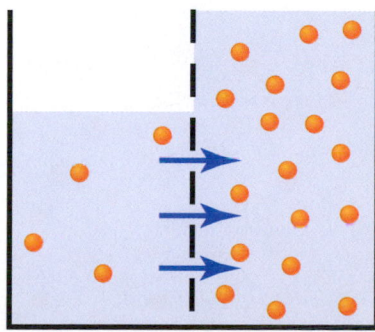

FIGURE 36-2 Osmosis is the movement of water across a membrane from a less concentrated solution to a more concentrated solution.

is expressed as milliosmoles per kilogram (mOsm/kg). Sodium is the greatest determinant of serum osmolality, and potassium is the greatest determinant of intracellular osmolality. Glucose and urea also contribute to osmolality in the ICF and ECF.

Another term for osmolality is **tonicity.** A fluid that is of the same osmolality as blood is called **isotonic.** An isotonic solution is often given by intravenous (IV) infusion if blood volume is low. Because the solution is the same concentration as blood, the fluid will remain in the vascular space, and no osmosis will occur. A **hypotonic solution** is of lower osmolality than blood. When a hypotonic solution is infused, water moves by osmosis from the vascular system into the cells. A **hypertonic solution** contains a higher concentration of solutes than does blood. When a hypertonic solution is given to a patient, water moves by osmosis from the cells into the ECF.

Diffusion

Diffusion is a passive process by which molecules of a solute move through a cell membrane from an area of higher concentration to an area of lower concentration. Movement occurs (Fig. 36-3) until the concentrations are equivalent on both sides of the membrane. For an example of diffusion, pour yourself a cup of coffee. Now add cream to the coffee. Initially, the cream is concentrated in the area where you have poured it. However, within a short time the cream is evenly dispersed throughout the coffee. If you stir the coffee, the cream disperses even more quickly. Fluids within the human body work on a similar principle; movement of the body speeds the diffusion of molecules.

The rate of diffusion varies according to the size of the molecules, the concentration of the solution, and the temperature of the solution. Small molecules move more rapidly than larger molecules. Large discrepancies in concentration require a longer period of time to reach equilibration. Higher temperatures cause molecules to move faster, so that diffusion occurs more rapidly.

Filtration

Filtration is the movement of both water and smaller particles from an area of high pressure to one of low pressure (Fig. 36-4). **Hydrostatic pressure** is the force created by fluid within a closed system; it is responsible for normal circulation of blood. In other words, blood flows from the high-pressure arterial system to the lower pressure capillaries and veins. As fluid (plasma) moves through the capillary membrane, only solutes of a certain size can flow with it. For example, the membrane pores of Bowman's capsule in the kidneys are very small, and only albumin, the smallest of the proteins, can be filtered through the membrane. By contrast, the membrane pores of liver cells are extremely large, so a variety of solutes can pass through and be metabolized.

Osmotic pressure is the power of a solution to draw water. A highly concentrated solution (with many molecules in solution) draws water and has a high osmotic pressure. The plasma proteins in the blood exert osmotic, or colloidal, pressure to help maintain fluid in the vascular space. However, when hydrostatic pressure exceeds osmotic pressure, fluid leaves the vessels. This difference, known as the **filtration pressure,** represents the net pressures that move fluid and solutes.

Active Transport

Active transport occurs when molecules (e.g., electrolytes) move across cell membranes from an area of low concentration to an area of high concentration. Active transport requires energy expenditure for the movement to occur against a concentration gradient (Fig. 36-5). Adenosine triphosphate (ATP) is released from the cell to enable certain substances to acquire the energy needed to pass through the cell membrane. For example, sodium concentration is greater in ECF; therefore, sodium tends to enter by diffusion into the intracellular compartment. This tendency is offset by the sodium-potassium pump, which is located on the cell membrane. In the presence of ATP, the sodium-potassium pump actively moves sodium from the cell into the ECF. Active transport is vital

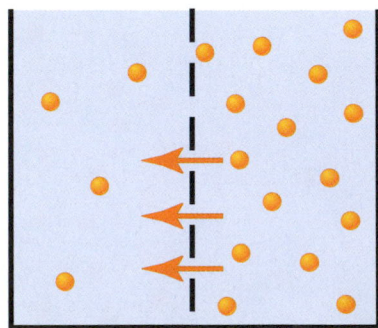

FIGURE 36-3 Diffusion is the movement of molecules of a solute through a cell membrane from an area of higher concentration to an area of lower concentration.

FIGURE 36-4 Filtration is the movement of water and smaller particles from an area of high pressure to an area of low pressure.

FIGURE 36-5 Active transport is the movement of electrolytes against a concentration gradient. For the movement to occur, active transport requires energy expenditure.

for maintaining the unique composition of both the extracellular and intracellular compartments.

Table 36-2 summarizes the processes of fluid and electrolyte movement.

KnowledgeCheck 36-2

Identify the appropriate mechanism: osmosis, diffusion, filtration, or active transport:

■ Molecules move across a membrane to equalize concentration.
■ Fluid moves across a membrane to equalize concentration.
■ Molecules move against a concentration gradient.
■ Molecules move to equalize pressure.

 Go to Chapter 36, **Knowledge Check Response Sheet and Answers,** on the Student Resource Disk or DavisPlus at http://davisplus.fadavis.com/Wilkinson2

How Does the Body Regulate Fluids?

A balance between fluid intake and output is essential to maintain homeostasis. Excesses or deficits of intake or output can lead to severe disorders.

Fluid Intake

You have undoubtedly been told to drink eight to ten glasses of water per day. Did you ever wonder where that recommendation came from or why that volume is important? Eight to ten 8-ounce glasses of water provide 1920 to 2400 mL of fluid. The Institute of Medicine (IOM) (2004), however, recommends a total fluid intake of 2700 mL per day for women and 3700 mL per day for men. This is higher than the previous recommendation of 2500 mL per day for the average adult engaged in moderate activity in moderate temperature, which you may have learned in a biology class. The IOM states we should obtain 80% of our intake from drinking fluids and the remaining 20% from food and cellular metabolism of foods. Prolonged exercise and heat exposure increase the requirements. The IOM did not set an upper limit on fluid intake.

Habit and culture influence fluid intake. However, thirst is the major regulator. Changes in plasma osmolality signal the thirst center in the hypothalamus, which leads to the urge to drink. Situations that increase plasma osmolality (and promote thirst) include excessive fluid loss, excessive sodium intake, and decreased fluid intake. Situations that inhibit the thirst mechanism include a high intake of fluids, fluid retention, excessive IV infusion of hypotonic solutions, and low sodium intake.

Fluid Output

Fluid loss occurs throughout the day, creating a constant need to replenish fluid. In a healthy state, fluid losses are equivalent to fluid intake. **Sensible fluid loss** is measurable and perceived (e.g., urine, diarrhea, ostomy, and gastric drainage). **Insensible fluid loss** is loss that we do not perceive and that is not easily measured. It occurs primarily by diffusion and evaporation through the skin, but also from the lungs, and accounts for about 900 mL per day. Insensible loss increases with open wounds, burns, or other breaks in the protective layer of the skin.

The following are common sources of fluid loss:

■ *Urine* (1500 mL/day). Urine accounts for the greatest amount of fluid loss. Urine output varies according to intake and activity, but should remain at least 30 to 50 mL/hour. The volume of urine increases as intake increases, and it decreases to compensate for other fluid losses (e.g., vomiting and excessive perspiration).
■ *Feces* (100 to 200 mL/day). Soft stools contain more water than hard stools. As stool frequency increases, water loss also increases.
■ *Skin* (about 600 mL/day). **Sensible (perceived) fluid loss** through the skin occurs through perspiration, at 300 to 600 mL/day. Perspiration varies based on temperature, skeletal muscle activity, and metabolic

Table 36-2 ▶ Processes of Fluid and Electrolyte Movement			
PROCESS	**WHAT MOVES**	**FROM AREA OF**	**TO AREA OF**
Diffusion	Molecules (solute)	High concentration	Low concentration
Active transport	Molecules (solute)	Low concentration	High concentration
Osmosis	Water	Low concentration	High concentration
Filtration	Water and small particles	High pressure	Low pressure

activity. Fever, exercise, and some disease processes increase metabolic activity and heat production, leading to increased fluid loss.

■ *Lungs* (about 300 mL/day). Insensible loss occurs through the lungs as water is exhaled with the breath. An increase in respiratory rate increases the amount of fluid lost.

Hormonal Regulation

The kidneys are the principal regulator of fluid and electrolyte balance. The following hormones are involved:

Antidiuretic Hormone. Pressure sensors in the vascular system stimulate or inhibit the release of **antidiuretic hormone (ADH)** from the pituitary gland. ADH causes the kidneys to retain fluid. If fluid volume within the vascular system is low, fluid pressures within the system decrease, and more ADH is released. If fluid volume (and therefore pressure) increases, less ADH is released, and the kidneys eliminate more fluid. ADH is also produced in response to a rise in serum osmolality, fever, pain, stress, and some opioids.

Renin–Angiotensin System. When extracellular (i.e., intravascular) fluid volume is decreased, receptors in the glomeruli respond to the decreased perfusion of the kidneys by releasing renin. **Renin** is an enzyme responsible for the chain of reactions that converts angiotensinogen to angiotensin II. **Angiotensin II** acts on the nephrons to retain sodium and water and directs the adrenal cortex to release aldosterone.

Aldosterone. When aldosterone is released, it stimulates the distal tubules of the kidneys to reabsorb sodium and excrete potassium. Sodium reabsorption results in passive reabsorption of water, thereby increasing plasma volume and improving kidney perfusion. When fluid excess is present, renin is not released, and this process stops.

Other Hormones. *(1) Thyroid hormone* affects fluid volume by influencing cardiac output. An increase in thyroid hormone causes an increase in cardiac output, thereby increasing glomerular filtration rate and urine output. A decrease has the opposite effect. *(2) Atrial natriuretic peptide (ANP), brain natriuretic peptide (BNP),* and *C-type natriuretic peptide (CNP)* are important in renal and cardiovascular regulation of fluid maintenance. **Natriuresis** (natriuretic) is the discharge of sodium through urine. BNP is actually released from both the brain and the right atrium. In clinical practice, BNP can be measured in the serum to help determine presence of heart failure with fluid excess and to distinguish heart failure from pulmonary edema. The test can be performed at the bedside.

Critical**Thinking** 36-2

Apply the information on fluid balance to the LaGuardia family ("Meet Your Patients"). What have you learned that helps you explain why some family members require hospitalization? What additional information do you need to be able to predict each person's fluid balance?

How Does the Body Regulate Electrolytes?

To maintain health, the body must balance electrolyte losses and intake. For example, potassium lost through diarrhea and vomiting must be replaced by dietary potassium or potassium supplements. Table 36-3 provides information about the function, regulation, and food sources of major electrolytes in the body. The body has various mechanisms for regulating electrolyte balance, which are discussed later in this chapter. Maintenance of normal serum levels also depends on dietary intake, discussed in the remainder of this section.

Sodium (Na⁺)

Sodium is the major cation in the ECF. Its primary function is to regulate fluid volume. When sodium is reabsorbed in the kidney, water and potassium are also reabsorbed, thereby maintaining ECF volume. According to the 2004 Dietary References Intake report, a healthy adult between the ages of 19 and 50 should consume 1.5 grams of sodium and 2.3 grams of chloride each day—or 3.8 grams of salt—to replace daily losses and maintain serum blood levels. Intake should not exceed 5.8 grams per day. However, among persons 31 to 50 years of age, more than 95% of American men, 90% of Canadian men, 75% of American women, and 50% of Canadian women regularly consume salt in excess of 5.8 g/day. In short, most people eat too much salt. Older adults; African Americans; and people with chronic diseases including hypertension, diabetes, and kidney disease are especially sensitive to the blood pressure raising effects of salt. As a result, they are advised to limit salt to 2.0 g/day (IOM, 2004), just about the amount needed to maintain serum blood levels.

Potassium (K⁺)

Potassium is the major cation of the ICF; only 2% of body potassium is found in the extracellular fluid. Potassium is a key electrolyte in cellular metabolism. The 2004 Dietary References Intake (DRI) report (IOM, 2004) recommends that adults consume at least 4.7 grams of potassium per day. However, most American and Canadian women ages 31 to 50 years consume less than half of the recommended amount of potassium, and intake is only moderately higher for men. In short, most people do not consume enough potassium. Moderate potassium deficiency is associated with increased blood pressure, increased salt sensitivity, increased risk of kidney stones, and increased risk of bone turnover. Because of its effect on blood pressure, low intake of dietary potassium is associated with increased risk of stroke.

The DRIs do not specify an upper limit of potassium intake because there is no evidence of problems associated with higher potassium intake (IOM, 2004). In a healthy person, a high potassium intake does not

Table 36-3 ➤ Major Electrolytes

ELECTROLYTE	FUNCTION	REGULATION	SOURCES
Sodium (Na⁺) Major cation in the ECF Normal serum level = 135–145 mEq/L	Regulates fluid volume. Helps maintain blood volume. Interacts with calcium to maintain muscle contraction. Stimulates conduction of nerve impulses.	Moves by active transport across cell membranes. Regulated by aldosterone and ADH levels Reabsorbed and excreted through the kidneys Minimal loss through perspiration and feces Low sodium may be caused by excess water intake.	Table salt, soy sauce, cured pork, cheese, milk, processed foods, canned products, and foods preserved with salt
Potassium (K⁺) Major cation in the ICF Normal serum level = 3.5–5 mEq/L	Maintains ICF osmolality. Regulates conduction of cardiac rhythm. Transmits electrical impulses in multiple body systems. Assists with acid–base balance.	Regulated by aldosterone Excreted and conserved through the kidneys Lost through vomiting and diarrhea Loss triggered by many diuretics	Common food sources include bananas, oranges, apricots, figs, dates, carrots, potatoes, tomatoes, spinach, dairy products, and meats.
Calcium (Ca²⁺) Most abundant electrolyte in the body Normal serum level = 8.5–10.5 mg/dL	Promotes transmission of nerve impulses. Major component of bone and teeth Regulates muscle contractions. Maintains cardiac automaticity. Essential factor in the formation of blood clots Catalyst for many cellular activities	Combines with phosphorus to form the mineral salts of the teeth and bones. Calcium and phosphorus levels inversely proportional Parathyroid hormone (PTH) stimulates release of calcium from bones and reabsorption from kidneys and intestines. Calcitonin (from the thyroid) blocks bone breakdown and lowers calcium levels. Absorption stimulated by vitamin D	See Table 36-4 for average daily requirements. Common food sources include milk, milk products, dark green leafy vegetables, and salmon, as well as calcium-fortified foods such as breads and cereals.
Magnesium (Mg²⁺) Present in skeleton and ICF; second most abundant cation in ICF Normal serum level = 1.6–2.6 mEq/L	Involved in protein and carbohydrate metabolism Necessary for protein and DNA synthesis within the cell Maintains normal intracellular levels of potassium Involved in electrical activity in nerve and muscle membranes, including the heart May have a role in regulating blood pressure and may influence the release and activity of insulin (IOM, 2004).	Ingested in the diet and absorbed through the small intestine Excreted by kidneys Loss may be triggered by diuretics, poorly controlled diabetes mellitus, and excess alcohol intake.	Average daily requirement is 18–30 mEq. Found in most foods, but high levels are present in green vegetables, cereal grains, and nuts.
Chloride (Cl⁻) Major anion in the ECF Normal serum level = 95–105 mEq/L	Works with Na⁺ to maintain osmotic pressure between fluid compartments. Essential for production of HCl for gastric secretions Functions as buffer in oxygen–carbon dioxide exchange in RBCs. Assists with acid–base balance.	Reabsorbed and excreted through the kidneys along with sodium Regulated by aldosterone and ADH levels Deficits lead to potassium deficits; potassium deficits lead to chloride deficits.	Found in foods high in sodium

Continued

Table 36-3 ➤ Major Electrolytes—cont'd

ELECTROLYTE	FUNCTION	REGULATION	SOURCES
Phosphate (PO_4^-) Major anion in the ICF Normal serum level = 1.7–2.6 mEq/L	Serves as a catalyst for many intracellular activities Promotes muscle and nerve action Assists with acid–base balance Important for cell division and transmission of hereditary traits	Combines with calcium to form the mineral salts of the teeth and bones Calcium and phosphorus levels inversely proportional Regulated by PTH; has inverse response to calcium Excreted and reabsorbed by the kidneys	Foods high in phosphorus are meat, fish, poultry, milk products, carbonated beverages, and legumes. Readily available in body as a result of metabolism
Bicarbonate (HCO_3^-) Major buffer in the body In ECF and ICF Normal serum level = 22–26 mEq/L	Maintains acid–base balance by functioning as the primary buffer in the body	Lost through diarrhea, diuretics, renal insufficiency Excess possible if person ingests quantities of acid neutralizers	Present in acid neutralizers (e.g., sodium bicarbonate)

result in a high serum potassium level (hyperkalemia) because the kidneys efficiently eliminate excess dietary potassium.

Calcium (Ca^{2+})

Calcium is responsible for bone health and neuromuscular and cardiac function. It is also an essential factor in blood clotting. About 99% of body calcium is located in the bones and teeth. The remaining 1% circulates in the blood and affects system functions. Because calcium is so vital for cardiac and muscle function, serum levels are tightly regulated. As serum levels drop, calcium leaches from the bones into the blood to compensate. If dietary intake is not sufficient to replace it, bone loss occurs; prolonged deficiencies lead to osteoporosis.

Half the women older than age 50 and 90% of women older than age 75 have osteoporosis; about 30% of men older than age 50 are affected. About half of all Caucasian women will suffer an osteoporosis-related fracture at some point in life, as will approximately one in five men. Because most Americans do not include the recommended amount of calcium in their diets, the chances of bone loss increase with age. Most calcium should be obtained from naturally calcium-rich foods, such as dairy products. Calcium-fortified foods and calcium supplements can be used as a secondary source. Calcium requirements are highest during childhood, adolescence, pregnancy, and breastfeeding. People who are immobile are at increased risk for reduced bone density. Older adults are at risk for calcium deficiencies because of reduced absorption that occurs with aging and chronic medical conditions (National Osteoporosis Foundation, 2008; U.S. Department of Health and Human Services, 2004, 2009). For recommended calcium intake by age group, see Table 36-4.

Magnesium (Mg^{2+})

Magnesium is a mineral used in more than 300 biochemical reactions in the body. Like calcium, only about 1% of magnesium is found in the blood. The remaining 99% is divided between the ICF and bone (in combination with calcium and phosphorus). Although magnesium deficiency is rare, you may find low levels in individuals who have a high alcohol intake. Some malabsorption disorders may also cause magnesium depletion.

Chloride (Cl^-)

Chloride is the most abundant anion in the extracellular fluid. It is usually bound with other ions, especially sodium or potassium (e.g., as sodium chloride, or salt). A healthy adult between the ages of 19 and 50 should consume 2.3 grams of chloride each day along with 1.5 grams of sodium to replace daily losses and maintain serum blood levels (IOM, 2004).

Phosphorus (Phosphate [PO_4^-])

Most phosphorus in the body is combined with oxygen, forming phosphate—mostly bound with calcium in teeth and bones as calcium phosphate. Phosphate is the most abundant intracellular anion. Phosphate and calcium exist in an inverse relationship; as one increases, the other one decreases. As a result, high blood phosphate levels decrease the movement of calcium from the bones. Phosphate in the ECF is known as **phosphorus.**

Bicarbonate (HCO_3^-)

Bicarbonate is present in both ICF and ECF. The kidneys regulate extracellular bicarbonate to maintain acid–base balance. When serum levels rise, the kidneys excrete

Table 36-4 ➤ Recommended Daily Calcium Intake

AGE	DIETARY REFERENCE INTAKE (DRI) FOR CALCIUM (MILLIGRAMS)	VITAMIN D* (INTERNATIONAL UNITS)
Birth to 6 months	210	200
6–12 months	270	200
1–3 years	500	200
4–8 years	800	200
9–18 years	1300	200
19–50 years	1000	200
51–70 years	1200	800–1000
Older than 70 years	1200	800–1000
Pregnant or Lactating Women		
18 years or younger pregnant or lactating	1300	200
19-50 years	1000	200

*Adequate intake of Vitamin D is necessary for absorption of calcium.
Source: National Guideline Clearinghouse (NGC) (2010). Screening for osteoporosis in the adult U.S. population: ACPM position statement on preventive practice. In: National Guideline Clearinghouse (NGC) [website]. Rockville, MD. Retrieved July 19, 2010, from http://www.guideline.gov/summary/summary.aspx?view_id=1&doc_id=15270; USDA (2004) Dietary Reference Intakes: Recommended Intakes for Individuals. National Academy of Sciences. Retrieved from http://www.iom.edu/Global/News%20Announcements/~/media/48FAAA2FD9E74D95BBDA2236E7387B49.ashx

excess bicarbonate. If serum levels are low, the kidneys conserve bicarbonate. Bicarbonate is not consumed in the diet but is produced by the body to meet current needs.

KnowledgeCheck 36-3

- Identify the major functions of sodium, potassium, calcium, magnesium, chloride, phosphate, and bicarbonate.
- What are the major concerns associated with sodium and potassium intake?
- Identify at least five potassium-rich foods.
- Identify the ideal calcium intakes for each member of the LaGuardia family ("Meet Your Patients").

  Go to Chapter 36, **Knowledge Check Response Sheet and Answers,** on the Student Resource Disk or DavisPlus at http://davisplus.fadavis.com/Wilkinson2

CriticalThinking 36-3

Based on the information you have learned about the major electrolytes of the body, which electrolytes are most likely to be out of balance in members of the LaGuardia family? Explain your answer.

How Is Acid–Base Balance Regulated?

Acids and bases are formed in the body as part of normal metabolic processes. An **acid** is any compound that contains hydrogen ions (H^+) that can be released. For this reason, acids are referred to as cation donors. A common strong acid is hydrochloric acid (HCl), which is present in gastric secretions. A **base** or **alkali** is a compound that combines with (accepts) hydrogen ions in solution. Therefore, bases are referred to as cation (a positively charged particle) acceptors. A strong base has a tendency to bind hydrogen ions, whereas a weak base binds only a small portion of the available hydrogen ions.

The amount of acid or base present in a solution is measured as **pH**. The pH is reported on a scale of 1 to 14: 1 to 6.9 is acidic, 7 is neutral, and 7.1 to 14 is basic, or alkaline. The stronger an acid, the lower the pH. In contrast, a strong base has a high pH. The pH is a *logarithmic* scale. For example, a pH of 4 is 10 times more acidic than a pH of 5. The body functions normally within a narrow range of pH values. Arterial blood and tissue fluid normally have a pH of 7.35 to 7.45; therefore, they are slightly alkaline. A serum pH below 7.30 or above 7.52 alters enzymatic activity and creates myocardial irritability. A serum pH below 6.9 or above 7.8 is usually fatal. Three complex mechanisms maintain acid–base balance: (1) buffers, (2) respiratory control of carbon dioxide, and (3) renal regulation of bicarbonate (HCO_3^-).

Buffers

Buffer systems prevent wide swings in pH. A buffer system consists of a weak acid and a weak base. Buffer molecules keep strong acids or bases from altering the pH either by absorbing or releasing free hydrogen ions.

Carbonic Acid–Sodium Bicarbonate System. Carbonic acid (H_2CO_3) and sodium bicarbonate ($NaHCO_3$) buffer almost 90% of metabolic processes in the ECF. Blood and tissue fluid depend on this buffer system to maintain a relatively constant pH. During normal metabolism, blood and tissue fluids tend to become acidic; therefore, more sodium bicarbonate is required than carbonic acid. The usual ratio of $NaHCO_3$ to H_2CO_3 is 20:1. As long as this ratio is maintained, the pH remains within its normal range. If bicarbonate is depleted while neutralizing a strong acid, the pH may drop below 7.35, resulting in a condition called **acidosis.** If a strong base is added to extracellular fluid and depletes carbonic acid, the pH may rise above 7.45, resulting in a condition called **alkalosis.**

Phosphate System. The phosphate system helps regulate acid–base balance in intracellular fluids. The phosphate system works in the same way as the bicarbonate system but converts alkaline sodium phosphate (Na_2HPO_4) to acid sodium phosphate (NaH_2PO_4).

Protein System. Plasma proteins and the globin portion of hemoglobin (in red blood cells) contain chemical groups that can either combine with or free up hydrogen ions. This system helps buffer intracellular fluid and plasma to maintain pH balance.

Respiratory Mechanisms

The lungs are the second line of defense to restore normal pH. They control the body's carbonic acid supply via carbon dioxide retention or removal. When the serum pH is too acidic (pH is low), the lungs remove carbon dioxide through rapid, deep breathing. This reduces the amount of carbon dioxide available to make carbonic acid. If the serum pH is too alkaline (pH is high), the lungs try to conserve carbon dioxide through shallow respirations. This system works with the carbonic acid–sodium bicarbonate buffer system to maintain the 20:1 ratio of base to acid.

Renal Mechanisms

The last line of defense is the kidneys, which regulate the concentration of plasma bicarbonate. They can neutralize more acid or base than either the respiratory system or the chemical buffers. If the serum pH is too acidic, the kidneys conserve additional bicarbonate to neutralize the acid. If the serum pH is too alkaline, the kidneys excrete additional bicarbonate to lower the amount of base and thereby decrease the pH. The kidneys also buffer pH by forming acids and ammonium (a base).

Although the renal system is very effective at altering pH, it is slow. It may take up to 3 days to return the pH to normal limits. This process is known as *compensation*. The pH returns to normal, but the carbon dioxide or bicarbonate level is abnormal. Over time, or when the original problem is corrected, these levels also return to normal.

KnowledgeCheck 36-4

- Briefly describe the three mechanisms used to maintain pH.
- Rank in order the acid–base balance mechanisms from the most rapidly acting to the slowest acting.

 Go to Chapter 36, **Knowledge Check Response Sheet and Answers,** on the Student Resource Disk or DavisPlus at http://davisplus.fadavis.com/Wilkinson2

Fluid, Electrolyte, and Acid–Base Imbalances

Illness or disease may lead to imbalances of fluid, electrolytes, or pH. These are discussed in the next sections. The "Practical Knowledge" section, later in the chapter, presents some interventions to correct these imbalances.

Fluid Imbalances

Fluid imbalances involve a deficit or excess in fluid volume or an alteration in distribution among the fluid compartments. You may hear nurses use the term *volume (-volemia)* when discussing fluid losses or gains regardless whether the fluid is blood or other body fluid (e.g., ICF or interstitial fluid). Fluid deficit, regardless of the cause, is referred to as *hypovolemia*, whereas fluid excess, usually not blood, is referred to as *hypervolemia*.

Deficient Fluid Volume

Deficient fluid volume (hypovolemia) occurs when there is a proportional loss of fluid and electrolytes from the ECF. Loss of blood volume is called hypovolemia (*hypo* = low, *vol* = volume, *emia* pertains to blood). Hypovolemia may occur with surgery, trauma, or uterine rupture.

Dehydration describes a state of negative fluid balance in which there is a loss of water (*hydra* = water) from the intracellular, extracellular or intravascular spaces. Dehydration can be categorized by three causes:

- Insufficient intake of fluids
- Excessive fluid loss (e.g., bleeding, vomiting, diarrhea, diaphoresis, diuresis)
- Fluid shifts (e.g., intravascular fluid may leak into body tissues).

When dehydration occurs from the loss of body fluids, electrolytes may also be lost. Loss of fluids can also lead to an increase is serum osmolarity.

The first symptom of volume loss is thirst. If the patient is able to recognize thirst and respond by drinking liquid, no further treatment may be required. If fluid is not available or the patient is unable to drink, or if blood loss continues faster than fluid is replaced (e.g., hemorrhage), fluid becomes deficient. Initially as fluid volume decreases, the heart rate increases and the blood vessels constrict. This increases the blood pressure, in order to continue to circulate the remaining fluid to meet the body's fluid demands. If volume continues to be lost, the heart pumps faster but not as powerfully, resulting in a rapid, weak pulse, and orthostatic hypotension. This is known as **hypovolemic shock**. Orthostatic blood pressure is measured when the patient is lying, sitting, and standing. A drop in the systolic blood pressure (from lying or sitting to standing) greater or equal to 20 mm Hg is called **orthostatic hypotension**. Low fluid volume is just one of its causes.

As fluid loss continues, water is pulled from the interstitial spaces and the ICF into the vascular system, resulting in dry skin and mucous membranes, decreased skin and tongue turgor, decreased urine output, and flat neck veins. Patients complain of muscle weakness, fatigue, and feeling warm. Temperature increases because the body is less able to cool itself through perspiration. In an older adult, temperature will rise but may not be elevated above normal body temperature.

Weight is a sensitive measure of fluid loss. A sudden 5% loss of body weight is considered clinically significant. When loss approaches 8%, fluid loss is severe. A sudden loss of 15% of body weight due to fluid loss is usually fatal. The patient with fluid volume deficit usually has elevated blood urea nitrogen (BUN)–to-creatinine ratio and elevated hematocrit. Both values increase because there is less water in proportion to the solid substances being measured. Specific gravity of the urine increases as the kidneys attempt to conserve water, resulting in more concentrated urine.

You can help prevent fluid volume deficit by identifying patients who have the highest risk for developing this condition. High-risk patients include older adults, infants, children, and any patients with conditions associated with fluid loss (e.g., diabetes insipidus, vomiting, diarrhea, fever). You will learn how to facilitate fluid intake and provide parenteral fluid replacement in the "Planning Interventions/Implementation" section.

Excess Fluid Volume

Excess fluid volume (hypervolemia) involves excessive retention of sodium and water in the ECF. Fluid volume excess can result from excessive salt intake, disease affecting kidney or liver function, or poor pumping action of the heart. The retained sodium increases osmotic pressure in the ECF. This pressure pulls fluid from the cells into the ECF.

The vital sign changes in a patient with hypervolemia are the opposite of those in a patient with hypovolemia. The blood pressure is elevated, pulse is bounding, and respirations are increased and shallow. The neck veins may become distended. Along with increased intravascular volume, excess ECF may accumulate in the tissues, especially in dependent areas, as *edema*. The skin is pale and cool. Urine output becomes dilute, and volume increases. The patient rapidly gains weight. In severe fluid overload, the patient develops moist crackles in the lungs, dyspnea, and ascites (excess peritoneal fluid).

Hemodilution causes BUN, hematocrit, and the specific gravity of the urine to decrease.

You can help prevent fluid overload by monitoring intake and output and observing patients for signs and symptoms of fluid overload. Electronic infusion pumps control the rate of infusion of intravenous fluid, thereby limiting the risk for patients receiving IV therapy (see "Planning Interventions/Implementation").

KnowledgeCheck 36-5

- Define *deficient fluid volume* and *excess fluid volume*.
- Identify the signs and symptoms of deficient fluid volume and excess fluid volume.
- Describe dehydration and hypervolemia.

 Go to Chapter 36, **Knowledge Check Response Sheet and Answers,** on the Student Resource Disk or DavisPlus at http://davisplus.fadavis.com/Wilkinson2

Electrolyte Imbalances

Any electrolyte may become imbalanced. Table 36-5 discusses the common causes; signs and symptoms; and treatment of sodium, potassium, calcium, magnesium, and phosphate imbalances. Disorders affecting chloride ions occur along with sodium disorders. As sodium levels rise, chloride levels also rise. Decreases also occur simultaneously. Clinical signs and treatments are identical to the treatments used for sodium imbalances. Because of the role of bicarbonate as a buffer, bicarbonate levels rise and fall to maintain pH. You will find further discussion of abnormal bicarbonate levels in the "Acid–Base Imbalances" section, which follows.

We can apply the information in Table 36-5 to the LaGuardia family ("Meet Your Patients"). Jackson LaGuardia has end-stage renal disease (ESRD), or renal failure. As a result, he is at risk for imbalances in all of his electrolytes. Now he is experiencing nausea, vomiting, and diarrhea. This will further aggravate the imbalance of potassium and sodium. Due to his complex imbalances, he is a candidate for admission to the hospital. He will need careful rehydration and monitoring of his electrolytes. The remaining family members are likely to be experiencing sodium, potassium, and fluid deficits.

 CriticalThinking 36-4

Martha LaGuardia is taking the following medications: atenolol (Tenormin) 50 mg daily at bedtime, alendronate sodium (Fosamax) 10 mg daily, furosemide (Lasix) 20 mg every morning, and calcium carbonate 500 mg three times per day. She takes her medications regularly and sees her primary care provider monthly. Using your reference books, look up her prescribed medications. Given that Ms. LaGuardia is now experiencing nausea and vomiting, she may be at risk for developing problems and side effects related to her medications. Which medications may cause problems and what problems might they cause? Explain your rationale.

Table 36-5 ➤ Electrolyte Imbalances

DISORDER	COMMON CAUSES	SIGNS AND SYMPTOMS	TREATMENT
Hyponatremia Na^+ <135 mEq/L	Diuretics GI fluid loss Adrenal insufficiency Excessive intake of hypotonic solutions, such as water or D_5W IV fluids Syndrome of inappropriate ADH	Anorexia, nausea, and vomiting Weakness Lethargy Confusion Muscle cramps or twitching Seizures	Monitor I&O. Monitor sodium level. Increase oral sodium intake. Administer IV saline infusion and take seizure precautions, if severe.

Hypernatremia Na^+ <145 mEq/L	Excessive sodium intake
	
	Water deprivation
	
	Increased water loss through profuse sweating, heat stroke, or diabetes insipidus
	
	Administration of hypertonic tube feeding
		Thirst
		
		Elevated temperature
		
		Dry mouth and sticky mucous membranes
		
		If severe:
		  Hallucinations
		  Irritability
		  Lethargy
		  Seizures
			Monitor I&O.
			
			Monitor sodium level.
			
			Monitor vital signs and level of consciousness.
			
			Restrict sodium in the diet.
			
			Beware of hidden sodium in foods and medications.
			
			Increase water intake.
			
			Administer IV solutions that do not contain sodium.

Hypokalemia K^+ <3.5 mEq/L	Diuretics GI fluid loss through vomiting, gastric suction, or diarrhea Steroid administration Hyperaldosteronism Anorexia or bulimia	Fatigue Anorexia, nausea, and vomiting Muscle weakness Decreased GI motility Dysrhythmias Paresthesia Flat T wave on ECG Increased sensitivity to digitalis	Monitor I&O. Monitor potassium level. If the client is taking digoxin, monitor pulse and observe for toxicity. Encourage intake of foods rich in potassium. Administer potassium supplements (Note: IV supplements must be well diluted and administered into a central vein slowly.)
Hyperkalemia K^+ >5.0 mEq/L	Renal failure Potassium-sparing diuretics Hypoaldosteronism High potassium intake coupled with renal insufficiency Acidosis Major trauma Hemolyzed serum sample produces pseudohyperkalemia	Muscle weakness Dysrhythmias Flaccid paralysis Intestinal colic Tall T waves on ECG	Monitor I&O. Monitor potassium level. Caution about potassium-rich food intake in patients with elevated creatinine levels.
Hypocalcemia Ca^{2+} <8.5 mq/dL	Hypoparathyroidism Malabsorption Pancreatitis Alkalosis Vitamin D deficiency	Diarrhea Numbness and tingling of extremities Muscle cramps Tetany Convulsions Laryngeal spasms Cardiac irritability Positive Trousseau's and Chvostek's signs	Monitor I&O. Monitor serum calcium. Encourage increased calcium intake. Administer calcium supplements. If severe, monitor patency of airway, institute seizure and safety precautions, and administer parenteral calcium.

VOL 2 Go to Chapter 36, **Clinical Insight 36-1: Assessing for Trousseau's and Chvostek's Signs,** in Volume 2.

Table 36-5 ➤ Electrolyte Imbalances—cont'd

DISORDER	COMMON CAUSES	SIGNS AND SYMPTOMS	TREATMENT
Hypercalcemia Ca^{2+} >10.5 mq/dL	Hyperparathyroidism Malignant bone disease Prolonged immobilization Excess calcium supplementation Thiazide diuretics	Muscle weakness Constipation Anorexia, nausea, and vomiting Polyuria and polydipsia Kidney stones Bizarre behavior Bradycardia	Monitor I&O. Encourage fluid intake to prevent stone formation. Encourage fiber to prevent constipation. Eliminate calcium supplements and limit calcium-rich foods. Avoid calcium-based antacids. Renal dialysis may be required.
Hypomagnesemia Mg^{2+} <1.3 mEq/L	Chronic alcoholism Malabsorption Diabetic ketoacidosis Prolonged gastric suction	Neuromuscular irritability Disorientation Mood changes Dysrhythmias Increased sensitivity to digitalis	Monitor I&O. Encourage foods high in magnesium. Avoid alcohol intake. If the client is taking digoxin, monitor pulse and observe for toxicity.
Hypermagnesemia Mg^{2+} <2.1 mEq/L	Renal failure Adrenal insufficiency Excess replacement	Flushing and warmth of skin Hypotension Drowsiness, lethargy Hypoactive reflexes Depressed respirations Bradycardia	Monitor vital signs and airway. Monitor reflexes. Avoid magnesium-based antacids and laxatives. Restrict dietary intake of foods high in magnesium.
Hypophosphatemia PO_4^- <1.7 mEq/L	Refeeding after starvation Alcohol withdrawal Diabetic ketoacidosis Respiratory acidosis	Paresthesia Joint stiffness Seizures Cardiomyopathy Impaired tissue oxygenation	Monitor serum phosphorus level. Monitor calcium levels as phosphate is replaced. Start TPN slowly to avoid drops in phosphate.
Hyperphosphatemia PO_4^- >2.6 mEq/L	Renal failure Hyperthyroidism Chemotherapy Excess use of phosphate-based laxative	Short term: tetany symptoms—tingling of extremities and cramping Long term: Calcification in soft tissue	Monitor serum phosphorus level. Monitor for tetany. If severe, administer aluminum hydroxide with meals to bind phosphorus.

Acid–Base Imbalances

The two broad types of acid–base imbalance are acidosis and alkalosis. **Acidosis** occurs when the serum pH falls below 7.35. **Alkalosis** occurs when the serum pH increases above 7.45 (Fig. 36-6). Arterial blood gases (ABGs) are used to monitor acid–base balance. **ABG analysis** measures pH, partial pressure of oxygen (Po_2), partial pressure of carbon dioxide (Pco_2), saturation of oxygen (Sao_2), and bicarbonate (HCO_3^-) level. Acid–base balance is reflected by the pH, Pco_2, and HCO_3 values.

A respiratory disturbance alters the carbonic acid portion of the buffering system, and the resulting imbalance is labeled **respiratory acidosis** or **respiratory alkalosis**. A metabolic disturbance alters the bicarbonate portion of the buffering system, so the resulting imbalance would be labeled as **metabolic acidosis** or **metabolic alkalosis**.

Metabolic and respiratory problems can coexist, resulting in disturbances of both sides of the buffering system. Compensatory mechanisms may also produce both bicarbonate and carbon dioxide abnormalities.

Interpreting ABGs

To determine acid–base balance, you must examine the ABG results. The pH, Pco_2, and HCO_3^- values are of primary importance (Table 36-6). The partial pressure of oxygen (Po_2) and saturation of oxygen (Sao_2) are also part of the ABG result, but they do not affect acid–base balance. Instead, they affect tissue oxygenation. For further discussion on those two measures, see Chapter 35. Table 36-7 describes the causes, manifestations, ABG results, and treatments of acid–base imbalances. Use the following steps to interpret acid–base balance.

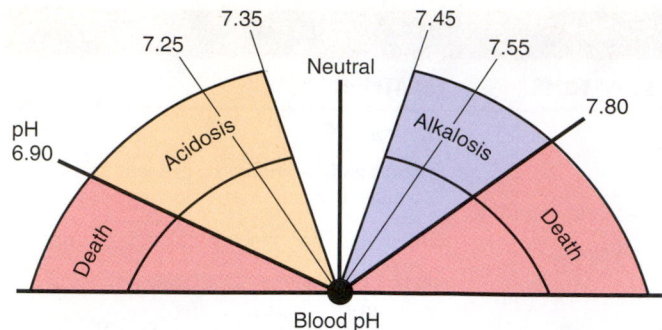

FIGURE 36-6 The pH scale ranges from 1 to 14. Normal blood pH is 7.35 to 7.45.

Step 1: Examine the pH. *(Is it acidotic, alkalotic, or normal?)* A pH value of 7.4 is neutral, or normal. However, the normal *range* for pH is 7.35 to 7.45. Values below 7.35 indicate acidosis; values above 7.45 indicate alkalosis. But, don't forget that neutral is 7.4. This will be very important when we discuss compensation.

Step 2: Examine the P_{CO_2} and HCO_3^-.

a. **Determine which value is abnormal.** Determine which value, P_{CO_2} or HCO_3^-, is responsible for the change in pH—that is, which one is not within normal limits. It helps to think of carbon dioxide (P_{CO_2}) as "acid" and bicarb (HCO_3^-) as base ("alkaline").

- Changes in the P_{CO_2} represent changes in acid: respiratory disorders.
- Changes in HCO_3^- represent changes in base: metabolic disorders.

b. **Determine the direction of change (too high or too low). Is it acidosis or alkalosis?**

- Normal P_{CO_2} is 35 to 45 mm Hg.
  <35 represents too little acid (respiratory alkalosis).
  >45 represents too much acid (respiratory acidosis).
- Normal HCO_3^- is 22 to 26 mEq/L.
  <22 represents too little base (metabolic acidosis).
  >26 represents too much base or (metabolic alkalosis).

Let's work through an example, using steps 1 and 2:

ABG values: pH = 7.30, P_{CO_2} = 50 mm Hg, HCO_3^- = 24 mEq/L

Step 1, Examine the pH:

pH = 7.30. Acidosis (The pH is below normal range of 7.35.)

Step 2a, Is it a respiratory or metabolic cause?

P_{CO_2} > 45 mm Hg (outside the normal range); HCO_3^- is normal. So it is a respiratory cause.

Step 2b, Is it acidosis or alkalosis?

P_{CO_2} > 45 mm Hg (too high, so it is acidosis). HCO_3^- is in the normal range of 22 to 26 mEq/L

Answer: Respiratory acidosis

Step 3: Determine Whether There is Compensation and if so, the Degree of Compensation.

In a respiratory problem, the renal system must compensate for the abnormal pH. In a metabolic problem, the respiratory system compensates. The respiratory system compensates early in the disorder, but it may take up to 3 days for the renal system to compensate fully. During that time, the ABGs will be changing as compensation occurs.

- **No compensation.** If the pH and only one ABG component are abnormal, no compensation has occurred, as in this respiratory acidosis example, in which the pH and the P_{CO_2} are abnormal. The following example shows *no compensation.*

Initial ABG values: pH = 7.30, P_{CO_2} = 50 mm Hg, HCO_3^- = 24 mEq/L

- **Partial compensation.** If the pH and one ABG component are abnormal, with the second ABG value starting to change and the pH beginning to move toward normal, partial compensation is taking place. In this same respiratory acidosis example the pH and P_{CO_2} are still abnormal in the ABG below. However, the HCO_3 has also become abnormal (high) and is pulling the pH toward normal. This example is *partially compensated respiratory acidosis.*

Second ABG values: pH = 7.32, P_{CO_2} = 50 mm Hg, HCO_3^- = 28 mEq/L

- **Full compensation.** Full compensation occurs when the pH returns to normal range and both other ABG components are abnormal. The initial causal component is still abnormal, and the second ABG

Table 36-6 ➤ Using ABGs To Assess Acid–Base Balance				
EXPLANATION OF CHANGES	**ABG COMPONENT**	**NORMAL RANGE**	**ACIDOSIS**	**ALKALOSIS**
Indicates acidosis, alkalosis, or normal acid–base balance	pH	7.35–7.45	Low	High
Carbon dioxide ("acid"). Signals respiratory cause	P_{CO_2}	35–45 mm Hg	High	Low
Sodium bicarbonate ("base"). Signals metabolic cause	HCO_3^-	22–26 mEq/L	Low	High

Table 36-7 ➤ Acid–Base Imbalances

DISORDER	CLINICAL MANIFESTATIONS	INTERVENTIONS
Respiratory Acidosis May be caused by conditions or medications that impair gas exchange at the alveolar–capillary membrane, depressed respiratory rate and depth, or injury to the respiratory center in the brain.	*Acute:* Increased pulse and respiratory rate Headache, dizziness Confusion, decreased level of consciousness (LOC) Muscle twitching ABGs: pH < 7.35; P_{CO_2} > 45 mm Hg; HCO_3^- normal or slightly elevated *Chronic:* Weakness Headache ABGs: pH ≤ 7.35; P_{CO_2} > 45 mm Hg; HCO_3^- >26 mEq/L—rises to compensate and return pH to near normal	Provide pulmonary hygiene. Institute measures to improve gas exchange, such as chest physiotherapy, bronchodilators, antibiotics possible. Provide supplemental oxygen. Maintain hydration.
Respiratory Alkalosis May be caused by hyperventilation due to anxiety, fever, sepsis, thyrotoxicosis, lesion in the respiratory center in the brain, or excessive ventilation with a mechanical ventilator.	Confusion, difficulty focusing Headache Tingling Palpitations Tremors ABGs: pH > 7.45; P_{CO_2} < 35 mm Hg; HCO_3^- < 22 mEq/L—falls to compensate and return pH to near normal	If caused by anxiety, encourage the patient to relax and breathe slowly. For other causes: Identify and treat the underlying disorder.
Metabolic Acidosis May be caused by retained acids in the blood due to renal impairment, poorly controlled diabetes mellitus, or starvation. Conditions that decrease bicarbonate, such as excessive GI loss, will also trigger metabolic acidosis. May be caused by excessive intake of acids, which may occur with aspirin poisoning, or by prolonged infusion of chloride-containing IV fluids.	Headache Confusion, drowsiness Weakness Peripheral vasodilatation Nausea and vomiting Kussmaul breathing (rapid and deep) ABGs: pH < 7.35; P_{CO_2} < 35 mm Hg—falls to compensate and return pH to near normal; HCO_3^- < 22 mEq/L Frequently associated with hyperkalemia	Treatment is directed at correcting the underlying problem. Bicarbonate may be ordered.
Metabolic Alkalosis May be caused by excessive acid loss due to vomiting or gastric suction, use of potassium-wasting diuretics, hypokalemia, excess bicarbonate intake, or hypoaldosteronism.	Dizziness Tingling of extremities Hypertonic muscles Decreased respiratory rate and depth ABGs: pH > 7.45; P_{CO_2} > 45 mm Hg—rises to compensate and return pH to near normal; HCO_3^- >26 mEq/L	Treatment is directed at correcting the underlying problem. Treatment often includes administration of NaCl-rich fluids.

component (that had the normal values) has changed enough to return the pH to normal. Using the same respiratory acidosis example, below, the pH is now in the normal range and the P_{CO_2} is still high. But the HCO_3 is now also high; it has moved enough to raise the pH into the normal range.

Third ABG values: *pH = 7.35, P_{CO_2} = 50 mm Hg, HCO_3^- = 30 mEq/L*

Now work through the steps again. Remember that the neutral pH is 7.4, so for this step you can consider anything above 7.4 to be alkalosis, even though the actual value (7.35 in this case) is within the normal range.

Step 1: pH < 7.4 (acidosis)

Step 2: The P_{CO_2} is still high, indicating a respiratory cause.

Step 3: The HCO_3^- has risen to 30 mEq/L, increasing the base and bringing the pH back into the normal range. This indicates that the problem is now *fully compensated respiratory acidosis*.

Here is another example:

ABG values: pH = 7.50, P_{CO_2} = 40 mm Hg, HCO_3^- = 30 mEq/L

Step 1, Examine the pH: pH = 7.50. Alkalosis (The pH is above normal range of .45.)

Step 2a, Is it a respiratory or metabolic cause? P_{CO_2} = 40 mm Hg (normal); HCO_3^- > 26 (abnormally high). So it is a metabolic cause (the "base" is the abnormal value).

Step 2b, Is it acidosis or alkalosis?

P_{CO_2} = 40 mm Hg (normal)
HCO_3^- > 26 (too high). Therefore it is alkalosis.
Conclusion from Steps 2a and 2b: Metabolic alkalosis

Step 3, Is there compensation? The pH is abnormal and only one ABG component is abnormal; therefore, no compensation has occurred. *This is uncompensated metabolic alkalosis.*

For a summary table to help you interpret ABGs in the clinical setting,

 Go to Chapter 36, **Clinical Insight 36-2: Interpreting ABGs,** in Volume 2.

KnowledgeCheck 36-6

Interpret the following ABG results:

pH = 7.53	P_{CO_2} = 26 mm Hg	HCO_3^- = 22 mEq/L
pH = 7.40	P_{CO_2} = 39 mm Hg	HCO_3^- = 25 mEq/L
pH = 7.30	P_{CO_2} = 70 mm Hg	HCO_3^- = 30 mEq/L
pH = 7.48	P_{CO_2} = 46 mm Hg	HCO_3^- = 30 mEq/L

 Go to Chapter 36, **Knowledge Check Response Sheet and Answers,** on the Student Resource Disk or DavisPlus at http://davisplus.fadavis.com/Wilkinson2

Practical Knowledge
knowing how

In the remainder of this chapter, you will learn to apply theoretical knowledge of fluids, electrolytes, and acid–base balance to patient care.

ASSESSMENT

Assessment of a client for fluid, electrolyte, and acid–base imbalances includes collecting a focused nursing history, performing a physical assessment, and reviewing pertinent laboratory tests. The purpose of the focused assessment is to identify clients at risk for or already experiencing imbalances, to identify the nature of the disorder, and to evaluate responses to treatments.

Focused Nursing History

The nursing history related to fluids, electrolytes, and acid–base balance includes questions about demographic data, past medical history, current health concerns, food and fluid intake, fluid elimination, medications, and lifestyle. For questions to use in obtaining this focused nursing history,

 Go to Chapter 36, **Assessment Guidelines and Tools, Focused Assessment for Fluid, Electrolyte, and Acid–Base Balance, Nursing History,** in Volume 2.

Focused Physical Assessment

Correlate physical assessment data with the nursing history and laboratory studies. You will need to assess the following:

- *Skin*. Assess for color, temperature, moisture content, continuity, turgor, and edema.
- *Mucous membranes.* Inspect the tongue and buccal mucosa; assess the color, moisture, and continuity of the mucous membranes, as well as tongue turgor. Tongue turgor is not affected by age, so it is useful for all age groups.
- *Cardiovascular system.* Pulse and blood pressure are affected by fluid and electrolyte status. Also assess for orthostatic hypotension, capillary refill, jugular venous distention, and peripheral edema.
- *Respiratory system.* Assess respiratory rate, depth, and pattern, as well as breath sounds.
- *Neurological system.* As described in Tables 36-5 and 36-7, neurological status (e.g., level of consciousness) provides cues to fluid, electrolyte, and acid–base imbalance.

In addition to the above assessments, you will track vital sign changes, monitor daily weights, and record intake and output. These are independent nursing assessments. They do not require a medical prescription. You may delegate these tasks to assistive personnel, but you remain responsible for evaluating the data. For complete guidelines for focused physical assessments and clinical observations,

 Go to Chapter 36, **Assessment Guidelines and Tools, Focused Assessment for Fluid, Electrolyte, and Acid–base Balance, Physical Assessments,** in Volume 2.

Vital Signs

All of the vital signs reflect information about fluid, electrolyte, and acid–base balance. These effects are briefly summarized below.

- *Temperature.* An elevated body temperature increases the loss of body fluids. In hypernatremia, body temperature rises because the fluid available for sweating decreases. In uncomplicated fluid volume deficit, body temperature decreases.

- *Pulse.* Tachycardia is an early sign of fluid volume deficit. Dysrhythmias can result from potassium, calcium, and magnesium imbalances. Fluid status directly affects the pulse volume: As fluid volume increases, the pulse volume also increases; similarly, a drop in fluid volume leads to a drop in pulse volume.
- *Respiratory rate.* Alterations in respiratory rate may cause acid–base imbalances or be associated with compensation for a metabolic disorder.
- *Blood pressure.* Blood pressure rises and falls with fluid volume. It is also affected by electrolytes. High sodium intake is a factor in hypertension, whereas high potassium and magnesium intake may lower blood pressure.

Daily Weights

Monitoring daily weight change is an accurate method of assessing fluid status. Weight changes over time are usually related to diet and exercise. In contrast, short-term changes usually indicate changes in fluid status. Each kilogram (2.2 lb) of weight is equivalent to 1 liter (1000 mL) of fluid. Thus, in a client with diarrhea, a sudden drop in weight of 5 pounds is equivalent to a fluid loss of almost 2300 mL.

For weight to accurately reflect fluid status, you must use the same balanced scale each time. Weigh the client at the same time each day, making sure that he is wearing the same amount of clothing. Clients undergoing hemodialysis (blood cleansing through an artificial kidney) are usually weighed before and after dialysis treatments. Many lose 3 to 4 kg (6.6 to 8.8 pounds) over the course of several hours of dialysis. As a result, hypotension, tachycardia, and feelings of lightheadedness are common after a dialysis treatment.

Weight monitoring is especially valuable data when it is impractical or impossible to measure intake and output. For example, it is not easy to know for sure how much fluid a breastfed infant receives with each feeding. If the infant is feeding well but experiencing diarrhea, weight monitoring will help the parents and pediatrician assess fluid status. Incontinence, draining wounds, and limited resources may also make it difficult to monitor intake and output. Weight monitoring is a practical solution that may be initiated as a nursing order.

Fluid Intake and Output

Intake and output (I&O) are monitored to assess fluid status. I&O are usually tallied at the end of each shift, as well as for each 24-hour period. In intensive care units, I&O are measured at least hourly. To monitor I&O, measure all fluids the client consumes or excretes. You must correlate I&O with daily weights to accurately determine overall fluid status (Pflaum, 1979, 2000, 2006).

- **Output.** Fluid output includes urine, liquid stools, emesis, gastrointestinal fluids (e.g., from suction devices), and drainage (e.g., from wounds and pressure ulcers). Output also includes insensible losses through perspiration and respiration, but these are not usually measured. For more information about intake and output, refer to Chapter 27, "Measuring Intake and Output." For procedure steps,

VOL 2 Go to Chapter 26, **Procedure 27-1: Measuring Urine,** in Volume 2.

- **Intake.** Include the following items as fluid intake: oral fluids, semiliquid foods, ice chips, parenteral fluids, enteral feedings, and irrigations instilled and not withdrawn immediately. For more information about measuring intake,

VOL 2 Go to Chapter 36, **Clinical Insight 36-3: Guidelines for Measuring Intake and Output (I&O),** in Volume 2.

Most healthcare facilities have standardized I&O forms for recording at the bedside and as a permanent part of the patient record (either paper or electronic). To see an electronic I&O record, see Figure 16-2 in Chapter 16. For an example of a paper I&O flow sheet,

VOL 2 Go to Chapter 16, **Forms: Intake and Output Record,** in Volume 2.

KnowledgeCheck 36-7
- Identify ten physical assessment components that can be used to monitor fluid, electrolyte, and acid–base balance.
- What aspects should be evaluated in a nursing history focused on fluid, electrolyte, and acid–base balance?

 Go to Chapter 36, **Knowledge Check Response Sheet and Answers,** on the Student Resource Disk or DavisPlus at http://davisplus.fadavis.com/Wilkinson2

 CriticalThinking 36-5

What vital sign changes would you expect to find when assessing Jackson LaGuardia ("Meet Your Patients")?

Laboratory Studies

Several laboratory tests are performed to evaluate fluid, electrolyte, and acid–base status.

Complete Blood Count. Fluid status is reflected in a **complete blood count (CBC),** which is a measure of red blood cells (RBCs), white blood cells (WBCs), and platelets. Included in the CBC is the hematocrit, a measure of the percentage of RBCs in whole blood. As fluid levels decrease, the percentage of blood made up by cells increases, and the hematocrit rises. As fluid levels increase, the hematocrit falls.

Serum Electrolytes. Venous blood samples are taken to measure sodium, potassium, chloride, and bicarbonate levels. In many labs, electrolyte panels also include blood urea nitrogen (BUN)/creatinine ratio and glucose. BUN and creatinine are sensitive measures of fluid status and kidney function.

Serum Osmolality. A measure of the solute concentration of the blood is **serum osmolality**. It is expressed as milliosmoles per kilogram (mOsm/kg). Sodium is the greatest determinant of serum osmolality. Glucose and urea also contribute to serum osmolality. Serum osmolality may be directly measured with venous blood or estimated by doubling the serum sodium level. A rise in serum osmolality indicates fluid volume deficit; a decrease indicates fluid volume excess. Changes in serum osmolality usually indicate alterations in sodium levels.

Urine Osmolality. The solute concentration of urine is measured by **urine osmolality**. The body excretes nitrogenous wastes as well as electrolytes. As a result, urine osmolality is substantially higher than serum levels. Fluid volume deficit increases urine osmolality; fluid volume excess decreases urine osmolality. This test may call for a 24-hour urine specimen, or for discarding the first morning specimen and collecting a clean-catch specimen 2 hours later.

Urinalysis. The routine screening test, **urinalysis**, includes a measure of urine pH and specific gravity. Urine pH normally ranges from 5.0 to 9.0, with an average of 6.0.

- *pH.* Urine becomes more acidic in respiratory or metabolic acidosis, starvation, or fluid volume deficit. Alkaline urine is associated with an alkaline state in the blood.
- *Specific gravity.* Specific gravity rises and falls in opposition to fluid status. A normal range is 1.001 to 1.029. A low specific gravity occurs when fluid is plentiful. When fluid levels decrease, urine becomes more concentrated, and specific gravity increases. For a procedure for testing specific gravity of urine,

 Go to Chapter 27, **Procedure 27-3B: Measuring Specific Gravity of Urine**, in Volume 2.

ABGs. Interpretation of ABGs was discussed earlier in this chapter. For a list of these values, along with other lab studies discussed earlier,

 Go to Chapter 36, **Diagnostic Testing: Assessing Fluid, Electrolyte, and Acid–Base Balance**, in Volume 2.

ANALYSIS/NURSING DIAGNOSIS

Nursing diagnoses directly related to fluid, electrolyte, and acid–base balance include the following: Deficient Fluid Volume, Excess Fluid Volume, Readiness for Enhanced Fluid Volume, Risk for Deficient Fluid Volume, Risk for Electrolyte Imbalance, Risk for Imbalanced Fluid Volume, and Risk for Vascular Trauma.

Impaired Gas Exchange is appropriate for a client with a disorder affecting gas exchange at the alveolar–capillary membrane in the lungs (see Chapter 35). This condition limits the effectiveness of the carbonic acid–bicarbonate buffer system and alters serum pH, predisposing the patient to acid–base imbalances.

Fluid, electrolyte, and acid–base imbalances (e.g., dehydration, metabolic acidosis, respiratory alkalosis) may be etiologies of other nursing diagnoses. Below are a few examples:

- Activity Intolerance related to excess fluid and electrolyte loss through Diarrhea
- Impaired Oral Mucous Membrane related to Deficient Fluid Volume
- Impaired Skin Integrity related to dehydration
- Decreased Cardiac Output related to hypovolemia

For other related NANDA-I diagnoses,

 Go to Chapter 36, **Standardized Language, NANDA-I Diagnoses Related to Fluid, Electrolyte, and Acid-Base Balance**, in Volume 2.

PLANNING OUTCOMES/EVALUATION

The overall goal for a client experiencing fluid, electrolytes, or acid–base imbalance is to restore balance. *NOC standardized outcomes* for describing fluid and electrolyte status include the following: Electrolyte & Acid/Base Balance, Fluid Balance, Fluid Overload Severity, and Hydration. For selected indicators for these outcomes,

 Go to Chapter 36, **Standardized Language; Selected NOC Outcomes and NIC Interventions for Fluid and Electrolyte Problems**, in Volume 2.

Individualized goals/outcome statements you might write for a client include the following examples:

- Maintains fluid balance, as evidenced by balanced 24-hour intake and output; good skin and tongue turgor; blood pressure and heart rate within normal limits; and no adventitious breath sounds.
- Electrolyte balance restored, as evidenced by alertness and cognitive orientation and no muscle cramping, seizures, or electrocardiogram changes.
- Drinks at least 2500 mL in 24 hours.
- Urine specific gravity within normal limits.

PLANNING INTERVENTIONS/IMPLEMENTATION

NIC standardized interventions related to fluid, electrolyte, and acid–base balance include Acid–Base Management, Electrolyte Management, and Fluid Management. For a listing of other interventions,

 Go to Chapter 36, **Standardized Language; Selected NOC Outcomes and NIC Interventions for Fluid and Electrolyte Problems**, in Volume 2.

Individualized interventions are aimed at correcting the underlying disorder that led to imbalance. Nursing care

focuses on preventing imbalances, modifying oral intake, providing parenteral fluids, and transfusing blood products, all of which are discussed in the rest of this chapter.

Preventing Fluid and Electrolyte Imbalances

It is better to prevent imbalances than to treat them. Use the data obtained from your assessment to plan how to help your client avoid imbalances. Common strategies are listed in the accompanying box, Self-Care: Teaching Patients to Prevent Fluid and Electrolyte Imbalances.

Dietary Changes

To promote fluid and electrolyte balance, most people need to limit their sodium intake and increase their

Self-Care

Teaching Patients to Prevent Fluid and Electrolyte Imbalances

➤ Teach the client about usual fluid needs and circumstances that increase fluid needs, such as high environmental temperature, fever, GI fluid loss, or draining wounds. Base your teaching on the client's current intake and the changes required to meet fluid goals.

➤ Identify medications or conditions that place the client at risk for imbalances. For example, if the client is receiving a potassium-wasting diuretic, she will need to increase potassium intake, either by taking a supplement or by altering the diet.

Also teach clients to do the following:

➤ Drink at least eight to ten 8-ounce glasses of water per day unless your healthcare provider has told you to limit fluids.

➤ Use thirst as a guide to fluid intake.

➤ Limit consumption of fluids high in salt, sugar, caffeine, or alcohol.

➤ Drink water before, during, and after strenuous exercise.

➤ Avoid routine use of laxatives, antacids, weight-loss products, or enemas. All of these products may cause imbalances of fluids and electrolytes such as sodium and potassium.

➤ Weigh yourself daily if fluid balance is critical or if you are experiencing excessive loss or gain.

➤ Contact a health professional if there is a sudden change of weight, decreased urine output, swelling in dependent areas (e.g., hands and feet), shortness of breath, or dizziness.

➤ Contact a healthcare provider if you experience prolonged vomiting, diarrhea, or inability to tolerate liquids or food.

➤ Eat a well-balanced diet, including dairy products rich in calcium.

dietary potassium and calcium. As previously discussed, most North Americans consume more sodium than they should and not enough potassium and calcium. Teach clients to eat foods rich in potassium and calcium every day and to avoid sodium-rich foods (e.g., processed foods) (see Chapter 26 to review foods, as needed). For example, instruct clients to read food labels, particularly when trying to limit sodium intake.

Oral Electrolyte Supplements

Many clients are unable to correct electrolyte disturbances with dietary changes alone. This is especially true for clients who have food intolerances, who rely on prepared meals, or who live in group settings. Such clients may need oral supplements to meet their dietary requirements. Potassium and calcium are among the most common supplements. Most adults, especially older adults, consume less dietary calcium per day than the recommended amount. Calcium supplements come in many forms, including tablet, liquid, and chewable form. Potassium supplements are available in pill and liquid form. Many have an unpleasant taste. The following are suggested nursing activities to help improve your patients' compliance with taking supplements:

- Encourage clients to take potassium supplements with juice to mask the taste.
- Teach clients to take supplements as prescribed to maintain electrolyte balance.
- Remind clients that supplements are medications and should be viewed as part of the treatment plan.
- If the client's medications are altered, review the continued need for supplements.
- Caution clients that salt substitutes contain potassium. If the client has been advised to use salt substitutes, review the need for potassium supplements.
- Encourage clients who take calcium supplements to consume at least 2500 mL of fluid per day to avoid constipation and reduce the risk of kidney stone formation.

KnowledgeCheck 36-8

- Identify laboratory tests that monitor fluid, electrolyte, and acid–base balance.
- Give at least five strategies to prevent fluid and electrolyte imbalance.

 Go to Chapter 36, **Knowledge Check Response Sheet and Answers,** on the Student Resource Disk or DavisPlus at http://davisplus.fadavis.com/Wilkinson2

Modifying Oral Fluid Intake

Clients experiencing fluid imbalances may need to restrict or increase their daily oral intake to correct the underlying disorder.

Facilitating Fluid Intake

Clients with actual or potential fluid volume deficit may need to increase their fluid intake. Whenever possible, clients should take fluids by mouth. You may provide replacement through a nasogastric or feeding tube if the client can tolerate fluids in the gastrointestinal tract but is unable to meet his needs independently. Parenteral fluid replacement is used only when enteral replacement cannot meet the client's fluid needs (for review, see Chapter 26).

To increase fluid intake successfully, you must establish the desired amount of fluid intake for the client. The daily fluid goal reflects the client's current fluid balance and underlying condition. For example, if a client is dehydrated, an order might read: "Force fluids: 2500 mL oral fluids per 24 hours." From this order you can develop a plan to increase fluids. Typically people drink more fluid during the day and early evening, when they are more likely to be active. A large volume of fluid late in the evening may interrupt sleep because it may prompt the need to urinate. Therefore, you should distribute fluids to reflect the time of day, for example:

```
0700 to 1500 —1300 mL
1500 to 2300 —1000 mL
2300 to 0700 —200 mL
```

Strategies to increase fluid intake include the following:

- Offer a variety of fluids throughout the day on a regular schedule. Vary hot and cold liquids, and offer a choice of juices and other drinks.
- Instruct nursing assistive personnel to make "fluids rounds" to offer and help with oral fluids.
- Each time you are at the bedside, remind the patient to drink.
- Break daily goals into hourly amounts. For example, in the preceding example, in the 8 hours between 0700 and 1500 have the patient drink 150 mL of fluid every hour. Give him a written schedule.
- Provide a glass or cup with milliliter markings on it so that the patient will know how much he is drinking.
- Always have fluid readily available to the patient. For example, keep a pitcher of water at the bedside.
- When possible, have the patient and family members participate in offering fluids and tracking fluid intake.
- Schedule diagnostic and surgical procedures to minimize the length of time the patient must fast.
- For ambulatory patients (e.g., residents in long-term care facilities) schedule "tea time" or "happy hour" to promote increased intake.

Facilitating Fluid Restriction

Patients may need to limit fluids for a variety of reasons (e.g., cardiovascular, liver, or renal impairment). Inform patients and caregivers of the reason for the restriction, as well as the amount of fluid allowed. This will help them to restrict fluids appropriately. Typically, fluid volume is divided into amounts allotted per shift. However, fluid restrictions usually include *all* forms of intake, not only oral. For example, an order might read: "Limit total fluid intake to 1500 mL per 24 hours." If the patient is receiving IV antibiotics four times per day, you must include that volume as a part of the total fluids. If 75 mL is infused with each administration, total IV fluids equal 300 mL. So, the oral intake must be limited to 1200 mL per day. This amount may be distributed as 700 mL on the day shift, 400 mL on the evening shift, and 100 mL at night. Strategies to restrict fluid intake include the following:

- Do not offer liquids with meals. Reserve liquids for between meals.
- Limit intake of dry, salty, or spicy foods; these foods increase thirst.
- Offer ice chips to help quench thirst.
- Provide frequent oral hygiene.
- Keep liquids away from the bedside.
- Provide diversional activities for the patient.

Parenteral Replacement of Fluids and Electrolytes

When fluid loss is severe or the client cannot tolerate oral or tube feedings, fluid volume is replaced parenterally. Intravenous therapy is the administration of fluids, electrolytes, medications, or nutrients by the venous route. Intravenous fluids are used to:

- Expand intravascular volume.
- Correct an underlying imbalance in fluids or electrolytes.
- Compensate for an ongoing problem that is affecting either fluid or electrolytes.

For instance, Martha LaGuardia ("Meet Your Patients") is being treated in the emergency department (ED) for gastroenteritis. She is experiencing fluid loss from vomiting and diarrhea, complicated by her use of a diuretic. IV therapy will allow her to receive fluid to expand her intravascular volume and to maintain her hydration until the vomiting and diarrhea subside. It will also provide electrolyte replacement based on her laboratory studies. Mrs. LaGuardia will remain on IV fluids until she can meet her fluid and electrolyte needs orally. All of the members of the LaGuardia family are experiencing fluid losses and would benefit from increasing their fluid intake. When fluid balance is fragile, or when the client cannot tolerate oral fluids, replacement may be supervised in an inpatient setting.

When initiating and maintaining intravenous infusions, always use careful aseptic technique. Remember that the IV catheter provides a portal of entry for pathogens directly into the bloodstream. Excellent nursing technique helps reduce the number of IV catheter-associated infections. You might be interested to know that Medicare will not reimburse a hospital for the expenses (e.g., antibiotics, extra hospital days) caused by catheter-related infections that occur during hospitalization.

Types of Intravenous Solutions

As we explained earlier, solutions are classified according to how they compare to the osmolality of blood serum. Intravenous fluids are these classified as isotonic, hypotonic, and hypertonic solutions.

Isotonic Fluids. Normal blood serum osmolality is 275 to 295 mOsm/kg. Isotonic solutions have similar tonicity, with a range of 250 to 375 mOsm/L. Therefore, when infused, isotonic solutions remain inside the blood vessels. As a result, they are useful for clients with hypotension or hypovolemia. Clients at risk for fluid volume excess due to congestive heart failure (CHF) must be closely monitored when they receive isotonic fluid replacement, because they may easily develop fluid overload. Examples of isotonic fluids are lactated Ringer's solution and 0.9% saline (normal saline [NS]).

Hypotonic Fluids. The osmolality of a hypotonic solution is less than that of serum. Therefore, when infused, these solutions pull body water from the intravascular compartment into the interstitial fluid compartment. As the interstitial fluid is diluted, its osmolarity decreases, drawing water into the adjacent cells. Hypotonic fluid is used for hyperglycemic conditions, such as diabetic ketoacidosis, in which high serum glucose draws fluid out of the cells and into the vascular and interstitial compartments. You must administer hypotonic fluids carefully to prevent a sudden fluid shift from the intravascular space to the cells. Examples of hypotonic fluids include 5% dextrose (D_5W) and 0.45% saline (½ NS). In the bag, D_5W is isotonic, with an osmolality of 253 mOsm/L, but in the body it becomes hypotonic.

Hypertonic Fluids. The osmolality of hypertonic fluids is higher than that of serum. When administered, they pull fluids and electrolytes from the intracellular and interstitial compartments into the intravascular compartment. Hypertonic fluids can help stabilize blood pressure, increase urine output, and reduce edema. Volume expanders are used to increase blood volume following severe loss of blood or plasma, such as in major burns or hemorrhage. Examples of hypertonic fluids include D_5 0.9% NaCl (D_5 NS), D_5 0.45% NaCl (D_5 ½ NS), and $D_{50\%}$ (50% dextrose in water). Volume expanders, such as dextran and serum albumin are also hypertonic.

To help you remember, here is a somewhat oversimplified summary. When infused:

- *Isotonic* fluids remain in the intravascular compartment.
- *Hypotonic* fluids pull body water *out* of the intravascular compartment.
- *Hypertonic* fluids pull body water *into* the intravascular compartment.

Peripheral Vascular Access Devices

Intravenous therapy requires placement of a vascular access device. You will choose the type of device on the basis of the client's condition, type of fluid that will be infused, and the anticipated length of treatment. IV catheters (and needles) are sized by their diameter, which is called the **gauge**. The smaller the diameter, the larger the gauge (e.g., a 16-gauge catheter is larger than a 21-gauge catheter). Therefore, the smaller the gauge, the more rapidly fluid can be delivered. Various types of catheters are used to access peripheral veins, including the following:

Over-the-Needle Catheters. These are also called **angiocaths,** short for angiocatheter (Fig. 36-7A). A polyurethane or Teflon catheter is threaded over a metal stylet (needle). You pierce the skin and vein with the needle, advance the catheter into the vein, and remove (or retract) the metal needle. In most cases, the plastic catheter is less than 7.5 cm (3 in.) in length. This type of access device is ideal for brief therapy. However, you cannot give highly irritating or hyperosmolar solutions through this type of catheter because it may cause severe damage to the vein. For an animated illustration of an over-the-needle IV catheter,

Go to **Animations: Insertion of an Over-the-Needle IV Catheter** on DavisPlus at http://davisplus.fadavis.com/Wilkinson2

Inside-the-Needle Catheters. This type of catheter is similar to the over-the-needle catheter; however, the polyurethane or Teflon catheter lies inside the metal needle (Fig. 36-7B). After you advance the catheter into the vein, you withdraw the needle.

Butterfly Needle. Also called a *scalp vein needle* or *wing-tipped catheter*, a **butterfly needle** is a short, beveled metal needle with flexible plastic flaps attached to the shaft

FIGURE 36-7 Typical IV access devices. *A,* An over-the-needle catheter. *B,* An inside-the-needle catheter.

(Fig. 36-8). You can pinch the flaps and hold them tightly together to facilitate insertion. After insertion, flatten them out and tape them against the skin to prevent dislodgement during the infusion process. These needles are commonly used for intermittent or short-term therapy for children and infants or for single-dose medications and drawing blood. Because the inflexible metal needle remains in the vein, a butterfly needle is more likely to **infiltrate** (damage the vein and allow fluid to leak into the interstitial spaces) than a plastic catheter.

Midline Peripheral Catheter. A **midline peripheral catheter** is a peripherally inserted flexible IV catheter, typically inserted into the antecubital fossa and then advanced into the larger vessels of the upper arm for greater hemodilution. It is 15 cm (6 in.) long, so it can be used for a longer period of time than a shorter, over-the-needle catheter. A midline peripheral catheter may remain in place for as long as 49 days, although the median length of use is 7 days (CDC, 2002). A midline catheter is still considered a peripheral line, so you cannot administer highly osmolar and irritating solutions through it.

In response to the Needlestick Safety and Prevention Act passed by Congress in 2000, the Centers for Disease Control and Prevention (CDC) and the Occupational Safety and Health Administration (OSHA) require the use of "needleless" systems. Therefore, you will usually have available access devices with safety features to prevent accidental "sticks." But if you find you must use an older, nonsafety device, do not attempt to recap the needle after removing it from the vein.

Peripheral Intravenous Lock

A **peripheral intravenous lock** (also called a saline lock, and sometimes a heparin lock) establishes a venous route as a precautionary measure for clients whose condition may change rapidly or who may require intermittent infusion therapy. Insert a peripheral IV catheter or butterfly wing-tipped catheter into a vein, and cap the hub with a lock port (Fig. 36-9). Maintain the patency of the lock by injecting normal saline or a dilute heparin solution, depending on agency policy.

Central Venous Access Devices

A **central venous access device (CVAD)** is an intravenous line inserted into a major vein. Typically, the subclavian or internal jugular vein is used. Using surgical asepsis, a catheter is advanced from the insertion site into the superior vena cava. CVADs are used to administer large volumes of fluid or highly irritating medications, when peripheral sites are unavailable, for monitoring central venous pressure, and for frequent blood draws. You will likely care for patients with central lines, and you may need to assist with inserting them. To learn how to care for patients with central lines, see the Critical Aspects box for a summary, and

VOL 2 Go to Chapter 36, **Clinical Insight 36-5: Caring for Patients with a Central Venous Access Device, Procedure 36-5B: Central Line Dressings,** and **Procedure 36-9: Assisting with Percutaneous Central Venous Catheter Placement,** in Volume 2.

Advantages of Central Lines. A central line offers several advantages:

- A central vein can accommodate highly irritating and hyperosmolar solutions because the blood and solution mix rapidly at the infusion site.
- Central veins are accessible even if the patient is experiencing severe fluid depletion.

FIGURE 36-8 The butterfly, or scalp vein, needle is commonly used for intermittent or short-term therapy for children and infants.

FIGURE 36-9 A peripheral intravenous lock establishes a venous route as a precautionary measure for clients whose condition may change rapidly or who may require intermittent infusion therapy.

- Some types of central lines may also be used to monitor central venous pressure.
- Central lines can be left in longer than peripheral IVs, ranging from a week to long term, depending on the type of central line used.
- Nutrition can be given parenterally.
- Phlebitis, extravasation, and infiltration are less likely to occur with central lines.
- Central lines with extra ports allow you to withdraw blood from a port to use for laboratory tests.

Disadvantages of Central Lines. Disadvantages of central lines include the following:

- Practitioners must have specialized training in order to insert the catheter.
- You must obtain patient consent.
- Placement must be confirmed by radiography.
- Placement is treated as a minor surgical procedure, requiring strict sterility.
- Dressing changes require strict sterile technique.
- When placed via the neck, especially though the subclavian vein, there is a risk of pneumothorax.
- There is a risk that the catheter will float into the right side of the heart, where it may cause ventricular dysrhythmias.
- There is a greater risk of air embolus and infection when compared to peripheral IVs.
- Associated costs are greater than with peripheral lines.
- The risk for sepsis is much higher than for peripheral sites. CVCs account for about 90% of catheter-related bloodstream infections.

Preventing Central Line-Associated Bloodstream Infections is one of The Joint Commission's national patient safety goals for 2009. The Institute for Healthcare Improvement (n.d.) recommends the following "bundle" of practices to help prevent CVC catheter-related infections:

Hand hygiene—Wearing gloves does not make handwashing unnecessary.
Maximal barrier precautions for insertion—Includes sterile drape for patient, hat, mask, and sterile gown and gloves.
Chlorhexidine skin antisepsis—Use 2% chlorhexidine gluconate in 70% isopropyl alcohol to prep the insertion site.
Optimal catheter site selection—The subclavian vein has the lowest rate of infection. The femoral vein should be avoided if possible.
Daily review of lines—The CVC should be removed as soon as it is no longer necessary. Risk of infection is closely related to the length of time the CVC is in place.

Types of Central Venous Catheters

There are four types of CVADs: peripherally inserted central catheters, nontunneled CVCs, tunneled CVCs, and implanted ports.

Peripherally Inserted Central Catheters (PICC lines)

PICCs are long, soft, flexible catheters inserted at the antecubital fossa through the basilic or cephalic vein of the arm. The catheter is then advanced into the superior vena cava (Fig. 36-10). A physician or specially trained registered nurse performs the insertion. PICC lines are most commonly used for prolonged IV antibiotic therapy, parenteral nutrition, and chemotherapy. A PICC line is intended for intermediate to long-term use and does not need to be replaced unless the site appears infected or the catheter is no longer patent.

Nontunneled Central Venous Catheters

Nontunneled CVCs are inserted by a physician, specially trained nurse practitioner, or physician assistant through the skin into the jugular, subclavian, and occasionally, femoral veins. They are sutured in place. Often these are referred to as single, double, triple or quadruple-lumen catheters, depending on the number of ports in the line (Fig. 36-11). These CVADs are intended for shorter use than a PICC line (less than 6 weeks); however, guidelines advise that nontunneled CVADs not be routinely replaced (CDC, 2002; National Guideline Clearinghouse, 2008). Blood can be drawn from a nontunneled CVAD for diagnostic studies. However, if parenteral nutrition or blood is running in a port, you cannot use that same port for blood draws.

Example: Suppose you have a frail elderly patient who needs two different kinds of IV fluid, parenteral nutrition, and frequent blood draws for lab tests. This patient has fragile peripheral veins and is also at high risk for infection and other complications. With a multiple-lumen central catheter, the patient needs only one insertion site. You can run both fluids and the parenteral nutrition fluids, and still reserve one port for drawing blood. The patient has less risk for the catheter to become dislodged or infiltrate, or for phlebitis to develop.

Long slim silastic catheter

Central veins

Entrance to vein

Exit site

FIGURE 36-10 A PICC line is a long, soft, flexible catheter inserted through a vein in the arm and threaded into a central vessel.

FIGURE 36-11 Nontunneled central venous catheters are inserted into the jugular, subclavian, and occasionally, femoral veins.

Nontunneled central catheters can also be used to measure central venous pressure (CVP). CVP measurements offer information on volume status, with a low reading indicating hypovolemia and a high reading, hypervolemia.

Tunneled Central Venous Catheters

Tunneled CVCs are intended for long-term use. The catheter is inserted by a surgeon through a 7.5- to 15-cm (3- to 6-in.) subcutaneous tunnel in the chest wall and then into the jugular or subclavian vein (Fig. 36-12). The catheter can either be sutured in place, with the sutures removed when fibrosis has developed around the catheter, or secured with an IV securing device, such as StatLock®. Because they are tunneled through the skin rather than through a vein,

the risk of infection is less than with PICCs or nontunneled central lines.

Implanted Ports

Implanted ports are devices made of a radiopaque silicone catheter and a plastic or stainless steel injection port with a self-sealing silicone-rubber septum. The catheter enters the internal jugular vein in the neck, and it may be tunneled or untunneled to a completely implanted subcutaneous reservoir (port) in the upper chest (Fig. 36-13). Implanted ports are placed by surgeons and only specially trained nurses are allowed to access an implanted port because of the risk of infiltration into the tissue if the needle placement is not correct. Implanted ports are also intended for long-term use.

✚ Blood pressures and blood draws should be avoided in the extremity of the side of the chest where the implanted port has been placed.

The Critical Aspects box summarizes steps for assisting with placement of a central venous catheter. For the full procedure,

VOL 2 Go to Chapter 36, **Procedure 36-9: Assisting with Percutaneous Central Venous Catheter Placement,** in Volume 2.

Intraosseous Devices

Designed for immediate access (within seconds) and short-term use (less than 24 hours), intraosseous (IO) access devices are used to administer fluids when a peripheral catheter cannot be inserted or when a central line insertion is not advisable, but especially in emergency situations. IOs are placed into the matrix of a bone. The venous sinusoids in the matrix can quickly absorb fluids

FIGURE 36-12 A tunneled central venous catheter is inserted through subcutaneous tissue in the chest wall into the jugular or subclavian vein.

FIGURE 36-13 An implanted venous access port (IVAD) is a CVAD that enters the internal jugular vein in the neck but is tunneled to a completely implanted subcutaneous reservoir (port) in the upper chest.

to send to the central circulation. The most common access site is the proximal tibia in both children and adults. The sternum and the head of the humerus can also be used in adults. Osteomyelitis is a rare complication, occurring in fewer than 1% of cases. Contraindications for IO use include obesity, fracture, recent surgery, infection, or evidence of poor circulation at the proposed insertion site.

KnowledgeCheck 36-9

- What is the purpose of intravenous fluids?
- Describe the types and functions of three IV solutions.
- Under what conditions would a central venous access device be preferable to a peripheral device?

  Go to Chapter 36, **Knowledge Check Response Sheet and Answers,** on the Student Resource Disk or DavisPlus at http://davisplus.fadavis.com/Wilkinson2

CriticalThinking 36-6

What type of venous access device would you expect Martha LaGuardia ("Meet Your Patients") to receive in the hospital? Why?

Starting an Intravenous Infusion

To start an IV infusion, you will need to gather equipment and supplies, set up the solution and administration set, select a venipuncture site, and perform venipuncture.

Obtain Equipment and Supplies

You will need venipuncture supplies and IV infusion equipment. Intravenous supplies are sterile, prepackaged, and disposable. They vary based on manufacturer, so familiarize yourself with what is available in your facility. Set up the solution and administration set before performing the venipuncture.

IV Catheter. Select the smallest diameter and the shortest length catheter that will accommodate the prescribed therapy (Infusion Nursing Society, 2006). Catheter sizes range from 16- to 24-gauge, depending on patient, type of fluid, and infusion rate. Nurses commonly use a 20- or 22-gauge catheter for adults. However, for most peripheral infusions, running at 50 to 175 mL per hour, a 24-gauge thin-walled catheter or a 22-gauge non–thin-walled catheter will deliver more than 1400 mL/hr if needed (Macklin, 2003). You will need a larger size for rapid infusions, viscous (thick) fluids, or surgical or trauma patients.

Administration Set (Infusion Kit). The administration set connects the fluid container to the catheter inserted in the patient. The set consists of tubing with a plastic insertion spike, a drip chamber, a roller clamp to regulate the flow, an injection port, and a catheter adapter (hub) (Fig. 36-14). Both ends of the infusion set (the spike and the hub) are sterile. Remove the protective caps just before use and avoid touching the spike and hub when connecting the tubing to the solution container and the IV catheter in the patient's vein.

FIGURE 36-14 A basic administration set, or infusion kit.

The drip chamber is calibrated to allow a predictable amount of fluid to be delivered in each drop. The drop factor is indicated on the package. A roller clamp on the tubing controls the rate of flow.

- A *macrodrip* delivers 10 to 20 drops per milliliter of solution, depending on the manufacturer; select a macrodrip for most adult infusions.
- A *microdrip* delivers 60 drops per milliliter; use a microdrip for very slow infusion rates or for children.

Extension Tubing and Filters. The end of the IV tubing contains an adapter that attaches to the inserted sterile IV catheter. This should be a locking or screw-on connection, if one is available. You may use extension tubing to lengthen the primary tubing (e.g., for active patients) or to provide additional Y-injection ports for administration of multiple IV solutions or medications.

Occasionally, a filter will be used to remove particulate matter from the solution (e.g., additives or medications that have a tendency to clump), or to filter microorganisms. Some administration sets have built-in filters, or you may attach one to the end of the tubing. The finer the filter size, the smaller the particles that are removed from the solution. Some studies have shown that IV filters reduce the rate of phlebitis and bacteremia by as much as 40%; however, at present, guidelines do not recommend using filters routinely for infection-control purposes (CDC, 2002; Infusion Nurses Society, 2006b).

Injection Port. Use the injection port to administer a secondary IV fluid or medication (see Chapter 23).

Solutions. Inspect the solution container to be certain that it contains the desired fluid, the fluid is clear, the bag is intact, and the solution has not expired. Glass containers were the first containers for IV fluids, but today most IV fluids are packaged in plastic. Fluids for continuous infusions are packed in 1-liter or 500-mL bags. Smaller solution bags (50 mL, 100 mL, and 250 mL) are used for intermittent infusions, such as antibiotics or other medications. Plastic containers collapse as fluid infuses, so you can use a nonvented administration set. Glass bottles do not collapse and therefore require a vented administration set.

Select a Peripheral Intravenous Site

As a rule, select the most distal site on an arm. To select a venipuncture site, consider the following:

- *Age.* For adults, you will usually use veins in the hand or arm (Fig. 36-15); for infants, veins in the scalp or dorsum of the foot.
- *Type of solution.* For hypertonic solutions, viscous solutions, or irritating medications, use a large vein to cause the least amount of trauma.
- *Speed of infusion.* The faster the rate, the larger the vein (and the larger the IV catheter) you will need. Use the largest vein available, keeping other selection criteria in mind.
- *Duration of infusion therapy.* To prevent bacterial colonization and phlebitis, national guidelines recommend changing short peripheral IV catheters every 72 to 96 hours. If the phlebitis rate in an agency is above 5%, catheters should be changed every 48 hours (CDC, 2002; Infusion Nurses Society, 2006b; National Guideline

Clearinghouse, 2008). A PICC line may be needed to extend the length of time the catheter can remain in the vein.

- *Presence of disease or previous surgery.* For example, avoid areas with scarring or with impaired circulation.

For more detailed guidelines for selecting an insertion site,

 Go to Chapter 36, **Clinical Insight 36-4: Guidelines for Selecting a Peripheral Venipuncture Site,** in Volume 2.

Perform Venipuncture

For a successful venipuncture, you need to be able to visualize or palpate the vein before attempting to insert the catheter. Your institution may have a vein viewer to aid in locating the vein. These instruments use infrared light and camera technology to project the patient's superficial veins onto the skin surface. For other suggestions for locating a vein,

 Go to Chapter 36, **Procedure 36-1: Initiating a Peripheral Intravenous Infusion** (the "What If..." section, especially), in Volume 2.

Procedure 36-1 also provides the "fine points" of venipuncture, such as how to stabilize the vein, the angle of insertion, and so on. The Critical Aspects box summarizes the procedure.

If you are not successful with the venipuncture, you can make a second attempt above the initial site or in the opposite extremity. But do not make more than two attempts to start an IV on a patient. Get help from a more experienced colleague.

A Superficial veins of the hand

B Superficial veins of the forearm

FIGURE 36-15 *A,* Superficial veins of the hand. *B,* Superficial veins of the forearm.

Regulating and Maintaining an Intravenous Infusion

Intravenous fluids can flow by gravity or be regulated by an electronic infusion control device ("pump"). You are responsible for maintaining the correct rate of flow and for monitoring the client's response to the infusion. Many factors can influence the flow rate of an IV solution, especially when using gravity flow.

- *The height of the solution container.* The greater the distance between the height of the container and the patient's heart, the faster the flow. Check the flow rate each time the client or IV solution is repositioned to ensure that it is correct.
- *Client position.* Pressure on the IV site decreases flow. If an IV is infusing in the right arm and the patient is positioned on his right side, the pressure on the right arm will be greater than if the client were positioned supine or on the left.
- *Blood pressure.* As blood pressure rises, more force is required to infuse into the vein.
- *The internal diameter of the IV catheter.* The smaller the diameter (the higher the gauge), the more you must open the roller clamp to achieve the flow rate desired.
- *Condition of the catheter and tubing.* If the catheter is dislodged from the vein, flow may stop entirely or continue at a slowed rate. A knot or kink at any point in the tubing will slow flow.

Gravity Flow

Most IV fluids are administered by a volume control pump. However, you may still encounter instances when you will need to regulate the rate with the roller clamp on the tubing. You should check gravity infusion rates hourly, and adjust the flow as needed. If the fluid is running too slowly, do not attempt to catch up by administering extra fluid rapidly. If the fluid is running too fast, slow the rate, and assess the client for signs of fluid volume excess.

If the client is ambulatory, attach the fluid container to a pole with wheels. Instruct the client to keep the solution container above the infusion site and to avoid pulling on the tubing or the infusion site. The Critical Aspects box summarizes how to regulate a gravity-flow IV. For the complete procedure,

 Go to Chapter 36, **Procedure 36-2: Regulating the IV Flow Rate,** Volume 2.

Volume-Control Set

A volume-control set (e.g., Buretrol, Soluset, Volutrol) is another method for regulating an IV infusion (see Fig. 23–34). You will drain a small amount of fluid from the larger IV solution container into the volume-control container. Typically, the volume placed in the volume-control container is equal to the prescribed hourly infusion rate. The rate is regulated in the same way as other administration sets (the drip factor is usually 60 gtts/mL);

however, the maximum amount of fluid that can enter a patient is limited to the volume in the volume-control set. You may use this type of equipment when the client is at risk for fluid volume excess and for infants and children, who require close supervision of fluid intake. However, more often, the policy will be to use an infusion pump for continuous infusions for such patients. An advantage of this system is that medications can be added to the volume-control set and diluted with IV fluid for intermittent administration.

Infusion Pump

If you are using an electronic volume-control device (pump), the machine will maintain the infusion rate after you program it. Most infusion pumps sound an alarm when the fluid bag is almost empty, when air is in the line, or when there is resistance to flow. Infusion control devices save time and prevent accidental delivery of large amounts of fluid. They do not, however, excuse you from regularly monitoring the flow rate and assessing the needle insertion site. ✚ You should know that absence of an alarm does not mean there is no problem. For example, if the IV is infiltrated, the pump may keep infusing fluid into the tissues. The Critical Aspects box describes how to regulate an IV using an infusion pump. For the complete procedure,

 Go to Chapter 36, **Procedure 36-3: Setting Up and Using Volume Control Pumps,** in Volume 2.

KnowledgeCheck 36-10

- What factors should you consider when selecting an insertion site for a peripheral IV line?
- What are the preferred locations for peripheral IV lines?
- What equipment is needed when inserting an IV and starting an IV infusion?
- Identify three ways to regulate the flow rate of IV fluid.

 Go to Chapter 36, **Knowledge Check Response Sheet and Answers,** on the Student Resource Disk or DavisPlus at http://davisplus.fadavis.com/Wilkinson2

Calculating Flow Rates

As you already know, intravenous administration sets are sized as microdrips or macrodrips. Microdrips deliver fluid at a rate of 60 drops/mL. Macrodrips deliver fluid at a rate of 10 to 20 drops/mL (depending on the manufacturer). To begin, you need to know the ordered infusion rate and the flow rate of the administration set in drops per minute. See Box 36-1 to learn how to calculate flow rates.

Managing Multiple Lines

When a patient has multiple IV solutions and multiple lines, you must label each line to identify what is infusing in it. Label the IV tubing close to the catheter so that it is easy to see which fluid is infusing the line. This is especially true when using double- and triple-lumen catheters. Multiple lines are often used because solutions are not compatible with each other (e.g., you

BOX 36-1 ■ Calculating IV Flow Rates

Microdrips = 60 drops/mL

Macrodrips = 10 to 20 drops/mL

You need to know drops per minute: the prescribed infusion rate and the flow rate of the administration set.

1. Multiply the hourly rate (number of mL to be infused in 60 minutes) by the drop factor (in drops per milliliter) to obtain the total drops per hour.

2. Then divide by 60 to get the drip rate in drops per minute. For example, an hourly rate of 100 mL multiplied by 15 drops per milliliter and divided by 60 equals the drip rate. Therefore, the drip rate equals 25 drops per minute.

Use this formula to calculate flow:

$$\frac{\text{Hourly rate in mL} \times \text{drop factor (drops/mL)}}{60 \text{ minutes}} = \text{drip rate}$$

Example:

$$\frac{100 \text{ (mL per hour)} \times 15 \text{ (gtts/mL)}}{60 \text{ minutes}} = 25 \text{ gtts/min}$$

can never infuse blood, parenteral nutrition, or lipids through a line with anything else; and you can never draw blood samples from these lines).

The name of each line should also be reflected in your nursing notes and the intake form. For peripheral IVs, use RA for right arm, LA for left arm, and so on; and designate a number for each site because there may be more than one line or site in each arm (e.g., RA 1, RA 1, LA 1). If the lines are in separate arms, it may seem unnecessary to give each one a number; however, over the course of therapy, some lines may need to be discontinued and new ones started.

For multiport central lines, label each port. For example, with a triple-lumen central catheter, you might have named each lumen as proximal, mid, and distal, or CVAD 1, CVAD 2, CVAD 3. The finished labeling and nursing record may indicate "CVAD 1 – TPN, CVAD 2 – D$_5$-½ NS, CVAD 3 – insulin."

✚ Also be sure to always keep the lines untangled and know where your main IV fluid is (e.g., the D$_5$-½ NS), so that if a crisis occurs or intermittent infusions are needed, you can quickly identify the correct solution and tubing for use.

Complications of Intravenous Therapy

Inserting an IV catheter breaks the body's first line of defense (the skin) and provides a portal of entry for microorganisms. In addition, trauma roughens the vein wall and predisposes the person to platelet clumping and thrombus formation. Minimize this effect by swiftly piercing the skin and anchoring the catheter and tubing to reduce tissue trauma. Complications at the IV site include infiltration, extravasation, infection, thrombus,

and thrombophlebitis. Systemic complications occur less frequently than local complications but may be life-threatening. They include fluid volume excess, sepsis, and embolus. Table 36-8 describes potential complications of IV therapy.

Changing Intravenous Solutions, Tubing, and Dressings

Follow practice guidelines and agency policies for changing IV solutions, tubing and dressings. As with IV insertion, use meticulous aseptic technique.

Changing IV Solutions. Hang a new container of fluid when the present container is nearly empty but fluid still remains at the appropriate level in the drip chamber. The infusion rate dictates how often you need to change the IV solution. For example, a liter of IV fluid infusing at 125 mL/hr must be changed every 8 hours; a liter infusing at 50 mL/hr will hang for 20 hours. Regardless of rate, The Infusion Nurses Society (2006b) recommends you not leave an intravenous solution hanging for more than 24 hours because the likelihood of contamination increases with time. There is not complete agreement about the allowable hang time for a container, though. The National Guideline Clearinghouse (2008) states that there is not enough evidence to make a recommendation about hanging time of parenteral fluids other than blood and parenteral nutrition. In any event, you will need to follow institutional policies. The Critical Aspects Box summarizes the procedure for changing solutions, tubing, and dressings. For full instructions,

VOL 2 Go to Chapter 36, **Procedure 36-4A: Changing the IV Solution, Procedure 36-4B: Changing the IV Solution and Tubing,** and **Procedure 36-5: Changing IV Dressings,** in Volume 2.

Changing Administration Sets. Administration sets for continuous peripheral and central infusions are usually changed every 72 hours (every 24 hours for total parenteral nutrition). Because most peripheral catheters are changed at least every 72 to 96 hours (CDC, 2002), changing the administration set often coincides with inserting a new intravenous catheter. As a rule, if you start an IV at a new site, use a new administration set. Reusing a set from a previous site increases the risk of contamination.

Changing IV Dressings. Change peripheral IV dressings routinely when the catheter is replaced, or at least weekly (CDC, 2002). CVCs usually remain in place for lengthy periods, but the dressing at the site must be changed periodically, usually every 72 hours in acute care settings. In home care, the dressing may be left in place for 1 week. Change any dressing, regardless of site, when it becomes soiled, damp, or loosened. It is best to dress both central and peripheral lines with transparent, semipermeable dressings. These dressings allow direct

Table 36-8 ➤ Complications of Intravenous Therapy

COMPLICATION	CAUSES	SIGNS AND SYMPTOMS	NURSING RESPONSE
Local Complications			
Hematoma—a localized mass of blood outside the blood vessel	Nicking the vein during an unsuccessful insertion, discontinuing an IV line without holding pressure over the site, or applying a tourniquet too tightly above a previously attempted venipuncture site	Ecchymosis, localized mass, discomfort	Be gentle with venipuncture technique. Apply pressure when discontinuing an IV.
*Infiltration—the seepage of nonvesicant solution or medication into surrounding tissues	IV catheter dislodges or the tip penetrates the vessel wall.	Slowed or stopped flow Swelling, tenderness, pallor, hardness and coolness at the site The patient may report a burning sensation in the area.	Stop the infusion immediately. Restart the IV infusion in a different vein, higher in the extremity or in another extremity. Elevate the affected arm on a pillow to promote absorption of excess fluid.
*Extravasation—seepage of a vesicant substance into the tissues. (A *vesicant* is a solution that causes the formation of blisters and subsequent tissue sloughing and necrosis.)	IV catheter dislodges, or the tip penetrates the vessel wall.	Slowed or stopped flow Pain, burning, and swelling at IV site, blanching and coolness of the surrounding skin Blistering is a late sign. If extravasation was due to vasoconstricting medication may see necrosis (death) of dermis.	Treatment depends on the severity of the infiltration. Stop the IV infusion immediately. Administer an antidote, if one is available. (Antidotes alter the pH, alter DNA binding, neutralize the drug, or dilute the extravasated drug.) Apply cold compresses, and elevate the extremity. Treatment depends on the severity of the infiltration. Stop the IV infusion immediately. Administer an antidote, if one is available. (Antidotes alter the pH, alter DNA binding, neutralize the drug, or dilute the extravasated drug.) Apply cold compresses, and elevate the extremity.
Phlebitis—inflammation of the vein	May be due to mechanical irritation, infusion of solutions that are irritating to the vessel, or sepsis. Dextrose solutions, potassium chloride, antibiotics, and vitamin C are associated with a higher risk of phlebitis.	Redness, pain, and warmth at the site, local swelling, palpable cord along the vein, sluggish infusion rate, and elevated temperature	Discontinue the IV infusion. Initially, apply cold compresses to the site. Thereafter, use warm compresses. Consult the primary care provider if there is streaking or erythema along the vein or a palpable cord. *Prevention measures:* Use the smallest catheter practical (usually 22-gauge or 24-gauge thin-walled catheter). Use polyurethane catheters instead of Teflon. Stabilize and secure the catheter to minimize movement in the vein. Rotate the site at least every 96 hours.

Continued

Table 36-8 ➤ Complications of Intravenous Therapy—cont'd

COMPLICATION	CAUSES	SIGNS AND SYMPTOMS	NURSING RESPONSE
	Trauma to the vessel, compression of the line by client movement, or a low flow rate	Slowed or stopped infusion, localized warmth at the site, inability to restart flow of IV	Discontinue the IV infusion, and restart in a new location. Apply cold compresses to the site if the site is warm and tender. Assess for circulatory impairment.
Thrombophlebitis—thrombosis and inflammation	Use of veins in the legs for infusion, use of a hypertonic or highly acidic solution; can be a result of untreated phlebitis	Sluggish flow rate, edema, tender and cordlike veins, warmth and erythema at site	Discontinue the IV infusion, and restart in the opposite extremity, using all new equipment. Apply warm, moist compresses. Consult the primary care provider.
Local infection—microbial contamination of the cannula or IV site	Using poor technique when inserting the catheter, leaving the catheter in place for longer than 72 hours, or direct contamination	Redness, swelling, exudate, elevated temperature	Remove the IV line. Apply a sterile dressing over the site. Administer antibiotics, if necessary.
Nerve injury—A nerve is inadvertently injured during venipuncture (direct) or is compressed	Using veins on inner surface of the wrist and forearm; not anchoring the vein for puncture; using a large needle; advancing the needle across instead of with the vein; "probing" (excessive redirection of the needle at insertion); inserting too deeply and through the back wall of the vein; too many venipuncture attempts; infiltration, extravasation, tourniquet too tight or left on too long	*Direct injury*—sharp acute pain at the site or up and down the arm; pins and needles or electric shock sensation; pain, numbness, or tingling in fingers; pain that persists after the needle is removed *Compression injury*—Pain and tingling typically appear 24 to 96 hours after venipuncture.	Do not make more than 2 venipuncture attempts. *If patient complains of symptoms:* Stop the procedure and withdraw the catheter. Apply pressure to prevent hematoma. Report to supervisor and physician. Do not start a new IV in the affected arm. Treat infiltration if it occurs. **Fasciotomy** (incisions around the area to let blood or fluid seep out) is the usual treatment; or fluid may be expressed.
Systemic Complications			
Septicemia—the presence of microorganisms or their toxic products in the circulatory system	A break in aseptic technique, or contaminated IV solution	Fluctuating fever, chills, tachycardia, confusion, hypotension, altered mental status, elevated WBC count	Discontinue the IV infusion immediately. Consult the primary care provider. Treatment often involves antibiotics, fluids, and medications to support vital signs.
Fluid overload	Infusing excessive amounts of IV fluids or administering fluid too rapidly.	Weight gain, edema, hypertension, shortness of breath, crackles, distended neck veins	Slow the IV flow rate. Place the client in high-Fowler's position. Monitor vital signs. Administer oxygen, if needed. If severe, diuretics may be ordered.
Air embolus—a rare complication involving the introduction of air into the vascular system	Loose connections, adding a new IV bag to a line that has run dry without clearing the line of air; air in tubing cassette of infusion pump	Palpitations, chest pain, lightheadedness, dyspnea, cough, hypotension, tachycardia, sudden change in mental status	Call for help. Place client in Trendelenburg's position on the left side. Administer oxygen. Have emergency equipment available.

Table 36-8 ➤ Complications of Intravenous Therapy—cont'd

COMPLICATION	CAUSES	SIGNS AND SYMPTOMS	NURSING RESPONSE
Catheter embolus— a piece of catheter breaks off and travels through the vascular system	Reinserting a catheter used in an unsuccessful insertion; removing and reinserting a stylet, causing shearing of the catheter; placing the catheter in a joint flexion	Sharp, sudden pain at IV site, jagged catheter end on removal, dyspnea, chest pain, tachycardia, hypotension	Apply a tourniquet above the site. Notify the physician and radiologist. Start a new IV line. Prepare the patient for radiographic examination.

*For more information about interventions for infiltration and extravasation,

 Go to Chapter 36, **Clinical Insight 36-6: Managing Infiltration and Extravasation,** in Volume 2.

Source: Phillips, L. D. (2010). *Manual of I.V. Therapeutics* (5th ed.). Philadelphia: F.A. Davis.

---

visualization of the site between dressing changes, permit evaporation of moisture, and provide a secure anchor for the catheter. You may still sometimes see tape securing a catheter at the insertion site. This trend has diminished, though, because of the risk of contamination of the site (Infusion Nurses Society, 2006b).

Converting to a Peripheral Intravenous Lock

Some clients require only intermittent infusion of medications or venous access for emergencies. They do not need the additional fluids provided by a constant infusion of solution. A peripheral intravenous lock is used for this purpose. The terms *peripheral lock, saline lock,* or *prn adapter* are used interchangeably. You may also hear the term *heparin lock*. A peripheral infusion can be easily converted to a peripheral lock when no further infusion is required.

To create a peripheral lock, remove the tubing from the IV catheter and replace it with a sterile injection cap (see Fig. 36-9). Some IV locks also contain a short segment of tubing. Each time you give a medication through the lock, you will need to disinfect and flush the lock before and after you administer the medication. Consult your agency policy regarding the type of solution to use (saline or a dilute heparin solution). Research has shown that saline is as effective as heparin in maintaining IV lock patency and that there is no difference in the incidence of phlebitis (LeDue, 1997; Niesen, Harris, Parkin, et al., 2006). Converting an IV line to an IV lock is described in the Critical Aspects box. For complete instructions,

 Go to Chapter 36, **Procedure 36-6: Converting a Primary Line to a Heparin or Saline Lock,** in Volume 2.

Discontinuing an Intravenous Line

Discontinue the IV line and IV catheter when IV fluids and medications are no longer needed or if the integrity of the line is compromised. Inspect the catheter to ensure that it is intact when you remove it. The Critical

Aspects box summarizes removal of an IV catheter. For the complete procedure,

 Go to Chapter 36, **Procedure 36-7: Discontinuing a Peripheral IV,** in Volume 2.

KnowledgeCheck 36-11

- The prescription reads, "5% dextrose in water/ 0.45% saline solution (D_5-½ NS) with 20 mEq KCl; infuse 1 liter in 5 hours." Calculate the hourly rate and the drip rate using (1) a macrodrip administration set with 15 drops/mL and (2) a microdrip set.
- Describe the difference between infiltration and extravasation as a complication of IV therapy.
- In general, how often are administration sets changed on peripheral IV lines? When TPN is infused?

Go to Chapter 36, **Knowledge Check Response Sheet and Answers,** on the Student Resource Disk or DavisPlus at http://davisplus.fadavis.com/Wilkinson2

Replacement of Blood and Blood Products

Intravenous fluids can replace fluid volume, but they do not restore oxygen-carrying capacity or replace clotting factors. Blood products are infused when the patient has experienced significant blood loss, diminished oxygen-carrying capacity, or a deficiency in one of the blood components. The American Association of Blood Banks (AABB) estimates that 8 million volunteers donate blood each year, for a total of 15 million units of whole blood and red blood cells (AABB, 2008a). Each unit of donated blood is separated into multiple components, such as red blood cells, plasma, platelets, and clotting factors. Thus, one unit of donated blood may be used in the care of four clients. Unfortunately, fewer than 5% of eligible persons donate blood each year. To be eligible to donate blood, a person must be in good health, at least 17 years of age (although some states permit younger people, with parental consent, to donate), have a hemoglobin of at least 12.5 gm/dL, and weigh at least 110 pounds. In

VOL 2 For steps to follow in *all* procedures, refer to the Universal Steps for All Procedures found on the inside back cover of Volume 2. Go to the full procedures in Volume 2 to practice and learn the procedure steps. Use these Critical Aspects later to help you review key points.

Procedure 36-1: Initiating a Peripheral Intravenous Infusion

➤ Prepare the intravenous solution and administration set, including extension tubing and volume control device if used. Prime the tubing.

➤ Label the IV solution container and place a time-tape on it with the infusion rate. Label the tubing with the date and time.

➤ Apply the tourniquet.

➤ Locate a vein. As a rule, select the most distal vein in an upper extremity. Then loosen the tourniquet.

➤ Don clean nonsterile gloves and open the catheter package. Keep the catheter sterile.

➤ Reapply the tourniquet and cleanse the site. Allow the antiseptic to dry on the skin.

➤ Inform the patient that you are about to insert the catheter.

➤ Use your nondominant hand to stabilize the vein.

➤ Hold the catheter bevel up at a 30° to 45° angle and pierce the skin.

➤ Watch for a flashback of blood. Lower the needle and catheter so they are parallel to the skin, and advance them into the vein.

➤ When the needle is at least halfway into the vein or when a steady backflow of blood occurs, gradually withdraw the needle while advancing the catheter fully into the vein.

➤ While holding the catheter in place with one hand, release the tourniquet with your other hand.

➤ Connect the IV administration set or extension tubing to the IV catheter.

➤ Adjust the flow rate according to the prescriber's order.

➤ Secure the connection; stabilize the catheter; and apply dressing to the IV insertion site.

➤ Label the dressing.

➤ Secure the tubing by looping and taping it to the skin.

➤ Place an arm board as needed.

Procedure 36-2: Regulating the IV Flow Rate

➤ When hanging a new container of IV solution:
  Check the solution to make sure that you have the proper IV fluid with the prescribed additives.
  Apply a time tape to the solution container. Mark the time the infusion was started.
  Open the roller clamp so that the IV fluid begins to flow.

➤ Verify the prescribed infusion rate.

➤ Calculate the drip rate.

➤ Hold a watch beside the drip chamber; count the number of drops for 1 minute.

➤ Adjust the roller clamp, increasing or decreasing the flow until you achieve the prescribed drip rate.

➤ Monitor manually regulated infusion rates closely for the first 15 minutes after you begin the infusion; then monitor the rate hourly.

Procedure 36-3: Setting Up and Using Volume Control Pumps

➤ Calculate the infusion rate.

➤ Attach the volume control pump to the IV pole, and plug it into the nearest electrical outlet.

➤ Take the administration set from the package, close the clamp, and spike the port of the solution container. Attach a filter if one is needed.

➤ Label the tubing and solution container.

➤ Hang the solution container on the IV pole.

➤ Fill the drip chamber halfway.

➤ Place the electronic eye on the drip chamber, if there is one. If not, consult the manufacturer's instructions.

➤ Prime the administration tubing, then close the clamp.

➤ Turn on the pump, and load the administration tubing into the pump.

➤ Program the pump with the hourly infusion rate, total hours, and the volume to be infused.

➤ Apply clean nonsterile gloves.

➤ Cleanse the injection port and check the IV site for patency.

➤ Connect the tubing adapter to the injection port.

➤ Unclamp the administration set tubing, and press the start button.

➤ Make sure that the alarms are turned on and audible.

➤ Check the pump regularly to make sure that the correct volume is infusing.

➤ At the end of your shift (or at the specified time), clear the pump and record the volume.

Procedure 36-4: Changing IV Solutions and Tubing

Procedure 36-4A: For Changing the IV Solution

➤ Prepare and label your next container of IV solution at least 1 hour before the present infusion is scheduled to finish.

➤ Close the roller clamp on the infusing (empty) administration set.

➤ Remove the old IV solution container from the IV pole. Remove the spike from the bag, keeping the spike sterile.

➤ Spike the new IV solution container.

➤ Hang the new IV solution, and inspect the tubing for air.

➤ Adjust the drip rate.

➤ Place the time tape on the new IV solution container. Mark the times.

Procedure 36-4B: Changing the IV Solution and Tubing

➤ Prepare and hang the new IV solution and tubing.

➤ Close the roller clamp on the old administration set.

➤ Wearing clean nonsterile gloves, stabilize the IV catheter while applying pressure over the vein just above the insertion site.

➤ Remove the protective cover from the distal end of the new administration set and connect the new tubing.

➤ Adjust the drip rate.

- Cleanse the IV site.
- Resecure the IV catheter and tubing connection; loop and tape the tubing.
- Label tubing and solution with date, initials, rate, and time tape.

Procedure 36-5: Changing IV Dressings

Procedure 36-5A: Peripheral IV Dressings

- Wearing clean procedure gloves, stabilize the catheter with your nondominant hand, and carefully remove the dressing.
- Inspect the insertion site.
- Don clean gloves. Cleanse the insertion site, following manufacturer's guidelines for product use
- Allow the antiseptic to dry on the skin.
- Don clean nonsterile gloves.
- Apply a new sterile catheter stabilization device and dressing.
- Secure the connection between the catheter and the tubing.
- Loop and tape the tubing to the patient's skin.
- Label the dressing with the date and time of insertion, catheter size, the date the dressing was changed, and your initials.

Procedure 36-5B: Central Line Dressings

- Obtain sterile central line dressing kit and mask for the patient. If there is no kit, you will need at least a mask, sterile gloves, antiseptic solution, dressing, and tape.
- Place the patient in a comfortable position. Some guidelines advise semi-Fowler's.
- Ask the patient to don a mask or turn his head to the opposite side if unable to tolerate a mask.
- Set up a sterile field and arrange your supplies.
- Don mask and clean nonsterile gloves.
- Carefully remove the old dressing and stabilization device.
- Inspect the site for signs of complications.
- Don sterile gloves contained in the kit.
- Scrub the site, using swabs contained in kit.
- Scrub the sutures (if any) and the catheter from insertion site to the hub or bifurcation with an antiseptic swab for at least 15 seconds.
- Allow the site to dry.
- Apply dressing that comes in the kit.
- Remove drape, if one was used.
- Apply the new catheter stabilization device, if one is used.
- Loop the catheter gently and secure it with tape to the skin. Avoid securing it to the dressing.
- Label the dressing with the date changed, time, and your initials.

Procedure 36-6: Converting a Primary Line to a Heparin or Saline Lock

- Don clean nonsterile gloves.
- Remove the IV lock from the package, and flush the adapter, according to agency policy. Do not contaminate the lock.
- Remove the IV dressing and the tape that is securing the tubing.

- Close the roller clamp on the administration set.
- With your nondominant hand, apply pressure over the vein just above the insertion site; stabilize the catheter hub with your thumb and forefinger.
- Disengage the used tubing from the IV catheter. Use a hemostat, if needed, to twist the lock and separate tubing from catheter.
- Quickly insert the lock adapter into the IV catheter and turn it to lock it in place.
- Scrub the adapter injection port and flush the lock again, using the "push, stop, push" technique.
- Apply a sterile transparent semipermeable dressing; do not cover the catheter-tubing connection.
- Label the dressing with date and initials.
- Discard used supplies.
- Maintain sterility of equipment throughout.

Procedure 36-7: Discontinuing a Peripheral IV

- Place a linen-saver pad under the extremity with the IV catheter.
- Don clean nonsterile gloves, and close the roller clamp on the administration set.
- Cleanse the catheter-skin junction with an alcohol pad.
- Place a sterile 2 × 2 in. gauze pad above the IV insertion site and gently remove the catheter. Do not press on the gauze pad while removing the catheter.
- Apply firm pressure with the gauze pad over the insertion site. Hold pressure for 1 to 3 minutes; hold longer if bleeding persists.
- Replace the soiled 2 × 2 in. gauze pad with a new sterile one. Secure it with tape or use a transparent dressing.

Procedure 36-8: Administering a Blood Transfusion

Procedure 36-8A: Administering Blood and Blood Products

- Verify that informed consent has been obtained.
- Verify the physician's order, noting the indication, and rate of infusion.
- Administer any prescribed pretransfusion medications.
- Obtain a blood administration set and 250 mL of IV normal saline solution.
- Obtain the blood product from the blood bank according to your institution's policy. Verify that the blood matches the order. Inspect it for abnormalities.
- With another qualified staff member and using two identifiers, verify the patient and blood product identification (e.g., date of birth, hospital identification number, blood type). Contact the blood bank immediately if there are discrepancies, and do not administer the blood product.
- Document on the blood bank form the date and time the transfusion is begun.
- Close all clamps on the blood administration set. Label the tubing.
- Hang the normal saline and prime the tubing.
- Gently invert the blood product container several times.
- Spike the blood product and hang the blood on the IV pole.

Continued

➤ Obtain a set of vital signs.

➤ Scrub the port with an alcohol swab or chlorhexidine/alcohol antiseptic product for at least 15 seconds before connecting to an existing line.

➤ Attach the administration set tubing to the IV catheter.

➤ Slowly open the roller clamp closest to the blood product. Infuse the first 50 mL slowly; if no reaction, set to the prescribed rate.

➤ Remain with the patient for the first 5 minutes. Measure vital signs in 5 minutes, 15 minutes, and 30 minutes; then hourly.

➤ Observe for and ask the patient to immediately report symptoms of transfusion reaction.

➤ When the blood has transfused, flush the line with the normal saline solution.

➤ Disconnect the tubing from the IV catheter, and dispose of the blood product container and tubing per agency policy.

➤ If a second unit of blood is to be transfused, the same administration set may be used.

➤ Administer any post-transfusion medications prescribed.

Procedure 36-8B: Managing a Transfusion Reaction

➤ If there are signs or symptoms of transfusion reaction, stop the transfusion immediately. Do not flush the tubing.

➤ Call for help and prepare for emergency care.

➤ Disconnect the administration set from the IV catheter.

➤ Call for help.

➤ Obtain vital signs, and auscultate heart and breath sounds.

➤ Maintain patency of the IV catheter by hanging a new infusion of normal saline solution, using new tubing.

➤ Notify the primary care provider.

➤ Place the administration set and blood product container, with the blood bank form attached, inside a biohazard bag. Send the bag to the blood bank immediately.

➤ Obtain blood (in the extremity opposite the transfusion site) and urine specimens according to your institution's policy.

➤ Continue to monitor vital signs frequently.

➤ Administer medications, as prescribed.

Procedure 36-9: Assisting with Percutaneous Central Venous Catheter Placement

➤ Perform meticulous hand hygiene.

➤ Use gowns and maximum barrier precautions.

➤ Obtain vital signs and verify informed consent.

➤ Gather and set up supplies and equipment.

➤ Prepare sterile field and add supplies.

➤ Position the patient (Trendelenburg with a rolled towel between the shoulders).

➤ Offer mask, gown, and sterile gloves to physician.

➤ Don sterile gloves and mask (or follow agency policy).

➤ Prep an 8×10-inch area around the site, using applicators of 2% chlorhexidine gluconate in 70% alcohol, per agency guidelines.

➤ Place the large sterile drape to cover patient's head and chest.

➤ Have the patient turn his head opposite the direction of insertion.

➤ Observe while the physician inserts and sutures the catheter.

➤ Apply sterile transparent dressing, close any lumen clamps, and place tape across the lumens near the injection caps.

➤ Monitor for complications (especially respiratory distress).

➤ Obtain a chest x-ray.

---

addition, each potential donor is screened for travel to certain countries and for a variety of disorders, such as hepatitis, HIV, and Creutzfeldt-Jakob disease (the human form of mad cow disease).

Blood Groups

Human blood is classified into four main groups based on the presence or absence of certain antigens and antibodies. The antigens are located on the surface of the red blood cells, and the antibodies are in the plasma. You inherit the blood group you belong to from your parents. The four main blood groups are A, B, AB, and O.

If you belong to blood group A, you have A antigens on the surface of your red blood cells (RBCs), and B antibodies in your plasma. The opposite is true for persons with blood group B. Blood group AB has both antigens on the surface of the red blood cells and no antibodies at all in the plasma. In contrast, blood group O has neither A or B antigens on the surface of the red blood cells but both A and B antibodies in the blood plasma (Table 36-9). Patients must receive only blood that is compatible with their own blood group.

An additional antigen, known as Rh factor, is also important with blood typing. If the antigen is present,

you are referred to as Rh positive (RH$^+$). If it is absent, you are Rh negative (Rh$^-$). Thus, you can belong to one of the following eight groups:

A Rh$^+$	B Rh$^+$	AB Rh$^+$	O Rh$^+$
A Rh$^-$	B Rh$^-$	AB Rh$^-$	O Rh$^-$

Blood Typing and Crossmatching

Once blood is donated, several tests are performed on the sample. First, the sample is tested for ABO group (blood type) and Rh type (positive or negative), as well as for any unexpected red blood cell antibodies that may cause problems in a recipient. Screening tests assess for evidence of donor infection with hepatitis B and C viruses, HIV, human T-lymphotropic viruses, West Nile Virus, and syphilis. If all disease screens are negative, the blood is acceptable for transfusion and is placed in the pool of available products.

When a potential donor is identified, crossmatching is performed. **Crossmatching** identifies possible minor antigens that will affect the compatibility of the donor blood in the recipient. RBCs from the donor blood are mixed with plasma from the potential recipient. A reagent is added, and the sample is observed for

Table 36-9 ➤ Blood Transfusions

BLOOD GROUP	ANTIGENS	ANTIBODIES	CAN GIVE BLOOD TO	CAN RECEIVE BLOOD FROM
AB	A and B	None	AB	AB, A, B, and O
A	A	B	A and AB	A and O
B	B	A	B and AB	B and O
O	None	A and B	AB, A, B, and O	O

clumping or agglutination. If no clumping is observed, the risk of transfusion reaction is low, and it is considered safe to transfuse the sample of blood. Table 36-9 summarizes blood group matching. As you can see, people with blood group O are considered universal donors, whereas people with blood group AB are considered universal recipients. In regard to Rh factor, people who are Rh$^+$ may receive blood with or without Rh factor. However, people who are Rh$^-$ may receive only Rh$^-$ blood.

When possible, **autologous** (self-donated) units of blood are given instead of blood from a donor. This negates the risk of a mismatch or exposure to undetected disease. Autologous blood is usually collected in the preoperative weeks for possible transfusion during elective surgery. Autologous donation is most often done with orthopedic, cardiac, and vascular surgery. The process of donating autologous blood stimulates the bone marrow to produce new blood cells. Given adequate time for recovery, the collected cells may be wholly or partially replaced prior to surgery.

Blood Products

Several blood products are available for transfusion:

- *Whole blood* contains red blood cells, white blood cells, and platelets suspended in plasma.
- *Red blood cells* are prepared from whole blood by removing the plasma. RBCs can raise the client's hematocrit and hemoglobin levels while minimizing an increase in volume. RBCs are available for transfusion as packed RBCs (PRBC).
- *Plasma* is the liquid portion of the blood. It is 90% water and makes up about 55% of blood volume. Plasma may be transfused whole or may be separated into specific products, such as albumin, clotting factor concentrates, and immune globulins.
- *Platelets* help the clotting process by sticking to the lining of blood vessels. Units of platelets are prepared by using a centrifuge to separate the platelet-rich plasma from the donated unit of whole blood. The platelet-rich plasma is then centrifuged again to concentrate the platelets further. Platelets are used to treat clients who have a shortage of platelets or have abnormal platelet function.
- *White blood cells (WBCs)*, specifically granulocytes, can be collected by centrifugation of whole blood. They

are transfused within 24 hours after collection and are used for infections that are unresponsive to antibiotic therapy. The effectiveness of WBC transfusion is still being investigated.

- *Plasma derivatives* are concentrates of specific plasma proteins prepared from many units of plasma. Plasma derivatives include a variety of clotting factors, immune globulins, and albumin.

Initiating a Transfusion

Before beginning a transfusion, verify the written prescription for the blood product, and obtain a set of vital signs. If the patient's temperature is elevated, inform the primary care provider before hanging the transfusion. Most patients experience a minor elevation in temperature after a transfusion is given. A preexisting elevated temperature may exacerbate this response. As a result, the premedication may be prescribed. Some patients will refuse a blood transfusion because of cultural, religious, or other beliefs. Be ready to discuss with them any available alternatives to whole blood administration.

It is critical to identify the patient and the blood product when transfusing blood. Also inspect the IV site to be sure it is patent before hanging the blood product. Nurses commonly use a 20-gauge catheter to infuse blood—and a larger size for rapid flow rates. There is evidence that a 22-gauge catheter can be used in adults without damage to the red blood cells (Infusion Nurses Society, 2006b; Macklin, 2003). Certainly, for children and the frail elderly, you will need a smaller, 22- or 24-gauge catheter. The Critical Aspects box summarizes the procedure for initiating and monitoring a blood transfusion. For the complete procedure,

 Go to Chapter 36, **Procedure 36-8A and B: Administering a Blood Transfusion** and **Managing a Transfusion Reaction,** in Volume 2.

Transfusion Reactions

Even though you use perfect technique, transfusion reactions can and do occur. Five types of reaction are possible: allergic, bacterial, febrile, or hemolytic reactions; and circulatory overload. Table 36-10 describes each of these reactions. To help prevent transfusion

Table 36-10 ➤ Transfusion Reactions

TYPE OF REACTION	SIGNS AND SYMPTOMS	NURSING RESPONSIBILITIES
Allergic—allergy to blood being transfused	Flushing, itching, wheezing, urticaria (hives); anaphylaxis, if severe	Stop the transfusion. Replace with a saline infusion. Notify the physician immediately. Administer prescribed antihistamine.
Bacterial—contamination of the blood	Fever, chills, vomiting, diarrhea, hypertension	Stop the transfusion. Replace with a saline infusion. Notify the physician. Administer antibiotics as ordered. Treat symptoms.
Febrile—temperature elevation due to sensitivity to WBCs, plasma proteins, or platelets	Fever, chills, warm, flushed skin, aches	Stop the transfusion. Replace with a saline infusion. Notify the physician. Treat symptoms.
Hemolytic reactions—destruction of RBCs as a result of infusing incompatible blood; occurs in 1 in 600,000 transfusions	Fever, chills, dyspnea, chest pain, tachycardia, hypotension; can be fatal	Stop the transfusion immediately. Replace with a saline infusion. Notify the physician immediately. Send the remaining blood, including tubing and filter; a sample of venous blood; and the first voided urine to the lab for analysis. Treat shock.
Circulatory overload—administering too great a volume or too rapidly	Persistent cough, crackles, hypertension, distended neck veins	Slow or stop the transfusion. Monitor vital signs. Place the client upright. Notify the physician.

Toward Evidence-Based Practice

Houck, D., & Whiteford, J. (2007). Transfusion with infusion pump for peripherally inserted central catheters and other vascular access devices. *Journal of Infusion Nursing, 30*(6), 341–344.

In a 500-bed community hospital, policy required that blood transfusions be infused by gravity flow. This policy necessitated that a peripheral IV be initiated if the patient had a peripherally inserted central catheter (PICC). Nurses sought to show that using a PICC line with an infusion pump was safe and efficient. A literature search indicated that one of the main concerns was exceeding the psi (pressure per square inch) tolerance of the catheter. Further literature review showed no increased risk of hemolysis of red blood cells when given via pump as compared to gravity. In the study, a total of 169 units of blood products were infused via various types of PICCs and infusion ports, some using a pump and some using gravity flow. All PICC lines remained patent during transfusion and no problems with using a pump were identified. The study also revealed that nursing time decreased by 30 minutes, using a pump—the time needed to start and maintain another IV site. Cost was decreased when using a pump because of the savings in nursing time and equipment needed for a new IV start. Based on the study, the policy for blood administration via PICC lines was changed.

1. Based on this study, how do you see nurses can affect institution policy and procedure?

2. Are there any other concerns related to infusing blood via an infusion pump that you might have, and why?

 Go to Chapter 36, **Toward Evidence-Based Practice Suggested Responses,** on the Student Resource Disk or DavisPlus at http://davisplus.fadavis.com/Wilkinson2

reactions, be extremely careful in identifying the patient and the blood, start the transfusion slowly, remain with the patient for the first 5 minutes of the transfusion, and assess again at 15 minutes (see Procedure 36-8, in Volume 2).

KnowledgeCheck 36-12

- Identify eight potential blood types.
- Describe the types of blood products that are available for transfusion.
- Identify and describe types of transfusion reactions.

 Go to Chapter 36, **Knowledge Check Response Sheet and Answers,** on the Student Resource Disk or DavisPlus at http://davisplus.fadavis.com/Wilkinson2

CarePlanning & MappingPractice

For Care Planning/Care Mapping practice,

 Go to Student Resources, **Care Planning & Care Mapping Practice,** at http://davisplus.fadavis.com/Wilkinson2

 Go to Chapter 36, **Resources for Caregivers and Health Professionals,** on the Student Resource Disk or DavisPlus at http://davisplus.fadavis.com/Wilkinson2

 Suggested Readings: Go to Chapter 36, **Reading More About Fluids, Electrolytes, and Acid–Base Balance,** on the Student Resource Disk or DavisPlus at http://davisplus.fadavis.com/Wilkinson2

 Bibliography: Go to Volume 2, Bibliography.

CHAPTER 37

Perioperative Nursing

Learning Outcomes

After completing this chapter, you should be able to:

➤ Discuss the importance of perioperative safety.

➤ List "never events" associated with surgery.

➤ Name and differentiate the three phases of the perioperative period.

➤ Describe the ways in which surgeries can be classified.

➤ Discuss factors that affect the degree of risk of surgery.

➤ Identify nursing actions associated with the preoperative phase, including physical preparations for surgery.

➤ Overview preoperative teaching.

➤ Describe the nurse's responsibilities with regard to surgical consent forms.

➤ Compare and contrast the roles of the circulating and scrub nurse.

➤ Compare and contrast general anesthesia, local anesthesia, regional anesthesia, and conscious sedation.

➤ Discuss common nursing interventions during the intraoperative phase, including skin preparation, positioning for surgery, and intraoperative safety measures.

➤ Describe nursing assessments appropriate for surgical clients on admission to the nursing unit.

➤ Identify potential postoperative complications.

➤ Provide nursing care to prevent postoperative complications, including application of sequential compression devices, use of incentive spirometry, and management of gastric suction.

➤ Use nursing diagnoses appropriately to describe a patient's unique needs during the preoperative, intraoperative, and postoperative periods.

Meet Your Patient

Nishad Singh is a 68-year-old man who came to the emergency department (ED) with sudden onset of rectal bleeding. He tells the ED nurse, "I've been real tired and dragging for several months. This morning I felt a little worse than usual. When I went to the bathroom, there was a lot of blood. I've never had that before, and it scared me. I've had to go to the bathroom a couple times this morning, and it's all blood." The ED nurse collects the following data:

BP: 138/88 mm Hg
Pulse: 104 beats/min and regular
Respiratory rate: 20 breaths/min
Temperature: 36.7°C (98.0°F)
Oxygen saturation: 98%

The ED nurse assesses that Mr. Singh is mildly anxious. His breath sounds are clear, but his abdomen is tender in the left lower quadrant (LLQ). The nurse draws blood to be sent to the lab. While they are waiting for the lab results, Mr. Singh tells the nurse, "My stomach is cramping down low, and I need to go to the bathroom." She provides him with a bed pan. He passes approximately 200 mL of bright red blood with a small amount of fecal material. He becomes sweaty and lightheaded after the BM. The nurse rechecks his vital signs and notes that his BP is

(continued on next page)

Meet Your Patient (continued)

now 120/76 mm Hg and that his pulse is up to 120 beats/min. The nurse shows the ED physician the bloody bowel movement and updates him on the change in vital signs. When the ED physician examines Mr. Singh, he tells Mr. Singh that he will need to be admitted to the hospital for further evaluation of the bleeding.

You are the nurse assigned to care for Mr. Singh on the medical–surgical unit. Mr. Singh has been sent from the ED directly to radiology for a computed tomography (CT) scan of his abdomen. The scan reveals a tumor in the sigmoid colon. Since leaving the ED, Mr. Singh has had three more bloody bowel movements. His blood pressure is 100/72 mm Hg, and his pulse rate is now 134 beats/min. The physician prescribes a bolus of 1000 mL of lactated Ringer's solution and a unit of packed red blood cells as soon as it is available. Mr. Singh is scheduled for colon resection surgery, which will occur as soon as the surgical team can be assembled and the room prepared.

In this chapter, we discuss how to prepare a client for surgery and the activities that occur before, during, and after surgery. We follow Mr. Singh through the stages of perioperative care.

Perioperative Nursing

Perioperative nursing involves the care of clients before, during, and after surgery and some other invasive procedures. Historically, perioperative nursing practice was called "operating room nursing" and was limited to transferring patients into and out of operating rooms and handing instruments to surgeons during surgical procedures. Now nurses in all phases of the operative experience actively provide and manage care, teach, and study the care of perioperative patients.

The Association of periOperative Registered Nurses (AORN) is one of the most highly organized and influential specialty organizations within the nursing profession. AORN *Standards and Recommended Practices* (2009) keep perioperative nurses up to date on current practice. For additional information about AORN,

 Go to the **AORN** Web site at www.aorn.org

Perioperative Safety

An important aspect of the perioperative nursing role is to help prevent complications of surgery. Hand hygiene is an important component of prevention (Box 37-1). Preventable perioperative errors cause 10% of surgery-related deaths, have an unfavorable financial impact on healthcare institutions, and result in physical and emotional harm to patients (Agency for Healthcare Research and Quality, 2008). Various government and private organizations stress the importance of patient safety.

- *The Association of periOperative Registered Nurses (AORN, 2009).* Perioperative Safety is one of the three domains under which AORN organizes its perioperative patient outcomes (the others are Physiological Responses and Patient and Family Behavioral Responses). Specific safety outcomes include prevention of injury and freedom from infection.
- *The Joint Commission.* The Joint Commission 2009 Patient Safety Goals (2008) applicable to surgery include preventing infection, improving the accuracy of patient identification, encouraging patients' active involvement in care as a safety strategy, and performing a time-out immediately before starting procedures.
- *The National Priorities Partnership (NPP, 2008).* The NPP National Quality Forum aims to eliminate harm, eradicate disparities, reduce disease burden, and remove waste in the American healthcare system. One

 BOX 37-1 ■ Recommended Practices for Hand Hygiene

- Perform hand hygiene:
  Immediately before and after each patient contact
  After removing gloves. Wearing gloves does not substitute for hand hygiene.
  Any time you may have come in contact with blood or potentially infectious substances
  Before and after eating
  After using the restroom
- Remove rings, watches, and bracelets before performing hand hygiene.
- Preferably, do not wear rings. They have been associated with a significant increase in skin microorganism count.
- Keep fingernails short and clean. They should not extend beyond the fingertips.
- Replace nail polish when it is chipped or at least every 4 days.
- Do not wear artificial nails. Fungal growth often occurs under them.
- Be certain there are no lesions or breaks in skin integrity on your hands.
- For handwashing and handrub procedures,

 Go to Chapter 20, **Procedure 20-1: Hand Hygiene,** in Volume 2.

Sources: Adapted from AORN (2009); Boyce & Pittet (2002); Siegel, Rhinehart, Jackson, et al. (2007).

of its six national priorities and goals is to improve the safety and reliability of healthcare, aiming for "zero" harm whenever possible.

- **Centers for Disease Control and Prevention (CDC).** Several years ago, the CDC issued seven healthcare safety challenges. One of the challenges was to reduce certain surgical adverse events and bacterial infections by 50% (CDC, 2001).
- **The Institute for Healthcare Improvement (IHI).** This is an independent, not-for-profit organization that works to reduce morbidity and death in American healthcare, including perioperative care. To see the entire list of IHI recommendations (IHI, n.d.),

 Go to Chapter 21, **ESG Box 21-1, The 100,000 Lives Campaign,** on the Student Resource Disk or DavisPlus at http://davisplus.fadavis.com/Wilkinson2

"Never Events"

"Never events" are serious and costly errors resulting in severe consequences for the patient, and that are mostly preventable. Believing these events are reasonably preventable and should never happen in a hospital, Medicare will no longer reimburse institutions for care related to such complications (Centers for Medicare and Medicaid Services, 2006, 2008). Several of the never events are also targeted by the national organizations listed earlier. Among the never events important to perioperative care are:

- Surgery on the wrong body part
- Surgery on the wrong patient
- Wrong surgery on a patient
- Deep vein thrombosis or pulmonary embolism after total knee or hip replacement
- Foreign body left in a patient after surgery (e.g., sponge, clip for draping)
- Surgical site infections after certain elective procedures (e.g., bariatric surgery for obesity). AORN, The Joint Commission, NPP, and IHI extend that to include all infections. The CDC targeted certain antimicrobial-resistant bacterial infections.

You will see those themes recur in the theoretical and practical knowledge in the remainder of this chapter and in Volume 2.

Preoperative Care

The **preoperative phase** begins with the client's decision to have surgery and ends when he enters the operating room.

Theoretical **Knowledge** knowing why

Nursing care during the preoperative phase focuses on identifying existing health concerns, planning for intraoperative and postoperative needs, and providing preoperative teaching. Preoperative nursing care is delivered in a variety of settings. More than two-thirds of surgeries in the United States are performed in outpatient settings, such as endoscopy suites, physicians' offices, and ambulatory surgery centers (CDC National Center for Health Statistics, 2009). The length of the preoperative period and the extent of the patient teaching depend on the type of surgery to be done and the patient's overall health status.

How Can Surgeries Be Classified?

Surgeries can be classified by body system, purpose, level of urgency, and acuity. The classifications often overlap. Knowing the type of surgery helps you identify the patient's perioperative needs and plan patient care.

By Body System

The body system classification is useful for determining the postoperative risk of infection. Surgical incisions that enter the gastrointestinal, respiratory, or genitourinary tracts have a higher risk for infection than does surgery of other body systems. However, if an organ ruptures or surgery is required to repair a penetrating injury, the risk of infection is very high regardless of the body system involved. Mr. Singh ("Meet Your Patient") will have surgery of the gastrointestinal system.

By Purpose

The following purposes are used to describe surgery. See whether you can identify the purpose that describes Mr. Singh's ("Meet Your Patient") surgery.

- **Ablative surgery** involves removal of a diseased body part. For example, a cholecystectomy removes a diseased gallbladder.
- **Diagnostic (exploratory) surgery** is undertaken to confirm or rule out a diagnosis. Examples include a biopsy, a fine-needle aspiration, or invasive testing, such as a cardiac catheterization.
- **Palliative surgery** is done to alleviate discomfort or other disease symptoms without producing a cure. Examples include nerve root destruction for chronic pain or tumor debulking (removal of a portion of a mass when complete excision is not possible).
- **Reconstructive surgery** is performed to restore function, for example, rotator cuff repair; repair of a torn ligament).
- **Cosmetic surgery** is done to improve appearance (e.g., a face-lift).
- **Transplant surgery** replaces a malfunctioning body part, tissue, or organ. Joint replacements and organ replacement procedures are included in this category. A related procedure, in which an organ or tissue is harvested from someone pronounced brain dead for transplantation into another person, is called **procurement surgery.**

By Degree of Urgency

Based on the following definitions, how would you describe the degree of urgency for Mr. Singh's surgery?

- **Emergency surgery** requires transport to the operating suite as soon as possible to preserve the patient's life or function. The surgical team is summoned and preparations are made rapidly. Internal hemorrhage, rupture of an organ, and trauma are common causes of emergency surgery.
- **Urgent surgery** is scheduled within 24 to 48 hours to alleviate symptoms, repair a body part, or restore function. Removal of a cancerous breast and internal fixation of a fracture are examples.
- **Elective surgery** is performed when surgery is the recommended course of action, but the condition is not time sensitive. The client may delay surgery to gather information, consider options, or organize care for the family. Examples include repair of a torn ligament, removal of rectal polyps, or a rhinoplasty (repair of the nose).

By Degree of Risk

There is an old adage that "the only minor surgery is someone else's surgery." This statement reflects the anxiety that often accompanies surgery. Nevertheless, surgery is defined as major or minor based on the degree of seriousness or risk associated with the procedure. The degree of risk varies with the condition of the client, as well as with the type of surgery.

Major surgery is associated with a high degree of risk. For example, it may be associated with the potential for significant blood loss, involve vital organs, be a prolonged or complicated procedure, or have significant potential for postoperative complications. Some examples of major procedures are coronary artery bypass graft (CABG), organ transplantation, nephrectomy (removal of a kidney), and colon resection.

Minor surgery, often performed on an outpatient basis, involves little risk and usually has few complications. Examples include arthroscopy, breast biopsy, and inguinal hernia repair.

What Factors Affect Surgical Risk?

The patient's age, general health, and personal habits can contribute to increased risk during any surgical procedure. Be sure to include parents and caregivers in your plan of care.

Age. The very young and very old are at greatest risk during surgical procedures. Infants have limited ability to regulate temperature and have immature immune, cardiovascular, liver, and renal systems. They are also at greater risk for infection. For infants, even minor blood loss may represent a substantial portion of the total blood volume. They are also at risk for volume overload. In addition, infants may have difficulty calming. They are unable to understand what is happening, so you cannot use verbal reassurance and explanations to comfort them. Toddlers understand simple explanations but may be anxious about separation from parents or caregivers. Many have fear of the dark. Preschoolers fear damage to body parts. Fear of pain or of needles is common for children of any age. Teens might fear disfigurement resulting from scars. Young adults commonly have anxiety about the cost associated with hospitalization or surgery.

Older adults are at increased risk because they have less physiological reserve and often have comorbid conditions (other illness not related to the surgery). Many of the physiological changes of aging predispose older adults to increased risk. Among these changes are decreased kidney function, diminished immune function, decreased bone and lean body mass, increased peripheral vascular resistance, decreased cardiac output, decreased cough reflex, and increased time required for wound healing.

Type of Wound. Both preexisting wounds (e.g., from trauma) and the wounds (incisions) created by the surgical procedure can pose a risk for infection (Table 37-1). Risk to the patient increases along with the risk for or presence of infection. Which type of wound will Mr. Singh have immediately after surgery?

Preexisting Conditions. The ideal surgical candidate is a healthy young adult who takes no medications. Unfortunately, many surgical clients have underlying acute or chronic disorders that increase surgical risk (Box 37-2).

Mental Status. Patients with altered cognition, from either physical or mental illness, may be unable to comprehend preoperative instructions or give informed consent for surgical procedures. They may also require medications (e.g., antipsychotic agents) that interact with anesthetics and analgesics given in the perioperative period. Surgery and anesthesia may aggravate preexisting dementia, confusion, and disorientation.

Medications. Both prescribed and over-the-counter medications may increase surgical risk (Box 37-3). For example, patients who self-prescribe high doses of vitamin E may be at increased risk for bleeding. Certain herbal and alternative medications can:

- Increase the risk for cardiac dysrhythmias secondary to potassium loss.
- Interfere with metabolism of anesthetics because of their effects on the liver.
- Increase the potential for excessive bleeding.
- Decrease cerebral blood flow.
- Cause hypertension.
- Increase the effects of opioids and sympathetic nervous system stimulants.

Table 37-1 ➤ Wound Type and Potential for Infection

WOUND TYPE	WOUND CHARACTERISTICS	EXAMPLES OF SURGERY ASSOCIATED WITH THE WOUND
Clean Wounds	Uninfected; minimal inflammation; little risk of infection AND Surgery does not involve the gastrointestinal, respiratory, or genitourinary tract.	Face lift, cataract surgery, joint replacement, breast biopsy, tonsillectomy
Clean-contaminated Wounds	Not infected, but carry increased risk for infection	Surgical incisions that enter the gastrointestinal, respiratory, or genitourinary tracts
Contaminated Wounds	Not infected, but carry high risk for infection	Surgery to repair trauma to open wounds, such as compound fractures; surgery in which a major break in surgical asepsis occurred
Infected Wounds	Evidence of infection, such as purulent drainage, necrotic tissue, or bacterial counts above 100,000 organisms per gram of tissue	A postoperative surgical incision of any type that has evidence of infection

---

BOX 37-2 ■ Preexisting Conditions that Increase Surgical Risk

Chronic Conditions

- *Cardiovascular diseases,* such as hypertension, congestive heart failure, and myocardial infarction, affect the ability of the heart to work as an efficient pump. If these disorders are well controlled (e.g., with blood pressure medications or cardiotonic medications), risk is limited.

- *Coagulation disorders* delay clotting and increase blood loss, placing the patient at risk for hemorrhage and hypovolemic shock. In contrast, a hypercoagulation state increases the risk of stroke, embolism, or intravascular clotting.

- *Chronic respiratory disorders,* such as emphysema, asthma, or bronchitis, decrease pulmonary function, increase the risk of respiratory infection, and may be exacerbated (made worse) by general anesthesia.

- *Renal disease* affects the patient's ability to excrete many medications, including anesthetic agents. It also affects the ability to regulate fluid and electrolytes.

- *Diabetes mellitus* delays wound healing and increases the risk of infection and cardiovascular disorders associated with diabetes.

- *Liver disease* affects the body's ability to metabolize amino acids, carbohydrates, and fat; to manufacture prothrombin

for clotting; and to detoxify medications. Therefore, the patient is at increased risk for poor wound healing, hemorrhage, and toxic reactions to anesthetics and medications.

- *Neurological disorders,* such as paralysis or spinal cord injury, increase the risk for vasomotor instability and thus create the potential for wide swings in blood pressure. In addition, patients with seizure disorders are more likely to have a seizure in the perioperative period.

- *Nutritional disorders* can affect surgical outcomes. Patients who are malnourished or obese are at risk for delayed wound healing, infection, and fatigue. Obese clients are also more prone to cardiovascular disorders and impaired pulmonary function.

Acute Conditions

- *Upper respiratory tract infections* are associated with increased risk of postoperative pneumonia, especially if the patient receives a general anesthetic.

- *Acute infections* tax the patient's energy and physiological reserves, increasing the risk for various postoperative complications.

For a list of herbal products and associated surgical risks,

Go to Chapter 37, **ESG Box 37-1,** on the Student Resource Disk or DavisPlus at http://davisplus.fadavis.com/ Wilkinson2

Personal Habits. Abusing alcohol, nicotine, or other substances can increase surgical risk. Smoking affects pulmonary function; long-term alcohol use contributes to liver disease, predisposing the patient to bleeding.

Alcohol and drugs interact with anesthetic agents and medications to create adverse effects. Also, habitual substance abusers may have a cross-tolerance to anesthetic and analgesic agents, causing them to need higher than normal doses.

Allergies. Patients may be allergic to medications (e.g., certain antibiotics, such as penicillins or cephalosporins), analgesics (e.g., codiene), tape, latex, and solutions used in surgery. Reactions range from unpleasant to life-threatening.

BOX 37-3 ■ Medications that Increase Surgical Risk

Antibiotics	May potentiate the action of anesthetic agents.
Anticoagulants	Increase risk for bleeding.
Antidysrhythmics	May impair cardiac function during anesthesia.
Antihypertensives	Increase the risk for hypotension during surgery; may interact with anesthetic agents to cause bradycardia and impaired circulation.
Aspirin	Increases risk for bleeding.
Corticosteroids	Delay wound healing and increase risk for infection.
Diuretics	Alter fluid and electrolyte balance (especially potassium balance).
Opioids	Increase the risk of respiratory depression.
NSAIDs	Inhibit platelet aggregation, increasing the risk for bleeding.
Tranquilizers	Increase the risk of respiratory depression.

KnowledgeCheck 37-1

- Define *preoperative phase.*
- What are four ways surgery can be classified?
- What factors affect surgical risk?

Go to Chapter 37, **Knowledge Check Response Sheet and Answers,** on the Student Resource Disk or DavisPlus at http://davisplus.fadavis.com/Wilkinson2

CriticalThinking 37-1

How would you evaluate Mr. Singh's ("Meet Your Patient") surgical risk? What additional information do you need to answer this question?

Practical Knowledge
knowing how

The nursing focus in the preoperative phase is to prepare the patient for surgery. You will use the nursing process to identify any unique nursing diagnoses a patient might have. However, many perioperative nursing interventions are routine preventive measures that you will use for *all* surgical patients.

Perioperative Nursing Data Set

In the late 1980s, AORN began to develop the Perioperative Nursing Data Set (PNDS), a standardized vocabulary specifically designed to describe the care of perioperative patients. The PNDS is derived from the Perioperative

Patient-Focused Model. The patient is at the center of the model and the focus of care. The perioperative nurse intervenes within the context of the healthcare system to assist the patient throughout the perioperative experience to achieve outcomes in the following domains:

Health System Domain
Patient-Centered Domains
- Safety
- Physiological responses to surgery
- Behavioral responses to surgery

The health system domain refers to the system in which perioperative care is given. It involves administrative and structural elements necessary for successful surgical outcomes—for example, equipment, supplies, staff, and policies (AORN, 2009).

The PNDS is the first nursing language developed by a specialty organization that has been recognized by the American Nurses Association. The PNDS includes terminology for nursing diagnoses, nursing interventions, and nurse-sensitive patient outcomes appropriate for use in any surgical setting.

In this chapter, we continue to use the NANDA-I, NOC, and NIC standardized languages, to which you have already been introduced in previous chapters.

ASSESSMENT

For patient safety, patient data must be correct and complete. To prevent omission of important information, many organizations have developed a preoperative checklist. Although the forms may vary at each institution, the areas for assessment are the same and are discussed in the sections that follow.

Focused Nursing History

It is essential to determine whether the client is physiologically, cognitively, and psychologically prepared for the intraoperative and postoperative phases of surgery. For an accurate nursing history, you will collect assessment data from the client, significant others, medical records, and other members of the healthcare team. Include the following topics in your preoperative assessment: health history, physical status, allergies, medications (including herbal products and over-the-counter medications), mental status, knowledge and understanding of the surgery and anesthesia, cultural and spiritual factors, access to social resources, coping strategies, and use of alcohol and drugs. To see an example of a preoperative assessment form developed by the AORN,

Go to Chapter 37, **Assessment Guidelines and Tools, Example of a Perioperative Checklist (AORN),** in Volume 2.

Additional assessments may be needed if the client is undergoing outpatient surgery or has a planned short stay after surgery (see the box, Home Care: Preoperative

Home Care

Preoperative Assessment for the Surgical Client Who Will Be Discharged to Home

The type of surgery, the client's condition, and the support system determine whether it is safe to discharge a client to home after surgery. Your assessment for home care should focus on these questions:

➤ What kind of care will be needed?

➤ Is the client able to take care of himself? If not, who is available to assist with care?

➤ Does the caregiver have the necessary skills to provide care?

➤ If not, can these skills be taught before the client is discharged?

➤ What features in the home environment will facilitate the client's progress? What features will inhibit progress? For example, can the client get to the bathroom? Can the client negotiate the stairs in the house?

➤ How will the client be followed after discharge? That is, how soon should he visit his physician? Will he receive home nursing care?

Assessment for the Surgical Client Who Will Be Discharged to Home).

Focused Physical Assessment

If you identify risk factors from the nursing history, focus on these aspects during your brief head-to-toe physical assessment. For example, if the patient states she had a cough last week, perform a focused assessment of the ear, nose, throat, and lungs to determine how the cough may affect the patient's risk. If the patient has lower airway congestion, as evidenced by rhonchi and productive cough, communicate these findings to the surgeon and the anesthesia team; if a general anesthetic is planned, it may be necessary to delay the surgery. For all patients, assess risk factors for thrombophlebitis, as venous thrombus is one of the never events that are important to prevent. For additional details on a brief (bedside) physical assessment, see Chapter 19.

Diagnostic Testing

Preoperative screening tests are usually prescribed before surgical procedures. The type of testing depends on the patient's age, health history, and facility policies. For example, most institutions require a complete blood count and urinalysis before surgery, as well as an electrocardiogram for patients older than age 50. Patients with chronic health problems may require additional testing.

 Go to Chapter 37, **Diagnostic Testing: Common Preoperative Screening Tests,** in Volume 2.

KnowledgeCheck 37-2

- List the information you should gather in the preoperative nursing history.
- What type of physical assessment is performed as part of the preoperative assessment?
- What laboratory tests are most commonly prescribed before surgery?

 Go to Chapter 37, **Knowledge Check Response Sheet and Answers,** on the Student Resource Disk or DavisPlus at http://davisplus.fadavis.com/Wilkinson2

CriticalThinking 37-2

- What factors will affect your preoperative assessment of Mr. Singh ("Meet Your Patient")?
- Describe how you might perform the assessment as well as provide physical care. What modifications, if any, should you make in his assessment?

■ ANALYSIS/NURSING DIAGNOSIS

As you learned in Chapter 4, nursing diagnoses describe the individualized needs of patients. Preoperative patients share a common set of needs, regardless of their individual differences and the type of surgery they are to have. Consider the following examples:

- All preoperative patients need preoperative teaching, so it's not necessary to write a nursing diagnosis of Deficient Knowledge for every patient. Agency protocols or critical pathways will almost certainly mandate teaching.
- Almost all surgical patients have at least mild anxiety, and many of your routine actions will help to relieve anxiety, so there is no need to always include a diagnosis of Anxiety.

Note: Do not put any nursing diagnosis on the care plan unless you plan to address it with something other than the routine preoperative interventions.

Individualized Nursing Diagnoses

Individualized nursing diagnoses for the preoperative patient evolve from your assessment. You should identify an actual nursing diagnosis only if the patient has the defining characteristics for it. Identify "risk" diagnoses only if the patient has an underlying condition that places him at higher risk than the average surgical patient. The following NANDA-I nursing diagnoses may be useful for certain preoperative patients:

- *Anxiety* may be mild, moderate, severe, or at panic level. In the preoperative client, anxiety may be related to the current change in health status or due to concerns about being unable to provide care for loved ones. Make this diagnosis only if the client has symptoms such as restlessness, trembling, increased pulse, and so on.

- **_Fear_** is a common reaction to surgery. Fear may be related to the unknown outcome of the surgery, to learning the diagnosis after a diagnostic procedure, and to the prospect of pain during and after surgery. Fear and Anxiety share several defining characteristics. Many of the routine preoperative interventions help to address Fear.

- **_Ineffective airway clearance_** may be used for patients who have a preexisting health problem, such as bronchitis or emphysema.

- **_Disturbed Sleep Pattern_** often results from anxiety about the upcoming surgery.

- **_Ineffective Coping_** may be appropriate for a patient with extreme anxiety and concerns about the outcomes of the surgery.

- **_Latex Allergy Response_** is appropriate for patients who have a known allergy to latex.

- **_Risk for Latex Allergy Response_** is appropriate for patients who have had multiple surgeries or urinary catheterizations; are in professions with daily exposure to latex; have a history of asthma; or are allergic to bananas, avocados, kiwi, chestnuts, or poinsettia plants. Do not use it routinely for all patients.

- **_Deficient Knowledge._** As you know, all patients need preoperative teaching, a routine intervention; so, you do not usually need a Deficient Knowledge diagnosis. If you believe the patient may not learn, or that the information is too complex to remember, then identify the problem likely to result from the Deficient Knowledge. For example:

Ineffective Management of Therapeutic Regimen related to Deficient Knowledge of postoperative medications and office visits

Risk for Infection related to Deficient Knowledge of wound care and asepsis.

Special Risks for Older Adults

Older adults, especially those older than age 70 and the frail elderly, are likely to need some individualized nursing diagnoses. They present unique risks because they often have other illnesses, but also because of certain physiological changes of aging. For example, older adults metabolize anesthetic agents differently from younger adults.

 Critical**Thinking** 37-3

Which, if any, of the preceding nursing diagnoses would be most appropriate for Mr. Singh ("Meet Your Patient")? Do not use the potential complications in Table 37-2. Explain your reasoning.

■ PLANNING OUTCOMES/EVALUATION

The overall nursing goal in the preoperative phase is to prepare the patient adequately for surgery and to deliver him to the operating suite in the best condition possible. Outcomes that provide evidence of achieving this goal, and that are appropriate for nearly all preoperative patients, are that the patient:

- Is able to describe his surgical procedure in a basic manner.
- Provides informed consent.
- When asked, states what he can expect in the postoperative period.
- States he has very little anxiety.

Table 37-2 ➤ Special Risks for Older Adults	
RISK FACTORS	**POTENTIAL COMPLICATIONS (PC) AND NURSING DIAGNOSES**
Most older adults have at least some degree of coronary artery disease.	■ PC: Hypotension ■ Risk for Falls secondary to postural hypotension
Age-related respiratory changes, such as decreased chest wall compliance, forced vital capacity, and diaphragmatic strength	■ PC: Pneumonia ■ PC: Atelectasis
Age-related skin changes: Dry, fragile skin; decreased turgor and elasticity	■ Risk for Impaired Skin Integrity ■ Risk for Impaired Tissue Integrity
Age-related musculoskeletal changes: Decreased bone mass and muscle fiber mass	■ Risk for Impaired Mobility ■ Risk for Falls
Comorbidities of the central nervous system are more common in older adults. Some conditions may be aggravated by surgery and anesthesia.	■ PC: Dementia ■ Risk for Acute Confusion
Age-related decrease in gastrointestinal motility	■ PC: Ileus ■ Risk for Aspiration secondary to vomiting
Age-related decreases in genitourinary function: decreased bladder tone, elasticity, and tone; decreased renal function	■ PC: Side effects of medications ■ PC: Renal complications ■ PC: Urinary tract infection ■ Risk for Impaired Skin Integrity r/t urinary incontinence

Associated NOC outcomes for the preoperative nursing client depend, of course, on the nursing diagnoses you identify. For outcomes and goals using NOC terminology for the diagnoses Anxiety, Fear, Deficient Knowledge, and Disturbed Sleep Pattern, and for *individualized goals/outcome statements* you might write for those diagnoses,

 Go to Chapter 37, **Standardized Language, Preoperative Patients—Selected Standardized Nursing Diagnoses, Outcomes, and Interventions,** in Volume 2.

PLANNING INTERVENTIONS/IMPLEMENTATION

For *NIC standardized interventions* designed to achieve the expected outcomes for the nursing diagnoses of Anxiety, Fear, Deficient Knowledge, and Disturbed Sleep Pattern,

 Go to Chapter 37, **Standardized Language, Preoperative Patients—Selected Standardized Nursing Diagnoses, Outcomes, and Interventions,** in Volume 2.

Many preoperative nursing activities are routine interventions to be used for *all* preoperative patients, regardless of their nursing diagnoses. NIC has a special Perioperative Care domain (category) for such interventions. The following are the preoperative NIC interventions in that domain:

- *Preoperative Coordination:* Facilitating preadmission diagnostic testing and preparation of the surgical patient. (Activity example: Notify the physician of abnormal diagnostic test results.)
- *Surgical Preparation:* Providing care to a patient immediately before surgery and verifying required procedures/tests and documentation in the clinical record. (Activity example: Complete the preoperative checklist.)
- *Teaching: Preoperative:* Assisting a patient to understand and mentally prepare for surgery and the postoperative recovery period. (Activity example: Correct unrealistic expectations of the surgery, as appropriate.)

The following sections explain in more detail how to carry out routine interventions such as obtaining informed consent for the surgery, providing preoperative teaching, communicating with the surgical team, and preparing the client physically.

Confirm that Surgical Consent Has Been Obtained

Before a surgical procedure is performed, professional standards and the law require the surgeon to obtain the patient's informed consent. Consent is nearly always obtained by having the patient sign a form provided by the healthcare agency. Once signed and witnessed, the consent form is part of the patient's record and accompanies him to the operating room.

The signed consent form verifies that the surgeon and patient have communicated adequately about the surgery (Dale, Rothrock, & McEwen, 2003). Informed consent helps protect patients from having a surgery they do not understand or want, and the signed document protects the healthcare agency and workers from later claims that the patient did not consent to have the procedure. Also see Chapters 44 and 45 regarding informed consent, if you would like more information.

Informed consent means that the physician presented information about the surgery and that the patient understood it and was not coerced (pressured) to consent. The patient must be alert, rational, mentally competent, and not sedated when he signs; and the information must be given to him in a language and vocabulary that he can understand. If a patient is not capable of giving informed consent (e.g., is unconscious or has dementia) or if the patient is a minor child, in most states a family member, conservator, or legal guardian may give consent for the procedure.

The surgical consent form includes the following information (The Joint Commission, 2008):

- The type of surgery being performed
- The name and qualifications of the person performing the surgery (e.g., Jason Esmar, MD) and the primary practitioner for the patient's care and treatment
- A statement that the risks and benefits of surgery, as well as reasonable alternatives, have been explained to the patient
- A statement of the relevant risks, benefits, and side effects of the alternatives
- The likelihood of achieving goals
- A statement that the patient has the right to refuse surgery or withdraw consent at any time
- When indicated, any limitations on the confidentiality of information about the patient

The surgeon is responsible for (1) giving the patient the necessary information and (2) determining the patient's competence to make an informed decision about the surgery. You are responsible for verifying that the surgical consent form is signed and witnessed. Often you will obtain the signature and document on the preoperative checklist that you have done so. As a patient advocate, you should first verify with the patient that the physician has explained the procedure and answered all his questions: Ask the patient to state what he was told during the consent process. If the patient has questions or if you have any questions about the patient's competence, notify the surgeon, and delay sending the patient to surgery. Be sure to document these conversations, and document in the nursing notes that the surgeon was notified of any additional questions or concerns.

KnowledgeCheck 37-3

- Who is responsible for obtaining informed consent for the surgical procedure?
- What are the nursing responsibilities related to informed consent?

Go to Chapter 37, **Knowledge Check Response Sheet and Answers**, on the Student Resource Disk or DavisPlus at http://davisplus.fadavis.com/Wilkinson2

Provide Preoperative Teaching

Preoperative teaching prepares the patient for the surgical experience, allays fears, and decreases the risks of postoperative complications. See Chapter 24 as needed to review patient teaching. The content of the teaching plan should focus on:

- Explaining what will happen before, during, and after surgery
- Explaining to patient's and families what they can do to help safeguard against surgical site infection.
- Instructing the patient or caregiver how to participate in the care
- Discussing common feelings and concerns that patients have about surgery. This helps the patient feel supported and less anxious.

What to Teach

The type of surgery influences the content of your teaching. For example, if the patient is scheduled for an outpatient knee arthroscopy (visualization of the joint) under spinal anesthesia, the teaching plan needs to describe the procedure and the anticipated discharge of the patient within hours after surgery. This is different from the teaching for a patient who will have cardiac surgery and spend a number of days in the hospital. It is important to teach patient's the content in the Self-Care box, Teaching Patients How to Help Prevent Surgical Site Infections. To learn the common content you need to discuss with *all* preoperative patients,

 Go to Chapter 37, **Clinical Insight 37-1: Preoperative Teaching,** in Volume 2.

The Critical Aspects box in this chapter summarizes the teaching of deep-breathing, coughing, moving in bed, and leg exercises. For the complete steps,

 Go to Chapter 37, **Procedure 37-1: Teaching a Patient to Cough, Deep-Breathe, Move in Bed, and Perform Leg Exercises,** in Volume 2.

How to Teach

You can use written instructions, video presentations, phone contact, or face-to-face discussion to provide preoperative teaching. Teach in a language the patient understands and at a level that is easily understood. Use terms the patient understands clearly, that is, avoid medical jargon that the patient could misunderstand. Read more information about health literacy in Chapter 24 (Teaching Clients). Obtain an interpreter for translation if the patient speaks a language that you do not speak. When possible, avoid using family members as translators in order to protect the patient's privacy or avoid a bias in translation (see Chapter 13 if you need more information about language differences).

Include family members in the teaching as much as possible and as much as desired by the patient; provide written materials to reinforce your instruction. If the patient is a child or dependent adult, be sure to include the parents or caregivers in the teaching and assessments. To facilitate a child's understanding, use dolls or age-appropriate toys, simple language (e.g., "Lie on your tummy, please"), and play (e.g., have the child give medicine to her doll with an empty syringe or listen to its "heart" with your stethoscope).

Self-Care

Teaching Patients How to Help Prevent Surgical Site Infections

Before Surgery

- If you smoke, stop. Those who smoke are more likely to get infections.
- Discuss your health problems with your surgeon (e.g., diabetes, allergies). These can affect incision healing.
- Ask your surgeon if you should have antibiotics before surgery.
- Don't shave near where you will have surgery. Not all procedures require hair removal, but if they do, it should be done with electric clippers. If someone starts to use a razor to shave you, speak up.

After Surgery

- Be sure family and friends wash their hands or use alcohol-based hand rub before and after they visit you.

- When anyone examines you or checks your incision ask them if they have washed their hands (or used alcohol-based hand rub).
- Wash your hands before and after caring for your own incision.
- Do not allow family and friends to touch your incision or the surgical dressing.
- Be sure you know how to care for your incision before you go home.
- If you have fever or redness, pain or drainage at the surgery site, call your physician right away.

Adapted from Centers for Disease Control and Prevention (updated 2010). Having surgery? What you should know before you go. Retrieved June 25, 2010, from http://www.cdc.gov/features/SafeSurgery/

VOL 2 For steps to follow in *all* procedures, refer to the Universal Steps for All Procedures found on the inside back cover of Volume 2. Go to the full procedures in Volume 2 to practice and learn the procedure steps. Use these Critical Aspects later to help you review key points.

Procedure 37-1: Teaching a Patient to Deep Breathe, Cough, Move in Bed, and Perform Leg Exercises

➤ Assess the patient's readiness to learn.

➤ Ensure that the patient is clear about the difference between coughing and merely clearing the throat.

➤ Demonstrate how to splint a potential chest or abdominal incision.

➤ Make sure the patient flexes her knees before turning on her side in bed.

➤ Use pillows to support the patient who is unable to maintain a side-lying position.

➤ Teach the patient to alternately flex and extend the knees.

➤ Teach the patient to alternately dorsiflex and plantar flex the foot.

➤ Teach the patient to rotate her ankles in a complete circle.

Procedure 37-2: Applying Antiembolism Stockings

➤ Measure the patient's legs to ensure that you select stockings of the correct size.

➤ Inspect the legs and feet for edema, abrasions, lesions, open areas, and circulatory changes.

➤ Elevate the patient's legs for at least 15 minutes before applying stockings.

➤ Insert your hand and turn the stocking inside out to the level of the heel.

➤ Insert the patient's foot into the stocking. Gradually pull the remaining portion of the stocking up and over the leg.

Keep knee-high stockings 2.5 to 5 cm (1 to 2 in.) below the joint.

Do not apply thigh-high stockings if the thigh circumference is greater than 100 cm (25 in.).

➤ Make sure the stocking is free of wrinkles and is not rolled at the top or bunched.

Procedure 37-3: Applying Sequential Compression Devices

➤ Determine whether elastic stockings are to be used concurrently with the sequential device. If so, apply them (see Procedure 37-2).

➤ Place the regulating pump for the sequential compression in a location that will ensure patient safety.

➤ Place the patient in a supine position.

➤ If you are using thigh-high compression sleeves or thigh-high pneumatic air stockings, measure the thigh.

➤ Place the lower extremity on the open sleeve, ensuring that the compression chambers are located over the correct anatomical structure (e.g., knee opening is at the level of the joint).

➤ Leave one to two fingerbreadths between the sleeve and the extremity.

➤ Set the regulating pump to the correct pressure, as prescribed.

➤ Instruct the patient to call for assistance in disconnecting the tubing from the sleeve.

Procedure 37-4: Managing Gastric Suction

Procedure 37-4A: Initial Equipment Setup

➤ Connect and secure the suction source, collection container, and drainage tubing.

➤ Don nonsterile gloves.

➤ Connect the suction drainage tubing to the nasogastric (NG) tubing.

➤ Secure the NG tube to the patient's nose and gown (if not already done).

➤ Turn on the suction.

Procedure 37-4B: Emptying the Suction Container

➤ Don nonsterile gloves.

➤ Turn off the suction; close the stopcock (or clamp the tubing).

➤ Empty the suction container and measure the contents.

➤ Empty and wash the graduated measuring container.

➤ Cleanse the suction container port and close the stopper; place the container back in the holder.

➤ Turn on the suction.

➤ Observe for proper functioning and tubing patency.

Procedure 37-4C: Irrigating the Nasogastric Tubing

➤ Prepare the irrigation set.

➤ Don nonsterile gloves.

➤ Check for NG tube placement.

➤ Fill the syringe with 30 to 50 mL of saline.

➤ Turn off the stopcock or clamp the NG tube.

➤ Disconnect the NG tube from drainage.

➤ Drain the suction tubing and turn off the suction source.

➤ Turn on the stopcock or unclamp the NG tube.

➤ Slowly instill and withdraw irrigant into the NG tube until fluid flows freely.

➤ Turn off the stopcock or reclamp the NG tube.

➤ Reconnect the NG tube.

➤ Turn on the stopcock or release the clamp.

Procedure 37-4D: Providing Comfort Measures

➤ Don nonsterile gloves.

➤ Provide mouth care.

➤ Remove nasal secretions.

➤ Apply water-soluble lubricant to the nostrils.

➤ Check that the tape or tube fixation device is secure.

When to Teach

For elective surgery, many patients have a scheduled preoperative assessment about a week before the surgery. The session may include preoperative testing, an appointment with the anesthesia staff, signing the consent form, and planned preoperative teaching.

Patients undergoing emergency surgery usually require extensive physical care preoperatively. You may need to give IV fluids, transfuse blood, treat for pain, and administer many medications, as in the case of Mr. Singh ("Meet Your Patient"). Because of the urgency of some surgeries, you may have limited time for preoperative teaching. However, you should always teach the patient as much as possible to prepare him for the surgical experience.

Prepare the Patient Physically for Surgery

Physical preparation of the patient for surgery involves several nursing concerns.

Maintaining Normothermia. Recent evidence-based guidelines stress that maintaining a normal body temperature helps produce good surgical outcomes (American Society of PeriAnesthesia Nurses, 2009). In addition to monitoring temperature, you can provide passive thermal care measures, such as providing blankets, socks, and head coverings; and keeping the room temperature at or above 75°F (24°C). Some agencies are using forced-air warming gowns or mattresses to pre-warm patients before surgery, as well as in the intraoperative and postoperative periods.

Nutritional Status. Anxiety and anesthesia reduce gastrointestinal motility. To decrease the risk of nausea and vomiting, patients usually fast, taking no food or liquids (NPO) for 8 hours before surgery. Stress to patients and family the importance of fasting to avoid the danger of aspiration.

Skin Preparation. Depending on the surgery and facility, patients may be asked to shower or scrub the surgical site with soap or an antibacterial solution (e.g., 4% chlorhexadine gluconate, Betadine) the evening before surgery and the morning of the surgery. Studies demonstrate that this reduces bacterial colonization on the skin, but do not clearly prove that it reduces surgical infection (National Guideline Clearinghouse [NGC], 2009; National Institute for Health and Clinical Excellence, 2008). Final skin preparation and hair removal, if done, should be completed before taking the patient into the surgical suite.

Bowel Preparation. Historically, clients received enemas before all surgeries. However, enemas are now used only for surgical procedures of the colon. To empty the colon of feces, patients are asked to consume a low-residue diet for several days before surgery and are given a regimen of medications and/or enemas to clear the bowel. Stress the importance of adhering to the regimen to limit the risk of contaminating the operative site with feces.

Urinary Elimination. Indwelling catheters are not routinely inserted for surgery. Catheterization may be prescribed if it is important to keep the bladder empty during surgery or if fluid status is being carefully monitored.

✚ If a catheter is not prescribed, have the patient void before receiving preoperative medications. The patient could fall if he gets out of bed to use the bathroom after being sedated or given opioids for pain.

Preoperative Medications. The anesthesiologist may prescribe preoperative medications to relax the patient, reduce respiratory secretions, or reduce the risk of vomiting and aspiration (Table 37-3). If the surgery time is known, the medication is prescribed at a prearranged time (e.g., at 0615). If the surgery time is likely to vary, the medication may be prescribed to give "on call." You will give the on-call medication when the surgical suite staff notifies you it is time to do so.

Antibiotics are often administered prophylactically to help prevent postoperative infections. You will usually administer the antibiotic intravenously, timed so that a bactericidal concentration of the drug will be present in serum and tissues by the time the incision is made (usually within the hour preceding incision) (Mangram, Horan, Pearson, et al., 1999; National Guideline Clearinghouse, 2008; NICE, 2008). Antibiotics are commonly given just as the patient is going to the surgical suite.

Routine Medications. Many routine medications are held (not administered) on the day of surgery. For example, an insulin-dependent diabetic patient may be instructed to hold her morning injection or administer half of the normal dose. The patient needs less insulin because her NPO status will keep her blood sugar lower than usual. The anesthesiologist will monitor the blood sugar in the operating room and give additional insulin if needed. Some patients may be instructed to stop routine medications several days before surgery. For example, a client receiving warfarin for anticoagulation may need to stop the medication 7 days before surgery.

Prostheses. Before being transported to the operating suite, the patient must remove all artificial body parts, such as dentures, artificial limbs, or contact lenses. Wigs, eyeglasses, makeup, and jewelry must also be removed.

Antiembolism Stockings. Also referred to as "TED hose," **antiembolism stockings** are elastic stockings that compress the veins of the legs and increase venous return to the heart (Fig. 37-1). They may be applied preoperatively to prevent venous pooling during surgery and decrease the risk of thrombus formation. Older adults and those with risk factors for venous thromboembolism are most in need of antiembolism

Table 37-3 ➤ Preoperative Medications

TYPE OF MEDICATION	USE	EXAMPLES
Antibiotics	Reduce the microbial burden of intraoperative contamination to a level that cannot overwhelm host defenses	Cephalosporins (e.g., cefazolin, cefoxitin), clindamycin, vancomycin
Anticholinergics (e.g., phenothiazines)	Reduce oral and pulmonary secretions, prevent laryngospasms, prevent bradycardia	Atropine (Atropisol), chlorpromazine (Thorazine), scopolamine (Hyoscine), glycopyrrolate (Robinul)
Anxiolytics (e.g., benzodiazepines)	Control anxiety, calming	Alprazolam (Xanax), clonazepam (Klonipin), diazepam (Valium), lorazepam (Ativan), midazolam (Versed)
Antihistamines	Provide sedation and antiemetic effects	Hydroxyzine (Vistaril), diphenhydramine (Benadryl)
Barbiturates	Provide sedation without significant cardiopulmonary depression	Secobarbital (Seconal), pentobarbital (Nembutal)
H_2 receptor antagonists	Reduce gastric acidity	Cimetidine (Tagamet), ranitidine (Zantac)
Hypnotics	Provide sedation and increase the duration of sleep	Temazepam (Restoril)
Neuroleptics	Provide sedative, antiemetic, and anticonvulsant effects	Droperidol (Inapsine), Innovar (fentanyl and droperidol)
Opioid analgesics	Provide pain relief and sedation; induce anesthesia	Fentanyl (Sublimaze), meperidine (Demerol), morphine (Duramorph)

FIGURE 37-1 Antiembolism stockings compress the veins of the legs and increase venous return to the heart.

stockings (Bartley, 2006). Risk factors include the following conditions:

- Venous stasis (such as occurs with bed rest, lengthy surgery, varicose veins, and heart failure)
- Vascular wall injury, which initiates clotting (e.g., surgery, IV catheter, irritating IV drugs, prior deep vein thrombus).
- Hypercoagulability (e.g., estrogen therapy, oral contraceptive use, cancer, dehydration, pregnancy)
- Older age, especially adults with other risk factors

Stockings are contraindicated for some patients (e.g., those with peripheral arterial disease) (The Joanna Briggs Institute, 2008a; Winslow & Brosz, 2008). Stockings may extend from foot to knee, or foot to thigh. Some have an opening at the toes that allows you to assess circulation in the feet. Stockings must be sized and applied correctly in order to be effective (see Critical Aspects). For the complete steps for applying antiembolism stockings,

 Go to Chapter 37, **Procedure 37-2: Applying Antiembolism Stockings,** in Volume 2.

Take Measures to Prevent Wrong Patient, Wrong Site, Wrong Surgery

✚ Include the following safety measures to help prevent patient misidentification and wrong-site surgery (Ridge, 2008; The Joint Commission, 2008):

- Use a preoperative checklist to confirm that appropriate documents are available and the appropriate activities have been performed.
- Verify the patient's identity before the patient leaves the preoperative area.
- Mark the surgical site before surgery. Use a permanent marker that will not be removed by the surgical skin prep, and involve the patient in the marking process.
- Take a time-out with all team members before starting the procedure (see "Perioperative Safety," near the beginning of this chapter).

Communicate with the Surgical Team

The most common root cause of medical errors is communication failure (AHRQ, 2003). For this reason, good communication is essential for patient safety in perioperative care. The following are elements of successful communication among the surgical team. Team members:

- Receive a summary of the plan of care (e.g., a short briefing by the surgeon) and develop a shared understanding of the plan.

- Speak up and are assertive with concerns about the procedure or decisions.
- Ask questions to clarify confusion.
- Acknowledge that they have heard and understood.
- Ask for and provide feedback (e.g., read back) on critical information.
- Use standard terminology (e.g., checklists). In one large, long-term study, use of surgical checklists was found to reduce the number of deaths from surgery by more than 40% (Haynes, Weiser, Berry, et al., 2009).

Surgical briefings encourage team members to talk when there is no problem, so they are more likely to speak up when they have misgivings of when problems occur (Hendrickson, Wadhera, & El Bardissi, 2008). Two-minute briefings led by the attending surgeon, using a standardized format, just before surgery have been found to improve communication and reduce delays and wrong-site surgery (Makary, Mukherjee, Sexton, et al., 2007).

KnowledgeCheck 37-4

- Identify topics that should be discussed in preoperative teaching.
- Describe the typical physical preparation of a client undergoing surgery.

 Go to Chapter 37, **Knowledge Check Response Sheet and Answers,** on the Student Resource Disk or DavisPlus at http://davisplus.fadavis.com/Wilkinson2

CriticalThinking 37-4

- What aspects of preoperative teaching should you stress when caring for Mr. Singh ("Meet Your Patient")?
- A bowel preparation is typically part of preoperative preparation for a client having colon surgery. Do you think this will be part of Mr. Singh's physical preparation? Why or why not?

Transfer to the Operative Suite

Once you have completed your preoperative care, the patient is ready for transport by stretcher to the operative area, usually to the surgical holding area (Fig. 37-2). The completed preoperative checklist and the patient's chart must accompany the patient. Lock up valuables according to agency policy, or have the patient's family keep them. Occasionally, especially if the patient has a significant sensory deficit, the patient can wear his hearing aid or glasses to the surgical suite. You will need to arrange this in advance with the surgical staff or anesthesia team.

Often children are permitted to bring a favorite toy with them to the OR to provide comfort. Children may fear being separated from their parents. Arrange for parents to spend time with the child immediately before the surgery and as soon as possible after the surgery. Keep the parents informed, and let them know what to expect.

If you transfer the patient to the surgical suite from a nursing unit in the hospital, you should prepare the

FIGURE 37-2 Surgical holding area.

room for the patient's return after surgery. Put clean linens on the bed and arrange the supplies and equipment you will need. For complete instructions,

 Go to Chapter 37, **Clinical Insight 37-2: Preparing a Room for a Patient's Return from Surgery,** in Volume 2.

Intraoperative Care

The **intraoperative phase** begins when the patient enters the operating suite and ends when she is admitted to the postanesthesia care unit.

Theoretical **Knowledge** knowing why

To provide intraoperative care, you will need theoretical knowledge of the roles of the various members of the intraoperative team and of the different types of anesthesia that are used.

Operative Personnel

The personnel who attend the client during the surgical procedure are called the *intraoperative team*. The team is divided into members who must use sterile technique and those who use clean technique (see Chapter 20 if you need to review medical and surgical asepsis). During the intraoperative phase, a registered nurse can function as the scrub nurse, circulating nurse, or registered nurse first assistant. Each of these roles contributes to the safe care of surgical clients.

Sterile Team

Members of the sterile intraoperative team include the surgeon, surgical assistant, and scrub person. Before beginning the surgery, they perform a surgical scrub of the hands and arms, dry with sterile towels, and don sterile gowns and gloves. (To review these procedures, see Chapter 20.)

The **scrub nurse** is a member of the sterile team. He can be an RN, LVN/LPN, or a surgical technician. The

Toward Evidence-Based Practice

Makary, M., Mukherjee, A., Sexton, J., et al. (2007). Operating room briefings and wrong-site surgery. *Journal of the American College of Surgeons, 204,* 236–243.

These researchers evaluated the impact of operating room briefings on coordination of care and the perceived risk for wrong-site surgery. A questionnaire was administered to 154 surgeons, anesthesiologists, and nurses before and after beginning an OR briefing program. The authors compared care provider perceptions before and after implementation of the briefings. The OR briefings were found to significantly (1) reduce perceived risk for wrong-site surgery and (2) improve perceived collaboration among the OR team.

Haynes, A., Weiser, T., Berry, W., et al. (2009). A surgical safety checklist to reduce morbidity and mortality in a global population. *New England Journal of Medicine, 360*(5), 491–499.

These researchers investigated whether using a surgical safety checklist designed to improve team communication and consistency of care would reduce complications and deaths associated with surgery. Using eight hospitals in eight cities globally, they collected data from 3733 patients 16 years of age and older before introduction of the checklist. They later collected data from similar patients

after the introduction of the checklist. The death rate was 1.5% before the use of checklist and 0.8% afterward. Inpatient complications fell from 11.0% before to 7.0% after.

Imagine that you are the OR nurse manager and that the incidence of wrong-site surgery in your hospital is higher than the national average. You want to introduce some changes in the OR, and need to "start small," by introducing changes gradually, one at a time. You are trying to decide whether to use an OR briefing program or a surgical safety checklist. In practice, you would have more studies to rely on, but pretend you must base your decision on just the two studies described here.

1. Before introducing an OR briefing program, what would you like to know about briefings that the first study does not tell you?

2. What information is missing from the summary of the second study that you will need in order to know if a surgical safety checklist would be helpful in your situation?

 Go to Chapter 37, **Toward Evidence-Based Practice Suggested Responses,** on the Student Resource Disk or DavisPlus at http://davisplus.fadavis.com/Wilkinson2

---

scrub nurse sets up the sterile field, prepares the surgical instruments, assists with the sterile draping of the patient, anticipates and responds to the surgeon's needs, and maintains the integrity of the sterile field. The **registered nurse first assistant (RNFA)** is an RN with additional education and training in surgical technique and is also part of the sterile team. The RNFA serves as an assistant to the surgeon, a role that has historically been filled by physicians. The RNFA works with the surgeon to perform the surgical procedure. The RNFA is employed by the surgeon or the hospital.

Sterile team members are the only persons allowed to enter the sterile field. The sterile field encompasses the client and the area immediately surrounding the client. Creation of the operative field is explained in:

 VOL 2 Chapter 37, **Clinical Insight 37-3: Creating an Operative Field,** in Volume 2.

Clean Team

Team members who abide by clean technique (medical asepsis) include the anesthesiologist or nurse anesthetist, the circulating RN, biomedical technicians, and radiology technicians. These personnel never enter the sterile field, but instead function around and beyond it.

An **anesthesiologist** or a **nurse anesthetist (CRNA)** induces amnesia, analgesia, and muscle relaxation or paralysis with anesthesia. His role is to continuously

monitor and evaluate the patient's responses to the anesthetic agent and the surgical procedure. CRNAs administer more than half of all anesthetics in the United States.

The **circulating nurse** is a registered nurse who applies the nursing process to coordinate all activities in the operating room. She is a strong client advocate who continuously monitors the client and the sterile field. The circulating nurse maintains a safe, comfortable environment, communicates with appropriate personnel outside the operating room, manages care of the intraoperative client, and responds to emergencies. An important aspect of the circulating nurse's role is to attend to the patient during the induction of anesthesia. In some cases, the circulating nurse administers sedation to the patient.

KnowledgeCheck 37-5

- Identify the intraoperative nursing roles that are part of the sterile intraoperative team and those that are part of the clean intraoperative team.
- Which nursing roles are always held by a registered nurse?

 Go to Chapter 37, **Knowledge Check Response Sheet and Answers,** on the Student Resource Disk or DavisPlus at http://davisplus.fadavis.com/Wilkinson2

Types of Anesthesia

During surgery, anesthesia is used to obtain analgesia (control of pain), muscle relaxation or paralysis, and amnesia (memory loss). Anesthesia is classified as general, conscious sedation, or regional.

General Anesthesia

General anesthesia produces rapid unconsciousness and loss of sensation. The anesthesiologist or nurse anesthetist administers inhaled and intravenous medications that depress the patient's central nervous system (CNS) and relax the musculature. Muscle relaxants, paralyzing agents, narcotics, barbiturates, and inhaled gases are some of the agents used during general anesthesia.

Advantages of General Anesthesia

- The patient is unconscious, so she experiences no anxiety that might affect cardiac and respiratory functioning.
- The muscles are relaxed, so the patient remains completely motionless during the surgical procedure.
- Anesthesia can be adjusted to accommodate the length of the procedure and the patient's age and physical condition. For example, an older adult may require less anesthetic than anticipated; if so, the anesthetist can decrease the dosage without interrupting the procedure. Also, if complications occur, the anesthesia can be continued for longer than originally planned.

Disadvantages of General Anesthesia

- The respiratory and circulatory muscles are depressed, so mechanical ventilation is needed while the patient is under the effects of the anesthetic agent(s). These effects predispose the patient to pneumonia and thrombophlebitis in the postoperative period.
- General anesthesia creates a risk for death, heart attack, stroke, and malignant hyperthermia. **Malignant hyperthermia** is a rare, often fatal, metabolic condition that can occur during the use of muscle relaxants and inhalation anesthesia. Metabolism increases in the skeletal muscles, and they become rigid. The temperature rises rapidly. Predisposition to this condition is inherited.
- Frequent minor complaints after general anesthesia include sore throat (from intubation), nausea and vomiting (from relaxation of gastrointestinal smooth muscle), headache, uncontrollable shivering, and confusion.

Conscious Sedation

Conscious sedation is an alternative form of anesthesia that provides intravenous sedation and analgesia without producing unconsciousness. The patient is aware of his surroundings and can talk with the surgical team during the procedure. During conscious sedation, the patient may feel sleepy but can be easily aroused by touch or speech. Nevertheless, blood pressure, heart rate, respiratory rate, and oxygen saturation are monitored, and the patient usually receives oxygen via nasal cannula during the procedure. Because of the amnesic effect of many of the medications, the patient may not recall aspects of the procedure afterwards. Advantages are that (1) pain and anxiety are adequately controlled without the risks of general anesthesia, and (2) recovery is rapid. Conscious sedation is used for procedures such as bronchoscopy and cosmetic surgery, but it is not practical for highly anxious patients.

Regional Anesthesia

Regional anesthesia prevents pain in the area of the procedure by interrupting nerve impulses to and from the area. The patient remains alert but is numb in the involved area. Regional anesthesia may be administered by infiltration of the surgical site and surrounding tissue with local anesthetics, such as lidocaine (Xylocaine) or bupivacaine (Marcaine). These medications may also be injected into and around specific nerves to depress the sensory, motor, and/or sympathetic impulses of a limited area of the body.

Regional anesthesia is low in cost, simple to administer, and requires a minimal recovery period. It is especially suitable for minor, ambulatory procedures. However, many patients are apprehensive about being able to see and hear the procedure. Regional anesthesia may not be practical if the patient is highly anxious or if adequate pain control cannot be achieved. Techniques for achieving regional anesthesia include the following.

Peripheral Nerve Block

A **nerve block** is the injection of an anesthetic into and around a nerve or group of nerves (e.g., the facial nerve, the brachial plexus). A **Bier (intravenous) block** is a nerve block technique in which the anesthetist places a tourniquet on an arm or leg, and then injects a local anesthetic agent intravenously below the level of the tourniquet. The tourniquet is maintained at a pressure that limits venous return but continues to allow arterial circulation. The patient feels no pain in the extremity as long as the tourniquet is in place. Advantages of the Bier block are its rapid onset and recovery time. Also, the tourniquet decreases bleeding during the surgical procedure and prevents systemic absorption of the local anesthetic. However, when the procedure is finished, the tourniquet is deflated, and there is potential for systemic absorption of the anesthetic. To prevent tissue damage, the tourniquet must not be left in place for more than 2 hours.

Spinal Anesthesia

Spinal anesthesia is the injection of an anesthetic into the cerebrospinal fluid (CSF) in the subarachnoid space (Fig. 37-3A). This injection blocks sensation and movement below the level of the injection. Spinal anesthesia is often used for surgical procedures in the lower abdomen, pelvis, and lower extremities. This technique allows the patient to remain conscious during the procedure and usually does not depress respirations. Occasionally a higher level of spinal anesthesia is achieved than intended—that is, the medication may migrate upward in the spinal fluid. This can depress respirations and cardiac rate. Placing the patient in Fowler's position may prevent respiratory paralysis.

Side effects of spinal anesthesia include hypotension, nausea, vomiting, urinary retention, or a headache from leakage of CSF. A headache after spinal anesthesia must be closely monitored and may require additional treatment by the anesthesia staff.

The blood pressure may also decrease suddenly due to pervasive vasodilatation—the anesthesia blocks the sympathetic vasomotor nerves, which normally maintain muscle tone in peripheral blood vessels. Patients with these complications often require ventilation and support of blood pressure during surgery, so they must be carefully monitored during surgery and in the recovery period.

Epidural Anesthesia

Epidural anesthesia requires insertion of a thin catheter into the epidural space (Fig. 37-3B). Anesthetic agents are infused through the catheter to produce loss of sensation. Epidural anesthesia can be used as a surgical anesthetic and to provide postoperative analgesia. Advantages and disadvantages of epidural anesthesia are similar to those of spinal anesthesia. Epidural anesthesia is safer than spinal anesthesia because the anesthetic does not enter the subarachnoid space and the depth of anesthesia is not as great. However, drugs intended for epidural administration are of a higher concentration than those for spinal administration; so if the medication is inadvertently injected too deeply (into the subarachnoid space), hypotension and respiratory paralysis occur, and temporary mechanical ventilation is necessary.

Epidural anesthesia is ideal for obstetrics procedures (e.g., cesarean birth or pain control with vaginal birth) because the mother is awake to bond with the newborn, and her mobility is limited for only a short time.

Local Anesthesia

Local anesthesia produces loss of pain sensation at the desired site (e.g., a wound to be sutured, a growth on the skin). Local anesthesia is typically used for minor procedures. However, after finishing a major surgery, the surgeon may infiltrate the operative area with local anesthetics to provide postoperative pain relief. Local anesthetics may be applied topically or injected. A **topical anesthetic** is applied directly to the skin and mucous membranes. Lidocaine (Xylocaine) and benzocaine (Orajel, T-caine) are commonly used because they are rapidly absorbed and rapid-acting.

KnowledgeCheck 37-6
- What is the purpose of anesthesia?
- Under what type(s) of anesthesia does the client remain conscious?

 Go to Chapter 37, **Knowledge Check Response Sheet and Answers,** on the Student Resource Disk or DavisPlus at http://davisplus.fadavis.com/Wilkinson2

 Critical**Thinking** 37-5

What form of anesthesia is Mr. Singh most likely to receive? Why?

Practical **Knowledge**
knowing how

When a patient arrives in the surgical suite, the nurse verifies the information on the preoperative checklist and assesses the patient. After that, the nursing focus is on safe and successful completion of the surgery.

FIGURE 37-3 A, Spinal anesthesia is the injection of a local anesthetic into the subarachnoid space to block sensation and movement. B, Continuous epidural anesthesia can be used to provide postoperative analgesia.

ASSESSMENT

The circulating nurse greets the client in the preoperative holding area and performs a brief assessment. The nurse first verifies that the surgical consent has been signed and witnessed and that the preoperative checklist is complete. The nurse then assesses the client's anxiety level and physical condition. The next steps are to measure the vital signs; examine the surgical site; and inspect IV lines, drainage tubes, and catheters. Often the circulating nurse or the anesthetist starts an IV line in the holding area if one is not already present. A preoperative medication may be given in the holding area. Vital signs are monitored often, or even continuously, during the intraoperative period.

For common interview questions to use in the intraoperative period,

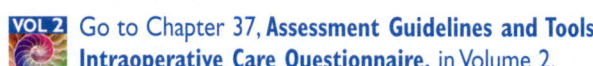 Go to Chapter 37, **Assessment Guidelines and Tools, Intraoperative Care Questionnaire,** in Volume 2.

In addition to the checklist completed in the preoperative period, the surgery team will also probably complete a checklist, with one staff member functioning as the checklist coordinator. The World Health Organization (WHO, 2008) checklist covers three phases of a surgical procedure:

- Sign in (before anesthesia is given)
- Time out (before the skin incision)
- Sign out (before the patient leaves the surgical suite).

To see the complete WHO checklist,

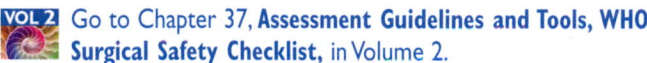 Go to Chapter 37, **Assessment Guidelines and Tools, WHO Surgical Safety Checklist,** in Volume 2.

ANALYSIS/NURSING DIAGNOSIS

The circulating nurse uses the assessment data to develop relevant nursing diagnoses. As in the preoperative phase, most intraoperative nursing care consists of standard activities to be used for all patients. Most intraoperative patients, regardless of the surgery, have the following potential complications (collaborative problems):

- Potential complications of surgery:
  Hypothermia
  Fluid and electrolyte imbalance
  Excessive bleeding or hemorrhage
  Musculoskeletal injury secondary to positioning
- Potential complications of anesthesia:
  Aspiration
  Vasomotor instability (and resultant hypotension and diminished peripheral perfusion)
  Respiratory depression
  Cardiovascular compromise

Except in unusual circumstances (e.g., a patient in poor nutritional status, a frail elderly patient), you may not need to identify nursing diagnoses for a patient because the standardized care addresses all the potential complications.

However, for nurses who prefer to organize care according to nursing diagnoses, the following potential diagnoses apply to most patients having major surgery:

- *Risk for Imbalanced Body Temperature* related to exposure in cool environment and administration of cool IV fluids. This applies especially to very young, very old, and very thin patients.
- *Risk for Aspiration* related to depressed respirations and reflexes. For patients who have weak muscles for coughing or a poor gag reflex, this diagnosis is especially relevant.
- *Risk for Imbalanced Fluid Volume* related to NPO status and blood loss from surgery. Some patients are at higher than normal risk, for example, patients with renal or cardiac problems.
- *Risk for Perioperative Positioning Injury* related to patient factors such as edema, emaciation, obesity, and sensory perceptual disturbances secondary to anesthesia.

Use the following nursing diagnoses only if the patient has the necessary defining characteristics or risk factors. Do not use them for all patients.

- *Risk for Latex Allergy Response* related to multiple exposures (e.g., multiple surgeries, catheterizations) or history of related allergies
- *Latex Allergy Response* (needs no etiology)

PLANNING OUTCOMES/EVALUATION

The overarching goals in the intraoperative phase are that the patient will:

- Be free from injury.
- Remain physiologically stable.
- Experience optimal surgical outcomes.

For *associated NOC standardized outcomes* for intraoperative patients, along with examples of goals created with NOC indicators and scales,

 Go to Chapter 37, **Standardized Language, Intraoperative Patients—Selected Standardized Nursing Diagnoses, Outcomes, and Interventions,** in Volume 2.

Notice that the goals are appropriate for nearly all surgical patients.

Individualized goals/outcome statements are formulated from the patient's nursing diagnoses. The following are examples:

- Maintains body temperature within the normal range.
- Has clear lung sounds and patent airway.
- Has urine output of at least 30 mL/hr.
- Will have no skin, tissue, or neuromuscular injury as a result of positioning.
- Will not acquire healthcare-related infection.

PLANNING INTERVENTIONS/IMPLEMENTATION

Intraoperative care focuses on maintaining a safe environment and assisting the surgery team to provide appropriate care for the client. The nurse anesthetist manages the interventions for most of the patient's potential problems, for example, fluid volume status, airway protection, and vital signs monitoring.

NIC standardized interventions for the intraoperative period come from the domain of Perioperative Care. They include interventions for all intraoperative patients, regardless of their individual nursing diagnoses. One intervention, Anesthesia Administration, must be performed by an anesthesiologist or nurse anesthetist. The nurse assists in implementing a number of interventions:

- Anesthesia Administration
- Autotransfusion
- Infection Control: Intraoperative
- Positioning: Intraoperative
- Surgical Assistance
- Surgical Precautions
- Surgical Preparation
- Temperature Regulation: Intraoperative

For *NIC standardized interventions* for specific intraoperative nursing diagnoses,

 VOL 2 Go to Chapter 37, **Standardized Language, Intraoperative Patients—Selected Standardized Nursing Diagnoses, Outcomes, and Interventions,** in Volume 2.

Notice, however, that most of the interventions apply to all surgical patients and are subsumed by (or fall under) the preceding NIC Perioperative Care interventions. As in all of healthcare, you should be always mindful of using hand hygiene. Sterile asepsis is an important focus in the intraoperative period; you can review that in Chapter 20.

The following sections explain in more detail how to carry out "routine" interventions, such as providing skin preparation, positioning, and intraoperative safety measures. Note that "routine" in this context means that the activities are planned and performed for all patients. Nursing interventions are *never* routine in the general sense; they must always be performed with thought and skill.

Skin Preparation

Surgical skin preparation reduces the risk of postoperative wound infection by reducing the microbial count at the operative site. Skin preparation may begin in the preoperative phase, when the client cleanses the skin with an antimicrobial solution the evening before and the morning of surgery. The intraoperative nurse provides additional skin preparation as follows.

Assess the Skin. Assess skin for signs of infection, rash, or other forms of skin irritation. Document the condition of the skin on the intraoperative record.

Remove Hair from the Site Only if Necessary. Historically, the surgical site was always shaved. Now, however, you will remove hair only if there is a large amount of it in the area of the surgery or if the surgeon specifies

a preference for hair removal. Hair removal increases the risk of abrasions or nicks in the skin, which can provide a portal of entry for bacteria. If you do remove hair, you will likely do it in the preoperative holding area immediately before surgery to reduce the time for bacterial growth. Use clippers or depilatory cream to trim hair because they are less likely than a razor to cause skin irritation (The Joanna Briggs Institute, 2007).

Cleanse the Surgical Site. In the operative suite, skin preparation precedes draping of the client. Cleanse the surgical site and a generous part of surrounding area with the recommended anti-infective solution. Povidone-iodine (Betadine) is commonly used for the scrub; then the skin is painted with Betadine solution. If the client has an allergy to iodine, use an alternative preparation solution.

Positioning

Five variables determine the position of the patient in the OR: the surgical site, access to the patient's airway, the need to monitor vital signs, comfort, and safety. A position that is ideal for accessing the surgical site may not be used if any of the other factors are compromised. If the patient has preexisting injuries or discomfort, this information is also factored into the decision about how to position. For example, a patient with chronic cervical spine pain may be positioned using a neck-roll.

The patient is usually positioned after anesthesia has begun. Use straps, wedges, pillows, and surgical table attachments to maintain the position during the surgery. To prevent shearing, lift—do not slide—the patient into position. In many cases, the surgical team assists with positioning.

The circulating nurse is responsible for preventing positioning injuries. Surgical patients often spend 3 to 4 hours, or even longer, in the same position. This places them at risk for pressure ulcer formation. Some anesthetic agents decrease tissue perfusion, further increasing the patient's risk for sustaining positioning injuries. Padding the bony prominences is one measure to protect the client during surgery. For nursing interventions to address the NANDA-I diagnosis Risk for Perioperative Positioning Injury,

VOL 2 Go to Chapter 37, **Standardized Language, Selected Standardized Nursing Diagnoses, Outcomes, and Interventions for Intraoperative Patients,** in Volume 2.

Intraoperative Safety Measures

As a part of their 2009 National Patient Safety Goals, the Joint Commission (2008) suggests that just before starting any surgical or invasive procedure, you conduct a final verification process to confirm the correct patient, procedure, and site. The circulating nurse is responsible for a variety of other measures that protect the patient in the intraoperative phase. These measures are briefly explained here.

Assist the Scrub Nurse to Prepare and Maintain the Sterile Field. The circulating nurse gathers surgical supplies and equipment for use during surgery. She then works with the scrub nurse to transfer the supplies to the sterile field.

Provide Supplies and Materials During Surgery. If additional supplies are needed during surgery, the circulating nurse obtains them and opens them onto the sterile field. Supplies may include dressings, surgical equipment, medications, irrigating solutions, or sutures.

Monitor Intake and Output of the Client. Together with the anesthetist, the circulating nurse monitors the fluid infused, urine output, drainage, and blood loss.

Handle Specimens. Often the surgeon will obtain a tissue sample that must be analyzed during the operative procedure. The circulating nurse receives the specimen; coordinates with the pathologist to review the sample; and reports the pathology findings to the surgeon. The circulator also handles specimens that will be sent for evaluation after the surgery is complete.

Perform Sponge, Sharps, and Instrument Counts. The circulating nurse and the scrub nurse count the material that is added to the sterile field. As the surgery comes to an end, a repeat count is performed to ensure that no instruments, sponges, or sharps are left inside the client. A retained sponge can lead to infection and additional surgeries. A major surgery, such as a heart surgery, can use several hundred sponges. Once soaked in blood, sponges can blend in with the body cavity and be difficult to see. Some agencies are now using sponges with barcodes, which the nurse scans before and after use. The system alerts the surgical team if they are left behind. In another system, chip-embedded sponges rely on radiofrequency identification technology to count sponges and locate any that are left behind.

Document. Record the care provided and the client's response to care on the surgical record. Usually you will use a graphic or a checklist form, perhaps with some space for narrative notes about anything the form does not address.

KnowledgeCheck 37-7

- For what activities is the circulating nurse responsible for in the surgical suite prior to the skin incision?
- Describe six intraoperative safety measures performed by the circulating nurse.

 Go to Chapter 37, **Knowledge Check Response Sheet and Answers,** on the Student Resource Disk or DavisPlus at http://davisplus.fadavis.com/Wilkinson2

CriticalThinking 37-6

What special concerns, if any, may affect Mr. Singh ("Meet Your Patient") during the intraoperative phase of care?

Postoperative Care

The postoperative phase begins when the client enters the postanesthesia care unit and ends when he has healed from the surgical procedure. This phase consists of two parts: recovery from anesthesia and recovery from surgery.

Theoretical **Knowledge** knowing why

When the surgical procedure is complete, members of the surgical team prepare the client for transfer to the postanesthesia care unit (PACU), also called the recovery room (Fig. 37-4).

Recovery from Anesthesia

The first postoperative phase is often known as the *postanesthesia phase* or the *immediate postoperative phase*. This phase begins when the client is transferred from the operating table to a bed (or gurney) for transport to the PACU. In the immediate postoperative phase, the client is at high risk for respiratory and cardiovascular compromise. As a precaution, the anesthetist and the circulating nurse accompany the client and attend to her needs during transport to the PACU. They are also responsible for giving a comprehensive report to the PACU nurse.

The PACU, located near the OR, is typically an open unit that allows nurses to observe clients easily. PACU nurses have specialized education and experience in caring for postoperative clients. Commonly, nurses working in the PACU have experience in critical care. The PACU nurse receives a comprehensive report from the anesthesia provider and circulating nurse (Box 37-4).

Recovery from Surgery

The second phase of postoperative care begins when the patient is discharged from the PACU and admitted to the

FIGURE 37-4 Postanesthesia care unit.

BOX 37-4 ■ Information Contained in the Report from the Surgical Suite

- Procedure performed
- Type of anesthesia
- Medications administered in the surgical suite
- Duration of the procedure and anesthesia
- Postoperative vital signs
- Pulse oximetery values
- Allergies
- Lab values
- Estimated blood loss
- Fluid intake and output, including urine, stool, gastric losses
- Preoperative mobility status, skin integrity, and sensory perception abilities
- Surgical complications
- Presence of tubes, drains, catheters
- Existing IV lines
- Postoperative prescriptions

surgical nursing unit. The patient is transported to the surgical unit only after he has recovered from anesthesia and his condition is stable. The goal of this phase is to facilitate healing and prevent postoperative complications.

Practical **Knowledge**
knowing how

In the next sections we discuss nursing care associated with both phases of postoperative care.

Nursing Care in the Postanesthesia Care Unit

The PACU nurse performs a quick, focused initial assessment of the surgical patient in the presence of the anesthesia provider and circulating nurse. After that, she assesses the patient every 5 to 15 minutes. AORN (2009) has identified the essential elements of assessment in the PACU. For that information,

 Go to Chapter 37, **Assessment Guidelines and Tools, Postanesthesia Assessments: Essential Elements,** in Volume 2.

NIC: Postanesthesia Care. The only postoperative intervention from NIC's Perioperative Care category is Postanesthesia Care. Postanesthesia Care encompasses the preceding assessments and adds measures such as providing for safety and administering oxygen. Many patients arrive in the PACU with an artificial airway or endotracheal tube in place. For most, the PACU nurse will remove the airway or tube once she determines that the patient is able to maintain his own airway.

An unconscious client is usually positioned on his side to help maintain an open airway. This decreases the likelihood of aspirating mucus or saliva by allowing it to drain out instead of back into the throat. Elevating the superior arm on a pillow allows for good chest expansion so the patient can breathe deeply and expand the lungs fully.

For *NIC interventions* for other postoperative nursing diagnoses,

VOL 2 Go to Chapter 37, **Standardized Language, Selected Standardized Nursing Diagnoses, Outcomes, and Interventions for Postoperative Patients,** in Volume 2.

The client remains in the PACU until he has recovered from the effects of anesthesia (Box 37-5).

Postoperative Nursing Care on the Surgical Unit

The assigned nurse admits the patient to the surgical unit. If the patient is transported by gurney, assist him to the bed. As soon as the patient has arrived, perform an assessment, and listen to a summary report from the PACU nurse.

BOX 37-5 ■ Evidence of Recovery from Anesthesia

Airway—The patient is able to maintain a patent airway independently and to deep-breathe, cough, and expectorate secretions.

Level of consciousness—The patient is conscious and easily reoriented. Often patients will drift off to sleep between arousals; however, they easily reorient and are generally aware of circumstances and surroundings.

Vital signs—Vital signs are stable and within an acceptable range. The blood pressure may be markedly different from that taken during the immediate preoperative measures, because BP is often elevated preoperatively. This can also be due to anxiety, pain, and not administering routine BP medications because of NPO status. The patient may require medication to control pain or BP before he can be discharged from the PACU.

Mobility and sensation—The patient is able to move all extremities that he could move preoperatively. The patient regains movement and sensation once spinal or epidural anesthesia has worn off.

Fluid balance (I & O)—The patient is urinating at least 30 mL/hr and is in relative fluid balance. Consider blood loss, urine output, gastric drainage, and emesis when calculating fluid balance.

Dressings and drains—Dressings are dry and intact, or wound drainage is considered appropriate for the procedure. The patient should have no overt signs of excessive blood or fluid loss before he is transferred to the surgical unit.

ASSESSMENT

The initial postoperative assessment is identical to the assessment performed by the PACU nurse. However, the patient has undergone a period of stabilization since surgery, so the frequency of assessment can be less than in the PACU, where the patient was assessed every 5 to 15 minutes. You may increase the frequency if the patient's condition changes. Of course agency protocols vary, but a common pattern is to assess the patient:

On arrival to the nursing unit
Every 15 minutes for the first hour
Every 30 minutes for the next 2 hours
Every hour for the next 4 hours
Then every 4 hours

KnowledgeCheck 37-8

- What are the two phases of the postoperative phase of care?
- How often is a patient typically assessed after surgery?
- What assessments are made?

 Go to Chapter 37, **Knowledge Check Response Sheet and Answers,** on the Student Resource Disk or DavisPlus at http://davisplus.fadavis.com/Wilkinson2

ANALYSIS/NURSING DIAGNOSIS

If healing proceeds normally and no complications develop, most postoperative patients have a common set of collaborative problems (Table 37-4), regardless of the type of surgery they underwent. You will not need to write potential ("risk for") nursing diagnoses, except in special situations (e.g., patients with comorbid conditions, such as diabetes or asthma).

Potential Nursing Diagnoses

Write potential nursing diagnoses (instead of collaborative problems) only if a patient has a higher risk for the problem than the average surgical patient. For example, you might use:

- *Risk for Ineffective Peripheral Tissue Perfusion* for patients who have a history of peripheral arterial disease or cardiac insufficiency.
- *Risk for Deficient Fluid Volume* for patients who have lost a large amount of blood in surgery or who are dehydrated on admission.

Table 37-4 ➤ Potential Postoperative Complications (Collaborative Problems)

POTENTIAL COMPLICATION	DESCRIPTION	CLINICAL SIGNS	INTERVENTIONS FOR PREVENTION AND EARLY DETECTION
Respiratory System			
Aspiration Pneumonia	Airway inflammation caused by inhaling gastric secretions (especially hydrochloric acid from the stomach) because of absent gag reflex secondary to anesthesia	Cough, fever, elevated WBC, decreased or absent breath sounds, decreased oxygen saturation (Sao_2), tachypnea, dyspnea, blood-tinged sputum.	*Preoperative:* Institute NPO for at least 8 hours prior to surgery. *Postoperative:* Continue NPO until intestinal motility returns; carefully monitor sedated patient and place in side-lying position.
Atelectasis	Collapse of alveoli due to hypoventilation, airways blocked by mucus plugs, opioid analgesics, immobility	Decreased or absent breath sounds, noisy respirations, decreased O_2 saturation (Sao_2), chest asymmetry, sternal retractions, accessory muscle use, trachea deviated from midline, fever, tachypnea, dyspnea, tachycardia, diaphoresis, pleural pain, increased restlessness, anxiety	■ Monitor for clinical signs (Column 3) ■ Monitor rate, rhythm, depth, and effort of respirations. ■ Monitor ability to cough effectively. ■ Determine need for suctioning by listening for crackles and rhonchi over major airways. ■ Suction, as needed. Auscultate lung sounds after suctioning, and other respiratory treatments to determine effectiveness. ■ Encourage deep breathing, coughing, moving in bed, ambulation, use of incentive spirometry. ■ See interventions for NIC category Respiratory Monitoring.

Continued

Table 37-4 ➤ Potential Postoperative Complications (Collaborative Problems)—cont'd

POTENTIAL COMPLICATION	DESCRIPTION	CLINICAL SIGNS	INTERVENTIONS FOR PREVENTION AND EARLY DETECTION
Pneumonia	Inflammation of the alveoli due to infection with bacteria or viruses, toxins, or irritants. Caused by hypoventilation secondary to anesthesia and opioid analgesics, and by poor cough effort as a result of aging or weakness.	Productive cough with blood-tinged or purulent sputum, fever, elevated WBC, decreased or absent breath sounds, decreased Sao$_2$, chest pain, tachypnea, dyspnea	■ Monitor for clinical signs. ■ Encourage and assist with deep breathing, coughing, moving in bed, ambulation, use of incentive spirometry.
Pulmonary Embolus	A clot that occludes blood flow to a portion of the lungs; usually a result of clot formation in the lower extremities, which breaks loose and migrates to the lungs. May also be due to venous injuries, hypercoagulable state, use of high-dose estrogen, preexisting circulatory disorders.	Sudden onset of dyspnea, shortness of breath, chest pain, hypotension, tachycardia, decreased Sao$_2$, cyanosis	■ Prevent thrombophlebitis: Encourage and assist with leg exercises, ambulation, antiembolism stockings, sequential compression devices, hydration. **VOL 2** Go to Chapter 37, **Procedure 37-2: Applying Antiembolism Stockings**, and **Procedure 37-3: Applying Sequential Compression Devices**, in Volume 2. ■ If thrombophlebitis occurs, position and immobilize the limb; do not massage calves.
Cardiovascular System			
Thrombophlebitis	Blood clot and inflammation of a vein or artery, usually in the legs. Results from increased coagulability and venous stasis due to immobility during and after surgery.	*Superficial:* Vein is red, hard, and hot to touch. *Deep:* Limb is pale and edematous; aching, cramping in limb; Homans' sign (pain in calf when foot is dorsiflexed).	Refer to "Pulmonary embolism" actions, above.
Embolus	■ Movement of a thrombus or foreign body from its original location. ■ Movement in the arterial system results in symptoms in the area affected (e.g., cerebrovascular accident (CVA), myocardial infarction (MI), or loss of circulation to an area). ■ In the venous system, often results in pulmonary embolus (see "Pulmonary Embolus," preceding).	See pulmonary embolus. For arterial emboli, symptoms depend on the location.	■ Monitor for clinical signs. ■ Prevent thrombophlebitis. If thrombophlebitis occurs, position and immobilize the limb. ■ Do not massage calves.
Hemorrhage	Bleeding may be internal or external. May be caused by slipped ligature, uncontrolled bleeder, or infection.	*If external:* Dressings saturated with bright red blood; increased output in drains or chest tubes *If internal:* Increased pain, increasing abdominal girth, ecchymosis or swelling around incision, tachycardia, hypotension	Frequently monitor vital signs, dressings, and wound drainage.

Table 37-4 ➤ Potential Postoperative Complications (Collaborative Problems)—cont'd

POTENTIAL COMPLICATION	DESCRIPTION	CLINICAL SIGNS	INTERVENTIONS FOR PREVENTION AND EARLY DETECTION
Hypovolemia	Decreased blood volume; may be due to blood loss during and after surgery, dehydration, or excess loss through vomiting, diarrhea, or drains	Hypotension, tachycardia, decreased urine output, fatigue, thirst, dehydration	▪ Monitor vital signs and I&O. ▪ Insert urinary catheter, if appropriate. ▪ Monitor skin color, temperature, and moistness; central and peripheral cyanosis. ▪ Identify possible causes of changes in vital signs. ▪ Administer IV therapy as prescribed. ▪ Promote oral intake when tolerated. ▪ Prepare to administer blood or blood products, as prescribed.
Gastrointestinal System			
Nausea and Vomiting	Stomach upset or vomiting related to pain, anxiety, anesthesia, medications, or oral intake before peristalsis returns	Vomiting, retching, stated nausea	▪ Have patient remain NPO until return of bowel sounds. ▪ Advance diet slowly. ▪ Treat pain.
Abdominal Distention (Tympanites)	Excess gas within the intestines; may be due to a slow return of peristalsis or from handling of the intestines during surgery	Abdominal discomfort, bloating, hypoactive or absent bowel sounds	▪ Encourage and assist to move in bed and ambulate. ▪ Maintain NPO until return of bowel sounds; avoid drinking with a straw. ▪ Provide fluids at room temperature.
Constipation	A decrease in the frequency of bowel movements, resulting in the passage of hard stool. Usually related to use of opioids, immobility, inadequate fluid intake, or low-fiber diet	Abdominal discomfort, bloating, hypoactive or absent bowel sounds	Encourage and assist the patient to move in bed, ambulate, and increase fluid and fiber intake after bowel sounds return.
Ileus	Loss of the forward flow of intestinal contents due to decreased peristalsis secondary to anesthesia, handling of the intestines during surgery, electrolyte imbalances, infection, or ischemic bowel	Abdominal pain, distention, absent bowel sounds, vomiting	There are few independent preventive measures. Observe for symptoms; notify the surgeon.
Genitourinary System			
Renal Failure	Decreased or absent urine output due to hypovolemia, shock, or toxic reaction to medications.	Urine output < 30 mL/hr; rising BUN and creatinine levels	Carefully monitor I&O and lab values.
Urinary Retention	Accumulation of urine in the bladder. May result from poor muscle tone as a result of anesthesia and anticholinergic medications, handling of tissues during surgery, or inflammation in the pelvic region.	Bladder distention, suprapubic pain, diminished urine output or output less than fluid intake, inability to void or small frequent voidings, hypertension, restlessness	▪ Monitor for clinical signs. ▪ Provide privacy and adequate time to urinate. ▪ Catheterize if needed.

Continued

Table 37-4 ➤ Potential Postoperative Complications (Collaborative Problems)—cont'd

POTENTIAL COMPLICATION	DESCRIPTION	CLINICAL SIGNS	INTERVENTIONS FOR PREVENTION AND EARLY DETECTION
Urinary Tract Infection	Infection in the urinary tract related to catheterization, stagnant urine in the bladder secondary to immobility or anticholinergic medications, or instrumentation of the urinary tract	Urinary frequency, suprapubic discomfort, burning on urination, cloudy urine	■ Monitor for clinical signs. ■ Monitor I&O. ■ Use aseptic technique with catherization and perineal care. ■ Provide adequate IV and oral fluids.
Surgical Incision			
Dehiscence	Separation of one or more layers of the wound due to poor nutritional status, obesity, or other strain on suture line, inadequate closure of the muscles, or wound infection	A pop or tearing sensation, especially with sudden straining from coughing, vomiting, or changing positions in bed. Usually an immediate increase in serosanguinous drainage occurs.	■ Provide adequate nutrition. ■ Use binders to support the incision. ■ Have client avoid strain. ■ Monitor for infection.
Evisceration	Protrusion of organs or tissues through the separated incision. For causes, see Dehiscence.	Visible protrusion of organs through incision	Same as for Dehiscence
Wound Infection	Inflammation or drainage from a wound due to growth of microorganisms secondary to poor aseptic technique or pathogens already present in surgical area	Localized swelling, redness, heat, pain, fever (>100.4°F or 38°C), foul-smelling drainage, or a change in the color of the drainage.	■ Effective skin prep in preoperative period ■ Surgical scrub according to guidelines in the intraoperative period ■ Monitor for systemic and localized signs and symptoms of infection. ■ Inspect incision and drain areas for redness and extreme warmth. ■ Inspect surgical dressings for drainage and odor. ■ Monitor vital signs, especially temperature. ■ Assess vulnerability to infection. ■ Maintain aseptic nontouch technique with surgical dressing changes. ■ Use and teach good hand hygiene. ■ Use sterile saline for wound cleansing up to 48 hours postop (NICE, 2008). ■ See interventions for NIC category Infection Protection. ■ Limit the number of visitors, as appropriate. ■ Obtain cultures as needed. ■ Encourage sufficient nutritional and fluid intake. ■ Teach client about signs of infection.

- *Risk for Ineffective Breathing Pattern* for patients with weak accessory muscles for breathing, with a decreased level of consciousness, or with a respiratory condition such as emphysema.
- *Risk for Infection* for patients who have compromised immune status or who may not be capable of managing their own wound care at home.

Actual Nursing Diagnoses

Of course, you will use a nursing diagnosis whenever a problem becomes actual instead of merely potential. Nursing diagnoses will vary based on the surgical procedure and the client situation. There is no need for a *Deficient Knowledge* diagnosis because patient teaching is a routine intervention for all postoperative patients. Two common postoperative nursing diagnoses are:

- *Delayed Surgical Recovery*, which is appropriate when the patient requires more days to recover than the anticipated length of stay for the surgery.
- *Acute Pain.* There are independent nursing interventions to relieve pain (e.g., teaching the patient to splint the incision). However, they do not usually provide adequate relief in the early postop period. You will nearly always need to administer analgesics, which require a medical prescription.

For other frequently used diagnoses,

 Go to Chapter 37, **Standardized Language, Selected Standardized Nursing Diagnoses, Outcomes and Interventions for Postoperative Patients,** in Volume 2.

▬ PLANNING OUTCOMES/EVALUATION

A comprehensive plan of care for common postoperative nursing diagnoses includes NOC standardized outcomes as well as individualized goals. Because of shortened hospital stays, the postoperative period now extends well past the patient's discharge from the hospital. Often, especially for those who have had major or complex procedures, a home health nurse continues to follow the patient at home to facilitate a smoother transition through the postoperative process.

For *NOC standardized outcomes and individualized goals,*

 Go to Chapter 37, **Standardized Language, Selected Standardized Nursing Diagnoses, Outcomes, and Interventions for Postoperative Patients,** in Volume 2.

▬ PLANNING INTERVENTIONS/IMPLEMENTATION

Most postoperative interventions focus on prevention and early detection of potential complications (collaborative problems). Many such interventions are done as a part of the preoperative teaching. Others are described

in Table 37-4. These are routines that are followed for all postoperative patients, regardless of type of surgery. For *NIC interventions for postoperative nursing diagnoses,*

 Go to Chapter 37, **Standardized Language, Selected Standardized Nursing Diagnoses, Outcomes, and Interventions for Postoperative Patients,** in Volume 2.

Specific nursing activities should be designed to relieve identified nursing diagnoses. In the next sections, we discuss pain management, routine postoperative teaching, and the use of sequential compression devices.

Pain Management

One systematic evidence synthesis has found that there is no strong evidence to support that any particular nursing intervention for relief of postoperative pain is better than any other. Interventions included medication administration, preoperative education, regular assessment and documentation of pain intensity, use of protocols and flow sheets, and nonpharmacological interventions (e.g., massage) in relieving postoperative pain (Crowe, Chang, Fraser, et al., 2008). Therefore, when interventions seem to be equally effective, you will need to weigh the potential benefits, possible adverse events, and patient preferences to decide which to use.

Postoperatively, a patient will usually receive analgesics by more than one route. For example, in the immediate postoperative period, the patient may receive intravenous or epidural medications, progress to oral opioids in a day or two and then to nonopioid analgesics (e.g., acetaminophen). For a complete discussion of types of pain relief, refer to Chapter 30, "Routes of Administration for Opioid Analgesics," and

 Go to Chapter 30, **Procedure 30-1: Connecting a Patient-Controlled Analgesia Pump,** and **Clinical Insight 30-1: Nursing Care of the Patient with an Epidural Catheter,** in Volume 2.

One recent development is a type of pain relief pump that administers a continuous, regulated flow of local anesthetic through a thin catheter directly into the patient's surgical site. A dressing holds the tubing in place, and the pump can be carried in a small bag and used after the patient returns home. It reduces the need for opioids, thus reducing complications, such as nausea, vomiting, and respiratory depression, and is said to hasten ambulation and the return to normal activities. The pump is intended for a single use. Depending on the type of pump, it is filled with 65 to 750 mL of medication and can remain in place for up to 5 days, depending on the amount of anesthetic included (Fig. 37-5).

FIGURE 37-5 A single-use pain relief pump delivers a local anesthetic directly into the patient's surgical site.

CAM for Pain and Anxiety

Reflexotherapy for Acute Postoperative Pain and Anxiety

Tsay, Chen, Chen, et al. (2008) collected data from, 61 patients in Taipei, Taiwan, who received surgery for gastric and liver cancer. Thirty of the patients received 20 minutes of foot reflexotherapy in addition to the usual pain management during postoperative days 2, 3, and 4. They reported less pain and less anxiety than the control group, who did not receive foot reflexotherapy.

Self-Care

Postoperative Patient Teaching Topics

➤ Postoperative treatment regimen (e.g., dressing changes, exercises), including rationale for the treatments

➤ Self-management of the treatment regimen

➤ Expected results and effects of the surgery

➤ The prescribed diet, and how to select foods on the diet

➤ Prescribed activity

➤ Signs and symptoms of complications that require the patient to notify the surgeon or primary care provider

➤ Return office or clinic visits

➤ Lifestyle changes that may be needed

➤ Community resources available (e.g., Reach for Recovery)

See also the complementary and alternative modalities box: Reflexotherapy for Acute Postoperative Pain and Anxiety for an alternative approach to pain management.

Postoperative Teaching

Teaching is especially important postoperatively because most patients must perform quite a bit of self-care. Postoperative teaching should reinforce content taught preoperatively. In addition, you should teach the patient about the topics in the box, Self-Care: Preoperative Patient Teaching. To use time efficiently, try to do some teaching each time you are at the bedside for other care. Be sure the patient is comfortable but alert. Do not attempt teaching when the patient is in pain, needs to void, or is drowsy from opioid analgesics.

Incentive Spirometry

Incentive spirometry may be prescribed for patients who are at high risk for atelectasis and pneumonia. Incentive spirometry is especially useful if the patient has a history of lung problems or smoking or will experience a prolonged period of inactivity. Incentive spirometry facilitates deep breathing, increases lung volume, and promotes coughing to clear mucus from the respiratory tree. The equipment varies in appearance, but all devices include a gauge to monitor the patient's progress visibly (Fig. 37-6).

If you know that the patient will be using an incentive spirometer postoperatively, include its use in your preoperative teaching (see the box, Self-Care: Teaching Your Patient About Incentive Spirometry). If it is prescribed postoperatively, explain to the patient that this is a method to monitor his deep breathing.

FIGURE 37-6 Incentive spirometry facilitates lung expansion and coughing to clear mucus from airways.

Antiembolism Stockings and Sequential Compression Devices

More than half of all hospitalized patients are at risk for venous thromboembolism, and surgical patients seem to be at higher risk than medical patients (Cohen, Tapson, Bergman, et al., 2008). Preventive measures include anticoagulant medications (so-called "blood thinners"), postoperative exercises, and anti-

embolism stockings. You may also hear these called TED (thromboembolic disorder) hose. You may recall that antiembolism stockings were discussed previously in this chapter in the interventions in the Preoperative Care section. Encourage postoperative patients to ambulate as soon and as much as possible to promote peripheral circulation and prevent thrombophlebitis. Antiembolism stockings are not a substitute for activity.

To learn how to apply antiembolism stockings,

 Go to Chapter 37, **Procedure 37-2: Applying Antiembolism Stockings,** in Volume 2.

In addition to the preceding measures, a sequential compression device (SCD) may be prescribed for patients at high risk for thrombophlebitis. The SCD is a plastic sleeve with chambers. The sleeve is wrapped around the patient's legs, and connecting tubes extending from the sleeve are attached to an air pump (Fig. 37-7). The sleeve may extend from ankles to knees or up to the top of the thighs. The SCD provides sequential pressure to the chambers of the plastic sleeve. Starting at the ankle, the first chamber is inflated. When the second chamber inflates, the first chamber deflates. This process continues up to the top of the sleeve and then resumes again at the base by the ankle. SCDs apply brief pressure to each segment of the leg. The pressure compresses the veins and promotes venous return to the heart. The Critical Aspects box summarizes application of sequential compression devices. For the complete steps,

 Go to Chapter 37, **Procedure 37-3: Applying Sequential Compression Devices,** in Volume 2.

Gastrointestinal Suction

Patients having certain surgeries, such as a laparotomy to close a bowel perforation or surgery to relieve

---

Self-Care

Teaching Your Patient About Incentive Spirometry

➤ Explain to the patient that the machine will enable him to monitor the depth of his breathing.

➤ Patients with abdominal or chest incisions may require pain medication to use the incentive spirometer.

➤ Assist the patient to an upright position in the bed or chair.

➤ Instruct the patient to do the following:

1. Breathe out normally.

2. Place the mouthpiece in the mouth and create a seal.

3. Breathe in slowly and as deeply as possible through the mouthpiece. Monitor the depth of inspiration by viewing the gauge. (Establish goals for the patient so that progress can be monitored.)

4. Hold your breath as long as possible, at least to a slow count of 3.

5. Remove the mouthpiece from your mouth, and exhale.

6. Rest for a few seconds

7. Repeat this process 10 times every hour while awake, if possible.

8. After each set of 10 deep breaths, cough to be sure lungs are clear. Support any incision when coughing by holding a pillow firmly against it.

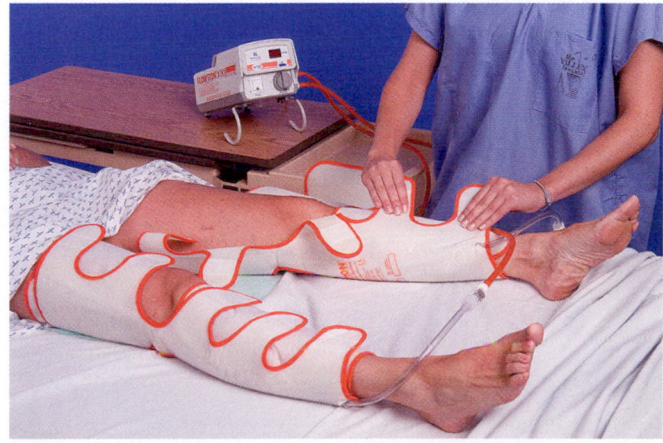

FIGURE 37-7 Sequential compression devices (SCDs) may be prescribed for clients at high risk for thrombophlebitis.

a bowel obstruction, are at high risk for abdominal distention. In addition to causing pain, distention can increase postoperative respiratory problems, place a strain on suture lines, and interfere with wound closure. Such patients will return from surgery with a nasogastric (NG) or nasointestinal tube in place for gastric or intestinal decompression. If prolonged intestinal decompression is anticipated, a gastrostomy may be performed instead of using a nasogastric tube.

Decompression tubes are typically connected to either intermittent or continuous suction to collect excess fluid and gas. Suction is continued until peristalsis resumes, bowel sounds are audible, and the patient is passing flatus. While suction is in place, the patient remains NPO. To review insertion and care of NG and nasoenteric tubes, see Chapter 26. To learn how to manage gastrointestinal suction, see the summary in the Critical Aspects Box and,

 Go to Chapter 37, **Procedure 37-4: Managing Gastrointestinal Suction,** in Volume 2.

KnowledgeCheck 37-9

- Identify six potential postoperative complications.
- Why are sequential compression devices used?

 Go to Chapter 37, **Knowledge Check Response Sheet and Answers,** on the Student Resource Disk or DavisPlus at http://davisplus.fadavis.com/Wilkinson2

CarePlanning & MappingPractice

For Care Planning/Care Mapping practice,

 Go to Student Resources, **Care Planning & Care Mapping Practice,** at http://davisplus.fadavis.com/Wilkinson2

 Go to Chapter 37, **Resources for Caregivers and Health Professionals,** on the Student Resource Disk or DavisPlus at http://davisplus.fadavis.com/Wilkinson2

 Suggested Readings: Go to Chapter 37, **Reading More About Perioperative Nursing,** on the Student Resource Disk or DavisPlus at http://davisplus.fadavis.com/Wilkinson2

 Bibliography: Go to Volume 2, Bibliography.

Nursing Functions

CHAPTER 38

Leading & Managing

Learning Outcomes

After completing this chapter, you should be able to:

➤ Distinguish leadership, followership, and management.

➤ Compare and contrast authoritarian, democratic and laissez-faire leadership styles.

➤ Explain the differences between transactional and transformational theories.

➤ Discuss the qualities and behaviors that contribute to effective leadership and followership.

➤ Discuss the qualities and activities that contribute to effective management.

➤ Explain how a SWOT analysis or a SOAR analysis can help you prepare to become a leader and manager.

➤ Discuss the qualities of preceptors and mentors.

➤ Present strategies for effective followership.

➤ Describe the challenges presented to nurse managers by the economy and the nursing labor market.

➤ Define power and empowerment.

➤ Describe several ways in which nurses can be empowered.

➤ Explain why communication skills are important to nurse leaders and managers.

➤ Describe the change process.

➤ Identify methods of dealing with change.

➤ Describe the major concepts of conflict, conflict resolution, and informal negotiation.

➤ Describe the major concepts of safe and effective delegation.

➤ Set short- and long-term personal and career goals.

➤ Organize your work to make effective use of time.

Portions of this chapter were taken from R. M. Tappen, S. A. Weiss, & D. K. Whitehead (2007). *Essentials of nursing leadership and management* (4th ed.). Philadelphia: F. A. Davis. Used with permission.

Meet Your Peer

Mary is a student in a nursing program. She considers herself a "pretty good test-taker" and has a GPA of 3.4. She received her first test grade in the Nursing Fundamentals class, and it was a C. Mary is sure that she will never pass this course and that her dream of becoming a nurse will vanish. When discussing the test with her classmates, she realized there are several other disappointed students who have been used to making As and Bs on exams. The nursing exams seem different, because they do not just ask students to recall memorized material but also apply what they have learned. Mary decides to get the group together and plan some strategies for study groups. She asks the instructor whether she will meet with them and go over their plan to make sure they are on the "right track." Mary has exhibited some leadership qualities.

Theoretical **Knowledge** **knowing** why

In this chapter, we define *leadership, management, followership,* and the relationships among them. We discuss the challenges to nurses today as they lead and manage others. Those challenges also involve the concepts of power and empowerment.

What Is Leadership?

You may be thinking, "I just started in my nursing program. How can you expect me to be a leader now?" As a student, you do need time to learn how nurses function in a work environment. However, you can begin to assume some leadership skills as a new student. The essence of **leadership** is the ability to influence other people. Effective leaders enable people to move "in the same direction, toward the same destination, at the same speed, not because they have been forced to, but because they want to" (Lansdale, 2002, p. 63). A leader in healthcare has three primary tasks:

- Set direction (i.e., help people develop vision, a mission, goals, and purpose).
- Build commitment (i.e., help people develop motivation, team spirit, and teamwork).
- Confront challenges that arise from innovation, change and turbulence (Drath, 2001).

Critical**Thinking** 38-1

1. Think of a goal your class might have. Obviously, each student wants to develop the skills necessary to provide excellent patient care and learn the theory content to pass the course and continue in the program. What other goals might you have, as a group? As a leader, how might you help the group meet their goals?

2. Brainstorm with your peers to identify some shared goals of professional nurses.

Leadership Theories

How does a person become a leader? What type of leader is most effective? Although much research has been done on these questions, no theory has yet emerged as the clear answer. The reason may be that different situations require different qualities and behaviors. In nursing, for example, some situations require quick thinking and fast action. Others require time to reflect on the best solution to a complicated problem. Let's look now at some of the best-known leadership theories, beginning with some of the older ones.

Trait Theories

Have you ever heard someone say, "Leaders are born, not made"? That implies some of us are natural leaders, but others of us are not. Much of the early leadership research was done in an attempt to identify the qualities, or **traits,** that distinguish a leader from a nonleader. The traits most often identified are intelligence and initiative. Other qualities that were found to be associated with leadership are excellent interpersonal skills, high self-esteem, creativity, willingness to take risks, and ability to tolerate the consequences of taking risks (White & Lippitt, 1960). Leadership may come more easily to some than to others, but everyone can be a leader, at least in certain areas, if she develops the necessary knowledge and skills.

Behavioral Theories

The trait theories were concerned with what a leader *is;* the behavior theories are concerned with what the leader *does*. One of the most influential of these behavioral theories is concerned with leadership style. Three styles have been identified (White & Lippitt, 1960).

Authoritarian Leadership. This is also called *autocratic, directive, controlling*. The authoritarian leader gives orders, makes decisions for the group as a whole, and bears most of the responsibility for the outcomes. For example, when a decision needs to be made, an authoritarian leader would say, "I've given this a great deal of thought and decided this is the way we're going to solve our problem." Authoritarian leadership may be either punitive or kind and compassionate. Although this type of leadership is an efficient way to run things, it usually inhibits creativity and motivation. However, group output tends to be high in quality and quantity.

Democratic Leadership. This is also called *participative leadership*. In contrast to the authoritarian leader, the democratic leader shares the planning, decision making, and responsibility for outcomes with other members of the group. A democratic leader tends to provide guidance rather than control. Although this is often a less efficient way to run things, it is more flexible and more likely to foster motivation and creativity. Group output tends to be of high quality.

Laissez-faire Leadership. Laissez-faire ("let it alone") is also called permissive or nondirective leadership. This leader has a relatively inactive style. She believes the best leader is distant from the action, and intervenes only when goals have not been met or a problem arises (Jones & Rudd, 2007). Laissez-faire leadership gives followers the majority of control in the decision-making process. For example, when a decision needs to be made, a laissez-faire leader may postpone making the decision or never make it at all. In most instances, the leader offers little feedback and support to the followers, leaving people feeling confused and frustrated because there is no goal, no guidance, and no direction. Some mature individuals thrive under laissez-faire leadership because they need little guidance. However, most people do not work effectively under this kind of leadership, and work output is inefficient and may be of poor quality.

Pavitt summed up the difference between these three leadership styles:

- A democratic leader tries to move the group toward its goals.
- An autocratic leader tries to move the group toward the leader's goals.
- A laissez-faire leader makes no attempt to move the group (Pavitt, 1999, p. 330).

KnowledgeCheck 38-1

Identify the three common styles of leadership in the behavioral theories of leadership.

Go to Chapter 38, **Knowledge Check Response Sheet and Answers,** on the Student Resource Disk or DavisPlus at http://davisplus.fadavis.com/Wilkinson2

Task versus Relationship Theories

Another important distinction in leadership style is the one between a *task* focus and a *relationship* focus (Blake, Mouton, & Tapper, 1981). Some leaders emphasize the tasks (e.g., keeping the nursing station neat, getting charting done) and fail to realize that interpersonal relationships (e.g., attitude of physicians toward nursing staff, treating housekeeping staff with respect) have considerable impact on employee morale and productivity. Others focus on the interpersonal aspects and ignore the quality of the job being done as long as people get along with each other. The most effective leader is able to balance the two, attending to both the task and the relationship aspects of working together.

Emotional Intelligence Theory

Emotional intelligence theory focuses on the relationship aspects of leadership. In part, what sets leadership "stars" apart from ordinary leaders is that they consciously address the effect of people's feelings on the team. This is done by leaders who:

- Learn how to recognize, understand, and manage their own emotions; and to stay clear-headed and suspend judgment until all the facts are in (Baggett & Baggett, 2005).
- Listen attentively to others, pick up unspoken concerns, and acknowledge others' perspectives.
- Bring people together in an atmosphere of respect and cooperation so they can direct their energies toward achieving team goals.

The emotionally intelligent leader's enthusiasm, caring, and support generates the same feelings throughout the team (Porter-O'Grady, 2003).

Situational Theories

We know now that people and leadership situations are far more complex than the early theories recognized. Furthermore, situations may change rapidly, requiring even more complex theory to explain people's responses. In recognition of this, less simplistic theories have evolved to replace the trait and behavioral theories.

Adaptability is the key to the situational approach (McNichol, 2000). Instead of assuming that one particular approach works in all situations, situational theories recognize the complexity of work situations and encourage the leader to consider a number of factors when deciding what action to take. Every situation is different. A change that is welcomed by one group may be strongly resisted by another group. Resistance to change is affected by the leadership approach and the type of organizational structure. Situational theories emphasize that it is important to (1) understand all of the factors that affect a particular group of people in a particular environment, and

(2) vary the type of leadership to meet the needs of the situation.

Transformational Theories

Although the situational theories were an improvement over earlier theories in recognizing how complex the process of influencing others really is, they were still missing something. They did not address meaning, inspiration, and vision, which are the distinguishing features of transformational leadership theory. According to transformational theory, people need a sense of mission that goes beyond good interpersonal relationships or the appropriate reward for a job well done (Bass & Avolio, 1993). This is especially true in nursing. Caring for people, sick or well, is the goal of our profession. Most of us chose nursing to do something for the good of humankind; this is our vision. One goal of nursing leadership should be to guide us toward achieving that vision.

Transformational leadership involves the ability to inspire and motivate followers. The transformational leader creates a supportive climate, listening to followers, and acts as a coach and mentor. Transformational leaders communicate their vision in a way that is so meaningful and exciting that it reduces negativity and inspires commitment in the people with whom they work (Leach, 2005; Trofino, 1995). Followers become motivated to go beyond their own self-interests for the good of the group or organization, often accomplishing more than what would normally be expected of them (Jones & Rudd, 2007).

The American Nurses Credentialing Centers (ANCC) Magnet Recognition® Program was developed to recognize healthcare organizations that provide the very best in nursing care. The ANCC expects leaders in Magnet organizations to demonstrate the transformational qualities listed in Table 38-1.

Transactional Theories

Whereas transformational leadership uses more of a "selling" style, transactional leadership uses more of a "telling" style. Transactional theory assumes that people are motivated by reward and punishment and that they work best within a clear chain of command. The leader creates structures to make clear what is required of subordinates and what the rewards are. The structure also usually includes formal systems of discipline. These leaders monitor behaviors closely to point out errors and make corrective criticisms. They enforce rules to avoid mistakes (Jones & Rudd, 2007). Transactional leadership is commonly used by managers, and in an organization, the "rewards" are salary and benefits (e.g., healthcare insurance). However, when the demand for a skill—or for workers of a particular type—is greater than the supply, the usual rewards may not be sufficient, and other types of leadership are more effective. Table 38-1 compares the traits of transactional and transformational leadership.

Table 38-1 ➤ Contrast of Traits in Transactional and Transformational Leadership	
TRANSACTIONAL LEADERSHIP	**TRANSFORMATIONAL LEADERSHIP**
Directive	Participative
Top down	Bottom up
Information	Conversation
Hierarchical communication	Matrix communication
Event oriented	Future oriented
Task-focused	Overall experience-focused
Directed	Facilitated
Rigid	Flexible
Here and now	Visions for the future
Traditional	Contemporary
Rules	Risk taking
Control	Creativity
Individual performance	Team and relationships
Responsibility	Accountability

Used with permission of Patricia Davis, RN, DNP, MS, NEA-BC, CNL; Concord, CA.

Critical Thinking 38-2

Observe a nurse in one of the healthcare agencies where you are doing a clinical rotation. What leadership qualities and behaviors do you see the nurse exhibiting? How do these behaviors help in planning nursing care?

What Is Management?

Whereas leaders may or may not have official appointments to the position, managers are usually officially appointed to a position that has power and authority to enforce decisions. A **manager** is an employee of an organization who has the power, authority, and responsibility for planning, organizing, coordinating, and directing the work of others. Every nurse should be a good leader and a good follower; however, not everyone can or should be a manager. You may notice the following discussion of management overlaps a great deal with the content on leadership you have just read. That is because managers must be leaders, and they have varying styles of leadership. To sum up: Not all leaders should be managers; but all managers should be leaders.

Management Theories

Although there are many management theories, there are two major schools of thought in management: (1) scientific management and (2) the human relations approach to management. As you will see, the first emphasizes the task aspects of managing people, and the second emphasizes the relationship aspects.

Scientific Management

Almost 100 years ago, Frederick Taylor argued that most jobs could be done more efficiently if they were thoroughly analyzed (Lee, 1980; Locke, 1982). Given a properly designed task and sufficient incentive to get the work done, workers would be more productive. For example, Taylor encouraged paying people "by the piece," that is, by the number of "widgets" made rather than by the number of hours worked. This encourages workers to get the most work done in the least amount of time, Taylor said. In healthcare, the equivalent of paying "by the piece" would be to pay for the number of clients bathed or monitored. In scientific management, the fastest way to do a job is usually thought to be the best way (Dantley, 2005).

Which do you think would take the least amount of time and manpower: bringing patients to the radiology department or bringing a portable x-ray machine to the bedside? What about physical therapy: taking patients to the physical therapy department or having the therapist come to the patient's room? In healthcare, there has been much discussion about these kinds of questions. This type of thinking is the basis for the emphasis on eliminating excess staff and increasing the productivity of remaining employees.

Human Relations–Based Management

McGregor's (1960) theory X and theory Y are good examples of the difference between scientific management and human relations–oriented management.

Theory X. Managers believe that most people really do not want to work very hard and that the manager's job is to make sure that they do work hard. According to theory X, a manager needs to use strict rules, constant supervision, and the threat of punishment (e.g., reprimands, withheld raises, and threats of job loss) to create industrious, conscientious workers. Theory X is similar to scientific management.

Theory Y. The opposite viewpoint, theory Y, is a human relations–oriented theory. Managers believe that work itself can be motivating, that people want to do their jobs well, and that they will work hard if their managers provide a supportive atmosphere. A theory Y manager emphasizes guidance rather than control, development rather than close supervision, and reward rather than punishment.

A theory Y nurse manager is concerned with keeping staff morale as high as possible, assuming that satisfied, motivated staff will do the best work. Employees' attitudes, opinions, hopes, and fears are important to this type of leader. Such a manager would make an effort to work out conflicts and promote mutual understanding among the staff to provide an atmosphere in which people can do their best work.

Servant Leadership

Despite its name, servant leadership applies more to supervisors and administrators than to nurses in staff positions. This type of management emphasizes interpersonal relationships, but goes one step further. The servant leadership manager believes people have value as people, not just as workers (Greenleaf, 2004; Spears & Lawrence, 2004). The manager's attitude is employee first, and the manager is committed to improving the way each employee is treated at work. The servant-leader manager is there to remove barriers, make the work easier, and provide employees with whatever they need to provide the best patient care possible.

Qualities of an Effective Manager

Two-thirds of people who leave their jobs say the main reason was an ineffective or incompetent manager (Hunter, 2004). With job turnover rates high, nurse managers are challenged to retain staff nurses. A review of the nursing administration literature indicates that effective leadership styles of nurse managers and administrators enhance staff nurse retention (Kleinman, 2004). An effective nurse manager has the qualities of leadership, clinical expertise, and business sense. None of these alone is enough; it is the combination that prepares a person for the complex task of managing a group of healthcare providers. Let's look at each quality:

Leadership. All of the "people skills" and other leadership qualities are the core skills the nurse needs to function as an effective manager.

Clinical Expertise. If a nurse manager is to help others develop their skills and evaluate how well they have done so, she needs a certain amount of clinical expertise. It is not necessary (or even possible) to know everything every other professional on the team knows, but it is important to be able to assess the effectiveness of their work in terms of client outcomes.

Business Sense. Nurse managers need to be concerned with the "bottom line," that is, with the cost of providing care, especially in comparison with the benefit received from that care. In other words, nurse managers need to be able to analyze how much time is spent to provide a given amount of client care, how effective that client care has been, how much will be paid to the institution for the care delivered, and who will pay for it (e.g., private insurance, government insurance, or the client). These are complex tasks that require knowledge of budgeting, staffing, and measurement of patient outcomes, most of which are beyond the scope of this textbook.

There is some controversy over the amount of clinical expertise versus business sense that is needed to be an effective nurse manager. Some argue that a person can be a "generic" manager—that the job of managing people is the same, no matter what tasks they perform. Others argue that the manager must understand the tasks better than anyone else in the work group. Our position is that both are needed, along with excellent leadership skills.

You may be saying to yourself, "I don't want to be a manager. I just want to take care of patients." However, as a registered nurse, you will manage groups of patients, and you will be responsible for supervising nursing assistants, licensed practical nurses, and other ancillary staff. Even as a staff nurse, you will be a manager of care. You may be interested to know that the NCLEX-RN Testing Plan has an entire section devoted to management of care, which is not necessarily about managing the nurses or the nursing unit but rather organizing and delivering (i.e., managing) care to the patient. Questions address nursing activities, such as assessing clients to prioritize care, making appropriate referrals to the community, and acting as a client advocate.

Activities of an Effective Manager

Mintzberg (1989) divides the manager's activities into three categories: interpersonal, decisional, and informational. Whitehead, Weiss, and Tappen (2007) build on that work:

Interpersonal Activities. Interpersonal activities are important to both leaders and managers. In fact, one might say that interpersonal skills are important to everyone! From the beginning of your career in nursing school, you will have many opportunities to develop positive working relationships with members of other disciplines, departments, and units within the organization. Can you see how Mary ("Meet Your Peer") would need interpersonal skills to accomplish her goals?

Interpersonal activities of managers include the following:

- *Networking.* Managers must clearly articulate nurses' roles and value to the institution.
- *Conflict negotiation and resolution*
- *Employee development.* This includes providing for continuing learning and upgrading employees' skills.
- *Rewards and punishments.* Examples include salary increases, time off, and praise.
- *Coaching.* The goal is to help the employee do a better job through learning. Some managers use a directive approach ("Let me show you how to do this"). Others use a nondirective approach ("How do you think we can improve our outcomes?").

Decisional Activities. From the very beginning of your career, you will be expected to develop critical-thinking, prioritizing, and decision-making skills in your clinical experiences. Even as a student, you will need to know what information to report to your instructor and when to provide it. Nurse managers' decisions include:

- *Employee evaluation,* including conducting formal performance appraisals
- *Resource allocation* (e.g., budgeting and how to use available funds wisely)
- *Hiring and terminating* employees
- *Planning* for future changes (e.g., in budgets or client populations)
- *Job analysis and redesign* (e.g., to make the units run as efficiently as possible)
- *Unit-based decisions* (e.g., staffing policies, space utilization)

What decisions did Mary ("Meet Your Peer") make?

Informational Responsibilities. Side by side with decisional responsibilities are the informational responsibilities of a manager.

- *Spokesperson.* The manager relays information from administration to staff members, and speaks to administration on behalf of staff members.
- *Monitoring.* Managers monitor the activities of their units or departments (e.g., the number of clients seen, length of stay), as well as the staff (e.g., absenteeism), and the budget (e.g., money spent).
- *Public Relations.* Nurse managers share information with clients, staff members, and employers, for example, regarding new developments in healthcare and policy changes.

What are some kinds of information Mary ("Meet Your Peer") would need to communicate to the students interested in forming a study group?

KnowledgeCheck 38-2

- How is transformational leadership different from the other theories of leadership?
- Define *manager*.
- In McGregor's management theory, which is more like scientific management: theory X or theory Y?

 Go to Chapter 38, **Knowledge Check Response Sheet and Answers,** on the Student Resource Disk or DavisPlus at http://davisplus.fadavis.com/Wilkinson2

How Can I Prepare to Become a Leader and Manager?

You may still be asking yourself, "What does all this leadership and management stuff have to do with me?" Besides learning the role of the registered nurse, you should begin right now to look at the skills employers think you need to be ready to work for them. Along with passing the NCLEX-RN examination to obtain nursing licensure, employers cite the skills listed in Box 38-1 as desirable in job candidates (Shingleton, 1994; Villarreal, 2002). Many of these skills have been identified in our

BOX 38-1 ■ Desirable Job Candidate Skills

- Ability to assume responsibility
- Computer knowledge
- Critical-thinking and analytical skills
- Interpersonal skills
- Leadership abilities
- Motivation, initiative, and flexibility
- Oral and written communication skills
- Organizational skills
- Problem-solving and decision-making abilities
- Proficiency in field of study or technical competence
- Self-discipline
- Teamwork ability
- Willingness to work hard
- Ability to teach others
- Ability to adapt equipment to serve user needs
- Flexibility to adjust action in relation to others

discussion of leading and managing. It is not too early to begin to develop your abilities in these areas. These skills will assist you as you go through your nursing program, and will also make your adjustment to the RN role much easier.

One of the first steps in identifying what skills you already possess and which you need to develop is to do a brief SWOT analysis. A SWOT (strengths, weaknesses, opportunities, threats) analysis plan, borrowed from the corporate world, can guide you through an analysis of your own internal strengths and weaknesses and reveal external opportunities and threats that may help or hinder your leadership and management skills (Ellis, 1999). Your SWOT analysis may include the factors listed as examples in Table 38-2, but certainly you will have others.

You might prefer to use the SOAR strategic planning model to help you prepare to become a leader and manager (Table 38-3). This model can be used to analyze any type of situation and create a plan to achieve personal and professional goals. With this model, you would use inquiry, imagination, innovation, and aspiration focus on strengths, opportunities, aspirations, and results (Stavros, Cooperrider, & Kelly, 2007).

CriticalThinking 38-3

Stop and think! Take some time to personalize the SWOT analysis in Table 38-2. What weaknesses do you need to minimize, or which strengths do you need to develop as you begin to develop your leadership and management skills?

How Can Mentors and Preceptors Help Me?

There are two aspects to consider as you get ready to become a leader and manager. The first part, discussed earlier, consists of developing self. The second part is really a combination of developing self and developing others: mentorship and preceptorship. A **mentor** is someone more experienced who provides career development assistance, such as coaching, sponsoring advancement, providing challenging assignments, protecting protégés from adversity, and promoting positive visibility. Mentors provide guidance to new students or graduates as they continue in the profession. They offer a constructive example as a role model to novices. Mentors can also fulfill psychosocial roles, such as personal support, friendship, acceptance, role modeling, and counseling.

Many organizations have preceptors for new employees. A **preceptor** is someone with more experience who provides practical teaching and guidance for a student or new employee. As a student, you may be assigned an RN preceptor in your clinical rotations. You may work side by side with a preceptor to provide patient care now and as a new graduate. In many instances, the preceptor will become your mentor. However, the mentor role is much more encompassing than the preceptor role. The mentor

Table 38-2 ➤ SWOT Analysis Plan—Examples			
STRENGTHS	**WEAKNESSES**	**OPPORTUNITIES**	**THREATS**
Relevant work experience	Poor communication and people skills	Changes in healthcare	Changes in healthcare
Advanced education	Inflexibility	Availability of mentors and preceptors	Lack of time
Good communication and people skills	Lack of interest in self-learning	Variety of experiences in clinical rotations	Competition from other students and other nursing programs
Computer skills	Difficulty adapting to change	Many leadership and management books and self-learning programs available	

Table 38-3 ➤ SOAR Strategic Planning

THE PROCESS: HOW TO SOAR	THE SOAR REPORT OR SUMMARY
To SOAR: Inquire, imagine, innovate, and inspire. **Inquiry:** Internal analysis of strengths and external analysis of opportunities	Use SOAR to report or tell your story. **Strengths.** My (or the group's) strengths are... (Examples of strengths may be a supportive environment, individual strengths, a product that others need, and so on.)
Imagination: Co-create vision, values, and mission. Imagine desired outcomes. Imagine the best pathway to achieve the outcomes.	**Opportunities.** My values are... (e.g., dedication, quality). As I imagine the future, my vision (for myself, for our group) is... (e.g., to become a transformational manager on a nursing unit).
Innovation: Create initiatives, strategies, structures, and systems. Create plans for tactics.	**Aspirations.** Here is how I believe I (or we) can achieve the desired outcomes.
Inspiration: Inspire action-oriented activities that achieve results. Implement a plan for continuous improvement.	**Results.** To achieve your desired outcomes, you must be motivated (and possibly need to inspire others) to take the necessary actions.

relationship is a voluntary one and is built on mutual respect and development of the mentee. Box 38-2 identifies responsibilities of the mentor and mentee in this relationship.

You should look for a mentor in the nursing program right now—someone to guide you as you grow into your professional role. A student who has already completed several semesters and appears to be a leader is a good choice. In some programs, you may be assigned a student preceptor while you are in the program. Although this student may or may not become your mentor, you will need to have leadership and management skills to work side by side effectively.

Will you assume the role of preceptor or mentor while you are still in school? We hope your response is yes. As you progress in the program, remember the feelings of uncertainly and anxiety that you may now have, and volunteer to mentor another new student. Through the mentoring process, you can continue to develop yourself as a leader. Mentoring and preceptoring are part of your professional responsibilities, as

the ANA Standard of Nursing Practice 13 (2010, in press) states:

> *Collegiality.* The registered nurse interacts with and contributes to the professional development of peers and colleagues.

How Will Leadership Grow in My Nursing Career?

As you begin your nursing clinical experiences, your nursing instructor will supervise most of your decisions. As you continue to develop your knowledge and skills, you will begin working more as a member of the team. You will be expected to prioritize patient care, work with a variety of team members and families, and provide care for groups of clients. You may go to community agencies and network with community groups. To be successful in your continued role development as a nurse, you must work on perfecting the skills discussed in this chapter.

BOX 38-2 ■ Mentor and Mentee Responsibilities

Mentor Responsibilities
- Demonstrate excellent communication and listening skills.
- Be sensitive to the needs of nurses, patients, and the workplace.
- Encourage excellence in others.
- Share and provide counsel.
- Exhibit good decision-making skills.
- Demonstrate an understanding of power and politics.
- Demonstrate trustworthiness.

Mentee Responsibilities
- Demonstrate eagerness to learn.
- Participate actively in the relationship by keeping all appointments and commitments.
- Seek feedback, and use it to modify behaviors.
- Demonstrate flexibility and an ability to change.
- Be open in the relationship with the mentor.
- Demonstrate an ability to move toward independence.
- Evaluate choices and outcomes.

Source: Whitehead, D., Weiss, S., & Tappen, R. (2007). *Essentials of nursing leadership and management* (4th ed.). Philadelphia: F. A. Davis, p. 224.

KnowledgeCheck 38-3

- Identify four skills that employers cite as desirable in job candidates.
- Identify three responsibilities of a mentor and three responsibilities of a mentee.

Go to Chapter 38, **Knowledge Check Response Sheet and Answers,** on the Student Resource Disk or DavisPlus at http://davisplus.fadavis.com/Wilkinson2

CriticalThinking 38-4

Think about how you are working with your peers at this time. What mentor responsibilities are you exhibiting? Is there someone who is already mentoring you? If so, what qualities does this person exhibit?

What Is Followership?

Leadership and followership are two separate concepts, two separate roles that are complementary, not competitive. Great leaders can create successful followers, and great followers create successful leaders. No one person can have the best strategy, have the clearest vision, or identify the most effective approaches to solve problems. All participants need to be recognized as full partners in the organizational venture. If we define **followers** as individuals who take another as a role model and who act in accordance with, imitate, support, and advocate the ideas and opinions of another (Grossman & Valiga, 2009), then we can define **followership** as the willingness to work with others toward accomplishing the group mission. This term also refers to those who show a high degree of teamwork and build cohesion among the group (Ruskin, 2007).

An organization is a community of many leaders and many followers, frequently changing places depending on the particular activity that is occurring. Blindly following a leader without question or taking a passive role in one's work or professional organization will do little to advance the profession, promote individual growth, or achieve quality patient care. To participate fully and provide significant feedback, followers need to demonstrate a number of important qualities and behaviors (Grossman & Valiga, 2009; Spreitzer & Quinn, 2001; Whitehead, Weiss, & Tappen, 2007):

- Suggest ways to improve client care.
- If you discover a problem, inform your team leader right away. Include a suggestion for solving the problem, if you can.
- Listen carefully and reflect on what the leader or manager says.
- Be truthful. Give honest feedback and constructive criticism, even if it means politely challenging the leader's ideas. Suggest alternative courses of action.
- If, after giving your input, you disagree with decisions that are, your job is then to support—not undermine—the leader.
- If you feel you must have a "heated" discussion with the leader, do so privately.

- Freely invest your interest and energy in your work and in finding best solutions for the group.
- Function independently; be a self-starter; take on extra tasks without being asked.
- Be actively involved.
- Be innovative and creative.
- Be responsible and hold up your end of the bargain; accept responsibility when it is offered.
- Be supportive of new ideas and directions suggested by others, but think critically about ideas that are proposed.
- When you disagree, explain why.
- Don't gossip.
- Think and act as a team; be cooperative and collaborative.
- Draw on and complement each other's and the leader's specialties, strengths, and areas of expertise.
- Work on behalf of the organization and the mutually agreed on vision and goals.
- Continue to learn as much as you can about your specialty area; share what you learn with others.
- Seek information so you can see the larger picture.
- Know your own strengths and what your unique contributions to the effort can be.
- Know how to assume the role of the leader when necessary.
- Have a positive sense of self-worth and a "can do" attitude.
- Take care of yourself and your family. If you and they are unhappy, your job performance will suffer.

If you need other, more specific, suggestions for developing your skills as a follower,

Go to Chapter 38, **ESG Box 38-1,** on the Student Resource Disk or DavisPlus at http://davisplus.fadavis.com/Wilkinson2

What Are the Challenges to Being an Effective Leader and Manager?

Even after you have developed the skills necessary to become an effective leader or manager, challenges exist in the healthcare environment. These challenges include the economic climate of healthcare and the nursing labor market.

Economic Climate of Healthcare

For many years, decisions about care were based primarily on providing the best quality care, whatever the cost. More recently, however, healthcare providers are pressured to seek methods of care delivery that achieve quality outcomes at lower cost. This economic perspective is rooted in three fundamental observations:

1. *Resources are scarce.* The scarcity of resources means that three decisions must be made:
   - How much do we spend on healthcare services, and what do those services consist of?

- How will those healthcare services be produced?
- How should, or can, we distribute healthcare? In other words, how are services apportioned within the population? For example, it is hard to believe that the healthcare needs of more than 47 million uninsured individuals in America are not being met because these people cannot afford to pay insurance premiums. But to change that, their healthcare and/or their insurance premiums must be paid for. Who will pay for that? Where will the money come from?

2. *Resources have alternative uses.* Because resources are limited, a choice to spend resources in one area eliminates the allocation of those same resources for another use. If we wish to build more nursing homes, for example, we must be willing to accept fewer hospitals or less housing, education, or other uses of those same resources. In healthcare, an expanded program of immunization may mean limiting care for certain chronic illnesses or for certain age groups.

3. *Individuals want different things or have different preferences.* Some people choose alternative treatment modalities, such as acupuncture, herbal therapy, or massage therapy, rather than traditional healthcare. The assumption exists that preferences for products and services can be influenced—hence, the extensive marketing of healthcare services.

Nursing Labor Market

Not so long ago, registered nurses made up 77% of the nurse workforce in the United States, with almost 60% employed in hospitals (Spratley, Johnson, Sochalski, et al., 2000). In 2001, the Bureau of Labor Statistics predicted there would be more than one million vacant positions for registered nurses by 2020 (American Association of Colleges of Nursing, 2005). However, more recently, depending on the source, the nationwide unemployment rate for RNs has been reported to be between 1% and 6%. After a 2-year surge of employment in the early 2000s, total employment fell slightly during 2004 and 2005, especially in hospitals, leading some to question whether the nursing shortage is over (Buerhaus, Auerbach, & Staiger, 2007).

The need for nurses is expected to increase even more dramatically as the Baby Boomers reach their 60s, 70s, and beyond. From now until 2030, the population aged 65 and older will double. The questions are (1) whether there will be enough nurses available to fill those jobs, and (2) even if nurses are available, whether it will be economically feasible for organizations to hire as many as they need. Government-proposed sweeping changes in the healthcare system in the United States will certainly affect the supply and demand of nurses, but until the changes are made more specific, it is difficult to predict what the effects will be.

As in the past, cost control and demand for nursing services will most likely involve changing nurse staffing patterns, the model of care, or professional nursing practice (Ritter-Teitel, 2002). All of these changes will affect you, the nurse. Regardless of the changes, healthcare system changes will likely demand that the RN lead and manage personnel delivering patient care while maintaining fiscal responsibility. Healthcare is big business, even though it is heavily regulated by government and other agencies. Nurses must juggle the needs of their patients with the needs of the organization. From time to time, think about how we might do that.

CriticalThinking 38-5

Identify changes in your community that will affect you as you embark upon your nursing career. What will you do to prepare for these changes?

What Are Power and Empowerment?

The leadership and management techniques discussed so far will help you to achieve your goals. However, there are times when your attempts to influence others are overwhelmed by other forces or individuals. Where does this power come from? Who has it? Who does not?

Although people at the top of an organization have most of the *authority* in the organization, they do not have all of the *power*. In fact, the people at the bottom of the hierarchy also have some power. **Power** is the ability to influence other people despite resistance from them. In other words, one person or group can impose its will on another person or group (Haslan, 2001). Power may be actual or potential, intended or unintended. It may also be used for good or for evil, for serious purposes or for selfish ones.

Sources of Power

There are many sources of power. Many of them are readily available to nurses, but some of them are not (Barraclough & Stewart, 1992).

- **Authority:** The power granted to an individual or a group by virtue of position (within the organizational hierarchy, for example)
- **Reward:** The promise of money, goods, services, recognition, or other benefits
- **Expertise:** The special knowledge an individual is believed to possess. As Sir Francis Bacon said long ago, "Knowledge is power" (Bacon, 1597, quoted in Fitton, 1997, p. 150).
- **Coercion:** The threat of pain or of harm, which may be physical, economic, or psychological

Let's look at various groups of people in a healthcare organization in terms of the types of power that may be available to them.

Managers are able to reward people with salary increases, promotions, and recognition. They can also use coercion—cause economic or psychological pain for the people who work for them, particularly through their authority to evaluate and fire people.

Patients at first appear to be relatively powerless in a healthcare organization. However, if patients refused to use the services of a particular organization, that organization would eventually cease to exist. Patients reward healthcare workers by praising them to their supervisors. They can also cause discomfort by complaining about them.

Registered nurses have expertise power, as well as authority to delegate appropriately to licensed practical nurses, NAPs, and other personnel by virtue of their position in the hierarchy and the Nurse Practice Act. Nurses are essential to the operation of most healthcare organizations and could cause considerable trouble if they refused to work, another source of power (coercion).

Assistants and technicians may appear to have less power because of their position in an organization's "top-down" hierarchy. Imagine, though, how the work of the organization (e.g., hospital, nursing home) would grind to a halt if all the nursing assistants failed to appear one morning. Therefore, they have both expertise and coercive power.

Fralic (2000) offered a good example of the power of information, or expertise, that nurses have always had: Florence Nightingale showed very graphically in the 1800s that wherever her nurses were, far fewer patients died; and wherever they were not, far more died. Think of the power of that information. Immediately people were saying, "What would you like, Miss Nightingale? Would you like more money? Would you like a school of nursing? What else can we do for you?" (p. 340). She had solid data, she knew how to collect it, and she knew how to interpret and distribute it in terms of things that people valued.

KnowledgeCheck 38-4

What are the sources of power available to nurses?

 Go to Chapter 38, **Knowledge Check Response Sheet and Answers,** on the Student Resource Disk or DavisPlus at http://davisplus.fadavis.com/Wilkinson2

Sources of Empowerment

How can nurses, either individually or collectively, maximize their power and increase their feelings of empowerment? To answer this question, you should first distinguish between the concepts of power and empowerment. Recall that power is the ability to influence other people despite resistance from them. **Empowerment** is a psychological state, a feeling of competence, control, and entitlement that a person experiences. Given these definitions, it is possible to be powerful and yet not feel empowered. Power refers to action, and empowerment refers to feelings. Both are of interest to

nursing leaders and managers. Feeling empowered includes the following:

- **Self-determination:** Feeling free to decide how to do your work
- **Meaning:** Caring about your work, enjoying it, and taking it seriously
- **Competence:** Confidence in your ability to do your work well
- **Impact:** Feeling that people listen to your ideas, that you can make a difference

Nurses, like most people, want to have some power and to feel empowered. They want to be heard, recognized, valued, and respected. They do not want to feel unimportant or insignificant to society or to the organization in which they work. The following contribute to nurse empowerment: (a) manageable, reasonable work assignments; (b) reward, recognition, and appreciation for a job well done; and (c) fair, consistent treatment of all staff.

Not all empowerment comes from others. You can become empowered by actively participating in professional nursing organizations, joining a collective bargaining unit, and seeking opportunities to be involved in decision making in your organization. Two other ways of empowering yourself are by enhancing and sharing expertise.

Enhancing Expertise

Nurses and other healthcare professionals are empowered to some degree by their own professional knowledge and competence. Following are some ways in which you can enhance your competence, thereby increasing your own sense of empowerment:

- Actively participate in interdisciplinary team conferences and patient-centered conferences on your unit.
- Attend continuing education activities to enhance your expertise. This might include local, regional, national, and international conferences sponsored by nursing organizations.
- Read journals and books in your specialty area.
- Participate in nursing research projects related to your clinical area.
- Discuss with colleagues in nursing and other disciplines how to handle a difficult clinical situation.
- Observe the practice of experienced nurses.
- Continue education by earning additional degrees and certifications in nursing.

Although you have just begun your nursing career, it is not too early to begin thinking of ways to become empowered.

Sharing Expertise

The second part, becoming empowered through expertise, is to share with others the knowledge and experience you have. This means not only using your knowledge to improve your own practice, but also communicating what you have learned to other students and, later, to your colleagues in nursing. It also means letting your instructors and supervisors know that you have enhanced your professional competence. You can share your knowledge with your clients, empowering them as well. In the future, you may even reach the point at which you have learned more about a particular subject than most nurses have and want to write about it for publication.

Practical **Knowledge** **knowing** how

As a leader or manager, you will need to get people to work together to make things happen. To do so, you will need to communicate effectively, delegate, deal with conflict and change, and manage your time appropriately.

Communicating

Leadership arises through relationships with other people, and leaders use communication to engage and support these relationships. One model views communication as a circular process that is affected by many factors. Communication in this model has both content and a relationship context. This means the activity is continuous, mutually interdependent, and influenced by the behaviors of each communicator. You need to use active listening (see Chapter 18) to pick up all levels of meaning in a communication. Surface listening, or inattention, often causes a misinterpretation of the message. A person's attitude also influences what he hears and how he interprets the message.

To manage client care effectively, it is important to keep the lines of communication open on all levels. As a professional nurse, you will need to communicate client information to other members of the nursing team, to members of other disciplines, to families, and to individual clients. Trust and sincerity enhance communication among team members. Congruence (agreement) between your words and your deeds promotes trust. If team members feel that you are trustworthy and sincere, they will be more likely to ask questions and seek clarification when they are uncertain of something.

A leader is responsible for providing frequent evaluative feedback. Done poorly, evaluation can be stressful, even injurious. Done well, it promotes growth and employee satisfaction. Evaluative feedback is important because it:

- *Reinforces constructive behavior.* Positive feedback lets people know which behaviors are most productive and encourages them to continue the behaviors.
- *Discourages unproductive behavior.* Negative feedback prompts the person to correct inappropriate behavior.
- *Provides recognition.* Praise is an excellent motivator.

Delegating

An important aspect of leadership and management is learning how to delegate. You can apply the nursing process to delegating to safely provide client care.

- *Assess and diagnose.* Before deciding who should care for a particular client, you must assess each client's particular needs.
- *Plan goals and interventions.* Set client-specific goals, and identify what interventions are required to achieve these goals. Mentally identify which staff member is best suited for the task or activities. Thinking this through before delegating helps prevent problems later.
- *Implement.* Next, determine which personnel have the knowledge and skills to care for the client, and assign the tasks to the appropriate person.
- *Evaluate.* You must still oversee care and determine whether client care needs have been met. Be sure to allow time for feedback during the day. This enables all personnel to see how they are doing and what they still need to do. If you must give negative feedback, do so privately.

You will find an extended discussion of delegation in Chapter 7. You might also find helpful the National Council of the State Boards of Nursing (NCSBN) (2009) checklist, *Five Rights of Delegation.* To use this checklist,

 Go to Chapter 7, **Implementation and Evaluation Tools, The Five Rights of Delegation-Checklist,** in Volume 2.

Often, a manager must first determine the mix of personnel (RN, LVN/LPN, or NAP) required to deliver care on a unit before being able to delegate tasks to individuals. By looking at the needs of each client, you can make an educated decision about which staff members have the appropriate education and skill to deliver safe, quality care.

What if I Lack the Experience to Delegate?

The added responsibility of delegation often causes discomfort for new graduates. You may be used to providing total patient care for one or more clients but lack the experience of organizing care for groups of clients with other team members. To overcome your discomfort, you need to observe how more experienced nurses delegate to others. Working with a preceptor will also give you experience in delegation.

Become familiar with nursing professional organization guidelines. The American Nurses Association (ANA) (2005) has specified that RNs may not delegate the following tasks:

- Initial nursing assessment; follow-up assessments if nursing judgment is indicated
- Nursing diagnosis
- Decisions and judgments about outcomes
- Formulation and approval of a patient plan of care

- Interventions that require professional nursing knowledge, decisions, or skills
- Decisions and judgments necessary for the evaluation of patient care

The ANA (2002, 2007) has issued a Position Statement on use of nursing assistive personnel. Box 38-3 lists examples of direct and indirect client care that may be delegated to NAPs. Figure 38-1 shows examples of the skills of various nursing personnel that can be used to meet patient care needs.

What Are the Concerns About Delegating?

Today's healthcare environment requires nurses to delegate. Many nurses voice concerns about the personal risk to their licensure if they delegate inappropriately. The courts have usually ruled that nurses are not liable for the negligence of other workers, provided that the nurse delegated appropriately. Delegation is within the scope of nursing practice, according to the ANA. If you would like further discussion of the legal aspects of delegation, see Chapter 45.

Nurses have also expressed concern over the effects of delegation on the quality of client care. When you delegate, you control the delegation. You decide to whom you will delegate the task. Remember that there are levels of acceptable performance and that not every task needs to be done perfectly.

KnowledgeCheck 38-5

Explain the relationship of delegation and the nursing process.

 Go to Chapter 38, **Knowledge Check Response Sheet and Answers,** on the Student Resource Disk or DavisPlus at http://davisplus.fadavis.com/Wilkinson2

Managing Change

Change is a naturally occurring phenomenon, a part of everyone's life. Every day, we have new experiences,

---

BOX 38-3 ■ Examples of Care that May Be Delegated to Nursing Assistive Personnel

Direct Client Care Activities
- Assisting with activities of daily living: feeding, drinking, ambulation, grooming, toileting, dressing
- Assisting with socializing
- Taking vital signs

Indirect Client Care Activities
- Providing a clean, safe environment
- Providing transport for noncritical clients
- Assisting with stocking nursing units
- Providing messenger and delivery services
- Making beds
- Ordering supplies

---

meet new people, and learn something new. We grow up, leave home, graduate from college, and begin a new career, perhaps a new family as well. Some of these changes are milestones in our lives, ones we have prepared for and anticipated for some time. Others are entirely unexpected—sometimes welcome and sometimes not. Many are exciting, leading us to new opportunities and challenges. When change occurs too rapidly or demands too much of us, though, it can make us very uncomfortable.

The Comfort Zone

The basic stages of the change process are unfreezing, change, and refreezing (Lewin, 1951; Mander, Gomes, & Castle, 2002). Figure 38-2 shows the relationship among those stages and the following concepts of comfort zone, the discomfort associated with change, and the establishing of a new comfort zone.

Let's assume that your daily routine was basically stable before you started nursing school. You took care of the family or worked during the day and took a class or two each term. You knew what to expect and how to

FIGURE 38-1 Patient care needs.

FIGURE 38-2 The change process. (Based on Farrell, K., & Broude, C. (1987). *Winning the change game: How to implement information systems with fewer headaches and bigger paybacks.* Los Angeles: Breakthrough Enterprises; and Lewin, K. (1951). *Field theory in social science: Selected theoretical papers.* New York: Harper & Row.)

deal with whatever problems arose in the course of a day. In other words, you were operating within your "comfort zone" (Farrell & Broude, 1987; Lapp, 2002). A big change is likely to move you out of this comfort zone into disequilibrium, possibly into discomfort. Now you are most likely attending a full-time nursing program and juggling changes in finances, child-care arrangements, and planning options. This first stage in the change process is called *unfreezing*. You are moving out of your comfort zone.

Resistance to Change

People resist change for a variety of reasons. For example, you may find that you can manage the change in class schedule, but that the child-care arrangements are more difficult. Resistance to change (and unfreezing) comes from three major sources: technical concerns, psychosocial needs, and threats to a person's position and power. For a student, so-called technical concerns may involve practical issues related to transportation to school or work, getting children to school, or managing household responsibilities.

Recall Maslow's (1970) hierarchy of needs, discussed in Chapters 3, 9, and 11. Maslow observed that the more basic needs (e.g., physiological and safety needs) must be at least partially met before a person is motivated to seek fulfillment of the higher-order needs. Change can make it more difficult for a person to meet any or all of these physiological and psychosocial needs. Once status, power, and influence are gained within families and organizations, they are hard to give up. You may be the one in charge in the family and in the office, yet be a novice in the nursing program.

Recognizing Resistance

It is easy to recognize resistance to a change when it is expressed directly. When a person says to you, "That's not a very good idea," "I am going to quit if I can't get better grades," or "There's no way I'm going to do that," there is no doubt that you are meeting resistance. When resistance is less direct, however, you may not recognize it unless you know what to look for.

Resistance may be active or passive. **Active resistance** can take the form of aggressive actions or outright refusals to comply (such as the statements in the previous paragraph), writing negative e-mails that attack and destroy the idea or the person who suggested it, quoting existing rules that make the change difficult or impossible to implement, or organizing resistance to the change (encouraging others to resist). **Passive approaches** involve avoidance: canceling appointments to discuss implementing the change; being "too busy" to make the change; agreeing to the change but doing nothing to effect it; and simply ignoring the entire process as much as possible.

Lowering Resistance

You can use various approaches to lower people's resistance to change. Strategies fall into four categories: commanding, disseminating information, refuting currently held beliefs, and providing psychological safety (Whitehead, Weiss, & Tappen, 2004).

Critical Thinking 38-6

Recall one change that you have experienced that was put into effect by a command (or a new rule, policy, or law).

- What effects did this change have on your life (e.g., work, school, home)?
- How did the command make you feel?
- What would have made this change easier for you?

Commanding Change. Obviously, the quickest way to implement change, if you have the authority to do so, is to issue a command. Dictating change is not necessarily the best strategy, but it is sometimes necessary when the change must be made quickly. Commanding a change may not be effective if there are ways for people to resist, for example, when:

- Passive resistance can undermine the change
- High motivational levels are necessary to make the change successful
- People can refuse to obey the order without negative consequences

Sharing Information. Much resistance is simply the result of misunderstandings about a proposed change. Sharing information is usually an effective way to reduce uncertainty and ease transition. Information about the change can be shared on a one-to-one basis, in group meetings, or through written materials distributed by print or electronic means. As a student, it is important that any changes in the program are communicated to you on a timely basis. You should also communicate any changes in your plans to the appropriate people, such as other students, your nurse team leader, or your instructor. As a student nurse or staff member, you should treat client resistance to change in the same manner. The more information that you give the client, the more likely she will be to cooperate with the change.

Refuting Currently Held Beliefs. Simply providing evidence that what people are doing or believing is inadequate, incorrect, or inefficient can sometimes increase their willingness to change. For example, patients may enter the hospital recalling horror stories from friends and family but may then find that there was no basis for the stories. As another example, how have your ideas about the nursing program changed since you first began? What happened, or what information did you receive, that caused you to change your beliefs?

Providing Psychological Safety. When a proposed change threatens basic human needs in some way, reducing that threat can lower resistance. This leaves people feeling more comfortable about the change. Although each situation poses different kinds of threats and requires different actions to reduce them, Box 38-4 identifies common strategies that help increase psychological safety and reduce resistance to change.

Implementing the Change

In planning for change, you will already have asked yourself these questions:

- What is the purpose of this change? What are we trying to accomplish?
- Is the change necessary?
- Is the change technically correct?
- Will the change work?
- Is there a better way to do this?

BOX 38-4 ■ Common Strategies to Increase Psychological Safety and Reduce Resistance to Change

- Point out similarities between old and new procedures.
- Suggest ways in which the change can provide new opportunities and challenges.
- Allow time for learning and practice of any new procedures, if possible, before a change is implemented.
- Recognize the competence and skill of the people involved.
- Involve as many people as possible in both the design and implementation of the change.
- Express approval of people's concern for providing the best care possible.
- Express the value of each individual's and group's contributions in general and to the proposed change.
- Provide a climate of trust and acceptance in which mistakes can be made without negative consequences for individuals.
- If possible, provide assurance that no one will lose his or her position because of the change.
- Provide opportunities for people to express their feelings and ask questions about the proposed change.

After employing some unfreezing strategies, you are ready to make the change that has been so carefully planned. In addition to employing strategies to lower resistance, increase motivation, and help people work well together, consider the following factors related to change. Consider the following characteristics of the change:

Magnitude of the Change. Is this a major change that affects almost everything people do, or is it a minor one with little impact on what people do every day?

Complexity of the Change. Is this a difficult change to make? Does it require much new knowledge or skills, or both? How long will it take for people to acquire the necessary knowledge and skills?

Pace of the Change. How urgent is this change? Can it be done gradually, or must it be implemented all at once?

Stress Level of Those Involved. What is the current stress level of the people involved in this change? Is this the only change that is taking place, or is it just one of many changes taking place? How stressful are these changes? How can I help people keep their stress levels within tolerable bounds?

As indicated earlier, some discomfort is likely to occur with almost any change, but it is important to keep it within tolerable limits. You need enough pressure to get people to pay attention to the change process, but not so much that they are overstressed by it. In other words, you want to raise the heat enough to get them moving, but not so high that they boil over (Heifetz & Linsky, 2002).

Integrating the Change

Integrating the change is the last step. After the change has been made, it is important to make sure that everyone has moved into a new comfort zone. Ask yourself:

- Is the change well integrated into everyday operations?
- Are people comfortable with it now?
- Is it well accepted and perceived as valuable? If not, why not? What can be done to increase acceptance?
- Is there any residual resistance that could still undermine full integration of the change? If there is, how can this resistance be overcome?

Change "sticks" when, instead of being the new way to do something, it has become "the way we always do things around here" (Kotter, 1999, p. 18).

Change is an inevitable part of living and working. Your leadership can influence how people respond to change, the amount of stress it causes, and the amount of resistance it provokes. Handled well, most changes can become opportunities for professional growth and development rather than just additional stressors for students, nurses, and their clients.

Toward Evidence-Based Practice

The Center for Health Design (2009). Pebble Project® Data Summary. Retrieved August 2, 2009, from http://www.healthdesign.org/research/pebble/data.php

Preliminary data from the Pebble Project® include the following studies:

Weill Cornell Medical College, New York, New York. Conducted studies at six ambulatory sites to examine how wait times affect perceived quality and anxiety. Key findings include:

- The more attractive the environment, the higher the perceived quality and the lower the anxiety
- There was no significant relationship between *actual* wait times and perceived quality or anxiety.
- There was a significant relationship between *perceived* wait times and perceived quality and anxiety.

Parrish Medical Center, Titusville, FL. Opened a new hospital in 2002. A 2004 survey of staff found:

- The majority of staff feel the design features (e.g., "homelike" room design) positively affect the quality of their work life and help them provide care more effectively.
- Since opening the new building, staff turnover decreased from 20% to 13%.

The Barbara Ann Karmanos Cancer Institute, Detroit, MI. Data collected on two inpatient units that opened in 1999 and 2000 include:

- 30% reduction in medical errors as a result of increased space in the medication room, location of the medication room, organization of medical supplies, standardized visual cues, and acoustical panels to decrease noise levels
- 6% reduction in patient falls, a result of better visualization of patients due to angle of doorway, improved lighting, and room layout

1. Imagine you are a nurse manager about to present at a budget meeting your ideas for why it would be cost-effective to remodel the clinic lobby, including addition of skylights, plants, and a small fountain. List your rationale and state which of the healthcare agency studies supports each item. Be sure to tie your rationale to cost effectiveness.

 Go to Chapter 38, **Toward Evidence-Based Practice Suggested Responses,** on the Student Resource Disk or DavisPlus at http://davisplus.fadavis.com/Wilkinson2

Conflict

Nursing education and working in healthcare bring together people of different ages, genders, income levels, statuses, ethnic groups, educational levels, lifestyles, and professions. They share the goal of maintaining people's health. Differences of opinion over how to best accomplish goals are a normal part of working with people of various skill levels and backgrounds. Each of us brings different experiences, beliefs, values, and habits to interactions with others. These differences are a natural part of our being unique individuals and members of different segments of our society. Various pressures and demands in the classroom, clinical setting, and workplace also generate problems and conflicts among people. Any or all of these can interfere with our ability to work together.

Conflicts Occur at All Levels

Conflicts can occur at any level and involve any number of people, including your boss, subordinates, peers, patients, or families. On the *individual level,* they can occur between two people working together on a classroom or clinical project, between two people in different departments, or even between a staff member and a client or family member. On the *group level,* conflict can occur between two or more teams, departments, or professional groups (e.g., nurses and social workers may conflict over who is responsible for discharge planning). On the *organizational level,* conflicts can occur between two or more hospitals, health agencies, or community organizations. *Gender-based* conflicts may involve equal pay for women and sexual harassment issues.

"Win–Win" Resolutions

Some people think about problems and conflicts in the same way as they think about a football game or tennis match: Someone has to win, and someone has to lose. There are some problems with this comparison to sports competition:

- In healthcare, our aim should be to work together more effectively, not to defeat the other party.
- The people who lose are likely to feel bad about losing. As a result, they may spend their time and energy preparing to win the next round, rather than on their work.
- A tie (neither side wins or loses) may be just a stalemate; no one has won or lost, but the problem is also still there and no gain is achieved.

So the answer to the question, "Win, lose, or draw?" is, "None of the above." Instead, a win-win result, in which both sides gain some benefit, is the best resolution (Haslan, 2001).

Conflict Resolution

When differences and disagreements first arise, problem-solving may be sufficient. If the situation has already developed into a full-blown conflict, however, formal or informal negotiation of a settlement may be necessary. Using a problem-solving process, the goal is to find a solution that satisfies everyone involved.

Step 1. Identify the problem or issue. Ask people what they want (Sportsman, 2005). Sometimes, if the issue is not a highly charged, or highly political one, it is easy to identify the real issue or problem. At other times, however, some discussion and exploration of the issues are necessary before the real problem emerges. "It would be relaxing if what other people were really saying was always obvious, if all their essential thoughts were clearly labeled for us . . . and if all knowledgeable people agreed about answers to important questions" (Browne & Kelley, 2010, p. 6). Of course, this is not what usually happens. People are often vague about what their real concern is; sometimes they are genuinely uncertain about what the real problem is. Emotional involvement may further cloud the issue. All of this needs to be sorted out so that the problem is clearly identified and a solution can be sought.

Step 2. Generate possible solutions. Here creativity is especially important. As a leader, begin the process of trying to find new, creative solutions. It is natural for people to try to repeat something that worked well for them in the past, but solutions that were previously successful may not work in the future. Instead, encourage people to spend some time searching for innovative solutions. Think outside the box for new and better ways to handle things.

Step 3. Evaluate suggested solutions. An open-minded, objective evaluation of each suggestion is needed, but you may find that this is not always easy to accomplish. When a group engages in problem solving, it is sometimes difficult to separate the suggestion from its source. For example, on a team, the status of the person who made the suggestion may influence whether the suggestion is judged to be useful. Judge the suggestion on its merits, not its source.

Step 4. Choose the best solution. Choose the solution that is most likely to work—one that will give you the best results with the fewest negative effects. A combination of suggestions is often the best solution.

Step 5. Implement the solution chosen. The true test of any solution is how well it actually works. Once a solution has been implemented, it is important to give it time to work. Impatience may lead you to abandon a good solution prematurely.

Step 6. Evaluate—Is the problem resolved? Not every problem is resolved successfully on the first attempt. If the problem has not been resolved, you need to resume the process with even greater attention to identifying the real problem and how it can be successfully resolved.

Informal Negotiation

If problem-solving does not resolve the conflict, you may have to move on to the next step—informal negotiation. The following steps may prove useful.

1. **Clarify the situation in your own mind**.
   What am I trying to achieve?
   What is the environment in which I am operating?
   What problems am I likely to encounter?
   What do both sides want?
2. **Set the stage**.
   This may involve confronting the two parties or groups with their behavior toward one another, making direct statements designed to open communication and challenge them to seek resolution of the situation.
3. **Conduct the negotiation**.
   Manage the emotions.
   Set the ground rules.
   Clarify the problem.
   Make your opening move.
4. **Continue with offers and counteroffers.**
5. **Agree on the resolution of the conflict.**

Conflict is inevitable within any large or diverse group of people who are trying to work together over an extended period of time. However, it does not have to be destructive, and it does not even have to be a negative experience if everyone handles it skillfully. In fact, conflict can stimulate people to learn more about each other and how to work together in more effective ways. Resolution of a conflict, when it is done well, can lead to improved relationships, more creative methods of problem solving, and higher productivity.

Time Management

Many of the personal management and organizational skills related to the workplace focus on time management and scheduling. Although new nurses may have the required job skills, many lack personal management skills, specifically, time management. You might be able to handle conflict and change, delegate appropriately, and be a strong leader among your peers, your faculty, and staff. But if you can't organize and manage your time, you will never gain your full potential.

Many nurses "punch a time clock" that records the minute they enter and leave work, and management accepts very few excuses for being late. Timesheets and schedules are part of most healthcare workers' lives. We are expected to follow precisely set schedules and meet deadlines for virtually everything we do, from distributing medications to getting reports done on time. Many agencies analyze computer-generated data to determine the amount of time spent on various activities. Consider how you can use the following suggestions to improve your time management.

Setting Your Own Goals

It is difficult to decide how to spend your time, because there are so many things that need time. A good first step is to get an overview of the situation. Then ask yourself, "What are my goals?" Goals help clarify what you want and give you energy, direction, and focus. Once you know where you want to go, set priorities. This is not an easy task. In Lewis Carroll's *Alice's Adventures in Wonderland*, the child heroine, Alice, becomes lost and asks for help from a fantasy creature, the "Cheshire Cat." They have this conversation:

"Would you tell me please, which way I ought to go from here?" asked Alice.
"That depends a good deal on where you want to go to," said the Cat.
"I don't care where," said Alice.
"Then it doesn't matter which way you go," said the Cat.

How can you get somewhere if you do not know where you want to go? It is important to explore your personal and career goals. This can help you make decisions about the future. You can apply these ideas to daily activities as well as to career decisions. Spend some time thinking about what you want to accomplish over a particular time period.

To help organize your time, you need to set both short- and long-term goals. **Short-term goals** are goals that you wish to accomplish within the near future. Setting up your day in an organized fashion is a short-term goal, and so is scheduling a time to study. **Long-term goals** are goals you wish to complete over a long period of time. Advanced education and career goals are examples. A good question to ask yourself is, "What do I see myself doing 5 years from now?" Every choice you make requires a different allocation of time.

Organizing Your Work

Many healthcare professionals are linear, fast-tempo, achievement-oriented people. However, working at a rapid pace is not necessarily the same as accomplishing a great deal. You can spend much energy in rushing around and stirring things up while actually achieving very little. Fast does not necessarily mean efficient or effective.

To "manage" time, you need to handle time with a measure of skill. Therefore, time management includes efficiently meeting client care needs during a nursing shift. Organizing your work can eliminate extra steps or serious delays in completing your work. It can also reduce the amount of time you spend doing things that are neither productive nor satisfying. As you begin your nursing program, you may care for only one or two patients. However, as you develop time management skills, you will be able to handle a workload of care for seven or eight inpatients. The following are some suggestions:

Time Inventory. Do a personal time inventory. To begin managing your time, you need to develop a clearer understanding of how you use your time. A personal time inventory helps you estimate how much time you spend in typical activities. Keeping the inventory for a week gives a fairly accurate estimate of how you spend your time. The inventory also helps identify "time wasters." Set up a time log and enter your activities every half hour. Keep this record for about 3 days so you can see a pattern emerging. You may be interested to know that one study of 36 hospitals found that medical–surgical nurses spend their time in the following ways (Hendrich, Chow, Sklerczynski, et al., 2008; Robert Wood Johnson, 2009):

Documentation	27.5%
Care coordination	16.0%
Patient care activities	15.1%
Medication administration	13.4%
Assessments/vital signs	5.8%
Nonclinical	12.6%
Waste [of time]	6.8%
Unit-related functions	2.8%

Energy Use. Work on the most difficult tasks when you have the most energy. This decreases frustration later in the day, when you may be more tired and less efficient. Also consider your energy levels when beginning a big task. Start when levels are high and not at, say, 4 o'clock in the afternoon, if that is when you find yourself winding down. For example, if you are a "morning person," plan your demanding work in the morning. If you get energy spurts later in the morning or early afternoon, plan to work on larger or heavier tasks at that time. Of course, this choice is not always within your control. Many nursing tasks are based on a schedule. If the wound care is due at 1 o'clock, you must carry out the task then, even if you would prefer to eat lunch and rest. Analyze your work to determine which tasks are fixed and what you can manipulate to match your energy.

Lists and Schedules. Make a "to do" list and prioritize the tasks in order of importance. Determine how much time each task will require, and when each must be completed. If you find yourself postponing an item for several days, decide whether to give it top priority the next day or drop it from the list altogether.

Daily Worksheet. To help organize your day, provide yourself with reminders of various tasks and when they need to be done. Without some type of schedule, you are more likely to drift through a day or shift from one activity to another in a disorganized fashion. The risk in using schedules, however, is that the more they divide the day into discrete segments, the more they fragment the work and discourage a holistic approach. Use the schedule as an organizational tool, but focus on your clients. For a worksheet you can use,

VOL 2 Go to Chapter 7, **Implementation and Evaluation Tools, Worksheet for Organizing Nursing Care,** in Volume 2.

Say "No." Take control to avoid time wasters. It is important to prevent endless activities and other people controlling you. Learn when to say no. Learn to say, "I would really like to help you; can it wait until I finish this?" Or, "I am sorry, I won't be able to help you with that."

Delegate. See previous discussions about delegation.

Multitasking. Studies show that people who do many things at once do none of them well, even though they believe they do. Do not check your voicemail while documenting in the patient record, for example. Finish one task, then move on to the next one.

Streamline Your Work. Many tasks cannot be eliminated or delegated, but they can be done more efficiently. Here are three wise sayings in time management:

- "Work smarter, not harder." This should appeal to nurses facing increasing demands on time (Box 38-5).
- "Never handle a piece of paper more than once." This philosophy can be used for patient care, as well as office work and school work. Handle an issue now rather than putting it off until later.
- "A stitch in time saves nine." Preventive action saves time in the long run.

BOX 38-5 ■ Work Smarter, Not Harder

- Gather materials, such as bed linens, for all of your clients at one time. As you go to each room, leave the linen so that it will be there when you need it.
- While giving a bed bath or providing other personal care, perform some of the aspects of the physical assessment, such as taking vital signs, skin assessment, and parts of the neurological and musculoskeletal assessment.
- If a client does not "look right," do not ignore your instincts. The client is probably having a problem.
- Prevention is always a good idea. If you are not sure about a treatment or medication, ask before you proceed. It is usually less time-consuming to prevent a problem than it is to resolve one.
- When you set aside time to do a specific task that has a high priority, stick to your schedule and complete it.
- Do not allow interruptions while you are completing any tasks (e.g., paperwork, medication administration). Focus on the task at hand.

Plan the Night Before. Take a few minutes before bedtime to lay out your clothing for the next day, set up the coffee pot, or whatever you need to do to avoid last-minute chaos in the morning.

Components of Time Management

Time can be your best friend or your worst enemy. It is important to identify how you feel about time and to assess your own time management skills. Nursing requires that you perform numerous activities within what often seems a very short period of time, so learn how to make the most of your day. Finally, remember that you should set aside 8 hours for sleep and a few more for personal or leisure time ("time off"). Use Table 38-4 to help you to review the necessary components of time management.

Table 38-4 ➤ Components of Time Management

ACTION	EXAMPLES
Prioritize	List tasks in order of importance.
	Remember that some tasks must be done at specific times, whereas others can be done at any time.
	Emergencies take precedence.
	Identify events you control and events others control.
	Use critical-thinking skills to assign priorities.
Question	
■ Effectiveness	■ Did the task produce the desired outcome?
■ Efficiency	■ How can I accomplish the plan with the least expenditure of time? Is there a way to break this down into simpler tasks?
■ Efficacy	■ Do I have the skill and ability to obtain the desired effect?
Recheck	Mentally and physically recheck an unfinished or delegated task.
Practice Self-reliance	Identify tasks that are within your control and those that are not.
	Use critical-thinking skills and adaptability to revise priorities
	"Go with the flow."
Treat	Treat yourself to a break when you can.
	Treat yourself to time off.
	Treat yourself to an educational experience: Commit yourself to excellence.
	Treat others with courtesy and respect.

KnowledgeCheck 38-6

- List the steps of conflict resolution.
- List several suggestions for organizing your work.
- State one "wise saying" to guide you in streamlining your work.

 Go to Chapter 38, **Knowledge Check Response Sheet and Answers,** on the Student Resource Disk or DavisPlus at http://davisplus.fadavis.com/Wilkinson2

Putting It All Together

You are just beginning your journey toward becoming a nurse. Undoubtedly you will want to function well within your organization and deliver high quality patient care. Begin now to examine and work on your own strengths and weaknesses. As you work with your classmates, your instructors, and the clinical facilities, focus on developing the traits of a good leader. You will soon recognize that conflict and change are a normal part of life and your clinical practice, so learn to become proactive as issues arise. You will observe how "real" nurses delegate and manage their time. Take what is useful, and learn from their examples. There will be opportunities to be mentored; watch for those and make time to mentor others. Above all, remember that you may be the most important person in the life of your client during the time you are with him or her—a very big responsibility, but one you will meet with honor and courage.

 Go to Chapter 38, **Resources for Caregivers and Health Professionals,** on the Student Resource Disk or DavisPlus at http://davisplus.fadavis.com/Wilkinson2

 Suggested Readings: Go to Chapter 38, **Reading More About Leading and Managing,** on the Student Resource Disk or DavisPlus at http://davisplus.fadavis.com/Wilkinson2

 Bibliography: Go to Volume 2, Bibliography.

CHAPTER 39

Nursing Informatics

Learning Outcomes

After completing this chapter, you should be able to:

➤ Define informatics and its four components.

➤ Describe the importance of computers in evidence-based nursing practice.

➤ Discuss the benefits of the electronic health record.

➤ Discuss the impact of legislative efforts to encourage electronic health record adoption.

➤ Describe the importance of protecting personal health information.

➤ Explain the relationship between computers and standardized nursing languages.

➤ Identify at least two ways that automation decreases error in health care.

➤ Explain how computers can reduce some of the barriers to evidence-based practice.

➤ Identify at least four online sources of nursing research.

➤ Describe the process of literature database searching.

➤ Outline a process for evaluating evidence and determining a solution.

Meet Your Nurse Role Model

Ted Samuels, 67, is a business executive who six weeks ago began experiencing headaches, occasional palpitations, blurred vision, and increased thirst. Mr. Samuels accesses the **patient web portal** of his **personal health record** (PHR) and sends an e-mail to his physician's scheduling service requesting an appointment The office clerk responds within an hour, confirming an appointment with the family nurse practitioner (FNP) the next day.

The physician's office has just installed an electronic health record system (EHR). At his appointment, the registrar explains to Mr. Samuels that the new system is **integrated** with the hospital record for seamless communication among his caregivers. She enters his insurance and personal contact information into the system, and explains that the system is **encrypted** (special security coding) to protect his personal information. In the exam room, the medical assistant weighs Mr. Samuels, takes his vital signs, and enters the information in the EHR. A few minutes later, Karen Shock, FNP, arrives. As she takes his

history and completes a physical examination, she updates the information in the computer. Noting Mr. Samuels' family history of diabetes, the increased thirst, and slight weight gain, she checks a random glucose via the office glucometer and finds a blood sugar level of 300 mg/dL. The **decision support algorithms** built into the software alert her that Mr. Samuels' blood pressure was also elevated at 170/98. The software suggests possible medical diagnoses of hyperglycemia and hypertension. Following the evidence-based care guidelines in the computer, Ms. Shock uses computerized provider order entry **(CPOE)** to enter requests for a basic metabolic profile, lipid profile, ECG, BUN, creatinine, and Hgb A1c. She asks that Mr. Samuels be fasting for the blood work, and prints patient education instructions. Ms. Shock

(continued on next page)

Meet Your Nurse Role Model (continued)

instructs Mr. Samuels to check his blood pressure two to three times daily for one week and to enter the results in the online log in his PHR. She asks Mr. Samuels to grant viewing rights to the log for her and Dr. Gregg.

The next morning Mr. Samuels arrives at the hospital for his lab work and ECG. His registration information is automatically updated from the information provided with a previous health visit. The **online order requisitions** Ms. Shock entered yesterday provide the technicians with the information needed, the tests are completed, and Mr. Samuels is quickly on the way back to his office. At the end of the day, he receives an e-mail notification that his lab results are available for review. He logs into the PHR portal to view the results. He also finds a message from Ms. Shock confirming the preliminary diagnosis of type 2 diabetes. Many providers would still want at least a phone consult when ordering a new medication. The office is scheduling diabetic instruction, and they have submitted a prescription to Mr. Samuels' pharmacy for metformin, an antidiabetes drug. An education leaflet explaining the medication and potential side effects is attached to the message. Mr. Samuels notices that metformin is now showing on his **medication list** in his PHR.

Over the course of the week, Ms. Shock monitors Mr. Samuels' blood pressure log entries. A **trending graph** shows consistently high blood pressure readings. She orders Lisinopril, an antihypertensive, 5 mg daily, and requests that

he continue to check his blood pressure frequently. A follow-up appointment is scheduled for 6 weeks.

A few weeks later, Mr. Samuels wakes up with severe chest pain and calls 911. En route to the emergency department (ED), the paramedic transmits an ECG tracing via satellite to the ED physician. By the time the ambulance arrives, the physician has interpreted the ECG, determined that Mr. Samuels is having a myocardial infarction, and has notified the cardiac catheterization team to be on standby. The ED physician sees that Mr. Samuels has recently completed tests at the hospital, and reviews his medication list, allergies, and medical history online. Within 30 minutes Mr. Samuels is sent to the cath lab for percutaneous transluminal coronary angioplasty.

Four hours later, Mr. Samuels is resting comfortably in the progressive care unit. Throughout the next 48 hours, the bedside nurse monitors Mr. Samuels' vital signs and cardiac rhythm. An **interface** between the physiological cardiac monitor and the EHR allows the nurse to directly import vital signs information into his electronic health record. Caregivers document electronically at the bedside, and the physician uses CPOE to manage Mr. Samuels' prescriptions. At discharge, the nurse gives Mr. Samuels a printed copy of his medication list, discharge instructions, and follow-up appointments are made with Dr. Gregg and the cardiologist.

Critical Thinking 39-1

Reflect on this "Meet Your Nurse Role Model" scenario. Identify how information was managed and processed.

- What mechanisms for gathering and disseminating information were used?
- How did automation assist decision making?
- How was evidence used in decision making?
- What characteristics make it more likely for patients to use personal health records?

Theoretical Knowledge
knowing why

Computers are becoming as much of a diagnostic tool as stethoscopes have been for the past century. The "Meet Your Nurse Role Model" scenario is an example of how healthcare professionals use these tools to make decisions in practice. This chapter gives you an overview of how this works.

What Is Nursing Informatics?

Whether you become a staff nurse, an administrator, a researcher, primary health care provider, or an educator, you will need current, accurate, and "best available"

information to do your job well. The good news is that plenty of information is available. MEDLINE, a vast medical literature database supported through the National Institutes of Health, currently contains more than 18 million citations and is growing at the rate of more than 670,000 new entries per year (National Institutes of Health, 2009). If a conscientious nurse reads two new articles every day, by the end of the year she would be 918 years behind in keeping up with the literature. The bad news (if you want to call it that) is that we are drowning in information while still lacking in knowledge. Do you ever feel that way as a student?

It is not possible to keep all the necessary information in your head. No one can. We need critical thinking and tools to manage the information to make it useful to us. If it is not possible to learn and retain all the information, then you must know how to find, process, and manage it to arrive at the best decisions for your practice. In essence, this is the definition of **informatics:** the managing and processing of information necessary to make decisions. **Nursing informatics** is informatics applied to nursing practice, education, and research. The first conceptual framework for informatics envisioned the elements ("stuff") of informatics as *data, information,* and *knowledge* (Graves & Corcoran, 1989). Full-spectrum nurses interact with all three of these elements in daily practice, so you need to understand how they interrelate.

The **nursing informatics specialist** (NIS) works with informatics technicians and others to provide clinical information and data analysis for effective patient care. In addition, the nursing informatics specialist works with computers, data analysis systems, and nursing knowledge and experience to be sure the best possible care is provided. This role involves good understanding of basic nursing techniques and standards. Data collection, analysis of different types of data, information sharing, and research dissemination are functions of the NIS. The nursing informatics specialist also acts as a manager or team leader to bring together all aspects of treatment options and best practice research. In sum, the NIS uses nursing science, computer science, and information science to manage and communicate data, information, knowledge, and wisdom in nursing practice. The sections that follow describe these four elements of informatics.

Data

Data are "discrete entities that are described objectively without interpretation" (American Nurses Association [ANA], 2007). In other words, data are raw, unprocessed numbers, symbols, or words that have no meaning by themselves. For example, what does 101 mean? It could indicate the movie title *101 Dalmatians*, a piece of programming language, or someone's body temperature, pulse rate, weight, or age. Without a context, data are meaningless.

In nursing, we speak of data as the primary facts and observations acquired when providing services, such as the numerical value of a blood pressure measurement, or facts such as, "Father died of prostate cancer." Notice that even this information has no meaning until the nurse interprets it: The meaning of "Father died of prostate cancer" changes if the client is a healthy 24-year-old female sharing this information versus a 74-year-old male experiencing blood in his urine.

Information

Information consists of groupings of data processed into a meaningful, structured form (ANA, 2001). If you combine 300 with a unit of measure, you know that the number represents a blood sugar result. If other data—gender (male), age (67), and family history—are grouped together, information is formed. You now know that this man has most likely developed type 2 diabetes.

Data:	300 mg/dL glucose, male, 67, thirst
Grouped data:	Male gender, age 67, family history of diabetes
Information:	Man with probable new onset of diabetes

In the opening scenario, what information did the FNP receive that triggered an alert?

Knowledge

In the "Meet Your Nurse Role Model" scenario, what *information* did the FNP use to create knowledge of Mr. Samuels's condition? Take a minute to write your answer.

The answer to the question is that the FNP received information on the blood sugar (300 mg/dL) and blood pressure (170/98). Grouping this with other information (e.g., the history of headaches, blurred vision, palpitations, family history of diabetes), the FNP created *knowledge* of the potential for a diagnosis of type 2 diabetes and hypertension.

Knowledge is formed when data are grouped, creating meaningful information and relationships, which are then added to other structured information (ANA, 2007). The knowledge can either be previously known or new. In the preceding scenario of the 67-year-old man with the blood sugar of 300 mg/dL, we can add information about pathophysiology, pharmacokinetics (how medications work), patient history, and physical assessment, providing the knowledge to make an informed decision about the patient's current condition and further treatment.

Figure 39-1 depicts the transformation of data into knowledge. As we have come to realize that the gathering of data and information to make decisions is never ending, the model has evolved to depict overlapping circles and both forward and backward movement.

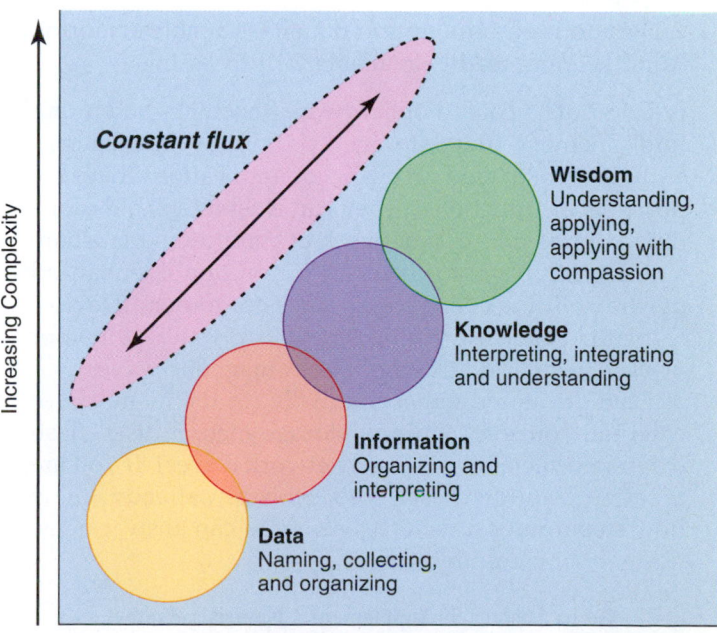

FIGURE 39-1 The relationship of data, information, knowledge, and wisdom. Each level increases in complexity. (Reprinted from Englebardt, S., & Nelson, R. *Health care informatics: An interdisciplinary approach.* Copyright 2002. With permission from Elsevier.)

Wisdom

Nelson and Joos (1989) added *wisdom* to the Graves and Corcoran model. **Wisdom** is defined as the *appropriate use* of knowledge in managing or solving human problems. As we discussed in Chapter 1, wisdom develops as an outcome of your clinical experience, theoretical knowledge, critical thinking, and intuition—as you progress from novice to expert in the practice of full-spectrum nursing.

KnowledgeCheck 39-1

- What is the difference between knowledge and wisdom?
- Define the following: *data, information, knowledge.*
- Give an example of each: data, information, knowledge.

 Go to Chapter 39, **Knowledge Check Response Sheet and Answers,** on the Student Resource Disk or DavisPlus at http://davisplus.fadavis.com/Wilkinson2

Understanding Computers

Computers are vital to the functioning in our daily lives. We rely on them for communication (e.g., e-mail, texting, blogs, social networking), access to information (e.g., personal and business contacts, education, general information), business operations (e.g., scheduling, purchasing), to name but a few. By definition, a **computer** is an electronic device with four main functions: input, process, output, and storage. Collectively, these operations are known as **information processing** (or *data processing*). The power of a computer is based on:

- The speed, accuracy, and reliability with which it operates
- The enormous amounts of data it is capable of storing and keeping readily available for processing

Computers consist of hardware (machines and monitors), memory (data storage), processors (translators), and software (coded programs or applications that support specific functions). They can exist as a stand-alone device, or as part of a network of computers that share a common purpose. Power in computing is enhanced by the ability to connect to other computers. Devices can either be *wired* (connected with physical wires) or *wireless* (connected through electromagnetic waves).

Data are stored either internally (in the memory) or externally on some form of storage media (discs, flash drives, portable hard drives, network drives). If you are a savvy computer user, you probably already know how a computer functions. See if you can answer questions about computer basics.

 Go to Chapter 39, **Supplemental Materials: Pretest Questions and Pretest Answer Key,** on the Student Resource Disk or DavisPlus at http://davisplus.fadavis.com/Wilkinson2

If you had difficulty answering the questions,

 Go to Chapter 39, **Supplemental Materials: How Does a Computer Work?** and **Tables, Boxes, Figures: ESG Figure 39-1,** on the Student Resource Disk or DavisPlus at http://davisplus.fadavis.com/Wilkinson2

Computers in the Workplace

Because computers are so important and so widely used in healthcare, it is essential that nurses develop a set of core computer competencies or skills (Hart, 2008). These include a basic understanding of computer logic, data entry, data retrieval, information literacy, and troubleshooting hardware and software issues. Additional skills may become necessary as your career develops and you transition into leadership roles.

In your work as a nurse, you will use computers to provide and manage patient care, for continuing education, and for communication. To give you an idea of the extent to which you will encounter computers consider the following examples.

Tools for Providing and Managing Care

As a nurse, you will be called on to use a wide variety of computerized devices in the workplace. Digital thermometers, cardiorespiratory monitors, glucometers, cell phones, smart IV pumps, barcode scanners, and electronic bedscales are all types of computers.

Some agencies are using **Real Time Location Systems** (RTLS) or Radio Frequency Identification Detectors (RFID) to assist in locating patient care equipment that may be scattered throughout the building. These systems save nurse time, discourage staff from storing equipment on a particular unit rather than a centrally accessible location, and decrease costs of lost equipment (Turisco & Rhoads, 2008). Other efficiency-enhancing devices include handsfree communication badges and wireless phones, which may be interfaced with alerts from bedside equipment. These devices can save nurses several minutes on a busy day.

Internet-based tools for staff scheduling, patient flow, access to evidence-based references, policy and procedures, and staff education are fast becoming the norm. Many hospitals have developed internal resources, special intranet pages of references specific to nursing.

Computers in Nursing Education

New trends in nursing education include the use of clinical simulation mannequins and Web programs (Cannon-Diehl, 2009) (Fig. 39-2). Research indicates that these methods are effective in teaching critical thinking, problem-solving, physical assessment, and some clinical skills. You may have already been using clinical simulation mannequins in your nursing program. Would it surprise you to know that practicing nurses

FIGURE 39-2 Human patient simulator offers practical experience before caring for patients or training special skills.

also use them in continuing education provided in their workplaces? What kind of computer programs and devices are available in your clinical setting?

Electronic Communication

Electronic communication can be very simple (e.g., text messaging), or very complex (e.g., long-distance telehealth) and can sometimes replace face-to-face interaction between people.

Electronic Mail and Text Messaging

In many facilities electronic mail (e-mail) is now the primary method for managers to communicate with staff. In many cases, leadership teams have widened their scope of responsibility to include multiple practice areas or programs. E-mail allows for rapid, simultaneous distribution of information and messaging to a large number of recipients. Nurses and other healthcare providers can use e-mail to interact with patients, consult with colleagues, and communicate with insurance industry representatives, pharmacies, and hospitals. E-mail and text offer convenient, up-to-the-minute patient updates among nurses, other providers, patients and their families. However, it is critical that these transmissions occur only on secure or encrypted sites if personal patient information is involved.

Be aware that privacy is not ensured with electronic mail. For example, it is entirely legal and not uncommon for employers to read incoming and outgoing employee messages when they are sent on company equipment. In addition, once a message has been sent, you have no control over who may actually read it or to whom it might be forwarded. You also don't know if other people receive a blind copy of the message without your knowledge. A patient's **protected health information** should never be shared in an e-mail. Protected information includes any individually identifiable health information, current, past, or potential physical or mental conditions, and any payment information,

such as social security numbers or insurance. For more information about e-mail security,

 Go to Chapter 39, **Supplemental Materials: E-mail Security,** on the Student Resource Disk or DavisPlus at http://davisplus.fadavis.com/Wilkinson2

Most facilities have policies governing use of company e-mail for personal use. You always check facility policies before sharing e-mail addresses with persons outside of the organization.

How was e-mail used to facilitate communication between the patient and providers in the "Meet Your Nurse Role Model" situation?

Web Conferencing and Webinars

Web conferencing is used to conduct or participate in live or synchronous meetings or presentations via the Internet. Attendees download a Web-based application onto their local computers. These interactions are most often two-way communication. To access the meeting, an e-mail is distributed to the attendee(s) that contains a link to enter the conference at the arranged time. A **webinar,** or **webcast,** is a specific type of Web conference that is one way from the speaker to the audience. These tools can be useful in helping staff obtain updated clinical information (e.g., continuing education, inservice) for patient care.

Listserv

Electronic mailing lists are an extension of e-mail use. The most common mailing list application is called a **listserv** (standing for *list server*). The names and addresses of the people on the mailing list, called **subscribers,** are stored by the listserv on a single server. A single address is then designated for the group to use. When a message is sent to that address, it is delivered to the listserv server, which then distributes the message via e-mail to all subscribers (Fig. 39-3).

Nearly all subspecialties and special interest groups in healthcare have a listserv. Interested professionals subscribe to the list and receive mailings from others on the list. Like e-mail, if you use a listserv, be aware that any message you send through the mailing list goes to *everyone* on the mailing list. So be careful when you hit the "Reply All" command!

Listservs are a powerful communication tool. Communication is global and almost instantaneous. Ideas and protocols can be shared, questions asked and answered, and surveys taken. Everyone on the list has an equal opportunity to share in the discussion. Numerous nursing listservs are available representing a wide variety of topics and health specialty areas. Use your favorite Web search engine and search using the key words "nursing listservs." Look for a site that interests you. What kind of information do you see? Visit one of the sites. What kind of information do you see?

Message sent to list manager

Message relayed to list members

FIGURE 39-3 A message sent to the listserv server is relayed to all list members.

Social Networking

Social networking tools allow people to connect interactively with others who have similar interests. This can be done through **blogging** (posting open messages that can be read by anyone with permissions to access the site), sharing pictures, videos, or **instant messaging** (real time conversations with another person who is online). Sites generally require you to register for the site, create a profile, and be granted access privileges by the Web page administrator. MySpace, Twitter, FaceBook, YouTube, and LinkedIn are examples of popular social networking sites. You can go to You-Tube to view video demonstrations showing nursing skills. You will need to be cautious about whether the source of information is expert and reliable; for example, some of the YouTube skills videos have errors in the demonstrations. To find nursing videos, often it's easiest to search the specific topic, not simply nursing videos.

As with many Web-based tools, social networking sites are searchable by anyone with access. Many employers now regularly include searching these sites as part of their applicant verification process. A wise rule of thumb is to not post anything on these sites that you would not want an employer to see. In addition, posting pictures or descriptions of patient information represents significant risk of violating federal privacy laws.

Another tool gaining popularity is a Wikipedia. **Wikis** are Web pages that can either be public or limited to specific groups through user name and passwords. Many schools have created Wikis to support communication among student groups. Support group Wikis are becoming common for use by patients with chronic health conditions, such as diabetes and congestive heart failure. It is important to note that anyone with access can add information to these sites, creating potential for finding inaccurate information. It is useful to know if support groups are being facilitated or at least monitored by a professional before recommending them to patients.

Second-Life is a virtual world, accessible via the Internet. Residents or participants in Second-Life, also called Avatars, can interact with one another in a social networking-type community the residents refer to as the Grid. This game-like environment is now being used to simulate a nurse–patient experience and clinical care. It will be interesting to see how this technology further evolves in student education.

Telehealth

Telehealth is the use of telecommunication to send healthcare information between patients and professionals at different locations (Fig. 39-4). It improves access to healthcare by providing long-distance clinical healthcare, patient and professional education, and health administration. For instance, the U.S. Department of Defense pioneered telehealth technology and now uses it to provide healthcare services to soldiers in combat and dependent families in outlying posts. The following are other examples of the use of telehealth.

Rural Healthcare. In rural healthcare sites when a patient needs to see a specialist, there may not be one located in the area. Telecommunications equipment at the rural site and the specialist's site allow the specialist and patient to see and talk to each other. The specialist can also view the health records, x-ray films, lab results, and so on. This reduces the cost of traveling to a distant site, and the stress on a patient who may not feel well enough to travel.

Home Health Monitoring. A more common use of telehealth is the use of home health monitoring devices. These devices allow the healthcare professional to monitor vital signs and other indicators without physically entering a home or requiring a patient to make a clinic trip. Therefore, patients can be monitored more frequently, providing better follow-up care, and earlier discharge from the hospital. See Home Care: Use of Informatics in Home Care.

Shortage of Healthcare Providers. In the hospital, large numbers of critically ill patients can be remotely monitored by a single **intensivist** and critical care nurses from a central location. These systems enhance patient safety and provide an extra set of eyes for a busy nurse who cannot remain constantly at a patient's bedside.

FIGURE 39-4 *A, B,* Telehealth improves access among healthcare providers at remote and central sites.

Emergency Care Triage. Some cities have incorporated telehealth nurse triage into their emergency 911 call system. Telenurses use a set of **protocols** to manage patient calls. These cities report a significant decrease in need for ambulance services and emergency room visits (Enrado, 2009).

Despite barriers, such as cost and issues surrounding licensing and reimbursement, telehealth applications will continue to expand in the future. For information about barriers that slow the growth of telehealth,

Go to Chapter 39, **Supplemental Materials: Barriers to Telehealth,** on the Student Resource Disk or DavisPlus at http://davisplus.fadavis.com/Wilkinson2

Critical Thinking 39-2

- As a patient, would you prefer a telehealth or a face-to-face consultation? Why?
- Now imagine that you are an accident victim brought to a rural clinic staffed only with paraprofessionals. Does your answer change? If so, why?

Use of Informatics in Home Care

A telephone application for documentation has been developed for home health aides. On arriving at a patient's home, the aide uses the patient's phone to dial in to a central number and keys in her identification. The time of the call, telephone number from which it came, and identification of the worker are automatically recorded. At the end of the visit, the aide again calls from the patient's phone. Again, the location, time, and identification of the caller are recorded. Using the telephone key pad, the aide then keys in codes indicating the tasks accomplished. She never has to physically write a documentation record; it is accomplished using the telephone. This reduces the amount of time the aide must spend in recording care, improves accuracy, and prevents lost documentation.

Computers and Healthcare Reform

The rising cost of healthcare affects nearly every sector of the population. As costs have steadily increased, consumers and third-party payers have expressed concerns about the quality of care and the outcomes associated with chronic health conditions. Government agencies and private organizations emerged to seek information technology solutions to assist in decreasing costs, improving efficiency, and improving patient outcomes.

Electronic Health Record Adoption

Western Europe has led the world in adopting electronic health record (EHR). The United States healthcare community has been slower to embrace EHR, due in large part to fears of loss of physician autonomy, purchase and installation costs, user adoption and systems training, and uncertainty about the ability of the EHR vendors to remain in business and support their software (Ford et al., 2009). Some people adopt early, some more slowly. If you would like to know the categories of how people tend to respond to innovation.

Go to Chapter 39, **Tables, Boxes, Figures: ESG Box 39-2, Adopters of Innovation** on the Student Resource Disk or DavisPlus at http://davisplus.fadavis.com/Wilkinson2

In 2004, a nationwide system for exchange of medical information through electronic health records was set in motion. **Interoperability** refers to the ability of computers to talk with each other through standard languages or formats without losing the meaning of the information. If information about heart rate is to be exchanged, for example, consistent languages are needed. For example the EHR system in Hospital A might refer to "heart rate," while the EHR system in a physician's office might refer to "pulse rate," which could interfere with clear communication. The computers need a language that allows each to recognize the other's terminology.

The rationale for government support of a nationwide interoperable system of health records is to:

- *Provide patient-focused health care.* Patient-focused health care is assumed to be higher quality and more cost efficient. It is to be accomplished through wider use (access) of electronic health information by care providers and patients.
- *Improve population health.* The nationwide interoperable system of EHR is expected to allow more timely access and use of patient information—information that would be used in research, quality improvement, and emergency preparedness.

In early 2009, healthcare reform was included in legislation intended to stimulate the U.S. economy. The Health Information Technology for Economic and Clinical Health (HITECH) Act designated a multibillion-dollar program for healthcare reform, and is expected to have an insignificant impact on promoting EHR adoption in hospitals and private physician practices. Initial phases of the Bill provide financial incentives for providers who adopt and use EHR by the end of 2011. Later phases begin to penalize providers who have not adopted this technology. The proposed goal is an EHR for all Americans by 2015. Hospitals and physician offices will need to devote considerable time and resources to meet this aggressive timeline.

Patients Are Using Computers Too

A 2008 Harris Poll found that roughly two-thirds of American adults have gone online to find healthcare-related information (Taylor, 2008). Patients who look for this information may be seeking information about conventional, alternative, or complementary therapies and treatments, or looking for shared experiences of others with similar conditions. In addition, friends or family members may seek information on the patient's behalf. Patients may not always share their findings from online searches with their healthcare providers, which can lead to confusion or adverse reactions to prescribed treatment.

You can help guide your patients in their searches by educating them about how to use online sources and choose reputable, trustworthy sites. You may also need to help interpret information that patients find. Many hospitals have patient education materials on their Web sites that provide links to reputable sources.

TIGER

The Technology Informatics Guiding Education Reform (TIGER) initiative was launched in 2006, when a think tank of nursing educators, government and industry leaders and representatives met to develop a shared vision, strategies, and specific actions to improve nursing education, nursing practice guidelines, and clinical care of patients through the use of health

information technology (DeLong, 2009). More than 70 professional nursing organizations drafted a vision statement to make healthcare safer, more effective and efficient, and more patient-centered and equitable.

The teams have begun sharing results of their work with the nursing community through national and local presentations and publications. Continuing activities focus on bringing the activities of the TIGER group into everyday nursing practice, and in getting more nurses involved in developing a stronger health information technology (IT) infrastructure. You may have already seen changes in your nursing school curriculum. What kinds of informatics skills are required in your program? Do you know how to do a literature search to find support for your nursing practice?

The Role of Informatics in Nursing Practice

You have been introduced to several ways in which computer information systems are used in nursing care. In this section, we describe the role of informatics and standardized nursing languages in communicating health information, promoting evidence-based practice, using health records, decreasing medical error, and protecting patient privacy and confidentiality. Table 39-1 summarizes the use of computers in practice, education, administration, and research.

Why Are Computers Important for Evidence-Based Practice?

Rapid access to the ever-increasing volume of knowledge changes the way decisions are made in healthcare. The *traditional model of healthcare decision-making* relies on each practitioner's personal experience and judgment. But healthcare is now so complex that problems routinely exceed the clinical decision-making capacity and reliability of individual practitioners. A better model of decision-making is *evidence-based practice.* As we discussed in Chapters 6 and 8, evidence-based practice uses a knowledge base of accumulated "best evidence" that can change quickly and continuously. To find the current *best* evidence, you must be able to locate the evidence, evaluate its quality and relevance to the problem, and apply the solution.

Critical Thinking 39-3

Analyze the "Meet Your Nurse Role Model" scenario. What example of evidence-based practice do you find in it?

What Are the Benefits of an Electronic Health Record?

Electronic health records (EHRs) as part of networked information systems software allows clinicians to create, store, edit, and retrieve patient charts on a computer. Figure 39-5 is an example of a computer screen using

Table 39-1 ➤ Use of Computer Information Systems in Nursing

NURSING PRACTICE	NURSING EDUCATION	NURSING ADMINISTRATION	NURSING RESEARCH
Literature access and retrieval (e.g., for evidence-based practice)	Literature access and retrieval	Quality assurance and utilization review	Literature review
Care planning	Computer-assisted instruction (CAI) programs	Employee records (e.g., to track licenses, immunizations)	Data collection
Client records (e.g., documenting, order entry, retrieving lab results)	Classroom technology	Staffing patterns, hiring	Data analysis (both qualitative and quantitative)
Telenursing (e.g., in home health)	Distance learning	Buildings and facilities management	Research dissemination
Case management	Testing and grading	Finance and budgets	Applying for grants
Documenting medications	Student records	Accreditation reviews (e.g., monitoring quality indicators for The Joint Commission)	
Transcribing orders	Development of electronic and learning communities using the World Wide Web		
Reordering medications			
Identifying drug interactions			
Warning practitioners about drug incompatibilities			

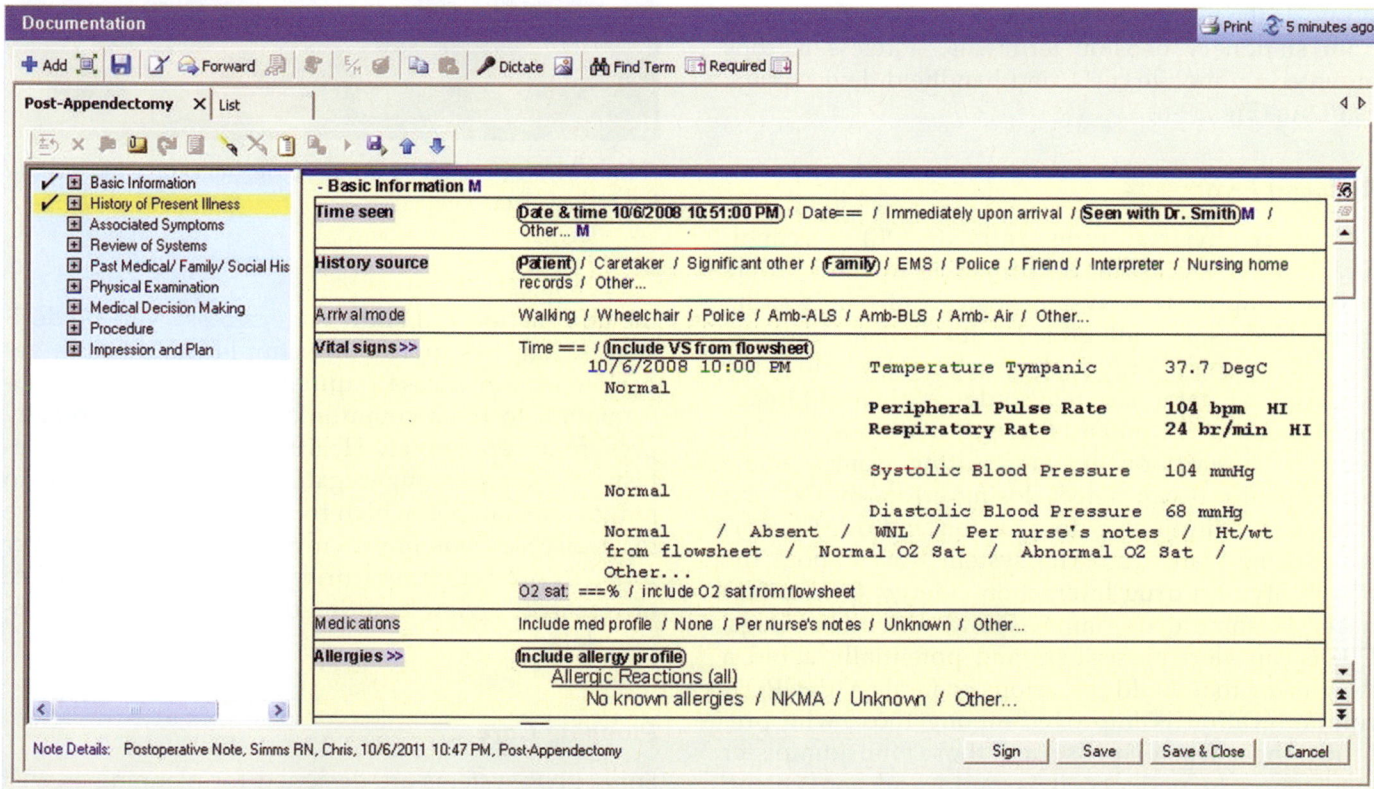

FIGURE 39-5 Computer screen from an electronic health record. (Courtesy of Cerner Corporation, Kansas City, MO.)

EHR software. Notice the electronic view uses combinations of tabs and icons to support logical navigation through the patient chart. These tabs are often named and arranged to match tabs from a traditional paper chart, including patients' clinical and personal data.

A successful EHR project allows an organization to replace paper charts and care plans with electronic health records. Other benefits of the EHR are discussed following (also see Box 16-1).

Improved Efficiency

Improved data access can increase efficiency, productivity, and continuity of care. A paperless health record conveniently stores all patient information in one location, rather than in bits and pieces in many different files and locations.

Privacy

Access to sensitive patient information can be limited only to individuals with proper authorization, and each retrieval of data can be logged electronically—a vast improvement over the folders and charts that can pass through many hands without a record of who examines them.

Accessibility

Have you ever needed to write your nursing notes before leaving the clinical setting, only to discover that the chart was in the x-ray department with the patient? Or that the physician was making rounds with it in her hands? In contrast, any number of people in different locations can access a computerized record—and all at the same time. A physician can view lab results from the office while a nurse views them in the hospital and a lab technician adds more data. A variety of hardware supports the need to access patient health information, from stationary bedside terminals, wireless laptops mounted on mobile carts, and handheld devices such as PDAs (Fig. 39-6).

Reduced Errors

Computer physician order entry (CPOE) is technology that allows healthcare providers to enter orders into a computerized system instead of handwriting them. Orders are integrated with patient information, including allergy history, laboratory, and other prescription data. The new order is then automatically checked for potential errors or problems. This reduces prescription errors resulting from illegible penmanship. It can detect dosing errors by flagging medication dilution or dosages that fall outside normal dosing standards. The system warns about the possibility of a drug interaction, allergy, or incorrect dose. As some drug names sound like other drugs, CPOE can alert prescribers and potentially avoid a drug error that could be serious or fatal. With CPOE, communication is improved among those who prescribe, those who dispense, and those who administer medication to patients. It is rapid and convenient, which make medication available to patients more quickly.

Research and Public Health Benefits

Many healthcare leaders find themselves overwhelmed with data but lack the information they need to make informed decisions. Computerized records place data in repositories (storage areas) so that the information can be sorted and collated to create

FIGURE 39-6 *A,* Handheld device. *B,* Terminal unit for accessing patient data.

the information and knowledge necessary to aid decision-making research. For example, state health departments can access population-based medical information to track communicable diseases, possibly preventing epidemics. Health researchers and analysts can also use **aggregate** health information to judge, for example, which treatment is most effective for a disease, thus improving patient outcomes over time. To protect patient privacy and ethical practice of research, review boards govern access to population data.

Planning Care

Some EHR systems are designed for planning as well as for documenting care. Standardized care plans are typically incorporated in EHR systems. Other applications are designed to support efficient patient care workflow. Studies demonstrate that nurses who understand the nursing process and are familiar with computers are more accepting of automated documentation (Kossman & Scheidenhelm, 2008). As more people are comfortable with computers and use them daily, nurses' acceptance of computers in the workplace also is increasing.

Unintended Consequences

Little research has been done on the *unintended consequences* of EHR implementations. Consider the following examples:

- Although the intent of computerization is to decrease cost through improved efficiency and communication, instituting EHR without addressing *changes in nursing workflow* and *communication patterns* can actually make unit operations less effective (Kossman & Scheidenhelm, 2008).
- *Software upgrade* and *periodic new releases* are inevitable, some of which may require more robust hardware than previous editions. New, expensive equipment to replace perfectly serviceable hardware, which has been rendered obsolete by your EHR, is a factor when considering the cost of an EHR.
- The *portability* of EHR can lead to *decreased face-to-face communication* among the healthcare team.

The nurse informatics specialist, a nurse who has gained additional education and experience in informatics, often provides guidance for clinicians in identifying gaps between how the EHR system functions and how clinical processes work. Successful changes from paper to electronic systems are those that provide opportunities for nurses to have a voice in choosing systems and planning the change.

KnowledgeCheck 39-2

- What are some of the benefits of EHR implementation?
- What is personal health information, and why is it important to protect it?
- How is a listserv different from regular e-mail?

 Go to Chapter 39, **Knowledge Check Response Sheet and Answers,** on the Student Resource Disk or DavisPlus at http://davisplus.fadavis.com/Wilkinson2

Why Are Standardized Nursing Languages Needed for EHRs?

Suppose you wanted to find out how many patients on your hospital unit had a nursing diagnosis of Impaired Skin Integrity during the past year. If the hospital uses paper medical records, how could you find out? If the records are computerized, would that make a difference?

You probably said something like: Pull all the charts, and look at the nursing notes. Or maybe, search for the words *Impaired Skin Integrity* in the computerized records. That's a beginning. But think about this: Nurses use a variety of terms to describe the same data. For example, in some charts you would find the term *skin breakdown;* in others, *a reddened area, bedsore,* or a *stage III pressure ulcer.* Would you count all of these as Impaired Skin Integrity? What if the nurses used some terms you didn't think to search for? Do you see how the lack of a uniform way to describe

patient problems can hamper efforts to create and retrieve nursing data from automated documentation systems? Recall the goal for interoperability among EHR systems discussed previously in the chapter. Standardized language—using the same terms to describe a phenomenon in all EHRs—helps to achieve that goal.

Nurses do not describe clinical interventions any more uniformly than they describe nursing diagnoses. Inconsistent language and meaning make it difficult to compare and research nursing contributions to patient care (Beyea, 2000). Use of standardized nursing languages helps to ensure that nursing activities are an integral component of any electronic health record. As research and teaching of standardized interventions promotes wider understanding of them, they will help to further define the scope of nursing practice. When nursing terminology is visible in the EHR, it becomes possible to recognize the importance of nurses make to achieving patient outcomes and organizational goals.

The first use of standardized nursing language began in the 1970s, with the NANDA-I classification of nursing diagnoses. Since then, several initiatives to develop standardized languages for nursing practice have arisen (Wilkinson, 2011, in press). By 2003, the American Nurses Association Committee for Nursing Practice Information Infrastructure had recognized 13 standardized languages.

 Go to Chapter 39, **Standardized Language, American Nurses Association Recognized Languages for Nursing,** in Volume 2.

Each of these languages makes a unique contribution to knowledge development in nursing. At this time, it appears that no single language has captured nursing practice in its entirety. Each language is currently in the process of revision and further development. This is, of course, true of *all* languages, including English and Spanish and other spoken languages.

This text primarily uses the NANDA-I, NIC, and NOC classifications for describing patient problems, outcomes, and interventions (see Chapters 4, 5, and 6 if you need a review). Other classifications, such as the Omaha system and Community Care Classification, were created for specific settings (i.e., community health and home health, respectively), but can actually be used in all settings. Adoption of a single standardized language system would enhance communication among nurses, with other healthcare professionals, and with the public. Because this does not appear likely, however, nurses are working to "map" terms from each system to their equivalents in other systems (e.g., Impaired Skin Integrity in NANDA-I might map to Integument in the Omaha system). This contributes to the interoperability mentioned earlier in the chapter.

How Does Computerization Decrease Error in Healthcare?

As healthcare becomes more complex, the opportunities for error increase exponentially. Misdiagnosing, overlooking an allergy, or erroneously transcribing a medication order can carry serious consequences. A hospital stay can be prolonged or death can result from a seemingly simple mistake.

 Illegible or confusing handwriting by clinicians can lead to medication errors and other sentinel events. Mistaken abbreviations or acronyms, look-alike, and sound-alike medication mixups are errors that can be prevented with computer-entry prescriptions. Other times errors result from faulty communication among healthcare providers, which, in some cases, can also be prevented by electronic prescribing.

The largest share of medication errors occur either in the prescribing step (39%) or the administration step (38%) (Bell, 2009). Barcode point-of-care scanning applications have been proven effective in decreasing errors associated with errors in checking medications. For a more extensive discussion on the use of automation to decrease medication errors,

Go to Chapter 39, **Supplemental Materials: How Does Automation Decrease Error in Healthcare?** on the Student Resource Disk or DavisPlus at http://davisplus.fadavis.com/Wilkinson2

In healthcare, building a safer system means designing processes of care to ensure patients are protected from accidental injury. Automation (EHR) provides a secure way for providers to quickly and efficiently communicate with each other regarding a patient's allergies, medications, or current health status, so that an emerging situation does not become deadly. A computerized record can be quickly accessed, updated, and forwarded simultaneously to all members of the healthcare team. For example, many different departments (e.g., x-ray, nursing, pharmacy) need to be alert to a patient's allergies. Rather than continually asking the patient to report his allergies, the computer can record the information one time and notify every department that needs it.

1. *Computerized physician order entry (CPOE)* helps prevent errors in reading and transcribing orders.
2. *Bar-coding medications at the unit-dose level* helps to prevent nurses from selecting an incorrect medication.
3. *Use of smart technologies (e.g., infusion devices) at the point of care* helps to ensure that the correct dose is delivered to the patient.

Critical**Thinking** 39-4

- How does automation contribute to or decrease errors in healthcare?

How Can I Use Electronic Health Records Ethically?

No information may be more sensitive than medical records. Patients confide in nurses and physicians, trusting that their information will remain private. Most facilities have disciplinary policies in place to manage security breaches and assign fines or prosecution when patient privacy is violated. Strong personal

---

Toward Evidence-Based Practice

Fowler, S. B., Sohler, P., & Zarillo, D. F. (2009). Bar code technology for medication administration: Medication errors and nurse satisfaction. *MEDSURG Nursing, 18*(2), 103–109.

A barcode administration system provides a safe mechanism for delivering medications to the unit for the nurse to administer. This study compared nurse satisfaction with this system pre-implementation, 3 months post-implementation, and 6 months post-implementation. The new barcode medication administration system was piloted in a 53-bed medical surgical unit. The sample studied was small and did not show significant differences in satisfaction between nurses trained without technology versus those recently trained with the use of other computer-based programs.

1. What is a barcode medication system? And how does it work?

2. What are a few of the major benefits of using a barcode medication system?

3. What drawbacks or risks can you think of when using this type of system?

4. At first glance, what conclusion might you draw about the study of nurses' satisfaction with the barcode system?

5. How might you explain why some of the nurses in the study did not express overwhelming satisfaction when using the barcode technology?

6. Before drawing conclusions about whether the barcode technology has merit or not, though, what questions do you need to ask about the group of nurses sampled in this study? Should further research be recommended?

Go to Chapter 39, **Toward Evidence-Based Practice Suggested Responses,** on the Student Resource Disk or DavisPlus at http://davisplus.fadavis.com/Wilkinson2

integrity and adherence to nursing and other codes of ethics are necessary to protect patient privacy within healthcare organizations.

Only one person at a time can view a paper record, and that person and the record must be in the same geographical location. With an automated record, many people can view the information at the same time, and they can be in many different locations. Still, in some ways the automated record is more secure than the paper record. Almost anyone in the clinical unit can view the paper record. There is no record to show who has seen the information. In contrast, several measures protect the confidentiality of the electronic health record.

Passwords

Passwords for all users are probably the most obvious protection. In most institutions, passwords are tied to the responsibilities of the job description. For example, the business office does not have access to clinical information, and nurses do not have access to data about the patient's bill-paying arrangement. Some simple rules for password management:

- Never share passwords with others.
- The more complex the password, the harder it is for hackers to break it. Use combinations of letters, numbers, and symbols for maximum protection.
- Don't use words that are easy to guess (e.g., pet names, birthdays).
- Change passwords frequently.
- Do not record passwords in easily accessible places.

Although it is important to protect the privacy of healthcare records from outside observers, professionals who have password access but are not assigned to the patient to provide care make most breaches of confidentiality. For instance, think about the number of times that health details of noted celebrities have made headlines.

Audit Trails

Organizations are required to have software that tracks each person who accesses information. This is called an **audit trail**. Anything a person adds to or changes in the record is recorded automatically on the audit trail and can be investigated.

HIPAA Regulations

Most health insurance plans and care providers must comply with the Department of Health and Human Services (HHS) Privacy Rule (also referred to as "the HIPAA regulations"). The Privacy Rule was mandated in response to the Health Insurance Portability and Accountability Act (HIPAA) of 1996. It was the first comprehensive federal protection for the privacy of individually

identifiable health information. The two important requirements are that health plans and providers must:

- Obtain consent before disclosing health information used for treatment or payment options.
- Limit disclosure of information to the minimum necessary to accomplish intended purposes.

These rules were extended as part of the HITECH Act discussed earlier. New rules increase fines to organizations for each reported breach of personal health information, and give authority to individual states to monitor compliance with the rules. These rules apply to all forms of communication: electronic, written, and oral. For full information,

 Go to the **U.S. Department of Health and Human Services** Web site at www.hhs.gov/ocr/hipaa/

If you would like further discussion of EHR privacy issues, review Chapter 16, "How Do I Maintain Confidentiality and Data Security?"

Knowledge Check 39-3

- List at least three ways in which computers can help reduce healthcare errors.
- Discuss at least three measures to protect the confidentiality of patients' electronic health records.

 Go to Chapter 39, **Knowledge Check Response Sheet and Answers,** on the Student Resource Disk or DavisPlus at http://davisplus.fadavis.com/Wilkinson2

Practical Knowledge
knowing how

Professional standards require accountable practitioners to keep up to date with research and new knowledge. For example, ANA Professional Performance Standard 3, Criteria 2 and 3, state the nurse should demonstrate a commitment to lifelong learning and seek experiences that reflect current practice to maintain skills and competence (ANA, 2010 in press).[1] You can accomplish this by knowing how to search literature databases efficiently and use Web resources discriminatingly to complement your use of the EHR in providing quality patient care.

Using Informatics to Support Evidence-Based Practice

As you have learned in previous chapters, evidence-based practice involves (1) identifying a clinical question or need for change, (2) searching the literature,

---

[1]*Caveat:* This material is from the draft for public comment (ANA, 2010, in press); its wording may be changed somewhat in the final published version. For that version of the ANA Standards of Professional Nursing Practice, go to www.nursingworld.org

(3) evaluating evidence, and (4) translating the results into practice (Pipe, Cisar, Caruso, et al., 2007). It is not enough to find one journal article in support of an intervention, but rather to search broadly for high-quality, scientific evidence. Managing and processing information are essential for these tasks. Nurses require the most current, best-quality information for making decisions in their practice. In hospital settings, nurses need information on a wide variety of topics including clinical nursing issues, drug therapy, improving patient outcomes, innovative practice changes, and leadership skills. But how do nurses use automated systems to access that information? See Box 39-1 for a profile of an information-literate person.

How Do Computers Reduce Barriers to Evidence-Based Practice?

Most nurses are action oriented, preferring to learn by looking, listening, and talking. It may seem easier to seek information from colleagues, rely on past experience, draw on knowledge of pathophysiology, and read whatever references are closest at hand. However, in the clinical setting, the closest reference book may not contain the most current information or the best possible evidence. Computers at the workplace help overcome this barrier to evidence-based practice by providing fast, easy access to current practice information from around the world. For example, when traditional methods have failed, you could quickly use a computer to look up the latest, tested interventions for a patient who is incontinent of urine. Because the Internet is available 24 hours a day, you can access online libraries and other information sources as your personal schedule allows.

How Do I Use Computers to Search the Literature?

Lack of literature-searching skills is another reason why many nurses fail to take advantage of automated information available to them to enrich their practice. There are several steps to conducting an automated search of the literature.

- **Identify the information.** When you clearly define the information you want to gather and how it will be used, it is easier and more efficient to search, locate, evaluate, retrieve, organize, and manage the resources required to answer your question.
- **Formulate a precise definition of the problem.** This is usually in the form of a question, for example, "What are the leading causes of falls in older adults?" This question guides your search for information.
- **Conduct a search** of the most recent literature and most relevant studies. To learn about or review the

---

BOX 39-1 ■ Profile of an Information-Literate Person

An information-literate person *accesses* information:
- Recognizes the need for information
- Understands accurate and complete information is the basis for intelligent decision making
- Formulates questions based on information needs
- Identifies potential sources of information and selects those with credibility
- Accesses print and technology-based sources of information

An information-literate person *evaluates* information:
- Accepts authoritative, current reliable information
- Sorts information based on accuracy and relevance
- Distinguishes opinion from factual knowledge
- Rejects inaccurate and misleading information
- Rejects biased information
- Creates new information to replace inaccurate or missing information as needed

An information-literate person *manages* information:
- Develops successful search strategies.
- Organizes information so the most important points are clear.
- Breaks complex information into understandable chunks.

- Sorts out language and technical points into meaningful terms.
- Tracks sources of information responsibly and credits appropriately.

An information-literate person *uses* information:
- Organizes information for practical application.
- Integrates new information into an existing body of knowledge.
- Applies information in critical thinking and problem-solving.

Other characteristics:
- A resourceful and independent learner
- Competent reader
- Confident in his or her ability to solve problems
- Able to function independently and work well in groups
- Creative and able to adapt to change

Adapted from: Doyle, C. S. (1992). *Final report to National Forum on Information Literacy.* (University of Calgary. Information Literacy Group, 1998); Krumsieg, K., & Baehr, M. (2000). *Foundations of learning* (3rd ed.). Corvallis, OR: Pacific Crest; U.S. Department of Health and Human Services. (n.d.). *Quick guide to health literacy.* Retrieved from http://www.health.gov/communication/literacy/quickguide/factsbasic.htm.

PICO method of defining and stating questions, go to Chapter 8, "Formulate a Searchable Question" and Box 8-4, "PICO Questions."

Critical Thinking 39-5

Before reading the next section, see whether you can puzzle out the answers to the following two questions. Consult with your classmates and instructors, if necessary, after finishing the chapter.

- Why must a question be formed before initiating the search?
- The suggested question in the preceding section was "What are the leading causes of falls in older adults?" Why can't you use a general topic such as "falls" for your search topic?

Online Sources of Nursing Research

You must evaluate the type of literature you need to answer the question. For instance, a research report provides better support for an intervention than does an opinion article. Although some information is classic and timeless, it is usually best to find the most current studies.

Textbooks. Textbooks are good for general information, but are not the most current source of information because of the time it takes to prepare the publication.

Printed Journal Articles. Printed journal articles are more current, but the information may still be 6 months to 2 years old by the time the article is published. Journals come in varying degrees of academic rigor. You must discriminate among scholarly, general interest, and popular periodical literature.

- *Scholarly Journals.* Scholarly journals contain tables and graphs, but are not as colorfully illustrated as general interest periodicals. A scholar, clinical expert, or scientific researcher in the field submits topical articles that adhere to professional standards, carefully footnoting and citing references. Articles submitted to scholarly journals are reviewed by a group of experts to determine if they are suitable for publication. This process is known as peer review. The main purpose of a scholarly journal is to report on original research to make the information available to others. Examples of scholarly journals include: *Journal of Nursing Scholarship, Journal of Nursing Administration, Nursing Research, Nurse Educator, and International Journal of Nursing Terminologies and Classifications.*
- *General interest periodicals.* General interest periodicals are usually attractive. Articles tend to be heavily illustrated, commonly with photographs. News and general interest periodicals sometimes cite sources, but not always. Articles may be written by a member of the editorial staff, a scholar, or a freelance writer and are often peer reviewed. The language is geared to any educated audience. A specialty is not assumed. Some examples of general interest nursing periodicals include the American Journal of Nursing, RN, and Nursing [current year].
- *Popular periodicals.* Popular periodicals are usually slick and attractive in appearance. They include many graphics and photographs. These publications rarely, if ever, cite sources. Information in such journals is often second- or third-hand, and the original source is sometimes obscure. Articles are usually short, lack depth, and are written in simple language and designed to meet a minimal education level. The main purpose is to promote a product or viewpoint. Examples include Parents, Women's Health, and Modern Healthcare.

The World Wide Web. The World Wide Web contains the most current information, including some well-respected nursing journals (e.g., *American Journal of Nursing, NurseWeek, Online Journal of Issues in Nursing,* and *Nursing Standard Online*). New health information can be published immediately on the Web for the entire world to see without the delay of print publishing.

Literature Databases

Literature databases are a powerful tool for finding information. Literature databases are catalogues of articles, usually sorted by discipline. Databases exist for engineering, education, law, medicine, nursing, and other disciplines. These databases often overlap—what is found in one database might also be found in another. For example, MEDLINE is the largest medical database and lists internationally published articles from journals in all areas of biomedicine. The Cumulative Index for Nursing and Allied Health Literature (CINAHL) is a smaller database covering nursing, allied health, biomedical, and consumer health journal articles. Most of the articles in CINAHL are also listed in MEDLINE. If, however, you are looking for a nursing-focused article, it is more efficient to use CINAHL because the search is already narrowed to nursing and allied health.

Each entry in a database contains an article citation, subject headings describing the article, and a text summary of the article called an **abstract.** Other information about the article may also be included, such as the name of the author(s), the name of the institution at which the research was done, and the language in which the article was published (Box 39-2). Many full-text journal articles are available online, some free and some for a fee. Some are available in the school or hospital's library for nurses to access. Table 39-2 includes descriptions of some commonly used databases in health care. Do not limit your

BOX 39-2 ■ Example of a Database Entry

Author(s):	Ward, Kathleen R. Koerner, Dianna K.
Title:	Sink or swim: the Titanic medication administration fair.
Source:	Journal of Continuing Education in Nursing. 39(4):179-84, 2008 Apr.
Standard No:	ISSN: 0190-535X Serial Identifier: 006740000
	NLM Unique Identifier: 7809033
Language:	English
Descriptor:	Medication safety
	Decision Making, Patient
Document Type:	Journal article; research; tables/charts
Database:	CINAHL

The search results may also contain an abstract of the article, and in some instances, the full-text article is available either for a fee or at no charge.

search to a single database. You will find valuable information in the databases of other disciplines (e.g., psychology, education, business, law, and engineering).

How Do I Evaluate Evidence and Determine a Solution?

Evaluating the evidence is sometimes as simple as reading a descriptive research study and applying the results to your current situation. For example, in the search for information about falls in older adults, you may find research to indicate a number of safety measures that can be easily implemented to create a safer

environment for your patients. However, other times evaluating evidence can also be very complicated, requiring an understanding of statistics and research methodologies. Just because one study indicates that sugar causes cancer does not mean that the study was valid or reliable; therefore, you must not base conclusions on the results of only one study. Experience and further study about research will increase your ability to evaluate your findings in the literature.

 Although an article you find on the Web may be quite current, it is not necessarily accurate, valid, or reliable. Many sites are created by individuals with questionable credentials or by companies attempting to sell their product or service. Such sites may not provide the best information to support your research; even worse, their information may be incomplete, inaccurate, biased, or unreliable. See Box 39-3 for suggestions on evaluating materials you obtain from a Web site. For ethical principles to guide health information Web sites,

 Go to Chapter 39, **ESG Box 39-1, Guiding Ethical Principles for Health Information Web Sites,** on the Student Resource Disk or DavisPlus at http://davisplus.fadavis.com/Wilkinson2

If you would like to review the process for evaluating the quality of research articles you find in your searches, or for a process to find the best evidence for a nursing intervention, refer to Chapter 8, "How Can I Base My Practice on the Best Evidence?"

CriticalThinking 39-6

What factors can make the Web an unreliable source of information? What factors can help you find reliable information?

Table 39-2 ➤ Selected Databases for Health Literature

DATABASE	DESCRIPTION
CINAHL (Cumulative Index for Nursing and Allied Health Literature)	Covers nursing, allied health, biomedical, and consumer health journals, publications of the American Nursing Association, and the National League for Nursing. Coverage with abstracts is from January 1986 to the present. Coverage with indexing from 1982 to the present. Updated monthly.
Cochrane Library	A regularly updated collection of evidence-based medicine databases, including systematic reviews, reviews of effectiveness, and a controlled-trials register. This is a source of reliable evidence about the effects of health care.
Health and Wellness Resource Center	Provides integrated access to medical, health, and wellness information from reference sources, magazine and journal articles, pamphlets, and some Web resources. Quick Start links include a medical encyclopedia, dictionary, drug and herb finder, health organization directory, health assessment links, health news, and a few select medical Web sites.
MEDLINE	Produced by the U.S. National Library of Medicine, MEDLINE is world's largest medical library in all areas of biomedicine and healthcare.
PsycINFO 1887	Covers worldwide literature in psychology and related disciplines, such as psychiatry, sociology, anthropology, education, linguistics, and pharmacology. Journal articles, technical reports, and dissertations are included. Coverage is from 1887 to the present. Updated weekly.

BOX 39-3 ■ How to Evaluate a Health Information Web Site

Remember, anyone can publish anything on the Web. The information you obtain may have been created by an expert, but most World Wide Web sites are authored by nonexperts. They may contain fact or opinion. Do not believe everything you read on the Web! Use the following questions to guide your evaluation.

Evaluate For	Questions to Ask
Authority	*Who is the author?* What are his credentials and qualifications to speak on this topic? Are the sources of information stated? Don't confuse the author with the webmaster.
	Check the URL domain (e.g., *www.nih.gov*). What institution published the document? The Web address provides clues to this:

.com—a company.   .mil—the U.S. military

.edu—a school or university   .net—a network of computers

.gov—the U.S. government   .org—a nonprofit organization

	The domain symbols ~ or % or a name (e.g., jsmith), "users," or "members" indicate a personal web page.
	Who is the sponsor? The name right after "www" will provide a clue (e.g., see "nih"), but the full name (e.g., National Institutes of Health) should be on the page.
	Can you contact the author for clarification or more information?
Currency	*When was it produced?* For some topics, you need current information.
	When was it updated? Note that the fact that the Web page was "updated" may not mean that the information was updated at the same time. It may simply mean that the physical file was changed in some way (e.g., a misspelled word corrected)
	Are the links up to date? Check the links to see whether they work.
Purpose	*Why was the page put on the Web?* Remember that many sites are designed to a product or an idea. Other purposes may be to entertain, to give facts, to share humor, or to provide a forum for ideas and opinions.
	Look for words like "about our company," "mission," "philosophy," "who am I," and so on.
	Who are the intended users of the page? Students, experts, patients?
	Are there advertisements on the page? This may be a clue.
Availability	*Can you view or download the information* without a special browser or special software?
	Are there fees for viewing the full content?
Content quality (accuracy, objectivity, coverage)	*Are the sources documented* with footnotes or links? Are they scholarly links or information sources?
	Is the information provided by the site, or is it reproduced from another source?
	Are there links to the original sources (if they are online)? Or a reason for not providing a link? Do they work?
	Look for bias (e.g., political or ideological), especially when you agree with it! Are there links to opposing views if it is an opinion page?
	Is the information reliable and error-free? Is there someone who verifies or checks the information?
	How in-depth is the material?
	What does the page offer that you can't find elsewhere?
	Look up the page in a directory that evaluates the website contents. For example:
	www.ipl.org (the Librarians' Internet Index)
	http://www.lib.umd.edu/guides/webcheck.html
Usability	Is it easy to read and navigate?
	Are HELP screens available?
	Is there a search engine on the site?
	Is it frequently offline or slow to load?

Go to Chapter 39, **Resources for Caregivers and Health Professionals,** on the Student Resource Disk or DavisPlus at http://davisplus.fadavis.com/Wilkinson2

Bibliography: Go to Volume 2, Bibliography.

Suggested Readings: Go to Chapter 39, **Reading More About Nursing Informatics,** on the Student Resource Disk or DavisPlus at http://davisplus.fadavis.com/Wilkinson2

CHAPTER 40

Holistic Healing

Learning Outcomes

After completing this chapter, you should be able to:

➤ Explain holism and holistic care.

➤ Recognize the beliefs that form the basis of holistic care.

➤ Compare and contrast complementary, alternative, integrative, and allopathic healthcare.

➤ Explain how the placebo response relates to holistic care.

➤ Discuss the trends in use of complementary and alternative modalities (CAM).

➤ Differentiate the five types of CAM as categorized by the National Center for Complementary and Alternative Medicine.

➤ Discuss the most commonly used CAM therapies.

➤ Discuss the importance of a holistic nursing assessment.

➤ Identify ways to integrate CAM into nursing care.

Meet Your Patient

When Lisa, a new graduate nurse, entered the room to assess Mrs. Riddell a few hours after her surgery, the patient was lying in bed, crying softly. Mrs. Riddell sobbed, "I don't think I can handle this pain. I'm so worried about cancer and I don't have any sick time left at work; how am I going to manage?" Lisa put her hand gently on the patient's arm and said, "It sounds like you're going through a lot right now. It must be very difficult for you." Mrs. Riddell reached for Lisa's hand and began sobbing, "I'm so afraid."

Just then the manager of the surgical unit walked in, speaking rapidly, "Lisa, you forgot to turn the call light off. Oh, Mrs. Riddell, you seem upset. Are you in pain?" Mrs. Riddell nodded her head yes. When the manager asked her to rate the pain on a scale of 1 to 10, Mrs. Riddell replied, "About a 5." The manager said, "Ms. Jackson will check when you can have your next dose of pain medication."

Outside the room, Lisa explained to her manager that Mrs. Riddell was worried about her diagnosis. "First things first, Lisa, get the patient's pain under control,"

replied the manager. Lisa wanted to spend a few moments with the patient to allow her to express her feelings and concerns. She believed it would be easier to relieve Mrs. Riddell's pain if it were not complicated by her anxious feelings. However, Lisa was new on the unit and decided to follow the manager's orders to address the physical pain.

When Lisa returned with the analgesic, Mrs. Riddell refused it. She was still tearful and distressed and said that she really just needed to have her bed straightened. Lisa closed the curtains and explained that she would get some fresh linens and help her get comfortable. The manager saw Lisa carrying linens, stopped her, and said, "We have NAPs for bed changes, which frees you up to do the professional nursing care. There are two new patients being admitted, and I want you to learn the admission process." Lisa shared her concerns about Mrs. Riddell's

(continued on next page)

psychosocial needs and explained that she wanted to help her relax and express her concerns. Lisa said, "She refused the pain medication, but I'd like to use therapeutic touch (an energy intervention) to treat her." The manager replied, "I wish we had more time to talk to patients and try new things, but we are short-staffed, and the admissions, charting, treatments, and other work will never be done by the end of shift if we don't do first things first.

I'm sorry to disillusion you, but welcome to the real world of nursing."

Lisa and Mrs. Riddell are experiencing some problems common to contemporary healthcare: inadequate staff, time, and resources for the care we know our patients deserve. Many patients and nurses feel caught in a model of sick care that emphasizes disease and fosters emotional neutrality on the part of professionals.

Theoretical Knowledge knowing why

Holistic healing and nontraditional healthcare are becoming more common. Approximately 40% of adults in the United States use some form of complementary or alternative modalities (CAM) (Barnes, Bloom, & Nahin, 2008). If the use of prayer for health reasons is included, the figure is even higher. The U.S. public spends around $40 billion out of pocket on CAM therapies each year. CAM accounts for 1.5% of all healthcare costs in the United States, but it makes up slightly more than 11% of all out-of-pocket healthcare costs (National Center for Complementary and Alternative Medicine [NCCAM], 2009a,b). Most of the money spent on CAM is spent on **self-care therapies**—things people can do on their own without having to see a healthcare provider. In this chapter, we explore holistic care and the use of various complementary and alternative therapies.

Holism

The concept of **holism** emphasizes the relationships among all living things. Holism was the dominant philosophy throughout early history, but it fell out of favor in the 17th century, when René Descartes and other influential philosophers introduced the notion that the mind and body are separate. Descartes' thinking strongly influenced the emerging discipline of medicine and is largely responsible for Western medicine's separate treatment of physical and mental health. However, in 1926, Jan Christian Smuts reinvigorated the belief in holism by declaring that living entities are more than the sum of their parts. To oversimplify an example of holism, this means that although the body is made up of a liver, a brain, a heart, and other individual organs, it is more than just cells and organs. Rather, a body is all of the various pieces and parts working separately and together and with the environment—all affecting each other. Add to the body spirituality, emotions, and external systems such as culture, relationships, and the geopolitical environment—all affecting and being affected

by each other—and you have a holistic view of a person or patient.

Biomedical and holistic approaches consider health and disease from different perspectives. Consider the case of a person with bacterial pneumonia. Conventional biomedical treatment would use antibiotics to kill the bacteria, an antipyretic to suppress fever and discomfort, an expectorant to liquefy secretions, increased fluids, and rest. Treatment is successful when the pathology (i.e., infection) and symptoms (e.g., fever) are gone. Conventional medicine is often referred to as **allopathy,** a term used to indicate medical practice that treats disease with remedies that counteract the effects of the disease.

A **holistic approach** expands the patient encounter to include methods of enhancing the person's resistance to the illness (e.g., rest, fluids, nutritional counseling, reduction of aggravating behaviors, and stress management). Holism emphasizes the need to change lifestyle behaviors that increase vulnerability to illness. Holistic treatment is complete when the person has healed into his best possible state of wellness (as defined by the individual), understands why the illness occurred, and adopts lifestyle changes.

What Is Holistic Healthcare?

Many people now use, or are interested in, holistic care. So regardless of where you work you need to have theoretical knowledge of holistic practices and their effects in order to best meet patient needs. Holistic healthcare is founded on the beliefs in Box 40-1.

A **modality** is a method of treating a disorder (e.g., therapeutic touch, antibiotics). *Holistic healthcare* is often used interchangeably with *complementary healthcare* and *alternative health care,* but the terms do not have the same meaning. A **complementary modality** is a treatment that is used together with traditional medical care. An **alternative modality** is used instead of traditional medical care. CAM encompass a range of philosophies, approaches, and therapies that the conventional healthcare system does not commonly use, accept, understand, study, or make available. Although a number of CAM treatments are holistic, many are narrowly focused.

BOX 40-1 ■ Holistic Health Beliefs

- Each person is unique.
- Each person is a whole in constant interaction with the environment. The body, mind, and spirit must come together to achieve harmony and healing.
- Disease is a result of multiple contributing factors rather than one cause.
- Factors essential to health are social support, health practices, family illness patterns, personality traits, culture, child-rearing practices, and relatedness to nature.
- All healing is self-healing.
- Hope, faith, and the will to live are important to maintaining health and recovering from illness.
- The patient's expectation that the treatment will be effective is part of the self-healing process. A positive state of mind is necessary to bring harmony to the body.
- Each person is interconnected to others, nature, and to the world.
- Health is achieved when there is balance, integration, and harmony in life.
- Healthcare resources are better used when they focus on health promotion and disease prevention.
- Illness is an opportunity for growth and has meaning within the context of the life experience.
- Illness occurs when there is a shift in an individual's balance in any dimension or with the environment.

The creation of the National Center for Complementary and Alternative Medicine (NCCAM), a division of the National Institutes of Health, has stimulated research in the area of the effectiveness of CAM therapies. As a result, the list of what is considered CAM is continually changing: therapies that are proven to be safe and effective are incorporated into conventional healthcare (**integrative modalities**), and new modalities emerge. Still, for most CAM therapies, more research is needed, because without an evidence base there is the risk that CAM practices may harm rather than help.

Integrative healthcare refers to coordinated care that encompasses all treatments and health practices a patient uses. To provide integrative care a practitioner must know about the interactive effects of conventional and CAM treatments and be able to coordinate all the care modalities. The practitioner must establish trust so that the patient will disclose CAM use, and must communicate with other health providers for referral and coordination of care. Integrative healthcare is holistic because it considers all aspects of the patient's care.

KnowledgeCheck 40-1

- Compare and contrast alternative, complementary, and integrative modalities.
- What is the relationship between allopathy and holistic healthcare?

 Go to Chapter 40, **Knowledge Check Response Sheet and Answers,** on the Student Resource Disk or DavisPlus at http://davisplus.fadavis.com/Wilkinson2

CriticalThinking 40-1

- Review the "Meet Your Patient" scenario. What kind of care is Mrs. Riddell receiving: allopathic, complementary, alternative, or integrative? Would you be comfortable offering CAM therapies to Mrs. Riddell?
- As a holistic healer, should Lisa administer pain medications to Mrs. Riddell if she agrees to take them? Why or why not?

The Placebo Response

A **placebo response** occurs as a result of the patient's expectation that a treatment will be effective. As an expression of mind–body unity, the placebo response is a basic underlying principle of holistic care. The stronger a person's belief in treatment efficacy, the stronger the placebo effect. Its opposite, the **nocebo effect,** is a demonstration of the power of the mind to create bodily distress. For example, expecting that a treatment will be painful tends to increase the discomfort the person experiences. These responses illustrate the powerful influence of the mind on states of health and disease.

In holistic care, treatment outcomes are enhanced if the practitioner and the patient believe that the treatment will be effective and if the practitioner establishes an empathetic and supportive relationship with the patient. The ideal relationship is mutual and based on equality, with the patient assuming an active role in the treatment plan. The practitioner acts as a role model and negotiates care that incorporates a number of healing modalities. Practitioners teach patients to strengthen their intent to heal by focusing their minds to influence the course of illness and recovery. Techniques such as visual imagery, affirmations, and relaxation techniques enhance treatment outcomes because the mind and body function as a unit. Holistic healers believe that all healing is self-healing, and the placebo response demonstrates this natural phenomenon.

Spirituality and Holism

To fully understand the experience of health and illness, you must include the spiritual dimension. **Spirituality** is the vital process of discovering meaning, purpose, fulfillment, and value in life. As such, it has tremendous influence on health and an individual's ability to heal. Absence of spirituality creates a sense of disconnection from one's true source, a loss of meaning to one's life, and a state of *dis*-ease (Levine, 1984). A holistic perspective incorporates the realities of the human condition—disease, disability, misfortune, aging, pain, and death—into the life experience. Illness and disease are viewed as opportunities for transformation and growth. Holism helps to answer some vital questions: Who am I? How do I choose to live? What is the value of my life? A holistic environment fosters maturation through illness, disability, deformity, and even the death process.

CriticalThinking 40-2

Holistic healthcare relies on the placebo effect. However, traditional therapy discourages the use of placebos for pain control (ethicists hold that placebos are deceptive and do not respect patient autonomy). Traditional researchers attempt to factor out the placebo effect when conducting clinical research trials. React to these two belief systems. Which belief is most congruent with your view of healthcare? How do you think these divergent views might affect research on CAM?

Who Is a Holistic Patient?

Women, people with higher income levels, and people who have been hospitalized in the past year are most likely to use CAM.

By Race and Ethnicity. Excluding prayer as a therapy, two studies indicate that non-Hispanic whites use CAM more often than Hispanics and non-Hispanic blacks, and are more likely to report CAM use to their healthcare provider (Graham, Ahn, Davis, et al., 2005; NCCAM, 2004a, 2009a).

By Age Group. CAM is used least by those younger than age 18 and most by middle adults. Use progressively declines after age 69 (MedlinePlus, updated 2009). However, one study found the following:

- Of adults older than age 65, 88% used CAM.
- Of adults older than age 80, 90% used CAM
- Among those adults, dietary supplements and chiropractic had the highest use.

These researchers considered all multivitamins as CAM, which partially explains the high rates (Ness, Cirillo, Weir, et al., 2005).

Many parents use CAM for their children. Two out of three do not tell the child's clinician about CAM use. Use of multivitamins, dietary supplements, and herbal preparations is common (Barclay & Murata, 2008).

Why Do People Use CAM?

In a nationwide study, Astin (1998) discovered that most people who use CAM do so because they find it more in harmony with their own values, beliefs, and philosophical orientation toward health and life. The current interest in holistic healing is probably the result of a combination of forces. For example, some people:

- Are dissatisfied with the impersonal nature of traditional healthcare, and wish for more personal attention.
- Wish to promote health and avoid illness. For example, they may believe that techniques such as yoga

can improve overall well-being. Western medicine, in contrast, tends to focus more on illness (although that is slowly changing).
- Fear adverse effects from traditional medical treatments and prescription drugs. CAM is usually low risk and free of serious side effects.
- Lack of access to medical practitioners (e.g., older adults who are confined to home).
- Lack insurance coverage. CAM is not often reimbursed by insurance, but for those who do not have good insurance coverage, CAM is generally low in cost and may be less expensive than conventional medical treatment.
- Use CAM when conventional care is not relieving their symptoms. They do not stop using conventional care, but use the CAM along with it, believing that the combination is superior to either type of therapy alone.

Cassidy (1994) identified characteristics of persons likely to benefit from holistic care. They:

- Have a high need for affiliation and relational style of healthcare.
- Wish to alleviate symptoms gently or with fewer side effects.
- Will not take "hopeless" for an answer.
- Wish to prevent disease or enhance wellness.
- Interpret the body-person as being more than just physical and want to address energetic, psychosocial, and spiritual needs.
- Are concerned with the invasiveness of typical biomedical care.

Which Health Conditions Prompt CAM Use?

Pain is by far the most common symptom prompting people to use CAM. Chronic pain is hard to treat with regular medical approaches. Of the 20 conditions for which people use CAM, 9 are associated with chronic pain, especially musculoskeletal and back pain (NCCAM, 2009). More than 60% of cancer patients use prayer, relaxation, meditation, and massage (Gansler, Kaw, Crammer, et al., 2008). Other conditions are anxiety, elevated cholesterol, the common cold, headache, and insomnia. Parents report using CAM for their children for pain, anxiety and stress disorders, enuresis, encopresis, sleep disorders, autonomic nervous system dysregulation, habitual disorders, attention and learning disorders, asthma, cancer, and diabetes (Barclay & Murata, 2008).

KnowledgeCheck 40-2
- How does holism incorporate spirituality?
- What type of person is most likely to use CAM?

 Go to Chapter 40, **Knowledge Check Response Sheet and Answers,** on the Student Resource Disk or DavisPlus at http://davisplus.fadavis.com/Wilkinson2

Critical Thinking 40-3

The NCCAM (2004a) findings identified people who have been hospitalized in the past year as more likely to use CAM. React to this finding. What do you think this finding suggests about traditional hospital care?

What Is Holistic Nursing?

Nursing, like medicine, has been fragmented by the demands of technology and the need for nurses to care for more, and sicker, patients. As we see in the case of Lisa Jackson and Mrs. Riddell ("Meet Your Patient"), nurses and patients feel the strain of hurried, disconnected, and unsatisfying contact. In fact, nurses often leave a workplace, and even the profession, when they feel that care is being dehumanized. Holistic nursing practice is a theory-based, relationship-centered, potent solution to such problems facing contemporary nursing and healthcare.

The American Holistic Nurses Association (AHNA) can be a major source of support for you. AHNA connects you with like-minded colleagues, provides opportunities for scholarly development, and offers an affiliation with others who have holistic nursing values.

Holistic Nursing Theory

Holistic nursing is not new. Principles of holistic nursing are found in Florence Nightingale's vision of health and nursing. She described the work of nursing as putting patients in the best condition for nature to act upon them, emphasizing touch and kindness along with the healing influences of fresh air, sunlight, warmth, quiet, and cleanliness. Nightingale thought of people as multidimensional and as a part of their environment. More recently, three prominent nursing theorists have contributed to the evolution of holistic nursing: Martha Rogers, Margaret Newman, and Jean Watson (Bright, 2002). See Chapter 8 if you wish to review these nursing theories.

- *In Rogers' view,* the environmental energy field is in constant and meaningful interaction with the human energy field. Nurses exert influence on these energy fields to effect change in health status.
- *Newman,* a student of Rogers, identified disease as disequilibrium, which stimulates the person toward growth and regaining wholeness. From a holistic perspective, disease is an inevitable part of the human condition and is necessary and beneficial for growth, adaptation, and maturation.
- *Watson's* theory of nursing identified caring as the primary focus of nursing. She described "authentic presencing," which facilitates the "caring moment" between the nurse and the patient.

Holistic Concepts

Among the concepts found in holistic nursing are meaning, therapeutic use of self, role modeling, and integrated lifestyle and practice.

Meaning. It is important to know the meaning inherent in a disease and its symptoms. **Meanings** are individual constructions that reflect a person's values, belief system, expectations, and the unique way in which the person experiences health and illness (Dossey & Keegan, 2008).

Therapeutic Use of Self. Conventional nursing education emphasizes the therapeutic use of self. Holistic nursing expands the therapeutic use of self to include awareness of the effects of *presence* and *intention* on the healing process. The presence of the nurse is an integral part of the patient's environment. The mutual energetic process that is present in every caring act enhances health outcomes.

Role Modeling. A holistic nurse role models healthy behaviors for her patients. Practically speaking, a holistic nurse understands that unless her own health is balanced, it is difficult to sustain the energy necessary to be a constructive presence and an effective practitioner.

Integrated Lifestyle and Practice. Healthful nutrition, sleep, rest, and relaxation benefit your function as a healthcare provider. In addition, a support network of like-minded colleagues serves as a resource.

What Healing Modalities Are Commonly Used?

A wide variety of alternative health traditions, practices, and therapies is available. Most require at least some advanced training, and often certification, before practice. NCCAM organizes CAM into five categories (Fig. 40-1), which we discuss in the remainder of this chapter. Figure 40-1 shows three examples in each of the following categories:

1. Alternative systems of medical practice
2. Mind–body interventions
3. Biologically based therapies
4. Manipulative and body-based methods
5. Energy therapies

In general, dietary, mind–body interventions (e.g., prayer), and relaxation techniques are used most. When categorized more specifically, the 10 CAM therapies most commonly used by adults in 2007 (excluding prayer) were as follows. They are listed from highest (17%) to lowest (1.8%):

Non-vitamin, non-mineral natural products
Deep breathing exercises
Meditation
Chiropractic or osteopathic manipulation
Massage
Yoga
Diet-based therapies
Progressive relaxation
Guided imagery
Homeopathic treatment (Barnes, Bloom, & Nahin, 2008)

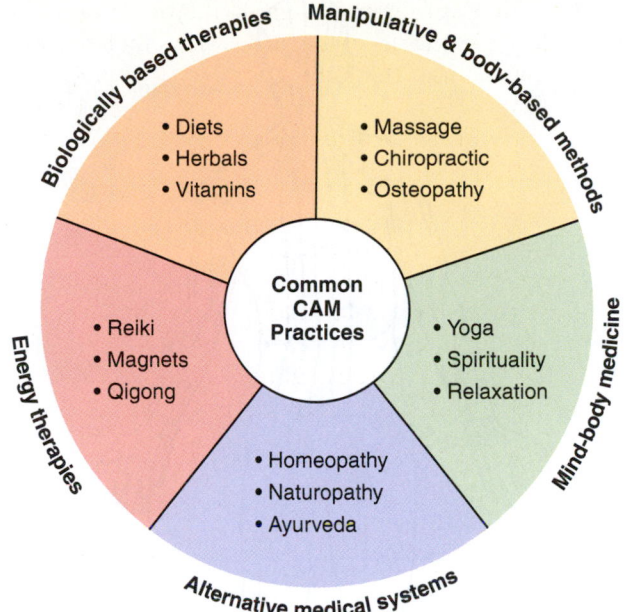

FIGURE 40-1 NCCAM organizes CAM into five categories.

Others have identified, from highest to lowest, the use of faith and spiritual healing, nutritional supplements, religious counseling and support groups, biofeedback, acupressure/acupuncture, and hypnosis. Notice that the most used are self-care therapies that do not require a visit to a practitioner.

KnowledgeCheck 40-3

- Identify the five categories of CAM identified by NCCAM.
- What are the most commonly used CAM therapies?

 Go to Chapter 40, **Knowledge Check Response Sheet and Answers,** on the Student Resource Disk or DavisPlus at http://davisplus.fadavis.com/Wilkinson2

Alternative Medical Systems

Alternative medical systems predate the traditional Western health system. They have been used for centuries throughout the world, and their use in Westernized countries is currently increasing. Alternative medical systems are built on complete systems of theory and practice, some vastly different from Western medicine. Examples include ayurveda, Chinese medicine, acupuncture, homeopathy, and naturopathy. Even though you may never use interventions from some of these alternative medical systems, you are likely to care for patients who use them; so it is a good idea to have an overview of the different approaches.

Ayurveda

Ayurveda, a healing system derived from ancient India, covers all aspects of health and wellness. Ayurveda's core belief is that a sense of harmony with nature and

our inner being produces health. Ayurveda attributes health to balance between three forces: creation (*kapha*), preservation (*pitta*), and destruction (*vata*). Imbalance between these forces leads to illness and disease. Humans have a physical and psychological constitution made up of those three forces. This constitution is known as a *dosha*.

The ideal *dosha* is *vata–kapha–pitta* in equal proportions. Imbalances may be caused by age; lifestyle; diet; too much or too little physical exertion; the seasons; or inadequate protection from weather, chemicals, or germs. During an ayurvedic consultation, the practitioner assesses the patient's *dosha* and uses diet, exercise, breathing, meditation, visualization, therapeutic massage, and herbs to treat illness and maintain health. Color therapy, sound therapy, and aromatherapy are also used to create balance.

✚ About one in five ayurvedic herbal remedies sold in stores and via the Internet contained potentially harmful levels of lead, mercury, and/or arsenic. Users of ayurvedic medicine may be at risk for heavy metal toxicity. The rate is 2 in 5 for rasa shastra medicines, which intentionally combine herbs with metals (Saper, Kales, Paquin, et al., 2004; Saper, Phillips, Sehgal, et al., 2008). Advise patients to avoid rasa shastra medicines and to purchase only ayurvedic products approved by ConsumerLab.com and the United States Pharmacopeia (USP).

Traditional Chinese Medicine

Chinese medicine is the oldest continuously practiced medicine in the world. **Traditional Chinese medicine (TCM)** is based on writings that originated between 200 B.C.E. and A.D.E. 200. TCM practitioners consider that each person has his own balance of *yin* and *yang* energies (complementary but opposing life forces) and the five elements of earth, water, wood, fire, and air/metal. If these balances are disturbed, ill health will result. Each element is associated with specific characteristics, such as color, smell, flavor, sound, and so on.

TCM practitioners base their therapies on information gathered from observing, asking questions, listening, and feeling the pulses. They may look closely at your face, mouth, tongue, skin, nails, and hair. They may listen to sounds you make through your voice, breathing, or digestive system. The characteristics of urine and stool are important. A major part of a diagnostic workup is the taking of pulses. TCM practitioners identify a large number of pulses and will almost certainly take three pulses (shallow, medium, and deep) at three points on each wrist.

They put this information together and determine your balance of *yin* and *yang*, of the five elements, and of the *qi* (sometimes written *chi*), or energy, flowing in your body. Finally, they will decide on the appropriate form of treatment. This will almost certainly involve lifestyle modifications and herbal remedies but may also involve massage, acupuncture, and **moxibustion** (the application of heat from burning the herb moxa at the acupuncture point). Your prescription, taken to a Chinese herbal pharmacy, will be written as weights of a variety of dried herbs. The herbalist will combine them and ask you to infuse and drink them as a tea. Research indicates that some TCM herbal remedies benefit people with asthma (Li & Brown, 2009).

Patients of various cultural backgrounds use TCM. Be sure to ask whether they are using any herbs or TCM products, because these may interact with prescribed therapies.

Acupuncture

Acupuncture is the penetration of the skin with thin metallic needles (Fig. 40-2) to stimulate anatomical structures of the body. Acupuncture was derived from TCM; however, some practitioners also use teachings from Japanese, Korean, and other medical systems. Energy, or *qi*, is believed to travel through the body along channels, known as *meridians*. A total of 72 meridians traverse the body (Fig. 40-3). Points along these meridians, known as *acupoints,* are centers of nerve and vascular tissue. The acupuncturist selects acupoints based on examination of the patient's pulses, appearance, tongue color, odors, and complaints. Stimulation of these points restores the flow of *qi* along the meridians.

Evidence. Acupuncture has been shown to be of value for nausea and dental pain. A systematic review concludes it is superior to medication in relieving chronic headache (Sun & Gan, 2008). Limited evidence suggests its potential for treating paralysis and numbness, depression, insomnia, and asthma. Scientific research does not fully explain how acupuncture works within the Western system of medicine (NCCAM, 2004b). However, it may cause physical responses in nerve cells, the pituitary gland, and the brain. These responses then cause the release of proteins, hormones, and brain chemicals that affect blood pressure and body temperature, boost immune system activity, and cause the body's natural analgesics (e.g., endorphins)

FIGURE 40-3 *Qi* travels through the body along 72 meridians. Acupuncture stimulates points along these meridians to restore health.

to be released (National Institutes of Health [NIH], n.d.). A 1997 NIH report concluded there was "sufficient evidence of acupuncture's value to expand its use into conventional medicine and to encourage further studies of its physiology and clinical value" (p. 6).

Homeopathy

Homeopathy is a complete system of medical theory and practice. It was developed in the 5th century B.C.E. by Hippocrates, the famous Greek physician. It was rediscovered in the late 18th century by Dr. Samuel Hahnemann. Homeopathy is based on an understanding of how the body heals itself and an acceptance that all symptoms represent the body's attempt to restore itself to health. The practice of homeopathy is based on the following three principles:

- *The law of similars,* or "like cures like." The substance that would cause the patient's symptoms in a healthy person is the substance that is most likely to produce a curative response in the patient who already has the symptoms.
- *The law of minimum dose.* Hahnemann developed his theory as a result of his own experience with the malaria treatment quinine, which in large doses causes

FIGURE 40-2 Acupuncture uses thin metallic needles to stimulate acupoints to restore the flow of *qi.*

symptoms of the disease in healthy individuals. He reasoned that if large doses can simulate disease, minute doses would stimulate the body's defenses against that disease. To limit side effects, practitioners use the smallest dose possible. Medicines are prepared by repeatedly diluting them in water or alcohol and mixing by **succussion**, a form of vigorous shaking. Hahnemann hypothesized that vigorous shaking potentiated the remedy's healing effect. Recent discoveries in quantum physics about the transfer of energy at the subatomic level appear to support the idea that succussion increases the energy of particles.

- *The single remedy.* This principle guides the homeopathic practitioner to select one remedy that encompasses the totality of the person's symptoms and constitutional characteristics. Thus, a homeopathic medication is person-specific rather than disease-specific.

One of the most frequently used homeopathic treatments is Rescue Remedy—a treatment derived from flower essences. It is believed to help alleviate stress.

Evidence. Overall, clinical trial results are contradictory, and systematic reviews have not definitively proven homeopathy treatment to be effective for any medical condition (NCCAM, 2004b).

Naturopathy

Naturopathic medicine is a system of healing based on the healing power of nature. Health is the outcome of understanding nature and allowing the body to heal itself. Diseases and aging result from ignoring the laws of nature. The principle belief behind naturopathy is that nature and each living being have the innate ability to establish, maintain, and restore health. Naturopathic practitioners support the ability of the body to heal itself through nutrition and lifestyle counseling, dietary supplements, medicinal plants, exercise, massage, and joint manipulation. Education and training in naturopathy vary widely.

Evidence. There is virtually no research on naturopathy as a complete system, although a few studies have been published on the use of herbs when used as a naturopathic treatment. For example, cranberry juice and cranberry tablets have been shown to decrease frequency of urinary tract infections (Di Martino, Agniel, David, et al., 2006; Stothers, 2002).

KnowledgeCheck 40-4

Which of the alternative systems of medical practice:
- Is based on the philosophy of restoring balance?
- Involves stimulation of points along meridians to restore *qi* flow?
- Involves medications given in very small doses?

 Go to Chapter 40, **Knowledge Check Response Sheet and Answers,** on the Student Resource Disk or DavisPlus at http://davisplus.fadavis.com/Wilkinson2

Mind–Body Interventions

Think back to the last time you experienced heartbreak—perhaps it resulted from the end of a relationship, the death of a loved one, or the realization that you cannot achieve something you aspired to. What kind of physical sensation did you experience? Most people report feeling physically exhausted, with tremors or even a painful feeling in the chest. This is an example of an emotion generating a physical sensation. **Mind–body therapies** are based on awareness of the unity of the mind and body and on the ability of social, familial, and economic factors to affect all aspects of health and illness. Interventions target the patient's mood and reaction to stress to enhance health. Illness is viewed as an opportunity for personal growth, and healthcare providers are thought of as guides in this process. Some mind–body techniques considered CAM have become a part of conventional healthcare (e.g., biofeedback and support groups). Several widely known practices are discussed in the sections that follow. In this section, we discuss prayer, meditation, imagery, humor, music therapy, and yoga.

Evidence. Strong evidence suggests that mind–body therapies combined with biofeedback may be the most effective CAM for migraine and tension headaches. They also appear to reduce low back pain and the pain of arthritis, as well as reducing pain, nausea, and vomiting for people with cancer. For older adults, relaxation exercises hold promise in treating depression, anxiety, and sleep disturbances (Hart, 2008; Meeks, Wetherell, Irwin, et al., 2007). Mind–body approaches have low emotional and physical risk, and most can be taught easily.

Prayer

Prayer, a dialogue with a spiritual being, is probably the most commonly used CAM modality. Prayer exists in all religions and all forms of spirituality, and may take the form of recited prose, meditation, or personal requests. People may pray for themselves or they may make a request on behalf of another.

Evidence. Studies have found that 35% to 45% of respondents used prayer for health concerns. Most prayed for wellness, but some also prayed about specific medical conditions. Individuals older than age of 33 and those with chronic health concerns were more likely to pray. Although prayer resulted in a high degree of satisfaction, only 11% of the participants informed their primary care provider of their use of prayer (McCaffrey, Eisenberg, Legedza, et al., 2004). Chapter 14 further discusses prayer and provides examples of prayers across many faiths, if you would like to review that information.

Meditation

Meditation uses practices that help to quiet and focus the mind and induce relaxation. There are two major forms of meditation: concentration meditation and mindfulness meditation. The two types are distinguished by their relationship to the object of meditation. In *concentration meditation*, the focus is on the breath, a sound *(mantra)*, or an object (e.g., a flower). *Mindfulness meditation* involves directing attention to thoughts, feelings, and sensations—opening up to all stimuli. Meditation can be practiced alone or with a group. Teaching and guidance from an experienced meditation teacher help establish effective practice.

Meditation is often incorporated into healing systems, such as ayurveda and even traditional Western medicine. Meditating for as little as 20 minutes per day can have positive effects on health. People who meditate report that they feel calmer, more focused, and more relaxed. Hospitalized patients may find that meditation helps control stress and promote relaxation. Health benefits include lowered blood pressure and metabolic changes that correlate with reduction in the effects of stress. To facilitate meditation, assist patients to a comfortable position, and create a quiet pleasant environment free of interruptions.

Evidence. Research demonstrates positive effects on various disease states (e.g., diabetes, asthma, fibromyalgia, premenstrual syndrome, Crohn's disease, psoriasis, cancer, and chronic pain) (Bright, 2002). Moreover, research suggests possible linkages among positive emotional states, localized brain responses, and improved immune function (Cohen, Doyle, Turner, et al., 2003; Smith & Nicholson, 2001). Small preliminary trials of Zen and Buddhist Insight meditation suggest that meditation may help reduce the cognitive decline of normal aging (NIH, 2009). At present, there is not enough evidence available from which to draw conclusions on the effects of meditation; however, analysis of evidence supports the value of future research in this area (Ospina, Bond, Karkhaneh, et al., 2007).

Imagery

Imagery, also known as *visualization,* uses the imagination to create a desired event or scenario. A successful visualization incorporates all the senses. As a nurse, you can use imagery to enhance your own energy state and performance. Visualizing yourself providing good care may increase your confidence and reduce stress. You may also use imagery with patients. For example, if you are caring for a patient experiencing pain and anxiety, ask the patient to imagine lying comfortably in the sun in a restful meadow. Successful visualization includes imagining sights, sounds, tastes, and feelings of warmth and comfort. Often this imagery allows patients to relax and sleep. You may offer suggestions to patients or recommend guided visualization tapes.

Evidence. Imagery has been used successfully to reduce pain, improve surgical outcomes, increase healing of joint injuries, enhance immune system function, reduce asthma symptoms, enhance breast milk production, decrease anxiety, and improve outlook among

patients with chronic illness (Astin, 2004; Bright, 2002; Sloman, 1995). The consistent use of imagery has also been shown to improve the performance of athletes.

Humor

Some hospitals have incorporated humor into their therapeutic strategies, for example, by making humorous literature, cartoons, and videos available to patients.

Evidence. Reading and telling jokes, viewing funny movies, and simply appreciating the humor of situations all help release tension and increase coping abilities (Johnson, 2002; Phipps, 2002). Laughter releases endorphins and relieves feelings of stress (Cousins, 1979). Laughter increases in pulse, respirations, muscle tension, and oxygenation; relaxation follows laughter. Despite a few positive studies, research has yet to prove that laughter has a measurable, positive effect on illness or injury.

Music Therapy

Music therapy is more than just listening to music to relax or perhaps energize you. Music therapy is more than self-help. **Music therapy** is the evidence-based use of music interventions within a therapeutic relationship to achieve individualized goals. It is relatively risk-free, but requires a credentialed professional who has completed an approved music therapy program. Music therapy can be designed to promote wellness, release emotions, manage stress, relieve pain, improve communication, and promote physical rehabilitation. It has been used to keep Alzheimer's patients calm and improve their memories; and it can also help depressed patients express their feelings. Music can activate the relaxation response (American Music Therapy Association, n.d.; Magill & Berenson, 2008). This in turn promotes deep breathing, lowers heart rate and blood pressure, reduces muscle tension, reduces stress, promotes better sleep, and relieves physical pain.

Patients do not need to have any musical ability to benefit from music therapy. This therapy is growing in acceptance in traditional medicine. When it meets the criteria for "active treatment" (e.g., is prescribed by a physician with a goal of improving functioning), Medicare will reimburse for music therapy under benefits for Partial Hospitalization Programs.

Yoga

Yoga is a 5000-year-old traditional art, science, and philosophy with origins in ancient Indian philosophy. The philosophy emphasizes a lifestyle of awareness, integrity, and compassion. Though many people practice yoga as exercise, it is designed to integrate body, mind, and spirit. Yoga typically combines physical postures, breathing techniques, and meditation or relaxation.

Popular images of yoga focus on postures, or *asanas,* that increase flexibility, strength, body alignment, stamina, balance, and concentration (Fig. 40-4). But the *asanas* are part of a practice intended to regulate the life force (called *prana* in the Hindu language) through breathing, meditation, reading sacred scriptures, and participating in a community of students who seek the teaching of yogi masters. As a result, many people classify yoga as an alternative medical system, although NCCAM lists as a mind-body medicine. The ultimate goal of yoga is to awaken the spiritual identity and experience happiness. A person of any age may practice yoga individually or as part of a group.

Yoga is useful for some types of chronic pain. However, because yoga can be physically rigorous, it has the potential to be harmful in chronic pain.

Evidence. One high-quality study found a 6-week program of *viniyoga* yoga therapy to be slightly better than exercise and moderately better than a self-care education for relief of chronic low-back pain (Sherman, Cherkin, Erro, et al., 2005). There is some evidence of positive effects for fatigue from multiple sclerosis, and for chronic insomnia (NIH, 2009).

Hypnosis

Hypnosis, another mind-body therapy, is a trance-like state characterized by relaxed brain waves, hypersuggestibility, and heightened imagination. A certified hypnotherapist may induce the state, or people can learn self-hypnosis. Although it is not clear how they work, hypnosis and self-hypnosis have been used to promote relaxation, weight loss, and smoking cessation and to suppress various symptoms (e.g., anxiety, pain). It has been used to modify pain in childbirth and as an adjunct to, or in place of, anesthesia for surgery.

Some myths about hypnosis have developed from the use of hypnosis for entertainment, as a stage act. The following are true statements about hypnosis (Mayo Clinic, 2007):

- You do not surrender your free will or lose your personality under hypnosis. It is a heightened state of concentration and focused attention.
- The hypnotherapist does not control you. You do hypnosis voluntarily for yourself. The hypnotherapist is merely a guide or facilitator.

- Under hypnosis, most people do not lose consciousness or have amnesia.
- You cannot be put under hypnosis against your will. Successful hypnosis depends on your willingness to experience it.

Evidence. There is some evidence to support the effectiveness of hypnosis (e.g., Jensen & Patterson, 2006; Lang, Berbaum, Faintuch, et al., 2006) and it is widely used in traditional psychiatric care. However, it is still not completely accepted in traditional Western medicine.

Biofeedback

Biofeedback, a mind-body therapy, is a technique by which some people can learn voluntary control over involuntary activities, such as heart rate. Biofeedback techniques use electronic instruments to measure body functions such as brain activity, blood pressure, muscle tension, heart rate, skin temperature, and sweat gland activity. Visual or auditory cues provide information to the patient in the form of sound or light. For example, as the heart rate slows, the feedback sound might become quieter. Immediate feedback helps the person become aware of and learn how to voluntarily control certain physiological responses, such as those produced by stress. We do not understand how people use the feedback to learn control, but in general it teaches them to achieve a state of relaxation in which the parasympathetic nervous system dominates.

Biofeedback practitioners require special training, and most are credentialed. A typical biofeedback session lasts 30 to 60 minutes. Biofeedback is generally considered safe, but should usually not be used by those with a major mental health disorder. Patients with diabetes or who are taking medications, such as insulin, should talk to their primary care provider before using biofeedback.

Evidence. Some traditional medical practitioners have been using biofeedback for many years. However, it is not completely accepted, even though there is evidence to support its effectiveness for certain purposes. For example, it has been used effectively for migraine headaches, to facilitate functioning and healing in various

FIGURE 40-4 Yoga combines physical postures, breathing techniques, and meditation or relaxation to regulate the life force.

anorectal disorders, to treat children with bladder dysfunction, and to treat attention deficit/hyperactivity disorder (Chiarioni, Whitehead, Pezza, et al., 2006; Friel, 2007; NIH, 2009; Yagci, Kibar, Akay, et al., 2005).

CriticalThinking 40-4

- Do you believe yoga is a mind–body intervention or an alternative system of healthcare?
- Which, if any of the alternative health systems or mind–body interventions would you be most comfortable facilitating for a patient?

Biologically Based Therapies

Biologically based therapies use substances found in nature, such as food, herbs, vitamins, and aromatherapy. These therapies are readily available and are often practiced as self-care measures and in conjunction with traditional healthcare and other CAM. For current information on the safety of particular biologically based products, check the "Dietary Supplements: Warnings and Safety Information" section on the U.S. Food and Drug Association (FDA) Web site, and the NCCAM Web site, respectively, at

 www.fda.gov/Food/DietarySupplements/Alerts/default.htm and www.nccam.nih.gov/news/alerts

A dietary supplement is a product that contains a dietary ingredient *intended to supplement the diet.* For example, stevia (a herb) is used as a sugar substitute to replace artificial sweeteners, which some believe are detrimental to health. However, in addition to supplementing the diet, people also take dietary supplements to prevent or treat diseases and injuries. Dietary ingredients may be herbal or nonherbal. They include vitamins, minerals, herbs or other plants; amino acids; and substances such as enzymes, organ tissues, glandulars, and metabolites.

Dietary supplements occur in many forms, such as tablets, capsules, softgels, gelcaps, liquids, or powders. A substantial number of older adults take multiple prescription drugs as well as multiple dietary supplements (Nahin, Pecha, Welmerink, et al., 2009), so be sure to include questions about dietary supplements in your assessments.

In the United States, the U.S. Food and Drug Administration (FDA) regulates biologically based therapies (e.g., dietary supplements, vitamins), and is developing guidelines for good manufacturing practices (GMPs). However, dosage and manufacturing processes are not standardized. The Federal Trade Commission monitors dietary supplements for truth in advertising. At present, it is difficult to know what dosage you are obtaining from a product, and safety cannot always be guaranteed.

Evidence. No biologically based therapy has been proven safe and effective for older adults in treating sleep problems, depression, and anxiety (Meeks, Wetherell,

Irwin, et al., 2007). In 2007, by far the most popular natural product used by adults was fish oil/omega-3 fatty acids. Also among the top 10, in order of frequency, were glucosamine, echinacea, flaxseed oil, combination herb pills, ginkgo biloba, chondroitin, garlic supplements, and coenzyme Q-10 (Barnes, Bloom, & Nahin, 2008). Some of these are discussed in the following sections.

Dietary Therapies

Dietary therapies are used in traditional healthcare as well as with CAM. For example, a low-sodium diet is part of the treatment plan for patients with hypertension. Dietary modifications may also be part of the treatment in alternative health systems. For example, in ayurvedic medicine, a patient with a *pitta dosha* is represented by the element of fire. Foods that are "cool" in nature are recommended to balance the patient's "fiery" nature. Traditional Chinese medicine also uses diet to treat disease. In TCM, illness results when there is an excess of wind, cold, fire, summer heat, dampness, or dryness. Foods that have opposite qualities are used to counteract these excesses. Naturopathy (previously discussed) stresses the importance of pure food (unprocessed), recommending generous servings of raw food to prevent disease and aging.

Evidence. Mainstream research has repeatedly demonstrated that as foods have become more processed, the incidence of chronic disease has increased. This is an example of a CAM approach that has been incorporated into traditional healthcare.

Herbal Products

People have used herbal preparations since the beginning of time. In fact, many prescription medications in use today are derived from herbs. Herbal products are often viewed as "natural" and, therefore, are sought out by people who wish to avoid exposure to chemicals. The sections that follow provide some evidence-based information about how people use herbal products:

Who Uses Herbs?

One study concluded that nearly one in five people in the United States report using an herb for health promotion or to treat a health condition. More than half of them did not disclose this to their conventional medical professional. People who use herbs tend to have the following characteristics (Gardiner, Graham, Legedza, et al., 2007; NCCAM, 2007):

- Age 45–64 years
- Uninsured
- Female
- Have a higher education
- Have a slightly higher income
- Live in the West or in a metropolitan area
- Self-identified as "non-Hispanic other"
- Have a specific disease, such as breast cancer

- Also use prescription or over-the-counter (OTC) medications. In fact, 84% of those who used herbs also used an OTC medication in the prior 12 months; 72% also used prescription medications.

Which Herbs Are Used Most?

One study found that among adults who use herbs, the following are mentioned most often (Gardiner, Graham, Legedza, et al., 2007): 41% used echinacea, 25% used ginseng, 22% used ginkgo, and 20% used garlic. These are among the top 10 natural products identified by Barnes, Bloom, and Nahin (2008).

Why Are Herbs Used?

Consumers state their primary reason for using herbal supplements is to promote overall health and wellness. However, they also report using them to improve performance and energy, treat and prevent illnesses (e.g., colds and flu), and alleviate depression. Specific conditions for which people used herbs reported in a recent study were:

Head or chest cold—30%
Musculoskeletal conditions—16%
Stomach or intestinal illness—11% (Gardiner, Graham, Legedza, et al., 2007)

What Risks Are Associated with Herb Use?

Although herbs are popular, they are not risk-free. Table 40-1 presents some of the pros and cons associated with herb use. The health benefits include lowered blood pressure and metabolic changes that correlate with reduction in the effects of stress. The following are some associated risks (most apply in at least some degree to all biologically based therapies):

- **Lack of Standardization.** One risk is that when you buy a product, you do not know for sure what you are getting. The FDA regulates herbs as dietary supplements,

so the manufacturing standards are not as strict as for medications. Different products may contain different amounts of the active ingredient, or they may even contain harmful contaminants. Many countries are scrutinizing herbal therapy intensely. Because most herbs contain several components, it is difficult to study their pharmacology. In addition, herbs may change based on the soil and weather conditions in which they grow.
- **Lack of a Formulary.** In some countries (e.g., Germany), a health commission has reviewed the safety and efficacy of many herbs and created a monograph or formulary detailing their findings. There is not yet a national formulary in the United States, but the United States Food and Drug Administration (FDA) has begun to investigate how to study and better regulate herbal products.
- **Interaction with Other Medications.** Many herbs are known to interact with medications and to adversely affect some disease processes (e.g., to aggravate hypertension) or lab results. For example:
  - Ginkgo extract is reported to inhibit platelet aggregation, and several cases have been reported of increased bleeding when used with anticoagulant drugs.
  - St. John's wort, garlic, glucosamine, ginseng, saw palmetto, soy, valerian, and yohimbe all either inhibit or potentiate the action of some prescription drugs.
- **Toxicity.** In addition to interacting with other drugs, some herbal supplements can be toxic. Misidentification, contamination, and adulteration may contribute to this, but other toxicities may result from the products themselves. For example, in 2001, extracts of kava were associated with fulminant (i.e., sudden, severe) liver failure. More recently, the FDA reinstituted a ban on the sale of ephedra after it was shown to be associated with an increased risk of adverse events (NCCAM, 2007).

Table 40-1 ➤ The Pros and Cons of Herbs		
ISSUE	**PRO**	**CON**
Safety	Many herbs are relatively safe.	Herbal products are not regulated by the FDA as medications so their dosage and safety cannot be guaranteed.
Effectiveness	Numerous pharmaceuticals have been derived from herbs (e.g., aspirin, digoxin, morphine).	Unregulated products may claim benefits they do not offer. The amount of active ingredient in products varies.
Cost	Herbs are readily available at health food stores; some (but not all) are less expensive than a medication prescribed for the same purpose. The patient does not need to pay for a visit to a medical care provider, however.	Inappropriate use of herbs may actually increase healthcare costs if they prove to be ineffective or harmful.
Convenience	Readily available without a prescription.	May discourage clients from seeking care from a practitioner when they truly need it.
Privacy Concerns	Allows clients to treat concerns privately.	May discourage clients from seeking care when they truly need it.

Because herbal products are readily available and widely used, you need to question your patients about their use. Advise patients to buy from reputable sources and seek advice from a credentialed practitioner to incorporate herbs into their care. The National Center for Complementary and Alternative Medicine (NCCAM) offers extensive material on herbal products for healthcare consumers and professionals, as do the Memorial Sloan-Kettering Cancer Center in New York City and the U.S. National Library of Medicine. To see these Web sites,

Go to Chapter 40, **Resources for Caregivers and Healthcare Professionals,** on the Student Resource Disk or DavisPlus at http://davisplus.fadavis.com/Wilkinson2

Evidence Base for Herbs. Although many studies have been done, the lack of consistently prepared and reliable herbal products has made it difficult to conduct reliable research on safety and effectiveness. However, the FDA and NCCAM have recently created a Botanical Review Team to provide direction to researchers, and studies have concluded or are in progress (NCCAM, 2007). If you would like to see some examples of research that have been done with various uses of specific herbs (e.g., echinacea for colds),

Go to Chapter 40, **ESG Table 40-1, Effectiveness and Safety of Specific Herbs—Examples of Evidence,** on the Student Resource Disk or DavisPlus at http://davisplus. fadavis.com/Wilkinson2

Aromatherapy

Herbs are used in ways other than as dietary therapies. **Aromatherapy** is the use of essential oils, which are concentrated extracts of roots, leaves, or blossoms, to enhance physical and mental well-being. It is one of the fastest growing CAM therapies. Essential oils are either inhaled; used as massage oils; or put into bath water, lotions, or dressings. Researchers believe the scent of essential oils activates the amygdala and hippocampus, the storage site for emotions and memories (Buckle, 2002).

People use aromatherapy for stress reduction, mood regulation, sleep enhancement, immune support, first aid, enhanced energy, reduction of pain, and accelerated wound recovery. Box 40-2 describes a number of commonly used aromatherapies.

Evidence. As with many biologically based therapies, research results are mixed (National Cancer Institute, last updated March 26, 2010; Stirling, Raab, Alder, et al., 2007; Woolard, Tatham, Barker, et al., 2007). Research is currently underway at several major universities on the effects of essential oils on inflammation, infection, depression, and dementia, as well as for alleviating side effects resulting from radiation treatment.

- Animal studies demonstrate the calming or energizing effects of essential oils, and their effects on behavior and immune responses.

BOX 40-2 ■ Common Aromatherapy Treatments

- *Basil:* Used to improve concentration, aid digestion, and relieve stress.
- *Eucalyptus:* Protects against respiratory problems, such as coughs, colds, and asthma; believed to boost the immune system and relieve muscle tension.
- *Ylang ylang:* Used to induce relaxation and reduce muscle tension.
- *Geranium:* Used to balance hormones in women and improve skin clarity. Can be both relaxing and uplifting.
- *Peppermint:* Extremely effective in treating digestive disorders, such as flatulence, nausea, and heartburn. A natural painkiller, peppermint can help treat headaches and general muscular aches. It also helps relieve morning sickness.
- *Lavender:* Used to induce relaxation and for superficial wounds, burns, and skin care.
- *Lemon:* An excellent essential oil for treating oily skin, acne, sluggish circulation, and digestive disorders. It is said to be emotionally uplifting, with a zingy, fresh scent. It is used to treat insomnia and nightmares. It is a diuretic and can be used in a spray as a disinfectant.
- *Clary sage:* A balancing oil that can lift depression. It is calming, restores tranquility, and can lower blood pressure.
- *Tea tree:* Used to treat fungal infections and clear the skin.
- *Chamomile:* Used to induce relaxation, reduce muscle tension, and promote sleep.
- *Rosemary:* Used for mental stimulation and stimulation of the digestive and immune systems.

- Clinical trials of aromatherapy are mixed. A few early studies indicate it may improve symptoms of nausea or pain and lower blood pressure, pulse, and respiratory rates in patients with cancer. One study found essential oils did not reduce anxiety in perioperative patients. Other than allergic reactions, very few risks have been found.

Topical Application of Herbs

Aloe vera is a base for nutritional drinks, moisturizers, lotions, and cosmetics. It is thought to have antioxidant and anti-inflammatory properties. Topical applications may help heal wounds, burns, and skin infections. Advise patients to not take aloe vera orally due to possible adverse effects and inconclusive clinical data. The FDA has ruled that it is not a safe stimulant laxative (NCCAM, 2006c; FDA, 2002).

Evidence. Some anecdotal data suggest that oral use of aloe vera can lower blood glucose; however, studies have not supported claims for its use in treating constipation, diabetes mellitus, and elevated lipid profiles. There is some evidence that it is effective in healing skin eruptions of psoriasis, genital herpes, and acne (Vogler

& Ernst, 1999). There is no evidence to support its use for treating minor burns, but the practice is not harmful (Sego, 2008).

Nonherbal Dietary Supplements

Recall that dietary supplements can be herbal and nonherbal. **Nonherbal dietary supplements** are those that are not plant products. Examples include hormones, probiotics, vitamins, and minerals.

Bioidentical Hormones

So-called **bioidentical hormones** are chemically compounded from wild yams and soy and customized for each person. Compounded bioidenticals are available by prescription only, but are not clearly classified as drugs and are not approved by the FDA. Manufactured bioidenticals do have FDA approval for use in treating postmenopausal symptoms. They are not intended to "replace" hormones in a woman's body (The North American Menopause Society [NAMS], 2007). Advertisements claim that they have anti-aging properties; allow your brain to work better; and defend against cancer, heart attack, and Alzheimer's disease. Some women report that these hormones relieve the hot flushes and night sweats associated with menopause. However, there is no evidence base for these claims (Lake, 2007). You should educate women who ask about bioidenticals, and if they insist on trying them, urge them to have regular physical exams, Pap tests, and mammograms.

Probiotics

Probiotics are live bacteria or yeasts that, when taken in sufficient amounts, have health benefits. They are found in foods such as yoghurt and dietary supplements. Hundreds of species of microbes live in the human intestines and nearly all are "good" (normal flora). The key is keeping them all in balance. Significant imbalance can lead to compromised health. Supplementing the diet with specific microorganisms (e.g., *Lactobacillus*) may be a cost-effective way to prevent diseases. For example, they are known to contribute to bowel regularity, they may alleviate symptoms of diarrhea and vaginitis, and may also help combat *Clostridium difficile* infections in patients taking antibiotics (Hickson, D'Souza, Muthu, et al., 2007).

As with herbs, there is little regulation and little attention has been paid to the quality of probiotics. Ongoing research is needed to resolve the following problems (NCCAM, 2007):

- When you buy a probiotic, you do not know for sure whether (and how long) the bacteria will live and be active.
- It is difficult to know for certain types and number of bacteria in the product and whether they are present in the recommended numbers.
- You do not know, for the different bacteria, how long they live under different storage conditions and in different types of product.

- You do not know exactly what protection the product will give you.

Teach patients that up to 25% of those who take probiotics will suffer diarrhea as a side effect. Teach patients how to read probiotic labels, and urge them to use reputable sources for their information. Remind them to check expiration dates. Probiotics are contraindicated for patients who are immunosuppressed and those taking certain drugs.

Vitamins and Minerals

Vitamin therapy, including minerals, is widely used. In fact, many people consider it a nutritional "insurance policy." Vitamin therapy ranges from taking a daily multivitamin to a full megavitamin regimen. Vitamin therapy receives mixed reviews. For example, there is widespread use of antioxidants (beta-carotene, vitamin C, and vitamin E) in efforts to limit heart disease and cancer, but there is little evidence to support megavitamin therapy for those purposes. Certainly people who do not eat a balanced diet should be advised to take a daily multivitamin so that they receive the recommended daily amounts (see Chapter 26 to review RDAs). This is an area of active research, so you can anticipate learning of new studies on a regular basis. For examples of single studies involving the use of vitamins and minerals for specific purposes,

Go to Chapter 40, **ESG Table 40-2, Individual Vitamins and Minerals—Examples of Evidence,** on the Student Resource Disk or DavisPlus at http://davisplus.fadavis.com/Wilkinson2

Other Nonherbal Biologically Based Products

The dietary supplements included in this section include fatty acids, hormones, and honey.

- **Fish Oil/Omega-3 Fatty Acids.** This is by far the most commonly used product reported by NCCAM. Dietary sources of omega-3 fatty acids include fish oil and certain plant/nut oils. Evidence from several studies suggests that fish oil slows the progress of atherosclerosis ("hardening of the arteries"), lowers the blood pressure, and may help prevent heart disease and abnormal heart rhythms. However, high doses may increase the risk of bleeding. Although flaxseed oil contains an essential fatty acid, its benefits are not the same as those of fish oil/omega-3 (Mayo Clinic, 2008).
- **Honey.** Over-the-counter cough medications are not safe for children younger than 4 years old. Their safety and effectiveness for children ages 5 through 11 years are still in question. At least one study has found buckwheat honey to be slightly superior to dextromethorphan in relieving cough frequency and severity in children (Paul, Beiler, McMonagle, et al., 2007). Advise parents not to give honey to children younger than one year of age because it has definitively been linked to infant botulism in laboratory and epidemiological studies.

■ **Melatonin.** Melatonin is a naturally occurring hormone found in animals (e.g., humans), and algae, but is usually made synthetically. Melatonin is a powerful antioxidant and is thought to control the circadian pacemaker and promote sleep. Animal studies suggest it may have some antitumor effects. People use melatonin to treat insomnia, jet lag, and cancer.

Evidence. As with herbs, study results are mixed for melatonin. The following are some research examples:

■ Melatonin appears to be relatively safe and effective as a sleep aid for people with uncomplicated sleep disorders and in alleviating jet lag that occurs from crossing multiple time zones (Herxheimer & Petrie, 2002).
■ In vitro and animal studies demonstrate antiproliferative effects on cancer cells. Clinical trials in patients with solid tumors suggest improvements in quality of life and survival (Memorial Sloan-Kettering Cancer Center, n.d.).
■ Evidence does not support the role of melatonin in managing dementia (Jansen, Forbes, Duncan, et al., 2006).
■ Side effects are rare, but may include headache, hypothermia, pruritus, abdominal cramping, elevated blood pressure, and tachycardia. Melatonin may interact with other medications (Memorial Sloan-Kettering Cancer Center, n.d.). Clients should consult their primary care provider before taking it.

KnowledgeCheck 40-5

■ Compare and contrast mind–body and biologically based therapies.
■ Identify at least four CAM interventions or therapies that could be easily practiced by a patient confined to bed.

 Go to Chapter 40, **Knowledge Check Response Sheet and Answers,** on the Student Resource Disk or DavisPlus at http://davisplus.fadavis.com/Wilkinson2

Manipulative and Body-Based Methods

Manipulative and body-based therapies focus on manipulating and moving the body to improve health. Several types of therapies are widely practiced. We discuss the most common therapies in the sections that follow: chiropractic, massage, and osteopathy.

Chiropractic

Chiropractic has recently come to be considered a conventional medical technique. It is an alternative medical system in that it takes a different approach from standard medicine in treating health problems. **Chiropractic** focuses on the relationship between the structure (mainly the spine) and the function of the human body. A basic concept is that the body has a powerful self-healing ability. The premise of chiropractic is that disease is caused by irritation of the nervous system. A total of 31 pairs of spinal nerves branch off the spinal cord to innervate all the organs in the body. *Subluxation* (loss of proper position or motion in a joint) of the vertebrae impinges on these nerves and leads to disease. Manipulation of body structures, especially the spinal column, realigns the vertebrae to allow nerve impulses to flow without interruption, thereby improving health. Realignment is referred to as an *adjustment*.

Chiropractors use health history, x-ray studies, and examination of the spine and posture to make a diagnosis. They treat primarily by performing adjustments; however, they may also use ice, heat, ultrasound, electrical stimulation, herbs, and nutritional supplements.

Evidence. Evidence indicates that spinal manipulation is generally safe and as effective as conventional treatments for low-back pain, neck pain, and headaches. Clinical trials have found no evidence that it is effective for asthma, hypertension, or dysmenorrhea (NCCAM, 2008b).

Massage

Massage involves the manipulation of muscles and other soft tissues. It is one of the oldest forms of healing. Massage works to control stress, improve mobility, and relieve pain in a number of ways: by promoting muscle relaxation, by increasing lymphatic circulation and thereby reducing inflammation, by breaking up scar tissue and adhesions, by promoting blood flow through the muscles, by enhancing parasympathetic nervous activity, and by promoting drainage of sinus fluids (Benjamin, 2010; Hart, 2008). Healthcare providers, family members, and friends can perform **simple massage. Therapeutic massage,** such as the following examples, is administered by certified therapists.

Swedish massage is used to induce relaxation and restore flexibility. It consists of five basic strokes: *effleurage* (touching lightly, with a gliding long stroke), *petrissage* (kneading for intensive work in small areas), *tapotement* (tapping with the fingertips), *vibration* (shaking), and *friction* (rubbing).

Sports massage is a specialized form of Swedish massage that facilitates maximum physical performance. Pressure, movement, and cross-fiber massage in a vigorous manner are used to warm up athletes before events, to relieve soreness after exertion, and to help repair athletic injuries.

Myofascial release restores balance, alignment, and mobility to the body by releasing tension in the soft connective fasciae through trigger point release, strumming, and muscle stretching. The therapist applies light pressure and stretching, but not to the point of pain. However, if the muscles are holding a great deal of tension and stress, myofascial release can be quite intense. It may produce more long-lasting effects than other forms of massage because fasciae surround, support, and interweave every muscle, organ, and bone in the body.

Rolfing is similar to myofascial release but is generally thought of as more intense. It is a type of deep tissue massage, also called structural integration. The practitioner manipulates connective tissue to allow the body to align itself so it is vertical in the field of gravity. Rolfing considers the effect of structure and gravity on human function, and patients may need to re-learn how to sit, stand, walk, and do daily activities. People get rolfed to relieve chronic pain, improve flexibility and posture, release emotional trauma, and strengthen the body–mind connection.

Shiatsu massage is a finger-pressure method that balances the energy force in the body. The therapist applies pressure to specific points that lie along energy meridians, the same meridian points used in acupuncture. Meridian points are thought to be areas of energy concentration that influence organ and neuromuscular functioning.

Reflexology is a massage technique that applies pressure to the feet (or sometimes the hands and ears) to promote unblocking a terminal nerve to improve function along that nerve pathway. Nerve endings on the hands and feet have been identified that relate to every structure of the body. Manipulating the reflex zones is thought to stimulate the same energy balancing that occurs when acupuncture points are used.

Although massage is relaxing, it is not advisable for everyone. People with a history of phlebitis or vascular disorders should not receive deep muscle massage because of the risk of dislodging a clot and causing an embolus (e.g., in the heart or a lung). As a nurse, you can provide simple massage (e.g., a back rub), but complex forms of massage require special training to perform. Massage therapists are licensed or credentialed in many states.

Evidence. Scientific research is limited, but there is some evidence to support massage therapy. Conclusions generally cannot be drawn about its effectiveness for specific health conditions (NCCAM, 2006d). The following are a few single studies regarding various uses of massage:

- Massage is more effective for pain management when performed by trained massage therapists with many years of experience (Chou & Huffman, 2007).
- There is insufficient evidence to conclude that massage and touch interventions are effective for anxiety, cognitive decline, and other problems associated with dementia (Hansen, Jorgensen, & Ortenblad, 2006).
- Massage is possibly effective for chronic low-back pain (Furlan, Imamura, Dryden, et al., updated 2008).
- Preterm and/or low birth-weight infants who received massage gained more weight each day, spent less time in the hospital, and had slightly fewer postnatal complications. There were no negative effects (Vickers, Ohlsson, Lacy, et al., 1998, updated 2004).

Osteopathy

Osteopathy is a hands-on, whole-body approach to medical care that emphasizes the role of the musculoskeletal system in health and disease. Because osteopaths (DOs) are licensed and granted the same privileges as MDs, they can also prescribe medicine and perform surgery. They may be considered part of the traditional healthcare system, and many function as mainstream providers. However, their training includes osteopathic manipulation, a method focused on normalizing joint function, eliminating strains, and facilitating the function of the primary respiratory mechanisms.

Energy Therapies

Energy therapies are widely used CAMs that involve the use of energy fields. **Biofield therapies** affect energy that surrounds and penetrates the body. The existence of biofields has not been scientifically proven. Examples include therapeutic touch, Reiki, and Qigong. **Bioelectromagnetic therapies** involve the use of electromagnetic fields (e.g., magnetic or electrical current fields) for healing. A review of research on touch therapies concluded that they have had no serious side effects (Engebretson & Wardell, 2007).

Therapeutic Touch

Therapeutic touch (TT), a biofield therapy, uses the hands on or near the body to provide comfort, pain relief, and healing. The premise of TT is that humans consist of energy fields that penetrate the body and extend 5 to 15 cm (2 to 6 in.) beyond the physical structure. In health, energy flows freely through the system in a balanced manner. But in illness or pain, the free flow of energy is disrupted. The TT practitioner's hands clear, energize, repattern, and balance the energy field to produce a more healthful state. TT is noninvasive and can be used as primary or adjunctive treatment in many settings, with clients of any age, and for a variety of conditions. To read instructions for using TT,

 Go to Chapter 40, **Clinical Insight 40-8: Performing Therapeutic Touch,** in Volume 2.

TT was co-developed by Delores Kreiger, RN, PhD, and Dora Kunz, a medical intuitive. It is now taught in 60 countries and practiced by thousands of nurses worldwide (Pumpkin Hollow Farm, 2004). Nurse Healers-Professional Associates International (NH-PAI), the official organization for TT, has developed guidelines, standard of practices, and a code of ethics for TT practitioners. NH-PAI also offers education and certification for TT practitioners. For more information,

 Go to the **Nurse Healers–Professional Associates International** Web site at www.therapeutic-touch.org and to the **Pumpkin Hollow Foundation** at www.therapeutictouch.org

Healing touch is also a biofield therapy. Developed more recently than TT, it includes a variety of techniques and interventions, including TT. For more information about healing touch,

 Go to the **Healing Touch Professional Association (HTPA)** Web site at http://www.htprofessionalassociation.com/

Evidence. TT and other healing touch therapies have been the subject of scientific inquiry for more than 25 years, yet conclusive evidence is still not available. Small studies have demonstrated various beneficial effects, including decreased anxiety, reduced pain, accelerated healing, enhanced immune functioning, reduced agitation among dementia patients, and enhanced well-being. However, meta-analyses and evidence reviews have found (1) no randomized control studies demonstrating that TT is effective in relieving anxiety, and (2) that it is of no benefit in wound healing after minor surgery. Although evidence is inconclusive, it does support the safety of TT, as well as its use for pain relief (So, Jiang, & Qin, 2008). If you would like to see summaries of integrative reviews of research and examples of some single TT studies,

 Go to Chapter 40, **Tables, Boxes, Figures: ESG Box 40-1, Therapeutic Touch—Examples of Evidence,** on the Student Resource Disk or DavisPlus at http://davisplus.fadavis.com/Wilkinson2

T'ai Chi and Qigong

The biofield therapies, t'ai chi and qigong are ancient Chinese practices that enhance health in many ways. **T'ai chi** (Fig. 40-5) is a nonaggressive martial art, and **qigong** is a series of movements, breathing, and meditation. Both modalities develop body strength and flexibility, improve balance, increase physical stamina, decrease pain and stiffness, improve sleep, and enhance mental alertness and muscular control.

There are many styles of t'ai chi and qigong. However, each strives to balance energy and cultivate the life force, known as *qi*, or *chi*. *Chi* cultivation involves relaxing the body, regulating or controlling breathing, and calming the mind. T'ai chi and qigong facilitate energy flow through the meridian system so that *qi* can be strong and balanced to support health. Consistent practice over time is said to have the most benefit. Because t'ai chi and qigong are gentle, they may be practiced throughout the life span.

Evidence. Most of the reports for qigong are published as abstracts in Chinese. The studies are mostly anecdotal case series, and there have been no large clinical trials (NCCAM, n.d.). However, there is some evidence that t'ai chi is effective for maintaining bone density in postmenopausal women, for enhancing the immune system, for improving range of motion in people with rheumatoid arthritis, and for reducing blood pressure. One database of more than 2000 records indicated that qigong has health benefits for a variety of conditions, including blood pressure and asthma (Sancier & Holman, 2004). If you would like to see citations of studies and evidence reviews,

FIGURE 40-5 T'ai chi strives to balance energy and cultivate the life force.

 Go to Chapter 40, **Tables, Boxes, Figures: ESG Box 40-2, Energy Therapies—Examples of Evidence,** on the Student Resource Disk or DavisPlus at http://davisplus.fadavis.com/Wilkinson2

Reiki

Reiki is a biofield energy therapy that originated in Japan. It seeks to balance energy to enhance the body's ability to heal itself. Like TT, it involves the laying on of hands. However, in Reiki, the patient draws the needed energy from the hands of the practitioner rather than the practitioner imparting energy (Fig. 40-6). Many Reiki treatments do not involve actual touching; instead, the hands are positioned a few inches away from the body.

Reiki is administered by practitioners who have undergone an initiation process in which the Reiki master employs ancient sounds and symbols to attune the nervous system to a higher level of energy. Reiki is also practiced as a form of self-care. People use it for relaxation, stress reduction, symptom relief, and improving

FIGURE 40-6 In Reiki, the patient draws energy from the practitioner's hands.

health and well-being. It is used for people who are dying to help them acquire a sense of peace.

Evidence. Reiki appears to be generally safe, with no serious side effects. Although there is impressive anecdotal evidence, there is little rigorous scientific research to support the claims that Reiki is beneficial for a wide range of problems, such as stress-related conditions, allergies, heart conditions, high blood pressure, and chronic pain (NCCAM, n.d.). As with many CAMs, more research is needed to establish effectiveness. If you would like to see summaries of other reviews and single studies,

 Go to Chapter 40, **Tables, Boxes, Figures: ESG Box 40-2, Energy Therapies—Examples of Evidence,** on the Student Resource Disk or DavisPlus at http://davisplus.fadavis.com/Wilkinson2

Magnet Therapy

Magnet therapy is an energy therapy that uses the property of magnetism to treat a variety of human conditions. The most widely claimed effect is improvement in musculoskeletal pain for patients with injury or arthritis. Magnet therapy operates on the premise that the iron in hemoglobin is attracted to a magnet placed on the skin. Application of a magnet to an injured or fatigued area increases blood flow, which is supposed to aid in healing. Many magnet products (e.g., mattresses, arm wraps) are available without prescription and without the need to consult a healer. The FDA and the Federal Trade Commission have not approved the marketing of magnets with claims of benefits to health (NCCAM, 2004c).

Evidence. Studies on the efficacy of magnet therapy show mixed findings and do not firmly support a conclusion that magnets can relieve pain. However, some people do experience some relief. If you would like to see summaries of reviews and single studies,

 Go to Chapter 40, **Tables, Boxes, Figures: ESG Box 40-2, Energy Therapies—Examples of Evidence,** on the Student Resource Disk or DavisPlus at http://davisplus.fadavis.com/Wilkinson2

KnowledgeCheck 40-6

Compare and contrast manipulative and body-based methods with energy therapies. How are they similar? How are they different?

 Go to Chapter 40, **Knowledge Check Response Sheet and Answers,** on the Student Resource Disk or DavisPlus at http://davisplus.fadavis.com/Wilkinson2

CriticalThinking 40-5

Which, if any, of the therapies previously discussed would be appropriate for use with Mrs. Riddell ("Meet Your Patient")? Do you believe that TT would be helpful for this patient? Explain your answers.

Practical Knowledge
knowing how

You may be wondering, "What do all these exotic therapies have to do with *me*? I certainly don't have time to get a massage therapy license or learn t'ai chi." Actually, there are three very practical applications to your practice.

1. You can, and should, facilitate communication about CAM between your patients and their healthcare providers.
2. You can use self-care practices to promote your own health and wholeness.
3. You can, with minimal training, use some of the less complex CAM therapies as independent nursing interventions.

We address these applications briefly in this section.

ASSESSMENT

Your approach to clients using CAM should be to:

- Protect them against dangerous practices.
- Permit harmless practices.
- Promote and use practices that are safe and effective.

A focused assessment will help you achieve those goals. You also need CAM information because of the possibility of interactions between the CAM and traditional biomedical interventions. People tend to assume CAMs are harmless and risk-free because (1) they are so widely used, (2) many of the products are "natural," and (3) some have been used for hundreds of years. However, studies show that many CAM products do interact with medications and that many clients do not tell their care providers about CAM use. To make a holistic assessment, inquire about CAMs the patient may be using.

- Ask the patient, "How do you usually take care of yourself at home when you are ill?" This will help you to obtain information about self-prescribed modalities.
- Ask the patient, "Many people see more than one kind of doctor or healer. Other than Dr. Jones [the traditional medical doctor], whom do you go to for advice and healing when you are ill?"
- When taking a medication history, add questions such as, "What nonprescription medications do you take? What natural or herbal remedies do you use? What nutritional supplements, vitamins, and minerals do you use?" Explain to the patient that some remedies might interact with prescribed medications or treatments.
- Inquiring about medications is especially important for older adults. Nearly 1 in 25 community-dwelling older adults use nonprescription and prescription drugs together, putting them at risk for drug–drug interactions (Qato & Jacobs, 2008).
- Above all, be neutral, accepting, and nonjudgmental in your interview. Patients may suspect that traditional caregivers will not approve of their alternative practices, so they must feel safe with you if they are to share information freely.

ANALYSIS/NURSING DIAGNOSIS

The NANDA-I taxonomy includes physical, cognitive, emotional, spiritual, individual, family, and community diagnoses. So taken as a whole, the NANDA-I *set* of diagnoses is holistic. However, the only diagnosis that might be interpreted specifically as a CAM diagnosis is Disturbed Energy Field, which is defined as "disruption of the flow of energy surrounding a person's being that results in disharmony of the body, mind, and/or spirit" (NANDA International, 2009, p. 132).

You need not fear that labeling a problem makes you less holistic. All CAM practitioners identify the patient's condition or status so that they can determine what treatment is needed. For example:

- An ayurvedic practitioner might diagnose an imbalance in the *dosha*.
- A TCM practitioner might diagnose an imbalance of emotion, or too much wind.
- A nurse might diagnose Chronic Pain before prescribing imagery.

It is your attitude, approach, and interventions that make you a holistic nurse, not the words you use to describe your patient's problem.

PLANNING OUTCOMES/EVALUATION

Patient outcomes, when achieved, should demonstrate resolution of the identified problem, regardless of whether you use traditional interventions or CAM. For example,

if you diagnose Acute Pain, the NOC outcome would be Pain Level, regardless of whether you treat the pain with narcotics or with imagery. One example of a holistic *individualized goal/outcome statement* is as follows:

> Freely shares information about folk practices and over-the-counter medications with the primary care provider.

NOC standardized outcomes for Disturbed Energy Field might include Personal Health Status, Personal Well-Being, and Spiritual Health.

PLANNING INTERVENTIONS/IMPLEMENTATION

NIC standardized interventions and activities that you may implement in the clinical setting include the following: Autogenic Training, Calming Technique, Humor, Meditation Facilitation, Simple Guided Imagery, Simple Massage, Simple Relaxation Therapy, and Therapeutic Touch. For descriptions and use of each of these techniques,

 VOL 2 Go to Chapter 40, **Clinical Insights 40-1 to 40-8,** in Volume 2.

Additional *NIC standardized interventions and activities* include the following, which require special training:

- *Aromatherapy* is the "administration of essential oils through massage, topical ointments or lotions, baths, inhalation, douches, or compresses (hot or cold) to calm and soothe, provide pain relief, enhance relaxation and comfort" (Bulechek, Butcher, & Dochterman, 2008, p. 141). You should have some education and training in the philosophy and use of essential oils. Assess for discomfort and nausea and obtain baseline vital signs before and after the treatment. Then monitor for contact dermatitis and exacerbation of asthma, as appropriate.
- *Biofeedback* requires special training. Once the patient has been taught about it, you can assist the patient to use instrumentation on which she has previously been instructed.
- *Hypnosis* is defined by NIC (Bulechek, Butcher, & Dochterman, 2008, p. 413) as "assisting a patient to achieve a state of attentive, focused concentration with suspension of some peripheral awareness to create changes in sensation, thoughts, or behavior." You will need advanced training to perform hypnosis. However, you can give your patient information about hypnosis.

Individualized interventions (non-NIC) you can perform independently include the following:

- *Self-care practices for nurse.* As you have learned, the vitality and health of the healer is a powerful force in the healing process. Holistic healing interventions are more effective when the healer is whole. Maintain your physical health by wise lifestyle choices; manage your stress; and develop a support network of colleagues,

Toward Evidence-Based Practice

Gooneratne, N. (2008). Complementary and alternative medicine for sleep disturbances in older adults. *Clinics in Geriatric Medicine, 24*(1), 121–138.

This literature review focused on CAM therapies for sleep disorders in older adults, specifically on the more common CAMs: acupuncture, ayurveda, melatonin, valerian, meditation, yoga, t'ai chi, and massage.

The results were as follows:

- By far, the most studies have been done on melatonin. Melatonin is an effective treatment of circadian phase disorders; however, its use for treating primary or secondary insomnia is not well established.
- Valerian has shown a benefit in some but not all clinical trials.
- T'ai chi, acupuncture, acupressure, yoga, and medication improved sleep parameters in a small number of early trials. These studies need to be replicated with more diverse patient groups.
- Most of the CAM therapies, with the limited data available, had no serious side effects.
- Most of the studies of massage therapy for sleep disorders were done on infants and children. Studies in adult populations were limited and tended to focus on patients with comorbid medical conditions. For example, massage therapy was found to reduce pain levels and increase sleep time in patients with fibromyalgia.
- More rigorous study designs and larger study sample sizes are crucial next steps for the field.

Paul, I., Beiler, J., McMonagle, A., et al. (2007). Effect of honey, dextromethorphan, and no treatment on nocturnal cough and sleep quality for coughing children and their parents. *Archives of Pediatrics & Adolescent Medicine, 161*(12), 1140–1146.

This randomized trial studied 130 children ages 2 to 17 years with untreated rhinorrhea and cough for 7 days or less. They were assigned randomly to receive honey, honey-flavored dextromethorphan, or nothing, to be given 30 minutes before sleep. Honey was found to be more effective than dextromethorphan or no treatment in decreasing the frequency and severity of cough. Sleep was also improved in those receiving honey.

For each of the following actions,

(a) State whether it is (W) well-supported, (S) somewhat supported, or (N) not supported by one of the two studies above.
(b) State which study (or both).
(c) Explain your thinking.

1. Giving honey to relieve the cough of an older adult

2. Performing massage therapy to relieve the pain of fibromyalgia in a middle-aged client

3. Performing massage therapy to promote sleep in healthy clients with sleep disorders

4. Using acupuncture to improve sleep in adults with sleep disorders

Go to Chapter 40, **Toward Evidence-Based Practice Suggested Responses,** on the Student Resource Disk or DavisPlus at http://davisplus.fadavis.com/Wilkinson2

---

family, and friends. Take satisfaction in your work, but balance it with a healthy personal life.

- *Music therapy* can be used to induce relaxation. Music can have a healing effect on the body, mind, and spirit. You will need some advanced knowledge of music therapy to use it to its fullest, but even now, you can suggest that patients listen to music, and you can help them obtain the type of music they prefer.
- *Pet therapy* has been used extensively in long-term care and is just beginning to be used in other settings. Pets induce a feeling of relaxation.
- *Evaluating credibility of information sources and providers.* Be sure patients are aware that not all practitioners who provide CAM therapy are equally qualified to do so. They should examine credentials and ask for referrals. The same is true of books and information taken

from Web sites. For suggestions on how to evaluate CAM information,

Go to the **National Center for Complementary and Alternative Medicine** Web site at http://nccam.nih.gov/health/webresources/

As with all interventions, you must obtain consent from your patient to use CAM and evaluate and document the patient's physiological and psychological responses.

As you learned in Chapter 13, a person's health practices can be helpful, neutral, harmful, or not known.

Promote and use practices that are safe and helpful.
Do not discourage practices that are neutral (safe) and that may help.

Discourage and protect the patient against practices that may be harmful.

If you do permit or promote a patient's CAM practices, document the patient's decision. Be sure to monitor for adverse side effects and for changes that indicate a need to reevaluate your decision to permit or promote the practice. Encourage the patient to communicate about the CAM and assist her to evaluate the outcomes.

Nurse practice acts are not always clear about which CAMs fall within a nurse's scope of practice, so it is important to be certain that any independent CAM therapies you perform are in accordance with agency policies.

 Go to Chapter 40, **Resources for Caregivers and Health Professionals,** on the Student Resource Disk or DavisPlus at http://davisplus.fadavis.com/Wilkinson2

 Suggested Readings: Go to Chapter 40, **Reading More About Holistic Healing,** on the Student Resource Disk or DavisPlus at http://davisplus.fadavis.com/Wilkinson2

 Bibliography: Go to Volume 2, Bibliography.

CHAPTER 41

Promoting Health

Learning Outcomes

After completing this chapter, you should be able to:

➤ Define *health, health promotion,* and *health protection.*

➤ Identify health prevention activities and categorize them as primary, secondary, or tertiary levels of prevention.

➤ Discuss the *Healthy People 2020* report in relation to leading causes of death and to health promotion strategies: nutrition, exercise, lifestyles, and environment.

➤ Apply Pender's Health Promotion Model to plan activities designed to change unhealthy behavior.

➤ Identify Prochaska and DiClemente's four stages of change.

➤ Identify specific health promotion strategies (including immunizations and screenings) across the life span.

➤ Discuss nurses' roles in health promotion, and list health promotion activities that a nurse may conduct in acute care facilities, in the workplace, in local communities, and schools.

➤ Identify the areas of assessment in relation to developing a health promotion plan.

➤ Assess a client's cardiorespiratory function, muscle strength and endurance, joint flexibility, and nutrition (body mass index or body fat percentage).

➤ Construct a health promotion plan of care using the nursing process, NANDA-I taxonomy, Nursing Outcomes Classifications, and Nursing Interventions Classifications.

Meet Your Peer

You have completed all your prerequisites and are now enrolled in your first nursing course. Aside from classroom work, you have a skills course and clinical rotation. You spend a lot of time reading, studying, preparing for clinical work, writing care plans, and completing follow-up assignments from your clinical rotation. You have other non-nursing course work and family responsibilities, as well. Often, you stay up late and get up early, usually getting about 5 or 6 hours of sleep. By the end of the week, you're exhausted. You don't have time to cook so you pick up fast food several times a week. Even though it is not the healthiest choice, at least this way you can get something to eat. You have little time to exercise, and when you do have time, you feel too tired and disinterested. You use cigarettes to relax you

and help you cope with stress. On the weekends, you let loose with friends, drinking beer and having a good time.

You spend most of your time learning about health and illness. Given your current lifestyle, do you consider yourself healthy? How did you make that decision? Your answer is based on your personal beliefs about health and what you have learned in your nursing course work. In this chapter, we explore health promotion. As you learn more about this topic, you may develop a plan to promote your own health as well as the health of clients.

Theoretical **Knowledge** **knowing** why

In Chapter 10, we considered the meaning of health, wellness, and illness. In this chapter, the emphasis is on strategies to promote health and prevent disease. To begin, we explore what others have written about the concepts. Various descriptions and definitions use the terms *health* and *wellness* interchangeably, and we do the same in this chapter.

What Is Health Promotion?

To promote health, we must first identify what we mean by *health* and *wellness*. The World Health Organization (WHO) defines health as "a state of complete physical, mental and social well-being and not merely the absence of disease or infirmity" (WHO, 1948). At the first conference for health promotion, WHO defined **health promotion** as the process of equipping people to have control over, and to improve, physical, emotional, and social health (WHO, 1986). Other professionals have also reflected on the meaning of health.

Jean Watson. This nursing theorist proposed in 1979 that health consists of three elements: (1) a high level of overall physical, mental, and social functioning; (2) a general adaptive-maintenance level of daily functioning; and (3) the absence of illness (or the presence of efforts that lead to its absence). She also refers to health as being a state of mind, the perception of the individual. A person may have a terminal illness and yet consider himself healthy.

Betty Neuman. In 1995 this nurse theorist contributed to nursing science with her theory describing health as an expression of living energy available to an individual. The energy is displayed as a continuum, with high energy (wellness) at one end and low energy (illness) at the opposite end. Individuals have varying levels of energy at various stages of life. When more energy is generated than expended, there is wellness. When more energy is expended than is generated, there is illness, possibly death.

Myers, Sweeney, and Witmer. In 2000 these theorists defined wellness as "a way of life oriented toward optimal health and well-being in which body, mind, and spirit are integrated by the individual to live more fully within the human and natural community" (p. 252). This definition includes lifestyles and habits as components of health and permits people who have been diagnosed with disease to be considered healthy.

Applying aspects of these reflections on health, **health promotion** means finding ways to help individuals develop a state of physical, spiritual, and mental well-being. Health promotion activities are useful to all individuals, whether well or sick, because they encourage optimal function. How does this compare to the WHO definition of health promotion you read earlier?

Health Promotion versus Health Protection

On the surface, it appears that activities that promote health also protect health; and, for the most part, that is true. Nevertheless, the ideas behind health promotion and health protection differ subtly but significantly. Pender, Murdaugh, and Parsons (2006) explain that motivation is what distinguishes the two activities. Health promotion is motivated by the desire to increase well-being, whereas health protection is motivated by a desire to avoid illness. For instance the 40-year-old who begins an exercise program to improve strength and endurance is motivated by the benefits of health promotion. If he starts exercising because his father died of a heart attack at age 50, he may be motivated by the need to protect his health.

Levels of Prevention

Leavell and Clark (1965) identified three levels of activities for health protection (illness prevention): primary, secondary, and tertiary. Interventions are classified according to where they occur in the disease process. This timing directs the types of interventions needed.

- **Primary prevention** activities are designed to prevent or slow the onset of disease. Activities such as eating healthy foods, exercising, wearing sunscreen, obeying seat belt laws, and immunizations are examples of primary level interventions.
- **Secondary prevention** involves screening activities and education for detecting illnesses in the early stages. Health activities such as breast self-examination, testicular exams, regular physical examinations, blood pressure and diabetes screenings, and tuberculosis skin tests are examples of secondary interventions.
- **Tertiary prevention** focuses on stopping the disease from progressing and returning the individual to the pre-illness phase. Rehabilitation is the main intervention during this level.

Patients and health providers move among these levels of prevention. For example, a patient hospitalized for a total hip replacement would receive tertiary prevention—care focused on helping her recover from surgery, preventing complications of surgery, and, later on, helping her regain her strength and learn to walk again. Secondary prevention strategies may have been used previously, for example, to screen for osteoporosis that leads to bone fragility and fractures. When she goes home, if she decides to limit her salt intake and eat a balanced diet that is low in fat, refined sugar, these activities would be primary prevention strategies.

Health Behaviors

For the population overall, life expectancy (at birth) reached a record high of 78.1 years, up from 75.4 years in 1990. The gap between men and women has narrowed from 7.0 years in 1990 to 5.3 years in 2006 (Centers for Disease Control and Prevention [CDC], 2009b). Health status is affected by health behavior, such as weight management, increasing physical activity, safer sex, and moderate alcohol use, avoidance of tobacco, and drugs.

Teen Pregnancy

Pregnant teenagers are less likely to receive early prenatal care. They are more likely to drop out of school and to live in poverty than are older pregnant women. In 2006, the birth rate for teenagers 15 to 19 years of age rose for the first time in 3 decades. Previously there was a 14-year downward trend for teen pregnancy (CDC, 2009b).

Abuse of Alcohol and Illicit Drugs

The risk of disease, injuries, and intentional death (suicide and homicide) increases with substance abuse.

- In 2006, one in five adults age 18 years and older reported drinking five or more alcoholic drinks on at least one day in the past year and almost one in ten reported five or more drinks on at least 12 days in the past year.
- In 2006, 6% of people age 12 years and older reported marijuana use in the past month, and 3% reported nonmedical use of prescription drugs. Use of illicit drugs was highest among young adults age 18 to 25 years (CDC, 2009b). Substance abuse in adolescents is associated with a greater frequency of suicide attempts, more medically lethal attempts, an increased seriousness of intent, and greater suicidal ideation.

Tobacco Use

Cigarette smoking increases the risk of lung cancer, tuberculosis, heart disease, emphysema, and other diseases.

- The percentage of high school students and adults who reported smoking cigarettes in the past month remained stable at 20% to 23%, after declining from 36% in the previous decade.
- Men were more likely to be current cigarette smokers than women (24% compared with 18%) (CDC, 2009b).
- The highest percentage of tobacco users are in the South (CDC, 2009a).
- Smoking as few as three cigarettes/day can increase the risk for cardiovascular disease by more than 60% (Pope, Burnett, Krewski, et al., 2009). The risk of active tuberculosis is nearly doubled with tobacco use (Linn, Ezzati, & Chang, 2009).

Obesity

The risk of heart disease, diabetes, and stroke increases with obesity.

- The prevalence of overweight preschool-age children increased by more than 50%. Among school-age children, the prevalence of overweight increased from 11% to 15% and among adolescents grew from 11% to 18%.
- Obesity rates among adults have nearly tripled between 1960 (13%) and 2006 (34%) (CDC, 2009b).
- With the U.S. obesity trend, only 7.5% of Americans now have five low-risk factors for cardiovascular disease—no tobacco use, normal blood pressure, normal weight, low blood cholesterol, no diabetes, and age younger than 75 years (Ford, van Dam, & Fonarow, 2009).

Sedentary Lifestyle

Exercise reduces the risk of disease and enhances mental and physical health.

- American adults have made no substantial progress toward achieving recommended levels of physical activity or strength training. Between 1995 and 2006, the percentage of adults 18 years of age and over engaged in regular leisure-time physical activity or strength training activities remained level.

KnowledgeCheck 41-1

- How does health promotion differ from health protection?
- Which level of prevention is represented by the following activities?
  Mumps, measles, rubella (MMR) vaccination
  Tuberculosis (TB) skin test
  Physical therapy after repair of a hip fracture

 Go to Chapter 41, **Knowledge Check Response Sheet and Answers,** on the Student Resource Disk or DavisPlus at http://davisplus.fadavis.com/Wilkinson2

Health Promotion Models

A model illustrates a system or framework to help explain what you see in clinical practice. The most common frameworks used for designing health promotion programs are described next.

Pender's Health Promotion Model

Pender's Health Promotion Model (HPM) (Fig. 41-1) identifies three groups of variables that affect health promotion: (1) individual characteristics and experiences, (2) behavior-specific cognitions and affect, and (3) behavioral outcome. The HPM is based on seven assumptions that reflect both nursing and behavioral science perspectives (Pender, Murdaugh, & Parsons, 2006).

Two general assumptions are about the interpersonal environment:

1. Health professionals constitute a part of the interpersonal environment, which exerts influence on persons throughout their life span.
2. Self-initiated reconfiguration of person–environment interactive patterns is essential to behavior change.

The other five assumptions are characteristics of people, whom they assume:

1. Seek to create conditions of living through which they can express their unique human health potential.
2. Have the capacity for reflective self-awareness, including assessment of their own competencies.
3. Value growth in directions viewed as positive and attempt to achieve a personally acceptable balance between change and stability.
4. Seek to actively regulate their own behavior.
5. In all their biopsychosocial complexity interact with the environment, progressively transforming the environment and being transformed over time.

Pender's model has been used extensively in several disciplines in research and professional practice focused on health promotion. As a nurse, you should find Pender's focus applicable to your work.

Critical Thinking 41-1

- How might peers influence health behaviors? At what age might peers have more influence?
- Apply Pender's model to a person trying to lose weight. What might be some perceived barriers (see Fig. 41-1)?

Wheel of Wellness

Several authors have likened the different facets of health to the spokes of a wheel (Hettler, 1984; Myers, Sweeney, & Witmer, 2000; Witmer & Sweeney, 1982). If one of the spokes is weak, the whole wheel is weak. The "spokes" of the health wheel represent the dimensions of health: emotional, intellectual, physical, spiritual, social/family, and occupational (Fig. 41-2). The level of wellness progresses from the center to the outer part of the wheel. The center represents the least amount of wellness, and the outer part represents optimal wellness. If one area of an individual's life is not functioning at optimal level, life will not be as fulfilling as it could be. As a nurse, you should assess each dimension for strengths and weaknesses.

Transtheoretical Model of Change

The transtheoretical model of change (Prochaska & DiClemente, 1982) may serve as a means to alter unhealthy behaviors. Health promotion and protection involve either changing the individual's response to the illness-producing stimuli or changing the environment so that the person will be less likely to encounter illness-producing stimuli. Either idea involves change. In this model, change occurs in four stages:

Stage 1   *Contemplation* involves the decision-making process.

Stage 2   *Determination* is the stage in which the person makes a decision to change a behavior and prepares a plan.

Stage 3   *The action stage* is the implementation of the plan.

Stage 4   *The maintenance stage* allows the changed behavior to be reinforced.

Ideally, the stages would progress in this order. Realistically, a person may progress and regress in any of the stages. The change process in persons with some unhealthy habits (e.g., cigarette smoking, substance abuse, and excessive eating) may best be described as a revolving door. An individual may exit at any point as the door goes around. If the exit occurs during or at the end of the maintenance period, the behavioral change is successful. If the exit occurs before the end of the maintenance period, relapse will occur, and the individual will return to the previous lifestyle.

Additional stages often precede and follow the change. The *precontemplation stage* precedes the change and identifies those who are not aware of having a particular problem and so are not ready to contemplate change. The *termination stage* completes the maintenance. A person who enters the termination stage has changed the behavior and is not in danger of relapse.

Health Promotion Programs

Health promotion programs help a person advance toward optimal health. In the sections that follow we discuss several types. For further discussion of individual activities that promote health,

 Go to Chapter 41, **Supplemental Materials: Individual Health Promotion Activities,** on the Student Resource Disk or DavisPlus at http://davisplus.fadavis.com/Wilkinson2

Disseminating Information. To recognize a problem and understand the options for change, people need information. Information may be disseminated at the individual, group, or community level. For example, teaching a client how to modify his personal dietary intake is a form of disseminating information to an individual. Group-level programs include classes offered at the local hospital, prenatal education programs, and worksite programs. Community-level health promotion programs are directed at the entire community. For instance, when you pass a billboard that presents the dangers of smoking, you are viewing a community-level health promotion program. Health blogs on the Internet and health fairs are other community-level strategies for disseminating health information.

Individual characteristics and experiences

Behavior-specific cognitions and affect

Behavioral outcome

Prior related behavior

Perceived benefits of action

Perceived barriers to action

Perceived self-efficacy

Activity-related affect

Personal factors
- Biological
- Psychological
- Sociocultural

Interpersonal influences
- Family, peers, providers
- Norms, support, models

Situational influences
- Options
- Demand characteristics
- Aesthetics

Immediate competing demands (low control)

and

Immediate competing preferences (high control)

Commitment to a plan of action

Health-promoting behavior

FIGURE 41-1 Pender's Health Promotion Model.

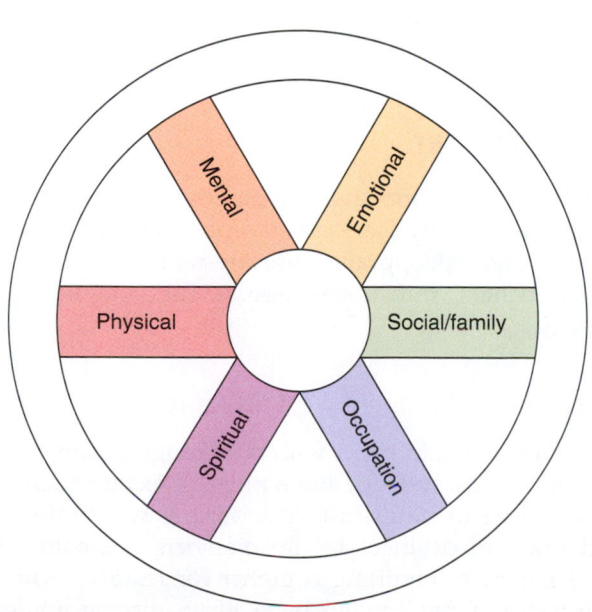

FIGURE 41-2 Wheel of Wellness.

Mental
Emotional
Physical
Social/family
Spiritual
Occupation

Changing Lifestyle and Behavior. These are group-level programs. They focus on such activities as weight loss, smoking cessation, exercise, nutrition, and stress management. These programs usually provide information and offer support. Many times, they include a maintenance program to help solidify the change.

Protecting the Environment. The term *environment* refers to air, water, and soil, as well as social and political surroundings. Environmental control programs promote health by working to create a healthy environment. Programs focus on air and water quality, toxic waste, healthy homes and communities, infrastructure and surveillance, and global environmental health.

Assessing Wellness and Appraising Health Risk. These programs focus on identifying behaviors that promote health and create the risk for disease. A wellness assessment tends to focus on the healthy behaviors. It supports positive change to improve health. A health risk appraisal identifies risky behaviors that promote disease. These programs are readily available on the Internet, in magazines, and at fitness centers.

KnowledgeCheck 41-2

- What are the six dimensions of health represented by the spokes on the wellness wheel?
- Identify the stages of change identified by Prochaska and DiClemente.
- Describe the four main types of health promotion programs.

 Go to Chapter 41, **Knowledge Check Response Sheet and Answers,** on the Student Resource Disk or DavisPlus at http://davisplus.fadavis.com/Wilkinson2

 CriticalThinking 41-2

J.T. drinks a vodka and tonic while eating lunch with his co-workers. He keeps a bottle of vodka in his office desk for use during the day. Later, he stops at a local bar for a drink on the way home. At home, he drinks a 6-pack of beer while watching the game. What information do you need to determine which of Prochaska and DiClemente's stages of change he is experiencing? How would you get this information?

Settings for Health Promotion Programs

The most common sites for health promotion programs are health facilities, worksites, and schools. Healthcare settings, such as clinics, physician offices, or hospitals, are natural settings for health promotion. Remember, each interaction between patient and healthcare provider is an opportunity for health promotion. Unfortunately, most interactions focus on the disease process and compliance with treatments. You will need to make a conscious effort to help clients focus on behaviors that prevent illness and promote health.

Nurses work in health clinics within large companies or may be contracted to provide specific health promotion programs, such as smoking cessation, stress management, weight reduction, and fitness training. Employers have found that health programs decrease work-related injuries and sick leave. For instance, Appleton Papers, Inc. is a fictitious example of a company that has an on-site wellness center aimed at reducing musculoskeletal injuries and illness. Staff at the center offer educational programs on topics, such as ergonomics, low back injuries, breast cancer awareness, and child car seat safety. There is a fitness center for strength and endurance training. The goal is to decrease injuries, illness, and costs while increasing productivity (Halls & Rhodes, 2002).

Another setting for community health promotion is the local school district. Health teaching can begin at an early age, and nurses and teachers can regularly reinforce healthy behaviors and redirect unhealthy behaviors. Schools provide a setting that allows for continued exposure to information. Interventions may be directed at general health promotion issues, such as physical activity, or they may focus on specific health risks, such as tobacco and alcohol use.

Ideally, parents and families are included in the learning. School nurses work closely with teachers and parents to provide health promotion services in the schools.

Health Promotion Throughout the Life Span

Health promotion is a lifelong process that begins at conception. Table 41-1 describes the focus of health promotion programs at each developmental stage, as well as the types of screenings recommended for each age group.

Practical Knowledge knowing how

Pender, Murdaugh, and Parsons (2006) summarized the health promotion process as a series of nine steps that involve the client and the nurse. Notice that many steps of this process are similar to the nursing process:

1. Review and summarize data from assessment.
2. Reinforce the client's strengths and abilities.
3. Identify health goals and related behavioral change options.
4. Identify behavioral or health outcomes that will indicate that the plan has been successful from the client's perspective.
5. Develop a behavior change plan based on the client's preferences, on the stages of change, and on "state-of-the-science" knowledge about effective interventions.
6. Reiterate benefits of change, and identify incentives for change from the client's perspective.
7. Address environmental and interpersonal facilitators and barriers to behavior change.
8. Determine a time frame for implementation.
9. Commit to behavior-change goals, and structure the support needed to accomplish them.

ASSESSMENT

A health promotion assessment involves obtaining a health history, physical examination, fitness assessment, lifestyle and risk appraisal, life stress review, analysis of health beliefs, nutritional assessment, and screening activities.

History and Physical Examination

Assessment should begin with a thorough health history, review of body systems, and a physical examination. Ask the client about family history of various health disorders and cause of death of family members. Keep in mind the accuracy of reporting is higher for relatives without, rather than those affected by, a given disease (Qureshi, Wilson, Santaguida, et al., 2009). Gather the history directly

Table 41-1 ➤ Health Promotion Throughout the Life Span

HEALTH PROMOTION FOCUS	HEALTH SCREENINGS	HEALTH PROMOTION FOCUS	HEALTH SCREENINGS
Conception to Birth		**Adolescence**	
Education about pregnancy	Alpha-fetoprotein level	Peer pressure	Growth and development
Abstinence from alcohol, cigarettes, and illicit drugs	Screening for gestational diabetes	Motor vehicle safety	Sexually transmitted infection (STI) screening
Nutrition, including folic acid and iron requirements	Prenatal care	Safety	Breast self-exam
	Abuse	Self-esteem	Testicular self-exam
Exercise to maintain strength and muscle tone and to control weight gain	Additional screenings that may be offered:	Physical activity	Mental health
	■ Ultrasound	Suicide and depression	Stress
	■ Amniocentesis	Firearm safety	Alcohol and drug use
Parenting education	■ Chorionic villus sampling	Violence	Abuse
Infancy		Sexuality	
Nutrition (breast versus bottle)	Hearing evaluation	Substance use and abuse	
Introduction of solid foods	Screening for birth defects	Limiting sun exposure	
Placing the infant on her back for sleep without a pillow to reduce the risk of sudden infant death syndrome (SIDS)	Blood work to rule out certain metabolic conditions	Update of immunizations	
	Monthly examinations until at least 6 months of age	Oral health	
	After age 6 months, visits every 2 or 3 months	**Young Adult**	
Sensory stimulation	Growth and development	Physical activity	Comprehensive exam at least every 3 years
Safety	Abuse	Motor vehicle safety	
Motor vehicle safety		Safety	Lifestyle
Oral health		Violence	Pap smear
Toddler and Preschool		Sexuality	STI screening
Adequate supervision	Annual examinations	Substance use and abuse	Breast self-exam monthly
Safety, including storage of poisons	Growth and development	Limiting sun exposure	Testicular self-exam monthly
Toilet training	Cognitive skills	Update immunizations	Mental health
Motor vehicle safety	Abuse	Oral health	Stress
Nutrition	Kindergarten readiness		Alcohol and drug use
Immunizations			Abuse
Oral health			
Sleep and rest		**Middle Adult**	
School-age		Physical activity	Comprehensive exam at least every 3 years to age 40, yearly after age 40
Nutrition	Annual examinations	Safety	
Physical activity	Growth and development	Obesity	BP screening
Safety	Cognitive skills	Sexuality	Lipid panel
Sexuality	Abuse	Lifestyle	Blood glucose
Stranger danger		Update of immunizations	Stress
Oral health		Oral health	Mammograms yearly and clinical breast exam for women over age 40
		Substance use and abuse	Digital rectal exam for prostate evaluation in men
			PSA for men yearly over age 50
			Annual eye exam
			Sigmoidoscopy or colonoscopy
			Stool for occult blood with comprehensive exam
			Bone density
			Abuse

Continued

Table 41-1 ➤ Health Promotion Throughout the Life Span—cont'd

HEALTH PROMOTION FOCUS	HEALTH SCREENINGS	HEALTH PROMOTION FOCUS	HEALTH SCREENINGS
Older Adult		**Older Adult**	
Physical activity	Functional skills (ADLs and IADLs)	Changes associated with aging	Mammograms and clinical breast exam
Nutrition			
Safety	Hearing		Digital rectal exam for prostate evaluation in men
Obesity	Falls risk		PSA for men who have a life expectancy of at least 10 years
Sexuality	Stress		
Lifestyle	Annual eye exam		Stool for occult blood
Update of immunizations	BP screening		Bone density
Oral health	Lipid panel		Follow-up sigmoidoscopy or colonoscopy
	Blood glucose		Mental health
			Abuse

from the client if possible; if not, gather information from the closest caregiver. As always, provide privacy and comfort while conducting the history and exam.

The level of detail of the physical examination depends on the health history. At a minimum, the exam should include vital signs, weight, body mass index (BMI) or waist circumference, auscultation and palpation of the chest and abdomen, inspection of the skin, and palpation of peripheral pulses. The exam may be accompanied by laboratory studies. Recommended lab work depends on the history and exam findings. For most adult clients, screening lab consists of a complete blood count, comprehensive metabolic panel (also known as a chem 20 panel), lipid panel, thyroid function panel, and urinalysis (American College of Sports Medicine [ACSM], 2009). In clients with known cardiac or pulmonary disease, additional disease-specific studies may be performed (e.g., electrocardiogram [ECG], carotid ultrasound, or pulmonary function tests).

Physical Fitness Assessment

Regular physical activity each week, sustained for months and years, can produce long-term health benefits. Regular physical activity is linked with a lower risk for heart disease, stroke, type 2 diabetes, hypertension, high cholesterol, metabolic syndrome, certain types of cancer, and depression. Regular physical activity also prevents weight gain; improves cardiorespiratory and muscular fitness; prevents falls by increasing muscle tone, strength and balance, and promotes better memory and cognition in older adults (American College of Sports Medicine [ACSM], 2009).

A physical fitness assessment includes the following:

- *Cardiorespiratory fitness* is reflected in the ability to perform large-muscle, moderate- to high-intensity exercise for prolonged periods of time (ACSM, 2009). There are many different modes of testing, such as field tests (walking or running), treadmills, stationary bicycles, and step testing. Results depend on age and gender.
- *Muscular fitness* refers to both muscle strength and endurance. Muscle strength is a measure of the amount of weight a muscle (or group of muscles) can move at one time. Muscle endurance refers to the ability of a muscle to perform repeated movements.
- Flexibility is the ability to move a joint through its range of motion. The most common assessment is to evaluate low back and hip (trunk) flexion.

For information and guidelines for assessing physical fitness,

 Go to Chapter 41, **Assessment Guidelines and Tools, Health Promotion: Physical Fitness Assessment,** in Volume 2.

Lifestyle and Risk Appraisal

Lifestyle refers to the manner in which a person conducts his life: physically, emotionally, spiritually, and mentally. Personal habits, recreation, and occupation are part of one's lifestyle. In the context of health and wellness, lifestyle includes all of the activities that promote optimal living, such as taking responsibility for one's health, physical activity, nutrition, interpersonal relations, spiritual growth, and stress management. You can gather this information by interview or by using a variety of questionnaires. A health risk appraisal (HRA) is a questionnaire that evaluates risk for disease based on current demographic data, lifestyle, and health behaviors. There are many HRA tools available; many are online. For one example of an HRA,

  Go to Chapter 41, **Assessment Guidelines and Tools, Lifestyle and Risk Assessment,** in Volume 2.

Critical Thinking 41-3

- Evaluate your own compliance with recommended health screenings for your age group. What activities should you incorporate into your own health promotion plan?
- Answer the questions in the "Lifestyle and Risk Assessment" in Volume 2. How did you score? What additional activities should be added to your health promotion plan?

Life Stress Review

In 1976, Hans Selye proposed that stress triggers physiological responses that may, over time, induce illness. Likewise, Richard Rahe (1974) identified some stress-inducing life change events and researched their possible effects on health. He attached numeric values for each change based on the degree of disruption or stress produced by the event. Rahe discovered that a high score on a life-change event scale is associated with a greater likelihood of a negative health change. To see and use a life-change event scale,

 Go to Chapter 25, **Assessment Guidelines and Tools, the Holmes–Rahe Social Readjustment Scale,** in Volume 2.

Other researchers have focused on daily stresses and their effects on actual health or on one's perception of health. Daily stresses involve travel to and from work, taking children to activities, daily chores, waiting in lines at shops, raising teenagers, and traffic jams. Researchers have found these stresses may gradually erode one's coping mechanisms, producing an inability to cope with daily events and an increased likelihood of illness.

Research has also demonstrated that in the face of life events, some people develop hardiness rather than vulnerability (Maddi, Koshaba, Fazel, et al., 2009). Kobasa (1979) identified hardiness as a quality in which an individual experiences high levels of stress yet does not fall ill. There are three general characteristics of the hardy person:

- **Control**—belief in the ability to control the experience
- **Commitment**—feeling deeply involved in the activity producing stress
- **Challenge**—the ability to view the change as a challenge to grow

These traits are associated with a strong resistance to negative feelings that occur under adverse circumstances (Sinha, 2009). If you need additional information on hardiness, review Chapter 10.

Critical Thinking 41-4

- Undoubtedly you are experiencing stress as a student in a nursing program. How would you rate your level of hardiness?
- What statements would demonstrate a hardy personality in each area (commitment, control, challenge)?

Health Beliefs

A health promotion assessment would not be complete without investigating an individual's health beliefs. Health beliefs are embedded in one's culture and personal experiences. Culture consists of characteristics, beliefs, and behaviors of an individual or group (Chapter 13)—all the experiences, biases, beliefs, and rituals. Culture influences beliefs and practices affecting wellness and disease prevention. For example, some people may use certain foods (e.g., garlic to prevent heart disease, orange juice to prevent a cold) or herbs to protect or restore health. It is important for you to respect cultural and religious views regarding health while working with clients to adopt personal health goals.

It will be helpful to know whether health outcomes are a result of actions the person takes, actions of powerful others, or chance. The Multidimensional Health Locus of Control scale (MHLC), developed by Wallston, Wallston, and DeVellis (1978), helps you obtain this information. The MHLC measures the person's perception of the extent of control from each source. The person rates her level of agreement with statements such as "I am in control of my health," "No matter what I do, if I am going to get sick, I will get sick" and "Regarding my health, I can only do what my doctor tells me to do." Identifying a patient's locus of control is of practical importance for several reasons:

- People who feel powerless about preventing illness are least likely to engage in health promotion activities.
- People who respond to direction from respected authorities often prefer a health promotion program that is supervised by a healthcare provider.
- Clients who feel in charge of their own health are the easiest to motivate toward positive change.

For a copy of the MHLC you can print out and use with your patients,

 Go to Chapter 41, **Resources for Caregivers and Health Professionals,** on the Student Resource Disk or DavisPlus at http://davisplus.fadavis.com/Wilkinson2

Nutritional Assessment

A nutritional assessment is a key component of an overall wellness assessment. Unhealthy eating habits occur across all ages, ethnicities, and socioeconomic classes. The assessment involves an evaluation of typical eating patterns correlated with physical examination findings and body mass index (BMI). Body composition is important in identifying health risks. The usual methods for determining body fat composition clinically are by measuring height, weight, circumferences, and skinfolds (see Chapter 26 to review these).

The pattern of body fat distribution is an important predictor of health risks. People with fat stored around the trunk and abdominal area have a higher incidence of metabolic syndrome, hypertension, hyperlipidemia, heart disease, type 2 diabetes, and premature death than those who have the fat stored in the extremities. Traditionally, the waist-to-height ratio has been used as a method for determining fat patterns in the body. More recently, the focus has shifted to waist circumference alone. The more fat stored in the abdominal area, the greater the risk for disease (Janssen, Katzmarzyk, & Ross, 2004).

Health Screening Activities

Health screening activities are secondary prevention activities designed to diagnose specific diseases at an early stage so that treatment can begin before there is an opportunity for the disease to spread or become debilitat-ing. Many of these screening activities are part of your usual care. For example, each time you check a client's blood pressure, you are performing a screen for hypertension. Table 41-1 identifies the typical health screening activities with each developmental stage. Box 41-2 provides further information about selected health screening activities.

Currently, there is some controversy about whether we should encourage breast self-examination (BSE). In studies around the world, breast self-examination was found not to reduce mortality due to breast cancer, and may even cause false security and delayed diagnosis when lumps are not detected. Because of the ongoing uncertainty raised by this and other studies and the fact some women do detect lumps that signal cancer, the American Cancer Society continues to advise women that BSE is an optional screening tool and plays only a small role in finding breast cancer (American Cancer Society, 2009c). However, BSE can be a useful screening strategy when used in combination with regular physical exams and mammography. So until evidence is conclusive, it seems reasonable to continue to encourage and teach BSE.

Toward Evidence-Based Practice

Maddi, S. R., Koshaba, D. M., Fazel, M., et al. (2009, July 1). The personality construct of hardiness, IV. *Journal of Humanistic Psychology, 49*(3), 292–305.

Hardiness is a personality trait involving a blend of commitment, control, and challenge. It is the characteristic of what a person relies on to turn hardship and stressful events into growth opportunities. Researchers studied a large group of college students and found hardiness associated with positive attitudes toward school and instructors. This trait was also linked to students' beliefs in their own inner capabilities and rated higher standards for living. Those rated as hardy expressed satisfaction with life. There was an opposite association of hardiness to depression, anxiety, and hostility.

Tindle, H. A., Chang, Y. F., Kuller, L. H., et al. (2009, August 10). Optimism, cynical hostility, and incident coronary heart disease and mortality in the Women's Health Initiative. *Circulation, 120*(8), 656. Retrieved from http://circ.ahajournals.org/cgi/content/abstract/CIRCULATIONAHA.108.827642v1

A large study of nearly 100,000 postmenopausal women compared the incidence of heart disease and cancer between those who showed optimism versus those who displayed cynical, hostile attitudes toward others. Study participants had no known cardiovascular disease or cancer before enrollment in the study. Optimists had lower rates of heart disease (CHD), cancer-related deaths, and total mortality. The most cynical, hostile women had higher rates of CHD and total mortality and cancer-related mortality.

Olson, M. B., Krantz, D. S., Kelsey, S. F., et al. (2005, July-Aug). Hostility scores are associated with increased risk of cardiovascular events in women undergoing coronary angiography: A report from the NHLBI-Sponsored WISE Study. *Psychosomatic Medicine, 67*(4), 546–552.

The National Heart, Lung, and Blood Institute conducted a large study to look at the occurrence of adverse cardiac events among women with suspected heart attack. They measured cynicism, hostility, and aggression. In the 6-year follow-up period, after accounting for coronary artery disease and other risk factors, researchers found a 35% increased risk of angina, nonfatal myocardial infarction, stroke, and congestive heart failure. This group who suffered adverse cardiovascular events also had poorer survival than those who scored lower on the hostility rating scale.

1. Based on these studies, how might you assess cynicism and hostility in your patient?

2. Why do you think people showing more hostility had poorer survival after suffering a heart-related problem than those rated as hardy?

3. In light of the research examining the impact of attitude on health outcomes, what would you do to promote optimism in your postmenopausal patient preparing for surgery?

 Go to Chapter 41, **Toward Evidence-Based Practice Suggested Responses,** on the Student Resource Disk or DavisPlus at http://davisplus.fadavis.com/Wilkinson2

BOX 41-2 ■ Selected Health Screening Activities

With regard to health screening guidelines, it is important to know:

1. Different agencies and groups generate different guidelines for type and frequency of screening. For example, the American Cancer Society has different Pap screening recommendations than the U.S. Preventive Services Task Force; ACOG may have yet another recommendation.

2. Most evidence-based guidelines make use of cost-benefit analysis to arrive at their recommendations.

3. Various third-party payors have different policies regarding the type and frequency of screening for which they will reimburse.

4. Guidelines and recommendations change often.

Clinicians must take all that into consideration when they decide which screening tests to offer to their patients.

Lipid screening. Adults age 20 years or older have a fasting lipid panel at least once every 5 years. If total cholesterol is 200 mg/dL or greater—or HDL is less than 40 mg/dL—frequent monitoring is required. Overweight children need to receive cholesterol screening, regardless of risk factors for cardiovascular disease (Daniels & Greer, 2009).

Dental health. Clients should have regular dental checkups to detect early signs of oral health problems such as tooth decay, gingivitis (gum disease), and oral cancers.

Colon cancer screening. Both men and women should have a fecal occult blood test every year beginning at age 50 and a screening colonoscopy based on risk factors. If there is a strong family history of colorectal cancer or polyps, screening should begin at an earlier age and be conducted more frequently (American Cancer Society, 2009d).

Breast cancer screening. Breast self-examination (BSE) is an option for women 20 years and older. Women between the ages of 20 and 39 should have a clinical breast examination by a health professional every 3 years. Women aged 40 and older should have a screening mammogram and a clinical breast examination by a healthcare professional every year.

The clinical breast examination should be scheduled close to and preferably before the scheduled mammogram (American Cancer Society, 2009c, 2009d). Thermal mammography shows promise for breast cancer detection without using radiation.

Cervical cancer screening. A Papanicolaou (Pap) smear is used to detect cellular changes in the cervix. Women older than 21 years (or 3 years after first vaginal intercourse) should be screened for cervical cancer every 2 to 3 years. Women with risk factors for cervical cancer (e.g., weakened immune system, those who have had abnormal Pap tests) should be screened more frequently. Women 70 years of age or older with no abnormal Pap test results in the last 10 years may choose to stop having cervical cancer screening (American Cancer Society, 2009d).

Testicular cancer screening. Given the low prevalence of testicular cancer and the limited accuracy of self-examination, routine clinical examination is not advised in symptom-free males.

Prostate screening. Prostate cancer can be detected early with a blood test called the prostate-specific antigen (PSA) test or a digital rectal examination (DRE) by a trained healthcare professional. The American Cancer Society does not support routine testing for prostate cancer. However, healthcare professionals may consider offering the PSA and DRE yearly to men age 50 years and older at risk for prostate cancer and with at least a 10-year life expectancy—if there are risk factors, testing should begin at age 40 to 45 years (American Cancer Society, 2009d).

Skin screening. During any health assessment or a specialized dermatologic exam, a general survey of the skin using the ABCD criteria is a useful approach for assessing for skin malignancy: **A**symmetry, **B**order irregularity, **C**olor variability, **D**iameter greater than 6 mm. Rapidly changing lesions are also associated with an increased risk for cancer. Any suspicious lesions should be biopsied (Agency for Healthcare Research and Quality [AHRQ], 2009a).

The issue of whether to perform mass prostate-specific antigen (PSA) screening for prostate cancer is also unsettled. The U.S. Preventive Services Task Force concludes that there is not sufficient evidence to recommend for or against routine PSA screening for prostate cancer. However, most experts and organizations agree that the most appropriate candidates for yearly screening are men older than age 50 and younger men who have increased risk factors (National Cancer Institute, 2009).

For points to include when teaching breast and testicular self examination,

 Go to the expanded discussion of Chapter 9, **Tables, Boxes, Figures: ESG Boxes 9-6, Breast Self-Examination (BSE), and 9-7, Testicular Self-Examination (TSE),** on the Student Resource Disk or DavisPlus at http://davisplus.fadavis.com/Wilkinson2

KnowledgeCheck 41-3

- Identify at least three common sites for health promotion activities.
- What assessments are part of a health promotion assessment?
- What role does stress play in health promotion?

 Go to Chapter 41, **Knowledge Check Response Sheet and Answers,** on the Student Resource Disk or DavisPlus at http://davisplus.fadavis.com/Wilkinson2

 CriticalThinking 41-5

Your 55-year-old aunt tells you she hasn't had a physical examination in 20 years. She is a registered nurse. "I don't need one because I feel fine and I can take care of myself." How would you respond?

ANALYSIS/NURSING DIAGNOSIS

Wellness diagnoses are appropriate for health promotion activities. Such diagnoses describe healthy responses in areas where you can intervene to promote growth or maintenance of the healthy response. NANDA-I defines a wellness diagnosis as describing "human responses to levels of wellness in an individual, family, or community that have a readiness for enhancement" (2009, p. 26). For specific NANDA-I labels you can use to describe wellness diagnoses,

 Go to Chapter 41, **Standardized Language, Examples of NANDA-I Wellness Diagnoses,** in Volume 2.

New NANDA-I wellness labels are preceded by the phrase *Readiness for Enhanced* and will be one-part statements (e.g., Readiness for Enhanced Parenting) with no etiology. Notice, however, that there are still some wellness labels that have different one-part formats (e.g., Effective Breastfeeding and Health-Promoting Behaviors).

PLANNING OUTCOMES/EVALUATION

NOC standardized outcomes related to health promotion vary depending on the focus area. For example, if the nursing diagnosis is Readiness for Enhanced Nutrition, a NOC outcome might be Nutritional Status. For examples of other NOC wellness outcomes,

 Go to Chapter 41, **Standardized Language, Examples of NOC Standardized Health Promotion Outcomes,** in Volume 2.

Individualized goals and outcomes might include losing 20 pounds or exercising for 30 minutes five times per week. The nurse's role in health promotion primarily is to motivate clients and facilitate change. Clients are independently responsible for most of their health promotion activities. You may need to help them identify goals, but it is essential that the goals be the clients', not yours.

Healthy People 2020 Goals. You may need aggregate wellness goals for groups as well as individualized goals. Four broad goals for the U.S. population set by the *Healthy People 2020* initiative (U.S. Department of Health and Human Services [U.S. DHHS], 2010, p. 2):

- Attain high quality, longer lives free of preventable disease, disability, injury, and premature death.
- Achieve health equity, eliminate disparities, and improve the health of all groups.
- Create social and physical environments that promote good health for all.
- Promote healthy development and healthy behaviors across every stage of life.

Interventions to achieve these goals are targeted at the 37 focus areas shown in Box 41-1. Public health agencies at the local, state, and federal levels use these focus areas as a blueprint to design programs aimed at

---

BOX 41-1 ■ Focus Areas of *Healthy People 2020*

1. Access to health services
2. Adolescent health
3. Arthritis, osteoporosis, and chronic back conditions
4. Blood disorders and blood safety
5. Cancer
6. Chronic kidney disease
7. Diabetes
8. Disability and secondary conditions
9. Early and middle childhood
10. Educational and community-based programs
11. Environmental health
12. Family planning
13. Food safety
14. Genomics
15. Global health
16. Health communication and health IT
17. Health-associated infections
18. Hearing and other sensory or communication disorders
19. Heart disease and stroke
20. HIV
21. Immunization and infectious diseases
22. Injury and violence prevention
23. Maternal, infant, and child health
24. Medical product safety
25. Mental health and mental disorders
26. Nutrition and overweight
27. Occupational safety and health
28. Older adults
29. Oral health
30. Physical activity and fitness
31. Public health infrastructure
32. Respiratory diseases
33. Sexually transmitted diseases
34. Social determinants of health
35. Substance abuse
36. Tobacco use
37. Vision

Source: U.S. Department of Health and Human Services, Office of Disease Prevention & Health Promotion and Human Services. (2009, October 30, revised). Proposed Healthy People 2020 objectives. Retrieved from http://www.healthypeople.gov/hp2020/Objectives/TopicAreas.aspx.

improving the health status of the community (U.S. DHHS, 2010). To view those objectives,

 Go to the **Healthy People 2020** Web site at www.healthypeople.gov/Search/objectives.htm

Whether standardized or individualized, expected outcomes for wellness diagnoses describe behaviors or responses that demonstrate health maintenance or achievement of an even higher level of health. For example:

Over the next year, Mr. Needham will continue to eat a balanced diet, with more emphasis on including whole grains and fiber.

By using the highest number (5) on the rating scale, you can use the NOC to write wellness outcomes. For example:

Nursing diagnosis: Readiness for Enhanced Nutrition
Expected outcome: Nutritional Status: (5) Not compromised

PLANNING INTERVENTIONS/IMPLEMENTATION

Nurses have been recognized as leaders in health promotion for a long time. Community and public health nurses focus on the problems contributing to disease, such as poor housing conditions, poor sanitation, poor nutrition, poverty, and substance abuse. Nurses in acute care focus on educating patients about health and disease.

Once the client identifies his goals, help him to identify the steps that he must take to reach the goals. Recall that change occurs in stages. To create positive change, the client will need to understand the benefits of change, overcome the barriers to change, and make a commitment to follow through on the plan.

For *NIC standardized interventions* for health promotion,

 Go to Chapter 41, **Standardized Language, Selected NIC Wellness Interventions,** in Volume 2.

NIC does not have a special domain, or grouping, for wellness interventions. Instead, they are found throughout all areas of the taxonomy, particularly in the Behavioral, Safety, Family, Health System, and Community domains.

Specific nursing activities for health promotion include those in the following four subsections. The remainder of the chapter provides some strategies to promote their use.

Nutrition. To guide people in making nutritional choices that promote health and prevent disease, the United States Department of Agriculture (USDA) and the U.S. Department of Health and Human Services (U.S. DHHS) updated the 2005 *Revised Dietary Guidelines for Americans* and the Food Guide and MyPyramid for Kids (you will find these in Chapter 26). *Canada's Food Guide* also offers guidelines for healthy nutrition. In short, this means eating a balanced diet and limiting the intake of fats, sugars, and salt.

Exercise. Physically active people have fewer healthcare visits and hospitalizations and use less medication than physically inactive people. Most health benefits occur with at least 150 minutes (2 hours and 30 minutes) a week of moderate-intensity physical activity, such as brisk walking. Additional benefits occur with more physical activity (U.S. DHHS, 2008). Children and teens should engage in at least one hour of age-appropriate, physical activity daily (Fig. 41-3). Activity should be vigorous-intensity and varied in type, not only to prevent boredom but mostly to promote muscle and bone-strengthening as well as flexibility. Programs, such as the President's Challenge, encourage the development of physical fitness lifestyle habits in people of all ages and abilities. For more information,

 Go to the **President's Challenge** Web site at www.presidentschallenge.org

Lifestyle Changes. Lifestyle changes focus on reducing tobacco and alcohol use, and substance abuse, promoting healthy sleep, and improving stress management.

Sleep. In general, adults need 6 to 9 hours of sleep a night. Children need more sleep (see Chapter 33). Inadequate sleep is linked with weight gain and obesity.

For an expanded discussion of these areas for health promotion,

 Go to Chapter 41, **Supplemental Materials: Individual Health Promotion Activities,** on the Student Resource Disk or DavisPlus at http://davisplus.fadavis.com/Wilkinson2

Role Modeling

A role model teaches by example, demonstrating the behaviors and/or attitudes to be learned. Models provide inspiration and strategies for health promotion behavior. For example, a morbidly obese female joins a weight loss group led by a woman who has lost nearly 100 pounds. She admires the leader for her determination and success and selects her as a role model.

Clients select their own role models, often without making a conscious decision to do so. But it may be helpful for you to facilitate the client's choice. When

FIGURE 41-3 Vigorous-intensity exercise promotes muscle and bone strength and improves cardiovascular health.

suggesting a model, consider the client's age, culture, values, and preferred activities. The model should be someone with whom the client identifies. Ideally, the role model should be someone accessible to the client during the early stages of change. This allows for interacting and for exchanging information. At times, however, a famous athlete or celebrity may be the model. The modeling is more likely to be effective if the celebrity has written about her success or speaks publicly about her positive change.

Nurses also serve as role models. As a result, we should provide an example of healthy behaviors. It is difficult to advocate for healthy behavior if you do not follow the behavior you recommend to clients. Imagine the trust a client loses when he finds out that the nurse who tells him not to smoke cigarettes has a two-pack per day habit. How compelling is a discussion of the importance of weight loss given by an overweight nurse? To what extent do you role-model healthy behaviors?

Providing Counseling

Counseling is an interpersonal communication process that helps a client to identify problems and make changes. In the context of health promotion, counseling promotes personal growth and helps clients change their lifestyle. Counseling may be formal one-to-one or small-group discussion, or it may be informal discussion with the client at a healthcare encounter. Each meeting with a client is a potential counseling session. In addition to face-to-face contact, counseling may be offered via telephone or even by e-mail.

Individual Counseling

Face-to-face interaction may be helpful when clients are attempting major lifestyle change. In an individual session, you can customize and map out the steps required to meet the client's goals. This may include writing a contract detailing the client's expected behaviors. Print out the contract, and have the client sign it to reinforce his commitment. Suggest the client post the plan in a location he sees often so that it serves as a frequent reminder.

During counseling sessions, remember to reinforce health-promoting behaviors that have already been established. For example, the client who uses tobacco may eat a balanced diet; reinforce the healthy habit to boost self-esteem. Stress to the client that although the behavior to be changed may be unhealthy, you believe the client can succeed in making the change.

Telephone Counseling

Telephone counseling may be used as a primary counseling approach or as follow-up. Many clients with hectic schedules find it easier to arrange telephone counseling than to schedule a face-to-face interaction. The disadvantage is that telephone counseling does not allow you to detect nonverbal communication.

When using telephone counseling, you will set goals and map out the strategy for change just as you would in face-to-face counseling. Make sure to inform the client about how and when you can be reached if questions arise. If you are using the telephone for follow-up counseling, it is best to schedule a time to speak. Having an appointment helps keep the patient accountable to the expected behavior and to reinforce the information.

Providing Health Education

Health education may focus on self-care strategies, caregiver concerns, or how to be an effective healthcare consumer. Self-care programs typically cover nutrition, exercise, stress management, or disease prevention. Programs may consist of lectures, printed material, billboards, or posters. For example, the accompanying box, Self-Care: Teaching Clients How to Prevent Upper Respiratory Infections, might be reproduced and posted in the lounge, rest rooms, or locker areas of a worksite during cold and flu season to decrease absenteeism. Caregiver education programs may teach caregivers how to perform nursing tasks or prevent injuries, or they may provide a list of community resources for respite care. Nurses can teach clients how to be effective healthcare consumers, how to interact with healthcare providers, and how to maneuver through the healthcare system. For a review of teaching and learning, see Chapter 24.

Providing and Facilitating Support for Lifestyle Change

Changing one's lifestyle is difficult. Most clients need support to make the change. You can provide support during your interactions and counseling sessions. You can also help the client to identify available support and resources within the community as well as from family, friends, coworkers, and others.

Group support exists for a variety of lifestyle changes. For example, Weight Watchers® is a group support program for clients who want to lose weight; Alcoholics Anonymous is a group support program for clients who want to become and stay sober; various cancer support groups help clients deal with the common issues and fears associated with dealing with a potentially life-threatening disease. Group support provides clients with a chance to meet people experiencing the same difficulties and perhaps to find a role model. As a nurse, you should be familiar with various programs available in your community and refer clients to them.

Self-Care

Teaching Clients How to Prevent Upper Respiratory Infections

➤ Maintain a healthy lifestyle. That means get adequate sleep, good nutrition and physical exercise. A balanced diet and physical fitness can boost your immune system to fight infection if it occurs.

➤ Wash your hands often; teach children to do so as well. This helps prevent spread of infection. When using public restrooms, wash your hands. Then, turn off the faucet with a paper towel. Also use a paper towel to open the door as you leave the room.

➤ Avoid touching your eyes, nose, and mouth, because doing so spreads any virus your hands have contacted (e.g., on doorknobs).

➤ Avoid crowds, especially when there is a cold or influenza epidemic.

➤ Throw away tissues as soon as you use them.

➤ When someone in the family has a cold, keep bathrooms and the kitchen very clean and do not drink from the same glass or use the same utensils.

➤ When someone at home or at work has a cold, wipe telephone receivers with soap and water or an antibacterial solution.

➤ If a child has a cold, wash his toys and commonly used items well.

➤ When choosing child care, look for a clean environment; ask what rules they have about keeping the children clean (e.g., washing hands before snack time).

➤ Don't smoke. Cigarette smoke can irritate the respiratory tract, making you more susceptible to colds and illness.

➤ Control stress. People experiencing emotional stress tend to have weakened immunity to fight infection.

➤ Consider taking echinacea, although conclusive evidence of its effectiveness does not exist at this time. Consult your primary healthcare provider.

Studies have found that group support works. The Task Force on Community Preventive Services (2005) found group-level interventions to be effective in promoting physical activity. These interventions included making changes in school-based physical education programs; conducting community-wide campaigns; improving access to places for physical activity; and offering individually adapted behavior change programs in group settings.

Family, friends, and caregivers may help or hinder the change process. Help clients identify who can offer support and who may be threatened by the client's proposed change. For example, when a woman begins to lose weight, an insecure husband may secretly feel concerned that she will become attractive to other men. Often you can provide information to family and friends that will help them support the physical and emotional changes the client is making.

KnowledgeCheck 41-4

Identify four strategies to help a client engage in positive lifestyle change.

 Go to Chapter 41, **Knowledge Check Response Sheet and Answers,** on the Student Resource Disk or DavisPlus at http://davisplus.fadavis.com/Wilkinson2

 Go to Chapter 41, **Resources for Caregivers and Health Professionals,** on the Student Resource Disk or DavisPlus at http://davisplus.fadavis.com/Wilkinson2

 Suggested Readings: Go to Chapter 41, **Reading More About Promoting Health,** on the Student Resource Disk or DavisPlus at http://davisplus.fadavis.com/Wilkinson2

 Bibliography: Go to Volume 2, Bibliography.

The Context for Nurses' Work

CHAPTER 42

Community Nursing

Learning Outcomes

After completing this chapter, you should be able to:

➤ Define a community.

➤ Identify at least four factors that make populations healthy.

➤ Identify at least four factors that make populations vulnerable.

➤ Identify the major differences between community nursing and acute care nursing.

➤ Compare and contrast community-based nursing, community health nursing, public health nursing, and community-oriented nursing.

➤ Distinguish primary, secondary, and tertiary interventions in regard to a community health scenario.

➤ Discuss the dimensions of a community that are included in a nursing assessment.

➤ Describe the roles of nurses in the community setting.

➤ Identify at least five career opportunities for community nurses.

➤ Discuss at least three strategies that nurses use to gather community data.

➤ Explain how NANDA-I, NIC, and NOC taxonomies are used when the client is a community.

➤ Describe how the Omaha classification system is used for community health nursing.

Meet Your Patient

You are nearing completion of your fundamentals course. One night while you are preparing for your next clinical, the telephone rings. It is your neighbor, Tanya. Her 5-year-old son, Jacob, attends kindergarten at the local public school. Jacob came home with a letter from the school nurse stating that another child in the class was ill with H1N1 influenza and that all the students in the class had been exposed to the disease.

Tanya is concerned about the risks to Jacob and the rest of the family. Tanya is 8 months pregnant, and the family has no health insurance. She states that because you are a nursing student, she thought you might know what she should do or where she might go for assistance.

Although you are flattered that your neighbor has consulted you, you need to consider whether you have the expertise to answer her questions. This complex situation requires knowledge from many aspects of nursing (e.g., immunizations, pregnancy, microbiology, pathophysiology). Though you may not have all of the information you need

to answer her questions, you should be able to help your neighbor resolve her concerns. You will need to consider the following questions:

- What is going on in the situation that may influence the outcome?
- Who should be involved to improve the outcome?
- What theoretical knowledge do I need to answer my neighbor's questions? Where would I find this information?
- What additional data do I need to collect from my neighbor?
- What suggestions and/or referrals should I offer to my neighbor?

In this chapter, we discuss community nursing, a facet of nursing that frequently deals with problems such as this.

Theoretical Knowledge
knowing why

Nurses working in community and public health regularly deal with concerns about communicable disease and immunization programs to prevent them. In this chapter, we discuss communities and community nursing care. We also explore the roles, interventions, and career opportunities for nurses who work within communities.

Understanding Communities

The word **community** comes from the Latin term *communis,* meaning the gift or fellowship of common relations and feelings. Historically, it meant a body of like-minded people or the inhabitants of a town. Then and now, the term suggests a general sense of selflessness, sharing, relationship, and doing good that comes from working together. Most members of a community share a common language, certain rituals, and special customs.

In contrast to community, a **population** is defined as all of the people inhabiting a specified area. For example, look at a map of Ohio and try to determine the approximate boundaries of the city of Dayton (Fig. 42-1). To accurately determine the physical boundaries of the city, you would need local maps showing exact roads, streets, rivers, and other landmarks. As you can imagine, the characteristics and concerns of the many people living within Dayton vary greatly—there are many communities within the larger city of Dayton.

The United States Bureau of the Census conducts a survey and count of the American people every 10 years. The most recent census is the one conducted in the year 2010. For results,

 Go to the **U.S. Census Bureau** Web site at http://2010. census.gov/2010census/

When the census is completed, the Bureau groups the data into sections of 1500 to 8000 people, known as **census tracts.** The area of individual census tracts varies

according to the density of the population. In urban centers, a census tract covers a small area. Rural census tracts are large. Census tracts are useful to public officials, market analysts, and anyone—including community nurses—who studies the characteristics and concerns of smaller sections of people.

Maps and census tracts show the *geopolitical* boundaries of a community. But as we noted earlier, a community can also be a group of people with a common purpose. They may live in different geographical areas, but they have a "sense of belonging" to their group (community). An **aggregate** is a group of individuals with at least one shared characteristic, either personal or environmental. For example, a community health nurse may work with a class of high school girls to reduce the incidence of adolescent pregnancy. The shared characteristics of this aggregate are that they are female, of child-bearing age, and attend a particular school. As another example, the nursing students in your school are an aggregate. What characteristics and goals do you share?

 Critical**Thinking** 42-1

- Why might the boundaries of a census tract change every 10 years?
- How could you figure out what census tract you live or go to school in?

Knowledge Check 42-1

- Give several examples of a community.
- How is a population different from a community?

 Go to Chapter 42, **Knowledge Check Response Sheet and Answers,** on the Student Resource Disk or DavisPlus at http://davisplus.fadavis.com/Wilkinson2

What Are the Components of a Community?

To understand a particular community and its needs, you will need information about its three components: structure, status, and processes.

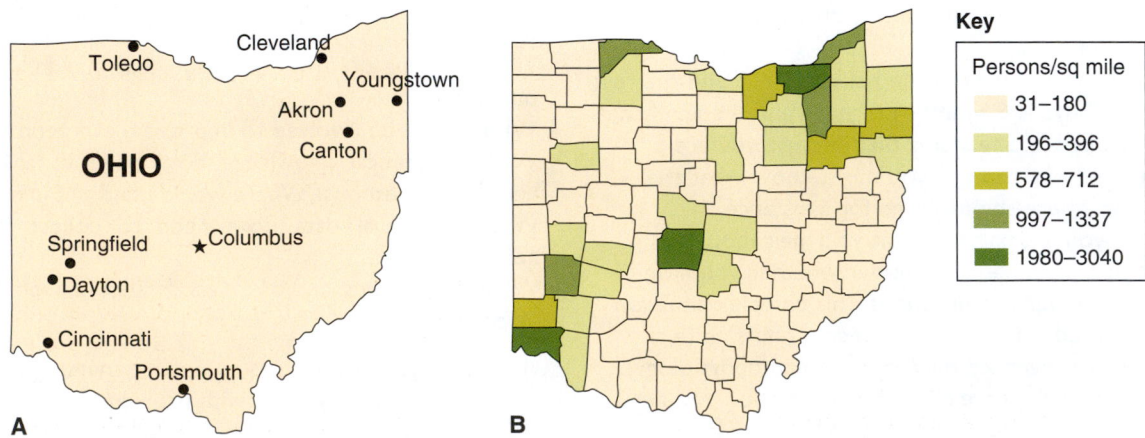

FIGURE 42-1 A, Geopolitical boundaries. B, Census tract data provide more detail about communities.

■ **Structure** refers to the general characteristics of a community. These include demographic data, such as gender, age, ethnicity, and educational and income levels, as well as data about healthcare services, such as the number of primary care providers or emergency departments in the area.

■ **Status** describes the biological, emotional, and social outcome components of a community. *Biological* data include morbidity (illness) and mortality (death) rates, life expectancy ratios, and risk factor profiles for the respective age groups within a community. *Emotional* data include general indications of mental health and consumer satisfaction survey results about various aspects of the community as compared to other locales. *Social* data include crime rates, citizenship involvement in community-wide activities, and general functioning levels of the community members.

■ **Process** describes the overall effectiveness level of the community. For example, do the members of the community perceive that they are part of a group with common interests? What is the extent of interaction among community members? Does the community have an established forum for conflict resolution?

What Makes a Community Healthy?

As with individuals, the meaning and perception of health varies among aggregates. For nurses, it is important to understand what a particular community defines (and values) as health rather than relying on personal definitions. Health is whatever the client community defines it to be.

When determining what makes a community healthy, the national consensus paper *Healthy People 2020* provides useful guidelines. The document (initially titled *Healthy People 2000* and now in another revised edition) was produced in response to a 1979 report from the surgeon general indicating that many of the health problems of Americans were preventable. *Healthy People 2020* identifies leading indicators for measuring the health of our nation. Some examples affecting community health include:

■ Physical activity
■ Overweight and obesity
■ Tobacco use
■ Substance abuse
■ Responsible sexual behavior
■ Mental health
■ Injury and violence
■ Environmental quality
■ Immunizations
■ Access to healthcare

For the complete list of indicators, see Box 41-1, Focus Areas of *Healthy People 2020*.

The four overarching goals of the *Healthy People 2020* initiative are: (1) increase years of healthy life; (2) eliminate health disparities among different populations, including

accessibility of healthcare; (3) create an environment conducive to social and physical health; and (4) promote healthy living for people across all life stages.

These aggregate goals are to be achieved through promoting healthy behaviors, increasing access to quality healthcare, and strengthening community health resources. For more information,

 Go to the *Healthy People 2020* Web site available at www.healthypeople.gov.

Note: Healthy People 2020 Proposed Objectives were available at the time of publication. Go to the Web site for most up-to-date information and final objectives.

KnowledgeCheck 42-2

■ What makes up the "structure" of a community?
■ What is community "status"?
■ What is community "process"?
■ Use the guidelines from *Healthy People 2020* to compile a list of several characteristics that make a community healthy.

 Go to Chapter 42, **Knowledge Check Response Sheet and Answers,** on the Student Resource Disk or DavisPlus at http://davisplus.fadavis.com/Wilkinson2

What Makes a Population Vulnerable?

A **vulnerable population** is defined as an aggregate that is at increased risk of adverse health outcomes. Members of vulnerable populations have a higher probability of developing illness than do members of the general population. For example, pregnant adolescents are more likely to develop complications than pregnant women of all ages taken as a whole. Because of their increased risk of health problems, vulnerable populations are a major focus of community health efforts. Vulnerability involves multiple factors:

Limited Economic Resources. Income is a major predictor of health risk. People with higher incomes typically have greater access to health services and greater selection of providers, treatment options, and location of health services. In contrast, the more limited a person's income, the more limited her healthcare options. Consequently, many persons of low income forego preventive or health maintenance care and seek healthcare services only when they are quite ill.

Limited Social Resources. Friends and family are valuable resources to help a person deal with day-to-day stress as well as the demands associated with illness. They provide feedback, listen to concerns, and offer emotional and physical assistance. Unfortunately, not everyone has social resources. Older adults who live alone and people with mental illness are examples of groups at increased risk because of social isolation.

Age. The very young and the very old are less able to adapt to physiological stress and are at increased risk of disease. They are more prone to infections and may not be able to protect themselves from environmental hazards, such as cold or heat. These age groups are also more likely to be living in poverty.

Chronic Disease and Obesity. People who have chronic diseases are at greater risk for many health problems. For example, people with obesity are at increased risk for heart disease, diabetes, impaired mobility, joint pain, and other complications. People with diabetes are at risk for blindness, impaired wound healing, and other complications.

History of Abuse or Trauma. People who have experienced abuse or traumatic events often feel they have limited control over their health and circumstances. They may experience powerlessness and/or hopelessness and be unable to initiate activities that promote health or lead to early treatment of illness. These circumstances also tax their reserves and place them at risk for mental health problems.

Other vulnerable populations include people who are poor or homeless, migrant workers, people with disabilities, premature infants, women with high-risk pregnancy, pregnant adolescents, people with communicable disease, people who abuse substances, members of certain ethnic/racial groups, and the untreated mentally ill.

Understanding Community Nursing

A community can be either a *site* for healthcare delivery or a *recipient* of healthcare services. Throughout history, most care was provided in or for the community. In fact, the first hospitals in the United States were established only in the late 1860s to protect society from contagious disease. Several decades passed before hospitals and their satellite clinics became the predominant settings for providing healthcare. However, as the technological advances of the last 30 years have escalated the costs of delivering health services, efforts to lower costs have created a move back to more community-based care, including complementary and alternative care.

Community-Based Care

Community-based care refers to acute care or rehabilitative services performed in clinics, offices, mobile care units, and other facilities in the community—rather than in acute care settings, such as hospitals (although acute care settings also exist within the community). For example, many surgeries and diagnostic procedures are now performed in surgicenters, clinics, and physicians' offices rather than in hospitals. People also receive mental, physical, cardiac, and pulmonary rehabilitation services in outpatient settings. Extended care facilities, or nursing homes, commonly provide rehabilitative care for patients after acute traumatic injuries, as well as continuous skilled care for older adults and people with chronic illness. The following sections describe three approaches

to community-based nursing care: community health nursing, public health nursing, and community-oriented nursing.

Community Health Nursing

Although many people use the terms *community health nursing* and *public health nursing* interchangeably, the two are not identical. **Community health nursing** focuses on how the health of individuals, families, and groups affects the community as a whole. Community health nurses strive to promote, protect, preserve, and maintain the health of the population through the delivery of personal health services to individuals, families, and groups. For example, a community health nurse may work in a prenatal clinic providing free services for low-income women. The nurse provides a direct service to each pregnant woman, yet she is doing that to improve the general health of the entire community. By encouraging the mother to eat balanced meals, exercise, and avoid harmful substances, the nurse improves the health of both mother and baby—who are members of the community—and, therefore, improves the overall health of the community.

Public Health Nursing

Public health nursing focuses on the community at large and the eventual effect of the community's health status on the health of individuals, families, and groups. The goal of public health is to prevent individual disease and disability, in addition to promoting and protecting the health of the community as a whole. For example, a public health nurse may be employed by a county health department to provide tuberculosis (TB) **surveillance** services. The nurse helps to protect the entire community by screening for TB at the local school, by testing high-risk individuals for TB, and by identifying and tracking clients with active disease to ensure that they complete the prescribed 6- to 9-month medication regimen.

Because public health focuses on large-scale programs that address the entire community, government-based agencies often provide these services. The United States Public Health Service (USPHS) is an example of a public health agency based within the federal government (Box 42-1).

For additional information on the USPHS,

 Go to Chapter 42, **Supplemental Materials: United States Public Health Service,** on the Student Resource Disk or DavisPlus at http://davisplus.fadavis.com/Wilkinson2

Community-Oriented Nursing

Community-oriented nursing combines components of community and public health, focusing on health promotion, illness prevention, early detection, and treatment

BOX 42-1 ■ Examples of Successful Public Health Programs

- Immunization
- Motor vehicle safety
- Safer workplaces
- Control of infectious diseases
- Decline in deaths from coronary heart disease and stroke
- Safer and healthier foods
- Healthier mothers and babies
- Family planning
- Fluoridation of drinking water
- Recognition of tobacco use as a health hazard
- Smoking cessation

FIGURE 42-2 Schematic relationship of community nursing approaches.

provided within the community setting. The practice is evidence-based and collaborative with other community health disciplines. The focus is a comprehensive look at the individual, family, group, and community at large. For example, a nurse with a community-oriented approach might work in a comprehensive adolescent prenatal program. The nurse provides individual care at the local clinic 2 days per week. While at the clinic, she gathers data from adolescent clients about the schools they attend; their knowledge of birth control, pregnancy, and childbirth; as well as the issues these girls face with pregnancy. On the remaining 3 days of the week, she engages in community-focused activities that are informed by her knowledge and experience with pregnant teens. For example, she meets with school officials to identify pregnant teens who need prenatal care, teaches a class about sexuality in the local high school, works with teachers to identify strategies to keep pregnant teens in school, provides parenting education to adolescents who have children, and advocates changing a bus route so that teens can easily get to the local clinic. Each aspect of care allows the nurse to gather more data about the needs of the individuals and the community as a whole. Figure 42-2 provides a schematic of the relationship of the various community-based nursing approaches identified in this section.

KnowledgeCheck 42-3

- What is the distinction between an aggregate population and a vulnerable population?
- Identify practice differences between a community-based nurse and an acute care nurse.
- How is public health nursing different from community health nursing? How is it the same?
- How is community-oriented nursing related to community health nursing and public health nursing?

 Go to Chapter 42, **Knowledge Check Response Sheet and Answers,** on the Student Resource Disk or DavisPlus at http://davisplus.fadavis.com/Wilkinson2

 Critical**Thinking** 42-2
Review the scenario of Tanya and Jacob ("Meet Your Patient"). Which form of community-based nursing would be most appropriate to address their concerns?

Who Were Some Pioneers of Community Nursing?

The following are some of the most notable people who have contributed to the development of community-based nursing care.

- *Florence Nightingale*—Established the importance of promoting health by manipulating the environment (e.g., light, warmth, sanitation, cleanliness) and nursing the whole person.
- *Lillian Wald*—Known as the first community health nurse; founded the first visiting nurses association in New York.
- *Clara Barton*—Founder of the American Red Cross.
- *Margaret Sanger*—Founded the International Planned Parenthood Federation. Pioneered the use of family planning and birth control education.

If you would like to learn more about the achievements of these community health pioneers,

Go to Chapter 42, **Supplemental Materials: Pioneers of Community-Based Nursing,** on the Student Resource Disk or DavisPlus at http://davisplus.fadavis.com/Wilkinson2

Working Within Communities

In the community setting, nurses' roles vary depending on the community and its identified needs. Community nursing care is by nature holistic, and it serves a large client population. Therefore, one of the most effective nursing interventions is **empowerment.** This means assisting the client (individual or community) to recognize and use available resources to achieve or maintain the desired level of health, achieve autonomy, and maintain positive self-esteem.

What Are the Roles of Community Nurses?

Community health nurses function as client advocates, educators, collaborators, counselors, and case managers. All of these roles require excellent written and oral communication skills. Although electronic health records and widespread use of e-mail, text messaging, and other forms of electronic communication have made it possible to communicate with large numbers of people, computer or Internet access might be a problem in some areas. In addition, there are still some people who do not have computer skills.

Client Advocate

The effective community health nurse consistently supports the identified or expressed concerns of the client and/or community. Advocating for a community often requires political involvement at the local, state, or national levels. The challenge is in knowing whom to approach for political support and how to gain their support. As a community health nurse you can effect change by getting involved in your local student nurses association, professional nursing organizations, school boards, citizen committees, or attending council meetings.

Educator

Because community nursing focuses on wellness and disease prevention, much of what the nurse does involves client education—of individuals, aggregates at risk of disease, politicians, or a community at large. However, it is difficult to evaluate the effect of the education because people may not act on the knowledge for months or years after the teaching moment. When planning teaching, you must be aware of the stage of development, educational level, and learning style of the community group you intend to educate. The best learning programs are short; provide relevant, practical information; and can be easily incorporated into the learner's daily routine. For more information, see Chapter 24.

Collaborator

A primary task of a community health nurse is to serve as a collaborator. Partnerships and coalitions can effectively address common concerns among different communities. Consider the following example: A community health nurse is concerned about poor compliance with recommended immunization schedules for 2-year-olds in a particular community. He surveys some of the parents to determine their reasons for not obtaining vaccinations. The nurse discovers that the clinic's operating hours are limited and the automated call routing system is frustrating for people trying to schedule an appointment. The nurse also discovers that some offices are not reminding clients to return for missed appointments. The community nurse schedules a meeting of clinic staff, practice managers, and patients to resolve these issues. At the meeting, some larger issues are revealed, such as failure of state Medicaid agencies to reimburse the providers adequately and in a timely manner. In addition, there are not enough Medicaid providers to serve the community.

Counselor

Once you have established rapport with a group, members may consult you about a variety of health and non–health-related concerns (Fig. 42-3). You must be careful to offer counsel only in areas within your scope of practice and make recommendations that are practical yet meet the needs of the community. Often, you may need only to serve as a witness to the group's concerns. Letting clients debate or work through issues empowers them and fosters self-reliance.

Case Manager

Community nurses commonly make referrals to or collaborate with other health and social agencies. Be cautious in referring clients to these resources, because agency policies and financing change frequently. Also, because community agencies often operate on grants and time-restricted funding, a program that is available at one time may be dissolved at another. As a nurse, you will need to remain in contact with agencies to which clients are referred so that you remain aware of the current restrictions and availability of services. For example, a local group has established a free healthcare program for resident children who are underinsured. Pediatricians and nurses volunteer their time to provide the care. Pharmaceutical representatives provide the medical supplies and routine

FIGURE 42-3 A community health nurse functioning in her counselor role.

medications. Local specialists (e.g., surgeons) provide services to those with complex or specialized needs. However, in such a clinic the appointment times fill up quickly, and often clients have to wait more than a month or two for an appointment. Before enrolling families in the program, you would need to be aware of these limitations and share this information with clients.

KnowledgeCheck 42-4

Give an example of a nursing activity involved in each of the following community health roles: educator, advocate, case manager, counselor, and collaborator.

 Go to Chapter 42, **Knowledge Check Response Sheet and Answers,** on the Student Resource Disk or DavisPlus at http://davisplus.fadavis.com/Wilkinson2

How Are Community Nursing Interventions Classified?

There are three basic levels of care in which nursing interventions can be classified: primary, secondary, and tertiary. Most community-oriented nursing practices are aimed at the primary (prevention) level.

Primary Interventions

The goal of primary (first-level) interventions is to promote health and prevent disease. Educating susceptible individuals with no known disease process is an example of a routine, primary intervention that community health nurses practice. For example, a nurse may educate high school freshman girls about the risk of hepatitis B and human papillomavirus (HPV), the benefits of vaccination, and strategies to reduce the likelihood of exposure to contaminated body fluids. Other examples include collaborating with local agencies to provide clean and secure temporary housing for migrant farm workers, and lobbying elected representatives for a ban on smoking in restaurants. Primary interventions are usually the least invasive and least expensive of the three levels of intervention.

Secondary Interventions

Secondary (second-level) interventions aim to reduce the impact of the disease process by early detection and treatment. For example, a community health nurse may screen a sexually active adolescent girl for hepatitis B and/or HPV. She has known risk factors for sexually transmitted infection but no apparent disease symptoms. The nurse will also teach the client how to protect herself from sexually transmitted infections, hepatitis B, and HIV in the future. Other examples of secondary interventions include providing outreach screening programs offering mammography, scoliosis

screening, lipid testing, or PSA testing for prostate cancer (Fig. 42-4).

Tertiary Interventions

The goal of tertiary (third-level) intervention is to halt disease progression and/or restore client functioning to the pre-disease state. The disease process is clinically apparent and client debilitation, including death, is likely without intervention. Tertiary level interventions are usually the most invasive and require the nurse to collaborate with members of other disciplines to provide treatment. For example, a student may report to a school nurse that she has been involved in unprotected sexual activities. The school nurse may refer the student to the public health clinic for a pelvic exam and lab testing to detect sexually transmitted infection (STI); and hepatitis B, HPV, and HIV screening. The student has an abnormal Pap smear, showing cells suggestive of HPV exposure. The nurse, in collaboration with the provider, provides medical treatment. There is no cure for HPV, so the teen also needs to learn how to prevent the spread of the disease to others and obtain regular Pap and pelvic exams to detect cervical cancer and other STIs.

CriticalThinking 42-3

What level of intervention is required to address the concerns of Tanya and Jacob ("Meet Your Patient")? Discuss your response.

KnowledgeCheck 42-5

For each of the nursing actions listed, identify the level of the nursing intervention as primary, secondary, or tertiary.

- Taking a client's blood pressure at a health fair
- Administering insulin to an elderly person at an extended care facility
- Teaching second-grade students to wash their hands correctly

 Go to Chapter 42, **Knowledge Check Response Sheet and Answers,** on the Student Resource Disk or DavisPlus at http://davisplus.fadavis.com/Wilkinson2

FIGURE 42-4 Secondary interventions. Early detection of heart disease with lipid screening.

Toward Evidence-Based Practice

Hicks, P., Tarr, G. M., & Hicks, X. P. (2007). **Reminder cards and immunization rates among Latinos and the rural poor in northeast Colorado.** *Journal of the American Board of Family Medicine, 20*(6), 581–586.

Reminder cards have been shown to increase immunization rates in urban settings. However, researchers wanted to investigate the effectiveness of reminder cards among impoverished Latino children living in rural areas. Language-appropriate reminder cards were mailed to patients with missing vaccines. These cards increased the rate of up-to-date immunization from 61.3% to 73.4%.

Moore, M. L., & Parker, A. L. (2006). **Influenza vaccine compliance among pediatric asthma patients: What is the better method of notification?** *Pediatric Asthma and Allergy Immunology, 19*(4), 200–204.

This study was conducted to find a better way to notify parents of changes in American Academy of Pediatrics vaccine requirements in order to improve compliance.

Researchers mailed a reminder card informing parents of asthmatic children at a military base about the need for influenza immunization. After the mailing the percentage of children ages 5 to 10 years receiving the vaccine increased significantly as compared to those receiving verbal reminders.

1. What would you anticipate to be patient-related obstacles to optimal vaccine coverage?

2. What would you anticipate to be some other factors in the medical clinic or office practice that could contribute to a less effective immunization program?

3. What are some ideas you have to improve the effectiveness of an immunization program in the setting where you might work?

Go to Chapter 42, **Toward Evidence-Based Practice Suggested Responses,** on the Student Resource Disk or DavisPlus at http://davisplus.fadavis.com/Wilkinson2

What Career Opportunities Are Available for Community-Based Nurses?

The following are only a few of the many career opportunities for nurses who want to practice from a community-based perspective.

School Nursing

Nursing practice in the school setting began when educators realized that children with health problems had more difficulty learning. School nurses provide direct care for children with chronic health conditions, such as asthma, hyperactivity disorder, and diabetes and for children who need routine procedures, such as catheterization, during the school day. School nurses perform mandated vision and hearing screenings. They also administer prescribed medication and ensure that age-appropriate immunizations are documented. Some school nurses offer health education on topics such as sexual and reproductive health. The nurse may also serve as a role model for students who lack parental support or who are struggling with peer pressure. For the most part, a school nurse is autonomous and must be capable of prioritizing and making decisions (American Nurses Association and the National Association of School Nurses, 2005).

Occupational Health

Occupational health nurses work primarily in industrial or corporate settings. Traditionally, occupational health nurses provided health teaching for employees and their families in an effort to reduce absentee hours and increase productivity. Few industries still use the occupational nurse in this manner. Instead, most employ nurses to fulfill union contracts and to complete required medical documentation for disability claims or occupational hazardous events. Thus, the responsibilities of the occupational health nurse may be limited to performing new-hire and annual screenings, providing care to injured workers, completing random drug testing, and filing worker's compensation claims. To reduce costs, most large industries hire a staffing agency to provide trained occupational health nurses. Nursing autonomy and responsibility vary with the employer and the negotiated contract.

Parish Nursing

Parish nursing, also known as faith community nursing, is a community-oriented nursing specialty, defined by the American Nurses Association (ANA) as "...the specialized practice of professional nursing that focuses on the intentional care of the spirit as part of the process of promoting holistic health and preventing or minimizing illness in a faith community" (ANA, 2005). The major accountabilities and job activities of the parish nurse role revolve around integrating faith with health. The parish nurse acts as health educator, and personal health counselor (Fig. 42-5). She develops support groups, trains of volunteers, and provides community referrals as needed (ANA and the Health Ministries Association, 2005). The level of autonomy and responsibility of parish nurses varies, depending on the faith community setting.

FIGURE 42-5 Parish nursing. Caring for an elderly woman in her home.

Nursing in Correctional Facilities

Corrections nurses deliver patient care within the criminal justice system, for example, in juvenile detention, substance abuse treatment facilities, and prisons. In this environment, the nurse provides primary care services to patients of all ages in an unbiased and nonjudgmental manner (ANA, 2007a). Correctional facilities have a medical team that provides routine examinations and acute and chronic healthcare on a scheduled or as-needed basis. The level of nursing autonomy is high in most correctional or substance rehabilitation facilities. The nurse also commonly performs occupational health duties for facility staff. For personal safety, nurses must meet certain physical requirements and complete special weapons training before working in most correctional facilities.

Public Health Clinics

Many community nurses practice within local and state departments of health, including public health clinics. Services offered by health departments can range from basic to comprehensive, based on financial constraints, such as the tax base of the community. Large cities tend to have many nurses who may specialize in an area, such as immunizations, prenatal health, school health, or epidemiological survey. Smaller communities may have only one full-time nurse providing all services. The autonomy and scope of practice of public health nurses are often limited by the philosophy of the political administration and availability of funding.

Disaster Services Nursing

A disaster is any event inflicting widespread loss of life and destruction of property. *Human-generated disasters* might be the result of activities, such as a terrorist attack, war, or use of nuclear energy to cause harm or fear. *Technological disasters* cause damage or disruption on a large scale (e.g., computer systems failure, mass power outage, explosion, or hazardous substance exposure). Examples of *natural or ecological disasters* include hurricanes, earthquakes, tsunamis, and floods. Community-oriented nursing emphasizes community assessment and education to prevent consequences in the aftermath of disasters when possible and to reduce the number of casualties when disasters occur.

Disasters affect the health status of a community in the following ways:

- Lead to premature death, illness or injury.
- Disrupt healthcare services offered within the community.
- Cause environmental issues, such as outbreaks of communicable disease or food/water-borne illness.
- Cause shortages of safe food and drinking water.
- Burden other healthcare systems when displaced populations shift to a host community for basic needs of living (Veenema, 2007).

If a disaster has been declared, the nurse may practice in any state under the direction of the American Red Cross. "Good Samaritan" laws protect nurses from liability provided they are performing care on a volunteer basis and in a manner considered reasonable and prudent and in accordance with standard practice. In large-scale disasters, nurses are typically needed to triage care, staff first-aid stations, assess casualties, assign priorities for care, administer treatment to stabilize the wounded, facilitate transport to local hospitals, and provide healthcare in temporary shelters. For additional information on disaster preparedness and preparation for terrorist attacks,

 Go to Chapter 42, **Supplemental Materials: Disaster Preparedness,** on the Student Resource Disk or DavisPlus at http://davisplus.fadavis.com/Wilkinson2

International Nursing

Nurses working in an international setting commonly provide relief services after a natural or man-made disaster. They may also offer health or human aid services through a medical clinic, faith-based mission, orphanage, or other international relief program. International nursing requires a high level of autonomy, flexibility, and ingenuity, depending on community needs and available resources. Common problems affecting the health of international communities are related to poor sanitation, contaminated food and water, waste management, limited or dangerous transportation, communicable disease, parasitic infections, cultural practices, and limited education. Nurses working globally commonly treat people with malnutrition, dehydration, mosquito and other insect-related illnesses, parasitic infestation, and HIV, to name a few (Fig. 42-6). Because of poor access to healthcare and limited or no resources to pay for medication, many people do not receive adequate healthcare.

Critical Thinking 42-4

Increase your self-knowledge: Assume you are going to be a community-based nurse. Of the many career opportunities available, which work do you think you would rather do? Explain why.

Practical Knowledge
knowing how

Community nursing care should be delivered in a practical, culturally sensitive manner. The nursing process follows the same steps you have studied in the previous chapters but uses different forms and different language when your client is a community.

The American Nurses Association, in the *Standards for Community Health Nursing*, defines the role of the community health nurse as it relates to theory, data collection, diagnosis, planning, intervention, evaluation, quality assurance and professional development, interdisciplinary collaboration, and research. If you need more information about community health nursing standards,

FIGURE 42-6 International nursing. Health and nutrition program for women and children at a Rwandan health clinic.

 Go to Chapter 42, **Resources for Caregivers and Health Professionals, Supplemental Materials,** on the Student Resource Disk or DavisPlus at http://davisplus.fadavis.com/Wilkinson2

ASSESSMENT

Community assessment is usually ongoing and requires the nurse to collaborate with and compile information from a variety of sources. The assessment approach is based on the type of community, the purpose of the assessment, and personal preference. Most beginning students elect to assess a geopolitical community because the data are more readily available than data from aggregate groups. Therefore, we focus on the geopolitical community assessment procedure.

Windshield Survey. Community assessment usually begins with a windshield survey. A **windshield survey** is performed by observing the community through your automobile window, on foot, or otherwise being physically present in the area. It is similar to general observation of the individual client in that it provides an overview and allows you to see the community in its natural state. As you observe, make note of the condition of buildings and public facilities, residences, religious facilities, streets and sewers, modes of transportation, lighting, outward signs of crime or violence, pollution, waste disposal, and other signs of the well-being of the community. Protective services, such as police and fire services, should be included. You may need to repeat the survey over a period of time at different times of the day, month, or year to get an accurate picture of the community.

- Begin by describing the neighborhood and the people you see in the community.
- Strive to remain objective in your observations. Avoid using personal opinions and prejudices.

For more reliable survey results, observers should be trained.

- Route your course prior to conducting the visit.
- Record your findings as soon as possible after your survey.
- Document the observation with photographs and videography when possible.

 Go to **CDC Web site for a sample Windshield Survey,** available at http://www.cdc.gov/dhdsp/library/seh_handbook/chapter_five.htm

Databases and Public Records. You can also obtain data from publicly available resources, such as birth records, marriage licenses, newspapers, and community Web sites. Internet search engines can help you obtain demographic information, morbidity and mortality data, vital statistics, educational levels, criminal activity, political leadership issues, and/or information about community resources.

Client Perceptions. You will also gather information about how individuals in the community perceive the community and its state of health. Through community forums and informal conversations, you can assess a cross-section of the population. This is not only an important part of your assessment, but also an excellent way to establish rapport, convey your concerns, and develop a working relationship with key community members. When you prepare to intervene in the community, you will find this time was wisely spent because community members are more likely to participate in the plan if they are involved from the beginning.

ANALYSIS/NURSING DIAGNOSIS

After a thorough assessment, you will analyze the complete set of data and compile a list of community strengths and limitations. Prioritize the list, considering priorities that have been identified by the client, availability of funding, and the political feasibility of addressing the issue.

In community practice, you need nursing diagnoses that describe the health status of individuals, families, groups, and entire communities. Recall from Chapter 4 that the NANDA-I taxonomy of nursing diagnoses can be used in any nursing setting or specialty. You would simply add the term *community* to other NANDA-I labels when creating a community-based diagnosis: for example, Decisional Conflict (Community) related to safety needs of the homeless population. In addition, the NANDA-I taxonomy includes three diagnoses that specifically describe the health status of a community:

- Ineffective Community Coping
- Readiness for Enhanced Community Coping
- Ineffective Management of Therapeutic Regimen: Community

The Omaha system was developed specifically for use in community settings (Martin & Norris, 1996). In addition to nursing diagnoses, it contains standardized terminology for outcomes and interventions. For a complete overview,

 Go to the **Omaha System** Web site at www.omahasystem. org/

For an expanded discussion of the Omaha problem classification scheme,

 Go to Chapter 42, **Standardized Language, Omaha Problem Classification Scheme,** in Volume 2.

PLANNING OUTCOMES/EVALUATION

In the community you will need to write goals and outcomes for aggregates. The *Healthy People 2020* goals are aggregate goals. The NOC and Omaha taxonomies provide standardized terms for stating community goals. For guidelines in using these two taxonomies,

 Go to Chapter 42, **Standardized Language, Using the NOC and Omaha Systems to Write Aggregate Goals,** in Volume 2.

PLANNING INTERVENTIONS/IMPLEMENTATION

As a community health nurse, you will need interventions to promote and preserve the health of individuals, aggregates, and communities. Both NIC and the Omaha system provide standardized vocabularies for aggregate interventions.

The NIC taxonomy includes 18 interventions specifically designed for community health. The Omaha taxonomy provides four intervention categories that can be used in community-oriented nursing practice. For guidelines,

 Go to Chapter 42, **Standardized Language, Using the NIC and Omaha Interventions Labels,** in Volume 2.

Putting It All Together

The process for conducting a community assessment may appear overwhelming. This final section applies the process to situations you are likely to encounter in the community.

As a community health nurse employed by the local health department within the immunization clinic, you have been hired into a new position created by federal and state grant monies to investigate why immunization levels are low among 2-year-olds in Census Tract 15. How you would approach your new nursing career?

Define the community. Determine the physical boundaries of Census Tract 15, a geopolitical community.

Learn the community. Start interacting with the community to build rapport. Begin the ongoing assessment by conducting windshield surveys, searching for information through reputable databases, and talking with community members.

Focus the data collection. Focus on the information that will help you determine possible causes of low immunization rates. In this case, the priority problem has already been defined by the financing agency.

Critical **Thinking** 42-5

What data would you want to look at? What are possible reasons for low immunization rates?

Analyze the data. Examine the characteristics of families failing to provide immunization for children, including:

- Family demographics
- Age of children
- Number of immunizations needed and the cost
- Beliefs about negative effects of vaccines
- Availability of transportation
- Public sites providing vaccinations
- Overall continuity of general healthcare for children

After working with the community for about 6 months, you have spoken at parenting classes about the need to vaccinate children. Several community members told you that they thought their child had already received all necessary vaccinations or that their doctor had said to wait until they have better insurance. You will need to arrange a meeting with the local providers to discuss low immunization status. They explain that many vaccinations are too expensive to provide, based on the reimbursement they receive from government funding sources.

Plan care. Using the Omaha system, you could generate a care plan to address some of the issues raised by the community members and the doctors.

Assess results, and follow up. Community assessment is never actually complete because the community itself is constantly changing. However, you need to define the identified needs and desired outcomes during a given period of time, based on best data available at the time of the as-

sessment. In this case, you would share with local healthcare providers, the health department, and local health policy committee your approach to addressing the suspected factors contributing to poor immunization compliance. An important part of the role of a community health nurse is need to continue to monitor and evaluate the data to provide updates to the appropriate groups.

Go to Chapter 42, **Resources for Caregivers and Health Professionals,** on the Student Resource Disk or DavisPlus at http://davisplus.fadavis.com/Wilkinson2

Suggested Readings: Go to Chapter 42, **Reading More About Community Nursing,** on the Student Resource Disk or DavisPlus at http://davisplus.fadavis.com/Wilkinson2

Bibliography: Go to Volume 2, Bibliography.

CHAPTER 43

Nursing in Home Care

Learning Outcomes

After completing this chapter, you should be able to:

➤ Identify the primary goal of home care.

➤ Describe ways in which home healthcare differs from hospital nursing.

➤ Categorize the various agencies that deliver home healthcare according to purpose, client served, and funding source.

➤ Identify four key roles of the nurse in home healthcare.

➤ Describe how the nurse's emphasis differs in hospice nursing as compared to home health nursing.

➤ List at least four criteria clients must meet in order for home care to be reimbursed by Medicare.

➤ Explain how clients are referred to home healthcare.

➤ Outline the steps required to prepare for a home visit, including considerations for the nurse's safety.

➤ Discuss ways in which the assessment process is unique in home care.

➤ State two standardized terminologies that can be used for stating home care nursing diagnoses.

➤ Explain the role of the nurse in helping clients and families manage medications.

➤ Describe how infection control measures differ in the home and in the hospital.

➤ Cite at least five examples of how care may be modified in the home setting.

➤ Describe the process for evaluating a home environment.

➤ State two important safety concerns in home care that arise out of The Joint Commission 2009 home care safety goals.

➤ Describe the nurse's role in treating caregiver strain.

Meet Your Patient

Flora Escobar is 78 years old. She lives at home with her 80-year-old husband, Roland. Both have enjoyed good health until Roland suffered a cerebrovascular accident (CVA, or stroke) 3 weeks ago. He was briefly hospitalized and then spent 2 weeks in a skilled nursing facility (SNF) for additional physical care and therapy. He returned home yesterday and will be followed by the local home health agency. You have been asked to make an initial visit today.

Flora Escobar greets you at the door. She opens the door with her left hand and carries a glass of water with her right. She is a petite woman who appears exhausted. Over her casual clothing, she is wearing an apron, the pockets stuffed with pill bottles. The narrow hallway is partially blocked with a bedside commode, walker, and tray table. Mr. Escobar is in a hospital bed in the living room. He is a tall, stocky man who is sitting up in bed but is slumped and leaning to the left. He is wearing pajamas and a robe.

After you introduce yourself, you start with an open-ended question to build rapport: "How have things been going since you came home yesterday?" Mrs. Escobar slowly nods, sighs, and says, "I'm worried that I'm doing things wrong. I have such a hard time helping him move. He is so much bigger than me, and I don't want to hurt him. He is frustrated with me, but he has difficulty talking and can't tell me what he needs." Tears fill Mrs. Escobar's eyes. Her husband turns away to avoid eye contact with you. To refocus their attention, you suggest that you go over some information and then begin to look at what additional services might be helpful.

Imagine how stressed Mrs. Escobar must feel. How do you think you could best help this family? In this chapter, as you read about home health nursing, you should find it easier to answer those questions.

Theoretical **Knowledge**
knowing why

The first true home care agencies in the United States were established in the 1880s. In fact, until the late 1920s, most nursing care was delivered in the home (National Association for Home Care & Hospice [NAHC], 2008). As the technical aspects of healthcare began to dominate, the hospital became the primary healthcare setting. By the early 1960s, there were just 1100 home care agencies in the United States. However, the enactment of Medicare in 1965 prompted new growth in the home-care field by making skilled nursing care and therapy available to older adults and disabled people in their homes. In the last two decades, home care has grown even more as the population has aged and hospital stays have become shorter in an effort to reduce costs. Early hospital discharges have led to increased use of the home as a site for care delivery. The technologies used in the hospital—in modified form—have followed the patient home (e.g., enteric feedings). The growing use of technology in the home has led to increasingly complex care and growing concerns about quality of life. Home care, like hospital-based care, has become a mix of high-tech and high-touch.

What Is Home Healthcare?

Home healthcare is the delivery of health-related services in the client's home. The NAHC reports that more than 17,000 providers deliver a variety of home care services to nearly 8 million clients each year in the United States. Seventy percent of home health clients are older than age 65. Older adults are expected to make up an even greater proportion of clients in the future, and fewer family members will be available to provide care.

Home healthcare is appropriate when a client needs ongoing care that exceeds the abilities of friends and family. It may supplement the skills a family member is providing or serve as a backup for safety or additional assessment. Older adults may use home healthcare services when they need ongoing care but want to avoid moving to a skilled nursing facility. People of any age may require home-care service when they are recuperating from illness or surgery or when they are terminally ill. Chronically ill adults and children may receive home healthcare for ongoing care or to avoid hospitalization.

Goals of Home Healthcare

The primary goal in home healthcare is to promote self-care. Nursing activities are directed at fostering the client's independence or teaching the family or other caregivers to assist the client with ongoing health needs. This approach may be very different from what you have experienced in other clinical settings. For example, in the hospital the nurses provided direct care for Mr. Escobar ("Meet Your Patient"). This included bathing, toileting, giving medications, and ongoing assessment. In home health, the focus is to help the couple manage Mr. Escobar's care at home independently. Initially you may work with Mrs. Escobar, showing her how to administer medicines and explaining their function. However, your goal is to move her toward handling this task independently. Similarly, you may show the Escobars strategies for turning and moving that are comfortable for both of them; but you must be certain they understand and are able to handle these tasks when you leave.

Distinctive Features of Home Healthcare

Home health nursing differs from hospital nursing in several ways. The hospital environment is controlled. Surfaces are regularly disinfected, supplies are stocked, and foods, medications, and other therapies are readily available. Computers on the unit store information about the patient that is almost immediately accessible. In addition, the hospital-based nurse can consult almost immediately with a large team of healthcare providers (i.e., other nurses, the primary care provider, various therapists, social workers, a pastoral care provider, and even a business office staff to ensure that reimbursement will be forthcoming).

In contrast, when you are in a patient's home, surprisingly little is within your control. The home may be spotless or filthy, food plentiful or scarce, and supplies readily available or unreliable. The television or music may be loud; a dog may bark continually; or several young children may be playing nearby and repeatedly interrupting your interactions with the client or caregiver. You will find nursing care in the home environment to be different from inpatient settings in the following ways:

- You are a guest in the client's home. The client and family determine whether they are willing to let you enter the home to deliver care.
- You are responsible for making the assessments and determining whether the primary care provider should be advised of client changes.
- You must bring all necessary supplies or arrange to have them predelivered.
- You must be able to distinguish between skilled services, which are eligible for reimbursement from Medicare, and homemaker services. **Skilled services** are services that must be performed or supervised by a licensed healthcare professional (Box 43-1). **Homemaker services** (e.g., cleaning, meal preparation) are available to clients only if the principal reason for home care is a skilled service. These services are provided by home health aides.
- You must be more self-sufficient and function more independently. Often there are no other team members immediately available for support, assistance, or consultation.
- You must be aware of and comfortable with the family observing as you provide care.
- You will need to adapt to varying family relationships and some home environments that are difficult or even dysfunctional.

BOX 43-1 ■ Skilled Nursing Services

Medicare defines *skilled nursing care* as services and care that can be done safely and correctly only by a licensed registered or practical nurse. The services must be reasonable and necessary for the treatment of the illness or injury.

- Patient assessment
- Ongoing monitoring of patient status
- Management and coordination of the patient's plan of care
- Evaluation of response to medications or treatment
- Medication instruction
- Teaching patients or caregivers to provide care or therapies
- Disease-related teaching (e.g., diabetes education)
- Complex tasks, such as injections, insertion of urinary catheters, infusion therapy, wound care, tube feedings, or ventilator management

---

- You will need to encourage the family to help in providing care and in taking over care when you leave the home. Overburdened caregivers may need your help as much as does the client.
- You must preplan your visit by figuring out the directions to sites in advance and arranging appointments efficiently.
- Your personal safety is more of a concern when making home visits. You must always be aware of the environment around you and alert to possible dangers.

One advantage of home healthcare is that it allows you to see the client differently. The home is a window into the client's life, through which you can see his personal environment—how he lives, eats, and negotiates his world (Fig. 43-1). The photos, mementos, personal belongings, and other things the client values and cherishes make cultural beliefs and practices more visible. These things provide clues to his lifestyle, strengths, resources, and motivation.

FIGURE 43-1 The home is a window into the client's life.

Home health nursing also differs from community healthcare. Community health nurses provide care for individuals, families, and groups with an emphasis on population-based care. In contrast, home health nursing focuses on the individual and his support system.

KnowledgeCheck 43-1

Identify at least four skilled services that may be provided in the home.

 Go to Chapter 43, **Knowledge Check Response Sheet and Answers,** on the Student Resource Disk or DavisPlus at http://davisplus.fadavis.com/Wilkinson2

Who Provides Home Healthcare?

Home healthcare is provided by a variety of healthcare professionals employed by or working in cooperation with home healthcare agencies.

Home Health Agencies

Home health agencies coordinate the services of various professionals and paraprofessionals. The various types of agencies may be categorized by purpose, by type of client served, or by funding source.

Purpose. In this category, **direct care agencies** are the most common. They focus on direct client interaction by providing skilled care, associated therapies and health services, home health aides, chore workers, and delivery of **respite care** (relief for family caregivers). **Indirect service agencies** also play a vital role in home healthcare. Examples of indirect home services include pharmaceutical and infusion companies and suppliers of durable medical equipment. **Durable medical equipment (DME)** is reusable equipment (e.g., walkers, wheelchairs, apnea monitors). Medicare pays for some, but not all, such devices. It is expensive, so before ordering it, be sure the DME is covered or the client is able to pay for it.

Type of Client Served. An important specialty home service agency is hospice care. This may be a separate agency or a division of a home health agency. Still other agencies specialize in caring for patients with complex diseases, such as AIDS, or ventilator-dependent clients, or patients of a certain age group (services for older adults or chronically ill children).

Funding Source. Agencies may take on many forms based on funding source, profit or nonprofit status, and relationship with other healthcare organizations.

- **Public agencies** are official or governmental agencies organized at the city, county, state, or national level. They are usually funded by taxes, along with reimbursement from insurance companies. The local health department is a good example of a public agency. Health departments focus chiefly on community needs, although they often also offer some home

health services, especially when tracking clients in some of their disease management programs.
- **Voluntary agencies** are prominent in the delivery of home healthcare. These agencies are normally governed by a board of directors and funded by donations, endowments, and third-party (insurance) reimbursement. Many **hospice organizations** (groups that provide care for people who are frail, terminally ill, dying, or not expected to improve) are voluntary organizations.
- **Proprietary organizations** are corporate or privately owned businesses that aim to make a profit. These agencies receive payment from insurance companies but also accept private-pay clients. Proprietary organizations may provide traditional home health services as well as private-duty care and other services that assist individuals to remain independent.
- **Hospital-based agencies** are an extension of the services provided by a hospital. Clients who no longer meet the criteria for continued hospitalization may be transferred to home care for continued services. A benefit of this type of home health agency is in the ease of transition between hospital and home.

The Home Health Team

In home healthcare, the registered nurse serves as the coordinator of health services, but other members of the healthcare team may also provide care. The team varies according to the needs of the client but is usually multidisciplinary. It may include physicians; nurse practitioners; registered nurses; licensed practical or vocational nurses; home health aides; physical, speech, occupational, or respiratory therapists; nutritionists; social workers; pharmacists; podiatrists; dentists; chaplains; and family members.

Home Health Nurses

To succeed in home healthcare, you must have the ability to work independently and collaboratively, be flexible and resourceful, and adapt to different home environments and family interactions. The American Nurses Association (ANA) asserts that because of the level of independence, knowledge, and expertise required to meet the demands of home care, baccalaureate nurses are better prepared for that role. However, they also say that the necessary knowledge and skills can be developed through formal orientation programs, structured preceptor programs, and guided clinical experiences (ANA, 2008, p. 8).

Home health nurses provide a broad range of services to clients of all ages. Your principal roles as a home health nurse (also called visiting nurse) are discussed in this section. Each of the roles requires you to function as a skillful communicator. Communication is crucial in home care because of the need to establish good rapport with the client and family and to communicate frequently with other members of the healthcare team.

Direct Care Provider. As a direct care provider, you may administer medications, dress wounds, or perform other skilled, complex tasks.

Client and Family Educator. Recall that the goal of home healthcare is to promote self-care. Instead of focusing on performing the procedures, you will be helping the client or family take over the care. You can easily see how you will need to communicate skillfully in this role. You must be able to clearly explain the care required, the rationale for the care, and how to safely perform the care. This requires patience, skill, and repetition.

Client Advocate. In home care, the client and family are directly in charge of the plan of care. As client advocate, you support the client's right to make healthcare decisions yet protect the client from harm if he is unable to make decisions. In the event family members disagree with the client's decisions, remember that as the client's advocate, you must try to see that his wishes are respected and his rights upheld. You must also advocate for services the client needs. This may mean trying to secure additional home health support to avoid hospitalization, or it may mean advocating for another level of service, such as referral to hospice or placement in the hospital, based on your assessment of the client and discussion with the client and family.

Care Coordinator. Patients at home may receive care from an array of healthcare providers. Therefore, home health nurses must manage and coordinate care. As the case manager, you will need to gather data at an initial visit and develop a plan of care that addresses the client's needs. Your plan may require you to make additional visits, as well as delivery of therapies and services by other professionals in the home.

KnowledgeCheck 43-2

What roles does the nurse assume in home care? List and describe them.

 Go to Chapter 43, **Knowledge Check Response Sheet and Answers,** on the Student Resource Disk or DavisPlus at http://davisplus.fadavis.com/Wilkinson2

Hospice Nurses

As you learned in Chapter 15, **hospice nursing** focuses on care of patients who are dying or whose condition is not expected to improve. Hospice services are provided in the home, in the hospital, in nursing homes, and in homes specifically designed as hospices. The goal of hospice care is to promote comfort and quality of life. For these reasons, the most hospice services are provided in the client's home. Because the client is not expected to recover, the focus of home hospice care is quite different from traditional home care. More than promoting self-care and independence, hospice care focuses on providing comfort and managing symptoms (Table 43-1).

Table 43-1 ➤	Home Healthcare and Home Hospice Care	
	HOME HEALTHCARE	**HOME HOSPICE CARE**
Purpose	To promote self-care	Promote comfort and quality of life
Focus of Nursing Interventions	Foster clients' independence or teach the family or other caregivers to assist the client with ongoing health needs	Provide comfort and manage symptoms

The roles of hospice nurse and home health nurse differ mainly in their emphasis. As a direct care provider, the hospice nurse assesses the client's condition and monitors responses to interventions aimed at relieving distress. As an educator, the hospice nurse teaches the client and family and how to adjust medications and care to control pain and other symptoms. The roles of communicator and client advocate assume prime importance as the client's condition deteriorates. The nurse shares these roles with the family and other home caregivers. Generally, there is less coordination of multiple services in home hospice care. Instead, there may be greater emphasis on pain management. (If you need more information on hospice care, see Chapter 15.)

Who Pays for Home Health Care?

Medicare, Medicaid, private insurance, and individual payments (private pay) help pay for home care services. **Medicare** is a federally funded healthcare system designed to provide health coverage for persons who are older than 65 years, disabled, or diagnosed with end-stage renal disease. Medicare and Medicaid are the largest payers for home healthcare. Keep in mind the federal healthcare act passed in 2010 will likely change reimbursement in a variety of ways over the coming years (111th Congress, 1st session, 2010).

Medicare Reimbursement

Reimbursement by Medicare for home care depends on the following strictly applied criteria:

- **The client must need skilled care.** Other services may also be provided, but the primary purpose for establishing care must be based on a skilled care need. This means that Medicare will not pay for personal care such as bathing and dressing when this is the only care the client needs.
- **The client must be homebound.** This means (1) the client must have a condition that restricts the ability to leave the home; and (2) leaving the home requires

special assistance, transportation, supportive devices, or an escort.

- *The client must require nursing care that is part-time and intermittent.* This means Medicare will pay for a limited number of hours per day or days per week that the client can get skilled nursing care or home health aide services.
- *The plan of care must be authorized by the physician and recertified every 62 days.* For the client to continue to receive care, there must be evidence of continued need that remains acute.
- *The care must be medically necessary and reasonable.* The plan of care must address the client's health concerns and have clearly delineated outcomes. The expectations of the patient must be reasonable.
- *Medicare will pay only for interventions identified on the treatment plan.* The payer may periodically request patient records to verify that the care was given.
- *The home health agency must be approved by Medicare.* An agency must show that it meets the Medicare definitions and requirements in order to become Medicare-certified.

Medicaid is a program sponsored jointly by the federal government and the states to provide services to people whose income is below a mandated level. In many states, the criteria for reimbursement are the same as those required by Medicare. However, each state presently determines what services will be part of its medical assistance plan.

Private Insurance and Private Payment

Private insurance companies may also offer home health services. The type and extent of covered services are specified in each separate insurance group and plan.

Many people require assistance in the home but do not meet criteria for reimbursement from Medicare, Medicaid, or their private insurer. Others simply do not have health insurance. (This was true when this book was published; but it is likely to change over the next few years as new healthcare regulations are gradually put into effect.) Frequently, older clients require home health assistance but may not need skilled services. For example, they may need assistance with grocery shopping, meal planning and preparation, or transportation. The client or family may contact an agency to provide chore worker assistance for these services. Services are billed directly to the client. Unfortunately, these services are usually available only to affluent clients and families. Those with limited income may be forced to do without needed services. This disparity may lead to inadequate care and illness, hospitalizations, and even death.

Critical Thinking 43-1

Review the scenario focused on Mr. Escobar. What members of the home health team may be required to provide care? Why?

What Is the Future of Home Healthcare?

Healthcare analysts have predicted several changes in home care over the next few decades:

Increased need for home healthcare. Over the next several decades, the demand for home care is expected to rise sharply. Considering the growing number of older adults in the United States, it is more cost effective to provide healthcare in the home than in an inpatient setting.

Increased use of the home for hospice care. Public acceptance of the home as a place of comfort and care, as well as concerns about the cost of inpatient care, has increased the number of persons who choose this compassionate option for end-of-life and palliative care.

Increased technology. Technological advances, such as online or telemedicine consultation, make it safer and more affordable to deliver complex care in the home and allow home health nurses to provide a growing array of services. Computerized monitoring and charting allow home health agencies to better coordinate care, receive needed supplies, and closely monitor costs.

Continued research. Research is needed in the area of strategies to improve the effectiveness of care, identify predictors of need for rehospitalization, and integrate home care into overall community-based services.

The home healthcare industry has grown into big business, and it is expected to continue its growth through 2015 (Borger, Smith, Truffer, et al., 2006), and perhaps beyond. However, the future of home care may depend mostly on the state of the U.S. economy, recent federal legislation that will change how healthcare is structured, and the portion of the federal budget that is allocated to healthcare in general. There is some indication that the healthcare act of 2010 provides less support for some home health services, which will shift older adults to the more expensive inpatient services (111th Congress, 1st session, 2010).

How Are Clients Referred to Home Healthcare?

Referrals to home healthcare come from a variety of sources. However, for home care to begin, there must be a medical prescription and a physician-approved treatment plan.

Hospital-based agencies have a built-in referral base. If the primary provider or nursing staff determine the client would benefit from home health services, they refer the patient to the agency for evaluation while he is still hospitalized. Many agencies have *intake coordinators* who work in the hospital and review clients for suitability of services, gathering information from the chart, the client, the family, and the hospital team. Home services are arranged before discharge from an inpatient facility.

Even if the hospital does not have its own home agency, the client may still be referred to home health services during a hospital stay. Ideally, a discharge planner gathers information, secures the prescription from the provider, and makes arrangements. In some smaller hospitals, this task falls to the staff nurse providing pre-discharge care.

Referrals may also come from doctors, nurses, primary care offices and clinics, mental health workers, and other healthcare providers in the community, as well as directly from families and clients. Most home health agencies evaluate clients to determine whether they are eligible for services that are reimbursable by insurance. They may also offer services that the client may pay for independently.

Practical **Knowledge** knowing how

As a home healthcare nurse, your days will vary quite a bit. Normally your caseload will be contained within a limited geographic boundary, so that you can schedule your visits efficiently, spending less time driving to visits, and have more time for delivering care. If you want to envision what it would be like to be a home health nurse, you need only to look at the list of services Medicare recognizes as skilled, in Box 43-1.

How Do I Make a Home Visit?

The home visit has three phases: preparation before the visit, nursing care during the visit, and evaluation after the visit. For a summary of the major activities in each phase,

VOL 2 Go to Chapter 43, **Clinical Insight 43-1: Conducting a Home Visit,** in Volume 2.

Before the Visit

You should first review the client's chart and referral form to determine why you are making the visit. You may also need to review material about the client's health problem, medications, or treatment plan. Then you can begin to plan for the visit. What supplies will you need? What teaching materials will you need? What are the goals of the visit? Does the agency require additional client information, such as insurance data, to provide care? The agency will probably have a set of forms (e.g., HIPAA privacy forms, billing information) for you to complete during the first visit. Be sure you have those with you.

Before the visit you will need to find the address, get directions to the home, and determine whether there are safety concerns. Contact the client to notify him of the planned date and time of the visit and to determine whether his health status has changed since the referral was made. This will allow you to bring additional equipment or personnel along if needed.

Prepare Supplies

Home health nurses usually carry a nursing bag (Fig. 43-2). The nursing bag is often customized to the needs of the clients in the nurse's case load, and normally contains the following:

- Hand-washing supplies (e.g., soap or antibacterial handrub, paper towels)
- Stethoscope
- Sphygmomanometers (with cuffs in a variety of sizes)
- Thermometers (oral and rectal)
- Small equipment (scissors, forceps, penlight, staple remover)
- Tape measure (with plastic coating that can be cleaned, or several disposable paper ones)
- Plastic apron
- Gloves, sterile and clean
- An assortment of gauze dressings, tape, and cotton balls
- Occupational Safety and Health Administration (OSHA) supplies: mask, protective eyewear, disinfectant spray, disposable gowns to protect clothing
- A variety of syringes and safety needles (this varies widely among agencies)
- Venipuncture supplies
- Airway and resuscitation mask
- Paper supplies (e.g., agency forms, business cards, local maps)

You may need other supplies, such as medications, a scale, and a transfer belt, depending on the requirements of the clients in your caseload. If the client needs frequent dressing changes or treatments that need supplies (e.g., tube feedings) it is best to have the supplies delivered directly to the client's house to reduce the number of materials you must carry. Note that in

FIGURE 43-2 The home health nursing bag contains some standard items but is usually customized according to the requirements of the clients in the nurse's case load.

some states, nurses are not permitted to carry medications because of safety concerns. You will need to check on the rules that apply to your state.

Provide for Your Safety

 As you drive to the home, begin to make your assessment. Locate the stores, hospital, and community resources. What is the overall character of the neighborhood? Does this appear to be a safe neighborhood? What are the conditions of the approach to the home?

Safety for yourself and the client is an essential consideration in home healthcare. Bring your impressions about neighborhood safety and home safety with you into the home. You should evaluate whether the environment contributes to the client's health problems. In addition, you must also assess the implications for your own safety. For suggestions about the safe delivery of home healthcare,

VOL 2 Go to Chapter 43, **Clinical Insight 43-3: Safety Considerations in Home Care,** in Volume 2.

KnowledgeCheck 43-3

What are the major tasks that must be completed before making a home visit?

 Go to Chapter 43, **Knowledge Check Response Sheet and Answers,** on the Student Resource Disk or DavisPlus at http://davisplus.fadavis.com/Wilkinson2

At the Visit

When you arrive at the home, you must remember this is the client's domain. Knock or ring the doorbell, and wait to be invited in. Home health nurses are guests of their clients. Observe common courtesies. Introduce yourself to the client and family. Be respectful of their home, as well as their beliefs, values, practices, and cultural preferences.

The first few minutes of the initial visit set the tone for the relationship among client, family, nurse, and agency. This is your opportunity to develop rapport and trust. Introducing yourself, waiting for permission to enter, and treating the client and family members with respect are ways to help to establish rapport (Fig. 43-3).

You should also offer your card to identify yourself, and provide contact information for the home health agency. Generally, agencies have information packets that include the client's bill of rights, client responsibilities, billing information, information on the frequency and duration of services, how to reach the agency, and the date and time of the next visit.

As you do all this, you also gather data. Who answered your questions? What is the relationship between the caregiver and the client? How do they interact? What other people live there? What is the condition of the home? If this is an initial visit, you may need to verify or complete client data on the referral form. In the

FIGURE 43-3 The first few minutes of the initial visit set the tone for the relationship among client, family, nurse, and agency.

hospital, admissions personnel usually gather admitting data and obtain consent for treatment. In home care you need to collect and document this information.

At a home visit, you might do a variety of things, such as performing physical care; drawing blood sample for lab work; checking weight; administering medication, IV fluid, or tube feedings; providing wound or ostomy care; or whatever is needed.

 ## CriticalThinking 43-2

Review the case of Mr. Escobar. What information did you gain from the first few minutes of the visit?

After the Visit

After you leave the home, there is still a lot of work for you to do. Often you will need to complete the documentation for the visit. In Chapter 16, you learned about documentation techniques, various forms of charting, and legal aspects of documentation. In home care all of these rules apply; however, some aspects of home care documentation are unique.

Home health agencies often use Medicare's Outcome and Assessment Information Set (OASIS) to record initial assessment data. To continue to provide needed services to the client, you must include in your documentation: (1) evidence of homebound status, and (2) evidence of continued need for skilled care.

Other post-visit activities include ordering supplies needed for the next visit, making referrals to additional services (e.g., occupational therapy), coordinating care among the various services, and scheduling the next visit.

Nursing Process in Home Care

The nursing process moves through the same phases in all patient care settings. The difference in home care is that you must use forms structured to satisfy Medicare and other insurance requirements. Nevertheless, you need to assess the client, the family, the home, and the community in order to identify nursing diagnoses and other health problems. You will work from a plan of care prescribed by a medical provider, but individualize it with suitable nursing diagnoses and interventions. Periodically, you must evaluate the client's continued homebound status and ongoing need for medical treatment and skilled nursing care.

◼ ASSESSMENT

On the initial visit, you need to perform an assessment to establish a baseline and determine the type of care required. This assessment includes a health history, review of all medications—prescribed, over-the-counter, and alternative—pertinent family and social history, mental status, functional ability, availability of family and informal support and caregivers, nutritional status, and assessment of the home environment. Often a full assessment requires multiple visits.

Medicare requires home health agencies to collect specific information for all Medicare clients they serve. This data set is called the Outcome and Assessment Information Set (OASIS). OASIS data must be collected at the start of care, with each recertification (every 60 days), and at the termination of care. Medicare uses these data to determine the effectiveness of care and to monitor client outcomes. In addition to the required OASIS information, many agencies use other assessment tools created specifically for their needs. For an example of the OASIS form,

Go to Chapter 43, **ESG Figure 43-1, OASIS Form,** on the Student Resource Disk or DavisPlus at http://davisplus.fadavis.com/Wilkinson2

It is also important to assess the needs of the caregivers—the family members, friends, and support system in the home. To be successful in home care, you must work *with* the caregivers. Take time at each visit to speak with them, making sure to include them in your assessment, plan of care, and teaching. Assessment of the caregivers often allows you to determine what services are needed in the home. Caregivers may have health problems of their own that affect their ability to provide care for another. This is common among older couples.

◼ ANALYSIS/NURSING DIAGNOSIS

As in any setting, the nursing diagnoses are based on the client's responses to illness and care. As a home healthcare nurse, you will work with clients with numerous medical and nursing diagnoses. Two frequent nursing diagnoses, Caregiver Role Strain and Deficient Knowledge, are discussed below. Safety and Risk for Infection, also key concerns in the home, are thoroughly discussed in Chapters 20 and 21. Infection control measures in the home are also presented in a following section, "Infection Control in the Home."

Caregiver Role Strain. Providing care to a loved one at home can be a challenge, especially when finances don't allow a family to hire home health aides. Around-the-clock caregiving duties can lead to physical exhaustion, social isolation, resentment, sadness, or depression. In addition, family members themselves may become seriously ill and no longer be able to function as caregiver. These role changes may be difficult for both the ill person and the caregiver. For example, imagine that your mother suddenly became very ill and you became her primary caregiver. This would be a reversal of the roles you both are used to, and it would be emotionally taxing, especially if you are already exhausted and isolated from your friends. In addition, a primary caregiver may worry that caring for the client interferes with other responsibilities (e.g., as a parent, spouse, friend, worker).

Given these factors, it is not surprising that the two nursing diagnoses most commonly applicable to loved ones providing care at home are Caregiver Role Strain and Risk for Caregiver Role Strain. These diagnoses identify those for whom the burden of delivering care has become—or is at risk for becoming—overwhelming. Common signs of caregiver role strain include difficulty adjusting to role changes, fatigue, isolation, depression, and difficulty in performing routine care for the client.

Deficient Knowledge. Client and family teaching is especially important in home care because most of the caregiving is performed by the client and significant others. You will spend much of your time teaching them the skills necessary for self-care (e.g., how to administer insulin, how to manage the oxygen equipment). Recall that to be eligible for home nursing care, clients must require skilled nursing care. Client education is a service that Medicare and other insurers will reimburse. You must be certain to include a Deficient Knowledge diagnosis on the care plan in order to ensure the client's continued eligibility and reimbursement for the service. In other chapters we caution against indiscriminate use of the Deficient Knowledge diagnosis. However, an exception must be made for home care.

KnowledgeCheck 43-4

- Why are the first few minutes of the initial visit so important?
- Identify five things that should be assessed at an initial home visit.

Go to Chapter 43, **Knowledge Check Response Sheet and Answers,** on the Student Resource Disk or DavisPlus at http://davisplus.fadavis.com/Wilkinson2

CriticalThinking 43-3

What, if any, evidence of caregiver strain does Mrs. Escobar exhibit?

Standard Terminology for Nursing Diagnoses

Recall from the nursing process chapters of this text that various disciplines, including nursing, have developed classifications of standardized terminology (also called taxonomies, vocabularies, and languages) for describing their work and for planning and documenting care. You are familiar with the NANDA-I taxonomy of nursing diagnoses; however, home care nurses more commonly use the Clinical Care Classification (CCC) because it is closely related to the OASIS reporting forms required by Medicare. If you need to review the concept of standardized nursing language, see Chapters 4, 5, and 6.

The CCC also contains 182 diagnostic concepts—59 major categories and/or 123 subcategories—that describe nursing diagnoses and patient problems (Saba, 2007, p. 159). Approximately 50 labels are also NANDA-I diagnostic categories. About 50 of the 182 terms are especially applicable to home healthcare. Common CCC nursing diagnoses used in the home include:

Activities of Daily Living (ADLs) Alteration
Caregiver Role Strain
Family Processes Alteration
Home Maintenance Alteration
Knowledge Deficit
Physical Mobility Impairment
Self-Care Deficit

The CCC system consists of 21 care components to classify diagnoses and interventions. An accompanying coding structure and framework parallels the steps of the nursing process and links the CCC diagnoses to interventions and outcomes. To see the CCC Care Components and other examples of CCC diagnoses, respectively,

VOL 2 Go to Chapter 43, **Standardized Language, CCC Care Components,** in Volume 2.

VOL 2 Go to Chapter 43, **Standardized Language, An Example of CCC Nursing Diagnoses and Interventions,** in Volume 2.

For complete information on the CCC and complete lists of diagnoses, outcomes, and interventions,

Go to the **Clinical Care Classification** Web site at www.sabacare.com

PLANNING OUTCOMES/EVALUATION

The CCC defines an outcome as "a measurable outcome of the therapeutic nursing care that alters the health status of the patient" (Saba, 2007, p. 154). Others conceptualize a CCC outcome as being "What really happened to the recipient of services in terms of the particular problem for which care was provided" (Head, Maas, & Johnson, 1997, p. 51). To formulate a goal/outcome in the CCC system, attach one of the three CCC "modifiers" (*improve, stabilize, deteriorate*) to the diagnosis. The outcome describes the *desired* client health status. To evaluate client progress, you again use one of the three modifiers to describe the client's *actual* health status. The following is an example:

CCC nursing diagnosis:	Knowledge Deficit
Goal/expected outcome:	Knowledge Deficit, Improve
Actual status on evaluation:	Knowledge Deficit, Stabilized

Medicare requires that the client's status be evaluated and coded as improved, stabilized, or deteriorated, the same as the CCC system. In your nursing notes, you would include additional narrative to support your evaluation.

The Nursing Outcomes Classification (NOC) can also be used in home health nursing (Moorhead, Johnson, Maas, et al., 2008). A few of the outcomes that pertain to home and families are Caregiver Home Care Readiness, Caregiver Performance: Direct Care, Caregiver Stressors, Family Coping, and Family Functioning. If you are using the NOC and need more information,

Go to the **Iowa Outcomes Project** Web site at http://www.nursing.uiowa.edu/excellence/nursing_knowledge/clinical_effectiveness/noc.htm

At least one study found neither OASIS data nor NOC outcomes to be sensitive or responsive to nursing interventions. Since nursing is the core service provided in home healthcare, it is important to use outcomes that can detect changes that result from nursing interventions. Further research is needed in this area (Stocker, 2004).

Do you remember the overall goal of home care? That goal has implications for the kinds of activities you will perform after completing your assessment. To prepare the client and family for self-care, inform them of the needs you have identified, and involve them in setting goals and planning care. They may be able to identify strategies to solve problems or to help you identify needs that are not readily apparent.

PLANNING INTERVENTIONS/IMPLEMENTATION

Medicare requires that the physician-prescribed plan of care include the following, as applicable:

- Parameters for notifying the primary provider of changes in vital signs and other clinical findings
- Diabetic foot care, including education

Toward Evidence-Based Practice

Inglis, S., Pearson, S., Treen, S., et al. (2006). Extending the horizon in chronic heart failure: Effects of multidisciplinary, home-based intervention relative to usual care. *Circulation,* 114(23), 2466–2473.

A total of 297 older adult patients with chronic heart failure were randomized to home-based intervention (HBI) or usual postdischarge care from the hospital, and followed for a minimum of 7.5 years (up to 10 years). The control group received typical follow-up: appointment with a primary physician and regular outpatient-review by a cardiologist. The HBI group received that care, as well as home visits from a nurse and a pharmacist. Visits included counseling, strategies to improve treatment adherence, a simple exercise regimen, and incremental monitoring by family caregivers; in addition, there was telephone follow-up over 6 months. Researchers concluded that HBI is, over the long term, a cost- and time-effective strategy for prolonging survival and reducing the frequency of recurrent hospitalization of patients with chronic heart failure.

Scherr, D., Kastner, P., Kollman, A., et al. and the **MOBITEL** investigators (2009). Original paper: Effect of home-based telemonitoring using mobile phone technology on the outcome of heart failure patients after an episode of acute decompensation: Randomized control trial. *Journal of Medical Internet Research,* 11(3):e34. Retrieved from http://www.jmir.org/2009/3/e34

This study evaluated the impact of home-based telemonitoring using Internet and mobile phone technology on the outcome of heart failure patients after an episode of acute decompensation. Subjects had a median age of 66 to 67 years. The control group received pharmacological treatment and the intervention group received pharmacological treatment with telemedical surveillance for 6 months (tele group). Physicians had continuous access to patient data via a secure Web portal. Data were analyzed for 108 patients. Researchers concluded that telemonitoring using mobile phones as patient terminals has the potential to reduce frequency and duration of heart failure hospitalizations.

1. Based on these two studies, home care for long-term management of heart failure seems reasonable. True or false? Explain your thinking.

2. What difficulty might you anticipate in implementing the intervention described in the Scherr, et al. study? That is, what could happen to interfere with its effectiveness?

 Go to Chapter 43, **Toward Evidence-Based Practice Suggested Responses,** on the Student Resource Disk or DavisPlus at http://davisplus.fadavis.com/Wilkinson2

- Falls prevention interventions
- Depression interventions
- Interventions to monitor and treat pain
- Interventions to prevent pressure ulcers
- Pressure ulcer treatments

Once the plan of care has been agreed on, you will document it and forward it to the client's physician for certification. At the first visit, you will determine the specific skilled care required and make referrals to other required services such as physical, occupational, or speech therapy, social services, nutritional support, or home health aide services.

Often a client has multiple services offered at the home. For example, Mr. Escobar ("Meet Your Patient") is recovering from a stroke. He may require physical therapy, occupational therapy, and speech therapy as well as skilled nursing care and the assistance of a home health aide. As the Escobars' home health nurse, you would serve as the coordinator of this complex care.

Standardized Nursing Interventions

The CCC contains 198 nursing interventions organized according to the care components. For an example,

 Go to Chapter 43, **Standardized Language: An Example of CCC Nursing Diagnoses and Interventions,** in Volume 2.

That list shows an example of an intervention for the Activity Component. An intervention consists of a label (e.g., Activity Care) and a definition (e.g., Actions performed to carry out physiological or psychological daily activities). In addition to the label, you must specify the type of intervention action from among four qualifiers:

Assess/Monitor/Evaluate/Observe
Care/Perform/Provide/Assist
Teach/Educate/Instruct/Supervise
Manage/Refer/Contact/Notify

The CCC nursing interventions include only skilled services, because this type of service is the only type of care reimbursed by Medicare and most insurers in home health. In the case of the Escobars, Mrs. Escobar is clearly experiencing Caregiver Strain. This is a nursing diagnosis under the Care Component of Coping. Several interventions are possible:

Coping Support: Actions to sustain a person dealing with responsibilities, problems, or difficulties Assess for Caregiver Strain.

Provide (perform) emotional support.
Refer to community services: caregiver support groups, Meals on Wheels, and respite care services.

The Nursing Interventions Classification (NIC) may also be used in home health nursing (Bulechek, Butcher, & Dochterman, 2008). A few of the interventions that pertain to home and families are Caregiver Support, Family Integrity Promotion, Home Maintenance Assistance, and Respite Care. If you will be using the NIC and need more information,

 Go to the **Iowa Interventions Project** Web site at http://www.nursing.uiowa.edu/excellence/nursing_knowledge/clinical_effectiveness/nic.htm

Assisting With Medication Management

One of The Joint Commission 2009 safety goals for home care is to improve the safety of using medications. This involves preventing errors with look-alike and sound-alike medications, educating patients about anticoagulant therapy, and keeping a list and reconciling medications when a client transfers from one agency to another.

Some patients, particularly older adults, have visual and motor deficits that limit their ability to read labels and manipulate bottle caps, syringes, and so on. Other reasons for noncompliance include lack of outward symptoms, inability to tolerate side effects, pain, forgetfulness, low motivation, and impaired mental capacity. Always investigate the patient's reasons for nonadherence so that you can take appropriate actions. You may need to teach clients and caregivers skills such as measuring dosages, giving injections, and managing intravenous therapy. Or they may need tips on how to take oral medications if the client has difficulty swallowing. For example, for some clients, pills may be crushed and mixed in a small amount of applesauce. Involve family members in the care of the older adult, including giving medication, providing they are competent in doing so (Hall & Maslow, 2007).

Older adults and caregivers may have difficulty remembering when to take their pills, remembering which ones to take, and even remembering whether they have already taken them. Suggest they use a medication organizer with a compartment for each day of the week. You may need to prepare a week's worth of oral medications for them during your visits. To help them remember which drug is used for each of their illnesses or symptoms, you can write the medical condition, names of medication, and doses on a large card. Then use clear tape to attach a sample of each drug next to its name on the card.

Infection Control in the Home

The Joint Commission 2009 safety goals for home care include reducing the risk of healthcare-associated infections. In the hospital, you have ready access to supplies that facilitate infection control. The home presents unique challenges. You will need to follow Standard Precautions but recognize how to modify infection control techniques for the home environment. The Centers for Disease Control and Prevention (CDC) has not yet developed guidelines for infection control in home care settings (CDC, modified 2008), but for suggestions to help you maintain infection control during a home visit,

VOL 2 Go to Chapter 43, **Clinical Insight 43-2: Infection Control in the Home**, in Volume 2.

Homes vary widely. Do not assume that a client lives in a clean residence or that running water and electricity are readily available. Some people with limited financial resources, especially in urban environments, live in single-room occupancy hotels (SROs). Residents of SROs live in a small room with shared bath and shower areas. Conditions can vary from clean and orderly to unclean and even detrimental to health. To provide optimal care, you need to bring infection control supplies and personal protective equipment to the visit or order them to be delivered to the home.

Barrier Precautions

Rationales for using barrier precautions differ from those in hospitals. As a rule, you will use gowns, gloves, and masks in home care to protect yourself, rather than the patient. You will need to use standard precautions, but will usually need a mask only when caring for clients who have pulmonary tuberculosis or multidrug-resistant infections. These organisms may be transmitted to other home-care patients through inanimate objects or hands, so use appropriate barrier precautions (Lescure, Locher, Eveillard, et al., 2009). See Chapter 20 if you need to review infection control.

Clean and Sterile Technique

Infection control in home care is different in many ways from that in acute care. In acute care, the patient is at risk from exposure to invasive interventions and environmental risks, including other patients and contaminated inanimate objects. Generally, patients have developed some resistance to the microorganisms in their own homes and are less likely to acquire infections there than in the hospital environment. You may find differences in how you handle home infusion therapy, urinary tract care, respiratory care, wound care, and enteral therapy. It is safe, in many instances, to replace sterile with clean technique, as in some of the following examples (Rhinehart, 2001):

Intravenous therapy. Sterile practices should be the same at home as in the hospital because the associated risk of asepsis is so high.

Insulin injections. Many people (e.g., those who have diabetes) must give themselves repeated injections, perhaps several each day. Supplies for home use are expensive. Insurance may or may not cover the cost, or the person may not have insurance. Therefore, although manufacturers recommend that disposable syringes and needles be used only once, and it is safest to do that, some people find it practical to reuse needles and syringes. For guidelines for patient teaching about this, see Clinical Insight 23-1.

Urinary catheters. Clients and family typically use clean, rather than sterile, gloves to perform catheterization. In the home, clients frequently interrupt the drainage system to empty a leg bag, or to change or disinfect the drainage bag. They may also disinfect and reuse urinary catheters.

Respiratory care. As an example, tracheostomy care in the home is nearly always performed using clean, not sterile, technique.

Wound care. Procedures for wound care should be based on the potential for contamination and infection. Usually clean technique is adequate. For example, a surgical site that is primarily closed and has no drains should be low risk for home-care-acquired infection. However, if the incision has drains or is open, the risk for infection increases, and your wound-care

procedures must address the risk. Also, you do not need to arbitrarily "always" discard irrigation fluids at set intervals (e.g., every 24 hours). Order, or guide caregivers to buy, small containers (e.g., no more than 500 mL) that can be used up in two or three visits. Teach them how to avoid contaminating the fluids (e.g., how to handle the cap, always recap the bottle, and store the bottle away from children and pets).

Enteral therapy. Emphasize the need to refrigerate the feedings after opening and store solutions until expiration. Teach caregivers to keep the kitchen appliances (e.g., blenders) and tools used in preparation meticulously clean. Sterilization of blender parts, measuring cups, and spoons is probably not necessary, but they should be washed in a dishwasher after use.

KnowledgeCheck 43-5

Identify three infection control supplies that you should bring in your nursing bag on a home health visit.

 Go to Chapter 43, **Knowledge Check Response Sheet and Answers,** on the Student Resource Disk or DavisPlus at http://davisplus.fadavis.com/Wilkinson2

BOX 43-2 ■ Ways to Help Caregivers

Provide a listening ear. Encourage caregivers to talk about what they do and how they feel, and listen actively to their concerns. Find time to focus on the caregiver's needs, rather than on those of the care recipient.

Give positive feedback and validate their importance to the client's health.

Help the caregiver identify people who may be able to help, for example, family members living outside the home, neighbors, church members, community support groups.

Talk with family and friends, if the caregiver wishes. Teach them how to support the caregiver, for example by telephoning regularly, visiting, sending cards, or staying with the client a few hours (or days) so the caregiver can rest or take a vacation. Encourage them to listen to the caregiver without giving advice, and to help her feel appreciated (e.g., "I really appreciate all you do for Dad.")

Arrange for a home health aide, if possible. This relieves the caregiver of housekeeping and grocery shopping.

Remind family members and significant others to take care of themselves. Explain that their health is important to both them and the patient. Even the most devoted and self-sacrificing person may understand when you explain, "You must take care of yourself in order to be able to take care of your loved one."

- Stress the need for the person to eat nutritious meals. Arrange for meals to be delivered to the home, if needed.

- Encourage the caregiver to rest as much as possible, perhaps while the home health aide is there; or ask family

members and acquaintances to take turns staying an hour or two with the patient while the caregiver rests or "gets away." Help contact these people and make a schedule, if needed.

- Stress the need for the caregivers to take some time for themselves, even if it is just an hour alone, or coffee with a neighbor.

- Encourage caregivers to take a vacation, if they can afford it. Reassure them that competent help can be obtained and that it is o.k. to delegate caregiving to others for a while.

- Some agencies have a weekend respite program for caregivers. The client is admitted to a skilled care unit for 2 or 3 days so the caregiver can have a break.

Encourage the caregiver to maintain spiritual connections, for example, to take time to go to church; or ask the spiritual adviser to visit the home.

Communicate medical updates about the client—lab results, new treatment plans, and so on.

Help the family understand the goals of care and solve problems when needed.

Teach the family what to expect with regard to medications, treatments, and signs of approaching death. If family members know what is normal, they will be less likely to panic or fear the inevitable.

Follow up with other healthcare team members promptly if the family has questions that are outside your scope of practice.

Safety in the Home

Two following Joint Commission 2009 home care safety goals are also important to keep in mind.

Reduce the risk of client harm resulting from falls. You will need to assess the client and the home for risk factors (e.g., dimly lit stairs, clutter on the floors) and teach caregivers falls reduction measures. You will find extensive discussion of falls prevention in Chapter 21 if you need more information about that.

■ *Identify risks associated with oxygen therapy* (e.g., fire). Be certain the home has working smoke detectors, fire extinguishers, and a fire safety plan. Assess the client and family's ability to understand and comply with fire prevention activities, and report any concerns to the physician.

If you need a checklist to use in assessing for safety hazards in the home,

VOL 2 Go to Chapter 21, **Assessment Guidelines and Tools, Home Safety Checklist,** in Volume 2.

Supporting Caregivers

Even when the client is receiving in-home care from an agency, it is not around-the-clock care. If the client cannot perform self-care, most of the duties fall to family members. One study found that even with short-term formal services, family caregivers provided three-fourths of the care of homebound patients. Half of the caregivers said they were not adequately prepared when it was time for their home health services to be discontinued. And at all stages, they expressed significant isolation, anxiety, and depression (Levine, Albert, Hokenstad, et al., 2006).

Recall that unrelieved caregiving duties are physically and emotionally taxing. Caregivers may become depressed, physically exhausted, isolated from friends, and neglect their own health. If the primary caregiver becomes unable to function, the client must be institutionalized. Clearly, it is important to provide caregiver support.

There is some evidence to indicate that caregiver support and training workshops can relieve depression, reduce the perceived burden of caregiving, and better prepare the caregivers for their role. However, the most improvement was shown by those with more independent lives, and social support. Furthermore, not everyone can—or will want to—attend a workshop. Some cannot leave their caregiving duties; others haven't the time or energy; and still others may not have transportation (Huynh-Hohnbaum, Villa, Aranda, et al., 2008; Leutz, Capitman, Ruwe, et al., 2002). See Box 43-2 for suggestions to help caregivers.

 Go to Chapter 43, **Resources for Caregivers and Health Professionals,** on the Student Resource Disk or DavisPlus at http://davisplus.fadavis.com/Wilkinson2

 Suggested Readings: Go to Chapter 43, **Reading More About Nursing in Home Care,** on the Student Resource Disk or DavisPlus at http://davisplus.fadavis.com/Wilkinson2

 Bibliography: Go to Volume 2, Bibliography.

CHAPTER 44

Ethics & Values

Learning Outcomes

After completing this chapter, you should be able to:

➤ Define *morals, ethics, bioethics,* and *nursing ethics.*

➤ Discuss what is meant by ethical agency.

➤ Identify at least four factors that contribute to the frequency of nurses' moral problems.

➤ Differentiate personal values and morality from professional values.

➤ Explain how developmental stages, values, moral frameworks, professional guidelines, and moral principles affect moral decisions.

➤ Describe five major ethical principles that are used in reasoning about healthcare.

➤ Compare and contrast four moral frameworks: consequentialism (e.g., utilitarianism), deontology, an ethics of care, and feminist ethics.

➤ Identify the moral issues and principles involved in a given ethical situation.

➤ Explain how nurses can use knowledge of values transmission and values clarification to facilitate the ethical decision-making of clients.

➤ Describe a systematic approach for resolving ethical dilemmas.

➤ Discuss the concept of an integrity-producing compromise.

➤ Describe the nurse's obligations in ethical decisions.

➤ Discuss the roles of the nurse as client advocate in the delivery of ethical nursing care.

➤ Apply the steps identified in the MORAL model for ethical decision-making to issues nurses encounter in patient care.

Meet Your Patients

Angie and Edward Frese are a couple with two teenaged children. They are a close and loving family with a large network of family and friends. Alan, 15 years old, has just been severely injured in a high school soccer game. Angie and Edward are summoned to the hospital, where they are told that Alan has multiple bone fractures and active internal bleeding.

The surgeon informs the distressed parents that Alan will need a blood transfusion to survive. Although genuinely devastated, the parents adamantly refuse to consent to a lifesaving blood transfusion, stating they are Jehovah's Witnesses and that receiving blood is against their religious beliefs. The surgeon asks you, Alan's nurse, to get the parents to change their minds right away. You talk with the couple, but they continue to refuse a blood transfusion. You immediately contact your charge nurse. Try to answer the following questions about Alan and his parents. You may not have the experience or theoretical knowledge to answer them all—you will acquire that in this and the following chapter—but do your best based on the background you have.

CriticalThinking 44-1

- Do Alan's parents have the right to refuse a blood transfusion based on their religious beliefs?
- Do you think the fact that Alan is a minor (under 18 years old) may make a difference in this situation?
- What actions do you think the charge nurse should take?
- Can an ethical conflict such as this be resolved to everyone's satisfaction?

Theoretical **Knowledge**
knowing why

The theoretical knowledge you will need to begin professional practice includes an understanding of the nature of morals and ethics (and especially nursing ethics) and basic information about factors that affect moral decisions (i.e., values, moral frameworks, professional guidelines, and ethical principles).

Ethics and Morals

Although the terms *ethics* and *morals* have similar meanings, in modern theory **morals** refers to private, personal, or group standards of right and wrong. **Moral behavior** is behavior that is in accordance with custom or tradition and usually reflects personal or religious beliefs. An example of morality might be a person's opposition to or support of abortion. Another example is the "golden rule," that you should treat others as you wish to be treated.

> Can you think of another example of moral behavior that you may have learned as a child?
>
> Can you identify any morals that are evident in the scenario about Alan at the beginning of the chapter?
>
> How do his parents' morals influence Alan's care?

Ethics, in contrast, is a systematic study of right and wrong conduct in situations that involve issues of values and morals. Ethics is a formal process for making logical and consistent moral decisions. Morals consider in a broad, general manner what is good or bad, right or wrong (e.g., "In general, it is wrong to steal"). Ethics answers the question "What should I do in a given situation?" (e.g., "Is it wrong to steal if you have to do it to feed your children?"). Ethics uses specific rules, theories, principles, and perspectives to inquire into the justification of an individual's actions in a particular situation. It seeks to discover what we "ought" to do in certain circumstances.

How are laws related to ethics and morals? Think about the following:

- *Law*: It is illegal to drive faster than the speed limit.
  Situation: A child is bleeding profusely and may have cut an artery. The driver drives very fast and even drives through a red light.
- *Question*: Was that illegal? Was it immoral?

- *Law:* In the United States, it is legal in certain situations to have an abortion.
  Fact: Although everyone would have to agree that the act is legal, people are about evenly divided as to whether they believe it is moral.

Ethics is rooted in the legal system and reflects the political values of a society. However, you should be able to see now that ethics is not the same as law, religion, institutional practices, or customs. An action that is legal or customary may not be morally right or ethically justifiable. The same holds true of religion. You cannot assume that an accepted practice of a certain religion is an ethical practice in every situation.

In the case of Alan and his family ("Meet Your Patients"), the ethical decision-making is quite different from the moral perspective of Alan's parents. The parents believe a blood transfusion is morally wrong; this fits with their religious beliefs. The surgeon and the nurse, however, believe withholding blood from Alan would be unethical.

Bioethics refers to the application of ethical principles to healthcare. Bioethics is concerned with every area of healthcare, including direct care of patients, allocation of resources, utilization of staff, and medical and nursing research.

What Is Nursing Ethics?

Nursing ethics is a subset of bioethics. It refers to ethical questions that arise out of nursing practice. The first things to come to your mind may be the dramatic questions such as, "Should we turn off the ventilator and allow this patient to die? Should this baby have surgery even though his quality of life will probably never be good? Is abortion moral?" And so on. In reality, you will not make the final decision in such situations. You may have some input, but the patient, physician, and family will decide. As a nurse, you are responsible for deciding the nature and extent of your own participation in each situation, and you must support patients who are making ethical decisions or perhaps coping with the results of decisions made by others. Consider the following true story paraphrased from Curtin and Flaherty (1982, pp. 3–4):

> A woman took her 6-year-old son to the emergency department (ED) to have a scalp laceration sutured. On the way to the hospital, she tried to calm him by telling him that the doctors would "numb" him and no one would hurt him "on purpose." When they arrived in the ED, they were placed in a cubicle next to another little boy who was awaiting treatment for a similar laceration. His father was also trying to reassure his son, as the woman had done.
>
> A nurse entered the cubicle of the father and son. She roughly cleansed the cut with no explanation or words of comfort. The physician came and sewed the laceration without a word and without waiting for the

local anesthetic to take effect. The boy screamed in pain and terror the whole time. The woman was horrified, and her son was scared. But when the very same nurse approached the woman and her son, she was kind and gentle. The same physician carefully injected a local anesthetic and waited for it to take effect before suturing.

Why do you think there was such difference in the treatment? Was it because the man and boy appeared to be of lower socioeconomic status? Was it the presence of a father rather than a mother? Was it because the father and son were from a minority group and the woman and son were not? Regardless of why it happened, what makes this case important? After all, both boys received medical treatment; both incisions will heal; no one's life or health was threatened; no life-and-death decisions were made. But the first child's humanity and dignity were violated, and the actions were not fair. An important thing for you to recognize from this case is that *this is a perfect example of nursing ethics*: questions that have to do with *the nurse's* actions, not the actions of others. The nurse did not need a medical order or permission from hospital administration to act ethically.

In the "Meet Your Patients" scenario, you, as the nurse, are not responsible for deciding the broad questions: "Is blood transfusion right or wrong?" or "Do the parents have a right to refuse blood transfusion?" Your decision is "What should *I* do? Should I try to persuade the parents to change their minds, as the surgeon directs, or not?" That is the *nursing ethics* question. And in that scenario, you will need to deal with the effects of the final decision on Alan. He may be frightened; he may be angry; he may die. The nurse is there for patients' most human and vulnerable moments.

Why Should Nurses Study Ethics?

Nurses should study ethics for a variety of reasons. This section will help you understand those reasons.

- *You will encounter ethical problems frequently in your work,* whether or not you are even aware of it. A consciously made, informed decision must surely be better than one made without awareness of the ethical issues involved. The most difficult question you will face as a nurse will not be "How do I do this," but "Should I do this?"
- *Ethics is central to nursing.* Commitment to caring for other human beings supports the claim that nursing is a moral art (Curtin & Flaherty, 1982). Traditionally, people have expressed idealism by attending the sick; health and compassion are central values in nursing.
- *Multidisciplinary input is important.* No one profession is responsible for an ethical decision. As situations become more complex, multidisciplinary input becomes increasingly important. For example, surgeons are responsible for knowing what surgery to perform and obtaining consent, but the nurse has a

part in being sure the patient is adequately informed so that true consent is obtained.
- *Ethical knowledge is necessary for professional competence.* Being a professional includes being accountable to others in the profession for the ethical conduct of your work. Using professional expertise for social good is one hallmark of a profession. Therefore, to conduct our work well and have it stand the test of public scrutiny, we need to be clear about the ethics of our work.
- *Ethical reasoning is necessary for nursing credibility among other disciplines.* For your opinion to be valued by others, you must be able to clearly express your moral position in a logical way. To be a truly accountable practitioner, you must be able to (1) understand your own values as they relate to basic morality and (2) use ethical reasoning to articulate your moral position.
- *Ethical proficiency is essential for providing holistic care.* Nurses deal with the whole person—that includes providing support for spiritual and moral concerns.
- *Nurses have a responsibility to be advocates for patients.* **Advocacy** is the communication and defense of the rights and interests of another. Since the 1960s, schools have socialized nurses to include patient advocacy in their role conceptions (Wilkinson, 1997). Currently, the American Nurses Association (ANA) Code of Ethics for Nurses (2001), provision 3, states: "The nurse promotes, advocates for and strives to protect the health, safety and rights of the patient."

 Advocacy includes protecting patients' legal or moral rights (e.g., taking appropriate action when the actions of a healthcare team member jeopardize the patient's rights or best interests). However, you can advocate for patients in everyday practice, for example by contacting a primary provider to request a new prescription when a pain medication is not effective. To advocate for patients in ethical situations, you must be able to identify the ethical issues and communicate the patient's wishes.
- *Studying ethics will help you to make better decisions.* The study of ethics prepares you to analyze moral problems from multiple perspectives rather than relying entirely on your personal values, intuition, and emotions. Practice in analyzing dilemmas will help you to become an informed decision maker, capable of understanding the perspectives of all the people in each situation—to understand, for example, why the Freses ("Meet Your Patients") are refusing a blood transfusion.

Most nursing problems have more than one acceptable answer. This is especially true of ethical problems. Each situation is unique in its details—for example, the people are different in how they evaluate what is and is not beneficial for themselves. By thinking it through critically from several different angles, you will be assured that you have done all that you can to provide your client with the highest quality of ethical care.

KnowledgeCheck 44-1

- Define *morals*, and give an example that is not in the text.
- Define *ethics*, and give an example that is not in the text.
- How is bioethics different from ethics?
- Why do nurses need to study ethics?

Go to Chapter 44, **Knowledge Check Response Sheet and Answers,** on the Student Resource Disk or DavisPlus at http://davisplus.fadavis.com/Wilkinson2

What Is Ethical Agency?

Moral agency or **ethical agency** for nurses is the ability to base their practice on professional standards of ethical conduct and to participate in ethical decision-making. Simply stated, it means that nurses have choices and are responsible for their actions. An ethical agent must be able to:

- Perceive the difference between right and wrong.
- Understand abstract moral principles.
- Reason and apply moral principles to make decisions, weigh alternatives, and plan sound ways to achieve goals.
- Decide and choose freely.
- Act according to choice (this assumes both the power and the capability to act).

For a more expanded discussion of ethical agency,

Go to Chapter 44, **Supplemental Materials: Elements of Ethical Agency,** on the Student Resource Disk or DavisPlus at http://davisplus.fadavis.com/Wilkinson2

CriticalThinking 44-2

Consider the five components of ethical agency. To what extent do you believe nurses possess those abilities? Explain your thinking.

Moral Distress

In practice, nurses often make but are unable to carry out their moral decisions. A seminal study by Wilkinson (1987/88) identified this as **moral distress**. Situational pressures (constraints) influence nurses' moral decisions as well as their ability to carry out their decisions (e.g., Corley & Minick, 2002; Erlen, 2001; Georges & Grypdonck, 2002; Hart, 2009; Hamric, Davis, & Childress, 2006; Jameton, 1984; Zuzelo, 2007). Whether these constraints are real or merely perceived, nurses in various studies have named the following as obstacles to carrying out their moral decisions: physicians, nurse administrators, other nurses, institutional policies, the law, threat of lawsuits, being socialized to follow orders, and doubting their own knowledge (Catlin, Volat, Hadley, et al., 2008; Glasberg, Eriksson, & Norberg, 2008; Schluter, Winch, Holzhauser, et al., 2008; Wilkinson, 1987/88).

The fact is that even if you make a well thought-out moral decision, you may not be able to do what you believe to be right. This problem is not unique to nurses, and recent studies describe moral distress among other healthcare professionals (e.g., Schwenzer & Wang, 2006). No one is 100% "free" to choose and act. Actions always have consequences: for you and for others. Nevertheless, if you are confident you have made a good decision and can express it logically and clearly to others, you can at least enter into a conversation with nurse administrators, physicians, and families about what ought to be done. Then you will be comfortable knowing that you have done all you could do, even if it is not all you wished to do.

If you would like an optional, expanded discussion of moral distress,

Go to Chapter 44, **Supplemental Materials: Moral Distress,** on the Student Resource Disk or DavisPlus at http://davisplus.fadavis.com/Wilkinson2

Whistleblowing

Nurses experience **moral outrage** when they perceive that others are behaving immorally (Wilkinson, 1987/1988). Moral outrage is similar to moral distress, except that in cases of moral outrage, nurses do not participate in the act. Therefore, they do not believe that they are responsible for doing wrong, but that they are powerless to prevent it (Burkhardt & Nathaniel, 2008). A nurse may respond to moral outrage by "blowing the whistle."

A **whistleblower** is specifically defined as a person "who identifies an incompetent, unethical, or illegal situation, or actions of others, in the workplace and reports it to someone who may have the power to stop the wrong" (Ahern & McDonald, 2002, p. 314; Wilmot, 2000). The "others" in question may be an individual or an entire organization. When the wrongdoing involves an organization, the whistleblower must hold the situation up to public scrutiny, for example, by going to the news media or pursuing legal recourse.

At some point in your nursing career, you may become aware that a health team member is doing something illegal, unethical, or incompetent. It is difficult to know what to do. You will need to consider the consequence of the action, the competence of the person involved, and the completeness of your data about the incident. Before deciding to report the person, you will want to be sure that the information has been confirmed through another source and that reporting the problem will be likely to correct the wrongdoing or prevent future problems (Attree, 2007; Peternelj-Taylor, 2003). Weigh the risks against the benefits.

Whistleblowing is difficult in the case of an impaired colleague. **Impaired nursing practice** occurs when the nurse's ability to perform the essential functions of nursing is diminished by chemical dependence on drugs or alcohol or by mental illness. Because such impairment is a threat to patients, and because the impaired nurse may have difficulty being accountable to herself or in assessing her self-competence, you would need to report your co-worker's questionable behavior. The Code of Ethics for Nurses and an American Nurses Association resolution propose that as a compassionate colleague, you must ensure that an impaired nurse receives assistance in regaining optimal function by reporting the behaviors to the appropriate entity within the employment setting (ANA, 2001, 2002).

KnowledgeCheck 44-2

- Define ethical agency.
- What five abilities must be present for ethical agency to exist?
- List at least three constraints that can keep nurses from carrying out their moral decisions.

 Go to Chapter 44, **Knowledge Check Response Sheet and Answers,** on the Student Resource Disk or DavisPlus at http://davisplus.fadavis.com/Wilkinson2

What Are Some Sources of Ethical Problems for Nurses?

Several factors contribute to the frequency of nurses' ethical problems, including societal factors, the nature of nursing work, and the nature of the nursing profession itself.

Societal Factors

Some ethical problems for nurses are created by the ever-changing nature of our dynamic, multicultural society. This section discusses some of those factors.

Increased Consumer Awareness. Historically, the healthcare system operated in a very paternalistic manner. Sick people sought the advice of a physician and then usually followed the physician's orders without question. Partly as a result of increased consumer awareness and availability of information online, professionals now are expected to share knowledge with patients and to obtain truly informed consent for treatments.

Technological Advances. With every new technology, new issues arise. For example, in vitro fertilization and embryo transfer methods have brought about questions of what should be done with embryos that are not implanted into a uterus. Can they be disposed of? What is their status as persons? Other ethical questions surround organ transplants, amniocentesis capable of revealing fetal defects, genetic engineering, human embryonic stem cell research, cryogenics, and technical advances that allow loved ones to be maintained on life support beyond what anyone might have imagined 20 years ago (Brock, 2006).

Multicultural Population. Not long ago, it was safe to assume that your values and beliefs would be similar to those of your patients; we had a fairly homogeneous society with a shared value system. We now live in a multicultural, multifaith society, and that assumption is no longer valid. You will work with patients and colleagues from a variety of cultural backgrounds, who probably hold very different sets of values. You will need to respect a variety of belief systems, and you will need to serve as a patient advocate even when the patient's value system is strikingly different from your own. There are nursing theories that can help you recognize various cultural values, for example, Leininger's (2002) theory of Cultural Care Diversity and Universality (for a review, see Chapters 8 and 14).

Cost Containment. The emphasis on cutting healthcare costs creates many morally questionable situations. For example, patients are being sent home from the hospital while they are still very ill. On being discharged, they may discover that insurance payments are limited for services outside the hospital, including specialists, home care, and medical supplies (e.g., bandages, walkers).

Cost containment efforts and the nursing shortage have led healthcare agencies to increase the number of patients each nurse is expected to care for. As a nurse, you will undoubtedly find yourself in situations where fewer nurses are available than patient acuity requires. You will have to make personal decisions about how far you will stretch your own resources.

Toward Evidence-Based Practice

Attree, M. (2007). Factors influencing nurses' decisions to raise concerns about care quality. *Journal of Nursing Management, 15*(4), 392–402.

Professional ethics require nurses to raise concerns about standards of practice; however, under-reporting is the norm. This qualitative study analyzed data from interviews with 142 nurses and found that nurses perceived reporting concerns to be a high-risk: low-benefit action. They lacked confidence in reporting systems. Nurses named fear of repercussions, retribution, labeling, and blame as reasons for not raising concerns, as well as the belief that nothing would be done about the concerns.

1. What type of moral situation (for the nurse) is best illustrated by this study: moral distress or whistleblowing? Explain your reasoning.

 Go to Chapter 44, **Toward Evidence-Based Practice Suggested Responses,** on the Student Resource Disk or DavisPlus at http://davisplus.fadavis.com/Wilkinson2

The Nature of Nursing Work

Ethical problems exist in all kinds of work. However, the nature of nursing work itself can create unique ethical problems.

Nurses' Moral Problems. Nurses' moral problems are immediate, serious, and frequent. In the classroom, you have the luxury to leave questions unsettled. In the real world, you must always decide: Either you take action, or you do not. But for a nurse, deciding *not* to act is, in effect, an act. For example, suppose the family wishes a patient to have aggressive Code Blue (resuscitation) efforts; however, you know the patient does not wish to be "coded." When the patient's heart stops, whether or not you know the "right" thing to do, you must decide immediately to carry out or not carry out the Code Blue. If you wait too long to ponder the ethical issues, it may be too late to carry it out. If you do not decide, the effect is the same as though you had decided *not* to code.

Nurses' Unique Position in Healthcare Organizations. Nurses have multiple obligations and relationships, and sometimes conflicting loyalties. They are employees (with a relationship with the agency) as well as professionals (with a special relationship with patients). In addition, they have peer relationships and a unique relationship with physicians. Although nurses are usually not employed by a physician, they are expected to follow physician prescriptions for patient care. In addition, in most organizations, physicians are higher on the power and status hierarchy than are nurses. Ethical questions arise when nurses experience conflicts among their loyalties to patients, families, physicians, employers, and other nurses. Consider the following example: A patient wants to know his test results; the physician is reluctant to tell him. What are the conflicting loyalties? Should the nurse give the patient the information or not? There are two options:

Tell. The nurse could honor the principle of personal autonomy and her obligation to the patient by telling him his test results. But this might harm the patient's relationship with the physician, which is important to the patient's well-being. Furthermore, if the nurse tells the patient his test results, it may create problems between the physician and the employer (e.g., the hospital). In addition, this action may in some instances violate hospital policies, and, therefore, harm the nurse's relationship with the hospital. It will certainly affect her relationship with the physician.

Don't tell. The nurse could preserve the patient–physician relationship by withholding the test results from the patient. This choice does not honor her relationship with the patient. Also, if the nurse does not tell the patient his test results, the patient may find out anyway and be angry with the hospital, the physician, and the nurse.

According to professional ethics, your first allegiance is to the patient. However, the patient's needs often conflict with institutional policies, family desires, or even laws of the state. There may also be conflicts in your relationships with the patient and his family. You can see an example of this in the "Meet Your Patients" scenario, wherein the nurse finds it impossible to honor the parents' autonomy and at the same time advocate for Alan. You may also encounter this type of conflict when a patient does not want any heroic measures and wishes only to die peacefully, but the family has not yet been able to accept the imminent death and are insisting on full resuscitation.

The Nature of the Nursing Profession

Some ethical problems arise because of value conflicts and a lack of clarity within the nursing profession. We have unresolved questions about the nature, scope, and goals of our practice, as well as our professional values (values are discussed later in the chapter). Notice the conflicts of values in the following items:

- *Caring versus time spent with patients.* Nursing values caring, humanistic care, and nurse–patient relationships—but nurses now spend less time at the bedside (with patients) than ever before. One reason is understaffing and heavier patient loads, but there are other factors: the use of technology; the need for careful documentation; and the nursing emphasis on leading, managing, and delegation instead of hands-on care.
- *Autonomy versus escaping hard choices.* On one hand, we believe nurses should have an equal status with other healthcare professionals—on the other hand, many nurses want to escape hard choices by "letting the doctor decide."
- *Higher pay versus cost effectiveness.* Most nurses believe we deserve higher pay—yet, we claim nurses are cost effective because we work less expensively than physicians.
- *Professionalism versus caring.* On one hand, we claim the nurse is a professional, citing critical thinking, knowledge, and management skills—on the other hand, we emphasize caring, with the nurse at the bedside offering comfort and doing hands-on tasks.

In most of those examples, we value both of the opposites. We would not wish to give up either one. But specific situations require us to choose between them, and that is one source of our discomfort.

What Factors Affect Moral Decisions?

By now, you should have an idea of the nature of morals and ethics and of the need to study nursing ethics. We turn our focus now to some basic theoretical knowledge about factors that are involved in making moral decisions: developmental stages, values, moral frameworks, ethical principles, and professional guidelines.

How Are Values, Morals, and Ethics Related?

Values and morals are learned in conscious and unconscious ways and become a part of your makeup. When we evaluate right and wrong, or good and bad, we are using moral judgment. Therefore, our individual preferences (values) of right or wrong become our moral values. Whether or not you are aware of it, your morals and values shape the manner in which you make ethical decisions in your nursing practice (Burkhardt & Nathaniel, 2008).

So, although ethics are based on a structured set of principles and theories, and ethical decisions are publicly stated in terms of possible alternative behaviors, such decisions are always influenced unconsciously by our own personal values and morals. It is important to clarify the influence of your values and morals each time you enter into a situation where you are called on to be objective in your decision-making. Later in this chapter, we will talk about practical strategies you can use to clarify your values and judge their influence on your ethical decisions.

Developmental Stage

A person's stage of moral development affects the way he reasons about moral issues. We learn and internalize our morals throughout the life span, beginning in childhood. Building on the classic developmental theory of Piaget (1932), Kohlberg (1968, 1981) theorized that moral development depends on a person's ability to think and reason at progressively higher levels. Kohlberg's studies led to his view that children go through a sequence of moral reasoning ability, proceeding through several stages to a final level in adulthood, in which they base moral principles on universal and impartial principles of justice (Table 44-1). If you would like to have an expanded version of Table 44-1 and examples of the stages,

 Go to Chapter 44, **Tables, Boxes, Figures: ESG Table 44-1, Stages of Moral Development,** on the Student Resource Disk or DavisPlus at http://davisplus.fadavis.com/Wilkinson2

People progress gradually through the stages as they mature and interact with the environment. The stages overlap. Kohlberg found that more than half of a person's thinking always reflects the stage he is in, with the remainder at the stage he is leaving or the stage into which he is moving. Although some people never achieve Kohlberg's highest levels, progression through the stages is always forward—except in extreme trauma, it is never backward—and people do not skip stages.

Gilligan (1993) challenged Kohlberg's perspective of moral development, citing it as male-biased. Gilligan found through her research that girls develop morally by paying attention to community and to relationships,

Table 44-1 ➤ Kohlberg's Stages of Moral Development	
LEVELS	**STAGES**
I. Preconventional Level The person conforms to cultural rules and labels of good and bad but interprets them in terms of (1) punishment and reward or (2) the physical power of those who enforce the rules. Children ages 4 to 10 years are usually at this level; some adults never progress beyond it.	**Stage 1**—Punishment–obedience orientation. (It is a right action if it avoids punishment.) **Stage 2**—Personal interest orientation. (It is a right action if it satisfies your personal needs.)
II. Conventional Level At this level, meeting family, group, or societal expectations is valuable in its own right, regardless of the consequences of the actions. The person goes beyond conforming to loyalty to the social order and identifying with those involved in it. Others set the standards, but the person is internally motivated to follow them.	**Stage 3**—Good boy–nice girl orientation. (It is a right action if it pleases others.) **Stage 4**—Law-and-order orientation. (It is a right action if it follows the rules.)
III. Postconventional, Autonomous, or Principled Level The person begins to define moral values and principles that have validity apart from society, groups, or persons in power. At this level, it becomes possible for the person to experience conflict between two socially accepted standards, and the person tries to decide rationally between them. Both the standards and the decision are internal. Moral principles have validity apart from the authority of groups and persons.	**Stage 5**—Legalistic, social contract orientation. (A right action is decided in terms of individual rights and standards agreed on by the whole society.) **Stage 6**—Universal ethical principles orientation. (A right action is determined by conscience and abstract principles such as the golden rule.)

Adapted from: Gibbs, J. (2009). *Moral development & reality: Beyond the theories of Kohlberg and Hoffman.* Upper Saddle River, NJ: Pearson Education (Allyn & Bacon imprint); Hoffman, M. (2000). *Empathy and moral development: Implications for caring and justice.* Cambridge, UK: Cambridge University Press; Kohlberg, L. (1968, 1981). *Essays on moral development.* Volumes 1–3. San Francisco: Harper & Row; Kohlberg, L. (1968). Moral development. In *International encyclopedia of social science.* New York: Macmillan; Power, F., Higgins, A., & Kohlberg, L. (1989). *Lawrence Kohlberg's approach to moral education,* New York: Columbia University Press; Waugh, D. (1978). Moral development: Theory and process. In *Teaching and evaluating the affective domain in nursing programs* (pp. 17–30). New York: Charles B. Slack.

whereas boys tend to process dilemmas through more abstract ideals or principles. If you need a review of Gilligan's three stages: caring for oneself, caring for others, and caring for self and others,

 Go to Chapter 9, **Expanded Discussion,** on the Student Resource Disk or DavisPlus at http://davisplus.fadavis.com/Wilkinson2

Values, Attitudes, and Beliefs

Your values influence what you think and do. This is important to know because values are entangled in all ethical situations. If asked, could you say what your values are? Could you explain how they affect your decisions about right and wrong in a given situation? If so, that's a great beginning. If not, you will learn more as you move through this section.

Values

A **value** is a belief you have about the worth of something; it serves as a principle or a standard that influences decision-making. Values are ideals, beliefs, customs, modes of conduct, qualities, or goals that are highly prized or preferred by individuals, groups, or society. You can value an idea, a person, a way of doing things, or even an object (e.g., money). People express their values through behaviors, feelings, knowledge, and decisions. For example, the nurse who values compassion will interact with patients in a sensitive, caring manner. Raths, Harmin, and Simon (1978) identified criteria by which to identify a value as a "full" value. A **full value** must be:

- Chosen freely from a list of alternatives after thoughtful consideration has been given to the consequences of each alternative
- Cherished and made known to other people
- Translated into behaviors that are consistent with the chosen value and integrated into the lifestyle

Some other characteristics of values are that they:

- Are often taken for granted
- Are learned in conscious and unconscious ways, through observation and experience in social groups (e.g., the family, school, church)
- Become a part of a person's makeup
- Can be individual or shared
- Vary from person to person
- Can change over time
- May be expressed overtly or manifested indirectly

Your **value set** is your "list" of values. It gives direction for your life and forms a basis for behavior. Your value system is your value set with the values ranked from most important to least important. The total number of values a person has is rather small. The number of significant ones is even smaller. It is easy enough to identify values—for example, love, freedom, courage, and responsibility—but how many of them have a consistent and predictable impact on your actions? Those are the significant values.

KnowledgeCheck 44-3
- What are values?
- What are three characteristics of values?

 Go to Chapter 44, **Knowledge Check Response Sheet and Answers,** on the Student Resource Disk or DavisPlus at http://davisplus.fadavis.com/Wilkinson2

Critical**Thinking** 44-3

- Think about what you value personally in your own life. What are the five ideals, principles, or things that are most important to you?
- Now refer back to Chapter 13, where you were asked to list five ideals, principles, or things that were most important to you. What did you list then? Is your list any different now that you have gained some clinical experience and theoretical knowledge?

Attitudes

Attitudes are mental dispositions or feelings toward a person, object, or idea. Attitudes can be cognitive (thinking), affective (feeling), and behavioral (doing). For example, you might have a positive attitude about cleanliness—that is, you may think it is a good thing (e.g., "The floor is clean. That's nice.") But if you *value* cleanliness, you would be willing to scrub the floor. You would also wash your hands at appropriate times, bathe regularly, and teach others about hygiene.

Beliefs

A **belief** is something that one accepts as true (e.g., "I believe that germs cause disease and that by washing my hands I remove germs"). Beliefs are sometimes based on faith and sometimes on facts. A belief may or may not be true. Beliefs may or may not involve values. Consider the following statements of belief. The first does not involve a value; the second one does.

"I believe the Earth is round."
"Working hard to achieve goals is important to me; therefore, I believe that I must work during the summer to save money for college."

From those examples, can you see how values, beliefs, and behaviors are related?

Critical**Thinking** 44-4

- Think about Alan and his family ("Meet Your Patients"). What do you think were the values of Alan's parents that influenced their behavior at the hospital? First, identify their behaviors specifically. Then speculate about the values underlying each behavior.
- How do you think values can influence health?

KnowledgeCheck 44-4
- Define *belief;* give a new example.
- Define *attitude;* give a new example

 Go to Chapter 44, **Knowledge Check Response Sheet and Answers,** on the Student Resource Disk or DavisPlus at http://davisplus.fadavis.com/Wilkinson2

Professional versus Personal Values

Your **personal value system** is a set of values that you have reflected on and chosen that will help you to lead a good life (Purtilo, 2005). You have internalized some *societal values* and have come to perceive them as your own (e.g., good manners, such as saying "Please" and "Thank you"). In addition, you probably have some *personal values* (e.g., friendship, fairness, creativity) that are important to you but may or may not be important to society at large.

As you move forward in your profession, you will integrate what you learn and experience and form **professional values**. Many of these will simply expand your personal values. The American Association of Colleges of Nursing (AACN) has identified six professional values. These are included in Table 44-2, along with other professional values. Personal and professional values are not always congruent, though. Consider the following situation:

> Alexandra Jensen is a 17-year-old pregnant woman who comes in to your ambulatory surgical center for a voluntary termination of an early pregnancy. You are assigned to admit her to your unit and get her ready for this procedure. Imagine that your personal value in this situation is that you do not believe in abortion but that your professional value is guided by the American Nurses Association (ANA) standards of professional practice, which state that the nurse "delivers care in a manner that preserves and protects patient autonomy, dignity, rights, values and beliefs" (ANA, 2010, in press, p. 41). It is difficult to hold a personal value in high regard while under pressure to assume a conflicting professional value. How might you feel in the situation just described?

Do you think that your personal and professional values need to be compatible in order for you to be a competent nurse? Do you think that you should have the absolute right to refuse to participate in a situation (such as the one above) that may violate your personal values?

 Critical**Thinking** 44-5

- Name some other examples of societal values.
- What groups and social experiences have helped to form your values?
- Examine your personal values to see whether they match the professional values in Table 44-2.
    Which of those values, if any, do you not share? Explain your thinking.
    Name a few of your personal values that are not found on this list of professional values.

Knowledge Check 44-5

- What is the difference between personal and professional values?
- What is an example of professional values?
- What are some other types of values?

 Go to Chapter 44, **Knowledge Check Response Sheet and Answers,** on the Student Resource Disk or DavisPlus at http://davisplus.fadavis.com/Wilkinson2

How Are Values Transmitted?

As you have learned, we acquire values from social interaction. So how does that work? How are values transmitted? Table 44-3 outlines the methods of value transmission. A recent study adds the information that values transmission between parents and adolescents can be reciprocal and that the presence of a receptive and supportive parent makes value transmission more likely (Pinquart & Silbereisen, 2004).

What Is Value Neutrality?

You have probably been taught that nurses need to be nonjudgmental in working with their clients. As a nurse, you have a duty to provide the best care to clients. You should not assume that your personal values are right, and you should not judge the client's values as right or wrong on the basis of whether they agree with your value system. Think back to the discussion regarding Alexandra, who was seeking to terminate her pregnancy. A nurse who does not believe in abortion could still provide competent nursing care to Alexandra even though his personal values regarding abortion are different from Alexandra's. **Value neutrality** means that we attempt to understand our own values regarding an issue and to know when to put them aside, if necessary, to become nonjudgmental when providing care to clients. However, you should know that some healthcare professionals believe value neutrality is not possible to achieve. Further, they say it is not even desirable because it obligates healthcare providers to suppress or modify their own deepest moral and religious beliefs (Balch, 2006; Beckwith & Peppin, 2000; Clark, 2006; Goldenberg, 2005; Pellegrino, 2000).

Knowledge Check 44-6

- What are some ways that values can be transmitted?
- What is value neutrality?

 Go to Chapter 44, **Knowledge Check Response Sheet and Answers,** on the Student Resource Disk or DavisPlus at http://davisplus.fadavis.com/Wilkinson2

Moral Frameworks

Moral (or **philosophical**) **frameworks** are systems of thought (theories) that are the basis for the differing perspectives people have in ethical situations. Many such frameworks are rooted in ancient works, for example, of the Greek philosophers Plato and Aristotle. No matter how well you know the theories, though, they will not provide answers for specific patient

Table 44-2 ➤ American Association of Colleges of Nursing (AACN) and Other Professional Nursing Values and Behaviors

VALUES	SAMPLE PROFESSIONAL BEHAVIORS
Altruism Concern for the welfare and well-being of others. Altruism is reflected by the nurse's concern for the welfare of patients, other nurses, and other healthcare providers. Includes patient advocacy.	■ Demonstrates understanding of cultures, beliefs, and perspectives of others. ■ Advocates for patients, particularly the most vulnerable. ■ Takes risks on behalf of patients and colleagues. ■ Mentors other professionals.
Autonomy The right to self-determination—to choose and act on that choice. Every competent person has the right to decide his own course of action.	■ Plans care in partnership with patients. ■ Honors the right of patients and families to make decisions about healthcare. ■ Provides information so that patients can make informed choices. ■ Informs patients about details of their care (e.g., test results).
Human Dignity Respect for the inherent worth and uniqueness of individuals and populations	■ Provides culturally competent and sensitive care. ■ Protects the patient's privacy. ■ Preserves the confidentiality of patients and healthcare providers. ■ Designs care with sensitivity to individual patient needs. ■ Values and respects colleagues and patients.
Integrity Acting in accordance with an appropriate code of ethics and accepted standards of practice. Includes honesty.	■ Provides honest information to patients and the public. ■ Documents care accurately and honestly. ■ Seeks to remedy errors made by self or others. ■ Demonstrates accountability for own actions.
Social Justice Upholding moral, legal, and humanistic principles. Treating others fairly regardless of race, age, citizenship, economic status, disability, or sexual orientation. This value is reflected in professional practice when the nurse works to ensure equal treatment under the law and equal access to quality healthcare.	■ Supports fairness and nondiscrimination in the delivery of care. ■ Promotes universal access to healthcare. ■ Encourages legislation and policy consistent with the advancement of nursing care and healthcare. ■ Works to ensure equal treatment under the law.

Additional professional values frequently cited for nursing include the following:

■ Caring
■ Diversity
■ Equality (having the same rights, privileges, or status)
■ Esthetics (qualities of objects or people that are pleasing)
■ Freedom (capacity to choose)
■ Truth (faithfulness to fact or reality)
■ Service (commitment to work useful to others)
■ Education (basic and lifelong continuing education for nurses)
■ Holism
■ Competence, excellence (skill, knowledge, performance of nursing work)
■ Loyalty (feeling of duty or attachment to other nurses)

Sources: American Colleges of Nursing Association (AACN). (2008). The essentials of baccalaureate education for professional nursing practice. Washington, DC: Author. Retrieved from http://www.aacn.nche.edu/Education/pdf/BaccEssentials08.pdf; Canadian Nurses Association (CNA). (2008). Code of Ethics for Registered Nurses. Retrieved from http://www.cna-nurses.ca/CNA/practice/ethics/code/default_e.aspx; Jameton, A. (1984). Nursing practice: The ethical issues. Englewood Cliffs, NJ: Prentice Hall; National League for Nursing (2007). Core values. Retrieved from http://www.nln.org/aboutnln/corevalues.htm; Watson, J. (1981, Summer). Socialization of the nursing student in a professional nursing education programme. Nursing Papers, 13, 19–24.

situations. They simply offer a lens through which you can examine an ethical problem. See Chapter 8 if you need to review the purposes and uses of theories.

There is no single "best" theory that will give you all the answers or provide the one "true" answer to an ethical problem. Each provides a different perspective. Using more than one framework to analyze a situation

Table 44-3 ➤ Modes of Value Transmission

MODE	DESCRIPTION
Modeling	Children learn values from a variety of role models (parents, peers, rock stars, significant others) by observation. This modeling may lead to socially acceptable or unacceptable behaviors.
Moralizing	"This way is the only way." Children are taught a complete set of values in an authoritarian approach. If the child does not conform, the parent may inflict guilt and fear on him. This approach by parents, teachers, church leaders, and other authorities may make it difficult for young people to make independent choices because they have no experience selecting values that are good for them.
Laissez-faire	"Doing your own thing." Children are allowed to explore differing sets of values on their own with little guidance or discipline. This may lead to conflict and confusion on the part of the child.
Reward and punishment	The child's behavior is controlled by offering rewards for certain valued behaviors and punishing the child who fails to comply. Rewards can strengthen behavior, whereas physical punishment may teach that violence is an acceptable behavior.
Responsible choice	A balance of freedom and restriction allows children to select the values, explore new behaviors, and experience the consequences. This can lead to personal satisfaction and parental support.

enables you to perform a more comprehensive analysis of the problem.

What Is Consequentialism?

In **consequentialist** theories, the rightness or wrongness of an action depends on the consequences of the act rather than on the act itself. Theories of this type are also called **teleology,** from the Greek word *telos,* meaning "end" or the study of ends (also called *final causes*) (Beauchamp & Childress, 2008). Utilitarianism is the most familiar consequentialist theory, and the one we will refer to in this chapter. **Utilitarianism** takes the position that the value of an action is determined by its usefulness. The *principle of utility* states that an act must result in the greatest good (positive benefit) for the greatest number of people. Any act can then become the ethical choice if it delivers "good" results. In healthcare, the principle of "first, do no harm," is consequentialist in nature. Because of this principle, we are always concerned about weighing the risks and benefits of our care (e.g., a medication may kill cancer cells, but side effects may harm the patient's quality of life).

Using utilitarianism to resolve an ethical problem, you would evaluate every alternative action for its potential outcomes, both positive and negative—similar to a technique you may already use when making other decisions, that is, making a list of pros and cons. You would then select the action that results in the most benefits for the greatest number of people involved in the situation. The following is an example of utilitarian reasoning: The practice of triage is used in a disaster when emergency workers sort patients to determine who will be treated first or who will receive limited resources (e.g., oxygen or intravenous therapy). If a victim

has little potential for survival, he may not be treated at all, or his treatment may be postponed to allow the healthcare team to treat those victims (i.e., "the greatest number") with the greatest potential to survive.

Critical Thinking 44-6

- Describe a time in your life when you used consequentialism to resolve a difficult situation.
- What types of clinical dilemmas might be best resolved using this model?

What Is Deontology?

Deontology is almost the opposite of the utilitarian model in that it considers an action to be right or wrong regardless of its consequences. Decisions are based on moral rules and unchanging principles. There are a variety of deontological theories, but you will commonly find they make use of the following, or similar, principles:

The Categorical Imperative. This principle, established by the philosopher Immanuel Kant (1724–1804), states that one should act only if the action is based on a principle that is universal—or in other words, if you believe that everyone should act in the same way in a similar situation.

Treat People as Ends and Never as Means. Treating people as an *end* means that the person is more important than the goal you may be trying to accomplish. Can you imagine the ethical concerns of research situations in which the research subjects were exposed to some amount of risk (e.g., a new surgical procedure) to find a drug or treatment that will benefit many other people?

Rules and Principles. When using a deontological model, you would critically examine a situation to determine which actions are right or wrong according to rules and principles such as justice, autonomy, doing good, and doing no harm. These principles are regarded as unchanging and absolute, and they come from the same universal values that underlie all major religions.

Rights and Duties. Deontological frameworks also emphasize rights (e.g., the right to freedom, the right of self-determination) and duties (obligations). For example, you must help someone in need because you have a duty to help others, not because helping will produce good consequences. In fact, you have a duty to help even if your helping may produce some bad consequences.

The following are two difficulties that may arise when using a deontology framework:

Conflict of Universal Principles. Sometimes you must choose between conflicting universal principles. It is not always clear which principle to honor. Allowing Alan's parents ("Meet Your Patients") to refuse to provide him with blood honors the principle of autonomy, but their decision may interfere with a right: Alan's right to life. Can you see that it might be difficult to decide which is the appropriate principle to honor?

It is Hard to Know Another's Motives. In deontological models, it is important to consider motives. It is one thing for Alan's parents to refuse a blood transfusion because they are honoring a religious principle; it would be quite another thing if they refused the transfusion because they stood to inherit a large trust fund left to Alan by his grandfather. Motives may place more weight on one of the conflicting universal principles over the other and make a decision clearer. Unfortunately, it is sometimes hard to recognize your own motives, much less to be sure about the motives of others.

 As a nurse, you will almost never be able to decide only on the basis of principles and rules; you will always need to consider the consequences of your actions.

KnowledgeCheck 44-7

- Describe utilitarianism.
- Define *deontology*.

Go to Chapter 44, **Knowledge Check Response Sheet and Answers,** on the Student Resource Disk or DavisPlus at http://davisplus.fadavis.com/Wilkinson2

What Is Feminist Ethics?

Feminist ethics is based on the belief that traditional ethical models provide a mostly masculine perspective, and that they devalue the moral experience of women (Bandman & Bandman, 2002). Traditional deontological models focus on abstract principles such as fairness, justice, and rights, which are more typical of male reasoning. In contrast, virtues such as love, relationships, caring, nurturing, and sympathy are more relevant to women but are rarely seen in traditional theories (Bandman & Bandman, 2002). Feminists assert that focusing on deontological principles distracts one from dealing with larger social issues. Feminist ethical reasoning uses relationships and stories rather than universal principles. Feminists argue that it is impossible to avoid being influenced by one's relationships. They see that influence as positive and believe it should not be lessened by an attempt to be objective—and in any case, that objectivity is impossible anyway.

Feminist theories do use principles and consequences, but they also ask you to look at social issues in the ethical situation to ensure that social facts are considered (Noddings, 2003). The point is to address issues of gender inequality within each situation. This means that part of your reasoning would be to think, "How is this decision affecting the woman?" Consider an example of deciding whether to allocate federally funded healthcare resources to younger people or to older adults. Feminist reasoning might say that, all other considerations being equal:

- In the United States there are more older women than older men.
- Older women tend to be poorer and are more likely to be alone than are men.
- Therefore, if healthcare for older adults were to be rationed, it would negatively affect women more than men.
- Therefore, it would be unfair and unethical to allocate more healthcare resources to younger people than to older people.

What Is an Ethics-of-Care?

The **ethics-of-care,** a nursing philosophy, directs attention to the specific situations of individual patients, viewed within the context of their life narrative. You would ask: "What is the story of this person's life? What is going on right now in his life? And what does that have to do with the morality of the action I'm considering?" Care theories grew directly out of feminist ethics and especially promote nurturing of patients and caregivers (i.e., caring) (Volbrecht, 2002). An ethics-of-care emphasizes the role of feelings, but also includes some of the principles that are part of traditional ethics, such as *autonomy* (self-determination) or *beneficence* (doing good).

In an ethics-of-care, nurses include a responsibility to care as a part of their professional behavior. Some aspects of care include the ability and duty to appreciate, understand, and even share the patient's pain or condition. Using a caring framework, your ethical analysis would focus on relationships and client stories. The following are specific ethics-of-care perspectives:

- Viewing caring as the central force in nursing (Leininger, 1988)
- Promoting dignity and respect for patients as people
- Attending to the particulars of each individual patient, especially the marginalized and disenfranchised members of society (Myhrvold, 2006).
- Cultivating responsiveness to others
- Redefining fundamental moral principles to include virtues such as kindness, attentiveness, empathy, compassion, and reliability

An advantage of including the caring perspective and patient stories in ethical dialogue is that it tends to focus discussion at the level where the relationships are located, rather than in an intellectual plane. Critics of the ethics-of-care suggest that the term *caring* can be misconstrued to become too sentimental and, therefore, ineffective. If nursing is sentimentalized through overemphasis on caring, nursing will be seen as less strong than medicine.

An ethics-of-care model does provide an alternative to the heavily intellectual camps of consequentialism and deontology. It can give a refreshingly new perspective into moral situations. Some questions that might reflect this model of discourse include the following:

- Should we provide free medical care to the homeless? An ethics-of-care position would probably say yes, even though it might not, for example, provide the greatest good for the greatest number of people.
- Our healthcare system uses discharge criteria that allow patients to be sent home from hospitals while they are still too ill to care for themselves. What does that say about caring in the healthcare system?

KnowledgeCheck 44-8

- How does feminist ethics affect ethical decision-making?
- What does the ethics-of-care model emphasize?

 Go to Chapter 44, **Knowledge Check Response Sheet and Answers,** on the Student Resource Disk or DavisPlus at http://davisplus.fadavis.com/Wilkinson2

Moral Concepts and Principles

Remember from Chapter 8 that theories are made up of concepts and principles. The same is true for moral theories. Moral concepts and principles are useful in ethical discussions because even if people disagree about which action is right in a situation, they may be able to agree about which principles apply. Agreement "in principle" may provide common ground for a compromise or other resolution of the

problem. Different moral frameworks use some of the same principles in ethical reasoning. We will discuss autonomy, nonmaleficence, beneficence, fidelity, veracity, and justice.

Autonomy

Autonomy refers to a person's right to choose and ability to act on that choice. Autonomy ties in with respect for human dignity. You demonstrate respect for autonomy when you treat patients with consideration, believe their stories about the course and symptoms of their illnesses, and protect those who are unable to decide for themselves.

The principle of autonomy underlies informed consent—the right of competent patients to decide for themselves whether to agree to a proposed treatment. You honor autonomy when you respect the patient's or surrogate decision-maker's right to decide, even when you believe those choices are not in the patient's best interest. You can help support autonomy by informing patients about advance directives and durable powers of attorney for healthcare.

In the "Meet Your Patients" scenario, if you believed autonomy to be the most important principle in the situation, what would you think about Alan's parents' refusing to allow him to receive blood products? If you believed that respecting their autonomy gives them the right to choose on the basis of their religious beliefs, would you still try to persuade them to change their minds?

Privacy and Confidentiality. The principles of **privacy** and **confidentiality** also partly derive from the principle of autonomy. An autonomous person has control over the collection, use, and access of her personal information. Many patients share sensitive information with nurses that they would not share with others, and it is important to maintain the patient's trust. This means that you should not discuss patients in the elevator, halls, lunchroom, or anywhere it can be overheard, even if the discussion is relevant to the patient's care. You should communicate to others only the information needed to provide healthcare. Share other information only with the patient's consent. If you would like more information about privacy and confidentiality, see Chapters 16 and 45; also

 Go to Chapter 44, **Supplemental Materials, Confidentiality and Privacy,** on the Student Resource Disk or DavisPlus at http://davisplus.fadavis.com/Wilkinson2

Nonmaleficence

The principle of **nonmaleficence** is the twofold duty to do no harm and to prevent harm. Nonmaleficence refers to both actual harm and risk of harm, as well as to intentional and unintentional harm. In nursing it is rare to find intentional harm, but unintentional harm due to lack of careful planning and consideration does occur (Beauchamp & Childress, 2008). Unintentional harm can also occur because of lack of knowledge, skill, or ability. Both the physicians' Hippocratic Oath and the nurses' Nightingale Pledge state that care providers have a duty to cause no harm to patients. When you are careful to prevent medication errors, or provide a walker, or use an ambulation belt for ambulating patients, you are honoring the nonmaleficence principle.

Nonmaleficence requires that you think critically about patient care and research situations, weighing the potential risks against the potential benefits. When using nonmaleficence to guide treatment regimens, ask the question, "Does this treatment cause more harm or more good to the patient?" Risk of harm is not always clear. Suppose you are about to get a patient out of bed for the first time after surgery. The benefit clearly is that this will prevent postoperative complications such as pneumonia and thrombophlebitis, but the risks, in terms of excessive pain or unintentional damage to the operative site, may be less clear. Weighing risks and benefits is a value-laden exercise. Who is to say what amount of pain is excessive—you or the patient? To honor the principle of nonmaleficence in this situation, you would need to be sure to premedicate the patient and carefully assess his status as you are helping him to ambulate.

Respect for Dignity. The value of respect for human dignity derives in part from the duty to do no harm. **Respect for dignity** refers to the nurse's respect for the intrinsic worth of each person, without respect to age, race, religion, or any other factors. It includes taking into account cultural and spiritual values, customs, and beliefs as well as their social and economic circumstances. Respect for dignity recognizes that patients are vulnerable; and that nurses should not abuse their relationships for personal gain, or enter into romantic, sexual, or other relationships with their patients.

Critical Thinking 44-7

Think about the "Meet Your Patients" scenario in terms of nonmaleficence. The parents refuse to allow a blood transfusion. You, the nurse, have tried to persuade them to change their minds. You do not need to decide what you ought to do; just analyze the situation in terms of the risks.

- What is it that creates the risk for harm to Alan?
- What is the risk for harm to Alan's parents because of the nurse's actions?

Beneficence

Beneficence is the duty to do or promote good. You can think of this principle as being on a continuum with nonmaleficence. At one end of the continuum is the duty to do no harm; beneficence, at the other end, is the duty to bring about positive good. The following examples illustrate the duties in priority order:

- Do no harm. (Don't push the man into the river.)
- Prevent harm when you can. (If the man is getting dangerously close to the river's edge, warn him that he is about to fall into the river.)
- Remove harm when it is being inflicted. (If you see a struggle and someone is trying to push the man into the river, interfere and try to stop it if you can do so without undue harm to yourself.)
- Bring about positive good. (If the man has fallen in the river, jump in and try to save him, or toss him a lifeline and call 9-1-1 if you can't swim.)

When weighing the risks and benefits of an action, you are actually balancing nonmaleficence with beneficence. Keep in mind that patients, family members, and other professionals may identify benefits and harms differently. A benefit to one may represent a burden to another. For example, in "Meet Your Patients," you may see a blood transfusion as a benefit to Alan, but to the parents it may represent harm. "Doing good" very much depends on the context and the rights of the person for whom the action is being taken.

Paternalism. Can you imagine that "doing good" might actually cause harm? Although beneficence seems like such a positive goal, it can have negative consequences. One such outcome is **paternalism** (treating others like children). This would occur, for example, if you think you know what is best for a competent client and then coerce the client to act as you wish rather than to act as she wishes. Saying to a patient, for example, "Trust us; we know what is best for you to do in this situation," may seem to be beneficent because you are trying to support the patient. But it is actually paternalistic behavior that lacks respect for the patient's autonomy.

Fidelity

Fidelity (faithfulness) is the duty to keep promises. It is a basic part of every patient care situation. Sometimes the promises are of major significance, such as promising not to share certain information with other members of the healthcare team. At other times it may be only a promise to come back to check the effectiveness of a pain medication or to bring a requested item back to the client's room. The duty to keep a promise is the same regardless of its level of importance.

In practice, you will often find that competing tasks prevent you from being able to deliver something exactly as you have promised. Make promises in a thoughtful, careful manner to maximize the likelihood that you can keep them. Instead of "I'll be right back with your medication," you might be a bit more vague and say, "I'll get back with your medication as quickly as I can" or "I must go help another patient for a few minutes, but I'll get here with your medication as quickly as I can."

Veracity

Veracity is the duty to tell the truth. This seems straightforward, and you may wonder why it even needs discussion. However, there are times when veracity presents a challenge. For example, should you tell the truth when you know that it might cause harm to the client? Would it be appropriate to tell a lie in order to relieve extreme patient anxiety? Most nurses would agree that it isn't hard to tell the truth, but at times it may be very hard to determine how *much* of the truth to tell. For example, healthcare professionals may feel uncomfortable giving families "bad news." So instead of saying, "Your father has a fatal illness and is unlikely to live for more than a month," they may say, "Your father is very ill, but we will do everything we possibly can for him." In this, as in most situations, the risk of losing patient trust outweighs any benefit of withholding the truth.

Although you always presume the value of telling the truth, there may be times when you are justified to withhold information. In some cultures, for example, families go to great lengths to protect a dying patient from the harsh truth of his prognosis, and the patient himself may not wish to know. In the United States, we tend to place a higher value on autonomy than in some cultures. In such a situation, you need to be culturally sensitive in order to act on the family's values, not the dominant cultural values. Always consider the context.

CriticalThinking 44-8

Review the "Meet Your Patients" scenario. Alan will not survive without a blood transfusion; the parents refuse. He asks the nurse, "Am I going to die?" You do not need to decide which response is best; just write an example that illustrates each of the following. What might the nurse say if she wishes to:

- Tell Alan the truth?
- Withhold or partially disclose the truth?
- Answer with an untruth?

Justice

Justice is the obligation to be fair. It implies equal treatment of all patients. Questions of justice will become a part of your everyday experience in patient care, from deciding how to allocate your time among patients to larger decisions, such as how to allocate limited healthcare resources.

Distributive Justice

Distributive justice requires fair distribution of both benefits and burdens (Husted & Husted, 2008). It is especially relevant to healthcare, as in the following issues.

- *Allocating resources.* Distributive justice questions come up when more than one person or group competes for the same resources. For example, in determining how to spend federal and state tax dollars, should more money be spent to fund AIDS research or to find better treatments for Alzheimer's disease? Or consider organ transplantation. Human organs are scarce re-

sources. How do we decide which patient should receive an available organ? Is an 18-year-old more deserving of a kidney than a 75-year-old? Is a person with liver disease due to alcoholism less deserving of a liver than someone with liver disease not caused by alcoholism? The decision of who should live and who may die is never an easy decision. In the United States, a national committee sets criteria for how organs will be distributed so the standard of justice can be considered.

- *Fair access to care.* Access to care is a specific kind of healthcare resource. The principle of distributive justice holds that we should provide equal access to healthcare for all. As the Baby Boomer generation ages, the federal budget will be strained. At the same time, the Baby Boomer nurses will be retiring. There are already fewer nurses to care for more aging patients at a time when national healthcare dollars are stretched very thin. How will the nation decide where to spend the limited dollars? How will nurse managers decide how to provide adequate care when they do not have enough nurses on their staff? The ability to develop sound criteria on which to base the allocation of resources is the challenge of distributive justice.

Compensatory Justice

Compensatory justice focuses on making amends for wrongs that have been done to individuals or groups. Malpractice suits consider this type of justice when they decide how much money to award a victim for being harmed. Groups of citizens may also be harmed. For instance, if a company's unintentional pollution of water was proven to cause cancer in members of the community, a monetary settlement might be made.

Procedural Justice

Procedural justice is important in processes that require ranking or ordering (Volbrecht, 2002). Often the unwritten rule of "first come, first served" is used as a basis for delivery of services. For example, institutional policies are written to ensure that the same procedures apply to all clients or employees in the same way (e.g., visiting hours, working on holidays, sick leave). Can you think of an example of procedural justice that you have experienced during your nursing education?

CriticalThinking 44-9

Look again at the emergency department situation described in "What Is Nursing Ethics?" at the beginning of this chapter. In this scenario, two little boys were treated for lacerations. Which principle of justice was violated: distributive, compensatory, or procedural? Explain your thinking.

KnowledgeCheck 44-9

List each of the six ethical principles and its definition.

Go to Chapter 44, **Knowledge Check Response Sheet and Answers,** on the Student Resource Disk or DavisPlus at http://davisplus.fadavis.com/Wilkinson2

Professional Guidelines

You should consult professional guidelines when making ethical decisions. Healthcare professionals have an obligation to society to be competent in their field; to allow only qualified persons entry into the profession; to discipline members of the profession who do not practice at an acceptable level; to do no harm; and to use high moral and ethical standards to resolve dilemmas (Husted & Husted, 2008). You can find ethical standards for nurses in codes of ethics, standards of practice, statements of patients' rights, and in various laws.

Nursing Codes of Ethics

Professional codes of ethics are formal statements of a group's expectations and standards for professional behavior generally accepted by members of the profession. Codes of ethics set forth ideal behaviors, but they are only as effective as the behaviors of the nurses who live up to the codes. The purposes of a nursing code of ethics are to:

- Inform the public about the profession's minimum standards.
- Demonstrate nursing's commitment to the public it serves.
- Outline major ethical considerations of nursing.
- Provide general guidelines for professional behavior.
- Guide the profession's self-regulating functions.
- Remind us of the special responsibility we assume in caring for the sick.

Nursing codes are not legally binding. However, they often exceed legal obligations. In most states, the state board of nursing uses the nursing code of ethics as the standard against which to evaluate a nurse's ethical

behavior. The board has the legal authority to censure or reprimand the nurse who does not practice within the boundaries of ethical practice.

The three following nursing organizations have had long-standing codes to guide nurses' ethical decision-making. The codes differ in specific details, but they are based on similar principles.

International Council of Nurses (ICN). The ICN first adopted its Code of Ethics for Nurses in 1953 as "a guide for action based on social values and needs" (ICN, 2006). The ICN Code has since served as the standard for nurses worldwide. The Code stresses respect for human rights, including cultural rights, the right to life and choice, the right to dignity, and right to be treated with respect. The code is designed to guide nurses in everyday choices, and it supports their refusal to participate in activities that conflict with caring and healing. If you wish to see the revised code,

 Go to Chapter 44, **Tables, Boxes, Figures: ESG Box 44-1, ICN Code of Ethics,** on the Student Resource Disk or DavisPlus at http://davisplus.fadavis.com/Wilkinson2

The American Nurses Association. The ANA revised their Code of Ethics for Nurses in 2001 (Box 44-1). ANA used input from a wide range of nurses and groups to ensure that the revised code would be relevant in many practice settings and reflect current ethical situations. The code has nine provisions, followed by interpretive statements to explain what is meant by each provision. If you would like more information about the ANA Code for Nurses,

 Go to the **ANA** Web site at www.nursingworld.org/ethics/ecode.htm

---

BOX 44-1 ■ American Nurses Association Code of Ethics for Nurses

1. The nurse, in all professional relationships, practices with compassion and respect for the inherent dignity, worth, and uniqueness of every individual, unrestricted by considerations of social or economic status, personal attributes, or the nature of health problems.

2. The nurse's primary commitment is to the patient, whether an individual, family, group, or community.

3. The nurse promotes, advocates for, and strives to protect the health, safety, and rights of the patient.

4. The nurse is responsible and accountable for individual nursing practice and determines the appropriate delegation of tasks consistent with the nurse's obligation to provide optimum patient care.

5. The nurse owes the same duties to self as to others, including the responsibility to preserve integrity and safety, to maintain competence, and to continue personal and professional growth.

6. The nurse participates in establishing, maintaining, and improving health care environments and conditions of

employment conducive to the provision of quality healthcare and consistent with the values of the profession through individual and collective action.

7. The nurse participates in the advancement of the profession through contributions to practice, education, administration, and knowledge development.

8. The nurse collaborates with other health professionals and the public in promoting community, national, and international efforts to meet health needs.

9. The profession of nursing, as represented by associations and their members, is responsible for articulating nursing values for maintaining the integrity of the profession and its practice, and for shaping social policy.

Source: Reprinted with permission from American Nurses Association, *Code of ethics for nurses with interpretive statements,* ©2001, Nursebooks.org, American Nurses Association, Washington, DC. Used with permission.

The Canadian Nurses Association (CNA). The CNA revised its Code of Ethics for Registered Nurses in 2008. As does the ANA code, it provides guidance for decision-making, serves as a means for self-evaluation and reflection regarding ethical practice, and provides a basis for peer review. The Canadian code is organized around seven values central to ethical nursing practice. To review those values, see Box 44-2. If you wish to see the full code with all of its interpretative statements,

 Go to www.cna-nurses.ca/cna/practice/ethics/code/default_e.aspx

ANA Standards of Care

In addition to its Code of Ethics, the American Nurses Association (ANA) sets standards for all aspects of clinical practice. In *Nursing: Scope and Standards of Practice* (2010, in press), standard 7 focuses on ethical practice. This standard (see Box 44-3) directs nurses to practice within the parameters described in the Code of Ethics for Nurses. Standard 7 speaks to the nurse's responsibilities to patients and directs nurses to manage ethical dilemmas and to report practices that are illegal, incompetent, or impaired.

The Patient Care Partnership

When patients are admitted to hospitals or to extended care facilities, they are entitled to specific rights in terms of their treatment: the right to make their own decisions, to be active partners in the treatment process, and to be treated with dignity and respect. Because rights are rooted in values, and because values are derived from culture, patient rights are different throughout the world. In the United

---

BOX 44-2 ■ Canadian Nurses Association Code of Ethics for Registered Nurses: Primary Values

1. Providing safe, compassionate, competent and ethical care
2. Promoting health and well-being
3. Promoting and respecting informed decision-making
4. Preserving dignity
5. Maintaining privacy and confidentiality
6. Promoting justice
7. Being accountable

This code is organized around the above described values. In the code, each value is further described by explanatory responsibility statements.

Source: Canadian Nurses Association. (2008). *Code of ethics for registered nurses.* Ottawa: Author, p. 3.

BOX 44-3 ■ American Nurses Association Standards of Professional Performance Standard 7. Ethics*

Definition: The registered nurse integrates ethical provisions in all areas of practice.

Measurement Criteria

The registered nurse:

- Uses the Code of Ethics for Nurses with Interpretive Statements (ANA, 2001) to guide practice.
- Delivers care in a manner that preserves and protects patient autonomy, dignity, and rights.
- Respects the centrality of the patient/family as core members of any health care team.
- Upholds and advocates for patient confidentiality within legal and regulatory parameters.
- Serves as a patient advocate assisting patients in developing skills for self-advocacy and informed decision-making.
- Maintains a therapeutic and professional patient–nurse relationship with appropriate professional role boundaries.
- Demonstrates a commitment to practicing self-care, managing stress, and connecting with self and others.
- Contributes to resolving ethical issues of patients, colleagues, community groups, systems and other stakeholders.
- Takes appropriate action regarding instances of illegal, unethical, or inappropriate behavior that can endanger or jeopardize the best interests of the patient or situation.
- Cooperates in an interprofessional team to make ethical decisions regarding the application of technologies and the acquisition and sharing of data.
- Demonstrates professional comportment (openness, honesty, integrity, and authenticity). (Mass. Board of Higher Education Nursing Initiative, 2007)
- Speaks up when appropriate to question health care practice when necessary for safety and quality improvement.

Source: Excerpted from American Nurses Association. (2010, in press). *Nursing: Scope and Standards of Practice* (2nd ed). Public Comment draft, January 2010. (To be published by August 2010). Silver Spring, MD: Nursebooks.org.
*Caveat: This material is from the draft for public comment (ANA, 2010 in press); its wording may be changed somewhat in the final published version. For that version of the ANA Standards of Professional Nursing Practice, go to www.nursingworld.org.

States, the American Hospital Association (AHA) published a document called *Patient Care Partnership* (2003). Instead of using "rights" language, this document is written in terms of patient expectations and responsibilities. The *Patient Care Partnership* encourages healthcare providers to be more aware of the need to treat patients in an ethical manner and to protect their rights. For a summary of the document, see Box 44-4.

Patients, when hospitalized, should expect the following:

- High-quality care, including the right to know the identity of caregivers

- A clean, safe environment, including safety, freedom from abuse and neglect, and discussion of any changes in care

- Respect for healthcare goals, values, and spiritual beliefs

- To be involved in making decisions about their care and treatment. This includes receiving information about:

  Health condition and treatments

  The benefits and risks of treatments, and whether a treatment is experimental or part of a research study

  What the patient and family will need to do regarding treatment follow-up after leaving the hospital

- Information about the right to make decisions and to refuse care, including advance directives and counselors or chaplains available to help with decision-making

- Protection of their privacy and confidentiality

- Help reviewing the bill and filing insurance claims

- Preparation and information when leaving the hospital, including:

  Identification of sources for follow-up care and whether the hospital has a financial interest in any of the referrals

  Coordination of hospital activities with caregivers outside the hospital

  Information and training about the self-care the person will need at home

Source: Excerpted and adapted from American Hospital Association. (2003). *The patient care partnership: Understanding expectations, rights and responsibilities.* Chicago: Author.
To see the complete brochure,

 Go to **The American Hospital Association Web site, "The Patient Care Partnership,"** at http://www.aha.org/aha/issues/Communicating-With-Patients/pt-care-partnership.html

The Joint Commission Accreditation Standards

The Joint Commission standards contain sections on organizational ethics and individual rights. The section on organizational ethics requires ethical behavior in care, treatment, services, and business practices. It includes a statement about the need to provide for meeting patient needs in the event care must be denied in the institution. The standards state that an organization should (2008, p. 145):

- Manage relationships with patients and the public in an ethical manner.
- Consider patients' values and preferences, including decisions surrounding discontinuing care, treatment, and services.

- Help patients understand and exercise their rights.
- Inform patients of their responsibilities in care, treatment, and services.
- Recognize the organization's legal responsibilities.

Knowledge Check 44-10

- How would the nurse use a professional guideline or code of ethics to assist in the ethical decision-making process?
- What are some examples of such resources?

 Go to Chapter 44, **Knowledge Check Response Sheet and Answers,** on the Student Resource Disk or DavisPlus at http://davisplus.fadavis.com/Wilkinson2

Ethical Issues in Healthcare

As a nurse, you are likely to encounter several ethical issues that occur in healthcare. For example, ethical questions arise in the following situations:

Acquired immune deficiency syndrome (AIDS)
Abortion
Allocation of healthcare goods and services
Confidentiality and privacy (e.g., reporting gunshot wounds and child abuse)
Advance directives
Do Not Attempt Resuscitation (DNAR) orders
Assisted suicide and euthanasia
Extraordinary (heroic) measures to prolong life
Withdrawing or withholding life-sustaining treatments (e.g., ventilators, artificial nutrition and hydration)
Informed consent
Organ transplantation
Reproductive technology (e.g., in vitro fertilization, surrogate mothering, sex preselection)
Compelling unwanted treatment

Extended discussion of those specific issues is best handled in an ethics text or an ethics course. However, if you wish to learn more about these situations and the ethical conflicts surrounding them,

 Go to Chapter 44, **Supplemental Materials: Ethical Issues in Healthcare,** on the Student Resource Disk or DavisPlus at http://davisplus.fadavis.com/Wilkinson2

Practical Knowledge knowing how

To fulfill your professional obligations for ethical practice, you will need practical knowledge of the processes of values clarification, moral decision-making, patient advocacy, and integrity-producing compromise.

■ ASSESSMENT/ANALYSIS/DIAGNOSIS

A holistic, comprehensive patient assessment will help you establish the context in which ethical decisions are made. For patients struggling with moral issues, the following diagnoses may apply:

- *Decisional Conflict*—Use this label when the patient is uncertain about which course of action to take. The patient may verbalize distress and uncertainty, may delay decision-making, may show physical signs of distress (e.g., increased heart rate), and may question moral rules and values, and personal beliefs.
- *Moral Distress*—Use this label when the patient has made a moral decision but is unable to carry out the chosen action. Cues include expressions of powerlessness, guilt, frustration, anxiety, self-doubt, and fear.

Values Clarification

Values clarification refers to the process of becoming conscious of and naming one's values (Burkhardt & Nathaniel, 2008). If you are clear about your values, you will be more able to make good decisions and to avoid imposing your values on others. Because each person has his own unique values set, it is important that you appreciate how others' values influence their decisions. Clarifying values should be a positive process of growth that results in more awareness, empathy, and insight (Seroka, 1994; Steele & Harmon, 1983). A values clarification process does not tell you what your values ought to be; it merely helps you discover what they are. Values change over time, so you may need to repeat the process more than once in your lifetime.

How Can I Clarify My Values?

As a nurse, you will need to examine your values regarding life, death, wellness, and illness. A good place to start is to ask yourself questions about situations that you think you may be uncomfortable with, such as caring for a substance abuser seeking drugs in the emergency department, an unwed adolescent mother pregnant for the second time in 11 months, or parents such as the Freses ("Meet Your Patients"), who refuse treatment for a child because of religious beliefs. Ask yourself questions such as:

- Could I take care of this person?
- Does this bother me?
- What would I do if confronted with such a situation?
- Could I provide the same quality care as for my other patients?

If you would like to use some exercises that can help you begin to clarify your values related to healthcare,

 Go to Chapter 44, **Tables, Boxes, Figures: ESG Box 44-2, Rank-Ordering Values** and **ESG Box 44-3, Values Preference Exercise,** on the Student Resource Disk or DavisPlus at http://davisplus.fadavis.com/Wilkinson2

Remember that there are no right or wrong answers to values clarification exercises. They are only to assist you as you identify your values and examine their relevance in your personal and professional life.

How Can I Help Clients to Clarify Their Values?

Some clients may exhibit behaviors that indicate that their values are not clear. Consider this example:

> Jon White is the chief executive officer of a large healthcare facility. Jon has had two myocardial infarctions (heart attacks) in the last 5 years. He also has hypercholesterolemia (high cholesterol) and hypertension (high blood pressure). Jon's physician has prescribed a heart medicine, low-dose aspirin, and medications to control his hypertension and cholesterol. Jon has repeatedly been taught about his diet, medications, and activity. He insists he is compliant. Jon's wife tells you that he has stopped exercising and is eating whatever he wants, including saturated fats. Jon tells her it is OK to eat what he wants because he is taking a "cholesterol-buster" pill.

The following patient behaviors may indicate that a patient needs values clarification:

- Ignoring the advice of a health professional
- Patient's words not consistent with his actions
- Numerous admissions to the agency for the same problem
- Uncertainty or confusion about which action to take

Which of those behaviors did Jon exhibit? To help Jon clarify his values, you might ask him to list the three things that are most important to him in life. Or you could help him work through the steps in Table 44-4 (choosing, prizing, and acting).

KnowledgeCheck 44-11
- What is values clarification?
- What are the steps in values clarification?

 Go to Chapter 44, **Knowledge Check Response Sheet and Answers,** on the Student Resource Disk or DavisPlus at http://davisplus.fadavis.com/Wilkinson2

Ethical Decision-Making

Decision models used in bioethics do not offer pat, easy decisions, but they do provide a guiding structure to follow to arrive at the best answer in specific situations. Decision models can help you decide on a course of action even if they do not tell you absolutely that the action is right or wrong.

Problem or Dilemma?

In the best of all possible worlds, you could easily apply moral principles and decide what to do. However, often in moral situations one ethical principle is at

Table 44-4 ➤ Values Clarification

STEP	DESCRIPTION	QUESTIONS TO ASK YOUR PATIENT
Choosing (cognitive)	**Beliefs are chosen:**	Do (did) you have any choice about what you do?
	Freely (allows you to cherish your choice)	Do you have any control over what happens?
		What have you decided to do?
	From alternatives	Can you list some alternative actions?
		What are your options?
	After considering all consequences (ensures that the alternative is right for you)	What could you do instead of . . . ?
		What do you think will happen if you do that?
		What will you gain by doing that?
		What is the disadvantage of doing that?
Prizing (affective)	**Beliefs and behaviors that are chosen are prized:**	How do you feel about your decision?
		People sometimes feel good after making such a decision. Others feel pressured. How is it for you?
	With pride (feeling good about your choice)	How do you intend to tell your family (friends) about this decision?
	With public affirmation	What will you say to your wife (friends, family)?
		When will you announce your decision to . . . ?
Acting (behavioral)	**Beliefs are acted on:**	Try to determine whether the client will act on the decision:
	By incorporating the choice into one's own behavior	■ How do you think your wife (significant other) will react when you do that?
		■ When will you actually carry out this decision?
	With consistency and repetition	Try to predict consistent behavior by asking:
		■ How many times in the past have you . . .?
		■ What kind of schedule have you worked out? How often and when will you . . . ?

Adapted from Raths, L. E., Harmin M., & Simon, S. B. (1978). *Values and teaching: Working with values in the classroom.* Columbus, OH: Merrill Publishing.

odds with another equally important principle. It is also possible for a philosophical framework to produce more than one acceptable option. An **ethical dilemma** is a situation in which a choice must be made between two equally undesirable actions. There is no clearly right or wrong option. Such situations are emotionally painful for everyone in the situation, as you can see from the "Meet Your Patients" scenario at the beginning of this chapter. If you support Alan's parents' right to refuse a blood transfusion, you honor the principle of autonomy, but at the expense of the principle of nonmaleficence, which says we should prevent harm to Alan.

Fortunately, not all moral problems are dilemmas. In fact, you will confront a true dilemma only occasionally (Cahn, 1987; Curtin & Flaherty, 1982; Levine, 1989; White, 1983; Wilkinson, 1997). Not all moral problems are complex and difficult. Some questions are easily answered (e.g., "Should I take the patient's morphine to relieve my back pain?"). It is probably more accurate, then, to talk about "moral questions," "moral problems," or "moral situations" and not use the term *di-*

lemma loosely. Only problems that pose a question between competing and equally valuable interests are true dilemmas.

Ethical behavior and decision-making do not deal only with dilemmas. They really involve choosing to be ethical in the everyday aspects of your practice: for example, treating colleagues and patients with respect, not passing up a room when you see a patient crying, or helping out a new graduate who is frustrated and anxious. The scenario about the two little boys in the emergency department is more representative of everyday ethics than is the "Meet Your Patients" scenario.

What Are Some Decision-Making Models?

Once you have identified an ethical problem, a decision model can help you think logically about the best action to take. Still, in the case of a true ethical dilemma, you will probably not be comfortable with any course of action, no matter how logically you think it through.

We have said it is important to be aware of the ethical issues in patient care situations, but how will you recognize them? The key is that there is usually a conflict. Conflict may occur:

- About the right action to take
- Among the duties and obligations of healthcare professionals (or they are unclear)
- Between the needs and interests of an individual and a group of clients
- Between what the family wants and what the client wants or needs
- Between the family and health professionals
- Among ethical principles or values (e.g., autonomy versus nonmaleficence, as in the "Meet Your Patients" scenario)

Ethical decision-making models will help you carefully consider several perspectives, guide your reasoning, and explain the reasons for your final action. As already mentioned, each approach may produce a different solution. One of the easiest to remember and use is the MORAL model. This model has been credited to two different authors: Thiroux (1977) and Crisham (in Scott, 1985). The letters MORAL will remind you of the steps in this model, which is described in the following section. To use the model in clinical settings,

 Go to Chapter 44, **Clinical Insight 44-1: Using the MORAL Model for Ethical Decision-Making,** in Volume 2.

How Do I Work Through an Ethical Problem?

Let's use the "Meet Your Patients" scenario to illustrate ethical decision-making.

First, Use Problem-Solving

As a first step in ethical decision-making, use the nursing process approach to describe the problem and alternative approaches:

Assessment—What are the relevant facts? Alan needs a blood transfusion to survive. Both the surgeon and the nurse (you) have tried to persuade the parents to consent, but they still refuse. The parents are Jehovah's Witnesses, a religion that prohibits blood transfusions. Alan is 15 years old (a minor), so you cannot administer a transfusion without his parents' consent.

Analysis/Diagnosis—Identify the problem; state the conflict. There is a values conflict: The healthcare professionals value preserving physical life; the parents place more value on preserving the soul. There is a moral dilemma, as well: If no transfusion is given, you violate the principle of nonmaleficence (harm to Alan); if you somehow coerce the parents to consent, you have violated the principle of autonomy (respect for their values and

their freedom to choose). So the decision to be made is whether to

- Follow the parents' wishes,
- Find a legal way to transfuse without their consent, or
- Find some compromise that will work.

Next, Use the MORAL Model

Now use the MORAL model to come up with alternative solutions for the Frese family.

M—Massage the Dilemma

1. *First identify and define the issues in the dilemma, and consider the values and options of all the major players:* Mr. and Mrs. Frese, Alan, the surgeon, possibly a clergyman, and you, the nurse. You have already identified the values in the problem-solving approach: physical life versus spiritual life. You and the surgeon also value the principles of autonomy and nonmaleficence

2. *Then identify the information gaps.* In massaging the situation, you should ask yourself:
   - Do I fully understand the situation that is causing the need for blood?
   - How much time is available to make this decision— do the parents have to decide within a few minutes, or do they have enough time to discuss this with their clergyman?
   - Does the physician know that the family are Jehovah's Witnesses?
   - Does the surgeon have any treatment that could be used to stabilize Alan while the parents discuss the situation?
   - Do Alan's parents fully understand the nature of Alan's physical emergency?
   - In the Freses' religious view, what is the consequence of receiving blood?
   - Do they understand what might happen if blood is not administered (i.e., do they understand the consequence of their action or inaction)?
   - Is this what Alan would want? Has Alan discussed in the past what he feels about blood transfusions? Have they ever had family discussions when other young Jehovah's Witnesses have been faced with such a decision? Where did Alan stand in those discussions?
   - How is this situation like other situations they have experienced in their lives?
   - Have they thought about their opposing duties: the duty to uphold their religious values and the duty to protect their son from harm?
   - Has everyone's voice been heard?
   - Have the parents contacted their clergyman and discussed the situation?
   - What emotions are coming into play in this situation?
   - How is this decision affecting the parents as individuals? Are they in agreement on the issue, or is

there dissension? If there is dissension, are both sides being supported fairly?

- Is there some common ground between what the surgeon wants and what the parents feel they need to do to uphold their religious convictions?

O—Outline the Options

At this step in the MORAL model, you (or the charge nurse or a member of the ethics committee) should outline all of the options to all parties, including those that are less realistic and conflicting. You might ask a member of the ethics committee or the hospital chaplain to help the family and the doctor understand the opposing viewpoints.

The surgeon needs to outline the state of emergency that exists for Alan and to explain what the limited medical options are: to transfuse blood or, if no blood is given, what other treatments are available (e.g., volume enhancers). The surgeon will need to say how soon the decision must be made, based on Alan's condition. He should clearly describe the consequences of each action. Carefully, and with as little emotion as possible, explain the consequences of each action to the parents. The physician should state whether one administration of blood will likely fix the situation or whether continued administration may be required.

The family (or a clergyman) should explain for the doctor and nurse the basis for their refusal to consent and what they believe the consequence would be if blood were given.

R—Resolve the Dilemma

Now carefully review the issues and options. Apply basic moral principles. If you can, also look at the situation using alternate ethical frameworks.

- **Autonomy.** By their refusing to give consent, the Freses are exercising their autonomy. How far will we go to honor their autonomy?
- **Beneficence and Nonmaleficence.** How are we defining "good" (beneficence) and "harm" (nonmaleficence) in this situation? The physician defines "good" as Alan receiving the needed blood. He defines "harm" as the outcome for Alan without the blood, even if he uses a less effective alternative. Alan's parents would define "good" as following their religious mandates and making sure their son will remain pure in the eyes of God. They might explain that a Jehovah's Witness who willingly accepts a blood transfusion might forfeit his or her eternal life. The Freses might believe the taking of blood to be more harmful than death, because they believe that would affect Alan's eternal life, not just his physical life.
- **Fidelity.** The surgeon is being loyal (exhibiting fidelity) to the principles of medicine and evidence-based practice, which mandate the administration of the blood. To the parents, their loyalty to their religious principles to ensure that Alan has eternal life may be more important than the loss of the physical life itself.
- **Veracity.** The principle of veracity holds that the surgeon should not exaggerate the need for the blood,

and he should be honest with the parents in terms of the consequences of the alternative actions. Another question of veracity involves the parents: Are they being honest with each other regarding their feelings?

Your role as a nurse is to be an advocate for the patient and the family. Talk with the family and their religious representative, if available, about what they are thinking about their opposing duties: the duty to uphold their religious values and the duty to protect their son from physical harm. Ensure that everyone's viewpoint has been respected and considered. This may be as important as the final decision that is reached. If you are in a position to do so, explain to the surgeon the reasoned position of Alan's parents. In this and other difficult situations, always look for the opportunity for a good compromise (to be discussed later in this chapter).

A—Act by Applying the Chosen Option

This step is the first one that actually requires action. The hospital is bound to follow the parents' decision because Alan is a minor. However, if there is time, many agencies might refer this situation to the hospital ethics committee. The hospital might also ask a legal court authority to resolve the situation. If an emergency requires an immediate decision, the only *legal* action is to follow the parents' decision, whether or not you consider it the best moral action.

Whatever happens, Alan's parents will need emotional support. If they decide to refuse the blood transfusion, you must remain nonjudgmental in supporting them, even if you do not agree with their decision. If they, or the court, decide that the blood will be given, they may need even more support. They may feel overwhelming guilt, and they may fear that Alan will be forever burdened with guilt at the realization that they violated church doctrine with the medical care. If their extended family is not present, you could volunteer to call in extended family, friends, and church members if they wish. They will need a quiet, private place to await the outcome of the treatment.

L—Look Back and Evaluate

This phase calls for evaluation of the entire process, not just the consequence of the decided action. How well did the process work? Were processes in place for the dilemma to be discussed respectfully without undue delay in treatment? Were all parties' expectations realistic? How are all of the affected parties feeling now (doctor, parents, family, Alan, you)? Regardless of the outcome of the decision, do all involved feel they had a voice and their views were respected? How well did you do in the situation? Did you act as an effective advocate for the rights of Alan and his parents? Were you unduly influenced by the power and authority of the physician or hospital in the situation? Were policies and procedures in place to guide you in the process of working out this situation? Has anything changed since the dilemma came to light? Has a greater good been achieved for future situations? Have future situations been made easier as a result of the things learned in this situation? Has any aspect of this ethical decision now become a universal policy at the institution? Are further actions required in terms of this or like situations?

For guidelines to help you avoid common errors when making moral decisions,

 Go to Chapter 44, **Supplemental Materials: Common Errors in Decision Making,** on the Student Resource Disk or DavisPlus at http://davisplus.fadavis.com/Wilkinson2

Look for a Good Compromise

Even if you believe you know the right thing to do, others may not agree with you, or there may be constraints that prevent you from doing it. For example, in the case of Alan, even if you decided the right thing to do is give him a blood transfusion, (1) his parents do not agree with you, and (2) the law says you cannot do so without his parents' consent. This will happen often—much more often than a true dilemma, in which you cannot *decide* the right thing to do. No matter how well we work together, there will always be ethical problems and disagreements. Many cases are full of complexity and uncertainty, and sometimes the price of acting on your beliefs is extremely high. For example, what might have happened if the surgeon had infused blood without the Freses' consent? What might have happened if you had refused to talk to the parents as the surgeon asked you?

Many times, it will be possible to reach a "good" compromise. A **good compromise** is one that preserves the integrity of all parties. This means that:

- The discussions are carried out in a spirit of mutual respect—that all viewpoints are respected and considered.
- The compromise solution itself is ethically sound; that is, you should be able to provide a principles-based rationale for the compromise, as well as for each of the opposing positions. In the case of Alan and his parents, there probably is no compromise position between "give blood" and "don't give blood." Perhaps the parents would agree to one, but no more than one, transfusion; but that is hard to justify ethically. If one transfusion is acceptable (to honor nonmaleficence), why not two or three? If two transfusions are against their religious beliefs, why would one be acceptable? Nevertheless, in many cases compromise is possible.

So how do you compromise without losing moral integrity? First, realize there is more at stake than the issue itself ("Is a blood transfusion right or wrong?"). There are some things that are inherently good in making a compromise.

- First, it is never good to settle things by force (as you would if you got a court order to transfuse Alan without his parents' consent). You have probably heard the old saying, "Might doesn't make right." A compromise can preserve the rights of the less powerful party in a disagreement.

- Keeping peace on a nursing unit is good for both the nurses and patients. When there is upheaval and moral suffering, care quality throughout the unit can suffer. A compromise can bring peace.
- There is intrinsic good in taking part in a process in which we must try to see things from others' points of view. It may make us more open-minded, more creative, and less judgmental.
- Keep in mind that most issues do contain room for reasonable differences of opinion. In the "Meet Your Patients" scenario, can you see that both sides are people of good will who have ethical reasons to justify their opinion? Also, there is often room for doubt, on your own part, about the morally best action to take.
- A compromise may achieve mutual respect. It is a significant thing to reach a settlement in which each party feels assured of the other's respect for its seriousness and sincerity.

Given all those ideas, a person of good will might want to reexamine and back off a very strong opinion. Remember, sometimes your position isn't all that strong, and the other position isn't all that weak (as in the case of Alan). There is also always the chance that you may have made an error in your reasoning or have not completely understood some facts of the case. Ethical disputes can be settled only if you are willing to engage in discussion and admit the other people might have a point! There may be cases in which you cannot compromise (perhaps Alan's case is one), but don't listen to people who say, "You can never reach agreement on ethical issues. They are too complex." It is possible to achieve integrity-producing compromises, and in nursing, it is often necessary.

What Are My Obligations in Ethical Decisions?

As you can see, in making ethical decisions, nurses rarely act alone. Usually you will be one of several healthcare professionals and family members who will jointly arrive at the best decision. Your role when an ethical decision is needed includes the following:

- *Be aware of and sensitive to issues,* so you can identify them when they arise. Educate yourself—attend workshops, read, and talk to other nurses.
- *Assume responsibility for your own moral actions.* Even if you do not have the "last word" about what happens to a patient or about what others do, you are always responsible for your own actions in every situation.
- *Function as a team member* when ethical problems arise. Realize you should have input—no one profession has full moral expertise—and realize that your input can be valuable.
- *Support the patient and family members* while they are making the decision and afterward. Listen. Ask questions. Provide unbiased information. Be helpful without being too directive or judgmental.

- *Support patients who are not being allowed to decide.* For example, in the "Meet Your Patients" scenario, you would want to be sure Alan's wishes were considered, if possible. However, if the parents insist on deciding for him, against his wishes, he may need a great deal of emotional support.
- *Use and participate in institutional ethics committees* if you are given the opportunity.
- *Most important, advocate for your client.* You may need to balance your client's autonomy with the wishes of family members or the responsibilities of other healthcare professionals to the patient. As an advocate, you may find yourself in conflict with other team members or family members. Frequently you and the others involved will have different ethical perspectives.

Use and Participate in Institutional Ethics Committees

There is no easy way to decide which principle should outrank another principle, or which person's values are best in a given situation. For this reason, many healthcare institutions have ethics committees. These typically interdisciplinary committees include nurses, doctors, clergy, ethicists, and lay representatives. Ethics committees develop guidelines and policies, provide education and counseling; and, in the case of ethical dilemmas, review the case and provide a forum for the expression of the diverse perspectives of those involved. Ethics committees usually follow one of three models when discussing a dilemma: the autonomy model, the patient benefit model, and the social justice model.

Autonomy Model. The **autonomy model** is useful when the patient is competent to decide. This model emphasizes patient autonomy and choice as the highest value. For example, if this committee knew Alan's ("Meet Your Patients") wishes, they might be inclined to try to persuade his parents to do as Alan wants.

Patient Benefit Model. The **patient benefit model** assists in decision-making for the incompetent patient by using substituted judgment (i.e., what the patient would want for himself if he were capable of making these issues known). If Alan is unconscious and cannot say what he wants, this committee would probably ask Alan's parents, family, and friends, "What do you think Alan would want? Have you ever heard him talk about a situation such as this?"

Social Justice Model. The **social justice model** focuses more on broad social issues involving the entire institution, rather than on a single patient issue (Yoder-Wise, 2007). Such a committee might consider whether, in general, an institution ought ever to seek a legal order to act against the wishes of the parents. Or they might discuss whether supporting parents' religious beliefs in this instance might have implications for supporting other types of religious beliefs in future cases.

KnowledgeCheck 44-12

- Define ethical dilemma.
- How can you recognize an ethical problem?
- What is an integrity-producing compromise?
- What are the functions of an ethics committee?
- What does the mnemonic MORAL stand for?

 Go to Chapter 44, **Knowledge Check Response Sheet and Answers,** on the Student Resource Disk or DavisPlus at http://davisplus.fadavis.com/Wilkinson2

Be a Patient Advocate

The role of advocates is to safeguard clients against abuse and violation of their rights. When you think of the rights and values described, for example, in the *Patient Care Partnership* and in nursing codes of ethics, you can see how important this role is. Be aware that advocacy in everyday clinical practice is less about the patient's legal rights and moral theory, and more about such seemingly "routine" measures as obtaining a new prescription when an analgesic is ineffective, even if it does mean telephoning the prescriber for the third time on your shift. The advocacy role requires you to be respectful, considerate, courageous, persistent, and concerned with justice.

Why do you think advocacy is so important? Why can't patients do these things for themselves? The following are some of the reasons.

You Have Special Knowledge that the Patient Does Not Have. Diseases, treatments, and the healthcare system are so complex that when clients become ill, they may not have the energy to deal with the complexity, even if they do have the necessary knowledge. You may need to help them to "jump through the necessary hoops" to get what they need. When patients' rights are denied or when patients do not have the ability to exert their rights, nurses have a responsibility to step in. "Without the advocacy and protection of rights there really are no rights" (Bandman & Bandman, 2002, p. 23).

One Aspect of Your Professional Role is to Defend Patients' Autonomous Decisions. Recall that the ANA Code of Ethics requires you to be a patient advocate (see Boxes 44-1, 44-2, and 44-3). As a nurse, you will be called on to defend your patient's autonomous decisions even if you do not agree with them and even if they conflict with the opinions of others involved in the patient's care. You may find yourself the sole supporter of a patient's right to choose for himself the direction of his care.

Nurses Have a Special Relationship with Patients. You may find that you are able to obtain information about a patient that is not available to professionals of other disciplines. In general, nurses interact with patients over longer time intervals and are involved in very personal activities, especially in inpatient settings. They often become the most trusted caregivers. Details about family life, coping styles, personal preferences, fears, and insecurities are all more likely to come out over the time involved in nursing interventions than in the brief minutes of interaction when a physician makes rounds. In addition, patients may perceive less social distance between themselves and the nurse and, therefore, feel more free to confide in them. The nurses' point of view can be a valuable asset to resolving an ethical problem satisfactorily. Of course, many providers have long-standing relationships with their patients; however, this does not negate the importance of the nurse's input, which may provide a different perspective.

Your Role as an Advocate is to Inform, Support, and Communicate. You should inform clients of their rights and provide the information they need to make informed decisions, if they are capable of doing so. Then you must remain objective and support them in the decisions they make, even when you believe it to be wrong. If others are not respecting client choices, you will need to intervene. This may simply be a matter of conveying information and clarifying the client's wishes to family or healthcare professionals (e.g., "I know how hard it is for you to let him go, but your dad says he has made peace and is ready to die. His treatments make him feel even more ill, and he simply does not want to fight anymore."). Advocacy may require you to arrange for the client to consult with a religious leader or an attorney for advice and support, or may require you to consult an institutional ethics committee.

Advance Directives. In 2004, three of every 10 U.S. nursing home residents did not have advance directives (Resnick, Schuur, Heineman, et al., 2008), so there is work to be done in this area. An important advocacy intervention is to ask patients whether they have an advance directive and to inform them about advance directives if they do not. Even people who have an advance directive do not always, or even often, understand the statements they have checked in the boxes on the form. Take the time to go over the form with them if they are able to do so. See Chapters 15 and 45 if you need further discussion of advance directives.

For guidelines that will help you to function effectively as an advocate,

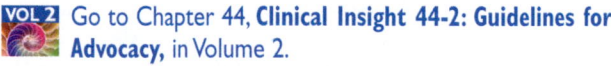 Go to Chapter 44, **Clinical Insight 44-2: Guidelines for Advocacy,** in Volume 2.

Improve Your Ethical Decision-Making

By now, you should understand that you cannot avoid making moral decisions in nursing. A recent study pointed out the need to promote nurses' development from the conventional (rules-bound) to the post-conventional (reasoning) stage of moral development. The study found that when nurses were faced with ethical dilemmas they tended to use conventions (e.g., rules, procedures) as criteria for decision-making rather than patients' personal needs and well-being (Dierckx de Casterlé, Izumi,

Godfrey, et al., 2008). As a full-spectrum nurse, you should use the following suggestions so you will be prepared when ethical issues arise.

Use Theoretical Knowledge. Review nursing and other literature for discussion of cases and experiences of other nurses. This will give you a broader view of the problems you may confront and the strategies for managing them. Become familiar with the various codes of ethics and the *Patient Care Partnership*, as well as the moral frameworks and principles.

Use Self-Knowledge. Examine your personal value system. Explore the influences of your religion, cultural beliefs, and personal experiences. This will help you to recognize your comfort zone with specific ethical issues.

Use Practical Knowledge. While still a student, you should ask to attend either ethical rounds or an ethics committee meeting. As a graduate nurse, you could benefit by volunteering to be a member of your institution's ethics committee or plan to attend nursing ethics rounds to familiarize yourself with the types of ethical problems that occur at your institution.

Consult Reliable Sources. Attend ethics education programs, and talk about issues with other healthcare providers. Attorneys, ethicists, and members of the clergy can provide helpful perspectives.

Share. Regularly engage in discussions with the staff on your unit to determine differences in value systems and to collaborate proactively to work out methods that can be used to resolve ethical dilemmas effectively. When you are faced with a difficult moral decision, consult with peers, co-workers, and teachers. Seek guidance and support.

Evaluate. After the situation is resolved, evaluate your decision and the effects of your actions. You should be able to learn from even the worst decision. And when everything goes well, you can file your strategies away to use in similar future situations.

KnowledgeCheck 44-13

- What are three reasons why patients may need a nurse advocate?
- Briefly describe the nurse's role as a patient advocate.

 Go to Chapter 44, **Knowledge Check Response Sheet and Answers,** on the Student Resource Disk or DavisPlus at http://davisplus.fadavis.com/Wilkinson2

 Go to Chapter 44, **Resources for Caregivers and Health Professionals,** on the Student Resource Disk or DavisPlus at http://davisplus.fadavis.com/Wilkinson2

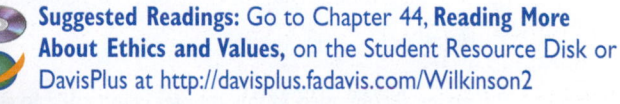 **Suggested Readings:** Go to Chapter 44, **Reading More About Ethics and Values,** on the Student Resource Disk or DavisPlus at http://davisplus.fadavis.com/Wilkinson2

 Bibliography: Go to Volume 2, Bibliography.

CHAPTER 45

Legal Issues

Learning Outcomes

After completing this chapter, you should be able to:

➤ Identify four basic sources of law.

➤ Discuss direct implications of the Bill of Rights to nursing practice.

➤ Explain the Health Insurance Portability and Accountability Act (HIPAA) and how it protects patients and affects healthcare workers.

➤ Discuss various aspects of the Patient Self-Determination Act affecting healthcare.

➤ Give examples of situations involving accommodation that conforms to the Americans with Disability Act (ADA).

➤ Present patient-care situations involving state mandatory reporting by a healthcare worker.

➤ Apply concepts of Good Samaritan laws to nurses outside the workplace.

➤ Discuss various types of practice guidelines that factor into providing reasonable and prudent nursing care.

➤ Present seven rights of nurses within the healthcare workplace.

➤ Discuss Nurse Practice Acts as it affects clinical nursing decisions and actions.

➤ Explain disciplinary actions for unacceptable nursing decisions or action and the impact on nursing licensure.

➤ Discuss basic principles of criminal law controlling nursing practice.

➤ Discuss basic principles of civil law controlling nursing practice, including different types of torts and medical–legal liability.

➤ Present the phases of the litigation process as it might occur with a nursing malpractice case.

➤ Discuss common causes of malpractice litigation.

➤ Identify measures to decrease the likelihood of committing nursing malpractice.

Disclaimer: The material contained in this chapter is intended to convey information on topics of interest to nursing students. Although prepared by a nurse attorney, this chapter should not be utilized as a substitute for legal counseling. No one should act upon the information contained in this chapter without professional guidance. These materials should not be considered legal advice or a legal opinion.

Meet Your Nurse Role Model

A nurse with 3 years' experience on a medical–surgical unit arrives to work and discovers that two of her colleagues called in sick, including the charge nurse. The nursing supervisor informs her that she will need to assume the charge nurse role, in addition to assuming care for three patients. Feeling frustrated, the nurse ponders whether she should just quit and find another job. She reasons that this is not the answer to resolve the situation and accepts the assignment. Two hours into the shift, one of her patients began to experience complications, requiring blood glucose checks every 2 hours and frequent monitoring. In addition, one of the nurses becomes ill and is replaced by a float nurse from the labor and delivery unit. The nurse contacts the nursing supervisor and requests additional assistance but is told no other nurse is available and she is involved with an emergency situation on another unit. The nurse begins to consider this situation from a legal perspective to determine the best course of action.

- Should the nurse have accepted the assignment? If yes, what factors should the nurse have considered before accepting the assignment?
- If the nurse should not have accepted the assignment, could she have been charged with abandonment?
- How should the nurse handle this situation?

Theoretical **Knowledge**
knowing why

Nurses in clinical practice are often confronted with situations that present legal issues. An understanding of the legal framework governing nursing practice is essential to protect yourself, your patients, your colleagues, and your employers. The theoretical knowledge in this chapter, combined with the critical thinking model in Chapter 2, will help you to answer questions related to this scenario.

The **law** is a binding practice, rule, or code of conduct that guides a community or society and is enforced by a controlling authority. The basic function of laws is to protect society by establishing acceptable patterns of behaviors. Nurses can use legal principles from the various sources of law to guide their actions, to minimize the possibility of lawsuits, and to promote defensible decisions. The legal framework that governs nursing practice consists of laws, regulations, and standards of practice. The common theme under this framework is that the nurse is legally responsible for his own actions, and this legal responsibility cannot be delegated.

What Are the Sources and Types of Law?

The United States Constitution establishes three branches of government: executive, legislative, and judicial. Each branch has specified powers that are designed to equalize power among the three and to provide a system of checks and balances.

- *Executive branch*—Identifies the powers given to the president of the United States at the federal level and

governor at the state level. This includes the power to execute and/or enforce laws.
- *Legislative branch*—Identifies the powers given to Congress to make or formulate laws.
- *Judicial branch*—Identifies the powers given to the United States Supreme Court. This includes the power to interpret statutory law and decide cases and controversies.

Laws are derived primarily from four sources: (1) the Constitution, (2) statutes, (3) administrative bodies, and (4) the courts (Table 45-1).

Constitutional Law. A **constitution** is a system of fundamental laws and principles that prescribes the nature, functions, and limits of a government. The U.S. Constitution is the superior law of the land and applies to all states throughout the United States. Thus, all state and federal laws must be consistent with the U.S. Constitution. The U.S. Constitution limits the powers of the federal government and gives each state the power to govern itself and to pass laws to promote the health, welfare, order, and security of its citizens (police power). Each state has a similar structure, beginning with a state Constitution that likewise establishes the governing system for the state. Any state or federal law that conflicts with the U.S. Constitution is considered invalid or void. If you would like to see the seven Articles of the Constitution,

Go to Chapter 45, **Tables, Boxes, Figures: ESG Box 45-1, The Bill of Rights, Amendments 1–10 of the Constitution,** on the Student Resource Disk or DavisPlus at http://davisplus.fadavis.com/Wilkinson2

Statutory Law. A **statute** is a law passed by a federal Congress or by a state legislative body. Congress passes

Table 45-1 ➤ Sources of Law and Common Questions that Apply to Nursing

TYPE/SOURCE OF LAW	EXAMPLE	QUESTION POSED
Constitutional Law	Freedom of speech	Can an employer prevent internationally-educated nurses from speaking in their native language in the work environment?
Statutory Law	Definition of nursing	What is the nurse's scope of practice (duties and responsibilities)?
Administrative Law	Delegation and supervision	Is the registered nurse legally responsible for tasks or assignments delegated to other nurses?
Common Law	Affirmative duty	Does a registered nurse have a responsibility to exercise an independent judgment to prevent harm to patients?

laws for the benefit of society as a whole; whereas states use their police power to pass laws to ensure the general health, safety, and welfare of their citizens. The Nurse Practice Act (NPA) is an example of statutory law. The legislative body of each state passes regulation (laws) that govern the profession of nursing, known as Nurse Practice Acts. These NPAs can be found in each state's Revised Statutes.

Administrative Law. Formally defined, **administrative law** refers to the laws that govern administrative agencies. Administrative agencies are created at the federal level by Congress and at the state level by its legislative bodies. As applied to nursing, administrative law comprises the rules and regulations passed by administrative bodies or agencies to fulfill their statutory missions. Within each state's Nurse Practice Act, the state legislative body has created a State Board of Nursing to enforce the NPA by passing the rules and regulations that are necessary to ensure compliance. These rules and regulations can be found in each state's Administrative Code.

Common (Judicial) Law. A compilation of laws made by judges or courts is known as **common law.** Also referred to as case law, common law is based on common customs and traditions. It comes from legal principles and guidelines that judges use to determine the outcome of legal cases.

What Laws and Regulations Guide Nursing Practice?

The practice of professional nursing requires nurses to understand the various laws and regulations that guide their practice. Laws and regulations at the federal and state levels have a direct impact on the nurse's actions and decisions.

Federal Law

State Nurse Practice Acts (NPAs) typically require you to have knowledge of federal laws affecting nursing practice.

Bill of Rights

The first ten Amendments to the United States Constitution are known as the *Bill of Rights*. The Bill of Rights clearly identifies, and in many ways limits, the role of government in individuals' lives. Many of these rights have direct implications for healthcare, including the rights of nurses and of patients. These include:

Amendment I: Freedom of religion, speech, press, and assembly

Amendment IV: Protection against *unreasonable search and seizures* (taking of property)

Amendment V: Protection from *double jeopardy* (being charged twice for the same crime); protection against self-incrimination; protection of property rights; and the right to due process of law in cases involving infringement on freedom, life, or property.

Amendment VI. The right to an attorney, a speedy public trial, and to be informed of the charges and to confront witnesses

Protecting patients' privacy rights is a fundamental role of the professional nurse and is derived from the Bill of Rights. If you would like to review the Bill of Rights,

Go to Chapter 45, **Tables, Boxes, Figures: ESG Box 45-1, The Bill of Rights, Amendments 1–10 of the Constitution,** on the Student Resource Disk or DavisPlus at http://davisplus.fadavis.com/Wilkinson2

Critical**Thinking** 45-1
- Develop a scenario illustrating how a nurse might protect a patient's right to privacy.
- What is one thing a nurse can do to respect a patient's property rights?

Go to Chapter 45, **Critical Thinking Response Sheet and Answers,** on the Student Resource Disk or DavisPlus at http://davisplus.fadavis.com/Wilkinson2

Health Insurance Portability and Accountability Act (HIPAA)

The Health Insurance Portability and Accountability Act (HIPAA) was passed by Congress in 1996 to:

- Protect health insurance benefits for workers who lose or change their jobs
- Protect coverage to persons with preexisting medical conditions
- Establish standards to protect the privacy of personal health information

The privacy regulations will be especially important in your practice. Nurses and other healthcare providers must protect the patient's right to privacy by not sharing patient information with unauthorized individuals. Under HIPAA rules, healthcare agencies and their employees must take steps to ensure the confidentiality of the patient information and medical records. In addition, HIPAA allows for patients to see, make corrections to, and obtain copies of their medical records.

Case: Violation of a Patient's Privacy

Patients at a state-operated psychiatric facility filed a lawsuit in the U.S. District Court for the Eastern District of New York challenging the facility's practice of supervising some of the patients' visitations by video (not audio) when ordered by the provider. The guard in this particular case was not close enough to hear conversations. Nor did he make an attempt to listen. The court ruled the patients' privacy rights were not being violated by the practice for prescribed supervised visits in effect at this facility.

Sparks v. Seltzer, __ F. Supp. 2d __, 2009 WL 1039886 (E.D. N.Y., April 20, 2009)

Emergency Medical Treatment and Active Labor Act (EMTALA)

The Emergency Medical Treatment and Active Labor Act (EMTALA) requires healthcare facilities to provide emergency medical treatment to patients who seek healthcare in the emergency department, regardless of their ability to pay, legal status, or citizenship status. The obligation is for the medical facility to provide medical screening to determine if an emergency exists and to stabilize the patient before transferring him or her to another healthcare facility.

Critical Thinking 45-2

A 54-year-old uninsured and unemployed woman arrives at the emergency department of a small private hospital complaining of chest pain and nausea. The triage nurse calls the on-call physician, who instructs the nurse to send the patient to the county hospital several blocks away. The nurse assesses the patient and contacts her supervisor, who tells her to contact the medical chief of staff to inform him that the patient is in need of emergency treatment.

- Discuss whether the nurse's action was appropriate or inappropriate.

Patient Self Determination Act (PSDA)

The Patient Self Determination Act (PSDA) of 1991 recognizes the patient's right to make decisions regarding his own healthcare, based on the information provided to him by the healthcare provider, regarding the medical or surgical treatment options available, the benefits, risks, and alternatives. Box 45-1 describes agency and healthcare workers' responsibilities under the PSDA.

There are two types of legal written advanced directives, the living will and the durable power of attorney for healthcare.

A **living will** is prepared by an alert and oriented (competent) individual that gives directions to others about the person's wishes regarding life-prolonging treatments if the person becomes unable to make those decisions. As a legal document, the requirements may vary from state to state. However, language common in the living will gives the person the opportunity to specify treatment in numerous areas (Box 45-2).

A **durable power of attorney for healthcare (DPOA)** identifies a person who will make healthcare decisions in the event the patient is unable to do so. The person given the right to make decisions is called the surrogate decision maker. The surrogate has the right to make the medical decisions for as long as the person is not able to do so for himself (incompetent).

Case: Durable Power of Attorney (DPOA)

Mr. Green was in a coma due to head trauma from a motor vehicle accident. In his DPOA, he had designated his brother, Joey, as his surrogate. Although Mr. Green is married with two adult children, Joey is the person legally recognized to make decisions

BOX 45-1 ■ The Patient Self-Determination Act

The Patient Self-Determination Act requires healthcare facilities to:

- Provide written information to each patient regarding the right to make decisions, including the right to accept or to refuse medical treatment, and the right to make advance directives.
- Document in the patient's medical record the presence or absence of advance directives.
- Provide education to the staff, healthcare providers, and community on advance directives.
- Follow state law as it relates to advance directives.
- Treat everyone the same regardless of the presence or absence of advance directives. (Do not discriminate).

BOX 45-2 ■ Sample Living Will Language

If I am in a terminal condition, irreversible coma, or in a persistent vegetative state, my wishes are as follows:

I ☐ **do** ☐ **do not** want to be in or taken to a hospital.

I ☐ **do** ☐ **do not** want pain medications to keep me comfortable.

I ☐ **do** ☐ **do not** want cardiac resuscitation, including drugs and electrical shock.

I ☐ **do** ☐ **do not** want mechanical respiration/artificial respiration.

I ☐ **do** ☐ **do not** want tube feeding or any other artificial or invasive form of nutrition (food).

I ☐ **do** ☐ **do not** want hydration (water), via tube or intravenous.

I ☐ **do** ☐ **do not** want blood or blood products.

I ☐ **do** ☐ **do not** want any form of surgery or invasive diagnostic tests.

I ☐ **do** ☐ **do not** want kidney dialysis.

I ☐ **do** ☐ **do not** want antibiotics.

---

regarding Mr. Green's healthcare. Two weeks later, Mr. Green came out of the coma and regained the ability to make decisions. At that point, Mr. Green no longer required Joey as a surrogate.

The American Nurses Association (ANA) highlighted the nurse's role in implementing the PSDA in a 1991 Position Statement. As a nurse, you have the following responsibilities:

- You must facilitate informed decision-making for patients making choices about end-of-life care.
- You should know the laws pertaining to advance directives in the state in which you are practicing.
- You should make sure the patient's advance directives are current and reflect the patient's desires.
- You should ask the following questions about advance directives as a part of the nursing admission assessment:

    Do you have basic information about advance care directives, including living wills and durable power of attorney?

    Do you wish to initiate an advance care directive? If you have already prepared an advance care directive, can you provide it now?

    Have you discussed your end of life choices with your family and/or designated surrogate and healthcare team worker? (ANA, 1991)

Case: Durable Power of Attorney

Mrs. Terry Schiavo collapsed in her Florida home in 1990 after a suspected potassium imbalance secondary to bulimia and was without oxygen for about 5 minutes. She suffered severe brain damage. Terry Schiavo did not have a living will. According to

Florida law, her husband became her legal guardian, and thus the decision-maker regarding her medical treatments. In November 1992, Mr. Schiavo won a medical malpractice lawsuit for $1 million dollars from her physician on the theory that he failed to diagnose Mrs. Schiavo's bulimia. In 2000, Mr. Schiavo petitioned the court to have Terri's feeding tube removed. Her parents opposed the action. Over the next five years, extensive legal battles ensued. Finally, the court ruled in favor of removing the feeding tube. Mrs. Schiavo died on March 31, 2005. It was lack of a living will that (1) allowed this to go on for so long and (2) made it impossible to know for sure what Terry Schiavo would have wanted. It's all guesswork without a living will (Quill, 2005).

Americans with Disabilities Act (ADA)

The Americans with Disabilities Act (ADA) of 1990 provides protection against discrimination of individuals with disabilities. A person has a *disability* if he has a physical or mental impairment that substantially limits one or more major life activities (EEOC, 1992). In general, the ADA provides that employers must provide reasonable accommodations within the work setting to allow employees with disabilities to perform their jobs.

Case: ADA Accommodations

- A nurse with a substance abuse addiction after rehabilitation was restricted from dispensing medication after she was caught using illegal drugs. Her employer had a policy allowing employees to participate in drug rehabilitation and return to work with a last-chance agreement. When the nurse returned to work after rehabilitation, she was reassigned to a job that did not require her to dispense medication. She was given periodic drug tests.
- An ICU nurse with leukemia had difficulty tolerating rotating schedules. The nurse manager accommodated her by assigning a permanent day schedule.
- A nurse with cerebral palsy works for an insurance company investigating medical claims. Her employer adapted the workstation by installing an adjustable keyboard tray, ergonomic chair, and room for mobility braces nearby. The employer also allowed regular rest periods. She was repositioned closer to the restroom to help reduce fatigue.
- A nurse with insulin-dependent diabetes has difficulty maintaining glucose control. Her employer provides consistent times for breaks and lunch and privacy to check blood sugars and administer insulin as needed (Job Accommodation Network, 2006).

For a list of additional strategies to accommodate various disabilities,

 Go to the **Job Accommodation Network** at http://www.jan.wvu.edu/media/nurses.html

KnowledgeCheck 45-1

- Which federal law requires healthcare agencies to provide patients with information about advance directives?
- Which federal law ensures that patients can receive emergency treatment regardless of their ability to pay?
- What protections are provided to patients by the Department of Health and Human Services "privacy rule" of the HIPAA?

 Go to Chapter 45, **Knowledge Check Response Sheet and Answers,** on the Student Resource Disk or DavisPlus at http://davisplus.fadavis.com/Wilkinson2

State Laws

In addition to federal law, many states have laws that directly impact nurses' actions and behaviors. These include mandatory reporting laws, Good Samaritan laws, Nurse Practice Acts, and medical malpractice statutes.

Mandatory Reporting Laws

The law in various states requires healthcare workers to report communicable diseases. You also have a duty to report physical, sexual, or emotional abuse or neglect of children, older adults, or the mentally ill, whether you suspect it or have actual evidence of it. The intent is to protect people who cannot protect themselves and to protect society against the spread of communicable diseases. Mandatory reporting laws also protect you when reporting abuse. In most instances, the identity of the reporter is kept confidential. If you fail to report certain communicable disease in a patient you are caring for in the clinic, or if you look the other way when you have reason to believe a child was abused, you are actually liable in a court of law and could be charged for criminal misdemeanor.

The duty to report is an act of protection that takes priority over the patient's right to privacy. Therefore, if you report abuse or neglect, you cannot be charged with violating a patient's right to privacy (e.g., under HIPAA). Since the mandatory reporting laws vary from state to state, you should be familiar with the law in your state.

Case: Mandatory Reporting

In Texas, two school administrators were charged with a misdemeanor for failing to report to police or to Child Protective Services that the mother of a student had twice reported seeing a teacher molest another student (Vaughn, 1998).

Good Samaritan Laws

Good Samaritan laws are designed to protect from liability those who provide emergency care to someone who has been injured. To successfully use the Good Samaritan defense, the following elements must be present:

- Care was provided in an emergency situation.
- Person(s) providing the care did not cause the emergency or injury.
- Care was provided in a reasonably competent manner.

- Care provided must be voluntary (not paid).
- Person receiving care did not object to receiving care.

Additional guidelines nurses should follow to ensure their protection by Good Samaritan laws are:

- Call 911, or have someone else call, as soon as you can.
- Do not leave the person unless you transfer care to an equally competent professional.
- Place the person under the care of emergency personnel, physicians, or advanced practice nurses as soon as possible and follow their instructions.
- Do not accept money or any other form of compensation for the services provided.

Good Samaritan laws vary from state to state. You should be familiar with the law in your state. A typical case involving Good Samaritan laws is as follows:

Case: Good Samaritan

A registered nurse is leaving the hospital after working a 12-hour shift, when she witnesses a single-person motor vehicle accident. She calls 911, stops, and approaches the accident scene, where she smells gasoline. Fearing that the car will explode, she pulls the accident victim from the car, lays him flat on the ground, and assesses his injuries. She puts pressures on his bleeding femoral artery and stays with him until the ambulance arrives. The victim has spinal cord injuries and sues the nurse for removing him from the car. The nurse is protected from liability by the Good Samaritan law.

Nurses working in healthcare environments may not be protected by Good Samaritan laws if they already have a responsibility to provide care to those in need.

Case: Good Samaritan

June, RN, was working in the emergency department (ED) when a patient walked in and collapsed. She started CPR until the medical treatment team arrived in the ED. June had a legal duty or obligation to provide care to the patient and cannot rely on the Good Samaritan law as a defense in any lawsuit.

Nurse Practice Acts

Nurse Practice Acts (NPAs) are statutory laws passed by each state's legislative body that define the practice of nursing. Nurse Practice Acts are designed to:

- Protect patients or society
- Define the scope of nursing practice
- Identify the minimum level of nursing care that must be provided to clients

The components of NPAs are discussed in more detail later in the chapter.

 Go to Chapter 45, **Tables, Boxes, Figures: ESG Box 45-2, Minimum Acceptable Standards of Care Required by a Typical State Nurse Practice Act,** on the Student Resource Disk or DavisPlus at http://davisplus.fadavis.com/Wilkinson2

Medical Malpractice Statutes

A primary function of the medical malpractice system is to encourage healthcare providers to follow standards of practice and perform their responsibilities in a competent manner. Medical malpractice refers to a lawsuit brought against a healthcare provider for damages due to the death, injury, or other loss of the person being treated. Laws governing medical malpractice vary from state to state, primarily regarding the time frame for bringing a lawsuit (statute of limitations) and the amount of monetary compensation allowed. To protect themselves from personal losses, many healthcare providers purchase malpractice insurance, which provides them with an attorney to defend against the claim and pay the damages (money) awarded to the claimant by a judge or jury. Malpractice is discussed in more detail later in this chapter.

Other Guidelines for Practice

Other practice guidelines may also factor into what constitutes reasonable and prudent nursing care.

Institutional Policies and Procedures

Institutional policies and procedures usually are more specific and detailed than standards set by professional organizations. They describe care that is reasonable, appropriate, and expected in the context of that facility. You must be familiar with these policies and procedures because they can be used as evidence of a violation of a standard of care if you failed to follow them. Agencies should review policies and procedures regularly to ensure compliance with the Nurse Practice Act, professional standards of practice, the ANA Code of Ethics for Nurses, and other documents that guide nursing practice. Healthcare facilities should not have policies and procedures that conflict with such standards. If you encounter any conflicts, or if a policy is not working well, you should bring the matter to your supervisor's attention and/or contact the board of nursing in your state for an advisory opinion.

American Nurses Association Code of Ethics

The American Nurses Association (ANA) Code of Ethics (2001) describes the standards of professional responsibility for nurses and provides insight into ethical and acceptable behavior. It describes nurses' obligations for safe, compassionate, nondiscriminatory, and quality care, while defining commitments to self, the patient, the employer, and the profession.

The Code of Ethics is not a law, and therefore you would not be charged with criminal offenses for violating the code's provisions. In many situations, there is a fine line between what is legal and what is ethical. When confronted with a situation, you should ask yourself, "Is there a law that relates to this situation?" You should also ask yourself, "What guidance is provided under the Code of Ethics?" Your action should then be consistent with the Code. The ANA Code guarantees the patient the right to dignity, privacy, and safety. The ANA Code also guarantees the nurse will:

- Be accountable and competent
- Use informed judgment
- Maintain employment conditions conducive to quality patient care
- Protect the client from misinformation and misrepresentation
- Collaborate with other healthcare professions to meet the patient's healthcare needs

A nurse who violates a provision of the Code of Ethics may have to defend her action to the state board of nursing. Likewise, in a malpractice suit, courts may look to these codes to judge whether the nurse's action was at the level expected by the profession. However, you must understand that the Code will not likely protect you if you break a law or fail to follow agency policies, regardless of your beliefs about the morality of the law. If you need more information on nursing codes of ethics, see Chapter 44.

Patient Care Partnership

The Patient Care Partnership (PCP) replaced the American Hospital Association's Patient Bill of Rights. The PCP brochure is available in eight languages that explain in detail to patients that during hospitalization, they should expect:

- High-quality care
- A clean and safe environment
- Involvement in care
- Protection of privacy
- Help when leaving the hospital
- Help with billing claims

Like the ANA Code of Ethics, these rights are not necessarily legally binding, but they can provide evidence by which to judge whether the patient's care and environment met reasonable and appropriate standards. For more information on the Patient Care Partnership, see Box 44-4.

American Nurses Association Bill of Rights for Registered Nurses

The Nurse's Bill of Rights is a policy statement adopted by the American Nurses Association (ANA) to identify the seven conditions nurses should expect from their workplace that are necessary for sound professional practice. It provides a framework for employers to understand what nurses need for a safe work environment and to support nurses as they address such issues as unsafe staffing, workplace violence, and mandatory overtime (ANA, 2009). The Bill of Rights highlights that nurses have the right to:

- Practice in a manner that fulfills their obligations to society and to those who receive nursing care
- Practice in environments that allow them to act in accordance with professional standards and legally authorized scopes of practice
- A work environment that supports and facilitates ethical practice in the Code of Ethics for Nurses
- Freely and openly advocate for themselves and their patients, without fear of retribution
- Fair compensation for their work, consistent with their knowledge, experience, and professional responsibilities
- A work environment that is safe for themselves and for their patients
- Negotiate the conditions of their employment, either as individuals or collectively, in all practice settings

American Nurses Association Standards of Practice

The American Nurses Association (2010, in press) has revised the Standards of Practice to provide guidelines for nursing practice, performance, and competence. The Standards have three components:

1. Professional standards of care that incorporate the nursing process in the diagnostic, intervention, and evaluation aspect of patient care
2. Professional performance standards that identify the various role functions of the nurse in direct patient care, quality of practice, ethics, education, communication, research, leadership, collaboration, resource management, collegiality, and environmental health
3. Practice guidelines for the various specialty areas that are developed by professional organizations (e.g., American Association of Critical Care Nurses).

If you need to review the ANA Standards of Clinical Nursing Practice, refer to Chapter 1, Table 1-4. Standards establish the minimum level of competency for nurses. Nurses are expected to follow the standards that apply to their specialty areas. For a list of the Scope and Standards of Practice for the various clinical areas published by ANA,

 Go to the **Resources for Caregivers and Health Professionals,** on the Student Resource Disk or DavisPlus at http://davisplus.fadavis.com/Wilkinson2

 Critical**Thinking** 45-3

Recall the opening scenario. You were asked: Did the nurse do the right thing when she decided not to accept the assignment and leave the nursing home facility immediately?

- What standards, guidelines, and laws would apply to determine whether the nurse's behavior was in accordance with standards of practice?
- Which statements in the ANA Bill of Rights for Registered Nurses might the nurse use to justify her actions?

Nurse Practice Acts

As you have learned, Nurse Practice Acts (NPAs) contain a provision that creates and empowers a state board of nursing to regulate the practice of nursing in that state. All 50 states, the District of Columbia, and the five United States territories have established boards of nursing. Although NPAs can vary from state to state, they all have common components, because states used American Nurses Association guidelines in developing their regulations. A state's Nurse Practice Act usually includes:

- The authority of the board of nursing, its composition and powers
- A definition of nursing and the boundaries of nursing practice
- Standards for the approval of nursing education programs
- The requirements for licensure of nurses
- Grounds for disciplinary action against a nurse's license

Case: Nurse Practice Act

Mejonus X Institute is advertising an associate degree nursing program that can be completed in 12 months at a cost of $45,000. You are interested in the program, but are not sure if the program is legitimate. Your initial investigation of the program should start with the state board of nursing, which approves nursing education programs. A list of approved nursing programs can usually be found on the state board of nursing Web site in many states.

Requirements for Licensure

Perhaps the most important function of state boards of nursing is establishing and enforcing the requirements for licensure. Unlicensed health providers pose a danger to the health, safety, and welfare of the general public because they have not met the specified standards to ensure a minimum level of competency to enter the nursing profession. In most states, the applicant for licensure must:

- Graduate from an approved or accredited nursing program
- Meet the established character criteria
- Undergo a criminal background check and fingerprinting
- Pass the NCLEX-RN® or -PN exam
- Pay an application fee
- Some states, such as Texas, may require applicants to pass a jurisprudence examination before receiving a permanent license.

Some states give a temporary license pending the outcome of the first attempt at the licensure exam.

Special Cases of Licensure

To protect the public, licensing is meant to ensure that practicing nurses have met the minimum competencies set by the state.

Mutual Recognition Model (MRM)/Multi-State Licensure Compact. Certain states, through a multistate agreement, allow nurses who are licensed to practice in one state to practice in all other states participating in the agreement. The nurse does not have to retake the NCLEX-RN® or –PN examination, but must apply to the new state and fulfill any of that state's application requirements such as fingerprinting, background check, transcripts, and fees.

Case: Multi-State Compact

Roberto is a clinical nurse residing in Overland Park, Kansas and originally licensed in the state of Kansas after passing the NCLEX-RN®. He is now employed at the Children's Hospital on the other side of the state line in Missouri. Roberto is required to maintain active licensure in the state where he is employed. He received an RN licensure in the state of Missouri by meeting the requirements of the Missouri State Board of Nursing, but did not have to retake the NCLEX-RN®.

When two states enter into the multistate licensure compact, you do not have to obtain a separate license to practice in either state.

Government/Military Personnel. Another special case of licensure involves nurses employed by the military, Veterans Administration, Public Health Service or other entities of the federal government. These nurses may practice in other states without obtaining a new license as long as they are practicing within the parameters or scope of their employment.

Case: Special Case of Licensure

Jane is a clinical nurse in the United States Air Force Reserve. She is licensed in the state of Texas, but is assigned to a military hospital in Nevada for her 2-week annual military tour. Jane will not need to obtain a license in the state of Nevada to practice at the military hospital.

Scope of Practice

The scope of nursing practice is found in the definition of nursing at the various levels. Nurses must be familiar with the definition of nursing at their level to appropriately plan and implement care that is consistent with their scope of practice. Any nurse who practices outside the scope of practice can be charged with violation of the Nurse Practice Act. Nurse Practice Acts vary slightly state by state. However, in most states, LPN scope of practice is limited in assessment privileges and interpretation of clinical data. Typically, LPN/LVNs do not have authority to alter nursing care plans.

Understanding the definition of nursing practice in your state is important, because it determines the legal limits of your practice, as illustrated in this landmark case.

Case: Scope of Practice

A physician delegated to an LPN the task of administering a polio booster to a 2-year-old boy. The nurse put the boy over her knee and proceeded to give the injection. The boy moved and the needle broke off in his buttocks, where it remained for 9 months despite attempts to surgically remove it. Since the Washington State Nurse Practice Act at that time did not allow LPNs to give injections, the nurse was in violation of the Nurse Practice Act by performing a task that was outside of her legal limits (*Barber v. Reinking*, 1966).

This case should make clear that no one, including an employer or physician, can increase a nurse's legal scope of practice. For a decision-making model on Scope of Practice,

 Go to Chapter 45, **Resources for Caregivers and Health Professionals,** on the Student Resource Disk or DavisPlus at http://davisplus.fadavis.com/Wilkinson2

Disciplinary Actions

The state board of nursing can take disciplinary actions against your license for violation of the Nurse Practice Act. A disciplinary action usually involves some or all of the following:

- The process begins with a complaint from an individual, employer, or professional organization that the nurse has engaged in unprofessional conduct.
- The complaint is then assigned to an investigator to determine its legitimacy or validity.
  If the investigator decides the complaint is invalid or does not constitute a violation of the NPA, it will be dismissed.
  If the complaint may violate the NPA, the investigator gathers additional information by contacting the nurse, interviewing witnesses, and reviewing documents and records.
- The case may be heard by the board of nursing, who will decide if the nurse violated the NPA and the appropriate punishment. To fulfill the due process requirements of the 14th Amendment, the board of nursing must provide you with:
  Notice of the charges against you
  The evidence that supports the charges
  A hearing in which you have the opportunity to cross-examine the witnesses and to present your own evidence and witnesses

- If you are not satisfied with the board's actions and punishment, you can appeal your case to the appropriate state court.
- At every stage during the disciplinary process, you have the right to have an attorney present. Questions that you should ask a potential attorney are: (1) How many of your cases were in the area of administrative law and procedures? (2) How many times have you represented clients in front of professional boards, such as the board of nursing?

For examples of nursing actions that constitute unprofessional conduct,

 Go to **Tables, Boxes, Figures: ESG Box 45-3, Actions, Behaviors, or Omissions that Constitute Unprofessional Conduct,** on the Student Resource Disk or DavisPlus at http://davisplus.fadavis.com/Wilkinson2

CriticalThinking 45-4

A registered nurse was assigned to care for a 76-year-old patient who had a stroke. Upon entering the room, the nurse found the patient surrounded by 10 family members. The nurse requested the family members leave the room so she could conduct her initial assessment and perform any related treatments. They did so. The nurse provided care in a professional, unhurried, and gentle manner. As she was leaving, the patient said, "Thank you. You are a wonderful nurse." Later, the nursing supervisor told her the patient told his family members that the nurse had spoken harshly to him and had yanked his arms. The family stated they would file a complaint with the hospital administrator and the board of nursing.

- Are there grounds for disciplinary actions? What should the nurse do?

KnowledgeCheck 45-2

How does each of the following protect patients?
- The Patient Care Partnership
- Nursing codes of ethics
- Mandatory reporting laws

 Go to Chapter 45, **Knowledge Check Response Sheet and Answers,** on the Student Resource Disk or DavisPlus at http://davisplus.fadavis.com/Wilkinson2

Credentialing

Many healthcare disciplines, including nursing, use a voluntary form of self-regulation called **credentialing**. In the legal sense, credentialing includes accreditation and certification. Having credentials implies that the person or agency has met higher standards than the minimum (e.g., licensure).

Accreditation. Most nursing boards establish educational requirements for nursing programs and continuing education courses within a given state. The board usually requires that for a nursing program to be **accredited**, it must meet the requirements for accreditation established by the National League for Nursing (NLN) or the American Association of Colleges of Nursing (ACCN) and by the state NPA. This helps ensure students receive education that meets the minimum standard for quality and that patients are cared for by safe practitioners.

Accreditation also applies to other than educational facilities; for example, hospitals seek accreditation by The Joint Commission. This is intended to ensure a minimum standard quality of care is provided.

Certification. Another form of credentialing is **certification**. Through certification and licensing, the board identifies nurses who are qualified for advanced practice (e.g., clinical nurse specialists, midwives, and nurse practitioners) or for certification in a subspecialty, such as emergency nursing or pediatric nursing. In some states, the board establishes the criteria for certification, including (1) educational preparation, (2) clinical experience, and (3) certification by other professional organizations. In other states, the nurse may obtain an advanced practice license only if she is first certified by a national organization, such as the American Nurses Credentialing Corporation (ANCC) or a specialty organization. Not all states require certification for advanced practice nurses.

What Is Criminal Law?

Criminal law deals with wrongs or offenses against society. It may result in prosecution (legal action) by the state or federal government for engaging in behavior that constitutes a crime. A **crime** is a violation of a law as defined by a legislative body. The legislature also specifies the punishments for the crime. State-level criminal laws vary from state to state.

There are two "levels" of crimes: misdemeanors and felonies. The primary difference is the possible punishment.

- **Felonies** involve crimes punishable by more than one year in jail (e.g., murder, assisted suicide, rape/sexual assault, stealing drugs and equipment, felony abuse). A person convicted of a felony loses the right to vote, hold public office, serve on a jury, and to possess firearms. The person may also lose any professional license.
- Compared to a felony, a **misdemeanor** is a minor charge. Misdemeanors involve less than a year in jail. They include crimes such as assault, battery, and petty theft. You may also lose your nursing license if you are convicted of a misdemeanor that involves crimes against persons or that can cause harm to others.

An emerging issue in the nursing profession is whether nurses who accidentally cause harm to patients should be charged with criminal offenses (e.g., a nurse accidentally administers the wrong drug to a patient and the patient dies). In the past, these cases have been dealt with under civil law and by the board of nursing. Now state prosecutors are beginning to bring felony and misdemeanor charges against these nurses.

Case: Criminal Law

Several patients complained that their pain medication was not working. A review of the medical records of the patients assigned to the nurse revealed that all but one of her patients who received pain medication had similar complaints. When confronted, the nurse admitted to stealing the patients' pain medication and giving them saline. She also admitted to using other nurses' passwords for stealing narcotics. The nurse was terminated and reported to the board of nursing. She refused to enter in the Impaired Nurse's Program. Her license was revoked after a hearing. She also faced criminal charges for theft of controlled substances.

Case: Criminal Law

Joan, RN, was arrested for stealing computer equipment and wound supplies from the hospital that were valued at $55,000. She was charged with grand larceny, a felony. Two weeks before her trial, she entered into a plea deal that reduced the charge to a misdemeanor with probation for 6 months.

For an expanded discussion of criminal law,

 Go to Chapter 45, **Supplemental Materials,** on the Student Resource Disk or DavisPlus at http://davisplus.fadavis.com/Wilkinson2

What Is Civil Law?

In contrast to criminal law, in which the state or federal government brings charges against a person, civil law involves a dispute between individuals or entities. A settlement in civil law often results in the guilty party paying monetary damages. The two types of civil law are contract law and tort law.

- **Contract law** involves a written or oral agreement between two parties in which one party accepts an offer made by the other party to perform (or not perform) certain acts in exchange for something of value. A breach of contract occurs if either party does not comply with the terms of the agreement. An example would be an employment contract.
- **Tort law**, on the other hand, deals with wrongs done to one person by another person that does not involve contracts. A tort is a civil wrong and there are three types of tort: quasi-intentional torts, intentional torts, and non-intentional torts.

What Are Quasi-Intentional Torts?

Quasi-intentional torts involve actions that injure a person's reputation. The overall concept for these torts is defamation of character. All four of the following essential elements of **defamation of character** must be present. The communication (written or oral) about the person:

- Was false
- Was made to another person or persons
- Caused the defamed person to experience shame and ridicule and had a negative impact on the person's reputation
- Was made as a statement of fact rather than as an opinion

Libel is the written or published form of defamation of character. **Slander** is the spoken or verbal form of defamation of character. A person is not guilty of defamation of character if the statement made about the other person is true or if the person has the protection of a "privilege," such as reporting possible child abuse.

Case: Quasi-Intentional Torts

The nursing supervisor calls you into an empty conference room and states, "I know that you have been stealing (diverting) narcotics from the unit and injecting yourself with it while at work. It shows, because your work is sloppy and you are falsifying your documentation. You are a poor excuse for a nurse." Before you can defend yourself, the supervisor turns and leaves. The statements are not true. The supervisor has committed slander.

What Are Intentional Torts?

An **intentional tort** is an action taken by one person with the intent to harm another person. The harm does not have to be violent, hostile, or cause a significant amount of pain or distress to the other person. The person must have merely intended to cause harm or known the action would bring about the harm. Intentional torts may also be prosecuted under criminal law. For example, a nurse who is sued for malpractice in civil court may also be charged with a homicide if a patient died because of the nurse's actions. Intentional torts most commonly encountered in nursing are assault, battery, false imprisonment, and invasion of privacy.

Assault

An assault occurs when a nurse intentionally places a patient in immediate fear of personal violence or offensive contact. An assault must include words expressing an intention to cause harm and some type of action. For example, a nurse has committed an assault if she says to the patient "I will slap you" and raises her hand as if to slap the patient. The combination of the words and action causes the patient to believe the threat will be carried out.

Battery

A **battery** is committed when (1) an offensive or harmful physical contact is made with the patient without his consent, or (2) there is unauthorized touching of a person's body by another person. To avoid charges of battery, always obtain informed consent before providing certain treatments. Upon admission to healthcare facilities, patients sign a general consent form, which usually covers routine aspects of nursing care, such as vital signs and patient assessments. However, when performing any invasive procedure, such as insertion of catheters or intravenous lines, you should always explain the procedure to the patient and obtain his consent before starting.

Assault and Battery

An **assault and battery** occurs when there is the intent to cause a person fear combined with an offensive or harmful contact.

> #### Case: Assault and Battery
>
> A patient admitted for an elective surgical procedure complained the automatic blood pressure cuff was causing her extreme pain and demanded it be removed. The nurse did not immediately remove the cuff as requested by the patient. The nurse was guilty of a battery, but no assault, because there was no evidence the nurse intended to create or cause fear or pain (*Coulter v. Thomas*, 33 S.W.3d 522 [Ky 2000]).

False Imprisonment

False imprisonment is the restraining of a person without proper legal authorization. It includes any type of unjustified restriction on a person's freedom of movement. Nurses may be accused of false imprisonment when they restrain patients without their permission or when patients are involuntarily committed to mental health units. False imprisonment can involve the use of physical restraints (e.g., vest or wrist restraints) or chemical restraints (e.g., sedative or narcotic medications). You may restrain patients who pose a threat or harm to themselves or others for safety. However, you must immediately obtain the proper authorization to continue the restraint. If a competent patient wishes to leave the healthcare facility, you should contact the nursing supervisor and the primary care provider. Inform the patient of the risks associated with leaving, and give her the choice to stay and receive treatment or to sign out against medical advice (AMA). You need to be aware of the hospital policy and procedures on AMA discharges.

Invasion of Privacy

Invasion of privacy violates a person's right to be left alone. The law recognizes that a person's personal life should not be opened up for public scrutiny and the person has the right to freedom from unwanted interference in her private affairs. A person has:

- The right to have her private information protected
- The right to not be falsely portrayed or intentionally misrepresented in character, beliefs, or actions

- The right to be free from unwanted intrusion (spying, eavesdropping).

Examples of violating right to privacy include discussing patients in public places (e.g., elevators, cafeterias), photographing patients without their permission, providing information to news media without consent, searching a patient's personal belongings without permission, and releasing medical information without the patient's consent.

Fraud

Fraud is the false representation of significant facts by words or by conduct. It can occur, through making false statements, falsifying documentation, or concealing information that should have been disclosed. It is intentionally misleading or deceiving another person to act (or not act) for the personal gain of the one committing the fraud.

> #### Case: Fraud
>
> A nurse admitted receiving more than $70,000 in Medicaid funds for private nursing services that she never provided. She submitted Medicaid reimbursement claims that falsely indicated that she provided nursing services to seven children and three young adults. The nurse entered a guilty plea to a felony (fraud) (*The Water Buffalo Press*, 2007).

What Are Non-Intentional Torts?

The most common type of non-intentional torts involving healthcare professionals are negligence or malpractice. **Negligence** is the failure to use ordinary or reasonable care or the failure to act in a reasonable and prudent (careful) manner. **Malpractice** has a similar definition, but applies only to professionals, such as nurses and physicians. It is defined as the failure of a professional person to act in a reasonable and prudent manner. A malpractice lawsuit may occur when such actions cause injury or death to the patient. The person bringing the lawsuit is the **plaintiff** and the person who must defend against the lawsuit is the **defendant**.

Malpractice/Negligence Liability

To win and recover damages (money) in a malpractice lawsuit, the plaintiff must prove four elements (duty, breach of duty, causation, and damages) by a "preponderance of the evidence," in other words, with enough evidence to tip the scale in his or her favor.

Duty. The nurse–patient relationship creates this legal obligation. A duty forms when the patient is assigned to the nurse or seeks treatment from the nurse, or when the nurse observes another person doing something that could harm the patient.

Breach of Duty. A breach of duty occurs when the nurse fails to meet standards of care. Attorneys look to several sources of information to identify the standards of care and to determine what a reasonable and prudent (careful) nurse would have done in the situation. These sources include the NPA, job descriptions, hospital policies and procedures, textbooks, professional standards and guidelines developed by professional organizations, and the nursing code of ethics.

The attorney will usually hire an expert witness who is a nurse with advanced education or experience. The purpose of an expert witness is to educate the judge and jury on the local practice of nursing and how the nurse's actions or omissions failed to meet acceptable practice for nurses.

Causation. The breach of duty or deviation from acceptable standards of care by the nurse must be the direct and proximate cause of the injury suffered by the patient. Causation is usually established based on the testimony of experts, such as physicians, advanced practice nurses, or other healthcare professionals, who can clearly show the connection between the nurse's action or omission and the resulting injury to the patient. Many cases claiming malpractice are lost because the plaintiff is unable to establish causation, which is often the most difficult element to prove.

Case: Causation

A nurse forgot to change the patient's dressing at the scheduled time, but changed it 3 hours later. The hospital policy reads that nurses must administer medications or perform prescribed treatments within 30 minutes before or 30 minutes after the scheduled time. The patient did not experience any harm or infection. In this case, there was the existence of a duty and a breach of duty, but the breach of duty did not cause any harm or injury to the patient. Therefore, if a malpractice action was brought, the plaintiff would

not receive an award. Nurses are encouraged to report medication and treatment errors as promptly as possible so that actions can be taken to prevent and/or minimize injury to the patient.

Damages. In civil cases, the remedy for the harm the patient suffered is money. The judge or jury will award the plaintiff money to compensate him for pain and suffering, lost wages, additional medical bills, and other losses. In some cases, the plaintiff may be awarded punitive damages for grossly negligent or wrongful behavior by the healthcare provider.

Case: Damages

A 16-year-old pregnant female went into labor and was admitted to the hospital. She was diagnosed with a strep infection and an intravenous (IV) antibiotic was prescribed. The nurse mistakenly administered an epidural pain medication into the IV line. The patient began having seizures and died; however, the baby was safely delivered by an emergency cesarean section. Several safeguards were in place to prevent medication errors, such as a computerized system that scans medications to ensure accuracy, and a bright pink label on the epidural pain medication warning against IV administration. A lawsuit was brought by the family (plaintiff) against the hospital and nurse (defendants).

Analysis of the case:
Duty: Based on the nurse–patient relationship
Breach of Duty: Administering an incorrect medication via the wrong route
Causation: Medication caused the female to have seizures and die.
Damages: In the above case, a settlement was reached with a present value of about $1.9 million.
(Frew, 2006; Nursing Service Organization [NSO], 2008).

Toward Evidence-Based Practice

Snyder, E. K. (2008, October). Psych: No fall-risk assessment done, negligence found. *Legal Eagle Eye Newsletter for the Nursing Profession, 16(10), 8.*

A 57-year-old woman was admitted for inpatient psychiatric care for suicidal ideation. The day before hospitalization she had fallen and fractured her right tibia and fibula. The nurses admitting the patient marked through the risk assessment and fall precautions section of the admission nursing assessment form with letters "N.A.," signifying the risk assessment and fall precautions were not relevant to the care of this patient. Yet her other nursing documentation noted the patient's unsteady gait, muscle weakness, confused mental state, and poor judgment. While hospitalized, the patient reportedly awoke during the night and alerted the nurse for help to the restroom. When she got no response, she attempted to get up on her own and

fell. The jury in the Supreme Court, Richmond County, New York awarded her $598,000 for negligence of the nurse.

Cifelli v. St. Vincent's, 2008 WL 4093163 (Sup. Ct. Richmond Co., New York, July 17, 2008).

1. The nurse noted the client to be unsteady on her feet, weak, confused, and making poor judgments. What do you think was the basis for the court decision that the patient's injury was due to negligence of the nurse?

Snyder, E. K. (2006, April). Falls: Court finds substandard precautions. Negligence found. *Legal Eagle Eye Newsletter for the Nursing Profession, 14(4), 8.*

The New York Supreme Court, Appellate Division, made note that the elderly patient had right-sided weakness,

Toward Evidence-Based Practice—cont'd

dementia, psychosis, and aphasia and was on multiple medications. After this patient had fallen numerous times during unassisted ambulation, the nurse reminded him repeatedly to ring the call bell and wait for assistance. The court ruled the nurse did not properly evaluate the patient's risk of falling in light of his medical history, medications, prior falls, and the fact that additional safeguards other than simple verbal reminders are necessary to ensure the patient's safety. Negligence was found.

Hranek v. United Methodist Homes, __ N.Y.S.2d __, 2006 WL 560208 (N.Y. App., March 9, 2006).

2. In this case, what was the basis for the court decision that the patient's injury was due to negligence of the nurse?

Snyder, E. K. (2006, June). Patient falls while nurses were busy with another patient: Court finds negligence. *Legal Eagle Eye Newsletter for the Nursing Profession, 14(6), 6.*

The patient, Mrs. McLaughlin, was admitted to an inpatient psychiatric facility for electroconvulsive therapy (ECT) as treatment of depression. Side effects of ECT can include headaches, memory difficulties, confusion, and hallucinations. In addition, the patient had a history of osteoarthritis, scoliosis, and Parkinson's disease that also make a falls-risk assessment appropriate while receiving hospital care. The psychiatrist ordered a vest restraint because the patient was combative with staff and hallucinating. The patient's antidepressant was increased and an anti-hallucinogen was added.

Meanwhile, another patient was admitted to the psychiatric unit who was in a highly agitated state. Nursing staff on the unit provided care to the newly admitted man with paranoid schizophrenia, leaving Mrs. McLaughlin unattended in her room. During this time she suffered a fall. No one had checked on Mrs. McLaughlin since the man was brought into the unit, although they were required to do so every 15 minutes.

The nurses were clearly aware of their duty toward the patient, who was in a highly confused state and had hallucinated for the past several days. She was at high risk for falling. The Court of Appeals of Ohio ruled that the hospital's psychiatric specialty nurses were negligent and that their negligence was the legal cause behind the patient's injuries resulting from a fall.

McLaughlin v. Firelands Community Hosp. 2006 WL 1047499 (Ohio App., April 21, 2006).

3. In the case where the nurse was caring for a patient at high risk for falls but got busy taking care of another patient at the time of the fall, what was the basis for the court decision that the patient's death was due to negligence of the nurse?

4. In retrospect, what could the nurse have done differently to protect the patient from injury?

 Go to Chapter 45, **Toward Evidence-Based Practice Suggested Responses,** on the Student Resource Disk or DavisPlus at http://davisplus.fadavis.com/Wilkinson2

KnowledgeCheck 45-3

- Distinguish negligence from malpractice.
- Distinguish civil from criminal law.
- Under which type of law (constitutional, statutory, administrative, or common law) does each of the following fall?
  A defendant claiming the right not to incriminate himself under the Fifth Amendment
  A nurse having her license revoked by the state board of nursing
  The wording of a state nurse practice act
- Define *plaintiff* and *defendant* in the context of civil law.

 Go to Chapter 45, **Knowledge Check Response Sheet and Answers,** on the Student Resource Disk or DavisPlus at http://davisplus.fadavis.com/Wilkinson2

 CriticalThinking 45-5

- Give one nursing example of each: negligence, malpractice, damages.
- Can you think of one nonfraudulent example of a nurse's being untruthful with a patient? Do you think that the circumstances described in your example make the untruthfulness justifiable?

- Can you think of an example of a nurse's committing assault, other than the one given in the text?

Vicarious Liability

A common legal principle that should guide your behavior is that you are legally accountable for your actions or inactions. This means that you can be sued for behavior or omissions that deviate from acceptable standards. In certain circumstances though, the law will assign liability to a person or entity that did not directly cause the injury, but with whom you have a special kind of relationship. This type of liability is known as **vicarious** or **substituted liability**. The various types of vicarious liability existing under common law are discussed below.

Captain of the Ship. This principle applies to situations where a physician (e.g., surgeon or obstetrician) is held liable for the negligence of another healthcare provider. *Captain of the Ship* usually applies to surgical suite situations. Many states no longer recognize it as protection for the nurse because the nurse is still liable for her own actions.

Borrowed Servant Doctrine. For situations involving liability for acts of a nonemployed worker, the *Borrowed Servant Doctrine*, relieves the primary employer of liability for the actions or omission of its employee when the employee was borrowed by another person. In theory, the borrower becomes liable for the actions of the employee. This would apply, for example, to agency nurses.

Respondeat Superior. The Latin term, **respondeat superior**, means "let the master answer." The employer must answer for the negligent acts or omissions of its employees, who are functioning within the scope of their employment. For example, a nurse is working within the scope of her practice as a labor and delivery nurse makes a medication error; the hospital can be sued for the nurse's error.

KnowledgeCheck 45-4

- Define these terms: *assault, battery, fraud, slander, libel, negligence, malpractice.*
- State the four elements of malpractice.

 Go to Chapter 45, **Knowledge Check Response Sheet and Answers,** on the Student Resource Disk or DavisPlus at http://davisplus.fadavis.com/Wilkinson2

Litigation in Civil Claims

Litigation is the formal process wherein the legal issues, rights, and duties between the parties are heard and decided (adjudicated). The litigation process follows several stages: (1) pleading and pretrial motions, (2) discovery, (3) alternative dispute resolution, (4) trial, and (5) appeal.

Pleading and Pretrial Motions

The litigation process starts when the plaintiff files a complaint. A **complaint** is a legal document outlining how the plaintiff has been harmed by another person. Once the case is filed with the court, the complaint is served on (delivered to) the defendant. The complaint identifies the plaintiff, the specific allegations of the timeframe involved, the behavior(s) or omissions, the persons (defendants) involved, and the harm suffered.

If you are served with a complaint, you must immediately notify your employer. In addition, if you have malpractice insurance, you must also notify your insurance company. You will need an attorney to defend you. Your attorney has a specified time within which to file an "answer" to the complaint. The answer addresses each of the allegations (unproven accusations). As a defendant, you should not contact the plaintiff or the plaintiff's attorney or discuss the case with co-workers or friends. The facility's risk manager and your attorney will advise you. Cooperate fully and be honest in all your answers.

Discovery Phase

The discovery process allows for both parties to gather facts and evidence about the case that can be used at trial. Discovery is designed to make sure there are no "surprises" during the trial. Attorneys may obtain discovery through written questions (*interrogatories*), requests for documents and other evidence, and by *depositions* (attorneys orally question parties to the lawsuit under oath, as though they were testifying in court). You may be deposed (questioned) as either a fact witness, a party to the lawsuit (defendant), or an expert witness. A *fact witness* is someone who was present when the incident occurred, whereas the defendant will testify as to the care provided and the actions taken.

Deposition may occur several years after the incident, so you may not remember specific information. You should prepare for the deposition by reviewing the medical records and any other evidence that may exist regarding the lawsuit. During the deposition, listen to your attorney, do not volunteer information, take your time before answering each question, and provide only objective information. Always tell the truth, but base your answers on facts; do not speculate. If your attorney objects to any question, immediately stop and do not provide an answer unless directed by your attorney.

Alternative Dispute Resolution

Lawyers and involved parties usually try to resolve disputes before going to trial. The three most common methods of alternative dispute resolution are as follows:

- **Negotiation** takes place informally between the lawyers for the plaintiff and the defendant in an attempt to settle the case prior to trial.
- **Mediation** is the attempt to resolve the dispute using a neutral third party. The primary role of the mediator is to help the parties focus on the issues and to facilitate communication to identify what is needed to reach a resolution.
- **Arbitration** involves a third party making a decision after hearing the evidence and information from both parties.

Trial Process

If the dispute cannot be resolved and is not dismissed by the court during pretrial motions, the case goes to trial. Malpractice cases are usually heard by a jury. After hearing all the evidence and reviewing submitted documents, the judge or jury makes a decision, which is either dismissal or the award of damages.

Appeal

After the judge or jury has made a decision, either party has the opportunity to present post-trial motions, move for a new trial, or appeal the verdict and/or damages to an appeals court. The Appeals Court will review the transcript and documents from the trial and determine if a correct verdict (decision) was made. The Appeals Court can uphold the verdict, dismiss the verdict, or remand (send back) the case to the trial court with special instructions.

KnowledgeCheck 45-5

- Identify the phases of the trial process.
- How is arbitration different from mediation?

 Go to Chapter 45, **Knowledge Check Response Sheet and Answers,** on the Student Resource Disk or DavisPlus at http://davisplus.fadavis.com/Wilkinson2

Practical **Knowledge**
knowing how

To decrease your chances of being involved in a malpractice suit, you should know the most common causes of malpractice claims and some practical preventive actions you can take. Keep in mind that causes are often difficult to categorize because they overlap; an error usually results from interlocking causes.

What Are the Most Common Malpractice Claims?

Nurses must use the nursing process to provide safe and efficient care to patients. The most common causes of nursing malpractice claims can be categorized according to where they fall in the nursing process; failure to assess and diagnose, failure to plan, failure to implement, and failure to evaluate (O'Keefe, 2001) (Box 45-3).

Failure to Assess and Diagnose

As the first step in the nursing process, the failure to conduct an adequate assessment can lead to numerous breaches of duty. Failure to analyze the data and make correct nursing diagnoses can lead to incorrect or no actions.

Case: Failure to Assess and Diagnose

In an actual case, the healthcare provider's failure to properly diagnose and treat status asthmaticus, intubate the patient, properly sedate, administer oxygen, administer the correct amounts of medication, and follow the hospital's protocols and standards of care resulted in the death of a 10-year-old child. The case resulted in a $3.5 million award of damages to the family (Nursing Service Organization [NSO], 2008, June).

Safe and competent assessment and diagnosis practices require the nurse to:

- Perform an admission assessment. This duty cannot be delegated to a nursing assistant.
- Analyze the assessment data to clearly identify problems.
- Apply theoretical knowledge to ensure a correct diagnosis. The presenting signs and symptoms should be consistent with the disease process or medical problem. Remember the nursing diagnosis consists of "Patient

---

BOX 45-3 ■ Common Causes of Malpractice Litigation

Failure to respond, such as not intervening to care for the patient's specific symptoms or expressed request for care.

Failure to educate, such as not answering questions, not teaching self-care measures, or not explaining procedures or equipment adequately on the patient's discharge.

Failure to follow standards of care and institutional policies and procedures. This most commonly occurs in the form of medication errors and failure to follow a provider's orders. It also frequently occurs from failure to use equipment responsibly. Among other reasons, a nurse may fail to follow standards of care when the unit is understaffed or the nurse is inexperienced.

Failure to communicate often comes up when a nurse fails to seek medical authorization for a treatment or fails to notify a physician in a timely manner when a patient's condition warrants action.

Failure to document the following in the patient's record: assessment data (e.g., drug allergies), patient injuries, medication administration details, patient progress and response to treatment, physicians' orders, and telephone conversations with physicians.

Failure to act as an advocate. Nurses must frequently intervene to prevent harm to the patient by other healthcare providers and by relatives and significant others. The following are examples of advocacy errors:

a. *Medical and discharge orders.* As an example of failure to advocate, suppose two physicians order the same drug for a patient, but under different brand names. The nurse does not recognize that two drugs are the same, so the patient receives twice the normal amount and has a toxic reaction. Other errors occur when the nurse does not question incomplete or illegible orders or does not question discharge orders when she believes the patient is not well enough to be discharged.

b. *Impaired nurses.* You have a duty under most state nursing practice acts to report impaired nursing practice (e.g., as a result of alcoholism or mental illness) to the appropriate licensing agency. Failure to do so is a failure to advocate for patients.

c. *Family and significant others.* Advocacy includes reporting neglect and intentional injuries to children, the elderly, and the disabled. Failure to do so may constitute negligence and/or violation of state statutes.

Response related to Etiology." When the assessment reveals adverse symptoms, the nurse must report the symptoms to the appropriate provider and carry out the standard nursing care and prescribed interventions.

- Conduct frequent focused assessments until the end of your shift or until the problem is resolved.

Failure to Plan

The American Nurses Association standards specifically require nurses to formulate a plan of care. The plan of care may be written or unwritten, depending on state regulations. Many agencies require nurses to complete nursing care plans or patient care tools as a means of measuring patient outcomes and progress. The plan of care should be consistent with standards of treatments acceptable for the given diagnosis or problem. Safe and competent practices in this category require the nurse to:

- Know the correct approach to treat patient actual or potential problems.
- Have the theoretical knowledge base to successfully plan nursing care for patients.
- Develop a plan of care that is individualized to the patient.

You must consider the whole patient based on your assessment data and not just the medical diagnosis. For example, if the plan of care involves teaching the patient about selecting high-protein foods, you would consider different selections for a vegetarian than for a non-vegetarian.

Failure to Implement a Plan of Care

Implementation is the nursing process step in which the nurse performs the care or nursing interventions. Failure to implement encompasses a variety of actions, shown in Box 45-3, Common Causes of Malpractice Litigation.

Failure to Evaluate

Evaluation is the last step in the nursing process. It requires you to make a decision or judgment about the success of your interventions in addressing the client's problems. The duty to evaluate requires an ongoing cycle of the following:

- *Observing for changes* after interventions and treatments. You must know the expected outcomes and side effects of medications and treatments, so you can accurately interpret and document anticipated and adverse responses.
- *Recognizing significance of the change.* For example, if Mr. Adkins's blood pressure (BP) is usually 140/88, a change to 150/90 after exercise would not be significant for him. But for Mrs. Jonas, whose BP is usually 100/64, a change to 150/90 would be cause for concern.

- *Documenting or reporting symptoms* to the appropriate person. If a change is significant, you have a legal duty to report the change to the appropriate provider and to document this change in the appropriate medical record.
- *Following up on patient responses* to nursing interventions requires you to know the expected outcomes and side effects of medications and treatments.

KnowledgeCheck 45-6

- State the four requirements of the nurse's duty to assess.
- State four ways in which the nurse may fail to implement a plan of care.
- Give one example of the duty to advocate for a patient.
- List the four components of the nurse's legal duty to evaluate.

 Go to Chapter 45, **Knowledge Check Response Sheet and Answers,** on the Student Resource Disk or DavisPlus at http://davisplus.fadavis.com/Wilkinson2

How Can You Minimize Your Malpractice Risks?

The best way to minimize your risk of malpractice is to practice in a safe and competent manner. You must have the appropriate body of theoretical knowledge for clinical practice, which you are already beginning to acquire. You should also be familiar with (1) your state's nurse practice act, (2) professional standards of practice, and (3) institutional policies and procedures. These provide the legal framework for your practice and help you to evaluate the quality of the care you deliver. Ignorance of the law and of practice standards is no excuse for failing to comply with the law, and it is no defense in a malpractice suit.

You may significantly reduce your risk exposures when you follow these three guidelines:

- Perform timely patient assessments and document your findings for every patient interaction.
- Communicate all changes in your patient's status to the primary healthcare provider and document those changes.
- Use the proper chain of command to ensure appropriate and timely care when the primary healthcare provider is not available (*Nursing 2009*, 2009; p. 21).

You will find discussion of other helpful suggestions in the remainder of this chapter. For more tips,

 Go to Chapter 45, **Clinical Insight 45-1: Tips for Avoiding Malpractice,** in Volume 2.

If you would like to see the typical standards of care found in a nurse practice act,

 Go to Chapter 45, **Tables, Boxes, Figures: ESG Box 45-2, Minimum Acceptable Standards of Care Required by a Typical State Nurse Practice Act,** on the Student Resource Disk or DavisPlus at http://davisplus.fadavis.com/Wilkinson2

Use the Nursing Process and Follow Professional Standards of Care

The nursing process provides you with a systematic approach to patient care and is the legally acceptable model of decision-making in nursing practice. Your documentation should reveal that you have assessed, diagnosed, planned, implemented, and evaluated care based on current and acceptable standards.

Avoid Medication and Treatment Errors

Medication errors are among the most common health-care errors. To accurately administer medications, you must know the rationale for administering the drug, safe dosage ranges, side effects of the medications, and relevant information to teach the patient about the medication. To prevent medication errors, you should:

- Follow the "rights of medication administration" (see Chapter 23).
- Investigate any patient concerns before giving the medication (e.g., the patient might say, "Is this a new medication? I have not taken this one before.")
- Question prescriptions that are incomplete or that seem inappropriate.
- Make sure the equipment used to administer drugs is working properly.
- Use the correct technique to provide patient treatment (e.g., failure to maintain a sterile field during wound care could lead to an infection).

For tips to help you use equipment properly and safely,

 Go to Chapter 45, **Clinical Insight 45-2: Using Equipment Safely,** in Volume 2.

Report and Document

For every suggestion for minimizing malpractice risk given in this section, add the reminder: "Document what happened." Remember the old adage: "If it isn't documented, it wasn't done." If you are ever required to appear in court the patient record may be the only proof you have of the care you gave. It is unlawful to make false entries or destroy entries in medical records, but do carefully record in detail all care you provide.

Charting

A basic principle of charting is that a third person should be able to read your documentation and form a mental picture of your patient and the care provided during your shift. Record all interactions with clients, as well as patients' refusal of or noncompliance with treatment. Document telephone conversations with primary care providers, including time, content of the conversation and the action you took. Document the

facts; do not editorialize (e.g., do not write, "I could not check on the patient as often as ordered because we were understaffed"). Refer to Chapter 16 for a review of your documentation responsibilities, and use the letters F-A-C-T as a reminder when charting (Helm, 2003).

  F—Your information must be **factual**: Don't chart your opinions.
  A—You must be **accurate**: For example, record the vital signs accurately.
  C—Stands for **complete**: Don't omit any important information.
  T—Stands for **timely**: Chart care as soon as possible after doing it; don't wait until end-of-shift and then try to remember everything that happened.

 Go to Chapter 45, **Clinical Insight 45-3: Guidelines for Documenting Patient Care,** in Volume 2.

Incident Reports

If a standard of care is breached or an unusual incident occurs (e.g., a visitor or patient falls or is injured), you should complete an **incident report** (also called variance report or occurrence report). These reports are used, in part, for quality improvement in the agency and should not be used to discipline staff members or be placed in employees' files. The goal is to prevent the incident from occurring again. In some states, an incident report must be made available as a part of discovery in litigation. In other states, only the chart may be subpoenaed. However, in those states if the incident report is mentioned in the chart, the otherwise confidential report may be used as evidence. Therefore, do not write "Incident report completed" in the patient record.

When reporting an incident, be sure to clearly identify the patient, date, time, and location. Briefly describe the incident in factual terms. Use the exact words of the patient or persons involved and put the information in quotes. Do not speculate, draw conclusions, or place blame. Identify any witnesses to the event or equipment involved.

For example:

1900 Demerol 50 mg given intramuscularly. Physician order: Demerol 15 mg.

1930 Patient's respirations: 8 breaths/minute; BP 100/60; skin pale.

2000 Called Dr. Smith. Orders for naloxone (Narcan) 1 mg IV STAT

2005 Narcan given as ordered. Resp 12 breaths/min, BP 118/70

You should be prepared to discuss the 30-minute delay between the patient's findings and contacting the physician. The standard of care would require that the physician be notified immediately. Chapter 16 presents additional information on occurrence reports.

Obtain Informed Consent

Informed consent is the permission for any and all types of care, given by the patient with full knowledge of the risks, benefits, costs, and alternatives. For hospital admission and for invasive or specialized treatments or diagnostic procedures, the consent must be written and signed by the patient or the person legally responsible for the patient. The law provides for implied or assumed consent in emergency situations; therefore, written consent is not necessary in an emergency if experts would agree that there was an immediate threat to life or health.

Elements of Consent

To be legally valid, the informed consent should fulfill the following requirements:

Completeness. Healthcare consumers need a great deal of information to make educated decisions. Be sure they get all the information needed to make decisions regarding the treatment. This includes the nature of the procedure, risks, benefits, post-procedure care and considerations, and alternatives.

Clarity and Comprehension. Language should be appropriate to the patient's educational level, so the patient (or his surrogate decision maker) can understand the explanation. Always ask the patient to describe in his own words the procedure to which he is consenting. If the patient asks, "What will the doctor do during surgery?" the nurse is aware that the patient does not understand the nature of the surgery. She could contact the surgeon.

Voluntariness. The patient must be free to accept or reject the treatment. He must not be pressured or coerced to give consent. There must be no actual or implied threat by anyone to force the patient into having the surgery (e.g., "Mom, if you don't let them do this, I'm never coming back to see you."). Otherwise, the consent is not valid.

Competence. The person must have the ability to understand the information and make a choice about the particular situation (e.g., the ability to decide what clothing to wear does not necessarily mean that the person is competent to decide whether to have surgery). If the person is confused and disoriented, you should contact the case manager or your supervisor for guidance. State law identifies the order of individuals who can make decisions for individuals who are judged incompetent. It is usually the spouse, then parents, then sisters and brothers, and so on. If the person does not have relatives, the court will appoint a legal guardian to make healthcare decisions.

Generally speaking, a competent adult has the legal right to consent to or refuse any treatment. However, this right does not always extend to situations where an adult is making the decision for a minor. A court sometimes will authorize treatment of a child against his parents' wishes. In some states, a minor who is married or living independently is considered emancipated and can make his/her own healthcare decisions.

The Nurse's Role

As a nurse, your legal role regarding written consent is to collaborate with the primary provider, usually a physician or advanced practice nurse. You may witness a patient's signature on a consent form, but you are not legally responsible for explaining the treatments and options, or for evaluating whether the provider has adequately explained them. You must, however, determine that the elements of a valid informed consent are in place, communicate the patient's needs for more information to the care provider, and provide feedback if the patient wishes to change her consent.

Be sure you have the patient's informal, verbal consent for nursing interventions that you perform (e.g., urinary catheterization). Coming to the agency for healthcare implies that the patient consents to usual treatment, such as injections and vital signs. However, you should explain all procedures to the patient before their implementation. If the patient objects, identify the reasons for the refusal, correct any misinformation, and explain the benefits of the treatment. If the patient still objects or refuses, do not proceed and contact the primary care provider.

In addition to state statutes, case law, and agency policy, The Joint Commission standards provide valuable guidance regarding informed participation in decision making. See Chapter 44 for discussion of informed consent from an ethical perspective.

Maintain Patient Safety

Falls are by far the most common incident reported in hospitals and long-term care facilities. On admissions to the facility, all patients should be assessed for risks of falls and "fall precautions" instituted when needed. Simply raising the siderails on the bed is not enough to prevent falls. You may still be found negligent if the patient falls because he called for help and no one came to assist him out of bed, or if the call bell was not placed within the patient's reach and he was unable to call for assistance. Several useful tools have been developed for assessing falls, including the Morse Fall Scale. See Chapter 21 for information about meeting patients' safety needs, including falls and use of restraints. For a falls risk tool,

 Go to Chapter 21, **Tables, Boxes, Figures: ESG Figure 21-1,** on the Student Resource Disk or DavisPlus at http://davisplus.fadavis.com/Wilkinson2

Maintain Confidentiality and Privacy

Always maintain patient confidentiality unless directed by law to do otherwise (e.g., when a patient is threatening to harm someone). Family members and significant others do not have an automatic right to information about the patient. For example, parents do not have an automatic right to see the medical records of their child if that child is married and/or declared legally competent to make independent decisions. Of course, you need to discuss clients' medical conditions with other health team members, but this does not include chatting about the client's personal life or talking about the patient in the lunchroom. The general nursing principle is that you should discuss the patient's health status with those who have a need to know (those involved in the patient's care).

Another aspect of privacy is to maintain the confidentiality of patient records (e.g., do not leave a patient's health record in locations that are accessible to visitors or nonauthorized staff). Do not give information about patients over the phone unless the agency has a system that enables you to know you are speaking to a person authorized by the patient. Refer to Chapter 39 if you require advice about maintaining confidentiality of electronic records. Also,

 VOL 2 Go to Chapter 16, **Clinical Insight 16-5: Guidelines for Documenting in the Electronic Health Record,** in Volume 2.

Provide Education and Counseling

Part of your role as a nurse is to provide information to patients and caregivers about their illness, medications, and other treatments. This helps to fulfill informed consent requirements and to involve patients in their own healthcare. Use teaching-learning principles to make sure the patient understands, retains the knowledge, and can demonstrate any skills. Ask the patient to repeat instructions to you or to provide a return demonstration of a skill, such as self-injection of insulin. To reinforce understanding, always review written information with the patient.

Assign, Delegate, and Supervise According to Guidelines

As a nurse, you are expected to make assignments and delegate tasks to ensure patients receive timely and quality care. To do this safely, you must know the education background, knowledge, experience, and physical and emotional capability of those to whom you delegate. In addition, you must consider the condition and requirements of the patient. For example, it would be negligent to assign a practical nurse to care for a patient on a ventilator without checking to ensure that the nurse has had training and experience with such patients.

The duty to delegate has a corresponding duty to supervise the care. For example, if you assign an aide to take vital signs, you must check periodically to see that the vital signs are taken, accurately reported, and

recorded. If you need to review specific guidelines for delegating, see Chapter 7. For the ANA and other relevant Web sites,

 Go to Chapter 45, **Resources for Caregivers and Health Professionals,** on the Student Resource Disk or DavisPlus at http://davisplus.fadavis.com/Wilkinson2

Accept Assignments for Which You Are Qualified

As a nurse, when you accept an assignment, you must consider whether the assignment is within your level of education, experience, and physical and emotional capability. The refusal to accept an assignment does not mean that you have abandoned the patient. Your duty to the patient begins once you accept the assignment. Remember the general principle that you are legally responsible for the assignment that you accept. If your assignment becomes overwhelming and unmanageable, immediately contact the charge nurse or nursing supervisor for assistance.

Nursing supervisors have a duty to ensure adequate staffing and patient coverage. This means that you must report to the nurse in charge when leaving the patient care unit. Failure to do this may result in charges of patient abandonment. A nurse should never leave the patient care unit without making certain there is another nurse available to provide care to the patient. This does not mean that you must work overtime (e.g., a double shift), as long as you follow established policies and procedures, which will include giving notice and explaining your reasoning (e.g., that you are too fatigued to provide safe care).

If you work a double shift or if a unit is understaffed, you are still liable for any malpractice that you commit. Unfortunately, being "busy" and overwhelmed is not a defense for error. In addition, you have the duty to tell supervisors that staffing is inadequate; be sure to do it in writing. You should know and follow agency policy on how to address short-staff issues.

Participate in Continuing Education

As a nurse, you have a duty to participate in ongoing education in your area of practice and to keep up with new laws, equipment, treatments, and procedures. Be sure to obtain documentation of your attendance. In some states, continuing education is mandatory for relicensure. In states where it is not mandatory, other standards of care still require that you obtain the education and training necessary to implement current nursing procedures and practices. In malpractice cases, the nurse's competency in providing nursing care is frequently an issue. Continuing education is available "for credit" through colleges and universities, other healthcare agencies, conferences, in some nursing journals (e.g., *The American Journal of Nursing*), and online.

Observe Professional Boundaries

Nurses must be careful to maintain professional boundaries, not only with the patient but also with other healthcare providers. Do not accept gifts from vulnerable patients or encourage attempts to have close personal relationships outside the healthcare setting. Violations of professional boundaries may be physical, sexual, emotional, or financial in nature. Cues to possible overstepped boundaries are listed in Box 45-4.

If you would like more specific information on professional boundaries,

 Go to the **National Council on State Boards of Nursing** Web site at: https://www.ncsbn.org/ProfessionalBoundariesbrochure.pdf.

Be aware of and report the behaviors of staff members who commit sexual harassment. **Sexual harassment** involves the use of power over people lower in the power structure of the organization. It is defined as "unwelcome sexual advances, requests for sexual favors, and other verbal or physical conduct of a sexual nature" if submission (1) is a condition of employment, (2) interferes with job performance, (3) is the basis for employment decisions, or (4) creates a hostile and intimidating work environment (Equal Employment Opportunity Commission [EEOC], 2002).

If you witness or experience sexual harassment, your first step is to consult the agency's sexual harassment policy. Every agency receiving federal funding must have such a policy in place. It will tell you how to file a grievance, what forms you need to use, to whom the

---

BOX 45-4 ■ Potential Boundary Violations Between Nurse and Client

Excessive Self-Disclosure—Discussing personal problems or intimate details with the client

Flirtation—Communication that is sexual in nature or reveals personal attraction between client and nurse

Secretive Behavior—When the nurse is defensive or guarded about the interaction between client and nurse

"Super Nurse" Attitude—The nurse that acts as though she is the only one who understands and can meet the client's needs

Excessive Attention to Client—When the nurse spends an unusually greater amount of time with a particular client than is required by his needs; personal gifts, off-duty visits, or trading assignments are signs of boundary violation

Unclear Communication—When only part of the story is told with client care. The client might repeatedly seek out the nurse, even when not assigned to his care.

Used with permission from: National Council of State Boards of Nursing (NCSBN). (n.d.). Professional boundaries: A nurse's guide to the importance of appropriate professional boundaries. Retrieved from https://www.ncsbn.org/ProfessionalBoundariesbrochure.pdf

---

incident is reported, and what the procedure is for hearing and resolution.

Observe Mandatory Reporting Regulations

As noted earlier in the chapter, most states have laws requiring the nurse to report communicable diseases, known or suspected abuse of patients, and impaired or unsafe professional practice. When you observe violations of the state's licensing regulations, you have a professional and legal responsibility to report them to the appropriate authority. The "authority" varies among states; it may be your immediate supervisor, the board of nursing, or a peer assistance program, often sponsored by the state nurses association. See the section "Mandatory Reporting Laws," earlier in the chapter. Also see the following discussion regarding impaired nurses.

Impaired Nurses

Nurses who come to work under the influence of alcohol or mind-altering substances pose a danger to the health, safety, and welfare of the patients. You have a legal obligation to protect patients from impaired nurses. Always pay attention to the possibility of a coworker using or stealing narcotics. Impaired nurses account for a major percentage of disciplinary actions against nurses. For example, the Kansas Board of Nursing reported that in a 2-year period, 325 cases were investigated that involved substance abuse by nurses. Of these cases, 72% involved drug use, 22% alcohol abuse, and 6% involved a combination of both alcohol and drugs (Sidlinger & Hornberger, 2008). See Box 45-5 for signs of chemical dependence in the workplace. To determine the magnitude of the problem in your state, go to the state board of nursing's Web site and click on *disciplinary actions*.

Unauthorized Practice

Your employer will require you to submit verification of current licensure in the state where you are working. If your license expires and you continue to practice nursing, you can be charged with unauthorized practice of nursing. You must report the unauthorized practice of nursing, which means reporting persons practicing nursing without a proper license. In addition, you must know the scope of practice for LPNs/LVNs and nursing assistive personnel to ensure that they practice within their professional boundaries. For example, unlicensed personnel cannot perform the initial patient assessment on a newly admitted patient.

Abuse and Communicable Diseases

State laws also require you to report known or suspected child, elder, and spousal abuse, and communicable disease. Since state laws may vary, you need to be

BOX 45-5 ■ Signs of Potential Chemical Dependence in the Workplace

Absenteeism

- Frequent unscheduled absences with improbable excuses
- Frequent late arrivals or early departures
- Absences after payday or days off
- Higher than average absences for cold, flu, and minor illnesses

Absent "On the Job"

- Long shift breaks
- "Locked door syndrome" (excessively long use of restroom)
- Frequent visits to Occupational Health Services for illness on the job

Difficulty Concentrating

- Errors, particularly involving medication or with taking and transcribing verbal orders
- Omitted, illogical, incomplete, or illegible charting
- Taking more time to carry out assignments than is expected given the nurse's skill and experience
- Deterioration of handwriting during the shift
- Overlooking the signs of patient's deteriorating condition

Inconsistent Work Patterns

- Alternating periods of high and low efficiency
- Minimal or substandard work compared to that of peers
- Frequent requests for help with patient assignments

Physical or Emotional Problems

- Nervousness, excessive sweating, tremors of the hands
- Physical or emotional condition changes during shift
- Deteriorating personal appearance, grooming, and hygiene

Decreasing Efficiency

- Omitting treatments; making bad decisions; showing poor judgment related to patient care
- Requests to be changed to a less supervised shift

Poor Relationships on the Job

- Mood swings, from isolation to angry outbursts
- Uncooperativeness
- Avoidance of contact with supervisors
- Patient complaints of irritability, roughness, or verbal abuse
- Lethargy and hyperactivity
- Emotional hypersensitivity

Medication-Centered Problems

- Excessive use of PRN psychoactive medications or narcotics recorded for patients
- Increased waste or breakage of controlled substances
- Missing drugs, unaccounted-for doses
- Omission of dates or times from narcotic sign-out sheets
- Patient complaints about lack of pain relief

Personal Life Interferes with Job

- Frequent or excessively long phone calls
- Visitors or unexplained errands during work shift
- Legal problems
- Increased number of accidents

Source: Georgia Nurses Association. (n.d.). Checklist for detecting potential chemical dependence in an employee. Retrieved from http://www.georgianurses.org/impaired_nurse.htm#pabi.

---

familiar with them in order to know what and to whom to report in your area. If you are working for a health-care agency when you suspect abuse, always report it to your supervisor. If you need to review signs of abuse,

 Go to Chapter 9, **Procedure 9-1: Assessing for Abuse,** in Volume 2.

Other Safeguards for Nurses

In addition to the Good Samaritan laws and the ANA Bill of Rights for Registered Nurses (previously discussed), safe harbor laws and professional liability insurance offer some legal protection for nurses.

Safe Harbor Laws

Safe harbor laws, found in the nurse practice act or other state laws, provide for exceptions to certain laws. They protect you from being suspended, terminated, disciplined, or discriminated against for refusing to do (or not do) something you believe would be harmful to

a patient. Under these laws, you also have a right to ask for peer review of either the situation or directives that you believe would violate the nursing practice act. You must follow the guidelines required under the safe harbor provisions.

Case: Prepping a Patient for a Surgical Procedure

The nurse cannot find documentation in the patient's medical record for informed consent. Knowing her legal role in informed consent, she refuses to assist with treatment when a patient has not given informed consent. Safe harbor laws protect her from dismissal for denying the surgeon's request for her to obtain it.

Professional Liability Insurance

If you are sued for malpractice, the insurance company pays for the attorney's fees and for any judgment or settlement, up to the limits. You should carefully review your insurance policy because most insurance policies have **exclusions** (items not covered by the policy). If the patient's claim arises out of excluded activities, the insurance company will not pay for the costs of litigation and damages. The following are examples of exclusions:

- Sexual abuse of a patient, assault and battery, and other intentional torts
- Injury caused while the nurse is under the influence of drugs or alcohol
- Criminal activity
- Transmission of acquired immunodeficiency syndrome (AIDS) from the nurse to a patient
- Actions that can lead to an award of punitive damages (damages awarded to punish the defendant for egregious acts or omissions)

Types of Coverage

There are two types of malpractice coverage. **Occurrence-type insurance** is most often recommended for nurses, because this policy covers malpractice claims for any injury or damage that occurred during the time the policy was in force, regardless of when the claim was reported and the lawsuit occurred. In contrast, **claims-made insurance** covers only those claims where the negligent action or omission occurred and the claim was filed or reported during the policy period. To maintain coverage under a claims-made policy after it has lapsed or been canceled, some insurers will offer "tail" insurance. You should consult an attorney to decide which type of policy is best for you.

As a rule, if you work for a hospital or other institution, you will be covered by the institution's insurance. However, it covers you only while you are working within the scope of your employment. For example, you would not be covered during the one day a week that you volunteer at a free clinic. Some legal experts recommend that you purchase individual liability insurance in addition to the coverage provided by your employer. Again, consult a lawyer before making a decision.

CriticalThinking 45-6

Susan, RN, was employed by Landold Nursing Service and assigned to Alvalup Hospital from June 1, 2007 to May 30, 2008. Susan carried her own professional liability claims-made policy during this time. She decided to attend real estate school and not renew her policy. On August 10, 2008, a medical malpractice claim was filed against Susan.

- Based on this scenario, would Susan have coverage under her policy? What kind of policy would she have to obtain in order to be protected from a claim made against her?

Student Responsibilities

As a student, you are held to the same standards of care as are licensed nurses. You must be familiar not only with your state's standards of practice, but also with the policies and procedures in the agency in which you have your clinical experiences. Your instructor is responsible for making assignments that are within your competence and for providing clinical supervision. However, this does not release you from your own legal responsibilities. To help protect yourself and your patients:

- Prepare carefully for each clinical experience.
- Never attempt a procedure or make a judgment about which you feel unsure. If you lack the theoretical or practical knowledge for an assignment, notify your clinical instructor immediately.
- Notify your instructor or a staff nurse if your patient's condition changes significantly.
- Unless otherwise arranged, take instructions only from your clinical instructor.

Your nursing school may require you to carry personal professional liability insurance. The school's policy will cover you only for the nursing care you give in your educational experiences. If you work, for example, as an aide, the school's policy will not provide coverage for you at work. Furthermore, you are legally permitted to perform only the procedures contained in your job description. For example, even though you administer injections in your student role, you are not licensed to do so in your role as an aide.

Summary

Ethical and legal issues are a major source of conflict for nursing practice. This chapter discusses only the legal aspects of the major issues. See Chapter 44 for ethical considerations. It is important to be clear in your mind that legal and ethical are not always the same thing. On the one hand, an act may be legal (e.g., abortion), even if you consider it unethical. On the other hand, you may believe an action (e.g., assisted suicide) is ethically necessary, but the law may forbid it. You should be aware of the legal consequences that your ethical decisions may bring about. For a more detailed discussion of some major legal issues in nursing (e.g., stem cell research, cloning, reproductive issues, life-sustaining medical treatment, etc.),

 Go to Chapter 45, **Supplemental Materials, What Are the Major Legal Issues in Nursing Practice?** on the Student Resource Disk or DavisPlus at http://davisplus.fadavis.com/Wilkinson2

 Go to Chapter 45, **Resources for Caregivers and Health Professionals,** on the Student Resource Disk or DavisPlus at http://davisplus.fadavis.com/Wilkinson2

 Suggested Readings, Go to Chapter 45, **Reading More About Legal Issues,** on the Student Resource Disk or DavisPlus at http://davisplus.fadavis.com/Wilkinson2

 Bibliography: Go to Volume 2, Bibliography.

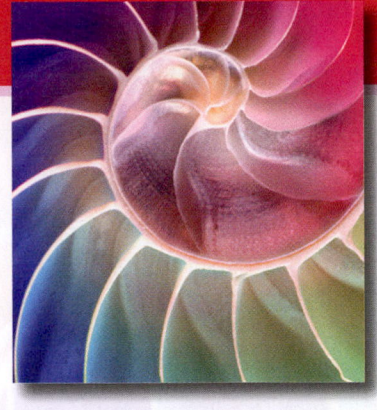

Credits

Note: Unless cited below, text credits appear within the text.

Chapter 1

Meet Your Patient 1-1: The National Library of Medicine

Meet Your Patient 1-2: Photo Copyright BananaStock

Figure 1-2: Jupiterimages Corporation/Getty Images/Photos.com

Figure 1-3: National Library of Medicine

Figure 1-4: © istockphoto.com/Kseniya Abramova

Table 1-4: From American Nurses Association. (2010, in press). *Standards of nursing practice.* Silver Spring, MD: Author.

Chapter 2

Meet Your Patient: Royalty-Free/Corbis

Figure 2-3: © istockphoto.com/mstay

Chapter 3

Meet Your Patient: Everyday Faces, Photo Copyright PhotoDisc

Figure 3-2: From Wilkinson, J. M. *Nursing process and critical thinking* (4th ed.). © 2007. Electronically reproduced by permission of Pearson Education, Inc., Upper Saddle River, NJ.

Figure 3-3: Comstock/Getty Images

Figure 3-4: Courtesy of Smith Northview Hospital, Valdosta, GA.

Figure 3-5: Courtesy of Shore Memorial Hospital, Somers Point, NJ.

Chapter 4

Meet Your Patient: Photo Copyright BananaStock

Figure 4-6: Adapted from Maslow, A. (1971). *The farther reaches of human nature.* New York: Viking Press; and Maslow, A., & Lowery, R. (Eds.). (1998). *Toward a psychology of being* (3rd ed.). New York: John Wiley & Sons.

Chapter 5

Meet Your Patient: Ryan McVay/Photodisc/Punchstock

Figure 5-3: Courtesy of Shawnee Mission Health System, Shawnee Mission, KS 66204.

Figure 5-4: Adapted from Genesis Medical Center, Davenport, IA 52804. Used with permission.

Figure 5-5: From Hospital of the University of Pennsylvania, Philadelphia, PA. Used with permission.

Chapter 6

Meet Your Patient: Ryan McVay/Photodisc/Punchstock

Figure 6-2: Courtesy of Fain, J. A. (2008). *Reading, understanding and applying nursing research: A text and workbook* (3rd ed.). Philadelphia: F. A. Davis.

Figure 6-4: Courtesy of Ergo Partners, L. D., 114 Balsam Lane, Boulder, CO 80304. Used with permission.

Chapter 7

Meet Your Patients: Thinkstock/Getty Images

Figure 7-2: Courtesy of Ergo Partners, L. D., 114 Balsam Lane, Boulder, CO 80304. All rights reserved. Used with permission.

Chapter 8

Figure 8-1: Courtesy of Jean Watson.

Box 8-2: From Marriner-Tomey, A., & Raille-Alligood, M. (2006). *Nursing theorists and their work* (6th ed.) St. Louis, MO: C. V. Mosby.

Figure 8-5: Adapted from Maslow, A. (1971). *The farther reaches of human nature.* New York: The Viking Press; and Maslow, A., & Lowery, R. (Eds.). (1998). *Toward a psychology of being* (3rd ed.). New York: John Wiley & Sons.

Chapter 9

Meet Your Patient: Photodisc Blue/Getty Images

The following figures appear only on the Electronic Study Guide:

Chapter 10

Meet Your Patient: Royalty-Free Corbis
Figure 10-4: Photo Copyright PhotoDisc

Chapter 12

Figure 12-3: Photo Copyright PhotoDisc, Senior Lifestyles
Figure 12-6: From Dillon, P. M. (2007). *Nursing health assessment: A critical thinking case studies approach* (2nd ed.). Philadelphia: F. A. Davis.

Chapter 13

Figure 13-1: Adapted from Hanson, S. (2001). *Family health care nursing: Theory, practice and research* (2nd ed.). Philadelphia, F. A. Davis. Data from *US Census Bureau News*, August 14, 2008, Washington, DC.
Figure 13-2: © istockphoto.com/RichLindle
Figure 13-3: © istockphoto.com/JerryPDX
Figure 13-5: © Jupiterimages Corporation
Figure 13-7: From Purnell, L., & Paulanka, B. (2007). *Transcultural health care: A culturally competent approach* (3rd ed.). Philadelphia: F. A. Davis. Reprinted with permission.

Chapter 14

Meet Your Patient: © Photodisc, Senior Lifestyles
Figure 14-4: Adapted from Millspaugh, C. D. (2005). Assessment and response to spiritual pain: Part II. *Journal of Palliative Medicine, 8*(6), 1110–1117.

Chapter 15

Figure 15-1: © istockphoto/clickhere
Figure 15-2: From U.S. Department of Health and Human Services. Retrieved from http://www.organdonor.gov
Passage in Critical Thinking 15-9: From Rando, T. (1984). *Grief, dying and death. Clinical interventions for caregivers.* Champaign, IL: Research Press.

Chapter 16

Meet Your Patient: © Photodisc/Getty
Figures 16-2 through 16-4, 16-6, and 16-7: Courtesy of Cerner Corporation.

Chapter 17

Meet Your Patient: Photo Copyright BananaStock

Chapter 19

Figures 19-1 and 19-3 through 19-8, 19-10 through 19-12, 19-14a–c, 19-16a–d, 19-17, 19-20, 19-22 through 19-24, and Figures a–c and f–i in Table 19-1: From Dillon, P. M. (2007). *Nursing health assessment: A critical thinking case studies approach* (2nd ed.). Philadelphia: F. A. Davis.
Figure 19-9: Courtesy of Tina S. Liang, DMD.
Figure 19-21: From Scanlon, V. C., & Sanders, T. (2003). *Essentials of anatomy & physiology* (4th ed.). Philadelphia: F. A. Davis.

Chapter 20

Meet Your Patient: © istockphoto.com/Maliketh
Figures 20-2 and 20-3: From Scanlon, V. C., & Sanders, T. (2003). *Essentials of anatomy & physiology* (4th ed.). Philadelphia: F. A. Davis.

Chapter 21

Meet Your Patient: Jay Fries/Digital Vision/Getty Images
Figure 21-4: © istockphoto.com/webking
Box 21-3: Courtesy of The Joint Commission.

Chapter 22

Meet Your Patient: Getty Images
Figure 22-2a and b: Courtesy of Invacare Corporation, Elyria, OH.
Figures 22-3 and 22-4: From Dillon, P. M. (2007). *Nursing health assessment: A critical thinking case studies approach* (2nd ed.). Philadelphia: F. A. Davis.

Chapter 23

Figure 23-16: Courtesy of Hospira, Lake Forest, IL.
Figures 23-17 and 23-30: Courtesy of Medi-Dose ®, Inc., EPS®, Inc.
Figure 23-19a–c: Courtesy of U.S. Department of Labor, Occupational Safety and Health Administration (OSHA).
Figure 23-29: Used by permission of the National Extravasation Information Service (UK). www.extravasation.org.uk

Chapter 24

Meet Your Patient: Photo Copyright BananaStock
Figure 24-3: Photos.com/Getty Images
Figure 24-4: Photo courtesy of Laerdal Medical Corporation.
Figure 24-5: Courtesy of Merck & Co., Inc. #994795(1)-05-COZ.

Chapter 25

Meet Your Patient: Digital Vision
Figures 25-3 and 25-5: From Scanlon, V. C., & Sanders, T. (2007). *Essentials of anatomy & physiology* (5th ed.). Philadelphia: F. A. Davis.
Figure 25-7: From Getty Images, Photodisc

Chapter 26

Figure 26-1: U.S. Department of Agriculture (2005).
Figure 26-2: © GC Nutrition Council, 2006, adapted from USDA 2005 Dietary Guidelines and www.mypyramid.gov
Figure 26-3: U.S. Department of Agriculture (2005).
Figure 26-4: Adapted from Scanlon, V. C., & Sanders, T. (2007). *Essentials of anatomy and physiology* (5th ed.). Philadelphia: F. A. Davis.
Figures 26-5 and 26-6: Adapted from Scanlon, V. C. & Sanders, T. (2003). *Essentials of anatomy and physiology* (4th ed.). Philadelphia: F. A. Davis.
Figures 26-7, 26-8a and b, and 26-11: Courtesy of Covidien, Mansfield, MA.
ALERT Acronym: © 2009 Nestlé HealthCare Nutrition, Inc. The Be A.L.E.R.T. poster is a joint effort of the American Society for Parenteral and Enteral Nutrition (A.S.P.E.N.) and Nestlé HealthCare Nutrition, Inc.

Chapter 27

Meet Your Patient: Photo copyright BananaStock
Figures 27-1 through 27-4: From Scanlon, V. C., & Sanders, T. (2007). *Essentials of anatomy & physiology* (5th ed.). Philadelphia: F. A. Davis.
Figure 27-7: Courtesy of Atago, USA, Inc.

Chapter 28

Meet Your Patient: © istockphoto.com/thelinke
Figures 28-1 and 28-2: From Scanlon, V. C., & Sanders, T. (2003). *Essentials of anatomy and physiology* (4th ed.). Philadelphia: F. A. Davis.
Figures 28-3 and 28-4: From Scanlon, V. C., & Sanders, T. (2007). *Essentials of anatomy and physiology* (5th ed.). Philadelphia: F. A. Davis.
Figure 28-8: Courtesy of Hollister Incorporated, Libertyville, IL.
Figure 28-9: Courtesy of ConvaTex, Skillman, NJ.
Figure 28-10: From Williams, L., & Hopper, P. (2007). *Understanding medical surgical nursing* (2nd ed.). Philadelphia: F. A. Davis.

Chapter 29

Meet Your Patient: © istockphoto.com/Aguru
Figures 29-1 and 29-2: From Scanlon, V. C., & Sanders, T. (2007). *Essentials of anatomy and physiology* (5th ed.). Philadelphia: F. A. Davis.

Chapter 30

Meet Your Patient: Photos.com/Jupiter Images
Figure 30-4: Developed by the World Health Organization. (1990). Cancer pain relief and palliative care: report of a WHO expert committee. WHO Tech Rep series, No. 804. Geneva, Switzerland. Author. Used with permission.
The Wong Baker FACES scale: From Hockenberry, M. J., & Wilson, D. (2009). *Wong's essentials of pediatric nursing* (8th ed.). St. Louis, MO: C. V. Mosby. Used with permission. Copyright Mosby. http://www1.us.elsevierhealth/FACES
Sedation Rating Scale: From Spies, C., Rehberg, B., Schug, S. A., & Jachnisen, G. (2009). *Pocket guide to pain management*. New York: Springer.

Chapter 31

Meet Your Patient: Jay Freis/Digital Vision/Getty Images
Figures 31-1 and 31-2: From Scanlon, V. C., & Sanders, T. (2007). *Essentials of anatomy and physiology* (5th ed.). Philadelphia: F. A. Davis.
Figure 31-5: From Williams, L., & Hopper, P. (2007). *Understanding medical surgical nursing* (2nd ed.). Philadelphia: F. A. Davis.
Figures 31-9, 31-10, 31-12a-c and 31-13: Courtesy of EZ Way, Inc. Clarinda, IA.

Chapter 32

Meet Your Patients: © istockphoto.com/CherylCasey, © istockphoto.com/SteveLuker and © istockphoto.com/cglade
Figures 32-1 through 32-4: From Scanlon, V. C., & Sanders, T. (2007). *Essentials of anatomy and physiology* (5th ed.). Philadelphia: F. A. Davis.
Figure 32-5: From photos.com, Getty Images
Figure 32-8: © istockphoto.com/iofoto

Chapter 33

Figure 33-5: From Guyton, A. C., & Hall, J. E. (2006). *Medical physiology* (10th ed.). Philadelphia: W. B. Saunders.

Chapter 34

Meet Your Patient: From PhotoDisc, Everyday Faces
Figure 34-1: From Scanlon, V. C., & Sanders, T. (2007). *Essentials of anatomy and physiology* (5th ed.). Philadelphia: F. A. Davis.
Figure 34-7b: Courtesy of Talley Group Limited, Premier Way, Abbey Park Industrial Estate, Romsey, Hampshire, S051 9DQ England.
Figure 34-9a: Courtesy of WoundEducators.com, LLC, Great River, NY.

Figure 34-10: Agency for Healthcare Policy and Research. (1994, December). Clinical Practice Guidelines: Pressure Ulcer.

Suspected Deep Tissue Injury: Courtesy of Laurie Swezey, RN, BSN, CWOCN, CWS, FACCWS, President, WoundEducators.com, LLC.

Chapter 35

Meet Your Patient: Photo Copyright BananaStock.

Figures 35-1 through 35-4 and 35-18 through 35-21: From Scanlon, V. C., & Sanders, T. (2007). *Essentials of anatomy and physiology* (5th ed.). Philadelphia: F. A. Davis.

Figures 35-6a and b, 35-7, 35-13a and b, and 35-15: From Williams, L., & Hopper, P. (2007). *Understanding medical surgical nursing* (2nd ed.). Philadelphia: F. A. Davis.

Chapter 36

Meet Your Patient: Getty Images, Photodisc

Figure 36-1a: From Scanlon, V. & Sanders, T. (2007). *Essentials of anatomy and physiology* (5th ed.). Philadelphia: F. A. Davis.

Figure 36-1b: From Williams, L., & Hopper, P. (2007). *Understanding medical surgical nursing* (2nd ed.). Philadelphia: F. A. Davis.

Chapter 37

Meet Your Patient: © istockphoto.com/Vikram Raghuvanshi

Figures 37-2 and 37-4: From Williams, L., & Hopper, P. (2007). *Understanding medical surgical nursing* (2nd ed.). Philadelphia: F. A. Davis.

Figure 37-5: Courtesy of I-flow Corporation, Lake Forest, CA.

Chapter 38

Figures 38-1 and 38-2: From Whitehead, D., Weiss, S., & Tappen, R. (2007). *Essentials of nursing leadership and management* (4th ed.). Philadelphia: F. A. Davis.

Chapter 39

Meet Your Patient: © istockphoto/sjlocke

Figure 39-1: Adapted from Englebardt, S., & Nelson, R. *Health care informatics: An interdisciplinary approach.* Copyright (2002). With permission from Elsevier.

Figure 39-2: Courtesy of Laerdal Medical Corp., Wappingers Falls, NY.

Figure 39-3: Courtesy of Global Media Group, LLC. Innovative Telemedic™ of Scottsdale, AZ.

Figure 39-4a and b: Courtesy of Doctors Telehealth Network, Newport Beach, CA.

Figure 39-5: Courtesy of Cerner Corporation.

Figure 39-6a: Courtesy of Corbis.

Figure 39-6b: © istockphoto.com/Adivin

Chapter 40

Meet Your Patient: © istockphoto.com/monkeybusinessimages

Figures 40-5 and 40-6: Courtesy of National Center for Complementary and Alternate Medicine.

Chapter 41

Meet Your Patient: © istockphoto.com/Thomas_EyeDesign

Chapter 42

Meet Your Patient: © istockphoto.com/PhotoEuphoria

Figure 42-3: From photos.com, Getty Images

Figure 42-5: © istockphoto.com/AlexRaths

Chapter 43

Meet Your Patient: From photos.com, Getty Images

Figure 43-5: © istockphoto.com/KLH49

Chapter 45

Meet Your Patient: © istockphoto.com/ntmw

Index

Note: Page numbers followed by *f* refer to figures; page numbers followed by *t* refer to tables; page numbers followed by *b* refer to boxes; page numbers followed by *p* refer to procedures.

Vascular system. *See also* Cardiovascular system
  assessment of, *(V1)* 395–396, *(V1)* 395f, *(V2)* 281p–288p
    critical aspects of, *(V1)* 406, *(V2)* 281
  central, *(V1)* 395–396, *(V1)* 395f
  peripheral, *(V1)* 396, *(V1)* 907
  risk for trauma to, *(V2)* 945
Vasectomy, *(V2)* 754
Vasocongestion, in sexual response cycle, *(V1)* 794
Vasodilators, *(V1)* 910
Vasomotor center, *(V1)* 902
Vastus lateralis muscle, injection into, *(V1)* 539, *(V1)* 539f, *(V2)* 492p, *(V2)* 494p
    critical aspects of, *(V1)* 546, *(V2)* 490
Vector, in infection transmission, *(V1)* 412, *(V1)* 441
Vedas, *(V1)* 4–5
Vegans, *(V1)* 620
Vegetarianism, *(V1)* 251, *(V1)* 252, *(V1)* 603f, *(V1)* 620–621
Vehicle accident. *See* Motor vehicle accidents
Vein(s), *(V1)* 900
  abdominal, *(V2)* 289
  access to. *See* Central venous access device; Venipuncture
  assessment of, *(V1)* 396, *(V2)* 287p
  hand, *(V2)* 938
  inflammation of, *(V1)* 941t–942t
  jugular, assessment of, *(V1)* 395f, *(V1)* 396, *(V2)* 282p
Venipuncture, for intravenous fluid and electrolyte administration, *(V1)* 938–939, *(V1)* 938f, *(V1)* 944, *(V2)* 903p–909p, *(V2)* 938
Venous hum, *(V2)* 284
Venous star, *(V2)* 329
Venous stasis
  immobility and, *(V1)* 764
  ulcers with, *(V1)* 835t, *(V1)* 842, *(V2)* 246
Ventilation
  impaired, *(V1)* 882, *(V2)* 894
  mechanical. *See* Mechanical ventilation
  minute, *(V1)* 873
  pulmonary, *(V1)* 336, *(V1)* 868–870, *(V1)* 869f. *See also* Lung(s); Pulmonary system; Respiration(s)
    adequacy of, *(V1)* 869–870
    mechanics of, *(V1)* 336–337, *(V1)* 337f
    in older adults, *(V1)* 872
    position for, *(V1)* 886
  room, *(V1)* 492
Ventilation-perfusion scan, *(V2)* 893
Ventilator-associated pneumonia, *(V1)* 893
Ventricles, *(V1)* 899, *(V1)* 899f
Ventricular dysrhythmia, *(V1)* 908
Ventrogluteal muscle, injection into, *(V1)* 538, *(V1)* 538f, *(V2)* 491p
    critical aspects of, *(V1)* 546, *(V2)* 490
Venules, *(V1)* 900
Veracity, *(V1)* 1097, *(V1)* 1104
Verbal communication. *See* Communication, verbal; Reporting
Verbal orders, *(V1)* 312, *(V2)* 179
Verbal prescription, *(V1)* 515–516, *(V1)* 516b
Vernix caseosa, *(V1)* 831
Vesicle, *(V2)* 244, *(V2)* 328
Vest restraint, *(V2)* 371p
Vestigial organ, *(V1)* 679

Vial technique, injection with, *(V1)* 531, *(V1)* 531f, *(V2)* 474p–480p
  clinical insights on, *(V2)* 513–514
  critical aspects of, *(V1)* 545, *(V2)* 471
Vibration, chest, *(V1)* 888, *(V2)* 279p, *(V2)* 844p–847p
  critical aspects of, *(V1)* 896, *(V2)* 844
Vibratory sensation, assessment of, *(V2)* 309p
Vicarious liability, *(V1)* 1121–1122
Vietnam War, *(V1)* 9, *(V1)* 9f
Villi, intestinal, *(V1)* 679, *(V1)* 679f
Violence. *See also* Abuse
  assessment for, *(V1)* 447–448
  domestic (intimate partner), *(V1)* 215, *(V1)* 798
  to healthcare workers, *(V1)* 446, *(V1)* 458, *(V1)* 462b, *(V2)* 1040–1041
  nursing diagnoses for, *(V2)* 35
  sexual, *(V1)* 798–799
Virchow's triad, *(V1)* 764
Visceral pain, *(V1)* 726, *(V1)* 727
Viscosity, blood, *(V1)* 341
Vision
  assessment of, *(V1)* 385–386, *(V2)* 252p–259p, *(V2)* 306p
    bedside, *(V2)* 694
    critical aspects of, *(V1)* 406, *(V2)* 252
  color, *(V1)* 385, *(V2)* 254p
  deficits in, *(V1)* 712, *(V1)* 712b
    client-nurse communication and, *(V2)* 691
    home care for, *(V1)* 722
    interventions for, *(V1)* 721, *(V2)* 695
    medication administration and, *(V1)* 524
  distance, *(V1)* 385, *(V2)* 253p
  near, *(V1)* 385, *(V2)* 253p
  peripheral, *(V1)* 385–386, *(V2)* 254p–255p, *(V2)* 306
  self-care for, *(V1)* 719
  stimulation of, *(V1)* 719
Visiting hours, *(V1)* 86
Visual Analog Scale, *(V2)* 707
Visual fields, *(V1)* 385–386, *(V2)* 254p–255p
Visual recognition, assessment of, *(V2)* 305p
Visualization techniques, *(V1)* 1026
  for stress, *(V1)* 594
Vital capacity, *(V2)* 892
Vital signs, *(V1)* 316–350, *(V2)* 192–219. *See also* Blood pressure (BP); Pulse; Respiration(s); Temperature
  critical thinking about, *(V2)* 216–218
  definition of, *(V1)* 316
  delegation of, *(V1)* 350
  documentation of, *(V1)* 318, *(V2)* 214
  in dying client, *(V2)* 161
  evaluation of, *(V1)* 350, *(V1)* 379, *(V2)* 239
  fifth, *(V1)* 317, *(V1)* 733–734. *See also* Pain
  frequency of, *(V1)* 318
  full-spectrum nursing and, *(V2)* 216
  knowledge map for, *(V2)* 219
  normal, *(V1)* 318, *(V1)* 318t, *(V2)* 239
  occasions for, *(V1)* 318
  postoperative, *(V1)* 970b
  racial variation in, *(V2)* 138
Vitamin(s), *(V1)* 609–612, *(V1)* 610t–611t
  cooking effects on, *(V1)* 620
  for infants, *(V1)* 617
  for older adults, *(V1)* 619
  oral contraceptive effects on, *(V1)* 620

Recommended Dietary Allowances for, *(V1)* 609, *(V1)* 610t–611t
  supplemental, *(V1)* 629–630, *(V1)* 1031
Vitamin A, *(V1)* 609, *(V1)* 610t
Vitamin B6, *(V1)* 611t, *(V1)* 612
Vitamin B12, *(V1)* 611t, *(V1)* 612
  supplemental, *(V1)* 630
  in vegetarian diet, *(V1)* 621
Vitamin C, *(V1)* 611t, *(V1)* 612
  cigarette smoking and, *(V1)* 620
  for common cold, *(V1)* 884
  evidence-based study of, *(V1)* 910
  fecal occult blood test interactions with, *(V1)* 688
  gastrointestinal effects of, *(V1)* 682
  for infants, *(V1)* 617
  skin effects of, *(V1)* 833
Vitamin D, *(V1)* 609, *(V1)* 610t, *(V1)* 612
  deficiency of, *(V1)* 762
  formation of, *(V1)* 470
  for infants, *(V1)* 617, *(V1)* 630
  in vegetarian diet, *(V1)* 621
Vitamin E, *(V1)* 609, *(V1)* 610t
  evidence-based study of, *(V1)* 910
Vitamin K, *(V1)* 609, *(V1)* 610t
  for infants, *(V1)* 629–630
Vitiligo, *(V2)* 328
Vocabulary, *(V1)* 354
Voice sounds, *(V1)* 392, *(V2)* 280p
Voiding. *See also* Urination
  scheduled, *(V1)* 669, *(V2)* 635
Volume (sound), in verbal communication, *(V1)* 355
Volume-control infusion set
  fluid and electrolytes, *(V1)* 939, *(V2)* 911p, *(V2)* 912p–915p
    critical aspects of, *(V1)* 944, *(V2)* 912
  medication, *(V1)* 542–543, *(V1)* 543f, *(V2)* 504p–505p
    critical aspects of, *(V1)* 547, *(V2)* 503
Voluntariness, for informed consent, *(V1)* 1126
Vomiting
  induction of, *(V1)* 438
  after medication administration, *(V2)* 449
  opioid-related, *(V1)* 741b
  postoperative, *(V1)* 973t
  during pregnancy, *(V1)* 683
  tube feeding and, *(V2)* 571
Vulnerable populations, *(V1)* 225
Vulva, *(V1)* 782
Vulvovaginitis, herpes, *(V2)* 331

W

Waddling gait, *(V1)* 766, *(V2)* 331
Waist circumference, measurement of, *(V1)* 1048, *(V2)* 583
Waist-to-hip ratio, *(V1)* 625, *(V2)* 583
Wald, Lillian, *(V1)* 10
  community nursing and, *(V1)* 1061
Walkers, *(V1)* 779, *(V1)* 779f
  sizing of, *(V2)* 733
  teaching for, *(V2)* 733
Walking. *See also* Gait
  assessment of, *(V1)* 398, *(V2)* 296p–297p
  assistance for, *(V1)* 777–780, *(V2)* 725p–728p
    conditioning exercises in, *(V1)* 777–778, *(V2)* 732
    critical aspects of, *(V1)* 774, *(V2)* 725